Textbook of
TUBERCULOSIS AND NONTUBERCULOUS MYCOBACTERIAL DISEASES

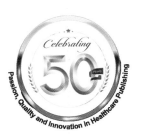

Textbook of
TUBERCULOSIS AND NONTUBERCULOUS MYCOBACTERIAL DISEASES

Third Edition

Editor
Surendra K Sharma
Former Senior Professor and Head
Department of Internal Medicine
[WHO Collaborating Centre for Research and
Training in Tuberculosis
Centre of Excellence for Extrapulmonary TB
Ministry of Health and Family Welfare, Government of India]
All India Institute of Medical Sciences
New Delhi, India

Adjunct Professor
Department of Molecular Medicine
Jamia Hamdard Institute of Molecular Medicine
Jamia Hamdard [Deemed to be University]
New Delhi, India

Adjunct Professor
Departments of General Medicine and Respiratory Medicine
Jawaharlal Nehru Medical College
Datta Meghe Institute of Medical Sciences [Deemed to be University]
Wardha, Maharashtra, India

Assistant Editor
Alladi Mohan
Chief, Division of Pulmonary and Critical Care Medicine
Professor and Head
Department of Medicine
Sri Venkateswara Institute of Medical Sciences
Tirupati, Andhra Pradesh, India

Foreword
Mario C Raviglione

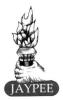

JAYPEE BROTHERS MEDICAL PUBLISHERS
The Health Sciences Publisher

New Delhi | London

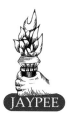

Jaypee Brothers Medical Publishers (P) Ltd.

Headquarters

Jaypee Brothers Medical Publishers (P) Ltd
4838/24, Ansari Road, Daryaganj
New Delhi 110 002, India
Phone: +91-11-43574357
Fax: +91-11-43574314
Email: jaypee@jaypeebrothers.com

Overseas Office

J.P. Medical Ltd
83 Victoria Street, London
SW1H 0HW (UK)
Phone: +44 20 3170 8910
Fax: +44 (0)20 3008 6180
Email: info@jpmedpub.com

Website: www.jaypeebrothers.com
Website: www.jaypeedigital.com

Textbook of Tuberculosis and Nontuberculous Mycobacterial Diseases

First Edition: 2001

Second Edition: 2009

Third Edition: **2020**

ISBN: 978-93-89129-21-2

Printed at Sanat Printers

Dedicated to

Our late parents for their encouragement
Our teachers and students for their inspiration
Anju and Himabala for their moral support
Abhishek, Animesh and Vikram Chandra for their cheerful enthusiasm

Contributors

SK Acharya
Former Professor and Head
Department of Gastroenterology and
Human Nutrition
All India Institute of Medical Sciences
New Delhi, India

SK Agarwal
Professor and Head
Department of Nephrology
All India Institute of Medical Sciences
New Delhi, India

AN Aggarwal
Professor and Head
Department of Pulmonary Medicine
Postgraduate Institute of Medical
Education and Research
Chandigarh, Punjab, India

Gautam Ahluwalia
Professor
Department of Medicine
Dayanand Medical College and Hospital
Ludhiana, Punjab, India

Vineet Ahuja
Professor
Department of Gastroenterology and
Human Nutrition
All India Institute of Medical Sciences
New Delhi, India

Jason Andrews
Assistant Professor
Department of Medicine-Infectious
Diseases
Stanford University
Stanford, California, USA

Minu Bajpai
Professor and Head
Department of Paediatric Surgery
All India Institute of Medical Sciences
New Delhi, India

VH Balasangameshwara
Former Chief Medical Officer
National Tuberculosis Institute
Directorate General of Health Services
Bengaluru, Karnataka, India

D Behera
Professor
Department of Pulmonary Medicine
Postgraduate Institute of Medical
Education and Research
Chandigarh, India

S Bhan
Former Professor and Head
Department of Orthopaedics
All India Institute of Medical Sciences
New Delhi, India

Deepali K Bhat
Department of Transplant Immunology
and Immunogenetics
All India Institute of Medical Sciences
New Delhi, India

Rajesh Bhatia
Former Director
Department of Communicable Diseases
WHO Regional Office for South-East Asia
New Delhi, India

Vineet Bhatia
Medical Officer–MDR-TB
Department of Communicable Diseases
World Health Organization
Regional Office for South-East Asia
New Delhi, India

Gregory Calligaro
Pulmonologist
Groote Schuur Hospital
Researcher at Lung Infection and
Immunity Unit
Division of Pulmonology and University
of Cape Town Lung Institute
Department of Medicine
University of Cape Town
Cape Town, South Africa

Abha Chandra
Professor and Head
Department of Cardiovascular and
Thoracic surgery
Sri Venkateswara Institute of Medical
Sciences
Tirupati, Andhra Pradesh, India

Rohan Chawla
Associate Professor
Dr Rajendra Prasad Centre for
Ophthalmic Sciences
All India Institute of Medical Sciences
New Delhi, India

Vatsla Dadhwal
Professor
Department Obstetrics and Gynaecology
All India Institute of Medical Sciences
New Delhi, India

Chandan J Das
Associate Professor
Department of Radiodiagnosis
All India Institute of Medical Sciences
New Delhi, India

Prasenjit Das
Additional Professor
Department of Pathology
All India Institute of Medical Sciences
New Delhi, India

Malika Davids
Lung Infection and Immunity Unit
Division of Pulmonology and
University of Cape Town Lung Institute
Department of Medicine
University of Cape Town
Cape Town, South Africa

Rodney Dawson
Professor and Head
UCT Lung Institute
Department of Medicine
University of Cape Town
Cape Town, South Africa

Sajal De
Associate Professor
Department of TB and
Respiratory Diseases
Mahatma Gandhi Institute of Medical
Sciences
Wardha, Maharashtra, India

Surendran Deepanjali
Associate Professor
Department of Medicine
Jawaharlal Institute of Postgraduate
Medical Education and Research
Puducherry, India

B Dey
Center for Tuberculosis Research
Johns Hopkins School of Medicine
Baltimore, MD, USA

Keertan Dheda
Professor of Respiratory Medicine
Head of the Lung Infection and
Immunity Unit
Division of Pulmonology and
University of Cape Town Lung Institute
Department of Medicine
University of Cape Town
Cape Town, South Africa

Samjot S Dhillon
Associate Professor of Oncology
Roswell Park Cancer Institute
Assistant Professor of Medicine
Department of Medicine
Pulmonary Medicine and Thoracic
Oncology
State University of New York [SUNY]
Buffalo, New York, USA

Alisgar Esmail
Lung Infection and Immunity Unit
Division of Pulmonology and
University of Cape Town Lung Institute
Department of Medicine
University of Cape Town
Cape Town, South Africa

Dennis Falzon
Medical Officer
Global TB Programme
World Health Organization
Geneva, Switzerland

Gaurav PS Gahlot
Assistant Professor
Department of Pathology
Army Hospital RR
New Delhi, India

SP Garg
Former Professor
Dr Rajendra Prasad Centre for
Ophthalmic Sciences
All India Institute of Medical Sciences
New Delhi, India

Haileyesus Getahun
Coordinator
TB/HIV and Community Engagement
[THC]
Global TB Programme [GTB]
World Health Organization [WHO]
Geneva, Switzerland

Marzieh Ghiasi
McGill International TB Centre
McGill University
Montreal, Quebec, Canada

Ankur Goyal
Assistant Professor
Department of Radiodiagnosis
All India Institute of Medical Sciences
New Delhi, India

KK Guntupalli
Professor of Medicine
Chief, Pulmonary
Critical Care and Sleep
Medicine Section
Baylor College of Medicine
Houston, Texas, USA

Arun K Gupta
Professor and Head
Department of Radiodiagnosis
All India Institute of Medical Sciences
New Delhi, India

Alisha Gupta
Department of Paediatric Surgery
All India Institute of Medical Sciences
New Delhi, India

Sanjay Gupta
Chief Medical Officer
Department of Tuberculosis and
Respiratory Diseases
National Institute of Tuberculosis and
Respiratory diseases
New Delhi, India

Siddhartha Datta Gupta
Professor
Department of Pathology
All India Institute of Medical Sciences
New Delhi, India

Nicola A Hanania
Associate Professor of Medicine
Section of Pulmonary and Critical Care
Medicine
Baylor College of Medicine
Houston, Texas, USA

J Harikrishna
Associate Professor
Department of Medicine
Sri Venkateswara Institute of
Medical Sciences
Tirupati, Andhra Pradesh, India

CV Harinarayan
Director
Institute of Endocrinology, Diabetes,
Thyroid and Osteoporosis Disorders
Sakra World Hospitals
Bengaluru, Karnataka, India

AK Hemal
Former Professor
Department of Urology
All India Institute of Medical Sciences
New Delhi, India

Md Khurshid Alam Hyder
Public Health Administrator
UN House Pulchowk
Lalitpur
Kathmandu, Nepal

R Jain
Center for Tuberculosis Research
Johns Hopkins School of Medicine
Baltimore, Maryland, USA

Manisha Jana
Associate Professor
Department of Radiodiagnosis
All India Institute of Medical Sciences
New Delhi, India

Babban Jee
Scientist C
Department of Health Research
Ministry of Health and Family Welfare
Government of India
New Delhi, India

SK Jindal
Former Professor and Head
Department of Pulmonary Medicine
Postgraduate Institute of Medical
Education and Research
Chandigarh, India

Thomas Joseph
Global TB programme
World Health Organization
Geneva, Switzerland

Shalini Joshi
Consultant
Department of Internal Medicine
Fortis Hospitals and Health Care
Bengaluru, Karnataka, India

SK Kabra
Professor
Department of Paediatrics
All India Institute of Medical Sciences
New Delhi, India

Tamilarasu Kadhiravan
Additional Professor
Department of Medicine
Jawaharlal Institute of Postgraduate
Medical Education and Research
Puducherry, India

Arvind Kumar Kairo
Assistant Professor
Department of ENT and Neck Surgery
All India Institute of Medical Sciences
New Delhi, India

DR Karnad
Professor and Chief
Medical-Neuro Intensive Care Unit
Department of Medicine
Seth GS Medical College and
KEM Hospital
Mumbai, Maharashtra, India

VM Katoch
Former Secretary
Department of Health Research [DHR]
Ministry of Health and Family Welfare
Government of India

Former Director General
Indian Council of Medical Research
New Delhi, India

NASI—ICMR Chair
Public Health Research
Rajasthan University of Health Sciences
Jaipur, Rajasthan, India

Sunil D Khaparde
Former Deputy Director General-
Tuberculosis
Central TB Division
Ministry of Health and Family Welfare
Government of India
New Delhi, India

Saurav Khatiwada
Department of Endocrinology and
Metabolism
All India Institute of Medical Sciences
New Delhi, India

MPS Kohli
National Consultant
Public Private Mix [Union SEA Office]
Central TB Division
Directorate General of Health Services
Ministry of Health and Family Welfare
Government of India
New Delhi, India

SS Kothari
Professor
Department of Cardiology
All India Institute of Medical Sciences
New Delhi, India

Amitabh Kumar
Chest Specialist
New Delhi Municipal Corporation
[NDMC] Charak Palika Hospital
New Delhi, India

Arvind Kumar
Former Professor
Department of Surgical Disciplines
All India Institute of Medical Sciences
New Delhi, India

Rajeev Kumar
Professor
Department of Urology
All India Institute of Medical Sciences
New Delhi, India

Shaji Kumar
Professor
Division of Hematology
Mayo Clinic
Rochester, Minnesota, USA

Sunesh Kumar
Professor
Department of Obstetrics and
Gynaecology
All India Institute of Medical Sciences
New Delhi, India

T Mohan Kumar
Head of the Department and Chief
Consultant
Institute of Pulmonary Medicine and
Research
Sri Ramakrishnan Hospital
Coimbatore, Tamil Nadu, India

Jason Limberis
Lung Infection and Immunity Unit
Division of Pulmonology and
University of Cape Town Lung Institute
Department of Medicine
University of Cape Town
Cape Town, South Africa

Rakesh Lodha
Professor
Division of Pulmonology, Intensive Care
and Tuberculosis
Department of Paediatrics
All India Institute of Medical Sciences
New Delhi, India

Knut Lönnroth
Professor of Social Medicine
Karolinska Institutet
Senior Consultant
Centre for Epidemiology and
Community Health
Stockholm County Council
Department of Public Health Sciences
Social Medicin
Stockholm, Sweden

Govind K Makharia
Professor
Department of Gastroenterology and
Human Nutrition
All India Institute of Medical Sciences
New Delhi, India

NK Mehra
Dr CG Pandit National Chair
Former Dean [Research]
Former Professor and Head
Department of Transplant Immunology
and Immunogenetics
All India Institute of Medical Sciences
New Delhi, India

DK Mitra
Professor and Head
Department of Transplant Immunology
and Immunogenetics
All India Institute of Medical Sciences
New Delhi, India

Alladi Mohan
Chief, Division of Pulmonary and
Critical Care Medicine
Professor and Head
Department of Medicine
Sri Venkateswara Institute of Medical
Sciences
Tirupati, Andhra Pradesh, India

Prasanta Raghab Mohapatra
Professor and Head
Department of Pulmonary Medicine and
Critical Care
All India Institute of Medical Sciences
Bhubaneswar, Odisha, India

SP Munigoti
Consultant
Department of Endocrinology and
Metabolism
Fortis Hospitals and Health Care
Bengaluru, Karnataka, India

Y Mutheeswaraiah
Professor and Head
Department of General Surgery
Sri Venkateswara Institute of Medical
Sciences
Tirupati, Andra Pradesh, India

HL Nag
Professor
Department of Orthopaedics
All India Institute of Medical Sciences
New Delhi, India

Sreenivas Achutan Nair
Stop TB Partnership
Geneva, Switzerland

Jai P Narain
Former Director
Department of Communicable Diseases
WHO Regional Office for South-East Asia
New Delhi, India

Madhukar Pai
Director
McGill Global Health Programs
Associate Director
McGill International TB Centre
Professor of Epidemiology
McGill University
Montreal, Quebec, Canada

CN Paramasivan
Senior Scientific Advisor
FIND, India

Tania Di Pietrantonio
McGill University Health Center
McGill University
Montreal, Quebec, Canada

John Porter
Professor
London School of Hygiene and Tropical
Medicine
London, UK

Jagdish Prasad
Former Director General of Health
Services
Ministry of Health and Family Welfare
Government of India
New Delhi
Head of Cardiothoracic and
Vascular Surgery Department
Safdarjung Hospital
New Delhi, India

Kurupath Radhakrishnan
Former Senior Professor
Department of Neurology and Director
Sree Chitra Tirunal Institute for Medical
Sciences and Technology
Thiruvananthapuram, Kerala, India
Senior Consultant
Avitis Institute of Medical Sciences
Palakkad, Kerala, India

AK Rai
Assistant Professor
Department of Biotechnology
Motilal Nehru National Institute of
Technology
Allahabad, Uttar Pradesh, India

M Ramam
Professor
Department of Dermatology and
Venereology
All India Institute of Medical Sciences
New Delhi, India

Mario C Raviglione
Professor
Department of Biomedical Sciences for
Health
University of Milan
Milan, Italy
Former Director
Global TB Programme
World Health Organization
Geneva, Switzerland

Ruma Ray
Professor
Department of Pathology
All India Institute of Medical Sciences
New Delhi, India

Divya Reddy
Pulmonary Division
Albert Einstein College of Medicine/
Montefiore Medical Center
Bronx, New York, USA

BB Rewari
Scientist–HIV/STI/HEP
World Health Organization Regional
Office for South-East Asia
New Delhi, India

A Roy
Professor
Department of Cardiology
All India Institute of Medical Sciences
New Delhi, India

KS Sachdeva
Deputy Director General–TB
Central TB Division
Directorate General of Health Services
Ministry of Health and Family Welfare
Government of India
New Delhi, India

Pournamy Sarathchandran
Former Assistant Professor
Department of Neurology
Sree Chitra Tirunal Institute for Medical
Sciences and Technology
Thiruvananthapuram, Kerala, India

Kavitha Saravu
Additional Professor
Department of Medicine
Kasturba Medical College
Manipal, Karnataka, India

Jussi Saukkonen
Director
Medical Intensive Care Unit
VA Boston Healthcare System
West Roxbury, MA, USA

Erwin Schurr
Leader
Infectious Diseases and Immunity in
Global Health
McGill University Health Centre
McGill University
Montreal, Quebec, Canada

Aparna Singh Shah
Regional Advisor
Blood Safety and Laboratory Technology
WHO Regional Office for South-East Asia
New Delhi, India

N Sarita Shah
Associate Chief
Science International Research and
Programs Branch
Division of Tuberculosis Elimination
National Center for HIV, Viral Hepatitis,
STD and TB Prevention
Centers for Disease Control and
Prevention
Atlanta, Georgia, USA

Aman Sharma
Professor
Rheumatology Services
Department of Internal Medicine
Postgraduate Institute of Medical
Education and Research
Chandigarh, India

Amit Sharma
Chest Specialist
Department of Tuberculosis and
Respiratory Diseases
National Institute of Tuberculosis and
Respiratory Diseases
New Delhi, India

Gaurav Sharma
Scientist I
Department of Transplant Immunology
and Immunogenetics
All India Institute of Medical Sciences
New Delhi, India

JB Sharma
Professor
Department of Obstetrics and
Gynaecology
All India Institute of Medical Sciences
New Delhi, India

K Aparna Sharma
Associate Professor
Department of Obstetrics and
Gynaecology
All India Institute of Medical Sciences
New Delhi, India

Kusum Sharma
Professor
Medical Microbiology
Postgraduate Institute of Medical
Education and Research
Chandigarh, India

SC Sharma
Professor and Head
Department of ENT and Neck Surgery
All India Institute of Medical Sciences
New Delhi, India

Surendra K Sharma
Former Senior Professor and Head
Department of Internal Medicine
[WHO Collaborating Centre for Research
and Training in Tuberculosis
Centre of Excellence for Extrapulmonary
TB, Ministry of Health and Family Welfare,
Government of India]
All India Institute of Medical Sciences
New Delhi, India

Adjunct Professor
Department of Molecular Medicine
Jamia Hamdard Institute of Molecular
Medicine
Jamia Hamdard [Deemed to be University]
New Delhi, India

Adjunct Professor
Departments of General Medicine and
Respiratory Medicine
Jawaharlal Nehru Medical College
Datta Meghe Institute of Medical
Sciences [Deemed to be University]
Wardha, Maharashtra, India

Amar Singh
Department of Transplant Immunology
and Immunogenetics
All India Institute of Medical Sciences
New Delhi, India

Divya Singh
Department of Radiodiagnosis
All India Institute of Medical Sciences
New Delhi, India

Rupak Singla
Head
Department of Tuberculosis and
Respiratory Diseases
National Institute of Tuberculosis and
Respiratory Diseases
New Delhi, India

Ramnath Subbaraman
Assistant Professor
Department of Public Health and
Community Medicine
Tufts University School of Medicine
Boston, MA, USA

Grant Theron
Lung Infection and Immunity Unit
Division of Pulmonology and University
of Cape Town Lung Institute
Department of Medicine
University of Cape Town
Cape Town, South Africa

Deanna Tollefson
Epidemiologist
International Research and Programs
Branch
Division of Tuberculosis Elimination
National Center for HIV, Viral Hepatitis,
STD and TB Prevention
Centers for Disease Control and
Prevention
Atlanta, Georgia, USA

Srikanth Tripathy
Scientist G and Director-in-charge
National Institute for Research in
Tuberculosis
Chennai, Tamil Nadu, India

AK Tyagi
Vice-Chancellor
Guru Gobind Singh [GGS]
Indraprastha University
Sector 16-C, Dwarka, New Delhi, India

Professor
Department of Biochemistry
University of Delhi [South Campus]
New Delhi, India

Mukund Uplekar
Former Senior Medical Officer
Policy, Strategy and Innovations Unit
Global TB Programme
World Health Organization
Geneva, Switzerland

Hon. Professor
Interdisciplinary School of
Health Sciences
Pune University
Pune, Maharashtra, India

Pradeep Venkatesh
Professor
Dr Rajendra Prasad Centre for
Ophthalmic Sciences
All India Institute of Medical Sciences
New Delhi, India

Andrew Vernon
Chief
Clinical Research Branch
Division of Tuberculosis Elimination
National Center for HIV, Viral Hepatitis,
STD and TB Prevention
Centers for Disease Control and
Prevention
Atlanta, Georgia, USA

Late VK Vijayan
Former Advisor
ICMR Bhopal Memorial Hospital and
Research Centre
National Institute for Research in
Environmental Health

Former Director
Vallabhbhai Patel Chest Institute
University of Delhi
Delhi, India

Kamini Walia
Scientist F
Indian Council of Medical Research
New Delhi, India

Diana Weil
Coordinator
TB Policy, Strategy and Innovations [PSI]
Global TB Programme [GTB]
World Health Organization [WHO]
Geneva, Switzerland

Ting-Heng Yu
McGill University Health Center
McGill University
Montreal, Quebec, Canada

Foreword

"Rarely has any epidemic tormented the humankind with the tenacity and destructive impact of tuberculosis [TB]...TB still constitutes a social, economic and political threat set to impede development of entire populations...". This is what I said in my foreword to the previous edition of this book in 2009. It is hardly surprising that the statements remain true nine years later. On the occasion of the publication of the new edition that will explore in-depth from all angles this ancient disease, I feel honoured to have been asked by Professor Surendra K Sharma, for a second time in a row, to write a foreword of his *Textbook of Tuberculosis and Nontuberculous Mycobacterial Diseases—3rd edition*, a book that is a true state-of-the-art manual on the disease. In the Global TB Report of the World Health Organization [WHO], published in October 2017 when I was still director of the Global TB Programme, we highlighted several important facts. First, thanks to recent intensive efforts to improve the collection and reporting of data through special surveys and surveillance, WHO now estimates that there may be over a million more cases of TB than previously believed. This translated into 10.4 million people developing TB in 2016 and 1.7 million dying of it. Second, the report stresses that, despite the rise in absolute numbers, the mortality rate from TB continues falling at about 3% per year. As a result of control efforts, an estimated 53 million lives have been saved since 2000. This is encouraging; however, the TB incidence rate is declining very slowly at an average of 1.5% a year. With such an enormous toll in terms of number of deaths, TB, remains the biggest killer from a single infectious agent. Thirdly, over 4 million people who develop TB are still being 'missed' by health systems each year: a large number of them are not diagnosed due to poor access to services or lack of capacity; and an even larger number is probably diagnosed and treated somehow outside the public sector but not notified. Fourth, the global multidrug-resistant TB [MDR-TB] crisis continues, with an estimated 600,000 new MDR-TB and rifampicin-resistant cases in 2016. A trend analysis revealed that the estimated percentage of new TB cases with MDR-TB globally remains roughly unchanged at 4%. However, severe epidemics still ravage some regions, particularly Eastern Europe and Central Asia. Extensively drug-resistant TB [XDR-TB], which is more expensive and difficult to treat than MDR-TB, has now been reported in most countries that are capable of detecting it. Unfortunately, the progress in the MDR-TB response has been far too slow: while there has been an increase of cases being diagnosed thanks to more laboratories rolling out rapid tests, only less than a quarter of the estimated cases are being detected and treated. In 2019, at the time of publication of the 3rd edition of this book, therefore, several major challenges remain to be faced. The first one is to ensure that all the cases are diagnosed, managed successfully and notified; the second is to respond effectively to the MDR-TB crisis; the third is to consolidate achievements in the response to HIV-associated TB; the fourth is to ensure research efforts are urgently intensified so that innovations emerge within years instead of decades; and the fifth is to ensure all financial gaps in both control and research efforts are filled. In May 2014, the World Health Assembly of WHO approved—through an historical resolution—a set of new and ambitious targets for 2030 and 2035 to be reached through a new global TB strategy. This new End TB Strategy, based on three pillars and four fundamental principles, incorporates all possible elements that are essential for a recipe towards TB elimination. The TB-specific interventions are included in the first pillar of the new strategy: it consists of a modern version of DOTS [1994-2005] and the Stop TB Strategy [2006-2015], which incorporates all technological innovations from early diagnosis of TB and universal drug susceptibility testing using rapid molecular tests to treatment of all types of TB and management of latent infection among people with a higher risk of getting TB. The second pillar consists of those broad health system policies that are essential to render any disease control effort successful: these include regulatory approaches such as mandatory case notifications and rational drug use, as well as essential far-reaching measures like universal health coverage and social protection to ensure that the poorest among the poor can access care. The third pillar emphasises the role of research and rapid intake and adaptation of all innovations in all countries world-wide. It is in this context that the publication of the 3rd edition of this book by Professor Surendra K Sharma is particularly important. Indeed, this edition represents a major advance over the previous ones as it is based on the feedback received from different categories of students and health professionals and adapted to the needs of such different audiences. As a result of a "client survey", the editor decided to develop a set of two different textbooks: an elaborate version for postgraduates and more advanced readers and a compact one providing the essentials for undergraduate students. The larger version, similar to the 2nd edition, although slimmer and more user-friendly, is a comprehensive and well-referenced textbook. It will contain chapters focused on clinical aspects—a true reference for clinicians managing patients with any variety of TB. It will also present the very basics of TB, from epidemiology to bacteriology, from genetics to immunology, and from diagnosis to treatment. In some cases, the old chapters have been merged to make them more easily accessible. For some new areas, such as the place of TB in the post Millennium Development Goal [MDG] agenda or the engagement of communities in TB care, new chapters have been added. Continuing its laudable trend, the inclusion of many chapters devoted to public health and control aspects in this edition makes this textbook an international reference in a broader sense. Above all, there are chapters that examine the delicate interface between public services and the private and non-state sector, an issue that must be faced with an innovative spirit given its challenging nature, and the fundamental infection control measures often neglected in many countries. Importantly, for every clinical and public health practitioner, the book contains a description of the WHO's new global strategy—the End TB Strategy 2016-2035—and the International Standards of TB Care including their adaptation in the Indian context. These chapters provide the most modern and innovative thinking about the way the TB epidemic must be addressed at the bedside, in the clinics, and in the health centres supervised by TB control programmes. The second compact version of the book is a practical "handbook" for young undergraduates to carry in the pockets of a coat. This will contain the essential information with additional sections made available "on-line". It is intended as a rapid reference to help quick learning and action. Naturally, to cover all needs and provide the best possible information to readers, a remarkable panel of authors has been put together by Professor Sharma; it includes both experts from India and international authorities. In conclusion, the two versions of this prestigious textbook, devoted to a major disease that has affected humanity since its beginning, have all the characteristics to consolidate the previous edition's reputation of an authoritative and international reference for all readers. The fact that it is conceived and produced in India, the country which not only has the highest TB burden in the world, but has also contributed to many of the major advances in TB care and control over the past decades, is symbolic. And the fact that it is published in the historical year during which TB will be the subject of a high-level meeting of leaders at the United Nations General Assembly adds value to a book that expresses the latest scientific knowledges about the crucial topic of TB. It is my hope that this modern and up-to-date textbook becomes a fundamental companion for all junior and senior practitioners tackling TB prevention, care and control in India, elsewhere in Asia, and world-wide so that our global fight against this ancient disease can be better informed and more effective.

Mario C Raviglione FRCP [UK] FERS Hon RSP [RF]

Professor

Department of Biomedical Sciences for Health

University of Milan

Milan, Italy

Former Director

Global TB Programme

World Health Organization

Geneva, Switzerland

Preface to the Third Edition

The first edition of *Tuberculosis* book in 2001 was widely acclaimed not only in India and South-East Asia, but also in several other parts of the world. Subsequently, the second edition of *Tuberculosis* was published in 2009 which was well received and established itself as a standard textbook on tuberculosis [TB]. The last decade has witnessed phenomenal changes in our understanding of TB and there have been overwhelming requests for updating this textbook. Further, major advances have also occurred in nontuberculous mycobacterial [NTM] diseases in the recent years. This prompted us to bring out the third edition of the book which is now titled *Textbook of Tuberculosis and Nontuberculous Mycobacterial Diseases* with an aim to provide a well referenced standard textbook on TB and NTM diseases that will chronicle the rich and vast experience of clinicians and researchers from across the globe.

This edition has several new contributors, all of them are leading authorities, from various parts of the world. All the chapters have been thoroughly re-written and updated, many of them are by new but renowned contributors. Several new high quality clinical, radiographic images, gross pathology specimen photographs, and photomicrographs have been included in this edition for the readers' convenience. This edition documents the rapid advances that have occurred at a blistering pace in TB diagnosis, universal drug-susceptibility testing [DST] and treatment of dug-susceptible and drug-resistant TB, including multidrug-resistant and extensively drug-resistant TB [M/XDR-TB], programmatic management of drug-resistant TB, public-private mix, the ENGAGE-TB approach, and END TB strategy, among others. The present edition includes recent classification of drugs and drug combinations including recent generation quinolones, bedaquiline and linezolid used in treating M/XDR-TB and a chapter detailing the latest developments in the field of laboratory diagnosis and management of NTM diseases.

We sincerely believe that the third edition will help undergraduate and postgraduate medical students and medical college faculty members in updating their knowledge. We hope that it will continue to be a valuable source of reference to researchers and enhance the understanding of practising physicians and contribute to patient management. The third edition is also envisaged to be a practical guide for health care workers, nurses, and other paramedical staff.

This effort would not have been possible but for the kind co-operation and magnanimity of our contributors who spared their valuable time and patiently went through endless series of revisions and constant updating. We would like to thank Shri Jitendar P Vij [Group Chairman], Mr Ankit Vij [Managing Director], Ms Chetna Malhotra Vohra [Associate Director–Content Strategy] of M/s Jaypee Brothers Medical Publishers [P] Ltd, New Delhi, India, for their encouragement and support, and excellent technical assistance. Our families have stood by us through these turbulent times and without their unstinting support and constant encouragement, this third edition would not have materialised.

Surendra K Sharma
Alladi Mohan

Preface to the First Edition

Tuberculosis is an ancient disease which continues to haunt us even as we step into the next millennium. Tuberculosis is the most common cause of death world over due to a single infectious agent in adults and accounts for over a quarter of all avoidable deaths globally. One-third of India's population is infected with *Mycobacterium tuberculosis,* there are 12 million active tuberculosis cases in India. One person dies of tuberculosis every minute in India. The deadly synergy between *Mycobacterium tuberculosis* and the human immunodeficiency virus [HIV] has resulted in a resurgence of tuberculosis world over. The impact of this "cursed duet" on human suffering has been enormous. With HIV making rapid inroads in India, the spectre of dual infection with HIV and tuberculosis is going to be a daunting prospect. In spite of this gloomy scenario, the treatment of tuberculosis is one of the most cost-effective methods of cure. Research work carried out in India has had a tremendous impact on tuberculosis control. The observations from the well-known, randomized controlled trial "The Madras Study" carried out at the Tuberculosis Research Centre [TRC], Chennai, Tamil Nadu, India, established the efficacy of the domiciliary treatment and has paved the way for the National Tuberculosis Programme in India and several other countries. Pioneering contributions from eminent clinicians, bacteriologists and epidemiologists from the TRC, Chennai; National Tuberculosis Institute, Bangalore; Sanatoria at Madanapalle, Kasauli, Dharampur, Bhowali, have greatly enhanced our understanding of tuberculosis.

The changing clinical presentation of tuberculosis, advances in laboratory and imaging diagnostic modalities and therapeutic measures such as directly observed treatment, short-course [DOTS] all suggest a pressing need to have a recent textbook of tuberculosis. Furthermore, while every doctor working in India encounters the disease in one or other form, very little has been documented regarding the Indian perspective of tuberculosis. Often, the medical students, postgraduates and researchers returning empty handed from libraries expressed their desire for a book which documents the Indian experience. Paucity of a well referenced, standard textbook of tuberculosis, which chronicles the rich and vast clinical experience of clinicians from India prompted us to undertake this venture. We have attempted to present a picture of tuberculosis as it is seen in India with contributions from experts who have vast experience in managing tuberculosis in the Indian setting. Our book contains chapters on History, Pathology, Epidemiology, Clinical Presentation, Diagnosis, Treatment, Prevention and Control of tuberculosis highlighting the Indian perspective of tuberculosis. We have also provided guidelines published by the authorities concerned with tuberculosis control, and other statements as useful appendices. Though we have made an effort to maintain a uniform style and format, we have been careful to preserve the views expressed by the contributors in their original form. As we step into the new millennium, it is obvious that the crusade against this ancient foe of mankind is still going on. Contrary to the wishful thinking in the 1980s, tuberculosis still remain to be a research priority of paramount importance and is an important component of curricula of medical schools. Keeping in mind the need of the hour, we have attempted to highlight the rationale behind DOTS and its importance in tuberculosis control. We believe that our book will help undergraduate and postgraduate medical students to update their knowledge. It will also be a source of reference to researchers and better the understanding of practising physicians and help in patient management. We also hope that the book can serve as a practical guide on the management of tuberculosis to health care workers, nurses and other paramedical staff.

A book of this magnitude would not have been possible but for the magnanimity and kindness of our contributors who took time off their busy schedule to prepare their manuscripts. We would like to thank Mr Jitendar P Vij, Chairman and Managing Director and Mr RK Yadav, Publishing Director, M/s Jaypee Brothers Medical Publishers Pvt Ltd., for their support, co-operation and technical excellence. Without the unstinting support, constant encouragement and help from our families this endeavour would not have been possible.

S.K. Sharma
A. Mohan

Acknowledgements

We would like to especially thank the M/s Jaypee Brothers Medical Publishers [P] Ltd, New Delhi, India, who have granted permissions to reproduce various items from their published work and these have duly acknowledged in the respective chapters. An invaluable help of the World Health Organization [WHO], Geneva, Switzerland for liberally granting permission to reproduce figures and tables from several publications is gratefully acknowledged.

We express our sincere gratitude to the following Drs Mario Raviglione, Dennis Falzon, Mukund Uplekar, Knut Lonnroth, Deanna Tollefson, N Sarita Shah, Andrew Vernon, Haileyesus Getahun, Mr Thomas Joseph, Drs Sreenivas A Nair, Md Khurshid Alam Hyder, Vineet Bhatia, Diana Weil, Divya Reddy, Jussi Saukkonen, Keertan Dheda, Erwin Schurr, Madhukar Pai and John Porter, for their excellent contributions. Special thanks are also due to Dr PC Hopewell, University of California, San Francisco, USA for his suggestions on the International Standards for Tuberculosis Care [ISTC].

We especially thank Dr Jai P Narain, Former Director, Department of Communicable Diseases, WHO Regional Office for South-East Asia, New Delhi, Dr Jagdish Prasad, Former Director General of Health Services [DGHS], Ministry of Health and Family Welfare, Government of India [MoH & FW, GoI], Dr LS Chauhan, Former Deputy Director General [Tuberculosis], Central TB Division, Directorate General of Health Services, Ministry of Health and Family Welfare, Government of India, for their valuable contributions, critical comments, stimulating discussions, constant support and encouragement. We would like to thank Dr VM Katoch, Former Secretary, Department of Health Research [DHR], MoH & FW, GoI, and Former Director General, Indian Council of Medical Research [ICMR], New Delhi, and Dr CN Paramasivan, Foundation for Innovative New Diagnostics [FIND], India, for their constant encouragement.

We thank Dr KS Sachdeva, Deputy Director General [Tuberculosis], Central TB Division, Directorate General of Health Services, MoH & FW, GoI, for his constant support and encouragement. We also wish to thank Directors of National Institute of Tuberculosis and Respiratory Diseases [NITRD], New Delhi; ICMR-National Institute for Research in Tuberculosis [NIRT], Chennai and National Tuberculosis Institute [NTI], Bengaluru, Karnataka, the administration of Arogyavaram Medical Centre, Madanapalle, Andhra Pradesh, and TB Sanatorium at Bhowali, Uttarakhand for permitting us to reproduce the images of these well known institutions.

We are grateful to the Departments of Pathology, All India Institute of Medical Sciences [AIIMS], New Delhi; Sri Venkateswara Institute of Medical Sciences [SVIMS], Tirupati, Andhra Pradesh; and Postgraduate Institute of Medical Education and Research [PGIMER], Chandigarh for providing gross pathology specimen figures and histopathology photomicrographs. We wish to thank the Departments of Radiodiagnosis, AIIMS, New Delhi and SVIMS, Tirupati for providing classic radiographic imaging figures. We sincerely thank Dr Ajay Garg, Department of Neuroradiology, Neurosciences Centre, All India Institute of Medical Sciences, New Delhi for providing radiographic images, Dr C Narasimhan, CARE Hospitals, Hyderabad, Telangana, India, Dr Tara Roshini Paul, Professor, Department of Pathology, Nizam's Institute of Medical Sciences, Hyderabad, for providing echocardiographic images, photomicrographs respectively.

We also wish to thank faculty members of AIIMS, New Delhi; SVIMS, Tirupati; and other medical colleges across India and several other parts of the world, several generations of undergraduate and postgraduate students, for their constructive criticism and useful suggestions during our discussions. These inputs were indeed useful for the Third Edition of the book.

Invaluable help rendered by Dr Krishna Srihasam, Boston, USA; and Dr Srinivas Bollineni, Dallas, USA, in getting full text references is also thankfully acknowledged. We also wish to thank Mr Alladi V Srikumar's timely help with broadband connectivity.

Contents

History

Alladi Mohan, Surendra K Sharma

INTRODUCTION

As a destroyer of mankind, tuberculosis has no equal...
VA Moore (1)

Tuberculosis [TB] has been a major cause of suffering and death since times immemorial. Thought to be one of the oldest human diseases, the history of TB is at least as old as the mankind. Over the years, not only the medical implications but also the social and economic impact of TB has been enormous.

There have been references to this ancient scourge in the *Vedas* [*vide infra*] and it was called "rajayakshma" [meaning "wasting disease"]. Hippocrates [460-377 B.C.] called the disease "pthisis", a Greek word which meant "to consume", "to spit" and "to waste away" (2,3). The word "consumption" [derived from the Latin word "consumere"] has also been used to describe TB in English literature. The Hebrew word "schachepheth" [meaning "waste away"] has been used in the Bible. J.L. Schonlein, Professor of Medicine at Zurich, is credited to have named the disease "tuberculosis" (1). The word "tuberculosis" is a derivative of the Latin word "tubercula" which means "a small lump" (2,4,5). Several names have been used to refer to TB in the years gone by. Acute progressive TB has been referred to as "galloping consumption". Pulmonary TB has been referred to as "tabes pulmonali". Tuberculosis cervical lymphadenitis has been called as "scrofula", "King's Evil", "stroma". Abdominal TB has been called as "tabes mesenterica". Cutaneous TB has been called "lupus vulgaris". Vertebral TB has been called as "Pott's disease". Oliver Wendell Holmes referred to the disease as "white plague" (6). While scores of other diseases like smallpox and plague killed millions of people, their reign has been relatively short-lived. Tuberculosis has been ever present and is resurging with a vengeance.

TUBERCULOSIS IN ANCIENT TIMES

It is thought that TB probably existed in cattle before its advent in man.

muncami tva havisa jivanayakam
agnatayaksmad uta rajayakshma...
[I deliver you by means of oblation so that you may live from the unknown disease and from the "rajayakshma"]
[RV, X,161,1]

In the *Krishna Yajurveda Samhita*, there is reference to how, Soma [Moon] had been affected by "yakshma". Since "Soma", who was the "King and Ruler" was affected by "yakshma", it came to be known as "rajayakshma" [Figure 1.1].

In Sanskrit, the disease has been called "rajayakshma", "ksayah", and "sosa".

Rajayakshma ksayah soso rogarad iti cha smritah
naksatranam, dvijanam cha rajno bhud yad aym pura
yach cha raja cha yakshma cha rajayakshma tato matah
[Vagabhatta, Ast-s and Ast-hrd, Nidana V, 1-2]

Krodho yakshma jvaro roga eko 'rtho dukhasamjnitah
yasmat sa rajnah prag asid rajayakshma tatomatah
[Charaka Samhita, Chikitsasthanam VIII, 11]

Changes resembling those caused by TB have been described in the skeletal remains of neolithic man (7). Terms such as "lung cough" and "lung fever" have been used in ancient Chinese literature to describe a disease which might have been TB (8). There have been references to what could have been TB in the Code of Hammurabi of the Babylonian era (6). Evidences of TB lesions of bone have also been found in Egyptian mummies dating back

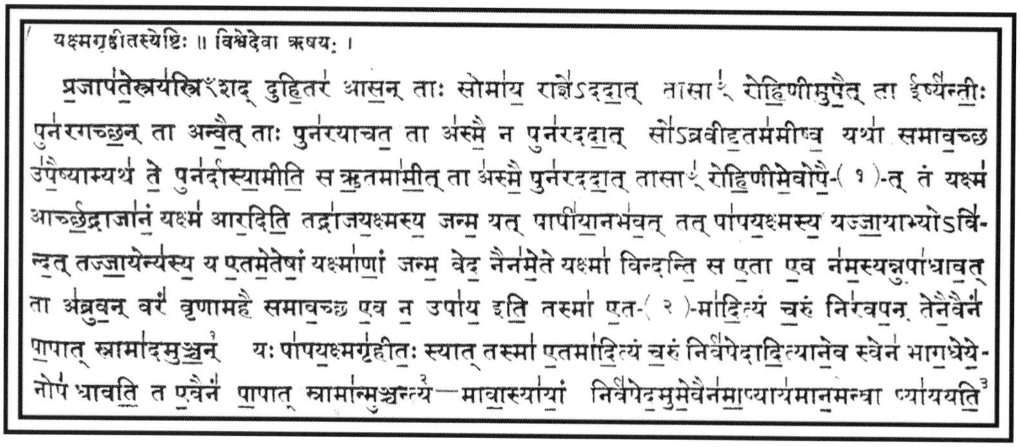
यक्ष्मगृहीतस्येष्टिः ॥ विश्वेदेवा ऋषयः ।

प्रजापतेस्त्रयस्त्रिꣳशद् दुहितर आसन् ताः सोमाय राज्ञेऽददात् तासाꣳ रोहिणीमुपैत् ता ईर्ष्यन्तीः पुनरगच्छन् ता अन्वैत् ताः पुनरयाचत ता अस्मै न पुनरददात् सोऽब्रवीदृतममीष्व यथा समावच्छ उपैष्याम्यथ ते पुनर्दास्यामीति स ऋतमामीत् ता अस्मै पुनरददात् तासाꣳ रोहिणीमेवोपै-(१)-त् तं यक्ष्म आर्च्छद्राजानं यक्ष्म आरदिति तद्राजयक्ष्मस्य जन्म यत् पापीयानभवत् तत् पापयक्ष्मस्य यज्जायाभ्योऽविन्दत् तज्जायेन्यस्य य एतमेतेषां यक्ष्माणां जन्म वेद नैनमेते यक्ष्मा विन्दन्ति स एता एव नमस्यन्नुपाधावत् ता अब्रुवन् वरं वृणामहै समावच्छ एव न उपाय इति तस्मा एत-(२)-मादित्यं चरुं निरवपन् तेनैवैनं पापात् स्रामादमुञ्चन् यः पापयक्ष्मगृहीतः स्यात् तस्मा एतमादित्यं चरुं निर्वपेदादित्यानेव स्वेन भागधेये-नोप धावति त एवैनं पापात् स्रामान्मुञ्चन्त्य-मावास्यायां निर्वपेदमुमेवैनमाप्यायमानमन्वा प्याययति[3]

Figure 1.1: *Krishna Yajurveda Samhita, II kanda, III prasna, V anuvaka, 25th stanza,* where the legend of "Soma" being afflicted with "rajayakshma" is described

to 3400 B.C. (7). *Mycobacterium tuberculosis* has been demonstrated microscopically in the mummy of a child of five years (8).

There are several references to conditions resembling TB in Greek literature by Homer [800 B.C.], Hippocrates, Aristotle [384-322 B.C.] and Plato [430-347 B.C.], Galen [129-199], Vegetius [420] were also familiar with consumption. Arabic physicians Al Razi [850-953], Ibn Sina [980-1037] correlated lung cavities with skin ulceration.

During the middle ages, there are records of healing touch of monarchs was being used to treat "scrofula" [King's Evil]. King Charles II bestowed the royal touch on an astounding 92,102 patients with "scrofula" (9). By around 1629, death certificates in London specified the disease as "consumption" which was a leading cause of death. By this time the contagious nature of TB was strongly believed though there were people who contested this opinion. The Republic of Lucca is credited to have passed the first legislative action aimed at controlling TB in the world (4,9). This was followed by similar measures in several Italian cities and Spain.

DIAGNOSIS

Why, when one comes near consumptives... does one contract their disease, while one does not contract dropsy, apoplexy, fever, or many other ills?....

Aristotle

In the early days, diagnosis of TB was based on symptoms and signs. In *Charaka Samhita* [*Nidanasthana, VI, 14*], heaviness in the head, coughing, dyspnoea, hoarseness of voice, vomiting of phlegm, spitting of blood, pain in the sides of the chest, grinding pain in the shoulder, fever, diarrhoea and anorexia have been described as the eleven symptoms of TB. Furthermore, a physician who is well versed in the aetiology, clinical presentation and premonitory symptoms of "consumption" was considered to be a "Royal Physician" [*Charaka Samhita, Nidanasthana, VI, 17*].

The earliest classical descriptions of TB in Greek literature date back to the writings by Hippocrates. Aretaeus the Cappodocian [50 B.C.], in his book *The causes and symptoms of chronic diseases* gave a very accurate description of TB and mentioned that fever, sweating, fatigue and lassitude were symptoms of the TB. He suggested testing the sputum with fire or water was of diagnostic value (7). Galen described that patients with "consumption" manifest cough, sputum, wasting, chest pain and fever and considered haemoptysis to be pathognomonic of the disease (6).

Following the pioneering efforts by Andreas Vesalius [1514-1564] post-mortem examination was performed frequently. This method of study facilitated understanding of pathological findings, such as, lung cavities, empyema among others. Franciscus de Boe [1614-1672] [also known as Sylvius] for the first time associated small hard nodules discovered in various tissues at autopsy with symptoms of "consumption" which the patients suffered during their life-time though his explanation for the same was not correct (7). John Jacob Manget in 1700 gave the description of classical miliary TB (10). The clinical presentation of consumption was described in detail by Thomas Willis [1621-1675]. Richard Morton [1637-1698] had described several pathological appearances of "pthisis" in his treatise *Pthisiologica* (4-6,7).

Meaningful clinical examination became possible with the description of the technique of percussion by Leopold Auenbrugger [1722-1809]. However, Auenbrugger's work was virtually ignored until the time of Jean Nicolas Covisart [1775-1821], who rediscovered and propagated the technique. Gaspard Bayle [1774-1816] accurately described many of the pathological changes of TB, but unfortunately succumbed to the disease which he probably contracted while performing autopsy studies (11). The technique of physical examination of the lung was further refined by the invention of stethoscope by Rene Theophile Hyacinthe Laënnec [1781-1826], who was a student of Corvisart and a friend of Bayle. Sadly, Laennec, his younger brother, mother and two uncles all succumbed to TB (6).

Fracastorius [1443-1553] is credited to have originated the "germ theory" and believed that TB was contagious. He also mentioned about antiseptics in his chapter on the treatment of TB. In 1720, the English physician Benjamin Marten conjectured, in his publication *A new theory of consumption*, that TB could be caused by "certain species of animalcula or wonderfully minute living creatures", which, once they had gained a foothold in the body, could generate the lesions and symptoms of the disease. He also stated that

> *"it may be therefore very likely that by an habitual lying in the same bed with a consumptive patient, constantly eating and drinking with him, or by very frequently conversing so nearly as to draw in part of the breath he emits from the lungs, consumption may be caught by a sound person...I imagine that slightly conversing with consumptive patients is seldom or never sufficient to catch the disease"* (12)

For unknown reason the work of Marten went into oblivion for a long time. The likely reason could be that he was thinking very much ahead of his time. Jean Antoine Villemin [1827-1892] in a series of experiments provided conclusive evidence that TB was indeed a contagious disease though some workers of that era did not accept these results. He presented his results to the Academie de Medcine on December 5, 1865 and stated that TB was a specific infection caused by an inoculable agent (3,6).

> *"During my wandering through medicine, I encountered sites where gold was lying around. It needs a lot of serendipity to distinguish gold from ignobility; this, however, is not a particular achievement."*
>
> Robert Koch (13)

Robert Heinrich Herman Koch [Figure 1.2], son of a mining engineer, was born on December 11, 1843 in Clausthal village in the Harz mountains (3,6,14,15). Koch pursued medical studies at the Gottingen University in 1862 and qualified maxima cum laude in 1866 with his M.D. thesis on succinic acid. On March 24, 1882 Koch announced the discovery of the tubercle bacillus during the monthly evening meeting of the Berlin Physiological Society. In 1884, he published a more comprehensive paper *Die aetiologic der tuberculose* in the second volume of the *Reports of the Imperial Health Office*. In 1905, he was awarded the Nobel Prize for his contributions in the field of TB research (3,5,6). In 1982, a century after Dr Koch's announcement, the World Health Organization [WHO] and the International Union Against Tuberculosis and Lung Disease [IUATLD], now called The Union proposed the 24th March as the "World TB Day" as a part of a year-long centennial effort under the theme "Defeat TB: Now and Forever." Thereafter, since 1996, 24th March is celebrated as "World TB Day" every year (16,17). The event was intended to educate the public about the devastating health and economic consequences of TB, and its continued tragic impact on the global health. Each "World TB Day" addresses a different theme [Table 1.1]. Robert Koch died on May 27, 1910, aged 66 years.

It was Robert Koch who finally demystified the secret of the cause of TB and after thousands of years, the organism finally revealed itself to humans. Though, Robert Koch was wrong in his belief that tuberculin would cure TB, tuberculin became an invaluable tool for the diagnosis of latent TB infection (18).

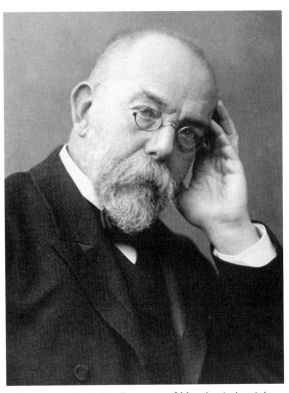

Figure 1.2: Robert Koch: the discoverer of *Mycobacterium tuberculosis Reproduced with permission from "Rubin SA. Tuberculosis. The captain of all these men of death. Radiol Clin North Am 1995;33:619-39 (reference 6)"*

Table 1.1: World TB Day themes	
Year	*World TB Day theme*
1997	Use DOTS more widely
1998	DOTS success stories
1999	Stop TB, use DOTS
2000	Forging new partnerships to stop TB
2001	DOTS: TB cure for all
2002	Stop TB, fight poverty
2003	DOTS cured me–It will cure you too!
2004	Every breath counts–stop TB now
2005	Frontline TB care providers: Heroes in the fight against TB
2006	Actions for life–Towards a world free of TB
2007	TB anywhere is TB everywhere
2008	I am stopping TB
2009	I am stopping TB
2010	On the move against TB: Innovate towards action
2011	On the move against TB: Transforming the fight towards elimination
2012	Call for a world free of TB
2013	Stop TB in my lifetime
2014	Reach the three million–A TB test, treatment and cure for all
2015	Gear up to end TB
2016	United to end TB
2017	Let's unite to end TB
2018	Wanted: Leaders for a TB-free world
TB = tuberculosis; DOTS = directly observed treatment, short-course	

With the advent of Wilhelm Conrad Roentgen [1845-1923], the technique of radiological imaging became available. Francis Williams in Boston, L. Bouchard and A. Beclere in France, John MacIntyre and David Lawson in Britain were pioneers in the use of radiography in the study of TB (3,6). By this time, the deep mystery that was TB became demystified to some extent in that basic concepts of the agent, the pathology as a result of it and its detection became established ushering in the era of definitive diagnosis of TB.

TREATMENT

In the *Yajurveda*, there are references to Soma performing a "yagna" [sacred offering] seeking cure from TB. Since ancient times amulets, invocations, charms, Royal touch and prayers have been used to treat TB. Chemicals such as arsenic, sulphur, calcium, several vegetable, plant and animal products including excreta of humans and animals, blood letting have been used over the centuries in the fond hope of curing TB. Robert Koch, soon after his discovery of the tubercle bacillus, ambitiously introduced the treatment using "Koch's lymph" with disastrous results. It was later known that the substance was a glycerin extract of the tubercle bacillus and was named as "tuberculin" (3,6).

During the 19th century, bed rest and change in environment emerged as important forms of treatment of TB. Hermann Brehmer, Peter Dettweiler, George Bodington, Edward Livingston Trudeau, were all pioneers of the sanatorium movement. Hermann Brehmer, a Botany student suffering from TB, was instructed by his physician to seek out a healthier climate. He travelled to the Himalayan mountains where he could pursue his botanical studies while trying to rid himself of the disease. He returned home cured and began to study medicine. In 1854, he presented his doctoral dissertation bearing the title, "Tuberculosis is a curable disease". In the same year, he built an institution in GÖrbersdorf where, in the midst of fir trees, and with good nutrition, patients were exposed on their balconies to continuous fresh air. This set up became the blueprint for the subsequent development of sanatoria (12). During this period, surgery was extensively used for the treatment of TB. The reader is referred to the chapter *"Surgery for pleuropulmonary tuberculosis" [Chapter 46]* for the details.

Efforts by Albert Calmette and his assistant Camille Guérin resulted in the introduction of bacille Calmette-Guérin [BCG] vaccine (19). Pioneering work of Selman Waksman led to the introduction of streptomycin as an effective anti-TB drug. Jorgen Lehman was instrumental in the discovery of para-amino salicylic acid [PAS]. With the availability of these drugs and isoniazid, the era of modern predictably effective treatment ushered in. With the introduction of rifampicin, the treatment duration could be further shortened to the present-day six-month short-course chemotherapy.

TUBERCULOSIS IN ARTS AND LITERATURE

Youth grows pale, and spectre thin, and dies

John Keats
Ode to a Nightingale

'Tis called the evil:
A most miraculous work in this good king;
Which often since my here-remain in England
I have seen him do. How he solicits heaven,
Himself best knows; but strangely visited people,
All swollen and ulcerous, pitiful to the eye,
The mere despair of surgery, he cures,
Hanging a golden stamp about their necks,
Put on with holy prayers; and 'tis spoken,
To the succeeding royalty he leaves
The healing benediction

William Shakespeare
Macbeth, IV, iii, 146

There have been references to TB in several works of fiction. There are references to TB in William Shakespeare's plays such as the "consumptive lover" of *Much Ado About Nothing* and "scrofula" in *Macbeth*. Charles Dickens describes the sufferings of Little Blossom in *David Copperfield*. Thomas Mann's *The Magic Mountain* contains one of the most well-known descriptions of TB sanatorium. Little Eva of Harriet Beecher Stowe's *Uncle Tom's Cabin*, Milly Theale in Henry James' *The Wings of the Dove*, Marguerite Gautier in Alexander Dumas' *La Dame aux Cameilas* also suffered from TB.

TB does not respect anybody. Several important personalities, statesmen, writers, poets, performing artists have been consumed by TB [Table 1.2]. John Keats and Percy Bysshe Shelley symbolised the era of the "romantic consumptive youths of the 19th century" (3). The image of John Keats conveyed by the writings of contemporaries of his era is that of a fragile poet who fell victim to TB because his sensitive nature had been unable to withstand contact with a crude world (3). In a well-known anecdote, when his friend John Brown discovers a drop of blood on the sheet while examining him, Keats says:

"I know the colour of that blood. It's 'arterial blood'...
That blood is my death warrant, I must die ... (3)

Shelley, a fellow poet also suffered from TB pleurisy but did not succumb to the disease. On hearing the passing of Keats, Shelley wrote:

From the contagion of the world's slow stain
He is secure, and now can never mourn
A heart grown cold, a head grown gray in vain;
Nor, when spirit's self has ceased to burn,
With sparkless ashes load an unlamented urn...

The Bronte family included six children all of whom succumbed to TB. Maria and Elizabeth died at a very young age. The son died of consumption, alcohol and opium. Emily *[Wuthering Heights]* and Charlotte *[Jane Eyre]* died aged 29 and 39 respectively. It was thought that, their father Rev. Patrick Bronte was the source of infection. The families of Ralph Waldo Emerson and Henry David Thoreau were also wiped out by consumption (3,6).

Several famous Indians had also succumbed to TB. The list includes the famous mathematician Srinivasa Ramanujan, writer Munshi Prem Chand, Kamala Nehru, among others.

Table 1.2: Well-known victims of tuberculosis

Mathematician
  Srinivasa Ramanujan
Doctors
  Rene Theophile Hyacinthe Laënnec
  Edward Livingston Trudeau
Writers and Poets
  Alexander Pope
  Samuel Johnson
  Jean-Jacques Rousseau
  Johann Wolfgang von Goethe
  Sir Walter Scott
  Percy Bysshe Shelley
  John Keats
  Leigh Hunt
  Elizabeth Barrett Browning
  Charlotte Brontë
  Emily Brontë
  Anne Brontë
  Fyodor Dostoevsky
  Robert Louis Stevenson
  Anton Chekhov
  Franz Kafka
  Katherine Mansfield
  George Orwell
  Munshi Prem Chand
Statesmen/Stateswomen
  Kamala Nehru
  Eleanor Roosevelt
  Mohammed Ali Jinnah
  Nelson Mandela
Musicians
  Frederic Francois Chopin
  Niccolo Paganini
  Carl Maria von Weber
Performing Artists
  Vivien Leigh
  Elisa Rachel Felix
  Amitabh Bachchan

RISK FACTORS

Historically, several genetic, social, environmental and biological determinants of health have been identified as risk factors for TB. Role of genetic factors in the causation of TB has been covered in the chapters *"Genetic susceptibility parameters in tuberculosis"* [Chapter 6] and *"Genetics of susceptibility to tuberculosis"* [Chapter 7]. No account of the history of TB would be complete without a reference to this modern foe. The impact of the twin disaster of human immunodeficiency virus [HIV] infection and TB on human suffering has been covered in the chapter *"Tuberculosis and human immunodeficiency virus infection"* [Chapter 35]. The deadly interaction between diabetes mellitus [DM] and TB is being increasingly recognised world over and has lead to the institution of bi-directional screening for TB and DM (20-22). Evidence has become available suggesting that use of immunomodulator drugs [biologicals] has been associated with the development of fatal TB in rheumatoid arthritis (22,23). Data are also emerging suggesting that tobacco smokers have about three-fold higher risk of TB than non-smokers; even after adjustment for other factors (24,25).

DRUG-RESISTANT TUBERCULOSIS

With the introduction of anti-TB drugs in the mid-1940s, the era of cure for TB became a reality. Within a short period of about a half-century, the menace of drug-resistant TB [DR-TB] became a serious threat to TB control. The 1990s witnessed mutlidrug-resistant TB [MDR-TB], then the early years of the new millennium have witnessed the menace of extensively drug-resistant TB [XDR-TB]. The impact of X/MDR-TB on TB control is covered in *"Drug-resistant tuberculosis"* [Chapter 42].

INDIA AND TUBERCULOSIS CONTROL

Research carried out in India has had a tremendous impact on TB and this experience has been of immense value in the control of TB worldwide. The first sanatorium in India was started in 1906 in Tilonia, Rajasthan. Subsequently, other sanatoria were set-up in Almora in 1908 and Pendra Road, Central Provinces in Madhya Pradesh, at about the same time. The first sanatorium outside the patronage of Christian missionary organisations, called Hardinge Sanatorium was established at Dharampur, near Shimla in 1909 with the help of donations from some Mumbai-based philanthropists, mainly Parsis, under the banner of the Consumptives' Homes Society. The first Government-run sanatorium [King Edward Sanatorium] was started at Bhowali in Uttarakhand [Figure 1.3]. The Union Mission Tuberculosis Sanatorium [UMTS] was established in Arogyavaram, Madanapalle, Chittoor district, Andhra Pradesh in 1915 [Figure 1.4A]. With the advent of the National Tuberculosis Programme [NTP] in 1962, the UMTS was converted to a general hospital called the Arogyavaram Medical Centre [Figure 1.4B] which is continuing to function even today. Till the mid-1950s, important TB research activity in India was pioneered by researchers [Figure 1.4C] at the UMTS sanatorium (26,27).

India became a member of the International Union Against Tuberculosis in 1929. From the funds generated in response to the appeal made on behalf of the government by the then Vicereine Lady Linithgow, and the King George V Thanksgiving [Anti-Tuberculosis] Fund, the Tuberculosis Association of India [TAI] was formed in February, 1939. In 1940, the TAI and Government of India jointly set-up the New Delhi Tuberculosis Centre as a model clinic. In 1951, the clinic was upgraded as first TB Training and Demonstration Centre in the country. In 1941, the Lady Linlithgow sanatorium was setup at Kasauli (26-29). The subsequent years saw the establishment of the Tuberculosis Chemotherapy Centre [TCC] at Chennai [then called Madras] and the National Tuberculosis Institute [NTI] at Bengaluru [then called Bangalore].

National Institute for Research in Tuberculosis, Chennai

In October 1955, on the request of the Government of India, the WHO sponsored the visit to India of three representatives of the British Medical Research Council [BMRC] to advise on studies designed to provide information on the mass

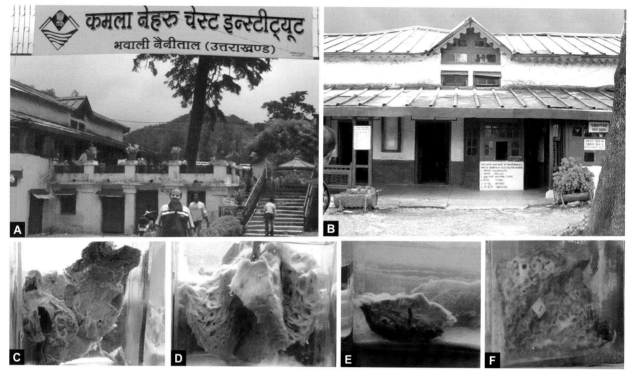

Figure 1.3: King Edward Sanatorium at Bhowali, Nainital, Uttarakhand state [A,B]. Late Dr Tarachand, originally a physician, who became a famous thoracic surgeon and his wife Dr Shanti Tarachand [expert in anaesthesiology] are well-known names at this Sanatorium. The museum in the sanatorium houses many of the surgically resected gross pathology specimens [C to F]

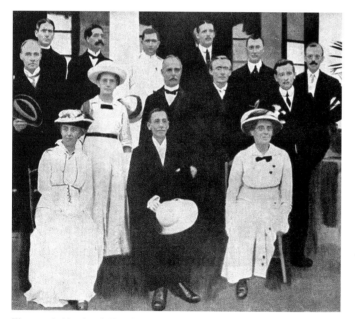

Figure 1.4A: Lord Pentland, Governor of the then Madras State opened the Union Mission Tuberculosis Sanatorium at Madanapalle on July 19, 1915, seen along with Dr Christian Frimodt-Moller, the first Medical Superintendent and members of the Governing Body
[Kind courtesy: Dr B Wesley, Director, Arogyavaram Medical Centre, Madanapalle]

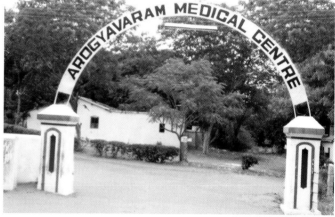

Figure 1.4B: The Union Mission Tuberculosis Sanatorium, at Arogyavaram, Madanapalle, Chittoor district, Andhra Pradesh, that later became the Arogyavaram Medical Centre

domiciliary application of chemotherapy in the treatment of pulmonary TB (30). This was particularly relevant as the number of patients with TB far outnumbered the number of beds available for their admission at that time. It was feared that outpatient treatment might prove inadequate for the treatment of the disease, and that a high proportion of patients so treated might become chronic excretors of drug-resistant organisms and might pose a serious public health risk if use of domiciliary chemotherapy was widespread. With the knowledge then available, it was agreed that it would be premature to begin mass domiciliary application of chemotherapy, even in a limited area. It was finally decided to undertake a controlled comparative study of the treatment of patients at home and in a sanatorium initially, and to follow up the family contacts. Patients were to be admitted to study from among those routinely diagnosed by the chest clinic service of a large city. In order to implement these decisions, the TCC was established at Madras [Chennai] in 1956 [Figure 1.5A] as a five-year project, under the joint auspices of the Indian Council of Medical Research [ICMR], the Government of Tamil Nadu, the WHO and the BMRC. This Centre started its activities with eight international staff members belonging to the WHO and a team of national staff members drawn from the ICMR and the Government of Tamil Nadu under the dynamic leadership of Dr Wallace Fox of the BMRC. The Centre was housed in two main blocks, in a one-and-a-quarter hectare campus on Spur Tank Road, Chetput, in the heart of Chennai city. The Centre, which had an initial lease of life of only five years and had faced the threat of closure in 1961, has evolved further. In keeping with the wide sphere of activities of the Centre, the ICMR in 1978 renamed the TCC as the "Tuberculosis Research Centre" [TRC] (30) [Figure 1.5B]. The TRC was renamed on August 1, 2011 as National Institute for Research in Tuberculosis [NIRT] [Figure 1.5C]. Presently, a permanent institute under the ICMR, the NIRT is an internationally recognized institution for TB research. It is a Supranational Reference Laboratory and a WHO Collaborating Centre for TB Research and Training [Figure 1.5D]. Recently, an International Centre for Excellence in Research [ICER], in collaboration with NIH, was established at the Centre.

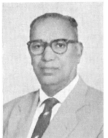
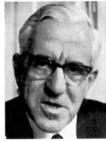
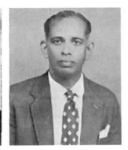

Figure 1.4C: Pioneers of research at Union Mission Tuberculosis Sanatorium, Arogyavaram, Madanapalle: Dr PV Benjamin [left panel], Dr Johannes Frimodt-Moller [middle panel], and Dr KT Jesudian [right panel]
[Kind courtesy: Dr B Wesley, Director, Arogyavaram Medical Centre, Madanapalle]

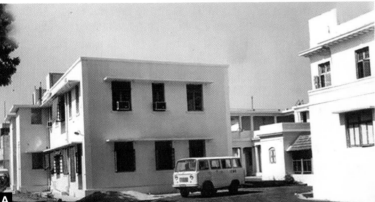
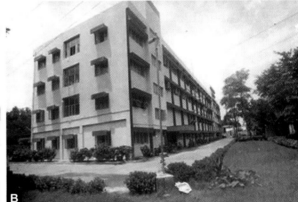
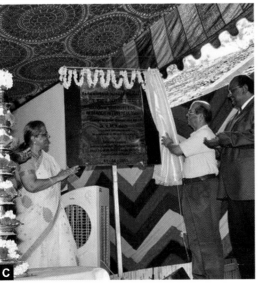
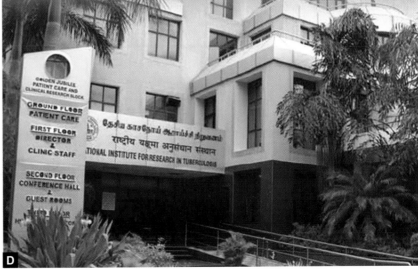

Figure 1.5: Tuberculosis Chemotherapy Centre, Madras [Chennai] [A]; Tuberculosis Research Centre, Madras [Chennai] [B]; renaming of Tuberculosis Research Centre as National Institute for Research in Tuberculosis [C,D]
[Kind courtesy: National Institute for Research in Tuberculosis]

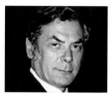
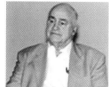
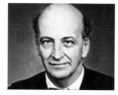

Figure 1.6: Pioneers of research at Tuberculosis Chemotherapy Centre, Madras [Chennai]: Dr Wallace Fox [left panel]; Professor D.A. Mitchison [middle panel]; and Dr Hugh Stott [right panel]
[Kind courtesy: National Institute for Research in Tuberculosis, Chennai]

The Madras Experiment

Pioneering researchers who worked at TCC, TRC, NIRT are shown in Figure 1.6. The findings of the "Home-Sanatorium study" conducted by the TRC, Madras [Chennai], have found their way into several journals and textbooks on TB. The finding that TB patients can be effectively treated as outpatients and continue to live in their homes without added risk to their family contacts has revolutionised the whole concept of the management of TB (30). These pioneering studies also form the conceptual basis for the modern-day "DOTS".

National Tuberculosis Institute

In order to formulate an effective strategy to control TB in India, the NTI was established under Directorate General of Health Services, Ministry of Health and Family Welfare, Government of India, at Bengaluru [then, called Bangalore] in 1959, and was formally inaugurated on September 16, 1960 by Pandit Jawaharlal Nehru, the first Prime Minister of India (31). The NTI is located in the northern part of the Bengaluru near Rajamahal Guttahally on a sprawling field of 23 acres of land [Figure 1.7A]. The main central old building of oriental architecture called *"Avalon"*, was a palace belonging the erstwhile Maharaja of Mysore [Figure 1.7B]. The NTI has grown rapidly and has been designated as the WHO Collaborating Centre for TB research and training since June 1985. The NTI plays an important role in organising training activities in TB control

for medical and paramedical personnel, in policies and procedures consistent with the WHO recommended DOTS strategy. Other functions of the NTI include monitoring and supervising TB control programme in the country, to plan, co-ordinate and execute research in TB epidemiology in India.

National Institute of Tuberculosis and Respiratory Diseases

The Lala Ram Sarup [LRS] TB hospital was established by TAI in 1952. It was upgraded into an autonomous institute, the LRS Institute of Tuberculosis and Respiratory Diseases under the Ministry of Health and Family Welfare in 1991 by the Government of India. The institute has recently been renamed in 2012 as National Institute of Tuberculosis and Respiratory Diseases [NITRD] (32). The LRS TB hospital functions in the NITRD. The WHO and the Global Laboratory Initiative [GLI] have recently recognised Microbiology Laboratory at NITRD as a National Centre of Excellence in 2014 for the WHO/GLI TB Supranational Reference Laboratory Network. The NITRD [Figure 1.8] has been designated by the WHO as a WHO Collaborating Centre [WHO CC] in TB Training [WHOCC No. IND-128] on November 6, 2014. The NITRD-WHO CC was opened on World TB Day 2015. The NITRD is a key player in TB control in India.

National JALMA Institute for Leprosy and Other Mycobacterial Diseases

The India Centre of Japanese Leprosy Mission for Asia [JALMA] was established in Agra by the Japanese in 1963 and was managed by a Tokyo based voluntary organisation JALMA (33). On April 1, 1976 the India Centre of JALMA was officially handed over to the Government of India and subsequently to the ICMR. This was named as Central JALMA Institute for Leprosy in 1976 and has been renamed as "National JALMA Institute for Leprosy and other Mycobacterial Diseases [NJILOMD]" in 2005 [Figure 1.9].

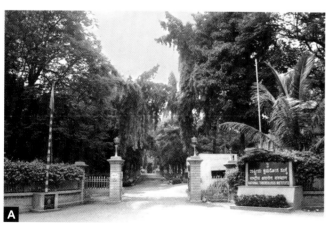
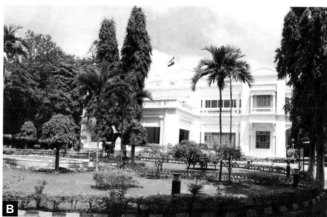

Figure 1.7: National Tuberculosis Institute, Bengaluru: Entrance [A]; *Avalon* building [B]

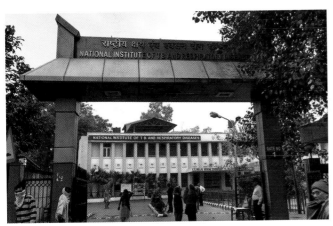

Figure 1.8: National Institute of Tuberculosis and Respiratory Diseases [NITRD], Lala Ram Sarup [LRS] TB hospital, New Delhi

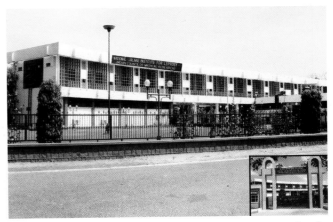

Figure 1.9: National JALMA Institute for Leprosy and other Mycobacterial Diseases, Agra. Inset: Main gate

The NJILOMD is equipped with the state-of-the art facilities such as well-equipped laboratories, modern hospital and well-set Field Programmes at Model Rural Health Research Unit [MRHRU] at Ghatampur and a satellite centre at Banda, serves as a National Reference Laboratory [NRL] for TB for 4 states [Assam, Himachal Pradesh, Uttarakhand and Eastern Uttar Pradesh] and repository centre for mycobacterial strains. The institute has a major thrust on research in TB and other mycobacterial diseases (33).

The history of TB and time line of various TB diagnostic tests are shown in Figures 1.10 and 1.11 respectively.

Revised National Tuberculosis Control Programme

Considered to be one of the most spectacular cost-effective health interventions ever conceived, the Revised National Tuberculosis Control Programme [RNTCP] of the Government of India, which began in 1997, now covers the whole country. The RNTCP has been the fastest expanding programme, and the largest in the world in terms of patients initiated on treatment. The reader is referred to the chapter *"The revised national tuberculosis control programme"* [Chapter 53] for details on this topic.

Involvement of Medical Colleges in Tuberculosis Control

The RNTCP has the unique distinction of involving medical colleges in TB control (34). This topic is covered in detail in the chapter *"The role of medical colleges in tuberculosis control"* [Chapter 48].

Tuberculosis Notification

In order to have complete information of all TB cases, the Government of India declared TB to be a notifiable disease on May 7, 2012 (35). Accordingly, all health care providers including government, private, non-governmental organisations, individual practitioners are expected to notify TB cases.

National Antituberculosis Drug-resistance Survey

The RNTCP, in collaboration with the NTI, Bengaluru; U.S. Centers for Disease Control and Prevention and the WHO; has initiated the first national anti-TB drug-resistance survey (36,37). In this survey covering 120 TB units in 24 states, 13 drugs including all first-line and most of second-line anti-TB drugs were tested. The survey was conducted in a representative sample of both newly diagnosed sputum smear-positive pulmonary TB cases [Category I] and previously treated sputum smear-positive pulmonary TB cases [Category II] (36,37).

Other New Innovations

Since the beginning, the RNTCP had provided thrice-weekly intermittent treatment (38-41). With more recent evidence accumulating, the programme has introduced daily treatment from 2016 and the entire country is being covered in a phased manner. The RNTCP is also scaling up the newer diagnostic modalities, namely, cartridge-based nucleic acid amplification tests [CBNAAT], such as, Xpert MTB/RIF and line probe assay [LPA] for early diagnosis of TB and molecular detection of drug susceptibility. The evidence-based Indian Extrapulmonary TB [INDEX TB] guidelines have been published in 2017 (42). Active case finding in vulnerable populations under the RNTCP is also being studied (43,44). Introduction of newer anti-TB drugs, such as bedaquiline and delamanid under conditional access program, under RNTCP is underway (45).

CHANGING GLOBAL FACE OF TUBERCULOSIS CONTROL

The recent paradigm shift in efforts directed at TB control globally is highlighted in the chapters *"Building partnerships for tuberculosis control"* [Chapter 50], *Integrating Community-based Tuberculosis Activities into the Work of Non-governmental and Other Civil Society Organisations [The ENGAGE-TB Approach]"* [Chapter 51] and *"WHO's new end TB strategy"* [Chapter 52].

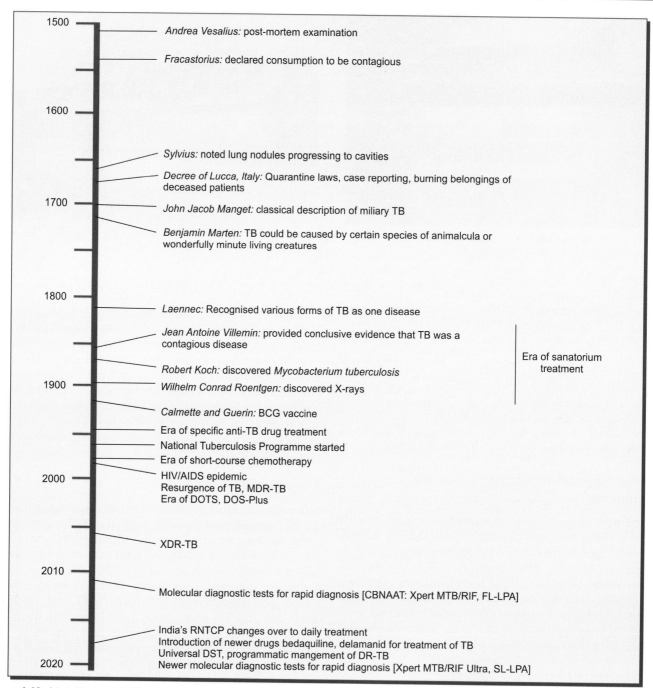

Figure 1.10: A brief history of TB

TB = tuberculosis; BCG = bacille Calmette-Guérin; HIV = human immunodeficiency virus; AIDS = acquired immunodeficiency syndrome; MDR-TB = multidrug-resistant tuberculosis; XDR-TB = extensively drug-resistant tuberculosis; CBNAAT = cartridge-based nucleic acid amplification tests; RNTCP = Revised National Tuberculosis Control Programme; FL-LPA = first-line line probe assay; DST = drug-susceptibility testing; DR-TB = drug-resistant tuberculosis; SL-LPA = second-line line probe assay

EPILOGUE

A look at the history of TB [Figure 1.10] and time line of various TB diagnostic tests [Figure 1.11] reveals that it took several thousands of years for humans to identify the causative organism, another 60 years to arrive at effective treatment. Towards the end of the twentieth century, the twin disaster of HIV and TB and X/MDR-TB seem to be on the verge of threatening to ruin the mankind. While it is heatedly debated that TB is "resurging", this may hold true for the industrialised countries. But in the third-world countries like India, TB never seems to have "disappeared" to "resurge" later. TB has always been with us, only revealing itself every now and then and making us wiser.

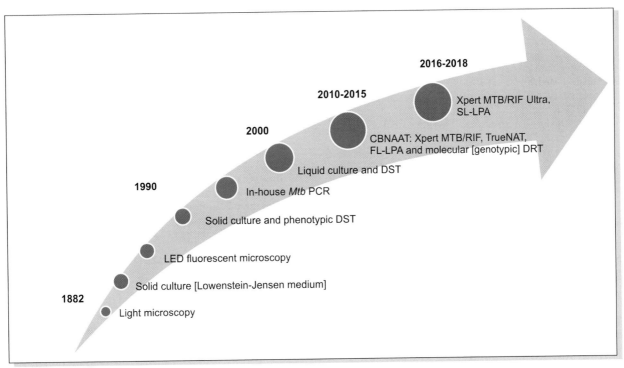

Figure 1.11: Time-line of various TB diagnostic tests
TB = tuberculosis; LED = light emitting diode; DST = drug-susceptibility testing; PCR = polymerase chain reaction; FL-LPA = first-line line probe assay; SL-LPA = second-line line probe assay; DRT = drug-resistance testing

ACKNOWLEDGEMENTS

The authors wish to acknowledge the help rendered by Vedic scholars K Gopala Ghanapatigal, Vedaparayandar, Tirumala Tirupati Devasthanams, Tirupati, and V Swaminatha Iyer, Retired Principal, Kendriya Vidyapeetha, Guruvayoor, Kerala, India, for their invaluable help in tracing the references to TB in the *Vedas*.

REFERENCES

1. Rosenblatt MB. Pulmonary tuberculosis: evolution of modern therapy. Bull NY Acad Med 1973;49:163-96.
2. Flick LF. Development of our knowledge of tuberculosis. Philadelphia: Wickersham; 1925.
3. Daniel TM. The history of tuberculosis. Respir Med 2006;100: 1862-70.
4. Dubos R, Dubos J. The white plague. Tuberculosis, man and society. Boston: Little, Brown and Company; 1952.
5. Waksman SA. The conquest of tuberculosis. Berkeley and Los Angeles: University of California Press; 1964.
6. Rubin SA. Tuberculosis. The captain of all these men of death. Radiol Clin North Am 1995;33:619-39.
7. Keers RY. Pulmonary tuberculosis. A journey down the centuries. London: Bailliere-Tindall; 1978.
8. Zimmerman MR. Pulmonary and osseus tuberculosis in an Egyptian mummy. Bull NY Acad Med 1979;55:604-8.
9. Evans CC. Historical background. In: Davies PDO, editor. Clinical tuberculosis. London: Chapman and Hall Medical; 1994.
10. Mangett JJ. Sepulchretum sive anatomica practice, vol 1. Observatio XLVII [3 vols]. London: Cramer and Perachon; 1700.
11. Duffin JM. Sick doctors: Bayle and Laennec on their own pthisis. J Hist Med Allied Sci 1988;43:165-82.
12. History of tuberculosis. Available from URL: http://globaltb. njms.rutgers.edu/abouttb/historyoftb.html. Accessed on July 15, 2018.
13. Kaufmann SHE. Robert Koch the Nobel Prize, and the ongoing threat of tuberculosis. N Engl J Med 2005;353:2423-6.
14. Sakula A. Robert Koch: centenary of the discovery of the tubercle bacillus, 1882. Thorax 1982;37:246-51.
15. Akkermans R. Robert Heinrich Herman Koch. Lancet Respir Med 2014;2:264-5.
16. Ulrichs T. The Berlin Declaration on tuberculosis and its consequences for TB research and control in the WHO-Euro region. Eur J Microbiol Immunol [Bp] 2012;2:261-3.
17. Zumla A, Maeurer M, Marais B, Chakaya J, Wejse C, Lipman M, et al. Commemorating World Tuberculosis Day 2015. Int J Infect Dis 2015;32:1-4.
18. Daniel TM. Robert Koch and the pathogenesis of tuberculosis. Int J Tuberc Lung Dis 2005;9:1181-2.
19. Calmette A. Tubercle bacillus infection and tuberculosis in man and animals [translated by Soper WB, Smith GB]. Baltimore: Williams and Wilkins; 1923.
20. Ronacher K, Joosten SA, van Crevel R, Dockrell HM, Walzl G, Ottenhoff TH. Acquired immunodeficiencies and tuberculosis: focus on HIV/AIDS and diabetes mellitus. Immunol Rev 2015;264:121-37.
21. Riza AL, Pearson F, Ugarte-Gil C, Alisjahbana B, van de Vijver S, Panduru NM, et al. Clinical management of concurrent diabetes and tuberculosis and the implications for patient services. Lancet Diabetes Endocrinol 2014;2:740-53.
22. Sharma SK, Mohan A. Tuberculosis: From an incurable scourge to a curable disease - journey over a millennium. Indian J Med Res 2013;137:455-93.

23. Scrivo R, Armignacco O. Tuberculosis risk and anti-tumour necrosis factor agents in rheumatoid arthritis: a critical appraisal of national registry data. Int J Rheum Dis 2014;17:716-24.

24. Bates M, Marais BJ, Zumla A. Tuberculosis comorbidity with communicable and noncommunicable diseases. Cold Spring Harb Perspect Med 2015;5[11] pii:a017889.

25. Dheda K, Barry CE 3rd, Maartens G. Tuberculosis. Lancet 2016;387:1211-26.

26. Leaves from history-12. Anti-tuberculosis movement in India. Indian J Tuberc 2002;49:132.

27. Leaves from history-15. The Union Mission Tuberculosis Sanatorium, Arogyavaram, Madanapalle. Indian J Tuberc 2003; 50:70.

28. Mahadev B, Kumar P. History of tuberculosis control in India. J Indian Med Assoc 2003;101:142-3.

29. The early days. Available from URL: http://www.tbcindia.nic.in/history.html. Accessed on July 9, 2018.

30. National Institute for Research in Tuberculosis. Available from URL: http://www.nirt.res.in/. Accessed on July 9, 2018.

31. National Tuberculosis Institute. Available from URL: http://ntiindia.kar.nic.in. Accessed on July 10, 2018.

32. Annual Report 2012-13. National Institute of Tuberculosis and Respiratory Diseases [erstwhile LRS Institute of Tuberculosis and Respiratory Diseases]. Available at URL: http://www.lrsitbrd.nic.in/. Accessed on July 10, 2018.

33. National JALMA Institute For Leprosy And Other Mycobacterial Diseases. Available at URL: http://www.jalma-icmr.org.in/. Accessed on December 15, 2017.

34. Sharma SK, Mohan A, Chauhan LS, Narain JP, Kumar P, Behera D, et al. Task Force for Involvement of Medical Colleges in Revised National Tuberculosis Control Programme. Contribution of medical colleges to tuberculosis control in India under the Revised National Tuberculosis Control Programme [RNTCP]: lessons learnt & challenges ahead. Indian J Med Res 2013;137: 283-94.

35. Central TB Division. Ministry of Health and Family Welfare, Government of India. Guidance for TB notification in India. Available at URL: http://tbcindia.nic.in/WriteReadData/l892s/ 2362168570 Guidance%20tool%20for%20TB%20notification%20 in%20India.pdf. Accessed on December 20, 2017.

36. WHO supports the first national anti-tuberculosis drug resistance survey. Available at URL: http://www.searo.who.int/india/mediacentre/events/2014/TBDR_survey/en/. Accessed on December 18, 2017.

37. National Drug Resistance Survey. Available at URL: http://ntiindia.org.in/ndrs/. Accessed on December 16, 2017.

38. Sharma SK, Solanki R, Mohan A, Jain NK, Chauhan LS; Pleural Effusion Study Group. Outcomes of Category III DOTS treatment in immunocompetent patients with tuberculosis pleural effusion. Int J Tuberc Lung Dis 2012;16:1505-9.

39. Jindal SK, Aggarwal AN, Gupta D, Ahmed Z, Gupta KB, Janmeja AK, et al. Tuberculous lymphadenopathy: a multicentre operational study of 6-month thrice weekly directly observed treatment. Int J Tuberc Lung Dis 2013;17:234-9.

40. Makharia GK, Ghoshal UC, Ramakrishna BS, Agnihotri A, Ahuja V, Chowdhury SD, et al. Intermittent directly observed therapy for abdominal tuberculosis: a multicenter randomized controlled trial comparing 6 months versus 9 months of therapy. Clin Infect Dis 2015;61:750-7.

41. Vashishtha R, Mohan K, Singh B, Devarapu SK, Sreenivas V, Ranjan S, et al. Efficacy and safety of thrice weekly DOTS in tuberculosis patients with and without HIV co-infection: an observational study. BMC Infect Dis 2013;13:468.

42. Sharma SK, Ryan H, Khaparde S, Sachdeva KS, Singh AD, Mohan A, et al. Index-TB guidelines: Guidelines on extrapulmonary tuberculosis for India. Indian J Med Res 2017;145:448-63.

43. Prasad BM, Satyanarayana S, Chadha SS, Das A, Thapa B, Mohanty S, et al. Experience of active tuberculosis case finding in nearly 5 million households in India. Public Health Action 2016;6:15-8.

44. Active case finding. Available at URL: https://tbcindia.gov.in/index1.php?sublinkid=4754&level=3&lid=3290&lang=1. Accessed on December 28, 2017.

45. Guidelines for use of bedaquiline in RNTCP PMDT in India. Available at URL: https://tbcindia.gov.in/index1.php?lang=1&level=2&sublinkid=4682&lid=3248. Accessed on December 28, 2017.

2

Epidemiology of Tuberculosis: Global Perspective

Dennis Falzon, Knut Lönnroth, Mario C Raviglione

INTRODUCTION

No country in the world today, rich or poor, can claim to be free of tuberculosis [TB]. In some high income countries, the rates of TB have been brought down to very low levels, but the demographic realities of aging and migration, shifts in host vulnerability, as well as the evolution of the organism itself, constantly threaten a comeback. The burden of TB morbidity and mortality in the world as a whole impinges most heavily on the people of developing countries, and disproportionately on the poor and other disadvantaged subpopulations of better resourced countries. In 2014, 9.6 million new TB cases were estimated by the World Health Organization [WHO] to have occurred globally, with 4 million in the South-East Asian Region [SEAR] of WHO and 2.2 million in India alone (1). Apart from posing a formidable burden of disease worldwide, TB ranks as the 10th leading cause of global deaths and 13th in terms of years of healthy life lost worldwide (2). It competes with human immunodeficiency virus [HIV] as the leading cause of death from an infectious disease. These staggering statistics jar with the fact that the large majority of TB patients could be cured and many TB deaths avoided with 6 months of treatment, which is generally well-tolerated, accessible and affordable in most settings. This chapter traces the historical imprint of TB upon humankind and looks at the major determinants of TB in the world today and the evolution of the epidemic in recent decades in different geographical regions. In conclusion, we outline the actions that need to be taken in future to consign TB to history, as the perspective for global health and development policy shifts beyond the 2015 horizon of the United Nations Millennium Development Goals [MDG] (3).

This Chapter uses findings from several published sources. In addition to those referenced throughout the text we use estimates derived by WHO based on notification and surveillance data reported by the national authorities responsible for TB control in their respective countries. The burden of disease is expressed as the TB incidence and prevalence; the burden of death as TB mortality. The background data are collected online in aggregated format by the Global TB Programme of WHO on an annual basis and are also supplemented periodically with data from special surveys [e.g., drug-resistance and disease prevalence]. Following collection, data undergo checks for internal consistency and are then consolidated into a central database. Modelled estimates are used when data are missing; the methodology employed to derive these estimates has been described elsewhere (1,4). The updated information is published each year in the annual Global Tuberculosis Reports that WHO has issued uninterruptedly since 1997 (5,6). The information is updated each year and the raw data can be downloaded free-of-charge or via interactive query tools [e.g., country profiles]. Mortality data are also collected by WHO through a separate mechanism from the one described above and estimates are also used to replace missing data in the countries where vital registration is not functional (7). The definitions and indicators in use in this Chapter have been revised and standardised over a number of years, and their latest update was released in 2013 (8). The countries included in the regional groupings in this Chapter are as defined by WHO (1).

HISTORICAL PERSPECTIVE

Deoxyribonucleic acid [DNA] studies of archaeological material show that TB has afflicted mankind since the Neolithic period (9). However, it is also likely that this host-pathogen relationship dates back much further than nine millennia (10). Hippocrates [c.460-c.377 BCE], the Father of Western Medicine, described the public health importance of what was referred to as phthisis at his time. Over the years, the disease acquired evocative names such as "galloping consumption", "the white plague" and "captain of all these men of death", all attesting to its tragic legacy (11,12). At the height of the epidemic in western Europe around the end of the 18th and start of the 19th centuries, TB was likely to be killing an astounding 1% of the population each year (13). Around this time, TB was the cause of one-fourth of deaths in London and of between one-third and one-sixth elsewhere in England and Wales (14). TB mortality declined during the 19th century in western Europe, albeit it remained a major killer even at the end of the century (15). This decrease is commonly ascribed to improvements in socioeconomic conditions (16), although it has been argued that the isolation of cases in sanatoria and possibly the evolution of natural immunity may have contributed to this trend (17). The decline in TB was disturbed during the period of the two World Wars in the 20th century but resumed immediately after their end. In countries like France, Great Britain, the Netherlands, and Norway, the annual risk of TB infection fell at the fastest rates ever documented in the decades after 1950 (18,19). Continued improvements in the economic situation, nutrition, and living conditions, effective preventive measures, and expanded curative services equipped with the newly introduced anti-TB medicines brought the burden of disease in European

countries to very low levels. Even if this decline was temporarily halted or even reversed in a number of industrialised countries from the late 1980s (20,21), rates have since continued to fall bringing the TB incidence lower than 10/100,000 in many of them today [Figure 2.1]. In western countries, the TB burden has now become largely concentrated in two broad age-bands in the population: [i] the elderly native patient with reactivation of TB infection contracted at a time when TB was rife and [ii] younger adults who have a higher risk of recent infection [e.g., homeless persons, migrants from high prevalence settings] or of progression [e.g., people living with HIV].

However, the TB caseload in the world today concentrates to a large extent in poorer countries where the disease remains an important public health threat. There is much less documentation about trends of TB in the developing world. In many low and lower-middle income countries the impact of control efforts on annual risk of TB infection has been less dramatic than in the richer ones (22).

NATURAL HISTORY, RISK AND DETERMINANTS OF TUBERCULOSIS

In humans, the natural course of TB from infection to disease shares some characteristics with other infectious conditions

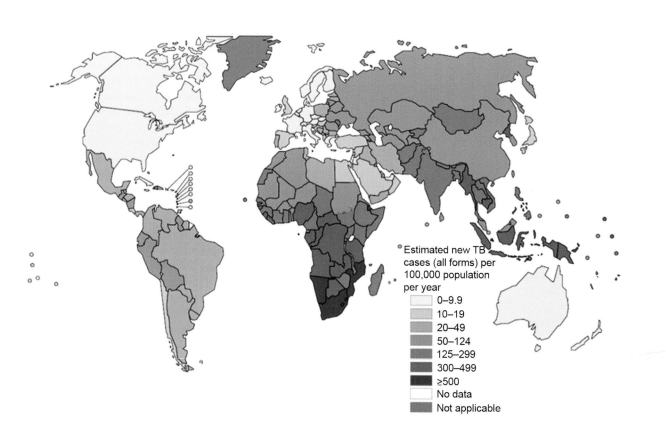

Figure 2.1: Estimated TB incidence rates by country, 2014
Reproduced with permission from "World Health Organization. Global tuberculosis report 2015. WHO/HTM/TB/2015.22. Geneva: World Health Organization; 2015 (1)"
The World Health Organization updates these data annually. The reader can access the updated information from the WHO report of the current year available at the URL: http://www.who.int/topics/tuberculosis/en/

caused by directly transmissible organisms. Exposure to the viable organisms, usually through respiratory droplets expelled during coughing, but also possible through infected milk can lead to implantation in the lung or other tissues. This normally results in asymptomatic [latent or persistent] infection. Progression to disease with the clinical manifestations may then ensue rapidly in the first 12-18 months post-exposure or after many decades. In up to half of cases, pulmonary forms of the disease develop which are infectious to their contacts; other individuals contract less infectious pulmonary or non-infectious extrapulmonary forms. The disease, if left untreated, results in death in over two-thirds of pulmonary sputum-smear positive cases within 10 years [without HIV infection], as was documented in the pre-antibiotic era (23). Alternatively, it may resolve spontaneously in a minority of cases or evolve towards a chronic form of disease that may last for years. Successful resolution of the disease does not confer a lasting immunity and the disease may later reactivate. Patients with chronic disease may survive for several years and be infectious until death or, rarely, spontaneous resolution. The propensity of TB to chronicity and to recurrence makes it different from many other infectious conditions.

Spontaneous mutations create strains of *Mycobacterium tuberculosis* [*Mtb*] which are resistant to different drugs used in their treatment (24). These events are rare, and have been estimated to occur at average rates of 2.56×10^8 and 2.25×10^{10} per bacterium per generation for isoniazid and rifampicin respectively (25). However, exposure to individual anti-TB medicines favours the selection and replication of drug-resistant strains within an affected individual. TB patients who acquire drug-resistance from treatment may transmit these strains to their contacts [primary drug-resistant infection].

A number of factors influence the natural history of TB at its different stages in an individual. Exposure to infection is more likely when the number of infectious cases is high in a particular setting, when the period of transmissibility is long, and when opportunities for effective contact between infectious and susceptible persons are high. In situations where population density is high such as during rapid urbanization and the expansion of slum settlements, the risk of exposure may also increase, as crowded and poorly ventilated settings are conducive to an intense exposure to the infectious agent. Once exposed, not all individuals have the same risk of infection and other factors come into play: these determinants are largely external to the host and include those related to the infecting inoculum [critical size of droplets, concentration of bacilli in sputum], environmental conditions which promote the persistence of infectious nuclei in the air, and virulence of the strain. Certain genotypes of the Beijing lineage of *Mtb* have been associated with rapid worldwide spread and an association with disease clustering, suggesting increased virulence even when drug-resistance is acquired by these strains, an added concern (26-28). It has been estimated in the past that, if left untreated, each person with active TB may infect on average between 10 and 15 people every year. TB patients infected with HIV are on average less infectious, albeit the overall transmission of TB is increased within a community where HIV prevalence is elevated.

In contrast to infection, the risk of progression to disease is largely determined by predisposing factors in the host. Many conditions which modulate the immune response can thus increase the likelihood of disease in a person infected with *Mtb*. HIV stands out as the most potent risk factor, increasing the relative risk for TB by more than 20, but others such as under-nutrition, silicosis, tobacco smoking, diabetes, harmful alcohol use, and immunomodulatory drugs such as anti-tumour necrosis factor agents also play a role. Age is also an important factor and risk appears higher in late adolescence and young adulthood. Finally, besides these risks, the likelihood that a person is cured or dies of TB is influenced also by an array of other factors, including the form of disease, for e.g., higher mortality in miliary TB and TB meningitis (29-31) and whether effective chemotherapy for TB is provided (32,33). If treated with combined, first-line anti-TB chemotherapy, the chances of cure may exceed 90% among patients with drug-susceptible bacilli. Patients treated for multidrug-resistant TB [MDR-TB], defined as isolates of *Mtb* resistant to rifampicin and isoniazid, with or without resistance to other anti-TB drugs, however, are less likely to have a successful outcome than those without, and success is less likely if additional resistance is present (34,35). The provision of anti-retroviral treatment [ART] to TB/HIV patients has been shown to significantly decrease the chances of unsuccessful outcomes (36-38).

The impact that different risks factors for TB infection, disease progression and unfavourable outcome have on TB epidemiology varies substantially across the world. The sum effect of the interplay of these risks on a population is a function of the potency of these factors at the individual patient level and their prevalence in the population. For instance, the overall population level effect of HIV is very pronounced in southern African countries, where infection is highly prevalent in contrast to countries of the Indian subcontinent, where less potent risk factors which occur more frequently are more important. The use of population attributable fractions [PAF] is useful to analyse this interaction in individual countries (39,40). There are sharp differences among the 22 highest TB burden countries which concentrate about 80% of TB incidence in the world in the relative contribution of each of these determinants to their TB incidence. For instance, in all countries except Thailand and those in Africa, the PAF for adult TB associated with smoking was higher than for HIV while in 14 of the 22 countries the total PAF related to under-nutrition was the highest. Problems of alcohol use and diabetes are important in certain countries but if their prevalence increases in the world, they may become more prominent in future. These risk factors for TB are eminently modifiable and, therefore, amenable to public health interventions; in contrast, other risk factors like age and genetic predisposition could serve to profile individuals and risk groups where action could be more meaningfully targeted.

THE GLOBAL BURDEN OF TUBERCULOSIS

Incidence

In 2014, there were an estimated 9.6 million [range 9.1-10 million] incident cases of TB in the world, equivalent overall to 133 cases per 100,000 population but with very extreme geographical variations [Figure 2.1] (1). One million incident cases were children and 3.2 million [range, 3.0-3.4 million] occurred among women. Fifty-eight percent of incident TB cases occurred in Asia and 28% in the African Region. India [23%], Indonesia and China [10% each] accounted for two-fifths of global cases in 2014. Over one third of the world's caseload was concentrated in the 11 countries of the South-East Asia Region, where the rate, at 211/100,000 population, was much higher than the global value [Table 2.1] (1).

In South Africa and Swaziland, about 1% of the population is estimated to develop TB each year, while many countries in western Europe, the US, Australia and New Zealand have rates about a 100 times lower than this. In 2014, 1.2 million [13%] of the 9.6 million new TB cases were HIV-seropositive globally, and 74% of TB cases among people living with HIV worldwide were in the African Region [Figure 2.2] (1). In parts of southern Africa, more than 50% of TB cases were co-infected with HIV. Globally, the estimated TB incidence rate was relatively stable from 1990 until around 2000, since when it has been slowly declining [Figure 2.3] achieving this MDG target far ahead of the 2015 deadline. The MDG target has also been met in all six WHO regions and in 16 of the 22 HBCs (1).

Table 2.1: TB incidence and case detection, South-East Asia Region of WHO, by country, 2014

Country	Incidence [in thousands; including HIV]	Case detection (%)
Bangladesh	360 [320-410]	53 [47-60]
Bhutan	1.3 [1.1-1.4]	85 [77-94])
DPR Korea	110 [100-120])	93 [87-100]
India	2200 [2000-2300]	74 [70-80]
Indonesia	1000 [700-1400]	32 [23-46]
Maldives	0.15 [0.130-0.170]	89 [78-100]
Myanmar	200 [180-220]	70 [64-78]
Nepal	44 [39-50]	79 [71-90]
Sri Lanka	13 [12-15]	69 [62-79]
Thailand	120 [61-190]	59 [36-110]
Timor-Leste	5.8 [4.8-6.9]	63 [53-77]
All S-E Asia Region	4000 [3700-4400]	62 [56-68]

TB = tuberculosis; WHO = World Health Organization; HIV = human immunodeficiency virus; S-E = South-East

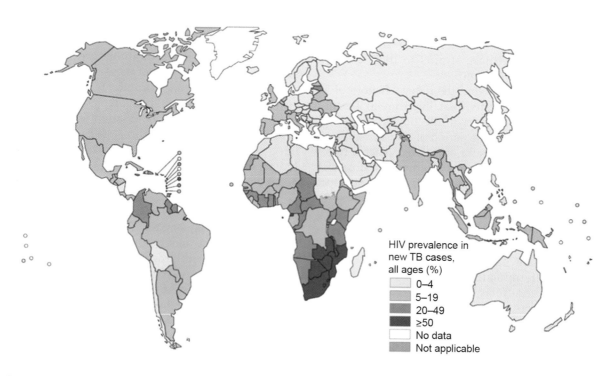

Figure 2.2: Estimated HIV prevalence in new and relapse TB cases, 2014
Reproduced with permission from "World Health Organization. Global tuberculosis report 2015. WHO/HTM/TB/2015.22. Geneva: World Health Organization; 2015 (reference 1)"
The World Health Organization updates these data annually. The reader can access the updated information from the WHO report of the current year available at the URL: http://www.who.int/topics/tuberculosis/en/

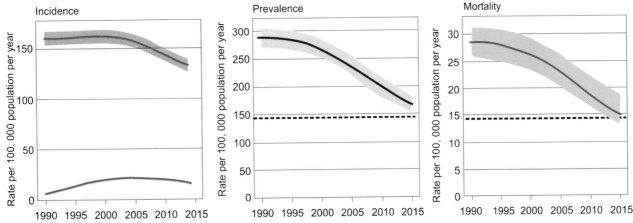

Figure 2.3: Global trends in estimated rates of TB incidence [1990-2014], and prevalence and mortality rates [1990-2015]. Left: estimated incidence rate including HIV-positive TB [green] and estimated incidence rate of HIV-positive TB [red]. Centre and right: The horizontal dashed lines represent the Stop TB Partnership targets of a 50% reduction in prevalence and mortality rates by 2015 compared with 1990. Shaded areas represent uncertainty bands. Mortality excludes TB deaths among HIV-positive people.
HIV = human immunodeficiency virus
Reproduced with permission from "World Health Organization. Global tuberculosis report 2015. WHO/HTM/TB/2015.22. Geneva: World Health Organization; 2015 (reference 1)"
The World Health Organization updates these data annually. The reader can access the updated information from the WHO report of the current year available at the URL: http://www.who.int/topics/tuberculosis/en/

Prevalence

There were an estimated 13 million prevalent cases [range, 11-14 million] of TB in 2014, equivalent to a rate of 174 cases per 100,000 population. TB prevalence rates are declining in all six WHO regions and by the end of 2015 and are estimated to have fallen by 42% globally since 1990 missing the international target of halving TB prevalence by 2015, compared with the baseline in 1990. However, the target has already been met by the Region of the Americas and the Western Pacific Region and SEAR (1).

Deaths

There were an estimated 1.5 million total TB deaths in 2014 or about 16 deaths per 100,000 population in the world. About 390,000 of these deaths were among people living with HIV. Approximately 90% of total TB deaths occurred in the African Region and SEAR, with India and Nigeria accounting for about one-third of the global TB deaths in 2014. TB mortality rate [excluding deaths among HIV-positive people] has fallen by 47% between 1990 and 2015 narrowly missing the target of a 50% reduction [Figure 2.4]. Mortality rates are declining in all six WHO regions but at a different pace (1).

Drug-resistant TB

The prospect of an increase in the number of drug-resistant cases among the TB burden remains a matter of concern, even if the overall number of TB patients is on the decline. Cases with drug-resistant TB need more resources and support to treat appropriately with regimens that are longer, more toxic and costly than those in general use for drug-susceptible disease (34,41,42). Representative data from surveys performed at least once or on routine surveillance of diagnostic drug susceptibility testing of TB patients is now available from 144 countries worldwide.

Based on these data, it is estimated that in 2014 there were 480,000 [360,000-600,000] newly emerging MDR-TB cases in the world, and 190,000 [120,000-260,000] MDR-TB deaths. Globally, 3.3% {95% confidence intervals [CI] 2.2% to 4.4%} of new [previously untreated] TB cases and 20% [95% CI 14% to 27%] of previously treated cases are estimated to have MDR-TB. These proportions, however, differ markedly between countries, showing low levels in the SEAR 2.2% [95% CI 1.9% to 2.6%] in new and 16% [14% to 18%] in previously treated patients and very high levels in eastern Europe and central Asia compared with the rest of the world [Figure 2.5]. Among new cases in Belarus MDR-TB is present in 34%, and in 23%-26% in Kazakhstan, Kyrgyzstan, the Republic of Moldova, and Uzbekistan; between 55% and 62% of previously treated patients in these countries had MDR-TB. Levels vary across the vast expanse of the Russian Federation but some regions have the highest proportions ever reported worldwide. The time trends in drug resistance levels vary substantially between countries (43), although comparable data from serial measurements over time are not available for many countries. Extensively drug-resistant TB [XDR-TB] or MDR-TB with additional resistance to both the fluoroquinolones and the second-line injectable drugs, the two most important classes of medicines in the treatment of MDR-TB, has now been reported by 105 countries globally, including all countries of the WHO SEAR except Sri Lanka and Timor-Leste. In countries with representative data, globally 9.7% [95% CI 7.4% to 12%] of MDR-TB cases have XDR-TB.

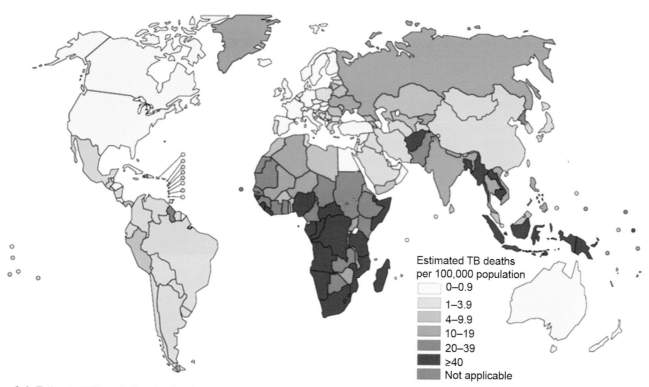

Figure 2.4: Estimated TB mortality rates [excluding TB deaths among HIV-positive people], 2014
Reproduced with permission from "World Health Organization. Global tuberculosis report 2015. WHO/HTM/TB/2015.22. Geneva: World Health Organization; 2015 (reference 1)"
The World Health Organization updates these data annually. The reader can access the updated information from the WHO report of the current year available at the URL: http://www.who.int/topics/tuberculosis/en/

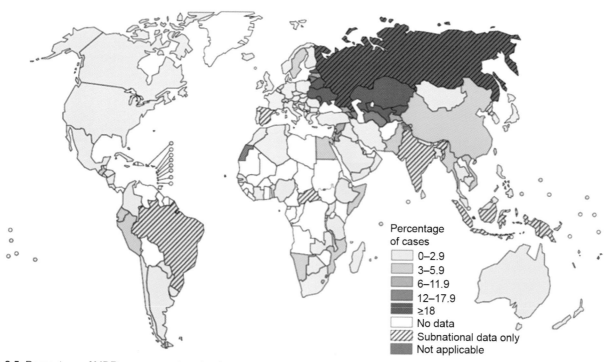

Figure 2.5: Percentage of MDR among new [previously untreated] TB cases. Figures are based on the most recent year for which data have been reported, which vary among countries. Data reported before the year 2000 are not shown.
Reproduced with permission from "World Health Organization. Global tuberculosis report 2015. WHO/HTM/TB/2015.22. Geneva: World Health Organization; 2015 (reference 1)"
The World Health Organization updates these data annually. The reader can access the updated information from the WHO report of the current year available at the URL: http://www.who.int/topics/tuberculosis/en/

A GLOBAL RESPONSE

In the early 1990s, after more than a decade of neglect, WHO published new estimates showing that millions of people were affected with TB and died from it (44). As a result, in 1993, WHO declared TB to be a global health emergency (45). It was realised back then that many countries were ill-prepared to counter the challenge that TB posed for the future. Political commitment was lacking, surveillance was neglected, and treatment regimens and diagnostic services varied greatly in effectiveness. In 1994, WHO proposed a basic package of interventions to address the emergency, which eventually acquired the term DOTS [originally an acronym for "directly-observed treatment, short course"] (46). In 2006, DOTS evolved into a more comprehensive framework—the Stop TB Strategy—with activities covering a larger set of dimensions important for TB care and prevention (47,48).

In 2000, an ambitious Global Plan to Stop TB was launched by WHO and the Stop TB Partnership with the long-term vision of eliminating TB as a public health problem (49). The planning became more elaborate over the following years and in its latest update, in 2010, it was estimated that US\$ 47 billion would be required to be spent between 2011 and 2015 in order to achieve the targets set for 2015 (50).

More than two decades after the WHO emergency announcement, TB remains one of the principal public health concerns due to an infectious condition in all countries in the world. But despite the plight of the millions of patients who have fallen ill with TB and died since 1993, much important progress has been registered. National programmes have been strengthened and learnt to adapt to the changes in the epidemic such as the challenges of HIV-associated TB and of drug-resistant strains as well as the environment around them, including the impact of migration, health sector reforms, financial crises and perennial pressure to integrate TB services in primary health care. As a result, about 43 million lives have been saved between 2000 and 2014 through effective diagnosis and treatment (1). The efforts of treatment programmes have thus had a profound impact on sustaining the substantial decline in TB incidence and mortality over the last decade in all regions of the world. TB/HIV interventions have progressed and by 2014, 51% of TB patients worldwide knew their HIV status [79% in the African Region where the TB/HIV burden is the highest]. Among known TB/HIV patients coverage of therapy with anti-retroviral drugs reached 77% in 2014, up from 49% in 2011. However, only 23% of countries globally reported provision of isoniazid preventive therapy [IPT] to people living with HIV in 2014.

In 2014, countries notified a total of 6.3 million TB cases, just over 6 million newly diagnosed and 261,000 on treatment [Table 2.2]. About 15% of newly emerging cases reported globally were extrapulmonary; the proportion of these cases varied substantially from 7% in the Western Pacific Region to 23% in the Eastern Mediterranean Region.

These differences may reflect geographical variations in TB epidemiology as well as diagnostic and reporting practices. The 5.7 million new and relapse cases notified in 2013 represent about 64% [range: 61-66%] of the estimated incidence that year. Case detection ratio [CDR] was highest in 2014 in the Region of the Americas [77%; range 75%-81%], the Western Pacific Region [85%; range 81%-90%] and the European Region [79%; range 75-83%]. All regions have improved their estimated CDRs since 1995, when the global estimate was 39% [range 38%-41%] and when DOTS started to be expanded in the world. However, in 2014, there still remained a gap of approximately 3.6 million people with TB who were "missed" [Table 2.1]. The gap between estimated TB incidence and notified cases is a result of either under-reporting of TB cases to the national surveillance systems of under-detection or both. Under-reporting of diagnosed TB cases may occur when the private sector providers fail to notify cases to the national TB programme or else when reporting from diagnostic facilities and laboratories within the national TB programmes is dysfunctional. Under-diagnosis of patients with TB may occur because of lack of awareness of TB among communities, poor access to the health care services to appropriate diagnostics for people who do present to health facilities seeking care or a low index of suspicion of TB among health professionals.

The detection and treatment of patients with rifampicin-resistant disease and MDR-TB, conditions requiring longer, more toxic and expensive treatment regimens, has also increased; in 2014, the number of new enrollments on MDR-TB treatment reached about one third of estimated cases that could potentially be detected among the pulmonary TB cases notified by the countries.

The World Health Assembly [WHA] in a resolution in 2009 urged countries to work towards providing universal access to care for drug-resistant TB patients (51). Drug-resistant strains have been detected in an increasing number of countries over the last two decades, and the widespread introduction and use of new, rapid molecular assays are destined to snowball this trend. The response of countries has varied but some of the countries with the highest burden are on track to achieve universal access to treatment for their population if they sustain the efforts put in place in the last few years (52).

As a result of the worldwide expansion of effective care, treatment success in new TB cases has reached 86% among patients placed on treatment in 2013 globally, a substantial increase from 2000 when it was 69%. The target of 85% success has thus been reached and sustained. Success rates are lower among retreatment patients [65%] and among MDR-TB patients [48%] attesting to the worse prognosis when the effectiveness of first line drugs is diminished [Figure 2.6]. Treatment of XDR-TB and forms of TB with additional resistance is fraught with difficulties and outcomes are generally poorer than in MDR-TB (35,53,54); patients with infectious forms of TB bearing such advanced patterns of resistance present a challenge to infection control.

Table 2.2: TB case notifications in the 22 high TB burden countries, WHO Regions and globally, 2014

	Total notified	New and relapse	Retreatment excluding relapse	New or previous treatment history unknown			Relapse			Percentage of pulmonary cases bacteriologically confirmed
				Pulmonary bacteriologically confirmed	Pulmonary clinically diagnosed	Extra-pulmonary	Pulmonary bacteriologically confirmed	Pulmonary clinically diagnosed	Extra-pulmonary	
Afghanistan	32,712	31,746	966	14,737	8,573	7,227	1,209			65
Bangladesh	196,797	191,166	5,631	106,767	42,832	37,406	2,989	863	309	72
Brazil	81,512	73,970	7,542	41,120	17,801	9,479	3,602	1,488	480	70
Cambodia	43,738	43,059	679	12,168	11,286	18,310	445	709	141	51
China	826,155	819,283	6.872	235,704	526,106	32,348	25,125			33
DR Congo	116,894	115,795	1,099	75,631	13,494	19,566	4,298	1,892	914	84
Ethiopia	119,592	119,592		40,087	41,575	37,930				49
India	1,683,915	1,609,547	74,368	754,268	343,032	275,502	124,679	112,066		66
Indonesia	324,539	322,806	1,733	193,321	101,991	19,653	6,449	1,391	1	66
Kenya	89,294	88,025	1,269	34,997	30,872	14,640	3,569	2,947	1,000	53
Mozambique	58,270	57,773	497	24,430	23,455	6,276	1,542	2,070		50
Myanmar	141,957	138,352	3,605	42,608	70,305	16,108	5,276	3,650	405	39
Nigeria	91,354	86,464	4,890	49,825	29,460	4,764	2,415		0	64
Pakistan	316,577	308,417	8,160	122,537	120,350	57,463	7,420	426	221	52
Philippines	267,436	243,379	24,057	92,991	139,950	4,161	6,277			41
Russian Federation	136,168	102,340	33,828	37,296	40,894	8,763	7,982	6,753	652	49
South Africa	318,193	306,166	12,027	155,473	106,482	33,522	7,430	2,693	566	60
Thailand	71,618	67,722	3,896	34,394	21,115	10,244	1,969	0	0	63
Uganda	46,171	44,187	1,984	26,079	11,854	4,180	1,499	468	107	69
UR Tanzania	63,151	61,571	1,580	23,583	23,380	13,600	1,008			51
Viet Nam	102,087	100,349	1,738	49,938	25,179	18 118	7,114			69
Zimbabwe	32,016	29,653	2,363	11,224	13,151	3,909	1,369			49
High-burden countries	5,160,146	4,961,362	198,784	2,179,178	1,763,137	653,169	223,666	137,416	4,796	56
AFR	1,342,400	1,300,852	41,548	635,560	399,155	212,057	39,782	11,217	3,081	62
AMR	228,476	215,243	13,233	127,864	40,746	32,501	10,193	2,918	1,021	76
EMR	465,677	453,393	12,284	183,630	151,696	103,959	12,368	866	874	56
EUR	321,421	266,058	55,363	112,416	76,759	39,175	23,935	11,483	2,290	61
SEAR	2,580,605	2,482,074	98,531	1,188,654	632,418	389,819	152,498	117,970	715	64
WPR	1,375,572	1,335,816	39,756	449,845	734,179	103,085	44,354	3,037	1,316	40
Global	6,314,151	6,053,436	260,715	2,697,969	2,034,953	880,596	283,130	147,491	9,297	58

TB = tuberculosis; WHO = World Health Organization; AFR = African; AMR = American region; EMR = Eastern Mediterranean region; EUR = European region; SEAR = South-East Asia region; WPR = Western Pacific region

Reproduced with permission from "World Health Organization. Global tuberculosis report 2015. WHO/HTM/TB/2015.22. Geneva: World Health Organization; 2015 (reference 1)"

THE FUTURE OF TB: A LONG-TERM PERSPECTIVE

The last 150 years have seen significant improvement in the social conditions of large swathes of the world's population. They have also been characterised by significant scientific discoveries and the broad scale application of interventions based on this knowledge. These two phenomena have contributed hugely to the gradual decline in global burden of TB in the world. However, these gains have not benefited the whole of humanity in an equitable manner and huge disparities have emerged within the globalised economies of today's world. TB remains a barometer of poverty, insecurity, malnutrition and low basic health coverage, risk factors that abound in poor and rich countries alike. The HIV-epidemic has influenced the TB dynamic in many countries in Africa and elsewhere over the last three decades.

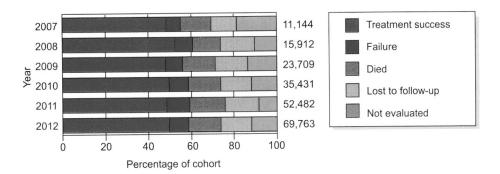

Figure 2.6: Treatment outcomes for patients diagnosed with MDR-TB by WHO Region, 2007-2012 cohorts. The total number of cases with outcome data is shown beside each bar
Reproduced with permission from "World Health Organization. Global tuberculosis report 2015. WHO/HTM/TB/2015.22. Geneva: World Health Organization; 2015 (reference 1)"
MDR-TB = multidrug-resistant tuberculosis; WHO = World Health Organization
The World Health Organization updates these data annually. The reader can access the updated information from the WHO report of the current year available at the URL: http://www.who.int/topics/tuberculosis/en/

For a disease that is largely curable, the fact that millions of people still develop it each year and that about 4,000 TB patients die each day is a sordid reminder of the sad inequities of today's world and the ability of the TB bacillus to elude modern medicine and public health measures. Nonetheless, recent advances in diagnostics, vaccine science and therapeutics bring fresh optimism to the future perspective of the TB pandemic. For the first time in four decades, new TB drugs are starting to become available with an express indication for TB (55,56). In addition, new compounds are being tested in clinical trials and other medicines are being repurposed for use in TB. About 10 vaccine candidates have now entered clinical trials (57), albeit the prospect of having an effective vaccine for the prevention of TB in adults in the near future remains uncertain.

For new technologies to make a difference to TB care and control they need to be effectively implemented in the target settings using, where possible, innovative methods. One illustrative example was the broad scale adoption of Xpert® MTB/RIF, a rapid, reliable molecular diagnostic method that the WHO endorsed in December 2010 (58,59). By September 2014, more than 3,500 machines and 8.8 million test cartridges had been procured by 110 low- or middle-income countries [http://www.who.int/tb/areas-of-work/laboratory/mtbrifrollout/en/]. This rapid, unprecedented transfer of technology and expanded adoption of a new test was made possible in these countries through a lowering of the price for the equipment and the consumables following negotiations with the manufacturers by its co-developer, Foundation for Innovative and New Diagnostics [FIND] [www.finddiagnostics.org], and the financial support of the US Government, the Bill and Melinda Gates Foundation [www.gatesfoundation.org] and UNITAID [www.unitaid.eu].

A new vision beyond 2015 has now been endorsed by the WHA (60). This strategy [End TB Strategy] envisages a reduction in the importance of TB as a public health priority worldwide, bringing down its burden to levels which have only been achieved by industrialized countries to date. Three key targets are aimed for by 2035, namely: [i] a 95% reduction of TB mortality [in comparison with 2015 levels]; [ii] a 90% reduction of TB incidence [down to <10 cases per 100,000 population]; and [iii] the elimination of catastrophic costs due to TB for all families affected by the disease. The reader is referred to the chapter *"WHO'S New end TB strategy [Chapter 52]"* for further details.

The activities encompassed by the new strategy will build upon the successes achieved up until now but will also embark upon new ones within territories that lie beyond the traditional confines of TB care programs. The activities are grouped under three pillars: [i] integrated, patient-centred care and prevention; [ii] bold policies and supportive systems; and [iii] intensified research and innovation. Components within all of the three pillars concern the practice of surveillance and epidemiology in one way or another. For instance, the drive to rapidly find and treat the 3.6 million TB patients who escape detection or reporting will involve a number of articulated actions to improve the coverage of reliable diagnostics, implement early diagnostic strategies, increase the awareness about TB of the public and health care workers, mandate the obligatory notification of TB, and ensure that this is matched by means to facilitate the reporting of cases and the capture of data from laboratories and diagnostic centers [e.g., wider use of information and communication technology], provide universal health coverage and build links with the private health care sector. Broad-scale interventions aimed at active and earlier case finding, increasing contact tracing and treatment of latently-infected persons (61), will require close measurement of the response. Health workers who are monitoring patients on treatment would likewise need to exploit better the communication technologies which are available even in low resource settings, particularly mobile phones and data services; more evidence is required on the interventions which are most effective in this promising field and how they can be best adopted by programmes (62). Drug-safety monitoring in the context of the early introduction of new medicines will be important to fully understand the potential toxicity of these agents (63). Many countries will need to invest on more effective vital registration systems to monitor deaths from TB and M-/XDR-TB. The increased use of surveys of TB prevalence and drug-resistance would be needed where appropriate to assess the size of the burden and to monitor response (64,65). Local knowledge of TB epidemiology, including social studies, will be important to adjust interventions accordingly; thus, for instance, the relevance of a focus on migration, vulnerable groups, cities and large settlements in the high- and in some middle income countries in particular (66,67). Research will be required to optimize the implementation of interventions and inform upon the direction of new interventions. Linkages and alliances with other global initiatives, such as the drive to address antimicrobial drug resistance, may represent added opportunities to increase the span of public health efforts (68).

In conclusion, while TB has been a formidable threat to the wellbeing of mankind for many millennia, the population-scale interventions which have truly made an impact on its progression- improvements in living conditions and in health care have only occurred in the last two centuries. The latter six decades have seen acceleration in technological advances never before experienced in the history of man. Some of these have benefited TB control and made it possible to start thinking seriously about the prospect of TB elimination. The WHA Resolution 67.1 of 2014 now reflects the reinvigorated will of the world's political establishment to take bold action (60). This is thus an opportunity for national and international actors to help secure more resources and focus towards the global control of TB and to change the common perception surrounding this disease from that of a shameful icon of global neglect into the biggest public health success story.

DISCLAIMER

ACKNOWLEDGEMENTS

This chapter relied heavily on the data collected for the production of the annual Global Tuberculosis Reports. We, therefore, thank the many WHO staff involved in this process, as well as national TB programmes and technical partners [a detailed list of individuals involved in recent years is available at pages v to viii in reference 1]. We are especially indebted to Dr Philippe Glaziou of the Global TB Programme at WHO/HQ for his help in the development of this chapter.

REFERENCES

1. World Health Organization. Global tuberculosis report 2015. WHO/HTM/TB/2015.22. Geneva: World Health Organization; 2015.
2. Institute for Health Metrics and Evaluation. The Global Burden of Disease: Generating Evidence, Guiding Policy. Seattle: Institute for Health Metrics and Evaluation; 2013.
3. United Nations Millennium Development Goals. Available from URL: http://www.un.org/millenniumgoals/. Accessed on December 29, 2017.
4. Glaziou P, Sismanidis C, Pretorius C, Timimi H, Floyd K. Global TB Report 2015: Technical appendix on methods used to estimate the global burden of disease caused by TB [available online only] Available from URL: http://www.who.int/tb/publications/global_report/gtbr15_online_technical_appendix.pdf. Accessed on January 5, 2017.
5. Raviglione MC, Dye C, Schmidt S, Kochi A. Assessment of worldwide tuberculosis control. WHO Global Surveillance and Monitoring Project. Lancet 1997;350:624-9.
6. World Health Organization. TB data. Available from URL: http://www.who.int/tb/country/en/. Accessed on December 28, 2017.
7. World Health Organization. WHO Mortality Database. Available from URL: http://www.who.int/healthinfo/mortality_data/en/. Accessed on January 5, 2017.
8. World Health Organization. Definitions and reporting framework for tuberculosis – 2013 revision. WHO/HTM/TB/2013.2. Geneva; World Health Organization; 2013. Available from URL: http://www.who.int/iris/bitstream/10665/79199/1/9789241505345_eng.pdf. Accessed on December 28, 2017.
9. Hershkovitz I, Donoghue HD, Minnikin DE, Besra GS, Lee OY-C, Gernaey AM, et al. detection and molecular characterization of 9000-Year-Old Mycobacterium tuberculosis from a Neolithic settlement in the Eastern Mediterranean. PLoS ONE 2008;3: e3426.
10. Comas I, Coscolla M, Luo T, Borrell S, Holt KE, Kato-Maeda M, et al. Out-of-Africa migration and Neolithic coexpansion of Mycobacterium tuberculosis with modern humans. Nat Genet 2013;45: 1176-82.
11. Dunglison R. Medical lexicon: a dictionary of medical science. Philadelphia: Lea and Blanchard; 1868.p.1031.
12. Bunyan J. The Life and Death of Mr. Badman. 1680. Available from URL: http://acacia.pair.com/Acacia.John.Bunyan/Sermons.Allegories/Life.Death.Badman/. Accessed on January 5, 2017.
13. Rieder H. Epidemiologic basis of tuberculosis control. 1st edition. Paris: UNION; 1999.
14. Chalke HD. The impact of tuberculosis on history, literature and art. Med Hist 1962;6:301-18.
15. Koch R. Die Aetiologie der Tuberculose. Berl Klin Wochenschr. 1882;15:221-30.
16. McKeown T. The role of medicine: dream, mirage or nemesis? The Nuffield Provincial Hospitals Trust; London: 1976. Available from URL: www.nuffieldtrust.org.uk/sites/files/nuffield/publication/The_Role_of_Medicine.pdf. Accessed on December 26, 2017.

17. Davies RP, Tocque K, Bellis MA, Rimmington T, Davies PD. Historical declines in tuberculosis in England and Wales: improving social conditions or natural selection? Int J Tuberc Lung Dis 1999;3:1051-4.

18. Styblo K, Meijer J. Recent advances in tuberculosis epidemiology with regard to formulation or adaptation of tuberculosis control programs. Bull Int Union Tuberc 1978;53:301-12.

19. Sutherland I, Stýblo K, Sampalík M, Bleiker MA. Annual risks of tuberculosis infection in 14 countries according to the results of tuberculosis surveys from 1948 to 1952. Bull Int Union Tuberc 1971;45:80-122.

20. Raviglione MC, Sudre P, Rieder HL, Spinaci S, Kochi A. Secular trends of tuberculosis in western Europe. Bull World Health Organ 1993;71:297-306.

21. Centers for Disease Control and Prevention. Tuberculosis morbidity–United States, 1992. MMWR Morb Mortal Wkly Rep 1993 Sep 17;42:696-7, 703-4.

22. Cauthen G, Pio A, ten Dam H. Annual risk of tuberculosis infection. Bull World Health Organ. 2002;80:503-11.

23. Tiemersma EW, van der Werf MJ, Borgdorff MW, Williams BG, Nagelkerke NJD. Natural history of tuberculosis: duration and fatality of untreated pulmonary tuberculosis in HIV negative patients: a systematic review. PLoS ONE 2011;6:e17601.

24. Silva PEAD, Palomino JC. Molecular basis and mechanisms of drug resistance in Mycobacterium tuberculosis: classical and new drugs. J Antimicrob Chemother 2011;66:1417-30.

25. David HL. Probability distribution of drug-resistant mutants in unselected populations of Mycobacterium tuberculosis. Appl Microbiol 1970;20:810-4.

26. European Concerted Action on New Generation Genetic Markers and Techniques for the Epidemiology and Control of Tuberculosis. Beijing/W Genotype Mycobacterium tuberculosis and Drug Resistance. Emerg Infect Dis 2006;12:736-43.

27. López B, Aguilar D, Orozco H, Burger M, Espitia C, Ritacco V, et al. A marked difference in pathogenesis and immune response induced by different Mycobacterium tuberculosis genotypes. Clin Exp Immunol 2003;133:30-7.

28. Toungoussova OS, Caugant DA, Sandven P, Mariandyshev AO, Bjune G. Impact of drug resistance on fitness of Mycobacterium tuberculosis strains of the W-Beijing genotype. FEMS Immunol Med Microbiol 2004;42:281-90.

29. Sharma SK, Mohan A, Sharma A, Mitra DK. Miliary tuberculosis: new insights into an old disease. The Lancet Infectious Diseases 2005;5:415-30.

30. Marx GE, Chan ED. Tuberculous meningitis: diagnosis and treatment overview. Tuberc Res Treat 2011:e798764.

31. Christensen A-SH, Roed C, Omland LH, Andersen PH, Obel N, Andersen ÅB. Long-Term Mortality in Patients with Tuberculous Meningitis: A Danish Nationwide Cohort Study. PLoS One 2011;6:e27900.

32. Pablos-Méndez A, Sterling TR, Frieden TR. The relationship between delayed or incomplete treatment and all-cause mortality in patients with tuberculosis. JAMA 1996;276:1223-8.

33. Velásquez GE, Becerra MC, Gelmanova IY, Pasechnikov AD, Yedilbayev A, Shin SS, et al. Improving outcomes for multidrug-resistant tuberculosis: aggressive regimens prevent treatment failure and death. Clin Infect Dis 2014;59:9-15.

34. Ahuja SD, Ashkin D, Avendano M, Banerjee R, Bauer M, Bayona JN, et al. Multidrug resistant pulmonary tuberculosis treatment regimens and patient outcomes: an individual patient data meta-analysis of 9,153 patients. PLoS Med 2012;9:e1001300.

35. Falzon D, Gandhi N, Migliori GB, Sotgiu G, Cox H, Holtz TH, et al. Resistance to fluoroquinolones and second-line injectable drugs: impact on MDR-TB outcomes. Eur Respir J 2013;42:156-68.

36. Abdool Karim SS, Naidoo K, Grobler A, Padayatchi N, Baxter C, Gray A, et al. Timing of initiation of antiretroviral drugs during tuberculosis therapy. N Engl J Med 2010;362:697-706.

37. Blanc F-X, Sok T, Laureillard D, Borand L, Rekacewicz C, Nerrienet E, et al. Earlier versus later start of antiretroviral therapy in HIV-infected adults with tuberculosis. N Engl J Med 2011;365:1471-81.

38. Padayatchi N, Abdool Karim SS, Naidoo K, Grobler A, Friedland G. Improved survival in multidrug-resistant tuberculosis patients receiving integrated tuberculosis and antiretroviral treatment in the SAPiT Trial. Int J Tuberc Lung Dis 2014;18:147-54.

39. Rockhill B, Newman B, Weinberg C. Use and misuse of population attributable fractions. Am J Public Health 1998;88:15-9.

40. Lönnroth K, Castro KG, Chakaya JM, Chauhan LS, Floyd K, Glaziou P, et al. Tuberculosis control and elimination 2010-50: cure, care, and social development. Lancet 2010;375:1814-29.

41. Falzon D, Jaramillo E, Schünemann HJ, Arentz M, Bauer M, Bayona J, et al. WHO guidelines for the programmatic management of drug-resistant tuberculosis: 2011 update. Eur Respir J 2011;38:516-28.

42. World Health Organization. Companion handbook to the WHO guidelines for the programmatic management of drug-resistant tuberculosis. WHO/HTM/TB/2014.11. Geneva: World Health Organization. 2014. Available from URL: apps.who.int/iris/bitstream/10665/130918/1/9789241548809_eng.pdf. Accessed on December 28, 2017.

43. Zignol M, van Gemert W, Falzon D, Sismanidis C, Glaziou P, Floyd K, et al. Surveillance of antituberculosis drug resistance in the world: an updated analysis, 2007-2010. Bull World Health Organ 2012;90:111-9D.

44. Sudre P, ten Dam G, Kochi A. Tuberculosis: a global overview of the situation today. Bull World Health Organ 1992;70:149-59.

45. World Health Organization. TB - a global emergency. WHO/TB/94.177. Geneva: World Health Organization; 1994. Available from URL: http://whqlibdoc.who.int/hq/1994/WHO_TB_94.177.pdf. Accessed on December 27, 2017.

46. World Health Organization. WHO Tuberculosis Programme: framework for effective tuberculosis control. WHO/TB/94.179. Geneva: World Health Organization; 1994.

47. World Health Organization. An expanded DOTS framework for effective tuberculosis control. WHO/CDS/TB/2002.297. Geneva, World Health Organization; 2002. Available from URL: http://whqlibdoc.who.int/hq/2002/WHO_CDS_TB_2002.297.pdf?ua=1. Accessed on December 29, 2017.

48. Raviglione MC, Uplekar MW. WHO's new Stop TB Strategy. Lancet 2006;367:952-5.

49. Global Plan to Stop TB. Phase 1: 2001-2005. Geneva, Stop TB Partnership and World Health Organization; 2001. Available from URL: http://www.stoptb.org/assets/documents/global/plan/GLOBAL_PLAN_TO_STOP_TB_2001_2005.pdf. Accessed on December 24, 2017.

50. World Health Organization. The Global Plan to Stop TB 2011-2015: transforming the fight towards elimination of tuberculosis. WHO/HTM/STB/2010.2. Geneva: World Health Organization; 2010. Available from URL: http://www.stoptb.org/assets/documents/global/plan/TB_GlobalPlanToStopTB2011-2015.pdf. Accessed on December 30, 2017.

51. World Health Organization. Resolution WHA62.15. Prevention and control of multidrug-resistant tuberculosis and extensively drug-resistant tuberculosis. In: Sixty-second World Health Assembly, Geneva, 18-22 May 2009, Resolutions and decisions; annexes. Geneva, World Health Organization, 2009 [WHA62/2009/REC/1]:25-9. Available from URL: apps.who.int/gb/ebwha/pdf_files/WHA62-REC1/WHA62_REC1-en.pdf. Accessed on December 30, 2107.

52. Falzon D, Mirzayev F, Wares F, Garcia Baena I, Zignol M, Linh N, et al. Multidrug-resistant tuberculosis around the world: what progress has been made? Eur Respir J 2015;45: 150-60.

53. Jacobson KR, Tierney DB, Jeon CY, Mitnick CD, Murray MB. Treatment outcomes among patients with extensively drug-resistant tuberculosis: systematic review and meta-analysis. Clin Infect Dis 2010;51:6-14.

54. Migliori GB, Sotgiu G, Gandhi NR, Falzon D, DeRiemer K, Centis R, et al. Drug resistance beyond extensively drug-resistant tuberculosis: individual patient data meta-analysis. Eur Respir J 2013;42:169-79.

55. World Health Organization. The use of bedaquiline in the treatment of multidrug-resistant tuberculosis. Interim policy guidance. WHO/HTM/TB/2013.6. Geneva: World Health Organization. 2013. Available from URL: http://apps.who.int/iris/bitstream/ 10665/84879/1/9789241505482_eng.pdf. Accessed on April 22, 2017.

56. European Medicines Agency. Human medicines - Deltyba. Available from URL: http://www.ema.europa.eu/docs/ en_GB/document_library/EPAR_-Summary_for_the_public/ human/002552/WC500166235.pdf. Accessed on April 22, 2017.

57. Kaufmann SHE, Hussey G, Lambert P-H. New vaccines for tuberculosis. Lancet. 2010;375:2110-9.

58. Boehme CC, Nabeta P, Hillemann D, Nicol MP, Shenai S, Krapp F, et al. Rapid molecular detection of tuberculosis and rifampin resistance. N Engl J Med 2010;363:1005-15.

59. World Health Organization. WHO endorses new rapid tuberculosis test. Available from URL: http://www.who.int/ mediacentre/news/releases/2010/tb_test_20101208/en/. Accessed on December 24, 2017.

60. World Health Organization. Resolution WHA67.1. Global strategy and targets for tuberculosis prevention, care and control after 2015. Geneva: World Health Organization; 2014. Available from URL: http://apps.who.int/gb/ebwha/pdf_files/WHA67/ A67_R1-en.pdf. Accessed on December 25, 2017.

61. World Health Organization. Guidelines on the management of latent tuberculosis infection. WHO/HTM/TB/2015.01. Geneva: World Health Organization. 2014. Available from URL: http:// apps.who.int/iris/bitstream/10665/136471/1/9789241548908_ eng.pdf. Accessed on December 21, 2017.

62. Nglazi MD, Bekker L-G, Wood R, Hussey GD, Wiysonge CS. Mobile phone text messaging for promoting adherence to anti-tuberculosis treatment: a systematic review. BMC Infect Dis 2013;13:566.

63. Active tuberculosis drug-safety monitoring and management [aDSM]. Framework for implementation. WHO/HTM/ TB/2015.28. Geneva, World Health Organization; 2015. Available from URL: http://apps.who.int/iris/. Accessed on December 27, 2017.

64. World Health Organization. Tuberculosis prevalence surveys: a handbook. The lime book. WHO/HTM/TB/2010.17. Geneva: World Health Organization. 2011. Available from URL: http:// whqlibdoc.who.int/publications/2011/9789241548168_eng.pdf. Accessed on December 26, 2017.

65. Guidelines for surveillance of drug resistance in tuberculosis. 5th ed. WHO/TB/2015.13. Geneva, World Health Organization. 2015. Available from: http://apps.who.int/iris/bitstream/ 10665/174897/1/9789241549134_eng.pdf. Accessed on December 28, 2017.

66. Van Hest NA, Aldridge RW, de Vries G, Sandgren A, Hauer B, Hayward A, et al. Tuberculosis control in big cities and urban risk groups in the European Union: a consensus statement. Euro Surveill 2014;19[9]. pii:20728.

67. Dara M, de Colombani P, Petrova-Benedict R, Centis R, Zellweger J, Sandgren A, et al. Minimum package for cross-border TB control and care in the WHO European region: a Wolfheze consensus statement. Eur Respir J 2012;40:1081-90.

68. World Health Organization. Antimicrobial drug resistance. Report by the Secretariat. A67/39. Geneva: World Health Organization; 2014. Available from URL: http://apps.who.int/ gb/ebwha/pdf_files/WHA67/A67_39-en.pdf. Accessed on December 27, 2017.

3

Pathology of Tuberculosis

Siddhartha Datta Gupta, Prasenjit Das, Gaurav PS Gahlot, Ruma Ray

"He becomes the true discoverer who establishes the truth; and the sign of truth is the general acceptance. In science, credit goes to the man who convinces the world, not to the man to whom the idea first comes".

> *Dubos RJ. The germ theory of tuberculosis.*
> In: The White Plague: tuberculosis, man and society (1)

INTRODUCTION

Tuberculosis [TB] has been known to mankind since ancient times (1,2). The aetiology, pathogenesis, clinical features and the treatment of TB have been the subject of controversy and myths for centuries. However, there was agreement on one score, that the disease was associated with poor prognosis. Robert Koch discovered the infectious agent of TB, on March 24, 1882. It was hoped that the discovery of TB bacilli will mark the end of the scourge, phthisis, struma, phyma, hectic fever, consumption, white death, the 'white plague', or the 'Captain of all these men of death', as remarked by the evangelist John Bunyon. Unfortunately that did not happen. The human immunodeficiency virus [HIV] mediated acquired immunodeficiency syndrome [AIDS] pandemic has also had a devastating effect on demography of TB.

The pathology of TB is essentially similar to most other infectious diseases, that is the consequence of interplay between the bacillus and host immunity. The relationship between the two can be varied, complex and can last life-long. The host can win over the bacillus or the bacillus can overwhelm the host. At times, the battle may stop for years, only to resume later on. All this is reflected in the gross and microscopic appearances of the different organs. The infectious agent is in the form of 1-5 micron diameter airborne particles [droplet nuclei], that contain 1-5 bacilli; the infectious dose being 1-10 bacilli. One bout of cough can produce 3,000 droplet nuclei and a sneeze produces up to a million. Once infected, further progression of disease depends upon immunity level of the individual. In healthy individuals, 90% will not progress disease and only 10% will develop active disease [50% of these within 2 years and other 50% later on in life] (3). Therefore, pulmonary TB (80%) is the predominant form of disease. The lung is indeed the primary site of infection in most instances. Extra-pulmonary TB [EPTB] is commonly a consequence or accompaniment of pulmonary TB. However, TB affects almost every organ in the body. It would be beyond the scope of this chapter to deal with the pathology of TB with reference to each and every organ in detail. Readers are, therefore, referred to the respective chapters concerned with different organ systems that supplement this chapter.

CLASSIFICATION

TB is classified into different clinic-pathological types depending on various factors [Table 3.1]. Though there may be some link in the relationship of age to the exposure and type of TB, terminology related to age such as "childhood TB" and "adulthood TB" should not be used. The natural history of TB is described in detail in the chapter *"Pulmonary tuberculosis [Chapter 10]."* Certain key aspects of the natural history of TB are described here briefly. Primary TB occurs in persons who have been exposed to *Mycobacterium tuberculosis [Mtb]* for the first time. In areas of the world where TB is highly endemic, primary TB usually occurs in children. Primary TB can also occur when acquired immunity to TB is lost due to senescence or immunedeficiency diseases. As pointed out by Rich, "resistance is a notoriously fluctuating condition and even though resistance may have been previously acquired, it may be overcome by new invasion of tubercle bacillus" (4). Progressive primary TB arises when there is

Table 3.1: Classification of tuberculosis

Based on sequence of events following the first exposure
Primary TB

    Disease caused by *Mtb* in a person with no previous exposure

Progressive primary TB

    Primary disease which is generally self-limiting may progress to give rise to larger lesions

Post-primary TB

    Disease which is the result of endogenous reactivaton [in a person previously exposed to *Mtb*] or exogenous reinfection

Based on location
Localised disease

    Pulmonary TB

    Extrapulmonary TB

Disseminated TB

TB disease process involving more than two non-contiguous sites. Disseminated TB can occur in primary [early generalised TB] and post-primary [late generalised TB] forms of the disease. When the lesions are uniform and are of the size of a millet seed, the term miliary TB is used

TB = tuberculosis; *Mtb* = *Mycobacterium tuberculosis*

inadequate immunity. It is most commonly seen in infants, adolescents and elderly.

Post-primary TB, is generally a disease of the adults due to endogenous reactivation or exogenous reinfection in a previously sensitised patient, who has retained some degree of acquired immunity. Haematogenous spread of the disease throughout the lungs and to multiple organs [miliary TB] may occur in both the primary and post-primary forms of the disease.

HISTOPATHOLOGICAL APPEARANCE

The histopathological hallmark of TB is a granuloma. In fact, TB is cited as the classical example of a granulomatous inflammation. It is, therefore, necessary to briefly discuss the features of a granuloma here.

Histology of Granuloma

The term granuloma [derived from the diminutive of the Latin term for a grain, *granulum*] was used by Rudolph Virchow [1818], to describe tumours that may ulcerate and give rise to granulation tissue (5,6). However, the present connotation is different. Granuloma can be defined as a focal, compact collection of inflammatory cells in which mononuclear cells predominate. Granulomas are the result of a persistent non-degradable *Mtb*, or the result of hypersensitivity to its antigen or both. Therefore, granulomas may be formed as a consequence of an immunological mechanism or otherwise. Granulomas which are due to a non-immunological mechanism generally do not reveal a peripheral lymphocyte response [e.g., some of the foreign body granulomas], whereas those due to an immunological

mechanism have a prominent lymphocyte component [Figure 3.1]. There is an almost sequential change due to interplay amongst the causative agent [identifiable or non-identifiable], macrophage activity, T-cell responses, B-cell overactivity and circulating immune complexes of biological mediators resulting in a granulomatous inflammation.

Granuloma is not a mere collection of inflammatory cells but an active site production of numerous enzymes and cytokines, which are involved in the very serious business of trapping and removing the causative agent (7). Morphologically, granulomas invariably show some degree of organisation. Macrophages are the essential constituent of most granulomas. These macrophages are usually activated, with abundant, pale to eosinophilic or foamy cytoplasm. The margins become indistinct so that adjacent macrophages seem to form a continuous sheet, akin to the surface squamous epithelium, hence they are called epithelioid histiocytes and these granulomas are termed as epithelioid cell granulomas. Not all granulomas are, however, of the epithelioid cell type. Epithelioid cells may fuse to form multinucleated giant cells. Generally, two types of giant cells are identifiable in TB. In one type, the nuclei are arranged along the periphery, almost forming a rosette around the central cytoplasmic area. This is called the Langhans' type of giant cell after Theodore Langhans [1868] who critically evaluated granulomas in TB [Figure 3.1B, arrow] (4). In the foreign-body type of giant cells, the nuclei do not show such a regular arrangement and are oriented haphazardly [Figure 3.1C, arrow]. The offending foreign-body may or may not be identified within this giant cell. In some lesions associated with multiple discrete granulomas, it appears as though each granuloma has a single giant cell. The foreign body type of giant cells though are the most common giant cells noted in TB granulomas, the Langhans' type of giant cells are pathognomic of this disease. Surrounding the macrophages is a variable cuff of lymphocytes which may be relatively more prominent in immunologically induced granulomas [Figure 3.1A, black arrow]. Other types of inflammatory cells such as eosinophils may also form a part of the granuloma. Older granulomas that are healing show fibrosis. Ultimately, the entire granuloma may undergo fibrosis, hyalinisation, calcification and even ossification. The presence of a central area of necrosis distinguishes a necrotising granuloma from a non-necrotising granuloma. The histopathological lesion of TB is the prototype of a necrotising epithelioid cell granuloma [Figure 3.1A, yellow arrow] while that of sarcoidosis is a classic example of a non-necrotising epithelioid cell granuloma. Therefore, it is not uncommon to refer to TB type and sarcoid type of granulomas, based on presence or absence of necrosis. The causes of granulomatous infection are numerous and are provided in Table 3.2 (8). Often the TB granulomas are reticulin poor, that means, sparse reticulin fibres can be identified around and inside the granulomas; while in sarcoidosis reticulin condensation can be noted around and inside the granulomas, with silver reticulin stain. However, practical utility of this feature is often debated.

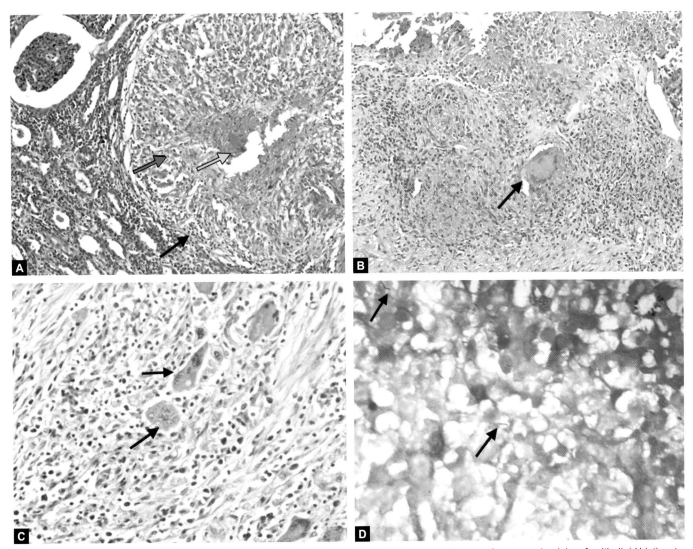

Figure 3.1: Histomorphology of an epitheloid cell granuloma with central granular necrosis [yellow arrow], an organized rim of epithelioid histiocytes [green arrow] and peripheral lymphocyte cuffing [black arrow] [A] *[Haematoxylin and eosin × 100]*. Langhans' giant cells [arrow] show peripheral nuclear garlanding [B] *[Haematoxylin and eosin × 100]*, on the other hand foreign body giant cells show irregular nuclear arrangement [arrow] [C] *[Haematoxylin and eosin × 100]*. Ziehl-Neelsen stain shows multiple beaded curved magenta coloured tubercle bacilli [D] *[Ziehl-Neelsen × 200]*.

Sometimes independent granulomas [if such a term can be used] appear to coalesce to form confluent granulomas. Presence of confluent granulomas, especially in intestinal biopsy, is a very useful histological feature to differentiate intestinal TB from Crohn's disease (9).

The diagnosis of the aetiology of granulomas, on histopathological grounds, can vary from "accurate" to "presumptive" to "impossible". If the cause is apparent, as in the case of a foreign body or a parasite or fungus or acid-fast bacilli [AFB], then the diagnosis can be made with reasonable certainty [Figure 3.1D, arrows]. Newer, sensitive molecular biological techniques may help resolve the issue, though, their specificity is variable. In other instances, the diagnosis is at the best presumptive or compatible with a clinical suspicion. In many cases, the cause of granulomatous inflammation may not be evident on histopathological examination.

Granulomatous Inflammation in Tuberculosis

As described, confluent necrotising granulomas characterise TB, though this feature is not always present (9). Broadly, the microanatomical lesions in TB are classified into exudative and proliferative lesions. Exudative lesions are less well-demarcated, comprise of neutrophils, lymphocytes, macrophages and epithelioid histiocytes arranged in a loose collection with little fibroblastic proliferation. These lesions are also described as soft granulomas and are likely to contain AFB. Proliferative lesions are well circumscribed with a lymphocyte cuff surrounding well-aggregated epithelioid histiocytes. Plasma cells may be found but neutrophils are scant. Surrounding fibroblastic profileration is also more marked [hard granuloma]. Acid-fast bacilli are less readily demonstrated. Langhans giant cells are seen in both types but are more common in the proliferative type.

Table 3.2: Aetiology of some granulomatous infections

Well-recognised agents	
Mycobacteria	Tuberculosis, leprosy, Buruli ulcer, swimming pool [fish tank] granuloma
Bacteria	Brucellosis, melioidosis, actinomycosis, nocardiosis, granuloma inguinale, listeriosis, tularemia
Chlamydiae	Lymphogranuloma venereum, trachoma
Rickettsiae	Q-fever [*Coxiella burnetii* infection], Spirochetes: syphilis, pinta, yaws Fungi: cryptococcosis, candidiasis, sporotrichosis, histoplasma, aspergillosis, blastomycosis, coccidioidomycosis, chromoblastomycosis, mycetoma
Protozoa	Leishmaniasis, toxoplasmosis
Nematodes	Visceral larva migrans [toxocariasis]
Trematodes	Schistosomiasis, paragonimiasis, fascioliasis, clonorchiasis
Viruses	Infectious mononucleosis, cytomegalovirus, measles, mumps
Foreign body	Talc, silica, zirconium
Recently recognised	
Bacterium	Cat-scratch disease [*Bartonella henselae*]
Actinomyces	Whipple's disease [*Tropheryma whipplei*]
Idiopathic or suspected but not established	
Measles virus	Crohn's disease
Mycobacterium	Primary biliary cirrhosis
Viral	Kikuchi's disease
?	Sarcoidosis
?	Chronic granulomatous disease of childhood, orofacial granulomatosis [Melkersson-Rosenthal syndrome]

These two types of granuloma are not specific to a particular type of TB and both can coexist. The number, size and extent of these granulomas depend upon the number of infecting bacilli, mode of spread and amount of tuberculo-protein discharged into the developing lesion. It may be mentioned that exudative lesions, sometime with a predominance of neutrophils, are seen more often in TB of serous surfaces, such as on the meninges, pleura and peritoneum. Sometimes, neutrophils may predominate in TB lesions in organs with a loose texture [e.g., TB bronchopneumonia] giving the appearance of a non-mycobacterial infection. It is in such instances that TB may be mistaken for an acute inflammation and the diagnosis can be missed if Ziehl-Neelsen [ZN] staining is not performed. Eosinophils are conspicuous by their absence in TB except in the gastrointestinal tract lesions.

Mathew Ballie in 1709 and subsequently, Alois Rudolph Vetter in 1803, compared some of the lesions in phthisis to cheese. This "cheese-like" necrosis, on gross examination of TB lesions is called the caseous necrosis. This term has been extended to microscopy also. Caseating granulomas are characteristically but not exclusively found in TB. Caseation necrosis is a structureless necrosis. It not only implies permanent tissue destruction, but is also a mechanism for destruction of *Mtb*. Within the caseum low oxygen tension, low pH and local accumulation of fatty acids inhibit bacillary replication. The caseum can become inspissated and encapsulated by fibrous tissue [fibrocaseous granuloma]. The caseous focus can become completely organised and converted to fibrous scar that is often calcified or ossified. It may undergo liquefaction and cavitation. Liquefaction probably involves proteolytic enzymes derived from neutrophils and macrophages which are present within or around the caseous focus. Unlike caseous debri, liquefied material is usually teeming with bacilli. Cavitation occurs when the liquefied area ruptures into an airway and is evacuated by coughing. Dissemination of bacilli in this manner contributes to the development of TB pneumonia. The caseous areas can become completely organised and converted to fibrous scar over a period of weeks. These areas may become calcified over several months. After several years, the foci may even be ossified. The presence of caseation necrosis generally implies that the lesion is active. However, it may be mentioned that tubercle bacilli may lie dormant for many years even in calcified lesions.

Of interest is the recent observation that instead of the usual reaction referred to, mycobacterium can give rise to a spindle cell-lesion. These pseudotumours are often loaded with bacilli (10). The typical lesions described above are responsible for the tiny tubercles that may be visible to the unaided eye. Galen noted tubercles in various animals [tubercle, Latin *tuberculum* meaning a diminutive of tuber, small swelling e.g., tuberosity] in the condition called hydrops thoracis. Sylvius noted that phthisis was accompanied by tubercles. Francisus Delaboe Sylvius in his Opera Medica in 1679 also made a description of tubercles. The name TB was derived for this disease because in 1839, JN Schonlein, Professor of Medicine at Zurich, suggested that TB be used as a generic term for all the manifestations of phthisis In 1869, Richard Morton in his book [Phthisiologica] named these lesions tubercles (1) and thus, this term has been in use ever since.

DIFFERENTIAL DIAGNOSIS

The histopathological diagnosis of TB lies essentially in the demonstration of the characteristic granulomatous inflammation and the causative organism. A presumptive diagnosis of TB can be made if a necrotising, confluent epithelioid cell granuloma is demonstrated. Unfortunately, not all TB granulomas are necrotising. Similarly in the list of granulomatous diseases [Table 3.2] there are conditions that reveal granulomas identical to TB. Comparison between TB and sarcoidosis granulomas is provided in Table 3.3.

It must be emphasised that there is no single appearance or combination of features that can distinguish TB and sarcoidosis histopathologically. Schaumann and Asteroid bodies within giant cells may be found in TB. Necrotising sarcoid granulomas are found especially in cutaneous sarcoidosis and are reported even in pulmonary lesions (11).

Table 3.3: Comparison between tuberculosis and sarcoidosis granulomas

Feature	Tuberculosis	Sarcoidosis
Epithelioid cells	Present	Present
Necrosis	Usual	Not common
Confluent granulomas	Usual	Discrete
Giant cells in granulomas	Multiple	Few
Reticulin within granulomas	Usually lost	Usually preserved
Acid-fast bacilli	May be present	Absent

Table 3.4: Methods of demonstration of mycobacteria in tissues

Culture
Modified Ziehl-Neelsen staining
Dieterle staining
Auramine-Rhodamine staining
Immunohistochemistry
Nucleic acid amplification tests

The preservation of reticulin in sarcoidosis can be attributed to the lack of necrosis and early fibrosis and is a useful distinguishing feature. Both reticulin-rich and reticulin-poor granulomas may be found in TB, there is nothing more rewarding than the demonstration of *Mtb*. Table 3.4 lists some of the possible methods of demonstrating *Mtb* in tissue samples.

Appropriate precautions are to be taken and protocols are to be followed for the collection and transport of tissue samples. It is always necessary to contact the laboratory for this purpose. Often invaluable information is lost because of improper collection and transport of samples. The most frequently employed method is the modified ZN staining. In May 1882, Paul Ehrlich published a paper indicating that tubercle bacilli are not decolourised by nitric acid following staining by a mixture of gentian violet and aniline oil. Hence, the expression "acid-fast" bacilli. Koch accepted this method. Franz Ziehl recommended that carbolic acid be used instead of aniline. Freidrich Neelsen recommended fuchsin and sulphuric acid instead of gentian violet and nitric acid. This is the ZN stain [1892] which is widely employed worldwide. Ironically, Paul Ehrlich diagnosed that he had TB by staining his own sputum sample. He spent a year resting in Egypt and returned to Germany in good health (1). The ZN staining is relatively simple, is applicable to paraffin sections and has been in use for many years throughout the world. However, with ZN stain, AFB are not always demonstrable and the species of the bacillus cannot be identified. In histopathological sections, to our experience, AFB can be demonstrated by ZN stain in 30%-40% cases; while in cytology smears, the positivity rate is up to 60%-70%. The typical AFB appreas as curved, beaded, purplish-red bacilli [Figure 3.1D], which may be confused with false positive staining of the *Nocardia*, *Legionella* and *M. leprae* with ZN stain. Hair shaft, dust particles and

other organisms, including a few fungal species can also show positivity. Less frequently used methods include fluorescence with Auramine-Rhodamine [AR] staining, Dieterle stain (12) and immunohistochemistry (13). All these methods are more sensitive than the conventional ZN staining and are applicable to paraffin sections and archival blocks. The former requires a fluorescence microscope for visualisation. Use of light emitting diodes for fluorescent microcopy, as an alternative to power consuming light microscopic examination in low resource setting may further popularize the use of AR stain in near future (14). The Dieterle stain is less specific due to morphologic similarities of organisms with *Nocardia* and those of cat-scratch disease (12). Immunohistochemical staining though is sensitive and specific, it lacks the simplicity of routine stains and is more expensive. Perhaps it would take some more time before this method gains as much popularity and acceptance for the demonstration of organisms as in diagnosis of tumours.

Direct detection of *Mtb*, rapidly, is perhaps one of the most significant landmarks in medicine. Molecular methods like use of cartridge-based nucleic acid amplification tests [CB-NAAT], line probe assay [LPA] (15,16) have made detection of *Mtb* and drug-susceptibility testing more rapid and specific. The reader is referred to the chapter *"Laboratory diagnosis"* [Chapter 8] for further details on this topic. In the authors' institution, due to high prevalence of cases of TB [and belief in the dictum: diagnose a rare disease and you will be rarely right!], in suspected cases, the demonstration of caseating epithelioid cell granulomas is considered sufficient evidence to strongly suggest TB even if AFB are not demonstrated. Therefore, it is not unusual to start appropriate therapy following a biopsy report "granulomatous lymphadenitis compatible with TB".

PATHOGENESIS OF TUBERCULOSIS

The lung is the predominant primary site of TB infection in postnatal life. *Mtb* is the most frequent pathogen. In the past *Mycobacterium bovis* was a significant pathogen but with the pasteurisation of milk and relative control over bovine TB, infection by *Mycobacterium bovis* is now rare. A variety of conditions are reported to render individuals susceptible or are associated with an increased risk of TB. Many of these result in decreased immunity. Some of these include silicosis, pulmonary alveolar proteinosis, malignant neoplasm (17) and immunodeficiency disorders among others [Table 3.5].

The key aspects related to the pathogenesis of TB are covered in the chapters *"Pulmonary tuberculosis"* [Chapter 10], *"Tuberculosis in children"* [Chapter 36], *"Immunology of tuberculosis"* [Chapter 5], *"Genetic susceptibility parameters in tuberculosis"* [Chapter 6], and *"Genetics of susceptibility to tuberculosis"* [Chapter 7].

PRIMARY TUBERCULOSIS

The following discussion focuses on the pathogenesis and pathology of primary TB in general. Primary pulmonary

Table 3.5: Conditions predisposing to the development of tuberculosis

Immunodeficiency disorders affecting CMI including HIV infection and AIDS

Immunosuppressive therapy

Malignant neoplasm [carcinomas of the head and neck, stomach, intestines and lungs; Hodgkin's disease, non-Hodgkin's lymphoma, acute lymphocytic and myelogenous leukaemia]

Silicosis

High dose, long-term corticosteroid treatment

Poorly controlled diabetes mellitus

Chronic kidney disease, haemodialysis

Connective tissue disorders

Organ transplantation

Intravenous drug abuse, heroin addiction

Tobacco smoking

CMI = cell-mediated immunity; HIV = human immunodeficiency virus; AIDS = acquired immunodeficiency syndrome

TB will be discussed a little later under "pulmonary TB." The earliest foundation of primary TB was actually laid by Marie-Jules Parrot [1829-1883] in 1876. At a time when the understanding of TB was based on several conjectures, primary TB in children was explained on the basis of what is known as the *Parrot's Law* which stated that: "pulmonary TB does not exist in the child without involvement of the tracheobronchial gland". In other words, this observation implies that primary TB includes a prominent lymph nodal involvement. The significance of this was not clear even after the discovery of the tubercle bacillus. In 1896, George Kuss [1867-1936] brought out a monograph on the pathology of TB due to aerogenous infections which included what is understood as primary TB. Once again his ideas did not receive much attention. Eugene Albrecht [1872-1908] in 1907 extended the concept of primary TB in childhood to adult TB and Hans Albrecht in 1909 confirmed the observations of Kuss and elaborated on *Parrot's law* (18). These studies formed the basis of the observations of Anton Ghon [1866-1936] (19).

The infection is carried along the lymphatics to the draining tracheobronchial lymph nodes that enlarge. The regional nodes are invariably involved and may be more prominent than the parenchymal lesion especially so in children. Spread of infection to the draining lymph nodes as well as vascular involvement, mentioned earlier, may lead to dissemination of bacilli from primary complex to almost all tissues through blood and lymphatics. A bacillaemia is, therefore, common at this stage (20,21). The initial infection is typically unrecognised though the tubercle bacilli disseminate throughout the body. Most primary TB infections heal spontaneously, with calcification in some of the cases. Repair begins with the resorption of caseous material, followed by fibrosis and dystrophic calcification. A typical primary parenchymal focus of TB in the lung is characterised by a nodular, often subpleural, area of necrosis surrounded by fibrosis. Hyalinisation and eventual calcification of this nodule is the routine. Microscopic calcification can occur as early as two months but radiologically visible calcification takes a year or longer. Calcification does not imply a sterile lesion. The most important aspect of primary TB is that the organisms remain dormant for a variable length of time. Resorption of calcium from the lung and lymph node lesions occurs subsequently in about one-third of children with primary complex [see below] over a period of years (22). Although, the above account of the sequence of events briefly describes primary TB in the lungs, the description in other organs is essentially similar.

Primary Complex

It can be appreciated that in primary TB there is usually a unit comprising the focus of primary TB and the infected draining lymph nodes. This is known as the *primary complex of Ranke*. Invariably the intervening lymphatics between the lesion and the lymph nodes are included as a constituent of the primary complex. The term primary complex as such is used in reference to TB and has the advantage that it can be used as a general term implying primary TB without any reference to a particular organ. A similar primary complex has been described in the case of cryptococcosis (23).

Over the years, the terms primary complex in the lung and Ghon's complex [named after Anton Ghon] are used synonymously. The focus of primary infection in the lung is usually subpleural, in the middle portion [upper region of the lower lobe or the lower portion of the middle lobe when on the right side] and is known as the Ghon's focus. Therefore, the unit of Ghon's focus and the draining tracheobronchial lymph nodes [with the intervening lymphatics, included by some] is the Ghon's complex. The term Ghon's complex should not be used to denote primary complex in organs other than the lung. More details regarding Ghon's complex will be discussed in the section on pulmonary TB.

In keeping with Koch's observations in guinea pigs, the lesion in primary TB is small, often not discernible; whereas the draining lymph nodes are appreciably enlarged. This is reflected in *Parrot's Law* mentioned earlier. This is opposite to what is seen in post-primary TB. Therefore, the presence of an enlarged lymph node with a correspondingly smaller parenchymal lesion is suggestive of primary TB and serves as a general guideline to distinguish primary and post-primary TB. In post-primary TB the parenchymal lesion usually overshadows the lesion in the draining lymph nodes. The importance of the lung being a common site of primary TB has already been mentioned. The mucosa of the gastrointestinal tract is another site of entry of tubercle bacilli. However, there are other routes of infection that are less common and less easily recognized (24).

Congenital and Perinatal Tuberculosis

The youngest possible contact of TB is the foetus of a mother with active TB. Fortunately, the foetus is less susceptible to

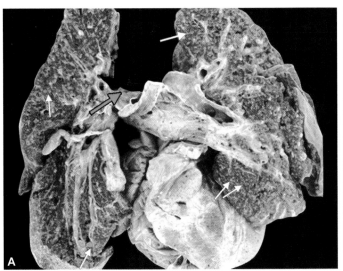
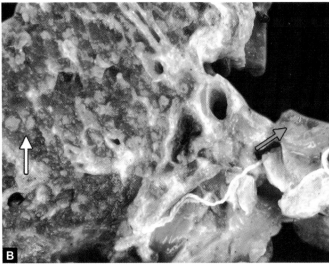

Figure 3.2: A heart-lung complex from an autopsy with congenital tuberculosis showing multiple millet-like tubercles [white arrows] in both lungs. In addition, one hilar necrotising lymph node is evident [blue arrow].

TB in utero in contrast to the vulnerability of the newborn infant. Although the cause for this is not apparent, a relative anoxia of foetal tissues may be a reason. Rarely, infection may occur in utero or at birth. There are over three hundred cases of congenital TB reported in the literature (25-28). The route of infection in congenital TB could be aspiration of the amniotic fluid in perinatal period [due to TB of the endometrium, genital tract] or placenta [late in pregnancy] or haematogenous spread. When the route of infection is haematogenous, the bacilli reach the foetus through the placenta along the umbilical vein so that a primary complex forms in the liver and accompanying portal lymph nodes.

The bacilli may sometimes bypass the liver and may be conveyed via the ductus venosus to the lungs. Widespread involvement of the lungs, hilar and mediastinal lymph nodes without an associated hepatic lesion indicates aspiration of the infected amniotic fluid (25), inhalation of tubercle bacilli from the genital tract or from the room air during or just after birth (26). Congenital TB is characterised by a non-immune, non-reactive response. Multiple primary foci or miliary distribution are common (27,28), and regional lymph node involvement occurs with emphasis on caseation and a large number of bacilli [Figure 3.2]. Microscopically, polymorphonuclear leucocytes predominate but lymphocytes, epithelioid cells and Langhans' giant cells are rare. The reader is referred to the chapter *"Tuberculosis in children" [Chapter 36]* for more details on this topic.

Skin

The skin when intact is the best form of protection from infections. Unfortunately, even a small breach in this seemingly impenetrable barrier exposes the individual to infections. Thus, the skin may provide a site of entry for tubercle bacilli. Usually there is a history of trauma at the site of infection ranging from a dog's scratch to a major road accident. Common sites include exposed areas such as the face, scalp, knees, legs, feet, hands and forearm. Persons with occupations which involve contact with potentially infective material, such as, pathologists, microbiologists, laboratory workers, necropsy attendants, butchers, slaughter house workers, cattle handlers and milkers are all at special risk. Due to its similarity to primary syphilis, cutaneous TB is also known as "tuberculosis chancre". Regional lymph node enlargement occurs as in the case of primary complex at other body sites (29). Primary cutaneous TB has been described in a doctor eight weeks after he administered mouth to mouth respiration to a comatose TB patient (30). TB has also been described following subcutaneous or intramuscular injection. Contaminated syringe, needle or fluid or exhaled tubercle bacilli by the medical attendant may be the sources of inoculation of bacilli into the patients' skin. A primary syringe-transmitted infection of a muscle should be distinguished from secondary infection of a muscular haematoma by TB bacilli, in a patient, who is already infected. There is a report of one hundred and two children developing primary TB at the site of typhoid and paratyphoid A and B [TAB] vaccination, transmitted by a school vaccinator who was found to have active TB (31). Primary cutaneous TB has also been reported following venipuncture (32). Despite, a clear clinical information, it may be difficult to differentiate primary TB of the skin from a secondary one (33). The histopathological spectrum can vary from a sequence of non-necrotising epithelioid cell granulomas with no AFB [high-immune], to the necrotising epithelioid granulomas with some AFB, to the necrotising lesions with abundant AFB [low-immune]. Lupus vulgaris stands at the high immune pole, whereas TB cutis orificiales and acute miliary TB form the low immune pole (34,35).

It would not be out of place to mention that bacille Calmette-Guérin [BCG] inoculation is in essence an iatrogenic primary infection (36). Primary inoculation TB has been reported following BCG vaccination as a form of immunotherapy for malignant melanoma (37). Therefore, it appears that in many countries where BCG vaccination is given to the newborn, the most common primary TB is cutaneous, and with the draining lymph nodes [axillary in most instances] accounts for a frequent primary complex in such cases (38).

Gastrointestinal Tract and Liver

The gastrointestinal tract is one of the sites of primary contact between the tubercle bacilli and the host. With a significant reduction in the number of cases due to contaminated milk, it is unlikely that the gastrointestinal tract would be a relatively frequent site for primary TB. It should be noted that the lack of evidence or inability to demonstrate another site of infection often results in a mistaken labelling a site of TB as "primary". Almost every organ in the gastrointestinal tract is reported to as a likely site of primary TB. An associated enlargement of regional lymph nodes may or may not have been observed.

Primary TB has also been described in the buccal mucosa (39). It may follow dental extraction and result in infection of the tooth socket (40). The primary focus is usually small or not easily recognizable, whereas the lymph node enlargement, mainly submandibular, is prominent. The tongue is rarely the site of primary infection (41-43). Secondary TB of the tongue is more frequent and invariably follows TB of the respiratory tract.

Isolated reports of primary TB of the oesophagus (44,45), stomach (46-48), duodenum (49), ileum (50), and the colon (51) are available. Primary TB of the vermiform appendix and stomach is rare. Most of the cases of TB of the appendix are secondary to TB of the ileocaecal region. Nevertheless, there are cases of apparently primary infection of the vermiform appendix reported in literature (24,52,53). An interesting report describes multiple sites of primary TB of the gastrointestinal tract (54).

It may be mentioned that earlier observations indicate that primary TB of the gastrointestinal tract due to bovine TB infrequently involves the lungs. The classical evidence of primary infection of the gastrointestinal tract by TB is provided by observations following the tragedy at Lubeck, in Germany. During the period of this disaster, a virulent TB bacillus of the bovine strain [BCG] was employed for immunisation by mouth.

Unfortunately, a contamination of the cultures led to the accidental administration of virulent human strain of TB bacillus to 251 newborn infants. The bacilli were administered orally on three separate occasions during the first 10 days of life. A total of 72 infants died of primary and fatal TB while 175 were reported to be alive with arrested lesions at the end of four years. An autopsy study revealed that the alimentary tract was involved in all the cases. The small intestine was most frequently affected [98.3%],while the upper alimentary tract and the cervical lymph nodes were affected in 78.3% of cases. Interestingly, pulmonary lesions were found in 15% of the autopsies. In all probability, these lesions were secondary to aspiration because simultaneous lesions were demonstrated in the mouth, pharynx or the intestine (4).

Primary TB of the liver is invariably congenital. This has already been discussed in the description of congenital and perinatal primary TB. Cases of primary hepatic TB are reported from time to time (55,56). It must be emphasised that in adults, the lack of evidence for a focus of TB elsewhere does not necessarily indicate that the lesion in the liver is primary TB.

Head and Neck

Cervical lymph nodes are frequently affected by TB. A proportion of these may reflect a constituent of a primary complex. The likely route of infection in the case of cervical lymph node is considered to be the tonsil (57). However, in most cases, the focus in the tonsil is microscopic and difficult to identify. Exceptionally, the tonsillar lesion may be readily apparent and ulcerated [Figure 3.3], and the mucosa over the lymphoid tissue at the pharyngeal entrance may be the site of primary infection (58). Similarly, the uvula (59) the pharynx (60) and the larynx (61,62) have been reported to be the sites of primary TB. In these instances the infection may follow the common mode of entry, that is through inhalation. It is, therefore, not surprising that the nose (63,64) and the nasopharynx have been infected primarily (65,66). This forms the basis of the Calmette test, where tuberculin was used to be dropped into the conjunctiva (4).

Primary TB can involve the middle ear (67-69). The bacilli are thought to enter the Eustachian tube by swallowing and regurgitation of the infected amniotic fluid by the foetus. In the Lubeck disaster, some of the victims developed middle ear infection probably by aspiration of vomited vaccine into the Eustachian tube (7).

Primary TB of the salivary glands is uncommon and source of infection may be transoral spread with retrograde extension along the salivary ducts from oral mucosa or

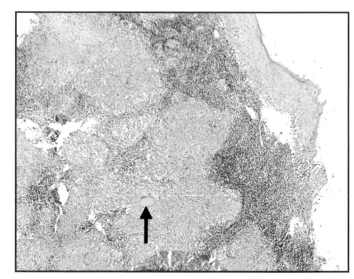

Figure 3.3: Photomicrograph showing tonsillar tissue covered by partially ulcerated stratified squamous epithelium with underlying evidences of confluent necrotising granulomas. A Langhans' giant cell is also noted [arrow] *[Haematoxylin and eosin × 40]*

haematogenous from primary site or lymphatic spread from infected tonsils. The parotid gland is thought to be involved, due to infection of the buccal mucosa at the site of the third molar tooth (70,71). Primary TB involving adenolymphoma [Warthin's tumour] of the parotid (4,24) has been described.

Genitourinary Tract

The skin of the penis is another rare site of primary TB (72-74). In some cases the infection is transmitted following circumcision (73) by operators suffering from TB. An interesting report (24), penile TB was described in 72 Jewish infants following ritual circumcision. As a part of haemostasis, the circumcised organ was sucked and in this manner the infection was supposedly transmitted from an infected rabbit to the infants. Some cases may occur following sexual transmission. Similarly an infected male may transmit the disease to the female partner (24). In general, it appears that the vagina is less often the site of primary TB than the penile skin. Infection of the vulva has also been reported.

Eye

Ocular TB can be classified into primary when there are no systemic manifestations, and secondary, when there is either haematogenous spread or direct invasion from adjacent tissue (75). Primary TB of the conjunctiva (76-79) and the lachrymal sac without the involvement of the conjunctiva have also been described. Most of the patients with conjunctival TB present with unilateral, chronic conjunctivitis without any systemic manifestations. Morphologically conjunctival lesions can be divided into four groups, as: [i] localised ulceration associated with lymphadenopathy; [ii] nodular-localised area of conjunctivitis containing multiple nodules that later ulcerate; [iii] hypertrophic granulomatous-massive flattened granulations commonly associated with lymphadenopathy [most common]; and [iv] pedunculated mass without lymphadenopathy (76). Lesions probably occur after some minor injury or abrasion. Enlarged regional lymph nodes [preauricular or submandibular] complete the primary complex (24). It may be mentioned that phlyctenular keratoconjunctivitis may appear as a consequence of hypersensitivity to proteins to which the individual has been previously exposed. Thus, phlyctenules may appear if droplets of coughed sputum containing bacilli or tuberculo-protein are deposited on the conjunctiva of such individuals. A rare instance of primary TB of the retina has been reported (80).

Whether it is necessary to catalogue and compile a list of sites of primary TB [Table 3.6] is open to debate. However, this gives an insight into the variety of possible locations through which the *Mtb* can enter the human body. It must be emphasised that the lung is perhaps the most frequent site of primary TB. The course of primary TB is generally benign especially with the advent of effective chemotherapy. In a majority no ill-effect is felt and infection is recognised by delayed type hypersensitivity [DTH] reaction

Table 3.6: List of some reported sites of primary tuberculosis
Common
Lung
BCG vaccination [when vaccination is successful in infancy]
Less common
Tonsil
Adenoids
Probably uncommon
Ileum [common in era when bovine type of infection was frequent]
Rare
Colon, pharynx, duodenum, stomach, uvula, skin, liver [in congenital infection], buccal mucosa, oesophagus, larynx, parotid gland, nasopharynx, tongue, nose, penile skin, conjunctiva, vulva, middle ear, injection site, lacrimal gland, retina
BCG = bacille Calmette-Guérin

to tuberculin skin test [TST]. There are two more aspects that need to be mentioned. Primary TB is invariably associated with haematogenous dissemination or generalisation. Subsequently, either disseminated/miliary TB may result or seeding of various organs may not be associated with concurrent disease. Later, depending on the relationship between the host immunity and the mycobacteria that may lie dormant for years, TB may manifest in one or more of these organs. In a small proportion of cases the primary infection may not heal but progress.

GENERALISED [DISSEMINATED] TUBERCULOSIS

Generalised TB is the occurrence of wide spread visceral tubercles due to haematogenous dissemination [Figure 3.2] of virulent TB bacilli from an active caseous source of infection (81-83). The reader is referred to the chapter *"Disseminated/miliary tuberculosis" [Chapter 29]* for further details.

The characteristic findings of miliary TB include small, discrete nodules, grey to reddish on cut surface, 1-2 mm in diameter, distributed evenly throughout the affected organ. Older lesions, that may be caseous, tend to be yellowish in colour. The lung, liver, spleen [Figures 3.2A and 3.4] and bone marrow are most frequently affected. Even in these organs, tubercles tend to be larger in the lung and spleen than in the liver and marrow. Miliary tubercles at the apical lobes of the lungs may be larger and more numerous especially in adults. Pleural and pericardial involvement is common with bilateral pleural effusions frequently associated with miliary TB. Miliary tubercles may be found studding other organs, such as, the kidney, intestine, fallopian tube, epididymis, prostate, adrenals, bone, meninges, brain, skin, eye and lymph nodes. Mediastinal lymph node enlargement occurs in a high percentage of infants. Patients may present with features that point to the involvement of only one organ, such as, meningitis, despite having disseminated disease.

All tubercles resulting from acute generalised dissemination are approximately of the same size and in the

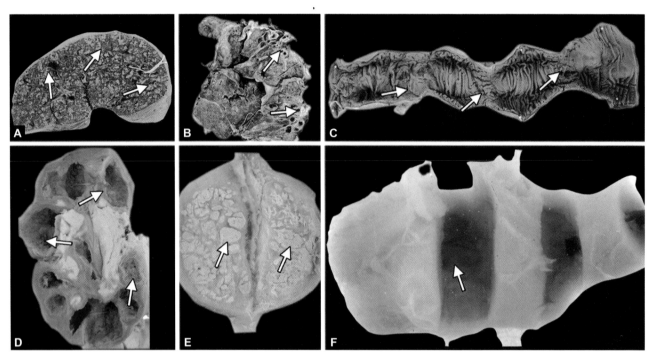

Figure 3.4: A specimen of spleen showing multiple yellowish white coalescent nodules on its cut surface [arrows] in a patient with miliary TB [A]. A lung specimen from a TB patient showing features of bronchiectasis [arrows] [B]. An excised small intestine specimen showing many transverse ulcers [arrows], in case of intestinal TB [C]. A nephrectomy specimen showing features of calyceal necrosis, cavity formation and a necrotic shaggy inner surface showing tubercles [arrows] [D]. A specimen of TB epididymo-orchitis showing multiple cohesive necrotic nodules [arrows] [E]. TB salpingitis with markedly thickened walls. The lumen is dilated and shows TB ulcer with shaggy base [arrow] [F]
TB = tuberculosis

same stage of histological spectrum. However, repeated showers of bacillemia may yield tubercles of different sizes. Histologically, miliary tubercles typically consist of a Langhans' giant cell with surrounding epithelioid cells. Depending on the compactness of the arrangement of epithelioid cells and necrosis, miliary tubercles are of two types: cellular and caseating. The cellular form consists of compact epithelioid and giant cells with very little or no caseation and are known as "hard" tubercles [ordinary miliary tubercles]. The caseating type consists of loosely formed tubercles with caseation necrosis. These are known as "soft" tubercles [acute caseating miliary tubercles]. AFB are more likely to be found in soft tubercles. It is not clear whether one type of granuloma is the precursor of the other.

Patients who survive for weeks may show a central area of caseation surrounded by satellite granulomas. Eventually healing takes place and the granulomas undergo progressive hyalinisation and calcification. This may give a fine mottling on chest radiographs. Some immunosuppressed patients with generalised [disseminated] TB may show granulomas that are softer than the soft tubercles. Giant cells are not found. The epithelioid cells are not well developed and are dispersed. On the other hand, there is prominent necrosis with numerous bacilli. This is also referred to as non-reactive TB.

PULMONARY TUBERCULOSIS

Pulmonary TB is the most frequent organ TB worldwide. Lungs account for a majority of both primary and post-

primary forms of TB. Miliary TB invariably affects both lungs symmetrically. Further, pulmonary TB is a major source of infection. The following account of the pathology of pulmonary TB may include certain features that have been described earlier. Although the intention is not to repeat, some aspects of primary TB are included with special reference to the lung as an organ and also to provide a basis for understanding further course of pulmonary TB.

The pathology of pulmonary TB has been elucidated by a number of studies that included a careful and detailed examination of lungs obtained at autopsies. In addition to the elegant studies of Rich (4) and Medlar (84), who studied nearly 1332 unexpected deaths in New York, with further evaluation of 17000 necropsy records with reference to pulmonary TB, Nayak and co-workers at New Delhi studied around 1680 autopsies (85,86).

Primary Pulmonary Tuberculosis

Primary TB has already been dealt with in detail earlier. Only certain relevant aspects shall be highlighted here. Classical features of a primary complex in the lung [Ghon Complex] are a small [usually < 1 cm] often inapparent parenchymal lesion [Ghon lesion or Ghon focus] coupled with enlarged, ipsilateral hilar and less commonly paratracheal nodes [Figure 3.2B]. The lymph nodes are generally much larger than the parenchymal focus. As has been repeatedly indicated, the location of the parenchymal lesion is usually towards the middle of the lung [upper part of the lower lobe or the lower region of the middle or upper lobe depending on the side]. Certain sites such as the apical and posterior segments of the upper lobe, apical segment of the lower lobe or upper portion of right middle lobe are described as likely sites of primary infection, however, no part of the lung is exempt (84). A single Ghon's complex was identified in 58% and multiple in 16% of cases studied by Medlar [84]. In one case, five foci were identified, one in each different lobe. In 26% cases, the complex was incomplete because either a parenchymal or lymph nodal component was not demonstrated. A typical primary or Ghon's focus is single, 2 mm or more in size and located within 1 cm of the pleura of the collapsed lung. Lesions within the lung are relatively uncommon. A majority of the primary foci calcify and a minority show caseous necrosis [85% and 15% respectively]. Lymph node enlargement is easily identified in a large majority [87%]. In order to demonstrate the tubercle, it may be necessary to make serial slices in about three-fourths of the cases whereas in the remaining, the lesions are readily apparent. Bilateral adenopathy is uncommon except with left-sided primary foci (87). Massive lymphadenopathy is reported (88) especially in the poorly nourished subjects.

Progression of Tuberculosis

The natural history of TB in the human host is influenced by age, sex, mycobacterial virulence, infecting dose, natural and acquired resistance, certain host factors resulting in a tendency of the disease to follow a pattern of progression according to Wallgren's timetable (89). Interplay of these factors and the likely mode of spread of the bacillus result in different manifestations.

Early in the course of disease, tuberculin conversion after primary infection may result in mild illness. In the first few years, there is an increased susceptibility to miliary spread and meningitis. Miliary disease and meningitis follow within two to nine months in 10% of children under two years of age although these forms can be seen at any age. Segmental large lesion [epituberculosis] is an early sequel of primary TB in infants and in a minority of adolescents and young adults, generally within two to nine months of primary infection. Though these lesions were large on chest radiograph, these used to disappear gradually over time. Pleural effusion, which follows primary TB, is also seen as a sequel of the post-primary pulmonary disease. Progression to post-primary TB is more likely if primary infection is acquired in the later years of young adulthood than in childhood. In childhood infection, the post-primary disease is delayed until adolescence. Extrapulmonary organ TB is variable. Cervical lymphadenitis may be early but, skeletal and renal TB usually present very late. This progression is only a broad direction and not absolute.

Further Changes of the Primary Complex

The primary complex may heal or progress further. Progression occurs in a small proportion of cases. Early dissemination is common but may not necessarily result in concurrent illness.

The spread of infection from the primary lesion is by a variety of ways, such as, direct extension into adjacent tissue or by endobronchial, lymphatic or vascular pathways for a disseminated spread. Endobronchial spread of liquefied caseous material is a cause of ipsilateral or contralateral acinar pneumonia. Implantation of mycobacterium in the mucosa of the upper airway can result in laryngotracheal, oral or middle ear TB. Swallowing infective sputum can also lead to TB and ulceration of the intestinal mucosa. Ipsilateral hilar lymph node spread is especially prominent in primary infections. Perforation of a bronchus by an enlarged caseous lymph node followed by endobronchial spread can result in massive segmental or lobular pneumonia. From regional lymph nodes, bacilli can disseminate through lymphatics to the pleura, spine and other viscera. Haematogenous dissemination can occur through the thoracic duct after lymph node involvement or by direct extension of the lesion into branches of the pulmonary vein.

Healing

Healing of the primary lesions is the rule. The caseous focus is gradually replaced by reticulin and collagen deposition. Eventually, hyalinisation, and calcification are common [up to 85%]. Subsequent demonstration of these lesions may be difficult. However, a minority of patients may demonstrate radiologically a residual hyalinised scar or calcification at the site of the primary [Ghon] lesion, in the lung parenchyma and in the hilar or paratracheal lymph nodes—a combination referred to as the healed primary [Ghon] complex.

Early Generalisation

Early generalisation or dissemination is an invariable accompaniment of primary pulmonary TB [detailed above]. The primary infection is accompanied by early lympho-haematogenous spread within hours or days from the site of initial implantation (90). It is felt that occult mycobacteraemia is probably common before acquired immunity, and thus, may seed many sites in the body especially where the bacillus is favoured to remain viable (20). While the sites of these seedings have already been mentioned, one aspect needs to be highlighted here. Huebschmann [1928] observed a group of nodular lesions in one or both apices of the lung that occasionally follow primary TB in children. These foci are so small that special techniques may be necessary to demonstrate them. These Huebschmann foci heal and cause no further disease. It is likely that Simon foci, which are larger, single or multiple apical caseous nodules with a tendency to calcify, are exaggerated form of these smaller foci. The importance of Simon foci lies in the pathogenesis of post-primary TB (4). In a minority of cases haematogenous dissemination results in miliary TB.

Liquefaction and Progressive Primary Tuberculosis

Liquefaction of solid caseous foci is thought to be related to the onset of delayed hypersensitivity with the release of hydrolytic enzymes by macrophages (91). Liquefaction may result in a caseous mass that may include the enlarged lymph nodes. Within the liquefied area there are multiplying tubercle bacilli and, therefore, there is a risk of transmission of disease. Due to the liquefactive necrosis there is extensive parenchymal destruction and cavitation, which is generally a little less than the size of the original caseous mass. The cavity may communicate with an airway, and thus, promote bronchial spread to other parts of the lung, larynx and the alimentary tract. An acute fatal bronchopneumonia may result. In some of these cases the inflammatory reaction is neutrophilic, like in the case of bacterial pneumonia, but AFB are demonstrable. Due to such a reaction, the diagnosis may be missed. Discharge of the liquefied material through the adjacent pleura results in pleural effusion, pneumothorax or empyema. Caseous lymph nodes may similarly discharge liquefied contents into the bronchus [Figure 3.5].

Progressive primary TB directly follows the primary lesion. There occurs an extended primary focus or TB bronchopneumonia. Cavitation may ensue. Cavitation and progressive primary disease are more likely in infancy, at puberty and in the elderly. There is a tendency for progressive primary TB to involve lesions that are apical. This location is similar to that of post-primary TB.

Lobar and Segmental Lesions

As a consequence of spread along the submucosal lymphatics of bronchi, tubercle formation with ulceration of bronchial mucosa at times, is followed by complete necrosis of the bronchus. Within the bronchus a cold abscess may develop and can be seen on the radiograph as a rounded or elongated shadow. Bronchial lesions are rare but may result in narrowing of the lumen. Extrinsic compression from enlarged lymph nodes is a relatively more likely cause of bronchial obstruction. The lobe or segment subtended by the obstruction may be the seat of obstructive hyperinflation, atelectasis, secondary [non-TB] pneumonia, TB pneumonia, and disseminated intra-alveolar epithelioid cell granulomas. Atelectasis most commonly affects the anterior segments of the upper lobes and the right middle lobe. Endobronchial TB is a complication of primary TB in children (92). Residual bronchostenosis and bronchiectasis [Figure 3.4B] may occur as late complications.

Hilar and mediastinal lymph nodes may very rarely cause impaired venous return, severe enough to cause superior mediastinal syndrome. Such lymph nodes may result in tracheal obstruction at the thoracic inlet, rupture into the mediastinum and pointing abscess into the supraclavicular fossa, erosion of blood vessel, invasion of pericardium, compression of or erosion into the oesophagus and the formation of various fistulae.

Epituberculosis

The term "Epituberculosis" was first coined by Eliasberg and Newland' in 1921 as a nontuberculous consolidation of TB lung (4). It is defined as the obstruction of adjacent lobar or segmental bronchus by the enlarged lymph nodes or primary pulmonary lesion resulting in accumulation of mucus, distal to the obstructed bronchus in the form of pulmonary infiltrate without any systemic manifestations. Epituberculosis is a rare but more frequent in infants and children than in adults. It is a benign lesion appearing as a dense homogeneous shadow on chest radiographs, typically wedge shaped, extending from the hilum to the pleura. The lesion is frequently large rather sharply defined and has the appearance of an area of consolidation. Clinical symptoms are few and the shadow generally clears after several months. Residual changes are infrequent and radiographs may show slight abnormal marking or calcifications. The radiographic appearance is relatively dramatic and sinister, in contradiction to clinical symptoms and the outcome. It has been suggested that this is a non-specific pneumonic consolidation that occurs in TB. The shape of the shadow is highly suggestive of involvement of a portion of lung tissue supplied by a bronchus. Rich (4) studied several of such cases and found that a caseous lymph node had perforated the bronchial wall, discharged its contents and resulted in aspiration of the material. It is understandable, that the caseous material is poor in bacilli, otherwise the lesion would be a progressive bronchopneumonia. The resulting consolidation could be partly due to a "hypersensitive" reaction to the contents of the lymph node [a positive "pulmonary tuberculin test", if such a term is acceptable]. The alveoli in such cases would resemble pneumonia with epithelioid cells and few or no AFB. There is also sufficient evidence to suggest the atelectasis theory and relief of atelectasis by interventional bronchoscopy (93). A combination of aspiration and obstruction by lymph nodal compression may occur. With continued treatment, the TB lymph nodes heal, obstruction is relieved, drainage is re-established, and resolution of the pulmonary infiltrate occurs. Often these lesions disappear on their own.

Primary Tuberculosis in Adults

The radiological and other features of adult primary TB are essentially similar to childhood primary disease (94,95). Prominent hilar and mediastinal glands and caseation are less frequent in adults except in patients with AIDS. Also, bronchial obstruction and dissemination are less common. As in children, endobronchial TB can complicate post-primary TB in adults. With increasing primary adult TB, endobronchial TB may occur as a sequelae of adjacent parenchymal disease from which submucosal lymphatic spread leads to mucosal ulceration, hyper-plastic polyp formation or fibrostenosis with atelectasis of the subtended lobe (96).

Post-Primary Pulmonary Tuberculosis

In contrast, to primary TB, the localisation of post-primary pulmonary TB is apical or sub-apical. This area has been referred to as the 'vulnerable region' by Medlar (84). This site probably relates to the relatively higher oxygen tension in the region resulting from the effect of gravity on the ventilation-perfusion ratio in the upright lung. Presently, evidence suggests that this is possibly because of better survival of the bacillus at this region as the higher oxygen tension has an unfavourable effect on the macrophage and thereby permits intracellular growth (97). This may also influence progressive primary disease that is more frequent in the apical and posterior segments of the upper lobe. Higher vascularity and consequently increased oxygen tension may determine the preferential multiplication of bacilli at other sites also, such as ends of long bones, vertebrae and the renal cortex. Similarly, mitral stenosis, which results in higher pulmonary arterial pressure and increased apical blood flow, confers a protective effect. The reverse is true for pulmonary stenosis (98). Lowered blood flow may also be associated with lower lymph flow, and thus, lesser antigen clearance.

The great majority of these cases represent recrudescence of dormant tubercle bacilli occurring several years after the primary infection or even decades after primary infection. As has been mentioned earlier, there is a haematogenous seeding of the apical and sub-apical regions of the lungs—following primary infection. This is the endogenous pathway resulting in reactivation TB (99). However, there is evidence to suggest that a bronchial spread from an index case may be the route of infection. This is the exogenous pathway resulting in reinfection TB. The organisms may reach by either pathways (4). Infection with other related species of mycobacteria may also have the same result. The pathological lesions seen in post-primary pulmonary TB are enumerated in Table 3.7 (84,85).

Early Lesions

The earliest lesion is probably an apical or subapical lobular pneumonia (85). These lesions are not well-documented because it is believed that the pneumonia gives way to a granuloma rapidly. An outline of the alveolar reticulin framework in the centre of some of these granulomas may suggest such a transition (85). It may be mentioned that in 1925, Assmann drew attention to the fact that the earliest lesion clearly visible in clinical TB consists of infiltrates not at the apex, but at the sub-apical and infraclavicular region. These infiltrates [Fruhinfiltrat] are known as *Assmann infiltrates* or *foci* (4). The histological counterpart of these lesions is not known.

Nodular Lesions

Nodular lesions [coin lesions, tuberculomas] are localised, well-defined areas of TB wherein the adjacent pulmonary parenchyma is usually normal or may show some scarring. A small nodule is less than a centimeter in diameter, whereas the large nodule is larger than a centimeter in diameter. Grossly, nodules are white to yellow in colour and may vary in consistency from soft lesions that are largely necrotic to firm or hard lesions that are fibrosed or calcified. Small nodules have a central area of caseation, are surrounded

Table 3.7: Lesions in post-primary pulmonary TB
Pulmonary lesions
Lobular pneumonia
Nodular TB
Small nodule
Large nodule
Healed nodules
Fibrocaseous TB
With cavity
Without cavity
Tuberculosis bronchopneumonia
Bronchial lesions
Bronchial inflammation
Endobronchial TB
Bronchiectasis
Whole lung TB
Miliary tuberculosis
Complications
Haemoptysis
Aspergilloma
Amyloidosis
Carcinoma
Oral cavity and upper respiratory tract TB
Pleural lesions
TB = tuberculosis
Based on references 85,86

by epithelioid cells and giant cells and are encapsulated by a fibrous wall. Large nodules are similar but show more caseation and less encapsulation [Figures 3.5A and 3.5B]. Healed nodules are of the size of small nodules and are fibrosed or hyalinised or calcified. Anthracotic pigment may be identified in any nodule (85).

Active nodules, especially of the small size are predominantly located in the apical and sub-apical regions and may be single or multiple. The reverse is true for healed nodules. It appears that small nodules give rise to larger ones and nodular TB may expand to form fibrocaseous lesions. It may be mentioned that these nodules are not related to Ghon's focus. The location and the absence of accompanying enlarged lymph nodes should provide a clue. AFB could be demonstrated in 7% of small nodules and 29% of large nodules [85].

Fibrocaseous Tuberculosis

Fibrocaseous TB includes lesions that reveal well-known features of TB such as caseation, consolidation, liquefaction and fibrosis. Grossly, various patterns are seen. The apical and posterior segments of the upper lobes are predominantly involved (100-102). Lymph node involvement is slight in comparison to primary TB. Retraction of lung parenchyma is associated often with pleural thickening. In some cases the lung may have an appearance of bronchopneumonia

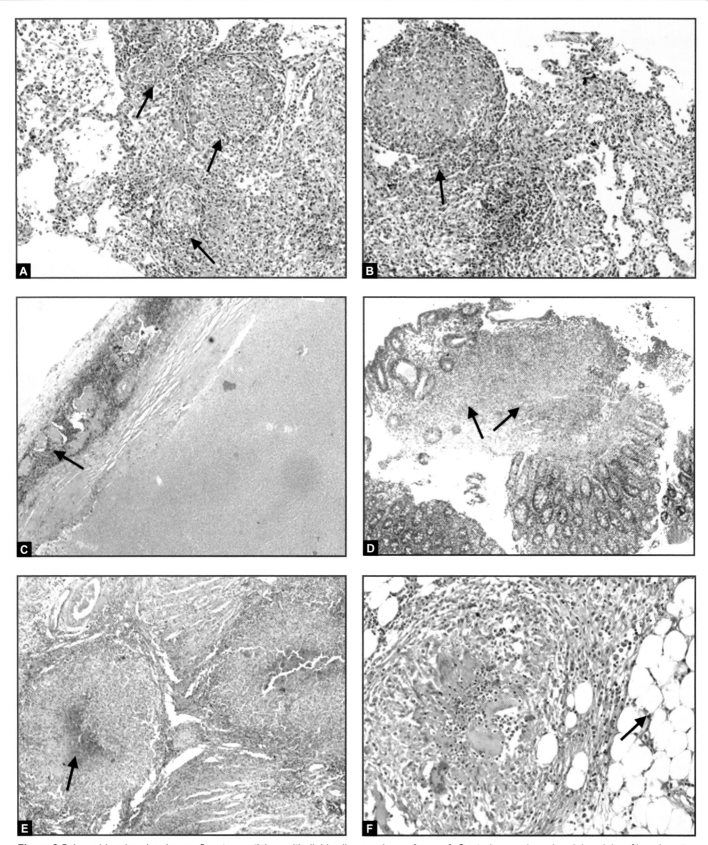

Figure 3.5: Lung biopsies showing confluent necrotising epithelioid cells granulomas [arrows]. Central necrosis and peripheral rim of lymphocytes are seen [A and B] *[Haematoxylin and eosin × 100]*. Extensive necrosis of lymph node with peripheral epithelioid cell granulomas [arrow] are noted [C] *[Haematoxylin and eosin × 40]*. Colonic biopsies showing submucosal large confluent necrotising epithelioid cell granulomas [arrows] [D], *[Haematoxylin and eosin × 40]*; [E] *[Haematoxylin and eosin × 100]*. Peritoneal biopsy showing necrotising epithelioid cell granulomas. Adjacent fat is marked with an arrow [F] *[Haematoxylin and eosin × 100]*

due to consolidation. At times, the caseous areas stand out amidst the black background of anthracotic pigmentation. The most striking feature is the presence of one or more cavities. Cavities may assume-varying sizes and may be so large as to result in a severe loss of lung parenchyma. The wall of the cavity may be lined by TB granulation issue or show varying fibrosis. Often the thick walls of cavities seen on radiographs are found to be accounted for by a rim of consolidation of the adjacent lung. Communication may or may not have been established with a bronchus. These findings have implications on auscultation of the chest. Traversing the wall or the lumen along fibrous bands, are bronchi and branches of pulmonary artery. Fortunately in most instances the chronic process allows the arteries to obliterate. The caseous material may soften the wall of the arteries giving rise to Rasmussen's aneurysms. These may give rise to haemoptysis that may be fatal.

Microscopically variable caseous necrosis, extensive fibrosis, numerous palisades of epithelioid cells and fibroblasts together with Langhans' giant cells are seen [Figure 3.5A]. Areas of consolidation may show caseous pneumonia or even a neutrophilic response. Microscopic cavities may be identified in such pneumonic foci. Cavities are lined by necrotic TB granulation tissue and show fibrosis. Occasional cavities may be lined in part by columnar or squamous epithelium. AFB can be demonstrated more frequently in fibrocaseous lesions than in nodular TB. Thus, in cavitary lesions AFB were found in 88% compared with 77% in non-cavitary lesions (4). Smaller cavities may heal. Healing in general results in fibrosis and cicatrisation extending between the upper pole of the hilum and the apex, thus elevating the hilum on that side. This causes volume loss on the ipsilateral side. Simultaneously the upper mediastinum would be pulled towards the side of the lesion distorting the trachea and giving a characteristic radiological appearance. Modern treatment, however, allows rapid closure of cavities, which leaves little evidence of disease on chest radiographs. Serious complications resulting from pulmonary TB are uncommon now except when the disease has been neglected and becomes chronic and progressive.

Other Lesions

The TB bronchopneumonia and miliary TB are a consequence of a large dose of virulent organisms disseminating through the bronchus or the blood stream respectively. It is obvious that the host immunity may be compromised. The lesions have been described earlier.

Bronchial Lesions

Despite being closely associated with the lung parenchyma, bronchi do not appear to be frequently affected in pulmonary TB (84). In a majority of cases, the inflammation is non-specific and typical granulomas may not be seen. In some cases endobronchial TB, as discussed under primary pulmonary TB, may follow post-primary lesions (103), and this is characterised by bronchial inflammation, ulceration,

granuloma, small pseudopolyps and eventual healing by fibrosis. Bronchostenosis may give rise to post-stenotic dilatation of the bronchus. This should not be confused with bronchiectasis. The reader is referred to the chapter *"Endobronchial tuberculosis" [Chapter 12]* for further details.

Bronchiectasis directly attributable to pulmonary TB is rare [Figure 3.4B] (84). In those instances when this is found, it usually occurs in the upper lobe and is relatively asymptomatic. Along with bronchostenosis it predisposes to secondary infection, haemoptysis and atelectasis. Extension of TB to the pleura is common. Pericardial TB may follow pleuritis or by lymphatic spread from a pulmonary focus.

Whole Lung Tuberculosis

Rarely TB can affect the whole lung. This condition has a high mortality and results due to diffuse bronchogenic spread or haematogenous dissemination (104).

Complications

The reader is referred to the chapter *"Complications of pulmonary tuberculosis [Chapter 31]* for details.

PLEURAL TUBERCULOSIS

Pleural effusion is a more frequent sequel to primary TB in adolescents and adults than in younger children. It can occur many years after primary infection as an extension of post-primary TB or as an isolated effusion. Pleural effusion may complicate any TB pathology of lung or rib cage where the pleura is an involved bystander.

Primary effusion usually occurs on the same side as the primary complex, and hence is a result of contiguous affliction. Bilateral pleural effusions or those on the side opposite to the primary complex should suggest miliary or disseminated TB. Pleural and subpleural granulomas, usually seen on both visceral and parietal surfaces, tend to follow the lymphatics on the visceral surface and may be discrete. Diffuse or focal fibrosis may follow.

Large caseous or cavitary lesions rupture into the pleural space more commonly in post-primary TB and cause bronchopleural fistula with empyema. Empyema may heal with a fibrothorax and sometimes as a calcified pleural plaque resulting in a trapped lung. These patients may present with functional disability. Histological diagnosis is based on the identification of granulomas [Figure 3.5A].

The volume and cellular nature of the exudate are dictated by the cell-mediated immunity. The fluid is exudative, serofibrinous and occasionally purulent. Predominant cell type is lymphocyte with a few mesothelial cells. Rarely, histiocyte clusters may be seen which strongly suggest TB pleural effusion. A neutrophilic response does not rule out TB, though it is necessary to demonstrate the organism unequivocally in such cases. Direct microscopy and culture studies often do not reveal tubercle bacilli. Primary pleural TB usually resolves without anti-microbial therapy but when it develops in adolescence and young adulthood, it may carry the risk of post-primary TB, usually pulmonary within five to ten years. Therefore, treatment of pleural effusion with antituberculosis drugs is fully justified.

ABDOMINAL TUBERCULOSIS

The term abdominal TB generally includes TB of the gastrointestinal tract and the peritoneum. It is customary to exclude TB of organs like the kidneys and adrenals from this list. Isolated TB of organs such as the liver is uncommon. The TB of the intestines accounts for a majority of such cases [65%-78%]. Disseminated abdominal TB has also been observed (105,106).

Intestinal Tuberculosis

The primary form of gastrointestinal TB is extremely rare and has been discussed earlier. Intestinal TB usually involves the ileum, ileocaecal region and the adjacent caecum. Although this disease is chronic and invariably presents with symptoms suggestive of an abdominal disorder. Recurrent intestinal obstruction is an important presentation. Around one-third to a quarter of the patients present with acute abdomen (107,108). Most cases of intestinal TB are due to post-primary TB.

Gross and Microscopic Pathology

The credit to the description of intestinal TB goes to F. Koenig, whose masterly description in 1892 resulted in the disease being called "Koenig's syndrome" (108). Grossly, intestinal TB is classified into three types: ulcerative [60%],

hypertrophic [10%] and ulcero-hypertrophic [30%]. Ulcerative lesions indicate a highly virulent process (109-111). The intestine is indurated with an increase in mesenteric fat. Ulcers are generally transverse to the long axis [Figure 3.4C]. Circumferential or annular ulcers are usually less than 3 cm in length (112,113). The ulcers are superficial and may have undermined edges. Apparently the disposition of the ulcers is a reflection of the direction of lymphatics around the intestine and vascular supply from the mesentery to the intestinal wall (114-116). The base of the ulcer is covered by necrotic sloughs. On the serosa small tubercles may be present, predominantly, seen over the areas of mucosal involvement. Authors feel that it is necessary to document these lesions in the serosa since in essence these are lesions of TB peritonitis. However, these are localised lesions and do not result in the usual manifestations of peritonitis that are discussed below. Perforation of the intestine when present is usually proximal to a stricture. The 'hypertrophic type' is characterised by scarring of the bowel loops and often mimics a carcinoma. The ulcero-hypertrophic type has features of the two types described earlier. Cobblestoning of mucosa and pseudopolypi may be seen due to mucosal fissuring ulcers. The ileocaecal region is distorted and the normal angle as seen on barium films becomes obtuse. It is important to note that in TB, both sides of the ileocaecal valve are involved leading to its incompetence. This is unlike the features seen in Crohn's disease (112,113). However, in practice, it is often not easy to differentiate ileal TB from Crohn's disease based on gross or endoscopic findings [Table 3.8]. Lymph nodes may be enlarged, but as in other

Table 3.8: Differentiating features between intestinal tuberculosis and Crohn's disease		
Features	*Tuberculosis*	*Crohn's Disease*
Macroscopic		
Anal involvement	Rare	Relatively common
Serosal tubercles	Usually present	Not seen
Length of strictures	Short [< 3 cm]	Long
Internal fistulae	Rare	Common
Perforation	Uncommon	Rare
Ulcers	Circumferential/transverse	Along mesenteric border/longitudinal serpiginous
Microscopic		
Granuloma in intestine/lymph node	Present in majority	Absent in a quarter
Lymph node granulomas	May be only site	Absent
Type of granuloma	Large, confluent	Small, discrete
Caseation	Present	Absent
Cuff of inflammatory cells	Common	Usually absent
Fibrosis/hyalinisation	Can be seen	Rare
Fissures beyond submucosa	Absent	Present
Transmural lymphoid aggregates	Not seen	Present
Submucosal widening	Absent	Present
Fibrosis of muscularis propria	May be present	Not seen
Pyloric gland metaplasia	May be seen	Absent
Adapted from reference 114		

cases of post-primary TB, these may not be prominent. Rarely lymph nodes may assume a large size, giving rise to the condition called *tabes mesenterica*. We have seen cases that have very little resemblance to the description provided above. Surely, if the abdomen is a magic box to the surgeon, intestinal TB has all the ingredients for a very successful show.

Microscopic appearance of intestinal TB is similar to that of TB elsewhere. Necrotising and non-caseating granulomas [Figures 3.5B, 3.5C and 3.5D] are the hallmark of intestinal TB. In addition, the intestinal mucosa shows features of chronic inflammation in the form of crypt architectural distortion, branching pyloric metaplasia, etc. Features of activity, in form of ulcer, cryptitis and crypt abscess may be noted. The granulomas in TB are mostly confluent, large, necrotising, with lymphocyte cuffing and Langhans' giant cells. While early lesions show granulomas in the mucosa and Peyer's patches, in later lesions these are mostly seen in the submucosa [Figures 3.5D and 3.5E]. Sometimes the granulomas may be elusive and certain specimens may not reveal any granuloma (117). In fact in some studies, granulomas have been demonstrated in only 40% of the resected intestinal specimens. Identification of granulomas in the mesenteric lymph nodes is a strong pointer of TB, however, the same may also be noted in Crohn's disease, up to 20%-25% cases (117). Demonstration of AFB in histological sections is very rare [10%-20% cases] (113). Hence, the pathologists must rely on overall histological appearance to convey a specific diagnosis. However, at times, based on mucosal pinch biopsies, a specific diagnosis is often not possible. In such scenarios, if the ancillary tests, such as, microbiological and molecular methods, also remain elusive, a therapeutic trial of anti-TB drugs are given. Clinical and radiological improvement confirms the diagnosis; if no improvement is seen, the diagnosis is reconsidered as Crohn's disease, and a repeat biopsy is obtained. Myco-bacterial culture of the biopsy material may increase the yield ten-fold. In the case of the colon, histopathological and bacteriological examinations can provide diagnosis in 60% of cases (118).

Complications

Haemorrhage, perforation, obstruction, fistula formation and malabsorption due to obstruction and blind-loop syndrome and massive enlargement of mesenteric lymph nodes [tabes mesenterica] can occur in intestinal TB.

Differential Diagnosis

Apart from Crohn's disease, ischaemic enteritis, *Yersinia enterocolitica*, amoebiasis and carcinoma caecum (113,115). Syphilis and lymphogranuloma venereum are curiosities of historical interest.

Peritoneal Tuberculosis

Peritoneal TB is post-primary and is the result of either haematogenous spread from a focus elsewhere or due to a spread from an abdominal organ, usually a ruptured TB lymph node. The lesions in peritoneal TB can be classified into two types: exudative or moist type, clinically characterised by ascites and the plastic or dry type that is responsible for the typical doughy abdomen. Cirrhosis may be associated in a small proportion [6%] of patients with peritoneal TB (119).

On gross examination, multiple, white tubercles are generally seen. With laparoscopic examination such lesions may resemble a metastatic carcinoma. In some cases numerous peritoneal adhesions are identified. Microscopic examination reveals typical granulomas [Figure 3.5F]. Ascitic fluid cytology shows a predominance of lymphocytes. It must be pointed out that on some occasions the reaction may be neutrophilic mimicking an acute bacterial peritonitis.

Tuberculosis of Liver

Hepatic involvement by TB is not rare and is usually associated in generalised TB spread. In a study of paediatric TB, only 12% of cases showed granulomas in the liver (120). This low incidence can be attributed to the inherent drawback of needle biopsy as it samples a very small portion of the liver. Examination of serial sections may yield better results with the presence of TB hepatic granulomas in 30% of cases with TB (121). The liver in TB can have specific and non-specific histopathological changes. Korn *et al* (122) have emphasised the occurrence of focal hyperplasia of Kupffer cells in TB. This refers to localised areas of Kupffer cell proliferation with dilated sinusoids. Although such lesions may be the forerunners of microgranulomas, they differ from microgranulomas in that these are composed of typical Kupffer cells, have a stellate rather than rounded configuration and lack characteristic epithelioid cells. On the other hand, microgranulomas are small aggregates of epithelioid cells, usually centrilobular in location and lack giant cells and caseation (122). In fatal cases of TB, actual involvement by granulomatous process is common; whereas in localised form, the non-specific changes predominate. The rarer forms of hepatic TB lesions include TB cholangitis, tuberculoma and TB of the lymph nodes at the porta hepatis. In TB, most of the hepatic granulomas are lobular, though, portal tract granulomas can be seen. Confluence of granulomas, Langhans' giant cells, lymphocyte cuffing, necrosis and poor reticulin fibers around the granulomas, if present, are indicators of possible TB aetiology [Figures 3.6A, 3.6B and 3.6C]. However, hepatic granulomas can be seen in sarcoidosis [portal tract predominant] [Figures 3.6D and 3.6E], parasitic infestation, fungal infections, steatosis associated granulomas [Figure 3.6F] or granulomas associated with hepatotrophic viral infections. Hence, the biopsy findings need to be correlated with clinical scenario and should be further investigated with ancillary techniques and special stains.

Genitourinary Tuberculosis

Genitourinary TB [GUTB] usually occurs in the reproductive age group with a considerable lag period of up to

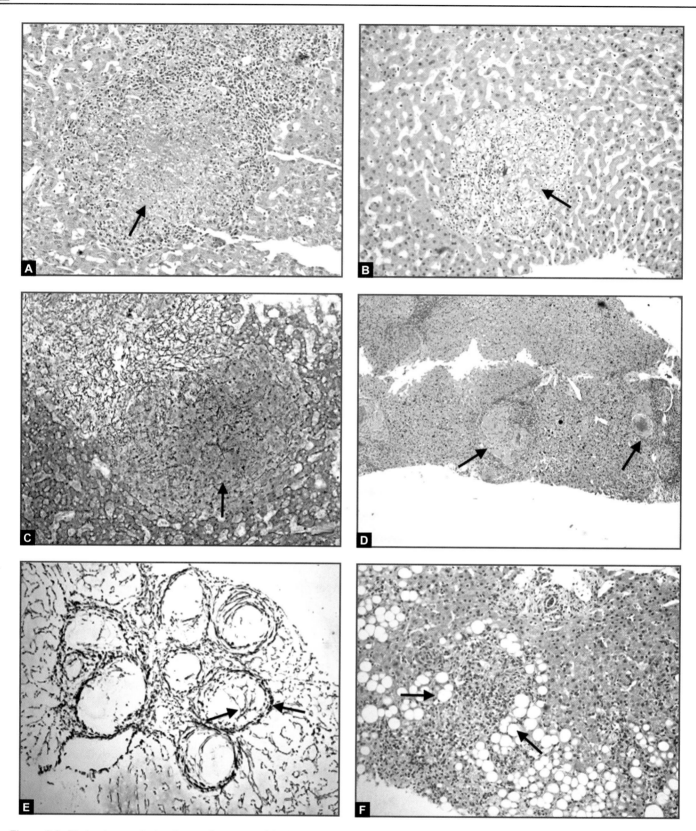

Figure 3.6: Photomicrograph showing confluent necrotising lobular epithelioid cell granulomas [arrows] [A and B] *[Haematoxylin and eosin × 100]*. Reticulin staining shows poor reticulin fibers around and inside the granuloma, suggesting TB [arrow] [C] *[Reticulin × 200]*. Portal based sarcoid granulomas with foreign body giant cells [arrows] [D] *[Haematoxylin and eosin × 100]*. Reticulin staining shows perigranuloma reticulin fibre condensation. Fibres are also seen inside the granuloma [arrows] [E] *[Reticulin × 200]*. A lobular fat granuloma in a case of nonalcoholic steatohepatitis. Fat droplets are noted inside the granuloma [arrows] [F] *[Haematoxylin and eosin × 100]*
TB = tuberculosis

two years in 90%-95% cases following the occurrence of primary TB (123). The disease involves the urinary tract and the genital tract either singly or in combination. Due to anatomical considerations, infection of the urinary tract and the male genital tract in combination is common.

Urinary Tract

Initially, renal TB granulomas are located in the cortex, which has a high perfusion rate. Cortical granulomas may remain dormant and if the host resistance is favourable, then fibrosis ensues. Highly virulent organisms or low resistance can cause progression of the lesion and the necrotic debri may lodge in the proximal tubule and loop of Henle. These produce medullary lesions which can enlarge, coalesce and produce papillary necrosis (124). The larger medullary lesions can persist as localised tuberculomas or discharge into the draining calyx. Sloughing of the necrotic contents into the calyx leads to cavity formation. Such cavities have shaggy necrotic walls with fibrosis of the adjacent renal parenchyma (125), or resulting in defunct, destroyed calcified kidney [autonephrectomy] [Figure 3.4D] (126). TB may result in changes of pyonephrosis with dilatation of calyces known as "putty" or "cement" or "chalk" kidney, which spreads down to affect ureters, bladder or urethera leading to ureteric strictures and segmental dilatation and obstruction (124). TB interstitial nephritis can only be diagnosed by presence of granuloma in interstitium, as kidney will be of normal size and smooth contour with sterile urine. Severe lesions may destroy the parenchyma fairly extensively [Figures 3.7A and 3.7B] (127).

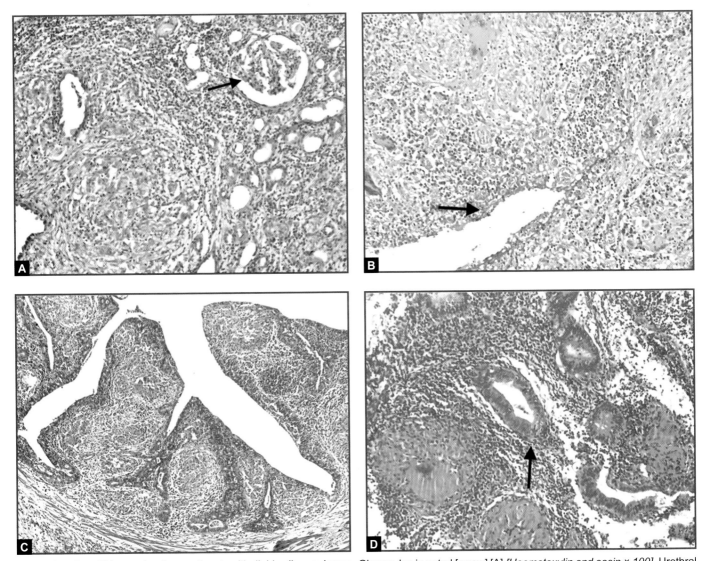

Figure 3.7: Renal biopsy showing confluent epithelioid cell granulomas. Glomerulus is noted [arrow] [A] *[Haematoxylin and eosin × 100]*. Urethral TB shows necrotising epithelioid cell granulomas with ulceration of urothelial lining [arrow] [B] *[Haematoxylin and eosin × 100]*. Fallopian tube section shows mucosal confluent granulomas [C] *[Haematoxylin and eosin × 100]*. Endometrial biopsy showing epithelioid cell granuloma in a proliferative endometrium [arrow] [D] *[Haematoxylin and eosin × 100]*
TB = tuberculosis

Some observers believe that kidneys can be involved by ascending infection from the bladder through the ureteral route. While such ascending infection is not very common, communication of the caseating granuloma with the collecting system is usually responsible for the spread of infection into the distal urinary system like pelvis, ureter and urinary bladder. Additionally, lymphatic spread can occur to contiguous structures. TB ureteritis initially appears as dilated and ragged irregular urothelium ["beaded" or "corkscrew" ureter]. Gradually it can lead to stricture formation leading to ureteral shortening and fibrous contraction that appears as "golf hole" orifice in the bladder. This can lead to obstruction, which in advanced cases, may result in TB pyonephrosis. There may be focal or diffuse calcification of the renal parenchyma.

Renal amyloidosis can occur in patients with pulmonary TB of long duration. Apart from specific TB process, kidney can show several non-specific changes in pulmonary TB. Shah et al (128) examined renal needle biopsy specimens from 30 patients with pulmonary TB. Of these, 70% had abnormal renal histopathology in the form of cloudy swelling of the tubular epithelial cells, focal lymphocytic aggregates, membranous glomerulonephritis, interstitial fibrosis and amyloidosis (128).

The initial lesions in the urinary bladder in TB are seen around the urethral orifices. Progressively, in advanced lesion the whole bladder wall may be involved. There is granulomatous inflammation and ulceration of the mucosa. Later on, fibrosis may lead to urethral stricture formation and and the bladder becomes small, contracted and calcified, finally resulting in nonfunctional bladder [autocystectomy] (129).

It may be mentioned that treatment of transitional cell carcinoma of the urinary bladder often involves instillation of BCG into the bladder. This may give rise to BCG granulomas, histologically indistinguishable from TB.

Male Genital Tract

If the infection proceeds from the urinary bladder, involvement of seminal vesicle, vas deferens and epididymis can occur (130). Isolated testicular TB is rare. All such cases are accompanied by epididymal infection through infected urine, lymphatics or haematogenous routes, resulting in TB epididymo-orchitis [Figure 3.4E]. TB epididymitis can lead to thickening of the vas by the granulomatous process and bilateral involvement has been noticed in 34% cases (131). Rarely cold abscess can also form near the epididymis (129). TB of the prostate can mimic a nodular or benign hyperplasia clinically. Involvement of multiple sites in the male genital tract is not uncommon, as reported in an autopsy series (124). As concurrent or previous renal TB is seen in many cases (132), genital TB is usually sequelae to a descending infection from the kidney (127).

Penile TB is very rare. As a form of skin TB, it can be acquired from sexual contact. It can also be a manifestation of either local or haematogenous spread.

Female Genital Tuberculosis

Female genital TB is usually secondary to a pulmonary TB. Modes of spread include haematogenous (90%), direct descending or lymphatic routes. It may be a component of generalised miliary TB. Transmission by sputum, used as a lubricant by an infected partner, has been reported (133). Sexual transport through semen in male patients with GUTB has been noticed in 3.9% cases (131).

Pathologically, the fallopian tube [95%-100%] is the most common site of involvement [Figures 3.4F and 3.7C] (134,135). The tubes are usually involved bilaterally. These get seeded during the primary infection. The lesions get reactivated or clinically manifested usually after a long latent period. Endometrial TB (50%-60%), myometrial TB (2.5%) are related to spread from the fallopian tubes (136). Less commonly, cervix [5%-15%] and vulva, vagina are involved, as an extension from the endometrial lesion. Ovarian infection [20%-30%] can also occur from the tubal source (137). Rarely sexual transmission can cause vulvar ulcers and inguinal lymphadenopathy in females (138). Frequently, more than one organ may be involved (127).

Gross lesions can be miliary, ulcerative, proliferative or a combination of these. Fistula formation has also been reported. Granulomas are identified usually in the mucosa of the affected organ. Histopathological confirmation by endometrial curettage with staining for AFB and culture are necessary for diagnosis. Curettage should ideally be done in the late menstrual cycle. However, it is not necessary to believe that granulomas are identified only in secretory endometrium. Granulomas can be found in any phase of the menstrual cycle and also in hyperplasia of the endometrium [Figure 3.7D]. Cervical biopsy is also useful. Identification of necrotising epithelioid cell granulomas with or without demonstration of AFB establishes the diagnosis in a considerable number of cases. Caseation has been reported to be more frequent in the elderly. Unfortunately, AFB are hardly identifiable in most instances (127).

NEUROTUBERCULOSIS

Neurotuberculosis includes TB of the meninges, the brain, spinal cord and the nerves. TB meningitis [TBM] is the most common form of neurotuberculosis and generally develops from the breakdown of a small initial focus in the superficial cortex or leptomeninges. This focus discharges caseous material into the cerebrospinal fluid [CSF] (139). Such a focus can destabilize following years of quiescence due to advanced age, trauma, malnutrition, chronic debilitation and immune suppression. TBM can also result from miliary spread of the disease. The miliary tubercles in the leptomeninges are most frequently seen on the lateral aspect of parietal and temporal lobes on either side of the Sylvian fissure and along the blood vessels at these sites.

There are six main parenchymal changes in neurotuberculosis. These are ventriculitis, border zone encephalitis, infarction, internal hydrocephalus, diffuse oedema and tuberculoma. Ventriculitis is less frequently encountered than meningitis. In this condition, the ependymal lining of the ventricles and choroid plexus show tubercles. Border zone encephalitis is caused by impingement of the meningeal exudate on the underlying brain parenchyma. Frequently, there is only a glial reaction. Occasionally the changes may be of inflammatory nature. Infarction is caused by vasculitis due to inflammation of the vessels in the meningeal exudate. The vessels commonly involved are branches of the middle cerebral artery, especially the perforating vessels to the basal ganglia (140). The vascular changes occur in the form of periarteritis, endarteritis, panarteritis, necrosis and thrombosis. Narrowing or total occlusion of the vessels results in infarction of the zone supplied by the artery.

In TBM, hydrocephalus evolves due to the following reasons: [i] blockage of the basal cisterns and medullocerebellar angles and obstruction to the flow of the CSF by the basal exudate; and [ii] interference in the absorption of CSF by arachnoid granulations.

Macroscopic Features

In TBM, the brain is heavier in weight due to cerebral oedema. The leptomeninges in the basilar area appear opaque as the underlying thick exudate fills up the cisterns [Figure 3.8A]. Sometimes, the exudate is found on the surface of the brain mimicking pyogenic meningitis. The gyri appear flattened with obliteration of sulci. Superficial blood vessels look congested. Serial slicing reveals ventriculitis with matted appearance of the choroid plexus. There may be ventricular dilatation and areas of infarction in the middle cerebral artery territory. Finding the parenchymal tubercles giving rise to TBM is difficult task because: [i] the tubercles are frequently of small size [commonly 3-5 mm in diameter]. Thus if the slices are thicker than 3 mm, the lesions may be missed; [ii] the site of origin is frequently a caseous meningeal plaque which is often masked macroscopically by the surrounding meningitis; and [iii] macroscopic visualisation of caseous nodules is often difficult.

Parenchymal tuberculoma is less frequently seen than TBM. This may be due to the difference in their pathogenesis. Usually small tubercles are found in association with TBM. While TBM is a typical leptomeningeal reaction to tubercle bacilli, tuberculoma is the manifestation of hypersensitivity to tuberculoproteins in the susceptible individual (141). Generally tuberculomas [Figure 3.8B] favour infratentorial location, the most frequent site being the cerebellum. The physical continuity between a tuberculoma and meningeal exudate is usually not evident, although this has been occasionally observed (142).

Microscopic Features

Large areas of caseous necrosis feature the leptomeningeal reaction with a cellular infiltrate consisting predominantly of lymphocytes and plasma cells. There may be focal epithelioid granulomas with giant cell reaction [Figure 3.9A]. Ependymal lining of the ventricles reveals ependymitis which resembles the inflammatory reaction of meningitis. Choroid plexitis may also be evident. In some cases the inflammatory reaction may be polymorphic giving the appearance of a pyogenic meningitis. However, in these cases, numerous AFB are demonstrable.

Immediately beneath the meningeal exudate, the brain shows oedema, perivascular inflammatory infiltrate and microglial reaction [Figure 3.9B]. In longstanding cases gliosis ensues. If the inflammation is caused by fewer bacilli, complete resolution of the exudate is possible with treatment. Residual well-circumscribed, small caseous foci may remain following treatment if the bacilli are abundant.

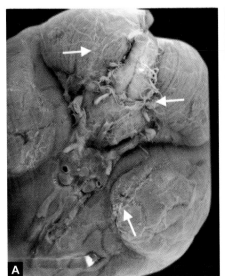
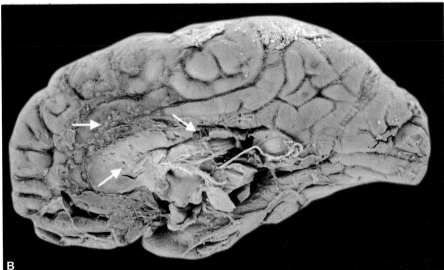

Figure 3.8: Gross specimen photograph of a brain base, showing thick exudate in TB meningoencephalitis [arrows] [A]. Cut-surface shows tubercles around the basal ganglia and corpus callosum [arrows] [B]

TB = tuberculosis

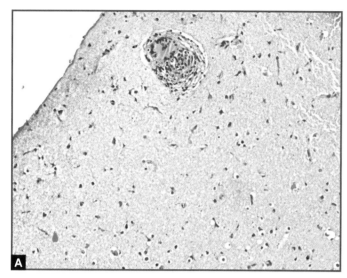
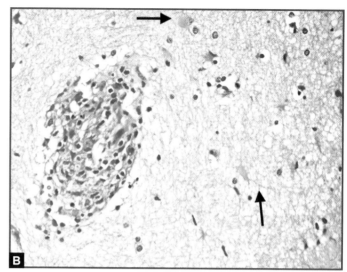

Figure 3.9: Photomicrographs showing perivascular epithelioid cell granulomas in TB encephalitis *[Haematoxylin and eosin × 100]* [A]. Cortical gliosis [arrows] is also noted *[Haematoxylin and eosin × 200]* [B]
TB = tuberculosis

Histopathologically, tuberculomas show epithelioid granulomatous response with chronic inflammatory cells and Langhans giant cells. There are areas of caseous necrosis. An occasional case shows focal calcification.

The TB abscess consists of pus-filled cavities containing tubercle bacilli. The wall of TB abscess shows granulation tissue with inflammatory cells. There is usually a paucity of epithelioid cells or giant cells and the lesion may be misdiagnosed clinically as pyogenic abscess. The content of the cavity usually shows numerous AFB.

Intracranial TBM often extends into the spinal meninges. Only in a few cases the inflammation starts in the sub-arachnoid space from a small subpial tubercle [Rich focus] or TB vertebral osteomyelitis. Rarely there can be spinal intramedullary tuberculomas similar to intracranial lesions.

MUSCULOSKELETAL TUBERCULOSIS

Bone and joint TB usually follows a primary pulmonary infection. Less commonly there can be contiguous spread from pleura, periaortic lymph nodes or haematogenous dissemination (143). The most frequently involved site is the vertebral body and this form of spinal TB is known as spondylitis, i.e., "Pott's disease". In this disease, the classical involvement is of two consecutive vertebrae with destruction of the intervertebral discs. The lower thoracic and upper lumbar areas are common sites of disease (144,145). It clinically presents as local pain, which increases in severity over weeks to months and the differential diagnoses include degenerative disc, spondyloarthropathy, facet joint disease, vertebral body collapse due to osteoporosis, osteopenia, subacute/chronic *Staphylococcus aureus* spinal infections, osteomyelitis and malignancies. Any other bone or joint can be involved by TB, but weight bearing ones like knee and hip joints are more prone to be affected (146). The next common form of skeletal TB is TB arthritis [Figure 3.10].

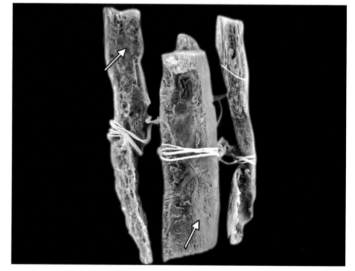

Figure 3.10: Gross specimen photograph of a long bone with evidences of TB osteomyelitis
TB = tuberculosis

Histopathologically, the presence of a granulomatous inflammation with necrosis is compatible with the diagnosis of TB. Histopathological evidence of mycobacterial infection has been documented in 94% of synovial biopsy samples (147). In general, mycobacterium load is 10^7-10^9 and less than 10^5 in pulmonary and osteoarticular lesions, respectively. In the case of the bone, the best material for microbiological assessment is centrifuged residue from large quantity of abscess, curettings from wall of cold abscess prior to secondary infections or curettings from the base of sinus tract lining. Direct smear examination of tuberculous material obtained during operation or obtained by aspiration of the infected synovium [from joints, bursae and tendon sheaths] or involved lymph nodes or the tuberculous osseous cavities may yield a positive result for tubercle bacilli. Special stains can demonstrate AFB in some cases (148,149). Mycobacterial culture positivity varies from 30.4%-87% of cases (150).

TUBERCULOSIS IN THE IMMUNOCOMPROMISED

TB is often the sentinel disease warning of HIV infection and the development of AIDS. When active TB occurs in patients with AIDS, pulmonary TB is almost always present and in up to 70% of the cases extrapulmonary disease is associated. The source of infection could be recrudescence of latent infection [the most common source], or accelerated progression of newly acquired disease or superinfection of those previously infected.

Impaired cell mediated immunity [CMI] due to the reduced number of T-cells, specifically, the CD4+ subset is considered to be the reason for the higher incidence of TB in AIDS. Macrophage and peripheral monocyte function is reduced and consequently there is reduced activation of lymphokines. The cellular arm of immunity is, thus, seriously impaired and the body's defences against intracellular pathogens such as mycobacteria and other organisms such as *Pneumocystis jiroveci* become defective. TB bacilli itself may also cause immunosuppression (151). Until a late stage has been reached in the immune impairment, TB presents the usual clinical and pathological patterns observed in immunocompetent persons. Post-primary TB is most often encountered. Only when the immune defect has become severe the presentation becomes atypical and resembles more the pattern of primary disease (152-154).

Hilar and mediastinal lymphadenopathy [often bilateral] can occur in up to 60% of adult TB cases co-infected with AIDS, while this is observed only in 3% patients without AIDS. Middle and lower zone involvement is more often observed than the usual upper lobe involvement. Diffuse infiltrates or a miliary pattern is apparent in 15% cases and distant haematogenous dissemination to unusual sites is common. Pleurisy commonly occurs. The disease, thus, resembles primary or progressive primary TB. Cavitation is less frequent. Therefore sputum is less frequently positive for AFB. Surprisingly even in the late stages of immunosuppression, typical compact or 'hard' tuberculoid granulomas with minimal necrosis and few bacilli, epithelioid cells and Langhans' giant cells can be seen. There is, however, the eventual tendency for the cell aggregates to become smaller. They are more loosely formed and the lymphocyte collar may not be evident. AFB are often found, giant cells are rare and karyorrhexis [nuclear fragmentation] is often seen (152-154).

Chest radiograph may be confusing. In a few cases, the chest radiograph may be normal even in patients with bacteriologically proven parenchymal TB. This is especially so in infections caused by *Mycobacterium avium-intracellulare* complex [MAIC]. Diffuse interstitial pattern on chest radiographs can be caused by *Pneumocystis jiroveci* infection in patients with AIDS and is easily confused with other diseases. A positive blood culture for *Mtb* has

been observed in up to about 26%-40% cases. Immune anergy with loss of tuberculin reactivity is common. The progressive loss of tuberculin reactivity appears to coincide with a CD4+ T-lymphocyte count below 300-400 per cubic millimeter, although very low counts may be associated with a significant tuberculin reaction at a level of 5 mm or greater particularly after boosting by a second test (152-154). In the terminal stages, when the immune defect is severe, there may be aggregates of macrophages with numerous intracellular organisms, but no granuloma formation. Disseminated, non-reactive TB with necrosis, much nuclear debris, many extracellular stainable AFB and minimal cellular reaction are also seen. Surrounded by a few histiocytes and lymphocytes areas of naked necrosis can be seen. The mechanisms of necrosis in the absence of significant numbers of inflammatory cells is unclear and so is the mechanism by which the cell response is excluded.

NONTUBERCULOUS MYCOBACTERIAL INFECTIONS OF LUNG

The focus of this section is on the pathogenesis and pathology of the infections caused by ubiquitously present [slow > rapid growing] nontuberculous mycobacteria [NTM]. Pulmonary involvement is most common [94%], other being lymphatics [3%] and skin/soft tissue/disseminated sites [3%]. Microbiological classification, characterisation and other details regarding NTM are dealt with elsewhere. The reader is referred to the chapters titled *"The mycobacteria"* [Chapter 4] and *"Nontuberculous mycobacterial infections"* [Chapter 41] for details.

Pathology

The gross and microanatomical knowledge regarding NTM disease is incomplete as the number of cases studied that have not been modified by previous treatment, are rare. Also many cases have not been studied, as they have been passed off as resistant TB or a nodular infiltrative disease. NTM disease differs from TB in not causing a defined sequence of primary and post-primary disease (155,156). Haematological dissemination occurs only in the immunosuppressed. Radiological patterns of *M. avium-intracellulare complex* [MAIC], *M. kansasii* disease and *M. xenopi* resemble post-primary TB. In *M. kansasii*, the cavities are thin walled. In NTM disease, the anterior segments of the upper lobes are more frequently affected. Spread to contiguous pleura and pericardium is rare and spread to the lymph nodes is uncommon. *M. genavense* is a new atypical agent in HIV patients. Study of an HIV-negative elderly female without other lung disease showed a wide distribution of the lesions, frequent bronchiectasis, patchy air-space disease, nodules and relative infrequency of cavities (157).

The histopathology of the lung in NTM infections can be summed up as a spectrum ranging from a collection of lymphocytes through aggregations of epithelioid cells and typical sarcoid-like tubercles to characteristic caseating granulomas (115,158). The nodular pattern seen on computed tomography [CT] consists of discrete peribronchial granulomas with focal caseating or multiple granulomas in a group. *M. kansasii* has been reported to have spread transplacentally.

Histopathologically the features are dimorphic displaying both loose granulomas with giant cells containing a central aggregation of polymorphs and areas of acute inflammation often with microabscesses within which clusters of AFB may sometimes be identified. Well-formed epithelioid granulomas are uncommon and caseous necrosis is not a feature. Disseminated disease from rapid growers is uncommon.

With more effective treatment of *Pneumocystis jiroveci*, there is an increasing evidence that the occurrence of NTM is growing. As NTM infection typically occurred in AIDS is a late feature [CD4+ T-lymphocyte count < 50/mm^3], these infections occur at a point when other opportunistic infections are present and this may complicate the histopathology of MAIC and other mycobacterial infections (159,160).

Radiological findings are frequently negative even when tissue evidence of pulmonary infection by MAIC is present (161,162). Macroscopically the organs are often enlarged and may be yellow because of the pigment. Recognisable granulomas may not be present or when present may be poorly formed. AFB may be plentiful with minimal or absent inflammatory reaction. A particular feature of MAIC infection is the occurrence of aggregates of macrophages filled with many AFB, so called multibacillary histiocytosis, a feature not seen in TB and AIDS. The use of antiviral therapy has permitted the repair of CMI which restores a more typical granulomatous response and an improved clinical response to antimycobacterial drug therapy. Diagnosis is achieved by blood culture, biopsy examination and culture of tissue from liver, bone marrow and other organs (159,162).

In the present era, mere identification of AFB in tissue sections would not suffice. It has become a goal of paramount importance to identify whenever possible the species of the *Mycobacterium* and its drug susceptibility patterns for diagnostic, prognostic, therapeutic and public health reasons.

ACKNOWLEDGEMENTS

The authors are grateful to members of the Department of Pathology who have taken photographs of the gross specimens.

REFERENCES

1. Dubos RJ, Dubos J. The white plague: tuberculosis, man and society. Boston: Little Brown and Company; 1952.
2. Bos KI, Harkins KM, Herbig A, Coscolla M, Weber N, Comas I, et al. Pre-Columbian mycobacterial genomes reveal seals as a source of New World human tuberculosis. Nature 2014;514:494-7.
3. Sharma SK, Mohan A. Tuberculosis: From an incurable scourge to a curable disease - journey over a millennium. Indian J Med Res 2013;137:455-93.
4. Rich AR. The pathogenesis of tuberculosis. 2nd edition. Illinois: Charles C. Thomas; 1951.
5. Skinner HA. The origin of medical terms. 2nd edition. Baltimore: The Williams and Wilkins Company; 1961.
6. Wain H. The story behind the word. Illinois: Charles C. Thomas; 1958.
7. Russell DG. Who puts the tubercle in tuberculosis? Nat Rev Microbiol 2007;5:39-47.
8. Zumla A, James GD. Granulomatous infections: etiology and classification. Clin Infect Dis 1996;23:146-58.
9. Rook GAW, al Attiyah R. Cytokines and Koch phenomenon. Tubercle 1991;72:13-20.
10. Morrison A, Gyure KA, Stone J, Wong K, Mc Evoty, Koeller K, et al. Mycobacterial spindle cell pseudotumor of the brain: a case report and review of the literature. Am J Surg Pathol 1999;23:1294-9.
11. Le Gall, Loeiullet L, Delaval P, Thoreux PH, Desrues B, Ramee MP. Necrotising sarcoid granulomatosis with and without extra-pulmonary involvement. Pathol Res Pract 1996;192:306-13.
12. Brady JG, Schutze GE, Seibert R, Horn HV, Marks B, Parham DM. Detection of mycobacterial infections using the Dieterle stain. Pediatr Dev Pathol 1998;1:309-13.
13. Gutierrez-Cancela MM, Garcia Marin JF. Comparison of Ziehl-Neelsen staining and immunohistochemistry for detection of Mycobacterium bovis in bovine and caprine tuberculous lesions. J Comp Pathol 1993;109:361-70.
14. Marais BJ, Brittle W, Painczyk K, Hesseling AC, Beyers N, Wasserman E, et al. Use of light-emitting diode fluorescence microscopy to detect acid-fast bacilli in sputum. Clin Infect Dis 2008;47:203-7.
15. Kaur R, Kachroo K, Sharma JK, Vatturi SM, Dang A. Diagnostic accuracy of Xpert test in tuberculosis detection: a systematic review and meta-analysis. J Glob Infect Dis 2016;8:32-40.
16. Eliseev P, Balantcev G, Nikishova E, Gaida A, Bogdanova E, Enarson D, et al. The impact of a line probe assay based diagnostic algorithm on time to treatment initiation and treatment outcomes for multidrug resistant TB patients in Arkhangelsk Region, Russia. PLoS One 2016;11:e0152761.
17. Kaplan MH, Armstrong D, Rosen P. Tuberculosis complicating neoplastic disease: a review of 201 cases. Cancer 1974;33:850-8.
18. Mettler CC. History of medicine. Philadelphia: The Blakiston Company; 1947.
19. Ghon A. The primary lung focus of tuberculosis in children [Translation by King DB]. London: Churchill; 1916.
20. Smith DW. Bacillemia in primary tuberculosis. Ann Intern Med 1971;75:479-80.
21. Stead WW, Bates JH. Evidence of a "silent" bacillemia in primary tuberculosis. Ann Intern Med 1971;74:559-61.
22. Morrison JBM. Resorption of calcification in primary pulmonary tuberculosis. Thorax 1990;25:643-6.
23. Salyer WR, Salyer DC, Baker RD. Primary complex of Crypto-coccus and pulmonary lymph nodes. J Infect Dis 1974;130:74-7.
24. Anonymous. Unusual tuberculosis. Tubercle 1965;46:420-6.
25. Lee LH, Le Vea CM, Graman PS. Congenital tuberculosis in a neonatal intensive care unit. Case report, epidemiological investigation and management of exposures. Clin Infect Dis 1998;27:474-7.
26. Kang GH, Chi JG. Congenital tuberculosis-report of an autopsy case. J Korean Med Sci 1990;5:59-64.
27. Hageman J, Shulman S, Schreiber M, Luck S, Yogev R. Congenital tuberculosis: critical reappraisal of clinical findings and diagnostic procedures. Pediatrics 1980;66:980-4.
28. Machin GA, Homore LH, Fanning EA, Molesky M. Perinatally acquired neonatal tuberculosis: report of two cases. Pediatr Pathol 1992;12:707-16.

29. Fisher I, Orkin M. Primary tuberculosis of the skin. Primary complex. JAMA 1966;195:314-6.

30. Hellman KM, Muschenhe C. Primary cutaneous tuberculosis resulting from mouth to mouth resuscitation. New Engl J Med 1965; 273:1035-6.

31. Tamura M, Ogawa G, Sagawa I, Amano S. Observations on an epidemic of cutaneous and lymphatic tuberculosis which followed the use of anti-typhoid vaccine. Am Rev Tuberc 1955; 71:465-72.

32. Irani A, Colaco P, Desai MP. Cutaneous primary complex following venepuncture. Indian Pediatr 1978;15:181-3.

33. Strikas R, Venezio FR O'Keefe JP. A case of cutaneous tuber- culosis: primary or secondary? Am Rev Respir Dis 1983;128: 316-8.

34. Lucas SB. Histopathology of leprosy and tuberculosis-an overview. Br Med Bull 1988;44:584-99.

35. Sehgal VN, Srivastava G, Khurana VK, Sharma VK, Bhalla P, Beohar PC, et al. An appraisal of epidemiologic, clinical- bacteriologic, histopathologic and immunologic parameters in cutaneous tuberculosis. Int J Dermatol 1987;26:521-6.

36. Maes RF. Tuberculosis II: the failure of the BCG vaccine. Med Hypotheses 1999;53:32-9.

37. Caplan SE, Kauflman CL. Primary inoculation tuberculosis after immunotherapy for malignant melanoma with BCG vaccine. J Am Acad Dermatol 1996;35:783-5.

38. Jakubikova J, Trupl J, Nevicka E, Drdos M, Zitnan D, Hrusovska F. Child's tuberculous lymphadenitis with fistula evoked by the BCG. Int J Pediatr Otolaryngol 1996;37:85-90.

39. Dimitrakopoulos I, Zoiloumis L. Lazarrdis N, Karkasis D, Trigonidis, Sichetidis L. Primary tuberculosis of the oral cavity. Oral Surg Oral Med Oral Pathol 1991;72:712-5.

40. Miller FJW. In: Health and Tuberculosis Conference. London: Chest and Heart Association, London; 1962.p.76.

41. Verma A, Mann SB, Radotra B. Primary tuberculosis of the tongue. Ear Nose Throat J 1989;68:718-20.

42. Hashimoto Y, Tanioka H. Primary tuberculosis of the tongue: report of a case. J Oral Maxillofac Surg 1989;47:744-6.

43. Gupta A, Shinde KJ, Bharadwaj I. Primary lingual tuberculosis: a case report. J Laryngol Otol 1998;112:86-7.

44. Eng J, Sabanathan S. Tuberculosis of the esophagus. Dig Dis Sci 1991;361:536-40.

45. Sood A, Sood N, Kumar R, Midda V. Primary tuberculosis of esophagus. Indian J Gastroenterol 1996;15:75.

46. Talib SH, Chawhan RN, Zaheer A, Talib VA. Primary tuber- culosis of the stomach [a case report]. J Assoc Physicians India 1975;23:291-3.

47. Sengupta P, Ghosh P, Mukherjee SD. Primary tuberculosis of the stomach. J Indian Med Assoc 1978;71:209-10.

48. Singh B, Moodley J, Ramdial P, Haffejee AA, Royeppen E, Maharaj J. Primary gastric tuberculosis. A report of 3 cases. S Afr J Surg 1996;34:29-32.

49. Ray JD, Sriram PV, Kumar S, Kochhar R, Vaiphei K, Singh K. Primary duodenal tuberculosis diagnosed by endoscopic biopsy. Trop Gastroenterol 1997;18:74-5.

50. Lanzieri CF, Keller RJ. Primary tuberculosis of the ileum: roentgen features. Mt. Sinai J Med 1980;47:596-9.

51. Deodhar SD, Patel VC, Bharucha MA, Vora IM. Primary tuber- culosis of the large bowel [a case report]. J Postgrad Med 1986;32:161-2.

52. Beibanaste M. Apparently primary tuberculosis of the vermiform appendix. Rass Clin Ther 1965;64:273-5.

53. Murali VP, Divakar D, Thachil MV, Raghu CG, Jacob MC. Primary tuberculosis of the appendix. J Indian Med Assoc 1989;87:162-3.

54. Stirk DI. Primary tuberculosis of the stomach, caecum, and appendix treated with antituberculous drugs. Br J Surg 1968;55:230-5.

55. Desai HG, Raman G, Lele RD. "Primary" tuberculosis of the liver. Indian J Gastroenterol 1983;2:14-6.

56. Essop AR, Moosa MR, Segal I, Posen J. Primary tuberculosis of the liver - a case report. Tubercle 1983;64:291-3.

57. Selimoglu E, Sutbeyaz Y, Ciftcioglu MA, Parlak M, Esrefoglu M, Ozturk A. Primary tonsillar tuberculosis: a case report. J Laryngol Otol 1995;109:880-2.

58. Mahindra S, Bazaz-Malik G, Sohail MA. Primary tuberculosis of the adenoids. Acta Otolaryngol Stockh 1981;92:173-80.

59. Murray A, Gardiner DS, McGuiness RJ. Primary mycobacterial infection of the uvula. J Laryngol Otol 1998;112:1183-5.

60. Sharma HS, Kurl DN, Kamal MZ. Tuberculoid granulomatous lesion of the pharynx-review of literature. Auris Nasus Larynx 1998;25:187-91.

61. Sinha SN, Dewan VK. Primary tuberculosis of the larynx. Ear Nose Throat J 1978;57:158.

62. Ali F. Primary tuberculosis of the larynx in children. Ear Nose Throat J 1985;64:139-40.

63. Sharan R. Primary tuberculosis of the nose. Practitioner 1981; 225:1506-7.

64. Purohit SD, Gupta RC. Primary tuberculosis of nose. Indian J Chest Dis Allied Sci 1997;39:63-4.

65. Sim J, Ong BH. Primary tuberculosis of the nasopharynx. Singapore Med J 1972;13:39-43.

66. Gnanapragasam A. Primary tuberculosis of the nasopharynx. Med J Malaysia 1972;26:3194-7.

67. Midholm A, Brahe-Pedersen C. Primary tuberculosis otitis media. J Laryngol Otol 1971;85:1195-200.

68. Sharan R, Isser DK. Primary tuberculosis of the middle ear cleft. Practitioner 1979;222:93-5.

69. Ozcelik, Ataman M, Gedikoglu G. An unusual presentation: primary tuberculosis of middle ear cleft. Tuber Lung Dis 1995;76:178-9.

70. Ustuner TE, Sensoz O, Kocer U. Primary tuberculosis of the parotid gland. Plast Reconst Surg 1991;88:884-5.

71. Kant R, Sahi RP, Mahendra NN, Agarwal PK, Shankhdhar R. Primary tuberculosis of the parotid gland. J Indian Med Assoc 1977;68:212.

72. Annobil SH, al-Hilfi A, Kazi T. Primary tuberculosis of the penis in an infant. Tubercle 1990;71:229-30.

73. Konohana A, Noda J, Shoji K, Hanyaku H. Primary tuberculosis of the glans penis. J Am Acad Dermatol 1992;26:1002-3.

74. Rossi R, Urbam F, Tortoli E, Trolta M, Zuccati G, Cappugi P. Primary tuberculosis of the penis. J Eur Acad Dermatol. 1999;12: 174-6.

75. Dunn JP, Helm CJ, Davidson PT. Tuberculosis. In: Pepose JS, Holland GN, Willhelmus KR, editors. Ocular infection and immunity. St Louis: Mosby; 1996.p.1421-9.

76. Archer D, Bird A. Primary tuberculosis of the conjunctiva. Br J Ophthalmol 1967;51:679-84.

77. Whitford J, Hansman D. Primary tuberculosis of the conjunctiva. Med J Aust 1977;1:486-7.

78. Charles V, Charles SZ. Primary tuberculosis of conjunctiva. J Indian Med Assoc 1980;74:74-5.

79. Rose JS, Arthur A, Raju R, Thomas M. Primary conjunctival tuberculosis in a 14-year-old-girl. Indian J Tuberc 2011;58:32-34.

80. Saini JS, Mukherjee AK, Nadkarni N. Primary tuberculosis of the retina. Br J Opthalmol 1986;70:533-5.

81. Slavin RE, Walsh TJ, Pokkack AD. Late generalised tuberculosis: a clinical, pathologic analysis and comparison of 100 cases in the pre-antibiotic and antibiotic eras. Medicine 1980;59:352-66.

82. Sharma SK, Mohan A, Sharma A, Mitra DK. Miliary tuberculosis: new insights into an old disease. Lancet Infect Dis 2005;5:415-30.

83. Sharma SK, Mohan A, Sharma A. Miliary tuberculosis: a new look at an old foe. J Clin Tuberc Oth Mycobact Dis 2016;3:13-27.

84. Medlar EM. The behaviour of pulmonary tuberculous lesion: A pathological study. Am Rev Tuberc 1955;71:1-244.

85. Nayak NC, Sabharwal BD, Bhathena D, Mital GS, Ramalingaswami V. The pulmonary tuberculous lesion in north India: a study in medicolegal autopsies. I. Incidence, nature and evolution. Am Rev Respir Dis 1970;101:1-17.

86. Bhathena D, Mohapatra LN, Mital GS, Ramalingaswami V, Nayak NC. The pulmonary tuberculous lesion in north India: a study in medicolegal autopsies. II. Bacteriologic aspects. Am Rev Respir Dis 1970;101:18-26.

87. Lincoln EM, Sewell BH. Tuberculosis in children. New York: McGraw-Hill; 1963.p.19-83.

88. Giammona ST, Poole CA, Zelkowitz P, Skrovan C. Massive lymphadenopathy in primary pulmonary tuberculosis in children. Am Rev Respir Dis 1969;100:480-9.

89. Wallgren A. The timetable of tuberculosis. Tubercle 1948;29: 245-51.

90. Bates JH. Transmission and pathogenesis of tuberculosis. Clin Chest Med 1980;1:167-74.

91. Dannenberg AM Jr, Sugimoto M. Liquefaction of caseous foci in tuberculosis. Am Rev Respir Dis 1976;113:257-9.

92. Altin S, Cikrikaogln S, Morgul M, Rosar T, Ozyurt H. Fifty endobronchial tuberculosis cases based on bronchoscopic diagnosis. Respiration 1997;64:162-4.

93. Jones EM, Rafferty TN, Willis HS. Primary tuberculosis complicated by bronchial tuberculosis with atelectasis. Trans Am Clin Climatol Assoc 1941;57:102-6.

94. Choyke PL, Sostman HD, Curtis AM, Ravin CE, Chen JT, Godwin JD, et al. Adult onset pulmonary tuberculosis. Radiology 1983;148:357-62.

95. Tead WW, Kerby GR, Schleuter DP, Jordahl CW. The clinical spectrum of primary tuberculosis in adults. Confusion with reinfection in the pathogenesis of chronic tuberculosis. Ann Intern Med 1968;68:731-45.

96. Smith LS, Schillaci RF, Sarlin RF. Endobronchial tuberculosis: Serial fiberoptic bronchoscopy and natural history. Chest 1987; 91:644-7.

97. Meylan PRA, Richman DD, Kornbluth RS. Reduced intracellular growth of mycobacteria in human macrophages cultivated at physiologic oxygen pressure. Am Rev Respir Dis 1992;145: 947-53.

98. Goodwin RA, Des Prez RM. Apical localisation of pulmonary tuberculosis, chronic pulmonary histoplasmosis and progressive massive fibrosis of the lung. Chest 1983;83:801-5.

99. Weigeshaus E, Balasubramanian V, Smith DW. Immunity to tuberculosis from the perspective of pathogenesis. Infect Immun 1989;57:3571-6.

100. Woodring JH, Vandiviere HM, Lee C. Intrathoracic lymphadenopathy in post-primary tuberculosis. South Med J 1988;81:992-7.

101. Lung AN, Muller NL, Pineda PR, Fitgerbld JM. Primary tuberculosis in childhood: radiographic manifestations. Radiology 1992;182:87-91.

102. Sweany HC, Cook CE, Kegeggereis R. A study of the position of primary cavities in pulmonary tuberculosis. Am Rev Tuberc 1931;24:558-82.

103. Van den Brande PM, Van de Mierop F, Verbeken EK, Demedts M. Clinical spectrum of endobronchial tuberculosis in elderly patients. Arch Intern Med 1990;150:2105-8.

104. Tsao TC, Juang YC, Tsai YH, Lan RS, Lee CH. Whole lung tuberculosis. A disease with high mortality which is frequently misdiagnosed. Chest 1992;101:1309-11.

105. Kapoor VK. Abdominal tuberculosis. Postgrad Med J 1998;74: 459-67.

106. Rasheed S, Zinicola R, Watson D, Bajwa A, McDonald PJ. Intra-abdominal and gastrointestinal tuberculosis. Colorectal Dis 2007;9:773-83.

107. Agarwal S, Gera N. Tuberculosis—an underestimated cause of ileal perforation. J Indian Med Assoc 1996;94:341,352.

108. Haddad FS, Ghossain A, Sawaya E, Netson AR. Abdominal tuberculosis. Dis Col Rectum 1987;30:724-35.

109. Benttey G, Webstar JHH. Gastrointestinal tuberculosis: a 10-year review. Br J Surg 1967;54:90-6.

110. McGee GS, Williams LF, Potts J, Barnwell S, Sawyers JL. Gastro-intestinal tuberculosis: resurgence of an old pathogen. Am Surg 1989;55:16-20.

111. Marshall JB. Tuberculosis of the gastrointestinal tract and peritoneum. Am J Gastroenterol 1993;88:989-99.

112. Tandon HD, Prakash A, Rao VB, Prakash O, Nair SK. Ulcero-constrictive disorders of the intestine in northern India: a pathologic study. Indian J Med Res 1966;54:129-41.

113. Tandon HD, Prakash A. Pathology of intestinal tuberculosis and its distinction from Crohn's disease. Gut 1972;13:260-9.

114. Shah P, Ramakantan R. Role of vasculitis in the natural history of abdominal tuberculosis—evaluation by mesenteric angiography. Indian J Gastroenterol 1991;10:127-30.

115. Kuwajerwala NK, Bapat RD, Joshi AS. Mesenteric vasculopathy in intestinal tuberculosis. Indian J Gastroenterol 1997;16:124-6.

116. Sarode R, Bhasin D, Marwah N, Roy P, Singh K, Panigrahi D. Hyperaggregation of platelets in intestinal tuberculosis. Am J Hematol 1995;48:52-4.

117. Makharia GK, Srivastava S, Das P, Goswami P, Singh U, Tripathi M, et al. Clinical, endoscopic, and histological differentiations between Crohn's disease and intestinal tuberculosis. Am J Gastroenterol 2010;105: 642-51.

118. Bhargava DK, Kushawaha AK, Dasarathy S. Endoscopic diagnosis of segmental colonic tuberculosis. Gastrointest Endosc 1992;82:511-4.

119. Manohar A, Simjee AA, Pettengill KE. Symptoms and investigative findings in 145 patients with tuberculous peritonitis diagnosed by peritoneoscopy and biopsy over a five-year period. Gut 1990;31:1130-32.

120. Shakil AO, Korula J, Kanel GC, Murray NGB, Reynolds TB. Diagnostic features of tuberculous peritonitis and presence of chronic liver disease. A case-control study. Am J Med 1996;100:179-85.

121. Sundervalli N, Karpagam CP, Raju B. Hepatomegaly in childhood tuberculosis. Indian Pediatr 1979;16:143-6.

122. Korn RJ, William FK, Paul H, Bernhard C, Hyman J, Zimmerman. Hepatic involvement in extra-pulmonary tuberculosis - histologic and functional characteristics. Am J Med 1959;27:60.

123. Kennedy DH. Extrapulmonary tuberculosis. In: Ratledge C, Stanford JL, Grange JM, editors. The biology of the mycobacteria. Vol. III. New York: Academic Press; 1989.p.245.

124. Eastwood JB, Corbishley CM, Grange J. Tuberculosis and the kidney. J Am Soc Nephrol 2001;12:1307-14.

125. Rosenberg S. Has chemotherapy reduced the incidence of genito-urinary tuberculosis? J Urol 1963; 90:317-23.

126. Jennette CJ, Olson LJ, Schwartz MM, Silva FG, editors. Heptinstall's pathology of the kidney. Sixth edition. Vol 2. Lippincott Williams and Wilkins; 2006.p.1010.

127. Das P, Ahuja A, Gupta SD. Incidence, etiopathogenesis and pathological aspects of genitourinary tuberculosis in India: a journey revisited. Indian J Urol 2008;24:356-61.

128. Shah PKD, Jain HK, Mangel HN, Singhi NM. Kidney changes in pulmonary tuberculosis—a study by kidney biopsy. Indian J Tuberc 1975;22:23.

129. Goel A, Seth A, Kumar R. Autocystectomy following extensive genitourinary tuberculosis: presentation and management. Int Urol Nephrol 2002;34:325-7.

130. Ekaterina K, Victor K. Male genital tuberculosis in Siberians. World J Urol 2006;24:74-8.

131. Alan JW, Louis RK, Andrew CN, Alan WP, Craig AP, editors. Campbell-Walsh Urology. Ninth edition. New York: Saunders, Elsevier; 2006.

132. Caorse CA, Belshe RB. Male genital tuberculosis—a review of the literature with instructive case reports. Rev Infect Dis 1985;7:511-24.

133. Roychowdhury NN. Overview of tuberculosis of the female genital tract. J Indian Med Assoc 1996;94:345-61.

134. Brown AB, Gilbent CRA, Te Linde RW. Pelvic tuberculosis. Obstet Gynecol 1953;2:476-83.

135. Sutherland AM. Tuberculosis of the female genital tract. Tubercle 1985;66:79-83.

136. Aliyu MH, Aliyu SH, Salihu HM. Female genital tuberculosis: a global review. Int J Fertil Womens Med 2004;49:123-36.

137. Gatoni DK, Gitau G, Kay V, Ngwenya S, Lafong C, Hasan A. Female genital tuberculosis. Obstet Gynecol 2005;7:75-9.

138. Lattimer JK, Colmore HP, Sanger CA, Robertson DB, McLellan FC. Transmission of genital tuberculosis from husband to wife via the semen. Am Rev Tuberc 1954;69:618-24.

139. Rich AR, Mc Cordock HA. Pathogenesis of tuberculous meningitis. Bull Johns Hopkins Hosp 1933;52:5-37.

140. Leonard JM, Des Prez RN. Tuberculous meningitis. Infect Dis Clin North Am 1990;4:769-87.

141. Dinakar I, Seetharam W, Ravilochan K. Tuberculoma of the brain with tuberculous meningitis. Indian J Tuberc 1983;30:101.

142. Barucha PE, Iyer CGS, Barucha EP, Deshpande DM. Tuberculous meningitis in children—a clinicopathological evaluation of 24 cases. Indian Pediatr 1969;6:282-90.

143. Tuli SM. Tuberculosis of the skeletal system [bones, joints, spine and bursal sheaths]. Third edition. New Delhi: Jaypee Brothers Medical Publishers; 2004.

144. Weaver P, Lifeso RM. The radiological diagnosis of tuberculosis of the adult spine. Skeletal Radiol 1984;12:178.

145. Lifeso RM, Weaver P, Harder EH. Tuberculous spondylitis in adults. J Bone Joint Surg Am 1985;67:1405.

146. Spiegel DA, Singh GK, Banskota AK. Tuberculosis of the muskuloskeletal system. Tech Orthop 2005;20:167-8.

147. Pertuiset E, Beaudreuil J, Horusitzky A, Lioté F, Kemiche F, Richette P, et al. Epidemiological aspects of osteoarticular tuberculosis in adults: retrospective study of 206 cases diagnosed in the Paris area from 1980 to 1994. Presse Med 1997;26:311-5.

148. Gorse GJ, Pais MJ, Kusske JA, Cesario TC. Tuberculous spondylitis: a report of six cases and a review of literature. Medicine 1983;62:178-93.

149. Tuli SM. Tuberculosis of the spine: An historical review. Clin Orthop Relat Res 2007;460:29-38.

150. Lakhanpal VP, Tuli SM, Singh H, Sen PC. The value of histology, culture and guinea pig exammation in osteoarticular tuberculosis. Acta Orthop Scand 1974;45:36-42.

151. Ellner JJ, Wallis RS. Immunologic aspects of mycobacterial infections. Rev Infect Dis 1989;2:5455-9.

152. Chaisson RE, Schecter GF, Theuer CP, Rutherford GW, Echenberg DF, Hopewell PC. Tuberculosis in patients with acquired immunodeficiency syndrome. Clinical features, response to therapy and survival. Am Rev Respir Dis 1987;136:570-4.

153. Hill AR, Premkumar S, Brustein S, Vadya K, Powell S, Li P-W, et al. Disseminated tuberculosis in the acquired immuno-deficiency syndrome era. Am Rev Respir Dis 1991;144:1164-70.

154. Sharma SK, Mohan A, Kadhiravan T. HIV-TB co-infection: epidemiology, diagnosis and management. Indian J Med Res 2005;121:550-67.

155. Khan K, Wang J, Marras TK. Nontuberculous mycobacterial sensitization in the United States: national trends over three decades. Am J Respir Crit Care Med 2007;176:306-13.

156. Griffith DE, Aksamit T, Brown-Elliott BA, Catanzaro A, Daley C, Gordin F, et al; ATS Mycobacterial Diseases Subcommittee; American Thoracic Society; Infectious Disease Society of America. An official ATS/IDSA statement: diagnosis, treatment, and prevention of nontuberculous mycobacterial diseases. Am J Respir Crit Care Med 2007;175:367-416.

157. Moore EH. Atypical mycobacterial infection in the lung: CT appearance. Radiology 1993;187:777-82.

158. Chapman JS. The atypical mycobacteria. Am Rev Respir Dis 1982;15:119-24.

159. El-Solh AA, Nopper J, Abdul-Khoudoud MR, Sherif SM, Aquilina AT, Grant BJ. Clinical and radiographic manifestations of uncommon pulmonary nontuberculous mycobacterial disease in AIDS patients. Chest 1998;114:138-45.

160. Andrejak C, Lescure FX, Douadi Y, Laurans G, Smail A, Duhaut P, et al. Non-tuberculous mycobacteria pulmonary infection: management and follow-up of 31 infected patients. J Infect 2007;55:34-40.

161. Turenne CY, Wallace R Jr, Behr MA. Mycobacterium avium in the postgenomic era. Clin Microbiol Rev 2007;20:205-29.

162. Appelberg R. Pathogenesis of Mycobacterium avium infection: typical responses to an atypical mycobacterium? Immunol Res 2006;35:179-90.

4

The Mycobacteria

Aparna Singh Shah, Rajesh Bhatia

INTRODUCTION

The generic name *Mycobacterium* was introduced by Lehmann and Neumann in 1896. The organisms were named so because of the mold like [myco: fungus; bacterium: bacteria] pellicular growth of these organisms in liquid medium (1). The true bacterial nature of these organisms was, however, soon established. The genus *Mycobacterium* is the only genus in the family *Mycobacteriaceae* and order *Actinomycetales*. The complete genome sequence of *Mycobacterium tuberculosis* [*Mtb*] comprises 4043 genes, 50 of which are responsible for encoding ribonucleic acids [RNAs] while remaining genes encode 3993 proteins. The guanine + cytosine [G+C] ratio in the deoxyribonucleic acid [DNA] of mycobacteria is 62-70 mol% and similar to that observed in Nocardia (2). High G+C ratio indicates strong aerobic requirements of organisms.

An important character of the *Mtb* is their ability to resist decolourisation by a weak mineral acid after staining with one of the aryl-methane dyes. This property of acid fastness is, however, not unique to mycobacteria because *Nocardia, Rhodococcus, Legionella micdadei*, bacterial spores and the protozoa *Isospora* and *Cryptosporidium* are also acid-fast. The genus is better defined on the chemical structure of the mycolic acids and its antigenic structure.

CLASSIFICATION

The genus *Mycobacterium* comprises of more than 197 species, of which several are non-pathogenic environmental bacteria. The different species of the *Mtb* complex show a 95%-100% DNA relatedness based on studies of DNA homology, and the sequence of the 16S rRNA gene are same for all the species. Mycobacteria has been classified in a variety

Table 4.1: Classification of mycobacteria
Group 1
Obligate pathogens
Mycobacterium tuberculosis
Mycobacterium leprae
Mycobacterium bovis
Group 2
Skin pathogens
Mycobacterium marinum
Mycobacterium ulcerans
Group 3
Opportunistic pathogens
Mycobacterium kansasii
Mycobacterium avium-intracellulare
Group 4
Non- or rarely pathogenic
Mycobacterium gordonae
Mycobacterium smegmatis
Group 5
Animal pathogens
Mycobacterium paratuberculosis
Mycobacterium lepraemurium

of ways. A clinical classification is more practical and is described in Table 4.1.

Mycobacteria other than human or bovine tubercle bacilli that cause human disease resembling tuberculosis [TB] are called nontuberculous mycobacteria [NTM]. These are also known as anonymous, unclassified, tuberculoid, paratubercle, *atypical mycobacteria*, mycobacteria other than *tuberculosis* [MOTT]. These have been classified by Runyon (2,3) in several groups [Table 4.2].

Table 4.2: Runyon classification of nontuberculous mycobacteria

Runyon group	Species	Disease in man
I. Photochromogens	Mycobacterium kansasii Mycobacterium marinum Mycobacterium simiae Mycobacterium asiaticum	Pulmonary disease Swimming pool granuloma
II. Scotochromogens	Mycobacterium scrofulaceum Mycobacterium gordonae Mycobacterium szulgai Mycobacterium flavescens	Lymphadenitis in children
III. Nonphotochromogens	Mycobacterium avium Mycobacterium intracellulare Mycobacterium xenopi Mycobacterium ulcerans Mycobacterium terrae Mycobacterium haemophilum	Pulmonary disease in immunocompromised hosts
IV. Rapid growers	Mycobacterium chelonae Mycobacterium fortuitum Mycobacterium abscessus	Superficial and systemic diseases

Source: reference 3

MYCOBACTERIUM TUBERCULOSIS

Morphology

The tubercle bacilli are slender, straight or slightly curved rod-shaped organisms measuring 2-4 µm in length and 0.2-0.8 µm in breadth occurring singly, in pairs or in small groups. The size depends on conditions of growth and long, filamentous, club shaped and branching forms may sometimes be seen. *M. bovis* is usually straighter, stouter and shorter. However, no distinction between *M. bovis* and *Mtb* can be made based on morphology. The bacilli are non-sporing, non-motile and non-capsulated. In suitable liquid culture media, virulent human and bovine tubercle bacilli form characteristic long, tight, serpentine cords in which organisms are aligned in parallel. Cord factor [trehalose 6, 6' dimycolate] is a glycolipid found in the cell walls of mycobacteria, which causes the cells to grow in serpentine cords. It is primarily associated with virulent strains of *Mtb*. It is known to be toxic to mammalian cells. Though its exact role in virulence is unclear, although it has been shown to induce granulomatous reactions identical to those seen in TB.

The bacilli are Gram positive though these do not take the stain readily. These organisms resist decolourisation by 25% sulphuric acid and absolute alcohol for 10 minutes and hence these are called acid and alcohol fast. Acid-fastness is based on the integrity of the cell wall. Beaded or barred forms are frequently seen in *Mtb* while *M. bovis* stains more uniformly. In younger cultures non acid-fast rods and granules have been reported.

Mycobacterial Cell Wall

The mycobacterial cell wall is complex in nature. It essentially distinguishes mycobacteria from other prokaryotes. Mycobacteria in general give a weakly positive response to Gram stain but are phylogenetically more closely related to Gram-positive bacteria (4). It has high lipid content which accounts for about 60% of the cell wall weight. *Mtb* has a tough cell wall that prevents passage of nutrients into and excreted from the cell, therefore giving it the characteristic of slow growth rate. The cell wall has several distinct layers. The inner layer, overlying the cell membrane is composed of peptidoglycan [murein]. External to the murein is a layer of arabinogalactan, which is covalently linked to a group of long chain fatty acids termed mycolic acid. The *Mtb* cell wall contains three classes of mycolic acids: alpha-, keto- and methoxymycolates. The cell wall also contains lipid complexes including acyl glycolipids and other complex, such as, free lipids and sulfolipids. There are porins in the membrane to facilitate trans-port (5). This complex structure confers low permeability to the cell wall, thus, reducing the effectiveness of antimicrobial agents. Lipoarabinomannan [LAM] present in the cell wall facilitates the survival of mycobacteria within macrophages. Diagnostic efficacy of detection of LAM is being studied especially for extra-pulmonary TB [EPTB] (6).

The unusually impermeable cell wall of mycobacteria is believed to be advantageous in stressful conditions of osmotic shock or desiccation. In addition, mycobacteria use other survival strategies including efflux pumps, response regulators, antibiotic-modifying or degrading enzymes such as β-lactamase, target-modifying enzymes, and decoys that mimic the drug target (7).

Culture Characters

Growth Requirements

Mycobacteria are obligate aerobes and derive energy from oxidation of many simple carbon compounds. Biochemical activities are not characteristic and growth rate is much slower than that of most bacteria. The generation time *in vitro* is about 18 hours. At the earliest, the growth appears in about two weeks but may be delayed up to six to eight weeks. Optimum temperature for growth is 37 °C and growth does not occur below 25 °C and above 40 °C. Optimum pH for growth is 6.4-7.0. Increased carbon dioxide [CO_2] tension [5%-10%] enhances growth. Human strains grow more luxuriantly in culture [*eugonic*] than do bovine strains [*dysgonic*]. The addition of a low percentage of glycerol to the medium encourages the growth of human strains but not that of bovine strains, which may infact be inhibited.

Culture Media

The reader is referred to the chapter *"Laboratory diagnosis"* [*Chapter 8*] for details on various types of media (8) that are commonly used for cultivation of mycobacteria.

Colony Characters

On solid media human type of tubercle bacilli give rise to discrete, raised, irregular, dry, wrinkled colonies which are creamy white to begin with and then develop buff colour. By contrast the bovine type grows as flat, white, smooth, moist colonies which "break up" more readily when touched.

Tubercle bacilli will grow on top of liquid medium as a wrinkled pellicle if the inoculum is carefully floated on the surface and flask left undisturbed, otherwise these will grow as floccules throughout the medium. However, a diffuse growth can be obtained by adding a wetting agent, such as, Tween 80. Virulent strains tend to form long serpentine cords in the liquid media while a virulent strains grow in a more dispersed fashion.

Virulence in Animals

Under natural conditions *Mtb* infects man, monkeys, cows, buffalo, pigs, dogs and occasionally parrots. Under experimental conditions, it is virulent to guinea pigs and mice and less virulent in rabbits and avirulent in chicken. Mice are most commonly used for reasons of cost, convenience, their amenability to genetic manipulations (9). Guinea pigs exhibit many pathological features similar to those seen in humans, but unlike humans these are exquisitely sensitive to a progressive pulmonary infection (10). Rabbits display pathogenicity more characteristic of human disease, ranging from spontaneous healing to caseous and cavitary pulmonary lesions (11).

Susceptibility to Physical and Chemical Agents

The best method to inactivate tubercle bacilli is by heat and chemical methods are all relative to it. The thermal death time at 60°C is 15-20 minutes. These are more resistant to chemical agents than other bacteria because of the hydrophobic nature of the cell surface and their clumped growth. Dyes, such as, malachite green or antibiotics such as penicillins can be incorporated into media without inhibiting the growth of tubercle bacilli. Acids and alkalies permit the survival of some exposed tubercle bacilli and are used for

concentration of clinical samples and partial elimination of contaminating organisms. These organisms can survive exposure to 5% phenol, 15% sulphuric acid, 3% nitric acid, 5% oxalic acid and 4% sodium hydroxide. Tincture iodine destroys it in five minutes while 80% ethanol does so in two to ten minutes. Thus, 80% ethanol is recommended as a disinfectant for skin, rubber gloves, and other such materials. The cultures of tubercle bacilli can be killed by exposure to direct sunlight for three hours while in sputum they can survive for 20-30 hours. In droplets these may survive for eight to ten days. Cultures can be stored for two years in a deep freezer at –20°C. The organisms are resistant to drying and can survive for long periods in dried sputum. Ordinary day-light even passing through glass has a lethal effect on bacteria.

Antigenic Structure

Mycobacteria being complex unicellular organisms, contain many antigenic proteins, lipids and polysaccharides. The exact number of antigenic determinants is unknown. The mycobacterial antigens have been broadly classified as: [i] soluble [cytoplasmic] and insoluble [cell wall lipid bound]; and [ii] carbohydrates or proteins. Antigens have been extensively used to classify, identify and type the mycobacteria.

Soluble Antigens

Up to 90 soluble antigens are demonstrated by sensitive techniques. Soluble antigens are divisible into four major groups designated as group I to IV [Table 4.3].

Polysaccharide Antigens

Polysaccharide antigens are responsible for the group specificity while type specificity is due to protein antigen. Following infection by tubercle bacilli, delayed hypersensitivity develops to the protein [tuberculin]. Tuberculins from *Mtb*, *M. bovis* and *M. microti* appear to be indistinguishable.

Biochemical Properties

Mtb has distinctive biochemical properties, some of which are utilised for identification of various species. The reader

Table 4.3: Soluble antigen sharing in mycobacteria		
Group	*Present in*	*Shared with*
Group I	All mycobacteria	Nocardia Corynebacterium Listeria
Group II	Slow growing mycobacteria	-
Group III	Rapid growing mycobacteria	Nocardia
Group IV	Individual species	None, unique

is referred to the chapter *"Laboratory diagnosis" [Chapter 8]* for further details.

Pathogenesis

The first event in the pathogenesis of TB, whether inapparent or overt, is the implantation of bacilli in tissues. The most frequent portal of entry is lungs, resulting from the inhalation of airborne droplets containing a few bacilli which are expectorated by an open case of TB. Less frequently the bacilli may be ingested and lodged, in the tonsil or in the wall of the intestine, which may follow consumption of raw contaminated milk. Finally, third but a rare mode of infection is direct implantation of bacilli into the skin, such as, in workers working with infected materials or handling cultures of tubercle bacilli. The reader is referred to the chapter *"Pathology" [Chapter 3]*, for further details on this topic.

Mycobacteria produce no recognised toxins. The various components of the bacillus have been shown to possess different biological activities which may influence pathogenesis, allergy and immunity in the disease [Table 4.4].

The production and development of lesions and their healing or progression are determined chiefly by the number of mycobacteria in the inoculum and their subsequent multiplication and resistance and hypersensitivity of the host. The essential pathology of TB consists of the production, in infected tissues of a characteristic lesion, the tubercle.

Mycobacteriophages

Mycobacteriophages have been used for subdivision of some species of mycobacteria. *Mtb* has been divided into four phage types-A, B, C and I [I stands for intermediate between A and B].

Mycobacteriophages have provided key tools for TB genetics. The advances in mycobacteriophage recombinants will facilitate postgenomic explorations into mycobacteriophage biology. More than 70 complete genome sequences are now available to facilitate better studies on mycobacterial genome (12).

Table 4.4: Mycobacterial components as determinants of pathogenicity

Cell component	Pathogenic effect
Cell wall	Induces resistance to infection Causes delayed hypersensitivity Can replace whole cell in Freund's adjuvant
Tuberculoprotein	Elicits tuberculin reaction Induces delayed hypersensitivity Induces formation of epitheloid and giant cells
Polysaccharides	Induce immediate hypersensitivity Causes exudation of neutrophils from blood vessels
Lipids	Cause accumulation of macrophages and neutrophils
Phosphatides	Induce formation of tubercles

Bacteriocins

There is limited evidence that some strains of mycobacteria liberate substances that inhibit the growth of other species. *Mtb* is divisible into 11 types by means of bacteriocins produced by rapidly growing mycobacteria.

Bacteriocins are being considered as new wave of potential therapeutic compounds, in particular type 1 bacteriocins known as lantibiotics. The gene encoded nature of these peptides facilitates their genetic manipulation and consequent activities as anti-microbial agents (13).

Molecular Typing

Molecular biological techniques provide valuable information for sub-classification or typing of Mycobacterium species–both *Mtb* and NTM. In past two decades several of these techniques have facilitated evaluation of relapse or reactivation of disease, reinfection with a different strain, epidemiological tracing or spread of infection, understanding dynamics of development of drug resistance and identification of different variants of mycobacteria that may predominantly infect high-risk populations.

A good typing method has to be robust, reproducible, capable of discriminating between strains of two different and based upon stable genetic structure. Strain specific pattern of DNA fragments can be demonstrated by splitting DNA strands into different fragments using restriction enzymes. The pattern of sliced fragments [genetic fingerprint] is strain specific and can be visualised using gel electrophoresis. A combination of this technique with hybridisation technology [Southern blot] has been applied to the analysis of the restriction fragment length polymorphism [RFLP]. The resolution of RFLP has been increased with the use of insertion sequences [IS] in construction of probes (14).

Mycobacteria have relatively large amount of repetitive DNA elements. These can be in the form of short sequences. A category of these are mobile genetic elements and called as insertion sequences. Multiple copies of these IS may be present within a strain. Most studied is IS6110 which may have one copy in *M. bovis* but multiple copies in different locations in *Mtb*, thus making it a reliable molecular marker for genotyping (15). IS6110-based typing is one of the most widely applied genotyping methods in molecular epidemiology of TB.

With the availability of polymerase chain reaction [PCR] technology which is economical, easy to perform and extensive automation, IS6110-based PCR fingerprinting has become popular. Major drawback is weak discriminatory power in strains with low copy numbers of IS6110 (16).

PCR technology is employed for spacer oligonucleotide typing, or spoligotyping. It is a rapid method for genotyping. Spoligotyping data can be represented in absolute terms [digitally], and the results can be readily shared among laboratories, thereby enabling the creation of large international databases. The method is highly reproducible, sensitive and cost-effective (17,18). Spoligotyping is fast, simple and robust method, but at times is less discriminatory.

Strain differences can be better determined by subjecting clusters obtained by spoligotyping to RFLP based on IS*6110* (19,20). Encouraged by the potential of these techniques, Ahmed and Hasnain (21) have advocated a systems biology approach.

Apart from IS genetic elements, mycobacteria may also have tandem repeats [TR] of genetic material, some of these are called as variable number of tandem repeats [VNTR]. Genotyping based on VNTR is also useful. A specific class of these VNTR is mycobacterial interspersed repetitive units [MIRUs]. A 24 MIRU-VNTR loci based typing system or IS*6110*-RFLP are considered as the gold standard in molecular typing of *Mtb* complex (22).

Commercial systems for the genotyping methods utilising PCR technology for repetitive DNA elements broadly called as repetitive sequence-based PCR are now becoming available, thus, enhancing access to this technology.

Immunity and Hypersensitivity

Infection with *Mtb* induces delayed hypersensitivity [allergy] and resistance to infection [immunity]. Unless a host dies during the first infection with tubercle bacilli, there is an increased capacity to localise tubercle bacilli, retard their multiplication, limit their spread and reduce lymphatic dissemination. This can be attributed to the development of cellular immunity during the initial infection.

In the course of primary infection the host also acquires hypersensitivity to the tubercle bacilli. This is made evident by the development of a positive tuberculin reaction. The reader is referred to the chapter *"Immunology of tuberculosis"* [Chapter 5] for further details.

Koch's Phenomenon

The contrast between primary infection and reinfection is shown experimentally in Koch's phenomenon. When a guinea pig is injected subcutaneously with virulent tubercle bacilli, the puncture wound heals quickly, but a nodule forms at the site of injection in two weeks. This nodule ulcerates and the ulcer does not heal. The regional lymph nodes develop tubercles and extensive caseation. When the same animal is later injected with tubercle bacilli in another part of the body, the sequence of events is quite different. There is a rapid necrosis of the skin and tissue at the site of injection, but the ulcer heals rapidly. Regional lymph nodes either do not become infected at all or do so only after a delay. These differences are attributed to immunity and hypersensitivity induced by the primary infection. The Koch's phenomenon has three components: [i] a local reaction; [ii] a focal response in which there occurs an acute congestion around the TB foci in tissues; and [iii] a "systemic" response of fever which may at times be fatal.

This effect is not caused exclusively by living tubercle bacilli, but also by killed ones, no matter whether they are killed by low temperatures or prolonged periods, or by boiling or by certain chemicals.

Although, the conventional tuberculin skin test [TST] and relatively advanced versions of interferon-γ release assays [IGRAs] are currently available for detection of latent TB infection [LTBI] detection, however, in the absence of gold standard neither of tests precisely identifies those infected (23). The accumulated evidence suggests either of the two tests alone or two step approach for LTBI detection in high-income countries, whereas, the low cost, simple technique based TST is the most preferred method in low-income countries (23,24).

Laboratory Diagnosis

Before TB can be treated, a diagnosis needs to be made in an efficient and timely manner. The laboratory diagnosis is based on demonstration and isolation of tubercle bacilli. The essential steps for diagnosis are: [i] collection of specimens; [ii] demonstration of organism; [iii] culture on suitable media; [iv] identification by various tests; [v] guinea pig inoculation; [vi] antibiotic sensitivity testing [wherever possible]; and [vii] nucleic acid amplification tests [NAATs].

Microscopy and culture are done in peripheral and intermediate laboratories, whereas identification of *Mtb* and antibiotic sensitivity testing are done in selected referral places. The reader is referred to the chapter *"Laboratory diagnosis"* [Chapter 8] for further details.

Global efforts are being made to develop an efficient and affordable point of care [PoC] test. PoC implies the ability to make a diagnosis at the point where patient consultation and presentation occurs. Nucleic acid amplification tests [NAATs] can rapidly detect small quantities of DNA through several different amplification methods, including the PCR. With their improved simplification and automation in recent years, NAAT is becoming increasingly attractive candidate for use at the PoC [24].

Sensitivity Testing

With the emergence of multidrug-resistance in mycobacteria, it is essential to perform sensitivity test on the tubercle bacilli isolates as an aid and guide to treatment. Drug-resistant mutants continuously arise at a low rate in any mycobacterial population. The purpose of sensitivity testing is to determine whether the great majority of the bacilli in the culture are sensitive to the anti-TB drugs currently in use. The sensitivity testing may be direct [performed on the original specimen] or indirect [performed on a subculture].

Four methods of drug-susceptibility testing [DST] have been standardised. These are: [i] the absolute concentration method; [ii] the resistance ratio method; [iii] the proportion method; and [iv] the BACTEC-460 radiometric method. However, the use of the BACTEC 460 radiometric method is phasing out due to the concerns of the radioactive waste disposal. This system is being replaced by the nonradiometric BACTEC MGIT 960 system (25).

In December 2010 WHO endorsed a new technology [cartridge-based NAAT, Xpert MTB/RIF] and recommended that this technology should be used as the initial diagnosis test in individuals suspected of having multidrug-resistant TB [MDR-TB], or human immunodeficiency virus [HIV] associated TB. They also suggested that it could be used as a follow-on test to microscopy in settings where MDR-TB and/or HIV is of lesser concern, especially in smear-negative specimens, because of the lack of accuracy of smear microscopy. This test does not eliminate the need for conventional microscopy culture and DST, as these are still required to monitor treatment progress and to detect resistance to drugs other than rifampicin (26). The reader is referred to the chapter *"Drug-resistant tuberculosis"* [*Chapter 42*] for details on this topic.

NONTUBERCULOUS MYCOBACTERIA

The NTM mycobacteria were initially grouped according to speed of growth at various temperatures and production of pigments (27). More recently individual species or complexes are defined by additional laboratory characteristics, e.g. nitrate reduction, production of urease, catalase and certain antigenic features (28,29). NTM have been classified in four groups by Runyon (2,3) based on production of pigment and rate of growth. The reader is referred to the chapter *"Nontuberculous mycobacterial infections"* [*Chapter 41*] for further details.

MYCOBACTERIA PRODUCING SKIN ULCERS

Two conditions where skin ulceration occurs are *M. ulcerans* infection causing what is known as *Buruli* ulcer and infection with *M. marinum* which causes swimming pool granuloma. In addition to these two, there are some other inoculation-associated infections.

Mycobacterium ulcerans

This was first described in Australia and the organism was named as *M. ulcerans* in year 1948. Later, a similar disease was seen in the Buruli county of Uganda, and hence, the name Buruli ulcer was given. Epidemiological investigations suggest that the organism is inoculated into the skin by thorny vegetation. The disease has an enormous socio-economic impact and is an important public health issue (30).

The earliest sign is a discrete firm nodule fixed to the skin but mobile over deep tissues. It is painless but very itching. If it does not resolve at this stage it progresses to the ulcerative stage which is full of bacilli. With further progress of the disease the overlying skin becomes anoxic and necrotic. Ulceration then occurs with escape of liquefied necrotic tissue and the formation of a deeply undermined ulcer. The lesions which may be single or multiple are more common on exposed parts of the body, especially, limbs.

The PCR is highly sensitive for diagnosis on both swab and biopsy samples of lesions due to *M. ulcerans*. The PCR approaches 100% specificity and 96% sensitivity for lesion swabs, and is considered as the test of choice for

its diagnosis. Mycobacterial cultures are less sensitive for diagnosis, although positive cultures are more commonly obtained from tissue biopsy than swab specimens (31).

The disease is progressive for about three years but then an effective immune response develops. Eventually the lesion heals but often with extensive fibrosis and contractures leading to crippling deformities. In general, chemotherapy has not proved very successful in treatment. Simple excision of the lesion early in the disease is curative. Physiotherapy is required to prevent deformities.

Mycobacterium marinum

M. marinum is a natural pathogen of cold-blooded animals. The skin disease produced is known as "swimming-pool granuloma" or "fish tank granuloma" or "fish fancier's finger". The organism was initially named as *M. balnei* but it was later found to be identical to the fish tubercle bacillus and was named as *M. marinum*. Lesions occur at sites of injury, which are usually the knees and elbows of swimming pool users and the hands of the fish fanciers.

The lesion commences as a solitary raised watery lesion, but secondary lesions develop along the draining lymphatics. Occasionally tenosynovitis may develop at back. Human infection may occur in epidemic form. Infection with *M. marinum* causes a low-grade tuberculin reaction. The reader is also referred to the chapter *"Cutaneous tuberculosis"* [*Chapter 21*] for further details.

SAPROPHYTIC MYCOBACTERIA

Saprophytic mycobacteria are non-pathogenic acid-fast bacilli found in milk, butter, water, manure, grass and smegma of human beings and animals. Important features of these mycobacteria are: [i] inability to set up a progressive infection in mammals or birds; [ii] profuse growth at room temperature, giving rise to growth in two to three days; [iii] optimum temperature is in the vicinity of 37 °C but growth at room temperature is also very good; and [iv] extracts and purified protein derivative [PPD] prepared from many of these mycobacteria may cross-react with PPD-S from *Mtb*, resulting in positive TST in persons who are tuberculin negative. High proportion of population becomes hypersensitive to mycobacteria acquired from the environment.

M. smegmatis is present in smegma and contaminates urine sample. It needs to be differentiated from tubercle bacilli. Smegma bacillus is acid-fast but not alcohol-fast. *M. smegmatis* with the esx-3 genes deleted has the potential to function as a novel vaccine vector with an enhanced innate immune-activating property. This vector, when engineered to express *Mtb* esx-3, may become a potent TB vaccine capable of a level of protection superior to that of BCG (32).

M. paratuberculosis [Johne's bacillus] causes chronic disease in cattle, characterised by massive infiltration of the intestinal tract.

REFERENCES

1. Grange JM. Mycobacterium. In: Greenwod D, Slack S, Peutherer J, editors. Medical microbiology. New York: Churchill Livingstone; 1997.p.200-14.

2. Runyon EH. Anonymous mycobacterial in pulmonary disease. Med Clin North Am 1959;43:273-90.

3. Wayne LG, Kubica GP. The Mycobacteria. In: Sneath PHA, Mair NS, Sharpe ME, Holt JG, editors. Bergey's manual of systematic bacteriology. Baltimore: Williams and Wilkinsons; 1989.p.1435-57.

4. Brennan PJ, Draper P. Ultrastructure of Mycobacterium tuberculosis. In: Bloom BR, editor. Tuberculosis: pathogenesis, protection and control. Washington: ASM Press; 1994.p.271-84.

5. Thomas ST, VanderVen, BC, Sherman DR, Russell DG, Sampson NS. Pathway profiling in Mycobacterium tuberculosis: elucidation of cholesterol-derived catabolite and enzymes that catalyze its metabolism. J Biol Chem 2011;286:43668-78.

6. Flores LL, Steingart KR, Dendukuri N, Schiller I, Minion J, Pai M. Systematic review and meta-analysis of antigen detection tests for the diagnosis of tuberculosis. Clin Vaccine Immunol 2011;18:1616-27.

7. Hett EC, Rubin EJ. Bacterial growth and cell division: a mycobacterial perspective. Microbiol Mol Biol Rev 2008;72: 126-56.

8. Petran EI, Vera HD. Media for selective isolation of mycobacteria. Health Lab Sci 1971;8:225-30.

9. Orme IM, Collins FM. Mouse model of tuberculosis. In: Bloom BR, editor. Tuberculosis: pathogenesis, protection and control. Washington: ASM Press; 1994.p.113-34.

10. McMurray DN. Guinea pig model of tuberculosis. In: Bloom BR, editor. Tuberculosis: pathogenesis, protection and control. Washington: ASM Press; 1994.p.135-47.

11. Cosma CL, Sherman DR, Ramakrishnan L. The secret lives of the pathogenic mycobacteria. Annu Rev Microbiol 2003;57:641-76.

12. Hatfull GF. Mycobacteriophages: genes and genomes. Annu Rev Microbiol 2010; 64:331-56.

13. Carrol J, O' Mahony J. Anti-mycobacterial peptides, made to order with delivery included. Bioeng Bugs 2011;2:241-6.

14. Eisenach KD, Crawford JT, Bates JH. Genetic relatedness among strains of the Mycobacterium tuberculosis complex. Analysis of restriction fragment heterogeneity using cloned DNA probes. Am Rev Respir Dis 1986;133:1065-8.

15. Soolingen D van, Hermans PW, de Haas PE, Soll DR, van Embden, JDA. Occurrence and stability of insertion sequences in Mycobacterium tuberculosis complex strains: evaluation of an insertion sequence-dependent DNA polymorphism as a tool in the epidemiology of tuberculosis. J Clin Microbiol 1991;29: 2578-86.

16. Sharma SK, Sethi S, Mewara A, Meharwal S, Jindal SK, Sharma M, et al. Genetic polymorphism among Mycobacterium tuberculosis isolates from patients with pulmonary tuberculosis in northern India. South-East J Trop Med Public Health 2012;43:1161-8.

17. Ross BC, Dwyer B. Rapid, simple method for typing isolates of Mycobacterium tuberculosis by using the polymerase chain reaction. J Clin Microbiol 1993;31:329-34.

18. Sougakoff W. Molecular epidemiology of multidrug-resistant strains of Mycobacterium tuberculosis. Clin Microbiol Infect 2011;17:800-5.

19. Kulkarni S, Sola C, Filliol I, Rastogi N, Kadival G. Spoligotyping of Mycobacterium tuberculosis isolates from patients with pulmonary tuberculosis in Mumbai, India. Res Microbiol 2005;156:588-96.

20. Purwar S, Chaudhari S, Katoch VM, Sampath A, Sharma P, Upadhyay P, et al. Determination of drug susceptibility patterns and genotypes of Mycobacterium tuberculosis isolates from Kanpur district, North India. Infect Genet Evol 2011;11:469-75.

21. Ahmed N, Hasnain SE. Molecular epidemiology of tuberculosis in India: moving forward with a systems biology approach. Tuberculosis 2011;91:404-13.

22. Oelemann MC, Diel R, Vatin V, Haas W, Rüsch-Gerdes S, Locht C, et al. Assessment of an optimized mycobacterial inter-spersed repetitive–unit-variable-number tandem-repeat typing system combined with spoligo-typing for population-based molecular epidemiology studies of tuberculosis. J Clin Microbiol 2007;45:691-7.

23. Miranda C, Tomford JW, Gordon SM. Interferon gamma release Assays. Interferon-gamma-release assays: better than tuberculin skin testing? Cleve Clin J Med 2010;77:606-11.

24. Dheda K, Ruhwald M, Theron G, Peter J, Yam WC. Point of care diagnosis of tuberculosis: past, present, and future. Respirology 2013;18:217-32.

25. Siddiqi S, Ahmed A, Asif S, Behera D, Javaid M, Jani J, et al. Direct drug susceptibility testing of Mycobacterium tuberculosis for rapid detection of multidrug resistance using the Bactec MGIT 960 system: a multicenter study. J Clin Microbiol 2012;50:435-40.

26. World Health Organization. Rapid implementation of the Xpert MTB/RIF diagnostic test. Technical and operational 'how-to'. Practical considerations. Geneva: World Health Organization; May 2011. Available at URL: whqlibdoc.who.int/publications/ 2011/9789241501569_eng.pdf. Accessed on December 14, 2017.

27. Griffith DE, Aksamit T, Brown-Elliott BA, Catanzaro A, Daley C, Gordin F, et al; ATS Mycobacterial Diseases Subcommittee; American Thoracic Society; Infectious Disease Society of America. An official ATS/IDSA statement: diagnosis, treatment, and prevention of nontuberculous mycobacterial diseases. Am J Respir Crit Care Med 2007;175:367-416.

28. Ryu YJ, Koh WJ, Daley CL. Diagnosis and treatment of nontuber-culous mycobacterial lung disease: clinicians' perspectives. Tuberc Respir Dis [Seoul] 2016;79:74-84.

29. Stout JE, Koh WJ, Yew WW. Update on pulmonary disease due to non-tuberculous mycobacteria. Int J Infect Dis 2016;45:123-34.

30. Sizaire V, Nackers F, Comte E, Portaels F. Mycobacterium ulcerans infection: control, diagnosis and treatment. Lancet Infect Dis 2006; 6:288-96.

31. Boyd SC, Athan E, Friedman ND, Hughes A, Walton A, Callan P, et al. Epidemiology, clinical features and diagnosis of Myco-bacterium ulcerans in an Australian population. Med J Aust 2012;196:341-4.

32. Jeyanathan M, Thanthrige-Don N, Xing Z. A novel genetically engineered Mycobacterium smegmatis-based vaccine promotes anti-TB immunity. Expert Rev Vaccines 2012;11:35-8.

5

Immunology of Tuberculosis

DK Mitra, AK Rai, Amar Singh

INTRODUCTION

Protective immunity and varied clinical manifestations of infection with *Mycobacterium tuberculosis* [*Mtb*] represent a delicate balance between the bacillus and magnitude and type of the host immune response. The latter is a broad term reflecting complex interactions among various arms of the immunity involving numerous cell types and molecules. This confers a homeostatic balance either in favour of the host, leading to containment of the infection, disease or in parasite's favour resulting in failure to contain infection. Immunity against *Mtb* needs to be understood not only in terms of sterilising immunity that eliminates *Mtb* infection at the initial exposure, but also with respect to immunity favouring granuloma formation that maintains the steady state control over the bacillary spread and prevents establishment of clinical disease. Both innate as well as adaptive immunity are involved at various levels following *Mtb* infection. In this chapter, first the innate and then the adaptive immunity will be discussed. It should be understood that this compartmentalised approach is only for the sake of better understanding of the complex cross-talk among diverse cell subsets and bio-molecules. However, *in vivo*, the innate and various components of adaptive immunity work synergistically in concert.

In this chapter, current understanding of the host immune response, various aspects of macrophage-mycobacterium interactions, with special emphasis on expansion and suppressive functions of CD4+ CD25+ Forkhead box P3 [FoxP3+] regulatory T-cells [T_{reg}]. Role of effector T-cells and the cytokine/chemokine mediated recruitment of accessory immune cells for local inflammatory response providing protective immunity is also discussed. Further, the ability of the organism to manipulate programmed cell death protein 1 [PD-1] pathway to establish chronic infection will also be discussed.

CHRONOLOGY OF IMMUNOPATHOGENESIS OF TUBERCULOSIS

Pathogenesis of pulmonary tuberculosis [TB] following infection with *Mtb* can be understood in four distinct phases [Figure 5.1]. Each phase is determined by homeostasis between bacillary factors and host's innate and adaptive immunity (1,2).

INITIAL ENCOUNTER AND INNATE IMMUNITY

Mycobacterium-Macrophage Interactions

Pathogenesis of TB starts with phagocytosis of bacilli by mononuclear cells including alveolar macrophages and dendritic cells [DCs] which play a crucial role during their initial encounter with *Mtb* by their intrinsic or innate defence mechanism[s]. A probable role of DC-specific intercellular adhesion molecule-3 [ICAM-3] grabbing no integrin [DC-SIGN], has been implicated in DC mediated dissemination of *Mtb* (3). Uptake of opsonised bacilli [coated with preformed humoral elements like antibodies or complement split products] is greatly facilitated by complement receptors [CR] expressed on macrophages, such as CR1, CR2, CR3 and CR4; and other cell surface receptor molecules (4). Non-opsonised bacilli are engulfed by macrophages through mannose receptors [MRs] recognising the terminal mannose moieties of mycobacteria. The interaction between MRs and mycobacteria seems to be mediated through the mycobacterial surface glycoprotein lipoarabinomannan [LAM] (4,5). Additionally, non-opsonised *Mtb* can be taken up by the macrophages through binding to scavenger receptor type A as blocking CRs and MRs was not able to completely abrogate the bacillary uptake. Cluster of differentiation 14 [CD14] receptor (6) and the scavenger receptors also play important role in mediating bacterial binding. Several other groups of molecules like collections

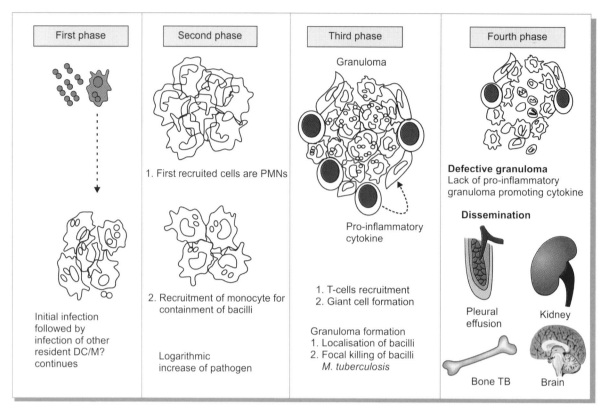

Figure 5.1: Events during TB infection. Broadly, TB infection is divided into four phases. The first phase includes an initial establishment of *Mtb* infection in the resident alveolar macrophages. This is followed by influx of PMNs, which prevents *Mtb* to escape from the innate immune factors. Subsequently, monocytes are recruited to the site of infection/ pathological site [second phase]. The third phase includes granuloma formation. Core of granuloma is made up of multi-nucleated giant cells and elongated epithelioid cells surrounded by T-cells. This is aimed at restricting the bacilli from spreading. The fourth and terminal phase includes dissemination of bacilli. Defective granuloma formation promotes release of bacilli from control of immune system. Organs/loci targeted by bacilli after dissemination are listed here

DC = dendritic cells; M = macrophages; PMNs = polymorphonuclear leucocytes; TB = tuberculosis; *Mtb* = *Mycobacterium tuberculosis*

of the innate immune system may also facilitate binding and uptake of *Mtb*. Surfactant protein A enhances the uptake while surfactant D blocks it. Fibronectins also facilitate uptake of *Mtb* by alveolar epithelial cells through binding to antigenic proteins (7). Thus, multiple mechanisms are operational in the uptake of *Mtb* by mononuclear phago-cytes giving cells chance to kill the bacilli. However, all these mechanisms only help in their uptake but fail to elicit optimal immune recognition leading to macrophage activation.

Recognition by Toll-like Receptors

Both the innate and adaptive response to *Mtb* infection depends to a large degree, on recognition of *Mtb* as a pathogen by the pattern recognition receptors. Toll-like receptors [TLRs] and myeloid differentiation primary response gene 88 [MyD88] pathway play a critical role in immune recognition of *Mtb* on the surface of macrophages and elicitation of an effective innate immune response and shaping the eventual T-cell responses. They are transmembrane proteins with leucine-rich repeat motifs in extracellular domain (8,9). Of the several TLRs discovered till date TLR2, TLR4, TLR3 and TLR9 appear to elicit cellular response to mycobacterial antigens including the 19-kDa

lipoprotein and LAM. In context of CD14, TLR2 binds to LAM, a heterodimer of TLR2 and TLR6 binds to CD19 kDa lipoprotein (10). TLR4 binds to yet undefined heat labile cell associated factor and TLR9 binds to mycobacterial DNA motifs. Engagement of TLRs by mycobacterial antigens leads to coupling of MyD88 and interleukin-1 receptor-associated kinase [IRAK] signalling molecules resulting in multiple signalling events that ultimately translocate transcription factor nuclear factor kappa-light-chain-enhancer of activated B cells [NFkB] from cytosol to nucleus to induce the production of various cytokines required for innate as well as adaptive immune events (11).

Phagolysosome Fusion

This highly regulated event during intracellular infection leads to degradation of phagocytosed microorganisms by intralysosomal acidic hydrolases (12,13). Prevention of phagolysosomal fusion is hypothesised to be the mechanism by which *Mtb* survives inside macrophages (14). Multiacylated trehalose 2-sulphate, a derivative of myco-bacterial sulphatides (15,16) and copious amount of ammonia generated during *in vitro Mtb* culture is thought to be responsible for the inhibitory effect (17).

IMMUNE EFFECTOR MECHANISMS AGAINST *MYCOBACTERIUM TUBERCULOSIS*

Free Radical-based Antimycobacterial Effector Functions of Macrophages

Macrophages are key player of host immune response against *Mtb* infection [Figure 5.2]. Phagocytosed microorganisms are subjected to degradation by intralysosomal acidic hydrolases upon phagolysosome fusion. This highly regulated event constitutes a significant antimicrobial mechanism of phagocytes. Upon activation, macrophages exhibit various degrees of anti-mycobacterial activity (18). Hydrogen peroxide [H_2O_2], one of the reactive oxygen intermediates [ROI] generated by macrophages via the oxidative burst, was the first identified effector molecule that mediated mycobacteriocidal effects of mononuclear phagocytes (19). *In vitro* infection of macrophages with *Mtb* leads to upregulation and excessive production of inducible nitric oxide synthase [iNOS2], which is required for the production of nitric oxide (20). Cytokines also play an important role in anti-mycobacterial effects of macrophages and interferon-gamma [IFN-γ] is key endogenous activating agent that triggers the anti-mycobacterial effects. Tumour necrosis factor-alpha [TNF-α], synergizes with IFN-γ induced anti-mycobacterial effects of murine macrophages *in vitro* (21). Together, they induce the production of nitric oxide and related reactive nitrogen intermediates [RNI] by macrophages via the action of the inducible form of nitric oxide synthase [NOS2] (22). Another potential mechanism involved in macrophage defence against *Mtb* is apoptosis or programmed cell death. Various research groups have demonstrated that (23,24) macrophage apoptosis results in

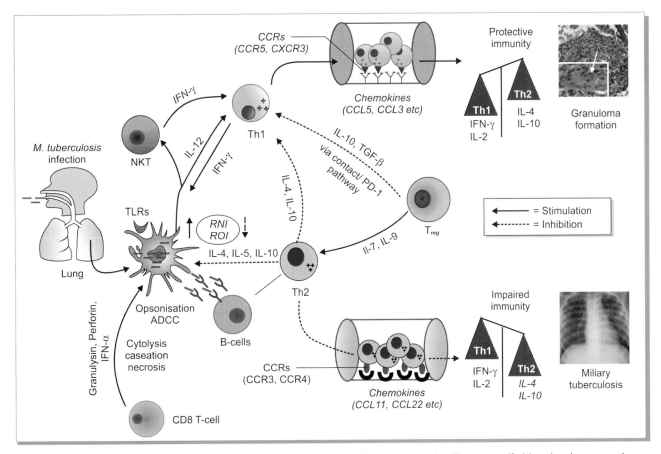

Figure 5.2: Key concepts in the immunopathogenesis of TB. In most individuals, inhaled bacilli are engulfed by alveolar macrophages and are contained by efficient microbicidal mechanisms [generation of ROI/RNI]. TLRs on the surface of macrophages recognise PAMPs and may elicit a robust innate immune response leading to bacillary elimination. Infected macrophages simultaneously process and present antigens to various T-cell subsets including polarised Th1/Th2 cells [CD4+ and MHC class II restricted], cytolytic [MHC class I restricted] T-cells, NKT [CD1 restricted], and CD4+CD25+FoxP3 regulatory T [T_reg] cells. Processed peptides, together with IL-12 secreted by the infected macrophage, trigger Th1 cells to secrete IL-2, IFN, and tumour necrosis factor to further activate the macrophages. Th1 cell activation, which is central to protective immunity, is under the control of other T-cell subsets. Effective generation of Th1 cytokine and appropriate recruitment of CCR5+, CXCR3+ T-cells particularly in local milieu leads to ensuing effective granuloma formation and containment of diseases. On the other side immune responses skewed towards Th2 [recruitment of CCR3+, CCR4+ T-cells] cross-inhibit protective responses, such as, granuloma formation and fails to limit the infection leading to miliary TB

TB = tuberculosis; ROI = reactive oxygen intermediates; RNI = reactive nitrogen intermediates; TLRs= toll-like receptors; PAMPs = pathogen-associated molecular patterns; IL = interleukin; IFN = interferon; NKT = natural killer T-cells

reduced viability of mycobacteria. In conclusion, it appears that macrophages play an important role both in early recognition of bacilli, thus shaping the effector immune response and mediating the terminal lytic events under the strong influence of orchestrated T-cells response.

MACROPHAGE T-CELL INTERACTION

Engulfed mycobacteria are transported to the draining lymph node via DCs/macrophages, where they get detected. DCs/macrophages are currently considered to be the most efficient inducers of activation in naïve T-cells. This efficiency stems from the fact that they provide not only the antigen-specific stimulus but also secondary and tertiary signals, via accessory molecules on macrophages, therefore, promoting efficient development of effector T-cells. Once bacteria arrive within the draining lymph node, naïve T-cells get activated, undergo proliferation, and differentiation into effector cells [CD4+ and CD8+ T-cells]. Activation of naïve T-cells occurs in the presence of live bacteria, and effector cells develop with expected kinetics and their phenotype depends on the availability of specific cytokines and types of co-stimulation provided by macrophages infected with bacilli (25). These effector cells eventually migrate to the lungs by chemokine driven process in response to inflammation and mediate protection by activating infected phagocytes, leading to granuloma formation (26).

ROLE OF CYTOKINES

Recognition of Mtb by phagocytic cells leads to cell activation and production of variety of cytokines, which in turn, induces further activation and cytokine production in a complex process of regulation and cross-regulation. Several cytokines are released, some of which take part in non-specific inflammation, and others, regulate the functional bias of the relevant T-cells. A brief account of the important cytokines produced by Mtb-infected macrophages is given in [Figure 5.2]. These cytokines induce further activation of immune cells and lead to a complex process of immune regulation. Among the pro-inflammatory cytokines TNF-α, interleukin-1β [IL-1β], interleukin-6 [IL-6], interleukin-12 [IL-12], interleukin-15 [IL-15] and interleukin-18 [IL-18] are important. Each one plays a distinctive role in immune response against TB.

Tumour Necrosis Factor-α

This prototype pro-inflammatory cytokine is produced by macrophages, DCs and Th1 like cells upon infection and stimulation with Mtb. It plays key roles in macrophage activation, immuno-regulation and particularly granuloma formation by induction of appropriate chemokine receptors on the effector T-cells and thus recruiting them at disease site (26). In mice, it has been shown to be involved in maintaining latency of TB infection and is found at disease site[s]. Its role in humans is best evidenced by increased incidence of TB among rheumatoid arthritis patients when treated with anti-TNF-α treatment. However, it is thought to be a "double-edged sword" causing bystander damage of the host tissue and cavity formation, particularly when present in relative excess in the milieu. Recently, it has been established that discrimination between latent infection versus active TB may be possible on the basis of preferential increase in the number of TNF-α+ Mtb-specific CD4+ T-cells (27).

Interleukin-1β and Interleukin-6

Interleukin-1β is another proinflammatory cytokine secreted by the Mtb infected macrophages and DCs and is found in excess at the pathologic site[s] of TB. An increased mycobacterial growth and a defective granuloma formation are observed in IL-1β knock out mice (28). IL-6, on the other hand, may serve as both pro- and anti-inflammatory cytokine and is increased in TB patients (29). Various reports suggest that it may antagonise either TNF-α or IFN-γ, both of which are believed to be critical for protective immune response against TB.

Interleukin-2

Interleukin-2 [IL-2] secretion by the protective CD4+ Th1 cells has a pivotal role in generating an immune response by inducing an expansion of pool of lymphocytes specific for an antigen. Several studies have demonstrated that IL-2 can influence the course of mycobacterial infections; either alone or in combination with other cytokines (30). Recent report suggests that IL-2 deprivation induces apoptosis of the effector T-cells. T$_{reg}$ cells are critically dependent on IL-2 for their survival, and therefore, strongly compete with effector T-cells for IL-2 available in the milieu. This may be one of the prominent mechanisms by which T$_{reg}$ cells inhibit effector T-cell response (31).

Interleukin-12 and Interleukin-18

Interleukin-12 is the most potent Th1 driving regulatory cytokine produced by infected or stimulated macrophages and DCs and thus, plays a crucial role in the development of protective Th1 type immunity in TB. In TB, IL-12 has been detected in disease sites like lung infiltrates, pleurisy and granulomas (32). Its receptor is also over-expressed in these sites. IL-18, another pro-inflammatory cytokine, is important for IFN-γ axis of the T-cell response. High susceptibility of IL-18 knockout mice to Mtb, bacille Calmette-Guérin [BCG] and M. leprae strongly suggests a protective role of this cytokine in TB (33). A close parallelism has been noted between the concentration of IL-18 and IFN-γ among patients suffering from TB pleural effusion. Protective effect of IL-18 may be mediated by enhanced production of IFN-γ.

Interferon-γ

The protective role of IFN-γ in TB is well recognized. But, it must be remembered that it is not the only terminal effector cytokine to confer protection in TB. Mycobacterial antigen specific *in vitro* production of IFN-γ by T-cells from patients represents a surrogate marker of immunity against TB. However, there exists a great deal of divergence of opinion in this respect among the researchers and clinicians. In TB, physiologically relevant sources of IFN-γ are natural killer [NK] cells, antigen specific T-cells [helper and cytotoxic], macrophages themselves, and other relatively rare fine T-cell subsets, such as, gamma-delta [γδ] T-cells and CD1d restricted NK T-cells (34,35). The IFN-γ is a potent activator of infected macrophages resulting in potentiation of lytic mechanism[s] responsible for killing of intracellular *Mtb* and enhancement of human leucocyte antigen [HLA] and co-stimulatory molecules which result in efficient presentation of macrophage processed mycobacterial antigens and elicitation of strong T-cell responses. In addition to the above proinflammatory cytokines, certain anti-inflammatory cytokines like IL-4, IL-10 and transforming growth factor-β [TGF-β] are produced as well in TB (36).

Interleukin-4

The deleterious influence of IL-4 in TB is well-known and is attributed to its suppressive effect on IFN-γ production. *Mtb* infected mice with progressive form of disease shows a significantly higher production of IL-4 (37). Disseminated form of TB, such as, miliary TB [MTB] is associated with a very high production of IL-4 by T-cells derived from peripheral blood and bronchoalveolar lavage [BAL] fluid following *in vitro* stimulation (38). It is widely believed that IL-4 production is responsible for suppression of Th1 type immune responses against TB, and thus, the host fails to contain the disease, leading to development of severe and disseminated forms of TB. In some recent elegant studies, a splice variant of IL-4 gene called IL-4δ has been detected. The IL-4δ gives rise to protein isoform, which inhibits the immunosuppressive Th2 like function of native IL-4. Expression of IL-4δ messenger ribonucleic acid [mRNA] was very minimal in the peripheral blood mononuclear cells of the healthy subjects while its expression was significantly higher in the thymocytes and BAL fluid in TB patients (39). Tissue specific expression of this splice variant and tight correlation with the disease severity suggests a potential immunoregulatory role in the pathogenesis of TB. Plausibly, IL-4δ functionally inhibits Th2 skewing of the host immune response by antagonising the effect of native IL-4, and thus, shifting the cytokine production profile towards Th1 response. Ratio of IL-4/IL-4δ may be useful in monitoring the cytokine polarised immune response among TB patients.

Interleukin-10

Interleukin-10 is produced by the macrophages after phago-cytosis of *Mtb* and also by the Th2 cells following recognition of duly processed mycobacterial antigens. Mononuclear cells from TB patients, particularly suffering from disseminated disease produce copious IL-10 *in vitro* in response to mycobacterial antigens (40). IL-10 transgenic mice supports better bacillary growth. Also in humans, IL-10 production is significantly higher patients who are purified protein derivative [PPD] anergic and in those with severe form of TB. Macrophages (40) and regulatory T-cells (41) from TB patients are suppressive for T-cell proliferation *in vitro*, and inhibition of IL-10 partially reversed this suppression. IL-10 directly inhibits CD4+ T-cell responses, and also inhibits antigen-presenting cell [APC] function of cells infected with mycobacteria (42). IL-10 is well-known for its ability to suppress IFN-γ, TNF-α and IL-12, all of which are critical for eliciting a desired Th1 type immune response in host's favour. Recent work on drug-resistant visceral leishmaniasis indicates IL-10 mediated upregulation of drug resistance genes in macrophages and parasites. Similar role of IL-10 may be a critical factor in the emergence of drug resistance due to biased host immune response (43).

Transforming Growth Factor-β

Transforming growth factor-β appears to inhibit protective immunity against *Mtb* and aggravates TB pathology. TGF-β is also produced in abundance by TB patients and its expression is observed at the pathologic site[s] (44). The TGF-β is a well-known inhibitor of T-cell proliferation, IFN-γ production, macrophage activation and antigen presentation. Moreover, it is also known for its potent host tissue damaging effect and fibrosis (45). TGF-β along with IL-10 potently suppresses the Th1 function during TB infection and is thought to contribute to the pathogenesis of TB.

ADAPTIVE IMMUNITY AND ROLE OF EFFECTOR T-CELLS

Cell-mediated adaptive immunity is critical in conferring protection against *Mtb* because antibodies fail to contain the infection due to its intracellular habitat. Upon initial exposure and recognition of immune dominant epitopes, naïve T-cells are primed and converted into effector and memory T-cells. Effector T-cells contain the initial infectious load. However, dormant foci of *Mtb* within macrophages persist and reactivation of the bacillary foci occurs in the event[s] of perturbation of a delicate balance of T-cell immunity that contained the foci so far (46). Additionally, a fresh exogenous infection may also take place. Whatever is the case, on these subsequent exposures, the memory T-cells generated during the primary infection elicit a strong Th1 response and migrate to the site of the pathogen. Several lines of evidences demonstrating that mice and human who lack T-cells, succumb to disease have elucidated the critical role of T-lymphocytes for protection against *Mtb* (47-49). These migrated T-cells are further activated by the processed antigens presented by the local infected macrophages and secrete key effector cytokines, such as, IFN-γ and TNF-α which help in activation as well as terminal differentiation of the macrophages into the giant cells and development of granuloma which is hallmark of TB.

CYTOKINE POLARISED TH1/TH2 EFFECTOR T-CELLS IN TUBERCULOSIS

Two broad categories of effector T-cells have been described: Th1 type and Th2 type, based on distinctively biased pattern of cytokines production.Th1-like response is critical for containment of *Mtb* infection, its robustness and balance between Th1 and Th2 type of response play an important role to dictate whether the disease will have limited extent, such as, pulmonary TB or dissemination to give rise to severe forms of disease such as MTB, multidrug-resistant TB [MDR-TB] [Figure 5.2] (38,50). Th1 cells secrete IL-2, IFN-γ and play protective role in intracellular infections. Th2 type cells secrete IL-4, IL-5 and IL-10 and are either irrelevant and/or exert a negative influence on the immune response. The balance between these two types of response determines host immune response against the pathogen. The differentiation of Th1 and Th2 from precursor unbiased Th0 cells may be under the control of cytokines, such as, IL-12. It has been reported that peripheral blood mononuclear cells [PBMCs] from TB patients, when stimulated *in vitro* with PPD, release lower levels of IFN-γ and IL-2, as compared to tuberculin-positive healthy subjects (51). Other studies have also reported reduced IFN-γ (52), increased IL-4 secretion or increased number of IL-4 secreting cells (53). To address the issue of Th1/Th2 paradigm in TB, investigators focussed attention to the cells producing the cytokines particularly the T-cells derived from the disease site. Cytokine profile of the pleural fluid revealed excess levels of IFN-γ and IL-12 relative to their levels in the peripheral blood compartment (28,54). Several investigators have demonstrated a Th1 biased response in the pleural compartment representing the site of a strong T-cell response of the local TB pathology. Study of T-cells from patients with MTB provided strong indication that extent and dissemination of TB tightly correlate with a strong Th2 bias demonstrated by the T-cells derived from BAL fluid representing the pathologic site of disseminated TB (38). Interestingly, IFN-γ production by the T-cells from the BAL fluid could be restored by supplementation with IL-12. These elegant recent studies with the patients diagnosed on stringent criteria and specimens from both peripheral as well as the local compartments representing the immune response at the local pathologic site[s] provide important insights in understanding the dynamics of Th1/Th2 paradigm in human TB.

CD4+ AND CD8+ T-CELLS IN TUBERCULOSIS

Existence of both CD4+ and CD8+ T-cells inside the granuloma and their participation in the host defence to contain the infection signifies the importance of these T-cells subsets (55,56). Mycobacteria-specific CD4+ T-cells are believed to be the primary cellular element involved in the pathogenesis of TB and are of Th1 like functional phenotype, as they produce IFN-γ and activate macrophages (25). Importance of CD4+ helper T-cells is best demonstrated by significantly higher incidence and occurrence of severe and disseminated forms of TB among patients co-infected with human immunodeficiency virus [HIV] and *Mtb* (57). Furthermore, various studies have demonstrated that CD4+ T-cells are required for activation and maintenance of CD8+ T-cells under many immunological conditions (58). Indeed, an abundant literature exists to support the important role of CD4+ T-cells in host defence against primary TB infection. The role of CD8+ T-cells in immunity against TB has drawn a relatively less attention from the investigators in the field. However, with recent studies demonstrating susceptibility of mice lacking major histocompatibility complex class I [MHC class I] expression to mycobacterial infection (59), alteration of CD4+/CD8+ ratio among TB patients, antigen specific *in vitro* proliferation indicate a definitive role of CD8+ T-cells in TB. Production of IFN-γ and TNF-α in response to mycobacterial antigens like early secretory antigenic target 6-kDa [ESAT-6] by the CD8+ T-cells derived from pleural fluid of patients with TB pleural effusion have substantiated the role of CD8 T-cells in the immunity of TB (60). CD8+ T-cells most probably play an important role in killing the *Mtb* infected target cells by initially [i] TNF receptor superfamily, member 6 [FAS] independent granule exocytosis pathway releasing lytic molecules, such as, granulysin (61); and then followed by [ii] FAS-FAS ligand dependent apoptosis of the infected target cells (62). In addition to the activation of macrophages by secreted cytokines, particularly IFN-γ, recent evidences indicate that CD8+ T-cells can kill the mycobacteria directly through the cytotoxic T-lymphocyte [CTL] activity (63). Therefore, a direct role of CTL in host immunity against TB, in addition to their macrophage activating property is well-established. However, their precise function still remains to be elucidated.

Cytokines, Chemokines and Granulomas Formation

The granulomas formation is pathologic hallmark of TB characterised by organised aggregation of mononuclear inflammatory cells or collection of modified macrophages, usually surrounded by a rim of lymphocytes and often containing multinucleated giant cells (64). TB granulomas form a focus that isolates the *Mtb* and promotes the development of protective immunity by allowing cross-talk between T lymphocytes and macrophages. These cells are generated through priming of resting memory T-cells by captured antigens presented on the surface of APCs in the draining lymphoid tissues and then released into the peripheral compartment. Subsequently, homing of effector and various other T-cell subsets is mediated by active process of well-orchestrated trafficking of T-cells mediated by the groups of molecules, such as, selectins, adhesion molecules and chemokines. Chemokines are largely responsible for such well-organised recruitment of T-cells involved in granuloma formation (65). A number of chemokines have been reported in TB. Interleukin-8 [IL-8] was found to be produced by macrophages infected with *Mtb* (66) and this could be blocked by neutralising antibodies against TNF-α and IL-1β, suggesting that IL-8 production was under the control of these cytokines and is produced during early course in TB patho-genesis (67). Another critical chemokine in TB and granulomas formation is monocyte chemoattractant protein-1 [MCP-1] which is produced by monocyte/macrophage and attracts the same (68). In murine models, deficiency of macrophage inflammatory protein 1-alpha [MIP1-α] inhibited the granuloma formation (69). Moreover, MIP1-α level was noted to be significantly elevated in the serum, BAL and pleural fluids in patients with TB. Expression of regulated on activation, normal T-cell expressed and secreted [RANTES], an important chemokine responsible for recruitment of T-cells particularly the Th1 like cells, is also increased in serum and pleural fluid of TB patients. Apart from these several other chemokines such as MIP1-α and MIP1-β, monokine induced by gamma interferon [MIG], IFN-γ-induced protein-10 [IP-10] and interferon-inducible T-cell alpha chemo-attractant [ITAC] are reported to be elevated in TB patients, particularly at the local disease site[s], such as, pleural effusion (50). Recent investigation in TB pleural effusion patients demonstrated that some of the chemokine receptors and/or chemokines can play a definitive hierarchical role in selective recruitment of Th1 cells at the disease site[s] and delineating such interaction is critical in designing molecular immunotherapeutic strategies. It was found that chemokine receptor chemokine [C-X-C motif] receptor 3 [CXCR3]-ITAC interaction was dominant in selective recruitment of IFN-γ producing Th1 cells in addition to regulated on activation, normal T-cell expressed and secreted RANTES-chemokine [C-C motif] receptor 5 [genep/pseudogene] [CCR5] and CD11a–ICAM interaction. All these observations indicate an important role of these chemokines in human TB (70).

ROLE OF B-LYMPHOCYTES

Role of B-lymphocytes in the pathogenesis of TB has not been critically evaluated. Existence of B220+ cells, which are likely B-cells in the lung granulomas, hints towards their important role in the pathogenesis of TB (71). Furthermore, the important role played by B-cells was highlighted by a study demonstrating that when B–cell deficient mice are challenged intravenously with a large dose of the bacilli, they are more susceptible to disease (72). Similarly, these findings were supported by recent elucidation that B-cells play an important role in immunity against the disease upon higher dose of aerosol infection (73).

FINE T-CELL SUBSETS WITH AN IMMUNOREGULATORY ROLE

These are regarded as non-classical T-cells in the sense that they either bear non-conventional T-cell receptors [TCRs] or do not recognise the antigens in context of classical MHC gene products. MHC non-restricted and exert an immunoregulatory influence on the rest of the T-cells including the effector T-cells. Important among them and worth mentioning are γδ T-cells [Tγδ cells], NK T-cells and the T_{reg} cells.

γδ T-cells

The γδ T-cells are fine T-cell subsets. Their functional TCRs is made of heterodimer of γ-δ chains. They are usually represented in the peripheral blood, less than 10% of total circulating T-cell population. Mice with severe combined immunodeficiency fail to form granuloma in response to challenge with BCG and succumb to death; they can survive such challenge when engrafted with syngeneic lymph node cells depleted of αβ T-cells, suggesting an important role for Tγδ cells (74). Recent data in patients also substantiate a possible role of Tγδ cells in TB. Mtb reactive Tγδ cells are increased in the peripheral blood of tuberculin positive healthy contacts (75,76). A 20%-30% increase in the Tγδ cells was noted in the peripheral blood of patients with a strong immune reactivity compared to the patients with disseminated forms of TB such as extensive pulmonary TB or MTB. Depletion of Tγδ cells results in less well-formed granulomas and increased infiltration of neutrophils. This indicates that Tγδ cells are recruited quite early in the infection with Mtb and direct granuloma formation.

Natural Killer T-cells

NK T-cells are non-conventional in the sense that they bear cell surface markers distinctive of NK cells in addition to functional TCRs. They represent a subset of T-cells with a distinct lineage and not restricted by MHC. They recognise lipid antigens in context of MHC like but relatively less polymorphic CD1 molecules (77). CD1 molecules are sub-grouped into group I consisting of CD1a, b and c whereas CD1d is the only member of group II so far known. CD1d restricted NK T-cells are heterogeneous in terms of their expression of CD4+/CD8+ markers and an important subset of NK T-cells uses restricted set of TCR chain pairs, namely Vα.24/Vβ.11. These are called invariant chain NK T-cells [iNKT]. The NK T-cells are one of the earliest T-cells to be triggered an immune response through several immunoregulatory cytokines [IFN-γ, IL-4, IL-10, and TGF-β etc.] and exert a strong regulatory effect on the effector T-cell response (78). The first reported non-protein mycobacterial antigen was mycolic acid. Several other lipid antigens of mycobacteria, such as, LAM, phosphatidyl inositol manoside [PIM], glucose monomycolate and isoprenoid glycolipids have been found to be recognised by NK T-cells when presented by CD1d molecules. Heterogeneity of NK T-cells in terms of release of either Th1 driving IFN-γ or Th2 driving IL-4 or immunosuppressive IL-10 and TGF-β determines the influence that NKT cell subsets may impose on the bulk T-cell responses. Selective expansion and/or activation of NK T-cell subset[s] may dictate their immunoregulatory role. Expansion and preferential homing of iNKT have been documented in granuloma formation. In addition to their prompt cytokine release, NK T-cells exhibit a potent cytolytic activity both by perforin/granzyme and FAS-FAS ligand dependent mechanisms. Cytotoxic NK T-cells may be relevant in immunity against intracellular microorganism including Mtb (77,78).

REGULATORY T-CELLS

These cells initially recognised as suppressor T-cells (79), were subsequently identified as regulatory T-cells (80). T_{reg} cells are initially defined on the basis of expression of CD25, the α-chain of the IL-2 receptor; they also share common markers with conventional, activated CD4+ T lymphocytes. T_{reg} cells are also characterised by some phenotypic markers like CTLA-4, glucocorticoids-induced TNF receptor [GITR], CD103 and glycoprotein A repetitions predominant [GARP] (80) etc. FoxP3 is most widely accepted as the definitive marker of T_{reg} cells (81). T_{reg} cells reportedly suppress the T_{eff} cells by release of suppressive cytokines [IL-10, TGF-β] or by a contact-dependent manner, or both (82-84). T_{reg} cells also express TLR2 (85,86) and TLR4 (87) which can bind to diverse mycobacterial pattern recognition molecules like lipids. Recent reports suggest that TLR2 engagement with mycobacterial component[s] may eliminate T_{reg} g cells thereby stimulating a Th1 response, while TLR4 engagement results in persistent expansion and activation of T_{reg} cells, thus, causing immunosuppression (87). T_{reg} cells express a distinct set of chemokine receptors, such as chemokine [C-C motif] receptor 4 [CCR4] and chemokine [C-C motif] receptor 8 [CCR8] (88,89), which recruit these to the pathological site[s] to interact and down regulate the function of T_{eff}. Involvement of T_{reg} cells in host defence against intracellular infections is well documented (83). Several recent studies on mice and human indicate T_{reg} cell expansion during TB (90-96) and viral infections (97,98). Expansion of T_{reg} cells in peripheral blood lymphocytes [PBL] as well as disease site[s] among patients with TB-pleural effusion and ascitic fluid has been reported (90). During active TB, suppression of Mtb specific T-cell response is evidenced by over production of suppressive cytokines such as IL-10 and TGF-β and decreased production of the cytokines such as IL-2 and IFN-γ. It has been reported that Foxp3+ regulatory T-cells are over-represented in TB and suppress the host effector T-cell response against Mtb (41,99). The higher ratio of T_{reg}/T_{eff} among these patients suggests the relative dominance of T_{reg} cells. These enriched T_{reg} cells were tightly associated with high bacillary load and that inversely correlated with the pathogen specific IFN-γ skewed effector T-cell response as measured by ratio of IFN-γ/IL-4. Higher frequency of T_{reg} cells among patients with higher bacillary load strongly hints towards the antigen induced T_{reg} cells generation among patients [Figure 5.3]. A significantly higher fraction of proliferating T_{reg} cells was observed *ex vivo*, suggesting their expansion during TB pathogenesis. This is further supported by markedly higher antigen induced *in vitro* proliferation of T_{reg} cells. These T_{reg} cells were preferentially expressing immune exhaustion marker PD-1 on their surface (99), which is involved in suppression of host immunity in addition to IL-10.

IMMUNE EVASION BY *MYCOBACTERIUM TUBERCULOSIS*

Mtb can evade and subvert various immune mechanisms adopted by the host to either eradicate or eliminate the infection. Even during the phase of latency, the bacilli use various immune evasion strategies to circumvent the effective host immune response that generally contains the infection but fails to eradicate them. Clearly such containing immune mechanism[s] is/are effective as any disruption in it results in reactivation of the persistent dormant infection, for example, in HIV infection. The ability of Mtb to survive the immune response clearly indicates existence of series of immune evasion mechanism[s]. Mycobacteria are capable of producing ammonia and sulphatides which inhibit the fusion between phagosomes with lysosomes. Inefficient phagolysosomes fail to process the antigens of mycobacteria and present to the cognate T-cells. This, in turn, fails to stimulate repertoire of T-cells optimally leading to weakening of immunity against the pathogen. Interestingly, cholesterol mediates the phagosomal association of tryptophan aspartate containing coat protein [TACO] and prevents their fusion with lysosomes. Also, by retaining TACO and intercepting the phagolysosomal fusion mycobacteria trigger their evasion mechanisms (100). Mtb-infected macrophages are relatively ineffective at optimally triggering the T-cell proliferation and cytokine production due to down-regulation of human leucocyte antigen [HLA] class II expression (101). Infected macrophages are also known to secrete immunosuppressive cytokines, such as, IL-10 and TGF-β (102). Experimental evidences suggest that Mtb- infected macrophages are relatively refractory to the effects of IFN-γ, which is a key mediator in macrophage activation. Recent studies suggest that recognition of mycobacterial antigens by TLR2 and TLR4 differentially regulates either pro- or anti-inflammatory cytokine production by macrophages and through these cytokines can suppress the immune recognition. Moreover, mycobacterial interaction with TLR2 and TLR4 can differentially expand or eliminate the T_{reg} cells which suppress the effector T cells (103). All these mechanism[s] help the ingested bacilli either to silence or to evade the immune effector function of the host and help the pathogen survival.

A number of microorganisms that cause chronic infection appear to exploit the PD-1-PD-ligand[s] [PD-1-PD-L] pathway to evade the immune responses and establish persistent infection (104). PD-1 and its ligand[s] have important roles in regulating immune defences against microbes that cause acute and chronic infections. Previously, it has been reported that PD-1-PD-L pathway inhibits T-cell effector functions during human TB (105). In addition, same group described the importance of PD-1-PD-L1 pathways during innate immunity against Mtb (106). Live infection of monocytes/macrophages with Mtb H37Rv upregulates PD-L1 expression on them and the PD-1 pathways actively involved in suppressing cytokine production, proliferation, CTL activity and in the apoptotic regulation of IFN-γ producing effector T-cells during active TB (107) [Figure 5.4]. These observations suggest that PD-1-PD-L pathway has been utilised by Mtb to dampen the host immune responses.

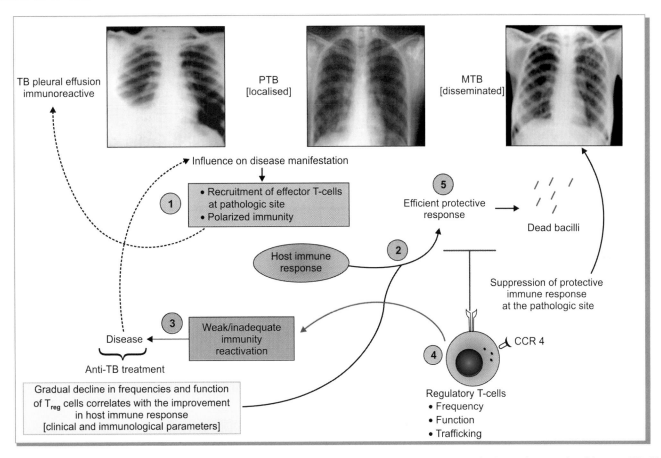

Figure 5.3: Tuberculosis: an immunologic spectrum. Model depicting the immunological spectrum in the pathogenesis of human TB. Host attempts to generate and recruit polarised immunity directed against the pathogen [①]. Elicitation of efficient immune response confers protection and abrogates progression of the disease [②]. Reactivation of the infection due to weak/inadequate host immunity facilitates the disease progression and its clinical manifestations [③]. Proportional imbalance of $T_{eff}:T_{reg}$ ratio towards selective enrichment of T_{reg} cells may lead to the suppression of effector immune response at the pathologic site and thereby influences [④]. Clinical manifestations of human TB as observed in the development of disseminated form of TB [MTB] [⑤]. Patient receiving successful anti-TB treatment are rescued from the adverse effects of the disease and observed to have improvement in their immunological and clinical status with commitment decline in the frequency of T_{reg} cells. TB = tuberculosis; T_{reg} = regulatory T-cells; PTB = pulmonary tuberculosis; MTB = miliary tuberculosis

IMMUNOMODULATORS IN TUBERCULOSIS

Several newer approaches to block certain key molecules responsible for tissue destruction are gaining attention for molecular therapy. Proinflammatory cytokines like TNF-α may be a target for healing of cavitary TB, while TGF-β is thought to be a good candidate for prevention of fibrosis, as it helps development of fibrotic lesions. Role of various other cytokines in the pathogenesis of TB makes them potential targets for intervention. Recent data support the role of aerosolised IFN-γ in disease resolution among patients with multidrug-resistant TB [MDR-TB]. Granulocyte, monocyte-colony stimulating factor [GM-CSF] has also been used simultaneously with IFN-γ (108). Daily low dose administration of recombinant IL-2 has been found to activate the immune system and may enhance the effect of the drugs in patients suffering from MDR-TB (109). Molecular strategies to modulate the immune response by means of changing the balance of cytokines and chemokines involved in TB are new fields and require further investigation.

Several agents have provoked interest as candidate adjuvant therapeutic elements. Heat killed preparation of *M. vaccae* (110) and *M. indicus pranii* [previously known as *Mycobacterium w*] have been co-administered with standard chemotherapy to enhance the immune response. It has been proposed that immunopotentiation by such adjuvant therapeutic vaccination may promote Th1 immunity while acting simultaneously with the drugs. Thalidomide and pentoxyfylline have been found to rescue the patients from excessive effect of TNF-α (111). Other agents like levamisole, inhibitors of IL-12, IFN-α have also been used in TB. However, further studies are definitely required to confirm their role.

HOST BIOMARKERS FOR TUBERCULOSIS

Identification of clinically relevant biomarkers is required for better diagnosis, treatment and prevention of TB. Emerging resistance to current TB drugs necessitates development of newer and better drugs. Hence, "biomarkers" indicating

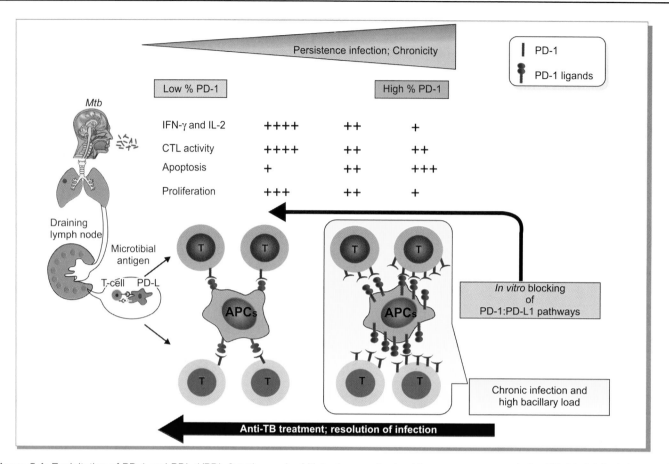

Figure 5.4: Exploitation of PD-1 and PDL-1/PDL-2 pathways by *Mtb* to dampen the host immune responses during TB. Model depicting manipulation of PD-1-PD-L1 pathway by *Mtb* during pathogenesis of human TB. During initial phase of infection APCs and T-cells have low expression of PD-L1 and PD-1 respectively and stimulate the proliferation, cytokine production and cytotoxic activity of antigen-specific naïve T-cells. During chronic infection or in the presence of persisting antigen, T-cells become 'exhausted' and lose the ability to proliferate. Exhausted T-cells have high expression of PD-1 and receive a strong co-inhibitory signal when engaging PD-L-expressing APCs. Blockade of interactions between PD-1 and its ligands can 'restore' T-cells to expand their populations and regain effector functions, including cytokine production, proliferation and cytolysis. Successful anti-tubercular therapy also leads to down-regulation of this inhibitory PD-1 receptor, and hence, restoring the T-cells functions

Mtb = *Mycobacterium tuberculosis;* T = T-lymphocytes; PD-1 = programmed cell death protein-1; IFN-γ = interferon-gamma; IL-2 = interleukin-2; CTL = cytotoxic T-lymphocyte; APCs = antigen presenting cells; PD-L1 = programmed cell death ligand 1

disease status would boost development of better drugs, vaccines and diagnostics (112,113). Research on transcriptomic and proteomic analysis in TB has picked up in recent years, leading to identification of several potential biomarkers for TB diagnosis, vaccine and drug development. Biomarker research in TB has been very effectively highlighted by quite a few research articles recently (113-116). Several potential host biomarkers in blood or blood cells in TB were identified in recent years and include IP-10, IL-6, IL-10, IL-4, FoxP3, PD-1, PD-L1 and IL-12. Similarly, IFN-γ, TNF-α, IL-2, IP-10, IFN-γ/TNF-α, IFN-γ/IL-2 and IL-13 were identified as strong candidate biomarkers [Table 5.1] that were upregulated in latent TB compared to healthy uninfected controls in stimulated blood samples (116-119). These biomarkers would again find an application in diagnosis of a latent TB infection. IL-6, IL-10, IP-10 and TNF-α are the most promising markers for active TB while FoxP3, IL-4 and IL-12 are identified as the most promising biomarkers for immunological correlates of

protection. Recently, therapy-induced decline of FoxP3$^+$ T$_{reg}$ cells was reported to parallel with decline of *Mtb*-specific IL-10 along with elevation of IFN-γ production, and IFN-γ/IL-4 ratio. Interestingly, persistence of T$_{reg}$ cells tightly correlated with MDR-TB (99). This finding further substantiates the utility of T$_{reg}$ cell monitoring as an important predictive biomarker for MDR-TB and response to chemotherapy. Recently, it was observed that PD-1 expressing T-cells were increased during active TB, and steadily declined in the PBL of PTB patients during successful anti-tuberculosis therapy. A tight correlation between the bacillary load and frequency of PD-1+ T-cells, and decrease of PD-1+ T-cell frequency was associated with increase in the *Mtb* specific IFN-γ/IL-4 among PTB patients (107). Thus, a potential role of PD-1+ T-cells as useful biomarker to monitor treatment outcomes during therapy and/or vaccine trial for TB patients can be considered. These biomarkers are important for two reasons: [i] discriminating TB disease and infection; and

Table 5.1: Potential biomarker candidates for TB

Denominator	Marker	
	Down-regulated	Up-regulated
Active TB versus healthy controls	Interferon-γ/Interleukin-4	Interferon-γ-inducible protein 10
	Interleukin-4δ2/Interleukin-4	Interleukin-2
		Interleukin-4
		Interleukin-6
		Interleukin-8
		Interleukin-10
		Tumour necrosis factor-α
		Monocyte chemoattractant protein-2
		Transforming growth factor-β1
		Interferon-γ
		Foxp3
		Programmed cell death protein 1
		Programmed cell death ligand 1
		T-cell immunoglobulin and mucin domain-containing molecule 3
Active TB versus latent TB infection	Interleukin-4δ2	Foxp3
	Interferon-γ	Tumour necrosis factor-α
	Interleukin-12	Interleukin-4
		Interleukin-12α, interleukin-12β
		Programmed cell death ligand 1

TB = tuberculosis

Based on references 116-120

[ii] identifying correlates of protective immunity. These protective immunological correlates would, in turn, be useful for vaccine studies. Validation of these biomarkers in large number of individuals across populations could identify a TB biosignature as well as "immune correlates of protective immunity" (120,121).

REFERENCES

1. Mitra DK, Rai AK. Immunology of tuberculosis. In: Sharma SK, Mohan A, editors. Tuberculosis. Second edition. New Delhi: Jaypee Brothers Medical Publishers; 2009.p.108-23.
2. North RJ, Jung YJ. Immunity to tuberculosis. Annu Rev Immunol 2004;22:599-623.
3. Van Crevel R, Ottenhoff TM, vander Meer JM. Innate immunity to tuberculosis. Clin Microbiol Rev 2002;15:294-309.
4. Schlesinger LS. Role of mononuclear phagocytes in M. tuberculosis pathogenesis. J Invest Med 1996;44:312-23.
5. Schlesinger LS, Hull SR, Kaufman TM. Binding of the terminal mannosyl units of lipoarabinomannan from avirulent strain of Mycobacterium tuberculosis to human macrophages. J Immunol 1994;152:4070-9.
6. Hoheisel G, Zheng L, Teschler H, Striz I, Costabel U. Increased soluble CD14 levels in BAL fluid in pulmonary tuberculosis. Chest 1995;108:1614-6.
7. Bermudez LE, Goodman J. Mycobacterium tuberculosis invades and replicates within type II alveolar cells. Infect Immun 1996;64:1400-6.
8. Takeda K, Akira S. TLR signaling pathways. Semin Immunol 2004;16:3-9.
9. Kleinnijenhuis J, Oosting M, Joosten LA, Netea MG, Van Crevel R. Innate immune recognition of Mycobacterium tuberculosis. Clin Dev Immunol 2011;2011:405310.
10. Xu Y, Jagannath C, Liu XD, Sharafkhaneh A, Kolodziejska KE, Eissa NT. Toll-like receptor 4 is a sensor for autophagy associated with innate immunity. Immunity 2007;27:135-44.
11. Underhill DM, Ozinsky A, Smith KD, Aderem A. Toll-like receptor-2 mediates mycobacteria-induced proinflammatory signaling in macrophages. PNAS 1999;96:14459-63.
12. Desjardins M, Huber LA, Parton RG, Griffiths G. Biogenesis of phagolysosomes proceeds through a sequential series of interactions with the endocytic apparatus. J Cell Biol 1994;124:677-88.
13. Cohn ZA. The fate of bacteria within phagocytic cells. The degradation of isotopically labeled bacteria by polymorphonuclear leucocytes and macrophages. J Exp Med 1963;117:27-42.
14. Hart PD, Armstrong JA, Brown CA, Draper P. Ultrastructural study of the behaviour of macrophages toward parasitic mycobacteria. Infect Immun 1972;5:803-7.
15. Goren MB, Brokl O, Das BC. Sulfatides of Mycobacterium tuberculosis: the structure of the principal sulfatide [SL-I]. Biochemistry 1976;15:2728-35.
16. Goren MB, Hart PD, Young MR, Armstrong JA. Prevention of phagosome lysosome fusion in cultured macrophages by sulfatides of Mycobacterium tuberculosis. Proc Natl Acad Sci USA 1976;73:2510-4.
17. Gordon AH, Hart PD, Young MR. Ammonia inhibits phagosome-lysosome fusion in macrophages. Nature 1980;286:79-81.
18. Chan J, Kaufmann SH. Immune mechanisms of protection. In: Bloom BR, editor. Tuberculosis: pathogenesis, protection and control. Washington: American Society of Microbiology; 1994.p.389-415.
19. Walker L, Lowrie DB. Killing of Mycobacterium microti by immunologically activated macrophages. Nature 1981;293:69-70.
20. Nozaki Y, Hasegawa Y, Ichiyama S, Nakashima I, Shimokata K. Mechanism of nitric oxide-dependent killing of Mycobacterium

bovis BCG in human alveolar macrophages. Infect Immun 1997;65:3644-7.

21. Flesch I, Kaufmann SH. Mycobacterial growth inhibition by interferon-gamma-activated bone marrow macrophages and differential susceptibility among strains of Mycobacterium tuberculosis. J Immunol 1987;138:4408-13.

22. Flynn J, Chan J. Immunology of tuberculosis. Annu Rev Immunol 2001;19:93-129.

23. Molloy A, Laochumroonvorapong P, Kaplan G. Apoptosis, but not necrosis, of infected monocytes is coupled with killing of intracellular Bacillus Calmette Guerin. J Exp Med 1994;180: 1499-509.

24. Placido R, Mancino G, Amendola A, Mariani F, Vendetti S, Piacentini M, et al. Apoptosis of human monocytes/macrophages in Mycobacterium tuberculosis infection. J Pathol 1997;181:31-8.

25. Cooper AM. Cell-mediated immune responses in tuberculosis. Annu Rev Immunol 2009;27:393-422.

26. Orme IM, Cooper AM. Cytokine/chemokine cascade in immunity to tuberculosis. Immunol Today 1999;20:307-12.

27. Harari A, Rozot V, Bellutti Enders F, Perreau M, Stalder JM, Nicod LP, et al. Dominant TNF-α+ M. tuberculosis–specific CD4+ T cell responses discriminate between latent infection and active disease. Nature Medicine 2011;17:372-6.

28. Bergeron A, Bonay M, Kambouchner M, Lecossier D, Riquet M, Soler P, et al. Cytokine patterns in tuberculosis and sarcoid granulomas: correlation with histopathologic features of the granulomatous response. J Immunol 1997;159:3034-43.

29. Hoheisel G, Izbicki G, Roth M, Chan CH, Leung JC, Reichenberger F, et al. Compartmentalisation of proinflammatory cytokines in tuberculous pleurisy. Respir Med 1998;92:14-7.

30. Blanchard DK, Michelini-Norris MB, Friedman H, Djeu JY. Lysis of mycobacteria infected monocytes by IL-2 activated killer cells: role of LFA-1. Cell Immunol 1989;119:402-11.

31. Pandiyan P, Zheng L, Reed J, Lenardo MJ. CD4+CD25+Foxp3+ regulatory T cells induce cytokine deprivation–mediated apoptosis of effector CD4+ T cells. Nature Immunol 2007;8: 1353-62.

32. de Jong R, Altare F, Haagen IA, Elferink DG, Boer T, van Breda Vriesman P, et al. Severe mycobacterial and Salmonella infection in interleukin-12 receptor deficient patients. Science 1998;280:1435-8.

33. Vankayalapati R, Wizel B, Weis SE, Samten B, Girard WM, Barnes PF. Production of interleukin-18 in human tuberculosis. J Infect Dis 2000;182:234-9.

34. Van Crevel R, Ottenhoff TH, van der Meer JW. Innate immunity to Mycobacterium tuberculosis. Clin Microbiol Rev 2002;15: 294-309.

35. Flynn JL, Chan J. Tuberculosis: latency and reactivation. Infect Immun 2001;69: 4195-201.

36. Hernandez-Pando R, Orozco H, Sampieri A, Pavon L, Velasquillo C, Larriva Sahd J, et al. Correlation between the kinetics of Th1/Th2 cells and pathology in a murine model of experimental pulmonary tuberculosis. Immunology 1996;89:26-33.

37. Sánchez FO, Rodríguez JI, Agudelo G, García LF. Immune responsiveness and lymphokine production in patients with tuberculosis and healthy controls. Infect Immun 1994;62:5673-8.

38. Sharma SK, Mitra DK, Balamurugan A, Pandey RM, Mehra NK. Cytokine polarisation in miliary and pleural tuberculosis. J Clin Immunol 2002;22:345-52.

39. Demissie A, Abebe M, Aseffa A, Rook G, Fletcher H, Zumla AI, et al. Healthy individuals that control a latent infection with Mycobacterium tuberculosis express high levels of Th1cytokines and the IL-4 antagonist IL-4delta2. J Immunol 2004;172:6938-43.

40. Boussiotis VA, Tsai EY, Yunis EJ, Thim S, Delgado JC, Dascher CC, et al. IL-10 producing T cells suppress immune responses in anergic tuberculosis patients. J Clin Invest 2000;105:1317-25.

41. Sharma PK, Saha PK, Singh A, Sharma SK, Ghosh B, Mitra DK. FoxP3+ regulatory T cells suppress effector T-cell function at pathologic site in miliary tuberculosis. Am J Respir Crit Care Med 2009;179:1061-70.

42. Rojas M, Olivier M, Gros P, Barrera LF, Garcia LF. TNF-α and IL-10 modulate the induction of apoptosis by virulent M. tuberculosis in murine macorphages. J Immunol 1999;162: 6122-31.

43. Mukherjee B, Mukhopadhyay R, Bannerjee B, Chowdhury S, Mukherjee S, Naskar K, et al. Antimony-resistant but not anti-mony-sensitive Leishmania donovani up-regulates host IL-10 to overexpress multidrug-resistant protein. Proc Natl Acad Sci 2013;12:110.

44. Toossi Z, Gogate P, Shiratsuchi H, Young T, Ellner JJ. Enhanced production of TGF-beta by blood monocytes from patients with active tuberculosis and presence of TGF-beta in tuberculous granulomatous lung lesions. J Immunol 1995;154:465-73.

45. Toossi Z, Ellner JJ. The role of TGF beta in the pathogenesis of human tuberculosis. Clin Immunol Immunopathol 1998; 87: 107-14.

46. Sharma SK, Mohan A, Sharma A, Mitra DK. Miliary tuberculosis: new insights into an old disease. Lancet Infect Dis 2005;5: 415-30.

47. Lefford MJ. Transfer of adopticve immunity to tuberculosis in mice. Infect Immun 1975;11:1174-81.

48. Mogues T, Goodrich ME, Ryan L, LaCourse R, North RJ. The relative importance of T cell subsets in immunity and immunopathology of airborne Mycobacterium tuberculosis infection in mice. J Exp Med 2001;193:271-80.

49. North RJ, Jung YJ. Immunity to tuberculosis. Annu Rev Immunol 2004;22:599-623.

50. Mitra DK, Sharma SK, Dinda AK, Bindra MS, Madan B, Ghosh B. Polarised helper T cells in tubercular pleural effusion: phenotypic identity and selective recruitment. Eur J Immunol 2005;35: 2367-75.

51. Huygen K, Van Vooren JP, Turneer M, Bosmans R, Dierckx P, De Bruyn J. Specific lymphoproliferation, gamma interferon production, and serum immunoglobulin G directed against a purified 32kDa mycobacterial protein antigen [P32] in patients with active tuberculosis. Scand J Immunol 1988;27:187-94.

52. Vilcek J, Klion A, Henriksen-DeStefano D, Zemtsov A, Davidson DM, Davidson M, et al. Defective gammainterferon production in peripheral blood leukocytes of patients with acute tuberculosis. J Clin Immunol 1986;6:146-51.

53. Surcel HM, Troye-Blomberg M, Paulie S, Andersson G, Moreno C, Pasvol G, et al. Th1/Th2 profiles in tuberculosis, based on the proliferation and cytokine response of blood lymphocytes to mycobacterial antigens. Immunology 1994;81: 171-6.

54. Zhang M, Gately MK, Wang E, Gong J, Wolf SF, Lu S, et al. Interleukin 12 at the site of disease in tuberculosis. J Clin Invest 1994;93:1733-9.

55. Caruso AM, Serbina N, Klein E, Triebold K, Bloom BR, Flynn JL. Mice deficient in CD4 T cells have only transiently, diminished levels of gamma interferon. J Immunol 1999;162:5407-16.

56. Tascon RE, Lukacs KV, Colstan MJ. Protection against M. tuberculosis infection by CD8 T cells requires production of gamma interferon, Infect Immun 1998;66:830-40.

57. Law KF, Jagirdar J, Weiden MD, Bodkin M, Rom WN. Tuberculosis in HIV-positive patients: cellular response and immune activation in the lung. Am J Respir Crit Care Med 1996;153:1377-84.

58. Serbina NV, Lazarevic, Flynn JL. CD4 T cells are required for the development of cytotoxic CD8+T cells during Mycobacterium tuberculosis infection. J Immunol 2001;167:6991.

59. Flynn JL, Goldstein MM, Triebold KJ, Bloom BR. Major histo-compatibility complex class I-restricted T cells are necessary for protection against M. tuberculosis in mice. Infect Agents Dis 1993;2:259-62.

60. Carranza C, Juarez E, Torres M, Ellner JJ, Sada E, Schwander SK. Mycobacterium tuberculosis growth control by lung macrophages and CD8 cells from patient contacts. Am J Respir Crit Care Med 2006;173:238-45.

61. Canaday DH, Ziebold C, Noss EH, Chervenak KA, Harding CV, Boom WH. Activation of human CD8+ alpha beta TCR+ cells by Mycobacterium tuberculosis via an alternate class I MHC antigen-processing pathway. J Immunol 1999;162:372-9.

62. Canaday DH, Wilkinson RJ, Li Q, Harding CV, Silver RF, Boom WH. CD4+ and CD8+ T cells kill intracellular M. tuberculosis by a perforin and Fas/Fas ligand-independent mechanism. J Immunol 2001;167:2734-42.

63. Stenger S, Mazzaccaro RJ, Uyemura K, Cho S, Barnes PF, Rosat JP, et al. Differential effects of cytolytic T cell subsets on intracellular infection. Science 1997;276:1684-7.

64. Saunders BM, Britton WJ. Life and death in the granuloma: immunopathology of TB. Immunol. Cell Biol 2007;85:103-11.

65. Nau GJ, Guilfoile P, Chupp GL, Berman JS, Kim SJ, Kornfeld H, et al. A chemoattractant cytokine associated with granulomas in tuberculosis and silicosis. Proc Natl Acad Sci 1997;94:6414-9.

66. Juffermans NP, Verbon A, van Deventer SJ, van Deutekom H, Belisle JT, Ellis ME, et al. Elevated chemokine concentrations in sera of human immunodeficiency virus [HIV]-seropositive and HIV-seronegative patients with tuberculosis: a possible role for mycobacterial lipoarabinomannan. Infect Immun 1999;67:4295-7.

67. Zhang Y, Broser M, Cohen H, Bodkin M, Law K, Reibman J, et al. Enhanced interleukin-8 release and gene expression in macrophages after exposure to Mycobacterium tuberculosis and its components. J Clin Invest 1995;95:586-92.

68. Kasahara K, Tobe T, Tomita M, Mukaida N, Shao Bo S, Matsushima K, et al. Selective expression of monocyte chemo-tactic and activating factor/monocyte chemoattractant protein 1 in human blood monocytes by Mycobacterium tuberculosis. J Infect Dis 1994;170:1238-47.

69. Lu B, Rutledge BJ, Gu L, Fiorillo J, Lukacs NW, Kunkel SL, et al. Abnormalities in monocyte recruitment and cytokine expression in monocyte chemoattractant protein 1-deficient mice. J Exp Med 1998;187:601-8.

70. Kurashima K, Mukaida N, Fujimura M, Yasui M, Nakazumi Y, Matsuda T, et al. Elevated chemokine levels in bronchoalveolar lavage fluid of tuberculosis patients. Am J Respir Crit Care Med 1997;155:1474-7.

71. Gonzalez-Juarrero M, Turner O, Turner J, Marietta P, Brooks J, Orme I. Temporal and spatial arrangement of lymphocytes within lung granulomas induced by aerosol infection with Mycobacterium tuberculosis. Infect Immun 2001;69:1722-8.

72. Vordermeier HM, Venkatprasad N, Harris DP, Ivanyi J. Increase of tuberculosis infection in the organs of B-cell deficient mice. Clin Exp Immunol 1996;106:312-6.

73. Maglione P, Xu J, Chan J. B-cells moderate inflammatory progression and enhance bacterial containment upon pulmonary challenge with Mycobacterium tuberculosis. J Immunol 2007;178:7222-34.

74. Munk ME, Gatrill AJ, Kaufmann SH. Target cell lysis and IL-2 secretion by gamma/delta T-lymphocytes after activation with bacteria. J Immunol 1990;145:2434-9.

75. North RJ, Izzo AA. Granuloma formation in severe combined immunodeficient [SCID] mice in response to progressive BCG infection: tendency not to form granulomas in the lung is associated with faster bacterial growth in this organ. Am J Pathol 1993;142:1959-66.

76. Barnes PF, Grisso CL, Abrams JS, Band H, Rea TH, Modlin RL. Gamma delta T-lymphocytes in human tuberculosis. J Infect Dis 1992;165:506-12.

77. Schaible UE, Kaufmann SH. CD1 and CD1-restricted T-cells in infections with intracellular bacteria. Trends Microbiol 2000;8:419-25.

78. Ulrichs T, Porcelli SA. CD1 proteins: targets of T-cell recognition in innate and adaptive immunity. Rev Immunogenet 2000;2:416-32.

79. Gershon RK, Kondo K. Cell interactions in the induction of tolerance: the role of thymic lymphocytes. Immunology 1970;18:723-37.

80. Sakaguchi S, Sakaguchi N, Asano M, Itoh M, Toda M, et al. Immunologic self-tolerance maintained by activated T cells expressing IL-2 receptor α-chains [CD25]. Breakdown of a single mechanism of self-tolerance causes various autoimmune diseases. J Immunol 1995;155:1151-64.

81. Sakaguchi S. Naturally arising Foxp3-expressing CD25 + CD4 + regulatory T-cells in immunological tolerance to self and nonself. Nat Immunol 2005;6:345-352.

82. O'Garra A, Vieira PL, Vieira P, Goldfeld AE. IL-10–producing and naturally occurring CD41 T_{regs}: limiting collateral damage. J Clin Invest 2004;114:1372-8.

83. Belkaid Y, Rouse BT. Natural regulatory T-cells in infectious disease. Nat Immunol 2005;6:353-60.

84. Fontenot JD, Rasmussen JP, Williams LM, Dooley JL, Farr AG, Rudensky AY. Regulatory T cell lineage specification by the forkhead transcription factor foxp3. Immunity 2005;22:329-41.

85. Sutmuller RP, den Brok MH, Kramer M, Bennink EJ, Toonen LW, Kullberg BJ, et al. Toll-like receptor 2 controls expansion and function of regulatory T-cells. J Clin Invest 2006;116:485-94.

86. Liu H, Komai-Koma M, Xu D, Liew FY. Toll-like receptor 2 signaling modulates the functions of CD4+ CD25+ regulatory T cells. Proc Natl Acad Sci 2006;103:7048-53.

87. Caramalho I, Lopes-Carvalho T, Ostler D, Zelenay S, Haury M, Demengeot J. Regulatory T cells selectively express toll-like receptors and are activated by lipopolysaccharide. J Exp Med 2003;197:403-11.

88. Iellem A, Mariani M, Lang R, Recalde H, Panina-Bordignon P, Sinigaglia F, et al. Unique chemotactic response profile and specific expression of chemokine receptors CCR4 and CCR8 by CD4+ CD25+ regulatory T-cells. J Exp Med 2001;194:847-53.

89. Baatar D, Olkhanud P, Sumitomo K, Taub D, Gress R, Biragyn A. Human peripheral blood T regulatory cells [T_{regs}], functionally primed CCR4+T_{regs} and unprimed CCR4-T_{regs}, regulate effector T cells using FasL. J Immunol 2007;178:4891-900.

90. Guyot-Revol V, Innes JA, Hackforth S, Hinks T, Lalvani A. Regulatory T-cells are expanded in blood and disease sites in patients with tuberculosis. Am J Respir Crit Care Med 2006;173:803-10.

91. Kursar M, Koch M, Mittrucker HW, Nouailles G, Bonhagen K, Kamradt T, et al. Regulatory T cells prevent efficient clearance of Mycobacterium tuberculosis. J Immunol 2007;178:2661-5.

92. Chen X, Zhou B, Li M, Deng Q, Wu X, Le X, et al. CD4[+] CD25[+]FoxP3[+] regulatory T-cells suppress Mycobacterium tuberculosis immunity in patients with active disease. Clin Immunol 2007;123:50-9.

93. Hougardy JM, Place S, Hildebrand M, Drowart A, Debrie AS, Locht C, et al. Regulatory T-cells depress immune responses to protective antigens in active tuberculosis. Am J Respir Crit Care Med 2007;176:409-16.

94. Scott-Browne JP, Shafiani S, Tucker-Heard G, Ishida-Tsubota K, Fontenot JD, Rudensky AY, et al. Expansion and function of Foxp3-expressing T regulatory cells during tuberculosis. J Exp Med 2007;204:2159-69.

95. Antas PR, Sampaio EP. Another round for the CD4+CD25+ regulatory T-cells in patients with tuberculosis. Am J Respir Crit Care Med 2007;176:214-5.

96. Burl S, Hill PC, Jeffries DJ, Holland MJ, Fox A, Lugos MD, et al. FOXP3 gene expression in a tuberculosis case contact study. Clin Exp Immunol 2007;149:117-22.

97. Shen T, Zheng J, Liang H, Xu C, Chen X, Zhang T, et al. Characteristics and PD- 1 expression of peripheral CD4+ CD127lo CD25hi FoxP3+ T_{reg} cells in chronic HCV infected-patients. Virol J 2011;8:279.

98. Punkosdy GA, Blain M, Glass DD, Lozano MM, O'Mara L, Dudley JP, et al. Regulatory T-cell expansion during chronic viral infection is dependent on endogenous retroviral superantigens. Pros Natl Acad Sci 2011;108:3677-82.

99. Singh A, Dey AB, Sharma PK, Mohan A, Mitra DK. Foxp3+ regulatory T-cells among tuberculosis patients: Impact on prognosis and restoration of antigen specific IFN-γ producing T-cells. PLoS ONE 2012;7:e44728.

100. Collins HL, Kaufmann SH. The many faces of host responses to tuberculosis. Immunology 2001;103:1-9.

101. Hmama Z, Gabathuler R, Jefferies WA, Dejong G, Reiner NE. Altenuation of HLA-DR expression by mononuclear phagocytes infected with Mycobacterium tuberculosis is related to intracellular sequestration of immature class II heterodimers. J Immunol 1998;161:4882-93.

102. Hirsch CS, Hussain R, Toossi Z, Dawood G, Shahid F, Ellner JJ. Cross-modulation by transforming growth factor beta in human tuberculosis: suppression of antigen-driven blastogenesis and interferon gamma production. Proc Natl Acad Sci 1996;93:3193-8.

103. Chang J, Huggett JF, Dheda K, Kim LU, Zumla A, Rook GA. Mycobacterium tuberculosis induces selective upregulation of TLRs in the mononuclear leukocytes of patients with active pulmonary tuberculosis. J Immunol 2006;176:3010-8.

104. Sharpe AH, Wherry EJ, Ahmed R, Freeman GJ. The function of programmed cell death 1 and its ligands in regulating autoimmunity and infection. Nat Immunol 2007;8:239-45.

105. Jurado JO, Alvarez IB, Pasquinelli V, Martínez GJ, Quiroga MF, Abbate E, et al. Programmed death [PD]-1:PD-ligand 1/PD-ligand 2 pathway inhibits T cell effector functions during human tuberculosis. J Immunol 2008;181:116-25.

106. Alvarez IB, Pasquinelli V, Jurado JO, Abbate E, Musella RM, de la Barrera SS, et al. Role played by the programmed death-1-programmed death ligand pathway during innate immunity against Mycobacterium tuberculosis. J Infect Dis 2010;202:524-32.

107. Singh A, Dey AB, Mohan A, Mitra DK. Inhibiting PD-1 pathway rescues M. tuberculosis specific IFN-γ producing T-cells from apoptosis in tuberculosis patients. J Infect Dis 2013;208:603-15.

108. Etemadi A, Farid R, Stanford JL. Immunotherapy for drug resistant tuberculosis. Lancet 1992;340:1360-1.

109. Raad I, Hachem R, Leeds N, Sawaya R, Salem Z, Atweh S. Use of adjunctive treatment with interferon-gamma in an immune compromised patient who had refractory multidrug resistant tuberculosis of the brain. Clin Infect Dis 1996;22:572-4.

110. Johnson JL, Nunn AJ, Fourie PB, Ormerod LP, Mugerwa RD, Mwinga A, et al. Effect of Mycobacterium vaccae [SRL172] immunotherapy on radiographic healing in tuberculosis. Int J Tuberc Lung Dis 2004;8:1348-54.

111. Strieter RM, Remick DG, Ward PA, Spengler RN, Lynch JP, Larrick J. Cellular and molecular regulation of tumor necrosis factor-alpha production by pentoxifylline. Biochem Biophys Res Commun 1988;155:1230-6.

112. Parida SK, Kaufmann SH. The quest for biomarkers in tuberculosis. Drug Discov Today 2010;15:148-57.

113. John SH, Kenneth J, Gandhe AS. Host biomarkers of clinical relevance in tuberculosis: review of gene and protein expression studies. Biomarkers 2012;17:1-8.

114. Wallis RS, Pai M, Menzies D, Doherty TM, Walzl G, Perkins MD, et al. Biomarkers and diagnostics for tuberculosis: progress, needs, and translation into practice. Lancet 2010;375:1920-37.

115. Walzl G, Ronacher K, Hanekom W, Scriba TJ, Zumla A. Immunological biomarkers of tuberculosis. Nat Rev Immunol 2011;11:343-54.

116. Petrucci R, Abu Amer N, Gurgel RQ, Sherchand JB, Doria L, Lama C, et al. Interferon gamma, interferon-gamma-induced-protein 10, and tuberculin responses of children at high risk of tuberculosis infection. Pediatr Infect Dis J 2008;27:1073-7.

117. Babu S, Bhat SQ, Kumar NP, Kumaraswami V, Nutman TB. Regulatory T cells modulate Th17 responses in patients with positive tuberculin skin test results. J Infect Dis 2010;201:20-31.

118. Nemeth J, Winkler HM, Karlhofer F, Selenko-Gebauer N, Graninger W, Winkler S. T-cells co-producing Mycobacterium tuberculosis-specific type 1 cytokines for the diagnosis of latent tuberculosis. Eur Cytokine Netw 2010;21:34-9.

119. Sutherland JS, de Jong BC, Jeffries DJ, Adetifa IM, Ota MO. Production of TNF-alpha, IL-12[p40] and IL-17 can discriminate between active TB disease and latent infection in a West African cohort. PLoS One 2010;5:e12365.

120. Wallis RS, Maeurer M, Mwaba P, Chakaya J, Rustomjee R, Migliori GB, et al. Tuberculosis-advances in development of new drugs, treatment regimens, host-directed therapies, and biomarkers. Lancet Infect Dis 2016;16:e34-46.

121. Cadena AM, Flynn JL, Fortune SM. The importance of first impressions: early events in Mycobacterium tuberculosis infection influence outcome. MBio 2016;7[2]pii:e00342-16.

6

Genetic Susceptibility Parameters in Tuberculosis

NK Mehra, Gaurav Sharma, Deepali K Bhat

INTRODUCTION

Most people exposed to tuberculosis [TB] develop effective immunity against the invading bacillus and do not develop disease. A strong host genetic influence has been proposed to be an important factor for the development of disease in a limited percentage of the population in a hyperendemic area (1,2). Evidence supporting the role of genetic factors influencing susceptibility/resistance to TB includes differences in the development of infection and disease among various human racial groups (3,4) and animal strains (5), concordance of the disease in monozygotic twins (6) and familial occurrence of the disease. Clinical manifestations of pulmonary TB are due to delayed type hypersensitivity [DTH] reaction against *Mycobacterium tuberculosis* [*Mtb*] rather than direct damage caused by the bacillus. Thus, final outcome of the disease is the result of interaction between the bacillus and host genes that govern immune response.

Available evidence indicate that susceptibility to TB is multifactorial. Host genetic factors explain, partly why some people are resistant and others susceptible to infection. Rare gene disruptions cause fatal vulnerability to certain pathogens, but more subtle differences are common and arise from minor variations in many genes. To predict how much our genetic make-up determines the different ways in which we respond to some infectious agents is a difficult task. This is especially because of the many contributory factors, such as, previous health status, acquired immunity and variability in the pathogen. Many immunogenetic loci influence susceptibility to several infectious agents. A genetic basis for inter-individual variation in susceptibility to human infectious disease is also explained through segregation analysis of human leucocyte antigen [HLA] linked genes as well as candidate gene studies (7-10).

The goal of identification of host genetic factors that underlie susceptibility to TB can be approached by two ways: [i] first, candidate gene studies can be carried out on genes of known function that have a possible biological role in the control of infection or disease; and [ii] the second approach utilises a non-targeted genome-wide linkage analysis, in which increased sharing of chromosomal regions by affected individuals leads to identification of positional candidates. Recently, development of high throughput genotyping technologies and identification of thousands of polymorphic microsatellite markers as well as genome-wide association studies [GWAS] has led to the identification of genes [candidate] not previously associated with the disease. A better understanding of the disease mechanisms and of the host-pathogen interplay could help to identify people at high or low risk of infection and provide a basis for early diagnosis and pre-emptive treatment of susceptible individuals. In this chapter, the role of genetic factors in influencing susceptibility to TB *per se* has been discussed.

GENETIC SUSCEPTIBILITY TO TUBERCULOSIS

Exposure to *Mtb* in a hyperendemic area does not always result in disease in all individuals. Though environmental and socio-economic factors are primarily related, numerous studies have emphasised the importance of host resistance and hereditary susceptibility. Although about one-third of the world's population is infected with the bacillus, only around 10% of those who get infected will ever develop clinical disease. Even in families with similar socio-economic and nutritional conditions, the disease develops only in a few children indicating the existence of host genetic factors regulating disease expression or resistance. Racial differences in susceptibility, family segregation analyses, immune response linked gene association studies, candidate gene studies and genome scan studies have all implicated host genetics as the major contributing factor in determining susceptibility and/or resistance to infectious diseases.

Racial Differences

Racial differences influence the degree of resistance to myco-bacterial diseases. For example, the African Americans (11) and certain African tribes have been reported to be parti-cularly more susceptible to pulmonary TB as compared to Jews, who are relatively immune. Similarly it has been reported that the non-White patients in the age group of 1–20 years had higher deaths rates from pulmonary TB as compared to the White children of the same age group (12). Also the disease prevalence in Gurkhas of Nepal has been found to be appreciably higher than in other ethnic groups residing in the same geographical area (4).

Twin Studies

Pulmonary TB has been reported to occur more commonly in twins even when they are living separately and in disparate environmental conditions (6). It has been suggested that the disease expression rate of TB is significantly higher in monozygotic twins [3.3%] than dizygotic twins [15.7%] (13). Among household contacts, the disease is more likely to occur in siblings than in the spouse despite closer physical contact in the latter.

ABO and Rh Blood Groups

There are reports indicating that Rh-negative persons are more susceptible to TB than their Rh-positive counterparts (14), although others failed to confirm this observation (15). Inci-dentally, Chinese with blood group 'O' have been found to be more resistant to develop pulmonary TB than those with other blood groups (16). A significant increase of pulmonary TB in persons with blood groups 'O' and 'AB' has also been reported in sputum positive Danish patients as compared to those with group 'A' or 'B' (17).

IMMUNE RESPONSE GENES

Genes within and associated with the major histocompatibility complex [MHC] have been shown to play a crucial role in governing susceptibility to intracellular mycobacterial infections. It is now recognized that MHC gene products play a crucial role in the immune response by not only providing a context for the recognition of foreign antigens by T-lymphocytes but also by controlling the immune regulatory processes and final elimination of the cell bound antigen. Some MHC gene products promote efficient T-cell function, whereas, others elicit a poor T-cell response or no response at all. These include immune response [*Ir*] genes and/or immune suppressive [*Is*] genes. In pulmonary TB, the host immune response to *Mtb* is responsible for clinical expression of the disease rather than damage by the mycobacteria. Therefore, an in depth study of MHC linked genes is essential for understanding mechanisms underlying disease susceptibility. A detailed description of the human HLA system, its gene organization, biological function of its various gene products and association studies with pulmonary TB as well as involvement of various non-HLA genes is given here.

MOLECULAR GENETICS AND ORGANISATION OF HUMAN MHC GENES

Human MHC gene cluster spans a region of about 4000 kb length [4×10^6 nucleotides] on the short arm of chromosome 6 in the distal portion of the 6p 21.3 band. Studies on the structural organisation of MHC molecules have helped in understanding the functional role of MHC gene products in the host immune response. In the MHC region, a total of 224 genes have been identified, of which 128 are assumed to be functional while the remaining 96 are pseudo genes. It is remarkable that greater than 40% of these genes have one or more assigned immune functions. The genes are arranged in three distinct sets of molecules, each comprising a cluster of *Ir* genes [Figure 6.1] (18). The most centromeric segment is the class II region that spans around 1100 kb and contains HLA-DP, DQ and DR loci, which are found as pairs, encoding the α- and β-chains. These chains encode the heterodimer class II protein molecules expressed at the cell surface of antigen presenting cells [macrophages, dendritic cells, Kupffer cells, Langerhans cells, B-cells, activated T-cells]. The class I region on the other hand, lies at the telomeric end and contains the classical HLA-A, B and C and related loci, spread over a region of approximately 2 Mb. The HLA class I molecules are expressed ubiquitously on almost all nucleated cells.

The HLA genes that are involved in immune regulation are mainly in the class I and class II region, which are structurally and functionally different. On the other hand, Class III genes, also referred to as the 'central genes' are placed between class I and class II regions and comprise of genes involved in the complement system, tumour necrosis factor [TNF], heat shock proteins [HSP] and a few others with non-immune functions, not directly related to antigen presentation.

Major Histocompatibility Complex Class I Genes

The class I region is the most telomeric part of the MHC complex. Although 36 genes have been defined so far in this region, HLA-A, B and C are the most important since their products have been well defined as 'classical transplantation antigens'. They are characterised by the high degree of polymorphism both in humans as well as most vertebrate species. Other human class I genes that show sequence homology to classical loci include HLA-E, F, G, H, and a set of 5 MHC class I chain related [MIC] genes, MIC A–E. These have reduced expression, restricted to certain tissues, such as, thymus, liver, intestine or placenta, and have low polymorphism. Of the five MIC genes, only MIC-A and MIC-B, situated between the TNF and HLA-B locus, are expressed. Closely related to these genes lies the hemochromatosis disease candidate gene [HFE].

HLA-A, B and C molecules are heterodimer glycoproteins consisting of a MHC-encoded α or the heavy chain of about 45 kDa and a non-MHC-encoded light chain, β2-microglobulin of 12 kDa molecular weight [Figure 6.2] (18). The α chain is some 350 amino acid residues long and can be divided

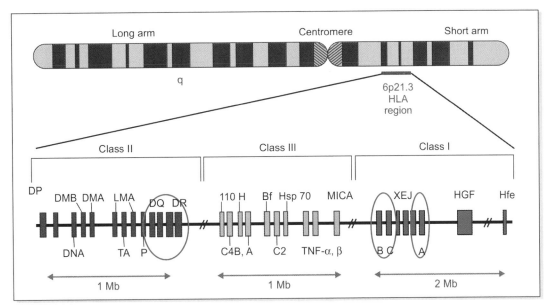

Figure 6.1: Chromosomal location and gene map showing multiple genes within the MHC region on the short arm of chromosome 6 [6p21.3] of man. Classical transplantation loci include HLA-A, B and C in class I and HLA-DR/DQ in the class II region [encircled]. These are highly polymorphic loci in the HLA system with hundreds of alleles already identified in each of them.
MHC = major histocompatibility complex; HLA = human leucocyte antigen
Reproduced with permission from "Mehra NK, Kaur G, editors. The HLA complex in biology and medicine; a resource book. New Delhi: Jaypee Brothers Medical Publishers; 2010 (reference 18)"

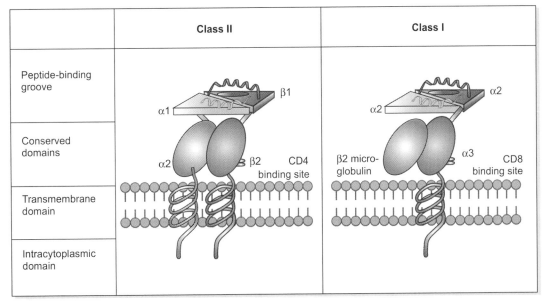

Figure 6.2: Schematic view of HLA class II and class I molecular structures showing the peptide-binding cleft formed between α1 and β1 domains in class II and α1 and α2 domains in class I molecules respectively. The membrane proximal domains [α2, b2 of class II and β2 microglobulin and α3 of class I] are conserved and nonpolymorphic
HLA = human leucocyte antigen
Reproduced with permission from "Mehra NK, Kaur G, editors. The HLA complex in biology and medicine; a resource book. New Delhi: Jaypee Brothers Medical Publishers; 2010 (reference 18)"

into three functional regions: external, transmembrane and intracytoplasmic. The extracellular portion of the heavy chain is folded into three globular domains, α1, α2 and α3, each of which contains stretches of about 90 amino acids encoded by separate exons. While the α1 and α2 domains take part in antigen binding [antigen-binding and presenting domains], the α3 domain is essentially conserved. It contains binding sites for the α chain of the CD8 glycoprotein, which is important for the recognition of antigens by cytotoxic T-cells. The outermost domains [α1 and α2] comprise of two long α helices separated by a cleft with a floor composed of a plane of eight antiparallel β-pleated sheets. The dimension of this cleft [2.5 × 1.0 × 1.1 nm] are suited to accommodate nonamers, but peptides ranging from 10–15 amino acids in length, can also bind, depending on how they fold.

The amino acid side chains of the peptides are accommodated in a series of pockets named from A to F. These peptide positions are critical for binding to specific pockets of a particular HLA class I molecule, hence termed anchors. Pockets A and F lie at the two ends of the peptide-binding groove, are highly conserved among various HLA class I molecules and accommodate the amino and carboxyl terminal residues respectively. Interaction of the peptide with conserved residues in A and F pockets, therefore, anchors it in the binding groove and the process is critical in stabilising the MHC-peptide complex. Although the peptide residues P2 and P9 serve as primary anchors, the residues P1, 3, 6 and 7 act as secondary anchors, and the P4, 5 and 8 interact with the T-cell receptor [TCR].

Major Histocompatibility Complex Class II Genes

The MHC class II region extends over 1000 to 1200 kb with at least six sub-regions, termed DR, DQ, DP, DO, DN and DM. Structurally, the class II molecules are similar to class I molecules and are expressed as heterodimers on the cell surface with one heavy α chain [molecular weight 34 kDa] and one β chain [molecular weight 29 kDa] of integral membrane glycoproteins [Figure 6.2] (18). Three-dimensional structural differences between the two include an altered position of the immunoglobulin-like 2 domain relative to that of the α3 domain of class I HLA, and considerable changes in the peptide-binding site. The α- and β-chains assemble non-covalently to create an antigen-binding cleft located above a conserved membrane proximal structure, which can interact with the CD4 molecule on T-cells. Found mainly on cells of the immune system, including B-cells, macrophages, dendritic cells [DCs] and thymic epithelium, class II molecules display a more limited distribution.

The DR region contains multiple, highly polymorphic β genes and only one invariant α gene. The conventional serologically defined DR molecules [DR1 to DR18] are coded for by the DRB1 gene, whereas the DR52 and DR53 specificities are encoded by the DRB3 and DRB4 genes respectively. DRB2, DRB6, DRB7, DRB8 and DRB9 are pseudogenes without a first domain exon. The DQ sub-region contains five genes, DQA1, DQA2, DQB1, DQB2 and DQB3, of which DQA2, DQB2 and DQB3 are not known to be expressed. In contrast, both DQA1 and DQB1 are functional and polymorphic, expressing four different types of DQ molecules by different 'cis' and 'trans' combinatorial events. The DP sub-region contains two α and two β genes, with DPA2 and DPB2 being pseudogenes. DPB1 shows extensive polymorphism, while DPA1 displays limited polymorphism. DO, DM and DN lie between the DQ and DP loci, and have very limited polymorphism, if any.

Three-dimensional structural analysis has demonstrated that peptides bind to HLA class II molecules in an extended conformation. By contrast to class I bound peptides, the N- and C-termini of class II bound peptides often extend beyond the binding groove. Three asparagine residues [α62Asn, α69Asn and β82Asn], β81His and β61Trp are conserved in all class II molecules and positioned to make hydrogen bonds with the peptide main chain. The α1 and β1 helical regions of most class II molecules are joined by a salt bridge formed between α76Arg and β57sp that stabilises the αβ dimer. Peptides bound by the class II groove twist along the length, progressing approximately three residues for each turn. Successive side chains project from the class II bound peptide at regular intervals, many of which are directed towards the class II molecule. The groove is lined by a series of pockets [P1-P9] that align the peptide to be read as a single unique determinant by the TCR. The size of the hydrophobic P1 pocket is controlled by the Gly/Val dimorphism at position 86 on the beta chain. The deepest and the most commonly used binding pockets are P1 and P9 followed by P4 and P6.

In addition to the above, two other groups of non-HLA genes exist in the MHC class II region. The first group is ABC transporter genes called transporter associated with antigen processing or transporter of antigen peptides 1 and 2 [TAP1 and TAP2] genes. TAP1 and TAP2 gene products associate as a heterodimer that is involved in the transport of antigen fragments produced in the cytoplasm, into the lumen of the endoplasmic reticulum. The second group is the set of proteasome-related genes that includes low molecular mass polypeptide or large multi-functional protease 2 and 7 [LMP2 and LMP7] genes. The products of LMP2 and LMP7 genes are large cytoplasmic proteolytic complex molecules that contain multiple catalytic sites. LMP complex is involved in the production of multiple peptides simultaneously from the same substrate to produce peptides better suited for MHC class I binding.

Major Histocompatibility Complex Class III or Central Genes

The central region of MHC has no structural or functional correlation with the class I or class II region. Presently, at least 39 genes have been located in a 680-kb stretch of deoxyribonucleic acid [DNA] within this region. This includes genes encoding proteins involved in the immune system: the complement genes C4, C2 and factor B [Bf], the TNF-α and TNF-β [lymphotoxin] genes and the HSP70 genes. Further, genes with no obvious association with the immune system have also been identified in this region. These include the valyl transfer ribonucleic acid synthetase [G7] gene. Further, two B-cell associated transcript genes, BAT2 [G2] and BAT3 [G3] are novel genes in the class III region that encode large proline rich proteins with molecular masses of 228 and 110k Da, respectively, while the RD gene encodes a 42-kDa intracellular protein.

Apart from the complement components, this region contains two genes coding for synthesis of the steroid hormone,

21-hydroxylase [CYP21] genes that associate very closely with the C4A and C4B genes. Of these, the CYP21B gene is more functional, and deficiency of this leads to congenital adrenal hyperplasia or salt-wasting disease. The CYP21A gene on the other hand, is most often deleted in certain specific HLA haplotypes, particularly the extended haplotype HLA-A1, B8, DR3, SCO1 in Western Caucasians. Such a haplotype is known to be associated with several autoimmune diseases including type 1 diabetes mellitus in these populations.

BIOLOGICAL FUNCTIONS OF THE HLA GENES

Determination of the crystal structure of the human MHC class I and class II molecules and the identification of the putative peptide binding cleft firmly established that MHC molecules are the principal antigen binding and presenting molecules to the T-cells. Thus, peptide antigens alter the HLA molecule by occupying the cleft to be scrutinised by the T-cell. Zinkernagel and Doherty (19) who were awarded the Nobel Prize for Medicine in 1996 for their epoch making discovery of the anti-viral T-cell recognition first put this concept forward. The fundamental difference in the above process is that whereas class I MHC molecules bind 'endogenous' peptides and eliminate them through the process of cytotoxic T-cell killing [inside out mechanism], the class II molecules, on the other hand, bind peptides derived from 'external' sources [exogenous] and present them to CD4+ helper T-cells [outside in mechanism].

The processing pathway in both situations utilises highly specialised cell machinery that works most effectively. The endogenous proteins in the cytoplasm of the cell are digested into nine to ten amino acid peptides by the LMP complex, a distinct subset of the cellular pool of proteasome. Peptides in the cytoplasm may gain access to the TAP transporter on the membrane of the endoplasmic reticulum [ER] via a specific transporter. Peptides transported into the ER lumen bind to class I molecules, inducing a conformational change that may facilitate their export to the cell surface. The CD8+ cytotoxic T lymphocytes see this MHC-peptide complex through the TCR and other co-receptors, subsequently causing killing of the target cell.

In the class II pathway, the proteolytic enzymes in the endosomal compartment help digest antigens taken from outside the cell into small peptide fragments by endocytosis. The MHC class II molecule with its α and β chains assembles in the ER with the invariant chain to form a stable trimolecular complex which inhibits binding of the endogenous or self-peptides in the ER. The trimolecular complex is efficiently transported out of the ER and is targeted to a post-Golgi compartment in the peripheral cytoplasm. The invariant chain is subsequently cleaved in endosomes, opening up the cleft for peptide occupancy.

The developments of accurate and reproducible high-resolution DNA-based HLA typing methods have significantly improved our ability to define HLA alleles at a single nucleotide difference. Further advanced technologies based on sequencing, mass spectroscopy and DNA chips have now opened up a whole new dimension of studying single nucleotide polymorphisms [SNPs]. Using these procedures, an appreciable number of 'novel alleles' and 'unique HLA haplotypes' have been discovered in the Indian population (20,21).

HLA and Disease Associations

Ever since the first successful demonstration in 1973 of a strong association between the presence of HLA-B27 and ankylosing spondylitis, a large number of diseases have been shown to be associated with variable HLA alleles. The strongest of these associations have been those involving HLA class II region genes with autoimmune and infectious diseases with definitive population based differences [Table 6.1] (22-32). A number of hypotheses have been put forward to explain these observed associations. HLA Class-I [A, B, C] and Class-II [DR, DQ and DP]

Table 6.1: Some of the prominent HLA associations with diseases

Disease	HLA allele
Ankylosing spondylitis	B*27:01 B*27:04 B*27:05
Addison's disease	DRB1*03:01–DQB1*02 and DRB1*04–DQB1*03:02
Behçet's disease	B*51, B*5701
Celiac disease	DQA1*05:01 – DQB1*02:01 DQA1*02:01 – DQB1*02:02 DQA1*03 – DQB1*03:02
Crohn's disease	DRB1*07, DRB1*01:03, DRB1*15:02
Graves disease	DRB1*03:01 – DQA1*05:01 – QB1*02:01 and DRB1*04:01–DQA1*03:01 – DQB1*03:02
HIV disease progression	HLA-B*27, B*57 [slow], B*35[Px] [fast]
Type 1 diabetes mellitus	DRB1*03:01, DQA1*05:01, DQB1*02:0 or DRB1*04:01, DQA1*03:01, DQB1*03:02
Multiple sclerosis	HLA – DRB1*15:01, DQA1*01:02, DQB1*06:02
Narcolepsy	DQB1*06:02, DRB1*15:01 – DQA1*01:02-DQB1*06:02
Psoriasis vulgaris	C*06
Rheumatoid arthritis	DRB1*01:01, DRB1*01:02, DRB1*04:01, DRB1*04:04, DRB1*04:05, DRB1*04:08, DRB1*10:01, DRB1*13:03, DRB1*14:02 and DRB1*14:06
Scleroderma	DRB1*11:04, DQB1*03:01, DRB1*15:02 DQB1*06:01, DQB1*05:01
Sjögren's syndrome	DRB1*03 – DQB1*02 – DQA1*05:01; DRB1*15 – DQB1*06 – DQA1*01:02
Systemic lupus erythematosus	DRB1*03:01, DQB1*02:01, DRB1*15:01, DQB1*06:02

HLA = human leucocyte antigen; HIV = human immunodeficiency virus

alleles could act directly as disease susceptibility agents by means of antigenic crossreactivity or mimicry between infectious agents and the particular HLA molecule ["molecular mimicry"] or by acting directly as receptors for microorganisms. Also, they can direct the immune response by acting as *Ir* genes since the latter are known to regulate immune response to the pathogen. The specific HLA gene may be physically very close to the chromosomal region that might carry a gene conferring susceptibility or resistance to a particular disease. This hypothesis may explain the lack of complete association, and geographical variation in the association accounting for the possible linkage disequilibrium. Further, genetic susceptibility may largely or in part may be due to the involvement of non-HLA genes. Though classical genetic studies in humans and experimental models have clearly documented the primary contribution of the MHC genes, information on the involvement of non-HLA genes in conferring susceptibility or resistance to various diseases is insufficient.

IMMUNOGENETICS OF TUBERCULOSIS

The demonstration that MHC acts as the T-cell restriction element with its linked Ir and/or Is genes has encouraged scientists to look for an association of HLA genes with various diseases at the population level. Several workers have demonstrated an association of HLA alleles [or their extended haplotypes] with diseases caused by known infectious agents. These include hepatitis B virus infection, infectious mononucleosis, viral capsid antigen in Epstein-Barr virus infection, human T-cell lymphotropic virus III [HTLV III] infection and development of Kaposi's sarcoma in patients with acquired immunodeficiency syndrome [AIDS], poliomyelitis, typhoid fever, congenital rubella, etc. In most cases, however, a clear relationship between HLA antigens and susceptibility to infectious diseases has not been established. Several explanations can be put forward to explain this lack of association. One of these relates to the complexity of *Ir* gene effects due to heterozygosity of the MHC gene products. Another contributing factor could be the 'disease heterogeneity' because of the multiplicity of epitope specific antigenic determinants on the infectious agents, which preclude the detection of the effects of HLA encoded factors as risk factors for infection. This antigenic complexity of the invading pathogen leads to an almost incomplete recognition of the relevant products of the HLA system, particularly those in the HLA class II region, which harbours majority of the genes relevant to antigen recognition and T-cell interaction.

Population-based Studies

Among the major infectious diseases, leprosy and TB have emerged as good examples of the role of HLA on susceptibility to infection. Like in leprosy, TB too follows a disease spectrum with the localised disease having limited lung involvement at one end of the spectrum and a more diffuse, disseminated infection at the other. The pathogenesis

of pulmonary TB appears to be due to a detrimental cell-mediated immune response to *Mtb*. Several investigators have searched for an association of the disease with either HLA class I [HLA-A, -B, -C] or class II [HLA-DR, DQ] molecules, both of which might play crucial roles in host susceptibility to pulmonary TB. Table 6.2 summarises the prominent immunogenetic association studies related to HLA and pulmonary TB (7-9,22-32). Majority of these studies point towards the influence of HLA class II region genes in governing susceptibility to the disease, suggesting a strong influence of HLA-DR or DQ linked genes in modulation of the immune response to *Mtb* infection, largely via the cell-mediated immunity (33).

Although only a few studies have addressed the question of the impact of HLA class I polymorphism on TB development, some HLA class I alleles have been reported to be associated with the disease *per se*. These include HLA-A1, HLA-B51, HLA-Cw6 and HLA-Cw7 in Indians (9,23) and HLA-B*1802 and HLA-B*4001 in Indonesians (22). Further analysis revealed that of the various HLA class I loci, alleles in the HLA-B locus play the most dominant role in pulmonary TB development as compared to A or C alleles. HLA-B is the most polymorphic locus within the human MHC and the fundamental genetic variation occurs within exons 2 and 3, known by its determinant function during the presentation of antigenic peptides. Using the interferon-γ [IFN-γ] enzyme linked immunospot [ELISPOT] assay system and following stimulation of T-cell clones with specific *Mtb* synthetic peptide arrays, it has been demonstrated that the immunodominant TB antigen presentation to the CD8+ T-cells is preferentially restricted by HLA-B molecules suggesting that majority of the epitope-specific CD8+ T-cells are HLA-B allele restricted in patients with pulmonary TB (34).

Studies conducted by our group on the population living around Delhi area revealed a significantly increased frequency of HLA-A2 and B44 in pulmonary TB patients as compared to healthy controls (10). Similar association of HLA-A2 with pulmonary TB has earlier been reported in Egyptian patients. Other studies have suggested an association between pulmonary TB and HLA-B15 in North American Blacks and Southern Chinese, HLA-B35 in Northern Chinese, HLA-B5 in Egyptians, HLA-B8 in Canadians and multiple HLA-A and HLA-B specificities in the Russian populations. However, no association of HLA class I antigens with pulmonary TB was reported in Mexican Americans, European Caucasians and Japanese subjects. Such a heterogeneity in HLA class I association in different populations may be due to the ethnic variability of the population groups tested, small number of study groups, poor documentation of their diagnosis. Further, batch variations in HLA antisera used in these studies may also account for the observed heterogeneity. It is also possible that the putative disease susceptibility gene lies in the HLA-class II region [DR/DQ locus] rather than the class I.

The study reported by Balamurugan *et al* (9) in the North Indian population is an attempt to delineate HLA

Table 6.2: Genetic association of important MHC gene variants with susceptibility and/or resistance to tuberculosis and with disease recurrence: summary of selected studies

Study [year] (reference)	HLA allele	Type of association	Population studied	Odds ratio	p-value
Balamurugan et al [2004] (9)	A1	Negative	Indian	ND	<0.001
Yuliwulandri et al [2010] (22)	B*1802	Disease recurrence	Indonesian	ND	<0.013
Yuliwulandri et al [2010] (22)	B*4001	Disease recurrence	Indonesian	ND	<0.015
Vijaya Lakshmi et al [2006] (23)	B51	Positive	Indian	18.5	<0.001
Vijaya Lakshmi et al [2006] (23)	B52	Negative	Indian	0	<0.003
Balamurugan et al [2004] (9)	Cw6	Negative	Indian	ND	<0.001
Balamurugan et al [2004] (9)	Cw7	Positive	Indian	ND	<0.001
Singh et al [1983] (7,8)	DR2	Positive	Indian	ND	<0.05
Brahmajothi et al [1991] (24)	DR2	Positive	Indian	0.29	0.01
Ravi Kumar et al [1999] (25)	DRB1*1501	Positive	Indian	2.68	0.013
Shi et al [2011] (26)	DRB1*15	Positive	Chinese	3.79	0.001
Dubaniewicz et al [2000] (27)	DRB1*16	Positive	Polish	9.7	<0.01
Lombard et al [2006] (28)	DQB1*0301-*0304	Positive	South Africa	2.58	0.001
Harfouch-Hammoud and Daher [2008] (29)	DRB1*04	Positive	Syrian	1.77	0.01
Harfouch-Hammoud and Daher [2008] (29)	DRB1*11	Negative	Syrian	0.51	0.003
Yuliwulandari et al [2010] (22)	DRB1*1101	Disease recurrence	Indonesian	ND	0.008
Yuliwulandari et al [2010] (22)	DRB1*1202	Disease recurrence	Indonesian	0.32	0.0008
Dubaniewicz et al [2000] (27)	DRB1*13	Negative	Polish	0.04	<0.001
Lombard et al [2006] (28)	DRB1*1302	Positive	South Africa	5.05	<0.001
Amirzargar et al [2004] (30)	DRB1*07	Positive	Iranian	2.7	0.025
Kim et al [2005] (31)	DRB1*0803	Disease recurrence	Korean	5.31	0.00009
Amirzargar et al [2004] (30)	DQA1*0301	Negative	Iranian	0.25	0.033
Vejbaesya et al [2002] (32)	DQA1*0601	Negative	Thai	ND	0.02
Vejbaesya et al [2002] (32)	DQB1*0301	Negative	Thai	ND	0.01
Vejbaesya et al [2002] (32)	DQB1*0502	Positive	Thai	2.06	0.01
Ravi Kumar et al [1999] (25)	DQB1*0601	Positive	Indian	2.32	0.008
Kim et al [2005] (31)	DRB1*0601	Disease recurrence	Korean	5.45	0.00003

MHC = major histocompatibility complex; ND = not described

class I association in TB on the basis of a shared 'sequence motif' in peptide-binding pockets of the HLA molecules. The rationale of such an analysis is that although HLA is highly polymorphic, small degree of genetic polymorphism may or may not affect peptide presentation and molecular function. Accordingly among the genetically related alleles, each HLA molecule could preferentially bind peptides with certain anchor residues and present the same to the CD8+ T-cells. However, within these allelic groups, there could be shared peptide epitopes and a considerable overlap in the peptide binding capacity. Therefore, there is a need to analyze functional differences in the variable peptide presenting HLA class I molecules. Based on the similarities of peptide binding pockets [B and F] and the preference of identical peptide motifs, nine different supertypes covering most if not all HLA class I alleles have been reported (35). The specificities of the anchor residues are determined by the amino acid sequences that constitute the peptide binding pockets as described by the crystallographic studies. In the Indian study (9), the class I supertypes were evaluated for their possible association with TB by comparing the data with a set of healthy controls belonging to the same ethnic background and socio-economic status. The data revealed a strong positive association of 'HLA-A3 like' and a negative association of 'HLA-A1 like' supertypes particularly in patients with more severe forms of the disease such as miliary, disseminated and/or multidrug-resistant TB [MDR-TB].

HLA Class II Association Studies

Beginning with studies representing a strong association of HLA-DR2 with pulmonary TB in the North Indian population (7,8), several workers have tried to search for similar association in other populations. The first such report came from north India (7) where a moderate increase of HLA-DR2 was demonstrated in sporadic patients with pulmonary TB. The same investigators while confirming these results using multiplex family studies further suggested an HLA-DR2 linked control of susceptibility to the disease (8). This association was later confirmed in several other populations, including south Indians and Chinese (24,36), Indonesians (37) and Russians (38). However, others could not confirm this association in studies carried out on Egyptians (39), North American Blacks (40), Mexican Americans (41), as well as in a study on South Indian patients (42). Except for the latter study, all other studies up until then were based on serological testing of expressed HLA antigens on the surface of lymphocytes. It may be mentioned that there is up to 25% discrepancy in DR typing results by serology when compared with the more sensitive molecular techniques of polymerase chain reaction-sequence specific oligonucleotide probe [PCR-SSOP] hybridisation. Besides being sensitive, these techniques allow definition of molecular subtypes of several serologically defined HLA-DR specificities, differing even at a single nucleotide level. Hence, HLA and disease association studies using molecular techniques provide the most relevant information on the critical amino acid residues in the peptide-binding groove of the MHC, rather than only an associated allele.

Studies in other populations revealed variable HLA allelic association with TB, for example HLA-DRB1*04 in the Syrian population (29), HLA-DRB1*07 and HLA-DQA1*0101 in Iranians (30), HLA-DRB1*11 in Indonesians (22), and HLA-DRB1*1302 in South Africans (28). Similarly, HLA-DRB1*0803 and HLA- DQB1*0601 were reported to be associated with pulmonary TB disease advancement in Koreans while a strong association with resistance to recurrent pulmonary TB was observed with HLA-DRB1*12 in Indonesians (22,31). A summary analysis of all these studies point towards HLA-DR2 or its major molecular subtypes, *1501 or *1502 as the main allelic variants that show a positive association with pulmonary TB in most populations. Taken together, HLA and TB association data suggests that amino acids present in the DRB1*15 molecule [but absent in DRB1*16 which is the other major subtype of HLA-DR2] could play an important role in disease development. Nevertheless, this data does not exclude the involvement of other immune associated or linked genes, either within or outside of the human MHC. The nucleotide sequence of peptides presented by DRB1*15 alleles are very different from those presented by DRB1*16 alleles. From the mechanistic point of view, the former set of peptides may be recognised by CD4+ T-lymphocytes in an inadequate form and consequently this situation could disturb the effective immune associated anti-TB response. At the more functional level, it has been suggested that both HLA-DRB1*1501 and *1502 may be associated with down-regulation of perforin positive cytotoxic cells [T-lymphocytes and natural killer] in pulmonary TB, supporting the potential role of theses alleles in the TB susceptibility (43). On the other hand,

HLA-DRB1*16 but not HLA-DRB1*15 is observed more frequently in Brazilian leprosy patients than in the controls group [9.0% vs 1.8%; p = 0.0016; odds ratio = 5.81; 95% confidence intervals = 2.05 to 15.45], underlying a difference in the impact of MHC polymorphism which may be related to the specificity of each pathology (44).

Almost all published studies on HLA association with TB have been performed in patients with pulmonary form of the disease, while no substantial data are available regarding the extrapulmonary disease. The authors' group had investigated HLA association with various clinical subgroups including pulmonary TB, MDR-TB, miliary, disseminated TB as well as lymph node TB. High resolution molecular subtyping of polymorphic DRB1 alleles revealed that in addition to the increased occurrence of *1501/*02 subtypes of HLA-DR2, a positive association was also observed with specific HLA-DR6 subtypes, in particular DRB1*1301 in patients with pulmonary TB and MDR-TB and DRB1* 1302 in extrapulmonary TB [miliary, disseminated TB and lymph node TB]. Although the DR2 associated haplotype association has been reported earlier also in pulmonary TB (45), the existence of additional DR6 associated haplotypes [both DRB1*13 and DRB1*14] in other clinical forms of TB indicates that alleles with similar 'sequence motif' in the peptide binding groove may influence susceptibility to *Mtb* infection and subsequent development of severe clinical disease.

Data on the clinical and immunogenetic association for the development of MDR-TB suggest that, in addition to poor past compliance to treatment and presence of higher number of cavities in the chest radiographs, presence of HLA-DRB1*14 allele in patients with pulmonary TB acts as an independent predictor for the development of MDR-TB (46). Also, the development of hepatotoxicity during anti-TB treatment was found to be asso-ciated with alleles in the DQ locus, namely DQA1*0102 and DQB1*020 (47).

Family Studies and Haplotypic Association

The observed variability of the associated HLA alleles in different ethnic groups indicates that genes controlling host response to mycobacteria may be 'linked' but not situated around the HLA class I and II molecules, and hence, reveal different linkage disequilibria in different populations. In order to understand the mode of inheritance or HLA-linked control of disease susceptibility, family studies particularly those with at least two affected sibs are most informative. Such studies conducted by us provided the first conclusive evidence for an important role of HLA-linked genes in governing susceptibility to pulmonary TB (7,8). Combined data from other populations also support an HLA-linked control of susceptibility to pulmonary TB with a dominant rather than a recessive mode of inheritance. This is in contrast to the situation in tuberculoid leprosy, where the data favours recessive mode of inheritance (48).

In a meta-analysis [1988 patients and 2897 controls], a lower risk of thoracic TB was found in carriers of HLA-B13,

DR3, and DR7 antigens, while patients positive for HLA-DR8 were at higher risk (33). The risk of thoracic TB tended to be higher in carriers of HLA-DR2 and its major molecular subtypes, although the results were not consistent between studies.

In the *Saharia* tribal population in central India, a significantly higher occurrence of pulmonary TB is evident compared with other tribal population in the same region. A three locus haplotype analysis of HLA-A, B and DR alleles in the *Saharia* tribal population revealed a significantly increased frequency of A24*-B40*-DRB1*15 haplotype and a significantly reduced frequency of A*02-B*40-DRB1*16 and A*02-B*40-DRB1*03 haplotype among TB patients compared to control subjects (49). Another two locus haplotype study involving HLA-MICA revealed a negative association of haplotype HLA-B*18-MICA*018 with the disease (50).

The mechanisms by which anti-TB drug resistance emerges is not completely understood. *In vitro* studies have identified several determinants of resistance to the main anti-TB drugs, but whole-genome analyses suggest that response to drug exposure might be much more complex than initially thought and involves a set of strategies developed by mycobacteria to enhance their ability to adapt and evolve. Recent research suggests that bacterial fitness might play a pivotal role in the spread of antibiotic-resistant *Mtb*. *In vitro*, bacterial fitness is determined by the interplay of numerous factors including the growth deficits incurred by resistance mutations, strain genetic background, and compensatory evolution. The involvement of HLA in TB drug-resistance has been evaluated in a study from Kazakhstan evaluating the HLA genes by sequence-based typing [SBT]. It was observed that HLA-DQA1*03:02 HLA-DRB1*08:01 and DRB1*08:03 occurred more frequently in patients with drug-resistant TB than in controls (51). The growing threat of MDR-TB and extensively drug resistant-TB [XDR-TB] highlights the need for a better understanding of the complexity of drug resistance following *Mtb* infection and the host susceptibility index determined by HLA genes. This shall allow the development of enhanced diagnostic tests to identify resistant strains, HLA-susceptible individuals and strategies to curb *Mtb* spread, and also help in the design of more potent anti-TB drugs.

High Resolution Analysis of Molecular Subtypes of HLA-DR2 in Mycobacterial Diseases

The frequency of HLA alleles in the North Indian population has revealed that two alleles, namely DRB1*1501 and DRB1*1502 constitute greater than 90% of the DR2 alleles in this population. Other alleles such as DRB1*1506 and DRB1*1602 are represented at much decreased frequencies. For example, DRB1*1601 occurs in only 4% of the DR2+ healthy individuals in this population. Studies carried out both in north as well as south India have indicated a population association of DRB1*1501 [rather than other subtypes of DR2] in patients with TB.

Sequence analysis of the DRB1 first domain residues has disclosed that only one amino acid variation can discriminate the products of DRB1*1501 from DRB1*1502 and DRB1*1601 from DRB1*1602. Particularly DRB1*1501 carries valine at amino acid position 86 while it is substituted with glycine in DRB1*1502. Similarly, DRB1*1601 subtype has the aromatic amino acid phenylalanine at position 67 which is substituted by aliphatic leucine in DRB1*1602. Studies on pulmonary TB did not favor a preferential involvement of any of these common subtypes of DR2 suggesting that the whole DR2 molecule or its closely linked gene[s] may be involved in governing susceptibility to pulmonary TB and the expression of its various clinical forms. However, analysis of DR2 subtypes and the differences in radiographic severity based on the extent of lung lesions unilateral limited [UL], unilateral extensive [UE], bilateral limited [BL] and bilateral extensive [BE] revealed an increased trend in the frequency of DRB1*1501 as the pulmonary severity increased from UL to BE lung lesions.

It has also been observed that the distribution of DR2 subtypes in TB based on the valine/glycine [V/G] dimorphism at codon $\beta86$ revealed an inverse association with V^{86} and G^{86} as the pulmonary severity increased from UL to BE lung lesions. Similar, inverse relationship of V^{86}/G^{86} has also been observed in leprosy as the disease severity progressed from paucibacillary to the borderline lepromatous [BL]/lepromatous [LL] multibacillary leprosy.

Knowledge on the three dimensional crystallography structure of the human class II HLA molecule has revealed that residues at position 67 and 86 of the α-helix of the β-chain are actively involved in the binding of a foreign peptide. Accordingly, the peptide binding and subsequent immune triggering capability of the host depends critically on these single amino acid variants. It is possible that DRB1*1501 and 1502 alleles may be selectively implicated in the presentation of pathogenic mycobacterial peptides leading to development of pulmonary TB.

The amino acid sequence analysis of the associated HLA-DRB1 genes in tuberculoid leprosy has yielded crucial information on critical sites in the peptide-binding groove of the DR molecule that affects peptide binding and/or T-cell interaction in immune response against mycobacteria. A large majority of patients [87%] carry specific alleles of DRB1 characterised by positive charged residues Arg^{13} or Arg^{70} or Arg^{71} as compared to 43% controls conferring a relative risk of 8.8. Thus, susceptibility to tuberculoid leprosy involves three critical amino acid positions of the β-chain, the side chains of which when modelled on the DR1 crystal structure, line 'pocket 4' accommodating the side chain of a bound peptide. Characteristically, 'pocket 4' is formed by the side chains of amino acids α^9, β^{13}, β^{70}, β^{71}, β^{74} and β^{78}. Substitutions of any of these can affect the local charge. For example, presence of positively charged Arg at position 13 and/or at position 70 or 71 will probably bind negatively charged residue of the same foreign peptide and stimulate particular T-cell clones leading to a detrimental immune response as seen in tuberculoid leprosy. Hence, identification of peptide motifs that bind disease associated HLA alleles would contribute significantly to the search for mycobacterial antigenic determinants. Similarly, sequence analysis of HLA class II alleles in TB could help identify critical amino acid residues for binding of *Mtb* derived pathogenic peptide[s] responsible for the detrimental/protective immune response. This has potential implications in immune interventions therapies in pulmonary TB.

NON-HLA GENES IN TUBERCULOSIS

Most of the classical genetic association studies in TB have targeted the HLA-associated immune response genes. Using the candidate gene-based approach; several risk, protection conferring non-HLA immune related genes have also been implicated with TB susceptibility in recent years. These include toll-like receptors [TLRs], vitamin D receptor [VDR], dendritic cell-specific intercellular adhesion molecule-3-grabbing non-integrin [DC-SIGN], solute carrier family 11 [proton-coupled divalent metal ion transporters], member 1 [SLC11A], formerly known as natural resistance associated macrophage protein 1 [NRAMP1] and others. A large number of variants in these genes show an association with susceptibility to TB infection with population specific genetic differences highlighted in various studies. Here, we have attempted to summarise some of these common associations with a brief description on each of them [Table 6.3] (52-102).

Chemokines and Cytokines

Chemokines play an important role in the recruitment of immune cells to the site of infection and the description of these immune regulatory molecules is beyond the scope of this chapter. The monocyte chemoattractant protein-1 which is encoded by the C-C chemokine ligand 2 gene [CCL2] is known to be involved in granuloma formation, and thereby, containment of *Mtb* infection in the lungs. Transition from adenine to guanine at position -2518 is known to increase the expression levels of this chemokine and the G allele has been shown to be associated with TB susceptibility in Mexicans and Koreans (53) but not in South African (54) and Brazilians (103). On the other hand, a protective effect of the -2518 G allele along with another allelic variant -362 C with resistance to TB has been reported in the population of Ghana (52). Similarly, chemokine [C-X-C motif] ligand 10 [CXCL10] and its -135 A allele has been shown to be associated with protection against TB infection (62).

Among cytokines, IFN-γ variant, +874A allele with reduced expression is associated with TB infection or severity in various studies (93). The regulatory cytokine interleukin [IL]-10 that suppresses the Th1 responses and its variant -1082 is associated with TB in the Turkish (72) and Colombian populations (89) but not in South Indians (82), Pakistanis (88) and Ghanians (104). TNF-α leads to inflammation in TB and a SNP at position -308 with G to A transition was found to be associated with resistance to TB infection in Colombians (77). However, no such association was observed in the Turkish (72), Thai (74), Cambodian (76)

and south Indian (75) populations. Another inflammatory cytokine, IL-1 showed an association of IL-1B +3953 C to T transition with resistance to TB in Colombians (78). In addition, an intronic variant rs 4252019 T allele and a microsatellite polymorphism in IL-1RA gene were found to influence susceptibility to TB in North Indian (80) and Ghana (79) populations respectively. In North Indians, risk conferring association of T allele of rs2070874 [C/T] variant of IL-4 [drives Th2 response], IL1-12 variants rs3212220 [G/T, T allele] and rs 2853694 [A/C, A allele] with pulmonary TB was also observed. Another commonly studied variant is IL-12B +1188A/C [rs3212227] that showed a positive association in the Chinese (84) but not in African-Americans, Caucasians (83) and South Indians (81,82).

Toll-like Receptors

Toll-like receptors are a family of pathogen recognition receptors [PRRs] consisting of 12 members in mammals. They are expressed on the surface of cell membrane or on the membrane of endocytic vesicles of mainly immune cells including macrophages and DCs. Although interaction of *Mtb* with TLRs leads to phagocytic activation, the interaction itself does not cause immediate ingestion of the mycobacteria. Following interaction of specific mycobacterial structures with TLRs, signalling pathways are triggered in which adaptor molecule, myeloid differentiation primary response protein 88 [MyD88] plays an important role. Subsequently, IL-1 receptor-associated kinases [IRAK], TNF receptor-associated factor 6 [TRAF6], transforming growth factor-beta [TGF-β] activated protein kinase1 [TAK1] and mitogen-activated protein [MAP] kinase are recruited in a signaling cascade leading to activation and nuclear translocation of transcription factors such as nuclear factor-κB [NF-κB]. This leads to transcription of genes involved in the activation of the innate host defense, mainly the production of proinflammatory cytokines, such as, TNF, IL1β, and IL-12 and nitric oxide.

The TLRs known to be involved in the recognition of *Mtb* including TLR2, TLR4, TLR9, and possibly TLR8. Several investigators have reported an association of various TLR variants with the TB infection and disease severity. Description of only some of these is discussed here. An association of the T allele of TLR2 variant Arg677Trp [2029 C/T, rs5743706] with TB infection in the Tunisian population (68) and of allele A of TLR2 Arg753Gln [rs5743708G/A] variant in the Turkish population with disease susceptibility (69) has been reported. Similarly an association of the short [≤16 GT] repeats of the microsatellite in intron II of the TLR2 gene with TB infection has been reported in the Koreans (70). In North Indians, the TLR4 variant 896A/G [Asp299Gly] revealed strong association with TB susceptibility (105). Further extensive genotyping of different TLRs revealed that the ins/ins genotype of ins/del variant -196 to -174 of TLR2 was protective against TB infection in the US Caucasian and West African TB cohorts but not in the African Americans (71).

Table 6.3: Summary of candidate gene studies of non-HLA immunogenetic variants and their associations with TB

Gene [Loci]	Function	Genetic variant	Population studied	Association	Study [year] (reference)
CCL2 [17q12]	Encodes monocyte chemoattractant protein involved in recruitment of immune cells and granuloma formation	−2518 A/G [rs 1024611]	Ghanaians	G allele associated with resistance to PTB	Thye et al [2009] (52)
			Mexican	G allele associated with TB susceptibility	Flores Villanueva et al [2005] (53)
			Korean	G allele associated with TB susceptibility	
			Russian	No association	Moller et al [2009] (54)
			South African	No association	
		−362 G/C rs2857656	Ghanaian	C allele associated with resistance to PTB	Thye et al [2009] (52)
CD209 [19p13]	Encodes DC-SIGN, a cell surface receptors for mycobacteria on dendritic cells	−871 A/G	South African	G allele associated with resistance to PTB	Barreiro et al [2006] (55)
			Tunisian	No association with TB	Ben-Ali et al [2007] (56)
		−336 A/G [rs 4804803]	Gambian	G allele protective in Gambian but variable outcome in other African populations. GG homozygosity associated with decreased risk of lung cavitatory TB	Vannberg et al [2008] (57)
			South Indian	No association with TB	Selvaraj et al [2009] (58)
			South African	A allele associated with resistance to PTB	Barreiro et al [2006] (55)
			Tunisian	No association with TB	Ben Ali et al [2007] (56)
			Colombian	No association with TB	Gomez et al [2006] (59)
CD14 [5q31]	CD14 plays a role in recognition of bacterial cell wall components and lipopolysaccharides by macrophages	−159 C/T [rs 2569190]	Mexican	TT homozygosity associated with higher risk of TB	Rosas-Taraco et al [2007] (60)
			Colombian	No association with PTB	Pacheco et al [2004] (61)
CXCL10 [4q21]	CXCL10 plays an important role in early immune response against respiratory tract pathogens	−1447 A/G [rs4508917]	Chinese	No association with TB	Tang et al [2009] (62)
		−872 G/A [rs4256246]	Chinese	No association with TB	
		−135 G/A	Chinese	A allele associated with protection against TB	
Gc [4q13]	Group specific component variants of vitamin D binding protein are involved in antimycobacterial immunity	Gc variants	UK [Gujarati]	Gc2/Gc2 genotype associated with TB susceptibility	Martineau et al [2010] (63)
			Brazil	No association with TB	
			South Africa	No association with TB	
PTPN22 [1p13]	PTPN22 gene encodes immunoregulatory molecule intracellular lymphoid specific phosphatase [Lyp]	788 G/A [rs 33996649]	Morocco	A allele associated with susceptibility to PTB	Lamsyah et al [2009] (64)
		1858 C/T [rs 2476601]	Morocco	T allele associated with resistance to PTB	
VDR [12q13]	VDR is the receptor for active form of vitamin D and has immunomodulatory effects	Taq1 T/C [rs 731236]	Gambians	TT homozygosity associated with protection against TB	Bellamy et al [1999] (65)

Contd…

Contd...

Gene [Loci]	Function	Genetic variant	Population studied	Association	Study [year] (reference)
		Taq1	Meta-analysis [Asia]	No association	Gao et al [2010] (66)
		Bsml	Meta-analysis [Asia]	bb genotype associated with protection against TB	
			Meta-analysis [Africa]	No association	
		Fokl	Meta-analysis [Asia]	If genotype associated with susceptibility to TB	
			Meta-analysis [Africa]	No association	
		Cdx-2 G/A	South Indian	G allele and GG homozygosity associated with protection against TB	Selvaraj et al [2008] (67)
TLR2 [4q32]	TLR2 is involved in recognition of mycobacteria by APCs	Arg677Trp [2029 C/T] [rs 5743706]	Tunisian	T allele associated with TB infection	Ben-Ali et al [2004] (68)
		Arg753Gln [G/A] [rs 5743708]	Turkish	A allele associated with TB infection	Ogus et al [2004] (69)
		Intron II [GT]n microsatellite	Korean	Association of shorter repeats with ≤16 GT with TB disease	Yim et al [2006] (70)
		Ins/del [−196 to −174]	USA [Caucasians]	Insertion/Insertion genotype associated with protection against PTB	Velez et al [2010] (71)
			USA [African-Americans]	No association	
			Guinea-Bissau	Insertion/Insertion genotype associated with protection against PTB	
TLR9 [3p21]	TLR9 regulates Th1 responses and cooperates with TLR2 in mediating resistance against TB	rs 352143 [G/A]	USA [African-Americans]	AA genotype associated with resistance to PTB	Velez et al [2010] (71)
			USA [Caucasians]	AA genotype associated with resistance to PTB	
			Guinea-Bissau	No association	
		rs 5743836 [C/T]	USA [African-Americans]	TT genotype associated with resistance to PTB	
			USA [Caucasians]	TT genotype associated with resistance to PTB	
			Guinea-Bissau	No association	
TNF-α [6p21]	TNF-α leads to inflammation in TB	−308 G/A [rs 1800629]	Turkish	No association with TB	Ates et al [2008] (72)
			Korean	No association with TB	Oh et al [2007] (73)
			Thai	No association with TB	Vejbaesya et al [2007] (74)
			South Indian	No association with TB	Selvaraj et al [2001] (75)

Contd...

Contd...

Contd...

Gene [Loci]	Function	Genetic variant	Population studied	Association	Study [year] (reference)
			Cambodian	No association with PTB	Delgado et al [2002] (76)
			Colombian	G allele associated with TB	Correa et al [2005] (77)
		-238 G/A [rs 361525]	Colombian	A allele associated with susceptibility to TB	
			Colombian	Protective effect of haplotype TNF-308A -238G	
IL-1 [2q14]	IL-1 mediates fever and inflammation in TB	IL-1B +3953 C/T [rs 1143634]	Colombian	T allele associated with protection	Gomez et al [2006] (78)
IL-1 RA [2q14]	IL-1 RA is a receptor antagonist which bind nonproductively to IL-1 receptor	Microsatellite	Gambian	Microsatellite alleles influence TB	Bellamy et al [1998] (79)
		Intronic variant rs 4252019 C/T	North Indians	T allele associated with higher risk of PTB	Abhimanyu et al [2012] (80)
IL-2 [4q27]	IL-2 is a mediator of the immune activation	-330 G/T [rs2069762]	South Indians	TT homozygosity associated with protection from PTB	Selvaraj et al [2008] (81)
IL-4 [5q31]	Drives and mediate Th2 response	rs 2070874 [C/T]	North Indians	T allele associated with higher risk of PTB	Abhimanyu et al [2012] (80)
IL-12 [5q33]	IL-12 drives a Th1 response	IL-12B +1188 A/C [rs 3212227]	South Indian	No association with PTB	Prabhu Anand et al [2007] (82), Selvaraj et al [2008] (81)
			African-American and Caucasians	No association with TB	Ma et al [2003] (83)
			Chinese	Associated with TB	Tso et al [2004] (84)
		rs 3212220 [G/T]	North Indians	T allele associated with PTB	Abhimanyu et al [2012] (80)
		rs 2853694 [A/C]	North Indians	A allele associated with PTB	
IL-12 RB1 [19p13]	IL-12 RB1 encodes a receptor chain for IL-12	-2 C/T	Moroccan	T allele associated with PTB	Remus et al [2004] (85)
			Indonesian	No association with TB	Sahiratmadja et al [2007] (86)
		+641 A/G, +1094 T/C and +1132 G/C	Japanese	+641, +1094 and +1132 associated with TB susceptibility and severity	Kusuhara et al [2007] (87)
IL-10 [1q32]	Suppress TNF and Th1 [IFN-γ] responses	-1082 A/G [rs 1800896]	Turkish	G allele associated with TB in Turkish population, no effects of -819 C/T and -592 C/A	Ates et al [2008] (72)
			South Indian	No association with PTB	Prabhu Anand et al [2007] (82)
			Pakistan	No association with PTB	Ansari et al [2009] (88)
			Colombian	AA homozygosity associated with pleural TB	Henao et al [2006] (89)
IFN-γ [12q15]	Activates monocytes to kill engulfed mycobacteria [mediates Th1 responses]	+874 T/A [rs 2430561]	Spanish	A allele associated with TB susceptibility	Lopez-Maderuelo et al [2003] (90)
			Pakistan	Associated with PTB	Ansari et al [2009] (88)

Contd...

Gene [Loci]	Function	Genetic variant	Population studied	Association	Study [year] (reference)
			Chinese	AA homozygosity associated with TB susceptibility	Ding et al [2008] (91)
				AA homozygosity associated with TB susceptibility	Tso et al [2005] (92)
				Associated with protection against TB in meta-analysis of different ethnicities	Pacheco et al [2008] (93)
			Colombian	T allele associated with pleural TB	Henao et al [2006] (89)
		Intronic SNP rs1861493 [A/G]	North Indian	A allele associated with higher risk of PTB	Abhimanyu et al [2012] (80)
		Intronic SNP rs1861494 [C/T]	North Indian	T allele associated with higher risk of PTB	Abhimanyu et al [2012] (80)
IFNγR1 [6q23]	IFNγR1 encodes ligand binding chain [alpha] of IFN-γ	−1616 G/A	West Africans	GG homozygosity associated with TB susceptibility	Cooke et al [2006] (94)
		+3234 T/C		TT homozygosity associated with TB susceptibility	
		−56 T/C		CC homozygosity associated with TB susceptibility	
		[CA]n microsatellite		Homozygosity of [CA] 12 allele associated protection	Sahiratmadja et al [2007] (86)
SLC11A1 [2q35]	SLC11A1 gene encodes a divalent cation transporter which is recruited to the phagolysosomal membrane on activation of macrophages	Intron 7 −81C/T rs 3731863	USA [Caucasians]	Associated with TB infection	Velez et al [2009] (95)
		Intron 4 +14G/C rs 3731865	USA [African Americans]	Associated with TB infection	
		G249G rs 17221959	USA [Caucasians]	Associated with TB infection	
		D543N [G/A] rs 17235409	Chinese	Associated with susceptibility to PTB	Leung et al [2007] (96)
				Heterozygosity associated with severe forms of PTB	Zhang et al [2005] (97)
			Gambian	Associated with susceptibility to PTB	Bellamy et al [1998] (98)
			Japanese	Associated with susceptibility to PTB	Gao et al [2000] (99)
			Cambodian	Associated with susceptibility to PTB	Delgado et al [2002] (76)
		3'UTR TGTG+/ del rs 17235416	Korean	Associated with TB pleurisy	Kim et al [2003] (100)
			Danish	No association with TB	Soborg et al [2002] (101)
NOS2A [17q11]	NOS2A gene encodes iNOS	Int G/T rs 2274894	USA [Caucasians]	No association with TB	Velez et al [2009] (102)
			USA [African-Americans]	Associated with susceptibility to TB	
		3'UTR C/T rs 7215373	USA [Caucasians]	No association with TB	
			USA [African-Americans]	Associated with susceptibility to TB	

HLA = human leucocyte antigen; TB = tuberculosis; CCL2 = C-C chemokine ligand 2; PTB = pulmonary tuberculosis; DC-SIGN = dendritic cell-specific intercellular adhesion molecule-3-grabbing non-integrin; CXCL10 = chemokine [C-X-C motif] ligand 10; PTPN22 = protein tyrosine phosphatase non-receptor type 22; VDR = vitamin D receptor; TLR = toll-like receptor; APCs = antigen presenting cells; TNF-α = tumour necrosis factor-alpha; IL = interleukin; IFN-γ = interferon-gamma; SLC11A1 = solute carrier family 11 [proton-coupled divalent metal ion transporters], member 1; NOS2 = nitric oxide synthase 2; iNOS = inducible nitric oxide synthase

Further, homozygosity for AA and TT in the TLR9 variants rs352143 [G/A] and rs 5743836 [C/T] respectively were found to be associated with resistance to infection in African-Americans and US Caucasians but not West Africans.

Nitric Oxide Synthase 2 Gene

Nitric oxide synthase 2 gene [NOS2A] gene encodes inducible nitric oxide synthase [iNOS], a cytoplasmic protein which is produced in response to cytokines and infection (106). Nitric oxide [NO] is a gaseous signalling molecule that plays an important role in host defense against TB and other infections. In South Africans, a haplotype consisting of rs9282799 and rs8078340 was found to be associated with TB (54). Others reported an association of rs2274894 and rs7215373 with TB in African Americans but not with Caucasians (102).

CD209 [DC-SIGN]

The CD209 gene encodes the C type lectin DC-SIGN which is the *Mtb* receptor on dendritic cells. An association of two promoter SNPs [-871G and -336A] with resistance to pulmonary TB was reported in South Africans (55). On the other hand, a -336G SNP was associated with protection in the Gambian population (57) while studies carried out in the Indian (58), Colombian (59) and Tunisian (56) populations showed no association of these variants with the disease.

Protein Tyrosine Phosphatase Non-receptor Type 22

The protein tyrosine phosphatase non receptor type 22 [PTPN22] gene encodes for an intracellular lymphoid specific phosphatase [Lyp] that regulates activation of T and B cells. The genetic variations influencing expression of this phosphatase affects the TB infection and the polymorphism 1858 T was found to be associated with resistance to TB in Morocco (64).

Vitamin D Receptor

Previous studies have found an association between vitamin D deficiency and susceptibility to active TB. The 1,25 dihydroxy vitamin D3 suppresses the growth of *Mtb* *in vitro* and its supplementation may enhance antimicrobial activity. A group specific component vitamin D binding protein [DBP] gene, called GC, encodes the DBP. This serum glycoprotein is involved in the transport of vitamin D and its metabolites to various tissues. On the basis of two SNPs in GC, three electrophoretic variants have been defined which differ in their binding affinity for active form of vitamin D. The GC2/GC2 genotype was reported to be associated with the susceptibility to TB in the Gujarati Asians but not in Brazilians and south Africans (63). Further, the VDR as a receptor for the vitamin D [active metabolite form] is known to have several immune regulatory effects. An association between Bsm1 and Fok1 genotypes in VDR and TB was observed in Asians but not in Africans or South Americans (66).

In a study from South India, the GG homozygosity of Cdx-2G/A variant was found to be associated with resistance to the TB infection (67).

Solute Carrier Family 11 Member 1

SLC11A1 [formerly known as natural resistance associated macrophage protein 1, NRAMP1] gene encodes a divalent cation transporter which is recruited to the phagolysosomal membrane on activation of macrophages. Genetic studies suggest that this transporter is associated with susceptibility to TB in humans (98). Genotyping of the various NRAMP1 polymorphisms revealed an association of at least one SNP in African Americans and of two in Caucasians with susceptibility to TB (95). In the Chinese population, variant D543N G/A showed an association with susceptibility to pulmonary TB and its presence in heterozygous state associated with severe forms of the disease (96,97). In another SNP study of the same gene conducted on the Gambians, Japanese and the Cambodian cohorts, patients carrying the SNP allele 2 were found to be susceptible for pulmonary TB (76,98,99). Similarly, an association of 3'UTR TGTG ins/del variant [rs17235416] with tuberculous pleurisy was observed in Koreans (100) while no such association was observed in the Danish population (101).

Genome-wide Association Studies

The GWAS involve unbiased [hypothesis free] analysis of thousands of genetic markers across the human genome for identification of disease association markers, and therefore, can identify new susceptibility loci for infectious diseases. Though evidence from twin studies suggests a strong genetic component to TB resistance; so far only a few statistically important loci have been identified in GWAS on TB. Thye and coworkers (107) combined two TB GWAS [from the Gambia and Ghana] with subsequent replication in a total of 11,425 individuals. In a gene-poor region on chromosome 18q11.2, a variant rs4331426 was found associated with disease {combined $P = 6.8 \times 10[-9]$, odds ratio = 1.19, 95% CI = 1.13-1.27} (107). Most of the genome-wide linkage and association studies have been performed in African populations. Recently, in an attempt to identify population specific novel targets, a multi-stage GWAS conducted in a cohort of the Indonesian [South-East Asia] population, 8 independent loci showed an evidence of association and these were located within or near the following signalling genes of the immune system: gene encoding protein-jagged 1 [JAG1], dynein, light chain, roadblock-type 2 [DYNLRB2], early B-Cell factor 1 [EBF1], transmembrane protein with EGF-Like and two follistatin-like domains 2 [TMEFF2], chemokine [C-C motif] ligand 17 [CCL17], HAUS Augmin-Like Complex, Subunit 6 [HAUS6], proenkephalin [PENK] and thioredoxin domain-containing protein 4 [TXNDC4] (108). In another study, a resistance locus was identified downstream of the gene encoding Wilms tumour 1 [WT1] on chromosome 11p13. Data from the 1000 Genomes Project was imputed into a genome-wide dataset of Ghanaian TB patients and healthy controls. One SNP, rs2057178 was found to be strongly associated and replication in Indonesian, Gambian and Russian case-control study cohorts also showed the same association (109). More recently, a study in South African coloured population confirmed the WT1 chr11 susceptibility locus [rs2057178] but did not show the earlier identified variants in the locus 18q11.2 and TLR8 gene (110).

Future Perspectives

The development of TB is the result of a complex interaction between the host and pathogen influenced by environmental factors. Numerous host genes are likely to be involved in this process. Recent developments in modern genetics and genomics have significantly enhanced our understanding of the pathogenic processes that underlie major infectious diseases by allowing a more systematic study of the genetic influences. Identifying HLA and non-HLA genes/products which are associated with susceptibility or resistance to TB could provide important genetic makers to predict the development or predisposition to disease. An understanding of the presence of risk conferring and/or protection genes in the human MHC will be useful for the development of new epitope-based vaccines. The number of candidate susceptibility genes is expanding rapidly. Moreover, genome-wide linkage analysis is also beginning to provide insights into complex diseases. Advances in SNP typing, microarray technology and bioinformatics will be helpful in the study of infectious diseases. Hence, these studies are expected to provide useful information for better management and control of the disease. Thus far, genes suggested to have a role in governing susceptibility to TB either act directly and modulate development of the adaptive immune response [HLA, TAP, VDR], or may bridge the innate and adaptive responses [SLC11A1, TLR 2, TLR 4, various cytokine genes and their receptors]. This is consistent with the idea that an appropriate cell-mediated immune response is critical in the control of mycobacterial infections. Many of the associations have only been found in a small series of patients, or in a single population, and should be repeated in larger studies. Lack of correlation in results between populations should not necessarily be regarded as negation of initial associations but may instead reflect heterogeneity in genetic susceptibility to this disease.

REFERENCES

1. Mehra NK, Singh M. Genetic susceptibility parameters in tuberculosis. In: Sharma SK, Mohan A, editors. Tuberculosis. Second edition. New Delhi: Jaypee Brothers Medical Publishers; 2009.p.127-45.
2. Wu UI, Holland SM. A genetic perspective on granulomatous diseases with an emphasis on mycobacterial infections. Semin Immunopathol 2016;38:199-212.
3. Opie EL. The epidemiology of TB in Negroes. Am Rev Tuberc 1930;22:603-28.
4. Large SE. Tuberculosis in the Gurkhas of Nepal. Tubercle 1964;45:320-35.
5. Nakamura RM, Tokunaga T. Strain difference of delayed-type hypersensitivity to BCG and its genetic control in mice. Infect Immun 1978;11:657-64.
6. Comstock GW. Tuberculosis in twins: a re-analysis of the Prophit survey. Am Rev Respir Dis 1978;117:621-4.
7. Singh SP, Mehra NK, Dingley HB, Pande JN, Vaidya MC. HLA-DR associated genetic control of pulmonary tuberculosis in north India. Indian J Chest Dis Allied Sci 1983;25:252-8.
8. Singh SP, Mehra NK, Dingley HB, Pande JN, Vaidya MC. Human leukocyte antigen [HLA]-linked control of susceptibility to pulmonary tuberculosis and association with HLA-DR types. J Infect Dis 1983;148:676-81.
9. Balamurugan A, Sharma SK, Mehra NK. Human leukocyte antigen class I supertypes influence susceptibility and severity of tuberculosis. J Infect Dis 2004;189:805-11.
10. Rajalingam R, Mehra NK, Mehra RD, Neolia S, Jain RC, Pande JN. HLA class I profile in Asian Indian patients with pulmonary tuberculosis. Indian J Exp Biol 1997;35:1055-9.
11. Bellamy R. Identifying genetic susceptibility factors for tuberculosis in Africans: a combined approach using a candidate gene study and a genome-wide screen. Clin Sci [Lond] 2000;98:245.
12. Brailey M. A study of tuberculosis infection and mortality in the children of tuberculosis households. Am J Hyg 1940;31:1-43.
13. Comstock GW. Frost revisited: the modern epidemiology of tuberculosis. Am J Epidemiol 1975;101:363-82.
14. Trobridge GF. Blood groups in tuberculosis. PhD Thesis. Birmingham: University of Birmingham; 1956.
15. Lewis JG, Woods AC. The ABO and Rhesus blood groups in patients with respiratory disease. Tubercle 1961;42:362-5.
16. Saha N, Banerjee B. Incidence of ABO and RH blood groups in pulmonary tuberculosis in different ethnic groups. J Med Genet 1968;5:306-7.
17. Viskum K. The ABO and rhesus blood groups in patients with pulmonary tuberculosis. Tubercle 1975;56:329-34.
18. Mehra NK, Kaur G, editors. The HLA complex in biology and medicine. A resource book. New Delhi: Jaypee Brothers Medical Publishers; 2010.
19. Zinkernagel RM, Doherty PC. Immunological surveillance against altered selfcomponents by sensitised T lymphocytes in lymphocytic choriomeningitis. Nature 1974;251:547-8.
20. Mehra NK, Jaini R, Rajalingam R, Balamurugan A, Kaur G. Molecular diversity of HLA-A*02 in Asian Indians: predominance of A*0211. Tissue Antigens 2001;57:502-7.
21. Jaini R, Kaur G, Mehra NK. Heterogeneity of HLA-DRB1*04 and its associated haplotypes in the North Indian population. Hum Immunol 2002;63:24-9.
22. Yuliwulandari R, Sachrowardi Q, Nakajima H, Kashiwase K, Hirayasu K, Mabuchi A, et al. Association of HLA-A, -B, and -DRB1 with pulmonary tuberculosis in western Javanese Indonesia. Hum Immunol 2010;71:697-701.
23. Vijaya Lakshmi V, Rakh SS, Anuradha B, Harisaipriya V, Pantula V, Jasti S, et al. Role of HLA-B51 and HLA-B52 in susceptibility to pulmonary tuberculosis. Infect Genet Evol 2006;6:436-9.
24. Brahmajothi V, Pitchappan RM, Kakkanaiah VN, Sashidhar M, Rajaram K, Ramu S, et al. Association of pulmonary tuberculosis and HLA in south India. Tubercle 1991;72:123-32.
25. Ravi Kumar M, Dheenadhayalan V, Rajaram K, Lakshmi SS, Kumaran PP, Paramasivan CN, et al. Associations of HLA-DRB1, DQB1 and DPB1 alleles with pulmonary tuberculosis in south India. Tuber Lung Dis 1999;79:309-17.
26. Shi GL, Hu XL, Yang L, Rong CL, Guo YL, Song CX. Association of HLA-DRB alleles and pulmonary tuberculosis in North Chinese patients. Genet Mol Res 2011;10:1331-6.
27. Dubaniewicz A, Lewko B, Moszkowska G, Zamorska B, Stepinski J. Molecular subtypes of the HLA-DR antigens in pulmonary tuberculosis. Int J Infect Dis 2000;4:129-33.
28. Lombard Z, Dalton DL, Venter PA, Williams RC, Bornman L. Association of HLA-DR, -DQ, and vitamin D receptor alleles and

haplotypes with tuberculosis in the Venda of South Africa. Hum Immunol 2006;67:643-54.

29. Harfouch-Hammoud EI, Daher NA. Susceptibility to and severity of tuberculosis is genetically controlled by human leukocyte antigens. Saudi Med J 2008;29:1625-9.

30. Amirzargar AA, Yalda A, Hajabolbaghi M, Khosravi F, Jabbari H, Rezaei N, et al. The association of HLA-DRB, DQA1, DQB1 alleles and haplotype frequency in Iranian patients with pulmonary tuberculosis. Int J Tuberc Lung Dis 2004;8:1017-21.

31. Kim HS, Park MH, Song EY, Park H, Kwon SY, Han SK, et al. Association of HLA-DR and HLA-DQ genes with susceptibility to pulmonary tuberculosis in Koreans: preliminary evidence of associations with drug resistance, disease severity, and disease recurrence. Hum Immunol 2005;66:1074-81.

32. Vejbaesya S, Chierakul N, Luangtrakool K, Srinak D, Stephens HA. Association of HLA class II alleles with pulmonary tuberculosis in Thais. Eur J Immunogenet 2002;29:431-4.

33. Kettaneh A, Seng L, Tiev KP, Tolédano C, Fabre B, Cabane J. Human leukocyte antigens and susceptibility to tuberculosis: a meta-analysis of case-control studies. Int J Tuberc Lung Dis 2006;10:717-25.

34. Lewinsohn DA, Winata E, Swarbrick GM, Tanner KE, Cook MS, Null MD, et al. Immunodominant tuberculosis CD8 antigens preferentially restricted by HLA-B. PLoS Pathog 2007;3:1240-9.

35. Sette A, Sidney J. Nine major HLA class I supertypes account for the vast preponderance of HLA-A and -B polymorphism. Immunogenetics 1999;50:201-2.

36. Mehra NK, Bovornkitti S. HLA and tuberculosis: a reappraisal. Asian Pac J Allergy Immunol 1986;4:149-56.

37. Bothamley GH, Beck JS, Schreuder GM, D'Amaro J, de Vries RR, Kardjito T, et al. Association of tuberculosis and M. tuberculosis-specific antibody levels with HLA. J Infect Dis 1989;159:549-5.

38. Khomenko AG, Litvinov VI, Chukanova VP, Pospelov LE. Tuberculosis in patients with various HLA phenotypes. Tubercle 1990;71:187-92.

39. Hafez M, el-Salab S, el-Shennawy F, Bassiony MR. HLA-antigens and tuberculosis in the Egyptian population. Tubercle 1985;66: 35-40.

40. Hwang CH, Khan S, Ende N, Mangura BT, Reichman LB, Chou J. The HLA-A, -B, and -DR phenotypes and tuberculosis. Am Rev Respir Dis 1985;132:382-5.

41. Cox RA, Downs M, Neimes RE, Ognibene AJ, Yamashita TS, Ellner JJ. Immunogenetic analysis of human tuberculosis. J Infect Dis 1988;158:1302-28.

42. Sanjeevi CB, Olerup O. Restriction fragment length polymorphism analysis of HLA-DRB, -DQA, and -DQB genes in south Indians and Swedish Caucasians. Transplant Proc 1992;24:1687-8.

43. Rajeswari DN, Selvaraj P, Raghavan S, Jawahar MS, Narayanan PR. Influence of HLA-DR2 on perforin-positive cells in pulmonary tuberculosis. Int J Immunogenet 2007;34:379-84.

44. Da Silva SA, Mazini PS, Reis PG, Sell AM, Tsuneto LT, Peixoto PR, et al. HLA-DR and HLA-DQ alleles in patients from the south of Brazil: markers for leprosy susceptibility and resistance. BMC Infect Dis 2009;9:1-7.

45. Mehra NK, Rajalingam R, Mitra DK, Taneja V, Giphart MJ. Variants of HLA-DR2/DR51 group haplotypes and susceptibility to tuberculoid leprosy and pulmonary tuberculosis in Asian Indians. Int J Lepr Other Mycobact Dis 1995;63:241-8.

46. Sharma SK, Turaga KK, Balamurugan A, Saha PK, Pandey RM, Jain NK, et al. Clinical and genetic risk factors for the development of multidrug-resistant tuberculosis in non-HIV infected patients at a tertiary care center in India: a case-control study. Infect Genet Evol 2003;3:183-8.

47. Sharma SK, Balamurugan A, Saha PK, Pandey RM, Mehra NK. Evaluation of clinical and immunogenetic risk factors for the development of hepatotoxicity during antituberculosis treatment. Am J Respir Crit Care Med 2002;166:916-9.

48. Mehra NK. Role of HLA linked factors in governing susceptibility to leprosy and tuberculosis. Trop Med Parasitol 1990;41:352-4.

49. Mishra G, Kumar N, Kaur G, Jain S, Tiwari PK, Mehra NK. Distribution of HLA-A, B and DRB1 alleles in Sahariya tribe of North Central India: an association with pulmonary tuberculosis. Infect Genet Evol 2014;22:175-82.

50. Souza CF, Noguti EN, Visentainer JE, Cardoso RF, Petzl-Erler ML, Tsuneto LT. HLA and MICA genes in patients with tuberculosis in Brazil. Tissue Antigens 2012;79:58-63.

51. Kuranov AB, Kozhamkulov UA, Vavilov MN, Belova ES, Bismilda VL, Alenova AH, et al. HLA-class II alleles in patients with drug-resistant pulmonary tuberculosis in Kazakhstan. Tissue Antigens 2014 ;83:106-12.

52. Thye T, Nejentsev S, Intemann CD, Browne EN, Chinbuah MA, Gyapong J, et al. MCP-1 promoter variant -362C associated with protection from pulmonary tuberculosis in Ghana, West Africa. Hum Mol Genet 2009;18:381-8.

53. Flores-Villanueva PO, Ruiz-Morales JA, Song CH, Flores LM, Jo EK, Montano M, et al. A functional promoter polymorphism in monocyte chemoattractant protein-1 is associated with increased susceptibility to pulmonary tuberculosis. J Exp Med 2005;202:1649-58.

54. Moller M, Nebel A, Valentonyte R, van Helden PD, Schreiber S, Hoal EG. Investigation of chromosome 17 candidate genes in susceptibility to TB in a South African population. Tuberculosis 2009;89:189-94.

55. Barreiro LB, Neyrolles O, Babb CL, Taileux L, Quach H, McElreavey K, et al. Promoter variation in the DC-SIGN encoding gene CD209 is associated with tuberculosis. PLoS Med 2006;3:e20.

56. Ben-Ali M, Barreiro LB, Chhabou A, Haltiti R, Braham E, Neyrolles O, et al. Promoter and neck region length variation of DC-SIGN is not associated with susceptibility to tuberculosis in Tunisian patients. Hum Immunol 2007;68:908-12.

57. Vannberg FO, Chapman SJ, Khor CC, Tosh K, Floyd S, Jackson-Sillah D, et al. CD209 genetic polymorphism and tuberculosis disease. PLoS One 2008;3:e1388.

58. Selvaraj P, Alagarasu K, Swaminathan S, Harishankar M, Narendran G. CD209 gene polymorphisms in South Indian HIV and HIV-TB patients. Infect Genet Evol 2009;9:256-62.

59. Gomez LM, Anaya JM, Sierra-Filardi E, Cadena J, Corbi A, Martin J. Analysis of DC-SIGN [CD209] functional variants in patients with tuberculosis. Hum Immunol 2006;67:808-11.

60. Rosas-Taraco AG, Revol A, Salinas Carmona MC, Rendon A, Caballero Olin G, Arce Mendoza AY. CD14 [-159] T polymorphism is a risk factor for development of pulmonary tuberculosis. J Infect Dis 2007;196:1698-1706.

61. Pacheco E, Fonesca C, Montes C, Zabaleta J, Garcia LF, Arias MA. CD14 gene promoter polymorphism in different clinical forms of tuberculosis. FEMS Immunol Med Microbiol 2004;40:207-13.

62. Tang NL, Fan HP, Chang KC, Ching JK, Kong KP, Yew WW, et al. Genetic association between a chemokine gene CXCL10 [IP-10, interferon gamma inducible protein 10] and susceptibility to tuberculosis. Clin Chim Acta 2009;406:98-102.

63. Martineau AR, Leandro AC, Anderson ST, Newton SM, Wilkinson KA, Nicol MP, et al. Association between Gc genotype and susceptibility to TB is dependent on vitamin D status. Eur Respir J 2010;35:1106-12.

64. Lamsyah H, Rueda B, Bassi L, Elaouad R, Bottini N, Sadki K, et al. Association of PTPN22 gene functional variants with development of pulmonary tuberculosis in Moroccan population. Tissue Antigens 2009;74:228-32.

65. Bellamy R, Ruwende C, Corrah T, McAdam KP, Thursz M, Whittle HC, et al. Tuberculosis and chronic hepatitis B virus

infection in Africans and variation in the vitamin D receptor gene. J Infect Dis 1999;179:721-4.

66. Gao L, Tao Y, Zhang L, Jin Q. Vitamin D receptor genetic polymorphisms and tuberculosis: updated systematic review and meta analysis. Int J Tuberc Lung Dis 2010;14:15-23.

67. Selvaraj P, Alagarasu K, Harishankar M, Vidyarani M, Narayanan PR. Regulatory region polymorphism of vitamin D receptor gene in pulmonary tuberculosis patients and normal healthy subjects of south India. Int J Immunogenet 2008;35: 251-4.

68. Ben-Ali M, Barbouche MR, Bousnina S, Chabbou A, Dellagi K. Toll like receptor 2 Arg677Trp polymorphism is associated with susceptibility to tuberculosis in Tunisian patients. Clin Diagn Lab Immunol 2004;11:625-6.

69. Ogus AC, Yoldas B, Ozdemir T, Uguz A, Olcen S, Keser I, et al. The Arg753Gln polymorphism of the human toll like receptor 2 gene in tuberculosis disease. Eur Respir J 2004;23:219-23.

70. Yim JJ, Lee HW, Lee HS, Kim YW, Han SK. The association between microsatellite polymorphisms in intron II of the human Toll-like receptor 2 gene and tuberculosis among Koreans. Genes Immun 2006;7:150-5.

71. Velez DR, Wejse C, Stryjewski ME, Abbate E, Hulme WF, Myers JL, et al. Variants in toll like receptors 2 and 9 influence susceptibility to pulmonary tuberculosis in Caucasians, African Americans and West Africans. Hum Genet 2010;127:65-73.

72. Ates O, Musellim B, Ongen G, Topal Sarikaya A. Interleukin 10 and tumor necrosis factor alpha gene polymorphisms in tuberculosis. J Clin Immunol 2008;28:232-6.

73. Oh JH, Yang CS, Noh YK, Kweon YM, Jung SS, Son JW, et al. Polymorphisms of interleukin-10 and tumor necrosis factor alpha genes are associated with newly diagnosed and recurrent pulmonary tuberculosis. Respirology 2007;12:594-98.

74. Vejbaesya S, Chierakul N, Luagtrakool P, Sermduangprateep C. NRAMP1 and TNF-alpha polymorphisms and susceptibility to tuberculosis in Thais. Respirology 2007;12:202-6.

75. Selvaraj P, Sriram U, Mathan Kurian S, Reetha AM, Narayanan PR. Tumor necrosis factor alpha [-238 and -308] and beta gene polymorphisms in pulmonary tuberculosis: haplotype analysis with HLA-A, B and DR genes. Tuberculosis 2001;81:335-41.

76. Delgado JC, Baena A, Thim S, Goldfeld AE. Ethnic specific genetic associations with pulmonary tuberculosis. J Infect Dis 2002;186:1463-8.

77. Correa PA, Gomez LM, Cadena J, Anaya JM. Autoimmunity and tuberculosis. Opposite association with TNF polymorphism. J Rheumatol 2005;32:219-24.

78. Gomez LM, Camargo JF, Castiblanco J, Ruiz-Narvaez EA, Cadena J, Anaya JM, et al. Analysis of IL-1b, TAP-1, TAP2 and IKBL polymorphisms on susceptibility to tuberculosis. Tissue Antigens 2006;67: 290-6.

79. Bellamy R, Ruwende C, Corrah T, McAdam KP, Whittle HC. Assessment of the interleukin 1 gene cluster and other candidate gene polymorphisms in host susceptibility to tuberculosis. Tuber Lung Dis 1998;79:83-9.

80. Abhimanyu, Bose M, Jha P; Indian Genome Variation Consortium. Footprints of genetic susceptibility to pulmonary tuberculosis: Cytokine gene variants in north Indians. Indian J Med Res 2012;135: 763-70.

81. Selvaraj P, Alagarasu K, Harishankar M, Vidyarani M, Nisha Rajeshwari D, Narayanan PR. Cytokine gene polymorphisms and cytokine levels in pulmonary tuberculosis. Cytokine 2008;43: 26-33.

82. Prabhu Anand S, Selvaraj P, Jawahar MS, Adhilakshmi AR, Narayanan PR. Interleukin 12 B and interleukin 10 gene polymorphisms in pulmonary tuberculosis. Indian J Med Res 2007;126:135-8.

83. Ma X, Reich RA, Gonzalez O, Pan X, Fothergill AK, Starke JR, et al. No evidence for association between the polymorphism in the 3' untranslated region of interleukin 12B and human susceptibility to tuberculosis. J Infect Dis 2003;188:1116-8.

84. Tso HW, Lau YL, Tam CM, Wong HS, Chiang AK. Associations between IL-12B polymorphisms and tuberculosis in the Hong Kong Chinese population. J Infect Dis 2004;190:913-9.

85. Remus N, El Baghdadi J, Fieschi C, Feinberg J, Quintin T, Chentoufi M, et al. Association of IL12B1 polymorphisms with pulmonary tuberculosis in adults in Morocco. J Infect Dis 2004;190:580-7.

86. Sahiratmadja E, Baak-Pablo R, de Visser AW, Alisjahbana B, Adnan I, van Crevel R, et al. Association of polymorphisms in IL-12/IFN-gamma pathway genes with susceptibility to pulmonary tuberculosis in Indonesia. Tuberculosis 2007;87:303-11.

87. Kusuhara K, Yamamoto K, Okada K, Mizuno Y, Hara T. Association of IL12RB1 polymorphisms with susceptibility to and severity of tuberculosis in Japanese: a gene based association analysis of 21 candidate genes. Int J Immunogenet 2007;34:35-44.

88. Ansari A, Talat N, Jamil B, Hasan J, Razzaki T, Dawood G, et al. Cytokine gene polymorphisms across tuberculosis clinical spectrum in Pakistani patients. PLoS ONE 2009;4:e4778.

89. Henao MI, Montes C, Paris SC, Garcia LF. Cytokine gene polymorphisms in Colombian patients with different clinical presentations of tuberculosis. Tuberculosis 2006;86:11-9.

90. Lopez-Maderuelo D, Arnalich F, Serantes R, Gonzalez A, Codoceo R, Madero R, et al. Interferon gamma and interleukin 10 gene polymorphisms in pulmonary tuberculosis. Am J Respir Crit Care Med 2003;167:970-5.

91. Ding S, Li L, Zhu X. Polymorphism of the interferon-gamma gene and risk of tuberculosis in a southeastern Chinese population. Hum Immunol 2008;69:129-33.

92. Tso HW, Ip WK, Chong WP, Tam CM, Chiang AK, Lau YL. Association of interferon gamma and interleukin 10 genes with tuberculosis in Hong Kong Chinese. Genes Immun 2005;6:358-63.

93. Pacheco AG, Cardoso CC, Moraes MO. IFNG +874T/A, IL10 -1082G/A and TNF-308G/A polymorphisms in association with tuberculosis susceptibility: a meta analysis study. Human Genet 2008;123:477-84.

94. Cooke GS, Campbell SJ, Sillah J, Gustafson P, Bah B, et al. Polymorphism within the interferon gamma/receptor complex is associated with pulmonary tuberculosis. Am J Respir Crit Care Med 2006;174:339-43.

95. Velez DR, Hulme WF, Myers JL, Stryjewski ME, Abbate E, Estevan R, et al. Association of SLC11A1 with tuberculosis and interactions with NOS2A and TLR2 in African Americans and Caucasians. Int J Tuberc Lung Dis 2009;13:1068-76.

96. Leung KH, Yip SP, Wong WS, Yiu LS, Chan KK, Lai WM, et al. Sex and age dependent association of SLC11A1 polymorphisms with tuberculosis in Chinese: a case control study. BMC Infect Dis 2007;7:19.

97. Zhang W, Shao L, Weng X, Hu Z, Jin A, Chen S, et al. Variants of the natural resistance associated macrophage protein 1 gene [NRAMP1] are associated with severe forms of pulmonary tuberculosis. Clin Infect Dis 2005;40:1232-6.

98. Bellamy R, Ruwende C, Corrah T, McAdam KP, Whittle HC, Hill AV. Variations in the NRAMP1 gene and susceptibility to tuberculosis in West Africans. N Engl J Med 1998;338:640-4.

99. Gao PS, Fujishima S, Mao XQ, Remus N, Kanda M, Enomoto T, et al. Genetic variants of NRAMP1 and active tuberculosis in Japanese populations. International Tuberculosis Genetics Team. Clin Genet 2000;58:74-6.

100. Kim JH, Lee SY, Lee SH, Sin C, Shim JJ, In KH, et al. NRAMP1 genetic polymorphisms as a risk factor of tuberculous pleurisy. Int J Tuberc Lung Dis 2003;7:370-5.

101. Soborg C, Andersen AB, Madsen HO, Kok-Jensen A, Skinhoj P, Garred P, et al. Natural resistance associated macrophage protein 1 polymorphisms are associated with microscopy positive tuberculosis. J Infect Dis 2002;186:517-21.

102. Velez DR, Hulme WF, Myers JL, Weinberg JB, Levesque MC, Stryjewski ME, et al. NOS2A, TLR4, and IFNGR1 interactions influence pulmonary tuberculosis susceptibility in African Americans. Human Genet 2009;126:643-53.

103. Jamieson SE, Miller EN, Black GF, Peacock CS, Cordell HJ, Howson JM, et al. Evidence for a cluster of genes on chromosome 17q11-q21 controlling susceptibility to tuberculosis and leprosy in Brazilians. Genes Immun 2004;5:46-57.

104. Thye T, Browne EN, Chinbuah MA, Gyapong J, Osei I, Owusu-Dabo E, et al. IL-10 haplotype associated with tuberculin skin test response but not with pulmonary TB. PLoS One 2009; 4:e5420.

105. Najmi N, Kaur G, Sharma SK, Mehra NK. Human Toll-like receptor 4 polymorphisms TLR4 Asp299Gly and Thr399Ile influence susceptibility and severity of pulmonary tuberculosis in the Asian Indian population. Tissue Antigens 2010;76: 102-9.

106. Burgner D, Rockett K, Kwiatkowski D. Nitric oxide and infectious diseases. Arch Dis Childhood 1999;81:185-8.

107. Thye T, Vannberg FO, Wong SH, Owusu-Dabo E, Osei I, Gyapong J, et al. Genome-wide association analyses identifies a susceptibility locus for tuberculosis on chromosome 18q11.2. Nat Genet 2010;42:739-41.

108. Png E, Alisjahbana B, Sahiratmadja E, Marzuki S, Nelwan R, Balabanova Y, et al. A genome wide association study of pulmonary tuberculosis susceptibility in Indonesians. BMC Med Genet 2012;13:5.

109. Thye T, Owusu-Dabo E, Vannberg FO, van Crevel R, Curtis J, Sahiratmadja E, et al. Common variants at 11p13 are associated with susceptibility to tuberculosis. Nat Genet 2012;44:257-9.

110. Chimusa ER, Zaitlen N, Daya M, Möller M, van Helden PD, Mulder NJ, et al. Genome-wide association study of ancestry-specific TB risk in the South African coloured population. Hum Mol Genet 2014;23:796-809.

7

Genetics of Susceptibility to Tuberculosis

Ting-Heng Yu, Tania Di Pietrantonio, Erwin Schurr

INTRODUCTION

The importance of host genetic factors in susceptibility to tuberculosis [TB] is supported by historical evidence. The variable pattern of TB incidence is thought to reflect, at least in part, the population history of exposure to *Mycobacterium tuberculosis [Mtb]*, the causative agent of TB. Like other infectious diseases entailing a high morbidity and mortality in early life, TB is expected to select for genetic variants that confer resistance/protection. Therefore, populations with a long history of exposure to *Mtb* [e.g., Europeans] display greater resistance than those who became only recently exposed [e.g., American natives and sub-Saharan Africans] (1-3). Generally, stronger genetic effects will be detected in younger, or early onset patients (3). For TB, numerous common genetic variants contributing moderately to susceptibility have been identified but their functional relevance and impact at the population level remain elusive (4-7). Since the pathogenesis of TB is only partly understood and clinical disease presents a complex disease syndrome rather than a single well-defined disease state, it is possible that different genes control different aspects of clinical disease. Hence, the genetic dissection of TB susceptibility will depend on additional careful investigation of disease pathogenesis in both animal and human models (8).

PATHOGENESIS AND GENETIC STUDIES

The natural history of TB is described in the chapter *"Pulmonary tuberculosis" [Chapter 10]*. Differentiating between infection and disease progression is crucial to dissect the genetic basis of TB (8). Exposure to mycobacteria usually does not lead to clinical disease. The outcome of exposure depends on a complex interaction between both host genetic and non-genetic factors, and environmental factors including the virulence, genetic make-up and mode of exposure to the infectious agent (9,10). For instance, host genetic susceptibility could involve a polymorphism impacting the function of a gene relevant in immunity to infection or progression from infection to clinical disease. Non-genetic factors might involve advanced age, human immunodeficiency virus [HIV] infection, acquired immunodeficiency syndrome [AIDS], alcohol abuse, diabetes mellitus, use of immunosuppressive drugs [e.g., corticosteroids], nutritional status or co-infection with other pathogens (11). Consequently, susceptibility to TB is dependent on the genetic background of the host and the tubercle bacilli, as well as epigenetic and ecological factors.

Host-Pathogen Interplay

Several studies have presented differences on how genetically heterogeneous *Mtb* strains interact with the host (12-15). A study investigating the impact of strain genetic diversity on the course of disease in a mouse model showed a noticeable difference in immunopathological events ranging from limited disease and 100% survival with Canetti strains to extensive disease and significant earlier mortality with Beijing strains (16). Another study showed that the overexpression of a lipid species produced by strains belonging to the W-Beijing family inhibited the release of the pro-inflammatory cytokines like tumour necrosis factor [TNF], interleukin-6 [IL-6], and IL-12 in murine monocyte-derived macrophages (9). Interestingly, there is a significant joint effect of strain and host genetic variation on extent of IL-12 and interferon-gamma [IFN-γ] production (17). The importance of strain-host interaction effects is further shown by the differences in the host genetic control of the closely related bacille Calmette–Guérin [BCG] Russia and BCG Pasteur strains of mycobacteria (18).

An analysis of TB patients from the cosmopolitan urban centre of San Francisco, California, showed stable associations between genetically distinct strains of *Mtb* and human host populations stratified by birthplace (19). The association was detected for both reactivation disease and recent transmissions occurring in San Francisco. It is likely that the important factors maintaining the association are biological and social (19). A subsequent study demonstrated that *Mtb* lineages tend to spread in patient populations originating from the same geographic area (14). Likewise, strains of the Beijing sublineage of *Mtb* preferentially associated with populations of a defined geographical setting (20). A more systematic analysis of the spread of Beijing strains suggested that virulence mutations under strong positive selection favoured the global spread of Beijing strains (21). In addition, results based on the comparative sequence analysis of a large number of geographically dispersed *Mtb* strains detected strong evidence for a co-expansion of the bacilli and their human hosts during the Neolithic period. This long co-evolutionary history may underlie the adaptation of different strains of *Mtb* to different ethnic groups (22,23). These broad population-based findings are further supported by the occurrence of distinct genetic lesions in *immunity-related guanosine triphosphatase family, M [IRGM]*, *arachidonate 5-lipoxygenase [ALOX5]*, and *mannose-binding lectin [protein C] 2 [MBL2]* for different strains of *Mtb* (24-26).

METHODS IN THE GENETIC DISSECTION OF COMPLEX INFECTIOUS DISEASES

Different approaches have been employed to identify the genetic control elements of infectious diseases. In the forward genetics approach [phenotype-to-genotype] Mendelian or complex inheritance in humans is a dissected using hypothesis-driven or -generating method both leading to candidate genes. Candidate genes can be identified, for example, by comparison with human hereditary disorders with a related clinical phenotype (11) or from linkage hits in whole-genome scans (27,28). Whole-genome scans using linkage analysis are most successful in pinpointing genes with strong effects on disease susceptibility. Linkage analyses search within families for regions of the genome that segregate preferentially with the phenotype of interest (29). Whole genome scans have been used to identify susceptibility loci in various human infectious diseases, including TB (30-32), schistosomiasis (33), visceral leishmaniasis and leprosy (5,34,35). Similarly, animal models [e.g., mice, zebra fish] have been successfully employed to generate candidate genes for study in human patients (36,37). Subsequently candidate genes are examined by association tests using population- or family-based case-control designs. Candidate genes are further analysed by mutation detection and functional studies to determine the impact of the polymorphism on gene function and on the phenotype of interest (11).

Single nucleotide polymorphisms [SNPs] have become the preferred markers for genetic studies. With the emergence of affordable high-density SNP arrays, the genome-wide study of common genetic variants [minor allele frequency > 5%] in complex human diseases has become popular in human genetic studies. Genome-wide association studies [GWAS] are a more powerful approach than linkage analysis to pinpoint common modest-risk genetic factors in complex diseases (29,38,39). Novel technologies such as next-generation sequencing [NGS] (40) will likely further improve our understanding of TB pathogenesis (41). For example, whole-exome sequencing [WES] has been employed to discover inherited *ISG15 ubiquitin-like modifier [ISG15]* deficiency in patients suffering from Mendelian susceptibility to mycobacterial disease [MSMD] and lead to the realization that ISG15 is a critical inducer of interferon-gamma [IFN-γ] (42).

In addition, epigenetic and transcriptomic studies have contributed to a better understanding of TB genetics. Epigenetic mechanisms are critical for functioning of the immune system (43), and related studies such as genome-wide analyses of methylation (44) may offer new insights into the genetic basis of TB (45). Interestingly, host and/or environmental factors such as diet or aging may affect epigenetic factors (46). As for transcriptomic studies, expression quantitative trait loci [eQTL] are critical genetic modifiers of the expression of genes and/or micro ribonucleic acids [microRNAs] in cell- or tissue-specific studies (47,48). Recently an interferon-inducible neutrophil-driven blood transcriptional signature was observed in TB, and the transcriptional profile in TB patients was significantly reduced after successful treatment (49-51). Likewise, transcriptional profiling offers promise for the diagnosis of paediatric TB (52).

GENETIC STUDIES IN MICE

Studies involving mouse models have played a key role for our understanding of susceptibility to TB. Although *Mtb* is not a natural mouse pathogen, infection of mice with *Mtb* gives rise to well-defined and reproducible phenotypes that reflect the genetic susceptibility of the host. Susceptible mice develop progressive lung disease, support rapid bacterial replication and succumb quickly to disease. Resistant mice restrict bacterial growth and limit tissue injury, although they eventually succumb to infection. At the time of death, lung pathology differs considerably between susceptible and resistant strains. Pulmonary lesions in resistant mice display large lymphocytic aggregates that penetrate the granuloma. Lesions in susceptible mice contain large foamy macrophages, degenerating neutrophils, and a few dispersed lymphocytes and are often necrotic (53-57).

Similar to human studies, two major genetic approaches have been applied in the mouse to identify the genetic factors that affect the host response to *Mtb* infection. In the reverse genetics approach, genetically engineered mice with targeted mutations [gene knock-out or knock-in] are infected to determine if absence or presence of the corresponding gene alters susceptibility (58). The forward genetics approach applies quantitative trait locus [QTL] analysis on infected informative F2 or backcross progeny resulting from crosses between inbred, recombinant, congenic or mutant strains. QTL analysis determines if genes impacting on phenotype expression are linked to the location of polymorphic markers, such as microsatellites and SNPs, distributed throughout the genome. Candidate genes or chromosomal regions identified through these studies can then be validated using genetically engineered or congenic mice (59). Congenic mice are produced by transferring a defined chromosomal segment from a donor strain onto a recipient background through marker-assisted backcrossing (60,61).

Reverse Genetic Studies of *Mtb* Infection

Gene-targeted mice have been used extensively to study the involvement of different molecules and cell types during *Mtb* infection. Activation of CD4+ T-cells by major histocompatibility complex [MHC] class II molecules is essential for the control of *Mtb* infection. Mice deficient in CD4 or MHC class II molecules had severely depleted levels of IFN-γ early in infection, which caused premature death of both types of mutant strains (62). Mice devoid of class II MHC molecules displayed a greater susceptibility to TB than mice lacking class I MHC molecules, demonstrating that CD4+ T-cell responses are dominant to CD8+ T-cell mediated immunity in the control of infection (63).

The rapid progression and death of mice lacking IFN-γ has provided indirect evidence that Th1-polarised CD4+ cells are more important than Th2 effector cells. Bacterial replication is essentially unrestricted in *Ifng* gene-deleted mice, and although granulomas develop, they become quickly necrotic (64). Macrophage activation is defective in IFN-γ-deficient mice and expression of *nitric oxide synthase 2 [Nos2]* is low (64,65), such that these mice cannot produce the reactive nitrogen intermediates necessary for the destruction of intracellular bacteria. However, the susceptibility of inducible nitric oxide synthase [iNOS] deficient mice is less severe than mice lacking IFN-γ, IFN-γ type I receptor [IFN-γR1], or the IFN-responsive, signal transducer and activator of transcription 1 [STAT-1] molecule, suggesting that there are iNOS-independent mechanisms of protection. A proposed alternative pathway involves LRG-47, a phagosomal protein involved in autophagy. A deficiency in LRG-47 caused early mortality similar to that of IFN-γR1 knockout mice, outlining a role for LRG-47 in the defense against *Mtb* infection (66).

Evidence for Th1-cell mediated protection against *Mtb* also arose from studies involving interleukin-12 [IL-12] knockout mice. Mouse strains with a double disruption of IL-12p35 and IL-12p40 [IL-12p70-deficient] were susceptible to a low dose aerosol *Mtb* infection and succumbed within 10 weeks. IL-12p70-deficient mice did not mount Th1 and cytotoxic T cell responses, resulting in severe lung pathology. These mutant mice exhibited greater susceptibility to *Mtb* compared to mice lacking only one of the two subunits (67). Mice lacking the IL-12p40 subunit were more susceptible than IL-12p35$^{-/-}$ mutant mice, as evidenced by increased bacterial burden, reduced IFN-γ production, and decreased survival time (68,69).

Given that Th1 cells antagonize Th2 cell functions, it was proposed that the absence or reduction of Th1 immunity in IFN-γ- and IL-12p40-deficient mice would lead to increased Th2 cell activation and IL-4 production. In both IFN-γ- and IL-12p40 mutant strains, however, a lack of mycobacterial-specific Th1 immunity did not trigger a Th2 response and IL-4 levels were not increased (64,69), suggesting that the increased susceptibility of these mice was caused by a defective Th1 response and not by an increased Th2 response.

Tumour necrosis factor [TNF] is essential for macrophage activation and for the formation and maintenance of granulomas. Mice devoid of TNF or TNF receptor-I [TNFRI] are highly susceptible to *Mtb* infection. Absence of TNF following a low aerosolised dose of *Mtb* caused mortality within 35 days (70). There were 10^5-fold more bacteria detected in TNF$^{-/-}$ mutant mice compared to wild-type controls. Mice lacking the TNFRI had a mean survival time of 20 days following an intravenous dose of *Mtb* [5 × 10^5 bacteria] and had 50- to 100-fold more bacilli than wild type mice (71). Mice devoid of both the TNF receptor-II [TNFRII] and TNFRI also succumbed within 28 days of aerosol infection and had larger bacterial burdens compared to control mice (72). The granulomatous response following *Mtb* infection was also defective in both TNF and TNFRI-deficient mice. Although a few activated macrophages were present, lymphocyte co-localisation with the macrophages was impaired, resulting in disorganised granuloma formation (70,71). Chemokine induction was also delayed in TNF-deficient mice, outlining a role for TNF in the regulation of chemokine expression (73).

Forward Genetic Studies of *Mtb* Infection

In the 1960s, Lynch and colleagues (74) speculated that the "gradation" across mouse strains in their susceptibility to TB argued for "existence of a number of genes, with different combinations or frequencies characterizing the different strains". They demonstrated, through interbreeding and backcrossing experiments between Swiss and C57BL strains, that genetic factors influenced the response of mice to infection with *Mtb* (74). F1 hybrids between the two strains exhibited over dominance, with F1 mice surviving longer than either parent strain. Informative backcross [F1 × C57BL] progeny resolved into two populations, resistant or susceptible, suggesting a major gene effect segregating in this cross. Thus, the authors concluded that susceptibility to TB in the mouse was a complex trait under multigenic control.

Modern genetic studies have confirmed that susceptibility to TB is under complex genetic control in the mouse. The first of these studies utilised the I/St and A/Sn mouse strains. The I/St mouse strain is particularly susceptible to *Mtb* infection compared to A/Sn mice with regard to survival time, bacterial load, lung pathology and body weight loss (75). The genetic basis for the differential susceptibility of I/St and A/Sn was investigated by whole genome scanning using weight loss as a proxy for TB susceptibility. Initial mapping studies in an informative [A/Sn × I/St] × I/St backcross indicated that weight loss induced by intravenous

Mtb H37Rv infection was controlled by two major loci on chromosomes 3 and 9 and two suggestive loci on chromosomes 8 and 17 in female mice (76). Suggestive loci in male mice were localised to chromosomes 5 and 10. A limited genome scan using weight loss and survival time as quantitative phenotypes in [A/Sn × I/St] F2 mice confirmed the loci that mapped to chromosome 3 [designated TB severity 1, *tbs1*], chromosome 9 [*tbs2*] and chromosome 17 in proximity to the H-2 complex (77). The effect of the H-2 locus has been attributed to a coding mutation in the *Tnfa* gene of the susceptible I/St strain. This polymorphism results in a larger secretion of TNF, which is speculated to contribute to the susceptibility of I/St mice by increasing lung pathology (78). The genes responsible for the *tbs1* and *tbs2* loci remain unknown.

The C3HeB/FeJ strain is exquisitely susceptible to *Mtb*. Premature death in C3HeB/FeJ mice is associated with progressive lung disease characterised by increased bacterial loads, extensive pneumonitis, and necrotic lesions. Classical linkage studies in [C3HeB/FeJ C57BL/6J] F2 mice intravenously infected with *Mtb* Erdman identified a major locus on chromosome 1 designated locus for susceptibility to TB 1 [*sst1*] (79). Congenic C3HeB/FeJ mice bearing a resistant C57BL/6J-derived allele of *sst1* [C3H.B6-*sst1*] survived two times longer and had a 50–100-fold lower pulmonary bacterial burden compared to the parental C3HeB/FeJ strain. Explanted bone-marrow derived macrophages from C3H.B6-*sst1* mice had an enhanced ability to restrict intracellular replication of *Mtb* and induced apoptosis following infection, whereas phagocytes from C3HeB/FeJ died by necrosis. A positional cloning strategy identified intracellular pathogen resistance 1 [*Ipr1*] as a strong candidate for *sst1*. The *Ipr1* encodes the interferon-induced protein 75 [Ifi75], a putative transcriptional regulator. *Mtb* infection induced expression of *Ipr1* in the lungs of C3H. B6-*sst1* mice and other C3H strains but not in susceptible C3HeB/FeJ mice. Restoration of a full-length *Ipr1* in C3HeB/FeJ mice limited *Mtb* replication in the lungs of mice and in macrophages infected *in vitro*, confirming that *Ipr1* was the gene underlying *sst1* (80). However, resistance and susceptibility alleles of *sst1* are not sufficient to confer full protection or susceptibility in congenic mice, indicating that genes outside of *sst1* also contribute to the phenotype of the C3HeB/FeJ and C57BL/6J parental strains. Indeed, a genome-wide scan in *sst1*-adjusted crosses [C3H.B6-*sst1* × C57BL/6J F2 hybrids] identified four loci which mapped to chromosomes 7, 12, 15 and 17, which overlaps the H-2 complex (81). The molecular identities of the loci on chromosomes 7, 12 and 15 are currently unknown.

A genetic study of TB susceptibility/resistance was also performed using susceptible DBA/2J and resistant C57BL/6J mouse strains. A genome-wide scan for loci affecting survival time following intravenous *Mtb* H37Rv infection was conducted in [C57BL/6J × DBA/2J] F2 hybrids. Two significant loci were detected on chromosomes 1 and 7, designated TB resistance locus-1 [*Trl-1*] and TB resistance locus-3 [*Trl-3*], respectively. A third suggestive locus TB resistance locus-2 [*Trl-2*] was identified on chromosome 3. Homozygosity for C57BL/6J-derived alleles was associated with resistance at each locus (82). A second genome scan analysed pulmonary replication in [C57BL/6J × DBA/2J] F2 mice 90 days following low dose aerosol infection. Strong linkage was detected on chromosome 19 designated TB resistance locus-4 [*Trl-4*] and suggestive linkages were localized to the *Trl-3* region as well as chromosomes 5 and 10. A strong additive effect was detected between *Trl-3* and *Trl-4* such that F2 mice homozygous for one parental allele at both loci had lung bacillary loads comparable to that parental strain (83). The genetic effect of *Trl-3* and *Trl-4* was further investigated using congenic strains. Transfer of a C57BL/6J-derived, *Trl-3* chromosome 7 segment onto a DBA/2J genetic background [D2.B6-Chr7] increased resistance to *Mtb* infection as evidenced by the decreased pulmonary load and longer survival time. In contrast, D2.B6-Chr19 congenic mice harboring a C57BL/6J-derived, *Trl-4* chromosome 19 segment did not have an altered resistance to *Mtb* infection relative to DBA/2J mice (84). This finding suggests that the effect of *Trl-4* involves genetic interactions with other unknown loci, further illustrating the genetic complexity of susceptibility to TB.

GENETIC STUDIES IN HUMAN POPULATIONS

Mendelian Susceptibility to Mycobacterial Disease [OMIM 209950]

Mendelian susceptibility to mycobacterial disease is a rare inherited condition represented by selective susceptibility to clinical disease caused by poorly virulent mycobacteria, such as BCG vaccines and nontuberculous mycobacteria [NTM], in otherwise healthy patients without obvious defects (85,86). The patients are also vulnerable to the more virulent *Mtb* (87,88) and approximately half also suffer from clinical disease caused by *Salmonella* (89,90).

Seven autosomal genes have been found to be mutated in patients with the syndrome: IFN-γ-receptor 1 [*IFNGR1*] and IFN-γ-receptor 2 [*IFNGR2*], which encodes the accessory chain of IFN-γ-receptor [IFN-γR]; *STAT1*, encoding signal transducer and activator of transcription 1; *IL12B*, encoding the p40 subunit of IL-12 and IL-23; *IL12RB1*, encoding the β1 chain common to the receptors for IL-12 and IL-23; interferon regulatory factor 8 [*IRF8*], a transcription factor inducible by IFN-γ, from the interferon regulatory factor [IRF] family; and *ISG15*, an IFN-γ-inducing molecule that acts in synergy with IL-12. Also, two X-linked genes, *NEMO*, encoding the nuclear factor-kappa B [NF-κB] essential modulator, which mediates signalling in the NF-κB pathway, and cytochrome B-245, beta polypeptide [*CYBB*], encoding the major component of the phagocyte nicotinamide adenine dinucleotide phosphate [NADPH] oxidase [PHOX] complex are MSMD genes (91). Interestingly, all nine MSMD-causing genes participate in IFN-γ-mediated immunity, controlling response to [*IFNGR1*, *IFNGR2*, *STAT1*, *IRF8*, *CYBB*], or the production of [*IL12B*, *IL12RB1*, *IRF8*, *ISG15*, *NEMO*] IFN-γ (91).

The extent to which cases with rare Mendelian mutations contribute to TB in areas of endemicity is unknown (92,93).

However, three children with loss of function mutation in *IL12RB1* were found to suffer from severe forms of TB (94). Moreover, sequencing of *IL12RB1* in 50 children with severe TB led to the discovery of two cases with *IL12RB1* loss of functional alleles. This result supports the suggestion that possibly a substantial proportion of severe childhood TB may arise from monogenic defects (94). Indeed, TB as only infectious disease has been described for 4 of the 9 MSMD loci (95).

CANDIDATE GENES

Interleukin-12/Interleukin-23/Interferon-γ [IL-12/IL-23-IFN-γ] Pathway

While the phenotype-genotype relationship for IFN-γ-mediated immunity against mycobacterial disease is relatively well-defined, the significance of genetic variation in the IL-12/IL-23-IFN-γ pathway at the population level is less well understood.

IL12RB1

Numerous sequence polymorphisms have been described for *IL12RB1* (96). The two most common haplotypes of the *IL12RB1* gene found in many populations are: 'QMG' and 'RTR', which are derived from the amino acids substitutions p.Q214R, p.M365T and p.G378R (96,97). The QMG haplotype is a better responder to IL-12 than RTR (97). Several *IL12RB1* polymorphisms were reported to be associated with increased susceptibility to TB disease. In two small samples of Japanese TB patients the frequencies of the QMG and RTR haplotypes were analysed, and carriage of the homozygous RTR haplotype was found to increase the risk of TB (98,99). Nine common polymorphisms, including two polymorphisms of the QMG/RTR haplotypes, were analysed in a Morrocan family-based study. A modest association with pulmonary TB was detected in two variants in the 5' untranslated region of the gene (92). However, this association has not been replicated in two ethnically distinct populations (92,98,99).

IL12B

A strong association between an *IL12B* intron 2 genetic variant and TB susceptibility was identified in a case-control study of Hong Kong Chinese TB patients. Homozygous carriers of the $[ATT]_8$ repeat variant had a 2.14-fold increased risk of developing TB (100). The effect of *IL12B* polymorphisms on TB susceptibility may strongly depend on the ethnic background of the study population. When studying samples of African and European ethnicity multiple association signals were characteristic for samples of African ancestry (101). By contrast, in a recent meta-analysis, no significant associations were observed for the *IL12B* promoter variant [rs17860508] and the 3' UTR A/C variant [rs3212227] (102). However, the C allele of the *IL12B* 3' UTR may be a TB risk factor in Caucasians but not in Asians or Africans (102).

IFNGR1

No associations were found in a Gambian population between *IFNGR1* polymorphisms, including one variant previously found associated in a Croatian population (103), and adult pulmonary TB (104). Two SNPs in the *IFNGR1* promoter region [G611A, T56C] influence expression but were not associated with increased susceptibility to pulmonary or disseminated NTM infection (93). By contrast, homozygosity at the -56 SNP [rs2234711] for the C-allele was a risk factor for TB in West Africa (105). This finding was replicated in an independent sample from Kampala, Uganda (106). In Uganda, the same SNP was associated with *Mtb* culture filtrate triggered production of TNF (106). In a meta-analysis, no significant association between the *IFNGR1* -56C/T polymorphism and TB susceptibility was detected (107). However, *IFNGR1* -56C/T is possibly associated with increased TB risk in Africans, but not in Asians or Caucasians (107).

Interferon-γ

The IFN-γ is a major TB susceptibility candidate gene considering the importance of IFN-γ-mediated immunity in MSMD and in animal models of TB. Two genetic variations are known to affect expression of *IFNG*: The first [rs3138557] is a polymorphic CA repeat, where allele #2 [12 repeats] drives high IFN-γ production when cells are stimulated (108-110). The T-allele of the second SNP in intron 1 [rs2430561, +874T/A] is in strong linkage disequilibrium [LD] with allele #2 of the CA repeat (111). The +874T/A SNP is located in an NF-κB binding site. The T-allele promotes while the A-allele reduces NF-κB binding and thus prevents IFN-γ expression in response to stimuli (111). The rs2430561 SNP is associated with various diseases like hepatitis (112-114), leprosy (115) and TB (6,109,110,116-120). In contrast, no association was identified between *IFNG* and TB in TB patients from the Karonga district of northern Malawi (121), Texas (122), Brazil (123) and Croatia (124).

Solute Carrier Family 11, Member 1

Solute carrier family 11A, member 1, [*SLC11A1*], earlier called natural resistance-associated macrophage protein 1 [*NRAMP1*] is the human homologue of the mouse *Nramp1* gene, which serves as a divalent cation pump across phagosomal membranes (125,126). *Nramp1*-altered cation fluxes are thought to abrogate pathogen-induced blockage of phagosome maturation (127-129). Initially *Slc11a1* [*Nramp1*] was identified in mice as a regulator of resistance to intracellular pathogens, and absence of mature *Nramp1* protein resulting from the G169D polymorphism causes increased susceptibility to several intracellular macrophage pathogens, including BCG, *Salmonella typhimurium,* and *Leishmania donovani* (130,131).

Polymorphisms within the human *SLC11A1* gene have been associated with TB in numerous studies (121,132-146). However, other studies failed to detect an *SLC11A1*-TB association (147-150) providing strong evidence for genetic heterogeneity in TB susceptibility. Because of this heterogeneity it has been suggested that *SLC11A1* accounts for only a small proportion of the total genetic contribution to TB susceptibility (5,151). An alternative explanation has been provided by a genetic study of TB susceptibility in a native Canadian community (152). A potent genetic effect [relative risk of 10] of the *SLC11A1* region on TB was only detected when gene-environment interactions were included into the analysis (152). Since the subjects in the Canadian study suffered from primary TB, a successful replication study was conducted in a pediatric TB sample from Texas (142). A major conclusion from this study was that *NRAMP1* is not a TB *per se* susceptibility gene but rather increases the speed of progression from infection to clinical disease.

Several studies aimed to establish a causal relationship between *SLC11A1* variants and increased TB susceptibility. The first study investigated the 5′ [CA] repeat allele that is associated with increased TB risk. Employing a whole blood assay the risk allele also directed higher lipopolysaccharide [LPS]-induced production of the anti-inflammatory cytokine IL-10 (153). Since mouse *Slc11a1* is expressed at the macrophage phagosomal membrane and its activity can be assayed by the relative acquisition of mannose 6-phosphate receptor [M6PR] in *Salmonella*-containing vacuoles (127), it was reasoned that recruitment of M6PR could be used to gauge the functional activity of NRAMP1 in human cells. Indeed, M6PR acquisition was significantly higher in human U-937 monocytic cell lines expressing *SLC11A1* as compared to non-expressing cells. Employing MDMs from paediatric TB patients, a significantly lower *SLC11A1* activity was detected in MDMs from individuals homozygous for the *SLC11A1* 274C/T [rs2276631] high-risk allele in comparison to heterozygous individuals (154).

Vitamin D Receptor

Vitamin D_3 is a major mediator of macrophage activity in response to pathogens such as *Mtb* (47). Prior to the discovery of antibiotics, vitamin D-rich cod liver oil was used as therapy for TB patients (155). TLR-1/2 stimulation of human macrophages by *Mtb* induces the expression of vitamin D receptor [VDR] and the enzyme CYP27B1, which catalyses the conversion of 1,25 [OH] vitamin D_3 to 1,25[OH]$_2$ vitamin D_3, which is the biologically active form. 1,25[OH]$_2$D$_3$ is an essential immunoregulatory molecule that participates in various immune processes: activating monocytes and cell-mediated immunity, controlling the Th1-Th2 host immune response, phagocytosis, and suppressing lymphocyte proliferation, immunoglobulin production and cytokine synthesis. *In vitro*, 1,25[OH]$_2$D$_3$ limits the growth of *Mtb* in human macro-phages (156,157). Additionally, data from epidemiologic studies indicate a link between a higher risk of TB and vitamin D defi-ciency (31,158). This is supported by reports of lower vitamin D serum levels and seasonal variation of TB incidence in untreated TB patients comparing to higher incidence of TB in individuals with relatively low serum vitamin D levels (7,159).

Since vitamin D exerts its effects via the VDR and the receptor is present on monocytes and lymphocytes a possible role of VDR genetic variants in TB susceptibility has been studied (160). Of the 22 SNPs in the *VDR* gene, those associated with TB susceptibility are the polymorphisms at the restriction sites Fok1, Apa1, Taq1, and Bsm1 (7,161). Of these, the 3′ UTR region SNPs Apa I, Bsm I and Taq I are assumed to affect messenger RNA [mRNA] stability, thus yielding variation in VDR activity (162,163). The minor alleles for Fok1, Apa1 and Bsm1 and the major allele for Taq1 have been implicated in diminished *VDR* function associated with TB (161). TaqI SNP [rs731236] in exon 9 is the best known polymorphism of the *VDR* gene (164). This SNP affects transcription and reduced VDR function (165). A number of studies across various ethnic populations have investigated the relationship between TaqI polymorphism and TB risk but yielded inconsistent results (7,39,133,137,166-182). A possible explanation for these inconsistencies is that the genetic effect of VDR polymorphisms is dependent on serum vitamin D levels (7).

Human Leucocyte Antigen

Since the 1970s (183), classical HLA loci have been recognized as leading candidates for infectious disease susceptibility. The extreme variability at the HLA loci was proposed to result from infectious diseases as the major selective force (184-186). Various attempts have been made to establish the association between HLA and TB susceptibility. Two genome-wide linkage scans of pulmonary TB in Africa (30,31) failed to detect a significant linkage signal at HLA, while weak association [p = 0.0017] with the HLA-DQ region was detected in a large GWAS for TB (187). There are more targeted studies investigating a possible role of Class II as compared to Class I alleles (188). Association of HLA-DR and HLA-DQ alleles was reported in samples from India (189), Korea (190), South Africa (172), Indonesia (191), China (192) and Cambodia (193). However, the specific alleles implicated were inconsistent and varied among populations. For example, a number of studies reported associations of HLA-DR2 alleles (194-196), *HLA-DQB1* 0501* (196), and *HLA-DQB1*0503* alleles (197) with TB, while others failed to detect those associations (198,199). More detailed functional studies led to the conclusion that specific alleles at the *HLA_DRB1* and *HLA_DQB1* genes modulate the human immune response to TB (193,200).

Mannose-binding Lectin

Secreted by the liver, mannose-binding lectin [MBL] is an acute-phase protein that is instrumental in innate immunity. MBL recognises microbial surface carbohydrates, particularly mannose- and N-acetylglucosamine-terminated glycoproteins. Intracellular pathogens, such as *Mtb*, partially exploit the complement system to invade and replicate within host cells. By binding to the mannose residues in the LAM covering *Mtb* (201,202). MBL acts as an opsonin, augments both complement-dependent and -independent phagocytosis, and promotes inflammation with the release of cytokines (203,204). The impact of MBL2 alleles on TB susceptibility is inconsistent. Studies in South African, Gabonese, Danish, Italian, Indian, Turkish, Brazilian, Chinese and African-American populations showed significant associations between *MBL2* genetic variants encoding low serum MBL levels and protection against active TB (131,205-212). However, these results could not be replicated in studies in Caucasian American, Tanzanian, Malawi, and the Polish TB patients (121,138,207,213,214).

Genome-wide Linkage Studies

Similar to candidate gene studies, results across genome-wide linkage studies have been inconsistent. In 2000, a study (31) was performed in sib-pairs with TB from Gambia and South Africa. The authors conducted a two-stage genome-wide linkage study to search for regions of the human genome containing TB-susceptibility genes. Suggestive evidence of linkage was found in chromosomes 15q and Xq (31). However, the genes causing the linkage peak could not be identified. A genome scan for TB in a Brazilian population identified four regions with suggestive evidence for linkage: 10q26.13, 11q12.3, 17q11-q21, 20p12.1 (32,215) without resulting in the identification of a susceptibility gene. Using a combined genome-wide and positional mapping approach, the melanocortin 3 receptor [*MC3R*] and cathepsin Z [*CTSZ*] genes were identified as TB susceptibility candidate genes (216). A genome-wide linkage study conducted in Moroccan multiplex families with pulmonary TB detected a susceptibility locus on chromosome 8q12-q13 (30). Association scanning of the linkage peak identified SNPs in the promoter region of the thymocyte selection-associated high mobility group box [*TOX*] gene as susceptibility factor for early onset pulmonary TB (27).

Two studies used resistance to infection by *Mtb* as phenotype. Resistance to infection was defined as persistently negative tuberculin skin test [PTST]. In a genome scan of *Mtb* infection and disease in Ugandans (217), suggestive linkage was observed on chromosome regions 2q21-2q24 and 5p13-5q22 for PTST (217). Nominal evidence for linkage of PTST was also observed at the *SLC11A1* [alias *NRAMP1*] gene.

A second genome-wide linkage analysis identified two loci relating to TST reactivity in 128 families from South Africa (218). The locus on chromosome region 11p14, termed *TST1*, controls TST = 0 mm versus TST greater than 0 mm, while a second locus on chromosome region 5p15, termed *TST2*, impacts on extent of TST reactivity. The most parsimonious explanation for individuals remaining TST negative despite documented exposure is that they are resistant to infection with *Mtb*. Importantly, the *TST1* locus was replicated in an independent household contact study in a suburb of Paris (219). In a subsequent study, a locus [*TNF1*] modulating TNF production by blood cells in response to BCG and BCG plus IFN-γ, and *TNF1* was genetically indiscernible from *TST1* (220). This suggested that resistance to *Mtb* infection may involve a TNF-mediated effector mechanism.

Genome-wide Association Scans

So far 4 GWAS in TB have been conducted. A first GWAS on pulmonary TB was conducted on two case control samples from Ghana and Gambia (187). Of the 17 SNPs associated with P less than 5×10^{-5} only rs4331426 located in gene desert on chromosome region 18q11.2 reached genome-wide significance after genotyping in additional samples from Ghana and Malawi. The chromosome 18 locus was replicated in sample of Han Chinese TB patients (221). Following imputation of a large number of additional SNPs in the Ghanaian discovery sample, a TB protective locus was identified on chromosome region 11p13. The signal comprised three highly correlated SNPs located 45 kb downstream of the Wilms' tumour 1 [*WT1*] gene of which one was located in a transcription factor binding site. The main protective SNP allele replicated well in the Gambian sample, but displayed borderline evidence for association in independent samples from Indonesia and Russia (222).

A GWAS in Thai and Japanese samples detected a TB risk locus on chromosome region 20q12 after stratification by age (223). Replication in additional samples is outstanding. A low marker density SNP was conducted in a sample from Indonesia (224). The results suggested the possible contribution of SNPs in the vicinity of several immune signalling genes but need to be replicated in a larger study. A fourth GWAS was conducted in the admixed South African coloured population residing in the Western Cape region (225). While the study failed to detect any markers with genome-wide significance, the chromosome 11 TB protective locus previously identified in the West African samples was confirmed (222). The study (222) demonstrated the value of genetic studies in admixed populations and established the locus on chromosome 11 as universal TB protective factor in African populations.

Genetic studies have contributed to the discovery of specific genes and immune pathways involved in anti-TB immunity. However, it is clear that a large proportion of the genes involved in genetic susceptibility remain to be discovered. This will require carefully planned studies with well-defined disease phenotypes (226). Furthermore, the contribution of rare genetic variants and epigenetic factors to TB risk deserves attention and replicated genetic associations with TB phenotypes need to be followed-up for their functional relevance. Only by linking genetic risk factors to biological functions will it be possible to fully exploit genetic results for improved tools of patient care and disease control.

REFERENCES

1. Motulsky AG. Metabolic polymorphisms and the role of infectious diseases in human evolution. Hum Biol 1989;61:835-69; discussion 870-7.
2. Daniel TM, Bates JH, Downes KA. History of tuberculosis. In: Bloom B, editor. Tuberculosis pathogenesis, protection and control. Washington: American Society of Microbiology; 1994.p.13-24.

3. Alcais A, Quintana-Murci L, Thaler DS, Schurr E, Abel L, Casanova JL. Life-threatening infectious diseases of childhood: single-gene inborn errors of immunity? Ann N Y Acad Sci 2010;1214:18-33.

4. Cervino AC, Lakiss S, Sow O, Bellamy R, Beyers N, Hoal-van Helden E, et al. Fine mapping of a putative tuberculosis-susceptibility locus on chromosome 15q11-13 in African families. Hum Mol Genet 2002;11:1599-603.

5. Shaw MA, Collins A, Peacock CS, Miller EN, Black GF, Sibthorpe D, et al. Evidence that genetic susceptibility to Mycobacterium tuberculosis in a Brazilian population is under oligogenic control: linkage study of the candidate genes NRAMP1 and TNFA. Tuber Lung Dis 1997;78:35-45.

6. Rossouw M, Nel HJ, Cooke GS, van Helden PD Hoal EG. Association between tuberculosis and a polymorphic NFkappaB binding site in the interferon gamma gene. Lancet 2003;361:1871-2.

7. Wilkinson RJ, Llewelyn M, Toossi Z, Patel P, Pasvol G, Lalvani A, et al. Influence of vitamin D deficiency and vitamin D receptor polymorphisms on tuberculosis among Gujarati Asians in west London: a case-control study. Lancet 2000;355:618-21.

8. Kaufmann SH. How can immunology contribute to the control of tuberculosis? Nat Rev Immunol 2001;1:20-30.

9. Reed MB, Domenech P, Manca C, Su H, Barczak AK, Kreiswirth BN, et al. A glycolipid of hypervirulent tuberculosis strains that inhibits the innate immune response. Nature 2004;431:84-7.

10. Abel L, Casanova JL. Genetic predisposition to clinical tuberculosis: bridging the gap between simple and complex inheritance. Am J Hum Genet 2000;67:274-7.

11. Casanova JL, Abel L. The human model: a genetic dissection of immunity to infection in natural conditions. Nat Rev Immunol 2004;4:55-66.

12. Asante-Poku A, Yeboah-Manu D, Octacher ID, Aboagye SY, Stucki D, Hattendorf J, et al. Mycobacterium africanum is associated with Patient Ethnicity in Ghana. PLoS Negl Trop Dis 2015;9:e3370.

13. Firdessa R, Berg S, Hailu E, Schelling E, Gumi B, Erenso G, et al. Mycobacterial lineages causing pulmonary and extrapulmonary tuberculosis, Ethiopia. Emerg Infect Dis 2013;19:460-3.

14. Gagneux S, DeRiemer K, Van T, Kato-Maeda M, de Jong BC, Narayanan S, et al. Variable host-pathogen compatibility in Mycobacterium tuberculosis. Proc Natl Acad Sci USA 2006;103:2869-73.

15. Hershberg R, Lipatov M, Small PM, Sheffer H, Niemann S, Homolka S, et al. High functional diversity in Mycobacterium tuberculosis driven by genetic drift and human demography. PLoS Biol 2008;6:e311.

16. López B, Aguilar D, Orozco H, Burger M, Espitia C, Ritacco V, et al. A marked difference in pathogenesis and immune response induced by different Mycobacterium tuberculosis genotypes. Clin Exp Immunol 2003;133:30-7.

17. Di Pietrantonio T, Correa JA, Orlova M, Behr MA, Schurr E. Joint effects of host genetic background and mycobacterial pathogen on susceptibility to infection. Infect Immun 2011;79:2372-8.

18. Di Pietrantonio T, Hernandez C, Girard M, Verville A, Orlova M, Belley A, et al. Strain-specific differences in the genetic control of two closely related mycobacteria. PLoS Pathog 2010;6:e1001169.

19. Hirsh AE, Tsolaki AG, DeRiemer K, Feldman MW, Small PM. Stable association between strains of Mycobacterium tuberculosis and their human host populations. Proc Natl Acad Sci USA 2004;101:4871-6.

20. Hanekom M, van der Spuy GD, Gey van Pittius NC, McEvoy CR, Ndabambi SL, Victor TC, et al. Evidence that the spread of Mycobacterium tuberculosis strains with the Beijing genotype is human population dependent. J Clin Microbiol 2007;45:2263-6.

21. Merker M, Blin C, Mona S, Duforet-Frebourg N, Lecher S, Willery E, et al. Evolutionary history and global spread of the Mycobacterium tuberculosis Beijing lineage. Nat Genet 2015;47:242-9.

22. Comas I, Coscolla M, Luo T, Borrell S, Holt KE, Kato-Maeda M, et al. Out-of-Africa migration and Neolithic coexpansion of Mycobacterium tuberculosis with modern humans. Nat Genet 2013;45:1176-82.

23. Gagneux S. Host-pathogen co-evolution in human tuberculosis. Philos Trans R Soc Lond B Biol Sci 2012;367:850-9.

24. Intemann CD, Thye T, Niemann S, Browne EN, Amanua Chinbuah M, Enimil A, et al. Autophagy gene variant IRGM -261T contributes to protection from tuberculosis caused by Mycobacterium tuberculosis but not by M. africanum strains. PLoS Pathog 2009;5:e1000577.

25. Herb F, Thye T, Niemann S, Browne EN, Chinbuah MA, Gyapong J, et al. ALOX5 variants associated with susceptibility to human pulmonary tuberculosis. Hum Mol Genet 2008;17:1052-60.

26. Thye T, Niemann S, Walter K, Homolka S, Intemann CD, Chinbuah MA, et al. Variant G57E of mannose binding lectin associated with protection against tuberculosis caused by Mycobacterium africanum but not by M. tuberculosis. PLoS One 2011;6:e20908.

27. Grant AV, El Baghdadi J, Sabri A, El Azbaoui S, Alaoui-Tahiri K, Abderrahmani Rhorfi I, et al. Age-dependent association between pulmonary tuberculosis and common TOX variants in the 8q12-13 linkage region. Am J Hum Genet 2013;92:407-14.

28. Mira MT, Alcaïs A, Nguyen VT, Moraes MO, Di Flumeri C, Vu HT, et al. Susceptibility to leprosy is associated with PARK2 and PACRG. Nature 2004;427:636-40.

29. Carlson CS, Eberle MA, Kruglyak L, Nickerson DA. Mapping complex disease loci in whole-genome association studies. Nature 2004;429:446-52.

30. Baghdadi JE, Orlova M, Alter A, Ranque B, Chentoufi M, Lazrak F, et al. An autosomal dominant major gene confers predisposition to pulmonary tuberculosis in adults. J Exp Med 2006;203:1679-84.

31. Bellamy R, Beyers N, McAdam KP, Ruwende C, Gie R, Samaai P, et al. Genetic susceptibility to tuberculosis in Africans: a genome-wide scan. Proc Natl Acad Sci USA 2000;97:8005-9.

32. Miller EN, Jamieson SE, Joberty C, Fakiola M, Hudson D, Peacock CS, et al. Genome-wide scans for leprosy and tuberculosis susceptibility genes in Brazilians. Genes Immun 2004;5:63-7.

33. Marquet S, Abel L, Hillaire D, Dessein H, Kalil J, Feingold J, et al. Genetic localization of a locus controlling the intensity of infection by Schistosoma mansoni on chromosome 5q31-q33. Nat Genet 1996;14:181-4.

34. Siddiqui MR, Meisner S, Tosh K, Balakrishnan K, Ghei S, Fisher SE, et al. A major susceptibility locus for leprosy in India maps to chromosome 10p13. Nat Genet 2001;27:439-41.

35. Mira MT, Alcaïs A, Van Thuc N, Thai VH, Huong NT, Ba NN, et al. Chromosome 6q25 is linked to susceptibility to leprosy in a Vietnamese population. Nat Genet 2003;33:412-5.

36. Lesley R, Ramakrishnan L. Insights into early mycobacterial pathogenesis from the zebrafish. Curr Opin Microbiol 2008;11:277-83.

37. Fortin A, Abel L, Casanova JL, Gros P. Host genetics of mycobacterial diseases in mice and men: forward genetic studies of BCG-osis and tuberculosis. Annu Rev Genomics Hum Genet 2007;8:163-92.

38. Risch N, Merikangas K. The future of genetic studies of complex human diseases. Science 1996;273:1516-7.

39. Abel L, Alcais A, Schurr, E. The dissection of complex susceptibility to infectious disease: bacterial, viral and parasitic infections. Curr Opin Immunol 2014;30:72-8.

40. Mardis ER. Next-generation DNA sequencing methods. Annu Rev Genomics Hum Genet 2008;9:387-402.

41. Hardy J, Singleton A. Genomewide association studies and human disease. N Engl J Med 2009;60:1759-68.

42. Bogunovic D, Byun M, Durfee LA, Abhyankar A, Sanal O, Mansouri D, et al. Mycobacterial disease and impaired IFN-gamma immunity in humans with inherited ISG15 deficiency. Science 2012;337:1684-8.

43. Suarez-Alvarez B, Rodriguez RM, Fraga MF, Lopez-Larrea C. DNA methylation: a promising landscape for immune system-related diseases. Trends Genet 2012;28:506-14.

44. Laird PW. Principles and challenges of genomewide DNA methylation analysis. Nat Rev Genet 2010;11:191-203.

45. Esterhuyse MM, Linhart HG, Kaufmann SH. Can the battle against tuberculosis gain from epigenetic research? Trends Microbiol 2012;20:220-6.

46. Kaelin W Jr, McKnight SL. Influence of metabolism on epigenetics and disease. Cell 2013;153:56-69.

47. Martineau AR, Wilkinson KA, Newton SM, Floto RA, Norman AW, Skolimowska K, et al. IFN-gamma- and TNF-independent vitamin D-inducible human suppression of mycobacteria: the role of cathelicidin LL-37. J Immunol 2007;178:7190-8.

48. Gregersen PK. Cell type-specific eQTLs in the human immune system. Nat Genet 2012;44:478-80.

49. Berry MP, Graham CM, McNab FW, Xu Z, Bloch SA, Oni T, et al. An interferon-inducible neutrophil-driven blood transcriptional signature in human tuberculosis. Nature 2010;466:973-7.

50. Blankley S, Berry MP, Graham CM, Bloom CI, Lipman M, O'Garra A. The application of transcriptional blood signatures to enhance our understanding of the host response to infection: the example of tuberculosis. Philos Trans R Soc Lond B Biol Sci 2014;369:20130427.

51. Bloom CI, Graham CM, Berry MP, Wilkinson KA, Oni T, Rozakeas FB, et al. Detectable changes in the blood transcriptome are present after two weeks of antituberculosis therapy. PLoS One 2012;7:e46191.

52. Anderson ST, Kaforou M, Brent AJ, Wright VJ, Banwell CM, Chagaluka G, et al. Diagnosis of childhood tuberculosis and host RNA expression in Africa. N Engl J Med 2014;370:1712-23.

53. Chackerian AA, Perera TV, Behar SM. Gamma interferon-producing CD4+ T lymphocytes in the lung correlate with resistance to infection with Mycobacterium tuberculosis. Infect Immun 2001;69:2666-74.

54. Medina E, North RJ. Genetically susceptible mice remain proportionally more susceptible to tuberculosis after vaccination. Immunology 1999;96:16-21.

55. Orme IM. The immunopathogenesis of tuberculosis: a new working hypothesis. Trends Microbiol 1998;6:94-7.

56. Turner J, Gonzalez-Juarrero M, Saunders BM, Brooks JV, Marietta P, Ellis DL, et al. Immunological basis for reactivation of tuberculosis in mice. Infect Immun 2001;69:3264-70.

57. Watson VE, Hill LL, Owen-Schaub LB, Davis DW, McConkey DJ, Jagannath C, et al. Apoptosis in Mycobacterium tuberculosis infection in mice exhibiting varied immunopathology. J Pathol 2000;190:211-20.

58. Buer J, Balling R. Mice, microbes and models of infection. Nat Rev Genet 2003;4:195-205.

59. Fisler JS, Warden CH. Mapping of mouse obesity genes: a generic approach to a complex trait. J Nutr 1997;127:1909S-1916S.

60. Boyse EA. The increasing value of congenic mice in biomedical research. Lab Anim Sci 1977;27:771-81.

61. Wakeland E, Morel L, Achey K, Yui M, Longmate J. Speed congenics: a classic technique in the fast lane [relatively speaking]. Immunol Today 1997;18:472-7.

62. Caruso AM, Serbina N, Klein E, Triebold K, Bloom BR, Flynn JL. Mice deficient in CD4 T cells have only transiently diminished levels of IFN-gamma, yet succumb to tuberculosis. J Immunol 1999;162: 5407-16.

63. Mogues T, Goodrich ME, Ryan L, LaCourse R, North RJ. The relative importance of T cell subsets in immunity and immunopathology of airborne Mycobacterium tuberculosis infection in mice. J Exp Med 2001;193:271-80.

64. Flynn JL, Chan J, Triebold KJ, Dalton DK, Stewart TA, Bloom BR. An essential role for interferon gamma in resistance to Mycobacterium tuberculosis infection. J Exp Med 1993;178: 2249-54.

65. Dalton DK, Pitts-Meek S, Keshav S, Figari IS, Bradley A, Stewart TA. Multiple defects of immune cell function in mice with disrupted interferon-gamma genes. Science 1993;259: 1739-42.

66. MacMicking JD, Taylor GA, McKinney JD. Immune control of tuberculosis by IFN-gamma-inducible LRG-47. Science 2003;302: 654-9.

67. Hölscher C, Atkinson RA, Arendse B, Brown N, Myburgh E, Alber G, et al. A protective and agonistic function of IL-12p40 in mycobacterial infection. J Immunol 2001;167:6957-66.

68. Cooper AM, Kipnis A, Turner J, Magram J, Ferrante J, Orme IM. Mice lacking bioactive IL-12 can generate protective, antigen-specific cellular responses to mycobacterial infection only if the IL-12 p40 subunit is present. J Immunol 2002;168:1322-7.

69. Cooper AM, Magram J, Ferrante J, Orme IM. Interleukin 12 [IL-12] is crucial to the development of protective immunity in mice intravenously infected with Mycobacterium tuberculosis. J Exp Med 1997;186:39-45.

70. Bean AG, Roach DR, Briscoe H, France MP, Korner H, Sedgwick JD. Structural deficiencies in granuloma formation in TNF gene-targeted mice underlie the heightened susceptibility to aerosol Mycobacterium tuberculosis infection, which is not compensated for by lymphotoxin. J Immunol 1999;162:3504-11.

71. Flynn JL, Goldstein MM, Chan J, Triebold KJ, Pfeffer K, Lowenstein CJ. Tumor necrosis factor-alpha is required in the protective immune response against Mycobacterium tuberculosis in mice. Immunity 1995;2:561-72.

72. Smith S, Liggitt D, Jeromsky E, Tan X, Skerrett SJ, Wilson CBS. Local role for tumor necrosis factor alpha in the pulmonary inflammatory response to Mycobacterium tuberculosis infection. Infect Immun 2002;70:2082-9.

73. Roach DR, Bean AG, Demangel C, France MP, Briscoe H, Britton WJ. TNF regulates chemokine induction essential for cell recruitment, granuloma formation, and clearance of mycobacterial infection. J Immunol 2002;168:4620-7.

74. Lynch CJ, Pierse-Chase CH, Dubos R. Genetic study of susceptibility to experimental tuberculosis in mice infected with mammalian tubercle bacilli. J Exp Med 1965;121:1051-70.

75. Nikonenko BV, Averbakh MM Jr, Lavebratt C, Schurr E, Apt AS. Comparative analysis of mycobacterial infections in susceptible I/St and resistant A/Sn inbred mice. Tuber Lung Dis 2000;80: 15-25.

76. Lavebratt C, Apt AS, Nikonenko BV, Schalling M, Schurr E. Severity of tuberculosis in mice is linked to distal chromosome 3 and proximal chromosome 9. J Infect Dis 1999;180:150-5.

77. Sánchez F, Radaeva TV, Nikonenko BV, Persson AS, Sengul S, Schalling M, et al. Multigenic control of disease severity after virulent Mycobacterium tuberculosis infection in mice. Infect Immun 2003;71:126-31.

78. Kähler AK, Persson AS, Sánchez F, Källström H, Apt AS, Schurr E, et al. A new coding mutation in the Tnf-alpha leader sequence in tuberculosis-sensitive I/St mice causes higher secretion levels of soluble TNF-alpha. Genes Immun 2005;6:620-7.

79. Kramnik I, Dietrich WF, Demant P, Bloom BR. Genetic control of resistance to experimental infection with virulent Mycobacterium tuberculosis. Proc Natl Acad Sci USA 2000;97:8560-5.

80. Pan H, Yan BS, Rojas M, Shebzukhov YV, Zhou H, Kobzik L, et al. Ipr1 gene mediates innate immunity to tuberculosis. Nature 2005;434:767-72.

81. Yan BS, Kirby A, Shebzukhov YV, Daly MJ, Kramnik I. Genetic architecture of tuberculosis resistance in a mouse model of infection. Genes Immun 2006;7:201-10.

82. Mitsos LM, Cardon LR, Fortin A, Ryan L, LaCourse R, North RJ, et al. Genetic control of susceptibility to infection with Mycobacte_ rium tuberculosis in mice. Genes Immun 2000;1:467-77.

83. Mitsos LM, Cardon LR, Ryan L, LaCourse R, North RJ, Gros P. Susceptibility to tuberculosis: a locus on mouse chromosome 19 [Trl-4] regulates Mycobacterium tuberculosis replication in the lungs. Proc Natl Acad Sci USA 2003;100:6610-5.

84. Marquis JF, Lacourse R, Ryan L, North RJ, Gros P. Genetic and functional characterization of the mouse Trl3 locus in defense against tuberculosis. J Immunol 2009;82:3757-67.

85. Al-Muhsen S, Casanova JL. The genetic heterogeneity of Mendelian susceptibility to mycobacterial diseases. J Allergy Clin Immunol 2008;122:1043-51.

86. Filipe-Santos O, Bustamante J, Chapgier A, Vogt G, de Beaucoudrey L, Feinberg J. Inborn errors of IL-12/23- and IFN-gamma-mediated immunity: molecular, cellular, and clinical features. Semin Immunol 2006;18:347-61.

87. Alcais A, Fieschi C, Abel L, Casanova JL. Tuberculosis in children and adults: two distinct genetic diseases. J Exp Med 2005;202:1617-21.

88. Ozbek N, Fieschi C, Yilmaz BT, de Beaucoudrey L, Demirhan B, Feinberg J. Interleukin-12 receptor beta 1 chain deficiency in a child with disseminated tuberculosis. Clin Infect Dis 2005;40:e55-8.

89. de Beaucoudrey L, Samarina A, Bustamante J, Cobat A, Boisson-Dupuis S, Feinberg J. Revisiting human IL-12R beta1 deficiency: a survey of 141 patients from 30 countries. Medicine [Baltimore] 2010;89:381-402.

90. Prando C, Samarina A, Bustamante J, Boisson-Dupuis S, Cobat A, Picard CP. Inherited IL-12p40 deficiency: genetic, immunologic, and clinical features of 49 patients from 30 kindreds. Medicine [Baltimore] 2013;92:109-22.

91. Bustamante J, Boisson-Dupuis S, Abel L, Casanova JL. Mendelian susceptibility to mycobacterial disease: Genetic, immunological, and clinical features of inborn errors of IFN-gamma immunity. Semin Immunol 2014;26:454-70.

92. Remus N, El Baghdadi J, Fieschi C, Feinberg J, Quintin T, Chentoufi M. Association of IL12RB1 polymorphisms with pulmonary tuberculosis in adults in Morocco. J Infect Dis 2004;190:580-7.

93. Rosenzweig SD, Schäffer AA, Ding L, Sullivan R, Enyedi B, Yim JJ. Interferon-gamma receptor 1 promoter polymorphisms: population distribution and functional implications. Clin Immunol 2004;112: 113-9.

94. Boisson-Dupuis S, El Baghdadi J, Parvaneh N, Bousfiha A, Bustamante J, Feinberg J. IL-12R beta1 deficiency in two of fifty children with severe tuberculosis from Iran, Morocco, and Turkey. PLoS One 2011;6:e18524.

95. Boisson-Dupuis S, El Baghdadi J, Parvaneh N, Bousfiha A, Bustamante J, Feinberg J. Inherited and acquired immuno-deficiencies underlying tuberculosis in childhood. Immunol Rev 2015;264:103-20.

96. van de Vosse E, Haverkamp MH, Ramirez-Alejo N, Martinez-Gallo M, Blancas-Galicia L, Metin A. IL-12R beta1 deficiency: mutation update and description of the IL12RB1 variation database. Hum Mutat 2013;34:1329-39.

97. van de Vosse E, de Paus RA, van Dissel JT, Ottenhoff TH. Molecular complementation of IL-12R beta1 deficiency reveals functional differences between IL-12R beta1 alleles including partial IL-12R beta1 deficiency. Hum Mol Genet 2005;14:3847-55.

98. Akahoshi M, Nakashima H, Miyake K, Inoue Y, Shimizu S, Tanaka Y. Influence of interleukin-12 receptor beta1 poly-morphisms on tuberculosis. Hum Genet 2003;112:237-43.

99. Kusuhara K, Yamamoto K, Okada K, Mizuno Y, Hara T. Association of IL12RB1 polymorphisms with susceptibility to and severity of tuberculosis in Japanese: a gene-based association analysis of 21 candidate genes. Int J Immunogenet 2007;34:35-44.

100. Tso HW, Lau YL, Tam CM, Wong HS, Chiang AK. Associations between IL12B polymorphisms and tuberculosis in the Hong Kong Chinese population. J Infect Dis 2004;190:913-9.

101. Morris GA, Edwards DR, Hill PC, Wejse C, Bisseye C, Olesen R. Interleukin 12B [IL12B] genetic variation and pulmonary tuberculosis: a study of cohorts from The Gambia, Guinea-Bissau, United States and Argentina. PLoS One 2011;6:e16656.

102. Liu G, Li G, Xu Y, Song N, Shen S, Jiang D. Association between IL12B polymorphisms and tuberculosis risk: a meta-analysis. Infect Genet Evol 2014;21:401-7.

103. Fraser DA, Bulat-Kardum L, Knezevic J, Babarovic P, Matakovic-Mileusnic N, Dellacasagrande J. Interferon-gamma receptor-1 gene polymorphism in tuberculosis patients from Croatia. Scand J Immunol 2005;57:480-4.

104. Awomoyi AA, Nejentsev S, Richardson A, Hull J, Koch O, Podinovskaia M. No association between interferon-gamma receptor-1 gene polymorphism and pulmonary tuberculosis in a Gambian population sample. Thorax 2004;59:291-4.

105. Cooke GS, Tosh K, Ramaley PA, Kaleebu P, Zhuang J, Nakiyingi JS. Polymorphism within the interferon-gamma/receptor complex is associated with pulmonary tuberculosis. Am J Respir Crit Care Med 2006;174:339-43.

106. Stein CM, Zalwango S, Chiunda AB, Millard C, Leontiev DV, Horvath AL. Linkage and association analysis of candidate genes for TB and TNF alpha cytokine expression: evidence for association with IFNGR1, IL-10, and TNF receptor 1 genes. Hum Genet 2007;121:663-73.

107. Wang W, Ren W, Zhang X, Liu Y, Li C. Association between interferon gamma receptor 1-56C/T gene polymorphism and tuberculosis susceptibility: a meta-analysis. Chin Med J [Engl] 2014;127:3782-8.

108. Pravica V, Asderakis A, Perrey C, Hajeer A, Sinnott PJ, Hutchinson IV. In vitro production of IFN-gamma correlates with CA repeat polymorphism in the human IFN-gamma gene. Eur J Immunogenet 1999;26:1-3.

109. Tso HW, Ip WK, Chong WP, Tam CM, Chiang AK, Lau YL. Association of interferon gamma and interleukin 10 genes with tuberculosis in Hong Kong Chinese. Genes Immun 2005;6:358-63.

110. Ding S, Li L, Zhu X. Polymorphism of the interferon-gamma gene and risk of tuberculosis in a southeastern Chinese population. Hum Immunol 2008;69:129-33.

111. Pravica V, Perrey C, Stevens A, Lee JH, Hutchinson IV. A single nucleotide polymorphism in the first intron of the human IFN-gamma gene: absolute correlation with a polymorphic CA microsatellite marker of high IFN-gamma production. Human Immunol 2000;61:863-6.

112. Huang Y, Yang H, Borg BB, Su X, Rhodes SL, Yang K. A functional SNP of interferon-gamma gene is important for interferon-alpha-induced and spontaneous recovery from hepatitis C virus infection. Proc Natl Acad Sci USA 2007;104:985-90.

113. Abbott W, Gane E, Winship I, Munn S, Tukuitonga C. Polymorphism in intron 1 of the interferon-gamma gene influences both serum immunoglobulin E levels and the risk for chronic hepatitis B virus infection in Polynesians. Immuno-genetics 2007;59:187-95.

114. Dai CY, Chuang WL, Hsieh MY, Lee LP, Hou NJ, Chen SC. Polymorphism of interferon-gamma gene at position +874 and clinical characteristics of chronic hepatitis C. Transl Res 2006;148:128-33.

115. Cardoso CC, Pereira AC, Brito-de-Souza VN, Dias-Baptista IM, Maniero VC, Venturini J. IFNG +874 T>A single nucleotide polymorphism is associated with leprosy among Brazilians. Hum Genet 2010;128:481-90.

116. Vallinoto AC, Graça ES, Araújo MS, Azevedo VN, Cayres-Vallinoto I, Machado LF. IFNG +874T/A polymorphism and cytokine plasma levels are associated with susceptibility to Mycobacterium tuberculosis infection and clinical manifestation of tuberculosis. Hum Immunol 2010;71:692-6.

117. Ansari A, Hasan Z, Dawood G, Hussain R. Differential combination of cytokine and interferon-gamma +874 T/A polymorphisms determines disease severity in pulmonary tuberculosis. PLoS One 2011;6:e27848.

118. Shen C, Jiao WW, Feng WX, Wu XR, Xiao J, Miao Q. IFNG polymorphisms are associated with tuberculosis in Han Chinese pediatric female population. Mol Biol Rep 2013;40:5477-82.

119. Lio D, Marino V, Serauto A, Gioia V, Scola L, Crivello A. Genotype frequencies of the +874T-->A single nucleotide polymorphism in the first intron of the interferon-gamma gene in a sample of Sicilian patients affected by tuberculosis. Eur J Immunogenet 2002;29:371-4.

120. Sallakci N, Coskun M, Berber Z, Gürkan F, Kocamaz H, Uysal G. Interferon-gamma gene+874T-A polymorphism is associated with tuberculosis and gamma interferon response. Tuberculosis [Edinb] 2007;87:225-30.

121. Fitness J, Floyd S, Warndorff DK, Sichali L, Malema S, Crampin AC, et al. Large-scale candidate gene study of tuberculosis susceptibility in the Karonga district of northern Malawi. Am J Trop Med Hyg 2004;71:341-9.

122. Moran A, Ma X, Reich RA, Graviss EA. No association between the +874T/A single nucleotide polymorphism in the IFN-gamma gene and susceptibility to TB. Int J Tuberc Lung Dis 2007;11: 113-5.

123. Leandro AC, Rocha MA, Lamoglia-Souza A, VandeBerg JL, Rolla VC, Bonecini-Almeida Mda G. No association of IFNG+874T/A SNP and NOS2A-954G/C SNP variants with nitric oxide radical serum levels or susceptibility to tuberculosis in a Brazilian population subset. Biomed Res Int 2013;901740.

124. Etokebe GE, Bulat-Kardum L, Johansen MS, Knezevic J, Balen S, Matakovic-Mileusnic N. Interferon-gamma gene [T874A and G2109A] polymorphisms are associated with microscopy-positive tuberculosis. Scand J Immunol 2006;63:136-41.

125. Gruenheid S, Pinner E, Desjardins M, Gros P. Natural resistance to infection with intracellular pathogens: the Nramp1 protein is recruited to the membrane of the phagosome. J Exp Med 1997;185:717-30.

126. Jabado N, Jankowski A, Dougaparsad S, Picard V, Grinstein S, Gros P. Natural resistance to intracellular infections: natural resistance-associated macrophage protein 1 [Nramp1] functions as a pH-dependent manganese transporter at the phagosomal membrane. J Exp Med 2000;192:1237-48.

127. Cuellar-Mata P, Jabado N, Liu J, Furuya W, Finlay BB, Gros P. Nramp1 modifies the fusion of Salmonella typhimurium-containing vacuoles with cellular endomembranes in macrophages. J Biol Chem 2002;277:2258-65.

128. Frehel C, Canonne-Hergaux F, Gros P, De Chastellier C. Effect of Nramp1 on bacterial replication and on maturation of Mycobacterium avium-containing phagosomes in bone marrow-derived mouse macrophages. Cell Microbiol 2002;4:541-56.

129. Hackam DJ, Rotstein O D, Zhang W, Gruenheid S, Gros P, Grinstein S. Host resistance to intracellular infection: mutation of natural resistance-associated macrophage protein 1 [Nramp1] impairs phagosomal acidification. J Exp Med 1998;188:351-64.

130. Vidal S, Tremblay ML, Govoni G, Gauthier S, Sebastiani G, Malo D. The Ity/Lsh/Bcg locus: natural resistance to infection with intracellular parasites is abrogated by disruption of the Nramp1 gene. J Exp Med 1995;182:655-66.

131. Vidal SM, Malo D, Vogan K, Skamene E, Gros P. Natural resistance to infection with intracellular parasites: isolation of a candidate for Bcg. Cell 1993;73:469-85.

132. Bellamy R, Ruwende C, Corrah T, McAdam KP, Whittle HC, Hill AV. Variations in the NRAMP1 gene and susceptibility to tuberculosis in West Africans. N Engl J Med 1998;338:640-4.

133. Delgado JC, Baena A, Thim S, Goldfeld AE. Ethnic-specific genetic associations with pulmonary tuberculosis. J Infect Dis 2002;186:1463-8.

134. Gao PS, Fujishima S, Mao XQ, Remus N, Kanda M, Enomoto T, et al. Genetic variants of NRAMP1 and active tuberculosis in Japanese populations. International Tuberculosis Genetics Team. Clin Genet 2000;58:74-6.

135. Cervino AC, Lakiss S, Sow O, Hill AV. Allelic association between the NRAMP1 gene and susceptibility to tuberculosis in Guinea-Conakry. Ann Hum Genet 2000;64:507-12.

136. Ryu S, Park YK, Bai GH, Kim SJ, Park SN, Kang S. 3'UTR polymorphisms in the NRAMP1 gene are associated with susceptibility to tuberculosis in Koreans. Int J Tuberc Lung Dis 2000;4: 577-80.

137. Liu W, Cao WC, Zhang CY, Tian L, Wu XM, Habbema JD, et al. VDR and NRAMP1 gene polymorphisms in susceptibility to pulmonary tuberculosis among the Chinese Han population: a case-control study. Int J Tuberc Lung Dis 2004;8:428-34.

138. Søborg C, Andersen AB, Range N, Malenganisho W, Friis H, Magnussen P, et al. Influence of candidate susceptibility genes on tuberculosis in a high endemic region. Mol Immunol 2007;44:2213-20.

139. Singh A, Gaughan JP, Kashyap VK. SLC11A1 and VDR gene variants and susceptibility to tuberculosis and disease progression in East India. Int J Tuberc Lung Dis 2011;15:1468-74.

140. van Crevel R, Parwati I, Sahiratmadja E, Marzuki S, Ottenhoff TH, Netea MG, et al. Infection with Mycobacterium tuberculosis Beijing genotype strains is associated with polymorphisms in SLC11A1/NRAMP1 in Indonesian patients with tuberculosis. J Infect Dis 2009;200:1671-4.

141. Hoal EG, Lewis LA, Jamieson SE, Tanzer F, Rossouw M, Victor T, et al. SLC11A1 [NRAMP1] but not SLC11A2 [NRAMP2] polymorphisms are associated with susceptibility to tuberculosis in a high-incidence community in South Africa. Int J Tuberc Lung Dis 2004;8:1464-71.

142. Malik S, Abel L, Tooker H, Poon A, Simkin L, Girard M, et al. Alleles of the NRAMP1 gene are risk factors for pediatric tuberculosis disease. Proc Natl Acad Sci USA 2005;102:12183-8.

143. Velez DR, Hulme WF, Myers JL, Stryjewski ME, Abbate E, Estevan R, et al. Association of SLC11A1 with tuberculosis and interactions with NOS2A and TLR2 in African-Americans and Caucasians. Int J Tuberc Lung Dis 2009;13:1068-76.

144. Zhang W, Shao L, Weng X, Hu Z, Jin A, Chen S, et al. Variants of the natural resistance-associated macrophage protein 1 gene [NRAMP1] are associated with severe forms of pulmonary tuberculosis. Clin Infect Dis 2005;40:1232-6.

145. Hsu YH, Chen CW, Sun HS, Jou R, Lee JJ, Su IJ, et al. Association of NRAMP 1 gene polymorphism with susceptibility to tuberculosis in Taiwanese aboriginals. J Formos Med Assoc 2006; 105:363-9.

146. Leung KH, Yip SP, Wong WS, Yiu LS, Chan KK, Lai WM, et al. Sex- and age-dependent association of SLC11A1 polymorphisms with tuberculosis in Chinese: a case control study. BMC Infect Dis 2007;7:19.

147. Liaw YS, Tsai-Wu JJ, Wu CH, Hung CC, Lee CN, Yang PC, et al. Variations in the NRAMP1 gene and susceptibility of tuberculosis in Taiwanese. Int J Tuberc Lung Dis 2002;6:454-60.

148. El Baghdadi J, Remus N, Benslimane A, El Annaz H, Chentoufi M, Abel L, et al. Variants of the human NRAMP1 gene and susceptibility to tuberculosis in Morocco. Int J Tuberc Lung Dis 2003;7:599-602.

149. Vejbaesya S, Chierakul N, Luangtrakool P, Sermduangprateep C. NRAMP1 and TNF-alpha polymorphisms and susceptibility to tuberculosis in Thais. Respirology 2007;12:202-6.

150. Ates O, Dalyan L, Müsellim B, Hatemi G, Türker H, Ongen G, et al. NRAMP1 [SLC11A1] gene polymorphisms that correlate with autoimmune versus infectious disease susceptibility in tuberculosis and rheumatoid arthritis. Int J Immunogenet 2009; 36:15-9.

151. Bellamy R. Susceptibility to mycobacterial infections: the importance of host genetics. Genes Immun 2003;4:4-11.

152. Greenwood CM, Fujiwara TM, Boothroyd LJ, Miller MA, Frappier D, Fanning EA, et al. Linkage of tuberculosis to chromosome 2q35 loci, including NRAMP1, in a large aboriginal Canadian family. Am J Hum Genet 2000;67:405-16.

153. Awomoyi AA, Marchant A, Howson JM, McAdam KP, Blackwell JM, Newport MJ, et al. Interleukin-10, polymorphism in SLC11A1 [formerly NRAMP1], and susceptibility to tuberculosis. J Infect Dis 2002;186:1808-14.

154. Gallant CJ, Malik S, Jabado N, Cellier M, Simkin L, Finlay BB, et al. Reduced in vitro functional activity of human NRAMP1 [SLC11A1] allele that predisposes to increased risk of pediatric tuberculosis disease. Genes Immun 2007;8:691-8.

155. Bell A. Calciferol for tuberculous adenitis. Lancet 1946;248:808.

156. Rook GA, Steele J, Fraher L, Barker S, Karmali R, O'Riordan J, et al. Vitamin D3, gamma interferon, and control of proliferation of Mycobacterium tuberculosis by human monocytes. Immunology 1986;57:159-63.

157. Rockett KA, Brookes R, Udalova I, Vidal V, Hill AV, Kwiatkowski D. 1,25-Dihydroxyvitamin D3 induces nitric oxide synthase and suppresses growth of Mycobacterium tuberculosis in a human macrophage-like cell line. Infect Immun. 1998;66: 5314-21.

158. Davies PD. A possible link between vitamin D deficiency and impaired host defence to Mycobacterium tuberculosis. Tubercle 1985;66:301-6.

159. Davies PD, Brown RC, Woodhead JS. Serum concentrations of vitamin D metabolites in untreated tuberculosis. Thorax. 1985;40: 187-90.

160. Provvedini DM, Tsoukas CD, Deftos LJ, Manolagas SC. 1,25-dihydroxyvitamin D3 receptors in human leukocytes. Science 1983;221:1181-3.

161. Selvaraj P, Chandra G, Kurian SM, Reetha AM, Narayanan PR. Association of vitamin D receptor gene variants of BsmI, ApaI and FokI polymorphisms with susceptibility or resistance to pulmonary tuberculosis. Curr Sci 2003;84:1564-8.

162. Schaaf MJ, Cidlowski JA. AUUUA motifs in the 3'UTR of human glucocorticoid receptor alpha and beta mRNA destabilize mRNA and decrease receptor protein expression. Steroids 2002; 67:627-36.

163. Chun RF, Adams JS, Hewison M. Immunomodulation by vitamin D: implications for TB. Expert Rev Clin Pharmacol 2011; 4:583-91.

164. Morrison NA, Qi JC, Tokita A, Kelly PJ, Crofts L, Nguyen T, et al. Prediction of bone density from vitamin D receptor alleles. Nature 1994;367:284-7.

165. Whitfield GK, Remus LS, Jurutka PW, Zitzer H, Oza AK, Dang HT, et al. Functionally relevant polymorphisms in the human nuclear vitamin D receptor gene. Mol Cell Endocrinol 2001;177:145-59.

166. Ates O, Dolek B, Dalyan L, Musellim B, Ongen G, Topal-Sarikaya A, et al. The association between BsmI variant of vitamin D receptor gene and susceptibility to tuberculosis. Mol Biol Rep 2011;38:2633-6.

167. Babb C, van der Merwe L, Beyers N, Pheiffer C, Walzl G, Duncan K, et al. Vitamin D receptor gene polymorphisms and sputum conversion time in pulmonary tuberculosis patients. Tuberculosis [Edinb] 2007;87:295-302.

168. Banoei MM, Mirsaeidi MS, Houshmand M, Tabarsi P, Ebrahimi G, Zargari L, et al. Vitamin D receptor homozygote mutant tt and bb are associated with susceptibility to pulmonary tuberculosis in the Iranian population. Int J Infect Dis 2010;14: e84-5.

169. Bellamy R, Ruwende C, Corrah T, McAdam KP, Thursz M, Whittle HC, et al. Tuberculosis and chronic hepatitis B virus infection in Africans and variation in the vitamin D receptor gene. J Infect Dis 1999;179:721-4.

170. Bornman L, Campbell SJ, Fielding K, Bah B, Sillah J, Gustafson P, et al. Vitamin D receptor polymorphisms and susceptibility to tuberculosis in West Africa: a case-control and family study. J Infect Dis 2004;190:1631-41.

171. Kang TJ, Jin SH, Yeum CE, Lee SB, Kim CH, Lee SH, et al. Vitamin D Receptor Gene TaqI, BsmI and FokI Polymorphisms in Korean Patients with Tuberculosis. Immune Netw 2011;11:253-7.

172. Lombard Z, Dalton DL, Venter PA, Williams RC, Bornman L. Association of HLA-DR, -DQ, and vitamin D receptor alleles and haplotypes with tuberculosis in the Venda of South Africa. Hum Immunol 2006;67:643-54.

173. Olesen R, Wejse C, Velez DR, Bisseye C, Sodemann M, Aaby P, et al. DC-SIGN [CD209], pentraxin 3 and vitamin D receptor gene variants associate with pulmonary tuberculosis risk in West Africans. Genes Immun 2007;8:456-67.

174. Roth DE, Soto G, Arenas F, Bautista CT, Ortiz J, Rodriguez R, et al. Association between vitamin D receptor gene polymorphisms and response to treatment of pulmonary tuberculosis. J Infect Dis 2004;190: 920-7.

175. Selvaraj P, Chandra G, Jawahar MS, Rani MV, Rajeshwari DN, Narayanan PR. Regulatory role of vitamin D receptor gene variants of Bsm I, Apa I, Taq I, and Fok I polymorphisms on macrophage phagocytosis and lymphoproliferative response to Mycobacterium tuberculosis antigen in pulmonary tuberculosis. J Clin Immunol 2004;24:523-32.

176. Selvaraj P, Kurian SM, Chandra G, Reetha AM, Charles N, Narayanan PR. Vitamin D receptor gene variants of BsmI, ApaI, TaqI, and FokI polymorphisms in spinal tuberculosis. Clin Genet 2004;65:73-6.

177. Selvaraj P, Prabhu Anand S, Harishankar M, Alagarasu K. Plasma 1,25 dihydroxy vitamin D3 level and expression of vitamin D receptor and cathelicidin in pulmonary tuberculosis. J Clin Immunol 2009;29:470-8.

178. Selvaraj P, Vidyarani M, Alagarasu K, Prabhu Anand S, Narayanan PR. Regulatory role of promoter and 3' UTR variants of vitamin D receptor gene on cytokine response in pulmonary tuberculosis. J Clin Immunol 2008;28:306-13.

179. Sharma PR, Singh S, Jena M, Mishra G, Prakash R, Das PK, et al. Coding and non-coding polymorphisms in VDR gene and susceptibility to pulmonary tuberculosis in tribes, castes and Muslims of Central India. Infect Genet Evol 2011;11:1456-61.

180. Vidyarani M, Selvara P, Raghava S, Narayana PR. Regulatory role of 1, 25-dihydroxyvitamin D3 and vitamin D receptor gene variants on intracellular granzyme A expression in pulmonary tuberculosis. Exp Mol Pathol 2009;86:69-73.

181. Wu F, Zhang W, Zhang L, Wu J, Li C, Meng X, et al. NRAMP1, VDR, HLA-DRB1, and HLA-DQB1 gene polymorphisms in susceptibility to tuberculosis among the Chinese Kazakh

population: a case-control study. Biomed Res Int 2013;2013: 484535.

182. Alagarasu K, Selvaraj P, Swaminathan S, Narendran G, Narayanan PR. 5′ regulatory and 3′ untranslated region polymorphisms of vitamin D receptor gene in south Indian HIV and HIV-TB patients. J Clin Immunol 2009;29:196-204.

183. Thorsby E. The human major histocompatibility system. Transplant Rev 1974;18:51-129.

184. Doherty PC, Zinkernagel RM. A biological role for the major histocompatibility antigens. Lancet 1975;1:1406-9.

185. Zinkernagel RM. Role of the H-2 gene complex in cell-mediated immunity to infectious disease. Transplant Proc 1977;9:1835-8.

186. Zinkernagel RM. Speculations on the role of major transplantation antigens in cell-mediated immunity against intracellular parasites. Curr Top Microbiol Immunol 1978;82:113-38.

187. Thye T, Vannberg FO, Wong SH, Owusu-Dabo E, Osei I, Gyapong J, et al. Genome-wide association analyses identifies a susceptibility locus for tuberculosis on chromosome 18q11.2. Nat Genet 2010;42: 739-41.

188. Blackwell JM, Jamieson SE, Burgner D. HLA and infectious diseases. Clin Microbiol Rev 2009;22:370-85.

189. Singh M, Balamurugan A, Katoch K, Sharma SK, Mehra NK. Immunogenetics of mycobacterial infections in the North Indian population. Tissue Antigens 2007;69 Suppl 1:228-30.

190. Kim HS, Park MH, Song EY, Park H, Kwon SY, Han SK, et al. Association of HLA-DR and HLA-DQ genes with susceptibility to pulmonary tuberculosis in Koreans: preliminary evidence of associations with drug resistance, disease severity, and disease recurrence. Hum Immunol 2005;66:1074-81.

191. Yuliwulandari R, Sachrowardi Q, Nakajima H, Kashiwase K, Hirayasu K, Mabuchi A, et al. Association of HLA-A, -B, and -DRB1 with pulmonary tuberculosis in western Javanese Indonesia. Hum Immunol 2010;71:697-701.

192. Shi GL, Hu XL, Yang L, Rong CL, Guo YL, Song CX. Association of HLA-DRB alleles and pulmonary tuberculosis in North Chinese patients. Genet Mol Res 2011;10:1331-6.

193. Delgado JC, Baena A, Thim S, Goldfeld AE. Aspartic acid homozygosity at codon 57 of HLA-DQ beta is associated with susceptibility to pulmonary tuberculosis in Cambodia. J Immunol 2006;176:1090-7.

194. Singh SP, Mehra NK, Dingley HB, Pande JN, Vaidya MC. Human leukocyte antigen [HLA]-linked control of susceptibility to pulmonary tuberculosis and association with HLA-DR types. J Infect Dis 1983;148:676-81.

195. Bothamley GH, Beck JS, Schreuder GM, D'Amaro J, de Vries RR, Kardjito T, et al. Association of tuberculosis and M. tuberculosis-specific antibody levels with HLA. J Infect Dis 1989;159:549-55.

196. Terán-Escandón D, Terán-Ortiz L, Camarena-Olvera A, González-Avila G, Vaca-Marín MA, Granados J, et al. Human leukocyte antigen-associated susceptibility to pulmonary tuberculosis: molecular analysis of class II alleles by DNA amplification and oligonucleotide hybridization in Mexican patients. Chest 1999;115:428-33.

197. Goldfeld AE, Delgado JC, Thim S, Bozon MV, Uglialoro AM, Turbay D, et al. Association of an HLA-DQ allele with clinical tuberculosis. JAMA 1998;279:226-8.

198. Sanjeevi CB, Narayanan PR, Prabakar R, Charles N, Thomas BE, Balasubramaniam R, et al. No association or linkage with HLA-DR or -DQ genes in south Indians with pulmonary tuberculosis. Tuber Lung Dis 1992;73:280-4.

199. Amirzargar AA, Yalda A, Hajabolbaghi M, Khosravi F, Jabbari H, Rezaei N, et al. The association of HLA-DRB, DQA1, DQB1 alleles and haplotype frequency in Iranian patients with pulmonary tuberculosis. Int J Tuberc Lung Dis 2004;8:1017-21.

200. Selvaraj P, Nisha Rajeswari D, Jawahar MS, Narayanan PR. Influence of HLA-DRB1 alleles on Th1 and Th2 cytokine response to Mycobacterium tuberculosis antigens in pulmonary tuberculosis. Tuberculosis [Edinb] 2007;87:544-50.

201. Turner MW. Mannose-binding lectin: the pluripotent molecule of the innate immune system. Immunol Today 1996;17:532-40.

202. Casanova JL, Abel L. Human mannose-binding lectin in immunity: friend, foe, or both? J Exp Med 2004;199:1295-9.

203. Takahashin K, Ezekowitz RA. The role of the mannose-binding lectin in innate immunity. Clin Infect Dis 2005;41 Suppl 7:S440-4.

204. Dommett RM, Klein N, Turner MW. Mannose-binding lectin in innate immunity: past, present and future. Tissue Antigens 2006;68:193-209.

205. Søborg C, Madsen HO, Andersen AB, Lillebaek T, Kok-Jensen A, Garred P. Mannose-binding lectin polymorphisms in clinical tuberculosis. J Infect Dis 2003;188:777-82.

206. Mombo LE, Lu CY, Ossari S, Bedjabaga I, Sica L, Krishnamoorthy R, et al. Mannose-binding lectin alleles in sub-Saharan Africans and relation with susceptibility to infections. Genes Immun 2003;4:362-7.

207. El Sahly HM, Reich RA, Dou SJ, Musser JM, Graviss EA. The effect of mannose binding lectin gene polymorphisms on susceptibility to tuberculosis in different ethnic groups. Scand J Infect Dis 2004;36:106-8.

208. Singla N, Gupta D, Joshi A, Batra N, Singh J, Birbian N. Association of mannose-binding lectin gene polymorphism with tuberculosis susceptibility and sputum conversion time. Int J Immunogenet 2012;39:10-4.

209. Capparelli R, Iannaccone M, Palumbo D, Medaglia C, Moscariello E, Russo A, et al. Role played by human mannose-binding lectin polymorphisms in pulmonary tuberculosis. J Infect Dis 2009;199: 666-72.

210. Cosar H, Ozkinay F, Onay H, Bayram N, Bakiler AR, Anil M, et al. Low levels of mannose-binding lectin confers protection against tuberculosis in Turkish children. Eur J Clin Microbiol Infect Dis 2008;27:1165-9.

211. da Cruz HL, da Silva RC, Segat L, de Carvalho MS, Brandão LA, Guimarães RL, et al. MBL2 gene polymorphisms and susceptibility to tuberculosis in a northeastern Brazilian population. Infect Genet Evol 2013;19:323-9.

212. Shi J, Xie M, Wang JM, Xu YJ, Xiong WN, Liu XS. Mannose-binding lectin two gene polymorphisms and tuberculosis susceptibility in Chinese population: a meta-analysis. J Huazhong Univ Sci Technolog Med Sci 2013;33:166-71.

213. Liu W, Zhang F, Xin ZT, Zhao QM, Wu XM, Zhang PH, et al. Sequence variations in the MBL gene and their relationship to pulmonary tuberculosis in the Chinese Han population. Int J Tuberc Lung Dis 2006;10:1098-103.

214. Druszczy?ska M, Strapagiel D, Kwiatkowska S, Kowalewicz-Kulbat M, Rózalska B, Chmiela M, et al. Tuberculosis bacilli still posing a threat. Polymorphism of genes regulating anti-mycobacterial properties of macrophages. Pol J Microbiol 2006;55:7-12.

215. Jamieson SE, Miller EN, Black GF, Peacock CS, Cordell HJ, Howson JM, et al. Evidence for a cluster of genes on chromosome 17q11-q21 controlling susceptibility to tuberculosis and leprosy in Brazilians. Genes Immun 2004;5:46-57.

216. Cooke GS, Campbell SJ, Bennett S, Lienhardt C, McAdam KP, Sirugo G, et al. Mapping of a novel susceptibility locus suggests a role for MC3R and CTSZ in human tuberculosis. Am J Respir Crit Care Med 2008;178:203-7.

217. Stein CM, Zalwango S, Malone LL, Won S, Mayanja-Kizza H, Mugerwa RD, et al. Genome scan of M. tuberculosis infection and disease in Ugandans. PLoS One 2008;3:e4094.

218. Cobat A, Gallant CJ, Simkin L, Black GF, Stanley K, Hughes J, et al. Two loci control tuberculin skin test reactivity in an area hyperendemic for tuberculosis. J Exp Med 2009;206: 2583-91.

219. Cobat A, Poirier C, Hoal E, Boland-Auge A, de La Rocque F, Corrard F, et al. Tuberculin skin test negativity is under tight genetic control of chromosomal region 11p14-15 in settings with different tuberculosis endemicities. J Infect Dis 2015;211: 317-21.

220. Cobat A, Hoal EG, Gallant CJ, Simkin L, Black GF, Stanley K, et al. Identification of a major locus, TNF1, that controls BCG-triggered tumor necrosis factor production by leukocytes in an area hyperendemic for tuberculosis. Clin Infect Dis 2013;57: 963-70.

221. Wang X, Tang NL, Leung CC, Kam KM, Yew WW, Tam CM, et al. Association of polymorphisms in the Chr18q11.2 locus with tuberculosis in Chinese population. Hum Genet 2013;132: 691-5.

222. Thye T, Owusu-Dabo E, Vannberg FO, van Crevel R, Curtis J, Sahiratmadja E, et al. Common variants at 11p13 are associated with susceptibility to tuberculosis. Nat Genet 2012;44:257-9.

223. Mahasirimongkol S, Yanai H, Mushiroda T, Promphittayarat W, Wattanapokayakit S, Phromjai J, et al. Genome-wide association studies of tuberculosis in Asians identify distinct at-risk locus for young tuberculosis. J Hum Genet 2012;57:363-7.

224. Png E, Alisjahbana B, Sahiratmadja E, Marzuki S, Nelwan R, Balabanova Y, et al. A genome wide association study of pulmonary tuberculosis susceptibility in Indonesians. BMC Med Genet 2012;13:5.

225. Chimusa ER, Zaitlen N, Daya M, Möller M, van Helden PD, Mulder NJ, et al. Genome-wide association study of ancestry-specific TB risk in the South African Coloured population. Hum Mol Genet 2014;23:796-809.

226. Grant AV, Sabri A, Abid A, Abderrahmani Rhorfi I, Benkirane M, Souhi H, et al. A genome-wide association study of pulmonary tuberculosis in Morocco. Hum Genet 2016;135:299-307.

Laboratory Diagnosis of Tuberculosis: Best Practices and Current Policies

Madhukar Pai, Marzieh Ghiasi, Kavitha Saravu

INTRODUCTION

Despite the progress made in tuberculosis [TB] control, the World Health Organization [WHO] estimated that 10 million people developed TB in 2017, and 1.3 million died (1). In 2014 [updated data as per WHO 2015], over 3.6 million cases were considered 'missing,' either because they were not diagnosed, or not notified to any national TB programme. India accounts for 1 of the 3 million missing cases, and accounts for 25% of the global incident cases. A recent systematic review has shown that a TB patient in India, on an average, faces a delay of nearly two months and visits to three healthcare providers before a diagnosis is made (2). Thus, diagnostic delays are common in the Indian context. Furthermore, a majority of Indian TB patients do not get tested for drug-resistance. Early and accurate diagnosis followed by rapid treatment is critical to break the cycle of transmission. The purpose of this chapter is to provide a summary of the best practices for diagnosis of active TB, drug-resistance, and latent TB infection [LTBI].

DIAGNOSIS OF ACTIVE TUBERCULOSIS

Active TB is a microbiological diagnosis, and every attempt should be made to get a bacteriological confirmation using a correct clinical specimen. According to the International Standards for TB Care [ISTC], all persons with cough lasting two weeks or more, or with abnormal chest radiographs should be evaluated for TB (3). All persons with previous history of TB treatment or with treatment failure must undergo drug-susceptibility testing [DST]. There are three methods that are recommended for the microbiological diagnosis of active TB disease [Table 8.1] (4-6). These are: [i] smear microscopy; [ii] nucleic acid amplification tests [NAAT]; and [iii] liquid cultures.

Role of Immunological Tests

Figure 8.1 shows the available immune-based tests for TB and their recommended use. The following tests are *not* recommended for active TB diagnosis: serological, antibody-based tests, such as enzyme-linked immune sorbent assay [ELISA] or rapid immunoglobulin G [IgG], immunoglobulin M [IgM] tests, and interferon-gamma release assays [IGRAs] such as QuantiFERON TB Gold and TB Platinum. Serological antibody tests are discouraged by the WHO, and banned by the Government of India. As with the tuberculin skin test [TST], IGRAs are meant for LTBI detection, and are not recommended for active TB diagnosis (7).

Role of Chest Radiology

Chest radiographs are an invaluable adjunct in the diagnosis and follow-up of TB. The sensitivity of the chest radiograph is high, but non-TB conditions may look like TB. Thus, chest radiographs do not have high specificity, and so remain a supplement to microbiological tests, such as, microscopy, polymerase chain reaction [PCR] and culture. Treatment of TB purely on the basis of radiological findings can result in significant over-treatment with adverse consequences and additional costs for patients. Therefore, all persons with chest radiographic findings suggestive of TB, should have sputum specimens submitted for microbiological examination.

Sample Collection Methods

Quality of samples can affect test results, and every effort should be made to ensure quality in specimen collection, transport and processing. Table 8.2 provides a summary of the samples required for the diagnosis of various types of TB (8). For pulmonary TB, sputum is the most important

Table 8.1: Methods recommended for diagnosis of active TB

Technology	WHO-endorsed tests	Advantages	Limitations	WHO policy recommendations
Smear microscopy: visualisation of acid-fast bacilli under microscope	LED fluorescence microscopy	Rapid, inexpensive and widely available technology; can rapidly identify infectious cases	Sensitivity is modest [50%-70%], specificity is very high [>98%]; cannot detect drug-resistance, and cannot distinguish between Mtb and NTM	At least two sputum samples, stained with a fluorescence stain, and read by a trained microscopist using LED microscopy, in a laboratory participating in EQA (4)
NAAT: molecular tests that amplify DNA/RNA targets specific to Mtb	Xpert MTB/RIF, based on the GeneXpert technology [Cepheid Inc, USA]	Rapid, 2-hour test. Used for detection as well as DST. Has a sensitivity 88% and specificity 98% when compared to culture; sensitivity of 68% in smear-negative cases. Can detect rifampicin resistance with a sensitivity of 95% and specificity of 98%	Cost and limited availability at decentralised or peripheral labs. NAAT cannot be used to monitor treatment response	Xpert MTB/RIF may be used rather than conventional microscopy and culture as the initial diagnostic test in all adults and children presumed to have TB. If this is not possible because of resource constraints, Xpert should be used rather than conventional microscopy, culture and DST as the initial diagnostic test in adults and children presumed to have MDR-TB or HIV-associated TB (5)
Liquid cultures: detects growing colonies of Mtb in liquid media	BACTEC MGIT® 960 [Becton Dickinson, USA], and BacT/ALERT 3D [bioMerieux, France]	Used for detection as well as DST. Gold standard for active TB diagnosis [highest sensitivity]. Can provide results within 10-14 days, and MGIT can provide phenotypic DST results for first-line and select second-line drugs	Reliability of second-line DST is limited. High cost and limited availability are other limitations	Liquid culture and DST is a key part of the diagnostic algorithm and should be routinely used in all patients with history of previous TB treatment or treatment failure. Liquid culture is also of help in paucibacillary TB cases [EPTB, smear-negative TB, and childhood TB] (6)

TB = tuberculosis; WHO = World Health Organization; LED = light-emitting diode; EQA = external quality assurance; NAAT = nucleic acid amplification tests; DNA = deoxyribonucleic acid; RNA = ribonucleic acid; DST = drug-susceptibility testing; MDR-TB = multidrug-resistant TB; HIV = human immunodeficiency virus; Mtb = Mycobacterium tuberculosis; NTM = nontuberculous mycobacteria; MGIT = mycobacteria growth indicator tube; EPTB = extra-pulmonary tuberculosis

sample for laboratory testing. Although peripheral venous blood is a popular sample in the Indian private sector, there is no accurate blood test for active TB. For extra-pulmonary TB [EPTB], it is important to obtain specimens from the site of disease, and this usually includes collection of tissue [biopsy] and/or body cavity fluids from the suspected disease site. For childhood TB diagnosis, sputum can usually be collected from older children. In younger children, fasting gastric aspirates can be collected. In all the above situations, clear instructions on specimen collection should be provided to patients as well as to laboratories and clinics.

Diagnosis of Extra-pulmonary TB

The ISTC emphasises the importance of seeking micro-biological and histopathological diagnosis of EPTB, and emphasises the need for collecting appropriate samples. ISTC recommends that all patients, including children, who are suspected of having EPTB, should have appropriate specimens obtained from the suspected sites of involvement for microbiological and histological examination. In clinical practice, this will mean collection of samples such as body fluids [cerebrospinal, pleural, ascitic fluid], lymph node

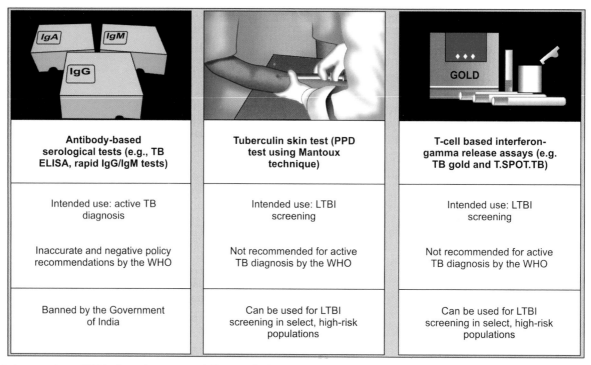

Figure 8.1: Immune-based TB tests and recommendations on their use
Ig = immunoglobulin; TB = tuberculosis; ELISA = enzyme-linked immunosorbent assay; PPD = purified protein derivative; WHO = World Health Organization; LTBI = latent tuberculosis infection

and other tissues [e.g., endometrial tissue], and aspirates [e.g., gastric aspirate]. Since no single test has high accuracy, it is important to perform microbiological [e.g., NAAT or cultures] as well as histopathological investigations.

Several recent studies and the WHO have endorsed the use of Xpert MTB/RIF® for TB meningitis, lymphadenitis, and pediatric TB [gastric aspirates] (5,9,10). In 2016, Xpert MTB/RIF® should be considered a central test in the work-up of EPTB, and should be used along with existing tools, such as, microscopy, liquid cultures which are the most sensitive technologies for detection of *Mycobacterium tuberculosis* [*Mtb*], and histopathology [biopsy] to arrive at the final diagnosis (11). Table 8.3 shows the data on accuracy of Xpert MTB/RIF® for EPTB, and the WHO recommendations on how it should be used (12). It is important to note that Xpert MTB/RIF® does not have high sensitivity for pleural samples. So, pleural biopsy and cultures are important tools for TB pleuritis.

In addition to Xpert MTB/RIF, there is a role for non-specific biomarkers such as adenosine deaminase [ADA] and unstimulated [free] interferon-gamma [IFN-γ] in sterile fluids such as pleural, peritoneal and ascitic fluid (13). These biomarkers can be used in combination with microbiological and histopathological investigations.

Drug Susceptibility Testing

The WHO recently announced the post-2015 "End TB Strategy" (14). A key component of this strategy is the push towards 'universal DST' which means that all TB patients should get a DST done at the time of their diagnosis. At the very least, all patients with history of previous TB treatment, treatment failure or recurrence must undergo DST.

DST can be done using two methods: genotypic and phenotypic. Genotypic methods are based on molecular tests that detect mutations that confer drug-resistance. For example, mutations in the rpoB gene of *Mtb* are strongly associated with rifampicin resistance. Examples of genotypic tests include Xpert MTB/RIF, and Hain Genotype MTBDRplus {commercial line probe assay [LPA]}. Phenotypic methods are based on detection of culture growth with and without TB drugs added to the culture media. Phenotypic methods include solid and liquid cultures. While solid cultures can take up to two months, liquid cultures can produce useful results within two weeks.

According to ISTC, DST should be performed at the start of therapy for all previously treated patients (3). Patients who remain sputum smear-positive at completion of the intensive phase of treatment and patients in whom treatment has failed, have been lost to follow-up, or relapsed following one or more courses of treatment should always be assessed for drug resistance. For patients in whom drug resistance is considered to be likely, an Xpert MTB/RIF® test should be the initial diagnostic test, as per the WHO policy. LPA or liquid culture and DST to at least isoniazid and rifampicin should be performed promptly if rifampicin resistance is detected. If multidrug-resistant TB [MDR-TB] is detected, DST to second-line anti-TB drugs especially fluoroquinolones and injectable drugs is required for correct management.

For DST, both the WHO and ISTC recommend Xpert MTB/RIF® test as the initial diagnostic test because it can rapidly detect rifampicin resistance within 90 minutes with

Table 8.2: Samples for TB detection

Site, purpose, or patient population	Specimen of choice	Comments
Active, pulmonary TB	Sputum [spontaneous or induced]	Sputum must be produced deep from within the lungs Saliva is not acceptable At least two sputum samples must be collected Blood is not acceptable as a sample for active, pulmonary TB Rarely, BAL fluid is used to collect lung secretions—this requires expertise and hospital care
Active, extra-pulmonary TB TB lymphadenitis	Lymph node aspirate or biopsy	Requires needle aspiration and/or excision biopsy Samples are then sent for smears for AFB, liquid culture, molecular [PCR] tests, and histopathological examination Histopathology and liquid culture are the most important tests; PCR may help, if positive
TB pleural effusion	Pleural fluid and pleural biopsy	Requires pleural tap and/or biopsy Samples are then sent for pleural fluid analysis, smears for AFB, liquid culture, molecular [PCR] tests, and histopathological examination; pleural fluid ADA or interferon-gamma is often helpful Histopathology and liquid culture are the most important tests; PCR may help, if positive
Peritoneal TB	Ascitic fluid and peritoneal biopsy	Requires ascitic tap and/or biopsy Samples are then sent for smears for AFB, ascitic fluid analysis, liquid culture, molecular [PCR] tests, and histopathological examination; ascitic fluid ADA or interferon-gamma is often helpful Histopathology and liquid culture are the most important tests; PCR may help, if positive
TB meningitis	CSF	Requires spinal tap for CSF collection Samples are then sent for smears for AFB, CSF analysis, liquid culture, molecular [PCR] tests; CSF fluid ADA or interferon-gamma may be helpful Liquid culture of CSF along with CSF analysis is most important; PCR may help, if positive
Bone and joint TB	Bone/synovial tissue via biopsy	Histopathology and liquid culture are the most important tests; PCR may help, if positive
Urinary tract and kidneys	Urine and tissue via biopsy	First voided morning urine sample; histopathology and liquid culture are the most important tests; PCR may help, if positive
Genitourinary tract	Tissue via biopsy [e.g., endometrial tissue in women]	Menstrual blood is not ideal; it is important to collect endometrial tissue Histopathology and liquid culture are the most important tests; PCR may help, if positive
Disseminated TB	Additional samples like bone marrow/ liver biopsy and blood cultures	Histopathology and liquid culture are the most important tests; PCR may help, if positive
Childhood TB	Sputum in older children; in younger children, gastric aspirates	Induced sputum may also be an option in older children
Latent TB infection	TST or whole blood for IGRAs	IGRAs are only meant for latent TB infection—they cannot separate latent infection from active disease TST must be correctly performed and read

TB = tuberculosis; BAL = bronchoalveolar lavage; AFB = acid-fast bacilli; PCR = polymerase chain reaction; CSF = cerebrospinal fluid; ADA = adenosine deaminase; IGRA = interferon-gamma release assay; TST = tuberculin skin test
Adapted from reference 8

high accuracy, and allow clinicians to initiate empiric MDR-TB therapy, pending confirmation with cultures (3,5). LPA [e.g., Hain Genotype MTBDRplus] or liquid culture and DST should then be performed promptly if rifampicin resistance is detected using Xpert MTB/RIF®. Once culture and DST results are obtained, MDR-TB therapy can be customised to the patient's drug-susceptibility profile, and must include a combination of at least 5 drugs to which the TB bacilli are still sensitive. The algorithm for DST is shown in Figure 8.2.

Mycobacterial culture [solid/liquid] remains the *gold standard* for the diagnosis of TB. In addition, for EPTB, a composite reference standard [CRS] is used for diagnosis. The CRS includes parameters like smear for acid-fast bacilli, mycobacterial culture, histopathology and cytology reports [for biopsy samples and aspirates, respectively], organ system specific ancillary diagnostic tests and response to treatment during follow-up visits. For DST, solid culture and phenotypic testing remains the *gold standard*.

Table 8.3: Accuracy of Xpert for EPTB samples and the WHO recommendations on how Xpert MTB/RIF should be used in each sample type

Sample	Sensitivity [compared to culture] [%]	Specificity [compared to culture] [%]	2013 WHO recommendations on the use of Xpert MTB/RIF (5)
Cerebrospinal fluid	81	98	Xpert is recommended as an initial diagnostic test in cerebrospinal fluid specimens for TB meningitis [strong recommendation given the urgency of rapid diagnosis]
Lymph nodes	83	94	Xpert is recommended as a replacement test for usual practice in specific non-respiratory specimens [lymph nodes and other tissues] for EPTB [conditional recommendation]
Pleural fluid	46	99	Pleural fluid is a suboptimal sample and pleural biopsy is preferred. While a positive Xpert result in pleural fluid can be treated as TB, a negative result should be followed by other tests
Gastric lavage and gastric aspirate	84	98	Xpert is recommended as a replacement test for usual practice in specific non-respiratory specimens [including gastric specimens] for EPTB [conditional recommendation]

EPTB = extra-pulmonary tuberculosis; WHO = World Health Organization
Adapted from reference 11; sensitivity and specificity estimates are derived from reference 12

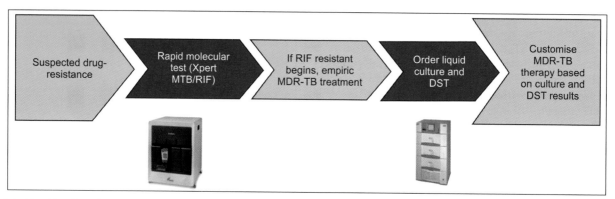

Figure 8.2: Algorithm for DST, based on International Standards for TB Care. Drug resistance must be suspected in all patients with history of TB treatment in the past. In addition, patients who remain smear-positive at completion of the intensive phase of treatment and patients in whom treatment has failed have been lost to follow-up or relapsed following one or more courses of treatment should always be assessed for drug-resistance
RIF = rifampicin; DST = drug-susceptibility testing; MDR-TB = multidrug-resistant tuberculosis; TB = tuberculosis
Source: reference 3

Diagnosis of Latent TB Infection

Most individuals, after exposure to *Mtb*, contain the infection using adaptive immune mechanisms, and the infection remains 'latent'. LTBI may progress to active TB disease in about 10% of those with infection, over a lifetime. Rate of progression to active disease is highest among patients who are also co-infected with human immunodeficiency virus [HIV]. Treatment of LTBI [earlier called preventive therapy, prophylactic treatment] can reduce the risk of progression to active disease by about 60%. For preventive therapy, treatment options include 6-9 months of isoniazid, 3-month regimen of weekly rifapentine plus isoniazid, or 3-4 months isoniazid plus rifampicin, or 3-4 months rifampicin alone.

Detection of LTBI, followed by treatment, is a useful strategy in specific high-risk groups. According to the WHO, the following groups should be prioritised for LTBI screening: people living with HIV, adult and child contacts of pulmonary TB cases, patients who are to be initiated on

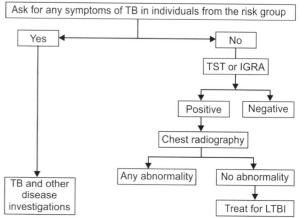

Figure 8.3: The WHO algorithm for latent TB infection testing and management
TST = tuberculin skin test; IGRA = interferon-gamma release assay; TB = tuberculosis; LTBI = latent tuberculosis infection; WHO = World Health Organization
Adapted from reference 14

anti-tumour necrosis factor [TNF] treatment, patients on dialysis, potential recipients of solid organ or haematologic transplantation, and patients with silicosis (15).

The algorithm for the management of LTBI as per the 2014 WHO guidelines is shown in Figure 8.3 (14). The WHO recommends that individuals should be asked about symptoms of TB before being tested for LTBI. Individuals with TB symptoms should be investigated further for active TB using microbiological tests. If TB symptoms are absent, either TST or an IGRA can be used to test for LTBI in high-

income and upper middle-income countries with estimated TB incidence less than 100 per 100,000. The IGRA should not replace TST in low-income and other middle-income countries (16).

It is important to note that there is no diagnostic gold standard for LTBI. Two tests are available currently: the TST performed using Mantoux technique and the IGRA [Table 8.4] (16,17). Evidence suggests that both TST and IGRA are acceptable but imperfect tests (18). These represent indirect immunological markers of *Mtb* exposure

Table 8.4: Comparison of TST with IGRAs

Characteristic	TST	IGRAs
Potential advantages or benefits	Simple, low-tech test Can be done without a laboratory No equipment necessary Can be done by a trained health worker even in remote locations Effect of BCG on TST results is minimal if vaccination is given at birth and not repeated Longitudinal studies have demonstrated its predictive value and systematic reviews of randomised trials show that treatment of LTBI is highly effective in those who are TST-positive	IGRAs require fewer visits than TST for test completion [follow-up visits will be needed for both tests for initiation of LTBI treatment] Potential for boosting test response eliminated with IGRA IGRA interpretation is objective whereas TST interpretation is affected by inter- and intra-reader variation IGRA results can be available within 24-48 hours [but are likely to take longer if done in batches] IGRA does not have cross-reactivity with BCG IGRA has less cross-reactivity than TST with NTM, though data are limited in low- and middle-income countries
Risks or undesired effects	TST may give false-negative reactions due to infections, live virus vaccines, and other factors TST may give false positive results because of BCG vaccination and NTM Requires an intra-dermal injection Can rarely cause adverse reactions [acute reactions, skin blistering and ulceration] Interpretation of serial TST is complicated by boosting, conversions and reversions TST interpretation is affected by inter- and intra-reader variation TST requires 48-72 hours for a valid result	IGRA requires a blood draw [which may be challenging in some populations, including young children] Risk of exposure to blood-borne pathogens Risk of adverse events with IGRA may be reduced compared to TST Interpretation of serial IGRA is complicated by frequent conversions and reversions, and lack of consensus on optimum thresholds for conversions and reversions Reproducibility of IGRAs is modest and influenced by several pre-analytical and analytical factors
Values and preferences	Patients may prefer to avoid visible reaction to TST Patients may prefer not to come back for repeat visit for reading the test result Patients with prior BCG may not trust TST results and may be reluctant to accept IPT Patients may self-read their TST results erroneously	Patients may prefer to avoid blood being drawn [for cultural or technical reasons] Patients with prior BCG may not trust TST results and prefer IGRA
Resource implications	Less expensive than IGRAs [reagent cost is substantially less than IGRA kit costs], but personnel time costs will have to be factored, along with time and cost for two patient visits No laboratory required Need to establish a programme with trained staff to administer and read TST results Staff training is needed to minimise reading errors and variability [under reading, within and between reader variability, digit preference, etc.] PPD must be stored at optimal temperatures Only standardised PPD must be used	Need to establish well-equipped laboratory with electricity, that can perform ELISA or ELISPOT Need to procure equipment and supplies for IGRA performance and quality assurance [IGRA reagents cost higher than TST reagents] Need for staff training, including blood-borne pathogen training Need for cold chain for transport of kits and reagents and for storing them Need for careful handling [e.g., tube shaking] and processing of blood samples [sample volume, time to incubation, etc.] to ensure reproducibility Availability of well-trained staff or staff to be trained

TST = tuberculin skin test; IGRA = interferon-gamma release assay; LTBI = latent tuberculosis infection; BCG = bacille Calmette-Guerin; NTM = nontuberculous mycobacteria; IPT = isoniazid preventive treatment; ELISA = enzyme-linked immunosorbent assay; ELISPOT = enzyme-linked immunospot assay; PPD = purified protein derivative
Source: references 20,21

and indicate a cellular immune response to MTB antigens. Neither TST nor IGRA can accurately differentiate between LTBI and active TB (19). In addition, both have reduced sensitivity in individuals with immune compromising conditions [e.g., HIV infection] (20). As well, both tests have low predictive value for progression to active TB (21,22).

In order to maximise the positive predictive value [PPV] of existing tests, LTBI screening should be reserved only for those who are at sufficiently high risk of progressing to disease to outweigh the known harms of LTBI treatment. Importantly, both TST and IGRAs should not be used for the diagnosis of active TB in high endemic settings like India (19). In children, these tests may have some value as a test for infection, in addition to chest radiograph, symptoms, history of contact, and other microbiological investigations [e.g., gastric aspirate smear for acid-fast bacilli and Xpert MTB/RIF®].

Every individual presenting with two weeks of cough or abnormal chest radiograph should be investigated for TB. The WHO-endorsed sputum tests [smears, Xpert MTB/RIF®, LPA and liquid cultures] should be used to diagnose TB and MDR-TB, and all cases must be notified to local public health authorities. Blood tests [antibody tests and IGRAs] are not recommended for active TB. For EPTB, samples from the site of the disease must be tested using Xpert MTB/RIF®, histopathology and cultures. Ideally, all TB patients should undergo DST. Persons with previous history of TB [or not responding to standard therapy] must undergo DST for first-line anti-TB drugs. For DST, tests like Xpert MTB/RIF, LPA and liquid cultures are recommended. Lastly, tests that are intended for detecting LTBI [e.g., TST and IGRAs] must only be used for LTBI diagnosis in select high-risk groups, and should not be used for detection of active disease.

REFERENCES

1. World Health Organization. Global tuberculosis report 2018. Geneva: World Health Organization; 2018.
2. Sreeramareddy CT, Qin ZZ, Satyanarayana S, Subbaraman R, Pai M. Delays in diagnosis and treatment of pulmonary tuberculosis in India: a systematic review. Int J Tuberc Lung Dis 2014;18:255-66.
3. TB CARE I. International Standards for Tuberculosis Care. Third edition. 2014. Available at URL: http://www.who.int/tb/publications/ISTC_3rdEd.pdf. Accessed on December 28, 2015.
4. World Health Organization. Fluorescent light-emitting diode [LED] microscopy for diagnosis of tuberculosis. Policy statement. 2011. Available at URL: http://whqlibdoc.who.int/publications/2011/ 9789241501613_eng.pdf. Accessed on December 28, 2017.
5. World Health Organization. Policy update: automated real-time nucleic acid amplification technology for rapid and simultaneous detection of tuberculosis and rifampicin resistance: Xpert MTB/RIF system for the diagnosis of pulmonary and extrapulmonary TB in adults and children 2013. Available at URL: http://www.stoptb.org/wg/gli/assets/documents/WHO%20Policy%20Statement%20on%20Xpert%20MTB-RIF%202013%20pre%20publication%2022102013.pdf. Accessed on December 28, 2017.
6. World Health Organization. Use of liquid TB culture and drug susceptibility testing [DST] in low and medium income settings. Summary report of the Expert Group meeting on the use of liquid culture media, Geneva 26 March, 2007. Available at URL:

7. World Health Organization. Policy statement. Use of tuberculosis interferon-gamma release assays [IGRAs] in low- and middle-income countries. 2011. Available at URL: http://whqlibdoc.who.int/publications/2011/9789241502672_eng.pdf. Accessed on December 29, 2017.
8. Pai M, Chedore P. Diagnosis of tuberculosis: importance of appropriate specimen collection. In: Pai M, editor. Let's talk TB. A supplement to GP Clinics. Second edition. 2016. Available at URL: http://www.ipaqt.org/images/ipaqt/latest_talk.pdf. Accessed on January 5, 2017.
9. Sharma SK, Kohli M, Chaubey J, Yadav RN, Sharma R, Singh BK, et al. Evaluation of Xpert MTB/RIF assay performance in diagnosing extrapulmonary tuberculosis among adults in a tertiary care centre in India. Eur Respir J 2014;44:1090-3.
10. Sharma SK, Kohli M, Yadav RN, Chaubey J, Bhasin D, Sreenivas V, et al. Evaluating the diagnostic accuracy of Xpert MTB/RIF assay in pulmonary tuberculosis. PLoS ONE 2015; 10:e0141011.
11. Pai M, Nathavitharana R. Extrapulmonary tuberculosis: new diagnostics and new policies. Indian J Chest Dis Allied Sci 2014;56: 71-3.
12. Denkinger CM, Schumacher SG, Boehme CC, Dendukuri N, Pai M, Steingart KR. Xpert MTB/RIF assay for the diagnosis of extrapulmonary tuberculosis: a systematic review and meta-analysis. Eur Respir J 2014;44:435-46.
13. Greco S, Girardi E, Masciangelo R, Capoccetta GB, Saltini C. Adenosine deaminase and interferon gamma measurements for the diagnosis of tuberculous pleurisy: a meta-analysis. Int J Tuberc Lung Dis 2003;7:777-86.
14. World Health Organization. The End TB Strategy. Global strategy and targets for tuberculosis prevention, care and control after 2015. URL: http://www.who.int/tb/post2015_TBstrategy.pdf?ua=12014. Accessed on December 29,2017.
15. World Health Organization. Guidelines on the management of latent tuberculosis infection. WHO/HTM/TB/2015.01. Geneva: World Health Organization; 2015.
16. Pai M, Menzies D. Interferon-gamma release assays for latent tuberculosis infection. Waltham, MA: UpToDate; 2014.
17. Pinto LM, Grenier J, Schumacher SG, Denkinger CM, Steingart KR, Pai M. Immunodiagnosis of tuberculosis: state of the art. Med Princ Pract 2012;21:4-13.
18. Pai M, Denkinger CM, Kik SV, Rangaka MX, Zwerling A, Oxlade O, et al. Gamma interferon release assays for detection of Mycobacterium tuberculosis infection. Clin Microbiol Rev 2014;27:3-20.
19. Metcalfe JZ, Everett CK, Steingart KR, Cattamanchi A, Huang L, Hopewell PC, et al. Interferon-gamma release assays for active pulmonary tuberculosis diagnosis in adults in low- and middle-income countries: systematic review and meta-analysis. J Infect Dis 2011;204: S1120-9.
20. Cattamanchi A, Smith R, Steingart KR, Metcalfe JZ, Date A, Coleman C, et al. Interferon-gamma release assays for the diagnosis of latent tuberculosis infection in HIV-infected individuals - a systematic review and meta-analysis. J Acquir Immune Defic Syndr 2011;56:230-8.
21. Rangaka MX, Wilkinson KA, Glynn JR, Ling D, Menzies D, Mwansa-Kambafwile J, et al. Predictive value of interferon-gamma release assays for incident active tuberculosis: a systematic review and meta-analysis. Lancet Infect Dis 2012;12:45-55.
22. Lewinsohn DM, Leonard MK, LoBue PA, Cohn DL, Daley CL, Desmond E, et al. Official American Thoracic Society/Infectious Diseases Society of America/Centers for Disease Control and Prevention Clinical Practice Guidelines: diagnosis of tuberculosis in adults and children. Clin Infect Dis 2017;64:e1-e33.

http://www.who.int/tb/laboratory/use_of_liquid_tb_culture_summary_report.pdf?ua=1. Accessed on December 31, 2017.

9

Roentgenographic Manifestations of Pulmonary and Extra-pulmonary Tuberculosis

Chandan J Das, Ankur Goyal, Divya Singh

INTRODUCTION

Tuberculosis [TB] continues to afflict large number of people in the developing countries (1). Human immunodeficiency virus [HIV] infection and acquired immunodeficiency syndrome [AIDS] have added fuel to the fire. TB affects all organ systems; however, lungs are most commonly affected and often are the first site of involvement. Imaging plays a pivotal role in screening, diagnosis as well as follow-up during treatment of pulmonary TB.

IMAGING MODALITIES

While a wide range of imaging modalities are available [Table 9.1], chest radiograph is the first imaging technique to be sought in patients suspected to have pulmonary TB.

Chest Radiograph

Postero-anterior [PA] radiograph of the chest is used as the initial imaging tool in patients suspected to have TB. It is an inexpensive, easily-available modality which is often sufficient for initial diagnosis and subsequent follow-up. Lateral view may be done to confirm the findings of

the PA view and better visualisation of certain 'hidden areas' [retrosternal, retrocardiac]. Apicogram facilitates visualisation of the lung apices that are partially obscured in PA view due to bony superimposition. Dual-energy subtraction radiography can also be employed to remove the overlapping bony shadows. A normal chest radiograph has a high negative predictive value for active TB. The frequency of false negative examination is approximately 1% in the adult immunocompetent population (2,3) and increases to 7%-15% in HIV-seropositive individuals (4-6).

Computed Tomography

Computed tomography [CT] generates multi-dimensional high resolution images and can detect small lesions which may be missed on radiograph. Miliary nodules in the lungs can be seen on CT even when the radiograph is normal. The pulmonary lesions are better characterised and disease activity is more accurately assessed. In a study from Korea (7), it was found that CT gave additional information in 37% cases which had a significant bearing on patient management. The mediastinum and hila are well visualised. The size and nature of lymphadenopathy [homogeneous,

Table 9.1: Advantages and disadvantages of various types of imaging modalities		
Modality	*Advantage*	*Disadvantage*
Radiography	Inexpensive, easily available	Radiation exposure, low sensitivity and specificity
Ultrasonography	Radiation free, portable, guide pleural sampling	Limited field of view [superficial structures]
Computed tomography	Excellent resolution, high sensitivity, guide sampling	Radiation, iodinated contrast, relatively expensive
Magnetic resonance imaging	Radiation free, accurate for lymphadenitis and associated spinal disease	Expensive, contraindications, less accurate for parenchymal lesions
PET or PET-CT	High sensitivity	Low specificity, radiation exposure
PET = positron emission tomography; PET-CT = positron emission tomography-computed tomography		

necrotic or calcified] is defined clearly. The trachea and bronchi can be evaluated for stenosis [site and extent]. Extraluminal causes of airway narrowing, e.g., lymph nodes [LNs] can be determined. Pleural pathology [effusion, empyema, thickening and calcification] and underlying chest wall involvement are well delineated. The pulmonary and bronchial vasculature is accurately evaluated with CT, thus providing a road-map for planning endovascular interventions.

Ultrasonography

Ultrasonography is an inexpensive, radiation free, portable imaging modality. It can assess pleural disease and facilitate diagnostic pleural fluid sampling and therapeutic drainage procedures. Ultrasonographic assessment of the abdomen can detect concomitant organomegaly and abdominal lymphadenopathy.

Magnetic Resonance Imaging

Magnetic resonance imaging [MRI] is a radiation free, but costly technique which can accurately assess mediastinal and hilar lymphadenopathy. Pulmonary parenchyma can also be evaluated, though to a lesser extent than CT. It can assess concomitant spinal involvement with high accuracy.

Positron Emission Tomography-Computed Tomography

The role of positron emission tomography-computed tomography [PET-CT] in TB is not clearly defined. However, due to increasing number of referrals for PET-CT in patients with pyrexia of unknown origin [PUO], many cases are being detected by PET-CT. Also, tubercular lymphadenopathy and parenchymal nodules may show intense 18-fluorodeoxy-glucose [FDG] uptake which can mimic malignancy (3,4).

IMAGING IN PULMONARY TUBERCULOSIS

The disease which develops after initial exposure to the pathogen is known as primary TB, whereas, the disease that develops as a result of reactivation of a previous endogenous focus of infection or less commonly, exogenous reinfection is known as post-primary TB. These two forms of TB differ in terms of the site of involvement, nature of involvement, presence of lymphadenopathy and pleural effusion. However, there may be variable degree of overlap in the radiologic manifestations. A recent study based on genotyping of *Mycobacterium tuberculosis* [*Mtb*] isolates has suggested that the radiographic features are often similar in patients who have a primary disease and those who have a reactivation TB. It has been proposed that, rather than the time lag from acquisition of infection to the development of clinical disease, it is the integrity of the host's immune system that predicts the radiographic appearance of TB (8,9). However, this result is preliminary and requires further validation.

PRIMARY TUBERCULOSIS

Primary TB is seen more commonly in children, however, it is being seen with increasing frequency in adults (10). Up to 60% of children with pulmonary TB are asymptomatic and found solely through contact investigation (11). Difficulty in obtaining a sputum sample further compounds the problem. Hence, diagnosis in such cases is based on presence of positive tuberculin skin test [TST] or radiographic abnormalities.

The structures involved in primary TB are, lymph nodes, pulmonary parenchyma, pleura and tracheobronchial tree. Table 9.2 enlists the various radiographic features of primary pulmonary TB.

Table 9.2: Radiologic features of primary pulmonary TB

Lymphadenopathy

Parenchymal consolidation

Tuberculoma

Miliary TB

Pleural effusion

Airway involvement

TB = tuberculosis

Lymphadenopathy

Lymphadenopathy is the hallmark of primary TB. Lymph node enlargement is seen in 83%-96% of paediatric cases (7,12,13). The frequency of lymphadenopathy ranges from 10%-43% in adults (14,15). The most common lymph node sites involved are right paratracheal and hilar region [Figure 9.1]. It is postulated that this right-sided preponderance is due to predominance of right-sided parenchymal lesions owing to higher probability of air-borne infection reaching the right lung through its shorter and wider bronchus and also because the right sided nodes drain the entire right lung along with the left lower lobe. Drainage of systemic lymph nodes to the right lymph duct and to the superior vena cava via thoracic duct also favour right side presentation. In a study (16) it was observed that the most frequently involved location was subcarinal [90%], followed by the hilar [85%], anterior mediastinum [79%], precarinal [64%] and right paratracheal [63%]. Nodes at all the sites simultaneously were present in 35% of patients. Bilateral lymphadenopathy is seen in 31% of cases (17,18). There is an age-related decline in the prevalence of lymphadenopathy. In a study (13), lymphadenopathy was seen in 100% cases between 0 and 3 years of age and in 88% of children between 4 and 15 years (13).

CT has a higher sensitivity than chest radiograph in detection of lymphadenopathy. Lymph nodes greater than 1 centimetre in short axis diameter [SAD] are considered enlarged. The lymph nodes show various patterns of enhancement [Figure 9.2] which can be characterised according to appearance on contrast-enhanced CT [CECT] [Table 9.3]. The CT appearance of lymph nodes reveals their pathologic appearance and correlates with clinical

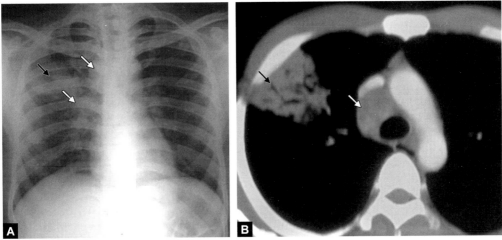

Figure 9.1: Chest radiograph [postero-anterior view] [A] and CECT chest [B] showing right parahilar consolidation [black arrow] with enlarged ipsilateral hilar and paratracheal lymph nodes [white arrows]
CECT = contrast-enhanced computed tomography

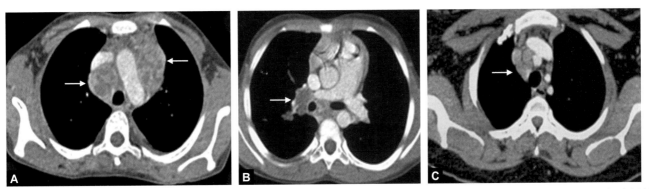

Figure 9.2: CECT chest of three different patients showing necrotic right paratracheal and prevascular nodes [arrows] [A], necrotic right hilar and subcarinal nodes with rim enhancement [arrow] [B] and homogeneously enhancing pretracheal nodes [arrow] [C]
CECT = contrast-enhanced computed tomography

Table 9.3: Characterisation of lymph nodes according to appearance in CECT

Appearance of TB lymphadenopathy on CECT	Pathology
Homogeneous enhancement	Lymphoid hyperplasia with TB granulomas without caseous necrosis
Heterogeneous enhancement with a small central non-enhancing area	TB granulomas, some caseous necrosis in the center and a complete capsule
Peripheral irregular thick wall enhancement with a central non-enhancing area and clear surrounding fat plane	TB granulomas, caseous necrosis in the center and a complete capsule
Peripheral thin rim enhancement with no central enhancement and clear surrounding fat plane	Few TB granulomas with a large amount of caseous necrosis in the centre
No obvious enhancement	Caseous necrosis with little tubercular granulomas
Peripheral irregular enhancement with central non-enhancement which obliterates surrounding fat plane	TB granulomas and caseous necrosis ruptured from the capsule
Peripheral irregular rim enhancement with central separate enhancement and an obliterated surrounding fat plane	Lymph nodes with liquefaction of caseous necrosis are adherent, the rim and separation are formed by TB granulomas
TB = tuberculosis; CECT = contrast-enhanced computed tomography	

symptoms (19). Pathologically, intrathoracic TB lymphadenitis passes through four stages. Stage 1 is characterised by lymphoid hyperplasia with formation of granulomas without caseous necrosis. In stage 2 caseous necrosis is evident in affected lymph nodes with complete capsule. In stage 3,

periadenitis without adhesions is seen. In stage 4 liquefaction followed by destruction of the capsules adhesion and confluence of multiple lymph nodes is observed. The lymph nodes in stage 1 show homogeneous enhancement. These patients often do not have clinical symptoms. Heterogeneous enhancement with a small central necrotic area is seen in early stage 2. Peripheral irregular thick enhancing wall with a central non-enhancing area and almost clear surrounding fat plane is seen in mid stage 2. Peripheral thin rim enhancement with no central enhancement and a clear surrounding fat plane is evident in late stage 2. In this stage, patients manifest clinical symptoms. Peripheral irregular enhancement with central non-enhancement which extends outside the lymph node capsule and obliterates surrounding fat plane is observed in stage 3. The irregular enhancement comprises of TB granulomas and caseous necrosis that have ruptured from the capsule. Peripheral irregular rim enhancement with central separate enhancement and an obliterated surrounding fat plane is observed in stage 4. The patients in stages 3 and 4 frequently manifest clinical symptoms. Peripheral rim enhancement with or without central low attenuation is the most common pattern and is considered fairly specific for TB in the appropriate clinical setting (20). However, microbiological, pathological or molecular confirmation of diagnosis is imperative as similar appearance has also been described in atypical mycobacterial infection (21), treated lymphoma (20), metastasis from testicular malignancy (22) and benign conditions like Whipple's and Crohn's disease (23).

Calcification is uncommon in primary disease [Figure 9.3]. It is seen in 10%-21% children with TB and never in infants

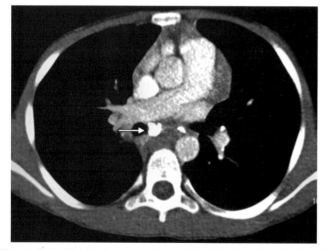

Figure 9.3: CECT chest showing calcification in subcarinal node [arrow]

less than six months of age (16,24). Central low attenuation and peripheral enhancement suggest active disease whereas homogeneous calcified nodes indicate inactive disease (25). In a study from New Delhi (26) in paediatric population, it was found that nodal enlargement, conglomeration and obscuration of perinodal fat were the major determinants of active disease (26).

Mediastinal sonography can be an inexpensive tool for monitoring response to treatment in children. In a retrospective study of 21 children with a positive TST, mediastinal sonography was performed through suprasternal and left parasternal approach (27). A comparison of pre-treatment mediastinal sonograms with those obtained after three months of anti-TB treatment showed a marked reduction of lymph node involvement in 17 [80.9%] patients.

MRI can also be used to accurately assess mediastinal and hilar lymphadenopathy [Figure 9.4]. Necrotic nodes appear bright on T2-weighted images. Three patterns of TB lymphadenitis have been described [Table 9.4]. Of these, the most common pattern is type 2, that is, inhomogeneous nodes with marked hyperintensity on T2-weighted images and peripheral enhancement in post-contrast images. This appearance is mostly seen in severely symptomatic patients and is due to caseation necrosis of the TB lymph nodes (28).

Table 9.4: MRI appearances of TB lymphadenopathy

Type 1	Homogeneous enhancement
Type 2	Inhomogeneous with a strong peripheral enhancement
Type 3	No contrast enhancement

MRI = magnetic resonance imaging; TB = tuberculosis

Parenchymal Lesions

Infection occurs when a susceptible person inhales droplet nuclei that contain *Mtb*. Ghon's focus refers to the initial site of lung parenchymal involvement at the time of first infection. The draining lymphatics and the involved lymph nodes together with Ghon's focus are referred to as the *Ghon's complex* [*primary complex*]. The Ghon's complex further evolves into the *Ranke complex* which is the combination of a Ghon's focus and enlarged or calcified lymph nodes. *Simon's foci* are apical nodules that are often calcified and result from haematogenous seeding at the time of initial infection (29).

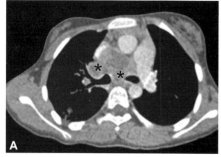
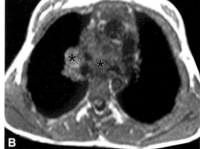
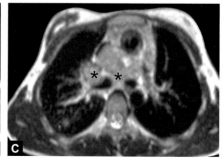

Figure 9.4: CECT chest [A] and MRI of thorax showing necrotic right hilar and subcarinal lymph nodes [asterisk] which are iso to hyperintense on T1 [B] and hyperintense on T2 weighted images [C]
CECT = contrast-enhanced computed tomography

Consolidation

Consolidation is the most common pattern of parenchymal involvement in pulmonary TB. On radiographs, it is seen as single homogeneous opacity with ill-defined margins [Figure 9.5]. There can be a mass-like consolidation which can involve an entire lobe with absent air-bronchogram. Consolidation abutting a fissure can have sharp margins. The radiographic picture of TB can often resemble that of bacterial pneumonia. However, lack of systemic toxaemia and non-responsiveness to standard antibiotic treatment can suggest the possibility of TB.

There is no predilection for a particular region of the lung, but a right-sided predominance has been noted (30). In adults with primary TB, the lesion is often seen in the lower lobe. Cavitation of the parenchymal lesion is rare in children but can be seen in 7%-29% adults with primary TB (15,31). Endobronchial spread is rare since cavitation is uncommon.

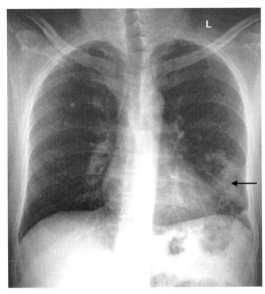

Figure 9.5: Chest radiograph [postero-anterior view] showing an ill-defined area of consolidation [arrow] in the left lower lobe in a patient with primary tuberculosis

CT has a higher sensitivity than radiographs in detecting the parenchymal changes. Consolidation is seen as a homogeneous soft tissue density lesion with air bronchogram or break down within it. Low-attenuation areas within the consolidation, representing caseating necrosis can be seen in 25% cases (7). CT is better than MRI in demonstration of parenchymal changes. In a series of 2677 patients visiting the paediatric TB Clinic from New Delhi, primary complex was seen in 50% cases of paediatric pulmonary TB. Of these, 32% had lymphadenopathy only, 29% had parenchymal and lymph node involvement and 39% had only parenchymal lesions (32).

Tuberculoma

A tuberculoma is a round or oval opacity which is seen in both primary and post-primary TB [Figure 9.6] in 7%-9% of patients. It can range in size from 0.5 cm-4 cm in diameter. Histologically, the central part of the tuberculoma consists of caseous material and the periphery, of epithelioid histiocytes and multinucleated giant cells with variable amount of collagen. It is commonly seen in the upper lobes, more often on right side. Cavitation can be seen in 10%-50% of the lesions (30). Small discrete nodules can be seen in the vicinity of the main lesion ["satellite lesions"] in 80% cases (33). Majority of tuberculomas remain stable over time. On CT, tuberculomas are seen as well-circumscribed soft tissue density nodules with smooth margin. Calcification is seen in the dominant nodule or the satellite lesions in 20%-30% cases. Tuberculomas can show ring-like and central curvilinear enhancement.

Miliary Tuberculosis

Haematogenous dissemination of the bacilli results in miliary TB in lungs and other organs (34). It is primarily a feature of primary TB although it may be seen in post primary disease. It is characterised by the presence of innumerable, 2 mm or less, non-calcified nodules scattered throughout both the lungs, with mild basilar predominance [Figure 9.7].

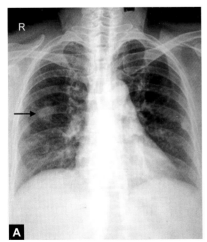
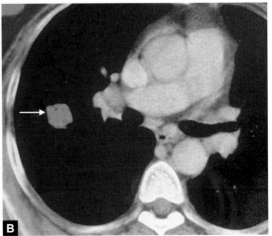

Figure 9.6: Chest radiograph [postero-anterior view] [A] and CECT chest [B], showing well-defined, single, oval lesion in right upper lobe [arrow] suggestive of a tuberculoma
CECT = contrast-enhanced computed tomography

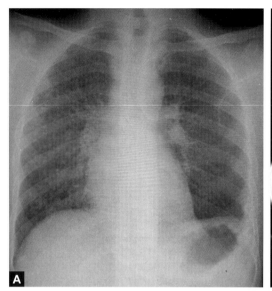
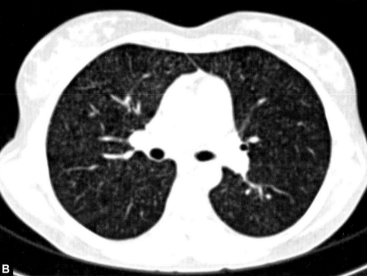

Figure 9.7: Chest radiograph [postero-anterior view] [A] and HRCT chest [B] showing bilateral, diffuse, tiny, discrete, pinpoint opacities, suggestive of miliary tuberculosis
HRCT = high resolution computed tomography

This basal predilection is attributed to the gravity dependent increase in blood flow to the lung bases. The chest radiograph can be normal in the early stages of disease in 25%-40% of persons (35-37). Typical miliary lesions are visible on radiographs after a latency of 3-6 weeks after haematogenous dissemination (38). Initially, the lesions are 1 mm in diameter. If left untreated, the nodules increase in size to 3-5 mm and coalesce to give a 'snow-storm' appearance. Uniform distribution of nodules is seen in 85% cases while 15% show asymmetric distribution (38). Associated lymphadenopathy is seen more commonly in children [95%] as compared to adults [11%]. The right paratracheal lymph nodes are involved most commonly. Associated parenchymal consolidation is also more common in children (12). In a study (32) miliary and broncho-pneumonic forms of TB were seen in 3% patients. Rarely, a diffuse alveolar pattern is observed in patients with associated acute respiratory distress syndrome [ARDS] (39,40).

High resolution computed tomography [HRCT] is highly sensitive for detecting miliary nodules (41). It can reveal randomly distributed, miliary nodules in the lung along with lymphadenopathy even if the radiograph is normal. Thickening of interlobular and intralobular septa is frequently evident. In the appropriate clinical setting where the clinical suspicion of miliary TB is high, if the chest radiograph is normal, it is advisable to obtain CT of the thorax.

Pleural Involvement

Pleural effusion is an uncommon manifestation of primary TB. Pleural effusion usually develops on the same side as the site of initial TB infection and is typically unilateral (42). Bilateral effusions occur in 12%-18% of cases (18,33).

Although usually observed in association with parenchymal and/or nodal abnormalities, pleural effusion is the only radiographic finding in primary TB in approximately 5% of adult cases.

Pleural effusion is most commonly non-loculated and moderate to large in quantity [Figure 9.8]. The effusion can sometimes be subpulmonary in location and cause elevation of ipsilateral hemidiaphragm. A lateral decubitus film can provide confirmation by showing the fluid shift along lateral chest wall. The effusion can become loculated when it demonstrates a convex medial margin towards the lung. Complications include empyema, bronchopleural fistula, *empyema necessitans* or bone erosion.

Ultrasonography is a useful modality for assessment and follow-up of pleural pathology [Figure 9.9]. The pleural effusion can be quantified, evaluated for septations, sampled and drained by ultrasonography. As little as 10 ml of fluid can be detected on ultrasonography when the chest radiograph is normal.

CT with its multi-dimensional capability helps in evaluating pleural involvement by delineating the site, extent of disease, presence of loculations, status of underlying ribs and chest wall involvement. It helps in planning further management. Empyema is visualised as fluid collection with diffuse enhancement of visceral and parietal pleura ['split pleura sign'] and extra-pleural fat proliferation [Figure 9.10]. Healing can result in residual pleural thickening and calcification [Figure 9.11].

Airway Involvement

Airway involvement may be extrinsic, due to compression by enlarged lymph nodes or intrinsic, due to endobronchial spread. Lymph node compression can lead to atelectasis

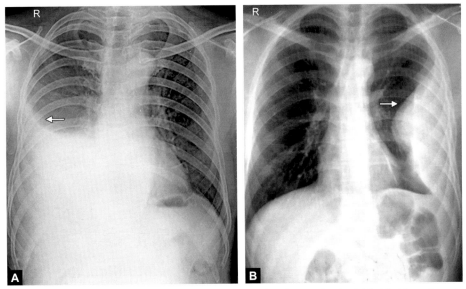

Figure 9.8: Chest radiograph [postero-anterior view] of two different patients showing moderate right-sided free pleural effusion [arrow] showing Ellis curve [A] and left-sided loculated pleural effusion [arrow] with a convex medial margin towards lung [B]

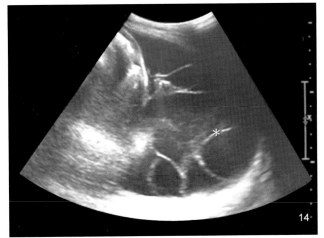

Figure 9.9: Ultrasonography of chest showing right sided pleural effusion with multiple septations [asterisk]

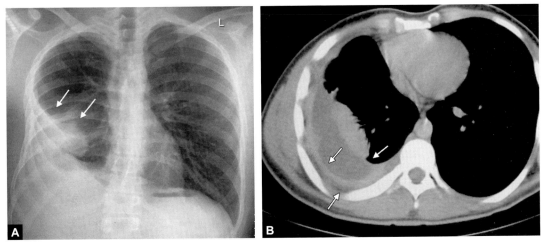

Figure 9.10: Chest radiograph [postero-anterior view] [A] showing an ill-defined opacity along the lateral chest wall [arrows] with loss of volume of right hemithorax. CECT chest of the same patient [B] showing loss of lung volume with thick enhancing pleura and proliferation of extra-pleural fat [arrows]

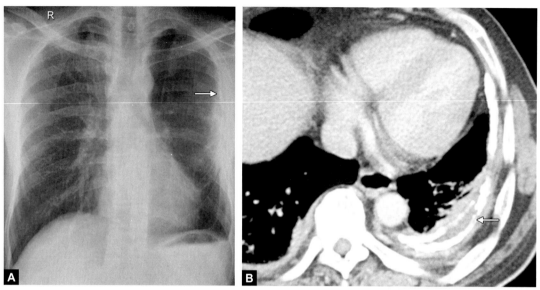

Figure 9.11: Chest radiograph [postero-anterior view] [A] and CECT chest [B] showing loss of volume, dense and thick, peripheral left pleural thickening with calcification [arrow] suggestive of chronic empyema

or hyperinflation. This is frequently seen in primary TB in children below two years of age and is less common in older children [9%] and adults [18%]. This is because of the larger calibre of airways and lower prevalence of lymphadenopathy in the older population. The involvement is right-sided with obstruction occurring at the level of the lobar bronchus or *bronchus intermedius*. Thus, atelectasis is commonly seen involving the anterior segment of upper lobe or the medial segment of the middle lobe. In adults, it can mimic bronchogenic carcinoma (43).

CT is the modality of choice for delineating the site, extent and the cause of airway involvement. CT can provide excellent reconstructions in any plane and endoscopic views to give a complete perspective of the tracheobronchial tree. Active airway disease is seen as long segment of circumferential wall thickening and irregularity causing luminal compromise. It can involve both main bronchi with equal frequency (44).

Follow-up of Primary Tuberculosis

Imaging is the main stay in the follow-up of patients with negative pre-treatment sputum examination results. It is of utmost value in children in whom bacteriological confirmation is not possible. Regression of radiographic abnormalities in pulmonary TB is a slow process. In the first three months of treatment, there may be worsening of radiographic findings in the form of progression of parenchymal involvement and enlargement of existing lymphadenopathy despite appropriate treatment (13,45-47). This occurs as a consequence of the hypersensitivity reaction that normally occurs two to ten weeks after initial infection (13). The parenchymal and nodal abnormalities usually regress in parallel. In a series of 252 paediatric patients with TB, consolidation resolved completely within

two years in all cases, 18% had parenchymal scarring, 11% had parenchymal calcification and nodal calcification was seen in 6% cases (13). Resolution of parenchymal abnormalities occurs within six months to two years on radiographs (13) and up to 15 months on CT (48). Lymphadenopathy may persist for several years after treatment (13).

POST-PRIMARY TUBERCULOSIS

Post-primary TB most often occurs due to reactivation of endogenous focus of infection acquired previously or exogenous reinfection. There are several patterns of involvement seen in post-primary TB [Table 9.5] which may be seen in isolation or in various combinations.

The radiographic features of post-primary TB which differentiate it from primary TB are: [i] predilection for apical and posterior segments of the upper lobes and the superior segment of the lower lobes; [ii] presence of cavitation; and [iii] rarity of lymphadenopathy.

Table 9.5: Radiographic features of post-primary TB
Cavitation
Local exudative lesion
Local fibroproductive lesion
Tuberculoma
Bronchogenic spread
Miliary TB
Bronchostenosis
Pleural disease
TB = tuberculosis

Parenchymal Disease

Exudative Lesion

The most common radiographic manifestation of reactivation TB is focal or patchy heterogeneous consolidation involving the apical and posterior segments of the upper lobes and superior segments of the lower lobes (25,47). Another common finding is the presence of poorly defined nodules and linear opacities, which are seen in approximately 25% of patients. Involvement of more than one segment is fairly common, seen in 88% cases [Figures 9.12 and 9.13]. Bilateral upper lobe involvement is seen in 32%-64% cases. Cavitation occurs in about 45% cases (31). If the disease is left untreated, additional opacities develop, that coalesce leading to lobar and total lung consolidation which can be associated with distortion of adjacent bronchovascular and mediastinal structures. In 3%-6% cases, tuberculomas are the predominant parenchymal manifestation. Lymphadenopathy is very uncommon and is seen in 5% cases (31).

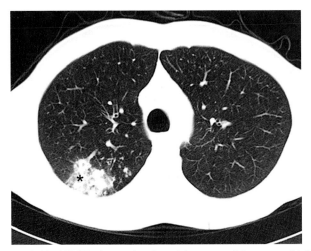

Figure 9.12: Chest radiograph [postero-anterior view] showing extensive consolidation in left lung

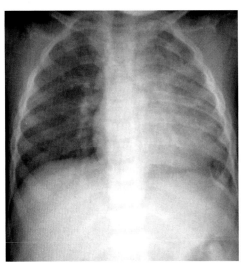

Figure 9.13: HRCT chest showing right upper lobe consolidation [asterisk]
HRCT = high resolution computed tomography

Fibroproductive or Fibroproliferative Lesion

Healing occurs by replacement of TB granulation tissue by fibrous tissue resulting in loss of volume. The fluffy ill-defined opacities of exudative lesions give way to well-defined reticular and nodular opacities [Figures 9.14 and 9.15]. Volume loss manifests as ipsilateral tracheo-mediastinal shift, elevation of diaphragm and retraction of hilum. In 41% cases, an apical opacity or apical cap results from pleural thickening, subpleural atelectasis and extra-pleural fat deposition. Mixed exudative and fibroproductive lesion is the most common finding seen in 79% cases. Pure exudative or fibroproductive lesions are uncommon (31).

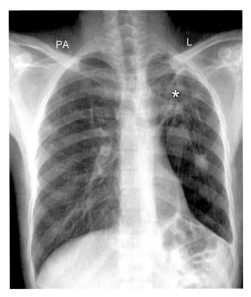

Figure 9.14: Chest radiograph [postero-anterior view] showing coarse, sharply defined opacities mainly in left upper lobe suggestive of parenchymal fibroproliferative lesion [asterisk]

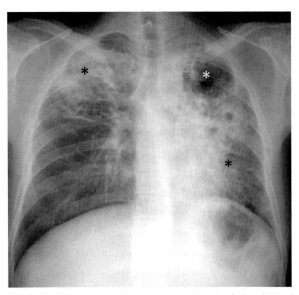

Figure 9.15: Chest radiograph [postero-anterior view] showing volume loss of left lung, extensive fibrosis both upper lobes, residual cavity [white asterisk] and bronchiectatic changes in both lungs [black asterisk].

Cavitation

Cavitation occurs when an area of caseous necrosis liquefies and communicates with the bronchial tree. The sputum of such patients is teeming with tubercle bacilli and cavity is an important sign of active disease. Cavities can be single or multiple. They may be evident radiographically in 40%–45% of patients with post-primary TB (31,48). Cavitation in an area of consolidation is a distinct feature of post-primary TB and indicates likely active disease. It involves the apical and/or posterior segments of the upper lobes in 83%–85% and the superior segments of the lower lobes in 11%–14% patients (49). The walls of cavities can vary from thin and smooth to thick and nodular [Figures 9.16 and 9.17]. The healing of cavitary lesions causes more cicatrisation than areas without cavitation (46).

Air-fluid levels are uncommon in TB cavities due to effective drainage and are evident in 9%-21% cases (33,50). The basal position of the entering bronchus, its downward course and its free communication with the cavity tend to keep the cavity empty (50). TB cavity may be complicated by intracavitary fungal ball ["mycetoma"]. The cavities may not be discernible on radiographs in the setting of dense fibrosis, consolidation, or architectural distortion. In such cases, CT is extremely helpful in detecting a cavity and intracavitary fungal ball.

Tuberculosis Bronchopneumonia

Bronchogenic spread of infection can be identified in 95% of cases with post-primary TB (51,52). This can occur due to communication of a TB cavity with the bronchial tree. Similar spread can occur due to intrabronchial rupture of caseous material of a lymph node. Endobronchial spread is evident in 19%-58% cases (3); with the use of HRCT this may be seen in up to 98% cases (43). The most common HRCT findings include 2-4 mm well-marginated centrilobular nodules and linear branching opacities (51). On pathologic correlation, these have been found to represent caseous necrosis within and around terminal and respiratory bronchioles.

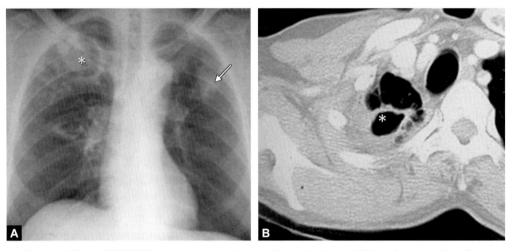

Figure 9.16: Chest radiograph [A] and HRCT [B] showing a large thick walled cavity [asterisk] in right apex with left upper zone consolidation [arrow] in a patient with post-primary tuberculosis

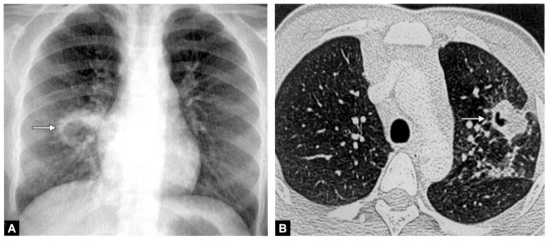

Figure 9.17: Chest radiograph [postero-anterior view] [A] showing a thick walled cavity [arrow] in the right upper lobe with surrounding fibroproliferative lesion. HRCT chest [B] showing another cavity [arrow] in left upper lobe with nodules in the vicinity

The pattern of distribution of nodules showing multiple branching linear structures of similar calibre that originate from a single stalk is known as "tree-in-bud" appearance [Figure 9.18]. These lesions result as a consequence of extensive endobronchial dissemination and are an important marker of disease activity. However, this appearance is non-specific and has been described in several other conditions [Table 9.6] in which there is plugging of small airways with fluid or exudates (53).

Another radiographic feature is the presence of multiple fluffy nodules approximately 5 mm in diameter, known as acinar nodules [Figure 9.19]. It is proposed that in most cases of acinonodose TB, small peribronchiolar nodules grow and coalesce into a larger nodule, by direct extension of inflammation through the pores of Kohn (54). The presence of a cavity and centrilobular nodules with or without *tree-in-bud pattern* can suggest the diagnosis of TB in such cases. While 70% cases of these lesions resolve completely, 30% can result in sequelae in the form of parenchymal scarring, residual nodules and calcification (33).

Two patterns of TB have been identified in adults recently using PET-CT. These include the "lung pattern" and the "lymphatic pattern". The lung pattern is seen in 67% patients with predominantly pulmonary symptoms. In these cases, mediastinal and hilar lymph nodes are slightly enlarged with moderate FDG uptake with a median maximum standardised uptake value [SUVmax] of 3.9 [range 2.5-13.3]. On the other hand, in the lymphatic pattern [Figure 9.20], patients have predominantly systemic symptoms with extra-thoracic involvement. The lymph nodes were larger in size and with higher FDG uptake [median SUVmax 6.8, range 5.7-16.8] (55).

Airway Involvement [Bronchostenosis]

Airway involvement can occur by direct extension from adjacent parenchymal infection due to cavitation, lymph node erosion, haematogenous spread, and extension to the peribronchial region *via* lymphatic drainage. The lesions evolve from submucosal sites of infection associated with ulceration to hyperplastic inflammatory polyps that heal

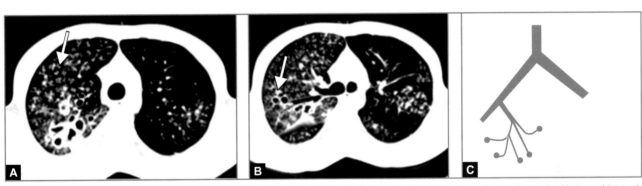

Figure 9.18: HRCT chest showing the typical "tree-in bud" nodules [arrow] [A] in a bronchovascular distribution [arrow] with bronchiectasis [B]. Line diagram [C] illustrating the "tree-in-bud" pattern

Table 9.6: Causes of "tree-in-bud" appearance
Peripheral airway disease
Infection
Bacterial
Mycobacterium tuberculosis, Mycobacterium avium-intracellulare complex, Staphylococcus aureus
Fungal
Aspergillus
Viral
Cytomegalovirus, respiratory syncytial virus
Congenital disorders
Cystic fibrosis, Kartagener's syndrome
Aspiration
Gastric contents, hydrocarbons, toxic fumes and gases
Immunologic disorders
Allergic bronchopulmonary aspergillosis
Connective tissue disorders
Rheumatoid arthritis, Sjögren's syndrome, peripheral pulmonary vascular disease
Neoplasms
Ewing's sarcoma, gastric, breast and renal cancer

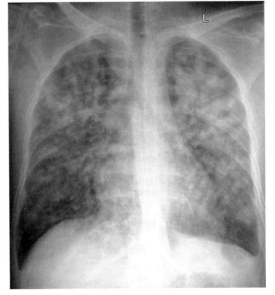

Figure 9.19: Chest radiograph [postero-anterior view] showing extensive bilateral bronchopneumonic tuberculosis

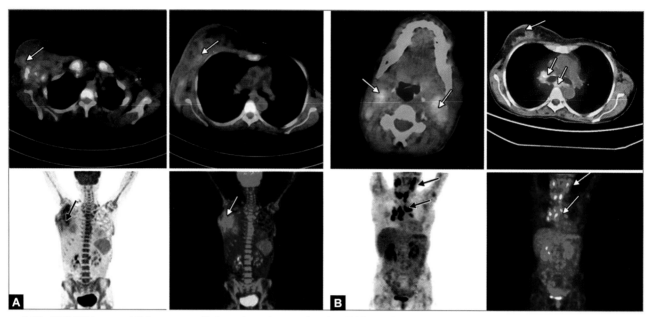

Figure 9.20: PET-CT images [A] in a case with breast carcinoma showing FDG uptake [arrow] in the right breast without any nodal uptake of FDG. Repeat PET-CT image [B] after completion of chemotherapy showing no uptake in the right breast lesion representing complete remission of the primary lesion. Multiple enlarged lymph nodes are seen in the neck and mediastinum showing FDG uptake which on FNAC showed multiple acid-fast bacilli suggestive of TB lymphadenitis

TB = tuberculosis; FDG = fluorodeoxyglucose; PET-CT = positron emission tomography-computed tomography; FNAC = fine needle aspiration cytology

Kind courtesy: Dr Rakesh Kumar, Department of Nuclear Medicine, All India Institute of Medical Sciences, New Delhi

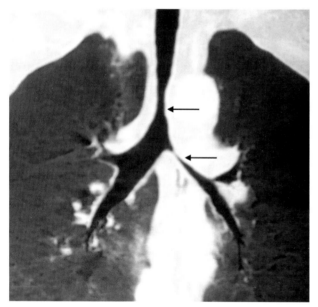

Figure 9.21: Coronal reformatted CT image showing smooth narrowing of the trachea and left main bronchus [arrows] in a patient with post-primary tuberculosis
CT = computed tomography

by fibrosis resulting in circumferential stenosis (56-60). Bronchostenosis occurs in 10%-40% patients. The main, upper, and lower lobe bronchi account for three-quarters of the involved sites (60). Segmental or lobar atelectasis is seen radiographically in 65%-75% and 18%-25% of cases,

respectively (56,58). On CT, endobronchial TB manifests as irregular [in active disease] or smooth [in fibrotic disease] circumferential bronchial narrowing associated with mural thickening [Figure 9.21].

Pleural Effusion

Tuberculous pleural effusion is usually regarded as a manifestation of primary disease. However, it may occur in association with post-primary disease in up to 19% cases (59). It is typically unilateral in distribution and often loculated. Residual pleural thickening or calcification may occur. Persistence of fluid in a calcified fibrothorax should raise concern regarding active disease, chronic TB empyema (60).

Evaluation of Activity of Tuberculosis on Imaging

The knowledge of imaging features of disease activity helps in evaluating response to treatment and detecting disease reactivation. Architectural distortion due to fibrosis and calcification are found in both active and healed disease. Also, small nodules and cavities may not be seen on radiographs. The exudative lesion may remain unchanged on serial radiographs despite adequate therapy and patient having negative sputum mycobacterial culture. Therefore, comment on disease status based on a single radiograph is unreliable. Radiographic stability for at least six months and repeated negative sputum cultures are the best indicators of disease inactivity. It is suggested that the cases should be termed as "radiographically stable" instead of "inactive" (31).

The HRCT has a significant role in determining activity of parenchymal lesions. It is particularly helpful in the detection of small foci of cavitation in areas of dense nodularity and scarring. In a series (61) 80% of patients with active disease and 89% of those with inactive disease were correctly differentiated on HRCT (61). Table 9.7 lists the CT features of active TB. Of these, presence of centrilobular nodules without fibrosis and bronchovascular distortion are the most common finding in active TB. Thin walled cavities, fibrotic bands and well-defined nodules are seen in inactive disease [Figure 9.22]. Sometimes, the CT picture may be equivocal. Hence, clinical correlation is a must.

Presence of necrosis is considered a pointer of active TB lymphadenitis. Since enhancement pattern of TB lymph nodes shows marked variation, evaluation of disease activity based on enhancement patterns has limited reliability. In pleural disease, presence of fluid in the presence of diffuse pleural thickening or enhancement suggests activity.

In a study (62) that assessed the role of PET-CT in patients with TB, all patients underwent PET-CT before and after one month of starting anti-TB treatment. The second PET-CT showed reduced radiotracer uptake intensity in 19 of 21 patients, with a median percentage decrease of SUVmax of 31% [range 2-84] (62). Thus, PET-CT can detect early response to therapy by quantification of reduction in FDG avidity of the lesions.

SEQUELAE AND COMPLICATIONS OF TUBERCULOSIS

A variety of sequelae and complications can occur due to pulmonary TB [Table 9.8]. The imaging features of some of these are described further.

Table 9.7: Features of active TB on CT

Centrilobular nodules; "tree-in-bud" appearance
Lobular consolidation
Cavitation
Bronchial wall thickening
Necrotic mediastinal and hilar lymphadenopathy
Pleural effusion
TB = tuberculosis; CT = computed tomography

Table 9.8: Complications and sequelae of pulmonary TB

Parenchymal complications
Acute respiratory distress syndrome
Aspergilloma
Extensive lung destruction and cicatrization
Multiple cystic lung lesions
Airway complications
Bronchiectasis
Bronchiolitis obliterans
Bronchostenosis
Broncholithiasis
Pleural complications
Bronchopleural fistula
Empyema
Fibrothorax
Hydropneumothorax, pneumothorax
Vascular complications
Bronchial and pulmonary arteritis and thrombosis
Bronchial artery pseudoaneurysm
Pulmonary artery pseudoaneurysm [Rasmussen's aneurysm]
Pulmonary artery hypertension
Mediastinal complications
Constrictive pericarditis
Oesophagobronchial fistula
Oesophagomediastinal fistula
Fibrosing mediastinitis
Chest wall complications
Chondritis
Empyema necessitatis
Osteomyelitis
Spondylitis
TB = tuberculosis

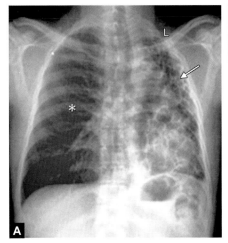 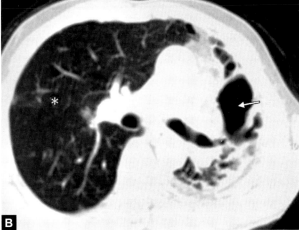

Figure 9.22: Chest radiograph [postero-anterior view] [A] and HRCT chest [B] showing extensive destruction of left lung with fibro-bullous changes [arrow] and contralateral hyperinflation [asterisk]
HRCT = high-resolution computed tomography

Parenchymal Complications

Parenchymal complications include acute respiratory distress syndrome [ARDS], thin-walled cavities, fibrotic bands, extensive lung destruction and aspergilloma. ARDS manifests radiologically as extensive bilateral areas of ground-glass opacity or consolidation superimposed on findings of miliary or endobronchial spread of TB. Thin-walled cavities can occur as a consequence of cicatrisation of previously active TB cavities after therapy or as sequelae of ARDS, in which case they are seen in the anterior portion of the lung. Residual fibrosis is characterised by calcification, architectural distortion and retraction of adjacent lung parenchyma. These changes when extensive can result in complete lung destruction making it defunct. An ectatic bronchus or, more commonly, a residual tuberculous cavity may be colonised by *Aspergillus* species. Haemoptysis is a life-threatening complication of aspergilloma and occurs in 50%-70% of affected patients (63). Radiographically, aspergilloma appears as a spherical nodule or mass separated by a crescent shaped area of decreased opacity from the adjacent cavity wall. The characteristic CT features consist of a mobile intracavitary nodule or mass that is usually surrounded by air but may completely fill the cavity [Figure 9.23]. On prone and supine CT images, the aspergilloma will gravitate to the dependent position.

Airway Complications

These include bronchiectasis, tracheobronchial stenosis and broncholithiasis. Bronchiectasis as a sequel of pulmonary TB typically involves the upper lobes [Figure 9.22]. Since bronchial drainage is adequate from these sites, symptoms are usually minimal [*bronchiectasis sicca*]. It occurs due to destruction and fibrosis of lung parenchyma, resulting in

retraction and irreversible bronchial dilatation or due to bronchostenosis leading to obstructive pneumonitis and distal bronchiectasis [Figures 9.24 and 9.25]. Bronchiectasis is seen in 71%-86% patients on HRCT. Bronchostenosis can result in persistent segmental or lobar collapse, lobar hyperinflation or obstructive pneumonitis. Broncholithiasis is an uncommon complication of pulmonary TB. It is characterised by calcified peribronchial nodes that erode into or cause distortion of an adjacent bronchus. Right-sided predominance has been observed (64). Other radiologic findings include segmental or lobar atelectasis, obstructive pneumonitis, branching opacities in a 'V' or 'Y' configuration [obstructive bronchocele] and focal hyperinflation (64,65).

Pleural Complications

The pleural complications are pleurisy, empyema, fibrothorax, pneumothorax and bronchopleural fistula [Figure 9.26]. Fibrothorax shows diffuse pleural thickening and calcification with volume loss of the hemithorax. Pnuemothorax can occur due to rupture of a cavity into the pleural space.

Vascular Complications

These include pulmonary and bronchial arteritis and thrombosis, bronchial artery dilatation [Figure 9.27] and pulmonary artery [Rasmussen's aneurysm]. These can result in massive haemoptysis. The ongoing inflammation in areas of active disease can cause vasculitis and thrombosis. Arteries in the vicinity of old cavities can show endarteritis obliterans. Rasmussen's aneurysm is a pseudoaneurysm that results from weakening of the pulmonary artery wall by adjacent cavitary TB [Figure 9.28]. It may form months to years after formation of the cavity and is seen

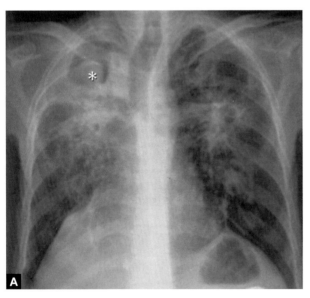
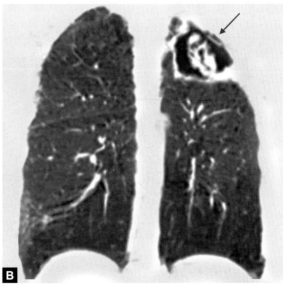

Figure 9.23: Mycetoma in TB cavity: Chest radiograph [postero-anterior view] [A] showing loss of volume of right upper lobe with a cavity having a fungal ball [asterisk] illustrating the 'air crescent' sign. CT chest [B] of another patient, showing soft tissue mass inside a cavity in left upper lobe caused by a fungus ball [arrow]

TB = tuberculosis; CT = computed tomography

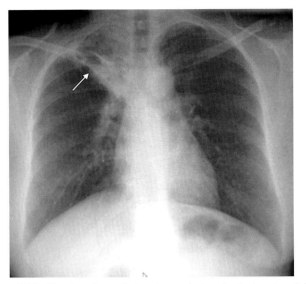

Figure 9.24: Chest radiograph [postero-anterior view] showing right upper lobe collapse with elevated minor fissure [arrow]

in 4%-5% autopsy cases (33). It may produce an 'air-crescent' on radiographs, thereby, mimicking a mycetoma. CT angiography can confirm the diagnosis. Arterial embolisation has been demonstrated as an effective method to achieve primary control of bleeding associated with chronic TB cavities.

Mediastinal Complications

These include oesophagomediastinal and oesophago-bronchial fistula, fibrosing mediastinitis and constrictive pericarditis. The mediastinal lymph nodes [especially subcarinal lymph nodes] can caseate to form fistula with the mid thoracic oesophagus. Fibrosis with formation of traction diverticula in the oesophagus may also develop. Fibrosing mediastinitis is seen as soft tissue in the mediastinum encasing the major vessels and airway, causing luminal compromise [Figure 9.29]. Involvement of the pericardium can cause diffuse pericardial thickening and calcification leading to constrictive pericarditis.

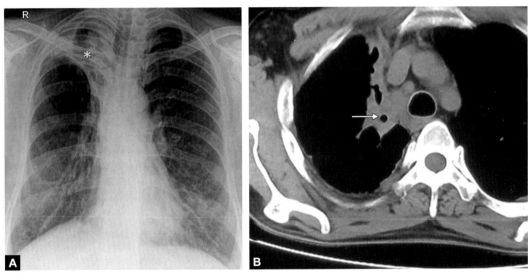

Figure 9.25: Chest radiograph [postero-anterior view] [A] showing volume loss of right upper lobe [asterisk]. HRCT chest of the same patient [B], revealing encasement of the right upper lobe bronchus [arrow] by soft tissue causing luminal narrowing
HRCT = high-resolution computed tomography

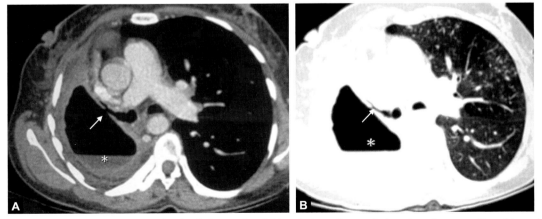

Figure 9.26: CECT chest [A] showing communication between the right main bronchus and pleural cavity suggestive of broncho-pleural fistula [arrow] with a thick-walled pleural collection having an air-fluid level [asterisk]. Multiple nodules are seen in left lung [B]
CECT = contrast-enhanced computed tomography

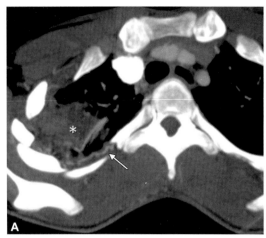 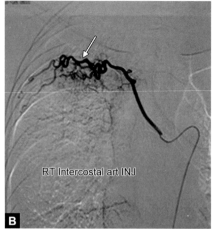

Figure 9.27: CT chest [A] showing consolidation in the right upper lobe [asterisk] with a hypertrophied intercosto-bronchial artery supplying the region [arrow]. Selective bronchial artery angiogram [B] illustrating the hypertrophied vessel [arrow]
CT = computed tomography
Kind courtesy: Dr Ashu Seith Bhalla, Department of Radiodiagnosis, All India Institute of Medical Sciences, New Delhi

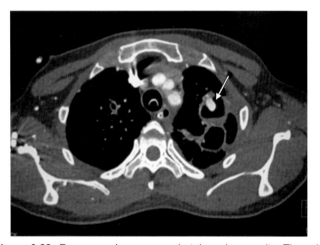

Figure 9.28: Rasmussen's aneurysm in tuberculous cavity: Thoracic CT angiogram showing fibro-cavitary changes in left upper lobe with a pseudoaneurysm [arrow] arising from pulmonary artery branch projecting in one of the cavities
CT = computed tomography

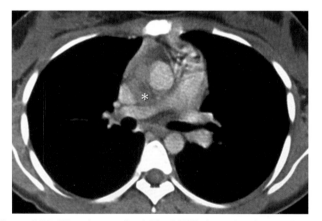

Figure 9.29: Fibrosing mediastinitis: CECT chest showing mediastinal soft tissue [asterisk] causing extrinsic compression and narrowing of right pulmonary artery
CECT = contrast-enhanced computed tomography

Chest Wall Complications

There can be involvement of the ribs, costal cartilage and dorsal vertebra. Also, the pleural collection can track exteriorly through the chest wall presenting as a subcutaneous lump. This is known as *empyema necessitans*.

TUBERCULOSIS AND HUMAN IMMUNODEFICIENCY VIRUS INFECTION

By suppressing cell-mediated immunity, HIV infection predisposes to development of progressive primary disease or reactivation of latent infection. HIV-TB co-infection is a common problem encountered by clinicians (66).

The radiographic manifestations of pulmonary TB in HIV-seropositive individuals depends on the level of immunosuppression. HIV-seropositive patients with a CD4+ T-lymphocyte count less than $200/mm^3$ have a higher prevalence of mediastinal or hilar lymphadenopathy, a lower prevalence of cavitation, and often extrapulmonary involvement (4). Miliary or disseminated disease is also associated with severe immunosuppression. Unusual or atypical manifestations of pulmonary TB are common in patients with very low CD4+ T-lymphocyte counts who are severely immunosuppressed. The reader is referred to the chapter '*Tuberculosis and human immunodeficiency virus infection*' [Chapter 35] for details.

Radiologic Manifestations of Multidrug-resistant Tuberculosis

Drug resistance is a major public health problem that threatens the success of global TB control. Bilateral involvement, multiple cavities and nodules and bronchial dilatation are more common in patients with multidrug-resistant TB [MDR-TB] (67). A correlation has been observed between the radiologic features of MDR-TB and the mode of acquisition of drug-resistance (68,69). In new patients with

MDR-TB, presentation with non-cavitary consolidation, pleural effusion, and a primary TB pattern of disease is seen (70). On the other hand, in previously treated patients with MDR-TB, cavitary consolidation and a reactivation pattern of the disease is evident. The CT findings in extensively drug-resistant TB [XDR-TB] are similar to MDR-TB. XDR-TB manifests as an advanced pattern of primary TB [extensive consolidation with or without lymphadenopathy] in AIDS patients or an advanced pattern of MDR-TB [multiple cavitary lesions in consolidative or nodular lesions] in non-AIDS patients.

FAMILY SURVEY

It is important to survey the family members who stay in close contact with a patient with pulmonary TB. All contacts should have a chest radiograph taken and children below 12 years of age should undergo TST to detect asymptomatic contacts with latent TB infection [LTBI]. In a study (32) conducted at New Delhi, with 2677 children with pulmonary TB, a positive family history of TB was evident in 30% patients. Radiographic screening of 300 adult contacts of children with primary pulmonary complex showed active pulmonary lesions in 4%-5% of those screened (32). The reader is referred to the chapter *"Tuberculosis in children"* [Chapter 36] for further details on this topic.

RADIOGRAPHIC FOLLOW-UP SCHEDULE

The American Thoracic Society [ATS] and Centers for Disease Control [CDC] (71) recommend the following radiographic schedule. In patients with a negative sputum mycobacterial culture, a repeat chest radiograph is indicated at two months of treatment; another chest radiograph is considered as desirable at the end of treatment. In patients with a positive sputum mycobacterial culture, repeat chest radiographs at two months and at the end of treatment are considered desirable [but not essential] (72).

EXTRA-PULMONARY TB

With the increasing prevalence of TB worldwide, there has been a similar rise in its extra-pulmonary TB [EPTB] manifestations as well (73). In the era before the HIV pandemic, EPTB constituted 15%-20% of all cases of TB (74-79). In HIV-seropositive individuals, EPTB accounts for more than 50% of all cases (80-85). The most common extrapulmonary site of TB in HIV-seropositive individuals is lymph node TB. However, genitourinary, neurological, pleural, pericardial, abdominal and musculoskeletal involvement has been described and virtually every organ system in the body can be affected. In studies (86,87) from India, EPTB constituted 45%-56% of all TB cases in AIDS patients.

Confirmation of diagnosis of EPTB is usually difficult. Positive findings on chest radiograph or a positive TST may support the diagnosis, but negative results do not exclude the possibility of EPTB (88-90). Systemic manifestations of TB can mimic a variety of neoplastic and non-neoplastic conditions including lymphoma, leukaemia, metastases, sarcoidosis, histoplasmosis, and pyogenic infections. Radiographs, ultrasonography, cross-sectional imaging with multidetector CT and MRI, all play an important role in the diagnosis and post-treatment follow-up of these patients.

LYMPH NODE TUBERCULOSIS

In India and other developing countries, lymph node TB is the most common form of EPTB. Nontuberculous mycobacteria [NTM] are the most common cause of lymphadenopathy in the developed world (91,92). Peripheral lymph nodes are usually affected, of which cervical and supraclavicular nodes are most commonly involved, followed by axillary and inguinal nodes (93,94). On ultrasound these nodes depict central hypoechoic areas corresponding to necrosis. CT demonstrates peripheral enhancement with low attenuation centres.

ABDOMINAL TUBERCULOSIS

Abdominal TB encompasses TB of the gastrointestinal [GI] tract, peritoneum, omentum, mesentery, abdominal lymph nodes, and solid visceral organs such as liver, spleen and pancreas. Only 15% of patients with abdominal TB have evidence of pulmonary involvement and chest radiograph may be normal in 50%-65% of these patients (95).

Gastrointestinal Tract Tuberculosis

Any segment of the GI tract may be involved and ileocaecal region is most commonly affected, seen in 80%-90% of patients with abdominal TB (96).

Oesophageal Tuberculosis

This is rare and usually secondary to advanced mediastinal or pulmonary disease. Barium swallow studies may show extrinsic compression by enlarged mediastinal nodes, strictures, ulceration, mucosal irregularity and traction diverticula. Sinus tracts and fistulous communications may develop with the mediastinum or tracheobronchial tree. CT can reliably demonstrate full extent of extramucosal disease but endoscopic biopsy is required for confirming the diagnosis.

Tuberculosis of Stomach and Duodenum

TB of stomach and duodenum can be ulcerative [most common], hypertrophic, or in the form of multiple or solitary tuberculomas, TB pyloric stenosis and TB lymphadenitis. Imaging features are non-specific, may mimic benign ulcers in ulcerative form and malignancy in hypertrophic form. Adenocarcinoma and lymphoma are important differential diagnosis (89,97). Duodenal involvement can be intrinsic or extrinsic. Intrinsic involvement can be ulcerative or hyperplastic while external lymphadenopathy may lead to duodenal C-loop widening.

TB Enteritis

TB is a common cause of small bowel obstruction in India. Ulcerative form is more common, the ulcers having stellate or linear shape. In addition, bowel loops can be matted and fixed by adhesions and fibrosis. In case of acute obstruction, plain radiograph of the abdomen shows dilated bowel loops with multiple air-fluid levels. Enteroliths, calcified lymph nodes and hepatosplenomegaly may be evident. There may be evidence of perforation, ascites or intussusception. In case of subacute bowel obstruction, barium-meal follow through or small bowel enterography study can be done. Per-oral pneumocolon can be employed for optimal distension of caecum and ileocaecal region in equivocal cases. Ultrasonography exhibits segments of circumferential bowel wall thickening, increased peristalsis proximal to obstruction and ascites. Latter may become loculated with multiple septations within. Imaging features of intestinal TB [Table 9.9] correlate with pathological stage of disease (98,99).

Ileocaecal TB

Ileocaecal region can be affected in a variety of ways [Figure 9.30]: [i] hyperplastic with long segments of narrowing, rigidity and loss of distensibility [pipe-stem colon]; [ii] ulcerative; [iii] ulcerohyperplastic; and [iv] carcinoma type, with short annular stenosis and overhanging edges. In the early stages, barium studies demonstrate spasm, hypermotility and thickening [oedema] of the ileocaecal valve. Focal or diffuse aphthous ulcers also occur in the early stages. These ulcers are larger than those seen in Crohn's disease and follow the orientation of lymphoid follicles [i.e., longitudinal in terminal ileum and transverse in colon]. A widely gaping ileocaecal valve with narrowing of terminal ileum [Fleischner sign, inverted umbrella sign] or a narrowed terminal ileum

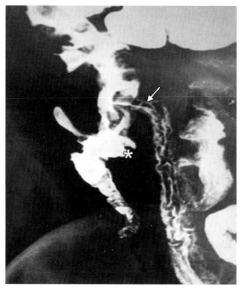

Figure 9.30: Barium-meal follow through study showing ileocaecal TB. Narrowing and mucosal irregularity of the terminal ileum [arrow] with thin stream of barium in its lumen is seen. Caecum is contracted, shrunken [asterisk] and pulled out of right iliac fossa. The normal acute angle of ileocaecal junction is distorted
TB = tuberculosis

with rapid emptying of the diseased segment through a gaping ileocaecal valve into a shortened, rigid, obliterated caecum [*Stierlin sign*] are considered characteristic (89). In advanced cases, symmetric annular napkin-ring stenosis and obstruction associated with shortening, retraction, and pouch formation may be seen. Caecum characteristically becomes conical, shrunken, and retracted out of the iliac fossa due to fibrosis within the mesocolon, and the ileocaecal valve becomes fixed, irregular, gaping, and incompetent (96,100,101). There is loss of the normal ileocaecal angle [which becomes obtuse] and the dilated terminal ileum appears suspended from a retracted amputated caecum [goose-neck deformity]. Localised partial stenosis opposite the ileocaecal valve with a rounded-off smooth caecum and a dilated terminal ileum resemble a 'purse-string stenosis'. Persistent narrow stream of barium indicates bowel stenosis and is called the 'string sign'. Terminal ileum may be fixed and narrowed due to stricture while the ileocaecal valve becomes fixed, irregular and incompetent. Stierlin sign and string sign are not specific for TB and may be seen in Crohn's disease also.

Ultrasonography shows wall thickening of caecum and terminal ileum, regional lymph nodes enlargement and mesenteric thickening. CT may show circumferential wall thickening of the caecum and terminal ileum with adjacent mesenteric lymphadenopathy. Asymmetric thickening of the ileocaecal valve, thickening of the medial caecal wall, exophytic extension and engulfment of the terminal ileum, and massive lymphadenopathy with central necrosis are more suggestive of TB. CT enteroclysis has greater sensitivity and specificity for detection of bowel wall abnormalities (102). TB wall thickening may show hyperintensity on T2-weighted

---

Table 9.9: Imaging features of intestinal TB
Stage 1 [superficial mucosal invasion]
Accelerated intestinal transit
Precipitation, flocculation or dilution of the barium suspension due to abnormal secretion
Hypersegmentation of the barium column [chicken intestine] because of abnormal tone and peristalsis
Mucosal pattern changes: fold irregularity and thickening
Irregular crenated intestinal contour
Stage 2 [ulceration]
Stellate ulcers are characterised by barium speck with converging mucosal folds
Linear ulcers are transversely oriented, resulting in spasm and circumferential strictures
Stage 3 [sclerosis, hypertrophy, stenosis and strictures]
Strictures are usually multiple and short with segmental dilation of bowel loops
Hour-glass stenosis: short stricture with smooth stiff contours
Fixity of bowel loops, matting and speculation
TB = tuberculosis

Table 9.10: Differentiating imaging features of ileocaecal involvement in TB and Crohn's disease

Imaging feature	TB	Crohn's disease
Wall thickening	Irregular asymmetric, especially medial caecal wall	Circumferential, more on mesenteric border
Omental and peritoneal thickening	Yes	No
Creeping fat [abnormal quantity of mesenteric fat]	No	Yes
Lymph node enlargement	Necrotic centres, calcification	Homogeneous
Pseudosacculations	No	Present on anti-mesenteric border
Positive findings on chest radiograph	Yes	No
Barium studies	Fleischner's sign	Cobblestone appearance
Enteroliths	Common	No
Perforations, fistulae	Less common	More common

TB = tuberculosis

MRI images and heterogeneous enhancement on post-gadolinium images.

The differential diagnoses for ileocaecal TB include Crohn's disease, amoebiasis and primary caecal malignancy. Differentiating imaging features of ileocaecal involvement in TB and Crohn's disease are listed in Table 9.10. Amputation of the caecum may be seen in amoebiasis, but small bowel is rarely involved. Caecal malignancy is always limited by the ileocaecal valve.

Appendiceal TB

Isolated involvement does not occur, rather it is usually affected in patients with active ileocaecal TB and clinically presents as chronic appendicitis.

Colonic and Anorectal TB

Colonic involvement can be segmental or diffuse and may manifest as ulcerations, rigidity, spasms, spiculations, perforations and pericolic abscesses. Ulcerating proctitis is another uncommon manifestation. Fistulae, strictures and chronic ischiorectal abscesses may occur. Anal TB, seen in paediatric patients, may present as ulcer, fissure, fistula, abscess. Differentials in colon include Crohn's disease, ulcerative colitis, ischaemic colitis and malignancy while those in anorectal region include Crohn's, malignancy, lymphogranuloma venereum and actinomycosis.

Peritoneal, Omental and Mesenteric TB

Classically three forms of peritoneal TB are described (89,103,104): [i] wet ascitic type [90% cases] characterised by a large amount of free or loculated viscous fluid; [ii] fibrotic-fixed type characterised by mesenteric and omental thickening, matted bowel loops; and [iii] dry or plastic type-fibrous peritoneal reaction, dense adhesions and caseous nodules.

Ultrasonography can detect even minimal amount of ascites. It may reveal multiple fibrin strands, septations and internal debris. The ascitic fluid demonstrates high attenuation at CT due to its high protein and cellular content. CT may also demonstrate tethering of bowel loops and mesenteric infiltration. Peritoneal thickening and nodules may be appreciated on ultrasonography or CT especially in the presence of ascites. Similarly, there can be omental thickening or caking along with thickening, increased vascularity and nodularity of mesentery. Fixed loops of bowel, standing out as spokes radiating out from thickened mesenteric root are described as 'stellate sign'. 'Club sandwich sign' or the 'sliced bread' appearance is due to alternating layers of echogenic bowel and anechoic inter-bowel loop fluid.

The radiographic differential diagnosis includes carcinomatosis, malignant mesothelioma, and non-TB peritonitis. Peritoneal mesothelioma manifests as multifocal peritoneal thickening, omental or mesenteric soft tissue masses, thick rigid peritoneal septae, fixed bowel loops and disproportionately small amount of ascites. Features suggestive of TB include smooth mild peritoneal thickening [< 5 mm], enhancement and multiple fine, mobile septae (97). TB has also been implicated in the aetiology of sclerosing encapsulated peritonitis [abdominal cocoon] [Figure 9.31]. Ultrasonography and CT show clustered bowel loops, loculated ascites and adhesions encapsulated within a thick membrane-like sac. Barium study may show concertina-like configuration of dilated small bowel loops in a fixed U-shaped cluster or "cauliflower sign" (105).

Abdominal Lymph Node TB

Lymph node enlargement is common in abdominal TB and may occur without any other evidence of abdominal involvement. The common lymph nodes involved are mesenteric, periportal, retroperitoneal and in omental regions [Figures 9.32 and 9.33]. There may be lymph node enlargement, increased number of normal-sized lymph nodes or conglomeration with matting resulting from adhesions due to periadenitis. On sonography, these nodes show central hypoechoic area in contrast to the homogeneous nodes seen in lymphoma [Figure 9.32]. Focal areas of

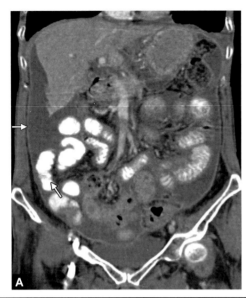

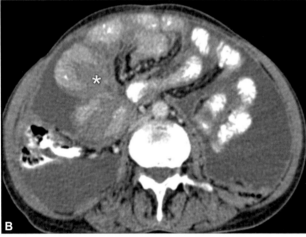

Figure 9.31: Sclerosing encapsulated peritonitis. Here is diffuse uniform peritoneal thickening [arrow] and ascites on coronal CECT image [A]. Axial CECT image shows that peritoneal thickening is forming a sac-like membrane around the ascites. Small bowel loops are arranged in concertina-like configuration [abdominal cocoon] [asterisk] [B]
CECT = contrast-enhanced computed tomography

calcification may also be evident on sonography or CT. Four different patterns of enhancement can be seen on CECT (106). Most frequent is peripheral rim enhancement with hypo-dense centre [Figure 9.33A]. This pattern seen in young patients reflects central liquefactive or caseous necrosis. Inhomogeneous enhancement is next common manifestation indicative of relatively less necrosis. Homogeneous enhancement and non-enhancement are less common patterns that may occasionally be seen. Lymphadenopathy, hypointense on T1-weighted [Figure 9.33B], hyperintense on T2-weighted images [Figure 9.33C], with perinodal hyperintensity, and predominant peripheral rim-like enhancement may suggest the diagnosis of TB (107).

Visceral TB

Hepatic and splenic involvement manifests in a micro-nodular [miliary] or macronodular [tuberculoma] form (36).

The micronodular form occurs in association with miliary pulmonary TB. On CT, multiple tiny, low-attenuating lesions may be seen. More frequently, these miliary nodules are not apparent, but the liver or spleen appear heterogeneous and enlarged (97). In the less common macronodular form, multiple hypo-attenuating lesions 1-3 cm in diameter or a single mass is seen in a diffusely enlarged liver or spleen [Figures 9.34 and 9.35] (89). These lesions may show heterogeneous enhancement and foci of calcification. These lesions are usually hypoechoic on ultrasound, hypointense on T1-weighted images, hyperintense on T2-weighted images with a less intense rim relative to the surrounding liver. The differential diagnosis of the miliary form includes metastases, fungal infection, sarcoidosis, and lymphoma. The macronodular form can be mistaken for metastases, primary malignant tumour, or pyogenic abscess.

Pancreatic TB is rare, may present as acute or chronic pancreatitis or may mimic malignancy (108,109). Lesions are commonly located in the head of pancreas, may have calcification and may be associated with peripancreatic lymph node enlargement. Multiple visceral abscesses have also been described in patients with HIV infections (109). TB can also affect the wall of abdominal vessels, resulting in formation of mycotic pseudoaneurysms.

GENITOURINARY TB

Genitourinary system is a common site of EPTB and kidneys are the most commonly involved organ [Table 9.11]. The kidneys, prostate and seminal vesicles are involved following hematogenous dissemination from the lungs. All other genital organs, including the epididymis and bladder, become involved by ascent or descent of mycobacteria. The testicle may become involved by direct extension from an epididymal infection.

Renal TB

Early findings are best detected on intravenous urography [IVU] while ultrasonography, CT and MRI depict the full extent of chronic changes. The earliest urographic abnormality is loss of definition of a minor calyx with indistinct feathery outline ["moth-eaten" calyx] due to erosion and irregularity of calyces or papillae. This is frequently followed by papillary necrosis, ulceration, wall thickening, and fibrosis of the collecting system. Pelvicalyceal system may get dilated due to a stricture of the ureteropelvic junction, or an infundibular stricture may cause localised hydrocalycosis. Cavitation within the renal parenchyma may be detected as irregular pools of contrast material on delayed phase images and may be seen to communicate with a deformed calyx. Cicatricial contractures of fibrotic parenchyma may lead to calyceal or renal pelvic traction. Infundibular stenosis may lead to incomplete opacification of the calyx [phantom calyx] due to failure of contrast excretion (110). Tiny infundibular stump may be seen in such cases [amputated calyx]. 'Hiked up pelvis' is the term used for cephalic retraction of the renal pelvis due to

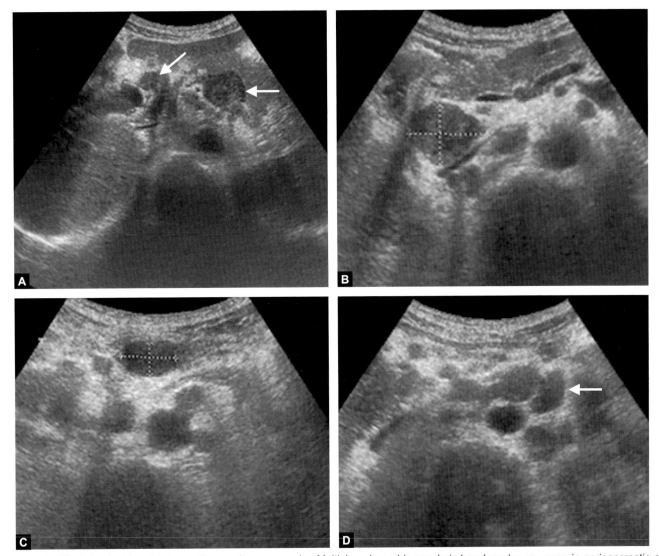

Figure 9.32: TB abdominal lymphadenopathy on ultrasonography. Multiple enlarged hypoechoic lymph nodes are seen in peripancreatic and periportal locations [A]. Large precaval lymph node and small retrocaval nodes [B], mesenteric [C] and retroperitoneal nodes in pre-aortic and left para-aortic locations [D] can also be seen.
TB = tuberculosis

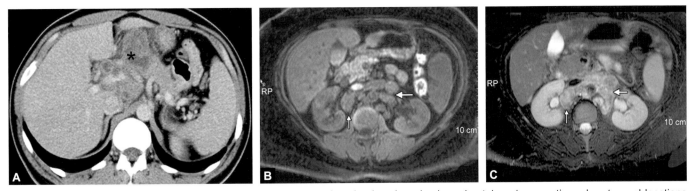

Figure 9.33: Axial CECT image showing multiple enlarged ring enhancing lymph nodes in periportal, peripancreatic and aortocaval locations with central necrosis within [asterisk]. [A] Axial T1-weighted [B] and T2-weighted [C] image showing multiple retroperitoneal lymph nodes around the aorta and IVC and in the renal hilum region [arrows]. The nodes are hypointense on T1 [B] and hyperintense on T2 [C] with central necrosis [arrow] within appearing more hyperintense on T2-weighted image [C]
CECT = contrast-enhanced computed tomography

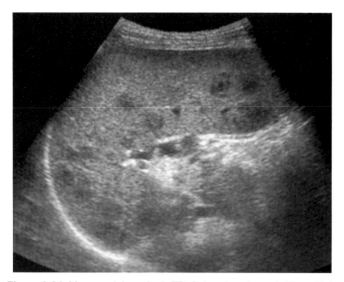

Figure 9.34: Macronodular splenic TB. Spleen is enlarged with multiple well-defined 1-3 cm hypoechoic nodules on ulrasonography
TB = tuberculosis

involvement of the inferior margin. 'Kerr's kink' refers to sharply angulated pelvic kink pointing in the direction of the involved calyx, strictured infundibulum. Calculi may be present within the renal collecting system. Characteristic calcifications in a lobar distribution are often seen in end-stage TB [putty kidney]. The calcifications may also be amorphous, granular or curvilinear, and may be seen on radiographs and CT. End-stage disease manifests as fibrosis and obstructive uropathy, produces autonephrectomy which may be of two types: [i] caseo-cavernous type characterised by an enlarged sac filled with caseous material; and [ii] calcified shrunken non-functioning kidney (110,111).

Various patterns of hydronephrosis may be seen depending on the site of the stricture and include focal caliectasis, caliectasis without pelvic dilatation, and generalised hydronephrosis (112). Other common findings include parenchymal scarring, low-attenuation parenchymal lesions and abscesses. CT is also useful in depicting the extension of disease into the extra-renal space. Ultrasonography findings of renal TB include hypoechoic parenchymal

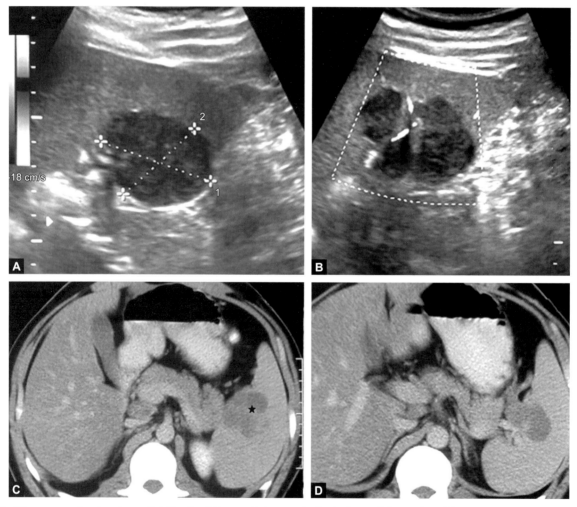

Figure 9.35: Ultrasonography showing well-defined solid hypoechoic mass lesion in the perihilar region of the spleen [A] with internal vascularity on colour Doppler [B]. Axial CECT images [C and D] show mild heterogeneous contrast enhancement in the lesion [asterisk]. Ultrasonography-guided FNAC revealed epithelioid granulomas with necrosis and stain for acid-fast bacilli was positive
CECT = contrast-enhanced computed tomography; FNAC = fine needle aspiration cytology

Table 9.11: Imaging features of TB of the urinary tract

Intravenous urography

   Renal calcifications [amorphous, granular, or curvilinear calcifications and putty kidney]
   Mesenteric lymph node and adrenal calcifications
   Fuzziness of minor calyces ["moth-eaten" calyces] - early finding
   Irregularity of the tips of medullary pyramids
   Infundibular stenosis and strictures
   Localised caliectasis or incomplete opacification of the calix [phantom calyx]
   Small parenchymal cavities communicating with PCS
   Generalised hydronephrosis or caliectasis without pelvic dilatation
   Kerr's kink and hiked-up renal pelvis
   Dilatation, strictures and wall irregularity of ureter [saw-tooth ureter]
   Rigid shortened ureter [pipe-stem ureter]
   Reduced bladder capacity [thimble bladder] with vesico-ureteric reflux

Ultrasonography

   Hydronephrosis with debris within
   Non-uniform caliectasis with filling defects
   Wall thickening of PCS [urothelial thickening]
   Hypoechoic parenchymal lesions

CECT + CT urography

   Renal, ureteric and nodal calcifications
   Hydronephrosis, irregular caliectasis, infundibular stricture, deformed renal pelvis
   Hypodense parenchymal lesions [ill-defined round or peripheral wedge-shaped]
   Urothelial thickening of PCS and/or ureter and/or bladder with strictures
   Parenchymal cavities, communicating with PCS, showing contrast pooling on delayed phase
   Parenchymal thinning, scarring, perinephric/periureteric fat stranding
   Thimble bladder
   Necrotic lymph nodes

MRI + MR urography

   Similar to CT, except for calcifications
   MR urogram gives excellent overview without administration of contrast
   Diffusion-weighted MRI can demonstrate focal pyelonephritis and evolving abscesses

TB = tuberculosis; PCS = pelvicalyceal system; CECT = contrast-enchanced computed tomography; CT = computed tomography; MRI = magnetic resonance imaging; MR = magnetic resonance

masses, dilated irregular calyces and hydronephrosis with debris (113). CT and MR urography demonstrate abnormal urothelial thickening and enhancement, uneven caliectasis, infundibular strictures and hydronephrosis [Figure 9.36]. The radiographic differential diagnosis for renal TB includes other causes of papillary necrosis, transitional cell carcinoma, acute focal bacterial nephritis and xanthogranulomatous pyelonephritis.

TB of the Adrenal Glands

TB of the adrenal glands is the most common cause of chronic adrenal insufficiency in developing countries where TB is highly endemic (114). Involvement is bilateral in 90% of cases and asymmetric soft tissue masses are usually seen (108). The appearance overlaps that of metastases, haemorrhage and primary neoplasms. Bilateral involvement, preserved contour and peripheral rim-enhancement favour TB rather than malignancy (115). The adrenal gland may undergo atrophy and calcification in the end stage of disease and show low signal on all MRI sequences.

TB of the Ureter

Ureter involvement [Figure 9.36] is almost always secondary to renal TB due to bacilluria. Dilatation and a ragged irregular appearance of the urothelium are the initial features, best appreciated on urography. In advanced disease, ureteral shortening, filling defects, strictures or wall calcifications may be seen (89,112). The sites of normal anatomic narrowing like pelviureteric junction, across the pelvic brim, and at the vesicoureteric junction are prone to develop strictures (104). A "beaded" or "cork-screw" appearance of the ureter has also been reported. Severe thickening of the wall produces a rigid shortened ureter with narrow lumen termed pipe stem appearance. Renal damage secondary to ureteral strictures may be more severe than the effect of the direct parenchymal involvement (116).

Urinary Bladder TB

The most common finding in TB cystitis is reduced bladder capacity which along with wall thickening and irregular contractures gives the appearance of 'thimble bladder'. Large tuberculomas in bladder wall can manifest as filling defects simulating malignancy. In advanced disease, the bladder is small, irregular, and calcified (89,112). Fibrosis in the region of the trigone produces gaping vesico-ureteric junction with free reflux. Calcified TB cystitis must be differentiated from schistosomiasis, cystitis due to cyclophosphamide, radiation-induced changes, and calcified bladder carcinoma.

Female Genital TB

Fallopian tubes are most commonly affected in female genital TB [in up to 94%] followed by the uterus. Salpingitis is often bilateral and results in infertility (89). Hysterosalpingography [HSG] is the mainstay for evaluating fallopian tube patency. HSG findings include tubal occlusion, strictures, hydrosalpinx, rigid pipe-stem tubes, endometritis with adhesions [causing Asherman syndrome] with obliteration and T-shaped distortion of the endometrial cavity (117). Ultrasonography and CT allow for adnexal evaluation, and may show tubo-ovarian abscesses, chronic calcifications and calcified lymph nodes in the adnexal region (89). Changes, such, as uterine adhesions, hydrosalpinx and tubo-ovarian abscess are better evident on MRI.

Male Genital TB

The most common finding in TB prostatitis is multiple hypoechoic areas in the peripheral zone of prostate on

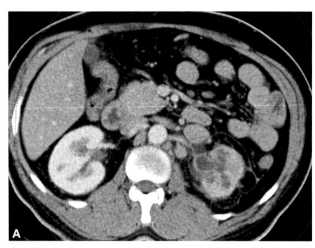
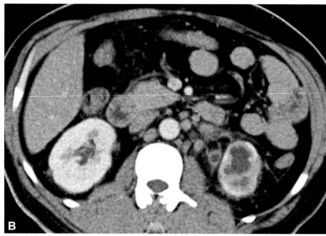

Figure 9.36: Renal TB. Axial CECT images [A and B] showing pelvi-calyectasis with urothelial wall thickening and ureteric dilatation with ureteric wall thickening on the left side. There is perinephric fascial thickening and multiple enlarged renal hilar and retroperitoneal lymph nodes
TB = tuberculosis; CECT = contrast-enhanced computed tomography

transrectal ultrasound. CECT may reveal hypoattenuating prostatic lesions, which likely represent foci of caseous necrosis and inflammation. At MRI, a prostatic abscess demonstrates peripheral enhancement. This finding helps differentiate an abscess from prostatic malignancy. In addition, MRI shows diffuse, radiating, streaks of low signal intensity in the prostate [*watermelon skin sign*] on T2-weighted images (118). TB epididymo-orchitis usually manifests as focal or diffuse areas of decreased echogenicity in testis and heterogeneous hypoechoic, enlarged, nodular epididymis at ultrasound (119). Urethral involvement leads to strictures, fistulas and periurethral abscesses.

NEUROLOGICAL TB

Haematogenous dissemination leads to subependymal or subpial focus of TB [Rich focus] which may be located in the meninges, brain, or spinal cord. Central nervous system TB may take a variety of forms, including meningitis, tuberculomas, abscess, cerebritis, ventriculitis and miliary involvement. TB meningitis is believed to be caused by rupture of a Rich focus into the cerebrospinal fluid [CSF]. However, tuberculoma may be secondary to haematogenous spread of systemic disease or evolve from extension of CSF infection into the adjacent parenchyma (120,121). Post-gadolinium MRI is superior to CECT for demonstration of meningeal disease as well as parenchymal abnormalities.

TB Meningitis

Meningeal involvement, the most common presentation of CNS TB, is seen more commonly in children and young adults [Figures 9.37 and 9.38]. On both CT and MRI, there is abnormal meningeal enhancement [corresponding to gelatinous exudates], typically more pronounced in the basal cisterns and sylvian fissures along with plaque like dural thickening. Even on non-contrast computed tomography [NCCT], there is obliteration of the basal cisterns by isodense-hyperdense exudates. Ependymal

involvement is seen as linear enhancement along the ventricular margins. Communicating hydrocephalus is the most common complication of cranial TB meningitis and has a poor prognosis. Also, ischaemic infarcts can be seen as complication of cranial tuberculous meningitis and are commonly bilateral. Majority are located in the basal ganglia and internal capsule, resulting from vascular compression and occlusion of middle cerebral artery and its branches especially small perforating vessels (120-122). Cranial nerves may also be involved.

The MRI features of spinal TB meningitis include cerebrospinal fluid [CSF] loculations and obliteration of the spinal subarachnoid space. There is loss of outline of the spinal cord especially in the cervico-thoracic spine and matting of the nerve roots in the lumbar region. Contrast-enhanced MRI reveals nodular, thick, linear intradural enhancement (122,123). Syringomyelia can occur as a complication of arachnoiditis, is seen as cord cavitation that demonstrates fluid signal intensity and does not show any enhancement (122).

Cerebral Parenchymal TB

Cerebral parenchymal disease [Figures 9.37 and 9.38] can occur with or without meningitis and usually manifests as tuberculomas while abscess and cerebritis are relatively rare (120). Multiple tuberculomas are usually evident. The frontal and parietal lobes are the most commonly affected regions with corticomedullary junction and periventricular location being the predisposed sites. On CT, tuberculomas appear as rounded or lobulated masses demonstrating homogeneous or ring enhancement and have irregular walls of varying thickness. The MRI features of a tuberculoma depend upon whether it is caseating or not. Non-caseating tuberculomas are often hyperintense on T2-weighted images with homogeneous [nodular] enhancement. Caseating solid granulomas are isointense to markedly hypointense on T2-weighted images and exhibit rim enhancement (120-122).

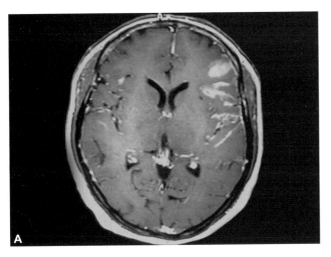

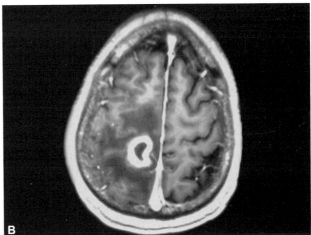

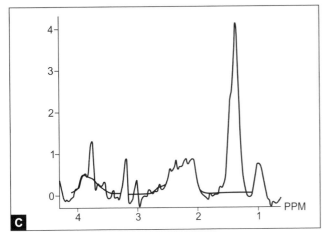

Figure 9.37: Axial contrast-enhanced MR image in patient of TB meningitis showing abnormal meningeal enhancement in bilateral [more prominent in left] sylvian fissure regions [A]. Axial contrast-enhanced MR image shows thick-walled ring enhancing lesion in the right high parietal lobe with significant amount of hypointense perilesional oedema [B]. MR spectroscopy shows lipid peak at 1.3 ppm, favouring the diagnosis of TB [C]

MR = magnetic resonance; TB = tuberculosis

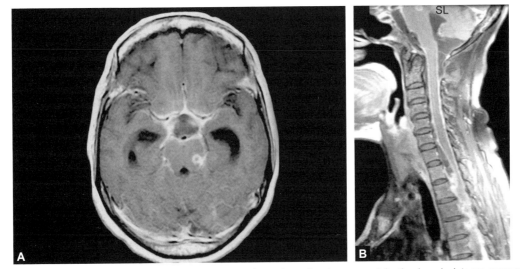

Figure 9.38: Axial contrast-enhanced MR image showing abnormal meningeal enhancement in the basal cisterns corresponding to basal exudates. Ring-enhancing tuberculomas are also seen in the left mid-brain region [A]. Sagittal contrast-enhanced MR image showing abnormal thick enhancement along the surface of spinal cord and also lining the CSF loculations anterior to the cord [B]

MR = magnetic resonance; CSF = cerebrospinal fluid

Table 9.12: Characteristic imaging features of neurological infections including TB

TB	Neurocysticercosis	Toxoplasmosis	Lymphoma
Lesions are larger than NCC	Individual lesion usually less than 2 cm	Basal ganglia and gray-while matter junction are favoured sites	Hyperdense on non-contrast CT
Thick irregular walls	Periphery is smooth and thin		T2 intermediate signal intensity
Perilesional oedema more than NCC	Clustering of lesions more common	Asymmetric nodular ring enhancement	Marked diffusion restriction
T2 hypointense central core favours TB	Eccentric scolex visible as hyperdensity or calcification on CT and T2 hypointensity on MR	Elevated lipid-lactate with diminished levels of all other metabolites on MR spectroscopy	Periventricular predominance
Associated TB meningitis may be seen			Elevated choline on MR spectroscopy
Lipid peak on MR spectroscopy	Central core is hyperintense on T2-weighted images [exception: calcification]	Haemorrhage may be detected on MR	Elevated relative cerebral blood volume on MR perfusion
Central core may show diffusion restriction	No diffusion restriction		Haemorrhage is rare

TB = tuberculosis; NCC = neurocysticercosis; CT = computed tomography; MR = magnetic resonance

Granulomas with central liquefaction appear centrally hyperintense on T2-weighted images with rim enhancement and surrounding oedema. Miliary tubercles appear as numerous round, homogeneously enhancing lesions less than 2 mm in diameter (122,124). Magnetic resonance [MR] spectroscopy shows prominent lipid peaks in tuberculomas. On imaging, TB abscess may be indistinguishable from pyogenic abscess. Thin smooth wall, large size [> 3 cm], presence of loculations and relatively less oedema favour TB.

The differential diagnosis for cranial and spinal TB includes other infectious or non-infectious inflammatory diseases [e.g., sarcoidosis, lymphoma, toxoplasmosis, neurocysticercosis, pyogenic and fungal infections], multicentric primary neoplasms [e.g., hemangioblastoma, gliomas], and metastases [Table 9.12] (122). Features favouring tuberculomas over neurocysticercosis include larger size [> 20 mm], thick irregular walls, central T2 hypointensity, lipid peak on MR spectroscopy, concomitant meningitis and relatively more perilesional oedema. In contrast, presence of eccentric scolex and clustering of lesions favour cysticercosis.

EXTRACRANIAL, EXTRANODAL HEAD AND NECK TB

In TB otomastoiditis, CT demonstrates soft-tissue opacification of the tympanic cavity and destruction of middle ear structures in the later stages. Associated retroauricular or epidural abscess can be seen. The differential diagnoses include pyogenic or fungal infections, sarcoidosis, cholesteatoma, and Wegener's granulomatosis.

Chorioretinitis and uveitis are the most common manifestations of ocular TB (125,126). On CT or MRI, ocular TB usually manifests as a unilateral choroidal mass with melanoma, metastasis, hemangioma, sarcoidosis, and fungal infection being the main differential diagnoses. Laryngeal TB manifests as soft-tissue thickening and infiltration of the pre-epiglottic and paraglottic spaces, without the presence of a focal mass. The laryngeal framework usually remains intact. Sinonasal cavity, thyroid gland, pharynx and skull base can also be rarely involved.

MUSCULOSKELETAL TUBERCULOSIS

Skeletal involvement occurs in approximately 1%–3% of patients with TB. Evidence of concurrent active intrathoracic TB is present in less than 50% of these patients (127).

TB Spondylitis

The spine is the most common site of osseous involvement [in up to 50% of cases] (128). The most common location is upper lumbar and lower thoracic spine. Usually two consecutive vertebrae are involved but several vertebrae may be affected; skip lesions and single-level involvement may also occur. The disease process usually begins in the anterior part of the vertebral body adjacent to the end plate. The disk space may then become involved *via* several routes. Extension may occur along the anterior or posterior longitudinal ligament or directly through the end plate. Disk involvement manifests as collapse of intervertebral disk space (129). However, disk space involvement occurs late and is less marked compared with pyogenic infection. Less often, posterior elements of the spine may get involved. Collapse of a vertebral body, particularly the anterior segment, may result in TB kyphosis. Depending upon the site of infection, four types of involvement can occur: paradiskal, anterior subperiosteal, central and appendiceal.

Paradiskal

Paradiskal involvement is the most common type wherein disease process begins in the anterior part of the vertebral body adjacent to the end plate. Two adjacent vertebral bodies are usually involved. There is demineralisation and loss of definition of their end plates. Reactive sclerosis or periosteal reaction in the adjoining vertebral bodies is typically absent. With spread of infection, there is narrowing of the intervertebral disk space. With disease progression, there is anterior wedging leading to varying degrees of kyphosis and gibbus formation.

Central

In the central type, a lytic region devoid of normal trabecular pattern is seen in the centre of vertebral body away from the disk margins. This gradually enlarges and the vertebral body may expand like a tumour. In late stages, concentric collapse occurs, just like vertebra plana.

Anterior Subperiosteal

In the anterior subperiosteal type, the infection begins at the anterior vertebral margin underneath the periosteum and spreads beneath the anterior longitudinal ligament producing anterior erosions of multiple vertebrae.

Appendiceal or Neural Arch

Isolated involvement of the neural arch is rare; usually it occurs in contiguity with vertebral body involvement. Unilateral pedicle involvement is the most common manifestation. Pedicular and laminar involvement favours TB whereas pyogenic spondylitis has a predilection for facet joints.

Paravertebral abscesses form early and are seen in the thoracic region as posterior mediastinal mass and in the cervical region as widening of prevertebral soft tissues. Paraspinal infection can also involve the psoas muscle, resulting in psoas abscess, which can extend into the groin and thigh. Calcification within the abscess is considered pathognomic of TB (130). In the dorsal spine, the posteromedial

pleura line is displaced laterally by the paravertebral abscess producing a fusiform 'bird's nest' appearance [Figure 9.39]. CT and MR imaging are of great value in demonstrating a small focus of bone infection, complete extent of the disease and treatment response [Figure 9.40]. However, the diagnosis of TB is favoured if a large, calcified paravertebral mass and absence of sclerosis or new bone formation is seen. Conversely, intervertebral disk destruction is more characteristic of a pyogenic infection.

TB Osteomyelitis

Isolated TB osteomyelitis in the absence of associated TB arthritis is relatively rare. When it does occur, however, femur, tibia and small bones of the hands and feet are most commonly involved. Typically, the metaphyses are affected. Radiographic findings [Figure 9.41] include osteopenia, osteolytic foci with ill-defined edges, and varying amounts of sclerosis (130). Sequestrum formation is more common in children. One specific type of TB osteomyelitis is cystic

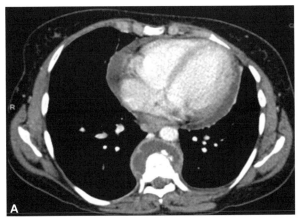

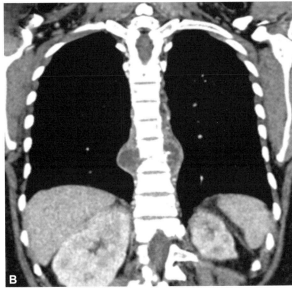

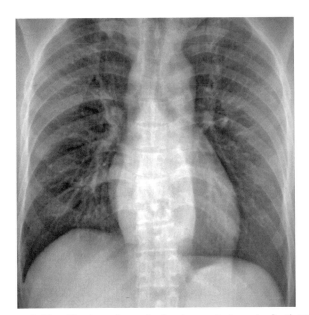

Figure 9.39: Chest radiograph [postero-anterior view] showing fusiform 'bird nest' paravertebral abscess in lower thoracic region with involvement of D9 and D10 vertebrae and intervening intervertebral disk space

Figure 9.40: Axial [A] and coronal [B] CECT images showing presence of prevertebral and paravertebral abscess with adjacent bone erosion. Note is made of mild pericardial effusion as well. Following anti-TB treatment, there was near-complete resolution of these findings
CECT = contrast-enhanced computed tomography; TB = tuberculosis

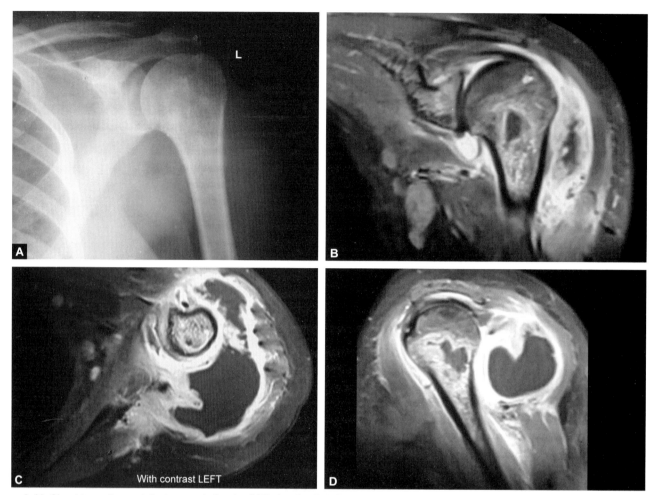

Figure 9.41: Shoulder radiograph [antero-posterior view] [A] showing ill-defined lytic lesion involving left proximal metaphysis with solid periosteal reaction and large soft tissue opacity lateral to it. Joint space is relatively preserved. No definite erosions are seen. Coronal [B], axial [C] and sagittal [D] contrast-enhanced MR images showing intra-osseous and large extra-osseous peripheral rim-enhancing TB abscesses involving proximal humerus, also extending into the gleno-humeral joint space; left axillary lymphadenopathy is also evident
MR = magnetic resonance; TB = tuberculosis

TB which affects diaphysis in children and young adults. On radiographs, the lesions are oval to round, radiolucent, well defined, and show variable amounts of sclerosis. The radiographic features of cystic TB resemble those of eosinophilic granuloma, sarcoidosis, cystic angiomatosis, multiple myeloma, chordoma, fungal infections, and metastases (130). TB involvement of short tubular bones of the hands and feet is termed TB dactylitis and is common in children. Fusiform soft-tissue swelling, bony expansion and periostitis are the most common radiographic findings. As underlying bone is destroyed, a cyst-like cavity forms and the remaining bone appears to be ballooned out. This appearance is termed *spina ventosa* ["wind-filled sail"] (130). A useful feature in distinguishing TB from pyogenic infection in immature skeleton is presence of trans-physeal spread; however, fungal infections can also extend across the physis. Other diseases, such as sarcoidosis, haemoglobinopathies, hyperparathyroidism, and leukaemia may produce changes similar to those of TB dactylitis (130).

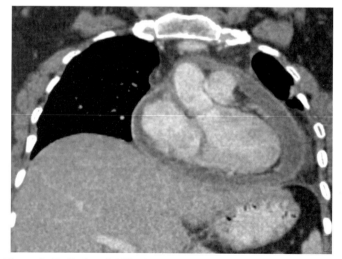

Figure 9.42: Pericardial TB. Coronal CECT image showing pericardial effusion and uniform, regular pericardial thickening
TB = tuberculosis; CECT = contrast-enhanced computed tomography

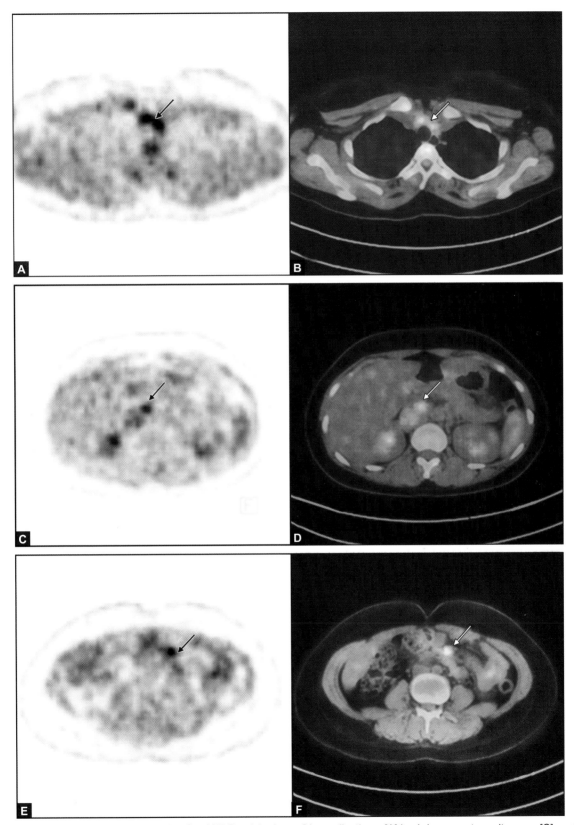

Figure 9.43: PET axial images [A, C, E] showing focal FDG uptake [arrow] in mediastinum [A] in abdomen, retroperitoneum [C], and mesentery [E]. Corresponding PET-CT fusion images aptly localising FDG uptake [arrow] in prevascular space of thorax [B], retroperitoneum [D] and mesentery [F]

PET = positron emission tomography; FDG = fluorodeoxyglucose; PET-CT = positron emission tomography-computed tomography

Kind courtesy: Dr Rakesh Kumar, Department of Nuclear Medicine, All India Institute of Medical Sciences, New Delhi

TB Arthritis

TB of the joints is characteristically a mono-articular disease with knees and hips being most frequently affected [Figure 9.41]. The triad of juxta-articular osteoporosis, peripherally located osseous erosions, and gradual narrowing of the joint space is called the *Phemister triad* and is characteristic of TB arthritis. However, these features can also be observed in rheumatoid arthritis [RA] (130). Relative preservation of the joint space is highly suggestive of TB arthritis; early loss of articular space is more typical of RA . MRI may be helpful in differentiating between RA and TB arthritis (131). Uniform synovial thickening, large size of bone erosions, rim enhancement at site of bone erosion, and extra-articular cystic masses favour TB arthritis (131). The eventual result in tuberculous arthritis is usually fibrous ankylosis of the joint whereas bony ankylosis favours pyogenic arthritis. Moreover, periostitis and osseous proliferation are generally more frequent and extensive in pyogenic arthritis than in tuberculous arthritis (130). Occasionally, wedge-shaped areas of necrosis [kissing sequestra] may be present on both sides of the affected joint. Necrosed cartilage and fibrinous material form rice bodies in synovial joints, tendon sheaths and bursae.

UNCOMMON BODY SITES

TB of the breast is extremely rare and affects young, multiparous, lactating women. Mass with or without ulceration is the usual presentation (132). Imaging findings are nonspecific and include abscesses, sinus tracts, cystic lesions and parenchymal asymmetry with enhancement.

Heart can also be rarely involved and pericardial involvement may be seen concomitant with mediastinal and pulmonary TB and is a cause of calcific pericarditis [Figure 9.42]. Myocardial involvement is even rarer and detected on post-mortem studies.

POSITRON EMISSION TOMOGRAPHY-COMPUTED TOMOGRAPHY

FDG-PET holds particular promise for monitoring response to therapy in cases of unsettled treatment duration such as multidrug-resistant TB or in EPTB and when other parameters are equivocal (133,134). It can appear as focal increase in FDG uptake in the various lymph nodes [Figure 9.43] although not specific. In a series of 30 patients with TB of the spine for instance, the percent change in SUVmax discriminated residual infection from successful treatment (135). But published evidence on routine use of PET-CT in distinguishing latent versus active disease is limited and also carries the risk of high radiation exposure.

REFERENCES

1. World Health Organization. Global tuberculosis report 2015. WHO/HTM/TB/2015.22. Geneva: World Health Organization; 2015.
2. Korzeniewska-Kosela M, Krysl J, Müller N, Black W, Allen E, FitzGerald JM. Tuberculosis in young adults and the elderly. A prospective comparison study. Chest 1994;106:28-32.
3. Hadlock FP, Park SK, Awe RJ, Rivera M. Unusual radiographic findings in adult pulmonary tuberculosis. AJR Am J Roentgenol 1980;134:1015-8.
4. Leung AN, Brauner MW, Gamsu G, Mlika-Cabanne N, Ben Romdhane H, Carette MF, et al. Pulmonary tuberculosis: comparison of CT findings in HIV-seropositive and HIV-seronegative patients. Radiology 1996;198:687-91.
5. Greenberg SD, Frager D, Suster B, Walker S, Stavropoulos C, Rothpearl A. Active pulmonary tuberculosis in patients with AIDS: spectrum of radiographic findings [including a normal appearance]. Radiology 1994;193:115-9.
6. Long R, Maycher B, Scalcini M, Manfreda J. The chest roentgenogram in pulmonary tuberculosis patients seropositive for human immunodeficiency virus type 1. Chest 1991;99:123-7.
7. Kim WS, Moon WK, Kim IO, Lee HJ, Im JG, Yeon KM, et al. Pulmonary tuberculosis in children: evaluation with CT. Am J Roentgenol 1997;168:1005-9.
8. Jones BE, Ryu R, Yang Z, Cave MD, Pogoda JM, Otaya M, et al. Chest radiographic findings in patients with tuberculosis with recent or remote infection. Am J Respir Crit Care Med 1997;156:1270-3.
9. Geng E, Kreiswirth B, Burzynski J, Schluger NW. Clinical and radiographic correlates of primary and reactivation tuberculosis: a molecular epidemiology study. JAMA 2005;293:2740-5.
10. Lee KS, Song KS, Lim TH, Kim PN, Kim IY, Lee BH. Adult-onset pulmonary tuberculosis: findings on chest radiographs and CT scans. Am J Roentgenol 1993;160:753-8.
11. Pineda PR, Leung A, Müller NL, Allen EA, Black WA, FitzGerald JM. Intrathoracic paediatric tuberculosis: a report of 202 cases. Tuber Lung Dis 1993;74:261-6.
12. Weber AL, Bird KT, Janower ML. Primary tuberculosis in childhood with particular emphasis on changes affecting the tracheobronchial tree. Am J Roentgenol Radium Ther Nucl Med 1968;103:123-32.
13. Leung AN, Müller NL, Pineda PR, FitzGerald JM. Primary tuberculosis in childhood: radiographic manifestations. Radiology 1992;182:87-91.
14. Stead WW, Kerby GR, Schlueter DP, Jordahl CW. The clinical spectrum of primary tuberculosis in adults. Confusion with reinfection in the pathogenesis of chronic tuberculosis. Ann Intern Med 1968;68:731-45.
15. Choyke PL, Sostman HD, Curtis AM, Ravin CE, Chen JT, Godwin JD, et al. Adult-onset pulmonary tuberculosis. Radiology 1983;148:357-62.
16. Andronikou S, Joseph E, Lucas S, Brachmeyer S, Du Toit G, Zar H, et al. CT scanning for the detection of tuberculous mediastinal and hilar lymphadenopathy in children. Pediatr Radiol 2004;34:232-6.
17. Lamont AC, Cremin BJ, Pelteret RM. Radiological patterns of pulmonary tuberculosis in the paediatric age group. Paediatr Radiol 1986;16:2-7.
18. Lee JY, Lee KS, Jung KJ, Han J, Kwon OJ, Kim J, et al. Pulmonary tuberculosis: CT and pathologic correlation. J Comput Assist Tomogr 2000;24:691-8.
19. Luo MY, Liu L, Lai LS, Dong YX, Liang WW, Qin J. Deepgoing study on intrathoracic tuberculous lymphadenitis in adults using multidetector CT. Chin Med J [Engl] 2010;123:1283-8.
20. Im JG, Song KS, Kang HS, Park JH, Yeon KM, Han MC, et al. Mediastinal tuberculous lymphadenitis: CT manifestations. Radiology 1987;164:115-9.
21. Hartman TE, Primack SL, Müller NL, Staples CA. Diagnosis of thoracic complications in AIDS: accuracy of CT. Am J Roentgenol 1994;162:547-53.
22. Scatarige JC, Fishman EK, Kuhajda FP, Taylor GA, Siegelman SS. Low attenuation nodal metastases in testicular carcinoma. J Comput Assist Tomogr 1983;7:682-7.

23. Pombo F, Rodríguez E, Mato J, Pérez-Fontán J, Rivera E, Valvuena L. Patterns of contrast enhancement of tuberculous lymph nodes demonstrated by computed tomography. Clin Radiol 1992;46:13-7.

24. Leung AN. Pulmonary tuberculosis: the essentials. Radiology 1999;210:307-22.

25. Moon WK, Im JG, Yeon KM, Han MC. Mediastinal tuberculous lymphadenitis: CT findings of active and inactive disease. Am J Roentgenol 1998;170:715-8.

26. Mukund A, Khurana R, Bhalla AS, Gupta AK, Kabra SK. CT patterns of nodal disease in pediatric chest tuberculosis. World J Radiol 2011;3:17-23.

27. Bosch-Marcet J, Serres-Créixams X, Borrás-Pérez V, Coll-Sibina MT, Guitet-Juliá M, Coll-Rosell E. Value of sonography for follow-up of mediastinal lymphadenopathy in children with tuberculosis. J Clin Ultrasound 2007;35:118-24.

28. Moon WK, Im JG, Yu IK, Lee SK, Yeon KM, Han MC. Mediastinal tuberculous lymphadenitis: MR imaging appearance with clinicopathologic correlation. Am J Roentgenol 1996;166:21-5.

29. Procop GW, Tazelaar HD. Tuberculosis and other mycobacterial infections of the lung. In: Churg AM, Myers JL, Tazelaar HD, Wright JL, editors. Thurlbeck's pathology of the lung. Third edition. New York: Thieme Medical; 2005.p.219-48.

30. McAdams HP, Erasmus J, Winter JA. Radiologic manifestations of pulmonary tuberculosis. Radiol Clin North Am 1995;33:655-78.

31. Woodring JH, Vandiviere HM, Fried AM, Dillon ML, Williams TD, Melvin IG. Update: the radiographic features of pulmonary tuberculosis. Am J Roentgenol 1986;146:497-506.

32. Mukhopadhyaya S, Gupta AK, Seith A. Imaging of tuberculosis in children. In: Seth V, Kabra SK, editors. Essentials of tuberculosis in children, Third edition. New Delhi: Jaypee Brothers Medical Publishers; 2006.p.375-404.

33. Fraser RG, Paré JA, Fraser RS, Genereux GP. Diagnosis of diseases of the chest. Vol.II. Third editon. Philadelphia: W.B.Saunders and Company; 1989.p.882-933.

34. Sharma SK, Mohan A, Sharma A, Mitra DK. Miliary tuberculosis: new insights into an old disease. Lancet Infect Dis 2005;5:415-30.

35. Kwong JS, Carignan S, Kang E, Müller NL, FitzGerald JM. Miliary tuberculosis: diagnostic accuracy of chest radiography. Chest 1996;110:339-42.

36. Gelb AF, Leffler C, Brewin A, Mascatello V, Lyons HA. Miliary tuberculosis. Am Rev Respir Dis 1973;108:1327-33.

37. Berger HW, Samortin TG. Miliary tuberculosis: diagnostic methods with emphasis on the chest roentgenogram. Chest 1970;58:586-9.

38. Reed MH, Pagtakhan RD, Zylak CJ, Berg TJ. Radiologic features of miliary tuberculosis in children and adults. J Can Assoc Radiol 1977;28:175-81.

39. Piqueras AR, Marruecos L, Artigas A, Rodriguez C. Miliary tuberculosis and adult respiratory distress syndrome. Intensive Care Med 1987;13:175-82.

40. Sharma SK, Mohan A, Banga A, Saha PK, Guntupalli KK. Predictors of development and outcome in patients with acute respiratory distress syndrome due to tuberculosis. Int J Tuberc Lung Dis 2006;10:429-35.

41. Pipavath SN, Sharma SK, Sinha S, Mukhopadhyay S, Gulati MS. High resolution CT [HRCT] in miliary tuberculosis [MTB] of the lung: Correlation with pulmonary function tests and gas exchange parameters in north Indian patients. Indian J Med Res 2007;126:193-8.

42. Wallgren A. The time-table of tuberculosis. Tubercle 1948;29:245-51.

43. Matthews JI, Matarese SL, Carpenter JL. Endobronchial tuberculosis simulating lung cancer. Chest 1984;86:642-4.

44. Moon WK, Im JG, Yeon KM, Han MC. Tuberculosis of the central airways: CT findings of active and fibrotic disease. Am J Roentgenol 1997;169:649-53.

45. Palmer PE. Pulmonary tuberculosis- usual and unusual radiographic presentations. Semin Roentgenol 1979;14:204-43.

46. Im JG, Itoh H, Shim YS, Lee JH, Ahn J, Han MC, et al. Pulmonary tuberculosis: CT findings—early active disease and sequential change with antituberculous therapy. Radiology 1993;186:653-60.

47. Krysl J, Korzeniewska-Kosela M, Müller NL, FitzGerald JM. Radiologic features of pulmonary tuberculosis: an assessment of 188 cases. Can Assoc Radiol J 1994;45:101-7.

48. Miller WT, Miller WT Jr. Tuberculosis in the normal host: radiological findings. Semin Roentgenol 1993;28:109-18.

49. Poppius H, Thomander K. Segmental distribution of cavities; a radiologic study of 500 consecutive cases of cavernous pulmonary tuberculosis. Ann Med Intern Fenn 1957;46:113-9.

50. Burrill J, Williams CJ, Bain G, Conder G, Hine AL, Misra RR. Tuberculosis: a radiologic review. Radiographics 2007;27:1255-73.

51. Im JG, Itoh H, Han MC. CT of pulmonary tuberculosis. Semin Ultrasound CT MR 1995;16:420-34.

52. Hatipoğlu ON, Osma E, Manisali M, Uçan ES, Balci P, Akkoçlu A, et al. High-resolution computed tomographic findings in pulmonary tuberculosis. Thorax 1996;51:397-402.

53. Rossi SE, Franquet T, Volpacchio M, Giménez A, Aguilar G. Tree-in-bud pattern at thin- section CT of the lungs: radiologic-pathologic overview. Radiographics 2005;25:789-801.

54. Itoh H, Tokunaga S, Asamoto H, Furuta M, Funamoto Y, Kitaichi M, et al. Radiologic- pathologic correlation of small lung nodules with special reference to peribronchial nodules. Am J Roentgenol 1978;130:223-31.

55. Soussan M, Brillet PY, Mekinian A, Khafagy A, Nicolas P, Vessieres A, et al. Patterns of pulmonary tuberculosis on FDG-PET-CT. Eur J Radiol 2012;81:2872-6.

56. Hoheisel G, Chan BK, Chan CH, Chan KS, Teschler H, Costabel U. Endobronchial tuberculosis: diagnostic features and therapeutic outcome. Respir Med 1994;88:593-7.

57. Smith LS, Schillaci RF, Sarlin RF. Endobronchial tuberculosis. Serial fiberoptic bronchoscopy and natural history. Chest 1987;91:644-7.

58. Lee KS, Kim YH, Kim WS, Hwang SH, Kim PN, Lee BH. Endobronchial tuberculosis: CT features. J Comput Assist Tomogr 1991;15:424-8.

59. Epstein DM, Kline LR, Albelda SM, Miller WT. Tuberculous pleural effusions. Chest 1987;91:106-9.

60. Schmitt WG, Hübener KH, Rücker HC. Pleural calcification with persistent effusion. Radiology 1983;149:633-8.

61. Lee KS, Hwang JW, Chung MP, Kim H, Kwon OJ. Utility of CT in the evaluation of pulmonary tuberculosis in patients without AIDS. Chest 1996;110:977-84.

62. Martinez V, Castilla-Lievre MA, Guillet-Caruba C, Grenier G, Fior R, Desarnaud S, et al. ^{18}F-FDG PET-CT in tuberculosis: an early non-invasive marker of therapeutic response. Int J Tuberc Lung Dis 2012;16:1180-5.

63. Fraser RS. Pulmonary aspergillosis: pathologic and pathogenetic features. Pathol Annu 1993;28:231-77.

64. Conces DJ Jr, Tarver RD, Vix VA. Broncholithiasis: CT features in 15 patients. Am J Roentgenol 1991;157:249-53.

65. Vix VA. Radiographic manifestations of broncholithiasis. Radiology 1978;128:295-9.

66. Central Tuberculosis Division, Directorate General of Health Services. TB India 2016. Revised National Tuberculosis Control Programme. Annual Report. New Delhi: Central Tuberculosis Division, Directorate General of Health Services, Government of India; 2016.

67. Yeom JA, Jeong YJ, Jeon D, Kim KI, Kim CW, Park HK, et al. Imaging findings of primary multidrug-resistant tuberculosis: a comparison with findings of drug-sensitive tuberculosis. J Comput Assist Tomogr 2009;33:956-60.

68. Kim HC, Goo JM, Lee HJ, Park SH, Park CM, Kim TJ, et al. Multidrug-resistant tuberculosis versus drug-sensitive tuberculosis in human immunodeficiency virus-negative patients: computed tomography features. J Comput Assist Tomogr 2004;28:366-71.

69. Chung MJ, Lee KS, Koh WJ, Kim TS, Kang EY, Kim SM, et al. Drug-sensitive tuberculosis, multidrug-resistant tuberculosis, and nontuberculous mycobacterial pulmonary disease in non-AIDS adults: comparisons of thin-section CT findings. Eur Radiol 2006;16:1934-41.

70. Fishman JE, Sais GJ, Schwartz DS, Otten J. Radiographic findings and patterns in multidrug-resistant tuberculosis. J Thorac Imaging 1998;13:65-71.

71. Abernathy RS. Tuberculosis in children and its management. Semin Respir Infect 1989;4:232-42.

72. Blumberg HM, Burman WJ, Chaisson RE, Daley CL, Etkind SC, Friedman LN, et al. American Thoracic Society/Centers for Disease Control and Prevention and the Infectious Diseases Society. American Thoracic Society/Centers for Disease Control and Prevention/Infectious Diseases Society of America: treatment of tuberculosis. Am J Respir Crit Care Med 2003;167:603-62.

73. Mehta JB, Dutt A, Harvill L, Mathews KM. Epidemiology of extrapulmonary tuberculosis: a comparative analysis with pre-AIDS era. Chest 1991;99:1134-8.

74. Goodman PC. Tuberculosis and AIDS. Radiol Clin North Am 1995;33:707-17.

75. Pitchenik AE, Fertel D, Bloch AB. Mycobacterial disease: epidemiology, diagnosis, treatment, and prevention. Clin Chest Med 1988;9:425-41.

76. Snider DE Jr, Roper WL. The new tuberculosis. N Engl J Med 1992;326:703-5.

77. Snider DE, Onorato M. Epidemiology. In: Rossman MD, MacGregor RR, editors. Tuberculosis: clinical management and new challenges. New York: McGraw-ill; 1995.p. 3-17.

78. Centers for Disease Control and Prevention. Reported tuberculosis in the United States, 1999. Atlanta: Centers for Disease Control and Prevention; 2000.

79. American Thoracic Society. Diagnostic standards and classification of tuberculosis in adults and children. Am J Respir Crit Care Med 2000;161:1376-95.

80. Raviglione MC, Narain JP, Kochi A. HIV-associated tuberculosis in developing countries: clinical features, diagnosis and treatment. Bull World Health Organ 1992;70:515-25.

81. Antonucci G, Girardi E, Armignacco O, Salmaso S, Ippolito G. Tuberculosis in HIV-infected subjects in Italy: a multicentre study. The Gruppo Italiano di Studio Tubercolosie AIDS. AIDS 1992;6:1007-13.

82. Jones BE, Young SMM, Antoniskis D, Davidson PT, Kramer F, Barnes PF. Relationship of the manifestations of tuberculosis to CD4 cell counts in patients with human immunodeficiency virus infection. Am Rev Respir Dis 1993;148:1292-7.

83. Lado Lado FL, Barrio Gomez E, Carballo Arceo E, Cabarcos Ortiz de Barron A. Clinical presentation of tuberculosis and the degree of immunodeficiency in patients with HIV infection. Scand J Infect Dis 1999;31:387-91.

84. Lee MP, Chan JW, Ng KK, Li PC. Clinical manifestations of tuberculosis in HIV-infected patients. Respirology 2000;5:423-6.

85. Poprawski D, Pitisuttitum P, Tansuphasawadikul S. Clinical presentations and outcomes of TB among HIV-positive patients. Southeast Asian J Trop Med Public Health 2000;31:140-2.

86. Sharma SK, Mohan A, Gupta R, Kumar A, Gupta AK, Singhal VK, et al. Clinical resentation of tuberculosis in patients with AIDS: an Indian experience. Indian J Chest Dis Allied Sci 1997;39:213-20.

87. Kumar P, Sharma N, Sharma NC, Patnaik S. Clinical profile of tuberculosis in patients with HIV Infection/AIDS. Indian J Chest Dis Allied Sci 2002;44:159-63.

88. Yao DC, Sartoris DJ. Musculoskeletal tuberculosis. Radiol Clin North Am 1995;33:679-89.

89. Leder RA, Low VHS. Tuberculosis of the abdomen. Radiol Clin North Am 1995;33:691-705.

90. Davidson P, Horowitz I. Skeletal tuberculosis. Am J Med 1970;48:77-84.

91. Dandapat MC, Mishra BM, Dash SP, Kar PK. Peripheral lymph node tuberculosis: a review of 80 cases. Br J Surg 1990;77:911-2.

92. White MP, Bangash H, Goel K, Jenkins PA. Nontuberculous mycobacterial lymphadenitis. Arch Dis Child 1986;61:368-71.

93. Hopewell PC. A clinical view of tuberculosis. Radiol Clin North Am 1995;33:641-53.

94. Bem C. Human immunodeficiency virus-positive tuberculous lymphadenitis in Central Africa: clinical presentation of 157 cases. Int J Tuberc Lung Dis 1997;1:215-9.

95. Bhansali SK. Abdominal tuberculosis, experiences with 300 cases. Am J Gastroenterol 1977;67:324-37.

96. Balthazar EJ, Gordon R, Hulnick D. Ileocecal tuberculosis: CT and radiologic evaluation. AJR Am J Roentgenol 1990;21:499-503.

97. Akhan O, Pringot J. Imaging of abdominal tuberculosis. Eur Radiol 2002;12:312-23.

98. Sharma MP, Bhatia V. Abdominal tuberculosis. Indian J Med Res 2004;120:354-76.

99. Prakash A. Abdominal tuberculosis. In: Gupta AK, Chowdhury V, Khandelwal N, editors. Diagnostic radiology: gastrointestinal and hepatobiliary imaging. 3rd edition. New Delhi: Jaypee Brothers Medical Publishers Private Limited; 2009.p.112-33.

100. Bargallo N, Nicolau C, Luburich P, et al. Intestinal tuberculosis in AIDS. Gastrointest Radiol 1992;17:115-8.

101. Denton T, Hossain J. A radiological study of abdominal tuberculosis in a Saudi population, with special reference to ultrasound and computed tomography. Clin Radiol 1993;47:409-14.

102. Boudiaf M, Jaff A, Soyer P, Bouchnik Y, Hamzi L, Rymer R. Small-bowel diseases: prospective evaluation of multi–detector row helical CT enteroclysis in 107 consecutive patients. Radiology 2004;233:338-44.

103. Batra A, Gulati MS, Sarma D, Paul SB. Sonographic appearances in abdominal tuberculosis. J Clin Ultrasound 2000;28:233-45.

104. Burril J, Williams CJ, Bain G, Conder G, Hine AL, Misra RR. Tuberculosis: a radiologic review. Radiographics 2007;27:1255-73.

105. Sieck JO, Cowgill R, Larkworthy W. Peritoneal encapsulation and abdominal cocoon: case reports and a review of the literature. Gastroenterology 1983;84:1597-601.

106. Yang ZG, Min PQ, Sone S, He ZY, Liao ZY, Zhou XP, et al. Tuberculosis versus lymphomas in the abdominal lymph nodes: evaluation with contrast-enhanced CT. AJR Am J Roentgenol 1999;172:619-23.

107. De Backer AI, Mortelé KJ, Deeren D, Vanschoubroeck IJ, De Keulenaer BL. Abdominal tuberculous lymphadenopathy: MRI features. Eur Radiol 2005;15:2104-9.

108. Engin G, Acunaş B, Acunaş G, Tunaci M. Imaging of extrapulmonary tuberculosis. Radiographics 2000;20:471-88.

109. Sharma SK, Mohan A. Extrapulmonary tuberculosis. Indian J Med Res 2004;120:316-53.

110. Brennan RE, Pollack HM. Nonvisualized ["phantom"] renal calyx: causes and radiological approach to diagnosis. Urol Radiol 1979;1:17-23.

111. Roylance J, Penry JB, Davies ER, Roberts M. Radiology in the management of urinary tract tuberculosis. Br J Urol 1970;42: 679-87.

112. Wang LJ, Wong YC, Chen CJ, Lim KE. CT features of genitourinary tuberculosis. J Comput Assist Tomogr 1997;21:254-8.

113. Matos MJ, Bacelar MT, Pinto P, Ramos I. Genitourinary tuberculosis. Eur J Radiol 2005;55:181-7.

114. Brooke AM, Monson JP. Addison's disease. Medicine 2005;33: 20-2.

115. Yang ZG, Guo YK, Li Y, Min PQ, Yu JQ, Ma ES. Differentiation between tuberculosis and primary tumors in the adrenal gland: evaluation with contrast-enhanced CT. Eur Radiol 2006;16: 2031-6.

116. Bhalla AS, Gupta AK, Sharma R. Tubercular infection of the urinary tract. In: Khandelwal N, Chowdhury V, Gupta AK, editors. Diagnostic radiology: genitourinary imaging. Third edition. New Delhi: Jaypee Brothers Medical Publishers; 2009.p.120-37.

117. Chavhan GB, Hira P, Rathod K, Zacharia TT, Chawla A, Badhe P, et al. Female genital tuberculosis: hysterosalpingographic appearances. Br J Radiol 2004;77:164-9.

118. Wang JH, Sheu MH, Lee RC. Tuberculosis of the prostate: MR appearance. J Comput Assist Tomogr 1997;21:639-40.

119. Harisinghani MG, McLoud TC, Shepard JA, Ko JP, Shroff MM, Mueller PR. Tuberculosis from head to toe. Radiographics 2000;20:449-70.

120. Whiteman MLH. Neuroimaging of central nervous system tuberculosis in HIV-infected patients. Neuroimaging Clin North Am 1997;7:199-214.

121. Castro CC, Barros NG, Campos ZMS, Cerri GG. CT scans of cranial tuberculosis. Radiol Clin North Am 1995;33:753-69.

122. Jinkins JR, Gupta R, Chang KH, Rodriguez-Carbajal J. MR imaging of central nervous system tuberculosis. Radiol Clin North Am 1995;33:771-86.

123. Sharma A, Goyal M, Mishra NK, Gupta V, Gaikwad SB. MR imaging of tubercular spinal arachnoiditis. Am J Roentgenol 1997;168:807-12.

124. Gee GT, Bazan C III, Jinkins JR. Miliary tuberculosis involving the brain: MR findings. Am J Roentgenol 1992;159: 1075-6.

125. Moon WK, Han MH, Chang KH, Im JG, Kim HJ, Sung KJ, et al. CT and MR imaging of head and neck tuberculosis. Radiographics 1997;17:391-402.

126. Helm CJ, Holland GN. Ocular tuberculosis. Surv Ophthalmol 1993;38:229-56.

127. Davidson P, Horowitz I. Skeletal tuberculosis. Am J Med 1970;48:77-84.

128. Moon MS. Tuberculosis of the spine. Spine [Phila Pa 1976] 1997;22:1791-7.

129. Boxer DI, Pratt C, Hine AL, McNicol M. Radiological features during and following treatment of spinal tuberculosis. Br J Radiol 1992;65:476-9.

130. Yao DC, Sartoris DJ. Musculoskeletal tuberculosis. Radiol Clin North Am 1995;33:679-89.

131. Choi JA, Koh SH, Hong SH, Koh YH, Choi JY, Kang HS. Rheumatoid arthritis and tuberculous arthritis: differentiating MRI features. AJR Am J Roentgenol 2009;193:1347-53.

132. Das CJ, Medhi K. Proton magnetic resonance spectroscopy of tubercular breast abscess: report of a case. J Comput Assist Tomogr 2008;32:599-601.

133. Heysell SK, Thomas TA, Sifri CD, Rehm PK, Houpt ER. 18-Fluorodeoxyglucose positron emission tomography for tuberculosis diagnosis and management: a case series. BMC Pulm Med 2013;13:14.

134. Gandhi NR, Nunn P, Dheda K, Schaaf HS, Zignol M, van Soolingen D, Jensen P, Bayona J. Multidrug-resistant and extensively drug-resistant tuberculosis: a threat to global control of tuberculosis. Lancet 2010;13:1830-43.

135. Kim SJ, Kim IJ, Suh KT, Kim YK, Lee JS. Prediction of residual disease of spine infection using F-18 FDG PET/CT. Spine [Phila Pa 1976] 2009;34:2424-30.

10

Pulmonary Tuberculosis

VK Vijayan, Sajal De

INTRODUCTION

Pulmonary tuberculosis [TB] is a chronic infectious disease of lung caused by *Mycobacterium tuberculosis* [*Mtb*] (1). Nontuberculous mycobacteria [NTM] exist in environment as saphrophyte and some can cause human disease especially in immunocompromised individuals (2). Pulmonary TB patients who have cavitary lesions in their lung are an important source of infection. These patients are usually sputum smear-positive. Coughing, sneezing or talking produces tiny infectious droplets. One bout of cough produces 3000 droplet nuclei and these can remain suspended in the air for a long period of time. Effective ventilation can dilute these infectious nuclei. *Mtb* can survive in the dark for several hours. Direct exposure to sunlight quickly kills these bacilli. Of the several factors, determining an individual's risk of exposure, two factors are important. These include the concentration of droplet nuclei in contaminated air and the length of time that air is breathed. The risk of transmission of infection from a person with sputum smear-negative pulmonary TB and miliary TB is low and with extra-pulmonary TB [EPTB] is even lower.

NATURAL HISTORY OF TUBERCULOSIS

The cardinal event in the pathogenesis of TB, whether inapparent or overt is the implantation of *Mtb* in the tissues. Lung is the most frequent portal of entry [Figures 10.1A and 10.1B]. The organism enters the lung from the inhalation of air-borne droplets, which have been coughed out by

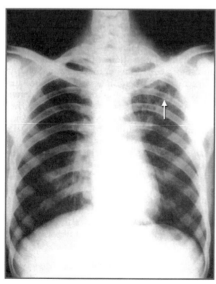

Figure 10.1A: Chest radiograph [postero-anterior view] showing a cavity in left upper zone [arrow]. Sputum culture was positive for *Mycobacterium tuberculosis*

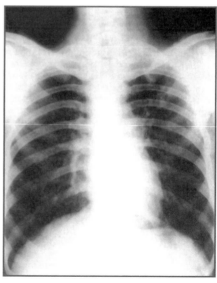

Figure 10.1B: Chest radiograph [postero-anterior view] of the same patient at 24 months of follow-up. The patient had received six months short-course chemotherapy. The left upper zone cavity has disappeared

'open' [sputum-positive] pulmonary TB patients who have received no treatment, or have not been treated fully. The initial contact with the organism results in few or no clinical symptoms or signs. The tubercle bacillus sets up a localised infection in the periphery of the lung. Four-to-six weeks later, tuberculin hypersensitivity along with mild fever and malaise develops. In the majority of patients, the process is contained by local and systemic defenses. Rupture of the sub-pleural primary pulmonary focus into the pleural cavity may result in the development of TB pleurisy with effusion.

Less commonly, tubercle bacilli may be ingested and lodged in the tonsil or in the wall of the intestine. This form of TB occurs following the ingestion of contaminated milk or milk products. Rarely, TB can occur as a result of direct implantation of the organisms into the skin through cuts and abrasions. This form of TB is a health hazard faced by health care workers and laboratory staff who handle materials infected with *Mtb*. These lesions were termed "prosector's warts" (2). Unfortunately, Laennec, the inventor of the stethoscope, acquired TB in this fashion which eventually led to his death (2).

Primary Tuberculosis

From the implantation site, the organisms disseminate via the lymphatics to the regional lymph nodes. The lesion at the primary site of involvement, draining lymphatics and the inflamed regional lymph node constitutes the *primary complex*. When the primary site of implantation is in the lung, it is called *Ghon's focus*. The draining lymphatics and the involved lymph nodes together with Ghon's focus constitute the *primary complex [Ghon complex]*. In children, the lymph node component may be much larger than the Ghon's focus.

Having secured entry, tubercle bacilli then disseminate *via* the haematogenous route to other parts of the lung and many organs of the body. Thus, TB widely disseminated during primary infection. Most of these metastatic foci heal at their own. However, some of these metastatic foci may remain dormant and may reactivate at a later date when the host resistance decreases. The subsequent course of the events varies considerably. In most of the patients, the primary complex resolves without becoming clinically apparent. This occurs when the immune status of the host is good, and healing occurs by fibrosis and calcification. In a minority of patients, progressive primary TB due to the extension of the inflammatory process at the site of the primary focus can occur. In the lung, this can present as an area of consolidation [TB pneumonia]. This form of the disease was often encountered in the pre-chemotherapeutic era and was termed "galloping consumption" or "pneumonia alba" [white pneumonia]. This form is encountered in the present era in patients with human immunodeficiency virus [HIV] infection. Caseation necrosis at the Ghon's focus may lead to liquefaction. Expectoration of the liquefied material can leave a cavity with shaggy margins in the pulmonary parenchyma which may be apparent on the chest radiograph.

Mediastinal and tracheobronchial lymphadenopathy may produce compression of the adjacent bronchus. If this obstruction is complete, the lung distal to the site of bronchial obstruction becomes atelectatic [epituberculosis] (3). If the obstruction is incomplete, it may act as a "ball-valve" and results in obstructive emphysema. The inflamed caseous lymph nodes may erode through the walls of the bronchus and result in bronchogenic dissemination. Bronchial mucosal involvement may result in TB bronchitis. In a patient with overwhelming infection, large number of *Mtb* may gain access to the circulation and result in miliary and meningeal TB. In majority of the patients, the initial focus of infection subsides. Cicatrisation, scar formation and often calcification develop. Repeated episodes of extension of infection followed by healing and fibrosis may result in the formation of "onion skin" or "coin lesion" (2).

Post-primary Tuberculosis

Rarely, the primary lesion may progress directly to the post-primary form characterised by extensive caseation necrosis and cavitation. More commonly, the primary lesion remains quiescent, and may remain so for decades or for the remainder of the individual's life time. The precise mechanism[s] underlying this phenomenon has not yet been clarified as yet. However, reactivation or reinfection TB may occur due to old age, malnutrition, malignant disease, HIV infection and acquired immunodeficiency syndrome [AIDS], use of immunosuppressive drugs and intercurrent infections.

While reactivation can occur at any site, post-primary TB classically involves the apical posterior segments of the upper lobes, or, the superior segment of the lower lobes in more than 95% of the cases. Balasubramanian *et al* (4) have critically reviewed the pathway to the apical localisation in TB and proposed the integrated model for the pathogenesis of TB.

Post-primary lesions are different from primary lesions in that, local progression and central caseation necrosis are much more marked in post-primary TB as compared to primary TB. TB cavities are abundant sites for the growth of *Mtb* as the temperature in them is optimal, there is abundance of oxygen and various nutrients derived from the cell wall are readily available. The bacilli in the wall of the cavity gain free access into the sputum and are expectorated. Such patients are said to have "open TB" and are infectious to the community. If these bacilli are aspirated from the cavity to other parts of the lung via the bronchi, many secondary pulmonary lesions develop. Early in the illness, TB cavities are moderately thick walled, usually have a smooth inner surface, lack an air-fluid level and are surrounded by an area of consolidation. Later, in the chronic phase of the disease, the wall may become thin, and the cavities may appear spherical.

SYMPTOMS

Pulmonary TB is a disease of protean manifestations and can mimic many diseases. Previous accounts referred to the development of erythema nodosum, phlyctenular conjunctivitis and fever at the time of tuberculin conversion (2). However, this presentation is uncommonly seen today. The patient may develop symptoms insidiously and some may remain asymptomatic. Usually patients with pulmonary TB present with constitutional and respiratory symptoms (3). Constitutional symptoms include tiredness, headache, weight loss, fever, night sweats and loss of appetite. Fever in TB usually appears in the late afternoon or evening, and is low-grade at the onset and becomes high-grade with the progression of disease. Some patients may remain afebrile. Weight loss may precede the other symptoms. The classic symptoms and signs of TB are observed more frequently among younger group than elderly: fever [62% *versus* 31%], weight loss [76% *versus* 34%], night sweats [48% *versus* 6%], sputum production [76% *versus* 48%], and haemoptysis [40% *versus* 17%] (5). Associated laryngeal TB can result in hoarseness of the voice. Amenorrhoea can occur in severe diseases. The most common respiratory symptom of pulmonary TB is cough which lasts for two or more weeks. Cough may be dry or productive. It is nearly impossible to differentiate cough due to pulmonary TB from cough due to other respiratory diseases including smoking and it is often passed off as a smoker's cough. Sputum may be mucoid, muco-purulent, purulent or blood-tinged and is usually scanty. Haemoptysis, although observed in many diseases, is an important and often the presenting symptom of pulmonary TB. Furthermore, TB is the most common cause of haemoptysis in India. Severity of haemoptysis in pulmonary TB varies from blood-stained sputum to massive haemoptysis. Massive haemoptysis usually results from rupture of a bronchial artery (1). Chest pain may be dull aching in character. Acute chest pain can occur in TB pleurisy or in pneumothorax; with severe pain occurring at the height of inspiration. In diaphragmatic pleurisy, pain is referred to the ipsilateral shoulder when central part of the diaphragm is involved. Occasionally chest pain can occur from fracture of ribs due to violent coughing. Breathlessness results from extensive disease or if complications such as bronchial obstruction, pneumothorax or pleural effusion occur. Localised wheeze can occur due to endobronchial TB or because compression of the bronchus by enlarged lymph nodes.

In addition to classical symptoms of cough and/or fever, paediatric patients may present with loss of body weight [defined as a loss of >5% of the highest weight recorded in the past three months]. Symptoms of pulmonary TB among immunocompromised host produces symptoms of combination of two diseases and symptoms of one disease often mimic the other. Clinical manifestations of TB in HIV-infected patients vary and generally depend upon the severity of immunosuppression. In early stages of HIV disease, clinical presentation of TB tends to simulate that observed in persons without immunodeficiency. Weight loss and fever are the most frequent symptoms seen in patients co-infected with HIV and TB (6). The reader is referred to the chapter *"Tuberculosis and human immunodeficiency virus infection"* [Chapter 35] for further details.

PHYSICAL SIGNS

A thorough general physical examination should be done in all patients with pulmonary TB. Anaemia and cachexia may be observed in severe cases. Tachycardia can occur and is usually proportional to the fever. Digital clubbing occurs rarely in advanced cases and with superadded suppuration. There can be an increase in the respiratory rate. EPTB foci such as cold abscess, enlarged cervical and mesenteric lymph nodes, deformity or localised immobility of the spine, epididymitis, etc., can be discovered on general physical examination. In addition, general physical examination may also reveal phlyctenular conjunctivitis or keratitis. Further, signs of meningeal irritation and focal neurological signs may be apparent in patients with extrapulmonary focus in the nervous system. Associated signs of protein-energy malnutrition such as anasarca, change in hair colour and leuconychia may occur. Adult patients with chronic disease can present with lower body mass index [BMI; kg/m^2].

Respiratory system examination may reveal displacement of the trachea and the heart depending on the underlying pathology. Asymmetrical abnormalities of the chest wall such as retraction, fibrosis or collapse and prominence in pleural effusion, emphysema or pneumothorax may be observed. Undue prominence of the clavicular head of the sternocleidomastoid muscle [*Trail's sign*] on one side may be indicative of apical fibrosis due to TB. Mobility of any part of the chest wall may be restricted on the affected side. A dull percussion note can occur as a result of consolidation, collapse of the lung, or thickened pleura or extensive infiltration of the lung due to TB. A stony dull note can be elicited over a pleural effusion or empyema. Hyperresonance on percussion is encountered in pneumothorax. Cracked-pot sound may be elicited in cases where percussion is practiced over a cavity which communicates with bronchus of moderate size and is most distinct when the mouth is open. It results due to a sudden expulsion of air through a constricted orifice. It has a hissing character, combined with a clinking sound like that produced by shaking coins together. It is a rare finding. Cracked-pot sound is often produced in healthy children when percussion is performed during crying. Myotactic irritability/myoedema can occur due to hyperirritability of malnourished muscles in front of the thorax. A light tap over the sternum produces fibrillary contractions, at some distance off, in the pectoral muscles.

High-pitched [tubular] bronchial breathing can be heard in patients with TB pneumonia. Bronchial breathing can be low-pitched [cavernous] if there is an underlying cavity in the lung or an open pneumothorax. A special type of high-pitched bronchial breathing with an "echo-like" quality [amphoric breathing] is indicative of a large cavity with smooth walls or of a pneumothorax communicating with a bronchus. It resembles the sound produced by blowing across the mouth of a bottle and consists of one or more low-pitched fundamental tones and a number of high-pitched overtones. Vocal fremitus is increased when lung is consolidated or contains a large cavity near the surface. Vocal fremitus is diminished when the corresponding bronchus is obstructed and is absent when there is pleural effusion or thickening. The presence of fine crepitations, especially post-tussive crepitations, is an important sign of TB infiltration. A pleural rub is characteristic of pleurisy.

Hippocratic succussion is the splashing sound which can be heard when a patient who has both air and fluid in the pleural cavity is shaken or moved suddenly. *Post-tussive suction,* a sucking noise resembling that produced by an India-rubber ball that is springing open again, can be heard after a coughing, over a cavity in the lung when its walls are not too rigid. It occurs due to re-entry of air.

DIAGNOSIS

The definitive diagnosis of pulmonary TB [primary and post-primary forms of the disease] involves detection and isolation of *Mtb*. In addition, identification of the mycobacterial species and drug-susceptibility testing may be required for the management.

Haematology

Haematological abnormalities in pulmonary TB include anaemia, leucocytosis, leucopaenia, purpura, leukaemoid reaction and polycythaemia vera. The erythrocyte sedimentation rate [ESR] is often [but not always] raised in TB and is commonly used as a surrogate marker of active TB by clinicians. However, due to wide range of normal value, raised ESR value should not be used as a diagnostic test for TB even among children (7).

Diagnostic Mycobacteriology

The definitive diagnosis of pulmonary TB is made by the isolation and identification of the *Mtb*. All patients presenting with cough and sputum for more than two weeks must have their sputum examined for *Mtb*. In addition, *Mtb* can be isolated from bronchial washings, bronchoalveolar lavage [BAL] fluid, pleural fluid, gastric aspirate, pus, cerebrospinal fluid [CSF], urine, blood, bone marrow biopsy and other tissue biopsy specimens. All diagnostic specimens should be collected before the patient is given anti-TB treatment.

Sputum microscopy is the earliest and quickest procedure for the preliminary diagnosis of pulmonary TB. Patients should be instructed that the material brought out from the lungs after a productive cough, not the nasopharyngeal discharge or saliva. The patient should rinse his/her mouth with water before specimen collection to remove materials that interfere with interpretation. Sputum collection should be done in an isolated, well-ventilated area. Sputum specimen should be collected in a wide-mouth, rigid container with tight-fitting screw tops. If the patient cannot produce sputum, deep coughing may be induced by inhalation of an aerosol of warm hypertonic [3% to 15%] saline or gastric lavage especially in children can be collected. The bacilli can be stained with basic fuchsin dyes [Ziehl-Neelsen or Kinyoun method] or with a fluoro-chrome [auramine-rhodamine] staining. The positive predictive value of a properly performed smear is more than 90% for pulmonary TB. In areas with low prevalence of NTM fluoresceindiacetate [FDA] vital staining of sputum can help in early diagnosis of rifampicin resistance (8).

Tuberculin Skin Test, Interferon-Gamma Release Assays

The reader is referred to the chapter *"Laboratory diagnosis of tuberculosis: Best practices and current policies" [Chapter 8]* for details on these topics.

Imaging

Imaging remains one of the important diagnostic modalities for diagnosing pulmonary TB. Sputum negativity does not exclude pulmonary TB especially when clinical symptoms and radiographic features are suggestive of TB. Standard posterior-anterior view of chest should be obtained in patients who have signs and symptoms suggestive of pulmonary TB. Initial radiological manifestations include parenchymal infiltration with ipsilateral lymph node enlargement. Hilar or mediastinal lymph node enlargement in TB is usually unilateral and this lymph nodal enlargement persists longer than the parenchymal lesions. Calcification of the lymph nodes and the lung lesions could occur several years after infection. In adults, the lesions may be patchy or nodular infiltrates and may occur in any segment. Dense and homogeneous lesions with lobar, segmental or subsegmental distributions are also encountered frequently [Figures 9.5, 9.12, 9.13, 10.1A, 10.1B, 10.2, 10.3A, 10.3B and 10.4]. Cavitation, often multiple, occurs in immunocompetent individuals, but is rare in immunocompromised individuals [Figures 9.16 and 9.17]. The radiographic features of pulmonary TB in HIV-positive patients are frequently atypical, particularly, in the late stage of HIV infection, with non-cavitary disease, lower lobe infiltrates, hilar lymph-adenopathy and pleural effusion. More typical post-primary TB with upper lobe infiltrates and cavitation is seen in the earlier stages of HIV infection.

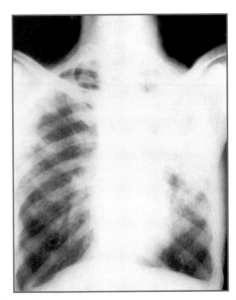

Figure 10.2: Chest radiograph [postero-anterior view] showing extensive parenchymal lesions in the left lung. Few scattered lesions are also seen in the right lung. The sputum smear and culture were positive for *Mycobacterium tuberculosis*

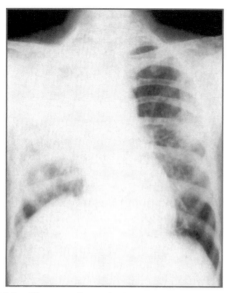

Figure 10.3A: Chest radiograph [postero-anterior view] showing extensive parenchymal infiltrates in the right lung. Few scattered infiltrates are also seen in the left lung. The patient had multidrug-resistant pulmonary tuberculosis

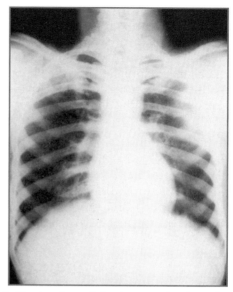

Figure 10.4: Chest radiograph [postero-anterior view] of a patient with sputum smear-negative and culture-positive pulmonary tuberculosis

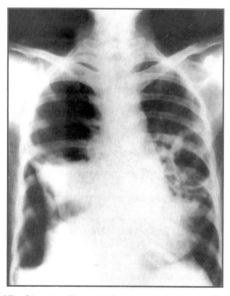

Figure 10.3B: Chest radiograph [postero-anterior view] of the same patient taken a year later showing pneumothorax on the right side and a large cavity in the left lung. The patient did not respond to treatment and died

Computed tomography [CT] is more sensitive than chest radiograph in detecting subtle parenchymal changes and mediastinal involvement. Primary TB typically appears as air-space consolidation with hilar or mediastinal lymphadenitis. Post-primary TB most commonly appears as nodular and linear opacities at the lung apex. High-resolution computed tomography [HRCT] findings of early bronchogenic spread of post-primary TB are centrilobular 2 to 4 mm nodules or branching linear structures and poorly defined nodules on CT scan correspond to caseous materials filling the bronchioles and this is referred as "tree-in-bud"

appearance [Figure 9.18]. Cavitations usually occur at the centrilobular area and may progress to a larger coalescent cavity. The CT scan can document miliary disease even when chest radiograph is normal. CT findings of early miliary dissemination commonly include ground-glass opacification with barely discernible nodules. On HRCT, miliary TB typically shows fine, nodular or reticulonodualr pattern with nodules involving both intralobular interstitium, interlobular septa and subpleural, and perivascular regions. Nodules are evenly distributed throughout the lung. CT more accurately defines the group of lymph nodes involved, their extent and size. The lymph nodes with central low attenuation and peripheral rim enhancement especially with contrast strongly suggest a diagnosis of mycobacterial infection. Complications of TB like post-TB bronchiectasis, aspergilloma etc., are better diagnosed with the help of a CT.

Other radiographic findings in pulmonary TB include atelectasis and fibrotic scarring with retraction of the hila and deviation of the trachea. Unilateral pleural effusion may be the only radiographic abnormality in pleural TB. Rarely, chest radiographs may be normal especially in patients with endobronchial TB and HIV infection. It is important to compare the current chest radiographs with the previous radiographs done months or years earlier so that subtle changes can be detected. Progression of lesions on serial chest radiographs indicates active disease.

Apical-lordotic or oblique view of chest may aid in visualisation of lesions obscured by bony structures or the heart. Contrast-enhanced computed tomography [CECT] and magnetic resonance imaging [MRI] of the chest may be useful in defining intrathoracic lymph nodes, nodules, cavities, cysts, calcification and vascular details in the lung parenchyma. Bronchial stenosis or bronchiectasis can be defined by bronchography and CT of the chest. Fluoroscopy may be useful in the detection of the mobility of thoracic structures.

Bronchoscopy

Microbiologic confirmation of TB among sputum smear-negative patients is important, especially in immuno-compromised hosts. Fibreoptic bronchoscopy is useful to collect various types of specimens [aspirate, brush, lavage fluid and biopsy] for diagnosis of TB among sputum smear-negative patients. An early diagnosis of TB is possible in nearly one-third of sputum smear-negative pulmonary TB, if different bronchoscopic procedures are employed instead of a single procedure alone (9-12). The overall yield of bronchoscopic sample is greater than 90% especially when cultures were included in the analysis (13). Smear examination and mycobacterial culture of post-bronchoscopy sputum had also high diagnostic yield [93%] (14). Lidocaine, the topical anaesthetic agent, that is used during bronchoscopy had inhibitory effect on myco-bacteria and, therefore, should be used carefully. Broncho-scopic examination in pulmonary TB may show normal bronchial mucosa to ulcerative lesions, granulomatous lesions, and ulcerative-granulomatous, tumour-like lesions and residual fibrotic stenosis. Because of high mortality in miliary TB, it is imperative that the diagnosis is confirmed as quickly as possible. In miliary TB, bronchoscopy is diagnostic in 73%-83% of cases (15). The yield of bronchoscopy for diagnosis of pulmonary TB in HIV-infected patients is similar to that in patients without HIV infection and transbronchial biopsy provides incremental diagnostic information (8). In paediatric patients, gastric lavage is superior to BAL for bacteriologic confirmation of pulmonary TB. The overall bacteriologic yield was 34% while gastric lavage alone was positive in 32% of the cases (16).

Bronchoscopy is useful to diagnose endobronchial TB. The reader is referred to the chapter *"Endobronchial tuberculosis" [Chapter 12]* for details. In addition to different endobronchial lesions, black pigmentation of bronchial mucosa with scarring [anthracofibrosis] or without scaring [anthracosis] can be seen (17). Indications for bronchoscopy as a diagnostic tool for pulmonary TB include: [i] patients suspected of having pulmonary TB with negative sputum smears and in whom treatment must be started due to clinical status; [ii] suspicion of cancer; [iii] selected patients with negative cultures; [iv] lack of material being obtained by simpler methods. However, it has been demonstrated that sputum induction is a safe procedure with a high diagnostic yield and high agreement with the results of fibreoptic bronchoscopy for the diagnosis of pulmonary TB in both HIV-seronegative and HIV-seropositive patients. Sputum induction was well tolerated, involved low-cost, and provided the same, if not better, diagnostic yield compared with bronchoscopy in the diagnosis of smear-negative pulmonary TB (18,19). In a decision analysis model to assess the overall utility of BAL in clinically suspected sputum smear-negative pulmonary TB, it has been suggested that, in a region of high TB prevalence, empirical treatment is the best course of action (12).

Point-of-Care Diagnostic Tests

Numbers of novel techniques are currently available as point-of-care diagnostic tests for TB. These tests are simple enough to be performed without the help of a specialized laboratory and the results are immediately available. These tests—will be useful as adjunctive diagnostic tests in difficult-to-diagnose TB especially persons infected with HIV and children, who are often smear-negative and also most adversely affected by delays in TB diagnosis. The reader is referred to the chapter *"Laboratory diagnosis of tuberculosis: Best practices and current policies" [Chapter 8]* for details.

Serological Tests

Several commercial serological tests using different antigen and antibody are available for diagnosis of TB. However, critical review of published evidence suggests that these tests are inaccurate, imprecise and lack of reproducibility. The use of serological tests in the diagnosis of TB has been discouraged by the World Health Organization [WHO], and banned by the Government of India (20).

Nucleic Acid Amplification Tests and Other Molecular Methods

The reader is referred to the chapter *"Laboratory diagnosis of tuberculosis: Best practices and current policies" [Chapter 8]* for details.

Breath Test

Detection of volatile organic compounds [electronic nose] and measurement of urease activity of exhaled air may be promising test to diagnose active pulmonary TB and currently they are under field evaluation (21,22).

DIFFERENTIAL DIAGNOSIS

TB can practically involve all organs of the body and can simulate most of the diseases. Diseases which are to be differentiated from pulmonary TB are listed in Table 10.1. However, by no means, this list is exhaustive.

Table 10.1: Differential diagnosis of pulmonary TB
Infections
Bacterial pneumonia
Lung abscess
Fungal and miscellaneous bacterial infections
Bronchogenic carcinoma
Bronchiectasis
Bronchial asthma
Sarcoidosis
Pneumoconiosis
Paragonimiasis
Congenital diseases
Other causes
Hyperthyroidism, diabetes mellitus
TB = tuberculosis

Bacterial Pneumonia

Bacterial pneumonia, especially occurring in the upper part of the lung, may mimic TB. In acute pneumonia, symptoms occur suddenly and a raised white blood cell count may point to the diagnosis. If sputum is negative for *Mtb*, antibiotics which have no effect on *Mtb* can be administered for seven-to-ten days. The patient may be re-evaluated after a course of antibiotics with a chest radiograph, which may show clearance of the lesions in acute pneumonia. However, it should be noted that shadows may look smaller after the antibiotic course if there is collapse of the part of the lung or pneumonia due to obstruction of a bronchus. Pneumonia due to *Pneumocystis jiroveci* is common in patients with AIDS. If the sputum examination is non-contributory, BAL fluid examination for *Mtb* and *Pneumocystis jiroveci* is indicated (23).

Lung Abscess

Patients with lung abscess often produce foul-smelling purulent sputum. Clubbing of fingers is a prominent feature in these patients. Peripheral blood examination reveals neutrophilic leucocytosis. Ziehl-Neelsen staining of sputum is negative for *Mtb*.

Fungal and Miscellaneous Bacterial Infections

The important fungal diseases of the lung that may mimic pulmonary TB include aspergillosis, blastomycosis, coccidioidomycosis, cryptococcosis, and histoplasmosis. Other miscellaneous bacterial infections can also simulate pulmonary TB and these include nocardiosis and actinomycosis. Nocardia are common bacterial inhabitants of soil. Examination of sputum or pus reveals crooked, branching, beaded, Gram-positive filaments. Most nocardia are weakly acid-fast. In TB endemic areas, fragments of nocardia can be mistaken as mycobcateria (24). Actinomycosis is an indolent, slowly progressive bacterial infection caused by a variety of Gram-positive, non-spore forming anaerobic or microaerophilic rods. The most characteristic feature of actinomycosis is the demonstration of "sulphur granules" in sputum, pus or tissue specimens. These are usually yellow and consist of aggregated microorganisms. Aspergillus is responsible for four types of pulmonary manifestations, viz: allergic broncho-pulmonary aspergillosis [ABPA], aspergilloma, chronic necrotising pulmonary aspergillosis and invasive aspergillosis. ABPA is characterised by asthma-like symptoms, eosinophilia, fleeting pulmonary infiltrates, a positive immediate skin test response to aspergillin, elevated serum IgE and anti-aspergillus IgG antibodies. Aspergilloma occurs in patients with pre-existing TB or other cavities and these patients can have high serum IgG antibody titres of aspergillus. Invasive aspergillosis usually occurs in immunocompromised patients. Blastomycosis can be diagnosed by demonstration of yeast-like organisms with a highly refractile cell wall and multiple nuclei in sputum samples. Patients with coccidioidomycosis can be diagnosed by showing spherules in the sputum stained with Gomori's or Papanicolaou's stains. Cryptococcosis can be identified by staining the specimens with India ink and demonstration of doubly refractile cell wall, the presence of budding and the clean capsule. Viable organisms in macrophages can be seen in histoplasmosis. Candidiasis can occur in the pulmonary TB patients with immunodeficiency.

Bronchogenic Carcinoma

A solid round tumour in the chest radiography may pose difficulty in distinguishing from a well-circumscribed TB lesion. Both bronchogenic carcinoma and pulmonary TB cause loss of weight, cough, blood-streaked sputum and fever. Bronchogenic carcinoma may also cavitate. Bronchogenic carcinoma can produce post-obstructive pneumonitis and lung abscess. The patient with bronchogenic carcinoma is usually a chronic smoker and sputum will be negative for *Mtb*. Confirmation of diagnosis requires bronchoscopic biopsy in these patients.

Bronchiectasis

Patients with bronchiectasis have long history of purulent sputum production. Clubbing of fingers is a prominent sign and coarse bubbling crepitations can be heard on auscultation. Sputum examination is negative for *Mtb*. The middle and lower lobes [or lingula on the left side] are commonly involved in bronchiectasis. The HRCT scan of the chest will confirm the diagnosis.

Bronchial Asthma

Bronchial asthma patients often present with complaints of wheezing. They often give history of allergy to inhalants or ingestants. However, localised wheeze can occur in TB if a bronchus is obstructed by an enlarged lymph node or if there is TB bronchitis. Bronchial asthma can be diagnosed by demonstrating obstructive lung function and reversibility after inhalation of bronchodilator.

Sarcoidosis

Sarcoidosis usually presents with bilateral hilar lymphadeno-pathy and pulmonary infiltration. It can also present with pulmonary infiltrates or nodular lesions without mediastinal lymphadenopathy. In these situations, it is difficult to differentiate these lesions from pulmonary TB, especially miliary TB. These patients have negative tuberculin skin test [TST] and the sputum is negative for *Mtb* (25). Almost every organ of the body can be involved in sarcoidosis and the tissue biopsy reveals non-caseating epithelioid cell granulomas.

Pneumoconiosis

Occupational exposure to silicon dioxide, asbestos, coal dust, beryllium, ferrous oxide etc., and hypersensitivity reactions to organic inhalants can cause pulmonary infiltration that may mimic pulmonary TB. Conglomerate masses and even cavitation can occur in silicosis. Sometimes TB develops in a patient with silicosis [silico-tuberculosis]. Coal miners suffering from rheumatoid arthritis can develop round shadows in the lung resembling TB. Some patients with pneumoconiosis develop progressive massive fibrosis. A carefully elicited occupational history and absence of *Mtb* in the sputum help in the diagnosis.

Paragonimiasis

Paragonimiasis is a food-borne parasitic infection caused by the lung fluke, most commonly, *Paragonimus westermani*. Humans are infected by ingestion of metacercariae present in undercooked crustaceans, contaminated water, among others. This disease is commonly seen in North-East region of India, South and South-East Asia, the Pacific Islands and West Africa. Initially, patients have low-grade fever and dry cough. Subsequently, viscous brown expectoration with rusty smell or frank haemoptysis may be present. Clinical and radiographic presentation of paragonimiasis is often indistinguishable from pulmonary TB especially in regions where TB is endemic. Presence of eggs in the sputum and peripheral blood eosinophilia should raise the suspicion of paragonimiasis (26).

Cardiovascular Diseases

Haemoptysis can occur in patients with mitral stenosis. In addition, hoarseness of voice occurs in mitral stenosis when enlarged left atrium compresses the left recurrent laryngeal nerve [Ortner's syndrome] and this may be mistaken for hoarseness due to TB. Radiographic abnormalities seen in haemosiderosis due to long-standing mitral stenosis can be confused with miliary TB. Haemoptysis can also occur in patients with primary or secondary pulmonary arterial hypertension and in severe pulmonic stenosis. Careful examination of the heart and appropriate investigations [electrocardiogram and echocardiogram] will help in the differential diagnosis.

Congenital Abnormalities

Dermoid cysts, arteriovenous fistulae and hamartomas may require differentiation from pulmonary TB. Sequestration of the lung may produce difficulty in diagnosis, if associated with bronchiectasis or purulent sputum and fever. Bronchoscopy, aortography and CT scan facilitate the diagnosis.

Other Diseases

Hyperthyroidism and diabetes mellitus can have symptoms such as loss of weight, easy fatigability and malaise which can be mistaken for the constitutional symptoms associated with TB. Appropriate investigations will confirm the diagnosis.

PRACTICAL APPROACH TO THE DIAGNOSIS OF ACTIVE PULMONARY TUBERCULOSIS

Even in a country like India where TB is highly endemic, diagnosis of active pulmonary TB can be a diagnostic dilemma. The following criteria would indicate active pulmonary TB: [i] clinical signs of infection and features of TB toxaemia [fever with evening rise, night sweats, malaise, weight loss etc.]; [ii] progressive radiographic changes; [iii] microbiological, molecular, histopathological, cytopathological evidence of TB; and [iv] response to therapeutic trial with anti-TB treatment. Of these, microbiological, molecular evidence is conclusive and the remaining are suggestive.

TREATMENT

The reader is referred to the chapter *"Treatment of tuberculosis"* *[Chapter 44]* for details.

REFERENCES

1. Kasaeva T, Baddeley A, Floyd K, Jaramillo E, Lienhardt C, Nishikori N, et al. Priorities for global political momentum to end TB: a critical point in time. BMJ Glob Health 2018;3:e000830.
2. Grange JM. Mycobacteria and human disease. London: Arnold; 1996.
3. Miller FJW. Tuberculosis in children. Edinburgh: Churchill Livingstone; 1982.
4. Balasubramanian V, Wiegeshaus EH, Taylor BT, Smith DW. Pathogenesis of tuberculosis: pathway to apical localisation. Tuber Lung Dis 1994;75:168-78.
5. Alvarez S, Shell C, Berk SL. Pulmonary tuberculosis in elderly men. Am J Med 1987;82:602-6.
6. Liberato IR, de Albuquerque Mde F, Campelo AR, de Melo HR. Characteristics of pulmonary tuberculosis in HIV-seropositive and seronegative patients in a Northeastern region of Brazil. Rev Soc Bras Med Trop 2004;37:46-50.
7. Al-Marri MR, Kirkpatrick MB. Erythrocyte sedimentation rate in childhood tuberculosis: is it still worthwhile? Int J Tuberc Lung Dis 2000;4:237-9.
8. Van Deun A, Maug AK, Hossain A, Gumusboga M, de Jong BC. Fluorescein diacetate vital staining allows earlier diagnosis of rifampicin-resistant tuberculosis. Int J Tuberc Lung Dis 2012;16:1174-9.
9. ennedy DJ, Lewis WP Barnes PF. Yield of bronchoscopy for the diagnosis of tuberculosis in patients with human immunodeficiency virus infection. Chest 1992;102:1040-4.
10. Vijayan VK, Paramasivan CN, Sankaran K. Comparison of bronchoalveolar lavage fluid with sputum culture in the diagnosis of sputum smear negative pulmonary tuberculosis. Indian J Tuberc 1996;43:179-82.
11. Chawla R, Pant K, Jaggi OP, Chandrashekhar S, Thukral SS. Fibreoptic bronchoscopy in smear negative pulmonary tuberculosis. Eur Respir J 1988;1:804-6.
12. Mohan A, Pande JN, Sharma SK, Rattan A, Guleria R, Khilnani GC. Bronchoalveolar lavage in pulmonary tuberculosis: a decision analysis approach. QJM 1995;88:269-76.
13. Baughman RP, Dohn MN, Loudon RG, Frame PT. Bronchoscopy with bronchoalveolar lavage in tuberculosis and fungal infections. Chest 1991;99:92-7.
14. de Gracia J, Curull V, Vidal R, Riba A, Orriols R, Martin N, et al. Diagnostic value of bronchoalveolar lavage in suspected pulmonary tuberculosis. Chest 1988;93:329-32.
15. Pant K, Chawla R, Mann PS, Jaggi OP. Fibrebronchoscopy in smear-negative miliary tuberculosis. Chest 1989;95:1151-2.
16. Somu N, Swaminathan S, Paramasivan CN, Vijayasekaran D, Chandrabhooshanam A, Vijayan VK, et al. Value of broncho-alveolar lavage and gastric lavage in the diagnosis of pulmonary tuberculosis in children. Tuber Lung Dis 1995;76:295-9.

17. De S. Effect of antitubercular treatment on tumorous endobronchial tuberculosis. J Bronchology Interv Pulmonol 2011; 18:171-5.

18. Conde MB, Soares SL, Mello FC, Rezende VM, Almeida LL, Reingold AL, et al. Comparison of sputum induction with fiberoptic bronchoscopy in the diagnosis of tuberculosis: experience at an acquired immune deficiency syndrome reference center in Rio de Janeiro, Brazil. Am J Respir Crit Care Med 2000;162:2238-40.

19. Anderson C, Inhaber N, Menzies D. Comparison of sputum induction with fiberoptic bronchoscopy in the diagnosis of tuberculosis. Am J Respir Crit Care Med 1995;152:1570-4.

20. World Health Organization. Commercial serodiagnostic tests for diagnosis of tuberculosis. Policy Statement. WHO/HTM/TB/2011.5. Geneva: World Health Organization; 2011.

21. Cheepsattayakorn A, Cheepsattayakorn R. Breath tests in diagnosis of pulmonary tuberculosis. Recent Pat Biotechnol 2014;8:172-5.

22. Nakhleh MK, Jeries R, Gharra A, Binder A, Broza YY, Pascoe M, et al. Detecting active pulmonary tuberculosis with a breath test using nanomaterial-based sensors. Eur Respir J 2014;43:1522-5.

23. Sharma SK, Pande JN. Fiberoptic bronchoscopy. Indian J Chest Dis Allied Sci 1988;30:163-5.

24. De S, Desikan P. Pulmonary nocardiosis mimicking relapse of tuberculosis. BMJ Case Rep 2009; 2009.pii.bcr06.2008.0233.

25. Sharma SK, Mohan A, Guleria R, Padhy AK. Diagnostic dilemma: tuberculosis? or, sarcoidosis? Indian J Chest Dis Allied Sci 1997;39:119-23.

26. Singh TN, Singh HR, Devi KhS, Singh NB, Singh YI. Pulmonary paragonimiasis. Indian J Chest Dis Allied Sci 2004;46:225-7.

11

Lower Lung Field Tuberculosis

Gautam Ahluwalia, Surendra K Sharma

INTRODUCTION

Post-primary pulmonary tuberculosis [TB] classically affects predominantly the upper lobes. Since Laennec's era, lower lung field TB was considered a rarity (1). Throughout the nineteenth century, most of the researchers were of the view that involvement of the lower lung field with TB was not an important issue (2,3). However, there was a school of thought holding a divergent view. In 1886, Kidd stated that "the apex of lower lobe is very prone to TB disease and may be attacked before the apex of the upper lobe" (4). Subsequently, two years later, Fowler stated that "the upper and posterior part of the lower lobe is a spot only second in point of vulnerability to the apex itself" (5). Except these two early documentations, the literature is silent over the occurrence of lower lung field TB till the first quarter of twentieth century. Subsequently, many authors concluded that lower lung field may be the site of pulmonary TB in specific situations encountered rather frequently by clinicians (6-11). Therefore, a high index of suspicion is key to the diagnosis of lower lung field TB.

TERMINOLOGY OF LOWER LUNG FIELD TUBERCULOSIS

It is important to understand the meaning of the term 'lower lung field TB'. In the earlier reports (4-11), the term 'basal TB' was frequently used. However, with the advent of lateral radiographs of the chest, the term 'lower lobe TB' had been used by various authors (12-16). In view of the proximity of the lesion to hilum, the term 'hilar and perihilar TB' was also used by few authors (17,18). However, Ostrum and Saber (16) suggested that various terms used by different authors were in fact referring to the same entity.

The lower lung field is defined as the area on the postero-anterior [PA] chest radiograph, which extends below an imaginary horizontal line traced across the hilum and includes the parahilar regions. A standard PA chest radiograph is ordinarily sufficient for the diagnosis of pulmonary TB. Since lateral films of the chest are available very infrequently, it is difficult to identify the exact topographic location of the lesion i.e., whether the disease is confined to the lower lobe only or is present in the middle lobe and lingula as well. Therefore, the term 'lower lung field TB' has come into vogue. In a PA radiograph of the chest, lower lung field includes the middle lobe on right side and lingula on left side in addition to the lower lobes.

PREVALENCE

The prevalence of lower lung field TB has ranged from 0.003%-18.3% [Table 11.1] (7,8,12,19-29). The reason for the wide variation in the prevalence is probably due to confusion in the terminology used [basal, parahilar, lower lobe, lower lung field] and selection bias [hospitalised or ambulatory patients].

In earlier medical literature, the prevalence of lower lung field TB in studies reported from India has been observed to be higher than that reported in western studies [Table 11.1]. This may be due to the fact that majority of Indians tie their clothes [women their sari and men their loin cloth] tightly around the upper abdomen and this results in impaired movement of diaphragm. This theory has been substantiated by Viswanathan (21) in the second quarter of the 20th century, who studied the diaphragmatic movements on the radiographic screen in subjects accustomed to tight lacing around their waists. It has been suggested that the resultant impaired movement of diaphragm leads to costal type of breathing [as in females], which leads to decreased ventilation, retarded blood circulation and lymphatic flow in lower lung fields, thus making them more vulnerable to TB.

Table 11.1: Prevalence of lower lung field TB

Study (reference)	Year of publication	No. of pulmonary TB cases	Prevalence of lower lung field TB [%]
Colton (7)	1928	2335	0.003
Ross (19)	1930	60	18.3
Du Fault (8)	1932	365	0.27
Reisner (20)	1935	4494	0.68
Hamilton and Freed (12)	1935	349	2.9
Viswanathan (21)	1936	638	6.4
Romendick et al (22)	1944	2354	2.7
Segarra et al (23)	1963	10962	0.85
Parmar (24)	1967	1455	3.4
Tripathy and Nanda (25)	1970	707	5.1
Mathur et al (26)	1974	5072	0.63
Berger and Granada (27)	1974	386	7.0
Chang et al (28)	1987	1276	5.1
Wang et al (29)	2006	520	15.8

TB = tuberculosis

PATHOGENESIS

Besides that above cited plausible mechanism (20,21), the other common pathogenetic mechanism of lower lung field TB is the ulceration of a bronchus by a lymph node affected by TB with spillage of TB material into the bronchus. Lower lung field TB occurs as a continuum of primary TB or soon after in the post-primary phase (23,24).

CLINICAL FEATURES

In various studies (9,19,23,30,31), female preponderance and predilection for patients under 40 years of age has been reported. Segarra et al (23) reported that 89% of patients with lower lung field TB were less than 40 years old and Parmar (24) reported that 46% of the patients were less than 20 years of age. However, Tripathy and Nanda (25) did not find a similar distribution in their study. In subsequent studies, it has been observed that lower lung field TB is no longer a disease of the young and afflicts the elderly more commonly (28,29,32).

Associated Conditions

Lower lung field TB appears to be more common in patients receiving corticosteroid treatment, patients with hepatic or renal disease, diabetes mellitus, pregnancy, silicosis kyphoscoliosis and human immunodeficiency virus [HIV] (23,27,28,33-35).

In fact, studies from Asia including India have revealed that in diabetic patients with TB not only lower lung field TB occurs more commonly at presentation, but diabetes also results in poor treatment outcome (36). Moreover, diabetic patients with TB are elderly and have a higher

mortality (36-38). It has also been observed that worsening glycosylated haemoglobin levels reflecting poor glycaemic control increase the relative risk of developing lower lung field TB (39). Furthermore, diabetic patients have a higher prevalence of positive acid-fast bacilli [AFB] sputum smears as compared to non-diabetic patients (36). With the increasing prevalence of diabetes in resource-limited countries like India, this may have implications for the TB control programme as diabetes-TB co-morbidity will add to the infectious burden of TB in the community.

Symptoms

The duration of symptoms may be less than two weeks, although the mean duration is 12 weeks (28). In most of the studies symptom duration of less than six months has been documented (23,27,28). Tripathy and Nanda (25) have observed that about 20% of patients reported within two weeks and 70% of patients within six months in their series of 36 cases.

Cough with variable amounts of expectoration is the most frequent symptom (21,23,25). Mathur et al (26) reported cough in 100% cases. Many authors have noted haemoptysis as an important symptom (8,11,12,20,21,23,24). Tripathy and Nanda (25) noted haemoptysis in nearly two-thirds of the cases and Romendick et al (22) noted it in 75% of cases.

The general toxaemic manifestations of TB infection, such as, fever, chills, malaise, weakness and anorexia are also frequently present. Segarra et al (23) reported these symptoms in about 40% of their cases, whereas Tripathy and Nanda (25) reported them in 86% of their cases. However, a recent study from east Asia has revealed that lack of fever more than 38 °C in lower lung field TB is an important discriminating symptom as compared to lower lung field bacterial pneumonia.

Signs

The physical signs vary with the extent and character of the lesions. Patients with extensive involvement of the lungs have pronounced signs of the underlying lesion. However, patients who have involvement of a relatively small area, especially those in whom the lesion is limited to the apical segment of lower lobe, physical signs may be scanty or even absent. However, physical signs are encountered more often in patients with lower lung field TB than in those with the classical upper lobe pulmonary TB (27).

INVESTIGATIONS

Sputum Examination

Although sputum examination is the simplest way to diagnose lower lung field TB, isolation of *Mycobacterium tuberculosis* [*Mtb*] is difficult on sputum smear or mycobacterial culture (27,28). However, the diagnostic yield of sputum examination is better in patients with cavitary lesions (22).

Chest Radiograph

More than half of the cases of lower lung field TB have right lung involvement, whereas one-third cases have left lung involvement. Bilateral lesions are reported in 10% of cases (24,25,30,33).

The radiographic findings in lower lung field TB differ significantly from those found in upper lobe disease (20). The most frequent radiographic finding is consolidation, which is more confluent and extensive than that found in upper lobe TB (22,30) [Figure 11.1]. Cavitary lesions are also frequently seen, which may be single or multiple and may lie within an area of consolidation (27,28) [Figure 11.2]. Cavities may be large [3-4 cm in diameter]. The presence of tension cavities [thin-walled with fluid] is also a radiological feature of lower lung field TB (22,23,25,41). Recently, it has been suggested that absence of air bronchogram in a chest radiograph is more common in patients with lower lung field TB as compared to lower lung field bacterial pneumonia (40). Other radiographic features include evidence of atelectasis or solitary mass with intrathoracic lymphadenopathy.

The radiographic features also have a prognostic value. The outcome is unfavourable in patients with lower lung field TB who have lung collapse or pulmonary consolidation in the chest radiograph (31,35).

Bronchoscopy

The early diagnosis of lower lung field TB is important for prevention of severe sequelae. Fibreoptic bronchoscopy [FOB] is the preferred diagnostic modality for the diagnosis of lower lung field TB. Abnormal bronchoscopic findings in lower lung field TB include ulcerative granuloma, mucosal erythema, submucosal infiltration and fibrostenosis [Figure 11.3].

FOB provides a higher diagnostic yield than sputum examination, especially in patients who present with radiographic findings of pulmonary consolidation, lung collapse or solitary mass (22,42). FOB is also important in assessing the severity of endobronchial lesions in lower lung field TB. The outcome is unfavorable in patients with lower lung field TB when FOB reveals fibrostenosis or ulcerative granuloma. If severe fibrostenosis is present, early surgical intervention should be considered to prevent damage of the lung distal to the obstruction (28,42).

Endobronchial Ultrasonography—Transbronchial Needle Aspiration

The role of endobronchial ultrasound [EBUS] in complement with FOB is also being evaluated to increase the diagnostic accuracy, especially in smear-negative TB suspects *per se*.

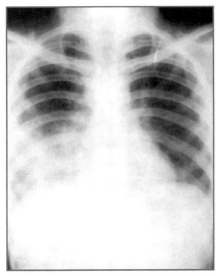

Figure 11.1: Chest radiograph [posteroanterior view] showing consolidation in the right lower zone

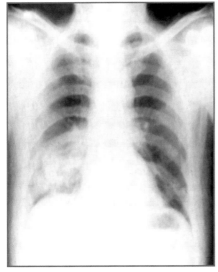

Figure 11.2: Chest radiograph [postero-anterior view] showing cavitary lesion in the right lower zone

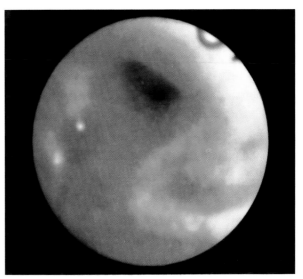

Figure 11.3: Mucosal erythema and submucosal infiltration observed during fibreoptic bronchoscopy in a patient with right lower lung field tuberculosis. Bronchoalveolar lavage revealed *Mycobacterium tuberculosis*

Additionally, combining EBUS with transbronchial needle aspiration [TBNA] of lymph nodes is another exciting development under evaluation. In resource-limited countries like India, these newer modalities will need to be validated for TB diagnosis as well as their cost effectiveness by indigenous operational research.

In a study (43) from China, it has been demonstrated that combining FOB with EBUS resulted in higher diagnostic accuracy of AFB smear in bronchoalveolar lavage [BAL] fluid [31.5% versus 12.5%, p = 0.018], Mycobacterium tuberculosis culture in BAL fluid [67.1% versus 47.9%, p = 0.024] and histopathology confirmation of TB in transbronchial lung biopsy [TBLB] specimens [32.9% versus 4.2%, p < 0.0001] as compared to FOB alone. Moreover, it was also observed that overall diagnostic accuracy for TB by using bronchoscopic procedures [smear and culture of BAL fluid and TBLB] with EBUS was higher than for FOB alone [80.8% versus 8.3%, p = 0.035]. The utility of EBUS in increasing the sensitivity of cartridge-based nucleic acid amplification tests for diagnosis of TB has also been demonstrated when compared to FOB alone (44).

Lymphadenopathy underlying a bronchus plays an important role in the pathogenesis of lower lung field TB. Combination of EBUS-TBNA as compared to conventional FOB is also being studied in patients of TB. The combination of EBUS-TBNA indicates that EBUS-TBNA results in higher diagnostic yield in pulmonary TB suspect patients with lymphadenopathy (45).

MANAGEMENT

Lower lung field TB presents a definite problem in diagnosis because of its location and radiographic findings. Moreover, when TB is confined to lower lung field, it often masquerades as pneumonia, lung cancer, bronchiectasis or lung abscess, thereby, delaying the correct diagnosis. The shift in age-distribution from the young to the aged and non-specific clinical features adds another challenge in the diagnosis of lower lung field TB (30,31,43). Therefore, TB should be considered a diagnostic possibility in patients with lower lung field lesions who have the following conditions: diabetes mellitus, advanced age, glucocorticoid treatment, renal or hepatic illness, malignancy or lesions with poor response to adequate antibiotic therapy (31,46). FOB should be performed early to ascertain the diagnosis of TB and assess the severity of the endobronchial lesions.

The patients with lower lung field TB show a favorable response to conventional anti-TB therapy. Delayed diagnosis affects the outcome in these patients (31,46). Significant resolution of chest radiograph findings and/or sputum negativity was observed with anti-TB treatment, if the diagnosis to treatment time was less than three months (43).

Treatment of lower lung field TB is similar to the treatment elsewhere in the body. The reader is referred to the chapter "Treatment of tuberculosis" [Chapter 44] for details. Long-term follow-up is recommended to diagnose possible relapse after the completion of treatment. In India, patients with lower lung field TB receive DOTS under the Revised National Tuberculosis Programme [RNTCP] of Government of India. The reader is referred to the chapter "The Revised National Tuberculosis Control Programme" [Chapter 53] for more details.

Tracheobronchial stenosis is an important complication of lower lung field TB leading to permanent damage of lung distal to the obstruction. Since the outcome is poor in patients with lower lung field TB, when FOB findings show fibrostenosis or ulcerative granuloma, these patients should be followed-up closely. The non-invasive methods such as chest radiograph and flow-volume loops on pulmonary function testing are insensitive for detecting or monitoring tracheobronchial stenosis. In these patients, close follow-up with FOB is necessary if chest radiograph shows no significant improvement or clinical features suggest progression of endobronchial lesions after anti-TB treatment for a few months. Surgical intervention is indicated if re-examination with FOB shows no significant improvement or worsening of endobronchial involvement. However, if severe fibrostenosis is present, early surgical intervention in the form of sleeve operation is indicated before permanent sequelae, such as, damage of lung distal to the obstruction and respiratory failure occur (28,29,42).

REFERENCES

1. Laennec RT. Treatise on the diagnosis and treatment of the diseases of the chest. New York: Haffner Publishing; 1962.
2. Landis HRM, Norris GW. Diseases of the chest. Second edition. Philadelphia: WB Saunders Company; 1921.
3. Fishberg M. Pulmonary tuberculosis. 3rd edition. Philadelphia: Lea and Febiger; 1922.
4. Kidd P. Basic tuberculous phthisis. Lancet 1886;2:616.
5. Fowler JK. The localization of lesions of phthisis. London: J and A Churchill; 1888.
6. Busby JF. Basal tuberculosis. Am Rev Tuber 1939;40:692-703.
7. Colton WA. Basal lesions in pulmonary tuberculosis with report of seven cases. US Vet Bureau Med Bull 1928;4:503.
8. Du Fault P. Basal pulmonary lesions. Am Rev Tuber 1932;25:17-23.
9. Dunham K, Norton W. Basal tuberculosis. JAMA 1927;89:1573-5.
10. Lander F. Selective thoracoplasty for persistent basal tuberculosis cavities. J Thorac Surg 1938;7:455.
11. Gordon BL, Charr R, Sokoloff MJ. Basal pulmonary tuberculosis. Am Rev Tuber 1944;49:432-6.
12. Hamilton CE, Freed H. Lower lobe tuberculosis-a review. JAMA 1935;105:427-30.
13. Jacob M. Lower lobe pulmonary tuberculosis. Med J Record 1929;129:32.
14. Middleton WS. Lower lobe pulmonary tuberculosis. Am Rev Tuber 1923;7:307.
15. Ossen EZ. Tuberculosis of the lower lobe. N Engl J Med 1944;230:693-8.
16. Ostrum HW, Saber W. Early recognition of lower lobe tuberculosis. Radiology 1949;53:42-8.
17. Bernard M, Lelong M, Renard G. La localisation perihilare de la tuberculose pulmonaire chronique de la adultae. Ann de Med 1927; 21:366.
18. Faber K. Perihilar pulmonary tuberculosis in adults. Acta Med Scand 1931;75:403.
19. Ross EL. Tuberculosis in nurses-a study of the disease in 60 nurses admitted to Manitoba sanatorium. Can Med Assoc J 1930; 22:347-54.

20. Reisner D. Pulmonary tuberculosis of the lower lobe. Arch Intern Med 1935;56:258-80.
21. Viswanathan R. Tuberculosis of the lower lobe. Br Med J 1936;2: 1300-2.
22. Romendick SS, Freidman B, Schwartz HF. Lower lung field tuberculosis. Dis Chest 1944;10:481-8.
23. Seggara F, Sherman DS. Rodriguez AJ. Lower lung field tuberculosis. Am Rev Respir Dis 1963;87:37-40.
24. Parmar MS. Lower lung field tuberculosis. Am Rev Respir Dis 1967; 96:310-3.
25. Tripathy SN, Nanda CN. Lower lung field tuberculosis in adults. J Assoc Physicians India 1970;18:999-1008.
26. Mathur KC, Tanwar KL, Razdan IN. Lower lung field tuberculosis. Indian J Chest Dis and Allied Sci 1974;16:31-41.
27. Berger HW, Granada MG. Lower lung field tuberculosis. Chest 1974;65:522-6.
28. Chang SC, Pui YL, Perng RP. Lower lung field tuberculosis. Chest 1987;91:230-2.
29. Wang JY, Heush PR, Lee CH, Chang HC, Lee LN, Liaw YS, et al. Recognizing tuberculosis in lower lung field: an age- and sex-matched controlled study. Int J Tuberc Lung Dis 2006;10: 578-84.
30. Kuaban C, Fotsin JG, Koulla-Shiro S, Ekono MR, Hagbe P. Lower lung field tuberculosis in Yaounde, Cameroon. Cent Afr J Med 1996;42:62-5.
31. Kobashi Y, Matsushima T. Clinical analysis of recent lower lung field tuberculosis. J Infect Chemother 2003;9:272-5.
32. Singh SK, Tiwari KK. Clinicoradiological profile of lower lung field tuberculosis cases among young adult and elderly people in a teaching hospital of Madhya Pradesh, India. J Trop Med 2015;2015:230720.
33. Sokoloff MJ. Lower lung tuberculosis. Radiology 1940;34: 589-94.
34. Fernandez MZ, Nedwicki EG. Lower lung field tuber. Mich Med 1969;68:31-5.
35. Morris JT, Seaworth BJ, McAllister CK. Pulmonary tuberculosis in diabetics. Chest 1992;102:539-41.
36. Wang CS, Yang CJ, Chen HC, Chuang SH, Chong IW, Hwang JJ, Huang MS. Impact of type 2 diabetes on manifestations and treatment outcome of pulmonary tuberculosis. Epidemiol Infect 2009;137:203-10.
37. Carreira S, Costeira J, Gomes C, André JM, Diogo N. Impact of diabetes on the presenting features of tuberculosis in hospitalized patients. Rev Port Pneumol 2012;18:239-43.
38. Rawat J, Sindhwani G, Biswas D. Effect of age on presentation with diabetes: Comparison of nondiabetic patients with new smear-positive pulmonary tuberculosis patients. Lung India 2011;28:187-90.
39. Chiang CY, Lee JJ, Chien ST, Enarson DA, Chang YC, Chen YT, et al. Glycemic control and radiographic manifestations of tuberculosis in diabetic patients. PLoS One 2014;9:e93397.
40. Lin CH, Chen TM, Chang CC, Tsai CH, Chai WH, Wen JH. Unilateral lower lung field opacities on chest radiography: a comparison of the clinical manifestations of tuberculosis and pneumonia. Eur J Radiol 2012;81:e426-30.
41. Perez-Guzman C, Torres-Cruz A, Villarreal-Velarde H, Salazar-Lezama MA, Vargas MH. Atypical radiological images of pulmonary tuberculosis in 192 diabetic patients: a comparative study. Int J Tuberc Lung Dis 2001;5:455-61.
42. Chang SC, Lee PY, Perng RP. The value of roentgenoand fiberbronchoscopic findings in predicting outcome of adults with lower lung field tuberculosis. Arch Intern Med 1991;151:1581-3.
43. Lin SM, Chung FT, Huang CD, Liu WT, Kuo CH, Wang CH, et al. Diagnostic value of endobronchial ultrasonography for pulmonary tuberculosis. J Thorac Cardiovasc Surg 2009;138: 179-84.
44. Patil S, Narwade S, Mirza M. Bronchial Wash Gene Xpert MTB/RIF in lower lung field tuberculosis: sensitive, superior, and rapid in comparison with conventional diagnostic techniques. J Transl Int Med 2017;5:174-81.
45. Ren S, Zhang Z, Jiang H, Wu C, Liu J, Liang L, et al. Combination of endobronchial ultrasound-guided transbronchial needle aspiration with standard bronchoscopic techniques enhanced the diagnosis yields of pulmonary tuberculosis patients with lymphadenopathy. Panminerva Med 2013;55:363-70.
46. Bacakoglu F, Basoglu OK, Cok G, Sayiner A, Ates M. Pulmonary tuberculosis in patients with diabetes mellitus. Respiration 2001;68:595-600.

12

Endobronchial Tuberculosis

Samjot S Dhillon, Nicola A Hanania

INTRODUCTION

Endobronchial tuberculosis [TB], which refers to the involvement of trachea and bronchi by TB, was first described in 1689 by an English physician, Richard Morton (1). However, it remained mainly a post-mortem diagnosis and was infrequently reported until the advent of bronchoscopy in the late 1920s (2-4). Subsequently, the natural history of endobronchial TB was described in large clinical and pathological series (2-4). Following the introduction of effective chemotherapy for TB, reports on endobronchial TB decreased dramatically to the extent that no cases were reported in several large studies on the bronchoscopic evaluation of patients with TB (5-9). The resurgence of TB in 1990s and recent advances in interventional pulmonary techniques have rekindled interest in endobronchial TB and the last two decades have seen several publications in this field (10-23).

EPIDEMIOLOGY

The exact prevalence of endobronchial TB is not known. In autopsy studies on patients with TB, the reported prevalence has ranged from 3% (24) to 72% (25) although most series report a rate of about 40% (26,27). This variation in prevalence rate may be due to the difference in severity of cases of TB studied and/or the extent of tracheobronchial tree evaluation (26). For e.g., in a study published in the pre-chemotherapy era, more than 30% of the patients with endobronchial TB had concomitant pulmonary TB for the duration of more than two years, a fact, that may explain the high prevalence of endobronchial TB noted (26).

Based on previously published bronchoscopic studies, endobronchial TB was reported in 10%-20% of patients with active TB (4,27-30). However, in recent studies, a lower prevalence rate has been reported, which is most likely due to the timely and more effective chemotherapy received by patients with TB (5-9). In fact, the current prevalence rate may be as low as 0.18% in areas where TB is not endemic (31). The difference in prevalence between autopsy and broncho-scopy studies is likely due to the inclusion of microscopic involvement of airways in autopsy data that is not detected by bronchoscopy (26). Bronchoscopy is also not done routinely in patients with TB due to concerns of spread of infection (32), and thus, most bronchoscopy studies likely underestimate its true prevalence. Endobronchial TB is mostly described in patients between 21-40 years of age (12,19,26), although similar prevalence has also been reported in the geriatric population (33). The majority of studies report a female preponderance (4,12,14,19,26,34,35). This may be due to the fact that the implantation of organisms from infected sputum occurs easily in women who tend to voluntarily suppress their cough because of socio-cultural and cosmetic issues (19,36,37). Small airways in women may also contribute to this difference in prevalence.

PATHOPHYSIOLOGY

Mechanisms of Endobronchial Infection

Endobronchial spread of TB can be via multiple mechanisms, which, alone or in combination, contribute to the development of endobronchial TB. Five potential mechanisms for the spread of endobronchial TB have been suggested (3).

Extension from the Lungs by Direct Infiltration

Direct spread probably occurs when bronchi in the immediate neighbourhood of an infected lung are involved. In general, tracheobronchial ulceration is more commonly seen adjacent to areas of extensive and progressive parenchymal TB (26).

Implantation of Organisms from Infected Sputum

The finding of endobronchial disease on the wall of bronchi opposite the opening of a diseased lobe is likely due to the implantation from infected material passing over the mucous membrane. Auerbach observed the presence of gross airways ulcerations on the same side where cavities in the lung were present (26). These cavities are a potential source of bacilli causing the endobronchial involvement. However, in some cases, cavity formation may follow the diagnosis of endobronchial TB, pointing to the possibility of other mechanisms (15). In addition, the absence of endobronchial involvement in cases where large cavities are present argues against this as the only mechanism (38).

Haematogenous Dissemination

Haematogenous spread is uncommon and endobronchial TB is infrequently described in miliary TB [MTB] (26,39).

Lymphatic Spread

This mechanism involves retrograde passage of the tubercle bacilli through lymphatics from bronchioles and sub-segmental bronchi to the main stem bronchus. Peribronchial infection of the lymphatics may be seen histologically in some cases. However, the data by Auerbach suggests that in most cases the infection starts in the submucosal region and progresses towards the adventitia (26). Only in few cases, infection is limited to or starts from the adventitia, where lymphatics are located. This fact argues against the lymphatic spread as a common mechanism.

As Part of the Primary Infection

In certain cases of primary TB, a lymph node erodes into a bronchus. The lymph node becomes attached to the bronchial wall because of the ongoing inflammatory changes, and thus, the infection spreads through the walls of the bronchus to the mucosal lining. This mechanism is predominantly seen in children (40,41). Chang *et al* (42) reported endobronchial involvement in 12 out of 16 patients with intrathoracic TB lymphadenopathy. Baran *et al* (43) also reported endobronchial abnormalities in 15 of 17 patients with intrathoracic TB lymphadenopathy in the absence of parenchymal lesions. Four of these patients had ulcerating endobronchial granulomas. Direct perforation of TB lymph nodes into the bronchi is relatively uncommon in adults, especially now in the post-chemotherapy era (44,45).

Macroscopic Appearance

The earliest bronchoscopic sign of endobronchial TB is the finding of erythematous mucous membranes. Discrete tubercles may have a rough granulated appearance to the naked eye or may lead to shallow ulcers of the mucous membrane that progress to deep ulcers involving the bronchial wall. Formation of extensive granulation tissue may occasionally result in a tumour-like growth into the lumen of the bronchus mimicking a neoplasm. In most cases where ulcers are deep, healing will be complicated by stenosis secondary to extensive fibrosis. Bronchial stenosis may also result from oedema or from extrinsic compression by a lymph node (26). On rare occasions, post-obstructive pneumonia, lung abscess, obstructive emphysema and subsequent bronchiectasis may develop distal to this stenosis (26).

Earlier autopsy studies suggested that ulcers are more common in region of the carina and posterior surface of the tracheobronchial tree (26). The size of these ulcers varies from 1-5 mm and their long axes are usually parallel to the cartilaginous rings (26). Ulcers may progressively coalesce leaving the cartilage partially exposed at the base of the ulcer (26).

Endobronchial TB may be an integral part of the parenchymal lung involvement with TB but this involvement is overlooked, as smaller airways cannot be accessed by bronchoscopy. Diffuse stenosis of small bronchi distal to the fourth generation mimicking bronchiolitis obliterans has been described (46).

Microscopic Appearance

Small, oval and round foci of epithelioid granulomas, with or without a central zone of caseation within the wall especially in the subepithelial region and in the region of mucous glands are the early microscopic findings with endobronchial TB. In advanced cases, these foci are also present in the adventitia and in rare occasions they may only seen in the adventitia (26). The involvement of the cartilage is usually limited to very extensive cases. Rupture of these submucosal foci results in ulceration and gradual destruction of the wall of bronchus. The zone of caseation is usually surrounded by vascular granulation tissue and is occasionally covered by a pseudo-membrane formed by fibrin exuded from capillaries in this granulation tissue. During the process of healing, granulation tissue replaces the inner zone of caseation and regenerating epithelium from all sides eventually covers the ulcer. Connective tissue ultimately replaces the cells and capillaries within the granulation tissue. If this process is extensive and involves most of the circumference of the airway, stenosis will eventually occur.

CLINICAL COURSE

The clinical presentation of endobronchial TB is variable. In adults, it may occur in primary or reactivation TB, however, in children, it is usually a complication of primary TB. The presentation of endobronchial TB may be acute respiratory failure requiring mechanical ventilation (47), subacute mimicking asthma, pneumonia, foreign body aspiration (3,31,48,49) or insidious, simulating lung cancer (10,33,50-53). Symptoms may start years after the diagnosis and treatment of pulmonary TB (54,55). A barking cough has been reported in majority of the patients. Dyspnoea, chest pain, fever, generalised weakness, weight loss and haemoptysis may also be present (10,12). Sputum production is variable; bronchorrhea [>500 mL/day] has been reported in rare cases (56). Physical examination may reveal diminished breath sounds or a localised fixed wheeze (3,34). Wheezing is classically low-pitched, constantly present, and heard over the same area of the chest wall (2) but may disappear as the airways become progressively narrowed. Partial airway obstruction may, on rare occasions, act as a one-way valve leading to tension pneumothorax (3). Unusual presentations include expectoration of bronchial cartilages (57,58) and fistula formation between the right and left main bronchi (59,60). In addition to usual chronic infections due to atelectasis and bronchiectasis, rare infectious complications, such as, pseudomembranous tracheobronchial aspergillosis on endobronchial TB stenotic area can occur (61).

Bronchial stenosis is the most significant complication of endobronchial TB. It may present with slowly progressive shortness of breath years after the diagnosis and treatment of pulmonary TB. Respiratory failure, difficult endotracheal intubation, need for tracheostomy and death by suffocation may occur as a consequence of tracheal stenosis (15).

Simultaneous involvement of other organs has been reported. Auerbach hypothesised that endobronchial TB represents a tendency towards the development of "tract TB". Concomitant intestinal and laryngeal involvement with TB was noted in 82% and 60% of autopsy cases, respectively (26). However, these findings have not been reported in more recent studies and were limited to older studies, which included patients with progressive TB of long duration.

LABORATORY AND RADIOLOGICAL INVESTIGATIONS

Sputum Examination

Sputum smear examination for acid-fast bacilli [AFB] has a low yield [15%-20%] (10,12) for the diagnosis of endobronchial TB. This may be because expectoration of sputum is difficult due to mucus entrapment by proximal bronchial granulation tissue (10). Furthermore, ulceration of the involved mucosa may be necessary for obtaining a positive sputum smear (12). Thus, a negative smear for AFB does not exclude the diagnosis.

Chest Radiograph

Endobronchial TB usually coexists with extensive pulmonary parenchymal or intrathoracic lymph node infection. However, 10%-20% of the patients have a normal chest radiograph (10,12,28,34,62-67). Chest radiograph may show patchy infiltrates (15), evidence of collapse [25%-35%] or consolidation [35%-60%] (10,12). Other radiographic features include hyperinflation, cavity formation, pleural effusion, miliary infiltrates and mediastinal lymphadenopathy (10,15).

Computed Tomography

Computed tomography [CT] of the chest is a very important tool in evaluating endobronchial TB. While the findings are non-specific, it may show endobronchial involvement of large, medium and small airways. In fact, in some studies the endobronchial involvement is more pronounced in small airways than large airway (68-71). These CT findings have been found to correlate well with corresponding pathological findings (70). Findings on CT of endobronchial disease in small airways may include: poorly defined nodules, centrilobular nodules, bronchial wall thickening and tree-in-bud appearance [Figure 12.1A] (68-70). All these findings are best visualised on high resolution CT [HRCT] (69). Centrilobular lesions reflect solid caseation material within or around the terminal or respiratory bronchioles. Terminal tufts of the "tree-in-bud" may represent the lesions within the bronchioles and alveolar ducts, while the stalk may represent a lesion that affects the last order bronchus within the secondary lobule [Figure 12.1B] (70). CT may show aneurysmal dilatation of

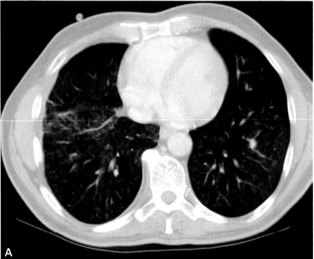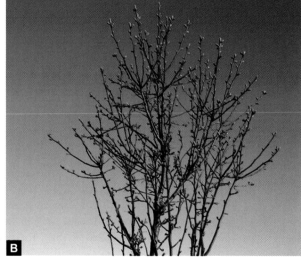

Figure 12.1: CT of the chest showing "tree-in-bud" pattern seen in endobronchial tuberculosis [A]. This pattern refers to peripheral, small centrilobular, and well-defined nodules that are connected to linear, branching opacities that have more than one contiguous branching site, thus resembling a *tree-in-bud* [B]. In histopathological studies, the tree-in-bud appearance correlates well with the presence of plugging of the small airways with mucus, pus, or fluid; dilated bronchioles; bronchiolar wall thickening; and peribronchiolar inflammation

medium sized bronchi due to endobronchial inflammatory tissue (72).

The CT may also show stenosis or obstruction of the major airways. A peribronchial cuff of soft tissue may be seen (71,73). During the active TB stage, irregular and circumferential luminal narrowing may be visualised. However, during the fibrotic stage, wall thickening is much less prominent and an equal distribution of smooth and irregular narrowing occurs (74,75). CT may on occasion show enlarged lymph nodes in the mediastinum and other parenchymal lesions, such as, segmental collapse, collapse with multiple low density areas, cavities and round low density lesions which most likely represent mucoid impaction distal to obstruction (71,73). An intra-luminal lower density polypoid mass with narrowing may, sometimes, be seen in a bronchus (71).

While the CT is extremely accurate in detecting focal bronchial lesions, it is inaccurate in predicting whether the lesion is endobronchial, submucosal or outside the airway (71,73). In addition, it may not be possible to accurately assess the thickness of the bronchial wall in many cases because of the loss of silhouette of the outer wall of the involved bronchus by the adjacent consolidation or of the inner wall by the absence of intraluminal air. It is often extremely hard to differentiate endobronchial TB from bronchogenic carcinoma by CT, and thus, broncho-scopy is ultimately needed. However, CT has the advantage of revealing areas of the airway beyond the stenosis as well as the length of stenosis and the extent of peri-bronchial soft tissue/lymph nodes involvement (20,76). Thus, CT complements bronchoscopy in evaluating these patients and can also be used to monitor response to treatment (76).

While it is very helpful, radiographic findings of endobronchial TB are non-specific and can be seen in other diseases. Conditions that may show bronchial wall thickening and luminal narrowing on CT like sarcoidosis, amyloidosis, relapsing polychondritis and tracheopathia osteochondroplastica should always be kept in mind (74). Newer radiographic techniques such as multi-planar and three-dimensional [3D] helical CT images with recon-struction [virtual bronchoscopy] allow a better assessment of tracheobronchial tree and can be helpful in evaluating endobronchial TB (74-79).

Spirometry

The most common abnormality seen on spirometry in endobronchial TB is restriction (20,35). Lee and Chung (20) evaluated spirometry findings in 68 patients and demon-strated a restrictive abnormality in 47%, obstructive abnormality in 5.9%, mixed in 23.5%, and normal spirometry in 23.5% of the patients. The flow volume loop abnormalities classically seen in patients with upper airway obstruction are rarely seen in endobronchial TB. Unlike patients with bronchial asthma, patients with endobronchial TB do not have increased bronchial hyper-reactivity to inhaled histamine (80).

Bronchoscopy

Bronchoscopy is the gold standard for the diagnosis of endobronchial TB. The diagnosis can be missed in some cases with normal chest radiograph if bronchoscopy is not considered (81,82). Unlike pre-chemotherapy era where tracheal ulcerations were commonly seen, most of the recent bronchoscopy series report more common involvement of the main stem and upper lobe bronchi (12,16) and some recent studies report left main stem as the most commonly involved site (35,47,83). Endobronchial biopsies usually reveal the classic histological features of TB. These range from non-necrotic epithelioid cell granulomas with no AFB to necrotic granulomas with abundant AFB. Bronchial brushings obtained along with biopsy increase the diagnostic yield (84). Cryobiopsy may aid in getting bigger samples and needs to be further explored (85).

Bronchoscopy has been useful in learning about the natural history and progression of endobronchial TB. Salkin *et al* presented one of the earliest serial follow-up data (27) and documented the progression of bronchial ulceration to polyp formation and stenosis in three to six months. Bronchostenosis develops in 50%-90% of patients despite effective therapy (10,19). This complication that can present years after diagnosis and therapy, may involve the trachea or mainstem bronchi. Ip *et al* (10) showed that stenosis developed in all but one of the 12 patients who had a follow-up bronchoscopy within eight to 49 months of completing anti-TB treatment. Eight of these patients were asymptomatic including one who had severe stenosis of the left main stem bronchus (10).

Several bronchoscopic classifications of endobronchial TB have been proposed (14,19,20,86). Chung and Lee (19) described seven forms of bronchoscopic findings [Figure 12.2]. In their report, they performed serial bronchoscopy on 81 patients with endobronchial TB to examine the predictive value of this classification. Bronchoscopic examination was initially performed every month until there was no subsequent change in the endobronchial lesions followed by an examination every three months until the completion of anti-TB treatment. The seven forms of bronchoscopic findings are described below.

Non-specific Bronchitic Endobronchial TB

Only mild mucosal swelling and/or hyperaemia are seen on bronchoscopy in this form. The prognosis is overall good and all cases resolve within two months of treatment.

Granular Endobronchial Tuberculosis

In granular endobronchial TB, the bronchoscopic appearance mimics scattered grains of boiled rice, and the underlying bronchial mucosa shows severe inflammatory changes. Only 20% of the cases develop fibrostenosis.

Oedematous Hyperaemic Endobronchial TB

In the oedematous-hyperaemic endobronchial TB, severe mucosal swelling with surrounding hyperaemia causing

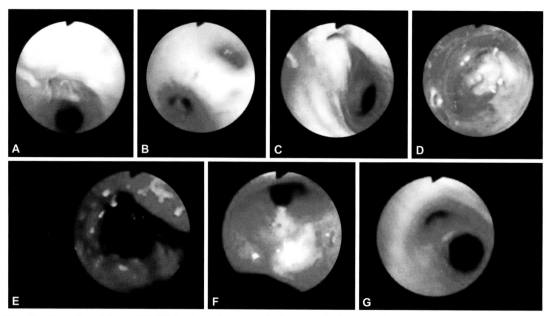

Figure 12.2: Classification of endobronchial TB by bronchoscopic findings: actively caseating type [A]; oedematous-hyperaemic type [B]; fibrostenotic type [C]; tumourous type [D]; granular type [E]; ulcerative type [F]; and non-specific bronchitic type [G]
Reproduced with permission from "Chung HS, Lee JH. Bronchoscopic assessment of the evolution of endobronchial tuberculosis. Chest 2000;117:385-92" (reference 19)

narrowing of the bronchial lumen is seen. Patients with these findings have poor prognosis as 60% of cases develop fibrostenosis within two to three months after treatment, and 30% progress to complete obstruction of the bronchial lumen.

Actively Caseating Endobronchial TB

Actively caseating endobronchial TB is the most commonly seen form and bronchoscopy shows swollen and hyperaemic mucosa that is diffusely covered with whitish cheese-like material. Luminal narrowing at diagnosis is usually seen whether granulation tissue is present or not. Significant improvement of bronchial stenosis is seen with treatment, although 65% of patients progress to fibrostenosis.

Ulcerative Endobronchial TB

Ulcerative endobronchial TB is characterised by the presence of ulcers in the tracheobronchial tree. The prognosis is generally good as most of the cases will completely resolve within three months of treatment.

Fibrostenotic Endobronchial TB

In firbostenotic endobronchial TB, marked narrowing of the bronchial lumen due to fibrosis is seen and patients show no response to treatment. Progression of fibrosis, despite treatment, may result in complete obstruction of the bronchial lumen two or three months after treatment.

Tumourous Endobronchial TB

Tumorous endobronchial TB is characterised by the presence of an endobronchial mass whose surface is often covered

with caseous material. This endobronchial mass may occlude the bronchial lumen and is frequently mistaken for lung cancer. The prognosis of tumourous endobronchial TB is grave and the most unpredictable; 70% of patients in this report had fibrostenosis at the end of treatment. More tumourous lesions can appear subsequently at different segmental bronchi.

The above classification closely correlates to the microscopic changes seen in endobronchial TB. Non-specific bronchitic endobronchial TB corresponds to the initial lesion, which presents as simple erythema and oedema of the mucosa with lymphocytic infiltration of the submucosa. This is followed by submucosal tubercle formation, which produces the erythema, granularity and partial bronchial stenosis seen at bronchoscopy caused by considerable congestion and oedema of the mucosa. These represent the granular and oedematous-hyperaemic type, respectively. With more progressive disease, caseous necrosis with formation of TB granulomas at the mucosal surface is seen and constitutes the actively caseating endobronchial TB. When the inflammation progresses through the mucosa, an ulcer, which may be covered by caseous material, is formed and this represents the ulcerative class. Finally, the bronchial mucosal ulcer may evolve into hyperplastic inflammatory polyps, and the endobronchial TB lesion heals by fibrostenosis, explaining the next two stages seen on bronchoscopy.

On rare occasions, TB lymph nodes may rupture into a bronchus (87). In the early stage, the lymph node may be seen as a greyish-yellow mass protruding through the mucosa sometimes obstructing the lumen. The bronchial wall may show haemorrhage and granulation tissue formation.

A fistula may subsequently develop in the bronchial wall with caseous material protrusion. The mucous membrane then becomes less inflamed and evacuation of the node occurs. The opening then gradually closes and fibrosis with scarring of the bronchial wall followed by bronchial stenosis may subsequently develop. Perforation of a lymph node into the lumen of a bronchus may present as a pigmented mass or stenotic bronchus with black pigmentation overlying the mucosa (11,45,51,53,88,89). This pigmentation is likely from the anthracotic material in lymph nodes and has been termed "anthracofibrosis" (89). Chung *et al* (89) demonstrated that 60% of patients whose bronchoscopy showed bronchial narrowing and black pigmentation had active TB. Endobronchial TB should be strongly considered when such findings are encountered on bronchoscopy.

All forms of endobronchial TB lie between the two ends of the spectrum of healing and fibrostenosis. Actively caseating, oedematous hyperaemic, and the granular subtypes are the most common (19). Different subtypes can be seen in the same patient and one subtype may transform into another except the fibrostenotic subtype (90). The extent of disease progression (14), formation of granulation tissue (11) and innate factors are important determinants of the different forms and outcome. Elevation of interferon-gamma [IFN-γ], transforming growth factor-beta [TGF-β] levels and increased metalloproteinase-1 activity is associated with increased risk of fibrosis and stenosis in endobronchial TB (91,92). Bronchial stenosis is inevitable in the presence of progressive disease. Therefore, prompt diagnosis including timely bronchoscopy and efficacious treatment are of paramount importance in order to minimise the progression to bronchial stenosis. The concern of worsening of TB and asphyxiation as a result of aspiration of caseous particles to opposite lung as a result of bronchoscopy should not be a limiting factor to perform a bronchoscopy. These complications have not been described recently despite the large number of bronchoscopies performed on such individuals (10,16). The importance appropriate air-borne precautions for TB while performing bronchoscopy cannot be overemphasised.

In addition to type of lesions founding bronchoscopy, additional risk factors for progression of bronchostenosis include age greater than 45 years and initiation of anti-TB treatment more than 90 days after initial symptoms (93,94).

Bronchography

Bronchography was once used for the definitive diagnosis and preoperative evaluation of bronchial stenosis (29,95). However, with improved CT imaging, this procedure is rarely performed now.

DIFFERENTIAL DIAGNOSIS

Prompt diagnosis requires a high-index of suspicion. Several cases can be misdiagnosed as bronchial asthma in the initial course (35). Endobronchial TB can imitate presentation of foreign body aspiration in children. Presence of an endobronchial mass should always raise the suspicion

of malignancy or TB coexisting with malignancy (96), atypical mycobacterium (97-103), sarcoidosis (104), actinomycosis (105) and papillomatosis (106). Presence of airway stenosis may be seen in other conditions. Focal stenosis may be a result of previous endotracheal intubation, or various systemic diseases that may involve the airways such as Crohn's disease and Behçet's syndrome (106). Diffuse stenosis of the central airways may be seen in Wegener's granulomatosis, relapsing polychondritis, tracheobronchopathia osteochondroplastica, amyloidosis, papillomatosis, and rhinoscleroma (106). Anthracofibrosis, typically described in non-smoking elderly woman exposed to biomass fuel, can also cause airway stenosis along with anthracotic pigmentation in the airway and peribronchial lymphadenopathy (89,107). Anthracofibrosis can pose as a diagnostic challenge as it can co-exist with TB and anthracotic airway pigmentation can also be seen in endobronchial TB. Bronchiostenosis due to anthracofibrosis usually involves multiple lobar or segmental bronchi and unlike endobronchial TB spares the central airways (107).

SPECIAL SITUATIONS

Lower Lung Field Tuberculosis

TB involving the right middle lobe, lingular division of left upper lobe and both lower lobes (108,109) occurs in 1%-7% of patients with pulmonary TB. It is more commonly seen in patients with diabetes mellitus, pregnancy, chronic renal disease and malignancies. Endobronchial involvement has been reported in up to 75% of these patients (108-114). Therefore, there should be a low threshold to perform a bronchoscopic examination in such patients. The reader is referred to the chapter *"Lower lung field tuberculosis"* [*Chapter 11*] for details.

Children

Endobronchial TB in children is a part of spectrum of primary TB. The incidence is high due to mediastinal lymph node involvement in primary TB and is reported to be 40%-60% (115-117). Lymph node erosion and subsequent drainage into the bronchus can spread infection and result in similar endobronchial findings as described in adult airways. Endobronchial TB can cause lobar collapse due to extrinsic compression (118) and can also masquerade foreign body aspiration (49,119). The most common finding on bronchoscopy is external bronchial compression followed by other similar lesions described in adults. Addition of gastric lavage sampling to bronchoscopy improves diagnostic yield (116). Small double-blinded studies of corticosteroid treatment in childhood endobronchial TB have shown a favourable response in the steroid treated group (120-122).

Elderly

At least 15% of elderly patients with pulmonary TB have concomitant endobronchial TB, although this is likely still an underestimation (33). Many of these cases are diagnosed during a work-up for lung cancer, or non-resolving pneumonia and delay in diagnosis is not uncommon (33,51,123). The pathogenesis of endobronchial TB in the elderly is considered to be similar as in other age groups. Cough is the most commonly observed symptom. Other symptoms, such as, dyspnoea, haemoptysis, chest pain and hoarseness of voice may be present. Constitutional symptoms, such as anorexia, weight loss and fatigue are usually present in most patients. In one series (124), almost 75% of the patients with right middle lobe syndrome due to endobronchial TB were elderly. Endobronchial findings on bronchoscopy are similar to those described in younger subjects. Bronchial stenosis occurs in about 60% of elderly patients with endobronchial TB (33).

Pregnancy

The hormonal and vascular changes in pregnancy result in airway oedema and increase secretions. This can unmask or worsen symptoms of airway stenosis. A recent report (125) describes a woman with asymptomatic post-tubercular tracheobronchial stenosis who became progressively symptomatic during pregnancy. Heliox was used due to the perceived high risk of airway interventions in late pregnancy and the patient underwent successful caesarean section under spinal anaesthesia. Heliox is a mixture of 79% helium and 21% oxygen and has lower density than room air and results in laminar flow and decreased airway resistance and thus, lower work of breathing. Patient's symptoms improved to baseline after delivery without any airway intervention. The hormonal changes of pregnancy may unmask underlying airway stenosis. Airway intervention should preferably be performed earlier in pregnancy as changes of pregnancy and the process of labour increases the work of breathing considerably.

Human Immunodeficiency Virus Infection

Endobronchial TB is not uncommon in patients with human immunodeficiency virus [HIV] infection. In one study (126), 6 out of 25 HIV-positive patients with TB had endobronchial TB on bronchoscopy. Endobronchial TB may be a part of primary infection in patients with HIV and hilar and mediastinal lymphadenopathy is commonly seen on chest radiograph (126-129). Other radiological findings described in these patients include a normal chest radiograph, a miliary pattern and a small pleural effusion. Pulmonary infiltrates are rare (126). The findings on bronchoscopy are similar to those observed in HIV-negative patients, although, the tumorous form has been more commonly reported (126-128) likely because the erosion of a lymph node into a bronchus causes the tumourous form. Lymph node perforation into the airway in HIV-associated TB has also been described by bronchoscopy (126,129). Progressive bronchostenosis was not reported in HIV-associated endobronchial TB (126,128). The differential diagnosis of endobronchial lesions in patients with HIV can be extensive including Kaposi's sarcoma, bacillary angiomatosis, lung cancer, lymphoma

and opportunistic infections including bacterial, viral and atypical mycobacterial infections (130).

Immune Reconstitution Inflammatory Syndrome

The immune reconstitution inflammatory syndrome [IRIS] is the paradoxical worsening of symptoms or appearance of new symptoms in immune compromised patients after restoration of immune functions due to therapy. The host's reinstated ability to mount an inflammatory response unmasks the subclinical manifestations and unabated inflammation results in multi-organ symptoms. Pulmonary manifestations include increasing mediastinal lymphadenopathy [with purulent aspirate and negative cultures for TB], pleural effusions, worsening pulmonary infiltrates and recurrent respiratory symptoms (131). IRIS is typically described in HIV patients with concomitant TB infection who get started on antiretroviral therapy, thus, resulting in improvement in immune functions (131-134). It is also reported in HIV patients with atypical mycobacterial infections and in patients without HIV including patients with TB, leprosy, solid organ transplant recipients, women after pregnancy, neutropenic patients and those on tumour necrosis factor [TNF] antagonists after restoration of immune function (135). Treatment is generally supportive and sometimes non-steroidal anti-inflammatory agents or corticosteroids are used. Endobronchial extension of inflammed mediastinal inflammatory lymph node due to IRIS in HIV positive patient with TB has been well documented in a recent case report (136). Similarly endobronchial lesions due to IRIS in TB patients without HIV have been described (137,138).

South-East Asian and Indian Experience

Several case reports and few case series have been published describing endobronchial TB in Indian adults (139-143). A study of bronchoscopic evaluation of 85 Indian children with active TB reported 9.4% prevalence of endobronchial TB in this cohort (144). Another series from Chandigarh, described 24 patients most of whom underwent bronchoscopy due to suspicion of malignancy (145). Two-thirds of these patients had right bronchial tree involvement and three patients had left vocal cord paralysis. All patients clinically improved with anti-TB treatment although follow up bronchoscopy was not done. In another older series, 42% of the 50 patients with lower lobe TB from a sanatorium in Amritsar were thought to have endobronchial TB based on clinical and radiographic findings, although it was confirmed in 5 out the 13 patients who underwent a bronchoscopic examination. In a study (146) assessing the usefulness of bronchioalveolar lavage in the diagnosis of sputum smear-negative pulmonary TB from New Delhi, endobronchial TB was not described in any of the 50 adult HIV-negative patients. A recent study of bronchoscopic evaluation of immigrants to Canada with diagnosis of TB revealed significant higher prevalence of associated anthracofibrosis in patients from Indian subcontinent as compared to other Asian countries [50% *versus* 3.7%; p<0.001] (147).

Endobronchial Involvement by Nontuberculous Mycobacteria

Endobronchial involvement with nontuberculous myco-bacteria is rare and mostly seen in patients with HIV (97-103). Most cases respond to therapy without any residual stenosis.

TREATMENT

Before the introduction of streptomycin and para-amino-salicyclic acid [PAS] for clinical use, the treatment of endobronchial TB lesions involved painting the small ulcers directly with caustic soda or silver nitrate to enhance fibrosis (3,148). These methods, however, caused more fibrosis due to their effect on the surrounding normal tissue (3,148). Salkin *et al* (27) demonstrated that many of the endobronchial TB ulcers heal when the parenchymal disease is adequately treated. Effective drug therapy and preventive measures have altered the natural history of endobronchial TB (149,150). A high clinical index of suspicion and prompt bronchoscopy are essential for the early diagnosis of this condition as it can present several years after the actual treatment of pulmonary TB (54,55,151).

Treatment options currently available for patients with endobronchial TB are described below.

Anti-TB Treatment

Chemotherapy of endobronchial TB is similar to that used for treatment of pulmonary TB. The reader is referred to the chapter *"Treatment of tuberculosis" [Chapter 44]* for details. Cases of endobronchial TB in patients with multidrug-resistant organisms have been reported only on rare occasion (83). The addition of inhaled streptomycin (150,152,153) and inhaled isoniazid (154) to the standard therapy has been reported to improve outcomes in some studies but their efficacy in large randomised, blinded trials has not yet been evaluated. Similarly efficacy of bronchoscopic injection of isoniazid and amikacin along with cryotherapy has been described in few cases of endobronchial TB (155,156) but need further validation with properly designed clinical trials.

Corticosteroids

Corticosteroids have used empirically with anti-TB medi-cations in some cases to prevent bronchial stenosis (10,12,19). Lee and colleagues (12) felt that corticosteroids may suppress the barking cough but may not alter the course of the disease or prevent bronchostenosis. Hypersensitivity reaction associated with anti-TB treatment is another situation where corticosteroid therapy may be beneficial (48,157,158). Local endoscopic injection of corticosteroids in endobronchial TB lesions with benefit has been described in one case report (159). Another group has advocated use of aerosolised streptomycin and dexamethasone for preventing progression of ulcerative endobronchial TB to fibrostenosis based on a small study with comparison to retrospective controls (153,160,161).

Some studies have suggested a positive role for corti-costeroid therapy in children with lymph node TB causing bronchial obstruction (120-122). However, the benefit of corticosteroids in this situation remains speculative (10,15,93) and a randomised trial in adults with endobronchial TB failed to show any beneficial effects from corticosteroid therapy (162). As of now, there is not enough evidence to suggest routine use of corticosteroids in endobronchial TB.

Bronchoscopic Modalities

A variety of bronchoscopic modalities are helpful in relieving airway stenosis if used alone or in combination with anti-TB treatment depending on the clinical situation in symptomatic patients. These techniques are useful in patients who are not surgical candidates due to comorbidities or have stenosis in both lungs or have multiple areas of stenosis or sometimes when an emergent airway intervention is needed. Due to advances and wider availability of interventional pulmonary techniques, the recent literature on endobronchial TB has focused significantly on these modalities (47,163-166). These modalities are briefly discussed below.

Mechanical Dilatation

Dilatation of the narrowed airway can be achieved with the barrel of a rigid bronchoscope or sequentially with the use of dilators, bougienage or balloons [balloon bronchoplasty]. A rigid scope can also help in securing the airway in emergent situation. Bougienage imparts a shearing force to airway wall as compared to radial force of balloon dilatation and causes more airway trauma (167). Balloon dilatation produces less mucosal trauma and granulation tissue as compared to the rigid scope (168). Balloon dilatation has been described successfully in cases of airway stenosis due to endobronchial TB (164,167,169,170). Balloon dilatation is usually successful when the stenotic segment is short (167,171). In general, the primary and secondary patency rates in benign strictures are low (163,172) and repeated dilatation of the stenotic segment are required. Balloon dilatation is mostly helpful to dilate a stenotic airway for stent placement. Potential complications of balloon bronchoplasty include airway malacia, airway laceration and sometimes rupture, bleeding, pneumothorax and pneumomediastinum (172-174).

Debulking

Debulking of tissue obstructing the airway can be achieved by using a rigid bronchoscope to core the tissue. Curettage with forceps during bronchoscopy for the removal of the pseudomembrane has been described (12).

Thermal Debulking Using Electrocautery and Argon Plasma Coagulation

Electrocautery uses an electric current to generate heat and destroy tissue while *argon plasma coagulation* [APC] causes superficial coagulative necrosis caused by ionised argon plasma. APC has minimal risk of airway perforation and also achieves excellent haemostasis. These modalities have to be used with caution in patients with pacemakers.

The fractional of inspired oxygen should be less than 40% to avoid airway fire. Effective use of APC in improving symptomatic obstruction has been described in few series of endobronchial TB (164,175).

Thermal Debulking Using Lasers

Lasers also use thermal energy for tissue destruction. The commonly used lasers are neodymium-yttrium aluminium garnet [Nd-YAG] or carbon dioxide [CO_2] laser. The Nd-YAG laser is preferred as it can achieve tissue vaporisation along with coagulation (172). CO_2 laser is a better cutting tool but has limited ability to coagulate tissue. Similar to APC and electrocautery, the fractional of inspired oxygen should be less than 40% to avoid airway fire during laser treatment. Several precautions including wearing protective eyeglasses specific to the laser being used are required. Thermal debulking therapies should not be attempted when the obstruction is purely extrinsic and caution should be exercised when using them to destroy and remove tissue in the vicinity of major blood vessels. Re-expansion of a segment collapsed for more than four weeks (83,176) or segment with chronic damage like bronchiectasis and parenchymal calcification (177) is typically not beneficial. Nd-YAG (47,163,164,166,178,179) and CO_2 laser (180,181) have been used to relieve stenosis in endobronchial TB although most of the data are about successful use of Nd-YAG laser.

Bronchoscopic Cryotherapy

Bronchoscopic cryotherapy involves a contact cryoprobe that utilises repeated freeze-thaw cycles for tissue destruction. It is comparatively safe as the fibrous tissue and cartilage are cryoresistant, thus minimising the risk of airway perforation (168). It is helpful in achieving haemostasis and there is no risk of airway fires. However effect is slow and usually a repeat clean-out procedure is needed. Few reports have descried favourable use of cryotherapy in cases of stenosis due to endobronchial TB (182,183). Recently, spray cryotherapy has been introduced that uses liquid nitrogen spray as a cryogen which comes in direct contact with tissue and delivers significant more energy than the catheter cryoprobe and causes immediate cell death without any risk of damage to deeper tissue (172). Spray cryotherapy use in the context of endobronchial TB has not yet been studied.

Airway Stents

Airway stents are tubular prosthesis placed in the airways to maintain patency of the airway. The stents also support weakened cartilage and can also close a airway fistula due to TB (164). Three main types of stents are available: metal stents, silicon stents and hybrid stents [covered metal stents].

Silicon stent Placement of silicon stent requires rigid bronchoscopy and has a higher migration rate but is easier to remove. Frequent bronchoscopic procedures for replacement may be needed. They seem to be the most successful stents in cases of endobronchial TB.

Metal stents Metal stents are relatively easier to place but are hard to extract. Granulation tissue can grow through spaces between metal struts. A review of 25 patients who underwent metal stent placement showed frequent complications at the time of removal including retained metal pieces, mucosal tear with bleeding, re-obstruction, tension pneumothorax and respiratory failure requiring mechanical ventilation (184). Similarly another study of 10 patients with benign strictures reported frequent occurrence of granulation tissue, one case of new subglottic stricture due to stent and a case each of broncho-pleural and tracheal-oesophageal fistula (185). Some patients who were deemed surgical prior to stent placement become non-operable. These complications have prompted a black-box warning from the United States Food and Drug Administration [FDA] in 2005, and thus, metal stents should be avoided in benign airway stenosis (186).

Hybrid stents Hybrid stents have a membrane covering the metallic cross-filaments and this avoids granulation ingrowth. They can be placed using flexible bronchoscopy, are easier to remove compared to uncovered metallic stents but have a higher migration rate. Just like other stents, mucous plugging remains a significant problem requiring repeat bronchoscopy procedures and sometimes stent replacement. They may have higher rate of complications necessitating removal in benign disease (187) although further studies are needed to evaluate their exact role in endobronchial TB.

The stents come in various sizes and shapes including the carinal Y-stent depending on the location of the lesion. Stents are most beneficial in trachea or main-stem bronchi although rarely stenting of subsegments has been described. There is a significant body of literature showing utility of silicone stents in endobronchial TB (47,164,170,188-190). Metal stents have been attempted (191) but do not fare comparatively well (164) and should be avoided (184). Successful placement of Y-stents (179) and Montgomery T-stent (192) have been described to alleviate symptoms of airway obstruction in cases of endobronchial TB in carina and long segmental tracheal stenosis.

A recent study of 17 patients with post-TB silicone stent placement showed that patients tolerated these stents well for long period [range 3-11 years] but the granulation tissue formation rate was 76%, migration rate was 70% and mucostasis rate was 17% (166). A total of 132 stents were inserted over 23 site requiring 1-32 rigid bronchoscopies [median 11] and 1-12 [median 3] flexible bronchoscopies showing that this is extremely health care resource intensive management. Other studies have reported slightly lower rate of complications *albeit* the rate is still high: granulation tissue 65%, migration 52% and mucostasis rate of 18% (83). Multi-detector row spiral computed tomography [MDCT] can be useful non-invasive method of detecting stent complications and reducing the number of invasive procedures (193).

Removal of a stent is another complex issue. The ideal time to remove an airway stent in endobronchial TB is not known. The stents are usually left in place for 6-18 months in cases of benign stenosis allowing the stenotic area to mature and stiffen (163,165). Stent should be removed when the stenotic segment has adequately healed to allow airway patency after stent removal. However, it is hard to determine when the stenosis has regressed. Stent removal can fail in 44%-76% of patients with endobronchial TB (83,165). Bronchoscopic features that can be used to make determination about stent removal include: improvement of mucosal inflammation, stabilization of wall at end of stents, loosening of device suggesting dilatation of airway lumen and stent dislocation due to loosening without residual stenosis (194). Non-invasive methods include measuring the length of air pockets between the outer wall of stent and tracheo-bronchial tree on a 3-D CT can be helpful as longer length of air pocket suggests improvement of stenosis (165). Damage to underlying cartilage as seen by radial probe ultrasound may suggest difficulty in stent removal (164). A recent analysis showed that absence of complete lobar collapse at presentation and bronchoscopic intervention within less than one month of atelectasis were associated with successful stent removal (83) at 6-12 months of clinical stabilization and this should be kept in mind at the time of stent placement and removal.

Endobronchial Ultrasound

Endobronchial ultrasound [EBUS] has been a revolution in the field of interventional pulmonary medicine. The curvilinear ultrasound is very useful in obtaining lymph node samples while the radial probe ultrasound with balloon is useful for visualizing the layers of the airway wall (164,195). The radial EBUS can show destruction of airway cartilage, which can aid in the decision to place a stent, as cases with damaged cartilage will not stay open just after dilatation or local debulking.

Special Situation: Endobronchial Tuberculosis without Critical Stenosis

Another group of patients that has received attention recently is the group that does not have a critical airway obstruction at presentation. Early intervention in this group is being advocated since a significant proportion of these patients eventually develop airway stenosis. Jin *et al* (196) demonstrated that utilizing APC with anti-TB treatment in patients with non-obstructive tumorous endobronchial TB accelerated the healing of lesions and prevented progressive airway stenosis as compared to similar patients who received anti-TB treatment alone. Similar benefit of cryotherapy along with anti-TB treatment was described in granular endobronchial TB (94).

Surgery

In the early part of last century, collapse therapy by inducing a pneumothorax, phrenic nerve paralysis or thoracoplasty [surgical removal of several rib bones from the chest wall in order to collapse a lung] for pulmonary TB was commonly performed. Endobronchial TB was noted to be an exception for the above procedures due to the high incidence of subsequent atelectasis, unexpandable lungs, empyaema and anaerobic infections (197). Pneumonectomy and lobectomy were commonly performed for endobronchial TB in the past, but became unpopular because of high operative mortality of about 27% (197). Recently, new surgical techniques have evolved and several series report very low mortality when resection along with surgical bronchoplasty [sleeve resection with end-to-end anastomosis] is done (198-203).

Surgery should ideally be performed when the patient is no longer considered to have active disease (202). Resection of lung parenchyma should be minimal, as the objective of the surgery is to restore pulmonary function to the hypo-ventilated lung. The mode of operation is determined by the location, extent and degree of stenosis (202). For lesions involving lobar or segmental bronchi, lobectomy may need to be performed. For lesion involving the trachea or main stem bronchus, bronchoplastic surgery along with lobectomy [if needed] is performed. Pneumonectomy should be left as the last resort when the involved lung has extensive bronchiectasis/damage from recurrent infections or when the main-stem bronchus is completely obliterated (203). Restenosis at the site of anastomosis may occur and repeated bronchoscopic dilatation may be needed (202). The reader is also referred to the chapter *"Surgery for pleuropulmonary TB"* [Chapter 46] for details on this topic.

MULTIDISCIPLINARY MULTIMODALITY MANAGEMENT

While most of the experts clearly feel that the prevalence of endobronchial component in pulmonary TB is high and a prompt diagnosis and management of endobronchial TB can prevent serious sequelae (19,90,204-211), yet there is no clear evidence to recommend routine bronchoscopy for all patients with pulmonary TB. There is also concern of significant risk of nosocomial spread of TB during bronchoscopy (32,212). The current approach is to perform bronchoscopy in TB suspect patients if they have three negative smears or if patients with diagnosed TB has intractable symptoms suggesting airway stenosis like refractory cough, localised wheezing, persistent or worsening dyspnoea, diminished breath sounds or radiographic evidence of atelectasis/collapse or tracheo-bronchial involvement or lack of clinical or radiological response to anti-TB treatment (90). Some of these clinical symptoms and findings are encountered late in course of endobronchial TB and timely treatment is not possible. Furthermore, even with timely anti-TB treatment, a significant proportion of patients have progression of endobronchial TB (11,12,15), thus needing airway interventions. Close surveillance, radiographic monitoring and timely bronchoscopic assessment of such patients is very important. A multidisciplinary team with expertise in multiple modalities is ideal for management of such complex patients. Patient factors, initial clinical presentation and findings [location, duration, degree and length of stenosis], local expertise and availability of equipment, determine the preferable method of management. Surgery, when possible is the desired modality but a significant proportion of patients may not be surgical candidates. Bronchoscopic interventions provide a valuable alternative but usually require multiple procedures as discussed above. MDCT can be very useful for initial evaluation, directing therapy including size of stents and recognizing procedural complications. Close coordination between interventional pulmonologist, radiologists, thoracic surgeons and infectious disease/TB specialist could be invaluable in appropriate management and follow-up of patients with endobronchial TB.

REFERENCES

1. Morton R. Phthisiologica, Seu Exercitationes de Phthisi. London: S Smith; 1689.
2. Cohen AG, Wessler H. Clinical recognition of tuberculosis of major bronchi. Arch Intern Med 1939;63:1132-57.
3. Smart J. Endo-bronchial tuberculosis. Br J Tuberc Dis Chest 1951;45:61-8.
4. Wilson NJ. Bronchoscopic observations in tuberculosis tracheobronchitis. Dis Chest 1945;11:36-59.
5. Danek SJ, Bower JS. Diagnosis of pulmonary tuberculosis by flexible fiberoptic bronchoscopy. Am Rev Respir Dis 1979;119: 677-9.
6. Jett JR, Cortese DA, Dines DE. The value of bronchoscopy in the diagnosis of mycobacterial disease. A five-year experience. Chest 1981;80:575-8.
7. Wallace JM, Deutsch AL, Harrell JH, Moser KM. Bronchoscopy and transbronchial biopsy in evaluation of patients with suspected active tuberculosis. Am J Med 1981;70:1189-94.
8. Willcox PA, Benatar SR, Potgieter PD. Use of the flexible fibreoptic bronchoscope in diagnosis of sputum-negative pulmonary tuberculosis. Thorax 1982;37:598-601.
9. Stenson W, Aranda C, Bevelaqua FA. Transbronchial biopsy culture in pulmonary tuberculosis. Chest 1983;83:883-4.
10. Ip MS, So SY, Lam WK, Mok CK. Endobronchial tuberculosis revisited. Chest 1986;89:727-30.
11. Smith LS, Schillaci RF, Sarlin RF. Endobronchial tuberculosis. Serial fiberoptic bronchoscopy and natural history. Chest 1987;91:644-7.
12. Lee JH, Park SS, Lee DH, Shin DH, Yang SC, Yoo BM. Endobronchial tuberculosis. Clinical and bronchoscopic features in 121 cases. Chest 1992;102:990-4.
13. Kurasawa T, Kuze F, Kawai M, Amitani R, Murayama T, Tanaka E, et al. Diagnosis and management of endobronchial tuberculosis. Intern Med 1992;31:593-8.
14. Kim YH, Kim HT, Lee KS, Uh ST, Cung YT, Park CS. Serial fiberoptic bronchoscopic observations of endobronchial tuberculosis before and early after antituberculosis chemotherapy. Chest 1993;103:673-7.
15. Hoheisel G, Chan BK, Chan CH, Chan KS, Teschler H, Costabel U. Endobronchial tuberculosis: diagnostic features and therapeutic outcome. Respir Med 1994;88:593-7.
16. Wang SY, Zhang XS. Endobronchial tuberculosis. Report of 102 cases. Chest 1994;105:1910-1.
17. Masotti A, Rodella L, Inaspettato G, Foccoli P, Morandini GC. Clinical and bronchoscopic features of endobronchial tuberculosis. Monaldi Arch Chest Dis 1995;50:89-92.
18. Altin S, Cikrikcioglu S, Morgul M, Kosar F, Ozyurt H. 50 endobronchial tuberculosis cases based on bronchoscopic diagnosis. Respiration 1997;64:162-4.
19. Chung HS, Lee JH. Bronchoscopic assessment of the evolution of endobronchial tuberculosis. Chest 2000;117:385-92.
20. Lee JH, Chung HS. Bronchoscopic, radiologic and pulmonary function evaluation of endobronchial tuberculosis. Respirology. 2000;5:411-7.
21. Ozkaya S, Bilgin S, Findik S, Kok HC, Yuksel C, Atici AG. Endobronchial tuberculosis: histopathological subsets and microbiological results. Multidiscip Respir Med 2012;7:34.
22. Miguel Campos E, Puzo Ardanuy C, Burgues Mauri C, Castella Riera J. A study of 73 cases of bronchial tuberculosis. Arch Bronconeumol 2008;44:282-4.
23. Qingliang X, Jianxin W. Investigation of endobronchial tuberculosis diagnoses in 22 cases. Eur J Med Res 2010;15:309-13.
24. Flance IJ, Wheeler PA. Postmortem incidence of tuberculous tracheobronchitis. Am Rev Tuberc 1939;39:633-6.
25. Sweany HC, Behm H. Tuberculosis of trachea and major bronchi. Dis Chest 1948;14:1-18.
26. Auerbach O. Tuberculosis of the trachea and major bronchi. Am Rev Tuberc 1949;60:604-20.
27. Salkin D, Cadden AV, Edson RC. The natural history of tuberculosis tracheobronchitis. Am Rev Tuberc 1943;47:351-69.
28. McIndoe RB, Steele JD, Samson PC, Anderson RS, Leslie GL. Routine bronchoscopy in patients with pulmonary tuberculosis. Am Rev Tuberc 1939;39: 617-28.
29. Jokinen K, Palva T, Nuutinen J. Bronchial findings in pulmonary tuberculosis. Clin Otolaryngol Allied Sci 1977;2:139-48.
30. So SY, Lam WK, Yu DY. Rapid diagnosis of suspected pulmonary tuberculosis by fiberoptic bronchoscopy. Tubercle 1982;63: 195-200.
31. Soni R, Barnes D, Torzillo P. Post-obstructive pneumonia secondary to endobronchial tuberculosis–an institutional review. Aust NZ J Med 1999;29:841-2.
32. Jensen PA, Lambert LA, Iademarco MF, Ridzon R. Guidelines for preventing the transmission of Mycobacterium tuberculosis in health-care settings, 2005. MMWR Recomm Rep 2005;54:1-141.
33. Van den Brande PM, Van de Mierop F, Verbeken EK, Demedts M. Clinical spectrum of endobronchial tuberculosis in elderly patients. Arch Intern Med 1990;150:2105-8.
34. Stone MJ. Clinical aspects of endobronchial tuberculosis. Dis Chest 1945;11:60-71.
35. Shim YS. Endobronchial tuberculosis. Respirology 1996;1:95-106.
36. Dhillon SS, Watanakunakorn C. Lady Windermere syndrome: middle lobe bronchiectasis and Mycobacterium avium complex infection due to voluntary cough suppression. Clin Infect Dis 2000;30:572-5.
37. Reich JM, Johnson RE. Mycobacterium avium complex pulmonary disease presenting as an isolated lingular or middle lobe pattern. The Lady Windermere syndrome. Chest 1992;101:1605-9.
38. Reichle HS, Frost TT. Tuberculosis of the major bronchi. Am J Pathol 1934;10: 651-63.
39. Tetikkurt C, Tetikkurt S, Bayat N, Ozdemir I. Endobronchial involvement in miliary tuberculosis. Pneumon 2010;23:135-40.
40. Jones EM, Rafferty TN, Willis HS. Primary tuberculosis complicated by bronchial tuberculosis with atelectasis. Trans Am Clin Climatol Assoc 1941;57:102-6.
41. Frostad S. Lymph node perforation through the bronchial tree in children with primary tuberculosis. Acta Tuberc Scan 1959; 47 Suppl:104-24.
42. Chang SC, Lee PY, Perng RP. Clinical role of bronchoscopy in adults with intrathoracic tuberculous lymphadenopathy. Chest 1988;93:314-7.
43. Baran R, Tor M, Tahaoglu K, Ozvaran K, Kir A, Kizkin O, Turker H. Intrathoracic tuberculous lymphadenopathy: clinical and bronchoscopic features in 17 adults without parenchymal lesions. Thorax 1996;51:87-9.
44. Schwartz P. The role of the lymphatics in the development of bronchogenic tuberculosis. Am Rev Tuberc 1953;67:440-52.

45. Arnstein A. Non-industrial pneumoconiosis, pneumoconio-tuberculosis and tuberculosis of the mediastinal and bronchial lymph glands in old people. Tubercle 1941;22:281-95.

46. Eloesser L. Bronchial stenosis in pulmonary tuberculosis. Am Rev Tuberc 1934;30:123-80.

47. Low SY, Hsu A, Eng P. Interventional bronchoscopy for tuberculous tracheobronchial stenosis. Eur Respir J 2004;24:345-7.

48. Williams DJ, York EL, Nobert EJ, Sproule BJ. Endobronchial tuberculosis presenting as asthma. Chest 1988;93:836-8.

49. Caglayan S, Coteli I, Acar U, Erkin S. Endobronchial tuberculosis simulating foreign body aspiration. Chest 1989;95:1164.

50. Matthews JI, Matarese SL, Carpenter JL. Endobronchial tuberculosis simulating lung cancer. Chest 1984;86:642-4.

51. Van den Brande P, Lambrechts M, Tack J, Demedts M. Endobronchial tuberculosis mimicking lung cancer in elderly patients. Respir Med 1991;85:107-9.

52. Lynch JP, Ravikrishnan KP. Endobronchial mass caused by tuberculosis. Arch Intern Med 1980;140:1090-1.

53. Yee A, Hardwick JA, Wasef E, Sharma OP. Pigmented polypoid obstructive endobronchial tuberculosis. Chest 1985;87:702-3.

54. Albert RK, Petty TL. Endobronchial tuberculosis progressing to bronchial stenosis. Fiberoptic bronchoscopic manifestations. Chest 1976;70:537-9.

55. Ito M, Yasuo M, Nakamura M, Tsushima K, Yamazaki Y, Kubo K. A case of tuberculous bronchial stenosis, diagnosed after 50 years of pulmonary and laryngeal tuberculosis. Nihon Kokyuki Gakkai Zasshi 2007;45:87-90.

56. So SY, Lam WK, Sham MK. Bronchorrhea. A presenting feature of active endobronchial tuberculosis. Chest 1983;84:635-6.

57. Park MJ, Woo IS, Son JW, Lee SJ, Kim DG, Mo EK, et al. Endobronchial tuberculosis with expectoration of tracheal cartilages. Eur Respir J 2000;15:800-2.

58. Memon AM, Shafi A, Thawerani H. Endobronchial tuberculosis-manifesting by coughing up of bronchial cartilage. J Pak Med Assoc 1996;46:86-8.

59. Yilmaz E, Akkoclu A, Sevinc C. CT and MRI appearance of a fistula between the right and left main bronchus caused by tracheobronchial tuberculosis. Br J Radiol 2001;74:1056-8.

60. Nemati A, Safavi E, GhasemiEsfe M, Anaraki MZ, Firoozbakhsh S, Khalilzadeh O, et al. Fistula formation between the right and left main bronchus caused by endobronchial tuberculosis. Am J Med Sci 2012;343:330-1.

61. Pornsuriyasak P, Murgu S, Colt H. Pseudomembranous aspergillus tracheobronchitis superimposed on post-tuberculosis tracheal stenosis. Respirology 2009;14:144-7.

62. Seiden HS, Thomas P. Endobronchial tuberculosis and its sequelae. Can Med Assoc J 1981;124:165-9.

63. Pierson DJ, Lakshminarayan S, Petty TL. Endobronchial tuberculosis. Chest 1973;64:537-9.

64. Volckaert A, Roels P, Van der Niepen P, Schandevyl W. Endobronchial tuberculosis: report of three cases. Eur J Respir Dis 1987;70:99-101.

65. Watson JM, Ayres JG. Tuberculous stenosis of the trachea. Tubercle 1988;69:223-6.

66. Shipman SJ. Diagnostic bronchoscopy in occult tuberculosis. Am Rev Tuberc 1939;39:629-32.

67. Golshan M. Tuberculosis bronchitis with normal chest X-ray among a large bronchoscopic population. Ann Saudi Med 2002;22:98-101.

68. Long R, Maycher B, Dhar A, Manfreda J, Hershfield E, Anthonisen N. Pulmonary tuberculosis treated with directly observed therapy: serial changes in lung structure and function. Chest 1998;113:933-43.

69. Gruden JF, Webb WR, Warnock M. Centrilobular opacities in the lung on high-resolution CT: diagnostic considerations and pathologic correlation. AJR Am J Roentgenol 1994;162:569-74.

70. Im JG, Itoh H, Shim YS, Lee JH, Ahn J, Han MC, Noma S. Pulmonary tuberculosis: CT findings—early active disease and sequential change with antituberculous therapy. Radiology 1993;186:653-60.

71. Lee KS, Kim YH, Kim WS, Hwang SH, Kim PN, Lee BH. Endobronchial tuberculosis: CT features. J Comput Assist Tomogr 1991;15:424-8.

72. Cha JH, Han J, Park HJ, Kim TS, Jung AY, Sung DW, et al. Aneurysmal appearance of medium-sized bronchi: a peripheral manifestation of endobronchial tuberculosis. AJR Am J Roentgenol 2009;193:W95-9.

73. Naidich DP, Lee JJ, Garay SM, McCauley DI, Aranda CP, Boyd AD. Comparison of CT and fiberoptic bronchoscopy in the evaluation of bronchial disease. AJR Am J Roentgenol 1987;148:1-7.

74. Kim Y, Lee KS, Yoon JH, Chung MP, Kim H, Kwon OJ, et al. Tuberculosis of the trachea and main bronchi: CT findings in 17 patients. AJR Am J Roentgenol 1997;168:1051-6.

75. Moon WK, Im JG, Yeon KM, Han MC. Tuberculosis of the central airways: CT findings of active and fibrotic disease. AJR Am J Roentgenol 1997;169:649-53.

76. Choe KO, Jeong HJ, Sohn HY. Tuberculous bronchial stenosis: CT findings in 28 cases. Am J Roentgenol 1990;155:971-6.

77. Finkelstein SE, Summers RM, Nguyen DM, Stewart JHt, Tretler JA, Schrump DS. Virtual bronchoscopy for evaluation of malignant tumors of the thorax. J Thorac Cardiovasc Surg 2002;123:967-72.

78. Lee KS, Yoon JH, Kim TK, Kim JS, Chung MP, Kwon OJ. Evaluation of tracheobronchial disease with helical CT with multiplanar and three-dimensional reconstruction: correlation with bronchoscopy. Radiographics 1997;17:555-67; discussion 568-70.

79. Rezaeetalab F, Farrokh D, Zandiee B. Multiplanar Reconstructed thoracic CT bronchoscopy in endobronchial tuberculosis. Iran J Radiol 2012;9:234-6.

80. Park CS, Kim KU, Lee SM, Jeong SW, Uh S, Kim HT, et al. Bronchial hyperreactivity in patients with endobronchial tuberculosis. Respir Med 1995;89:419-22.

81. Schmidek HH, Hardy MA. Pulmonary tuberculosis with normal chest radiographs: report of eight cases. Can Med Assoc J 1967;97:178-80.

82. Husen L, Fulkerson LL, Del Vecchio E, Zack MB, Stein E. Pulmonary tuberculosis with negative findings on chest X-ray films: a study of 40 cases. Chest 1971;60:540-2.

83. Lim SY, Park HK, Jeon K, Um SW, Koh WJ, Suh GY, et al. Factors predicting outcome following airway stenting for post-tuberculosis tracheobronchial stenosis. Respirology 2011;16:959-64.

84. Fang X, Ma B, Yang X. Bronchial tuberculosis. Cytologic diagnosis of fiberoptic bronchoscopic brushings. Acta Cytol 1997;41:1463-7.

85. Chou CL, Wang CW, Lin SM, Fang YF, Yu CT, Chen HC, et al. Role of flexible bronchoscopic cryotechnology in diagnosing endobronchial masses. Ann Thorac Surg 2013;95:982-6.

86. Rikimaru T, Kinosita M, Yano H, Ichiki M, Watanabe H, Shiraisi T, et al. Diagnostic features and therapeutic outcome of erosive and ulcerous endobronchial tuberculosis. Int J Tuberc Lung Dis 1998;2:558-62.

87. Kraan JK, Muller S. Perforation of tuberculous glands into a bronchus. Acta Tuberc Scand 1950;24:88-102.

88. Cohen AG. Atelectasis of the right middle lobe resulting from perforation of tuberculous lymph nodes into bronchi in adults. Ann Intern Med 1951;35:820-35.

89. Chung MP, Lee KS, Han J, Kim H, Rhee CH, Han YC, et al. Bronchial stenosis due to anthracofibrosis. Chest 1998;113:344-50.

90. Xue Q, Wang N, Xue X, Wang J. Endobronchial tuberculosis: an overview. Eur J Clin Microbiol Infect Dis 2011;30:1039-44.

91. Kim Y, Kim K, Joe J, Park H, Lee M, Choi Y, et al. Changes in the levels of interferon-gamma and transforming growth factor-beta influence bronchial stenosis during the treatment of endobronchial tuberculosis. Respiration 2007;74:202-7.

92. Kuo HP, Wang YM, Wang CH, He CC, Lin SM, Lin HC, et al. Matrix metalloproteinase-1 polymorphism in Taiwanese patients with endobronchial tuberculosis. Tuberculosis [Edinb] 2008;88:262-7.

93. Um SW, Yoon YS, Lee SM, Yim JJ, Yoo CG, Chung HS, et al. Predictors of persistent airway stenosis in patients with endobronchial tuberculosis. Int J Tuberc Lung Dis 2008;12:57-62.

94. Mu D, Nan D, Li W, Fu E, Xie Y, Liu T, et al. Efficacy and safety of bronchoscopic cryotherapy for granular endobronchial tuberculosis. Respiration 2011;82:268-72.

95. Rose RM, Cardona J, Daly JF. Bronchographic sequelae of endobronchial tuberculosis. Ann Otol Rhinol Laryngol 1965;74: 1133-43.

96. Gopalakrishnan P, Miller JE, McLaughlin JS. Pulmonary tuberculosis and coexisting carcinoma: a 10-year experience and review of the literature. Am Surg 1975;41:405-8.

97. Connolly MG Jr, Baughman RP, Dohn MN. Mycobacterium kansasii presenting as an endobronchial lesion. Am Rev Respir Dis 1993;148:1405-7.

98. Quieffin J, Poubeau P, Laaban JP, Brechot JM, Capron F, Rochemaure J. Mycobacterium kansasii infection presenting as an endobronchial tumor in a patient with the acquired immune deficiency syndrome. Tuber Lung Dis 1994;75:313-5.

99. Asano T, Itoh G, Itoh M. Disseminated Mycobacterium intracellulare infection in an HIV-negative, nonimmunosuppressed patient with multiple endobronchial polyps. Respiration 2002; 69:175-7.

100. Shih JY, Wang HC, Chiang IP, Yang PC, Luh KT. Endobronchial lesions in a non-AIDS patient with disseminated Mycobacterium avium-intracellulare infection. Eur Respir J 1997;10:497-9.

101. Cordasco EM Jr, Keys T, Mehta AC, Mehle ME, Longworth DL. Spontaneous resolution of endobronchial Mycobacterium avium-intracellulare infection in a patient with AIDS. Chest 1990;98:1540-2.

102. Mehle ME, Adamo JP, Mehta AC, Wiedemann HP, Keys T, Longworth DL. Endobronchial Mycobacterium avium-intracellulare infection in a patient with AIDS. Chest 1989;96: 199-201.

103. Lambert GW, Baddour LM. Right middle lobe syndrome caused by Mycobacterium fortuitum in a patient with human immunodeficiency virus infection. South Med J 1992;85:767-9.

104. Hsu JT, Cottrell TS. Pulmonary sarcoidosis: unilateral hilar adenopathy presenting as an endobronchial tumor. Case report. Radiology 1971;98:385-6.

105. Lee SH, Shim JJ, Kang EY, Lee SY, Jo JY, In KH, et al. Endobronchial actinomycosis simulating endobronchial tuberculosis: a case report. J Korean Med Sci 1999;14:315-8.

106. Prince JS, Duhamel DR, Levin DL, Harrell JH, Friedman PJ. Nonneoplastic lesions of the tracheobronchial wall: radiologic findings with bronchoscopic correlation. Radiographics 2002;22:S215-30.

107. Park HJ, Park SH, Im SA, Kim YK, Lee KY. CT differentiation of anthracofibrosis from endobronchial tuberculosis. Am J Roentgenol 2008;191:247-51.

108. Chang SC, Lee PY, Perng RP. Lower lung field tuberculosis. Chest 1987;91:230-2.

109. Chang SC, Lee PY, Perng RP. The value of roentgenographic and fiberbronchoscopic findings in predicting outcome of adults with lower lung field tuberculosis. Arch Intern Med 1991;151:1581-3.

110. Rothstein E. Pulmonary tuberculosis involving the lower lobes. Am Rev Tuberc 1949;59:39-49.

111. Segarra F, Sherman DS, Rodriguez-Aguero J. Lower lung field tuberculosis. Am Rev Respir Dis 1963;87:37-40.

112. Parmar MS. Lower lung field tuberculosis. Am Rev Respir Dis 1967;96:310-3.

113. Pratt-Johnson JH. Observations on lower lobe tuberculosis. Br J Dis Chest 1959;53:385-9.

114. Khan MA, Kovnat DM, Bachus B, Whitcomb ME, Brody JS, Snider GL. Clinical and roentgenographic spectrum of pulmonary tuberculosis in the adult. Am J Med 1977;62:31-8.

115. de Blic J, Azevedo I, Burren CP, Le Bourgeois M, Lallemand D, Scheinmann P. The value of flexible bronchoscopy in childhood pulmonary tuberculosis. Chest 1991;100:688-92.

116. Cakir E, Uyan ZS, Oktem S, Karakoc F, Ersu R, Karadag B, et al. Flexible bronchoscopy for diagnosis and follow up of childhood endobronchial tuberculosis. Pediatr Infect Dis J 2008;27:783-7.

117. Chan S, Abadco DL, Steiner P. Role of flexible fiberoptic bronchoscopy in the diagnosis of childhood endobronchial tuberculosis. Pediatr Infect Dis J 1994;13:506-9.

118. Lincoln EM, Harris LC, Bovornkitti S, Carretero RW. Endobronchial tuberculosis in children, a study of 156 patients. Am Rev Tuberc 1958;77:39-61.

119. Park AH, Fowler SS, Challapalli M. Suspected foreign body aspiration in a child with endobronchial tuberculosis. Int J Pediatr Otorhinolaryngol 2000;53:67-71.

120. Nemir RL, Cardona J, Vaziri F, Toledo R. Prednisone as an adjunct in the chemotherapy of lymph node-bronchial tuberculosis in childhood: a double-blind study II. Further term observation. Am Rev Respir Dis 1967;95:402-10.

121. Nemir RL, Cardona J, Lacoius A, David M. Prednisone therapy as an adjunct in the treatment of lymph node-bronchial tuberculosis in childhood. A double-blind study. Am Rev Respir Dis 1963;88:189-98.

122. Toppet M, Malfroot A, Derde MP, Toppet V, Spehl M, Dab I. Corticosteroids in primary tuberculosis with bronchial obstruction. Arch Dis Child 1990;65:1222-6.

123. Burke HL, Haponik EF. Endobronchial tuberculosis in the elderly: a case report and review of the literature. J Bronchology Interv Pulmonol 1997;4:132-5.

124. Kim HC, Kim HS, Lee SJ, Jeong YY, Jeon KN, Lee JD, et al. Endobronchial tuberculosis presenting as right middle lobe syndrome: clinical characteristics and bronchoscopic findings in 22 cases. Yonsei Med J 2008;49:615-9.

125. Shojaee S, Tilluckdharry L, Manning H. Tuberculosis-induced Tracheobronchial Stenosis During Pregnancy. J Bronchology Interv Pulmonol 2012;19:211-5.

126. Calpe JL, Chiner E, Larramendi CH. Endobronchial tuberculosis in HIV-infected patients. AIDS 1995;9:1159-64.

127. Maguire GP, Delorenzo LJ, Brown RB, Davidian MM. Endobronchial tuberculosis simulating bronchogenic carcinoma in a patient with the acquired immunodeficiency syndrome. Am J Med Sci 1987;294:42-4.

128. Wasser LS, Shaw GW, Talavera W. Endobronchial tuberculosis in the acquired immunodeficiency syndrome. Chest 1988;94: 1240-4.

129. Alame T, Dierckx P, Carlier S, Sergysels R. Lymph node perforation into the airway in AIDS-associated tuberculosis. Eur Respir J 1995;8:658-60.

130. Kumar T, Epstein M, Markovskaya Y, Narasimhan M, Rosen M, Talwar A. Bronchoscopy and endobronchial disease in patients with human immunodeficiency virus infection. Indian J Chest Dis Allied Sci 2011;53:99-105.

131. Leone S, Nicastri E, Giglio S, Narciso P, Ippolito G, Acone N. Immune reconstitution inflammatory syndrome associated with Mycobacterium tuberculosis infection: a systematic review. Int J Infect Dis 2010;14:e283-91.

132. Hill AR, Mateo F, Hudak A. Transient exacerbation of tuberculous lymphadenitis during chemotherapy in patients with AIDS. Clin Infect Dis 1994;19:774-6.

133. Narita M, Ashkin D, Hollender ES, Pitchenik AE. Paradoxical worsening of tuberculosis following antiretroviral therapy in patients with AIDS. Am J Respir Crit Care Med 1998;158:157-61.

134. Breen RA, Smith CJ, Bettinson H, Dart S, Bannister B, Johnson MA, et al. Paradoxical reactions during tuberculosis treatment in patients with and without HIV co-infection. Thorax 2004;59: 704-7.

135. Sun HY, Singh N. Immune reconstitution inflammatory syndrome in non-HIV immunocompromised patients. Curr Opin Infect Dis 2009;22:394-402.

136. Steinfort DP, Smallwood D, Antippa P, Irving LB. Endobronchial extension of granulomatous lymphadenitis in an HIV-positive man with immune reconstitution syndrome. Respirology 2009; 14:1064-6.

137. Bloch S, Wickremasinghe M, Wright A, Rice A, Thompson M, Kon OM. Paradoxical reactions in non-HIV tuberculosis presenting as endobronchial obstruction. Eur Respir Rev 2009;18: 295-9.

138. Liju A, Sharma N, Milburn H. An unusual cause of bronchial obstruction. Lung India 2012;29:393-4.

139. Guleria R, Behera D, Dhaliwal RS, Jindal SK. Tracheo-bronchial stenosis–report of 3 cases. Indian J Chest Dis Allied Sci 1991;33:165-70.

140. Guleria R, Gupta R, Pande JN. Endobronchial tuberculosis simulating lung cancer. Indian J Chest Dis Allied Sci 1997;39: 251-4.

141. Gupta A, Narasimhan KL. Endobronchial tuberculosis and the surgeon. Indian Pediatr 2002;39:977.

142. Roy PP, Dey SK, Sarkar A, Dwari AK, Banerjee A, Banerjee R. Diagnosis of three cases of endobronchial tuberculosis presenting as unresolved pneumonia, following fiberoptic bronchoscopic biopsy. Lung India 2010;27:185-8.

143. Ramya I, Mathews KP, Pichamuthu K, Keshava SN, Balamugesh T, Ramamani M, et al. Endotracheal tuberculous stenosis: ventilation rescue and bronchography guided stenting. Indian J Chest Dis Allied Sci 2010;52:55-8.

144. Joshi S, Malik S, Kandoth PW. Diagnostic and therapeutic evaluation of bronchoscopy. Indian J Pediatr 1995;62:83-7.

145. Aggarwal AN, Gupta D, Joshi K, Behera D, Jindal SK. Endobronchial involvement in tuberculosis: a report of 24 cases diagnosed by flexible bronchoscopy. J Bronchology Interv Pulmonol 1999;6:247-50.

146. Mohan A, Pande JN, Sharma SK, Rattan A, Guleria R, Khilnani GC. Bronchoalveolar lavage in pulmonary tuberculosis: a decision analysis approach. QJM 1995;88:269-76.

147. Hwang J, Puttagunta L, Green F, Shimanovsky A, Barrie J, Long R. Bronchial anthracofibrosis and tuberculosis in immigrants to Canada from the Indian subcontinent. Int J Tuberc Lung Dis 2010;14:231-7.

148. Judd AR. Tuberculous tracheobronchitis: a study of 500 consecutive cases. J Thorac Surg 1947;16:512-23.

149. Medical Research Council. Streptomycin treatment of tuberculous lesions of the trachea and bronchi. Lancet 1951;1:253-7.

150. Brewer LA, 3rd, Bogen E. Streptomycin in tuberculous tracheobronchitis. Am Rev Tuberc 1947;56:408-14.

151. Tse CY, Natkunam R. Serious sequelae of delayed diagnosis of endobronchial tuberculosis. Tubercle 1988;69:213-6.

152. Rikimaru T, Tanaka Y, Ichikawa Y, Oizumi K. Endoscopic classification of tracheobronchial tuberculosis with healing processes. Chest 1994;105:318-9.

153. Rikimaru T, Koga T, Sueyasu Y, Ide S, Kinosita M, Sugihara E, et al. Treatment of ulcerative endobronchial tuberculosis and

154. Yokota S, Miki K. Effects of INH [Isoniazid] inhalation in patients with endobronchial tuberculosis [EBTB]. Kekkaku 1999;74:873-7.

155. Xu Ru J, Yuping L, Chengshui C. Interventional bronchoscopy in the management of active bronchial tuberculosis: a case report. Chest. 2012;142:879A.

156. Zhang JX, Bai C, Huang HD, Li Q, Wang Q. Bronchoscopic cryotherapy combined with drugs infusion in the treatment of transbronchial tuberculous. Zhonghua Jie He He Hu Xi Za Zhi 2011;34:898-903.

157. Chan HS, Pang JA. Effect of corticosteroids on deterioration of endobronchial tuberculosis during chemotherapy. Chest 1989;96:1195-6.

158. Chan HS, Sun A, Hoheisel GB. Endobronchial tuberculosis–is corticosteroid treatment useful? A report of 8 cases and review of the literature. Postgrad Med J 1990;66:822-6.

159. Verhaeghe W, Noppen M, Meysman M, Monsieur I, Vincken W. Rapid healing of endobronchial tuberculosis by local endoscopic injection of corticosteroids. Monaldi Arch Chest Dis 1996;51: 391-3.

160. Rikimaru T. Endobronchial tuberculosis. Expert Rev Anti Infect Ther 2004;2:245-51.

161. Rikimaru T. Therapeutic management of endobronchial tuberculosis. Expert Opin Pharmacother 2004;5:1463-70.

162. Park IW, Choi BW, Hue SH. Prospective study of corticosteroid as an adjunct in the treatment of endobronchial tuberculosis in adults. Respirology 1997;2:275-81.

163. Ryu YJ, Kim H, Yu CM, Choi JC, Kwon YS, Kwon OJ. Use of silicone stents for the management of post-tuberculosis tracheobronchial stenosis. Eur Respir J 2006;28:1029-35.

164. Iwamoto Y, Miyazawa T, Kurimoto N, Miyazu Y, Ishida A, Matsuo K, et al. Interventional bronchoscopy in the management of airway stenosis due to tracheobronchial tuberculosis. Chest 2004;126:1344-52.

165. Verma A, Park HY, Lim SY, Um SW, Koh WJ, Suh GY, et al. Post-tuberculosis tracheobronchial stenosis: use of CT to optimize the time of silicone stent removal. Radiology 2012;263:562-8.

166. Verma A, Um SW, Koh WJ, Suh GY, Chung MP, Kwon OJ, et al. Long-term tolerance of airway silicone stent in patients with post-tuberculosis tracheobronchial stenosis. ASAIO J 2012;58:530-4.

167. Chhajed PN, Malouf MA, Glanville AR. Bronchoscopic dilatation in the management of benign [non-transplant] tracheobronchial stenosis. Intern Med J 2001;31:512-6.

168. Ernst A, Feller-Kopman D, Becker HD, Mehta AC. Central airway obstruction. Am J Respir Crit Care Med 2004;169:1278-97.

169. Nakamura K, Terada N, Ohi M, Matsushita T, Kato N, Nakagawa T. Tuberculous bronchial stenosis: treatment with balloon bronchoplasty. Am J Roentgenol 1991;157:1187-8.

170. Nomori H, Horio H, Suemasu K. Bougienage and balloon dilatation using a conventional tracheal tube for tracheobronchial stenosis before stent placement. Surg Endosc 2000;14:587-91.

171. Ball JB, Delaney JC, Evans CC, Donnelly RJ, Hind CR. Endoscopic bougie and balloon dilatation of multiple bronchial stenoses: 10 year follow up. Thorax 1991;46:933-5.

172. Fernando HC, Sherwood JT, Krimsky W. Endoscopic therapies and stents for benign airway disorders: where are we, and where are we heading? Ann Thorac Surg 2010;89:S2183-7.

173. Kim JH, Shin JH, Shim TS, Oh YM, Song HY. Deep tracheal laceration after balloon dilation for benign tracheobronchial stenosis: case reports of two patients. Br J Radiol 2006;79:529-35.

174. Kim JH, Shin JH, Song HY, Shim TS, Ko GY, Yoon HK, et al. Tracheobronchial laceration after balloon dilatation for benign strictures: incidence and clinical significance. Chest 2007;131: 1114-7.

bronchial stenosis with aerosolized streptomycin and steroids. Int J Tuberc Lung Dis 2001;5:769-74.

175. Erelel M, Yakar F, Yakar A. Endobronchial tuberculosis with lobar obstruction successfully treated by argon plasma coagulation. South Med J 2009;102:1078-81.

176. Mehta AC, Khan SU. Nd-YAG Laser photoresection through a flexible bronchoscope. J Bronchology Interv Pulmonol 1997;4: 68-72.

177. Lee JY, Yi CA, Kim TS, Kim H, Kim J, Han J, et al. CT scan features as predictors of patient outcome after bronchial intervention in endobronchial TB. Chest 2010;138:380-5.

178. Liu AC, Mehta AC, Golish JA. Upper airway obstruction due to tuberculosis. Treatment by photocoagulation. Postgrad Med 1985;78:275-8.

179. Nam HS, Um SW, Koh WJ, Suh GY, Chung MP, Kwon OJ, et al. Clinical application of the Natural Y stent in the management of benign carinal stenosis. Ann Thorac Surg 2009;88: 432-9.

180. Tong MC, van Hasselt CA. Tuberculous tracheobronchial strictures: clinicopathological features and management with the bronchoscopic carbon dioxide laser. Eur Arch Otorhinolaryngol 1993;250:110-4.

181. Mariotta S, Guidi L, Aquilini M, Tonnarini R, Bisetti A. Airway stenosis after tracheo-bronchial tuberculosis. Respir Med 1997; 91:107-10.

182. Marasso A, Gallo E, Massaglia GM, Onoscuri M, Bernardi V. Cryosurgery in bronchoscopic treatment of tracheobronchial stenosis. Indications, limits, personal experience. Chest 1993;103: 472-4.

183. Li Y, Yao XP, Bai C, Huang Y, Wang Q, Zhao LJ, et al. Therapeutic efficacy analysis of bronchoscopic interventional therapy on severe tuberculous main bronchial stenosis complicated with unilateral atelectasis. Zhonghua Jie He He Hu Xi Za Zhi 2011;34:454-8.

184. Lunn W, Feller-Kopman D, Wahidi M, Ashiku S, Thurer R, Ernst A. Endoscopic removal of metallic airway stents. Chest 2005;127:2106-12.

185. Gaissert HA, Grillo HC, Wright CD, Donahue DM, Wain JC, Mathisen DJ. Complication of benign tracheobronchial strictures by self-expanding metal stents. J Thorac Cardiovasc Surg 2003;126:744-7.

186. Lund ME, Force S, Chest ftI, Committee DPS. The FDA Advisory: a call for restraint and training in airway stent placement. J Bronchology Interv Pulmonol 2007;14:223-6.

187. Dooms C, De Keukeleire T, Janssens A, Carron K. Performance of fully covered self-expanding metallic stents in benign airway strictures. Respiration 2009;77:420-6.

188. Wan IY, Lee TW, Lam HC, Abdullah V, Yim AP. Tracheobronchial stenting for tuberculous airway stenosis. Chest 2002;122:370-4.

189. Nomori H, Horio H, Suemasu K. Granulation stenosis caused by a Dumon stent placed for endobronchial tuberculous stenosis. Surg Laparosc Endosc Percutan Tech 2000;10:41-3.

190. Yim AP, Abdullah V, Izzat MB, van Hasselt CA. Video-assisted interventional bronchoscopy. The Hong Kong experience. Surg Endosc 1998;12:444-7.

191. Han JK, Im JG, Park JH, Han MC, Kim YW, Shim YS. Bronchial stenosis due to endobronchial tuberculosis: successful treatment with self-expanding metallic stent. AJR Am J Roentgenol 1992;159:971-2.

192. Huang YK, Liu YH, Ko PJ, Liu HP. Successful treatment of long-segmental tuberculous tracheal stenosis with combined Montgomery T-stent and Hood stent. Interact Cardiovasc Thorac Surg 2004;3:349-51.

193. Dialani V, Ernst A, Sun M, Lee KS, Feller-Kopman D, Litmanovich D, et al. MDCT detection of airway stent complications: comparison with bronchoscopy. AJR Am J Roentgenol 2008;191:1576-80.

194. Schmidt B, Olze H, Borges AC, John M, Liebers U, Kaschke O, et al. Endotracheal balloon dilatation and stent implantation in benign stenoses. Ann Thorac Surg 2001;71:1630-4.

195. Dhillon SS, Dexter EU. Advances in bronchoscopy for lung cancer. J Carcinog 2012;11:19.

196. Jin F, Mu D, Xie Y, Fu E, Guo Y. Application of bronchoscopic argon plasma coagulation in the treatment of tumorous endobronchial tuberculosis: historical controlled trial. J Thorac Cardiovasc Surg 2012;145:1650-3.

197. Overholt RH, Wilson NJ. Pulmonary resection for tuberculosis complicated by tuberculous bronchitis: preliminary report. Chest 1945;11:72-91.

198. Caligiuri PA, Banner AS, Jensik RJ. Tuberculous main-stem bronchial stenosis treated with sleeve resection. Arch Intern Med 1984;144:1302-3.

199. Natkunam R, Tse CY, Ong BH, Sriragavan P. Carinal resection for stenotic tuberculous tracheitis. Thorax 1988;43:492-3.

200. Mellem H, Boye NP, Arnkvaern R, Fjeld NB. Stenotic tuberculous tracheitis treated with resection and anastomosis. Eur J Respir Dis 1986;68:224-5.

201. Watanabe Y, Murakami S, Iwa T. Bronchial stricture due to endobronchial tuberculosis. Thorac Cardiovasc Surg 1988;36: 27-32.

202. Kato R, Kakizaki T, Hangai N, Sawafuji M, Yamamoto T, Kobayashi T, et al. Bronchoplastic procedures for tuberculous bronchial stenosis. J Thorac Cardiovasc Surg 1993;106:1118-21.

203. Watanabe Y, Murakami S, Oda M, Hayashi Y, Ohta Y, Shimizu J, et al. Treatment of bronchial stricture due to endobronchial tuberculosis. World J Surg 1997;21:480-7.

204. Casali L, Crapa ME. Endobronchial Tuberculosis: a peculiar feature of TB often underdiagnosed. Multidiscip Respir Med 2012;7:35.

205. Tetikkurt C. Current perspectives on endobronchial tuberculosis. Pneumon 2008;21:239-45.

206. Lee P. Endobronchial tuberculosis. Indian J Tuberc 2015;62:7-12.

207. Jung SS, Park HS, Kim JO, Kim SY. Incidence and clinical predictors of endobronchial tuberculosis in patients with pulmonary tuberculosis. Respirology 2015;20:488-95.

208. Faisal M, Harun H, Hassan TM, Ban AY, Chotirmall SH, Abdul Rahaman JA. Treatment of multiple-level tracheobronchial stenosis secondary to endobronchial tuberculosis using bronchoscopic balloon dilatation with topical mitomycin-C. BMC Pulm Med 2016;16:53.

209. Kizilbash QF. Mechanical complication of endobronchial tuberculosis. Respir Med Case Rep 2015;16:128-30.

210. Panigrahi MK, Pradhan G, Mishra P, Mohapatra PR. Actively caseating endobronchial tuberculosis successfully treated with intermittent chemotherapy without corticosteroid: a report of 2 cases. Adv Respir Med 2017;85:322-7.

211. Abdullah H, Quek CZ. Undiagnosed acute phase endobronchial tuberculosis with progression to irreversible tracheobronchial stenosis. BMJ Case Rep 2017;2017.pii:bcr-2017-219877.

212. Agerton T, Valway S, Gore B, Pozsik C, Plikaytis B, Woodley C, et al. Transmission of a highly drug-resistant strain [strain W1] of Mycobacterium tuberculosis. Community outbreak and nosocomial transmission via a contaminated bronchoscope. JAMA 1997;278: 1073-7.

13

Tuberculosis Pleural Effusion

AN Aggarwal

INTRODUCTION

The frequency of tuberculosis [TB] as a cause of pleural effusion depends on the prevalence of TB in a particular population. In many regions of the world where TB is more common, TB pleural effusion maintains its position as the leading inflammatory pleural disease (1-9). In fact, pleural disease is one of the most common form of extra-pulmonary TB in developing countries (10-12). The increasing prevalence of human immunodeficiency virus [HIV] infection in some of these geographical locations may be an additional factor explaining the higher frequency of TB pleural effusion (4,7). The entity is relatively uncommon in the developed world where prevalence of TB is low (13-16). For example, the annual incidence of TB pleural effusion in the United States is only about 1000 patients. Approximately 1 in every 30 cases of TB is TB pleuritis, and this ratio has remained constant even after the advent of the acquired immunodeficiency syndrome [AIDS] epidemic (14,17). In other areas, the incidence of TB pleural effusion has significantly declined over the years (18). However, there is some evidence to suggest that that these low figures may be an underestimation of the true disease burden in the general population (19).

PATHOGENESIS AND IMMUNOLOGY

TB may affect the pleura at different stages of pulmonary or systemic disease and by a number of different mechanisms. TB pleural effusion may represent a manifestation of either primary infection or reactivation of latent disease, the latter being more common (20). Pleural effusion is believed to occur secondary to the rupture of a subpleural caseous focus in the lung [or less commonly a lymph node] into the pleural space. Supportive evidence comes from the operative findings of Stead and coworkers (21), who could

demonstrate such a focus in lung contiguous to the pleura in 12 of 15 patients with TB pleuritis; the remaining patients had parenchymal TB, although this focus was not adjacent to the pleura. More recently, such foci have been demonstrated on thoracic computed tomography [CT] in patients with TB pleural effusion (22). Possibly, rupture of such a focus allows the TB protein to enter the pleural space and generate hypersensitivity responsible for most clinical manifestations. Pleural effusions may also be seen with direct contiguous spread of the disease to the pleura or by haematogenous spread (13). Occasionally, it can also occur as a complication of tubercle infested thoracic vertebra with paravertebral abscess (23). TB osteitis of the rib may also be associated with pleural effusion.

One might speculate that the intense pleural inflammation and consecutively increased vascular permeability would provide an obvious and satisfying explanation for fluid retention. However, at least in animal models, no significant alterations in vascular permeability have been demonstrated (24). It is now believed that the intense inflammatory reaction obstructs the lymphatic pores in the parietal pleura, causing proteins to accumulate in pleural space with subsequent retention of fluid (24,25).

Delayed-type hypersensitivity [DTH], rather than TB infection *per se*, plays an important role in the development of TB pleural effusion. This explains the poor rate of isolation of mycobacteria from pleural fluid samples from these patients [*vide infra*]. Pleural effusion has been shown to develop in non-sensitised animals who have received cells from immunized animals, and shown not to develop in sensitised animals if they are administered anti-lymphocyte serum (24,26). TB pleural fluid is also rich in several potentially immunoreactive cells and substances that contribute to the vigorous local cell mediated immune response (27,28). Mycobacterial antigens enter the pleural space and interact with T-lymphocytes previously sensitised to mycobacteria, resulting in DTH reaction and accumulation of fluid. There is a general increase in the proportion of total CD3+ and CD4+ T-cell subsets in pleural fluid, as compared to peripheral blood. Several investigators have demonstrated T-lymphocytes specifically sensitised to TB protein in TB pleural fluid (29-33). The concentration of such lymphocytes in pleural fluid is nearly eight-fold than that found in peripheral blood (31). It is not clear whether this represents sequestration of these cells from peripheral blood into pleural space, or local expansion in the pleural cavity. In addition, these lymphocytes show greater responsiveness to purified protein derivative [PPD], and when co cultured with PPD, produce far greater levels of cytokines than do peripheral blood lymphocytes (30,34). The ratio of CD4+ [helper-inducer] to CD8+ [suppressor/cytotoxic] lymphocytes is also much higher in TB pleural fluid as compared to peripheral blood [3:4 versus 1:7] (27,35). These CD4+ T-cells are predominantly of effector and effector memory phenotypes, and are most poised to generate a polyfunctional inflammatory response and also to contain mycobacterial infection (36). Patients with TB pleural effusion have significantly higher gamma interferon [IFN-γ] levels in their pleural fluid than in peripheral blood, thus exhibiting localisation of predominantly T-helper cell type 1 [Th1] type immunity in the pleural space (35,37). More recently, there is experimental evidence to link other T-cell subpopulations as well [e.g. Treg cells, etc.] in pleural inflammation (38).

According to current views and based on experimental evidence the sequence of immunological processes involved in TB pleuritis follows a recently described three-stage pattern of cellular and granulomatous tissue reactions. Experimental data suggests that neutrophils are the first cells responding to mycobacterial protein in the pleural space. When intrapleural bacille Calmette-Guerin [BCG] is administered to previously BCG-sensitised animals, the resultant pleural fluid is rich in neutrophils in the first 24 hours (39). The accumulation of pleural fluid and inflammatory cells is markedly decreased in neutropenic animals, and appears to be restored by intrapleural injection of neutrophils. Any trigger mechanism that allows access of mycobacterial protein to the pleura will set off a rapid mesothelial-cell initiated and interleukin-8 [IL-8] mediated polymorphonuclear neutrophil cell influx, within a few hours. In addition macrophages and blood-recruited monocytes determine this early stage with the predominant expression of pro-inflammatory chemokines interleukin-1 [IL-1], interleukin-6 [IL-6] and tumour necrosis factor [TNF]. In animal models, after the initial neutrophil-rich phase, macrophages predominate in the pleural fluid from second to fifth days (39). Neutrophils in pleural space appear to secrete a monocyte chemotaxin that recruits monocytes to the pleural space and helps in granuloma formation (39). In addition, mesothelial cells may also play an important role (40). Animal models have shown that mesothelial cells stimulated with BCG or IFN-γ produce macrophage

inflammatory protein and monocyte chemotactic peptides, and that these two proteins account for more than 75% of the mononuclear chemotactic factor in the TB pleural fluid (41,42). After 3-4 days, in the following intermediary stage, lymphocytes are the prominent cell in the pleural fluid (43). They are mostly T-cells comprising CD4+ helper cells as well as CD8+ cytotoxic [natural killer, NK] cells with a CD4+/CD8+ ratio of about 4.3, and so-called unconventional cells including T-cell receptor double negative [DN] αβ T-cells and γδ-T cells (44,45). IFN-γ, a strong promoter of macrophage activation and granuloma formation [together with TNF], is the predominant IL at this stage. Initially, these lymphocytes do not respond to PPD. However, reactivity is restored over the next few days, and parallels the reactivity of lymphocytes in the peripheral blood (46). Lymphocyte activation can occur in the pleura of some patients who fail to react to cutaneous PPD, a fact that is explained by the presence in the circulation of suppressor cells that inhibit response in the skin; these suppressor cells are apparently lacking in the pleural fluid (29). Helper T-cells in pleural fluid express a battery of homing receptors, such as, cluster of differentiation [CD] 11a, c-C chemokine receptor type-5 [CCR5] and chemokine receptor CXCR3, which are important in modulating cell trafficking and recruitment in pleural space and tissue (45). The late phase of TB pleural effusion is characterized by an equilibrated and sustained CD4+/CD8+ cell-based response with continued IFN-γ release and consecutive granuloma formation that is modulated by the release of Th1-cells supporting interleukin-12 [IL-12] and counter-regulatory anti-inflammatory cytokines like interleukin-10 [IL-10] and transforming growth factor-beta [TGF-β]. Toll-like receptors [TLRs] may have a role in enhancing this antigen-specific Th1-cell function (47).

Recent studies have improved our understanding of the immunological pathways involved in TB pleuritis. After phagocytosing mycobacteria, macrophages act as antigen presenting cells and present TB antigen to T-lymphocytes. This results in activation of T-lymphocytes and subsequent promotion of macrophage differentiation and granuloma formation. Some components of the mycobacterial cell wall, such as protein/proteoglycan complex and lipoarabinomannan, can stimulate macrophages to produce TNF, which is a regulator of granuloma formation (48). Activated pleural macrophages can also produce IL-1, which along with TNF, is involved in lymphocyte activation (49). On exposure to mycobacterial antigens, pleural T-lymphocytes produce IFN-γ, which is an important activator of macrophage killing capacity, as well as interleukin-2 [IL-2] which is a regulator of T-cell proliferation (49-51). Cytotoxic cell activity could be an additional defense mechanism. CD4+ and NK cells present in pleural fluid of these patients demonstrate cytotoxic activity when stimulated with PPD (52,53).

On the other hand, there is also strong evidence that infectious invasion of the pleural space actually occurs at a substantial, *albeit* variable degree. At thoracoscopy, even with negative fluid studies, extensive inflammatory granuloma formation and fibrin deposits with unexpected abundant mycobacteria recovery are a common finding (54). Also the increasingly emerging evidence of a preferred association of TB pleurisy with reactivated TB in Western populations may be interpreted in favour of true infectious mechanisms (20). Thus the concept of exudative pleurisy representing exclusively delayed type hypersensitivity [DTH] may not hold true. Infectious as well as immunological mechanisms are obviously closely interrelated and operative in complex patterns.

CLINICAL MANIFESTATIONS

TB pleural effusion is typically a disease of young men (55,56). Patients with post-primary TB pleural effusion tend to be older than those with post-primary TB pleural effusion (20). The clinical presentation of TB pleural effusion may vary from an acute illness simulating bacterial pneumonia to an indolent disease first suspected on a chest radiograph in a patient with minor constitutional symptoms. TB pleuritis occurs as an acute illness in about two-thirds of cases, with symptoms often of less than a month duration (57-59). In fact, the illness often mimics bacterial pneumonia with parapneumonic effusion (59), as a general rule an acute illness is more likely to occur in younger and the immunocompetent patients. Older patients more frequently present with an insidious onset of symptoms (48). Non-productive cough [70%] and chest pain [75%] are the two most common symptoms at presentation (59). If both cough and pleuritic chest pain is present, the pain usually precedes the cough (58). Despite the frequency of pleuritic chest pain, a pleural friction rub is unusual. The patient is usually febrile, but a normal temperature does not rule out the disease (59). Other systemic manifestations, such as, night sweats, weakness, weight loss, anorexia and fatigue are also common. On physical examination, non-specific signs of pleural effusion, including mediastinal shift, stony dullness to percussion and the occasional demonstration of a pleural rub at auscultation may be evident. Untreated, this pleural effusion will usually resolve spontaneously.

IMAGING

TB pleural effusion is unilateral in more than 90% instances, and usually small to moderate in size, although it may occupy the entire hemithorax [Figure 9.8] (56,59,60). Although conventionally regarded as a rare cause of massive pleural effusion, recent data suggests that TB may represent more than 10% of all cases of large pleural effusion in high prevalence areas (61,62). In up to half of these patients, co-existing parenchymal disease can be demonstrated by conventional chest radiographs (56,59,63). In such patients, the pleural effusion is almost always on the side of the parenchymal infiltrate and usually indicates active parenchymal disease [Figure 13.1] (63). In three-fourths of such cases, the parenchymal disease is located in the upper lobe, suggestive of reactivation TB (64). In the remaining patients, the parenchymal disease involves the lower lobe and resembles primary disease. It is likely that even in cases with no radiographic evidence of parenchymal involvement; the effusion is associated with a subpleural focus of infection. If carefully searched for, thoracic CT can demonstrate this subpleural focus in many such patients (22,65-67). CT is more sensitive than chest radiography, showing parenchymal disease in over 80% of cases. Almost half of these patients have smooth pleural thickening exceeding 1 cm on a thoracic CT; involvement of mediastinal pleura is uncommon (65). Uncommonly, pleural-based nodular masses [pseudotumours] can also be identified (68-70).

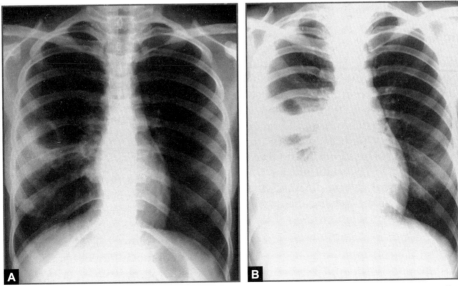

Figure 13.1: Chest radiograph of a woman being investigated for pulmonary TB [A]. Sputum examination was non-contributory, but bronchoalveolar lavage showed presence of acid-fast bacilli. During the course of her evaluation, she developed ipsilateral exudative pleural effusion [B]. Both pulmonary and pleural lesions responded to anti-TB treatment

TB = tuberculosis

Positron emission tomography-CT [PET-CT] may document high metabolic activity in the affected pleura (71).

Classically, TB effusion associated with acute symptoms and the absence of radiographically evident parenchymal lung disease has been felt to represent primary infection. By contrast, TB effusion that is associated with an indolent course and with parenchymal lung disease on the chest radiograph has been seen more frequently in older patients and has been considered to be a manifestation of post-primary [reactivation] disease [Figure 13.1]. However, such a clear-cut distinction between primary and reactivation disease cannot always be made with confidence based solely on chest radiography.

On conventional chest radiography, presence of at least 200 mL of pleural fluid becomes detectable as blunting of the costophrenic angle in standard projections. Thoracic ultrasonography may detect much smaller effusions. Specific advantages of thoracic ultrasonography are a more precise volumetry than by chest radiography, localisation of septae, membranes and pleural thickening, along with its clinical versatility for bedside diagnosis and in addition intervention guidance on demand [Figure 9.9].

DIAGNOSIS

The step-wise diagnosis of TB pleural effusion is essentially the same as for any other pleural exudate. An initial diagnostic thoracentesis is always indicated. The diagnosis of TB pleural effusion can be difficult because of the low sensitivity of the various diagnostic tools. No single laboratory test has 100% sensitivity and specificity for diagnosis of TB pleural effusion. Most patients undergo a battery of investigations, and the diagnosis is often established after careful consideration of clinical features and results of several laboratory parameters (72-76). Despite a comprehensive evaluation, almost 20% of TB pleural fluids will defy a definitive diagnosis.

Sputum Examination

Only a minority of patients with TB pleural effusion demonstrate sputum smear-positivity for acid-fast bacilli [AFB]. Sometimes, AFB can be demonstrated in the sputum even in patients with no radiographic evidence of pulmonary involvement (77). Sputum mycobacterial culture yield ranges from 30%-50% in patients having both pulmonary and pleural TB (59,78). However, yield of mycobacterial culture is less than 5% of patients with isolated TB pleural effusion (79). The yield of sputum mycobacterial culture obtained after sputum induction may be much higher even in patients with no apparent radiological parenchymal lesions (80).

Tuberculin Skin Test

In populations with a low prevalence of TB infection, a positive tuberculin skin test [TST] in a patient with exudative pleural effusion strongly suggests the diagnosis of TB, whereas, the diagnostic value of a positive test in countries with a high prevalence of TB is lower. A TST is positive in majority of patients, but a negative test does not rule out the diagnosis. Up to 30%-50% patients can manifest a negative TST at the time of initial evalu-ation (56,59,81). Such negative tests may be even more common in HIV infected patients (82). This anergy to PPD appears to be due to an antigen-specific extra-pleural immunosuppression. Although pleuritis is considered to be related to a DTH, circulating adherent cells in the acute phase of the disease may suppress the specifically sensitised T-lymphocytes in the peripheral blood and in the skin [but not in the pleural fluid], accounting for the negative results in these patients (29). Anergy may occasionally result from pleural compart-mentalisation of PPD-sensitised lymphocytes occurring in the early phase of infection, resulting in a relative depletion of these cells in the circulation. If the patient is not anergic or immunosuppressed, the skin test will almost always become positive within eight weeks of the development of the symptoms.

Pleural Fluid Analysis

The pleural fluid in TB pleuritis is often a serous exudates; the pleural fluid may be serosanguinous in less than 10% cases. Frequently, the pleural fluid protein level exceeds 5 g/dL (81,83,84). Biochemical analysis of the pleural fluid is otherwise of limited value. Although in the past it was observed that pleural fluid glucose was reduced in most patients of TB pleural effusion (85), more recent studies (59,79) show that majority of patients have a pleural fluid glucose of more than 60 mg/dL. A low pleural fluid pH was once thought to be suggestive of TB pleural effusion, but subsequent reports have not confirmed this (86-88). Glucose and pH values are in general not substantially different from exudates due to other aetiologies, and their diagnostic significance has probably been overestimated in the past.

In most patients, the pleural fluid differential white blood cell count reveals more than 50% lymphocytes, with a reported median of 82% in a recent large series (84). In another study, only 11% had a polymorphonuclear-rich pleural fluid; however, these patients showed a higher yield on sputum or pleural fluid mycobacterial culture (89). In another series [n = 49], only 5 patients had fewer than 50% lymphocytes in the pleural fluid (59). In fact, the overwhelming predominance on lymphocytes on pre-parations examined cytologically can sometimes result in a misdiagnosis of lymphoma (90). The percentage and absolute numbers of CD4+ T-lymphocytes in pleural fluid are higher than in the blood (91-94); by contrast, the percentage and number of B-lymphocytes are significantly lower (30,31,95). However, the separation of lymphocytes into T- and B-subsets is not useful diagnostically. In patients with symptoms of less than two-week duration, the pleural fluid may reveal predominantly polymorphonuclear leucocytes (58). If serial thoracenteses are performed, the differential count will reveal a shift to predominantly small lymphocytes (59). The fluid rarely contains more than 5% mesothelial cells, although the finding is not diagnostic (96,97). Several other disorders associated with pleural inflammation and infiltration are associated with decreased shedding of mesothelial cells in the pleural cavity, and numerous mesothelial cells can sometimes be found in some patients with pleural TB (98). Presence of eosinophils in a significant number in the fluid makes the diagnosis of TB unlikely, except in patients having a hydropneumothorax due to previous thoracentesis (99,100). It is reasonable to assume that effusions containing more than 50% of these cells are of a non-TB aetiology.

Pleural fluid smear for AFB is positive in less than 10% instances in most reports, while mycobacteria can be cultured from pleural fluid in 10%-70% cases (57,60,78,79,81,84,90,101-103). Corticosteroid use, concurrent TB involving another site, increased neutrophils and decreased glucose levels in pleural fluid are some of the predictive factors associated with culture positivity (104,105). Sensitivity of mycobacterial cultures is improved, if pleural fluid is transported in heparinised containers, bedside inoculation of pleural fluid is substituted for laboratory inoculation, large fluid volumes are cultured, or if liquid culture media and/or BACTEC system are used (106-109).

Pleural Biopsy

Closed parietal pleural biopsy can be performed using a Cope or Abram needle. The demonstration of parietal pleural granulomata on histopathological examination is suggestive of TB pleuritis; caseous necrosis and AFB are often not evident (83). Although other disorders, such as, fungal diseases, sarcoidosis and rheumatoid arthritis may produce granulomatous pleuritis, more than 95% of patients with this histopathology on pleural biopsy have TB pleural effusion. The initial biopsy reveals granulomas in 50%-97% patients with TB pleural effusion (60,78,79,81,84,101,102,110,111). The yield increases if multiple biopsies are performed (112-114). However, if properly obtained, even a single high quality sample should be enough to obtain a diagnosis (114,115). Mycobacteria can be cultured from pleural biopsy specimens in 33%-80% cases (60,78,79,81,84,102,110,116). When culture of biopsy specimen is combined with microscopic examination, the diagnosis can be established in up to 95% instances (117). Even when granulomata are not demonstrated, the biopsy specimen should be examined for AFB. In less than 10% of cases, organisms may still be demonstrated when no granulomas are present in the biopsy (59,78). Visceral pleural biopsy can sometimes yield diagnosis in patients with a negative parietal pleural biopsy (118). CT or ultrasonographic guidance may improve the yield and safety of closed pleural biopsy (119).

Adenosine Deaminase

Adenosine deaminase [ADA] is an enzyme involved in the purine catabolism. It catalyses the deamination of adenosine to inosine and of deoxyadenosine to deoxyinosine. ADA is found in most cells, but its chief role concerns the proliferation and differentiation of lymphocytes, especially T-lymphocytes. For that reason ADA has been looked on as a marker of cell-mediated immunity, which encompasses the DTH. ADA activity correlates with CD4+ T-lymphocyte cell infiltration in the pleura and the pleural fluid (120). Determination of pleural fluid ADA level appears to be a promising marker in the diagnosis of TB pleural effusion because of the ease, rapidity, and cost-effectiveness of the ADA assay (121). ADA estimation is performed using a simple colorimetric method that is quite suitable for use in the field setting (122). Adequately frozen and stored pleural fluid samples maintain ADA activity for more than 2.5 years (123). However, haemolysed blood in the fluid sample may cause false underestimation of ADA activity using colorimetric method (124).

Meta-analyses of published literature has shown that ADA estimation is reasonably accurate in diagnosing TB pleural effusion (125,126). It appears that pleural fluid ADA in excess of 70 U/L is highly suggestive of TB pleuritis, whereas as a level below 40 U/L virtually rules out the diagnosis (127-129). In addition, higher the pleural fluid ADA, the more likely the diagnosis of TB. However, very high pleural fluid ADA activity may also be seen in empyema or lymphoma (130). Essentially, observations from the developed countries (131) and more recent reports from Asia (132) have found that pleural fluid ADA level is useful diagnostically. It is not clear whether these differences represent methodologic differences or true ethnic variation. Some of the differences could also be explained by differences in methodology used for ADA estimation, as well as delays in transportation and processing of pleural fluid samples. It is well known that ADA levels in pleural fluids maintained at ambient temperatures, and without the use of specific additives, decrease with passage of time (133). In fact, in properly refrigerated and stored samples, pleural fluid ADA estimates remain stable up to four weeks after collection (134). Several investigators have reported the use of pleural fluid ADA in the diagnosis of TB effusions in India (135-159). Overall, the sensitivity and specificity of the test in diagnosis of TB have not been as good as that observed in Western datasets [Table 13.1]. However, based on epidemiological and Bayesian considerations, positive predictive value of pleural fluid ADA in diagnosis of TB pleural effusion should be far better in geographical regions with a higher prevalence of TB as a cause of pleural effusion (125). Hence elevated ADA can provide a reliable basis of diagnosing TB pleural effusion in such areas (160). It also appears that ADA is a poor discriminator when used as a single investigation, but may be more useful when results are interpreted in conjunction with clinicoradiograhic data and results of other investigations (161,162)

There are several isoforms of ADA, but the prominent ones are ADA1 and ADA2, which are coded by different gene loci (163). ADA1 isoenzyme is found in all cells, with the highest concentration found in lymphocytes and monocytes, whereas ADA2 isoenzyme is found only in monocytes (164). ADA2 is the predominant isoform

Table 13.1: Performance of ADA estimation in the diagnosis of TB pleural effusion in Indian patients

Study [year] (reference)	Cases/Controls	Cut-off [U/L]	Sensitivity	Specificity
Raj [1985] (135)	30/25	40	1.000	–
Sinha [1985] (136)	22/14	30	1.000	1.000
Sinha [1987] (137)	37/16	30	1.000	1.000
Chopra [1988] (138)	37/27	–	0.892	0.852
Gilhotra [1989] (139)	30/43	40	1.000	0.907
Gupta [1990] (140)	36/57	50.75	1.000	0.941
Subhakar [1991] (141)	62/18	38	0.984	1.000
Kaur [1992] (142)	21/52	30	0.667	0.923
Prasad [1992] (143)	21/26	30	1.000	1.000
Nagaraja [1992] (144)	30/18	50	1.000	1.000
Maldhure [1994] (145)	83/42	40	1.000	0.348
		60	0.806	0.623
		80	0.417	0.812
Singh [1998] (146)	41/43	–	0.902	0.870
Ghelani [1999] (147)	54/27	40	0.722	0.593
Parandaman [2000] (148)	25/09	47.3	0.760	0.714
Sharma [2001] (149)	48/27	35	0.833	0.666
		100	0.400	1.000
Nagesh [2001] (150)	20/40	50	0.550	0.550
Dil [2006] (151)	48/34	–	0.583	–
Bandyopadhyay [2008] (152)	34/15	30	0.588	0.600
Verma [2008] (153)	34/16	36	1.000	0.777
Gupta [2010] (154)	56/40	40	1.000	0.974
Pandit [2010] (155)	20/42	70	0.500	1.000
Ambade [2011] (156)	48/33	71	0.875	0.697
Kalantri [2011] (157)	50/50	44.8	0.980	0.880
Kelam [2013] (158)	39/18	40	0.897	0.500
Mehta [2014] (159)	49/73	40	0.857	0.808

ADA = adenosine deaminase; TB = tuberculosis

in the TB pleural fluid, accounting for approximately 90% of total ADA activity, whereas ADA1 is elevated in empyema (165). This would suggest that ADA2 is a more efficient marker of TB pleural effusion. ADA2 has been shown to be increased in TB pleural effusions (165-168). In pleural fluids with a high ADA level, a ADA1:ADA2 ratio less than 0.45 is highly suggestive of TB, whereas a ratio greater than 0.45 may be seen in malignancy, empyema, and other conditions (146,169). Although determination of this ratio may increase the diagnostic accuracy of ADA estimation in TB pleural fluids, in clinical practice the difference in the use of total ADA and isoform ADA2 may not be significant (170). In fact, there may be an advantage in the measurement of total ADA because of its low cost and rapid turnover. ADA1 activity is determined by subtracting ADA2 from total ADA. The measurement of ADA2 is almost 10 times more expensive than estimation of total ADA.

IFN-γ

IFN-γ is produced by the CD4+ lymphocytes in patients with TB pleural effusion in response to mycobacterial antigens (51,171). In fact, the concentration of tubercle bacilli in pleural liquid correlates with the amount of IFN-γ (172). Patients with pleural effusion may have up to 25-fold higher IFN-γ levels in the pleural fluid as compared to their peripheral blood, suggesting homing of Th1 cells in the pleural fluid from the peripheral blood and enrichment of pleural space with Th1 cytokines (37). IFN-γ can be estimated either by enzyme-linked immunosorbent assay [ELISA] or radioimmunoassay [RIA] methods. Estimation of pleural fluid IFN-γ levels is reported to be useful in differentiating TB pleural effusion from other causes (125,173). A number of reports have demonstrated that IFN-γ levels in patients with TB pleurisy are high, with sensitivity and specificity ranging from 90%-100% (51,129,172,174-188). However, proper comparison of results from different studies is not possible due to variability in methods of estimation and units used for quantification. Although the test is promising, it is expensive and still not widely available. The cost of performing a single test in India is, in fact, equivalent to the cost of a complete course of anti-TB treatment for six patients, and therefore does not appear to be a cost-effective investigation for differentiating TB from non-TB pleural effusions (189).

Interferon Gamma Release Assays

Interferon Gamma Release Assays [IGRAs] were developed as *in vitro* whole blood tests to assess a person's cellular immune reactivity by quantifying gamma-IFN production by T cells after stimulation with specific mycobacterial antigens. Two systems, with established protocols for test performance and reporting, are commercially available (190). The ELISA-based Quantiferon-TB Gold assay uses early secretory antigen-6 [ESAT-6], culture filtrate protein-10 [CFP-10] and TB7.7 as antigens, and the ELISpot-based T-Spot TB test uses ESAT-6 and CFP-10 as antigens. Much like the TST, positive IGRA results point more to TB infection rather than active disease.

Over the past few years, some investigators have explored the use IGRAs as a diagnostic marker for TB pleural effusion (191-208). In addition to the whole blood tests, IGRAs have also been adapted for use on pleural fluid specimens with mixed results [Table 13.2]. Overall test performance does not look encouraging. A meta-analysis (209) of seven studies reported an overall sensitivity and specificity of 75% and 82%, respectively for pleural fluid, and 80% and 72%, respectively for whole blood. In low prevalence settings, pleural fluid responses appear to be greater than whole blood responses (210,211). However, in high prevalence settings, the reverse seems true, and the sensitivity is also much inferior (210,211).

Specific problems have been noted with pleural fluid IGRAs. For one, IGRAs are standardised for whole blood, and not pleural fluid T-cell responses. Sample volumes, antigen concentrations, and response cut-off values are therefore not clearly defined for pleural fluid. Secondly, background IFN-γ levels may be high in pleural fluid, especially in TB, resulting in poorer stimulation on antigenic stimulation. Both these factors can result in frequent negative or indeterminate responses (210,211). In addition, pre-sensitised circulating T-cells can passively enter into non-TB pleural effusions, giving rise to false-positive results (210).

Table 13.2: Performance of IGRAs for diagnosis of TB pleural effusion*

Study [year] (reference)	Technique	Whole blood		Pleural fluid	
		Sensitivity	Specificity	Sensitivity	Specificity
Wilkinson [2005] (191)	ELISpot	1.000	–	1.000	0.875
Ariga [2007] (192)	ELISA	0.778	0.702	0.964	0.978
Losi [2007] (193)	ELISpot	0.900	0.667	0.950	0.762
Baba [2008] (194)	ELISA	0.708	1.000	0.444	1.000
Chegou [2008] (195)	ELISA	0.727	0.706	0.565	0.867
Nishimura [2008] (196)	ELISA	0.600	0.923	–	–
Dheda [2009] (197)	ELISpot	0.811	0.800	0.826	0.800
	ELISA	0.867	0.692	0.793	0.632
Lee [2009] (198)	ELISpot	0.778	0.857	0.947	0.905
Liao [2009] (199)	ELISpot	0.737	0.846	0.857	0.333
Katiyar [2010] (200)	ELISA	0.904	0.860	–	–
Ates [2011] (201)	ELISA	0.698	0.517	0.488	0.793
Chung [2011] (202)	ELISA	0.741	0.611	–	–
Losi [2011] (203)	ELISA	0.788	0.633	0.833	0.533
Eldin [2012] (204)	ELISA	0.700	0.778	0.600	0.833
Gao [2012] (205)	ELISA	0.931	0.900	–	–
Kang [2012] (206)	ELISpot	0.857	0.571	0.714	0.727
	ELISA	0.476	0.500	0.235	0.538
Keng [2013] (207)	ELISpot	–	–	0.387	0.553
Liu [2013] (208)	ELISpot	0.927	0.628	0.945	0.929

* Both confirmed and probable TB patients were considered as having disease. For sensitivity calculations, any indeterminate test was regarded as being a 'false negative'. For specificity calculations, any indeterminate test was excluded

IGRAs = interferon-gamma release assays; TB = tuberculosis; ELISpot = enzyme-linked immunospot assay; ELISA = enzyme-linked immunosorbent assay

As a result, IGRAs cannot be recommended for diagnostic use, especially in high prevalence settings. This is consistent with the World Health Organization [WHO] policy statement on use of IGRAs (212).

Serodiagnosis

Several studies are available on the immunodiagnosis of TB pleural effusion (146,213-233). Both mycobacterial antigens and their antibodies have been estimated in pleural fluid and/or serum using ELISA based [or similar] techniques to assess their utility in the diagnosis [Table 13.3]. The sensitivity reported in most studies is much less than desirable. The problem of false-positive results has also been troublesome in other studies (147,217,218,224,226,228,230). The kaolin agglutination test, which detects anti-tuberculophospholipid antibodies, may also provide equivalent sensitivity and specificity, while being much simpler (234). Recently, a multi-antigen and antibody assay developed in-house at Sevagram [SEVATB ELISA using a cocktail of mycobacterial

Table 13.3: Evaluation of antigens and antibodies in the diagnosis of TB pleural effusion

Study [year] (reference)	Target	Sensitivity	Specificity
Antibody in pleural fluid			
Samuel [1984] (213)		0.683	1.000
Murate [1990] (214)	Anti-PPD IgG	0.226	0.949
Caminero [1991] (215)	Anti-A60 IgG	0.500	1.000
Caminero [1993] (216)	Anti-A60 IgG	0.500	1.000
Ghelani [1999] (147)	Anti-A60 IgG	0.907	0.333
Chierakul [2001] (217)	IgG to five purified antigens	0.254	0.904
Kunter [2003] (218)	Anti-A60 IgM	0.841	0.730
Yokoyama [2005] (219)	Anti-lipoarabinomannan IgG	0.500	0.938
Kaisermann [2005] (220)	Anti-MPT64/MPT10.3 IgA	0.764	0.963
Morimoto [2006] (221)	Anti-mycobacterial glycolipid	0.526	0.957
Trajman [2007] (222)	Anti-MPT64/MPT10.3 IgA	0.817	0.941
Araujo [2010] (223)	Anti-MPT64/MPT10.3 IgA	0.814	0.955
Limongi [2011] (224)	Anti-HspX IgA	0.690	0.830
Antibody in serum			
Caminero [1991] (215)	Anti-A60 IgG	0.550	1.000
Caminero [1993] (216)	Anti-A60 IgG	0.533	1.000
Arora [1993] (225)	Anti-A60 IgM	0.900	0.950
Chierakul [2001] (217)	IgG to five purified antigens	0.463	0.596
Kunter [2003] (218)	Anti-A60 IgM	0.591	0.811
Limongi [2011] (224)	Anti-HspX IgA	0.300	0.840
Fernandez [2011] (226)	Anti-PPD IgG	0.500	0.725
	Anti-PPD IgA	0.900	0.300
Kaushik [2012] (227)	Anti-HspX IgG + IgA	0.633	0.947
Antigen in pleural fluid			
Samuel [1984] (213)	Soluble antigens	0.488	1.000
Baig [1986] (228)	Soluble antigens	0.600	0.800
Ramkisson [1988] (229)	Soluble antigens	1.000	0.983
Dhand [1988] (230)	Soluble antigens	0.800	0.381
Banchuin [1990] (231)	Soluble antigens	0.115	1.000
Anie [2007] (232)	Mycobacterial glycolipid	0.855	1.000
Feng [2011] (233)	ESAT-6	0.868	–
	CFP-10	0.763	–
Antigen in serum			
Banchuin [1990] (231)	Soluble antigens	0.000	1.000

TB = tuberculosis; PPD = purified protein derivative; Ig = immunoglobulin; ESAT-6 = early secretory antigen-6; CFP-10 = culture filtrate protein-10

antigens ES-31 and ESAT-6 and their specific antibodies] showed 100% specificity and 83% sensitivity in pleural fluid, and 78% specificity and 92% sensitivity in serum, in patients with TB pleural effusion (235). In view of the rampant misuse of serodiagnostic tests in several developing countries, despite documented suboptimal diagnostic performance, WHO has recommended that these tests should not be used in persons suspected to have active TB (236). The Government of India has also issued an advisory against the use of these tests and has banned import of commercial serodiagnostic kits.

The origin of antibodies to mycobacterial antigens in pleural fluid of these patients is not clear. Levy and coworkers (237) found close correlation between pleural fluid and serum levels, reflecting passive diffusion. Other investigators have demonstrated higher titres of antibodies in pleural fluid, indicating local accumulation (238). Assays based on detection of tuberculostearic acid in pleural fluid have not yielded encouraging results (239). Further work needs to be done before immunodiagnostic techniques can be recommended for routine use in the diagnosis of TB pleural effusions.

Thoracoscopy

Thoracoscopy, often considered the 'gold standard procedure' for the diagnosis of TB pleuritis, may have a role in evaluation of pleural effusions undiagnosed by less invasive investigations (240-242). The diagnostic accuracy of this procedure is greater because multiple selected biopsies can be obtained, which have a higher yield both on microbiological as well as histopathological examination (243-245). The endoscopic appearance of pleural TB is well described (246). It is characterised by greyish-white granulomata blanketing the whole parietal and diaphragmatic pleura, and in particular, the costovertebral gutter (247,248). However, lesions have often lost their specific appearance by the time of thoracoscopy and may mimic a simple inflammatory process. Rarely, mass-like lesions mimicking malignancy may be seen (68). In addition, the examination itself may be difficult because of numerous bands and adhesions. Complication rates for thoracoscopically guided pleural biopsy are minimal, and similar to closed pleural biopsy (245,247,248). Apart from cost concerns, the performance of thoracoscopy is limited by availability of equipment, and of personnel with expertise to perform this procedure.

Nucleic Acid Amplification Tests

The various nucleic acid amplification tests [NAAT] that have been used in the diagnosis of mycobacterial infection include target amplification techniques, such as, polymerase chain reaction [PCR], strand displacement amplification, and transcription mediated amplification, as well as probe/primer amplification techniques, such as, ligand chain reaction and Q-Beta replicase amplification. PCR, the most widely used of these techniques, is based on the amplification of

mycobacterial deoxyribonucleic acid [DNA]. In respiratory specimens, PCR can be performed rapidly and has a diagnostic yield comparable to that of culture (249). PCR offers the option of referring the sample, rather than the patient, to a specialised centre or laboratory. This procedure has also been used to detect mycobacterial DNA in pleural fluid (148,150-152,157,206,222,232,250-276). The Xpert MTB/RIF [Cepheid, Sunnyvale, CA, USA], another promising automated, real-time PCR assay used for the detection of TB pleural effusion (277). The sensitivity of the PCR in the diagnosis of TB pleural effusion ranges from as low as 17% to as high as 100%, depending on the patients selected, genomic sequence amplified, and the procedure used in the extraction of DNA [Table 13.4]. Specificity ranges from 61%-100%. The parameter that determines the sensitivity of PCR is probably the number of bacilli in the sample of pleural fluid analysed. Series with a pleural fluid culture positivity of as high as 69% report more than 80% sensitivity of PCR (253). PCR may be positive in 100% of culture positive TB pleural fluids and only in 30%-60% of culture negative pleural fluids (250-252,255-257,260,263,265). The lower sensitivity is most likely attributable to the inefficient recovery of genomic DNA from the characteristically low number of mycobacteria in patients with pleural TB. Genomic sequences present in multiple copies in mycobacteria give better results than sequences present in only a single copy (250-252). Contamination of samples by mycobacterial DNA in the laboratory environment is partly responsible for the low specificity. In general, use of commercial assays [such as, Amplicor or Xpert MTB/Rif] have shown poor sensitivity (257,262,263,266). In particular, Xpert MTB/Rif assay has poor sensitivity in patients clinically diagnosed as TB pleural effusion and a slightly better sensitivity [although still not useful clinically] using culture as gold standard (278). Based on available data WHO considers pleural fluid as a sub-optimal specimen for such testing, but recommends initiation of therapy based on a positive Xpert MTB/Rif result (279). The recently published Guidelines for extrapulmonary TB for India [INDEX-TB Guidelines] (280a), also suggest that Xpert MTB/RIF should not be used to diagnose pleural TB [strong recommendation, low quality evidence for sensitivity estimate, high quality evidence for specificity estimate]. A recent systematic review (280b), reported that, while the sensitivity of Xpert MTB/RIF in the pleural fluid was low overall, the sensitivity was higher in areas with higher TB prevalence.

Other approaches such as transcription-mediated amplification of 16S ribosomal ribonucleic acid [RNA], using the commercially available Amplified *Mtb* Direct [AMTD] test, have also shown poor results (281). Few investigators have also evaluated the value of various nucleic acid extraction and amplification techniques in formalin-fixed and paraffin-embedded pleural tissue samples (282-288). Although specificity of these techniques is high, approaching 100% in several instances, sensitivity was seen to be low [47%-90%]. However, in these studies,

Table 13.4: Pleural fluid polymerase chain reaction in the diagnosis of TB pleural effusion

Study [year] (reference)	Sequence amplified	Sensitivity	Specificity
de Wit [1992] (250)	336 bp repetitive sequence	0.811	0.774
de Lassence [1992] (251)	IS6110 sequence	0.600	1.000
	Gene coding 65 kD antigen	0.200	1.000
Verma [1995] (252)	150 bp sequence	0.632	0.931
Querol [1995] (253)	IS6110 sequence	0.809	0.977
Tan [1995] (254)	IS6110 sequence	0.700	1.000
	MPB64 fragment	0.700	1.000
Villena [1998] (255)	IS6110 sequence	0.424	0.990
Seethalakshmi [1998] (256)	IS6110 sequence	0.409	–
Parandaman [2000] (148)	IS6110 sequence and TRC4	1.000	0.850
Mitarai [2000] (257)	Amplicor kit	0.273	0.976
Martins [2000] (258)	MPB64 fragment	0.684	0.909
Villegas [2000] (259)	IS6110 sequence	0.738	0.898
Reechaipichitkul [2000] (260)	16S-23S rRNA gene spacer sequence	0.500	0.613
Nagesh [2001] (150)	150 bp sequence	0.700	1.000
Lima [2003] (261)	IS6110 sequence	0.313	0.966
Kim [2004] (262)	Amplicor kit	0.333	1.000
Moon [2005] (263)	Amplicor kit	0.175	0.981
Dil [2006] (151)	MPB64 gene	0.667	1.000
Trajman [2007] (222)	IS6110 sequence	0.821	0.852
Anie [2007] (232)	IS6110 sequence	0.870	0.930
Liu [2007] (264)	IS6110 sequence	0.434	0.955
Bandhopadhyay [2008] (152)	IS6110 sequence, dnaJ gene and 65 kD antigen gene	0.824	0.750
Kumar [2010] (265)	hupB gene	0.517	1.000
Kalantri [2011] (157)	16S rRNA gene	0.649	0.980
Friedrich [2011] (266)	Xpert MTB/RIF Assay	0.250	1.000
Maurya [2011] (267)	IS6110 sequence	0.607	–
Rosso [2011] (268)	IS6110 sequence	0.428	0.942
Gao [2012] (205)	IS6110 sequence and MPB64 fragment	0.948	0.900
Alvarez-Uria [2012] (269)	Xpert MTB/RIF Assay	0.320	–
Porcel [2013] (270)	Xpert MTB/RIF Assay	0.152	1.000
Christopher [2013] (271)	Xpert MTB/RIF Assay	0.121	1.000
Montenegro [2013] (272)	IS6110 sequence	0.333	0.944
Meldau [2014] (273)	Xpert MTB/RIF Assay	0.225	0.980
Trajman [2014] (274)	COBAS TaqMan MTB assay	0.160	0.860
	Xpert MTB/RIF Assay	0.030	1.000
	Detect-TB assay	0.020	0.970
Maheshkumar [2014] (275)	IS6110 sequence	0.240	–
Lusiba [2014] (276)	Xpert MTB/RIF Assay	0.287	0.966

TB = tuberculosis

nucleic acid amplification techniques resulted in a similar or higher positivity as compared to histological examination or culture of pleural biopsy specimens. PCR of pleural biopsy specimens can thus be useful when employed in combination with microbiological and histological examinations (287).

However, Xpert MTB/Rif testing was negative on all TB pleural tissues tested in a recent study from India (271).

Although these techniques are promising, the high cost and the technology involved in the procedure do not permit the routine diagnostic use of PCR at present (289).

Other Biomarkers

Lysozyme is a low molecular weight bacteriolytic protein distributed extensively in organic fluids. Mean lysozyme levels in TB pleural fluid have been reported to be higher than in other exudative effusions (128,290-293). However, there is so much overlap that the levels themselves are not diagnostic. Pleural fluid to serum lysozyme ratio of more than 1.0 or 1.2 can differentiate better between TB and non-TB pleural fluids (290,292,293). All studies have, however, not duplicated these good results (129).

A preliminary study showed that pleural fluid leptin levels were reduced in patients of TB effusion, as compared to those with other exudative effusions [82.4% sensitivity and 82.1% specificity, at a cut-off of 9.85 ng/mL] (294). A subsequent study (295) from Chennai confirmed these findings, but concluded that the decrease in leptin level was influenced by reduction in body mass index [BMI], rather than disease status *per se.*

Pleural fluid levels of IFN-γ inducible 10 kDa protein [IP-10] have been studied by some investigators. Three studies have demonstrated a relatively high sensitivity (188,296,297). Another study (296) concluded that although IP-10 has a suboptimal specificity, it might still be a useful investigation to rule out TB. Combining pleural IP-10 measurement with estimation of other cytokines can improve the diagnostic performance of this test (189,298).

Few investigators have shown high levels of matrix metalloproteinases [MMP] in TB pleural effusion. Pleural fluid MMP-9 concentrations are substantially elevated in these patients, more so in those showing granulomatous inflammation on pleural biopsy (299,300). Both blood and pleural fluid levels of MMP-1, MMP-8, MMP-9 were found elevated in patients with TB pleural effusions in another study and showed positive correlation with other inflammatory cytokines (301).

Levels of neopterin, a marker of Th1 immune response, have been shown to be elevated in pleural fluid of patients with TB (302-304). However, high levels are also seen in uraemic pleural effusions, suggesting poor specificity (305).

One study (300) has shown higher levels of pleural fluid angiotensin converting enzyme [ACE] in patients of TB effusion (300). High pleural D-dimer levels, measured by immunonephelometry assay, had a sensitivity and specificity of 84.4% and 85.5%, respectively in another study (306). Isolated reports have also indicated elevated levels of other cytokines, such as, interleukin-1B [IL-1B], IL-2, IL-12, IL-18, and TNF-alpha in pleural fluid, but the sensitivity and specificity are inadequate for clinical use (185,307,308).

Composite Algorithms and Predictive Models

As none of the individual diagnostic investigations is a good discriminator for identifying [or excluding] TB pleural effusion, scoring systems based on more than one pleural fluid parameters have been proposed. A recent large study, from a medium TB prevalence setting, showed that a combination of high pleural fluid protein [> 5 g/dL], lymphocyte proportion [> 80%] and ADA [> 45 U/L] were diagnostic of TB with a specificity of 100% (84). Another group demonstrated improvement in sensitivity and specificity using a combination of pleural fluid ADA, IFN-γ, and NAAT, as compared to single tests alone (261). A Brazilian study developed a predictive model using pleural fluid ADA, globulins and absence of malignant cells to differentiate TB from malignant effusions with greater than 95% sensitivity and specificity (309). More recently, an artificial neural network model based on results of pleural fluid investigations has been developed to support the diagnosis of pleural TB (310). Recently it has been reported that medical thoracoscoy, ADA and T-SPOT.TB together can rapidly and accurately detect TB pleural effusion (311).

Considering clinical and other laboratory parameters may also be helpful. A study from Brazil found that a combination of symptom duration, blood leucocyte count, and pleural fluid protein, lymphocytes proportion and ADA yielded greater than 95% sensitivity and specificity (312). A Spanish study (313) developed a decision tree for differentiating TB from malignant effusions using age, fever, and pleural fluid ADA and lactate dehydrogenase [LDH] as predictors. Another Spanish study (314) developed two regression models—one based on pleural fluid lymphocyte proportion and ADA level, and another based on fever, cough and pleural fluid lymphocyte proportion—in diagnosing TB in young patients. A Turkish study (315) also proposed a similar simple model based on age and pleural fluid ADA. The role of interleukin-33 [IL-33] along with ADA have also been identified in the diagnosis of TB pleural effusion (316). A composite algorithm showing the diagnostic approach is outlined in Figure 13.2.

NATURAL HISTORY

In the short-term, TB pleural effusion seems to be a self-limited inflammatory process in most instances. The natural history of untreated TB pleuritis and effusion is usually complete absorption of fluid and apparently complete restoration of the patient's health to normal [although some degree of pleural fibrosis may be evident pathologically or radiographically]. However, the likelihood of the subsequent development of pulmonary TB is high; for example, in a study from the pre-chemotherapy era conducted in 2816 members of the Finnish army with pleural effusion followed-up for seven years, 43% developed active TB during the follow-up period (317). Confirmatory evidence was provided in another study on 141 American military personnel who had presented with pleural effusion and a positive TST; nearly two-third subsequently developed some form of TB (318). In this study, isolation of mycobacteria from pleural fluid or size of pleural effusion was not correlated with subsequent appearance of active TB. Thus, the long-term prognosis in patients who have TB pleurisy is determined by its prompt recognition and the early initiation of effective therapy, which lowers the risk of subsequent disease (319).

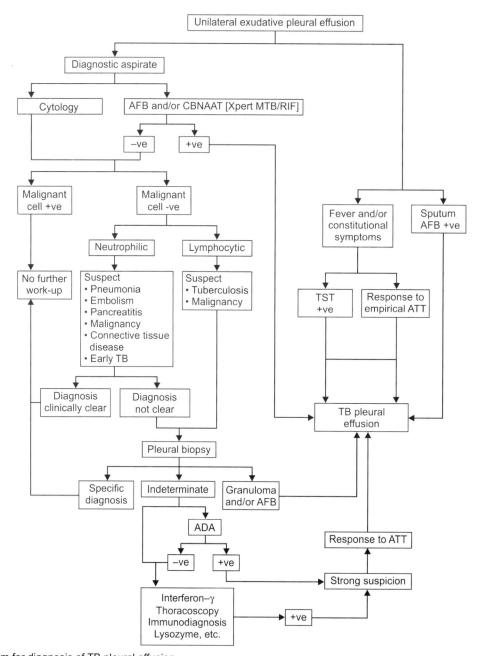

Figure 13.2: Algorithm for diagnosis of TB pleural effusion
TB = tuberculosis; AFB = acid-fast bacilli; CBNAAT = cartridge-based nucleic acid amplification test; TST = tuberculin skin test; +ve = positive; –ve = negative; PCR = polymerase chain reaction; ADA = adenosine deaminase; ATT = anti-TB treatment

TREATMENT

The goals of therapy in patients with TB pleural effusion are [i] prevention of subsequent development of active TB; [ii] relief from symptoms; and [iii] minimising the occurrence of pleural fibrosis.

Patients with TB pleural effusion respond well to treatment with standard short-course anti-TB treatment (320,321). Under the Revised National Tuberculosis Control Programme [RNTCP] of Government of India, new patients with TB pleural effusion are treated with thrice-weekly intermittent DOTS Category I treatment. Although the thrice-weekly intermittent Category III treatment regimen used earlier is no longer currently being used, it has earlier been shown to be effective and safe under programme conditions for unilateral small effusions in immunocompetent patients (322). The Category I DOTS treatment is well accepted by patients, and has a relapse rate of less than 3% (323). As per the recently published INDEX TB Guidelines (280), six months treatment with rifampicin, isoniazid, pyrazinamide and ethambutol administered for the first two months followed by rifampicin and isoniazid for the subsequent four months is considered adequate for pleural TB. Significant improvement in pleural effusion is usually evident by 6-8 weeks. The INDEX-TB guidelines (280) suggest a follow-up chest radiograph at eight weeks after starting anti-TB treatment to assess progress. An increase in the size of pleural effusion despite treatment may be due to paradoxical reaction, or an alternative diagnosis requiring further work-up and investigation.

Because patients with TB pleural effusion have low mycobacterial burden, less intensive regimens may also prove effective (324,325). With treatment, patients generally become afebrile within about two weeks, and the pleural effusion resolves within two months (326). Lung functions continue to improve even after completion of therapy (327). There appears no medical reason to confine these patients to bed, and patients need to be isolated, only if their sputum examination demonstrates AFB.

In some patients, the pleural effusion may worsen after anti-TB treatment is initiated. In this situation, the possibility of a wrong diagnosis must be considered, but paradoxical worsening can also occur with a correct diagnosis and appropriate anti-TB medications (328-330). One hypothesis is that these paradoxical responses are related to isoniazid-induced lupus pleuritis (331-333). New pleural effusion may occasionally arise on the contralateral side as well (334-337). Similarly, new parenchymal lesions may also be noticed within three months of start of medications, which eventually resolve on the same treatment (338).

Even after successful completion of treatment, nearly 10% patients may have a residual restrictive ventilatory defect on pulmonary function testing (339). Mild degrees of pleural fibrosis may be present on chest radiographs a year after therapy is begun in up to 50% of patients (81). With the strict definition of fibrothorax as a pleural membrane of at least 5 mm thickness extending across major portions of the hemithorax, a figure of around 5% is perhaps the more realistic and widely accepted rate of this complication. The presence of fibrosis is not related to the initial pleural fluid findings and is of limited clinical significance, although a higher pleural fluid glucose or IFN-γ may be associated with increased residual pleural thickening (340-342). A faster resolution of pleural effusion during the initial phase of treatment may decrease the occurrence of significant pleural thickening (343). The correlation between radiographic and functional sequelae [as assessed by pulmonary function testing] is poor (339).

Evidence regarding efficacy of systemic corticosteroids in the treatment of TB pleuritis remains insufficient (344-346). Three randomised, double-blind, placebo-controlled trials have been completed, but all had important methodologic differences. There were no benefits with the use of systemic corticosteroids in two controlled studies in which therapeutic thoracentesis was also performed (347,348). However, the duration of fever and the time required for fluid resorption were decreased in a third study in which no therapeutic thoracentesis was performed (349). Administration of corticosteroids did not influence residual pleural thickening in any of these studies. As per the recently published INDEX TB Guidelines (280), corticosteroids are not routinely recommended in pleural TB. Corticosteroids are occasionally to be used only in selected patients if acute symptoms, such as fever, chest pain, or dyspnoea, are disturbing to the patient. If needed, corticosteroids should be prescribed only after the institution of appropriate anti-TB treatment. Oral prednisolone 0.5-0.75 mg/kg [or equivalent alternate day doses] are administered until acute symptoms have subsided, with rapid tapering thereafter (350).

In general, surgical procedures have no place in the routine management. Therapeutic thoracentesis is only indicated if the patient has a moderate-sized or larger pleural effusion producing significant breathlessness. In fact, routine serial therapeutic thoracentesis, or continuous pigtail catheter drainage, does not alter the course of illness or development of residual pleural fibrosis (351,352). Early surgery for pleural thickening is also not recommended, as the thickening decreases with treatment. A recent study also suggests that instillation of a fibrinolytic agent into a loculated collection may help in subsequent reduction of pleural thickening (353). Although medical thoracoscopy can open intrapleural loculations, completely evacuate the pleural fluid, and to some extent produce effective debridement, no controlled study has so far proven the value of these efforts.

HUMAN IMMUNODEFICIENCY VIRUS CO-INFECTION

It appears that co-infection with HIV is the main factor responsible for the increase in TB pleurisy in the West and in Africa (354,355). Pleural effusion is seen in 6%-28% of HIV-infected patients with TB (355-358). Affected patients tend to develop pleural effusion in early stages of immunosuppression and the frequency of pleural effusion is higher in patients with CD4+ lymphocyte counts exceeding 200 cells/mm^3 (359). Pooled estimates from several reports reveal that TB is responsible for almost a quarter of all pleural effusions seen in patients with HIV infection, and that the condition is second only to bacterial parapneumonic effusions in terms of frequency (356). In addition to the DTH persistence of mycobacteria in the pleural space as result of failure of immune system has been proposed as an alternative explanation for the higher incidence of pleural disease in these patients (360). It is not clear if the higher rate of pleural disease reflects a greater burden of pleural mycobacteria or dysregulation of immune function in the pleural space. TB effusions may similarly also occur in patients immunodeficient because of other reasons (361).

Affected patients usually are symptomatic for longer periods, have additional symptoms [fever, dyspnoea, night sweats, fatigue, diarrhoea, etc.] and more commonly have hepatomegaly, splenomegaly and lymphadenopathy than patients who are seronegative (362-364). The diagnostic approach in patients with HIV infection is largely similar to other patients with TB pleural effusion, although the performance of some of the diagnostic tests is different. Patients are more likely to be anergic to TST (362,365).

AFB can be demonstrated in the pleural fluid smears in 6%-15%; and on pleural biopsy specimens in 44%-69% cases (82,359,363). AFB smears are more likely to be positive when CD4+ T-lymphocyte counts fall below 200 cells/mm^3 (233). Pleural fluid and/or biopsy cultures grow mycobacteria in 30%-50% cases (82,360,365,366). Despite the impaired T-lymphocyte function, pleural biopsy specimens show granulomatous inflammation in 44%-88% cases (82,360,366). The role of PCR, and measurements of ADA, lysozymes, or IFN-γ in the diagnosis of TB pleural effusion in HIV-seropositive patients is still not clear (364).

Management guidelines for these patients are similar to those for other patients, and standard four-drug anti-TB treatment is the treatment of choice (367). The clinical and microbiologic response to treatment in these patients appears to be similar to that in patients not infected with HIV. Most HIV-infected patients with TB pleural effusion respond favorably to standard treatment, with mortality rates less than 10% after an average follow-up of more than two years (360,368). Patients with poor or absent tissue reaction on pleural biopsy histology appear to have a less favorable response to therapy and higher mortality (365). The reader is referred to the chapters *"Treatment of tuberculosis"* [Chapter 44]; and *"Tuberculosis and human immunodeficiency virus infection"* [Chapter 35] for details.

PLEURAL EFFUSION DUE TO NONTUBERCULOUS MYCOBACTERIA

As with pulmonary disease, the vast majority of cases of pleural mycobacterial infection are caused by *Mycobacterium tuberculosis* [Mtb]; only occasional cases are related to nontuberculous mycobacteria [NTM] (369-376). Pleural effusions without parenchymal disease analogous to the post-primary pleural effusion with *Mtb* do not occur. Approximately 5% of patients with parenchymal disease due to either *Mycobacterium intracellulare* or *Mycobacterium kansasii* have an associated small pleural effusion (377). About 15% patients with parenchymal disease due to *Mycobacterium. intracellulare* have marked pleural thickening as well (377). In patients with AIDS and disseminated disease due to *Mycobacterium intracellulare* or *Mycobacterium avium* [collectively referred to as *Mycobacterium avium intracellulare* complex or MAIC], pleural fluid cultures are sometimes positive for MAIC (378). However, it is not clear whether these atypical mycobacteria are actually responsible for the pleural effusion. Even in immunocompetent patients one must be cautious regarding the interpretation of isolation of atypical mycobacteria from pleural fluid. It has been suggested that NTM cultured from pleural fluid should not be considered aetiologic, unless there is evidence of the same organism infecting other tissues (379).

TB EMPYEMA

TB empyema is an entity distinct from, and much less common than, TB pleural effusion. In contrast to DTH leading to pleural fluid accumulation in a TB pleural effusion, TB empyema is characterized by chronic, active mycobacterial infection of the pleural space. It usually represents the failure of a primary TB effusion to resolve and subsequent progression to a chronic suppurative form, and may develop in fibrous scar tissue resulting from pleurisy, artificial pneumothorax, or thoracoplasty (380). In addition, TB empyema can also occur due to extension of infection from intrathoracic lymph nodes or a sub-diaphragmatic focus, or haematogenous spread (381). In TB empyema, the pleural fluid is purulent, and it is common to find mycobacteria on direct smear examination or culture of pleural fluid (382). TB empyema represents nearly 20%-35% of all cases of empyema seen in high TB prevalence countries like India (383,384).

In many patients with chronic TB empyema, the inflammatory process may be present for years with a paucity of clinical symptoms (380,385). This prolonged asymptomatic course is largely related to the marked pleural thickening that isolates the tubercle bacilli to the empyema cavity. Patients are often diagnosed only after a routine chest radiograph or after development of complications such as bronchopleural fistula or empyema necessitans (386). Other patients may present with low-grade fever, night sweats and constitutional symptoms, such as fatigue and weight loss. Patients often have respiratory symptoms for several months prior to diagnosis (384,387).

The typical radiological findings of chronic TB empyema include a moderate to large loculated pleural effusion with pleural calcification and thickening of the overlying ribs [Figures 9.10, 9.11] (22). Diagnosis is confirmed after thoracentesis by finding grossly purulent fluid that is smear positive for AFB and subsequently grows mycobacteria on culture. Pleural fluid cell counts usually exceed 100,000/mm^3, with virtually all cells being neutrophils (382). The pleural fluid has low glucose [usually below 20 mg/dL] and high protein concentration [usually more than 5 g/dL], and is acidic [with pH usually below 7.20]. Anaerobic and aerobic cultures should also be performed to exclude concomitant bacterial and mycobacterial infection.

The principles of treatment, pleural space drainage, and antimicrobial chemotherapy are similar for bacterial and TB empyema. Difficulties specific to management of TB empyema include the inability of the trapped lung to re-expand adequately and failure to achieve therapeutic drug levels in pleural fluid, which can lead to drug resistance (382,388). It is therefore important to use multiple drugs at their maximum tolerated dosages. Pleural drainage is indicated for large empyemas and mixed empyemas, especially if there is a bronchopleural fistula. Because intensive chemotherapy coupled with serial thoracentesis can be curative at times, this approach should be attempted initially (389). In addition to standard anti-TB treatment, patients usually require surgery (390). Surgical procedures include standard decortication, decortication limited to the parietal sides of the empyema collection, thoracoplasty, muscle flap, plombage, parietal wall collapse, open drainage, or resection of the entire lung along with the empyema (381). Most patients have associated significant pulmonary parenchymal involvement (382,247).

The status of the underlying lung should be determined before planning any surgery, because presence of massive fibrotic lesions, cavities, or bronchiectasis can make surgery difficult or inadvisable. Ideally, anti-TB medications are given for two to four months preoperatively and the sputum should be negative for AFB for two months prior to surgery. Morbidity and mortality related to surgery continue to be high (382,391,392). It must be stressed that such surgery is extremely complex and challenging, and should only be undertaken by experienced thoracic surgeons to improve outcomes (393). As with other forms of chronic empyema, surgery can help in post-operative improvement of lung function (394). Presence of bronchopleural fistula, chronicity of the lesion and presence of disease in the underlying and/or contralateral lung contribute to a poorer outcome with treatment (390). The relative lung volume of the affected side, as well as the volume of empyema, can help predict the quantum of improvement in lung function after surgery (395). The reader is also referred to the chapter *"Surgery for pleuropulmonary tuberculosis"* [Chapter 46] for details.

PSEUDOCHYLOTHORAX AND CHYLOTHORAX

The term pseudochylothorax refers to thickened [and often calcified] pleura that contains cholesterol rich fluid. The pleural fluid cholesterol levels are greater than 200 mg/dL and cholesterol crystals are evident (396). The precise mechanism of cholesterol accumulation has not been elucidated, though it probably results from accumulation of cellular inflammatory debris secondary to local degeneration of red and white blood cells. TB is the main aetiological cause of pseudochylothorax, accounting for more than half of all reported cases (397). There is a remarkable correlation with previous collapse therapy and long-standing pleural effusions [typically 5 or more years]. Pseudochylothorax can develop even after, and despite, successful anti-TB treatment (398). Pleural fluid is usually sterile (396,397). However, anti-TB treatment should be administered to patients in whom mycobacteria are demonstrated on pleural fluid analysis or pleural biopsy histology, and those with enlarging effusions of suspected TB origin (397). Drainage is recommended only in symptomatic patients. Pulmonary decortication should be reserved for recurrent and symptomatic patients not responding to medical measures.

In contrast to pseudochylothorax, chylothorax is an acute effusion formed by accumulation of chyle in pleural space secondary to damage of thoracic duct. Triglyceride levels in pleural fluid are always greater than 50 mg/dL and usually higher than 110 mg/dL, but the main diagnostic criterion is the presence of chylomicrons in pleural fluid (392). TB is a rare cause of chylothorax (399-405). The genesis of chylothorax in TB is not clear, but may be related either to lymph nodes obstructing and eroding into the cisterna chyli or thoracic duct, or to direct involvement of lymphatic channels by tubercle bacilli.

REFERENCES

1. Al-Alusi F. Pleural effusion in Iraq: a prospective study of 100 cases. Thorax 1986;41:492-3.
2. Xiong Y, Gao X, Zhu H, Ding C, Wang J. Role of medical thoracoscopy in the treatment of tuberculous pleural effusion. J Thorac Dis 2016;8:52-60.
3. Vorster MJ, Allwood BW, Diacon AH, Koegelenberg CF. Tuberculous pleural effusions: advances and controversies. J Thorac Dis 2015;7:981-91.
4. Batungwanayo J, Taelman H, Allen S, Bogaerts J, Kagame A, Van de Perre P. Pleural effusion, tuberculosis and HIV-1 infection in Kigali, Rwanda. AIDS 1993;7:73-9.
5. Skouras VS, Kalomenidis I. Drug resistance in patients with tuberculous pleural effusions. Curr Opin Pulm Med 2018;24:374-9.
6. al-Qorain A, Larbi EB, al-Muhanna F, Satti MB, Baloush A, Falha K. Pattern of pleural effusion in Eastern Province of Saudi Arabia: a prospective study. East Afr Med J 1994;71:246-9.
7. Richter C, Perenboom R, Swai AB, Kitinya J, Mtoni I, Chande H, et al. Diagnosis of tuberculosis in patients with pleural effusion in an area of HIV infection and limited diagnostic facilities. Trop Geogr Med 1994;46:293-7.
8. Valdes L, Alvarez D, Valle JM, Pose A, San Jose E. The etiology of pleural effusions in an area with high incidence of tuberculosis. Chest 1996;109:158-62.
9. Udwadia ZF, Sen T. Pleural tuberculosis: an update. Curr Opin Pulm Med 2010;16:399-406.
10. Yoon HJ, Song YG, Park WI, Choi JP, Chang KH, Kim JM. Clinical manifestations and diagnosis of extrapulmonary tuberculosis. Yonsei Med J 2004;45:453-61.
11. Ilgazli A, Boyaci H, Basyigit I, Yildiz F. Extrapulmonary tuberculosis: clinical and epidemiologic spectrum of 636 cases. Arch Med Res 2004;35:435-41.
12. Prakasha SR, Suresh G, D'Sa I P, Shetty SS, Kumar SG. Mapping the pattern and trends of extrapulmonary tuberculosis. J Glob Infect Dis 2013;5:54-9.
13. Sahn SA. State of the art. The pleura. Am Rev Respir Dis 1988;138:184-234.
14. Mehta JB, Dutt A, Harvill L, Mathews KM. Epidemiology of extrapulmonary tuberculosis: a comparative analysis with pre-AIDS era. Chest 1991;99:1134-8.
15. Menzies R, Charbonneau M. Thoracoscopy for the diagnosis of pleural disease. Ann Intern Med 1991;114:271-6.
16. Marel M, Stastny B, Melinova L, Svandova E, Light RW. Diagnosis of pleural effusions. Experience with clinical studies, 1986 to 1990. Chest 1995;107:1598-603.
17. Baumann MH, Nolan R, Petrini M, Lee YC, Light RW, Schneider E. Pleural tuberculosis in the United States: incidence and drug resistance. Chest 2007;131:1125-32.
18. Valdes L, Ferreiro L, Cruz-Ferro E, Gonzalez-Barcala FJ, Gude F, Ursua MI, et al. Recent epidemiological trends in tuberculous pleural effusion in Galicia, Spain. Eur J Intern Med 2012;23:727-32.
19. Bouros D, Demoiliopoulos J, Panagou P, Yiatromanolakis N, Moschos M, Paraskevopoulos A, et al. Incidence of tuberculosis in Greek armed forces from 1965-1993. Respiration 1995;62:336-40.
20. Moudgil H, Sridhar G, Leitch AG. Reactivation disease: the commonest form of tuberculous pleural effusion in Edinburgh, 1980-1991. Respir Med 1994;88:301-4.
21. Stead WW, Eichenholz A, Stauss HK. Operative and pathologic findings in twenty-four patients with syndrome of idiopathic pleurisy with effusion, presumably tuberculous. Am Rev Tuberc 1955;71:473-502.

22. Hulnick DH, Naidich DP, McCauley DI. Pleural tuberculosis evaluated by computed tomography. Radiology 1983;149:759-65.

23. Malhotra HS, Garg RK, Raut TP. Pleural involvement in spinal tuberculosis. Am J Trop Med Hyg 2012;86:560.

24. Allen JC, Apicella MA. Experimental pleural effusion as a manifestation of delayed hypersensitivity to tuberculin PPD. J Immunol 1968;101:481-7.

25. Leckie WJ, Tothill P. Albumin turnover in pleural effusions. Clin Sci 1965;29:339-52.

26. Leibowitz S, Kennedy L, Lessof MH. The tuberculin reaction in the pleural cavity and its suppression by antilymphocyte serum. Br J Exp Pathol 1973;54:152-62.

27. Ellner JJ, Barnes PF, Wallis RS, Modlin RL. The immunology of tuberculous pleurisy. Semin Respir Infect 1988;3:335-42.

28. Kroegel C, Antony VB. Immunobiology of pleural inflammation: potential implications for pathogenesis, diagnosis and therapy. Eur Respir J 1997;10:2411-8.

29. Ellner JJ. Pleural fluid and peripheral blood lymphocyte function in tuberculosis. Ann Intern Med 1978;89:932-3.

30. Shimokata K, Kawachi H, Kishimoto H, Maeda F, Ito Y. Local cellular immunity in tuberculous pleurisy. Am Rev Respir Dis 1982;126:822-4.

31. Fujiwara H, Tsuyuguchi I. Frequency of tuberculin-reactive T-lymphocytes in pleural fluid and blood from patients with tuberculous pleurisy. Chest 1986;89:530-2.

32. Lorgat F, Keraan MM, Ress SR. Cellular immunity in tuberculous pleural effusions: evidence of spontaneous lymphocyte proliferation and antigen-specific accelerated responses to purified protein derivative [PPD]. Clin Exp Immunol 1992;90:215-8.

33. Qiao D, Yang BY, Li L, Ma JJ, Zhang XL, Lao SH, et al. ESAT-6- and CFP-10-specific Th1, Th22 and Th17 cells in tuberculous pleurisy may contribute to the local immune response against Mycobacterium tuberculosis infection. Scand J Immunol 2011; 73:330-7.

34. Mehra V, Gong JH, Iyer D, Lin Y, Boylen CT, Bloom BR, et al. Immune response to recombinant mycobacterial proteins in patients with tuberculosis infection and disease. J Infect Dis 1996;174:431-4.

35. Jalapathy KV, Prabha C, Das SD. Correlates of protective immune response in tuberculous pleuritis. FEMS Immunol Med Microbiol 2004;40:139-45.

36. El Fenniri L, Toossi Z, Aung H, El Iraki G, Bourkkadi J, Benamor J, et al. Polyfunctional Mycobacterium tuberculosis-specific effector memory CD4+ T cells at sites of pleural TB. Tuberculosis [Edinb] 2011;91:224-30.

37. Sharma SK, Mitra DK, Balamurugan A, Pandey RM, Mehra NK. Cytokine polarization in miliary and pleural tuberculosis. J Clin Immunol 2002;22:345-52.

38. Tong ZH, Shi HZ. Subpopulations of helper T lymphocytes in tuberculous pleurisy. Tuberculosis [Edinb] 2013;93:279-84.

39. Antony VB, Sahn SA, Antony AC, Repine JE. Bacillus Calmette-Guerin-stimulated neutrophils release chemotaxins for monocytes in rabbit pleural spaces and in vitro. J Clin Invest 1985;76: 1514-21.

40. Li X, Zhou Q, Yang WB, Xiong XZ, Du RH, Zhang JC. Pleural mesothelial cells promote expansion of IL-17-producing CD8+ T cells in tuberculous pleural effusion. J Clin Immunol 2013;33: 775-87.

41. Antony VB, Hott JW, Kunkel SL, Godbey SW, Burdick MD, Strieter RM. Pleural mesothelial cell expression of C-C [monocyte chemotactic peptide] and C-X-C [interleukin 8] chemokines. Am J Respir Cell Mol Biol 1995;12:581-8.

42. Mohammed KA, Nasreen N, Ward MJ, Mubarak KK, Rodriguez-Panadero F, Antony VB. Mycobacterium-mediated chemokine expression in pleural mesothelial cells: role of C-C chemokines in tuberculous pleurisy. J Infect Dis 1998;178:1450-6.

43. Widstrom O, Nilsson BS. Pleurisy induced by intrapleural BCG in immunized guinea pigs. Eur J Respir Dis 1982;63:425-34.

44. Baganha MF, Pego A, Lima MA, Gaspar EV, Cordeiro AR. Serum and pleural adenosine deaminase. Correlation with lymphocytic populations. Chest 1990;97:605-10.

45. Mitra DK, Sharma SK, Dinda AK, Bindra MS, Madan B, Ghosh B. Polarized helper T cells in tubercular pleural effusion: phenotypic identity and selective recruitment. Eur J Immunol 2005;35: 2367-75.

46. Widstrom O, Nilsson BS. Low in vitro response to PPD and PHA in lymphocytes from BCG-induced pleurisy in guinea pigs. Eur J Respir Dis 1982;63:435-41.

47. Prabha C, Rajashree P, Sulochana DD. TLR2 and TLR4 expression on the immune cells of tuberculous pleural fluid. Immunol Lett 2008;117:26-34.

48. Barnes PF, Fong SJ, Brennan PJ, Twomey PE, Mazumder A, Modlin RL. Local production of tumor necrosis factor and IFN-gamma in tuberculous pleuritis. J Immunol 1990;145:149-54.

49. Kurasawa T, Shimokata K. Cooperation between accessory cells and T lymphocytes in patients with tuberculous pleurisy. Chest 1991;100:1046-52.

50. Nathan CF, Murray HW, Wiebe ME, Rubin BY. Identification of interferon-gamma as the lymphokine that activates human macrophage oxidative metabolism and antimicrobial activity. J Exp Med 1983;158:670-89.

51. Ribera E, Espanol T, Martinez-Vazquez JM, Ocana I, Encabo G. Lymphocyte proliferation and gamma-interferon production after "in vitro" stimulation with PPD. Differences between tuberculous and nontuberculous pleurisy in patients with positive tuberculin skin test. Chest 1990;97:1381-5.

52. Lorgat F, Keraan MM, Lukey PT, Ress SR. Evidence for in vivo generation of cytotoxic T cells. PPD-stimulated lymphocytes from tuberculous pleural effusions demonstrate enhanced cytotoxicity with accelerated kinetics of induction. Am Rev Respir Dis 1992;145:418-23.

53. Ota T, Okubo Y, Sekiguchi M. Analysis of immunologic mechanisms of high natural killer cell activity in tuberculous pleural effusions. Am Rev Respir Dis 1990;142:29-33.

54. Loddenkemper R, Boutin C. Thoracoscopy: present diagnostic and therapeutic indications. Eur Respir J 1993;6:1544-5.

55. Aktogu S, Yorgancioglu A, Cirak K, Kose T, Dereli SM. Clinical spectrum of pulmonary and pleural tuberculosis: a report of 5,480 cases. Eur Respir J 1996;9:2031-5.

56. Valdes L, Alvarez D, San Jose E, Penela P, Valle JM, Garcia-Pazos JM, et al. Tuberculous pleurisy: a study of 254 patients. Arch Intern Med 1998;158:2017-21.

57. Sibley JC. A study of 200 cases of tuberculous pleurisy with effusion. Am Rev Tuberc 1950;62:314-23.

58. Levine H, Szanto PB, Cugell DW. Tuberculous pleurisy. An acute illness. Arch Intern Med 1968;122:329-32.

59. Berger HW, Mejia E. Tuberculous pleurisy. Chest 1973;63:88-92.

60. Seibert AF, Haynes J, Jr., Middleton R, Bass JB, Jr. Tuberculous pleural effusion. Twenty-year experience. Chest 1991;99:883-6.

61. Maher GG, Berger HW. Massive pleural effusion: malignant and nonmalignant causes in 46 patients. Am Rev Respir Dis 1972;105: 458-60.

62. Porcel JM, Vives M. Etiology and pleural fluid characteristics of large and massive effusions. Chest 2003;124:978-83.

63. Seiscento M, Vargas FS, Bombarda S, Sales RK, Terra RM, Uezumi K, et al. Pulmonary involvement in pleural tuberculosis: how often does it mean disease activity? Respir Med 2011;105: 1079-83.

64. Arriero JM, Romero S, Hernandez L, Candela A, Martin C, Gil J, et al. Tuberculous pleurisy with or without radiographic evidence of pulmonary disease. Is there any difference? Int J Tuberc Lung Dis 1998;2:513-7.

65. Yilmaz MU, Kumcuoglu Z, Utkaner G, Yalniz O, Erkmen G. Computed tomography findings of tuberculous pleurisy. Int J Tuberc Lung Dis 1998;2:164-7.

66. Antonangelo L, Vargas FS, Puka J, Seiscento M, Acencio MM, Teixeira LR, et al. Pleural tuberculosis: is radiological evidence of pulmonary-associated disease related to the exacerbation of the inflammatory response? Clinics [Sao Paulo] 2012;67:1259-63.

67. Kim HJ, Lee HJ, Kwon SY, Yoon HI, Chung HS, Lee CT, et al. The prevalence of pulmonary parenchymal tuberculosis in patients with tuberculous pleuritis. Chest 2006;129:1253-8.

68. Patel A, Choudhury S. Pleural tuberculosis presented as multiple pleural masses: an atypical presentation. Lung India 2013;30:54-6.

69. Arul P, Varghese RG, Ramdas A. Pleural tuberculosis mimicking inflammatory pseudotumour. J Clin Diagn Res 2013;7:709-11.

70. Kim JS, Shim SS, Kim Y, Ryu YJ, Lee JH. Chest CT findings of pleural tuberculosis: differential diagnosis of pleural tuberculosis and malignant pleural dissemination. Acta Radiol 2014; 55: 1063-8.

71. Shinohara T, Shiota N, Kume M, Hamada N, Naruse K, Ogushi F. Asymptomatic primary tuberculous pleurisy with intense 18-fluorodeoxyglucose uptake mimicking malignant mesothelioma. BMC Infect Dis 2013;13:12.

72. Aggarwal AN, Gupta D, Jindal SK. Diagnosis of tuberculous pleural effusion. Indian J Chest Dis Allied Sci 1999;41:89-100.

73. Diacon AH, Van de Wal BW, Wyser C, Smedema JP, Bezuidenhout J, Bolliger CT, et al. Diagnostic tools in tuberculous pleurisy: a direct comparative study. Eur Respir J 2003;22:589-91.

74. Ghanei M, Aslani J, Bahrami H, Adhami H. Simple method for rapid diagnosis of tuberculosis pleuritis: a statistical approach. Asian Cardiovasc Thorac Ann 2004;12:23-29.

75. Neves DD, Dias RM, da Cunha AJ, Preza PC. What is the probability of a patient presenting a pleural effusion due to tuberculosis? Braz J Infect Dis 2004;8:311-8.

76. Gopi A, Madhavan SM, Sharma SK, Sahn SA. Diagnosis and treatment of tuberculous pleural effusion in 2006. Chest 2007;131: 880-9.

77. Ghosal AG, Ghosh S, Guhathakurta R, Sinha A, Banerjee AK, Chakrabarti AK. Sputum AFB positivity in tuberculous pleural effusion with no radiologically apparent parenchymal lung lesion. Indian J Tuberc 1997;44:13-5.

78. Escudero Bueno C, Garcia Clemente M, Cuesta Castro B, Molinos Martin L, Rodriguez Ramos S, Gonzalez Panizo A, et al. Cytologic and bacteriologic analysis of fluid and pleural biopsy specimens with Cope's needle. Study of 414 patients. Arch Intern Med 1990;150:1190-4.

79. Epstein DM, Kline LR, Albelda SM, Miller WT. Tuberculous pleural effusions. Chest 1987;91:106-9.

80. Conde MB, Loivos AC, Rezende VM, Soares SL, Mello FC, Reingold AL, et al. Yield of sputum induction in the diagnosis of pleural tuberculosis. Am J Respir Crit Care Med 2003;167:723-5.

81. Chan CH, Arnold M, Chan CY, Mak TW, Hoheisel GB. Clinical and pathological features of tuberculous pleural effusion and its long-term consequences. Respiration 1991;58:171-5.

82. Relkin F, Aranda CP, Garay SM, Smith R, Berkowitz KA, Rom WN. Pleural tuberculosis and HIV infection. Chest 1994; 105:1338-41.

83. Light RW. Tuberculous pleural effusions. In: Light RW, editor. Pleural diseases. Fourth edition. Philadelphia: Lippincott Williams and Wilkins; 2001.p.182-95.

84. Sahn SA, Huggins JT, San Jose ME, Alvarez-Dobano JM, Valdes L. Can tuberculous pleural effusions be diagnosed by pleural fluid analysis alone? Int J Tuberc Lung Dis 2013;17:787-93.

85. Barber LM, Mazzadi L, Deakins DD, Reese CN, Rogers WL. Glucose level in pleural fluid as a diagnostic aid. Dis Chest 1957;31:680-7.

86. Light RW, MacGregor MI, Ball WC, Jr, Luchsinger PC. Diagnostic significance of pleural fluid pH and PCO_2. Chest 1973;64:591-6.

87. Chavalittamrong B, Angsusingha K, Tuchinda M, Habananananda S, Pidatcha P, Tuchinda C. Diagnostic significance of pH, lactic acid dehydrogenase, lactate and glucose in pleural fluid. Respiration 1979;38:112-20.

88. Good JT Jr, Taryle DA, Maulitz RM, Kaplan RL, Sahn SA. The diagnostic value of pleural fluid pH. Chest 1980;78:55-9.

89. Bielsa S, Palma R, Pardina M, Esquerda A, Light RW, Porcel JM. Comparison of polymorphonuclear- and lymphocyte-rich tuberculous pleural effusions. Int J Tuberc Lung Dis 2013;17:85-9.

90. Spieler P. The cytologic diagnosis of tuberculosis in pleural effusions. Acta Cytol 1979;23:374-9.

91. Kapila K, Pande JN, Garg A, Verma K. T lymphocyte subsets and B lymphocytes in tubercular pleural effusion. Indian J Chest Dis Allied Sci 1987;29:90-3.

92. Lucivero G, Pierucci G, Bonomo L. Lymphocyte subsets in peripheral blood and pleural fluid. Eur Respir J 1988;1:337-40.

93. Albera C, Mabritto I, Ghio P, Scagliotti GV, Pozzi E. Lymphocyte subpopulations analysis in pleural fluid and peripheral blood in patients with lymphocytic pleural effusions. Respiration 1991; 58:65-71.

94. Gambon-Deza F, Pacheco Carracedo M, Cerda Mota T, Montes Santiago J. Lymphocyte populations during tuberculosis infection: V beta repertoires. Infect Immun 1995;63:1235-40.

95. Pettersson T, Klockars M, Hellstrom PE, Riska H, Wangel A. T and B lymphocytes in pleural effusions. Chest 1978;73:49-51.

96. Light RW, Erozan YS, Ball WC Jr. Cells in pleural fluid. Their value in differential diagnosis. Arch Intern Med 1973;132:854-60.

97. Hurwitz S, Leiman G, Shapiro C. Mesothelial cells in pleural fluid: TB or not TB? S Afr Med J 1980;57:937-9.

98. Lau KY. Numerous mesothelial cells in tuberculous pleural effusions. Chest 1989;96:438-9.

99. Adelman M, Albelda SM, Gottlieb J, Haponik EF. Diagnostic utility of pleural fluid eosinophilia. Am J Med 1984;77:915-20.

100. Lakhotia M, Mehta SR, Mathur D, Baid CS, Varma AR. Diagnostic significance of pleural fluid eosinophilia during initial thoraco-centesis. Indian J Chest Dis Allied Sci 1989;31:259-64.

101. Onadeko BO. Tuberculous pleural effusion: clinical patterns and management in Nigerians. Tubercle 1978;59:269-75.

102. Kumar S, Seshadri MS, Koshi G, John TJ. Diagnosing tuberculous pleural effusion: comparative sensitivity of mycobacterial culture and histopathology. Br Med J [Clin Res Ed] 1981;283:20.

103. Enarson DA, Dorken E, Grzybowski S. Tuberculous pleurisy. Can Med Assoc J 1982;126:493-5.

104. Liu SF, Liu JW, Lin MC. Characteristics of patients suffering from tuberculous pleuritis with pleural effusion culture positive and negative for Mycobacterium tuberculosis, and risk factors for fatality. Int J Tuberc Lung Dis 2005;9:111-5.

105. Ruan SY, Chuang YC, Wang JY, Lin JW, Chien JY, Huang CT, et al. Revisiting tuberculous pleurisy: pleural fluid characteristics and diagnostic yield of mycobacterial culture in an endemic area. Thorax 2012;67:822-7.

106. Maartens G, Bateman ED. Tuberculous pleural effusions: increased culture yield with bedside inoculation of pleural fluid and poor diagnostic value of adenosine deaminase. Thorax 1991; 46:96-9.

107. Cheng AF, Li MS, Chan CY, Chan CH, Lyon D, Wise R, et al. Evaluation of three culture media and their combinations for the isolation of Mycobacterium tuberculosis from pleural aspirates of patients with tuberculous pleurisy. J Trop Med Hyg 1994;97: 249-53.

108. Cheng AF, Tai VH, Li MS, Chan CH, Wong CF, Yew WW, et al. Improved recovery of Mycobacterium tuberculosis from pleural aspirates: bedside inoculation, heparinized containers and liquid culture media. Scand J Infect Dis 1999;31:485-7.

109. von Groote-Bidlingmaier F, Koegelenberg CF, Bolliger CT, Chung PK, Rautenbach C, Wasserman E, et al. The yield of different pleural fluid volumes for Mycobacterium tuberculosis culture. Thorax 2013;68:290-1.

110. Scharer L, McClement JH. Isolation of tubercle bacilli from needle biopsy specimens of parietal pleura. Am Rev Respir Dis 1968;97:466-8.

111. Hira HS, Ranjan R. Role of percutaneous closed needle pleural biopsy among patients of undiagnosed exudative pleural effusion. Lung India 2011;28:101-4.

112. Levine H, Metzger W, Lacera D, Kay L. Diagnosis of tuberculous pleurisy by culture of pleural biopsy specimen. Arch Intern Med 1970;126:269-71.

113. Suri JC, Goel A, Gupta DK, Bhatia A. Role of serial pleural biopsies in the diagnosis of pleural effusions. Indian J Chest Dis Allied Sci 1991;33:63-7.

114. Kirsch CM, Kroe DM, Azzi RL, Jensen WA, Kagawa FT, Wehner JH. The optimal number of pleural biopsy specimens for a diagnosis of tuberculous pleurisy. Chest 1997;112:702-6.

115. Jimenez D, Perez-Rodriguez E, Diaz G, Fogue L, Light RW. Determining the optimal number of specimens to obtain with needle biopsy of the pleura. Respir Med 2002;96:14-7.

116. Katiyar SK, Singh RP, Singh KP, Upadhyay GC, Sharma A, Tripathi LK. Cultivation of Mycobacterium tuberculosis from pleural tissue and its histopathology in suspected cases of tuberculous pleural effusion. Indian J Pathol Microbiol 1997;40: 51-4.

117. Prakash UB, Reiman HM. Comparison of needle biopsy with cytologic analysis for the evaluation of pleural effusion: analysis of 414 cases. Mayo Clin Proc 1985;60:158-64.

118. Jain NK, Guhan AR, Joshi N, Dixit R, Singh V, Meena RP. Comparative study of visceral and parietal pleural biopsy in the etiological diagnosis of pleural diseases. J Assoc Physicians India 2000;48:776-80.

119. Koegelenberg CF, Diacon AH. Image-guided pleural biopsy. Curr Opin Pulm Med 2013;19:368-73.

120. Gaga M, Papamichalis G, Bakakos P, Latsi P, Samara I, Koulouris NG, et al. Tuberculous effusion: ADA activity correlates with CD4+ cell numbers in the fluid and the pleura. Respiration 2005;72:160-5.

121. Onyenekwu CP, Zemlin AE, Erasmus RT. High pleural fluid adenosine deaminase levels: a valuable tool for rapid diagnosis of pleural TB in a middle-income country with a high TB/HIV burden. S Afr Med J 2014;104:200-3.

122. Sharma SK, Mohan A. Adenosine deaminase in the diagnosis of tuberculosis pleural effusion. Indian J Chest Dis Allied Sci 1996;38:69-71.

123. Bielsa S, Esquerda A, Palma RM, Criado A, Porcel JM. Influence of storage time on pleural fluid adenosine deaminase activity. Clin Lab 2014;60:501-4.

124. Coitinho C, Rivas C. Auxiliary tools in tuberculosis. The hemolysis in pleural fluids underestimate the values of adenosine deaminase activity determined by the method of Giusti. Rev Argent Microbiol 2008;40:101-5.

125. Greco S, Girardi E, Masciangelo R, Capoccetta GB, Saltini C. Adenosine deaminase and interferon gamma measurements for the diagnosis of tuberculous pleurisy: a meta-analysis. Int J Tuberc Lung Dis 2003;7:777-86.

126. Liang QL, Shi HZ, Wang K, Qin SM, Qin XJ. Diagnostic accuracy of adenosine deaminase in tuberculous pleurisy: a meta-analysis. Respir Med 2008;102:744-54.

127. Ocana I, Martinez-Vazquez JM, Segura RM, Fernandez-De-Sevilla T, Capdevila JA. Adenosine deaminase in pleural fluids. Test for diagnosis of tuberculous pleural effusion. Chest 1983;84:51-3.

128. Fontan Bueso J, Verea Hernando H, Garcia-Buela JP, Dominguez Juncal L, Martin Egana MT, Montero Martinez MC. Diagnostic value of simultaneous determination of pleural adenosine deaminase and pleural lysozyme/serum lysozyme ratio in pleural effusions. Chest 1988;93:303-7.

129. Valdes L, San Jose E, Alvarez D, Sarandeses A, Pose A, Chomon B, et al. Diagnosis of tuberculous pleurisy using the biologic parameters adenosine deaminase, lysozyme, and interferon gamma. Chest 1993;103:458-65.

130. Porcel JM, Esquerda A, Bielsa S. Diagnostic performance of adenosine deaminase activity in pleural fluid: a single-center experience with over 2100 consecutive patients. Eur J Intern Med 2010;21:419-23.

131. Perez-Rodriguez E, Jimenez Castro D. The use of adenosine deaminase and adenosine deaminase isoenzymes in the diagnosis of tuberculous pleuritis. Curr Opin Pulm Med 2000;6:259-66.

132. Light RW. Clinical manifestations and useful tests. In: Light RW, editor. Pleural diseases. Fourth edition. Philadelphia: Lippincott Williams and Wilkins; 2001.p.42-86.

133. Miller KD, Barnette R, Light RW. Stability of adenosine deaminase during transportation. Chest 2004;126:1933-7.

134. Antonangelo L, Vargas FS, Almeida LP, Acencio MM, Gomes FD, Sales RK, et al. Influence of storage time and temperature on pleural fluid adenosine deaminase determination. Respirology 2006;11:488-92.

135. Raj B, Chopra RK, Lal H, Saini AS, Singh V, Kumar P, et al. Adenosine deaminase activity in pleural fluids: a diagnostic aid in tuberculous pleural effusion. Indian J Chest Dis Allied Sci 1985;27:76-80.

136. Sinha PK, Sinha BB, Sinha AR. Diagnosing tuberculous pleural effusion: comparative sensitivity of mycobacterial culture, histo-pathology and adenosine deaminase activity. J Assoc Physicians India 1985;33:644-5.

137. Sinha PK, Sinha BB, Sinha AR. Adenosine deaminase activity as a diagnostic index of pleural effusion. J Indian Med Assoc 1987;85:11-3.

138. Chopra RK, Singh V, Lal H, Saini AS, Chawla RK, Raj B. Adenosine deaminase and T-lymphocyte levels in patients with pleural effusions. Indian J Tuberc 1988;35:22-4.

139. Gilhotra R, Sehgal S, Jindal SK. Pleural biopsy and adenosine deaminase enzyme activity in effusions of different aetiologies. Lung India 1989;7:122-4.

140. Gupta DK, Suri JC, Goel A. Efficacy of adenosine deaminase in the diagnosis of pleural effusions. Indian J Chest Dis Allied Sci 1990;32:205-8.

141. Subhakar K, Kotilingam K, Satyasri S. Adenosine deaminase activity in pleural effusions. Lung India 1991;9:57-60.

142. Kaur A, Basha A, Ranjan M, Oommen A. Poor diagnostic value of adenosine deaminase in pleural, peritoneal and cerebrospinal fluids in tuberculosis. Indian J Med Res 1992;95:270-7.

143. Prasad R, Tripathi RP, Mukerji PK, Singh M, Srivastava VM. Adenosine deaminase activity in pleural fluid: a diagnostic test of tuberculous pleural effusion. Indian J Chest Dis Allied Sci 1992;34:123-6.

144. Nagaraja MV, Ashokan PK, Hande HM. Adenosine deaminase in pleural effusions. J Assoc Physicians India 1992;40:157-9.

145. Maldhure BR, Bedarkar SP, Kulkarni HR, Papinwar SP. Pleural biopsy and adenosine deaminase in pleural fluid for the diagnosis of tubercular pleural effusion. Indian J Tuberc 1994;41:161-5.

146. Singh V, Kharb S, Ghalaut PS, Janmeja A. Serum adenosine deaminase activity in pleural effusion. Thorax 1998;53:814.

147. Ghelani DR, Parikh FS, Hakim AS, Pai-Dhungat JV. Diagnostic significance of immunoglobulins and adenosine deaminase in pleural effusion. J Assoc Physicians India 1999;47:787-90.

148. Parandaman V, Narayanan S, Narayanan PR. Utility of poly-merase chain reaction using two probes for rapid diagnosis of

tubercular pleuritis in comparison to conventional methods. Indian J Med Res 2000;112:47-51.

149. Sharma SK, Suresh V, Mohan A, Kaur P, Saha P, Kumar A, et al. A prospective study of sensitivity and specificity of adenosine deaminase estimation in the diagnosis of tuberculosis pleural effusion. Indian J Chest Dis Allied Sci 2001;43:149-55.

150. Nagesh BS, Sehgal S, Jindal SK, Arora SK. Evaluation of polymerase chain reaction for detection of Mycobacterium tuberculosis in pleural fluid. Chest 2001;119:1737-41.

151. Dil A, Sharma D, Dhobi GN, Shah S, Eachkoti R, Hussain I, et al. Evaluation of polymerase chain reaction for rapid diagnosis of clinically suspected tuberculous pleurisy. Indian J Clin Biochem 2006;21:76-9.

152. Bandyopadhyay D, Gupta S, Banerjee S, Gupta S, Ray D, Bhattacharya S, et al. Adenosine deaminase estimation and multiplex polymerase chain reaction in diagnosis of extra-pulmonary tuberculosis. Int J Tuberc Lung Dis 2008;12:1203-8.

153. Verma SK, Dubey AL, Singh PA, Tewerson SL, Sharma D. Adenosine deaminase [ADA] level in tubercular pleural effusion. Lung India 2008;25:109-10.

154. Gupta BK, Bharat V, Bandyopadhyay D. Role of adenosine deaminase estimation in differentiation of tuberculous and non-tuberculous exudative pleural effusions. J Clin Med Res 2010;2:79-84.

155. Pandit S, Chaudhuri AD, Datta SB, Dey A, Bhanja P. Role of pleural biopsy in etiological diagnosis of pleural effusion. Lung India 2010;27:202-4.

156. Ambade V, Arora MM, Rai SP, Nikumb SK, Basannar DR. Markers for differentiation of tubercular pleural effusion from non-tubercular effusion. Med J Armed Forces India 2011;67:338-42.

157. Kalantri Y, Hemvani N, Chitnis DS. Evaluation of real-time poly-merase chain reaction, interferon-gamma, adenosine deaminase, and immunoglobulin A for the efficient diagnosis of pleural tuberculosis. Int J Infect Dis 2011;15:e226-31.

158. Kelam MA, Ganie FA, Shah BA, Ganie SA, Wani ML, Wani NUD, et al. The diagnostic efficacy of adenosine deaminase in tubercular effusion. Oman Med J 2013;28:417-21.

159. Mehta AA, Gupta AS, Ahmed S, Rajesh V. Diagnostic utility of adenosine deaminase in exudative pleural effusions. Lung India 2014;31:142-4.

160. Valdes L, Alvarez D, San Jose E, Juanatey JR, Pose A, Valle JM, et al. Value of adenosine deaminase in the diagnosis of tuber-culous pleural effusions in young patients in a region of high prevalence of tuberculosis. Thorax 1995;50:600-3.

161. Kataria YP, Khurshid I. Adenosine deaminase in the diagnosis of tuberculous pleural effusion. Chest 2001;120:334-6.

162. McGrath EE, Anderson PB. Diagnostic tests for tuberculous pleural effusion. Eur J Clin Microbiol Infect Dis 2010;29:1187-93.

163. Hirschhorn R, Ratech H. Isozymes of adenosine deaminase. In: Rattazzi MC, Scandalios JG, Whitt GS, editors. Isozymes: current topics in biological and medical research. Vol. 4. New York: Liss; 1980.p.131-57.

164. Ungerer JP, Oosthuizen HM, Bissbort SH, Vermaak WJ. Serum adenosine deaminase: isoenzymes and diagnostic application. Clin Chem 1992;38:1322-6.

165. Ungerer JP, Oosthuizen HM, Retief JH, Bissbort SH. Significance of adenosine deaminase activity and its isoenzymes in tuberculous effusions. Chest 1994;106:33-7.

166. Gakis C, Calia GM, Naitana AG, Ortu AR, Contu A. Serum and pleural adenosine deaminase activity. Correct interpretation of the findings. Chest 1991;99:1555-6.

167. Valdes L, San Jose E, Alvarez D, Valle JM. Adenosine deaminase [ADA] isoenzyme analysis in pleural effusions: diagnostic role, and relevance to the origin of increased ADA in tuberculous pleurisy. Eur Respir J 1996; 9:747-51.

168. Zemlin AE, Burgess LJ, Carstens ME. The diagnostic utility of adenosine deaminase isoenzymes in tuberculous pleural effusions. Int J Tuberc Lung Dis 2009;13:214-20.

169. Gakis C. Adenosine deaminase [ADA] isoenzymes ADA1 and ADA2: diagnostic and biological role. Eur Respir J 1996;9:632-3.

170. Carstens ME, Burgess LJ, Maritz FJ, Taljaard JJ. Isoenzymes of adenosine deaminase in pleural effusions: a diagnostic tool? Int J Tuberc Lung Dis 1998;2:831-5.

171. Barnes PF, Mistry SD, Cooper CL, Pirmez C, Rea TH, Modlin RL. Compartmentalization of a CD4+ T lymphocyte subpopulation in tuberculous pleuritis. J Immunol 1989;142:1114-9.

172. Soderblom T, Nyberg P, Teppo AM, Klockars M, Riska H, Pettersson T. Pleural fluid interferon-gamma and tumour necrosis factor-alpha in tuberculous and rheumatoid pleurisy. Eur Respir J 1996;9:1652-5.

173. Jiang J, Shi HZ, Liang QL, Qin SM, Qin XJ. Diagnostic value of interferon-gamma in tuberculous pleurisy: a metaanalysis. Chest 2007;131:1133-41.

174. Kim YC, Park KO, Bom HS, Lim SC, Park HK, Na HJ, et al. Combining ADA, protein and IFN-gamma best allows discrimi-nation between tuberculous and malignant pleural effusion. Korean J Intern Med 1997;12:225-31.

175. Ribera E, Ocana I, Martinez-Vazquez JM, Rossell M, Espanol T, Ruibal A. High level of interferon gamma in tuberculous pleural effusion. Chest 1988;93:308-11.

176. Shimokata K, Saka H, Murate T, Hasegawa Y, Hasegawa T. Cytokine content in pleural effusion. Comparison between tuberculous and carcinomatous pleurisy. Chest 1991;99:1103-7.

177. Villena V, Lopez-Encuentra A, Echave-Sustaeta J, Martin-Escribano P, Ortuno-de-Solo B, Estenoz-Alfaro J. Interferon-gamma in 388 immunocompromised and immunocompetent patients for diagnosing pleural tuberculosis. Eur Respir J 1996;9:2635-9.

178. Ogawa K, Koga H, Hirakata Y, Tomono K, Tashiro T, Kohno S. Differential diagnosis of tuberculous pleurisy by measurement of cytokine concentrations in pleural effusion. Tuber Lung Dis 1997;78:29-34.

179. Yamada Y, Nakamura A, Hosoda M, Kato T, Asano T, Tonegawa K, et al. Cytokines in pleural liquid for diagnosis of tuberculous pleurisy. Respir Med 2001;95:577-81.

180. Aoe K, Hiraki A, Murakami T, Eda R, Maeda T, Sugi K, et al. Diagnostic significance of interferon-gamma in tuberculous pleural effusions. Chest 2003;123:740-4.

181. Wong CF, Yew WW, Leung SK, Chan CY, Hui M, Au-Yeang C, et al. Assay of pleural fluid interleukin-6, tumour necrosis factor-alpha and interferon-gamma in the diagnosis and outcome correlation of tuberculous effusion. Respir Med 2003;97:1289-95.

182. Hiraki A, Aoe K, Matsuo K, Murakami K, Murakami T, Onoda T, et al. Simultaneous measurement of T-helper 1 cytokines in tuberculous pleural effusion. Int J Tuberc Lung Dis 2003;7:1172-7.

183. Prabha C, Jalapathy K, Matsa RM, Das SD. Role of TNF-alpha in host immune response in tuberculous pleuritis. Curr Sci 2003;85:639-42.

184. Hiraki A, Aoe K, Eda R, Maeda T, Murakami T, Sugi K, et al. Comparison of six biological markers for the diagnosis of tuberculous pleuritis. Chest 2004;125:987-9.

185. Sharma SK, Banga A. Diagnostic utility of pleural fluid IFN-gamma in tuberculosis pleural effusion. J Interferon Cytokine Res 2004;24:213-7.

186. Liu YC, Lee S-J, Chen YS, Tu HZ, Chen BC, Huang TS. Differential diagnosis of tuberculous and malignant pleurisy using pleural fluid adenosine deaminase and interferon gamma in Taiwan. J Microbiol Immunol Infect 2011;44:88-94.

187. Khan FY, Hamza M, Omran AH, Saleh M, Lingawi M, Alnaqdy A, et al. Diagnostic value of pleural fluid interferon-gamma and adenosine deaminase in patients with pleural tuberculosis in Qatar. Int J Gen Med 2013;6:13-8.

188. Wang H, Yue J, Yang J, Gao R, Liu J. Clinical diagnostic utility of adenosine deaminase, interferon-gamma, interferon-gamma-induced protein of 10 kDa, and dipeptidyl peptidase 4 levels in tuberculous pleural effusions. Heart Lung 2012;41:70-75.

189. Sharma SK, Banga A. Pleural fluid interferon-gamma and adenosine deaminase levels in tuberculosis pleural effusion: a cost-effectiveness analysis. J Clin Lab Anal 2005;19:40-6.

190. Mazurek GH, Jereb J, Vernon A, LoBue P, Goldberg S, Castro K, et al. Updated guidelines for using Interferon Gamma Release Assays to detect Mycobacterium tuberculosis infection - United States, 2010. MMWR Recomm Rep 2010;59[RR-5]:1-25.

191. Wilkinson KA, Wilkinson RJ, Pathan A, Ewer K, Prakash M, Klenerman P, et al. Ex vivo characterization of early secretory antigenic target 6-specific T cells at sites of active disease in pleural tuberculosis. Clin Infect Dis 2005;40:184-7.

192. Ariga H, Kawabe Y, Nagai H, Kurashima A, Masuda K, Matsui H, et al. Diagnosis of active tuberculous serositis by antigen-specific interferon-gamma response of cavity fluid cells. Clin Infect Dis 2007;45:1559-67.

193. Losi M, Bossink A, Codecasa L, Jafari C, Ernst M, Thijsen S, et al. Use of a T-cell interferon-gamma release assay for the diagnosis of tuberculous pleurisy. Eur Respir J 2007;30:1173-9.

194. Baba K, Sornes S, Hoosen AA, Lekabe JM, Mpe MJ, Langeland N, et al. Evaluation of immune responses in HIV infected patients with pleural tuberculosis by the QuantiFERON TB-Gold interferon-gamma assay. BMC Infect Dis 2008;8:35.

195. Chegou NN, Walzl G, Bolliger CT, Diacon AH, van den Heuvel MM. Evaluation of adapted whole-blood interferon-gamma release assays for the diagnosis of pleural tuberculosis. Respiration 2008;76:131-8.

196. Nishimura T, Hasegawa N, Mori M, Takebayashi T, Harada N, Higuchi K, et al. Accuracy of an interferon-gamma release assay to detect active pulmonary and extra-pulmonary tuberculosis. Int J Tuberc Lung Dis 2008;12:269-74.

197. Dheda K, van Zyl-Smit RN, Sechi LA, Badri M, Meldau R, Meldau S, et al. Utility of quantitative T-cell responses versus unstimulated interferon-gamma for the diagnosis of pleural tuberculosis. Eur Respir J 2009;34:1118-26.

198. Lee LN, Chou CH, Wang JY, Hsu HL, Tsai TH, Jan IS, et al. Enzyme-linked immunospot assay for interferon-gamma in the diagnosis of tuberculous pleurisy. Clin Microbiol Infect 2009;15:173-9.

199. Liao CH, Chou CH, Lai CC, Huang YT, Tan CK, Hsu HL, et al. Diagnostic performance of an enzyme-linked immunospot assay for interferon-gamma in extrapulmonary tuberculosis varies between different sites of disease. J Infect 2009;59:402-8.

200. Katiyar SK, Sampath A, Bihari S, Mamtani M, Kulkarni H. Using a whole-blood interferon-gamma assay to improve diagnosis of tuberculous pleural effusion. Eur Respir J 2010;36:679-81.

201. Ates G, Yildiz T, Ortakoylu MG, Ozekinci T, Erturk B, Akyildiz L, et al. Adapted T cell interferon-gamma release assay for the diagnosis of pleural tuberculosis. Respiration 2011;82:351-7.

202. Chung JH, Han CH, Kim CJ, Lee SM. Clinical utility of QuantiFERON-TB GOLD In-Tube and tuberculin skin test in patients with tuberculous pleural effusions. Diagn Microbiol Infect Dis 2011;71:263-6.

203. Losi M, Bocchino M, Matarese A, Bellofiore B, Roversi P, Rumpianesi F, et al. Role of the quantiferon-TB test in ruling out pleural tuberculosis: a multi-centre study. Int J Immunopathol Pharmacol 2011;24:159-65.

204. Eldin EN, Omar A, Khairy M, Mekawy AH, Ghanem MK. Diagnostic value of ex vivo pleural fluid interferon-gamma

205. Gao Y, Ou Q, Huang F, Wang S, Shen L, Shen Y, et al. Improved diagnostic power by combined interferon-gamma release assay and nested-PCR in tuberculous pleurisy in high tuberculosis prevalence area. FEMS Immunol Med Microbiol 2012;66:393-8.

206. Kang JY, Rhee CK, Kang NH, Kim JS, Yoon HK, Song JS. Clinical utility of two interferon-gamma release assays on pleural fluid for the diagnosis of tuberculous pleurisy. Tuberc Respir Dis [Seoul] 2012;73:143-50.

207. Keng LT, Shu CC, Chen JY, Liang SK, Lin CK, Chang LY, et al. Evaluating pleural ADA, ADA2, IFN-gamma and IGRA for diagnosing tuberculous pleurisy. J Infect 2013;67:294-302.

208. Liu F, Gao M, Zhang X, Du F, Jia H, Yang X, et al. Interferon-gamma release assay performance of pleural fluid and peripheral blood in pleural tuberculosis. PLoS One 2013;8:e83857.

209. Zhou Q, Chen YQ, Qin SM, Tao XN, Xin JB, Shi HZ. Diagnostic accuracy of T-cell interferon-gamma release assays in tuberculous pleurisy: a meta-analysis. Respirology 2011;16:473-80.

210. Hooper CE, Lee YC, Maskell NA. Interferon-gamma release assays for the diagnosis of TB pleural effusions: hype or real hope? Curr Opin Pulm Med 2009;15:358-65.

211. Joshi R, Pai M. Can pleural tuberculosis be diagnosed using interferon-gamma release assays? Respiration 2008;76:128-30.

212. World Health Organization. Use of tuberculosis interferon-gamma release assays [IGRAs] in low- and middle-income countries: policy statement. Geneva: World Health Organization; 2011.

213. Samuel AM, Kadival GV, Ashtekar MD, Ganatra RD. Evaluation of tubercular antigen and antitubercular antibodies in pleural and ascitic effusions. Indian J Med Res 1984;80:563-5.

214. Murate T, Mizoguchi K, Amano H, Shimokata K, Matsuda T. Antipurified-protein-derivative antibody in tuberculous pleural effusions Chest 1990;97:670-3.

215. Caminero JA, Rodriguez de Castro F, Carrillo T, Cabrera P. Antimycobacterial antibodies in tuberculous pleural effusions: reliability of antigen 60. Chest 1991;99:1315-6.

216. Caminero JA, Rodriguez de Castro F, Carrillo T, Diaz F, Rodriguez Bermejo JC, Cabrera P. Diagnosis of pleural tuberculosis by detection of specific IgG anti-antigen 60 in serum and pleural fluid. Respiration 1993;60:58-62.

217. Chierakul N, Damrongchokpipat P, Chaiprasert A, Arjratanakul W. Antibody detection for the diagnosis of tuberculous pleuritis. Int J Tuberc Lung Dis 2001;5:968-72.

218. Kunter E, Cerrahoglu K, Ilvan A, Isitmangil T, Turken O, Okutan O, et al. The value of pleural fluid anti-A60 IgM in BCG-vaccinated tuberculous pleurisy patients. Clin Microbiol Infect 2003;9:212-20.

219. Yokoyama T, Rikimaru T, Kinoshita T, Kamimura T, Oshita Y, Aizawa H. Clinical utility of lipoarabinomannan antibody in pleural fluid for the diagnosis of tuberculous pleurisy. J Infect Chemother 2005;11:81-3.

220. Kaisermann MC, Sardella IG, Trajman A, Coelho TL, Kampfer S, Jonas F, et al. IgA antibody responses to Mycobacterium tuberculosis recombinant MPT-64 and MT-10.3 [Rv3019c] antigens in pleural fluid of patients with tuberculous pleurisy. Int J Tuberc Lung Dis 2005;9:461-6.

221. Morimoto T, Takanashi S, Hasegawa Y, Fujimoto K, Okudera K, Hayashi A, et al. Level of antibodies against mycobacterial glycolipid in the effusion for diagnosis of tuberculous pleural effusion. Respir Med 2006;100:1775-80.

222. Trajman A, Kaisermann C, Luiz RR, Sperhacke RD, Rossetti ML, Feres Saad MH, et al. Pleural fluid ADA, IgA-ELISA and PCR sensitivities for the diagnosis of pleural tuberculosis. Scand J Clin Lab Invest 2007;67:877-84.

223. Araujo LS, Maciel RM, Trajman A, Saad MH. Assessment of the IgA immunoassay diagnostic potential of the Mycobacterium tuberculosis MT10.3-MPT64 fusion protein in tuberculous pleural fluid. Clin Vaccine Immunol 2010;17:1963-9.

224. Limongi LC, Olival L, Conde MB, Junqueira-Kipnis AP. Determination of levels of specific IgA to the HspX recombinant antigen of Mycobacterium tuberculosis for the diagnosis of pleural tuberculosis. J Bras Pneumol 2011;37:302-7.

225. Arora BR, Saini V, Prasad R, Kaur J, Arora K, Lal H. ELISA technique for the serodiagnosis of tuberculous pleural effusion. Lung India 1993;11:87-90.

226. Fernandez de Larrea C, Duplat A, Giampietro F, de Waard JH, Luna J, Singh M, et al. Diagnostic accuracy of immunological methods in patients with tuberculous pleural effusion from Venezuela. Invest Clin 2011;52:23-34.

227. Kaushik A, Singh UB, Porwal C, Venugopal SJ, Mohan A, Krishnan A, et al. Diagnostic potential of 16 kDa [HspX, alpha-crystalline] antigen for serodiagnosis of tuberculosis. Indian J Med Res 2012;135:771-7.

228. Baig MM, Pettengell KE, Simjee AE, Sathar MA, Vorster BJ. Diagnosis of tuberculosis by detection of mycobacterial antigen in pleural effusions and ascites. S Afr Med J 1986;69:101-2.

229. Ramkisson A, Coovadia YM, Coovadia HM. A competition ELISA for the detection of mycobacterial antigen in tuberculosis exudates. Tubercle 1988;69:209-12.

230. Dhand R, Ganguly NK, Vaishnavi C, Gilhotra R, Malik SK. False-positive reactions with enzyme-linked immunosorbent assay of Mycobacterium tuberculosis antigens in pleural fluid. J Med Microbiol 1988;26:241-3.

231. Banchuin N, Wongwajana S, Pumprueg U, Jearanaisilavong J. Value of an ELISA for mycobacterial antigen detection as a routine diagnostic test of pulmonary tuberculosis. Asian Pac J Allergy Immunol 1990;8:5-11.

232. Anie Y, Sumi S, Varghese P, Madhavi LG, Sathish M, Radhakrishnan VV. Diagnostic approaches in patients with tuberculous pleural effusion. Diagn Microbiol Infect Dis 2007;59:389-94.

233. Feng TT, Shou CM, Shen L, Qian Y, Wu ZG, Fan J, et al. Novel monoclonal antibodies to ESAT-6 and CFP-10 antigens for ELISA-based diagnosis of pleural tuberculosis. Int J Tuberc Lung Dis 2011;15:804-10.

234. Sarnaik RM, Sharma M, Kate SK, Jindal SK. Serodiagnosis of tuberculosis: assessment of kaolin agglutination test. Tuber Lung Dis 1993;74:405-6.

235. Wankhade G, Majumdar A, Kamble PD, De S, Harinath BC. Multi-antigen and antibody assays [SEVA TB ELISA] for the diagnosis of tuberculous pleural effusion. Indian J Tuberc 2012;59:78-82.

236. World Health Organization. Commercial serodiagnostic tests for diagnosis of tuberculosis. Policy Statement: 2011. Geneva: World Health Organization; 2011.

237. Levy H, Wayne LG, Anderson BE, Barnes PF, Light RW. Antimycobacterial antibody levels in pleural fluid as reflection of passive diffusion from serum. Chest 1990;97:1144-7.

238. Van Vooren JP, Farber CM, De Bruyn J, Yernault JC. Antimycobacterial antibodies in pleural effusions. Chest 1990;97:88-90.

239. Yew WW, Chan CY, Kwan SY, Cheung SW, French GL. Diagnosis of tuberculous pleural effusion by the detection of tuberculostearic acid in pleural aspirates. Chest 1991;100:1261-3.

240. Prabhu VG, Narasimhan R. The role of pleuroscopy in undiagnosed exudative pleural effusion. Lung India 2012;29:128-30.

241. Mootha VK, Agarwal R, Singh N, Aggarwal AN, Gupta D, Jindal SK. Medical thoracoscopy for undiagnosed pleural effusions: experience from a tertiary care hospital in north India. Indian J Chest Dis Allied Sci 2011;53:21-4.

242. Nattusamy L, Madan K, Mohan A, Hadda V, Jain D, Madan NK, et al. Utility of semi-rigid thoracoscopy in undiagnosed exudative pleural effusion. Lung India 2015;32:119-26.

243. Harris RJ, Kavuru MS, Mehta AC, Medendorp SV, Wiedemann HP, Kirby TJ, et al. The impact of thoracoscopy on the management of pleural disease. Chest 1995;107:845-52.

244. Mathur PN, Boutin C, Loddenkemper R. "Medical" thoracoscopy: techniques and indications in pulmonary medicine. J Bronchol 1994;1:1153-6.

245. Loddenkemper R. Thoracoscopy—state of the art. Eur Respir J 1998;11:213-21.

246. Kong XL, Zeng HH, Chen Y, Liu TT, Shi ZH, Zheng DY, et al. The visual diagnosis of tuberculous pleuritis under medical thoracoscopy: a retrospective series of 91 cases. Eur Rev Med Pharmacol Sci 2014;18:1487-95.

247. Mathur PN, Loddenkemper R. Medical thoracoscopy. Role in pleural and lung diseases. Clin Chest Med 1995;16:487-96.

248. Boutin C, Astoul P. Diagnostic thoracoscopy. Clin Chest Med 1998;19:295-309.

249. Chin DP, Yajko DM, Hadley WK, Sanders CA, Nassos PS, Madej JJ, et al. Clinical utility of a commercial test based on the polymerase chain reaction for detecting Mycobacterium tuberculosis in respiratory specimens. Am J Respir Crit Care Med 1995;151:1872-7.

250. de Wit D, Maartens G, Steyn L. A comparative study of the polymerase chain reaction and conventional procedures for the diagnosis of tuberculous pleural effusion. Tuber Lung Dis 1992;73:262-7.

251. de Lassence A, Lecossier D, Pierre C, Cadranel J, Stern M, Hance AJ. Detection of mycobacterial DNA in pleural fluid from patients with tuberculous pleurisy by means of the polymerase chain reaction: comparison of two protocols. Thorax 1992;47:265-9.

252. Verma A, Dasgupta N, Aggrawal AN, Pande JN, Tyagi JS. Utility of a Mycobacterium tuberculosis GC-rich repetitive sequence in the diagnosis of tuberculous pleural effusion by PCR. Indian J Biochem Biophys 1995;32:429-36.

253. Querol JM, Minguez J, Garcia-Sanchez E, Farga MA, Gimeno C, Garcia-de-Lomas J. Rapid diagnosis of pleural tuberculosis by polymerase chain reaction. Am J Respir Crit Care Med 1995;152:1977-81.

254. Tan J, Lee BW, Lim TK, Chin NK, Tan CB, Xia JR, et al. Detection of Mycobacterium tuberculosis in sputum, pleural and bronchoalveolar lavage fluid using DNA amplification of the MPB 64 protein coding gene and IS6110 insertion element. Southeast Asian J Trop Med Public Health 1995;26:247-52.

255. Villena V, Rebollo MJ, Aguado JM, Galan A, Lopez Encuentra A, Palenque E. Polymerase chain reaction for the diagnosis of pleural tuberculosis in immunocompromised and immunocompetent patients. Clin Infect Dis 1998;26:212-4.

256. Seethalakshmi S, Korath MP, Kareem F, Jagadeesan K. Detection of Mycobacterium tuberculosis by polymerase chain reaction in 301 biological samples: a comparative study. J Assoc Physicians India 1998;46:763-6.

257. Mitarai S, Shishido H, Kurashima A, Tamura A, Nagai H. Comparative study of amplicor Mycobacterium PCR and conventional methods for the diagnosis of pleuritis caused by mycobacterial infection. Int J Tuberc Lung Dis 2000;4:871-6.

258. Martins LC, Paschoal IA, Von Nowakonski A, Silva SA, Costa FF, Ward LS. Nested-PCR using MPB64 fragment improves the diagnosis of pleural and meningeal tuberculosis. Rev Soc Bras Med Trop 2000;33:253-7.

259. Villegas MV, Labrada LA, Saravia NG. Evaluation of polymerase chain reaction, adenosine deaminase, and interferon-gamma in pleural fluid for the differential diagnosis of pleural tuberculosis. Chest 2000;118:1355-64.

260. Reechaipichitkul W, Lulitanond V, Sungkeeree S, Patjanasoontorn B. Rapid diagnosis of tuberculous pleural effusion using polymerase chain reaction. Southeast Asian J Trop Med Public Health 2000;31:509-14.

261. Lima DM, Colares JK, da Fonseca BA. Combined use of the polymerase chain reaction and detection of adenosine deaminase activity on pleural fluid improves the rate of diagnosis of pleural tuberculosis. Chest 2003;124:909-14.

262. Kim SY, Park YJ, Kang SJ, Kim BK, Kang CS. Comparison of the BDProbeTec ET system with the roche COBAS AMPLICOR System for detection of Mycobacterium tuberculosis complex in the respiratory and pleural fluid specimens. Diagn Microbiol Infect Dis 2004; 49:13-8.

263. Moon JW, Chang YS, Kim SK, Kim YS, Lee HM, Kim SK, et al. The clinical utility of polymerase chain reaction for the diagnosis of pleural tuberculosis. Clin Infect Dis 2005;41:660-6.

264. Liu KT, Su WJ, Perng RP. Clinical utility of polymerase chain reaction for diagnosis of smear-negative pleural tuberculosis. J Chin Med Assoc 2007;70:148-51; discussion 146-7.

265. Kumar P, Sen MK, Chauhan DS, Katoch VM, Singh S, Prasad HK. Assessment of the N-PCR assay in diagnosis of pleural tuberculosis: detection of M. tuberculosis in pleural fluid and sputum collected in tandem. PLoS One 2010;5:e10220.

266. Friedrich SO, von Groote-Bidlingmaier F, Diacon AH. Xpert MTB/RIF assay for diagnosis of pleural tuberculosis. J Clin Microbiol 2011;49:4341-2.

267. Maurya AK, Kant S, Kushwaha RA, Nag VL, Kumar M, Dhole TN. The advantage of using IS6110-PCR vs. BACTEC culture for rapid detection of Mycobacterium tuberculosis from pleural fluid in northern India. Biosci Trends 2011;5:159-64.

268. Rosso F, Michelon CT, Sperhacke RD, Verza M, Olival L, Conde MB, et al. Evaluation of real-time PCR of patient pleural effusion for diagnosis of tuberculosis. BMC Res Notes 2011;4:279.

269. Alvarez-Uria G, Azcona JM, Midde M, Naik PK, Reddy S, Reddy R. Rapid diagnosis of pulmonary and extrapulmonary tuberculosis in HIV-infected patients. Comparison of LED fluorescent microscopy and the GeneXpert MTB/RIF assay in a district Hospital in India. Tuberc Res Treat 2012;2012:932862.

270. Porcel JM, Palma R, Valdes L, Bielsa S, San-Jose E, Esquerda A. Xpert® MTB/RIF in pleural fluid for the diagnosis of tuberculosis. Int J Tuberc Lung Dis 2013;17:1217-9.

271. Christopher DJ, Schumacher SG, Michael JS, Luo R, Balamugesh T, Duraikannan P, et al. Performance of Xpert MTB/RIF on pleural tissue for the diagnosis of pleural tuberculosis. Eur Respir J 2013;42:1427-9.

272. Montenegro LM, Silva BC, Lima JF, Cruz HL, Montenegro Rde A, Lundgren FL, et al. The performance of an in-house nested-PCR technique for pleural tuberculosis diagnoses. Rev Soc Bras Med Trop 2013;46:594-9.

273. Meldau R, Peter J, Theron G, Calligaro G, Allwood B, Symons G, et al. Comparison of same day diagnostic tools including Gene Xpert and unstimulated IFN-gamma for the evaluation of pleural tuberculosis: a prospective cohort study. BMC Pulm Med 2014;14:58.

274. Trajman A, da Silva Santos Kleiz de Oliveira EF, Bastos ML, Belo Neto E, Silva EM, da Silva Lourenco MC, et al. Accuracy of polimerase chain reaction for the diagnosis of pleural tuberculosis. Respir Med 2014;108:918-23.

275. Makeshkumar V, Madhavan R, Narayanan S. Polymerase chain reaction targeting insertion sequence for the diagnosis of extrapulmonary tuberculosis. Indian J Med Res 2014;139:161-6.

276. Lusiba JK, Nakiyingi L, Kirenga BJ, Kiragga A, Lukande R, Nsereko M, et al. Evaluation of Cepheid's Xpert MTB/Rif test on pleural fluid in the diagnosis of pleural tuberculosis in a high prevalence HIV/TB setting. PLoS One 2014;9:e102702.

277. Sharma SK, Kohli M, Chaubey J, Yadav RN, Sharma R, Singh BKharma, et al. Evaluation of Xpert MTB/RIF assay performance in diagnosing extrapulmonary tuberculosis among adults in a tertiary care centre in India. Eur Respir J 2014;44:1090-93.

278. Denkinger CM, Schumacher SG, Boehme CC, Dendukuri N, Pai M, Steingart KR. Xpert MTB/RIF assay for the diagnosis of extrapulmonary tuberculosis: a systematic review and meta-analysis. Eur Respir J 2014;44:435-46.

279. World Health Organization. Automated real-time nucleic acid amplification technology for rapid and simultaneous detection of tuberculosis and rifampicin resistance: Xpert MTB/RIF assay for the diagnosis of pulmonary and extra-pulmonary TB in adults and children. Policy update. Geneva: World Health Organization; 2014.

280a. Sharma SK, Ryan H, Khaparde S, Sachdeva KS, Singh AD, Mohan A, et al. Index-TB guidelines: Guidelines on extrapulmonary tuberculosis for India. Indian J Med Res 2017;145:448-63.

280b. Kohli M, Schiller I, Dendukuri N, Dheda K, Denkinger CM, Schumacher SG, et al. Xpert[®] MTB/RIF assay for extrapulmonary tuberculosis and rifampicin resistance. Cochrane Database Syst Rev 2018;8:CD012768.

281. Lin CM, Lin SM, Chung FT, Lin HC, Lee KY, Huang CD, et al. Amplified Mycobacterium tuberculosis direct test for diagnosing tuberculous pleurisy: a diagnostic accuracy study. PLoS One 2012;7:e44842.

282. Takagi N, Hasegawa Y, Ichiyama S, Shibagaki T, Shimokata K. Polymerase chain reaction of pleural biopsy specimens for rapid diagnosis of tuberculous pleuritis. Int J Tuberc Lung Dis 1998;2:338-41.

283. Salian NV, Rish JA, Eisenach KD, Cave MD, Bates JH. Polymerase chain reaction to detect Mycobacterium tuberculosis in histologic specimens. Am J Respir Crit Care Med 1998;158:1150-5.

284. Marchetti G, Gori A, Catozzi L, Vago L, Nebuloni M, Rossi MC, et al. Evaluation of PCR in detection of Mycobacterium tuberculosis from formalin-fixed, paraffin-embedded tissues: comparison of four amplification assays. J Clin Microbiol 1998;36:1512-7.

285. Palacios JJ, Ferro J, Ruiz Palma N, Roces SG, Villar H, Rodriguez J, et al. Comparison of the ligase chain reaction with solid and liquid culture media for routine detection of Mycobacterium tuberculosis in nonrespiratory specimens. Eur J Clin Microbiol Infect Dis 1998;17:767-72.

286. Ruiz-Manzano J, Manterola JM, Gamboa F, Calatrava A, Monso E, Martinez C, et al. Detection of Mycobacterium tuberculosis in paraffin-embedded pleural biopsy specimens by commercial ribosomal RNA and DNA amplification kits. Chest 2000;118:648-55.

287. Hasaneen NA, Zaki ME, Shalaby HM, El-Morsi AS. Polymerase chain reaction of pleural biopsy is a rapid and sensitive method for the diagnosis of tuberculous pleural effusion. Chest 2003;124:2105-11.

288. Baba K, Pathak S, Sviland L, Langeland N, Hoosen AA, Asjo B, et al. Real-time quantitative PCR in the diagnosis of tuberculosis in formalin-fixed paraffin-embedded pleural tissue in patients from a high HIV endemic area. Diagn Mol Pathol 2008;17:112-7.

289. Aggarwal AN. Polymerase chain reaction for the diagnosis of tuberculous pleural effusion. Natl Med J India 2004;17:321-3.

290. Piras MA, Gakis C, Budroni M, Andreoni G. Adenosine deaminase activity in pleural effusions: an aid to differential diagnosis. Br Med J 1978;2:1751-2.

291. Rajpal AS, Sharma GS, Gupta PK, Nanawati V. Value of pleural fluid lysozyme estimation in tubercular and non-tubercular pleural effusions. Indian J Tuberc 1981;28:205-8.

292. Asseo PP, Tracopoulos GD, Kotsovoulou-Fouskaki V. Lysozyme [muramidase] in pleural effusions and serum. Am J Clin Pathol 1982;78:763-7.

293. Verea Hernando HR, Masa Jimenez JF, Dominguez Juncal L, Perez Garcia-Buela J, Martin Egana MT, Fontan Bueso J. Meaning and diagnostic value of determining the lysozyme level of pleural fluid. Chest 1987;91:342-5.

294. Celik G, Kaya A, Poyraz B, Ciledag A, Elhan AH, Oktem A, et al. Diagnostic value of leptin in tuberculous pleural effusions. Int J Clin Pract 2006;60:1437-42.

295. Prabha C, Supriya P, Das SD, Sukumar B, Balaji S. Leptin response in patients with tuberculous pleuritis. Indian J Med Res 2008;128:721-7.

296. Supriya P, Chandrasekaran P, Das SD. Diagnostic utility of interferon-gamma-induced protein of 10 kDa [IP-10] in tuberculous pleurisy. Diagn Microbiol Infect Dis 2008;62:186-92.

297. Sutherland JS, Garba D, Fombah AE, Mendy-Gomez A, Mendy FS, Antonio M, et al. Highly accurate diagnosis of pleural tuberculosis by immunological analysis of the pleural effusion. PLoS One 2012;7:e30324.

298. Dheda K, Van-Zyl Smit RN, Sechi LA, Badri M, Meldau R, Symons G, et al. Clinical diagnostic utility of IP-10 and LAM antigen levels for the diagnosis of tuberculous pleural effusions in a high burden setting. PLoS One 2009;4:e4689.

299. Sheen P, O'Kane CM, Chaudhary K, Tovar M, Santillan C, Sosa J, et al. High MMP-9 activity characterises pleural tuberculosis correlating with granuloma formation. Eur Respir J 2009;33:134-41.

300. Hsieh WY, Kuan TC, Cheng KS, Liao YC, Chen MY, Lin PH, et al. ACE/ACE2 ratio and MMP-9 activity as potential biomarkers in tuberculous pleural effusions. Int J Biol Sci 2012;8:1197-205.

301. Sundararajan S, Babu S, Das SD. Comparison of localized versus systemic levels of Matrix metalloproteinases [MMPs], its tissue inhibitors [TIMPs] and cytokines in tuberculous and non-tuberculous pleuritis patients. Hum Immunol 2012;73:985-91.

302. Baganha MF, Mota-Pinto A, Pego MA, Marques MA, Rosa MA, Cordeiro AJ. Neopterin in tuberculous and neoplastic pleural fluids. Lung 1992;170:155-61.

303. Tozkoparan E, Deniz O, Cakir E, Yaman H, Ciftci F, Gumus S, et al. The diagnostic values of serum, pleural fluid and urine neopterin measurements in tuberculous pleurisy. Int J Tuberc Lung Dis 2005;9:1040-5.

304. Cok G, Parildar Z, Basol G, Kabaroglu C, Bayindir U, Habif S, et al. Pleural fluid neopterin levels in tuberculous pleurisy. Clin Biochem 2007;40:876-80.

305. Chiang CS, Chiang CD, Lin JW, Huang PL, Chu JJ. Neopterin, soluble interleukin-2 receptor and adenosine deaminase levels in pleural effusions. Respiration 1994;61:150-4.

306. Shen Y, Yang T, Jia L, Wang T, Chen L, Wan C, et al. A potential role for D-dimer in the diagnosis of tuberculous pleural effusion. Eur Rev Med Pharmacol Sci 2013;17:201-5.

307. Hua CC, Chang LC, Chen YC, Chang SC. Proinflammatory cytokines and fibrinolytic enzymes in tuberculous and malignant pleural effusions. Chest 1999;116:1292-6.

308. Valdes L, San Jose E, Alvarez Dobano JM, Golpe A, Valle JM, Penela P, et al. Diagnostic value of interleukin-12 p40 in tuberculous pleural effusions. Eur Respir J 2009;33:816-20.

309. Sales RK, Vargas FS, Capelozzi VL, Seiscento M, Genofre EH, Teixeira LR, et al. Predictive models for diagnosis of pleural effusions secondary to tuberculosis or cancer. Respirology 2009;14:1128-33.

310. Seixas JM, Faria J, Souza Filho JB, Vieira AF, Kritski A, Trajman A. Artificial neural network models to support the diagnosis of pleural tuberculosis in adult patients. Int J Tuberc Lung Dis 2013;17:682-6.

311. He Y, Zhang W, Huang T, Wang X, Wang M. Evaluation of a diagnostic flow chart applying medical thoracoscopy, adenosine deaminase and T-SPOT.TB in diagnosis of tuberculous pleural effusion. Eur Rev Med Pharmacol Sci 2015;19:3563-8.

312. Neves DD, Dias RM, Cunha AJ. Predictive model for the diagnosis of tuberculous pleural effusion. Braz J Infect Dis 2007;11:83-8.

313. Porcel JM, Aleman C, Bielsa S, Sarrapio J, Fernandez de Sevilla T, Esquerda A. A decision tree for differentiating tuberculous from malignant pleural effusions. Respir Med 2008;102:1159-64.

314. Valdes L, San Jose ME, Pose A, Gude F, Gonzalez-Barcala FJ, Alvarez-Dobano JM, et al. Diagnosing tuberculous pleural effusion using clinical data and pleural fluid analysis: A study of patients less than 40 years-old in an area with a high incidence of tuberculosis. Respir Med 2010;104:1211-7.

315. Li D, Shen Y, Fu X, Li M, Wang T, Wen F. Combined detections of interleukin-33 and adenosine deaminase for diagnosis of tuberculous pleural effusion. Int J Clin Exp Pathol 2015;8:888-93.

316. Demirer E, Miller AC, Kunter E, Kartaloglu Z, Barnett SD, Elamin EM. Predictive models for tuberculous pleural effusions in a high tuberculosis prevalence region. Lung 2012;190:239-48.

317. Patiala J. Initial tuberculous pleuritis in the Finnish armed forces in 1939-1945 with special reference to eventual postpleuritic tuberculosis. Acta Tuberc Scand Suppl 1954;36:1-57.

318. Roper WH, Waring JJ. Primary serofibrinous pleural effusion in military personnel. Am Rev Tuberc 1955;71:616-34.

319. Patiala J, Mattila M. Effect of chemotherapy of exudative tuberculous pleurisy on the incidence of postpleuritic tuberculosis. Acta Tuberc Pneumol Scand 1964;44:290-6.

320. Bass JB Jr, Farer LS, Hopewell PC, O'Brien R, Jacobs RF, Ruben F, et al. Treatment of tuberculosis and tuberculosis infection in adults and children. American Thoracic Society and The Centers for Disease Control and Prevention. Am J Respir Crit Care Med 1994;149:1359-74.

321. Ormerod LP, McCarthy OR, Rudd RM, Horsfield N. Short-course chemotherapy for tuberculous pleural effusion and culture-negative pulmonary tuberculosis. Tuber Lung Dis 1995;76:25-7.

322. Sharma SK, Solanki R, Mohan A, Jain NK, Chauhan LS, Pleural Effusion Study Group. Outcomes of Category III DOTS treatment in immunocompetent patients with tuberculosis pleural effusion. Int J Tuberc Lung Dis 2012;16:1505-9.

323. Dhingra VK, Rajpal S, Aggarwal N, Aggarwal JK. Treatment of tuberculous pleural effusion patients and their satisfaction with DOTS: one-and-half year follow up. Indian J Tuberc 2004;51:209-12.

324. Dutt AK, Moers D, Stead WW. Tuberculous pleural effusion: 6-month therapy with isoniazid and rifampin. Am Rev Respir Dis 1992;145:1429-32.

325. Canete C, Galarza I, Granados A, Farrero E, Estopa R, Manresa F. Tuberculous pleural effusion: experience with six months of treatment with isoniazid and rifampicin. Thorax 1994;49:1160-1.

326. Cohen M, Sahn SA. Resolution of pleural effusions. Chest 2001;119:1547-62.

327. Singla R. Pulmonary function tests in patients of tuberculous pleural effusion before, during and after chemotherapy. Indian J Tuberc 1995;42:33-41.

328. Al-Majed SA. Study of paradoxical response to chemotherapy in tuberculous pleural effusion. Respir Med 1996;90:211-4.

329. Jeon K, Choi WI, An JS, Lim SY, Kim WJ, Park GM, et al. Paradoxical response in HIV-negative patients with pleural tuberculosis: a retrospective multicentre study. Int J Tuberc Lung Dis 2012;16:846-51.

330. Jung JW, Shin JW, Kim JY, Park IW, Choi BW, Seo JS, et al. Risk factors for development of paradoxical response during anti-tuberculosis treatment in HIV-negative patients with pleural tuberculosis. Tohoku J Exp Med 2011;223:199-204.

331. Hiraoka K, Nagata N, Kawajiri T, Suzuki K, Kurokawa S, Kido M, et al. Paradoxical pleural response to antituberculous chemotherapy and isoniazid-induced lupus. Review and report of two cases. Respiration 1998;65:152-5.

332. Singh SK, Ahmad Z, Pandey DK, Gupta V, Naaz S. Isoniazid causing pleural effusion. Indian J Pharmacol 2008;40:87-8.

333. Khattri S, Kushawaha A, Dahal K, Lee M, Mobarakai N. Isoniazid [INH]-induced eosinophilic exudative pleural effusion and lupus erythematosus: a clinical reminder of drug side effects. Bull NYU Hosp Jt Dis 2011;69:181-4.

334. Vilaseca J, Lopez-Vivancos J, Arnau J, Guardia J. Contralateral pleural effusion during chemotherapy for tuberculous pleurisy. Tubercle 1984;65:209-10.

335. Raj B, Chawla RK, Chopra RK, Gupta KB, Kumar P. Development of contralateral pleural effusion during tuberculosis chemotherapy. Indian J Tuberc 1987;34:164-5.

336. Al-Ali MA, Almasri NM. Development of contralateral pleural effusion during chemotherapy for tuberculous pleurisy. Saudi Med J 2000;21:574-6.

337. Chopra V, Singh U, Chopra D. Contralateral paradoxical pleural effusion during antituberculous chemotherapy. Lung India 2008;25:124-5.

338. Choi YW, Jeon SC, Seo HS, Park CK, Park SS, Hahm CK, et al. Tuberculous pleural effusion: new pulmonary lesions during treatment. Radiology 2002;224:493-502.

339. Candela A, Andujar J, Hernandez L, Martin C, Barroso E, Arriero JM, et al. Functional sequelae of tuberculous pleurisy in patients correctly treated. Chest 2003;123:1996-2000.

340. Barbas CS, Cukier A, de Varvalho CR, Barbas Filho JV, Light RW. The relationship between pleural fluid findings and the development of pleural thickening in patients with pleural tuberculosis. Chest 1991;100:1264-7.

341. Kunter E, Ilvan A, Kilic E, Cerrahoglu K, Isitmangil T, Capraz F, et al. The effect of pleural fluid content on the development of pleural thickness. Int J Tuberc Lung Dis 2002;6:516-22.

342. Gerogianni I, Papala M, Tsopa P, Zigoulis P, Dimoulis A, Kostikas K, et al. Could IFN-gamma predict the development of residual pleural thickening in tuberculous pleurisy? Monaldi Arch Chest Dis 2008;69:18-23.

343. Wong CF, Leung SK, Yew WW. Percentage reduction of pleural effusion as a simple predictor of pleural scarring in tuberculous pleuritis. Respirology 2005;10:515-9.

344. Dooley DP, Carpenter JL, Rademacher S. Adjunctive corticosteroid therapy for tuberculosis: a critical reappraisal of the literature. Clin Infect Dis 1997; 25:872-87.

345. Matchaba PT, Volmink J. Steroids for treating tuberculous pleurisy. Cochrane Database Syst Rev 2000:CD001876.

346. Engel ME, Matchaba PT, Volmink J. Corticosteroids for tuberculous pleurisy. Cochrane Database Syst Rev 2007:CD001876.

347. Galarza I, Canete C, Granados A, Estopa R, Manresa F. Randomised trial of corticosteroids in the treatment of tuberculous pleurisy. Thorax 1995;50:1305-7.

348. Wyser C, Walzl G, Smedema JP, Swart F, van Schalkwyk EM, van de Wal BW. Corticosteroids in the treatment of tuberculous pleurisy: A double-blind, placebo-controlled, randomized study. Chest 1996;110:333-8.

349. Lee CH, Wang WJ, Lan RS, Tsai YH, Chiang YC. Corticosteroids in the treatment of tuberculous pleurisy: a double-blind, placebo-controlled, randomized study. Chest 1988;94:1256-9.

350. Light RW. Update on tuberculous pleural effusion. Respirology 2010;15:451-8.

351. Large SE, Levick RK. Aspiration in the treatment of primary tuberculous pleural effusion. Br Med J 1958;1:1512-4.

352. Lai YF, Chao TY, Wang YH, Lin AS. Pigtail drainage in the treatment of tuberculous pleural effusions: a randomised study. Thorax 2003;58:149-51.

353. Kwak SM, Park CS, Cho JH, Ryu JS, Kim SK, Chang J, et al. The effects of urokinase instillation therapy via percutaneous transthoracic catheter in loculated tuberculous pleural effusion: a randomized prospective study. Yonsei Med J 2004; 45:822-8.

354. Mlika-Cabanne N, Brauner M, Mugusi F, Grenier P, Daley C, Mbaga I, et al. Radiographic abnormalities in tuberculosis and risk of coexisting human immunodeficiency virus infection. Results from Dar-es-Salaam, Tanzania, and scoring system. Am J Respir Crit Care Med 1995;152:786-93.

355. Mlika-Cabanne N, Brauner M, Kamanfu G, Grenier P, Nikoyagize E, Aubry P, et al. Radiographic abnormalities in tuberculosis and risk of coexisting human immunodeficiency virus infection. Methods and preliminary results from Bujumbura, Burundi. Am J Respir Crit Care Med 1995;152:794-9.

356. Afessa B. Pleural effusions and pneumothoraces in AIDS. Curr Opin Pulm Med 2001;7:202-9.

357. Deivanayagam CN, Rajasekaran S, Senthilnathan V, Krishnarajasekhar OR, Raja K, Chandrasekar C, et al. Clinico-radiological spectrum of tuberculosis among HIV sero-positives: a Tambaram study. Indian J Tuberc 2001;48:123-7.

358. Debnath J, Sreeram MN, Sangameswaran KV, Panda BN, Tiwari SC, Mohan R, et al. Comparative study of chest radiographic features between HIV seropositive and HIV seronegative patients of pulmonary tuberculosis. Med J Armed Forces India 2002;58:5-8.

359. Jones BE, Young SM, Antoniskis D, Davidson PT, Kramer F, Barnes PF. Relationship of the manifestations of tuberculosis to CD4 cell counts in patients with human immunodeficiency virus infection. Am Rev Respir Dis 1993;148:1292-7.

360. Frye MD, Pozsik CJ, Sahn SA. Tuberculous pleurisy is more common in AIDS than in non-AIDS patients with tuberculosis. Chest 1997;112:393-7.

361. Madan K, Singh N, Das A, Behera D. Pleural tuberculosis following lung cancer chemotherapy: a report of two cases proven pathologically by pleural biopsy. BMJ Case Rep 2013;2013.

362. Richter C, Perenboom R, Mtoni I, Kitinya J, Chande H, Swai AB, et al. Clinical features of HIV-seropositive and HIV-seronegative patients with tuberculous pleural effusion in Dar es Salaam, Tanzania. Chest 1994;106:1471-5.

363. Heyderman RS, Makunike R, Muza T, Odwee M, Kadzirange G, Manyemba J, et al. Pleural tuberculosis in Harare, Zimbabwe: the relationship between human immunodeficiency virus, CD4 lymphocyte count, granuloma formation and disseminated disease. Trop Med Int Health 1998;3:14-20.

364. Aljohaney A, Amjadi K, Alvarez GG. A systematic review of the epidemiology, immunopathogenesis, diagnosis, and treatment of pleural TB in HIV-infected patients. Clin Dev Immunol 2012;2012:842045.

365. Kitinya JN, Richter C, Perenboom R, Chande H, Mtoni IM. Influence of HIV status on pathological changes in tuberculous pleuritis. Tuber Lung Dis 1994;75:195-8.

366. Gil V, Cordero PJ, Greses JV, Soler JJ. Pleural tuberculosis in HIV-infected patients. Chest 1995;107:1775-6.

367. Centers for Disease Control and Prevention. Prevention and treatment of tuberculosis among patients infected with human immunodeficiency virus: principles of therapy and revised recommendations. MMWR Recomm Rep 1998;47:1-58.

368. Arora VK, Gowrinath K, Rao RS, Rao RS. Extrapulmonary involvement in HIV with special reference to tuberculous cases. Indian J Tuberc 1995;42:27-32.

369. Repo UK, Nieminen P. Tuberculosis pleurisy due to Mycobacterium fortuitum in a patient with chronic granulocytic leukemia. Scand J Respir Dis 1975;56:329-36.

370. Sauret J, Jolis R, Ausina V, Castro E, Cornudella R. Human tuberculosis due to Mycobacterium bovis: report of 10 cases. Tuber Lung Dis 1992;73:388-91.

371. Huang HC, Yu WL, Shieh CC, Cheng KC, Cheng HH. Unusual mixed infection of thoracic empyema caused by Mycobacterium

tuberculosis, nontuberculosis mycobacteria and Iasteroides in a woman with systemic lupus erythematosus. J Infect 2007;54: e25-28.

372. Lee HT, Su WJ, Chou TY, Chen WS, Su KY, Huang DF. Mycobacterium avium complex-induced pleurisy in a patient with amyopathic dermatomyositis and interstitial lung disease after prolonged immunosuppressive therapy. J Clin Rheumatol 2009;15:193-4.

373. Domfeh AB, Nodit L, Gradowski JF, Bastacky S. Mycobacterium kansasii infection diagnosed by pleural fluid cytology: a case report. Acta Cytol 2007;51:627-30.

374. Haider A, Schliep T, Zeana C. Nontuberculous mycobacterial disease with pleural empyema in a patient with advanced AIDS. Am J Med Sci 2009;338:418-20.

375. Fabbian F, De Giorgi A, Pala M, Fratti D, Contini C. Pleural effusion in an immunocompetent woman caused by Mycobacterium fortuitum. J Med Microbiol 2011; 60:1375-8.

376. Lim JG, O SW, Lee KD, Suk DK, Jung TY, Shim TS, et al. Mycobacterium intracellulare pleurisy identified on liquid cultures of the pleural fluid and pleural biopsy. Tuberc Respir Dis [Seoul] 2013;74:124-8.

377. Christensen EE, Dietz GW, Ahn CH, Chapman JS, Murry RC, Anderson J, et al. Initial roentgenographic manifestations of pulmonary Mycobacterium tuberculosis, M. kansasii, and M. intracellularis infections. Chest 1981;80:132-6.

378. Aronchick JM, Miller WT Jr. Disseminated nontuberculous mycobacterial infections in immunosuppressed patients. Semin Roentgenol 1993;28:150-7.

379. Gribetz AR, Damsker B, Marchevsky A, Bottone EJ. Non-tuberculous mycobacteria in pleural fluid. Assessment of clinical significance. Chest 1985;87:495-8.

380. Mancini P, Mazzei L, Zarzana A, Biagioli D, Sposato B, Croce GF. Post-tuberculosis chronic empyema of the "forty years after". Eur Rev Med Pharmacol Sci 1998;2:25-9.

381. Sahn SA, Iseman MD. Tuberculous empyema. Semin Respir Infect 1999;14:82-7.

382. Bai KJ, Wu IH, Yu MC, Chiang IH, Chiang CY, Lin TP, et al. Tuberculous empyema. Respirology 1998;3:261-6.

383. Gupta SK, Kishan J, Singh SP. Review of one hundred cases of empyema thoracis. Indian J Chest Dis Allied Sci 1989;31:15-20.

384. Malhotra P, Aggarwal AN, Agarwal R, Ray P, Gupta D, Jindal SK. Clinical characteristics and outcomes of empyema thoracis in 117 patients: a comparative analysis of tuberculous vs. non-tuberculous aetiologies. Respir Med 2007;101:423-30.

385. Reeve PA, Seaton D. Tuberculous empyema: a case history extending over 30 years. Tubercle 1986;67:147-50.

386. Magness DJ. Empyema necessitans caused by Mycobacterium tuberculosis in an immunocompetent patient. WMJ 2013;112: 129-30.

387. Al-Kattan KM. Management of tuberculous empyema. Eur J Cardiothorac Surg 2000;17:251-4.

388. Elliott AM, Berning SE, Iseman MD, Peloquin CA. Failure of drug penetration and acquisition of drug resistance in chronic tuberculous empyema. Tuber Lung Dis 1995;76:463-7.

389. Neihart RE, Hof DG. Successful nonsurgical treatment of tuberculous empyema in an irreducible pleural space. Chest 1985;88:792-4.

390. Khanna BK. Management of tuberculous empyema. Indian J Tuberc 1987;34:147-9.

391. Mouroux J, Maalouf J, Padovani B, Rotomondo C, Richelme H. Surgical management of pleuropulmonary tuberculosis. J Thorac Cardiovasc Surg 1996;111:662-70.

392. Lahiri TK, Agrawal D, Gupta R, Kumar S. Analysis of status of surgery in thoracic tuberculosis. Indian J Chest Dis Allied Sci 1998;40:99-108.

393. Bagheri R, Haghi SZ, Rajabi MT, Motamedshariati M, Sheibani S. Outcomes following surgery for complicated tuberculosis: analysis of 108 patients. Thorac Cardiovasc Surg 2013;61:154-8.

394. Choi SS, Kim DJ, Kim KD, Chung KY. Change in pulmonary function following empyemectomy and decortication in tuberculous and non-tuberculous chronic empyema thoracis. Yonsei Med J 2004;45:643-8.

395. Kim DJ, Im JG, Goo JM, Lee HJ, You SY, Song JW. Chronic tuberculous empyema: relationships between preoperative CT findings and postoperative improvement measured by pulmonary function testing. Clin Radiol 2005;60:503-7.

396. Light RW. Chylothorax and pseudochylothorax. In: Light RW, editor. Pleural diseases. Fourth edition. Philadelphia: Lippincott Williams and Wilkins; 2001.p.327-43.

397. Garcia-Zamalloa A, Ruiz-Irastorza G, Aguayo FJ, Gurrutxaga N. Pseudochylothorax. Report of 2 cases and review of the literature. Medicine [Baltimore] 1999;78:200-7.

398. Hamm H, Pfalzer B, Fabel H. Lipoprotein analysis in a chyliform pleural effusion: implications for pathogenesis and diagnosis. Respiration 1991;58:294-300.

399. Vennera MC, Moreno R, Cot J, Marin A, Sanchez-Lloret J, Picado C, et al. Chylothorax and tuberculosis. Thorax 1983;38: 694-5.

400. Menzies R, Hidvegi R. Chylothorax associated with tuberculous spondylitis. Can Assoc Radiol J 1988;39:238-41.

401. Anton PA, Rubio J, Casan P, Franquet T. Chylothorax due to Mycobacterium tuberculosis. Thorax 1995;50:1019.

402. Singh S, Girod JP, Ghobrial MW. Chylothorax as a complication of tuberculosis in the setting of the human immunodeficiency virus infection. Arch Intern Med 2001;161:2621.

403. Gupta D, Maheswari U, Aggarwal AN. Tuberculous chylothorax. Lung India 2004; 21:54-5.

404. Ananthan VS, Siva KK. A rare case of acid-fast bacilli in chylothorax. Lung India 2012;29:166-8.

405. Kim KJ, Park DW, Choi WS. Simultaneous chylothorax and chylous ascites due to tuberculosis. Infect Chemother 2014;46: 50-3.

14

Silicotuberculosis

Prasanta Raghab Mohapatra

INTRODUCTION

Silicosis is an occupational fibrotic lung disease caused by inhalation of respirable free crystalline silicon dioxide or silica. Tuberculosis [TB] frequently accompanies silicosis as a comorbid condition particularly in TB endemic countries and contributes significantly towards mortality of patients with silicosis (1,2). Silicotuberculosis is a major occupational comorbid lung disease in both industrialised and developing countries.

SILICOSIS

Silicosis, one of the most common forms of pneumoconiosis, caused by the inhalation of crystalline silicon dioxide or silica is an ancient occupational disease worldwide (1). Environmental settings posing the greatest occupational risk include the following: mining and processing of stone; mining of gold and precious stones; well drilling, sandblasting; ceramic and glass production; and iron smelting (3,4). Workers involved in mining, rock breaking, sandblasting, construction and the founding of ferrous and non-ferrous metals are at risk of silicosis. The disorder is reported in all countries, but is more prevalent in low- and middle-income countries, where the burden is often under-reported because of a poor surveillance system. China has the most reported patients with silicosis, with nearly 6000 new cases and more than 24000 deaths reported annually (5). In the Brazilian gold-mining area in Minas Gerais alone, more than 4500 workers were reported to have had silicosis between 1978 and 1998 (6). Less than100 cases were reported every year in the UK between 1996 and 2009. In the USA, overall age-adjusted mortality rates declined from 8.9 per million in 1968 to 0.7 in 2004 (7,8). Protective measures [e.g., dust control and respirators] have caused a steady decline in death rates due to silicosis in the past few decades

in developed countries (8,9), but new outbreaks still occur occasionally (2,10).

The exact prevalence of silicosis in India is not known. Majority of these studies have utilised radiographic findings to make a diagnosis of silicosis. Studies (11,12) from Rohtak in Haryana state have shown radiographic evidence of silicosis in 35.2% of 227 stone-cutters. In Madhya Pradesh, silicosis was reported in 57% slate pencil workers (13). A report from Gujarat cited the prevalence of silicosis as 14% to 30.4% amongst 85 female workers in a quartz mill and 56 employees of open silica-grinding stones, respectively (14,15). Silicosis was also commonly reported from central India and mid-western states, such as, Madhya Pradesh, Chhattisgarh, Jharkhand, Gujarat and Rajasthan. Prevalence of silicosis was reported to be very high amongst unorganised sectors in India (16,17). India has witnessed rapid industrialisation and growth in the construction of buildings, roads, bridges in the last decades and it has been an ongoing process. The problems of dust exposure and prevalence of silicosis are, therefore, increasingly anticipated (2,18).

Pathophysiology

Pathological diversities of silicosis include simple [nodular] silicosis, progressive massive fibrosis, silicoproteinosis, and diffuse interstitial fibrosis and discrete hard nodules, usually with upper-lobe predominance (19). Hilar and peribronchial lymph nodes are often enlarged. Microscopically, the characteristic silicotic nodules are seen in hilar lymph nodes and lung parenchyma. Under polarised light microscopy, bi-refringent particles are often seen in the centre of silicotic nodules. In progressive massive fibrosis [PMF], lung nodules become confluent, resulting in lesions nearly a centimeter or bigger in diameter. Inhaled respirable silica dusts usually are deposited in distal airways. Reactive oxygen species being activated by silica can produce directly on freshly cleaved particle surfaces or indirectly through its effect on the phagocytic cells (20). Macrophage receptor expressed in alveolar macrophages help in the recognition and uptake of silica (21). The interleukin-1 [IL-1] signalling pathway and other inflammatory cytokines, such as tumour necrosis factor [TNF] play crucial roles in subsequent inflammation and fibrosis (2,22).

Clinically, silicosis can remain present in three different forms: acute; accelerated; and chronic.

Acute Silicosis

Acute silicosis also called silicoproteinosis, occurs rarely after exposure to high concentrations of respirable crystalline silica for a few weeks to five years. It commonly affects sandblasters. In addition to dyspnoea and cough, constitutional symptoms could be present, such as fatigue, fever, and weight loss. Respiratory failure and death often occur within a few months.

Acute silicosis occurs after exposure to a very high concentration of dust over a few months and is usually rapidly fatal within years (23). Currently, sandblasters and silica flour mill workers are the two groups considered at high risk of developing acute silicosis (2).

Chronic Silicosis

Chronic silicosis, the commonest form of silicosis, usually develops after at least a decade long exposure at low concentrations of silica (24). It is usually seen in industries with rigorous environmental control procedures. The patients with simple silicosis are usually asymptomatic in early stages and diagnosed by the way of radiological examination. Shortness of breath is more common at later stages than it is initially, especially with progression of

massive fibrosis. Other patients with chronic silicosis could present with comorbidity like TB and lung cancer (2).

Accelerated Silicosis

Accelerated silicosis occurs after a few years of exposure to silica. Accelerated silicosis develops 5-10 years after initial exposure and is associated with rapidly progressive features of dyspnoea and pulmonary fibrosis. Clinically it is similar to chronic silicosis, but progresses rapidly (1,2).

Radiographic Findings

Chest radiograph is the primary method of diagnosis. The radiographic features of silicosis are varied and range from diffuse, fine, rounded, regular nodularity resembling miliary TB to coarse irregular nodules [Figures 14.1 and 14.2] or extensive fibrosis resembling progressive massive fibrosis [Figures 14.3 and 14.4]. In simple silicosis, chest radiography

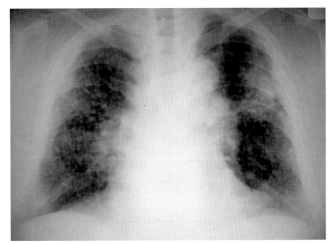

Figure 14.1: Chest radiograph [postero-anterior view] showing coarse irregular nodules and fibrosis in a patient with silicosis

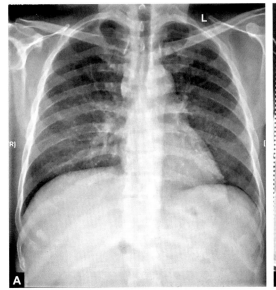
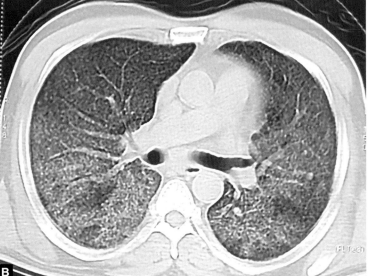

Figure 14.2: Chest radiograph [posetro-anterior view] [A] and CT chest [B] in a patient with silicosis showing nodular pattern

usually shows small round opacities, often symmetrically distributed with upper-zone predominance. With extensive fibrotic structure, hilar structures are usually pulled up, leaving hyper translucent zones of lung in the periphery and lower-lung zones, often with several bullae. The involvement of lymph nodes by chronic silicosis is fairly characteristic, with a tendency towards peripheral calcification, which produces the so-called *egg-shell* appearance [Figures 14.3 and 14.4]. The hilar and mediastinal groups are often affected, but other thoracic and extra-thoracic nodes may also be affected. The visceral pleura when involved are often diffusely thickened by fibrosis with occasional focal

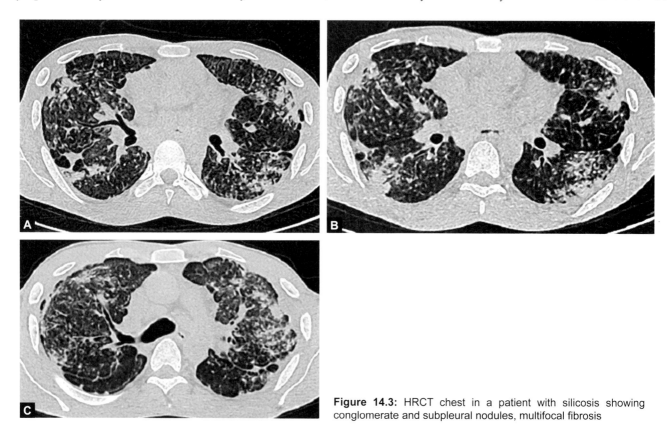

Figure 14.3: HRCT chest in a patient with silicosis showing conglomerate and subpleural nodules, multifocal fibrosis

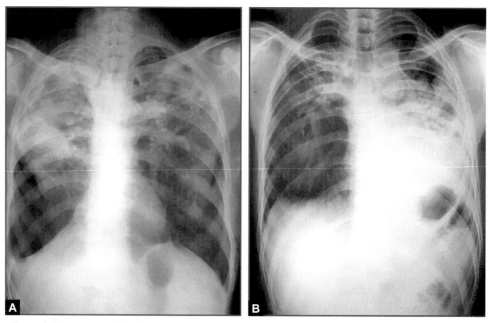

Figure 14.4: Chest radiograph [posetro-anterior view] [A] in a patient with complicated silicosis showing extensive fibrosis, *egg shell* calcification. Chest radiograph [postero-anterior view] [B] in another patient with complicated silicosis showing extensive fibrosis, *egg shell* calcification, bulla formation

calcification. Involvement of the middle and lower zones of the lungs is more frequent in accelerated silicosis (25,26).

Management

No curative treatment for silicosis exists. There is no evidence of benefit of using corticosteroid treatment for long-term benefit for patients with chronic or accelerated silicosis, and such treatment could increase the risk of TB. Silicosis patients should generally be removed from further exposure. Empirical treatment with bronchodilators should be considered for symptomatic patients with airflow obstruction. Cough suppressants and mucolytics could be useful for symptomatic relief. Antibiotics should be given as necessary for intercurrent chest infections. Complications, such as, pneumothorax, chronic cor pulmonale, and respiratory failure should be managed accordingly (1).

SILICOTUBERCULOSIS

Epidemiology

The coexistence of silicosis and TB has been called silico-tuberculosis. This has been reported since the early part of the twentieth century (23). Prolonged exposure to silica dust, even in the absence of radiological silicosis, also predisposes individuals to TB (27,28). On the other hand, TB may complicate simple silicosis to advanced disease (29). As an end result of inflammation, TB can contribute to the further development of fibrosis in patients with silicosis (30). With poor environmental conditions, the prevalence of silicosis and silicotuberculosis is shown to be higher (31).

Even after exposure ceases, there is increased life-long risk of both pulmonary and extra-pulmonary TB [EPTB] (27). In endemic area, the TB rates in advanced simple silicosis is up to three-fold higher and the relative risk of death from TB is three- to six-fold greater in patients with silicosis than in the general population. The risk is higher in patients with acute and accelerated silicosis (32). The pre-valence of pulmonary TB is correlated with age and service duration of the workers as well as the severity of underlying silicosis (33,34). There is 27% incidence of TB over five years among a group of 679 patients with silicosis in Hong Kong (35). TB were diagnosed in 43% patients with silicosis in a Chinese study with a follow up over a period of 18 years (36). TB was attributed to 11.8% deaths in patients with silicosis of 595 workers in Italy (37).

From India, available studies have shown 3-7 times higher incidence of TB in persons with silicosis compared to matched control (11,12). The fraction of silicosis suffering from TB has been reported in earlier reports from 4.8% to up to 60% and on average; it appears that TB occurs in 20%-25% of all silicosis patients in their lifetime. The mortality risk is higher if TB develops among silicosis (38).

Mycobacterium kansasii and *Mycobacterium avium-intra-cellulare* were reported in 12 of the 22 cases of silicosis with mycobacterial infection (39). Also nontuberculous myco-bacteria [NTM] were detected in 14% of 234 gold miners studied (34). NTM may account for a large proportion of the mycobacterial disease in some populations (13,40), *M. kansasii* being the most common type (13,41). When compared to the healthy control, the risk of developing pulmonary TB is reported to be 2.8-39 times higher and EPTB is also as much as 3.7 times more for patients with silicosis (13).

Pathogenesis

Several pathogenetic processes are common to TB and silicosis which are synergistic in producing more fibrosis and in enhancing susceptibility to mycobacterial infection or reactivation of a latent focus of infection [Figure 14.5, Table 14.1] (30). Evidence from experimental studies suggests that silica alters the immune response of the lungs, impairs

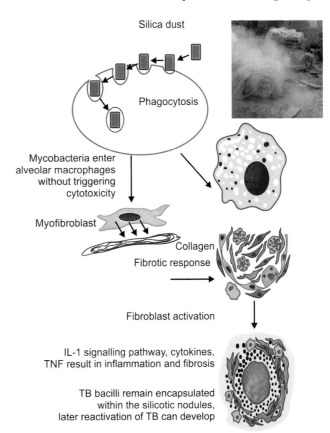

Figure 14.5: Pathogenesis of silicotuberculosis
IL-1 = interleukin-1; TNF = tumour necrosis factor; TB = tuberculosis

Table 14.1: Influence of TB on silicosis
Exposure of silica has an unfavourable influence on the course of induced TB
There is more fibrosis produced by the combination
Synergistic effect of silicosis and TB—proliferative fibrous reaction
TB may complicate simple silicosis as well as advanced disease
It may develop massive fibrosis
Exposure of silica has an unfavourable influence on the course of induced TB
TB = tuberculosis

the function of pulmonary macrophages, and, with frequent exposure, causes macrophage apoptosis (8,13). The silica particles are phagocytosed by the alveolar macrophages. Phagocytosis of crystalline silica in the lung causes lysosomal damage, activating the NALP3 inflammasome and triggering the inflammatory cascade with subsequent fibrosis. Silica has the capacity to cause damage to the cell membranes which leads to the death of the macrophages with re-exposure of the other macrophages to the same particles. Prior to the death, the macrophages become activated and secrete interleukin 1β [IL-1β] and TNF-α (42). These cytokines are responsible for fibroblast activation and fibrosis. The TNF-α also stimulates neutrophils to release oxidants which produce local damage.

It has been seen that surfactant protein A are present at high levels in the broncho-alveolar lavage [BAL] fluid of patients with silicosis. An excess of this protein seems to be associated with higher susceptibility to TB, possibly because it allows mycobacteria to enter the alveolar macrophages without triggering cytotoxicity and inhibits the formation of reactive nitrogen species by the activated microphages (43,44). It is also believed that the bacilli can remain encapsulated within the silicotic nodules, which would be responsible for the reactivation of TB in such patients (13). Impairment of lung function increases with disease progression, even after the patient is no longer exposed.

Lung fibrosis occurs in both diseases and may interfere with the clearance of dust-laden alveolar macrophages or mycobacteria-laden material from the lung. Lymphatic obstruction causes macrophages to accumulate in the interstitial tissues resulting in local fibrosis (45). Another hypothesis for the unexplained incidence of pulmonary TB in patients with silicosis is through the surface coordination of iron by dust particles (45). By this process, the body iron is absorbed by the silica crystals in the lung. Indeed, low serum iron has been observed among people exposed to silicates (46). Evidence that iron is complexed on the silicate dust can be found by the use of specific stains for iron or by measurement of the iron content of lungs in which silicate content is increased (47). This iron can be mobilised from the silicate surface by a strong iron chelator. Mycobacteria are dependent on iron for growth and produce the iron chelators, namely, *mycobactin* and *exochelin* to mobilise the metal from body stores; indeed iron is considered a virulence factor for mycobacteria. It has been hypothesised that silicate particles act as a reservoir of iron which can be used by the mycobacteria, thereby explaining the increased incidence of TB among those who inhale silica dust (45). The iron made available from silicato-iron complexes may activate dormant tubercle bacilli by a mechanism similar to the effect of iron repletion (48).

Clinical Features

The manifestations of TB in patients with silicosis are similar to those in general population. However, since weakness, fatigability, dyspnea and night sweats occur in silicosis also, at times, it may be difficult to detect concomitant TB clinically.

Diagnosis

Early diagnosis of active TB not only helps limiting own disability by early treatment but also stops spreading of the bacilli to silica-affected co-workers and the community. The diagnosis of active TB in patients with silicosis demands a high degree of suspicion and primarily on the basis of a history of exposure, clinical symptomatology and chest radiographic appearances [Table 14.2]. It is difficult to differentiate abnormalities in the chest radiograph of a patient with silicosis who has superimposed TB. The radiographic abnormalities are seen in the apical area of either of the lungs. These radiographic abnormalities are usually poorly demarcated infiltrates of variable size that do not cross the lung fissures (49). These opacities may surround pre-existing silicotic nodules. Presence of a cavity in a nodule is usually indicative of TB (30,49) although fluid-filled cavities can be found in silicosis also (50). TB cavities in patients with silicosis are usually not traversed by large vessels possibly due to vascular obstruction frequently seen in these patients (51). Additional suggestive findings include rapid changes in the radiographic picture, development of pericardial or pleural effusion, or onset of bronchial stenosis, especially of the right middle lobe (49). Computed tomography [CT] of the chest is useful in some patients [Figure 14.6].

Establishing the diagnosis of pulmonary TB in a patient with silicosis by bacteriological methods is often difficult (49,52). Therefore, more frequent sputum smear examination for acid-fast bacilli [AFB] is recommended (52a). The need for mycobacterial culture is more important in areas where there is a high prevalence of NTM infection. Occurrence of human immunodeficiency virus [HIV] infection and silicosis can result in profound susceptibility to *Mycobacterium kansasii* disease (52b). The reader is referred to the chapter *"Nontuberculous mycobacterial infections"* [Chapter 41] for further details. Differentiating silicosis from other conditions [Table 14.3] is important. Establishing the diagnosis of miliary TB in patients with silicosis is

---

Table 14.2: Features suggestive of TB in patients with silicosis

Radiographic abnormalities in the apical area of either lungs
Coalescence of nodules to form focal opacity of >1 cm, fibrotic mass, conglomerate massive shadowing
Poorly demarcated infiltrates of variable size that do not cross the lung fissures
Opacities surrounding pre-existing silicotic nodules
Adjacent emphysema with abrupt sharp border, presence of a cavity in a nodule
Radiographic abnormalities in the apical area of either lungs
Poorly demarcated infiltrates of variable size that do not cross the lung fissures
Distortion of lung parenchyma due to fibrosis, bronchial stenosis which may be irregular
TB = tuberculosis

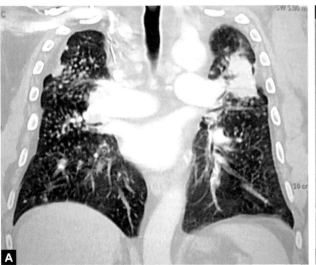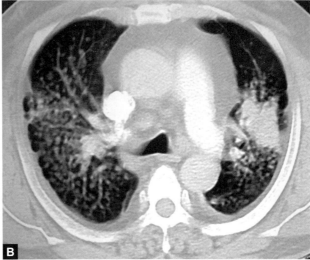

Figure 14.6: CT chest coronal section [A] and axial section [B] in a patient with silicotuberculosis showing bilateral coarser irregular nodules with fibrosis, conglomerate masses and calcification

Table 14.3: Differential diagnosis
Tuberculosis
Sarcoidosis
Coal worker pneumoconiosis
Welder's pneumoconiosis
Pulmonary alveolar proteinosis
Talcosis

Table 14.4: Complications of silicosis, silicotuberculosis
Cor-pulmonale
Spontaneous pneumothorax
Broncholithiasis
Tracheobronchial obstruction
Lung cancer
Hypoxaemic ventilatory failure

important as some patients can have both conditions. In some cases if diagnosis remains uncertain about active TB, BAL and transbronchial lung biopsy wherever possible; biopsies significantly increase the diagnostic yield of the test, even in patients whose sputum and BAL are negative for mycobacteria (53). These should be performed routinely if the diagnosis from sputum is inconclusive to facilitate accurate diagnosis and management (54).

Treatment

The silicosis *per se* is incurable, but TB is treatable; the management goals are aimed at early detection of silicosis, disability limitation and treating associated TB at the earliest opportunities. Careful monitoring of both recently and formerly exposed workers to establish surveillance programmes, to prevent TB and to reduce disability remains the important aspects of the management. The success rates of the treatment of TB in patients with silicosis were lower than that in patients without silicosis (52,55,56). It has been postulated that the deep fibrotic lung tissue and vascular obstruction seen in patients with silicosis make it difficult for the drugs to reach the target. However, it was shown later that once the febrile phase of the disease subsides on treatment with anti-TB drugs, the return to underground work has not adversely affected the treatment outcome in regards to the relapse rate which may be same (57,58), as in pulmonary TB, maximum relapses in patients with silicotuberculosis occur

within first two years after completion of treatment but the risk of relapse likely to continue indefinitely after completion of treatment (58). In several recent trials, the efficacy of a short-course chemotherapy has been established in patients with silicotuberculosis (40,57,58). However, a few studies have suggested the need for a longer duration of anti-TB treatment (41). Treatment of silicotuberculosis is similar to the treatment of TB elsewhere in the body. Long-term follow-up is recommended to diagnose possible relapse after the completion of treatment. In India, patients with TB receive DOTS under the Revised National Tuberculosis Control Programme [RNTCP] of the Government of India. The reader is referred to the chapter *"Revised National Tuberculosis Control Programme" [Chapter 53]* for details.

Generally a longer duration of anti-TB treatment is required for these patients and the outcome is often unsatisfactory due to irreversibility of lung fibrosis due to silica deposition. It is important to implement smoking cessation programmes in the work-place. The environmental factors and living conditions, those that predispose to TB and diseases must be taken care of. Complications in patients with silicosis and silicotuberculosis are listed in Table 14.4.

Recommendations for Prevention

As the TB is reasonably common in patients with silicosis, there is a strong opinion as per literature available on anti-TB treatment in patients with silicosis (59). Accordingly those who have periods of exposure to silica longer than 10 years, irrespective of silicosis disease, should have periodic chest radiographs and tuberculin skin test [TST] in the initial evaluation (60). If TST is positive [induration ≥10 mm], a 6-month course of isoniazid at 300 mg/day [or 10 mg/kg/day] should be instituted (61-63). If the TST is negative [induration <10 mm], the test may be performed again in two weeks for confirmation, considering that exposure to the TST can stimulate the immunological memory against the TB bacillus. If the negative result still persists, the test should be done annually (63). There is a strong evidence to support the concept that silica dust control is associated with a major reduction in risk TB in silica-exposed patients (64). Systematic testing and treatment of latent TB infection [LTBI] should be performed in people with silicosis (65). Short course prophylactic regimens using rifampicin alone have not demonstrated higher rates of active TB when compared with long-term isoniazid. A weekly regimen of rifapentine and isoniazid has higher completion rates, and less liver toxicity (66). An active surveillance of the workers should be carried out in both pre-employment and post-employment periods. Careful individualised clinical evaluations and close follow-up of tuberculin converters are essential to reduce the risk of developing TB. There is also a need for evolving a comprehensive policy for the prevention, treatment, rehabilitation, compensation and follow-up in patients with silicotuberculosis (67).

REFERENCES

1. Greenberg MI, Waksman J, Curtis J. Silicosis: a review. Disease-a-month: DM 2007;53:394-416.
2. Leung CC, Yu IT, Chen W. Silicosis. Lancet 2012;379:2008-18.
3. Barboza CE, Winter DH, Seiscento M, Santos Ude P, Terra Filho M. Tuberculosis and silicosis: epidemiology, diagnosis and chemoprophylaxis. J Bras Pneumol 2008;34:959-66.
4. Terra Filho M, Santos Ude P. Silicosis. J Bras Pneumol 2006;32:S41-7.
5. Tse LA, Li ZM, Wong TW, Fu ZM, Yu IT. High prevalence of accelerated silicosis among gold miners in Jiangxi, China. Am J Ind Med 2007;50:876-80.
6. Carneiro AP, Barreto SM, Siqueira AL, Cavariani F, Forastiere F. Continued exposure to silica after diagnosis of silicosis in Brazilian gold miners. Am J Ind Med 2006;49:811-8.
7. Kreiss K, Danilovs JA, Newman LS. Histocompatibility antigens in a population-based silicosis series. Br J Ind Med 1989;46:364-9.
8. Sluis-Cremer GK, Maier G. HLA antigens of the A and B locus in relation to the development of silicosis. Br J Ind Med 1984;41:417-8.
9. Ziskind M, Jones RN, Weill H. Silicosis. Am Rev Respir Dis 1976;113:643-65.
10. Seaton A, Legge JS, Henderson J, Kerr KM. Accelerated silicosis in Scottish stonemasons. Lancet 1991;337:341-4.
11. Gupta SP, Garg AK, Gupta OP. Silicosis amongst stone-cutters [a clinical and radiological study]. J Assoc Physicians India 1969;17:163-72.
12. Gupta SP, Bajaj A, Jain AL, Vasudeva YL. Clinical and radiological studies in silicosis: based on a study of the disease amongst stone-cutters. Indian J Med Res 1972;60:1309-15.
13. Jain SM, Sepaha GC, Khare KC, Dubey VS. Silicosis in slate pencil workers. A clinicoradiologic study. Chest 1977;71:423-6.
14. Tiwari RR, Narain R, Sharma YK, Kumar S. Comparison of respiratory morbidity between present and ex-workers of quartz crushing units: Healthy workers' effect. Indian J Occup Environ Med 2010;14:87-90.
15. Tiwari RR, Sharma YK. Respiratory health of female stone grinders with free silica dust exposure in Gujarat, India. Int J Occup Environ Health 2008;14:280-2.
16. Saiyed HN, Ghodasara NB, Sathwara NG, Patel GC, Parikh DJ, Kashyap SK. Dustiness, silicosis & tuberculosis in small scale pottery workers. Indian J Med Res 1995;102:138-42.
17. Jindal SK. Silicosis in India: past and present. Curr Opin Pulm Med 2013;19:163-8.
18. Tiwary G, Gangopadhyay PK. A review on the occupational health and social security of unorganized workers in the construction industry. Indian J Occup Environ Med 2011;15:18-24.
19. van Zyl Smit RN, Pai M, Yew WW, Leung CC, Zumla A, Bateman ED, et al. Global lung health: the colliding epidemics of tuberculosis, tobacco smoking, HIV and COPD. Eur Respir J 2010;35:27-33.
20. Hamilton RF, Jr., Thakur SA, Holian A. Silica binding and toxicity in alveolar macrophages. Free Radic Biol Med 2008; 44:1246-58.
21. Thakur SA, Hamilton R Jr, Pikkarainen T, Holian A. Differential binding of inorganic particles to MARCO. Toxicol Sci 2009;107:238-46.
22. Huaux F. New developments in the understanding of immunology in silicosis. Curr Opin Allergy Clin Immunol 2007;7:168-73.
23. Mazurek JM, Attfield MD. Silicosis mortality among young adults in the United States, 1968-2004. Am J Ind Med 2008;51:568-78.
24. Cocco P. The long and winding road from silica exposure to silicosis and other health effects. Occup Environ Med 2003;60:157-8.
25. Arakawa H, Fujimoto K, Honma K, Suganuma N, Morikubo H, Saito Y, et al. Progression from near-normal to end-stage lungs in chronic interstitial pneumonia related to silica exposure: long-term CT observations. Am J Roentgenol 2008;191:1040-5.
26. Arakawa H, Johkoh T, Honma K, Saito Y, Fukushima Y, Shida H, et al. Chronic interstitial pneumonia in silicosis and mix-dust pneumoconiosis: its prevalence and comparison of CT findings with idiopathic pulmonary fibrosis. Chest 2007;131:1870-6.
27. Hnizdo E, Murray J. Risk of pulmonary tuberculosis relative to silicosis and exposure to silica dust in South African gold miners. Occup Environ Med 1998;55:496-502.
28. teWaternaude JM, Ehrlich RI, Churchyard GJ, Pemba L, Dekker K, Vermeis M, et al. Tuberculosis and silica exposure in South African gold miners. Occup Environ Med 2006;63:187-92.
29. Westerholm P, Ahlmark A, Maasing R, Segelberg I. Silicosis and risk of lung cancer or lung tuberculosis: a cohort study. Environ Res 1986;41:339-50.
30. Ng TP, Chan SL. Factors associated with massive fibrosis in silicosis. Thorax 1991;46:229-32.
31. Huang J, Shibata E, Takeuchi Y, Okutani H. Comprehensive health evaluation of workers in the ceramics industry. Br J Ind Med 1993;50:112-6.
32. American Thoracic Society Committee of the Scientific Assembly on Environmental and Occupational Health. Adverse effects of crystalline silica exposure. Am J Respir Crit Care Med 1997;155:761-8.
33. Kleinschmidt I, Churchyard G. Variation in incidences of tuberculosis in subgroups of South African gold miners. Occup Environ Med 1997;54:636-41.
34. Cowie RL. The epidemiology of tuberculosis in gold miners with silicosis. Am J Respir Crit Care Med 1994;150:1460-2.

35. Hong Kong Chest Service/Tuberculosis Research Centre, Madras/British Medical Research Council. A double-blind placebo-controlled clinical trial of three antituberculosis chemoprophylaxis regimens in patients with silicosis in Hong Kong. Am Rev Respir Dis 1992;145:36-41.

36. Lou JZ, Zhou C. The prevention of silicosis and prediction of its future prevalence in China. Am J Public Health 1989;79:1613-6.

37. Forastiere F, Lagorio S, Michelozzi P, Perucci CA, Axelson O. Mortality pattern of silicotic subjects in the Latium region, Italy. Br J Ind Med 1989;46:877-80.

38. Ng TP, Chan SL, Lee J. Predictors of mortality in silicosis. Respir Med 1992;86:115-9.

39. Bailey WC, Brown M, Buechner HA, Weill H, Ichinose H, Ziskind M. Silico-mycobacterial disease in sandblasters. Am Rev Respir Dis 1974;110:115-25.

40. Lin TP, Suo J, Lee CN, Lee JJ, Yang SP. Short-course chemotherapy of pulmonary tuberculosis in pneumoconiotic patients. Am Rev Respir Dis 1987;136:808-10.

41. Hong Kong Chest Service/tuberculosis Research Centre, Madras/British Medical Research Council. A controlled clinical comparison of 6 and 8 months of antituberculosis chemotherapy in the treatment of patients with silicotuberculosis in Hong Kong. Am Rev Respir Dis 1991;143:262-7.

42. Piguet PF, Collart MA, Grau GE, Sappino AP, Vassalli P. Requirement of tumour necrosis factor for development of silica-induced pulmonary fibrosis. Nature 1990;344:245-7.

43. Hughes JM, Weill H, Rando RJ, Shi R, McDonald AD, McDonald JC. Cohort mortality study of North American industrial sand workers. II. Case-referent analysis of lung cancer and silicosis deaths. Ann Occup Hyg 2001;45:201-7.

44. Sharma SK, Pande JN, Verma K. Effect of prednisolone treatment in chronic silicosis. Am Rev Respir Dis 1991;143:814-21.

45. Ng TP, Allan WG, Tsin TW, O'Kelly FJ. Silicosis in jade workers. Br J Ind Med 1985;42:761-4.

46. Niculescu T, Dumitru R, Burnea D. Changes of copper, iron, and zinc in the serum of patients with silicosis, silicotuberculosis, and active lung tuberculosis. Environ Res 1981;25:260-8.

47. Guest L. The endogenous iron content, by Mossbauer spectroscopy, of human lungs--II. Lungs from various occupational groups. Ann Occup Hyg 1978;21:151-7.

48. Murray MJ, Murray AB, Murray MB, Murray CJ. The adverse effect of iron repletion on the course of certain infections. BMJ 1978;2:1113-5.

49. Barras G. Silicotuberculosis in Switzerland. Schweizerische medizinische Wochenschrift 1970;100:1802-8.

50. Malik SK, Behera D, Awasthi GK, Singh JP. Pulmonary silicosis in emery polish workers. Indian J Chest Dis Allied Sci 1985;27:116-21.

51. de la Hoz RE, Rosenman K, Borczuk A. Silicosis in dental supply factory workers. Respir Med 2004;98:791-4.

52a. Snider DE, Jr. The relationship between tuberculosis and silicosis. Am Rev Respir Dis 1979;119:515.

52b. Corbett EL, Hay M, Churchyard GJ, Herselman P, Clayton T, Williams BG, et al. Mycobacterium kansasii and M. scrofulaceum isolates from HIV-negative South African gold miners: incidence, clinical significance and radiology. Int J Tuberc Lung Dis 1999;3:501-7.

53. Charoenratanakul S, Dejsomritrutai W, Chaiprasert A. Diagnostic role of fiberoptic bronchoscopy in suspected smear negative pulmonary tuberculosis. Respir Med 1995;89:621-3.

54. Grobbelaar JP, Bateman ED. Hut lung: a domestically acquired pneumoconiosis of mixed aetiology in rural women. Thorax 1991;46:334-40.

55. Morrow CS. The results of chemotherapy in silicotuberculosis. Am Rev Respir Dis 1960;82:831-4.

56. Allison AC, Hart PD. Potentiation by silica of the growth of Mycobacterium tuberculosis in macrophage cultures. Br J Exp Pathol 1968;49:465-76.

57. Escreet BC, Langton ME, Cowie RL. Short-course chemotherapy for silicotuberculosis. S Afr Med J 1984;66:327-30.

58. Cowie RL, Langton ME, Becklake MR. Pulmonary tuberculosis in South African gold miners. Am Rev Respir Dis 1989;139:1086-9.

59. Sharma SK, Mohanan S, Sharma A. Relevance of latent TB infection in areas of high TB prevalence. Chest 2012;142:761-73.

60. Corbett EL, Churchyard GJ, Clayton T, Herselman P, Williams B, Hayes R, et al. Risk factors for pulmonary mycobacterial disease in South African gold miners. A case-control study. Am J Respir Crit Care Med 1999;159:94-9.

61. Gottesfeld P, Murray J, Chadha SS, Rees D. Preventing tuberculosis with silica dust controls. Int J Tuberc Lung Dis 2011;15:713-4.

62. Rees D, Murray J. Silica, silicosis and tuberculosis. Int J Tuberc Lung Dis 2007;11:474-84.

63. Balaan MR, Weber SL, Banks DE. Clinical aspects of coal workers' pneumoconiosis and silicosis. Occup Med 1993;8:19-34.

64. Lowrie DB. What goes wrong with the macrophage in silicosis? Eur J Respir Dis 1982;63:180-2.

65. World Health Organization. Guidelines on the Management of latent tuberculosis infection. Geneva: World Health Organization; 2015.

66. Sharma SK, Sharma A, Kadhiravan T, Tharyan P. Rifamycins [rifampicin, rifabutin and rifapentine] compared to isoniazid for preventing tuberculosis in HIV-negative people at risk of active TB. Cochrane Database Syst Rev 2013;7:CD007545.

67. Sharma N, Kundu D, Dhaked S, Das A. Silicosis and silicotuberculosis in India. Bull World Health Organ 2016;94:777-8.

15

Abdominal Tuberculosis

Govind K Makharia

INTRODUCTION

While one-third of the world's population is infected with *Mycobacterium tuberculosis [Mtb]*, only about 10% of them ever develop active TB (1-3). Extra-pulmonary tuberculosis [EPTB] accounts for approximately 20% of all cases with TB in immunocompetent individuals; of these 3%-5% have abdominal TB (4-6). While abdominal tuberculosis [TB] still remains an important disease in countries where TB is still endemic; increasing population migration and epidemic of human immunodeficiency virus [HIV] infection and acquired immunodeficiency syndrome [AIDS] have led to resurgence of this disease in regions where TB had previously been largely controlled (4-10).

Table 15.1: Classification of abdominal TB

Gastrointestinal TB

  Small and large intestinal TB
  Gastroduodenal TB
  Oesophageal TB

Peritoneal TB

  Chronic peritoneal TB

    Ascitic form
    Encysted [loculated] form
    Dry type

TB of the solid viscera

  Hepatobiliary TB
  TB of the spleen
  TB of the pancreas

TB of the abdominal lymph nodes

  TB mesenteric lymphadenitis
  TB of lymph nodes at porta hepatis
  TB retroperitoneal lymphadenitis

TB = tuberculosis

Mtb can affect many organs including gastrointestinal [GI] tract, peritoneum, hepatobiliary system and pancreas [Table 15.1]. Marshall *et al* (11), after pooling data from six studies [n = 596] reported that 42%, 50% and 8% had peritoneal, GI and lymph node TB, respectively (11). While GI and peritoneal TB usually do not co-exist, in some patients with peritoneal TB intestinal involvement may be observed on cross-sectional imaging such as contrast-enhanced computed tomography [CECT].

INTESTINAL TUBERCULOSIS

Site of Involvement

While any part of GI tract may be involved by *Mtb*, the most common site of involvement is ileocaecum [ileum, ileocecal valve and caecum] (11). Other common sites of involvement include the colon [where the frequency decreases segmentally from the ascending colon to the rectum], jejunum, stomach, duodenum and oesophagus (11-18). The ileocaecal region is the preferred site of involvement by TB because of abundance of lymphoid tissue, relative physiologic stasis, and minimal digestive activity permitting greater contact time of acid-fast bacilli [AFB] with the mucosal surface of the ileocaecum, among others (11).

Pathogenesis

TB can develop primarily within the intestinal tract or secondary to a focus elsewhere in the body. There are four possible ways by which an infection can reach the GI tract: [i] direct invasion by the ingested *Mtb*; [ii] transport by the way of infected bile; [iii] extension from adjacent diseased organs or tissues; and [iv] haematogenous spread. Intestinal involvement is probably related to the number and virulence of the ingested organisms and the nutritional status of the patient (7,11,13).

Pathological and Clinical Correlation

The diameter of a normal intestine decreases from the duodenum to jejunum and then to the ileum. The diameter of the jejunum is 3 cm and that of the ileum is 2.5 cm (18,19). The content which flows through the intestine is mostly liquid chyme. At what diameter of the intestinal lumen the obstruction to the flow of chyme occurs, is not well-established. In a rat model, it was observed that the pressure in the intestine started rising and the flow of the contents started decreasing when the luminal diameter decreased to 60% (20). Therefore, in the early stage intestinal TB, when the lesions are superficial and there is no cicatrisation of the lumen, the flow of chyme is not affected and patients may not have any intestinal symptoms. As the disease progresses, the effective diameter of the intestinal lumen decreases, resulting in obstruction to the flow of contents. The severity of symptoms increases as the intestinal luminal diameter decreases. The initial symptoms of intestinal colic are usually episodic and are precipitated by episodes of GI involvement resulting in temporary mild intestinal wall oedema and further decreasing the diameter of the already compromised intestinal lumen. As disease progresses, the interval between the episodes of symptoms decreases. Ultimately, the symptoms of intestianl colic become more frequent and patients develop partial intestinal obstruction. The ulcerations and nodularity caused by the tissue destruction can lead to oozing of blood from the ulcers, resulting in anaemia.

After effective treatment of the disease, there is resolution of active inflammation and healing of ulcers, which results in the improvement in symptoms. As it is well-known that chronic inflammatory process heals with fibrosis, the healing of ulcers and inflammation of the intestine leads to scarring of the intestinal lumen, and thus, compromise the normal intestinal diameter (21). There is a fundamental difference in the diseases affecting solid or spongy organs and luminal organs. In spite of residual changes in a part of the solid or spongy organ, there still may be sufficient volume to maintain the functions of the organ. On the contrary, healing of the intestinal lesions may result in the fibrotic stricture and may continue to be symptomatic. The resulting intestinal stricture or narrowing mostly remains sufficient to allow the passage of intestinal contents. A superimposed infection can precipitate intestinal colic or even partial intestinal obstruction, which mostly can be treated conservatively. On occasions, healing of lesions can result in a critical stricture resulting in frequent symptoms and may require resection.

It is important to differentiate an active unresponsive stricture caused by treatment failure or multidrug-resistant TB [MDR-TB] from the fibrotic stricture. An active ulcerated lesion on colonoscopic examination confirms non-healing of lesion at the end of the therapy. CECT enterography is also useful to differentiate between the two conditions. While active inflammatory lesions will show contrast enhancement, fibrotic strictures will show no enhancement of CT enterography (22-24).

Pathology

Traditionally, intestinal TB is described to be of three types, namely, ulcerative, hypertrophic and ulcero-hypertrophic. The ulcerative form of the disease is mainly due to deprivation of blood supply, because of endarteritis. In GI TB, ulcerogenesis is relatively slow, and an inflammatory wall develops ahead of the advancing ulcer. Thus, if perforation occurs, it will remain contained. There is an accumulation of collagenous tissue during the process of ulcer healing that subsequently contracts and results in circumferential stricture of the intestinal lumen. The diseased segment is moderately indurated and the serosa is studded with nodules. Mesenteric lymph nodes are usually enlarged. The mucosal surface may show single or multiple ulcers, and skip areas may be present with normal appearing mucosa between the involved segments. The ulcers are characteristically transverse and circumferential, but may be round, stellate, or longitudinal. The ulcers are deep, however, they generally do not penetrate the muscularis propria. In the acute phase, there may be a functional stenosis of the involved segment because of the spasm of a segment of intestine. In the more chronic phase, circumferential strictures may develop. In hypertrophic form of the disease, there is a marked inflammatory fibroblastic reaction in the submucosa and subserosa of the involved segment, mostly ileocaecum (12,13,25). Caseating granulomas [*vide infra*] are the histologic hallmark of TB (12,13,26,27)

Clinical Features

Intestinal TB is commonly seen in persons aged between 20 and 40 years; however, it can occur at any age (11,12,28-30). Both genders are equally affected. The symptoms in a patient with intestinal TB arise because of [i] intestinal ulcero-constrictive disease [intestinal colic, abdominal distension, nausea, vomiting, constipation, bleeding manifestations]; [ii] chronic inflammatory process [fever, weakness, weight loss, night sweats]; [iii] associated adjacent tissue involvement [ascites, lymph node enlargement or tubo-ovarian symptoms]; and [iv] coincident pulmonary TB [chronic cough, expectoration, haemoptysis].

Intestinal TB should be suspected in patients presenting with recurrent intestinal colic, partial or complete intestinal obstruction. Intestinal TB should also be suspected in patients having weight loss and pyrexia of unknown origin. There should be a high index of suspicion for intestinal TB in immunocompromised individuals.

The symptoms of GI TB depend upon the site[s] of involvement of the GI tract and also the type of lesions. The ileocaecal area is the most common site of involvement in patients with intestinal TB, and most of the lesions are ulcerative or ulcero-constrictive type. Abdominal pain is the most common manifestation and can occur because of a stricture of the intestinal lumen, mesenteric inflammation and peritoneal involvement. While pain arising from the intestine is mostly colicky in nature, pain arising from the mesentery or the peritoneum is mostly diffuse and non-specific. As disease advances with time, the severity and frequency of painful episodes increase and the patient may develop partial intestinal obstruction [abdominal distension, gurgling in the abdomen, partial or complete cessation of flatus, vomiting or movement of ball of wind in the abdomen] or even complete intestinal obstruction. Diarrhoea is seen in 20%-30% of patients and can be because of both small and large intestinal involvement. Patients with intestinal TB can also have malabsorption which results from [i] decrease in small intestinal mucosal surface; [ii] lymphatic obstruction; [iii] fistula formation between the small and large intestine; [iv] deconjugation of bile salts secondary to bacterial overgrowth; and [v] decreased bile salt pool because of impaired active absorption in the distal ileum. While lower GI bleeding is seen in 10%-15% of patients, the bleeding is rarely massive. Almost half of the patients with intestinal TB report having constipation. Constitutional symptoms in the form of fever, malaise, night sweats, anorexia, and weight loss are common. A few patients may have active TB elsewhere, especially lungs (11,12,28-30).

There are no very specific clinical signs in patients with GI TB. They may have poor nutritional status and anaemia. One-half to two-thirds of patients have low-grade fever. Abdominal tenderness is frequently present in the right lower quadrant. A mass may be palpable in 10%-20% of patients and is because of a conglomerate of adhered bowel loops, lymph nodes and, sometimes, mesentery. Extensive fibro-adhesive inflammation in the peritoneum can make the dough consistency of the abdominal wall. Complications of intestinal TB are listed in Table 15.2 (7,9-11,29-31).

Table 15.2: Complications of intestinal TB

Partial or complete intestinal obstruction
Lower GI bleeding
Intra-abdominal abscess
Malnutrition
Intestinal perforation
TB = tuberculosis; GI = gastrointestinal

Laboratory Investigations

Laboratory investigations in patients suspected to have intestinal TB aim at detection of site, extent, and type of lesion[s]; associated complication[s]; confirming the diagnosis of TB histopathological, microbiological and molecular methods; and documenting active or healed TB elsewhere in the body. In a patient suspected to have intestinal TB, haematological and biochemical investigations are non-diagnostic. However, these should be done to estimate the effects of the disease and also as a baseline for monitoring the effects or complications of the therapy (7,11,12,28,29-35). All patients suspected to have intestinal TB should be screened for HIV infection.

The imaging studies of the intestine include: luminal imaging [endoscopic, barium studies], imaging of the wall and extra-intestinal structures, which is detected by cross-sectional imaging, such as computed tomography [CT] and magnetic resonance imaging [MRI]. Combined imaging modalities, such as, CT-enteroclysis or magnetic resonance [MR-] enteroclysis is also helpful.

Imaging

Pulmonary lesions, either active or healed, may be evident in a quarter of subjects on the chest radiograph. In a patient with ulcero-constrictive disease of the intestine where intestinal TB is a differential diagnosis, presence of an active pulmonary lesion may point towards intestinal TB as a cause of ulceroconstrictive disease (28-30,36). In patients presenting with abdominal pain, where a diagnosis of intestinal obstruction cannot be ruled out, a plain radiograph of the abdomen may, sometimes, provide an important clue to the clinical diagnosis.

Although there are many suggestive features on radiographic investigations, none of them are diagnostic for intestinal TB. The radiological features depend upon stage of the disease, site of involvement and severity of the disease. In the early stage of mucosal invasion and ulceration, barium findings of ileocaecal TB are non-specific and include spasm and hyper-motility of the intestinal segment, oedema of the ileocaecal valve and mucosal thickening (37-41). TB ulcers are circumferential or transverse in orientation. With progression of the disease, the ulcers become confluent. The features on barium imaging are more definitive in advanced stages of the disease. There is a thickening of the ileocaecal valve with narrowing of the terminal ileum [Fleischner's sign or inverted umbrella sign]. In further advanced disease, the characteristic deformities include symmetric, annular stenosis with obstruction, and shortening of the intestine and the colon. The caecum classically becomes conical, shrunken, and pulled up from the iliac fossa due to contraction of the mesocolon. There may be a loss of the normal ileocaecal angle (37-41). The ileocaecal valve classically becomes incompetent, rigid and fixed with an irregular outline [Figure 15.1]. TB strictures are typically short and multiple, separated by unaffected segments [Figure 15.2]. Enteroliths may form proximal to the strictures and may vary from a single large lamellated calculus to multiple small stones visible on the radiograph (37-41).

Contrast-enhanced CT [CECT] or CT-enteroclysis, MR-enteroclysis are essential for the evaluation of extra-luminal, peritoneal, nodal and visceral involvement. CECT is more accurate than ultrasonography in detecting most of these manifestations including peritoneal and intestinal involvement. CT-enteroclysis may show intestinal wall thickening [unifocal or multifocal], a stricture with proximal dilation of the intestine, and regional lymphadenopathy. The pattern of lymphadenopathy in TB may vary widely, including increased number of normal sized nodes, mildly enlarged nodes to large confluent nodal masses (42-46). The involved lymph nodes typically show hypodense centre and peripheral enhancement which reflects central necrosis [Figure 15.3] in 40%-70% cases. Since intestine

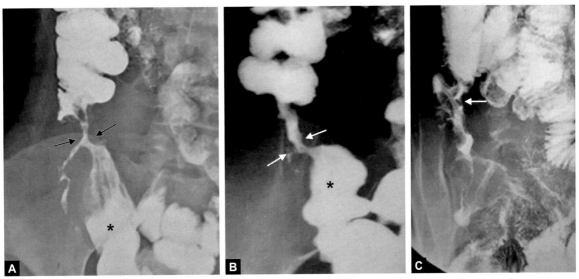

Figure 15.1: Barium meal follow-through examination showing ulcerations, contracted caecum, and stricture in the terminal Ileum [arrows] with proximal dilatation of the terminal ileum [asterisk] [A and B]; barium meal follow-through examination in another patient showing contracted caeum and terminal ileum, giving an appearance of swan-neck deformity [arrow] [C]

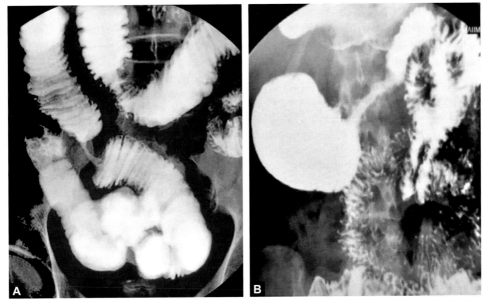

Figure 15.2: Barium enterography showing eccentric stricture in the jejunum [A]; barium meal follow-through examination showing long stricture in the duodenum [B]

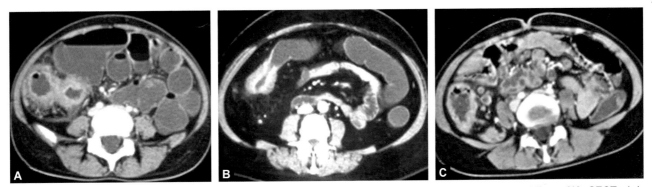

Figure 15.3: CECT abdomen [sagittal section] showing thickening and enhancement of caecum and terminal ileum [A]; CECT abdomen [sagittal section] showing markedly enhancing and thickening with narrowing of the terminal ileum [B]; CECT abdomen showing mesenteric lymphadenopathy with central hypodensity and caecal thickening [C]

remains collapsed, imaging of the luminal component of the intestine is not complete unless the intestine is distended. In CT-enterography or MR-enterography, intestinal lumen is distended using a negative contrast, such as, polyethylene glycol which allows simultaneous cross-sectional imaging of the intestinal lumen, the intestinal wall and the surrounding tissues. Therefore, CT-enterography or MR-enterography are preferable imaging technique to CECT or MRI for imaging of the small intestine (44-46).

Endoscopy

Since ileocaecal area is involved in majority of the patients with intestinal TB, colonoscopy with retrograde ileoscopy is the investigation of choice (14-17,42,47-52). Colonoscopic examination provides an opportunity to visualise the lesion directly and one can obtain biopsies from the lesions at the same time. The morphological appearance of intestinal TB depends upon the stage of the disease. The lesions may vary from mild lesion[s], such as loss of vascular pattern, erythema, small ulcerations and superficial ulcerations, to more advanced lesions including deep ulcerations, nodularity and strictures. The evolution of intestinal TB may take months to years; therefore, timely identification of the early lesions can help in preventing the progression of the disease. Intestinal TB classically causes ulceration [50%-80%], short strictures, marked thickening of the bowel wall due to inflammation, fibrosis and adhesions, or a combination of these (14-17,42,47-52). The ulcers [Figure 15.4] are transverse, often circumferential, with ill-defined, sloping or overhanging edges (14-17,42,47-52). The surrounding mucosa may show flattening of folds, ulcers, erosions and pseudopolyps. Multiple biopsies are obtained from the lesions histopathological examination, staining for AFB, mycobacterial culture, as well as for molecular diagnostic tests [*vide infra*].

For small intestinal lesions, newer endoscopic techniques such as single and double balloon enteroscopic examination can be done (53-56). Capsule endoscopic examination is generally not done for those patients where obstructive lesion such as intestinal TB is suspected (57).

Microbiological Tests Isolation of *Mtb* using mycobcacterial culture is the most specific method for the diagnosis of active TB. *Mtb* can be cultured from 10%-30% of mucosal biopsies in patients with colonic TB (58-61). However, this method has a low sensiti-vity (58-61). A presumptive diagnosis of TB may be considered by demonstrating AFB on intestinal biopsies which may be evident in 25%-36% in patients with intestinal TB (39,62,63).

Polymerase chain reaction [PCR] using *Mtb* specific primer shows a positivity varying from 20%-64%. Detection of *Mtb* by PCR has a high sensitivity and the positive results should be interpreted cautiously (40,63-65). PCR may be reported positive because of contamination in laboratories. Presence of saprophytic mycobacteria may also result in a positive test result in colonic biopsies. In one study (58), *in situ* PCR for TB in mucosal biopsies tested positive in six of the 20 intestinal TB patients.

Mucosal Biopsy With the increasing use of endoscopic procedures to visualise the intestinal lumen and obtain targeted biopsies from diseased areas, endoscopic mucosal biopsy has now mostly replaced the surgical biopsies for microscopic examination. Granulomas are found in 50%-80% of intestinal mucosal biopsies from patients with clinically confirmed TB (7,14,15,26,27,50,66-70). Presence of caseation and AFB, the diagnostic features of TB, are found in only 18%-33% of cases and in as low as 5% of cases, respectively (7,14,27,66-70). Other suggestive features include confluent granulomas, presence of a lymphoid cuff around granulomas. Further, granulomas larger than 400 μm in diameter, presence of five or more granulomas in biopsies from one segment, granulomas located in the submucosa or in granulation tissue, often as palisaded epithelioid histiocytes, and disproportionate submucosal inflammation [Figure 15.5] are all considered features suggestive of intestinal TB (27,66-70). In a recent meta-analysis (71), three histopathological features, namely, caseation, confluent granuloma and presence of a lymphoid cuff around the granulomas were found to be specific for TB.

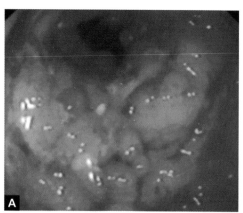 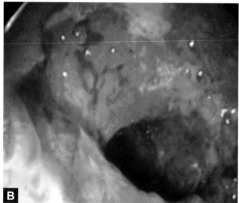 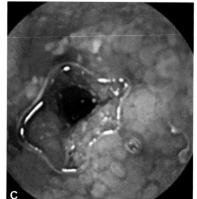

Figure 15.4: Colonoscopic image showing marked nodularity, ulceration and stricture in the ascending colon [A]; colonoscopic image showing ulceration and stricture in the caecum and ileocaecal valve [B]; enteroscopic examination showing ulcerations and stricture in the jejunum [C]

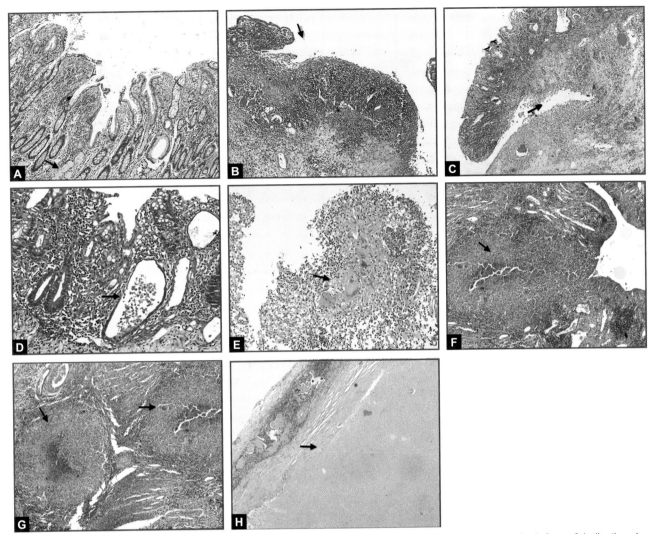

Figure 15.5: Photomicrograph showing an ileum with broad drum stick like villi, crypt branching and pyloric metaplasia [arrow], indicating changes of chronic ileitis [A] [Haematoxylin and eosin × 40]. Both broad superficial [B] and deep rail track like ulcers [C] [arrows] can be seen in TB [Haematoxylin and eosin × 40]. Photomicrograph of the mucosa showing cryptitis and crypt abscess [arrow] [D], [Haematoxylin and eosin × 100]. TB granulomas [arrows] are large and can be seen in the mucosa [E], submucosa [F] and in the deeper layers [G]. These are mostly confluent; central necrosis [G] and Langhans' giant cells [arrow] [E] are also seen [Haematoxylin and eosin × 100]. Presence of granulomas and necrosis [arrow] in abdominal lymph nodes is characteristic of TB [H] [Haematoxylin and eosin × 100]

TB = tuberculosis

Serological Tests

Antibody to *Saccharomyces cerevisiae* antigens [ASCA] is often used to distinguish Crohn's disease from ulcerative colitis, being positive in the former. In India, the diagnostic difficulty usually lies in distinguishing intestinal TB from Crohn's disease. However, antibody to *Saccharomyces cerevisiae* antigens has not been found to be helpful in studies from India (72-74). A study (72) from New Delhi, India, that included 59 patients with Crohn's disease and 30 patients with intestinal TB reported ASCA to be positive in 61% of Crohn's disease patients compared to 66% of intestinal TB patients. In another study (73) 8 of the 16 patients with intestinal TB and 10 of the 16 patients with Crohn's disease had tested positive for ASCA antibodies (73).

Diagnostic Criteria for Abdominal Tuberculosis

As per the recently published Guidelines for extrapulmonary TB for India [INDEX-TB Guidelines] (75), a "bacteriologically confirmed case" of abdominal TB is defined as a patient who has a microbiological diagnosis of abdominal TB, based on positive microscopy, culture or a validated PCR-based test [e.g., Xpert MTB/RIF]. A patient with negative microbiological tests for TB [microscopy, culture and validated PCR-based tests], but with strong clinical suspicion and other evidence of EPTB, such as compatible imaging findings, histopathological findings, ancillary diagnostic tests or response to anti-TB is designated as a "clinically diagnosed case" of abdominal TB.

While a positive culture, demonstration of AFB on smear and histopathological evidence of a caseating granuloma are "gold standard" tests for the definitive diagnosis of TB, the sensitivity of the combination of these tests is approximately 30%-50% (63). In rest of the patients, the diagnosis is considered presumptive based on clinical, endoscopic, radiographic and histopathological evidences. Good response to anti-TB treatment supports the diagnosis of TB in these patients. It should be emphasised that adherence to treatment is extremely important in those with presumptive diagnosis of TB who are receiving anti-TB treatment empirically. Non-response to treatment may occur because of non-adherence of the treatment, an alternative diagnosis, or MDR-TB.

Differential Diagnosis

The closest differential diagnosis for intestinal TB is Crohn's disease (14,27,39,41,42,63,70-72,76). Both intestinal TB and Crohn's disease are granulomatous diseases of the intestine. The clinical, morphological and histopathological features of intestinal TB and Crohn's disease are so similar that it becomes difficult to differentiate between these two entities (14,27,39,41,42,63,70-72). In geographical regions like Asia where both intestinal TB and Crohn's disease are prevalent, differentiating these two conditions may be challenging. In Asia, intestinal TB is common, but Crohn's disease is also being increasingly reported (77-80). Natural history of Crohn's disease is quite different from that of intestinal TB. While intestinal TB gets cured by appropriate anti-TB treatment, Crohn's disease has a remitting/relapsing or persistent course and usually stays lifelong. Because of similarity in the clinical presentation and morphology of these two entities, at times, such patients are treated empirically with anti-TB drugs (14).

The clinical, endoscopic and histopathological features which can differentiate these two diseases as reported are summarised in Table 15.3 (14,27,39,51,52,63,70-72,76). It is obvious that almost all the features are present in these two conditions and not many are diagnostic feature of one or another. However, with the use of a combination of these features, one is able to make a diagnosis of either TB or Crohn's disease in almost half of the patients.

There are often situations where a differentiation between intestinal TB and Crohn's disease remains unclear despite extensive investigation. Under these circumstances, both the Asia Pacific Association of Gastroenterology [APAGE] and Indian Society of Gastroenterology [ISG] consensus on Crohn's disease suggest a trial with anti-TB treatment (81,82). This is based on the rationale that the treatment of TB is finite, whereas treatment for Crohn's disease continues indefinitely (80,81). Further, there is a risk in treating patients diagnosed to have Crohn's disease with corticosteroids if there is a possibility that the diagnosis may actually be TB. Obviously, the decision to treat for one disease or the other would take into account other clinical considerations including the nature of presentation of the patient, whether acutely ill and requiring immediate definitive therapy or not. It would also be accompanied by a complete discussion with the patient of the possibilities and therapeutic alternatives.

Table 15.3: Clinical, endoscopic and histological differentiation between intestinal TB and Crohn's disease

Variables	Intestinal TB [% present]	Crohn's disease [% present]
Symptoms		
Chronic diarrhoea	20-40	60-80
Blood in the stools	10-20	50-70
Abdominal pain	90	60-80
Constipation	50	10-30
Partial intestinal obstruction	50-60	20-30
Perianal disease	5	30-80
Fever	40-70	30
Loss of appetite	40-80	40-60
Weight loss	60-90	50-60
Extra-intestinal manifestations	10	20-50
Involvement of intestine		
Anal canal	<5	15-50
Rectum	10-20	40-60
Sigmoid colon	5-10	10-50
Descending colon	5-10	10-50
Ascending colon	40-60	50-70
Ileocaecal area	70-90	60
Ileum	10-20	20-40
Endoscopic features		
Aphthous ulcers	5-10	30-50
Linear ulcers	5	20-30
Deep ulcers	50-70	30-40
Nodularity	50	20
Cobblestoning	ND	15-20
Histopathological features		
Granuloma	30-60	30
Necrosis in the granuloma	10-30	ND

TB = tuberculosis; ND = not described

In patients treated for intestinal TB, it is expected that there will be a complete resolution of the lesions, detectable by endoscopy or by imaging, following therapy. It is, therefore, appropriate to subject the patients who were treated empirically for intestinal TB to endoscopy once again to establish complete mucosal healing at the end of six months of treatment (81,82).

The problem of differentiation between intestinal TB and Crohn's disease is also further compounded by the fact that a proportion of patients with Crohn's disease have also been observed to respond to with anti-TB at least symptomatically (63,83,84).

PERITONEAL TUBERCULOSIS

Peritoneal TB is a subacute disease and its symptoms evolve over a period of several weeks to months (36,85). Peritoneal

TB frequently complicates patients with underlying end-stage renal or liver disease. The disease can present in three different forms, such as ascitic form [wet type], encysted [loculated] form and dry form. All of them have almost similar clinical manifestations except for abdominal distension which does not occur in dry type TB peritonitis. Abdominal pain [60%-70%] is a common presenting symptom and is frequently accompanied by abdominal distension. Abdominal pain in peritoneal TB is usually non-localised and non-specific in nature. The pain is largely due to the inflammation of the peritoneum and the mesentery. Less often, it could be due to involvement of the intestine. Tenderness on palpation is common in peritoneal TB and occurs in almost half of the patients. Rebound tenderness is rare as the presence of ascitic fluid prevents approximation of the parietal with the visceral peritoneum. A smaller percentage of patients [5%-10%] present with the classical 'doughy' abdomen. This is described as dry or plastic type of TB peritonitis (31,32,36,85,86).

Ascitic Fluid Analysis

The ascitic fluid is usually straw coloured. While red blood cells are seen frequently on microscopic examination, frank haemorrhagic ascites is uncommon. The ascitic fluid white blood cells [WBC] in peritoneal TB varies widely from less than 100 cells/mm^3 to 5000 cells/mm^3. However, most patients have cell counts between 500 and 1500 cells/mm^3. The WBCs are predominantly lymphocytes with the possible exception of patients with underlying renal failure where, for unknown reasons, the cells are mostly neutrophils. The protein content of ascitic fluid is high [>2.5 g/dL] and the ascitic fluid glucose levels are low. The serum ascites albumin gradient [SAAG] has more diagnostic yield than ascitic fluid total protein measurement. It is calculated by measuring both serum and ascitic fluid albumin on the same day and subtracting the ascitic albumin from the serum albumin concentration. While the SAAG is usually low [<1.1 g/dL] in TB peritonitis, a high SAAG [>1.1 g/dL] suggests portal hypertension.

Adenosine deaminase [ADA] is an enzyme that converts adenosine to inosine and its activity is more in activated T-lymphocytes than in B-lymphocytes. There is an increase in the number of activated T-cells in closed cavity infection, such as TB ascites or pleural effusion. With attrition of these lymphocytes, ADA along with other enzymes and end products are released in the closed compartment and, therefore, there is an increase in the ADA levels. A high value of ADA in any fluid cavity, in fact is a reflection of high T-cell activity. An ADA value of more than 32 IU/L in ascitic fluid has been reported to have high sensitivity and specificity for the diagnosis of TB ascites (85,87,88). High ADA may be seen in malignant ascites and even ascites due to cirrhosis. Interferon-gamma [IFN-γ] has also been reported to be higher in TB ascites compared to malignant and cirrhotic ascites (89). The clinical significance and utility of estimating IFN-γ in ascitic fluid for diagnostic purposes is not very clear.

While at least 5000 bacilli/mL of specimen is required for a positive smear, only a few bacilli/mL may be sufficient for a positive culture and for detection by molecular methods. Ziehl-Neelsen staining of the ascitic fluid for mycobacterial detection has a very low yield [3%-5%] in proven patients with peritoneal TB. In order to increase the yield, it is recommended that a larger volume of ascitic fluid should be sent to the laboratory and that the fluid should be centrifuged before staining (85). Cartridge-based nucleic acid amplification tests [CBNAAT] are increasingly being used to diagnose peritoneal TB (75,90a). In a recently published systematic review (90a), Xpert MTB/RIF was found to have a high pooled specificity in peritoneal fluid [97.9%] as well as peritoneal tissue [92%]; however, the pooled sensitivity was low both in peritoneal fluid [59.2%] as well as in peritoneal tissue [50%].

Elevation of cancer antigen [CA]-125 has been documented in majority of the patients with peritoneal TB mimicking advanced ovarian carcinoma. The levels of CA-125 fall rapidly with anti-TB treatment paralleling clinical response and resolution of ascites (85).

Imaging Studies

Ultrasonography of abdomen is generally the first diagnostic test in patients with ascites. Ultrasonography reveals echogenic debris seen as fine mobile strands or particulate matter within the ascitic fluid in patients with peritoneal TB. An encysted fluid can also be detected by ultrasonography (90b). The thickened and nodular peritoneum due to TB can be detected well by CECT [Figure 15.6]. The attenuation value of ascitic fluid in tubercular fluid on CT scan is high ranging from 20-45 Hounsfield units [HU]. The fibrotic type of peritoneal TB is characterised by a hypervascular peritoneum, matting of the loops, and omental masses. CECT can also show thickened mesentery [>15 mm] with mesenteric lymph node enlargement. One of the most important reasons to perform CECT in patients with high protein ascites is to differentiate TB peritonitis from the peritoneal carcinomatosis. While symmetrical thickening of the peritoneum with enhancement suggests peritoneal TB, nodular and irregular peritoneal thickening suggests carcinomatosis (91). The fine needle aspiration cytology [FNAC] or biopsies can be done under ultrasonography or CT guidance.

Laparoscopy

In those patients with suspected diagnosis of peritoneal TB, where a diagnosis cannot be confirmed on imaging, direct inspection and biopsy of the peritoneum are perhaps the most effective methods of diagnosing peritoneal TB. Three forms of features have been described in patients with peritoneal TB such as thickened, hyperaemic peritoneum with ascites and whitish miliary nodules [<5 mm] scattered over the parietal peritoneum, omentum and bowel loops [66%]; thickened and hyperaemic peritoneum with ascites and adhesions [21%]; markedly

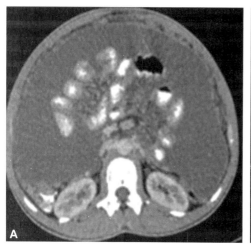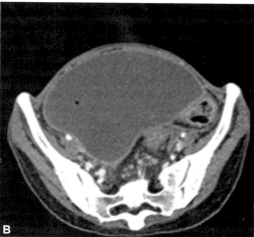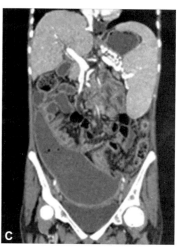

Figure 15.6: CECT abdomen, sagittal section showing thickened peritoneum and ascites [A]; loculated ascites [B]; and coronal section showing loculated ascites [C]

thickened parietal peritoneum with possibly yellowish nodules and cheesy material along with multiple thickened adhesions [fibro-adhesive type] [13%] (35). The diagnostic yield of laparoscopic examination is very high with a sensitivity of the macroscopic appearances approaching 93%. The cumulative data of 402 patients from 11 studies showed sensitivity and specificity rates of 93% and 98%, respectively when the macroscopic appearances were combined with the histological findings [epithelioid granulomata with caseation or mycobacterial identification] (92). Peritoneal biopsies should always be examined whenever possible for culture and sensitivity. Differential diagnosis of TB of peritoneum include peritoneal carcinomatosis, sarcoidosis, starch peritonitis, fungal peritonitis and chlamydial peritonitis.

In a patient with lymphocytic, exudative ascites with low SAAG and high ADA; TB peritonitis is the most likely cause. However, one should remember the possibilities of fungal peritonitis, and malignant ascites in such patients. Some of the patients with abdominal TB have marked thickening of the peritoneum which may grow so much so that the intestinal loops get encased in the cocoon (93).

OESOPHAGEAL TUBERCULOSIS

Oesophageal involvement in TB occurs mostly due to direct extension of infection from adjacent affected structures, such as mediastinal lymph nodes or the lung and isolated TB of the oesophagus is unusual. Upper part of the oesophagus is more often involved than the lower part. TB of the oesophagus as in the other parts of GI tract leads to formation of ulcerations and strictures. Therefore, main presenting features in them are dysphagia, odynophagia, chest discomfort/pain, and systemic symptoms (93-95). Some of these patients may develop tracheo-oesophageal or broncho-oesophageal fistula (96). Upper GI endoscopy is the first investigation in patients with mechanical type of dysphagia, which shows ulcerations and strictures. There are no specific characteristics of these lesions and they may mimic malignancy. Multiple biopsies should be

obtained from the lesions both for histopathological and microbiological tests including culture. TB of the oesophagus, although uncommon, should be suspected in persons presenting with dysphagia and oesophageal ulcerations or strictures. The extent of the disease can be assessed using endosonography which also allows indentification of mediastinal lymphadenopathy. If endoscopic biopsies are inconclusive, fine needle aspiration cytology [FNAC] of the lymph nodes can be done using endosonography (97). All these patients should also undergo a cross-sectional imaging of the abdomen, such as CECT or MRI for evaluation of the extent. If a definitive diagnosis of TB is not achieved, malignancy must be ruled out before initiating such patients on a therapeutic trial with anti-TB drugs. Patients receiving therapeutic trial with anti-TB drugs must be carefully monitored at periodic intervals. An endoscopic examination should also be done at the end of anti-TB treatment to see if the lesions have healed. A response is defined if the ulcers have healed completely. The healing process, however, can leave behind some fibrotic nodules and even a stricture, which can be dilated endoscopically if need ever arises.

GASTRODUODENAL TUBERCULOSIS

Because of acidic environment, stomach and duodenum are generally spared by *Mtb* infection. The TB lesions produce ulcerations and strictures in the duodenum and rarely in the stomach. Therefore, symptoms include abdominal pain, nausea, vomiting, GI bleeding, fever and weight loss (98-100). Once luminal obstruction occurs because of the lesion, the patient presents with obstructive features such as copious vomiting of stale food ingested four hours or more earlier. Endoscopic examination is the best investigation, wherein, the lesion can be visualised and biopsies can be obtained. The extent and characteristics of the stricture can be assessed using barium meal or barium meal follow-through examination. Cross-sectional imaging should also be done to evaluate completely the extent of the disease. Presence of surrounding lymph node enlargement with central necrosis makes the diagnosis of TB more likely. The gastro-duodenal stricture, if symptomatic, can be dilated using endoscopic balloon dilator (101). Endoscopic mucosal resection has also been done which yields a larger tissue for diagnosis. While the inflammatory component heals well with anti-TB treatment; it may leave behind a scarred antroduodenal area or duodenum. Most of these scarred lesions remain either asymptomatic or mildly symptomatic. If the narrowing produced by the healed lesions remain symptomatic, one can resort to endoscopic balloon dilatation or even surgery.

HEPATOBILIARY TUBERCULOSIS

The term hepatobiliary TB refers to either isolated hepatic, biliary, or hepatobiliary involvement with other organ system involvement. Liver is involved in *Mtb* in two major forms. The more common involvement of the liver in TB is as a part of a miliary or a disseminated disease (101-105). In such type of involvement, there may not be any specific signs or symptoms related to the liver except for the presence of hepatomegaly. Liver biopsy in such patients may show the presence of granulomas. The second form, which is seen less often, is a localised form of TB involving the liver and the biliary ducts. Localised hepatobiliary TB may occur as the following: [i] localised solitary or multiple nodules, tuberculoma and TB hepatic abscess without bile duct obstruction; [ii] bile ductal epithelium involvement producing inflammatory strictures resulting in obstructive jaundice; and [iii] enlarged lymph nodes at porta causing obstruction to the bile duct. Obstructive jaundice is more common in those having biliary system involvement. In most patients, an increase in alkaline phosphatase, gamma glutamyl transferase, and a mild rise in serum transaminases is evident. Ultrasonography and subsequently CECT are required for complete imaging. In suspected patients, the bile ductal abnormality [stricture, unifocal or multifocal; ductal irregularity] can be seen by magnetic resonance cholangiopancreatography [MRCP] or endoscopic retrograde cholangiopancreatography [ERCP] (101-105).

PANCREATIC TUBERCULOSIS

TB of pancreas is uncommon and most often occurs due to lymphatic or haematogenous dissemination or direct spread from other adjacent organs. The involvement of pancreas by TB infection can occur as part of miliary or disseminated form of TB or as isolated pancreatic TB. The usual lesion in such patients is a pancreatic mass, and therefore, symptoms depend upon the type and site of the mass (106,107). As other sites, anorexia, malaise, low-grade fever, weight loss, night sweats are seen in majority of the patients. The specific symptoms include abdominal pain and obstructive jaundice if the pancreatic head is involved. Imaging shows mass in the pancreas which is a conglomerate of lesions in the pancreas and peri-pancreatic lymph nodes. Therefore, pancreatic TB mimics a pancreatic malignancy (108). FNAC and a radiographically guided biopsy and mycobacterial culture helps in differentiating TB from pancreatic malignancy.

The lesion can also be approached using endoscopic ultrasound (109).

SPLENIC TUBERCULOSIS

As the liver, spleen can also be involved by tuberculous infection in two ways, mostly as a part of disseminated or miliary form of the disease and occasionally as isolated splenic TB. Most of these patients are immunocompromised; splenic TB, however, has been reported in otherwise immunocompetent individuals too (110). Most of the patients of splenic TB are recognised on imaging and sometimes, as a surprise on operated splenectomy specimen. In those with disseminated form of the disease, there are enough clinical clues in other organs; there is no specific feature in isolated splenic TB to suggest a clinical diagnosis of splenic TB. Fever, left upper quadrant abdominal pain, weight loss, splenomegaly and/or hepatomegaly are usual features. On abdominal ultrasonography or CT, spleen may be enlarged and there may be one or multiple lesions (111). The treatment is similar as elsewhere except that a splenectomy may be required in a few patients where the spleen is studded with tubercular abscesses.

TREATMENT

In general, patients with intestinal strictures should be advised to avoid high fibre diets. All these patients should undergo a nutritional assessment and nutritional deficiencies should be addressed.

All patients with TB should receive anti-TB drugs (112-115). Whether the optimal duration of treatment for gastrointestinal TB and peritoneal TB should be six months or longer has been debated (116-118). As per the recent INDEX-TB guide-lines (75), six months daily treatment with a standard first-line regimen using a combination of rifampicin, isoniazid, ethambutol, and pyrazinamide for two months, followed by rifampicin, isoniazid and ethambutol for the subsequent four months is recommended for abdominal TB [strong recommendation, very low quality evidence]. The reader is referred to the chapters *"Treatment of tuberculosis"* [*Chapter 44*] and *"Revised National Tuberculosis Control Programme"* [*Chapter 53*] for further details.

Since the treatment of TB is prolonged, adherence to treatment is a major problem in many parts of the world including India (119,120). A study from Kerala in South India showed that daily treatment and thrice-weekly intermittent DOTS [where treatment was directly observed to ensure treatment adherence], were equally effective for treating ileocaecal and colonic TB (121). In a multicentre randomised controlled trial [RCT] (122) in patients with abdominal TB [n = 197] evaluated thrice-weekly intermittent DOTS, no difference was observed in the complete clinical response rate both on per protocol analysis [91.5% versus 90.8%] and intention-to-treat analysis [75% versus 75.8%] in groups randomised to six months and nine months of treatment. Only one patient in the nine months treatment group and none in six months group had recurrence of the disease.

Side effects occurred in 21.3% and 18.2% patients in six months and nine months treatment groups respectively (122). There is a paucity of data on the optimal duration of treatment in patients with hepatic and pancreatic TB.

Patients with gastroduodenal TB, with obstructing lesions, should be fed a liquid diet. These patients with obstructing lesions may not be able to tolerate oral anti-TB treatment. Endoscopic dilatation of the obstructing lesions can help in restoring patency. Strictures elsewhere such as colon, and small intestine may also be dilated endoscopically (123).

Since simultaneous use of corticosteroids along with anti-TB treatment is thought to prevent or reduce the occurrence of post-inflammatory fibrosis, use of corticosteroids has been advocated by some workers in patients with abdominal TB. However, based on the available evidence at present, there appears to be no role for adjunctive corticosteroid treatment in patients with abdominal TB.

Surgical Treatment

Surgery is required only in a small number of patients with intestinal TB and other solid organ TB. The indications for surgery in intestinal TB are generally for the complications of the disease such as free perforation, confined perforation with abscess or fistula formation, intestinal obstruction not responding to usual conservative measures, and massive haemorrhage. A subset of patients, despite effective anti-TB therapy, continue to have episodes of intestinal obstruction which may occur because of two reasons, namely, treatment failure, or occurrence of residual tight fibrotic strictures. Stricturoplasty or resection of the diseased segment with end-to-end anastomosis is helpful. Surgical procedures such as bypass surgery [entero-enterostomy, ileotransverse colostomy] are not recommended for obstructive lesions as these procedures may facilitate the formation of blind loops leading to obstruction, malabsorption, or both. Strictures at ileocaecal region may be treated by limited ileocaecal resection with a 5 cm margin from a visible abnormal tissue or a limited right hemicolectomy and end-to-end anastomosis. Perforating ulcers are treated by excision of the perforated segment with primary anastomosis. Wherever appropriate, elective surgery should be performed after four to six weeks of anti-TB treatment. Even after surgery, the course of anti-TB treatment should be completed.

Follow-up and Monitoring

Patients receiving treatment for TB should be counselled regarding the adverse effects of drugs, especially hepatotoxicity (124-127) and should be assessed periodically for clinical improvement. While fever and constitutional symptoms may start improving within a few weeks, they may take up to eight-weeks for resolution. As the inflammatory component of the intestinal lesions starts resolving, the luminal narrowing improves and diameter widens the frequency and severity of abdominal pain improves. The reader is also referred to the chapter *"Hepatotoxicity associated with anti-tuberculosis treatment"* [Chapter 45] for details.

REFERENCES

1. Barry CE 3rd, Boshoff HI, Dartois V, Dick T, Ehrt S, Flynn J, et al. The spectrum of latent tuberculosis: rethinking the biology and intervention strategies. Nat Rev Microbiol 2009;7:845-55.
2. Achkar JM, Jenny-Avital ER. Incipient and subclinical tuberculosis: defining early disease states in the context of host immune response. J Infect Dis 2011;15:204:S1179-86.
3. Corbett EL, Charalambous S, Moloi VM, Fielding K, Grant AD, Dye C, et al. Human immunodeficiency virus and the prevalence of undiagnosed tuberculosis in African gold miners. Am J Respir Crit Care Med 2004;170:673-9.
4. Sharma SK, Mohan A. Extrapulmonary tuberculosis. Indian J Med Res 2004;120:316-53.
5. Golden MP, Vikram HR. Extrapulmonary tuberculosis: an overview. Am Fam Physician 2005;72:1761-8.
6. Rieder HL, Snider DE Jr, Cauthen GM. Extrapulmonary tuberculosis in the United States. Am Rev Respir Dis 1990;141:347-51.
7. Lazarus AA, Thilagar B. Abdominal tuberculosis. Dis Mon 2007;53:32-8.
8. Kapoor VK, Sharma LK. Abdominal tuberculosis. Br J Surg 1988;75:2-3.
9. Patel B, Yagnik VD. Clinical and laboratory features of intestinal tuberculosis. Clin Exp Gastroenterol 2018;11:97-103.
10. Bhansali SK. Gastrointestinal perforations: clinical study of 96 cases. J Postgrad Med 1967;13:1-12.
11. Marshall JB. Tuberculosis of the gastrointestinal tract and peritoneum. Am J Gastroenterol 1993;88:989-99.
12. Pimparkar BD, Donde UM. Intestinal tuberculosis I. Clinical and radiological studies. J Assoc Physicians India 1974;22:205-18
13. Tandon HD, Prakash A. Pathology of intestinal tuberculosis and its distinction from Crohn's disease. Gut 1972;13:260-9.
14. Makharia GK, Srivastava S, Das P, Goswami P, Singh U, Tripathi M, et al. Clinical, endoscopic, and histological differentiations between Crohn's disease and intestinal tuberculosis. Am J Gastroenterol 2010;105:642-51.
15. Shah S, Thomas V, Mathan M, Chacko A, Chandy G, Ramakrishna BS, et al. Colonoscopic study of 50 patients with colonic tuberculosis. Gut 1992;33:347-51.
16. Bhargava DK, Tandon HD. Ileocaecal tuberculosis diagnosed by colonoscopy and biopsy. Aust N Z J Surg 1980;50:583-5.
17. Bhargava DK, Tandon HD, Chawla TC, Shriniwas, Tandon BN, Kapur BM. Diagnosis of ileocecal and colonic tuberculosis by colonoscopy. Gastrointest Endosc 1985;31:68-70.
18. Leder RA, Low VH. Tuberculosis of the abdomen. Radiol Clin North Am 1995;33:691-705.
19. Jarman BT. Small bowel imaging. Surg Clin North Am 2011;91:109-25.
20. Morel P, Alexander-Williams J, Rohner A. Relation between flow-pressure-diameter studies in experimental stenosis of rabbit and human small bowel. Gut 1990;31:875-8.
21. Anand BS, Nanda R, Sachdev GK. Response of tuberculous stricture to antituberculous treatment. Gut 1988;29:62-9.
22. Grand DJ, Beland M, Harris A. Magnetic resonance enterography. Radiol Clin North Am 2013;51:99-112.
23. Ilangovan R, Burling D, George A, Gupta A, Marshall M, Taylor SA. CT enterography: review of technique and practical tips. Br J Radiol 2012; 85:876-86.
24. Mullan CP, Siewert B, Eisenberg RL. Small bowel obstruction. Am J Roentgenol 2012;198:W105-17.
25. Das P, Shukla HS. Abdominal tuberculosis: demonstration of tubercle bacilli in tissues and experimental production of hyperplastic enteric lesion. Br J Surg 1975;62:610-9.
26. Pulimood AB, Ramakrishna BS, Kurian G, Peter S, Patra S, Mathan VI, et al. Endoscopic mucosal biopsies are useful in

distinguishing granulomatous colitis due to Crohn's disease from tuberculosis. Gut 1999;45:537-41.

27. Pulimood AB, Peter S, Ramakrishna B, Chacko A, Jeyamani R, Jeyaseelan L, et al. Segmental colonoscopic biopsies in the differentiation of ileocolic tuberculosis from Crohn's disease. J Gastroenterol Hepatol 2005;20:688-96.

28. Bhansali SK. The challenge of abdominal tuberculosis in 310 cases. Indian J Surg 1978;40:65-77.

29. Das P, Shukla HS. Clinical diagnosis of abdominal tuberculosis. Br J Surg 1976;63:941-6.

30. Singh V, Jain AK, Agrawal AK, Khanna S, Khanna AK, Gupta JP. Clinicopathological profile of abdominal tuberculosis. Br J Clin Pract 1995;49:22-4.

31. Tandon RK, Bansal R, Kapur BM, Shriniwas. A study of malabsorption in intestinal tuberculosis: stagnant loop syndrome. Am J Clin Nutr 1980;33:244-50.

32. Singh MM, Bhargava AN, Jain KP. Tuberculosis peritonitis: an evaluation of pathogenic mechanisms, diagnostic procedures and therapeutic measures. N Engl J Med 1969;289:1091-4.

33. Dineen P, Homan WP, Grafe WR. Tuberculous peritonitis: 43 years' experience in diagnosis and treatment. Ann Surg 1976;184:717-22.

34. Manohar A, Simjee AE, Haffejee AA, Pettengell KE. Symptoms and investigative findings in 145 patients with tuberculous peritonitis diagnosed by peritoneoscopy and biopsy over a five-year period. Gut 1990;31:1130-2.

35. Bhargava DK, Shriniwas, Chopra P, Nijhawan S, Dasarathy S, Kushwaha AK. Peritoneal tuberculosis: laparoscopic patterns and its diagnostic accuracy. Am J Gastroenterol 1992;87:109-11.

36. Bevin J, Dalton S, Wakeman C, Perry W. Diagnosis of abdominal tuberculosis in Christchurch New Zealand: a case series. N Z Med J 2018;131:48-52.

37. Nagi B, Kochhar R, Bhasin DK, Singh K. Colorectal tuberculosis. Eur Radiol 2003;13:1907-12.

38. Nagi B, Sodhi KS, Kochhar R, Bhasin DK, Singh K. Small bowel tuberculosis: enteroclysis findings. Abdom Imaging 2004;29: 335-40.

39. Lundstedt C, Nyman R, Brismar J, Hugosson C, Kagevi I. Imaging of tuberculosis. II. Abdominal manifestations in 112 patients. Acta Radiol 1996;37:489-95.

40. Suri S, Kaur H, Wig JD, Singh K. CT in abdominal tuberculosis-comparison with barium studies. Indian J Radiol Imaging 1993;3:237-42.

41. Balthazar EJ, Gordon R, Hulnick D. Ileocecal tuberculosis: CT and radiologic evaluation. Am J Roentgenol 1990;154:499-503.

42. Mao R, Liao WD, He Y, Ouyang CH, Zhu ZH, Yu C, et al. Computed tomographic enterography adds value to colonoscopy in differentiating Crohn's disease from intestinal tuberculosis: a potential diagnostic algorithm. Endoscopy 2015;47:322-9.

43. Epstein BM, Mann JH. CT of abdominal tuberculosis. AJR Am J Roentgenol 1982;139:861-6.

44. Park YH, Chung WS, Lim JS, Park SJ, Cheon JH, Kim TI, et al. Diagnostic role of computed tomographic enterography differentiating Crohn's disease from intestinal tuberculosis. J Comput Assist Tomogr 2013;37:834-9.

45. Kalra N, Agrawal P, Mittal V, Kochhar R, Gupta V, Nada R, et al. Spectrum of imaging findings on MDCT enterography in patients with small bowel tuberculosis. Clin Radiol 2014;69: 315-22.

46. Park MJ, Lim JS. Computed tomography enterography for evaluation of inflammatory bowel disease. Clin Endosc 2013;46:327-66.

47. Jeong SH, Lee KJ, Kim YB, Kwon HC, Sin SJ, Chung JY. Diagnostic value of terminal ileum intubation during colonoscopy. J Gastroenterol Hepatol 2008;23:51-5.

48. Misra SP, Misra V, Dwivedi M. Ileoscopy in patients with ileocolonic tuberculosis. World J Gastroenterol 2007;13:1723-7.

49. Amarapurkar DN, Patel ND, Rane PS. Diagnosis of Crohn's disease in India where tuberculosis is widely prevalent. World J Gastroenterol 2008;14:741-6.

50. Patel N, Amarapurkar D, Agal S, Baijal R, Kulshrestha P, Pramanik S, et al. Gastrointestinal luminal tuberculosis: establishing the diagnosis. J Gastroenterol Hepatol 2004;19: 1240-6.

51. Li X, Liu X, Zou Y, Ouyang C, Wu X, Zhou M, et al. Predictors of clinical and endoscopic findings in differentiating Crohn's disease from intestinal tuberculosis. Dig Dis Sci 2011;56:188-96.

52. Lee YJ, Yang SK, Byeon JS, Myung SJ, Chang HS, Hong SS, et al. Analysis of colonoscopic findings in the differential diagnosis between intestinal tuberculosis and Crohn's disease. Endoscopy 2006;38:592-7.

53. Tsujikawa T, Saitoh Y, Andoh A, Imaeda H, Hata K, Minematsu H, et al. Novel single-balloon enteroscopy for diagnosis and treat-ment of the small intestine: preliminary experiences. Endoscopy 2008;40:11-5.

54. Yamamoto H, Sekine Y, Sato Y, Higashizawa T, Miyata T, Iino S, et al. Total enteroscopy with a nonsurgical steerable double-balloon method. Gastrointest Endosc 2001;53:216-20.

55. Pasha SF, Leighton JA, Das A, Harrison ME, Decker GA, Fleischer DE, et al. Double-balloon enteroscopy and capsule endoscopy have comparable diagnostic yield in small-bowel disease: a meta-analysis. Clin Gastroenterol Hepatol 2008;6:671-6.

56. Nakamura M, Niwa Y, Ohmiya N, Arakawa D, Honda W, Miyahara R, et al. Small bowel tuberculosis diagnosed by the combination of video capsule endoscopy and double balloon enteroscopy. Eur J Gastroenterol Hepatol 2007;19:595-8.

57. Reddy DN, Sriram PV, Rao GV, Reddy DB. Capsule endoscopy appearances of small-bowel tuberculosis. Endoscopy 2003;35:99.

58. Balamurugan R, Venkataraman S, John KR, Ramakrishna BS. PCR amplification of the IS6110 insertion element of Mycobacterium tuberculosis in fecal samples from patients with intestinal tuberculosis. J Clin Microbiol 2006;44:1884-6.

59. Morgan MA, Horstmeier CD, DeYoung DR, Roberts GD. Comparison of a radiometric method [BACTEC] and conventional culture media for recovery of mycobacteria from smear-negative specimens. J Clin Microbiol 1983;18:384-8.

60. Ye BD, Yang SK, Kim D, Shim TS, Kim SH, Kim MN, et al. Diagnostic sensitivity of culture and drug resistance patterns in Korean patients with intestinal tuberculosis. Int J Tuberc Lung Dis 2012;16:799-804.

61. Wilson ML. Rapid diagnosis of Mycobacterium tuberculosis infection and drug susceptibility testing. Arch Pathol Lab Med 2013;137:812-9.

62. Leung VK, Law ST, Lam CW, Luk IS, Chau TN, Loke TK, et al. Intestinal tuberculosis in a regional hospital in Hong Kong: a 10-year experience. Hong Kong Med J 2006;12:264-71.

63. Pulimood AB, Amarapurkar DN, Ghoshal U, Phillip M, Pai CG, Reddy DN, et al. Differentiation of Crohn's disease from intestinal tuberculosis in India in 2010. World J Gastroenterol 2011;28:17:433-43.

64. Anand BS, Schneider FE, El-Zaatari FA, Shawar RM, Clarridge JE, Graham DY. Diagnosis of intestinal tuberculosis by polymerase chain reaction on endoscopic biopsy specimens. Am J Gastroenterol 1994;89:2248-9.

65. Gan HT, Chen YQ, Ouyang Q, Bu H, Yang XY. Differentiation between intestinal tuberculosis and Crohn's disease in endo-scopic biopsy specimens by polymerase chain reaction. Am J Gastroenterol 2002;97:1446-51.

66. Gaffney EF, Condell D, Majmudar B, Nolan N, McDonald GS, Griffin M, et al. Modification of caecal lymphoid tissue and

relationship to granuloma formation in sporadic ileocaecal tuberculosis. Histopathology 1987;11:691-704.

67. Pettengell KE, Larsen C, Garb M, Mayet FG, Simjee AE, Pirie D. Gastrointestinal tuberculosis in patients with pulmonary tuberculosis. QJM 1990;74:303-8.

68. Pulimood AB, Peter S, Rook GW, Donoghue HD. In situ PCR for Mycobacterium tuberculosis in endoscopic mucosal biopsy specimens of intestinal tuberculosis and Crohn's disease. Am J Clin Pathol 2008;129:846-51.

69. Alvares JF, Devarbhavi H, Makhija P, Rao S, Kottoor R. Clinical, colonoscopic,and histological profile of colonic tuberculosis in a tertiary hospital. Endoscopy 2005;37:351-6.

70. Kirsch R, Pentecost M, Hall Pde M, Epstein DP, Watermeyer G, Friederich PW. Role of colonoscopic biopsy in distinguishing between Crohn's disease and intestinal tuberculosis. J Clin Pathol 2006;59:840-4.

71. Du J, Ma YY, Xiang H, Li YM. Confluent granulomas and ulcers lined by epithelioid histiocytes: new ideal method for differentiation of ITB and CD? A meta analysis. PLoS One 2014;9:e103303.

72. Makharia GK, Sachdev V, Gupta R, Lal S, Pandey RM. Anti-Saccharomyces cerevisiae antibody does not differentiate between Crohn's disease and intestinal tuberculosis. Dig Dis Sci 2007;52:33-9.

73. Ghoshal UC, Ghoshal U, Singh H, Tiwari S. Anti-Saccharomyces cerevisiae antibody is not useful to differentiate between Crohn's disease and intestinal tuberculosis in India. J Postgrad Med 2007;53:166-70.

74. Kim YS, Kim YH, Kim WH, Kim JS, Park YS, Yang SK, et al. Diagnostic utility of anti-Saccharomyces cerevisiae antibody [ASCA] and interferon-gamma assay in the differential diagnosis of Crohn's disease and intestinal tuberculosis. Clin Chim Acta 2011;412:1527-32.

75. Sharma SK, Ryan H, Khaparde S, Sachdeva KS, Singh AD, Mohan A, et al. Index-TB guidelines: Guidelines on extrapulmonary tuberculosis for India. Indian J Med Res 2017;145:448-63.

76. Almadi MA, Ghosh S, Aljebreen AM. Differentiating intestinal tuberculosis from Crohn's disease: a diagnostic challenge. Am J Gastroenterol 2009;104:1003-12.

77. Makharia GK. Rising incidence and prevalence of Crohn's disease in Asia: is it apparent or real? J Gastroenterol Hepatol 2006;21:929-31.

78. Makharia GK, Ramakrishna BS, Abraham P, Choudhuri G, Misra SP, Ahuja V, et al. Indian Society of Gastroenterology Task Force on Inflammatory Bowel Disease. Survey of inflammatory bowel diseases in India. Indian J Gastroenterol 2012;31:299-306.

79. Ahuja V, Tandon RK. Inflammatory bowel disease in the Asia-Pacific area: a comparison with developed countries and regional differences. J Dig Dis 2010;11:134-47.

80. Ooi CJ, Hilmi I, Makharia GK, Gibson PR, Fock KM, Ahuja V, et al. Asia Pacific Association of Gastroenterology [APAGE] Working Group on Inflammatory Bowel Disease. Asia Pacific Consensus Statements on Crohn's disease. Part 1: Definition, diagnosis, and epidemiology. Asia Pacific Crohn's Disease Consensus–Part 1. J Gastroenterol Hepatol 2016;31:45-55.

81. Ooi CJ, Hilmi I, Makharia GK, Gibson PR, Fock KM, Ahuja V, et al. Asia Pacific Association of Gastroenterology [APAGE] Working Group on Inflammatory Bowel Disease. Asia-Pacific consensus statements on Crohn's disease. Part 2: Management. J Gastroenterol Hepatol 2016;31:56-68.

82. Ramakrishna BS, Makharia GK, Ahuja V, Ghoshal UC, Jayanthi V, Perakath B, et al. Indian Society of Gastroenterology consensus statements on Crohn's disease in India. Indian J Gastroenterol 2015;34:3-22.

83. Goel A, Dutta AK, Pulimood AB, Eapen A, Chacko A. Clinical profile and predictors of disease behavior and surgery in Indian patients with Crohn's disease. Indian J Gastroenterol 2013;32: 184-9.

84. Dutta AK, Sahu MK, Gangadharan SK, Chacko A. Distinguishing Crohn's disease from intestinal tuberculosis—a prospective study. Trop Gastroenterol 2011;32:204-9.

85. Sanai FM, Bzeizi KI. Systematic review: tuberculous peritonitis—presenting features, diagnostic strategies and treatment. Aliment Pharmacol Ther 2005;22:685-700.

86. Sohocky S. Tuberculous peritonitis: a review of 100 cases. Am Rev Respir Dis 1967;95:398-401.

87. Tao L, Ning HJ, Nie HM, Guo XY, Qin SY, Jiang HX. Diagnostic value of adenosine deaminase in ascites for tuberculosis ascites: a meta-analysis. Diagn Microbiol Infect Dis 2014;79:102-7.

88. Tuon FF, Higashino HR, Lopes MI, Litvoc MN, Atomiya AN, Antonangelo L, et al. Adenosine deaminase and tuberculous meningitis—a systematic review with meta-analysis. Scand J Infect Dis 2010;42:198-207.

89. Su SB, Qin SY, Guo XY, Luo W, Jiang HX. Assessment by meta-analysis of interferon-gamma for the diagnosis of tuberculous peritonitis. World J Gastroenterol 2013;19:1645-51.

90a. Kohli M, Schiller I, Dendukuri N, Dheda K, Denkinger CM, Schumacher SG, Steingart KR. Xpert[®] MTB/RIF assay for extrapulmonary tuberculosis and rifampicin resistance. Cochrane Database Syst Rev 2018;8:CD012768.

90b. Jain R, Sawhney S, Bhargava DK, Berry M. Diagnosis of abdominal tuberculosis: sonographic findings in patients with early disease. Am J Roentgenol 1995;165:1391-5.

91. Ha HK, Jung JI, Lee MS, Choi BG, Lee MG, Kim YH, et al. CT differentiation of tuberculous peritonitis and peritoneal carcinomatosis. Am J Roentgenol 1996;167:743-8.

92. Reddy KR, DiPrima RE, Raskin JB, Jeffers LJ, Phillips RS, Manten HD, et al. Tuberculous peritonitis: laparoscopic diagnosis of an uncommon disease in the United States. Gastrointest Endosc 1988;34:422-6.

93. Solak A, Solak İ. Abdominal cocoon syndrome: preoperative diagnostic criteria, good clinical outcome with medical treatment and review of the literature. Turk J Gastroenterol 2012;23:776-9.

94. Gordon AH, Marshall JB. Esophageal tuberculosis: definitive diagnosis by endoscopy. Am J Gastroenterol 1990;85:174-7.

95. Eng J, Sabanathan S. Tuberculosis of the esophagus Dig Dis Sci 1991;36:536-40.

96. Robbs JV, Bhoola KD. Aorto-oesophageal fistula complicating tuberculous aortitis: a case report. S Afr Med J 1976;50:702-4.

97. Bhatia V. Endoscopic ultrasound: imaging techniques and applications in the mediastinum. Trop Gastroenterol 2010;30: S4-19.

98. Tandon RK, Pastakia B. Duodenal tuberculosis as seen by duodenoscopy. Am J Gastroenterol 1976;66:483-6.

99. Palmer ED. Tuberculosis of the stomach and the stomach in tuberculosis: a review with particular reference to gross pathology and gastroscopic diagnosis. Am Rev Tuberc 1950;61:116-30.

100. Talukdar R, Khanna S, Saikia N, Vij JC. Gastric tuberculosis presenting as linitis plastica: a case report and review of the literature. Eur J Gastroenterol Hepatol 2006;18:299-303.

101. Puri AS, Sachdeva S, Mittal VV, Gupta N, Banka A, Sakhuja P, et al. Endoscopic diagnosis, management and outcome of gastroduodenal tuberculosis. Indian J Gastroenterol 2012;31:125-9.

102. Chaudhary P. Hepatobiliary tuberculosis. Ann Gastroenterol 2014; 27:207-11.

103. Bandyopadhyay S, Maity PK. Hepatobiliary tuberculosis. J Assoc Physicians India 2013;61:404-7.

104. Alvarez SZ. Hepatobiliary tuberculosis. J Gastroenterol Hepatol 1998;13:833-9.

105. Kochar R, Fallon MB. Pulmonary diseases and the liver. Clin Liver Dis 2011;15:21-37.

106. Nagar AM, Raut AA, Morani AC, Sanghvi DA, Desai CS, Thapar VB. Pancreatic tuberculosis: a clinical and imaging review of 32 cases. J Comput Assist Tomogr 2009;33: 136-41.

107. Singh DK, Haider A, Tatke M, Kumar P, Mishra PK. Primary pancreatic tuberculosis masquerading as a pancreatic tumor leading to Whipple's pancreaticoduodenectomy. A case report and review of the literature. JOP 2009;10:451-6.

108. Rana SS, Chaudhary V, Gupta N, Sampath S, Mittal BR, Bhasin DK. Pancreatic tuberculosis presenting as an unusual head mass. Endoscopy 2013;45:E317-8.

109. Gupta P, Guleria S, Agarwal S. Role of endoscopic ultrasound guided FNAC in diagnosis of pancreatic TB presenting as mass lesion: a case report and review of literature. Indian J Tuberc 2011;58:120-4.

110. Sharma SK, Smith-Rohrberg D, Tahir M, Mohan A, Seith A. Radiological manifestations of splenic tuberculosis: a 23-patient case series from India. Indian J Med Res 2007;125:669-78.

111. Buxi TB, Vohra RB, Sujatha Y, Chawla D, Byotra SP, Gupta PS, et al. CT appearances in macronodular hepatosplenic tuberculosis: a review with five additional new cases. Comput Med Imaging Graph 1992;16:381-7.

112. Sia IG, Wieland ML. Current concepts in the management of tuberculosis. Mayo Clin Proc 2011;86:348-61.

113. Fonseca JD, Knight GM, McHugh TD. The complex evolution of antibiotic resistance in Mycobacterium tuberculosis. Int J Infect Dis 2015;32:94-100.

114. World Health Organization. Guidelines for the programmatic management of drug-resistant tuberculosis, 2011 update. Geneva: World Health Organization; 2011.

115. Nahid P, Dorman SE, Alipanah N, Barry PM, Brozek JL, Cattamanchi A, et al. Official American Thoracic Society/Centers for Disease Control and Prevention/Infectious Diseases Society of America Clinical Practice Guidelines: treatment of drug-susceptible tuberculosis. Clin Infect Dis 2016;63:e147-e195.

116. Kim SG, Kim JS, Jung HC,Song IS. Is a 9-month treatment sufficient in tuberculous enterocolitis? A prospective, randomized, single-centre study. Aliment Pharmacol Ther 2003;18: 85-91.

117. Park SH, Yang SK, Yang DH, Kim KJ, Yoon SM, Choe JW, et al. Prospective randomized trial of six-month versus nine-month therapy for intestinal tuberculosis. Antimicrob Agents Chemother 2009;53:4167-71.

118. Balasubramanian R, Nagarajan M, Balambal R, Tripathy SP, Sundararaman R, Venkatesan P, et al. Randomised controlled clinical trial of short course chemotherapy in abdominal tuberculosis: a five-year report. Int J Tuberc Lung Dis 1997;1: 44-51.

119. Kulkarni P, Akarte S, Mankeshwar R, Bhawalkar J, Banerjee A, Kulkarni A. Non-adherence of new pulmonary tuberculosis patients to anti-tuberculosis treatment. Ann Med Health Sci Res 2013;3:67-74.

120. Bagchi S, Ambe G, Sathiakumar N. Determinants of poor adherence to anti-tuberculosis treatment in Mumbai, India. Int J Prev Med 2010;1:223-32.

121. Tony J, Sunilkumar K, Thomas V. Randomized controlled trial of DOTS versus conventional regime for treatment of ileocecal and colonic tuberculosis. Indian J Gastroenterol 2008;27:19-21.

122. Makharia GK, Ghoshal UC, Ramakrishna BS, Agnihotri A, Ahuja V, Chowdhury SD, et al. Intermittent directly observed therapy for abdominal tuberculosis: a multicenter randomized controlled trial comparing 6 months versus 9 months of therapy. Clin Infect Dis 2015;61:750-7.

123. Misra SP, Misra V, Dwivedi M, Arora JS, Kunwar BK. Tuberculous colonic strictures: impact of dilation on diagnosis. Endoscopy 2004;36:1099-103.

124. Sonika U, Kar P. Tuberculosis and liver disease: management issues. Trop Gastroenterol 2012;33:102-6.

125. Saigal S, Agarwal SR, Nandeesh HP, Sarin SK. Safety of an ofloxacin-based antitubercular regimen for the treatment of tuberculosis in patients with underlying chronic liver disease: a preliminary report. J Gastroenterol Hepatol 2001;16:1028-32.

126. Sharma P, Tyagi P, Singla V, Bansal N, Kumar A, Arora A. Clinical and biochemical profile of tuberculosis in patients with liver cirrhosis. J Clin Exp Hepatol 2015;5:8-13.

127. Ibrarullah M, Mohan A, Sarkari A, Srinivas M, Mishra A, Sundar TS. Abdominal tuberculosis: diagnosis by laparoscopy and colonoscopy. Trop Gastroenterol 2002;23:150-3.

16

Granulomatous Hepatitis

Vineet Ahuja, SK Acharya

INTRODUCTION

Granulomas in the liver may be found incidentally and perplex the clinician, but more often reflect an underlying clinically relevant disease. The search for an aetiology of granulomas usually suggests a systemic disorder rather than primary liver disease. Granulomas represent the inflammatory response of the mononuclear phagocytic system to the presence of a foreign antigen. An extremely diverse array of inciting agents can result in the formation of granulomas in the liver. These granulomas often have a common histopathological pattern but may sometimes differ in detail (1-4). However, in spite of an extensive work-up and evaluation, the aetiology remains obscure in 10%-25% patients with hepatic granulomas and these patients have been labelled as having "granulomatous hepatitis" (2-6).

The word "hepatitis" implies that there is hepatic cell destruction. However, in most patients with hepatic granulomas, hepatic destruction is seldom seen. Therefore, several workers have proposed that the term "granulomatous hepatitis" should be avoided and have suggested "hepatic granulomatous disease" or "hepatic granulomas" as alternatives (3,4,7).

AETIOLOGY

Hepatic granulomas have varied aetiology and show considerable geographic variation. There are numerous causes of hepatic granulomas, both infective and non-infective. While the occurrence of sarcoidosis, primary biliary cirrhosis and fungal disease is high in the Western hemisphere, tuberculosis [TB] is the most common cause in India.

Hepatic granulomas usually represent a generalised disease process and have been described in 5%-10% of needle liver biopsy specimens (2,4). The causes of hepatic

Table 16.1: Common causes of hepatic granulomas
Infections
Bacterial: Brucella, Salmonella Mycobacterial: Tuberculosis, Leprosy, NTM Rickettsiae: Q fever Spirochaetal: Syphilis Fungal: Histoplasma, Coccidioidomycosis, Cryptococcosis Parasitic: Schistosomiasis Viral: Hepatitis C, Cytomegalovirus
Sarcoidosis
Primary biliary cirrhosis
Hodgkin's disease
AIDS related opportunistic infections
Drugs: Carbamazepine, chlorpromazine, chlorpropamide, phenylbutazone, procainamide
NTM = nontuberculous mycobacteria; AIDS = acquired immunodeficiency syndrome

granulomas are listed in Table 16.1. However, this list is by no means exhaustive. The relative frequency of occurrence of hepatic granulomas in some of the published studies is shown in Table 16.2. In many studies, TB and sarcoidosis have been the two most common causes of hepatic granulomas. With the advent of the human immunodeficiency virus [HIV] infection and the acquired immunodeficiency syndrome [AIDS], hepatic granulomas due to rare causes such as nontuberculous mycobacteria [NTM], cryptococcosis etc., are being increasingly encountered (1-4).

PATHOLOGY

Hepatic granulomas are the result of a cell mediated immune response by hepatic reticuloendothelial system to antigen/foreign substances (1-4).

Table 16.2: Major causes of hepatic granulomas in various case series

Variable	Guckian and Perry (8) [n = 63]	Neville et al (1) [n = 54]	Klatskin (9) [n = 565]	Cunnigham et al (10) [n = 77]	Ferrell (11) [n = 35]*	Kanel and Reynolds (3) [n = 202]	Sabharwal et al (12) [n = 51]
Tuberculosis	53	2	12.4	10.4	2.5	25.2	55
Sarcoidosis	12	54	38	10.4	20	27.2	1.9
Primary biliary cirrhosis	ND	19	10.4	6.5	22.8	0†	0
Malignancy	5	1.4	4.4	7.8	8.5	3.5	7.8
Unknown	20	10	6.5	31.2	20	17.3	12

All values are shown as percentages
ND = not described
* Patients with epithelioid cell granulomas only
† Patients with primary biliary cirrhosis were excluded

Histopathological features of hepatic granulomas depend on the aetiology. Generally, hepatic granulomas consist of pale-staining epithelioid cells with surrounding lymphocytes. Sometimes, the foreign body/infecting organism can be identified with the granuloma. Central area of caseation necrosis, foreign body and Langhans' giant cells can also be seen. Fibrous capsule and hyaline change representing healing may also be found.

Six basic morphological types of hepatic granulomas have been described [Table 16.3]. *Epithelioid granulomas* are often encountered in patients with TB [Figure 16.1], sarcoidosis,

Table 16.3: Morphological types of hepatic granulomas

Epithelioid cell granulomas

    Caseating [necrotising] granulomas
    Non-caseating granulomas

Fibrin ring granulomas

Granulomatoid reactions with poorly formed granulomas

Bile granulomas

Lipogranulomas

Microgranulomas

primary biliary cirrhosis among other conditions. *Caseating [necrotising] granulomas* have been classically associated with TB. *Fibrin ring granulomas* with a characteristic "doughnut" appearance occur in Q fever and have been described in several other conditions (13-15). *Granulomatoid reaction* with poorly formed granulomas occurs in patients with haematological malignancies and AIDS (3). *Bile granulomas* have been described in areas of cholestasis. *Lipogranulomas* can be seen in fatty liver. *Microgranulomas* can sometimes occur in patients with AIDS, cytomegalovirus [CMV] hepatitis and can occur along with other types of granulomas.

Klatskin (9) estimated that in a patient with one granuloma in the needle biopsy specimen, the entire liver would contain about 15 million granulomas assuming that there is a generalised distribution. Hepatomegaly is, therefore, commonly observed in patients with granulomatous liver disease (1-4,16-18).

CLINICAL PRESENTATION

Clinical presentation of patients with hepatic granulomas depends on the causative disorder. These patients often present with pyrexia of unknown origin [PUO]. Mild to

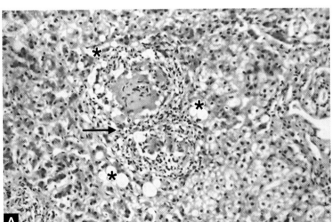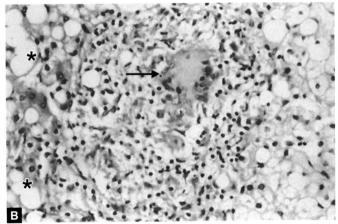

Figure 16.1: Granulomatous hepatitis. Photomicrograph showing a well-defined epithelioid granuloma [arrow], Langhans' giant cells, ballooning and fatty degeneration [asterisk] of hepatocytes [A], [Haematoxylin and eosin × 200]. Epithelioid granuloma and Langhans' giant cells [arrow] are also seen amidst hepatocytes showing ballooning degeneration [B] [Haematoxylin and eosin × 400]

moderate hepatomegaly, which is usually non-tender, is common. When the disease is due to TB, sarcoidosis, associated peripheral mediastinal lymphadenopathy, erythema nodosum, clinically apparent jaundice may be found. In some conditions, such as, Hodgkin's lymphoma and primary biliary cirrhosis where hepatic granulomas are an incidental finding, jaundice may be prominent.

LABORATORY ABNORMALITIES

In a patient with PUO, marked elevation of serum alkaline phosphatase [SAP] [three to six times the normal] with mild elevation of serum transminases [two to six times normal], well preserved hepatic synthetic function, normal prothrombin time, serum albumin and a normal to slight increase in serum bilirubin should arouse a suspicion regarding the presence of hepatic granulomas (2-4). Anaemia and elevated erythrocyte sedimentation rate [ESR] may be found. Peripheral blood eosinophilia may suggest Hodgkin's disease, parasitic infestation and drug sensitivity (2-4).

DIFFERENTIAL DIAGNOSIS

Hepatobiliary Tuberculosis

TB involvement of the hepatobiliary system can occur in several ways [Table 16.4]. Liver involvement in TB, though common both in pulmonary and extra-pulmonary TB [EPTB], is usually clinically silent. Occasionally, local signs and symptoms may be prominent in hepatic TB, and may constitute the initial or sole presenting feature of the disease. Using needle biopsy specimen, epithelioid granulomas can be demonstrated in hepatic TB in 80%-100% of cases; caseation necrosis in 30%-83% and acid-fast bacilli [AFB] on smear examination in up to 59% of cases (2-4).

Congenital Tuberculosis

Hepatic involvement is very common in congenital TB and has been recently incorporated into the diagnostic criteria for this condition (19). When an infant born to a mother with active TB manifests hepatomegaly, jaundice and failure to thrive, congenital TB should be considered in the differential diagnosis. The reader is referred to the chapter "*Tuberculosis in pregnancy*" [Chapter 25] for details on this topic.

Table 16.4: Clinical syndromes of hepatobiliary tuberculosis
Congenital tuberculosis
Primary hepatic tuberculosis
Disseminated/miliary tuberculosis
Tuberculoma
Tuberculosis of the biliary tract
Drug induced hepatic failure
Granulomatous hepatitis
Tuberculosis pylephlebitis

Primary Hepatic Tuberculosis

Primary hepatic TB is said to occur when there is involvement of the hepatobiliary tract by TB without apparent involvement elsewhere, or, only with local lymph node and splenic involvement (18). Some workers have called this condition "local hepatic TB" (18,19). Cinque *et al* (20) suggested that the tubercle bacilli reach the liver via the portal vein as opposed to miliary TB, where the organism reaches the liver via the hepatic artery. Alvarez and Carpio (21) reported clinical and histopathological features of 130 patients with localised hepatic TB seen over a 20-year period at Manila, Philippines. The disease was more common in males and most patients were in the 11-30 years age range. Most of them were symptomatic for one to two years prior to the time of confirmation of the diagnosis. The paper described two major forms of clinical presentation. A hard, nodular liver with fever and weight loss mimicking cancer was observed in 65% of the patients. In the remaining 35% patients, chronic recurrent jaundice mimicking extra-hepatic obstruction was observed. Percutaneous liver biopsy [positive in 48 of 71 patients; 67%] and laparoscopy [positive in 49 of the 53 patients; 92%] were the main methods of confirmation of the diagnosis. On laparoscopy, hepatic lesions appeared as cheesy white, irregular nodules. Hepatic calcification was evident in 49% of the patients. In patients with jaundice, serum aminotransferases were elevated in more than 90% and SAP was elevated in all patients. In those without jaundice, serum aminotransferases were elevated in about 5% and SAP was elevated in 60% patients. Overall, 12% patients died in this series (21).

In another series (22), hepatic TB was confirmed in 96 patients presenting with the features of liver disease, only 14 of whom had other concomitant hepatic pathology. Although respiratory symptoms occurred in 74% of cases, these were overshadowed by the abdominal manifestations which included pain in the right hypochondrium, abdominal distension, firm, tender hepatomegaly, splenomegaly and ascites. Icterus was observed in 11 cases [only one of whom had concurrent hepatic pathology] and liver failure was found in 10 patients. A surgical presentation occurred in three patients. Coagulation abnormalities were noted in 26 patients [24 with low prothrombin index and 2 with moderately raised fibrinogen degradation products]. The characteristic serum profile included hyponatraemia [64%], raised SAP [3%] and γ-glutamyl transferase [77%], hypoalbuminaemia [63%] and hypergammaglobulinaemia [83%]. Transaminase levels were moderately elevated in 78% of the cases. Hepatic imaging techniques were frequently misleading. Chest radiographs were normal in 25% of cases. Liver biopsy was the most useful aid to correct diagnosis, which was suspected clinically in only 47% of cases. Histopathologically, AFB, caseation [Figure 16.2] and granulomas were seen in 9%, 83% and 96% of cases, respectively. The overall morality was 42% (22).

Yu *et al* (23) have described computed tomography [CT] in hepatic TB in 12 cases. The patterns described by

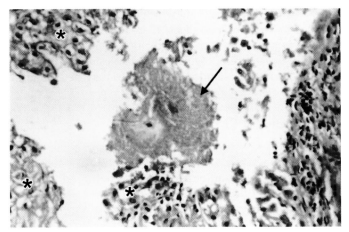

Figure 16.2: Granulomatous hepatitis. Photomicrograph showing ballooning degeneration of hepatocytes [asterisk] and caseation necrosis [arrow] [Haematoxylin and eosin × 400]

them include [i] multiple nodular lesions in the subcapsule of liver; [ii] multiple, miliary, micronodular and low-density lesions with military calcifications; [iii] singular, low-density mass with multiple flecked calcifications; [iv] multiple cystic lesions; and [v] multiple micronodular and low-density lesions fusing into multiloculated cystic mass or "cluster" sign. Balci *et al* (24) reported the spectrum of magnetic resonance imaging [MRI] features in 18 patients with a histopathological diagnosis of granulomatous hepatitis. Diffuse nodular liver involvement was visualised in all patients. Nodules were consistent with granulomas and were 0.5-4.5 cm in diameter. Caseating granulomas were intermediate and high signal on T2-weighted, low signal on T1-weighted images. Non-caseating granulomas revealed intermediate signal on T1, and T2-weighted images and increased enhancement on arterial phase images with persisting enhancement in late phase images.

Most patients respond to anti-TB treatment. For patients with obstructive jaundice, in addition to anti-TB treatment, biliary decompression should be performed either by stent insertion during endoscopic retrograde cholangiopancreatography, by percutaneous transhepatic biliary drainage or by surgical decompression whenever feasible (25).

Disseminated and Miliary Tuberculosis

Hepatic involvement is a common finding in patients with disseminated and miliary TB (17). Granulomas has been reported in 75%-100% patients in autopsy series (26-28) and in 25%-100% needle biopsy specimens in patients with miliary TB (17,29,30). Miliary lesions are small 1-2 mm epithelioid granulomas. The reader is also referred to the chapter *"Disseminated and miliary tuberculosis" [Chapter 29]* for details on this topic.

Pulmonary Tuberculosis

Up to two-thirds of the patients with pulmonary TB have been shown to have evidence of hepatic involvement (2,4,16).

In patients with pulmonary TB, hyperglobulinaemia is frequently present and mild hyperbilirubinaemia may occasionally be present (30). Serum aminotransferase levels are usually normal. Kupffer cell hyperplasia is often present (16,31,32).

Tuberculoma

Sometimes, hepatic TB lesions can present as masses larger than 2 mm in diameter (33). Symptoms of fever, malaise and loss of weight are common. Occasionally, abdominal pain and diarrhoea may occur. Hepatomegaly is frequently present. Jaundice and a palpable abdominal mass are uncommon presenting signs. Obstruction to bile flow due to compression at the porta hepatis by a tuberculoma has been postulated to be the cause of jaundice. Bleeding into a solitary tuberculoma presenting as an acute abdomen and progressive anaemia have also been reported (34). Consistent with a pattern characteristic of space occupying lesions of the liver, serum transaminases are normal or only slightly elevated; SAP levels are moderately elevated. On liver scan and arteriography, these lesions may mimick the appearance of a primary or metastatic carcinoma. They may also be confused with pyogenic or amoebic liver abscess (31,35). While blind percutaneous needle biopsy was not very helpful in the diagnosis (31,36), aspiration cytology at the time of laparoscopy was more useful in confirming the diagnosis (37). Most often these lesions resolve with effective anti-TB treatment.

Tuberculosis of Bile Ducts

TB of the bile ducts is uncommon. The disease is thought to result from rupture of tubercles in the periportal region into the walls of contiguous biliary ductules or by primary infection of bile ducts (38). Stemmerman (39) found TB of the biliary ducts in 45 of 1500 autopsies and estimated the incidence to be 3%. In these patients, symptoms and signs attributable to the biliary ducts are seldom found. Only three of the 45 patients [6.7%] reported by Stemmerman (39) manifested clinical jaundice, and hepatomegaly was evident only in one-third of them. However, evidence of TB of other organ systems draining into the portal circulation [e.g., caseous mesenteric lymph node TB, intestinal TB, and TB peritonitis] was observed in 41 of the 45 patients this series (39). Biliary stricture (40) and cholangitis (2) due to TB have also been described.

Tuberculosis of Gallbladder

Gallbladder is an uncommon site of involvement by TB. Most cases occur in association with other organ involvement. Rarely, isolated TB of the gallbladder can occur (41,42) and is usually a retrospective diagnosis, becoming evident on histopathological examination of the cholecystectomy specimen. Management consists of administration of anti-TB treatment (2,31,41,42).

Hepatobiliary Tuberculosis in Patients with Human Immunodeficiency Virus Infection and Acquired Immunodeficiency Syndrome

Hepatobiliary involvement is very common in patients with HIV infection and AIDS (7). Both, *Mycobacterium tuberculosis* [*Mtb*] and NTM can cause the disease (2,31). In patients with AIDS, it is important to distinguish hepatic granulomas due to TB from other causes.

Other Hepatic Lesions

Granulomatous hepatitis has been described in 12%-28% patients receiving bacille Calmette-Guérin [BCG] vaccination (43-45). Clinically, constitutional symptoms, hepatomegaly, mildly elevated serum transaminases, bilirubin and moderately elevated SAP levels are present. Focal defects or non-homogeneous uptake on technetium liver scan may be present. On histopathological examination, granulomas, hepatocellular necrosis, lymphohistiocytic aggregates and Kupffer cell hyperplasia have been described (43-45). Direct effect of viable BCG bacilli and hypersensitivity reaction have been proposed as the underlying pathogenetic mechanisms (46).

Amyloidosis has been described in 10% of patients with concomitant hepatic TB which may occasionally present as marked hepatomegaly (28). Most of these patients have long standing advanced disease frequently involving the intestinal tract (28,47). Nodular regenerative hyperplasia had been described in TB and several other disorders, such as, collagen vascular disorders [e.g., systemic lupus erythematosus, rheumatoid arthritis, progressive systemic sclerosis], antiphospholipid syndrome, macroglobulinemia, among others (48,49). In Bantus of Africa, haemosiderosis of the liver has often been described (50). Whether these are mere associations or the cause/effect of TB needs further clarification.

Hepatobiliary TB can rarely present as hepatic failure (51). Severe degree of immunosuppression following liver transplantation also predisposes to the development of TB (52).

Sarcoidosis

Sarcoidosis is a multi-system granulomatous disorder of unknown aetiology. In patients with sarcoidosis, hepatic granulomas are widely distributed in the liver; very often in the portal and periportal regions. Often, hepatic involvement seems incidental, but a few patients may present with signs and symptoms of hepatic dysfunction. In some patients, the clinical presentation may resemble primary biliary cirrhosis (52).

The granulomas are numerous enough to make it unlikely that could be missed in a liver biopsy sample of even moderate size (53). Central necrosis in these granulomas is less frequent than in TB and they contain abundant reticulin. The granulomas are made of epithelioid cells [often with a thin rim of lymphocytes] and giant cells, some of them containing stellate [asteroid] bodies. The granulomas may show characteristic clustering which is also seen in the lymph nodes. As the granuloma ages, there may be deposition of collagen in a lamellar manner at the periphery of granuloma. Sarcoidosis may present with chronic cholestasis, destruction of interlobular ducts and limiting plates may be evident in liver biopsy specimens (54-56).

Primary Biliary Cirrhosis

In the early stages, the hepatic granulomas in patients with primary biliary cirrhosis may be indistinguishable from sarcoidosis. The granulomas are epithelioid and are most often found in the portal tracts. Lymphocytes are scattered within the granuloma. Plasma cells are often present in perigranulomatous location. Multinucleated giant cells are not common and necrosis is not present. Sometimes epithelioid cells may surround the interlobular bile ducts undergoing non-suppurative destruction. Liver granulomas may also be seen in primary sclerosing cholangitis (14).

Drugs

Many drugs have the potential to produce hepatic granulomas that may be eosinophil rich (57). Pyrazinamide which is given for the treatment of TB has also been implicated as a cause of granulomatous liver disease (58,59).

Chronic Hepatitis

Hepatitis C Infection

Chronic hepatitis C virus [HCV] infection has recently been recognised as an aetiological cause of hepatic granulomas (60). Hepatic granulomas have been described in up to 10%, patients with chronic HCV infection. Development of hepatic granulomas following interferon treatment has been reported in patients with HCV infection (61). A recent multicentre study (60) evaluated a total of 725 liver biopsies from 605 patients with chronic HCV infection to identify an association between the presence of granuloma and response to interferon treatment and also to see whether interferon treatment leads to the formation of hepatic granulomas. In eight patients, hepatic granulomas were detected in the initial liver biopsies. Four patients had repeat biopsies, and all had hepatic granulomas again. The prevalence of hepatic granulomas in patients with chronic HCV was calculated to be 1.3%. The presence of granulomas was not found to be a predictor of response to interferon therapy. The development of hepatic granulomas during interferon therapy was also not found to be a common phenomenon in this study. Hence, the clinical relevance of finding hepatic granulomas in HCV infected patients still needs further studies. Development of systemic sarcoidosis many years after interferon-α treatment for chronic HCV infection has also been documented (62).

Hepatitis B Infection

Tahan *et al* (63) studied the prevalence of hepatic granulomas in 663 patients with chronic hepatitis B virus [HBV] infection, to determine its significance regarding treatment outcome. Hepatic granulomas were found in 10 cases [1.5%]. Of these 10 patients with hepatic granulomas, four responded to interferon therapy, two dropped out, and four were non-responders. This study (63) concluded that hepatic granuloma is a rare finding in chronic HBV infection and its presence does not seem to predict the response to interferon therapy.

Brucellosis

Brucella suis, Brucella abortus, Brucella melitensis and *Brucella canis* cause granulomatous reaction in the liver. Brucellosis is acquired by contact with cattle, goats, dogs or by ingestion of unpasteurised dairy products. The infection presents as undulating fever with remissions and relapses. Excessive weakness and depression are present during the acute illness. The diagnosis is made by brucella serology and positive reactions in titres of 1:320 or more are considered diagnostic. The most reliable method of establishing the diagnosis is by blood or bone marrow culture.

Systemic Mycoses

Histoplasma capsulatum and *Coccidioides immitis* usually infect humans by inhalation of organisms with primary infection occurring in the lungs. Chronic pulmonary lesions develop in a few and rarely there is widespread dissemination to other organs including the liver. The hepatic reaction to these fungi is usually by granuloma formation (2-4).

Histoplasma usually colonises in immunosuppressed patients but occasionally immunocompetent individuals may also be affected. The disease usually manifests as fever with hepatosplenomegatly and oral ulcers. Commonly there is associated adrenal involvement with Addison's disease. Liver usually contains granulomatous lesions, sometimes with central caseation necrosis resembling TB. Use of specials stains like methenamine silver, Hotchkiss-McManus stain makes identification easier, although the organism can often be found in the granuloma by haematoxylin and eosin staining. Diagnosis is best confirmed by culture of the organisms from blood, bone marrow, sputum and oral ulcer scrapings (2,4).

Leprosy

Three types of granulomas have been described in patients with leprosy (3). The tuberculoid type, consists of abundant epithelioid cells with scattered lymphocytes. Multinucleated cells may be present and these granulomas are most often present in the parenchyma. It is seldom possible to identify the bacilli even when special stains are used. The lepromatous type granuloma is inflammatory in nature and consists of histocytes with clear to foamy cytoplasm. Lymphocytes are infrequent and multinucleated giant cells are not present. These granulomas can be seen within the portal tracts or the parenchyma and contain abundant numbers of acid-fast organisms identified by Fite stain.

The intermediate type granulomas consist of epithelioid cells with only scanty number of lymphocytes. Giant cells are seldom seen.

Schistosomiasis

Hepatic granulomas are caused by *Schistosoma mansoni* and *Schistosoma japonicum*. The granulomas are quite disease specific and ova may be seen in the centre of the granuloma. Presence of eosinophils may point to parasitic aetiology (4).

Hodgkin's Lymphoma

Hepatic granulomas have been described in 8%-17% patients with Hodgkin's disease (64,65). The presence of hepatic granulomas does not appear to be related to disease outcome or prognosis in Hodgkin's lymphoma.

Typhoid Fever

Hepatic granuloma is a rare complication of typhoid fever. A report has described two cases of typhoid fever with hepatic, splenic and bone marrow granulomas (66).

Q Fever

Fibrin ring granulomas are often present in patients with Q fever. These granuloma contain a ring-like array of fibrin [stainable with phosphotungstic acid-haematoxylin] producing a "halo" effect around a central empty space (2-4). These granulomas have also been described in allopurinol hypersensitivity, cytomegalovirus hepatitis, leishmaniasis, toxoplasmosis, hepatitis A and systemic lupus erythematosus (2-4).

Acquired Immunodeficiency Syndrome

Several conditions result in hepatic granulomas in patients with AIDS (4,15,16,57). These are listed in Table 16.5. The diagnosis is confirmed with histopathological and microbiological examination of the liver biopsy specimen.

Table 16.5: Causes of hepatic granulomas in patients with acquired immunodeficiency syndrome
Mycobacterium tuberculosis
Mycobacterium avium-intracellulare complex
Cytomegalovirus
Histoplasmosis
Toxoplasmosis
Cryptococcosis
Neoplasms
Hodgkin's lymphoma   Non-Hodgkin's lymphoma
Drugs
Adapted from references 2-4

Idiopathic Granulomatous Hepatitis

Despite extensive investigations, 10%-25% of patients are labelled as having "idiopathic" hepatic granulomas (2-6,67). Idiopathic granulomatous hepatitis is a condition characterised by recurrent fever and granulomas in the liver and other organs where other causes of hepatic granulomas have been carefully excluded (5,68,69). Patients are usually in the age range of 16 to 60 years. The prominent symptom is fever, which is often relapsing in character although continuous and remittent fever patterns have also been described. In one series (5) 44% of patients first presented as PUO. Other symptoms, include malaise, chills, weight loss, abdominal pain, anorexia, night sweats, nausea, jaundice, diarrhoea and abdominal distension. The natural history of the disease is marked with multiple remissions and exacerbations. Response to corticosteroids is usually dramatic (5,68,69).

DIAGNOSIS

Patients with hepatic granulomas must be thoroughly investigated for a possible aetiological cause. Detailed history must be obtained specifically focusing on exposure to an infectious source, and occupational or environmental agents including drugs. Several laboratory tests are often employed in the work up of a patient with granulomatous hepatitis. Cultures of blood, body fluids and biopsy material must be done keeping in mind the common infectious causes of hepatic granulomas. Ant-mitochondrial antibodies may be helpful in the diagnosis of primary biliary cirrhosis. Elevated serum angiotensin converting enzyme [ACE] levels may suggest a diagnosis of sarcoidosis.

Liver biopsy is essential for the diagnosis. Biopsy material must be subjected to microbiological and histopathological examination. Type and location of granulomas may offer a clue to the aetiology. Special stains may be required to identify infectious agents. Examination under polarised light may help in visualising foreign bodies.

TREATMENT

When the investigations are conclusive, treatment should be directed towards the aetiological agent. In a country like India, when the aetiological cause of granulomatous hepatitis is unclear, a therapeutic trail with antituberculosis agents is often given. If this fails, then corticosteroid treatment may be tried (70).

In a study on idiopathic granulomatous hepatitis (5), the disease resolved spontaneously in seven patients, two patients responded with less than three months of oral corticosteroids or indomethacin treatment and seven patients required steroid treatment for two years or longer to maintain asymptomatic state.

PROGNOSIS

Outcome of hepatic granulomatous disease depends on the underlying cause. In a study on TB hepatitis (22), age below 20 years, acute presentation, presence of coagulopathy and a high mean caseation score were found to be predictors of a poor outcome. Drug related granulomas often resolve when the offending agent is withdrawn (59). The presence of hepatic granulomas in patients with Crohn's disease, Hodgkin's disease and primary biliary cirrhosis is thought to indicate a better prognosis (69,71-74).

REFERENCES

1. Neville E, Piyasena KH, James DG. Granulomas of the liver. Postgrad Med J 1975;51:361-5.
2. Sherlock S, Dooley J. Diseases of the liver and biliary system. Oxford: Blackwell Scientific Publications; 1993.p.461-7.
3. Kanel GC, Reynolds TB. Hepatic granulomas. In: Kaplowitz N, editor. Liver and biliary disease. Baltimore: Williams and Wilkins; 1992.p.455-62.
4. Lefkowitch JH. Hepatic granulomas. In: Haubrich WS, Schaffner F, Berk JE, editors. Bockus gastroenterology. Philadelphia: W.B. Saunders Company; 1995.p.2317-24.
5. Zoutman DE, Ralph ED, Frei JV. Granulomatuous hepatitis and fever of unknown origin. An 11-year experience of 23 cases with three years' follow-up. J Clin Gastroenterol 1991;13:69-75.
6. Simon HB, Wolff SM. Granulomatous hepatitis and prolonged fever of unknown origin–a study of 13 patients. Medicine [Baltimore] 1973;52:1-21.
7. Tobias H, Sherman A. Hepatobiliary tuberculosis. In: Rom WN, Gray SM, editors. Tuberculosis. Boston: Little, Brown and Company; 1996.p.599-608.
8. Guckian JC, Perry JE. Granulomatous hepatitis. An analysis of 63 cases and review of the literature. Ann Intern Med 1966;65:1081-100.
9. Klatskin G. Hepatic granulomata: problems in interpretation. Mt Sinai J Med 1977;44:798-812.
10. Cunnigham D, Mills PR, Quigley EM, Patrick RS, Watkinson G, MacKenzie JF, et al. Hepatic granulomas: experience over a 10-year period in the West of Scotland. Q J Med 1982;202:162-70.
11. Ferrell LD. Hepatic granulomas: a morphologic approach to diagnosis. Surg Pathol 1990;3:87-106.
12. Sabharwal BD, Malhotra N, Garg R, Malhotra V. Granulomatous hepatitis: a retrospective study. Indian J Pathol Microbiol 1995;38:413-6.
13. Bernstein M, Edmondson HA, Barbour BH. The liver lesion in Q fever. Clinical and pathologic features. Arch Intern Med 1965;116:491-8.
14. Hoffmann CE, Heaton JW. Q fever hepatitis: clinical manifestations and pathological findings. Gastroenterology 1982;83:474-9.
15. Marazuela M, Moreno A, Yebra M, Cerezo E, Gomez-Gesto C, Vargas JA. Hepatic fibrin-ring granulomas: a clinicopathologic study of 23 patients. Hum Pathol 1991;22:607-13.
16. Bowry S, Chan CH, Weiss H, Katz S, Zimmerman HJ. Hepatic involvement in pulmonary tuberculosis. Am Rev Respir Dis 1970;101:941-8.
17. Sharma SK, Mohan A, Prasad KL, Pande JN, Gupta AK, Khilnani GC. Clinical profile, laboratory characteristics and outcome in miliary tuberculosis. QJM 1995;88:29-37.
18. Essop AR, Moosa MR, Segal I, Posen J. Primary tuberculosis of the liver-a case report. Tubercle 1983;64:291-3.
19. Cantwell MF, Shehab ZM, Costello AM, Sands L, Green WF, Ewing EP Jr, et al. Brief report: congenital tuberculosis. N Engl J Med 1994;330:1051-4.
20. Cinque TJ, Gary NE, Palladino VS. "Primary" miliary tuberculosis of the liver. Am J Gastroenterol 1964;42:611-9.
21. Alvarez SZ, Carpio R. Hepatobiliary tuberculosis. Dig Dis Sci 1983;28:193-200.
22. Essop AR, Posen JA, Hodkinson JH, Segal I. Tuberculosis hepatitis: a clinical review of 96 cases. QJM 1984;53:465-77.

23. Yu RS, Zhang SZ, Wu JJ, Li RF. Imaging diagnosis of 12 patients with hepatic tuberculosis. World J Gastroenterol 2004;10:1639-42.

24. Balci NC, Tunaci A, Akinci A, Cevikbas U. Granulomatous hepatitis: MRI findings. Magn Reson Imaging 2001;19:1107-11.

25. Alvarez SZ. Hepatobiliary tuberculosis. J Gastroenterol Hepatol 1998;13:833-9.

26. Saphir O. Changes in the liver and pancreas in chronic tuberculosis. Arch Pathol 1929;7:1025-39.

27. Torrey RG. The occurrence of miliary tuberculosis of the liver in the course of pulmonary tuberculosis. Am J Med Sci 1916;151:549-56.

28. Ullom JT. The liver in tuberculosis. Am J Med Sci 1909;137:694-99.

29. Sharma SK, Mohan A, Sharma A, Mitra DK. Miliary tuberculosis: new insights into an old disease. Lancet Infect Dis 2005;5:415-30.

30. Sahn SA, Neff TA. Miliary tuberculosis. Am J Med 1974;56:495-505.

31. Lewis JH, Zimmerman HY. Tuberculosis of the liver and biliary tract. In: Schlossberg D, editor. Tuberculosis. New York: Springer Verlag; 1988.p.149-69.

32. Arora MM, Ali A, D'Souza AJ, Pawar KN. Clinical, function and needle biopsy studies of the liver in tuberculosis. J Indian Med Assoc 1956;26:341-4.

33. Achem SR, Kolts BE, Grisnik J, MacMath T, Monteiro CB, Goldstein J. Pseudotumoral hepataic tuberculosis. Atypical presentation and comprehensive review of the literature. J Clin Gastroenterol 1992;14:72-7.

34. Prochazka M, Vyhnanek F, Vorreith V, Jirasek M. Bleeding into solitary hepatic tuberculoma. Report of a case treated by resection. Acta Chir Scand 1986;152:73-5.

35. Tahiliani RR, Parikh JA, Hegde AV, Bhatia SJ, Deodhar KP, Kapadia NM, et al. Hepatic tuberculosis simulating hepatic amoebiasis. J Assoc Physicians India 1983;31:679-80.

36. Duckworth WC. Tuberculosis of the liver. S Afr Med J 1964;38:945.

37. Bhargava DK, Verma K, Malaviya AN. Solitary tuberculoma of the liver; laparoscopic, histologic and cytologic diagnosis. Gastrointest Endosc 1983;29:329-30.

38. Rosenkranz K, Howard LD. Tubular necrosis of the liver. Arch Pathol 1936;22:743-54.

39. Stemmerman M. Bile ductal tuberculosis. Q Bull Sea View Hosp 1941;6:316-24.

40. Fan ST, Ng IO, Choi TK, Lai EC. Tuberculosis of the bile duct: a rare cause of biliary stricture. Am J Gastroenterol 1989;84:413-4.

41. Wang CT. Hepatobiliary tuberculosis. Chin J Tuberc Respir Dis 1991;14:40-1.

42. Leader SA. Tuberculosis of the liver and gallbladder with abscess formation. Ann Intern Med 1951;37:594-605.

43. Bodurtha A, Kim YH, Laucius JF, Donato RA, Mastrangelo MJ. Hepatic granulomas and other hepatic lesions associated with BCG immunotherapy for cancer. Am J Clin Pathol 1974;61:747-52.

44. Ersoy O, Aran R, Aydinli M, Yonem O, Harmanci O, Akdogan B, et al. Granulomatous hepatitis after intravesical BCG treatment for bladder cancer. Indian J Gastroenterol 2006;25:258-9.

45. Hristea A, Neacsu A, Ion DA, Streinu-Cercel A, Stăniceanu F. BCG-related granulomatous hepatitis. Pneumologia 2007;56:32-4.

46. Obrien TF, Hysolp NE Jr. Case records of the Massachusetts General Hospital, Weekly clinicopathological exercises. Case 34-1975. N Engl J Med 1975;293:443-8.

47. Jones K, Peck WM. Incidence of fatty liver in tuberculosis with special reference to tuberculosis enteritis. Arch Intern Med 1944;75:371-4.

48. Rougier P, Degott C, Rueff B, Benhamou JP. Nodular regenerative hyperplasia of the liver. Report of six cases and review of the literature. Gastroenterology 1978;75:169-72.

49. Foster JM, Litwin A, Gibbs JF, Intengen M, Kuvshinoff BW. Diagnosing regenerative nodular hyperplasia, the "great masquerader" of liver tumors. J Gastrointest Surg 2006;10:727-33.

50. Hersch C. Tuberculosis of the liver: a study of 200 cases. S Afr Med J 1964;38:857-63.

51. Sharma SK, Shamim SQ, Bannerjee CK, Sharma BK. Disseminated tuberculosis presenting as massive hepatosplenomegaly and hepatic failure: case report. Am J Gastroenterol 1981;76:153-6.

52. Sharma SK, Mohan A. Sarcoidosis: global scenario & Indian perspective. Indian J Med Res 2002;116:221-47.

53. Devaney K, Goodman ZD, Epstein MS, Zimmerman HJ, Ishak KG. Hepatic sarcoidosis. Clinicopathologic features in 100 patients. Am J Surg Pathol 1993;17:1272-80.

54. Rudzki C, Ishak KG, Zimmerman HJ. Chronic intrahepatic cholestasis of sarcoidosis. Am J Med 1975;59:373-87.

55. Bass NM, Burroughs AK, Scheuer PJ, James DG, Sherlock S. Chronic intrahepatic cholestasis due to sarcoidosis. Gut 1982;23:417-21.

56. Sharma SK, Mohan A. Uncommon manifestations of sarcoidosis. J Assoc Physicians India 2004;52:210-4.

57. Ishak KG. Granulomas of the liver. In: Ioachim HL, editor. Pathology of granulomas. New York: Raven Press; 1993.p.307-70.

58. Knobel B, Bunyanowsky G, Dan M, Zaidel L. Pyrazinamide induced granulomatous hepatitis. J Clin Gastroenterol 1997;24:264-6.

59. McMaster KR, Hennigar GR. Drug–induced granulomatous hepatitis. Lab Invest 1981;44:61-73.

60. Ozaras R, Tahan V, Mert A, Uraz S, Kanat M, Tabak F, et al. The prevalence of hepatic granulomas in chronic hepatitis C. J Clin Gastroenterol 2004;38:449-52.

61. Fiel MI, Shukla D, Saraf N, Xu R, Schiano TD. Development of hepatic granulomas in patients receiving pegylated interferon therapy for recurrent hepatitis C virus post liver transplantation. Transpl Infect Dis 2008;10:184-9.

62. Tortorella C, Napoli N, Panella E, Antonaci A, Gentile A, Antonaci S. Asymptomatic systemic sarcoidosis arising 5 years after IFN-alpha treatment for chronic hepatitis C: a new challenge for clinicians. J Interferon Cytokine Res 2004;24:655-8.

63. Tahan V, Ozaras R, Lacevic N, Ozden E, Yemisen M, Ozdogan O, et al. Prevalence of hepatic granulomas in chronic hepatitis B. Dig Dis Sci 2004;49:1575-7.

64. Abt AB, Kirschner RH, Belliveau RE, O'Connell MJ, Sklansky BD, Green WH, et al. Hepatic pathology associated with Hodgkin's disease. Cancer 1974;33:1564-71.

65. Kadin ME, Donaldson SS, Dorfman RF. Isolated granulomas in Hodgkin's disease. N Engl J Med 1970;283:859–61.

66. Mert A, Tabak F, Ozaras R, Ozturk R, Aki H, Aktuglu Y. Typhoid fever as a rare cause of hepatic, splenic, and bone marrow granulomas. Intern Med 2004;43:436-9.

67. Sartin JS, Walker RC. Granulomatous hepatitis: a retrospective review of 88 cases at the Mayo Clinic. Mayo Clin Proc 1991;66:914-8.

68. Telenti A, Hermans PE. Idiopathic granulomatosis manifesting as fever of unknown origin. Mayo Clin Proc 1989;65:44-50.

69. Beswick DR, Klatskin G, Boyer JL. Asymptomatic primary biliary cirrhosis. A progress report on long-term followup and natural history. Gastroenterology 1985;89:267-71.

70. Sonika U, Kar P. Tuberculosis and liver disease: management issues. Trop Gastroenterol 2012;33:102-6.

71. O'Connell MJ, Schimpff SC, Kirschner RH, Abt AB, Wiernik PH. Epithelioid granulomas in Hodgkin's disease. A favorable prognostic sign. JAMA 1975;233:886-9.

72. Gaya DR, Thorburn D, Oien KA, Morris AJ, Stanley AJ. Hepatic granulomas: a 10 year single centre experience. J Clin Pathol 2003;56:850-3.

73. Flamm SL. Granulomatous liver disease. Clin Liver Dis 2012;16:387-96.

74. Ozaras R, Yemisen M, Balkan II. More on hepatic granulomas. Diagn Pathol 2015;10:203.

17

Neurological Tuberculosis

Pournamy Sarathchandran, Kurupath Radhakrishnan

INTRODUCTION

Involvement of the central nervous system [CNS] is one of the most dreaded complications of tuberculosis [TB]. Autopsy studies have revealed that 5%-15% of individuals exposed to *Mycobacterium tuberculosis [Mtb]* develop active pulmonary TB; and of these, 5%-10% develop neurological TB (1). The burden of neurological TB is largely borne by resource-poor regions of the world (2). Neurological TB disproportionately afflicts children and human immunodeficiency [HIV] infected persons (3-7). Even with modern-day anti-TB treatment, neurological TB carries a high morbidity and mortality.

Last two decades have witnessed major changes in several aspects of neurological TB. These include a change in the clinical picture of neurological TB with an increasing number of cases with atypical presentation and an alarming increase in the number of patients with multidrug-resistant TB [MDR-TB]. Widespread availability and utilisation of computed tomography [CT] and magnetic resonance imaging [MRI] have facilitated early diagnosis of neurological TB and detection of complications. Research on reliable molecular markers for early diagnosis of neurological TB is being intensively pursued both in resource-rich and resource-poor countries.

However, considerable barriers in the diagnosis and treatment of neurological TB still exist, especially in resource-poor countries. While the most consistent factor that determines the outcome for neurological TB is early diagnosis and prompt institution of treatment (3-7), the protean nature of the symptoms and lack of sensitive diagnostic methods poses a huge challenge for early diagnosis. A majority of the patients with neurological TB in developing countries are diagnosed and treated too late because of the non-availability, inaccessibility and/or inability to afford quality medical care. Late diagnosis of neurological TB occurs in developed countries as well because this diagnosis is seldom suspected as TB is rare in these regions. For example, in the United States, compared to nearly 4000 cases of bacterial meningitis, only 100 to 150 cases of TB meningitis [TBM] are seen annually (8). However, as a consequence of a large scale immigration of infected people from developing countries, neurological TB is being encountered increasingly in industrialised countries.

Neurological TB may be classified into three major clinic-pathological categories: TBM, tuberculoma, and TB radiculo-myelitis [TBRM] [Table 17.1]. In addition, there are less common clinicopathological entities, such as, TB abscess and TB optochiasmatic arachnoiditis. Despite the considerable advances that have been made during the last few years with regard to the diagnosis and treatment of TB, following questions on neurological TB have largely remained unanswered: How can we rapidly diagnose neurological TB? What is the optimum treatment of neurological TB? How can we minimise the significant morbidity among the survivors of neurological TB? In this chapter, we intent to address these questions with respect to TBM, intracranial tuberculoma and TBRM. In addition, diagnosis and management of chronic meningitis are also described. Spinal TB is covered in the chapter *"Skeletal tuberculosis" [Chapter 19].*

Table 17.1: Classification of neurological TB
TB meningitis
TB arachnoiditis
Basal
Opticochiasmatic
Spinal
Tuberculoma
Intracranial
Spinal
TB abscess
TB = tuberculosis

TUBERCULOSIS MENINGITIS

Sir Robert Whytt, the Scottish physiologist, is credited with the first clinical description of TBM in the late eighteenth century (9); this was even prior to isolation of *Mtb* by Robert Koch in 1882 (10). TBM, which accounts for 70%-80% of cases of neurological TB, is still an important public health problem in developing countries (2,4). The challenges in the management of TBM are listed in Table 17.2. Despite the common occurrence, extensive research and widespread public awareness, there is often a delay in the diagnosis and institution of specific therapy for TBM. The average duration of symptoms before presentation in patients with TBM has varied widely from 11-72 days (11,12). This delay in diagnosis is unfortunate as the promptness with which anti-TB treatment is initiated is the single most important physician-controlled factor influencing the prospects for recovery without serious neurological sequelae (3-7).

Table 17.2. Challenges in the management of TB meningitis

Variable clinical history and clinical features

Lack of sufficient sensitivity and specificity of existing diagnostic methods

Incomplete knowledge on the value of new rapid diagnostic methods

Unsuitability of most of the improved diagnostic methods for low income countries

Missed and delayed diagnosis

Uncertain duration of chemotherapy

Noncompliance to long duration of anti-TB treatment

Emergence of multiple drug resistance

Uncertainties with respect to timing of anti-retroviral therapy in HIV-associated disease

TB = tuberculosis; HIV = human immunodeficiency virus

Pathogenesis

A majority of cases of TBM are caused by *Mtb*. Isolated cases of TBM caused by bovine, avian mycobacteria and nontuberculous mycobacteria [NTM] have also been documented (13). Infection with specific mycobacterial genotypes may predispose to neurological TB (14,15). TBM is invariably secondary to TB elsewhere in the body. It is generally believed that the critical event in the development of TBM is the rupture of a subependymally located tubercle [Rich focus] resulting in the delivery of infectious material into the subarachnoid space (16). In the bacteraemic phase of primary lung infection, metastatic foci can get established in any organ, which can become active after a variable period of clinical latency. Whether the critical subependymal tubercle develops during primary haematogenous dissemination or due to secondary haematogenous spread from an area of extra-cranial extra-pulmonary TB [EPTB] is still a matter of dispute. Conditions such as intercurrent viral infections,

advanced age, malnutrition, alcoholism, HIV/acquired immunodeficiency syndrome [AIDS], use of corticosteroids and other immunosuppressive drugs may compromise cellular immunity of the host leading to reactivation of a latent infection (3-7,13). However, a majority of cases of TBM occur in the absence of any clinically demonstrable extra-cranial infection or overt disturbance in host immune function.

Pathology

The pathology of TBM comprises [i] inflammatory meningeal exudate; [ii] ependymitis; [iii] vasculitis; [iv] encephalitis; and [v] disturbance of cerebrospinal fluid [CSF] circulation and absorption [Table 17.3]. The leptomeningeal reaction is characterised by a serofibrinous exudate lying between the pia and arachnoid intermixed with areas of caseous necrosis. The cellular exudate consists predominantly of lymphocytes and plasma cells with infrequent epithelioid cells and giant cells. The proliferative arachnoiditis is most marked at the base of the brain, most prominent in the area of the optic chiasma. As the process of optico-chiasmatic arachnoiditis becomes more chronic, it may progress and encircle the brainstem to involve the function of other cranial nerves. For a detailed description of the pathology of TBM, the reader is referred to the chapter *"Pathology of tuberculosis" [Chapter 3]*.

Table 17.3: Pathology of TB meningitis

Meningitis
    Inflammatory leptomeningeal exudate
    Caseous necrosis
    Proliferative opticochiasmatic arachnoiditis

Vasculitis
    Arteritis
    Phlebitis

Ependymitis and choroid plexitis

Encephalitis
    Cortical
    Subependymal
    Vasculitis and infarction
    Encephalopathy

Hydrocephalus
    Communicating
    Obstructive

TB = tuberculosis

Ependymitis is almost a constant feature of TBM and may even be more severe than the meningeal reaction. The choroid plexus may show varying degrees of inflammatory process. The terminal portion of the internal carotid artery and proximal middle cerebral artery in the sylvian fissure are the vessels most frequently involved by vasculitis with inflammation, spasm, constriction and thrombosis. The meningeal veins traversing the inflammatory exudate show varying degrees of phlebitis and thrombosis. The brain parenchyma immediately underlying the meningeal exudate as well as the subependymal region shows a variable degree of oedema, perivascular inflammation and microglial reaction. A majority of infarcts occur in the territory of the middle cerebral artery.

Hydrocephalus develops in the majority of patients with TBM who have been symptomatic for more than 2-3 weeks (17,18). In the majority, it is a communicating hydrocephalus due to the blockage of the basal cisterns by the exudate in the acute stage and adhesive leptomeningitis in the chronic stage. Less frequently, the hydrocephalus is obstructive due to either narrowing or occlusion of aqueduct by ependymal inflammation or by a strategically placed brainstem tuberculoma, or at the outlet foraminae of the fourth ventricle. Hydrocephalus is more frequent and severe in children than in adults.

A pathological entity predominantly seen in the paediatric age group, designated as TB encephalopathy, characterised by diffuse brain oedema, perivascular myelinolysis and haemorrhagic leucoencephalitis with little evidence of meningitis has been described from India (19). This syndrome is ascribed to hypersensitivity reaction to tuberculoproteins. Clinical and pathological distinction of this entity from Reye's syndrome, acute disseminated encephalomyelitis and acute haemorrhagic leucoencephalitis will be difficult. There is little pathological evidence for the existence of TB encephalopathy without TBM.

Clinical Features

In developing countries, TBM is still a disease of childhood with the highest incidence in the first three years of life (3-7,20). Recent contact with TB, when elicited, can be found in 70%-90% of children with TBM (21). The disease usually evolves gradually over 2-6 weeks although an acute onset of illness can occur in 50% of children and in 14% of adults (21). The prodromal phase is non-specific and usually lasts 2-3 weeks with a history of vague ill-health, apathy, irritability, anorexia and behavioural changes. As a part of the prodrome, headache, vomiting or fever may occur in 13%-30% of patients and herald the onset of meningitis. Focal neurological deficits and features of raised intracranial tension may precede signs of meningeal irritation. Focal or generalised convulsions are encountered in 20%-30% of patients sometime during the course of illness and are particularly common in children and the elderly (3-7,13). The underlying mechanism could include hydrocephalus, tuberculoma, cerebral oedema, and hyponatraemia due to the syndrome of inappropriate antidiuretic hormone [SIADH] secretion. Cranial nerve palsies can occur in 20%-30% of patients, the sixth nerve involvement being the most common (3-7,13).

Exudate around the optic chiasma is the central feature of the pathology in TBM. Hence, complete or partial loss of vision is a major complication of the disease. The other mechanisms for vision loss may include arteritis or compression of the anterior visual pathways due to hydrocephalus or tuberculoma. Ethambutol toxicity too may contribute to the visual impairment. The frequency of optic nerve involvement in clinical reports varies from 4%-35% (13,22). Visual evoked potentials testing has shown disturbance in over 50% of patients examined in the acute stage of the disease (23).

In untreated cases, adhesions in the basal brain progress and result in expensive cranial nerve palsies, internal carotid constriction and stroke, increasing hydrocephalus with tentorial herniation, pupillary abnormalities, pyramidal signs and progressive deterioration in the consciousness state. The terminal illness is characterised by deep coma and decerebrate or decorticate posturing. Without treatment, death usually occurs in five to eight weeks.

According to the severity of the illness, patients with TBM can be categorised into three to five clinical stages (24-26). One of the clinical staging systems is shown in Table 17.4. The clinical staging helps to optimise therapy [e.g., addition of dexamethasone to anti-TB drugs] and to predict the prognosis. The prognosis of TBM is determined by the clinical stage at the time of initiation of treatment.

During the last two decades, the picture of TBM has changed in developed countries with an increasing number of atypical cases (3-7). Atypical presentations of TBM include acute meningitis syndrome simulating pyogenic meningitis, progressive dementia, status epilepticus, psychosis, stroke syndrome, locked-in-state, trigeminal neuralgia, and infantile spasm and movement disorders (13,22,27). The factors that are thought to be responsible for this changing pattern include delay in the age of onset of primary infection, immunisation, problems related to immigrant populations and HIV infection (3,5,6).

Table 17.4: Clinical staging system for TB meningitis	
Stage	Description
1	Conscious and rational, with or without neck stiffness, but no focal neurological signs or signs of hydrocephalus
2	Conscious but confused or has focal signs such as cranial nerve palsies or hemiparesis
3	Comatose or delirious with or without dense neurological deficit
4	Deeply comatose with decerebrate or decorticate posturing

TB = tuberculosis
Source: references 24-26

Tuberculosis Meningitis and Human Immunodeficiency Virus Infection

HIV-associated TB accounts for nearly 25% of global HIV/AIDS deaths each year (28).The risk of neurological TB is 5 times more frequent in HIV-seropositive compared to HIV-seronegative patients (28-31). Berenguer et al (29) reported that 10% of 455 patients co-infected with both TB and HIV-developed TBM. Yechoor et al (31) observed that 20 of the 31 patients [65%] identified as definite or probable TBM over a 12-year period were co-infected with

HIV. Neurological TB, either alone or associated with other opportunistic infections [OIs], was found in 35 of the 100 HIV-seropositive patients seen over seven years at the National Institute for Mental Health and Neurosciences [NIMHANS] in Bengaluru [earlier called Bangalore], in south India (32).

Although HIV-infected patients are at an increased risk for TBM, the HIV status generally does not alter the clinical manifestations, CSF findings and response to therapy (28-31). However, CSF examination may frequently be normal in HIV-seropositive subjects with TBM. In such patients, radiographic clues to the diagnosis of neurological TB include multiloculated abscess, cisternal enhancement, and basal ganglia infarction and communicating hydrocephalus, which are not the findings associated with the more commonly encountered CNS lymphoma or toxoplasma encephalitis. Extra-meningeal TB is seen more often [65%-77%] in patients co-infected with HIV and TB compared to HIV-seronegative individuals [9%] (29,33). Likewise, an associated tuberculoma may be present in more than half of HIV-infected patients with TBM (34). Neurological TB can also be the initial presentation of AIDS. Bishburg *et al* (30) noted that intravenous drug abusers with AIDS were more likely to develop TB of the CNS and TB brain abscesses.

Diagnosis

TBM should be differentiated from other causes of subacute and chronic meningitis [Table 17.5]. Early and accurate diagnosis of TBM can substantially reduce the morbidity and mortality, especially in children (3-6,13). Diagnosis of TBM is based on history, neurological symptoms, signs and CSF findings. Supporting features include radiological evidence from CT or MRI, such as, basal exudates, hydrocephalus, infarcts, tuberculomas and gyral enhancement. However, a definite diagnosis of TBM is fraught with difficulties because demonstration of *Mtb* in CSF is difficult and is often time-consuming.

Exposure to TB is important supportive evidence, especially in children. Evidence of TB outside the CNS with appropriate microbiological, molecular, radiographic or histopathological proof, a positive tuberculin skin test [TST] in the absence of a previous sub-clinical infection or bacille Calmette-Guérin [BCG] vaccination, and a resolution of the symptoms and signs of TBM after initiation of anti-TB treatment are also important supportive features for a diagnosis of TBM.

Laboratory Investigations

Routine laboratory studies are rarely helpful in establishing the diagnosis of TBM. Elevated erythrocyte sedimentation rate [ESR], anaemia and lymphocytosis are not seen in majority of the patients.

Imaging Studies

Chest radiograph The chest radiographs reveal findings consistent with pulmonary TB in 25%-50% of adult patients and 50%-90% of children with TBM seen in western countries (35).

Neuroimaging The CT or MRI of the brain may reveal thickening and enhancement of basal meninges, hydrocephalus, infarction, oedema [often periventricular], and mass lesions due to associated tuberculoma or TB abscess [Figures 9.37, 9.38]. Common sites of exudates are basal cisterna ambiens, suprasellar cistern and sylvian fissures [Figures 17.1, 17.2 and 17.3]. Bhargava *et al* (36) classified exudates as [i] mild, when cisterns were obliterated but not enhanced; [ii] moderate, when the cisterns were outlined by enhancing exudates and [iii] severe, when enhancing exudates enlarge the cisterns. Hydrocephalus is the single most common abnormality and is reported in 50%-80% of cases. The degree of hydrocephalus generally correlates with the duration of disease. Enhancements of basal meninges [60%] followed by cerebral infarction [28%], most frequently in the middle cerebral artery territory are other common findings. Bhargava *et al* (36) demonstrated the presence of hydrocephalus [83%], cerebral infarction [28%] and

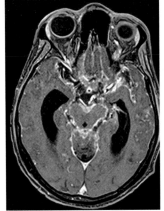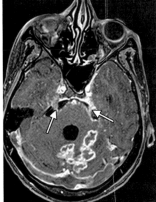

Figure 17.1: Contrast-enhanced axial fat saturated MR images of the brain showing meningeal enhancement in the interpeduncular cistern, perimesencephalic cistern and sylvian fissure. The temporal horns of the lateral ventricles, aqueduct and fourth ventricle are dilated, indicating a communicating hydrocephalus. Also, conglomerate irregular ring enhancing lesion in the cerebellum [tuberculoma] and enhancing V cranial nerves [arrows] are seen
MR = magnetic resonance

Table 17.5: Differential diagnosis of TB meningitis
Partially-treated bacterial meningitis
Cryptococcal meningitis
Viral meningoencephalitis
Carcinomatous meningitis
Parameningeal infection
Neurosarcoidosis
Neurosyphilis
TB = tuberculosis

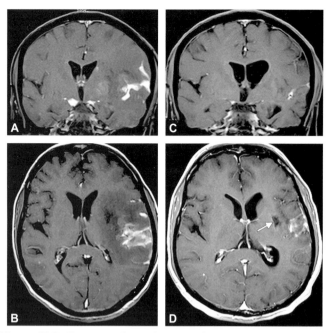

Figure 17.2: Contrast-enhanced coronal fat saturated [A] and axial [B] T1-weighted MR images of a 43-year-old male, who presented with fever, headache, vomiting of two months duration followed by acute onset aphasia and right hemiplegia, showing thick enhancing exudates in the left sylvian fissure and suprasellar cistern. Surrounding parenchymal oedema and mass effect are noted. Post-contrast coronal fat saturated [C] and axial [D] T1-weighted images three months after anti-TB treatment show decrease in enhancement, oedema and mass effect. Lateral putaminal infarct [arrow] secondary to vasculitis can be seen
MR = magnetic resonance

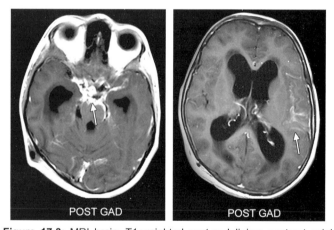

Figure 17.3: MRI brain, T1-weighted post-gadolinium contrast axial images showing ventricular dilatation and meningeal enhancement [arrows]
MRI = magnetic resonance imaging

tuberculoma [10%] on CT in patients with TBM. Vasculitis and thrombosis associated with TBM are seen on CT as multiple areas of hypodensity secondary to ischaemia. Serial CT are very helpful in assessing the course of tuberculomas and hydrocephalus. Gadolinium-enhanced MRI is superior to the CT scan in detection of basal meningeal enhancement and small tuberculomas. Contrast-enhanced MRI has been found to be superior to contrast-enhanced CT [CECT] in the detection of diffuse and focal meningeal granulomatous lesions. The MRI is also superior to CT in delineating focal infarcts of the basal ganglia and diencephalon [Figure 17.2]. Furthermore, MRI is superior to CT in defining the presence, location and extent of associated brainstem lesions.

Tuberculin Skin Test

TST with purified protein derivative [PPD] has been reported to be positive in 40%-65% adults and in 85%-90% children with TBM in western studies (21,35,37). However, TST lacks specificity in developing countries because of the possibility of previous sensitisation to environmental mycobacteria and BCG vaccination.

Interferon Gamma Release Assays

Interferon gamma release assays [IGRAs] have been used for detecting infection with *Mtb* (38). The reader is referred to the chapter *"Laboratory diagnosis of tuberculosis: best practices and current policies" [Chpater 8]* for details.

Cerebrospinal Fluid Study

Cytology and biochemistry Clear CSF with moderately raised cells and protein and low glucose constitute the typical CSF picture of TBM. However, these characteristics are shared by other forms of chronic meningitis and partially treated pyogenic meningitis. In TBM, the leucocyte count is usually between 100 and 500 cells/µL, but rarely can exceed 1000 cells/µL. Median leucocyte counts in various reports range from 63-283 cells/µL. Predominantly, lymphocytes are increased in the CSF, although in the acute stage, a polymorphonuclear response is not unusual. This response is transient and is replaced by lymphocytic reaction in the course of days to weeks. Occasionally the cell count may be normal. Rarely, the CSF may be haemorrhagic because of fibrinoid necrosis of vessels. A negative cytology for malignant cells in the CSF is an essential criterion for the diagnosis of TBM.

The CSF protein is generally between 100-200 mg/dL. In the presence of coexisting spinal meningitis and spinal block, the values can exceed 1 g/dL and the fluid may be xanthochromic. If allowed to stand, a pellicle or cobweb may form, indicating the presence of fibrinogen. The pellicle is highly suggestive but not pathognomonic of TBM. The CSF protein has been reported to be normal in some patients with AIDS and TBM (29,39).

The CSF glucose level is abnormal in majority of cases, being less than 40% of the corresponding blood glucose level. Median glucose levels are reported to be between 18-45 mg/dL. In patients with TBM, CSF glucose levels are never undetectable as in patients with pyogenic meningitis. Low CSF chloride level was previously considered to be a non-specific marker for TBM. It is actually a reflection of co-existent serum hypochloraemia and is presently not considered to be helpful in discriminating between TBM, bacterial and viral meningitis. Thomas et al (22) observed the classical TB pattern in 66.8% of cases; pseudopyogenic pattern in 14.5% patients and normal CSF in 5% cases.

Patients with miliary TB and CNS involvement can, sometimes, present with a normal CSF profile and absence of neurologic signs. An acellular CSF may also be found in elderly patients suffering from TBM (33). In a report, Raman spectroscopy of the CSF demonstrating silicates was found to be highly sensitive and specific test for the diagnosis of TBM (40).

Microbiological tests A negative Gram's stain, negative India ink stain and a sterile culture for bacteria and fungi are pre-requisites for the diagnosis of TBM. Demonstration of acid-fast bacilli [AFB] in the CSF by microscopy is the most crucial part of the investigation and the rate of detection varies in different reports from 12.5%-69% (37,41). The yield of CSF smears by Ziehl-Neelsen staining and auramine staining is low, ranging from 4%-40% in various reports and is found to be a function of the volume and the number of samples of CSF. Centrifuging the CSF [10-20 mL] for 30 minutes and thick smear examination from the pellicle and repeat CSF examination enhance the detection rate. Kennedy and Fallon (25) in a series of 52 patients with TBM reported a higher yield of AFB with examination of four CSF smear samples [37% in the first, and a further 25%, 19% and 3% in the second, third and fourth samples, respectively].

Lowenstein-Jensen [LJ] culture of CSF takes four to eight weeks to isolate the organisms because of the slow growth of *Mtb*. The reported positivity of CSF culture ranges from 25%-70% of cases, but is less than 50% in most reports (3-7). In many Indian reports, the yield has been much lower, around 20% (13,22). The yield can be increased by using liquid culture media, such as, Septi-Chek AFB system, and Middlebrook 7H9 instead of the conventional LJ medium. The isolation rate of *Mtb* is higher from cisternal and ventricular CSF than lumbar CSF (42), but in routine practice, CSF is seldom collected from the ventricles. Similar to AFB smear examination, repeated cultures of CSF samples increased the sensitivity from 52% for the first culture up to 83% after four cultures (25). In patients with disseminated and miliary TB with CNS involvement, cultures from extra-neural sites such as the sputum, lymph node and bone marrow may be positive.

Immunological tests As the CSF picture in patients with TBM can be variable and non-specific, there is urgent need for a reliable and rapid test to diagnose TBM. In the Indian context, the difficulty in differentiating TBM from partially treated pyogenic meningitis is an added problem.

Several tests have been devised for these reasons and they are broadly divided into direct tests that measure the chemical components or antigens of *Mtb* and indirect tests that measure the components of the host response to *Mtb*. The specificity of immunodiagnosis depends on the specificity of the antigens or antibodies used. Non-availability of a clear cut "gold standard" has hampered the validation of the usefulness of newer diagnostic tests for the

diagnosis of TBM. As the yield of conventional methods, such as, culture is low when applied to the CSF in patients with suspected TBM, these methods cannot be considered to be a gold standard against which immunodiagnosis or other tests can be compared. In tests, such as, enzyme-linked immunosorbent assay [ELISA], a significant overlap between the results of patients with and without TBM necessitates specification of a cut-off point to separate positive from negative test results. When establishing such a cut-off, there is usually a trade-off between sensitivity and specificity. With regards to immunoassays, it is also important to understand that the sensitivity of any immunoassay depends on standardisation and evaluation of the assay system, whereas specificity depends on the type of the probe employed in the system. Furthermore, false-negative results of antigen detecting immunoassays can also result from masking of the antigens by specific circulating antibodies.

Mycobacterial antibodies Antibodies against glycolipids and proteins isolated from *Mtb*, BCG, PPD, antigen 5, and lipo-arabinomannan [LAM] have all been used as a supporting test in the diagnosis of TBM. Radioimmunoassay [RIA], ELISA, and immunoblot methods have all been used to detect these antibodies. Various authors have reported sensitivity ranging from 61%-90% and specificity ranging from 58%-100% with these antibodies (43-48). Assay of antibodies against *Mtb* antigens has a better sensitivity and specificity than PPD or BCG. Recent antibody targets have included antibodies against A-60 antigen. They have shown a greater sensitivity in sera [95%] compared to CSF and a greater specificity in the CSF [100%] compared to the sera (49,50).

Mycobacterial antigens There are many reports of detection of mycobacterial antigens using ELISA and latex particle agglutination (51-54). Antigen detection has been shown to be more specific than antibody assays. Rabbit immunoglobulin G [IgG] raised against BCG, culture filtrate antigen, antigen 5, and immunoabsorbent affinity column-purified antigen have all been used for antigen detection. The diagnostic yield is considerably improved by performing both antigen and antibody assays (46,55). Other mycobacterial antigen targets have included the 35kDa antigen (56). Unfortunately, many assays showing early promise in highly controlled studies do not perform with high sensitivity and specificity in clinical practice.

Circulating immune complexes Circulating immune complexes in the serum and CSF of patients have been used in the diagnosis of TBM by isolating these complexes and confirming the presence of mycobacterial antigens and antibodies by ELISA test. Mathai et al (46) demonstrated antigen 5 in the immune complexes of CSF in 30% of their patients with TBM. The antigen concentration in the immune complexes declined during the course of treatment. Though antimycobacterial antibodies were present in 70% patients, the immune complexes were not formed probably because of the non-availability of antigen 5 in optimal concentration.

Patil *et al* (55) detected immune complexes in the CSF in 60% and antimycobacterial antibodies in 55% and both in 82% patients with suspected TBM.

Other indirect measures of host response Adenosine deaminase [ADA], an enzyme produced by T-lymphocytes, is elevated in the CSF of 60%-100% of patients with TBM (57-59). However, false-positive results have been reported in other forms of meningitis. The CSF lymphocyte transformation assay, detection of anti-BCG secreting cells in CSF, leucocyte migration inhibition assay, and T-cell immunoblotting are other tests used as indirect evidence of host response to *Mtb*.

Biochemical detection of mycobacterial products Detection of tuberculostearic acid [TSA], a structural component of *Mtb* has been reported to have a sensitivity of about 75% and specificity of 96% (60). Requirement of complex instrumentation is a major limitation to its wide application. Detection of 3-[2-ketohexyl] indoline has also been used as an evidence of *Mtb* infection (61).

Molecular methods Amplification of the *Mtb* specific deoxyribonucleic acid [DNA] sequences by polymerase chain reaction [PCR] is one of the most frequently used means for rapid diagnosis of neurological TB (62-66). The use of primers derived from the insertion sequence IS*6110*, which is a multiple repetitive element in the genome of the *Mtb* complex, has yielded amplification of high analytical sensitivity. One-step amplification used in conventional methods has a low sensitivity, which is attributed to the low copy numbers of the DNA template that could be extracted from CSF samples of patients with TBM. In comparison, two-step nested amplification can enhance the sensitivity by several folds. Using this technique, Liu *et al* (64) detected *Mtb* genome in 19 of the 21 [90.5%] patients with clinically suspected TBM.

Cartridge-based nucleic acid amplification tests [CBNAAT] [e.g., Xpert MTB/RIF] are increasingly being used for the diagnosis of TB meningitis. The CSF Xpert MTB/RIF has the advantage of being the only available technique besides AFB smear test, which can confirm the diagnosis of TB on the same day. The Xpert MTB/RIF is not affected by the presence of other infecting bacteria as may occur in an immunocompromised host. In the recently published Guidelines for extrapulmonary TB for India [INDEX-TB Guidelines] (67a), pooled sensitivity and specificity of CSF Xpert MTB/RIF against culture were found to be 80.5% and 97.8% respectively. In a recently published systematic review (67b) the sensitivity and specificity of CSF Xpert MTB/RIF were found to be 71.1% and 98% respectively. The INDEX-TB guidelines recommended that Xpert MTB/Rif may be used as an adjunctive test for the diagnosis of TB meningitis. A negative Xpert MTB/RIF test result on a CSF specimen does not rule out TB meningitis. The decision to give anti-TB treatment should be based on clinical features and CSF profile [conditional recommendation, low quality evidence for sensitivity estimate, high quality evidence for specificity estimate].

Comparative value of different tests It can be concluded that even though there are many recently introduced rapid diagnostic methods for TBM, most of them lack the required combination of reproducibility, high sensitivity and specificity. Thus, a negative test does not exclude TBM and many immunodiagnositc tests show false-positive results in other forms of meningitis. Unless stringent measures are adopted to prevent cross-contamination in laboratories, false-positive results could limit the use of commercial available NAAT assays.

In the developing countries, confirmation of the diagnosis, either by molecular methods or by immunological methods is seldom possible in every case, because of the limited facilities available. Apart from the investigations, there are indirect evidences of the disease being TBM, especially in countries with a high prevalence of TB infection. These include clinical diagnosis of chronic meningitis, a history of pulmonary TB, especially if inadequately treated, exposure to a patient with pulmonary, a positive TST and CT or MRI evidence of basal meningitis and/or its sequelae. Though none of the above information in isolation is sufficient, a combination of these factors should raise the suspicion of a diagnosis of TBM.

Treatment

If suspicion of TBM is high, anti-TB treatment should be initiated at the earliest. The *pros* and *cons* of initiating anti-TB treatment before the confirmation of the diagnosis should be carefully weighed in each patient. However, the most important principle of therapy is that anti-TB treatment should be initiated when the disease is suspected. It should not be delayed until proof of diagnosis of TBM has been obtained.

The following situations can be considered as separate management issues in TBM.

Uncomplicated Tuberculosis Meningitis

It is important to stage TBM patients according to one of the clinical stages described earlier before the initiation of treatment (24-26). Primary management of this condition is with first-line anti-TB agents. There are no convincing randomised, controlled clinical trials to suggest that any particular regimen is superior in the treatment of TBM. However, enormous clinical experience has accumulated over the past many years to recommend some treatment regimens (1,3-7,13). It is advisable to commence a four-drug regimen. The recommended drugs are isoniazid, rifampicin, pyrazinamide and ethambutol or streptomycin. Though a drug susceptibility result is preferred prior to, or soon after starting the treatment, it is seldom practical, especially in developing countries. Unless there is a very high suspicion of drug-resistant organism in a particular patient, the proposed four-drug regimen is generally effective. After two months of intensive phase of treatment, pyrazinamide, streptomycin are stopped. In the continuation phase, rifampicin, isoniazid and ethambutol are continued. Pyridoxine is usually administered along with anti-TB treament to reduce the risk of isoniazid-induced peripheral neuropathy. However, there is no consensus regarding the optimal dose of pyridoxine; a wide dosage range [10 mg/day to 100 mg/day] of pyridoxine has been used to prevent peripheral neuropathy in high-risk groups.

A recently published randomised, double-blind, placebo-controlled trial (68) in patients with TBM compared a standard, 9-month anti-TB treatment regimen [that included rifampicin 10 mg/kg/day] with an intensified regimen [that included a higher-dose rifampicin, 15 mg/kg/day] and levofloxacin [20 mg/kg/day] for the first 8 weeks of treatment. Occurrence of death by 9 months of randomisation was defined as as the primary outcome. In this study (68), intensified anti-TB treatment was not associated with a higher rate of survival.

The reader is referred to the chapters *"Treatment of tuberculosis"* [*Chapter 44*] and *"Revised National Tuberculosis Control Programme"* [*Chapter 53*] for further details.

Duration of Treatment

The optimum duration of treatment for TBM is unknown. Longer duration of treatment possibly lowers the relapse rates, though the cost, risk of toxicity and chances of poor compliance are greater. In a large series of 95 children treated with a four-drug regimen, with 96% of cases presenting in Medical Research Council [MRC] stage 2 or 3, a high rate of success and a mortality of as low as 16% was achieved with 6 months treatment (69). In another large series [n = 781] of TBM, nearly all patients with relapse had received less than 6 months of therapy (70). The maximum duration of treatment has varied. The British Thoracic Society [BTS] (71), the American Thoracic Society [ATS], Centers for Disease Control and Prevention [CDC] and Infectious Diseases Society of America [IDSA] (72) prescribe 12 months of treatment for uncomplicated TBM. Although 18 to 24 months treatment was recommended in the past (70), there is substantial evidence to suggest that a duration ranging between 6 to 12 months may be adequate (73,74). As per the recently published evidence-based INDEX-TB guidelines (67a), TB meningitis should be treated with standard first-line anti-TB treatment for at least 9 months. These guidelines also indicate that extension of anti-TB treatment may, sometimes, be indicated and this should be assessed by the treating clinician on a case-by-case basis.

Additional factors that need to be considered prior to the initiation of treatment include age, co-existent renal or hepatic disease and pregnancy. One of the most common drug-induced side effects during the treatment of TB is the development of hepatotoxicity (75). It is practically impossible to differentiate drug-induced hepatotoxicity [DIH] from coincidental viral hepatitis that is highly prevalent in developing countries. The reader is referred to the chapter *"Hepatotoxicity associated with anti-tuberculosis treatment"* [*Chapter 45*] for further details.

Role of Corticosteroids

The role of corticosteroids in the treatment of TBM has been a subject of intense and interesting debate for many decades, with both proponents (76,77) and opponents (78,79) for its use. Administration of corticosteroids has been found to be most beneficial in patients with complications of TBM. The common indications for use of corticosteroids in TBM are listed in Table 17.6.

Seven trials of various degrees of rigour have investigated the effects of corticosteroids on TBM (80-86). Five of these seven trials, including the best-analysed one (80), clearly demonstrated an advantage of adjunctive corticosteroid therapy over standard therapy for survival, frequency of sequelae or both. The CSF abnormalities and elevated pressures resolved significantly faster in corticosteroid recipients. Two of the studies (80,83) stratified participants by severity and found no benefit in either mild or severe disease, but significant benefit for patients with intermediate disease. Studies with longer regimens [4 weeks to several 'months'] demonstrated significant beneficial effects while those with shorter regimens [2-4 weeks] did not. Dexamethazone at 8 to 12 mg/day (80,81,83) or prednisolone of equivalent dose (86,87) was effective and had fewer side effects than higher doses. The recommended daily dose of prednisolone is 0.75 to 1 mg/kg in adults and 1 to 2.5 mg/kg/day in children.

In a randomised prospective study of 47 patients, Kumaravelu *et al* (88) reported that the addition of dexamethasone to anti-TB treatment resulted in better outcome in those who had severe disease. In a randomised, double-blind, placebo-controlled trial [n = 545] from Vietnam, Thwaites *et al* (89) studied whether adjunctive treatment with dexamethasone reduced the risk of death or severe disability after nine months of follow-up. In this study, patients were randomly assigned to groups that received either dexamethasone [n = 274] or placebo [n = 271]. It was observed that treatment with dexamethasone was associated with a reduced risk of death [p = 0.01]. However, dexamethasone treatment did not result in a significant reduction in the proportion of severely disabled patients [18.2% among survivors in the dexamethasone group versus 13.8% in the placebo group, p = 0.27] or in the proportion of patients who had either died or were severely disabled

---

Table 17.6: Possible indications for corticosteroids in TB meningitis

Clinical
    Clinical stages 2 and above
    Evidence of raised intracranial pressure
    Focal neurological deficits suggesting arteritis

Radiological
    Cerebral/perilesional oedema
    Hydrocephalus
    Infarcts
    Opticochiasmatic pachymeningitis

TB = tuberculosis

after nine months of treatment. The treatment effect was consistent across subgroups that were defined by disease severity grade and by HIV status.

As per the recently published evidence-based INDEX-TB guidelines (67a), corticosteroids are recommended for TBM in HIV-seronegative persons; the duration of corticosteroid treatment to be for at least 4 weeks with tapering as appropriate [strong recommendation]. In HIV-seropositve individuals with TBM, corticosteroids may be used where other life-threatening opportunistic infections are absent.

Drug-resistant Tuberculosis Meningitis

TBM caused by multidrug-resistant and extensively drug-resistant *Mtb* is a serious condition and several newer drugs and treatment regimens are available to treat drug-resistant TBM (90-92). The reader is referred to the chapter *"Drug-resistant tuberculosis" [Chapter 42]* for details.

Treatment of Tuberculosis Meningitis Associated with Human Immunodeficiency Virus Infection

The management of HIV-seropositive patients co-infected with TBM requires a combination of anti-TB treatment, anti-retroviral therapy [ART], and trimethoprim-sulphamethoxazole prophylaxis against other opportunistic injections (93). Because of the concern of immune reconstitution disease with rapid ART initiation (94,95), which is particularly severe when associated with neurological TB, the optimal time to initiate ART during TB treatment is still being debated (96). The recent revision of the 2010 WHO ART guidelines recommended to start ART as soon as possible after TB treatment is tolerated, but not later than 8 weeks of anti-TB treatment (97). Treatment of neurological TB in patients with HIV infection is the same as in patients without HIV infection (98). The reader is referred to the chapter *"Tuberculosis and human immunodeficiency virus infection"* [Chapter 35] for further details.

Monitoring Therapy

Once anti-TB treatment is initiated, the mononuclear pleocytosis in CSF may briefly become polymorphonuclear. At two months of anti-TB treatment, CSF glucose levels normalise in almost all, patients. Normalisation of CSF protein levels takes between 4 to 26 months, with a median period of eight months (21). The CSF cell counts normalise in one-third of the patients by 16 months and in almost all patients by three years (21).

Clinical improvement in the form of abatement off ever and decrease in meningeal signs occurs over a variable period of time. However, clinical improvement may not be reflected in the improvement in CSF parameters. Any clinical worsening during treatment warrants neuroimaging to rule out complications, such as, hydrocephalus, tuberculoma, TB abscess or arteritis leading to infarction. Vigilance should also be maintained to detect the development of anti-TB DIH, ethambutol-induced optic neuritis and streptomycin-

induced vestibulopathy. These complications develop at varying intervals and are dose related.

A repeat CSF examination may not be required in patients showing a steady clinical improvement. However, in patients, showing neither clinical improvement nor deterioration, CSF parameters should be monitored along with neuroimaging, if required. In those patients showing deterioration in clinical status, neuroimaging should precede a CSF examination.

Complications of Tuberculosis Meningitis

TBM is a devastating disease with about 30% mortality in the severe forms of the disease and neurological sequelae in a majority of the survivors (3-7). In a series from a teaching hospital from North-west India (22), only 58 of the 170 surviving patients [34%] with TBM were left with no sequelae. In the west, permanent neurological sequelae was noticed in 47%-80% of children with TBM, with motor disorders [25%-27%], visual loss [20%] and cognitive and behavioural changes [17%-40%] being the three most common consequences in long-term follow-up studies (37,99). In a study of 65 patients from Lucknow, India (100), neurological sequelae were observed in 78.5% patients [cognitive impairment in 55%, motor deficit in 40%, optic atrophy in 37% and other cranial nerve palsy in 23%]. The complications, sequelae of TBM are listed in Table 17.7.

Table 17.7: Complications and sequelae of TB meningitis
Raised intracranial pressure, cerebral oedema, stupor
Basal meningitis with cranial nerve palsies
Focal neurological deficits
Hydrocephalus
Tuberculoma
TB abscess
Opticochiasmatic pachymeningitis resulting in visual loss
TB arteritis and stroke
Endocrine disturbances
Hypothalamic disorder leading to loss of control of blood pressure and body temperature
Diabetes insipidus
SIADH
Internuclear ophthalmoplegia
Hemichorea
Psychiatric and psychological disturbances
Hearing defects
Intracranial calcifications
Seizures and epilepsy
Spinal block
Spinal arachnoiditis
TB = tuberculosis; SIADH = syndrome of inappropriate antidiuretic hormone secretion

Hydrocephalus

Hydrocephalus is common in TBM, occurring in about two-thirds of patients and is more common in children (17,18). The most frequent cause for hydrocephalus, in almost 75% of cases, is obstruction to CSF flow by exudates in the basal cisterns, known as communicating hydrocephalus. In the remaining 25%, the hydrocephalus is due to a block at the outlet foramina of the fourth ventricle or at the aqueduct causing obstructive [non-communicating] hydrocephalus.

The management of hydrocephalus in TBM is still associated with considerable uncertainties and controversies. The clinical grade of the patient appears to be one of the most important determinants of how to manage these patients. The grading system of patients with TBM with hydrocephalus evolved at the Christian Medical College, Vellore, India is shown in Table 17.8 (101). Medical management with furosemide, acetazolamide, steroids and weekly, or more frequent lumbar punctures has been reported to be successful in a significant proportion of patients with communicating hydrocephalus in clinical stages I and II (17). Patients with altered sensorium [grades III and IV] will require CSF diverting procedures to reduce the raised intracranial pressure. Surgical measures available are ventricular tap, external ventricular drainage [EVD], ventriculoperitonial [VP] shunt and endoscopic third ventriculostomy [ETV]. Ventricular tap and EVD are emergency short-term procedures for patients in poor condition who require reduction in CSF pressure immediately. Because of the inherent risk of infection, EVD cannot be used for long periods. In patients who require EVD for more than 4 or 5 days, it is better to place an Ommaya reservoir and do regular tapping of the ventricles till meningitis subsides and decision on shunt surgery taken (102). The choice between VP shunt and ETV varies between centers depending upon their experience. Most of the centers recommend ETV as the first choice for patients with TBM and hydrocephalus, with VP shunts reserved for failed ETV cases (17,18). Even children with clinical grade IV with TBM may benefit from VP shunts (103).

Hyponatraemia

Hyponatraemia is common in TBM and is an independent risk factor for poor outcome (104). Although two conditions have been implicated in the development of hyponatraemia

Table 17.8: Clinical grading system for patients with TB meningitis with hydrocephalus

Grade	Description
I	No neurological deficit and normal sensorium [GCS 15]
II	Neurological deficit present, normal sensorium [GCS 15]
III	Neurological deficit present, altered sensorium, but easily arousable [GCS 9-14]
IV	Comatose [GCS 3-8], decerebrate or decorticate posturing

TB = tuberculosis; GCS = Glasgow coma scale
Adapted from reference 101

in TBM, namely the syndrome of inappropriate anti-diuretic hormone secretion [SIADH] and cerebral salt wasting [CSW], the distinction between them is often difficult to make (105,106). Given the difficulty of making a definitive diagnosis of the cause of hyponatraemia, fluid restriction as a treatment for hyponatraemia should be avoided in patients with TBM. Cautious treatment with hypertonic saline and fludrocortisone is advised (106,107). The reader is referred to the chapter "Endocrine implications of tuberculosis" [Chapter 34] for more details on SIADH and diabetes insipidus.

Vasuclitis stroke occurs in 15%-57% of patients with TBM, especially in advanced and severe disease (108,109). Most of the infarcts in TBM are multiple, bilateral and located in the basal ganglia, especially in the caudate, anterior thalamus and internal capsule. These are related to the involvement of perforating arteries which are embedded in exudates. Major territorial infarcts can occur due to involvement of proximal portions of the middle, anterior and posterior cerebral arteries as well as the supraclinoid portion of the internal carotid artery [Figure 17.2].

Opticochiasmatic Arachnoiditis

Early institution of anti-TB treatment may help in preventing the occurrence optico-chiasmatic arachnoiditis causing visual loss. Although steroids have been recommended for its prevention, treatment of established optico-chiasmatic arachnoiditis is disappointing.

CHRONIC MENINGITIS

Definition and Aetiology

Chronic meningitis is defined as the clinical syndrome characterised by symptoms and signs of meningitis or meningoencephalitis developing in a subacute or chronic fashion associated with CSF abnormalities and persisting for at least four weeks (110-112). In general, chronic meningitis has an insidious evolution and a gradual progressive course. Sometimes chronic meningitis may begin relatively acutely and may become chronic later on. Chronic meningitis is a potential manifestation of several infectious and non-infectious diseases (110-112) [Table 17.9].

As the aetiology of chronic meningitis is diverse, these patients require a thorough diagnostic evaluation to establish the cause. Partially treated pyogenic meningitis often needs to be differentiated from chronic meningitis. In India, majority of patients with chronic meningitis are presumed to have TBM and are treated accordingly. A detailed account of various aetiological causes of chronic meningitis is beyond the scope of this chapter. The diagnostic and therapeutic approach in patients with chronic meningitis will be discussed briefly.

TB is the most common cause of chronic meningitis in the developing world, where TB is highly endemic. By contrast, in areas with a low prevalence of TB, the scenario may be different. In a study from Mayo Clinic (113), sarcoidosis [31%] and metastatic adenocarcinoma [25%] were the most frequent causes of chronic meningitis.

Table 17.9: Causes of chronic meningitis

Infectious causes
    Mycobacterium tuberculosis
    Partially-treated bacterial meningitis
    Cryptococcus neoformans
    Treponema pallidum
    Borrelia burgdorferi
    Candida
    Brucella
    Leptospira icterohaemorrhagiae
    Coccidioides immitis
    Histoplasma capsulatum
    Aspergillus
    Toxoplasma gondii
    Actinomyces
    Nocardia
    Zygomycetes
    Larva migrans

Non-infectious causes
    Neoplasms
    Sarcoidosis
    Vasculitis
    Connective tissue disorders: SLE, Behcet's disease
    Vogt-Koyanagi-Harada syndrome
    Chronic benign lymphocytic meningitis
    Mollaret's meningitis
    Drug/chemical exposure: iodophendylate dye, sulphonamides, isoniazid, ibuprofen, and tolmentin

TB = tuberculosis; SLE = systemic lupus erythematosus

Clinical Evaluation

The history is critical to distinguish partially treated pyogenic meningitis and TBM [which may present as acute onset chronic meningitis], chronic meningitis with remission and exacerbations, and recurrent meningitis [Mollaret's meningitis]. Useful aetiological clues such as a known systemic disease, immunocompromised state, exposure to drugs and infectious agents [such as *Borrelia*, *Treponema*, *Leptospira* and *Brucella*] can be obtained from a carefully taken history. Physical examination may reveal a systemic disease, erythema nodosum [EN] which may occur in TB, sarcoidosis, histoplasmosis, coccidioidomycosis, erythema chronicum migrans [Lyme disease], oral and genital ulcers [Behcet's disease], pulmonary abnormalities [suggestive of TB, sarcoidosis, fungal infections], heart murmurs [bacterial endocarditis] and splenomegaly [lymphoproliferative diseases, brucellosis]. Ophthalmoscopic examination may show choroid tubercles, sarcoid granulomas or uveitis [Behcet's disease, Vogt-Koyanagi-Harada syndrome]. Granulomatous myositis [tender, nodular muscles and proximal weakness] may be found in sarcoidosis.

Diagnostic Evaluation

Chest radiograph, bronchoscopy with transbronchial lung biopsy, open lung biopsy, and lymph node or liver biopsy may help in identifying systemic diseases. Neutrophilic CSF pleocytosis may occur in chemical meningitis, systemic lupus erythematosus [SLE], bacterial [*Actinomycetes, Listeria, Nocardia*] and fungal [*Aspergillus, Candida, Zygomycetes*] meningitis. Eosinophilic CSF pleocytosis favours a parasitic aetiology. Low glucose in the CSF is non-specific and can occur in a variety of infectious and non-infectious causes of chronic meningitis. The CSF should be exhaustively searched for specific aetiologic clues utilising the currently available facilities.

Contrast-enhanced CT or MRI of the head, in addition to revealing hydrocephalus and parenchymal lesions, may demonstrate meningeal enhancement. In the study from the Mayo Clinic (113), MRI with gadolinium contrast was the most useful diagnostic imaging technique demonstrating meningeal enhancement in 15 of 32 patients [47%] while CT showed meningeal enhancement only in 2 of 32 [6%].

Despite numerous diagnostic advances, the cause of chronic meningitis frequently remains a diagnostic dilemma. Few patients eventually require a leptomeningeal biopsy, with or without sampling of underlying cortex through suboccipital and pterional craniotomy. In a study (113), a definitive aetiological diagnosis of chronic meningitis was made in 16 of 41 biopsies [39%]. In patients in whom meningeal enhancement was present on CT or MRI, a diagnosis was obtained in 80%, while in contrast only 9% of non-enhancing regions were diagnostic. Therefore, CECT or MRI findings provide valuable assistance in predicting the yield and selecting the site for biopsy.

Management

In patients with inconclusive clinical and laboratory data concerning the aetiology of chronic meningitis, the decision between empirical therapeutic trial and meningeal biopsy is critical. The clinical presentation, especially the pace of progression of course of the disease, will often dictate the choice. Anti-tuberculosis treatment is indicated early in the course of chronic meningitis in a patient whose clinical condition shows deterioration. If PCR, serological tests and culture of the CSF for *Mtb* are all negative, TST continues to remain non-reactive even after re-testing at two weeks, and no clinical response occurs, then anti-TB treatment may be stopped after six weeks. The decision to empirically use potentially toxic antifungal drugs such as amphotericin-B in chronic meningitis is more difficult. In the absence of a positive proof for a fungal aetiology, the following situations may warrant such a strategy: [i] a host with neutropenia or compromised cell-mediated immunity; [ii] presence of unequivocal clinical evidence or culture or biopsy proven systemic fungal disease, and [iii] a patient with obscure chronic meningitis, hypoglycorrhachia and progressive neurological deterioration in spite of anti-TB treatment.

A well-preserved patient with undiagnosed chronic meningitis and a static or slowly progressive course is a candidate for meningeal biopsy, especially when the neuro-imaging studies suggest an enhancing lesion accessible through a pterional or suboccipital craniotomy. Empirical corticosteroid therapy in chronic meningitis is inappropriate because it can result in the rapid progression of an undiagnosed fungal disease. Of the 168 patients with chronic meningitis who were treated with anti-TB drugs at the Sri Chitra Tirunal Institute for Medical Sciences and Technology [SCTIMST], Thiruvananthapuram [earlier called Trivandrum], India (114,115), 19% required ventriculo-peritoneal shunt for symptomatic hydrocephalus. At one and half years follow-up, 20% patients had died, 44% were fully functional, the remaining 36% of patients had significant neurological sequelae.

INTRACRANIAL TUBERCULOMAS

Definition and Pathology

Tuberculoma is a mass of granulation tissue made up of a conglomeration of microscopic small tubercles. A tubercle consists of a central core of epithelioid cells surrounded by lymphocytes. Giant cells are scattered among epithelioid cells. The centre of the tuberculoma becomes necrotic, forming caseous material, while the periphery tends to be encapsulated with fibrous tissue. There may be liquefaction of the caseous material resulting in the formation of a TB abscess.

The size of cerebral tuberculomas is highly variable. In most cases their diameters range from a few millimeters to three to four centimeters (116). Intracranial tuberculomas in patients under the age of 20 years are usually infratentorial, but supratentorial lesions predominate in adults. Solitary tuberculomas are more frequent than multiple lesions.

Epidemiology

In the early decades of the twentieth century, cerebral tuberculoma was a common lesion, accounting for 20%-40% of all intracranial tumours (116,117). In 1972, Maurice-Williams (118) from Great Britain reported a frequency of 0.15%. Ramamurthi and Varadarajan (119) noted that the tuberculomas formed 20% of all intracranial tumours at Chennai [then called Madras] in the 1950s. Although the frequency has decreased in the last two to three decades, tuberculomas still constitute about 5%-10% of intracranial space occupying lesions in the developing world (13,120).

Diagnosis

The CT and MRI have facilitated the diagnosis and assessment of intracranial tuberculomas. The characteristic CT and MRI finding is a nodular enhancing lesion with a central hypointensity (36,119) [Figures 17.4, 17.5 and 17.6]. The pattern of enhancement can be quite variable; homogeneous, patchy, serpentine and ring enhancement, have all been observed. A lipid peak on proton MR spectroscopy is characteristic of tuberculoma (121) [Figures 17.4, 17.7]. The spinal cord is less frequently involved by tuberculoma [Figure 17.7]. Unless treated with steroids, oedema is nearly always present and can be quite marked. These CT findings are non-specific and may simulate the appearance of gliomas, metastasis, abscess, cysticercosis and fungal granulomas. In a study from Saudi Arabia (120), the initial diagnosis, based on

the CT appearance, was wrong in 80% of cases. The rupture of a parenchymal tuberculoma or tuberculoma en plaque of the meninges can result in TBM. In a study reported by Bhargava et al (36), tuberculomas occurred in 10% of patients with TBM. Brainstem tuberculomas, although uncommon, constitute 2%-8% of all intracranial tuberculomas and are more commonly seen in children (122). Ventricles form a relatively rare site for tuberculomas (123).

The characteristic CT features of neurocysticercosis are shown in Figure 17.8, 17.9 and 17.10. The imaging features of intracranial tuberculomas are shown in Figures 17.11, 17.12, 17.13, 17.14, 17.15 and 17.16. The features differentiating various types tuberculomas are listed in Table 17.10. Comparison of salient imaging findings of tuberculomas and neurocysticercosis is shown in Table 17.11.

Management

In the past, management of tuberculoma was mainly surgical (114-117,124). With the availability of CT and MRI, therapeutic trial with anti-TB treatment in patients with a solitary lesion suspicious of a tuberculoma is a widely accepted option (125,126). Short-course chemotherapy may be adequate for the treatment of tuberculoma (125) although its efficacy is not yet established. Corticosteroids are helpful in selected patients who have cerebral oedema and are symptomatic. Tuberculomas begin to decrease in size within the first two months of anti-TB treatment. Choudhury (125) reported that 17 [68%] of 24 patients treated conservatively showed complete recovery, while only 2 patients [8%] had significant residual neurological problems. Paradoxical expansion of intracranial tuberculomas during anti-TB treatment for neural or extra-neural TB has been observed rarely (127-129). This phenomenon is thought to have an immunological basis similar to immune reconstitution inflammatory syndrome [IRIS]. Surgery is still indicated for large lesions producing midline shift and severe intracranial hypertension, expanding lesions during anti-TB treatment, when clinical and neuroimaging findings favour alternate possibilities, such as, glioma or metastasis, and when the expected improvement is not forthcoming in the clinical and CT picture during follow-up of medical treatment.

TUBERCULOSIS ABSCESS

TB abscess is an uncommon manifestation of neurological TB [Figure 17.7], most often occurring as a complication in immunosuppressed patients receiving anti-TB treatment for systemic or neurological TB. It is characterised by an encapsulated collection of pus that contains viable TB bacilli without evidence of the classic TB granuloma. The differentiation between tuberculoma and TB abscess is often difficult by conventional MR images. Diffusion-weighted images may show diffusion restriction that favours abscess (130); however, even this finding may not be reliable (131). TB abscess develops in the brain parenchyma although intraventricular (132) and subdural (133) sites have also been reported. Differentiation from pyogenic abscess can

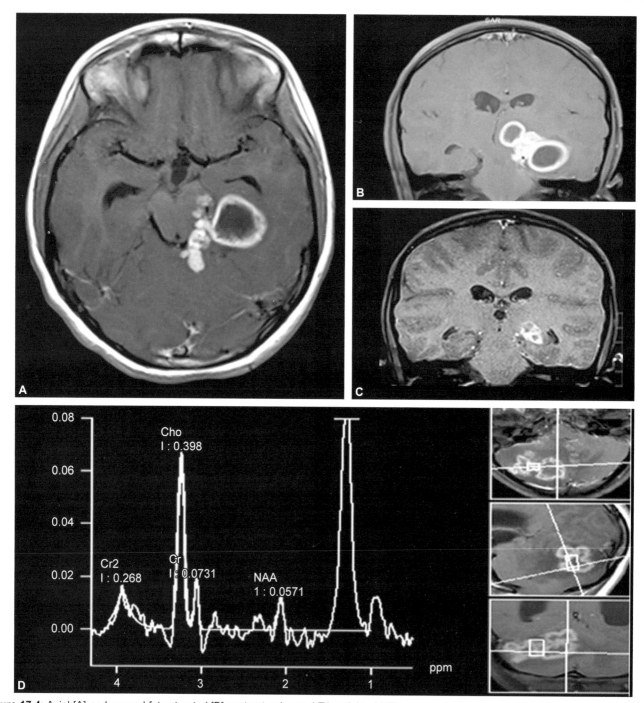

Figure 17.4: Axial [A] and coronal fat saturated [B] contrast-enhanced T1-weighted MR images of a 9-year old child, who presented with fever, headache, encephalopathy showing conglomerate ring enhancing lesions in the left temporal lobe and thalamus extending to left ambient cistern. Abdominal ultrasonography revealed matted abdominal nodes. Tuberculin skin test was positive. Coronal post-contrast T1-weighted fat saturated image [C] three months after anti-TB treatment shows a decrease in the size of the ring enhancing lesions. Single voxel MR spectroscopy [D] at TE of 135 ms reveals a large lipid peak at 1.2 ppm, related to the predominant lipid content in the cell wall of *Mycobacterium tuberculosis*
MR = magnetic resonance; TE = echo time; ppm = parts per million

often be difficult and presence of indirect evidence of TB, mycobacterial culture of the aspirate or response to anti-TB treatment may be needed. Elevated lipid and lactate levels if accompanied by an elevated amino acid levels favour a pyogenic abscess over a TB abscess on MR spectroscopy (134). A significantly higher magnetisation transfer ratio has also been observed in the wall of the pyogenic abscess compared to that in the TB abscess (134). Imaging features that help differentiating TB abscess from pyogenic and fungal abscesses is shown in Table 17.12.

Surgical aspiration of the abscess or excision of a multi-loculated abscess may be required as these lesions harbour

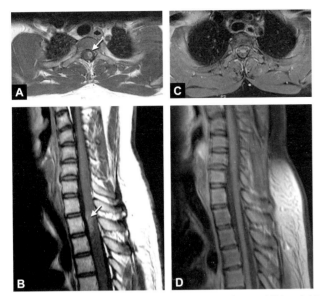

Figure 17.5: Axial [A] and sagittal [B] contrast-enhanced T1-weighted MR images of the cervico-dorsal spine of a 28-year-old male, who presented with low-grade fever, weight loss and progressive myelopathy with bladder involvement, showing intramedullary ring enhancing conglomerate lesions [arrow] at T2 vertebral level. Four months after anti-TB treatment axial [C] and sagittal [D] post-contrast T1-weighted fat saturated images reveal complete resolution of the lesion
MR = magnetic resonance; TB = tuberculosis

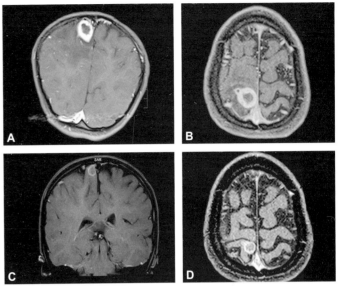

Figure 17.6: Contrast-enhanced T1-weighted fat saturated coronal [A] and axial [B] MR images of a 5-year old child, who presented with simple partial seizures involving left lower limb, showing a thick ring enhancing lesion with surrounding oedema behind the right motor cortex. Physical examination revealed cold abscess in the neck. Tuberculin skin test was positive. Coronal [C] and axial [D] T1-weighted fat saturated post-contrast images three months after anti-TB treatment show a decrease in size of the lesion and the oedema surrounding the lesion
MR = magnetic resonance; TB = tuberculosis

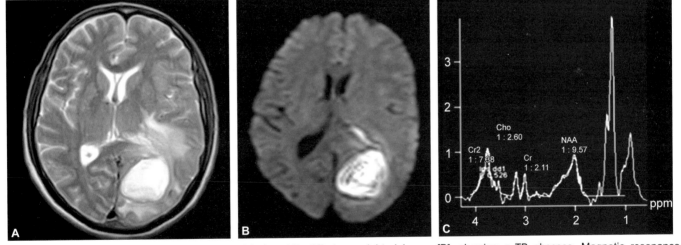

Figure 17.7: MRI of the brain, T2-weighted, axial view [A], diffusion weighted image [B], showing a TB abscess. Magnetic resonance spectroscopy [C] of the lesion showing a large lipid peak at 1.2 ppm suggestive of TB abscess
MRI = magnetic resonance imaging; TB = tuberculosis

TB bacilli and their thick capsules are often impervious to anti-TB agents. Draining the abscess decreases the myco-bacterial load. Development of fulminant TBM following surgical excision of TB abscess remains a problem (135).

SINGLE, SMALL, ENHANCING BRAIN LESION ON COMPUTED TOMOGRAPHY AND SEIZURES

Patients, who present with new onset focal seizures and ring enhancing single CT lesions [single, small, enhancing lesions, SSEL], have been described almost exclusively from India (136). These enhancing lesions are less than 2 cm in size, but may show considerable oedema around it. Epidemiologically, the occurrence of SSEL corresponds to the endemicity of cysticercosis. For example, in Kerala state in India, where cysticercosis is not endemic, SSEL are encountered only in subjects who have lived outside Kerala. Rajashekhar *et al* (137) compared clinical and CT data of six consecutive patients with histologically proven tuberculomas and 25 consecutive patients with histologically verified

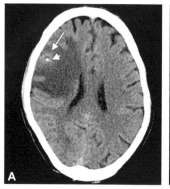
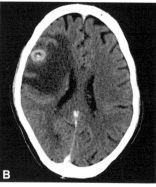

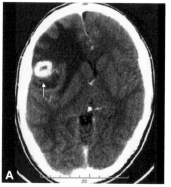
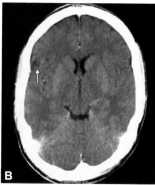

Figure 17.8: Neurocysticercosis [arrow] with scolex [arrow head]. NCCT head, axial view [A], showing single small lesion in the right fronto-parietal region, eccentric nodule, perilesional oedema. CECT head, axial view [B] of the same patient showing ring enhancement
NCCT = non-contrast computed tomography; CECT = contrast-enhanced computed tomography

Figure 17.10: CECT head, axial view in a patient with neurocysticercosis showing a contrast-enhancing ring lesion [arrow] in the right fronto-parietal region with perilesional oedema. Midline shift is also seen [A]. Post-treatment image of the same patient showing significant resolution of the lesion [arrow] [B]
CECT = contrast-enhanced computed tomography

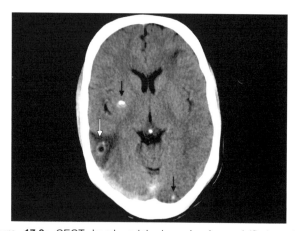

Figure 17.9: CECT head, axial view showing calcified nodules [black arrows] and a ring lesion with perilesional oedema [white arrow]
CECT = contrast-enhanced computed tomography

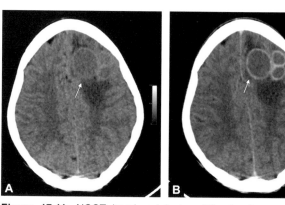

Figure 17.11: NCCT head, axial view [A], showing conglomerate tuberculomas. CECT head, axial view of the same patient [B] showing riming-enhancement
NCCT = non-contrast computed tomography

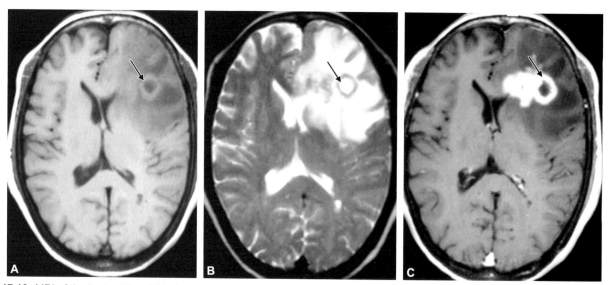

Figure 17.12: MRI of the brain, T1-weighted, axial view [A], T2-weighted, axial view [B], post-gadolinium T1-weighted, axial view [C], showing caseating tubercuolma with liquefied centre [arrow]
MRI = magnetic resonance imaging

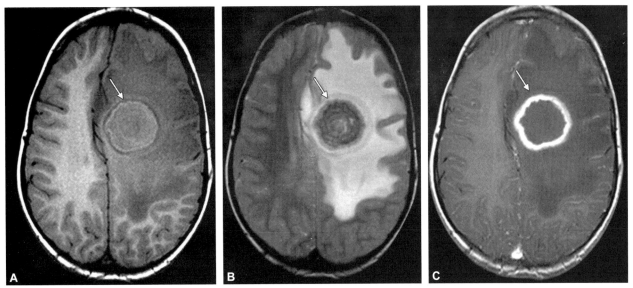

Figure 17.13: MRI of the brain, T1-weighted, axial view [A], T2-weighted, axial view [B], post-gadolinium T1-weighted, axial view [C], showing tubercuolma with caseation [arrow]. Perilesional oedema is also seen
MRI = magnetic resonance imaging

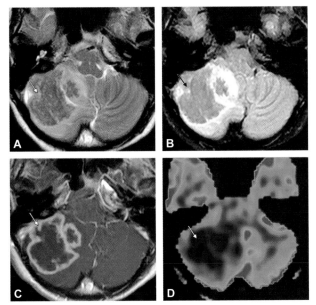

Figure 17.14: MRI of the brain, T2-weighted, axial view [A], T2-weighted, gradient echo sequence [B], post-gadolinium T1-weighted, axial view [C], showing tubercuolma in the cerebellum [arrow]. Perfusion image shows no perfusion in the lesion [arrow] [D]
MRI = magnetic resonance imaging

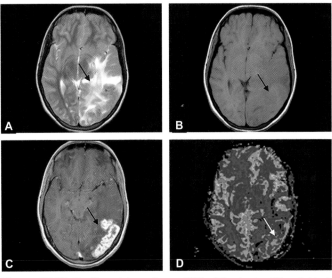

Figure 17.15: Gyriform tuberculoma. MRI of the brain, T2-weighted, axial view [A], showing gyriform hypointensity with perilesional oedema left parieto-occipital region. The lesion appears isointense in T1-weighted axial view [B]. Post-gadolinium T1-weighted, axial view [C], shows gyriform enhancement in left, parieto-occipital lesion. Perfusion image showing low perfusion in the lesion [arrow] [D]
MRI = magnetic resonance imaging

Table 17.10: MRI findings in different types of intracerebral tuberculomas

Type of tuberculoma	T1-weighted images	T2-weighted images	T1-weighted post-gadolinium contrast images
Non-caseating granuloma	Isointense/hypointense	Hyperintense	Homogeneous enhancement
Caseating granuloma with solid centre	Hypointense/isointense	Isointense/hypointense	Rim-enhancement
Caseating granuloma with liquid centre	Hypointense	Hyperintense; rim hypointense	Rim-enhancement
MRI = magnetic resonance imaging			

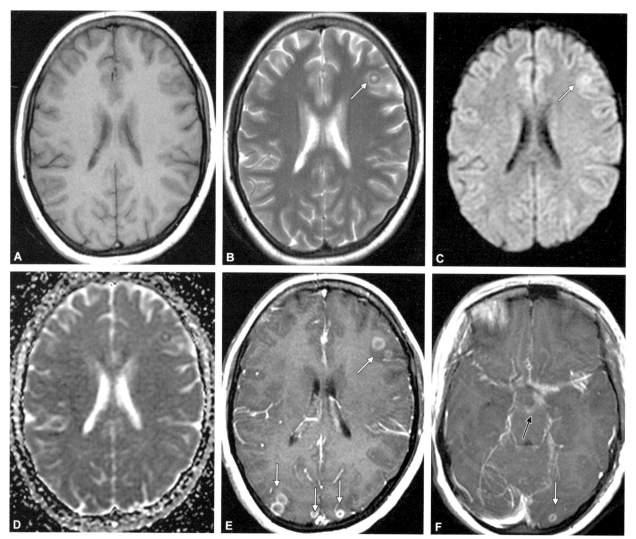

Figure 17.16: MRI of the brain, axial view, T1-weighted image [A], T2-weighted image [B], diffusion weighted image [C], apparent diffusion coefficient image [D], post-gadolinium T1-weighted image [E and F] showing multiple ring lesions [white arrows] and meningeal enhancement [black arrow, F]

MRI = magnetic resonance imaging

Table 17.11: Imaging features helpful in differentiating neurocysticercosis from intracerebral tuberculoma*

Variable	Neurocysticercosis	Intracerebral tuberculoma
Size	Usually <20 mm	Usually >20 mm
Scolex	Present, seen as eccentric hyperdensity on CT or hypointensity in T2-weighted image on MRI; not seen in racemose neurocysticercosis	Absent
Core of ring lesion on FLAIR images	May get suppressed in vesicular stage of neurocysticercosis [differential diagnosis arachnoid cyst, neurenteric cyst]	Never gets suppressed
MR spectroscopy	Difficult to get good spectrum in smaller lesions; large lesions have succinate and acetate peaks; succinate peak larger than acetate peak	Core: lipid-lactate peak; wall: increased choline may be seen
Leptomeningeal disease	Seldom seen	More common
Multiple lesions	Multiple lesions are seen in different stage of evolution	Multiple lesions are seen in same stage of evolution

*Degree of oedema, location, presence of mass effect or presence of midline shift may not be a differentiating feature in differentiating neurocysticercosis from intracerebral tuberculoma

CT = computed tomography; MRI = magnetic resonance imaging; FLAIR = fluid-attenuated inversion recovery; MR = magnetic resonance

Table 17.12: Imaging features helpful in differentiating pyogenic abscess, TB abscess and fungal abscess

Type of abscess	Morphology on conventional images	Intra-cavitary projections	Contrast enhancement	Diffusion weighted imaging	MR spectroscopy
Pyogenic abscess	Ring lesion T1 hypointense/T2 hyperintense core with T2 hypointense wall	Absent	Rim-enhancement	Restricted in core	Elevated succinate, acetate, cytosolic aminoacids
TB abscess	Ring lesion T1 hypointense/T2 hyperintense core with T2 hypointense wall	Absent	Rim-enhancement	Restricted in core	Lipid lactate peak with absence of other metabolites within core. Wall may show increased choline
Fungal abscess	Ring lesion T1 hypointense/T2 hyperintense core with T2 hypointense wall	Present [T2 hypointense]	Rim-enhancement with non-enhancing projections	Projections cause diffusion restriction; Variable in core	Lipid lactate peak with trehalose peak

TB = tuberculosis; MR = magnetic resonance

cysticercus granulomas. Evidence of raised intracranial pressure and a progressive focal neurological deficit was seen only in patients with tuberculomas. On CT, all tuberculomas were greater than 2 cm in size and majority were irregular in outline. In contrast, all cysticercous granulomas were less than 20 mm and majority were regular in outline. Only tuberculomas were associated with a midline shift on CT. The authors (137) concluded that based on clinical findings [evidence of raised intracranial tension and a progressive neurological deficit] and CT appearance [size, shape and association with a midline shift], it is possible to distinguish between tuberculoma and neurocysticercosis in a majority of patients presenting with SSEL and seizures.

PROGNOSIS AND OUTCOME OF NEUROLOGICAL TUBERCULOSIS

The two most important factors determining the outcome of TBM are early diagnosis and prompt initiation of treatment (3-7,138). The factors contributing to poor outcome are listed in Table 17.13.

Table 17.13: Factors contributing to poor outcome of TB meningitis

Advanced clinical disease at presentation

Delayed diagnosis and initiation of therapy

Extremes of age

Infection with drug-resistant mycobacterial strains

HIV infection, AIDS associated with a low CD4+ T-lymphocyte count

Hydrocephalus

Raised intracranial pressure

Brain ischaemia due to vasculitis

Direct parenchymal injury

Hyponatraemia

Seizures

TB = tuberculosis; HIV = human immunodeficiency virus; AIDS = acquired immunodeficiency syndrome

Clinical Stage of the Disease

When anti-TB treatment and corticosteroids are initiated in clinical stage 1 or early stage 2 diseases, high cure rates ranging from 85%-90% have been observed. Clinical stages 3 and 4 are usually accompanied by very high morbidity and mortality. A multivariate analysis of 199 Chinese patients with TBM (138) showed that only the age and the stage of presentation affected the outcome and with respect to the disease stage and the mortality raises from none to 4% in stage 1, to 22%-30% in stage 2, to 78%-79% in stages 3 or 4.

Age

The outcome of TBM, particularly in children, is often poor irrespective of the region where they live. Extremes of age have poorer outcome; children below 3 years and adults above 50 years of age generally have a poor prognosis (37,139).

Cerebrospinal Fluid Parameters

Though earlier studies suggested that lower glucose levels in CSF had a poorer outcome, studies with larger number of patients have failed to show any correlation between CSF sugar levels and the clinical outcome (21). The only CSF parameter that correlated with a poor outcome was high protein levels [greater than 2 g/L], as it was associated with a more advanced stage of the disease at presentation.

Neuroimaging

Patients with dense exudates in the basal cisterns and visual loss due to organised exudates over optico-chiasmatic region respond poorly to treatment (36). Similarly, patients with diencephalic infarcts and angiographic evidence of narrowing in the middle or anterior cerebral arteries have higher morbidity (17,109). It is also important to note that diencephalic infarcts give rise to SIADH, which is a poor prognostic indicator.

Others Variables

Poor outcome has also been associated with raised intracranial pressure with hydrocephalus and infection with drug-resistant mycobacterial strains. Children who have not received BCG vaccination also have a poor outcome. Infection with HIV does not seem to alter the prognosis of TBM except in patients with CD4+ lymphocyte counts below 0.2×10^9/L (29,31).

TUBERCULOSIS RADICULOMYELITIS

TB radiculomyelitis [TBRM] is a form of spinal TB and may develop in one of the three ways: [i] as a primary TB lesion; [ii] as a downward extension of TBM; and [iii] as a secondary extension from vertebral TB. The first two varieties of TBRM are discussed here briefly. Wadia and Dastur (140) suggested TBRM as a generic term to include cases designated as arachnoiditis, intradural spinal tuberculoma or granuloma and spinal cord complications of TBM.

Pathology and Clinical Features

Pathologically, it is characterised by extensive, copious and tenacious exudates that may occupy the entire space between the spinal dura mater and the leptomeninges that may encase the cord and impinge on the roots. Clinical features include a subacute to chronic progressive flaccid paraparesis, often in the presence of a positive Babinski's sign, that is frequently preceded by root pains, paraesthesias, bladder disturbances and focal muscle wasting. Secondary TBRM may follow TBM during the acute stage but can also occur after a variable periods of months to years (140). Furthermore, it is known

to occur in patients with TBM on inadequate or adequate anti-TB treatment regimens (140,141). Lumbosacral region is the most commonly affected site in TBRM, although cervical involvement is not unknown [Figure 17.17]. In contrast, TBRM secondary to vertebral TB is relatively more common in the dorsal region.

Investigations

In most patients with TBRM, if the lumbar puncture is not a dry tap, CSF shows lymphocytic pleocytosis, hypoglycorrhachia and characteristically, a very high protein level [probably secondary to a CSF flow block]. These findings may persist despite sterilisation of CSF. Although in practice, CT myelography or contrast MRI of the spine is often preferred over the conventional spinal myelography in patients with TBRM, a study (141) comparing these modalities of imaging found conventional myelography to be the primary radiographic method for diagnosis of suspected TBRM, particularly in those cases that are characterised by chronic adhesive changes. In patients with active intrathecal inflammatory process or with myelopathy, gadolinium-enhanced MRI was found to be the optimal choice. In contrast to this observation, MRI was favoured as the primary imaging modality for screening patients with suspected intraspinal TB, regardless of the stage of the disease, in another study (142), an opinion that may find wider acceptance in view of the non-invasive nature of the investigation and the recent advances in spinal MRI technology. CT myelography has no superiority over contrast-enhanced MRI, except perhaps in cases with extensive vertebral TB. The MRI features of TBRM include

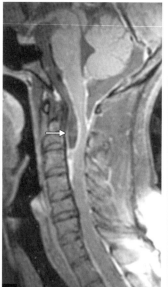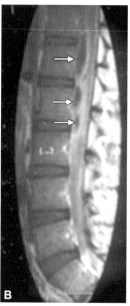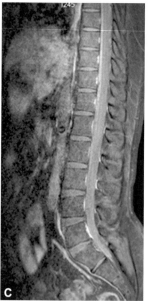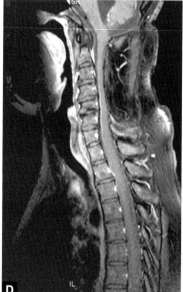

Figure 17.17: Contrast-enhanced sagittal fat saturated cervical [A] and lumbar [B] spine MR images of a 35-year-old male, who presented with fever, headache, radicular pains and quadriparesis, show enhancement of the meninges with CSF loculations anterior to the cord [arrows] suggestive of arachnoiditis. Post-contrast fat saturated sagittal lumbar [C] and cervical [D] spine MR images one year after anti-TB treatment along with corticosteroids reveal marked reduction of the enhancement of the meninges. The CSF loculations are no longer evident

MR = magnetic resonance; CSF = cerebrospinal fluid; TB = tuberculosis

loculation and obliteration of the spinal subarachnoid spaces, loss of outline of the spinal cord in the affected region, clumping or matting of the nerve roots in lumbar region, a syringomyelic cavity [as a late complication] and nodular, thick, linear intradural and meningeal enhancement on gadolinum-enhanced MRI. Spinal meningeal enhancement in the cervical and thoracic region is highly suggestive of TBRM, if a clinical suspicion exists. It must, however, be noted that in chronic TBRM, enhancement may be conspicuous by its absence.

Management

Some researchers consider TBRM as a form of paradoxical reaction to TB treatment, which might represent a delayed hypersensitivity response in a recovering patient to myco-bacterial antigens liberated after anti-TB treatment. Although this view might support the use of corticosteroids to prevent and treat TBRM, reports on the efficacy of corticosteroids for this condition are conflicting (143-145) and the studies are handicapped by lack of randomisation. In view of vasculitis of the spinal vessels, most clinicians consider the use of corticosteroids in conjunction with anti-TB treatment, as beneficial in the prevention and treatment of TBRM. Except in cases with vertebral TB that need vertebral stabilisation, the role of decompressive spinal surgery in the treatment of TBRM is very limited, and often fails to arrest the relentless progression of the related neurological deficits.

ACKNOWLEDGMENTS

The authors are grateful to Dr C Kesavadas and Dr Bejoy Thomas of the Department of Imaging Sciences and Interventional Radiology, Sree Chitra Tirunal Institute of Medical Sciences and Technology, Thriuvananthapuram, Kerala, India, for providing the figures, and Mr Liji and Mrs S Vasanthy of the Medical Illustrations Division for processing them. Kind help rendered by Dr Ajay Garg, Department of Neurology, All India Institute of Medical Sciences, New Delhi, in providing Figures and Tables is thankfully acknowledged.

REFERENCES

1. Zuger A. Tuberculosis. In: Scheld WM, Whitley RJ, Marra CM, editors. Infections of the central nervous system. Third edition. Philadephia: Lippincott Williams & Wilkins; 2004.p.441-60.
2. World Health Organization. Global tuberculosis report 2018. WHO/CDS/TB/2018.20. Geneva: World Health Organization; 2015.
3. Thwaites G, Chau TT, Mai NTH, Drobniewski F, McAdam K, Farrar J. Tuberculous meningitis. J Neurol Neurosurg Psychiatry 2000;68:289-99.
4. Sharma SK, Mohan A. Extrapulmonary tuberculosis. Indian J Med Res 2004; 120:316-53.
5. Rock RB, Olin M, Baker CA, Molitor TW, Peterson PK. Central nervous system tuberculosis: pathogenesis and clinical aspects. Clin Microbiol Rev 2008;21:243-61.
6. Sinner SW. Approach to the diagnosis and management of tuberculous meningitis. Curr Infect Dis Rep 2010;12:291-8.
7. Delfino LN, Fariello G, Lancella L, Marabotto C, Menchini L, Devito R, et al. Central nervous system tuberculosis in non-HIV-positive children: a single-center 6-year experience. Radiol Med 2012;117:669-78.
8. Thigpen MC, Whitney CG, Messonnier NE, Zell ER, Lynfield R, Hadler JL, et al. Bacterial meningitis in the United States, 1998-2007. N Engl J Med 2011;354:2016-25.
9. Whytt R. Observations on the nature causes and cure of those disorders which are commonly called nervous hypochondriac or hysteric. In: Robinson DN, editor. Significant contribution to the history of psychiatry. Washington: University Publications of America; 1978.
10. Koch R. Classics in infectious diseases. The etiology of tuberculosis: Robert Koch. Berlin, Germany 1882. Rev Infect Dis 1982;4:1270-4.
11. Katrak SM, Shembalkar PK, Bijwe SR, Bhandarkar LD. The clinical, radiological and pathological profile of tuberculous meningitis in patients with and without human immune deficiency virus infection. J Neurol Sci 2000;181:118-26.
12. Tan EK, Chee MWL, Chan LL, Lee YL. Culture positive tuberculous meningitis: clinical indicators of poor prognosis. Clin Neurol Neurosurg 1999;101:157-60.
13. Tandon PN, Bhatia R, Bhargava S. Tuberculous meningitis. In: Harris AA, editor. Handbook of clinical neurology [revised series]. Amsterdam: Elsevier Science; 1988.p.195-226.
14. Pando RH, Aguilar D, Cohen I, Guerrero M, Ribon W, Acosta P, et al. Specific bacterial genotypes of Mycobacterium tuberculosis cause extensive dissemination and brain infection in an experimental model. Tuberculosis [Edinb] 2010;90:268-77.
15. Faksri K, Drobniewki F, Nikolayevskyy V, Brown T, Prammananan T, Palittapongarnpim P, et al. Epidemiological trends and clinical comparisons of Mycobacterium tuberculosis lineages in Thai TB meningitis. Tuberculosis [Edinb] 2011;91: 594-600.
16. Rich AR, Mc Cordock HA. Pathogenesis of tuberculous meningitis. Bull John Hopkins Hosp 1933;52:5-37.
17. Figaji AA, Fieggen AG. The neurosurgical and acute care management of tuberculous meningitis: evidence and current practice. Tuberculosis [Edinb] 2010; 90:393-400.
18. Tandon V, Mahapatra AK. Management of post-tubercular hydrocephalus. Childs Nerv Syst 2011;27:1699-707.
19. Udani PM, Dastur DK. Tuberculous encephalopathy with and without meningitis. Clinical features and pathological correlations. J Neurol Sci 1970;10:541-61.
20. Principi N, Esposito S. Diagnosis and therapy of tuberculous meningitis in children. Tuberculosis [Edinb] 2012; 92:377-83.
21. Kent SJ, Crowe SM, Yung A, Lucas CR, Mijch AM. Tuberculous meningitis: a 30-year review. Clin Infect Dis 1993;17:987-94.
22. Thomas MD, Chopra JS, Walia BN. Tuberculous meningitis. A clinical study of 232 cases. J Assoc Physicians India 1977;25: 633-9.
23. Sridharan R, Krishnamurthy L. Visual evoked potentials in tuberculous meningitis. Neurol India 1984;32:27-33.
24. Medical Research Council. Streptomycin treatment of tuber-culous meningitis: report of the committee on sterptomycin in tuberculosis trials. Lancet 1948;1:582-97.
25. Kennedy DH, Fallon RJ. Tuberculous meningitis. JAMA 1979; 241:264-8.
26. Bhagwati S, Mehta N, Shah S. Use of endoscpic third ventriculotomy in hydrocephalus of tubercular origin. Childs Nerv Syst 2010;26:1675-82.
27. Kocen RS, Parsons M. Neurological complications of tuber-culosis: some unusual manifestations. QJM 1970;39:17-30.
28. Lawn SD, Churchyard G. Epidemiology of HIV-associated tuberculosis. Curr Opin HIV AIDS 2009; 4:325-33.

29. Berenguer J, Moreno S, Laguna F, Vicente T, Adrados M, Ortega A, et al. Tuberculous meningitis in patients infected with the human immunodeficiency virus. N Engl J Med 1992;326:668-72.

30. Bishburg E, Sunderam G, Reichman LB, Kapila R. Central nervous system tuberculosis with the acquired immunodeficiency syndrome and its related complex. Ann Intern Med 1986;105:210-3.

31. Yechoor VK, Shandera WX, Rodriguez P, Cate TR. Tuberculous meningitis among adults with and without HIV infection. Experience in an urban public hospital. Arch InternMed 1996;156:1710-6.

32. Satishchandra P, Nalini A, Gourie-Devi M, Khanna N, Santosh V, Ravi V, et al. Profile of neurologic disorders associated with HIV/AIDS from Bangalore, south India [1989-96]. Indian J Med Res 2000;111:14-23.

33. Karstaedt AS, Valtchanova S, Barriere R, Crewe-Brown HH. Tuberculous meningitis in South African urban adults. QJM 1988;91:743-7.

34. Dube MP, Holtom PD, Larsen RA. Tuberculous meningitis in patients with and without human immunodeficiency virus infection. Am J Med 1992;93:520-4.

35. Wang YY, Xie BD. Progress on diagnosis of tuberculous meningitis. Methods Mol Biol 2018;1754:375-86.

36. Bhargava S, Gupta AK, Tandon PN. Tuberculous meningitis - a CT study. Br J Radiol 1982;55:189-96.

37. Farinha NJ, Razali KA, Holzel H, Morgan G, Novelli VM. Tuberculosis of the central nervous system in children: a 20-year survey. J Infect 2000;41:61-8.

38. Fan L, Chen Z, Hao XH, Hu ZY, Xiao HP. Interferon-gamma release assays for the diagnosis of extrapulmonary tuberculosis: a systematic review and meta-analysis. FEMS Immunol Med Microbiol 2012;65:456-66.

39. Laguna F, Adrados M, Ortega A, Gonzalez-Lahoz JM. Tuberculous meningitis with acellular cerebrospinal fluid in AIDS patients. AIDS 1992;6:1165-7.

40. Satyavathi R, Dingari NC, Barman I, Prasad PSR, Prabhakar S, Rao DN, et al. Raman spectroscopy provides a powerful, rapid diagnostic tool for the detection of tuberculous meningitis in ex vivo cerebrospinal fluid samples. J Biophotonics 2013;6:567-72.

41. Verdon R, Chevret S, Laissy JP, Wolff M. Tuberculous meningitis in adults: review of 48 cases. Clin Infect Dis 1996;22:982-8.

42. Radhakrishnan VV, Mathai A. Correlation between the isolation of Mycobacterium tuberculosis and estimation of mycobacterial antigen in cisternal, ventricular and lumbar cerebrospinal fluids of patients with tuberculous meningitis. Indian J Pathol Microbiol 1993;36:341-7.

43. Chandramuki A, Bothamley GH, Brennan PJ, Ivanyi J. Levels of antibody to defined antigens of Mycobacterium tuberculosis in tuberculous meningitis. J Clin Microbiol 1989;27:821-5.

44. Ashtekar MD, Dhalla AS, Mazarello TB, Samuel AM. A study of Mycobacterium tuberculosis antigen and antibody in cerebrospinal fluid and blood in tuberculous meningitis. Clin Immunol Immunopathol 1987;45:29-34.

45. Behari M, Raj M, Ahuja GK, Shrinivas. Soluble antigen fluorescent antibody test in the serodiagnosis of tuberculous meningitis. J Assoc Physicians India 1989;37:499-501.

46. Mathai A, Radhakrishnan VV, Sehgal S. Circulating immune complexes in cerebrospinal fluid of patients with tuberculous meningitis. Indian J Exp Biol 1991;29:973-6.

47. Park SC, Lee BI, Cho SN, Kim WJ, Lee BC, Kim SM, et al. Diagnosis of tuberculous meningitis by detection of immunoglobulin G antibodies to purified protein derivative and lipoarabinomannan antigen in cerebrospinal fluid. Tuber Lung Dis 1993;74:317-22.

48. Srivastava L, Prasanna S, Srivastava VK. Diagnosis of tuberculous meningitis by ELISA test. Indian J Med Res 1994;99:8-12.

49. Ghoshal U, Kishore J, Kumar B, Ayyagari A. Serodiagnosis of smear and culture-negative neurotuberculosis with enzyme linked immunosorbent assay for anti A-60 immunoglobulins. Indian J Pathol Microbiol 2003;46:530-4.

50. Maheshwari A, Gupta HL, Gupta S, Bhatia R, Datta KK. Diagnostic utility of estimation of mycobacterial antigen A-60 specific immunoglobulins in serum and CSF in adult neurotuberculosis. J Commun Dis 2000;32:54-60.

51. Radhakrishnan VV, Mathai A. Detection of mycobacterial antigen in cerebrospinal fluid: diagnostic and prognostic significance. J Neurol Sci 1990;99:93-9.

52. Kadival GV, Mazarelo TB, Chaparas SD. Sensitivity and specificity of enzyme-linked immunosorbent assay in the detection of antigen in tuberculous meningitis cerebrospinal fluids. J Clin Microbiol 1986;23:901-4.

53. Wagle N, Vaidya A, Joshi S, Merchant SM. Detection of tubercule antigen in cerebrospinal fluids by ELISA for diagnosis of tuberculous meningitis. Indian J Pediatr 1990;57:679-83.

54. Desai T, Gogate A, Deodhar L, Toddywalla S, Kelkar M. Enzyme-linked immunosorbent-assay for antigen detection in tuberculous meningitis. Indian J Pathol Microbiol 1993;36:348-55.

55. Patil SA, Gourie-Devi M, Anand AR, Vijaya AN, Pratima N, Neelam K, et al. Significance of mycobacterial immune complexes [IgG] in the diagnosis of tuberculous meningitis. Tuber Lung Dis 1996;77:164-7.

56. Mathai A, Radhakrishnan VV, Shobha S. Diagnosis of tuberculous meningitis confirmed by means of an immunoblot method. J Infect 1994;29:33-9.

57. Ribera E, Martinez-Vazquez JM, Ocana I, Segura RM, Pascual C. Activity of adenosine deaminase in cerebrospinal fluid for the diagnosis and follow-up of tuberculous meningitis in adults. J Infect Dis 1987;155:603-7.

58. Gautam N, Aryal M, Bhatta N, Bhattacharya SK, Baral N, Lamsal M. Comparative study of cerebrospinal fluid adenosine deaminase activity in patients with meningitis. Nepal Med Coll J 2007;9:104-6.

59. Coovadia YM, Dawood A, Ellis ME, Coovadia HM, Daniel TM. Evaluation of adenosine deaminase activity and antibody to Mycobacterium tuberculosis antigen 5 in cerebrospinal fluid and the radioactive bromide partition test for the early diagnosis of tuberculosis meningitis. Arch Dis Child 1986;61:428-35.

60. Mårdh PA, Larsson L, Høiby N, Engbaek HC, Odham G. Tuberculostearic acid as a diagnostic marker in tuberculous meningitis. Lancet 1983;1:367.

61. Brooks JB, Choudhary G, Craven RB, Alley CC, Liddle JA, Edman DC, et al. Electron capture gas chromatography detection and mass spectrum identification of 3-[2'-ketohexyl] indoline in spinal fluids of patients with tuberculous meningitis. J Clin Microbiol 1977;5:625-8.

62. Kaneko K, Onodera O, Miyatake T, Tsuji S. Rapid diagnosis of tuberculous meningitis by polymerase chain reaction [PCR]. Neurology 1990;40:1617-8.

63. Shankar P, Manjunath N, Mohan KK, Prasad K, Behari M, Shriniwas, et al. Rapid diagnosis of tuberculous meningitis by polymerase chain reaction. Lancet 1991;337:5-7.

64. Liu PY, Shi ZY, Lau YJ, Hu BS. Rapid diagnosis of tuberculous meningitis by a simplified nested amplification protocol. Neurology 1994;44:1161-4.

65. Thwaites GE, Caws M, Chau TT, Dung NT, Campbell JI, Phu NH, et al. Comparison of conventional bacteriology with nucleic acid amplification [amplified mycobacterium direct test] for diagnosis of tuberculous meningitis before and after inception of antituberculosis chemotherapy. J Clin Microbiol 2004;42:996-1002.

66. Pai M, Flores LL, Pai N, Hubbard A, Riley LW, Colford JM. Diagnostic accuracy of nucleic acid amplification tests for

tuberculous meningitis; a systematic review and meta-analysis. Lancet Infect Dis 2003;3:633-43.

67a. Sharma SK, Ryan H, Khaparde S, Sachdeva KS, Singh AD, Mohan A, et al. Index-TB guidelines: Guidelines on extrapulmonary tuberculosis for India. Indian J Med Res 2017;145:448-63.

67b. Kohli M, Schiller I, Dendukuri N, Dheda K, Denkinger CM, Schumacher SG, et al. Xpert[®] MTB/RIF assay for extrapulmonary tuberculosis and rifampicin resistance. Cochrane Database Syst Rev 2018;8:CD012768.

68. Heemskerk AD, Bang ND, Mai NT, Chau TT, Phu NH, Loc PP, et al. Intensified antituberculosis therapy in adults with tuberculous meningitis. N Engl J Med 2016;374:124-34.

69. Donald PR, Schoeman JF, Van Zyl LE, De Villiers JN, Pretorius M, Springer P. Intensive short course chemotherapy in the management of tuberculous meningitis. Int J Tuberc Lung Dis 1998;2:704-11.

70. Goel A, Pandya SK, Satoskar AR. Whither short-course chemotherapy for tuberculous meningitis? Neurosurgery 1990;27:418-21.

71. National Institute for Health and Care Excellence. Tuberculosis. Clinical diagnosis and management of tuberculosis, and measures for its prevention and control. NICE clinical guideline 117. Issued: March 2011. Available at URL: https://www.nice.org.uk/guidance/cg117. Accessed on January 12, 2018.

72. Nahid P, Dorman SE, Alipanah N, Barry PM, Brozek JL, Cattamanchi A, et al. Official American Thoracic Society/Centers for Disease Control and Prevention/Infectious Diseases Society of America Clinical Practice Guidelines: treatment of drug-susceptible tuberculosis. Clin Infect Dis 2016;63:e147-e195.

73. Phuapradit P, Vejjajiva A. Treatment of tuberculous meningitis: role of short course chemotherapy. QJM 1987;239:249-58.

74. Acharya VN, Kudva BT, Retnam VJ, Mehta PJ. Adult tuberculous meningitis: comparative study of different chemotherapeutic regimens. J Assoc Physicians India 1985;33:583-5.

75. Sharma SK, Balamurugan A, Saha PK, Pandey RM, Mehra NK. Evaluation of clinical and immunogenetic risk factors for the development of hepatotoxicity during antituberculosis treatment. Am J Respir Crit Care Med 2002;166:916-9.

76. Wasz-Hockert O. Late prognosis in tuberculous meningitis. Acta Paediatr 1962;51:1-119.

77. Lorber J. Treatment of tuberculous meningitis. Br Med J 1960;1:1309-12.

78. Smith H. Tuberculous meningitis. Int J Neurol 1964;4:134-57.

79. Hockaday JM, Smith HM. Corticosteroids as an adjuvant to the chemotherapy of tuberculous meningitis. Tubercle 1966;47:75-91.

80. Girgis NI, Farid Z, Kilpatrick ME, Sultan Y, Mikhail IA. Dexamethasone adjunctive treatment for tuberculous meningitis. Pediatr Infect Dis J 1991;10:179-83.

81. Grigis NI, Farid Z, Hanna LS, Yassin MW, Wallace CK. The use of dexamethazone in preventing ocular complications in tuberculous meningitis. Trans R Soc Trop Med Hyg 1983;77:658-9.

82. Ashby M, Grant H. Tuberculos meningitis treated with cortisone. Lancet 1955;1:65-6.

83. Voljarec BF, Corpe RF. The influence of corticosteroid hormones in the treatment of tuberculous meningitis in Negroes. Am Rev Respir Dis 1960;81:539-45.

84. Lepper MH, Spies HW. The present system of the treatment of tuberculosis of the central nervous system. Ann NY Acad Aci 1963;106:106-23.

85. O'Toole RD, Thronton GF, Mukherjee MK, Nath RL. Dexamethasone in tuberculosis meningitis: relationship of cerebrospinal fluid effects to therapeutic efficacy. Ann Intern Med 1969;70:39-48.

86. Escobar JA, Belsey MA, Duenas A, Medina P. Mortality from tuberculous meningitis reduced by steroid therapy. Pediatrics 1975;56:1050-5.

87. Dooley DP, Carpenter JL, Rademacher S. Adjunctive corticosteroid therapy for tuberculosis: a critical reappraisal of the literature. Clin Infect Dis 1997;25:872-87.

88. Kumaravelu S, Prasad K, Khosla A, Behari M, Ahuja GK. Randomized controlled trial of dexamethasone in tuberculous meningitis. Tuber Lung Dis 1994;75:203-7.

89. Thwaites GE, Nguyen DB, Nguyen HD, Hoang TQ, Do TT, Nguyen TC, et al. Dexamethasone for the treatment of tuberculous meningitis in adolescents and adults. N Engl J Med 2004;351:1741-51.

90. Andries K, Verhasselt P, Guillemont J, Gohlmann HW, Neefs JM, Winkler H, et al. A diaryl quinoline drug active on the ATP synthase of Mycobacterium tuberculosis. Science 2005;307:223-7.

91. Sánchez F, López Colomés JL, Villarino E, Grosset J. New drugs for tuberculosis treatment. Enferm Infec Microbiol Clin 2011;29:47-56.

92. Vinnard C, Winston CA, Wileyto EP, MacGregor RR, Bisson GP. Multidrug resistant tuberculous meningitis in the United States, 1993-2005. J Infect 2011;63:240-2.

93. Harries AD, Zachariah R, Corbett EL, Lawn SD, Santos Filho ET, Chimzizi R, et al. The HIV-associated tuberculosis epidemic—when will we act? Lancet 2010;375:1906-19.

94. Lawn SD, Bekker LG, Miller RF. Immune reconstitution disease associated with mycobacterial infections in HIV-infected individuals receiving antiretrovirals. Lancet Infect Dis 2005;5:361-73.

95. van Toorn R, Rabie H, Dramowski A, Schoeman JF. Neurological manifestations of TB-IRIS: a report of 4 children. Eur J Pediatr Neurol 2012;16:676-82.

96. Lawn SD, Wood R. Poor prognosis of HIV-associated tuberculous meningitis regardless of the timing of antiretroviral therapy. Clin Infect Dis 2011;52:1384-7.

97. World Health Organization. Antiretroviral therapy for HIV infection in adults and adolescents. Recommendations for public health approach [2010 revision]. Geneva: World Health Organization; 2010.

98. Croda MG, Vidal JE, Hernandez AV, Molin TD, Gualberto FA, de Oliveira ACP. Tuberculous meningitis in HIV-infected patients in Brazil: clinical and laboratory characteristics and factors associated with mortality. Int J Infect Dis 2010;14:e586-91.

99. Schoeman J, Wait J, Burger M, van Zyl F, Fertig G, van Rensburg AJ, et al. Long-term follow-up of childhood tuberculous meningitis. Dev Med Child Neurol 2002;44:522-6.

100. Kalita J, Misra UK, Ranjan P. Predictors of long-term neurological sequelae of tuberculous meningitis: a multivariate analysis. Eur J Neurol 2007;14:33-7.

101. Palur R, Rajshekhar V, Chandy MJ, Joseph T, Abraham J. Shunt surgery for hydrocephalus in tuberculous meningitis: a long-term follow-up study. J Neurosurg 1991;74:64-9.

102. Lin J, Zhou H, Zhang N, Yin B, Sheng HS. Effects of the implantation of Ommaya reservoir in children with tuberculous meningitis hydrocephalus: a preliminary study. Childs Nerv Syst 2012;28:1003-8.

103. Peng J, Deng X, Omran A, Zhang C, Yin F, Liu J. Role of ventriculoperitoneal shunt surgery in grade IV tubercular meningitis with hydrocephalus. Childs Nerv Syst 2012;28:209-15.

104. Murthy JMK. Management of intracranial pressure in tuberculous meningitis. Neurocrit Care 2005;2:306-12.

105. Moller K, Larsen FS, Bie P, Skinhoj P. The syndrome of inappropriate secretion of antidiuretic hormone and fluid restriction in meningitis – how strong is the evidence? Scand J Infect Dis 2001;33:13-26.

106. Sterns RH, Silver SM. Cerebral salt wasting versus SIADH: what difference? J Am Soc Nephrol 2008;19:194-6.

107. Camous L, Valin N, Zaragoza JL, Bourry E, Caumes E, Deray G, et al. Hyponatremic syndrome in a patient with tuberculosis – always the adrenals? Nephrol Dial Transpl 2008;23:393-5.

108. Misra UK, Kalita J, Maurya PK. Stroke in tuberculous meningitis. J Neurol Sci 2011;303:22-30.

109. Javaud N, Certal Rda S, Stirnemann J, Morin AS, Chamouard JM, Aurier A, et al. Tuberculous cerebral vasculitis: retrospective study of 10 cases. Eur J Intern Med 2011;22:e99-104.

110. Anderson NE, Willoughby EW. Chronic meningitis without predisposing illness—a review of 83 cases. QJM 1987;63:283-95.

111. Ellner JJ, Bennett JE. Chronic meningitis. Medicine [Baltimore] 1976;55:341-69.

112. Wilhelm C, Ellner JJ. Chronic meningitis. Neurol Clin 1986;4:115-41.

113. Cheng TM, O'Neill BP, Scheithauer BW, Piepgras DG. Chronic meningitis: the role of meningeal or cortical biopsy. Neurosurgery 1994;34:590-5.

114. Radhakrishnan K, Kishore A, Mathuranath PS. Neurological tuberculosis. In: Sharma SK, editor. Tuberculosis. First edition. New Delhi: Jaypee Brothers Medical Publishers; 2001.p.209-28.

115. Mathuranath PS, Radhakrishnan K. Neurological tuberculosis. In: Sharma SK, editor. Tuberculosis. First edition. New Delhi: Jaypee Brothers Medical Publishers; 2009.p.304-29.

116. Dastur HM, Desai AD. A comparative study of brain tuberculomas and gliomas based upon 107 case records of each. Brain 1965;88:375-96.

117. Armstrong FB, Edwards AM. Intracranial tuberculoma in native races of Canada: with special reference to symptomatic epilepsy and neurologic features. Can Med Assoc J 1963;89:56-65.

118. Maurice-Williams RS. Tuberculomas of the brain in Britain. Postgrad Med J 1972;48:678-81.

119. Ramamurthi B, Varadarajan MG. Diagnosis of tuberculomas of brain. Clinical and radiological correlation. J Neurosurg 1961;18:1-7.

120. Naim-Ur-Rahman. Intracranial tuberculomas: diagnosis and management. Acta Neurochir [Wien] 1987;88:109-15.

121. Gupta RK, Roy R, Dev R, Husain M, Poptani H, Pandey R, et al. Fingerprinting of Mycobacterium tuberculosis in patients with intracranial tuberculoma by using in vivo, ex vivo and in vitro magnetic response spectroscopy. Magn Reson Med 1996;36:829-33.

122. Kumar R, Jain R, Kaur A, Chhabra DK. Brain stem tuberculosis in children. Br J Neurosurg 2000;14:356-61.

123. Desai K, Nadkarni T, Bhatjiwale M, Goel A. Intraventricular tuberculoma. Neurol Med Chir [Tokyo] 2002;42:501-3.

124. Arseni C. Two hundred and one cases of intracranial tuberculoma treated surgically. J Neurochem 1958;21:308-11.

125. Choudhury AR. Non-surgical treatment of tuberculomas of the brain. Br J Neurosurg 1989;3:643-53.

126. Tandon PN. Brain biopsy in tuberculoma: the risks and benefits. Neurosurgery 1992;30:301.

127. Rajeswari R, Sivasubramanian S, Balambal R, Parthasarathy R, Ranjani R, Santha T, et al. A controlled clinical trial of short course chemotherapy for tuberculoma of the brain. Tuber Lung Dis 1995;76:311-7.

128. Teoh R, Humphries MJ, O'Mahony G. Symptomatic intracranial tuberculoma developing during treatment of tuberculosis: a report of 10 patients and review of the literature. QJM 1987;63:449-60.

129. Chambers ST, Hendrickse WA, Record C, Rudge P, Smith H. Paradoxical expansion of intracranial tuberculomas during chemotherapy. Lancet 1984;2:181-4.

130. Sadeghi N, Rorive S, Lefranc F. Intracranial tuberculoma: is diffusion-weighted imaging useful in the diagnosis? Eur Radiol 2003;13:2049-50.

131. Gupta RK, Prakash M, Mishra AM, Husain M, Prasad KN, Husain N. Role of diffusion weighted imaging in differentiation of intracranial tuberculoma and tuberculous absecess from cysticercus granuloma—a report of more than 100 lesions. Eur J Radiol 2005;55:384-92.

132. Vajramani GV, Devi BI, Hegde T, Santosh V, Khanna N, Vasudev MK. Intraventricular tuberculous abscess: a case report. Neurol India 1999;47:327-9.

133. van Dellen A, Nadvi SS, Nathoo N, Ramdial PK. Intracranial tuberculous subdural empyema: case report. Neurosurgery 1998;43:370-3.

134. Gupta RK, Vatsal DK, Husain N, Chawla S, Prasad KN, Roy R, et al. Differentiation of tuberculous from pyogenic brain abscesses with in vivo proton MR spectroscopy and magnetization transfer MR imaging. AJNR Am J Neuroradiol 2001;22:1503-9.

135. Kumar R, Pandey CK, Bose N, Sahay S. Tuberculous brain abscess: clinical presentation, pathophysiology and treatment [in children]. Childs Nerv Syst 2002;18:118-23.

136. Rajshekhar V. Etiology and management of single small CT lesions in patients with seizures: understanding a controversy. Acta Neurol Scand 1991;84:465-70.

137. Rajashekhar V, Haran RP, Prakash GS, Chandy MJ. Differentiating solitary small cysticercus granulomas and tuberculomas in patients with epilepsy. Clinical and computerized tomographic criteria. J Neurosurg 1993;78:402-7.

138. Humphries MJ, Teoh R, Lau J, Gabriel M. Factors of prognostic significance in Chinese children with tuberculous meningitis. Tubercle 1990;71:161-8.

139. Hsu PC, Yang CC, Ye JJ, Huang PY, Chiang PC, Lee MH. Prognostic factors of tuberculous meningitis in adults: a 6-year retrospective study at a tertiary hospital in Northern Taiwan. J Microbiol Immunol Infect 2010;43:111-8.

140. Wadia NH, Dastur DK. Spinal meningitides with radiculo-myelopathy.1. Clinical and radiological features. J Neurol Sci 1969;8:239-60.

141. Chang KH, Han MH, Choi YW, Kim IO, Han MC, Kim CW. Tuberculous arachnoiditis of the spine: findings on myelography, CT, and MR imaging. AJNR Am J Neuroradiol 1989;10:1255-62.

142. Gupta RK, Gupta S, Kumar S, Kohli A, Misra UK, Gujral RB. MRI in intraspinal tuberculosis. Neuroradiology 1994;36:39-43.

143. Naidoo DP, Desai D, Kranidiotis L. Tuberculous meningomyelo-radiculitis—a report of two cases. Tubercle 1991;72:65-9.

144. Fehlings MG, Bernstein M. Syringomyelia as a complication of tuberculous meningitis. Can J Neurol Sci 1992;19:84-7.

145. John JF Jr, Douglas RG Jr. Tuberculous arachnoiditis. J Pediatr 1975;86:235-7.

18

Tuberculosis and Heart

SS Kothari, A Roy

INTRODUCTION

Cardiovascular involvement is a relatively uncommon manifestation in patients with tuberculosis [TB] and has been described in 1%-2% of patients (1). It mainly effects pericardium, but very rarely myocardium, valves or large arteries are involved. Although cardiovascular involvement is always secondary to TB elsewhere in the body, it may be the sole clinical manifestation of TB. *Mycobacterium tuberculosis [Mtb]* is the usual infective agent. Cardiovascular TB caused by nontuberculous myocobacteria [NTM] has been documented in patients with human immunodeficiency virus [HIV] infection (2).

TUBERCULOSIS PERICARDITIS

Pericardial TB may present as acute pericarditis, chronic pericardial effusion, cardiac tamponade or pericardial constriction. Hence, TB should always be considered in the differential diagnosis of pericardial disease. In developing countries where the disease is endemic, TB is an important cause of pericardial disease (3-5). In India, TB is responsible for nearly two-thirds of the cases of constrictive pericarditis (3,4). Over all, TB accounts for 60%-80% of cases of acute pericarditis in the developing countries. However, recently published literature suggests that, in the developed world, TB is a relatively rare cause of pericardial disease and it occurs in HIV negative, immunocompetent persons and accounts for 2% of the cases of acute pericarditis (6,7), 2% of cardiac tamponade (8) and less than 1% of constrictive pericarditis (9,10). TB pericarditis has been described in 1%-8% of patients with pulmonary TB (11).

Pericarditis is the predominant form of cardiovascular TB. Before the advent of anti-TB treatment, TB pericarditis carried a grave prognosis. The reported mortality rate in TB pericarditis was more than 80% during the acute phase of illness and still more at a later stage due to constrictive pericarditis (12-14). Even with the advent of modern anti-TB treatment, the mortality rate in patients with TB still remains worrisome with reported death rates of 3%-17% in the pre-HIV era (15,16) and as high as 27%-40% in patients with HIV infection, acquired immunodeficiency syndrome [AIDS] (17).

Pathogenesis

Pericardial involvement most commonly results from direct extension of infection from adjacent mediastinal lymph nodes or through lymphohaematogenous route from a focus in lungs, kidneys, or bones. The TB pericarditis has following stages: [i] dry stage; [ii] effusive stage; [iii] absorptive stage; and [iv] constrictive stage (18). The disease may progress sequentially from first to fourth stage or may present at any of the stages. The factors that lead to a dominant exudative inflammation in some patients and fibrosis in others are not known (19). While acute pericarditis appears to be a primary hypersensitivity response to tuberculoprotein[s], chronic effusion and constriction reflect granuloma formation and fibrosis. Epithelioid granulomas, Langhans' giant cells and caseation necrosis are evident on histopathological examination (20). The T-lymphocytes, in addition to activated macrophages, are important in granuloma formation. The accompanying exudative pericardial fluid may contain polymorphonuclear leucocytes in the initial 1-2 weeks, but later on, it is predominantly lymphocytic with high protein content. In 80% of the cases, the fluid is straw coloured or sero-sanguinous, and may be grossly bloody resembling venous blood at times (1). Very rarely, severe inflammation may result in pyopericardium due to TB (21). The amount of pericardial fluid may vary from 15-3500 mL (22).

Development of cardiac tamponade due to TB pericarditis depends on the rapidity of collection of pericardial fluid. It may occur even with a slowly accumulating large pericardial effusion. Fibrinous exudates, pericardial effusion and thickening of pericardium from fibrosis [especially the visceral layer] result in features of effuso-constrictive pericarditis within weeks of development of TB pericarditis. Continued inflammation and fibrotic activity may lead to chronic constrictive pericarditis [CCP]. With effective anti-TB treatment, the pericardial effusion may resolve without development of CCP in nearly half the patients (5). Many patients with CCP, however, have no history of previous TB pericarditis. Complete obliteration of pericardial space by a fibrotic constricting shell results in impairment of cardiac function. In chronic cases, the inflammatory process may extend into myocardium resulting in myonecrosis and muscle atrophy. The constriction, at times, may be patchy and localised to certain areas like mitral or tricuspid annulus (23). The space around transverse and oblique sinus is often spared from fibrosis, and, therefore, some degree of left atrial enlargement commonly occurs in CCP.

Clinical Features

TB pericarditis can develop at any age but commonly occurs in the middle ages. In the series, reported by Strang et al (16) more than 80% patients were older than 35 years with nearly half of them being more than 55 years old. Like other forms of TB, it is more common in patients who are immunosuppressed. However, the majority of patients do not have any other co-morbid conditions. It is more common among the black race as compared to whites in the western world (1,23,24). The clinical features depend on the stage and severity of the disease. The pericarditis is often insidious in onset and presents with fever, malaise and weakness. Attention to the diagnosis is drawn by the presence of pericardial rub, vague chest pain or cardiomegaly on chest radiograph. Dyspnoea, non-productive cough and weight loss are common symptoms. Chest pain, orthopnoea and ankle oedema occur in nearly 40%-70% of patients (1,22,25). Chest pain is usually pleuritic in nature and is characteristically relieved by sitting up and leaning forward. This manoeuvre relieves increased pericardial tissue tension due to inspiration and truncal extension and also splints the diaphragm (26). Pain radiation to shoulder and jaw can mimic angina rarely. Radiation of pain to trapezius ridge though the phrenic nerve is virtually pathognomonic of pericardial pain (26). However, TB pericarditis may also present with an acute illness in 20% of the cases (5). The reported frequency of various symptoms in different series is shown in Tables 18.1 and 18.2 (1,24,25,27-29).

Pericardial Effusion

Patients with TB pericarditis may develop chronic pericardial effusion with mild or severe constitutional symptoms (1,25). Patients may also present acutely with cardiac tamponade and may manifest severe distress, retrosternal compress, tachycardia and raised jugular venous pressure [JVP] with blunted descent. In patients with cardiac tamponade, the heart sounds are usually distant. A pericardial rub may be heard despite significant pericardial effusion. Pulsus paradoxus [inspiratory decline of systolic blood pressure of more than 10 mmHg] is the hallmark of bedside diagnosis of cardiac tamponade.

Subacute Effusive-Constrictive Pericarditis

This subacute stage of TB pericarditis is also termed as subacute "elastic" pericarditis. It has features of both pericardial effusion and constriction. The fluid-fibrin layer leads to relatively elastic compression of heart, which has been compared to "wrapping the heart tightly with rubber bands" (30). The haemodynamics of the non-rigid fibroelastic form of constrictive pericarditis resembles tamponade because the fibroelastic constriction compresses the heart throughout the cardiac cycle, and respiratory changes in intra-thoracic pressure are transmitted to the cardiac chambers (30). Thus, the pattern of ventricular filling is similar to cardiac tamponade rather than constrictive pericarditis and includes a systemic venous waveform with a predominant x descent or equal x and y descent, an inconspicuous early diastolic dip in the ventricular waveforms, an inspiratory dip in systemic venous and right atrial pressures, and presence of pulsus paradoxus.

Table 18.1: Clinical symptoms in patients with tuberculosis pericarditis

Variable	Hageman et al (24) [n = 44]	Rooney et al (25) [n = 35]	Fowler (1) [n = 19]	Komsuoglu et al (27) [n = 20]	Yang et al (28) [n = 19]	Reuter et al (29) [n = 162]
Weight loss	ND	85	40	ND	32	79
Night sweats	14	37	58	10	ND	62
Chest pain	39	57	76	40	37	27
Cough	48	85	94	50	47	90
Haemoptysis	ND	17	14	ND	ND	ND
Dyspnoea	80	74	88	60	84	86
Orthopnoea	39	66	53	ND	ND	38

All values are shown as percentages
n = number of patients; ND = not described

Table 18.2: Physical signs in patients with tuberculosis pericarditis

Variable	Hageman et al (24) [n = 44]	Rooney et al (25) [n = 35]	Fowler (1) [n = 19]	Komsuoglu et al (27) [n = 20]	Yang et al (28) [n = 19]	Reuter et al (29) [n = 162]
Fever	73	97	83	ND	58	75
Tachycardia [> 100/min]	68	94	83	73	47	74
Pulsus paradoxus	45	23	71	33	11	27
Ankle oedema	64	49	39	24	42	38
Raised JVP	70	46	61	47	68	78
Pericardial rub	41	37	84	ND	32	ND
Cardiomegaly	90	85	95	98	79	ND
Pleural effusion	ND	71	58	10	42	38
Hepatomegaly	68	63	65	67	26	62
Ascites	34	3	ND	ND	26	ND
Pulmonary infiltrates	ND	ND	ND	ND	42	ND

All values are shown as percentages
n = number of patients; JVP = jugular venous pressure; ND = not described

This stage can develop within weeks of TB pericarditis. With effective anti-TB treatment the disease may resolve in some patients, but commonly chronic constriction supervenes (5,16).

Chronic Constrictive Pericarditis

In hearts with CCP, the inflow of blood is impeded due to thickened unyielding pericardium, especially in the late diastole. Thus the patients usually present with predominant symptoms of systemic and pulmonary venous congestion. Abdominal swelling [from ascites or hepatomegaly] and peripheral oedema are the most common presenting symptoms. Dyspnoea and orthopnoea are also present in nearly half the patients requiring surgical intervention (31). Cardiac output is mildly reduced at rest. These patients have compensatory tachycardia to maintain cardiac output. Since more than 75% of diastolic filling occurs in the first 25% of the diastole, shortening of diastole does not reduce stroke volume much but helps in augmenting cardiac output. Other clinical signs seen are raised JVP with rapid y descent [Friedreich's sign], which increases further on inspiration [Kussmaul's sign]. Pulsatile hepatomegaly, ascites with an impalpable apex or systolic retraction of precordium [Broadbent's sign] are also seen commonly. A pericardial knock that occurs 0.11-0.12 sec after the second heart sound may be present; murmurs are uncommon. In one Indian study (32), atrio-ventricular regurgitation was present in 78% of patients with CCP on Doppler examination, but an audible murmur was present in only 2 of the 33 patients. In general, presence of cardiomegaly, third and fourth heart sounds, significant mitral or tricuspid regurgitation, and severe pulmonary hypertension favour restrictive cardio-myopathy rather than CCP.

Other atypical manifestations include clinical presentation with ascites disproportionate to the peripheral oedema [ascites precox] which may be mistaken for primary liver disease. Sometimes, patients may also present with subtle signs like fatigue, without obvious clinical findings of CCP. These patients with "occult" constrictive pericarditis often manifest pericardial thickening on radiological imaging. The clinical signs of constrictive pericarditis often manifest pericardial thickening on radiological imaging. The clinical signs of constrictive pericarditis may become evident on fluid challenge in such patients. These patients improve with pericardiectomy. Other patients may present with congestive splenomegaly and protein losing enteropathy resulting in hypoproteinemia. Rarely, nephritic syndrome due to CCP has been described (31). Cardiac cirrhosis may also develop after many years of hepatic venous congestion.

The disease worsens gradually and in chronic cases, significant myocardial atrophy occurs due to extension of inflammation and possibly disuse of muscle. These patients have suboptimal results and high mortality with pericardiectomy (23).

Differential Diagnosis

The differential diagnosis of TB pericarditis includes a number of conditions like idiopathic, viral, or, infectious pericarditis and pericarditis due to neoplasia, collagen vascular disorders and uraemia among others. The aetiological diagnosis in pericarditis is often established on the basis of "guilt by association".

Majority of patients with idiopathic or viral pericarditis have acute onset with characteristic chest pain. Pericardial effusion may be small or absent. Idiopathic or viral pericarditis is a self-limited illness lasting two to three weeks (33). However, a more protracted course, large pericardial effusion or cardiac tamponade are not infrequent in idiopathic or viral pericarditis. On the other hand, TB pericarditis may have an acute onset. The differentiation of TB pericarditis from idiopathic or viral pericarditis may present a diagnostic dilemma.

Diagnosis

Chest Radiograph

Cardiomegaly has been commonly reported in various published series on TB pericarditis. It was present in 40 of 44 patients described in one study (24) and in 190 of the 193 patients in another (16). Active pulmonary TB has been reported in nearly 30% patients with TB pericarditis (1,16,34,35). However, pericarditis may be the only manifestation of extra-pulmonary TB [EPTB] in several patients. Reduced cardiac pulsations on fluoroscopy have been reported in 76% patients (24). Pleural effusion has also been frequently described and may be bilateral in some patients (25). Pericardial calcification [Figure 18.1] commonly occurs around the annulus and has been observed in 15% patients in western series (3,23).

Electrocardiogram

The most common electrocardiogram [ECG] findings in patients with TB pericarditis are presence of low voltage complexes and T-wave inversion with or without ST-segment changes [Figure 18.2]. One of these findings is present in over 90% patients (24,25). In a recent study (36) of 88 patients with TB pericarditis, presence of low voltage in the extremity and/or precordial leads correlated with the presence of greater than 750 mL of pericardial fluid. However, no ECG parameters were predictive of cardiac tamponade (36). The presence of classical ST-segment elevation of acute pericarditis is rare and is seen in 2%-9% of patients (24,25).

Pericardial Fluid

The pericardial fluid is usually straw coloured or serosanguinous and has high protein content. The cell count is high with predominance of lymphocytes and monocytes. In the initial weeks, predominantly polymorphonuclear leucocytes may be seen and very rarely TB may cause purulent pericarditis (21). A smear of pericardial fluid rarely identifies acid-fast bacilli [AFB] on Ziehl-Neelsen [Z-N] staining. Fluorochrome staining is a more sensitive technique for identifying mycobacteria than conventional Z-N staining (37). Culture of pericardial fluid grows *Mtb* in about 50%-60% cases using Lowenstein-Jensen [LJ] or double strength Kirchner medium (16,25). However, the major drawback is that six to eight weeks are needed for the conventional mycobacterial cultures to yield results. Newer radiometric culture techniques like BACTEC yield quicker results. Molecular diagnostic methods like cartridge-based nucleic acid amplification tests [CBNAAT], especially Xpert MTB/RIF® has been found to be useful in the diagnosis of TB pericarditis (38). In a recently published systematic review (39) pooled sensitivity and specificity of pericardial fluid Xpert MTB/RIF were found to be 65.7% and 96.0%, respectively. Pericardial fluid adenosine deaminase [ADA] levels above 70 IU/L has been shown to be highly sensitive and specific for the diagnosis of TB pericarditis (27). However, ADA which is produced by activated macrophages and lymphocytes may also be raised in malignant effusions. Simultaneous measurement of lysozyme, which is raised in TB effusions, along with ADA may help in distinguishing TB pericardial effusion from malignant pericardial effusion (40).

Pericardial Biopsy

Pericardial biopsy, though rarely done, is another useful method for confirming the aetiology of pericarditis and it gives results earlier than pericardial fluid culture. Tissue can be obtained by open biopsy or percutaneously using a

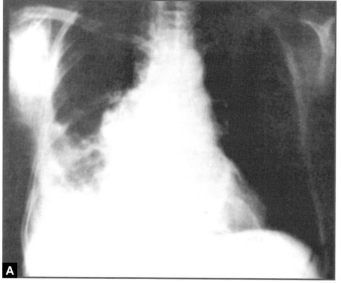
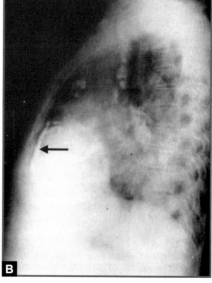

Figure 18.1: Chest radiograph [postero-anterior view] [A] showing moderate cardiomegaly, dense, plaque-like calcification of the pericardium in the anterior and inferior atrioventricular groove. Right basal pneumonitis and pleural effusion are also seen. Extensive calcification of hilar, anterior mediastinal and right paratracheal lymph nodes is seen. Chest radiograph [lateral view] of the same patient [B]. Pericardial calcification [arrow] is better appreciated in this view

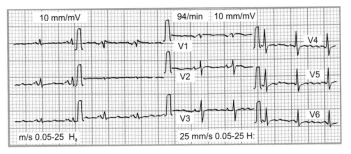

Figure 18.2: Three-channel recording of a 12-lead electrocardiogram at 25 mm/s in a child with chronic constrictive pericarditis. Limb leads show a low-voltage graph and non-specific T-wave inversion in leads V4-V6. Left atrial enlargement is also evident

bioptome (41,42). Percutaenous biopsy is taken from multiple sites and has been shown to be safe in a selected group of patients, including children. Histopathological examination of pericardial tissue may be diagnostic of TB in 70% of cases when performed prior to initiation of therapy (16). However, it is important to note that in some patients with culture positive TB, histopathology may show non-specific changes. Thus, a non-specific histopathological change in the pericardial biopsy does not exclude TB (16). The pericardial tissue culture also provides an additional source for isolating *Mtb* and increases the diagnostic yield (16,42).

Echocardiogram

The echocardiogram is highly sensitive and specific for the diagnosis of pericardial effusion and cardiac tamponade [Figures 18.3, 18.4, 18.5, 18.6 and 18.7]. When 1 cm of posterior echo-free space is evident in systole and diastole, with or without fluid accumulation elsewhere, the pericardial effusion is classified as 'small'. When a posterior clear space of 1-2 cm is maintained in systole and diastole, the effusion is classified as 'moderate'. In 'large' pericardial

effusions, a clear space of 2 cm or more is evident; or when an anterior and posterior clear space can be seen in systole and diastole (43).

Collapse of right atrial and right ventricular free wall in diastole by pericardial fluid and exaggerated respiratory variation in atrio-ventricular valve flow velocities are diagnostic of tamponade and may precede clinical evidence. Pericardial fluid often contains fibrinous exudates. Rarely, these exudates may appear as a fleshy tumour that disappears with anti-TB treatment (44). Thickened pericardium and pericardial effusion are seen in the effusive-constrictive stage [Figures 18.8, 18.9, 18.10, 18.11, 18.12 and 18.13]. Pericardial thickening is best visualised anteriorly over the right ventricular free wall. Transoesophageal echocardiography is

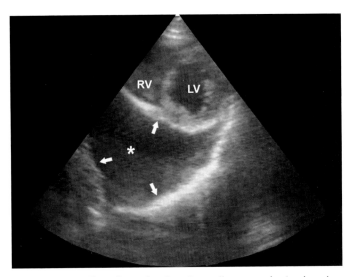

Figure 18.4: Two-dimensional echocardiogram short-axis view showing thickened pericardium [arrows] and massive pericardial effusion [asterisk]
RV = right ventricle; LV = left ventricle

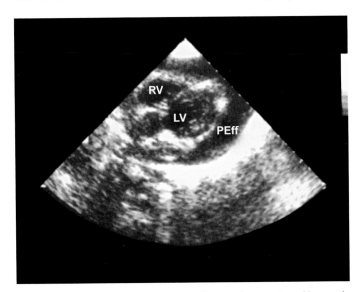

Figure 18.3: Two-dimensional echocardiogram in parasternal long axis view of a child with tuberculosis pericardial effusion
RV = right ventricle; LV = left ventricle; PEff = pericardial effusion

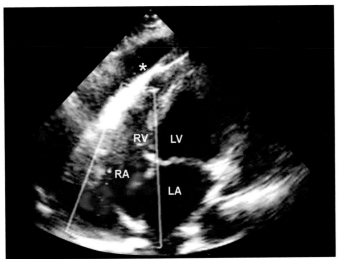

Figure 18.5: Two-dimensional echocardiogram, apical four-chamber view showing diastolic compression of RA and RV in a patient with pericardial effusion [asterisk] and cardiac tamponade
LA = left atrium; LV = left ventricle; RA = right atrium; RV = right ventricle

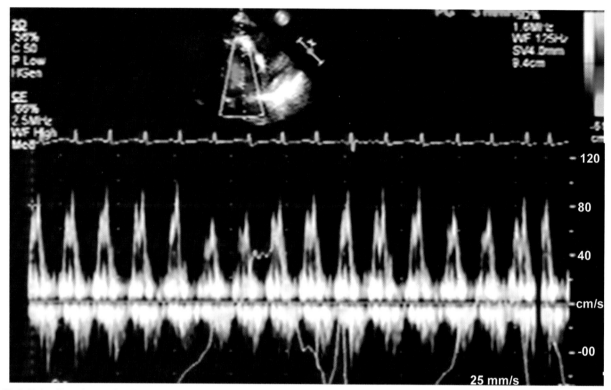

Figure 18.6: Pulse Doppler study of mitral valve in a patient with cardiac tamponade showing significant respiratory variation [>25%] in mitral inflow

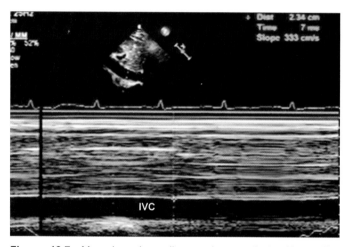

Figure 18.7: M-mode echocardiogram in a patient with cardiac tamponade showing IVC plethora with no respiratory variation
IVC = inferior vena cava

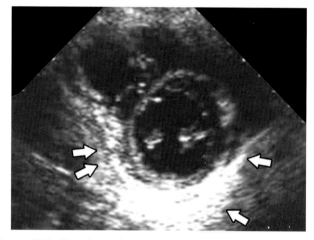

Figure 18.8: Two-dimensional echocardiogram, short-axis view, in a patient with chronic constrictive pericarditis. Thickened calcified pericardium [arrows] can be seen along basal ventricles and AV groove. The pericardium was 4.7 mm thick
AV = atrio-ventricular

superior to transthoracic echocardiography in the detection of pericardial thickening. The normal pericardium is a thin, bright line of 1.2 ± 0.8 mm. In one study (45), the pericardium in patients with constrictive pericardtis measured 9.8 ± 1.6 mm. Pericardial thickness as measured by transoesophageal echocardiography was found to have an excellent correlation with computed tomography [CT] (46). When a value of 3 mm was used as a cut-off for defining pericardial thickness as measured by transoesophageal echocardiography, the sensitivity and specificity of this technique for CCP were calculated to be 95% and 86% respectively (46).

The other findings in CCP include abrupt flattening of mid to late diastolic movement of the left ventricular posterior wall on M-mode, reflecting a sudden decline in diastolic filling (47). Other M-mode features include rapid early closure of the mitral valve and, uncommonly, premature pulmonary valve opening from increased right-sided diastolic pressures. A diastolic septal bounce is also commonly seen. Diastolic septal motion is controlled by the pressure gradient across the septum. The abrupt bounce may be caused by sudden changes in the trans-

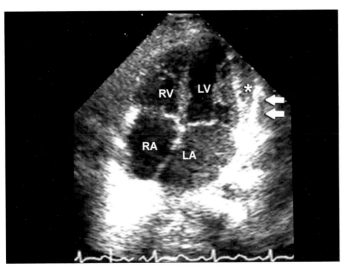

Figure 18.9: Two-dimensional echocardiogram, apical four-chamber view, in a patients with effusive-constrictive pericarditis showing thickened pericardium adjacent to the basal lateral LV [arrows], biatrial enlargement. Moderate pericardial effusion [asterisk] is also present LA = left atrium; LV = left ventricle; RA = right atrium; RV = right ventricle

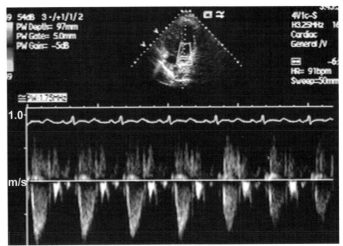

Figure 18.11: Continuous Doppler study of aortic valve in a patient with chronic constrictive pericarditis showing significant respiratory variation in aortic flow demonstrating ventricular interdependence

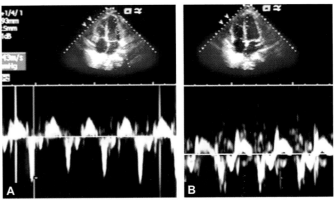

Figure 18.12: Tissue Doppler study showing increased excursion velocity of lateral [A] and septal [B] mitral annulus suggestive of constrictive pericarditis

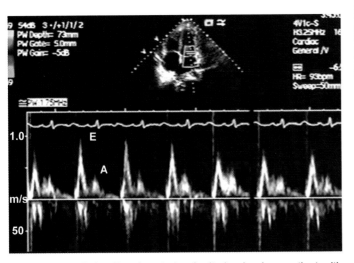

Figure 18.10: Pulse Doppler study of mitral valve in a patient with constrictive pericarditis showing restrictive pattern of mitral filling with E/A >2. Also demonstrated is the significant respiratory variation [> 20%] in mitral inflow characteristic of ventricular interdependence E = mitral valve flow velocity during early diastole; A = during late diastole

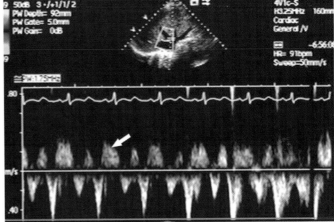

Figure 18.13: Pulse Doppler study of hepatic vein in a patient with constrictive pericarditis showing diastolic flow reversal [arrow]

septal gradient during diastole, when filling is particularly rapid (48). Additional echocardiographic abnormalities include mild atrial dilatation and dilatation of inferior vena cava [IVC].

Doppler studies also help in diagnosing CCP and differentiating it from restrictive cardiomyopathy [Figures 18.10, 18.11, 18.12 and 18.13]. The mitral flow velocities show more than 25% respiratory variation [decrease with inspiration], most pronounced in the first heartbeat after inspiration from apnoea (49). Similarly, an expiratory increase in diastolic flow reversal [>25%] of the hepatic venous flow velocities is suggestive of CCP. Tissue Doppler velocities are usually preserved in CCP [Figure 18.12] and this feature helps to distinguish it from restrictive cardiomyopathy wherein tissue velocities are commonly impaired.

Cross-sectional Imaging

Cross-sectional imaging with CT or magnetic resonance imaging [MRI] can reveal pericardial effusion [Figures 9.42, 18.14], are very useful in the diagnosis of CCP and in distinguishing it from restrictive cardiomyopathy. The diagnostic hallmark is the presence of pericardial thickening with or without calcification [Figure 18.15]. Additionally, CT scan is useful in demonstrating mediastinal lymphadenopathy [Figure 18.16]. While CT scores over MRI in detection of minimal amounts of pericardial calcification, MRI provides better soft tissue characterisation (50), this may be useful in distinguishing restrictive cardiomyopathy from CCP. Pericardial thickening of more than 3 mm is usually considered abnormal. Often a localised process, pericardial thickening is most frequently seen over the right ventricle. In a study of 29 patients (51), MRI was found to be 88% sensitive and 100% specific, with a diagnostic accuracy of 93% for detecting CCP. However, pericardial thickening can be seen without constrictive physiology. Similarly, in a small proportion of patients with constrictive physiology, no pericardial thickening can be identified. Therefore, it is important to search for additional findings suggestive of CCP like tubular shaped ventricles, enlarged atria, focal contour abnormalities of the ventricles, dilated IVC, ascites and pleural effusion on CT or MRI (50).

Positron Emission Tomography–Computed Tomography

Positron emission tomography–computed tomography [PET-CT] using ¹⁸F labelled 2-deoxy-D-glucose [FDG] is increasingly being used in the evaluation of patients with EPTB, including TB pericarditis and has been found to be useful in disease localisation and assessing response to treatment on follow-up [Figure 18.17].

Cardiac Catheterisation

Cardiac tamponade or CCP due to any cause produces a similarly elevated right, left atrial [or pulmonary arterial wedge], right and left ventricular end-diastolic pressures. These pressures are within 5 mmHg of each other [Figure 18.18]. The other classical haemodynamic criteria favouring CCP over restrictive cardiomyopathy (52) are a right ventricular systolic pressure less than or equal to 50 mmHg and a ratio of right ventricular end-diastolic pressure to right ventricular systolic pressure greater than or equal to 1:3. If all these three haemodynamic criteria are met, the probability of CCP is over 90%. If one or none of these criteria are present, then probability of CCP is less than 10%. However, one-fourth of patients may not be classified by these haemodynamic criteria (53).

Measuring respiratory variation in ventricular haemodynamics during catheterisation is another useful criteria for the diagnosis of CCP (49,53). As a manifestation of ventricular interdependence, respiratory discordance occurs in peak right ventricular systolic pressure and left ventricular systolic pressure. In CCP, right ventricular systolic pressure increases with inspiration while left ventricular systolic pressure simultaneously decreases. Wedge pressure declines more than the left ventricular pressure leading to reduction in mitral flow, which translates into the observed reduction in left ventricular systolic pressure. This criterion has 100% sensitivity and 95% specificity for diagnosis of CCP (53). In restrictive cardiomyopathy, both right and left ventricular systolic pressures decrease concordantly with inspiration (53).

Treatment

Once diagnosis of TB pericarditis is established, prompt initiation of anti-TB treatment is mandatory (54). Recommended therapy consists of four-drug regimen containing isoniazid, rifampicin, pyrazinamide and ethambutol for two months followed by isoniazid, rifampicin and ethambutol for next four months. Some physicians prefer to administer longer duration of treatment. However, no randomised controlled trial has compared different durations of anti-tuberculosis drug regimens in TB pericarditis. Similar duration of treatment is recommended for HIV-positive patients. As per the recently published evidence-based

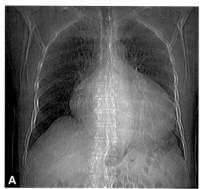 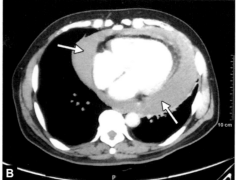 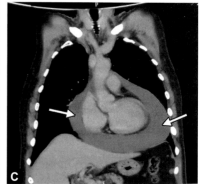

Figure 18.14: CT chest in a patient with TB pericardial effusion [topogram] [A] showing cardiomegaly [known as "money bag" or "water bottle" sign]. CECT chest of the same patient axial view [B], coronal reconstruction [C] showing pericardial effusion [arrows]
CECT = contrast-enhanced computed tomography

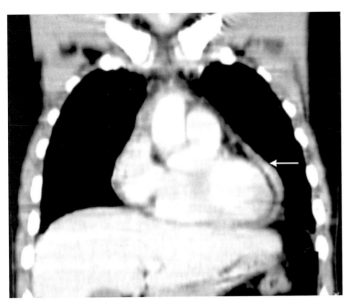

Figure 18.15: Sagittal reconstruction of a contrast-enhanced CT of the chest showing shell-like thickening [11 mm] of the pericardium [arrow] in a patient with tuberculosis pericardial effusion. Echocardiography did not reveal any evidence of constriction

Guidelines for Extrapulmonary TB for India [INDEX-TB Guidelines] (55), a treatment duration of 6 months is considered adequate for TB pericarditis. The reader is referred to the chapter *"Treatment of tuberculosis" [Chapter 44]* for details. Under the Revised National Tuberculosis Control Programme [RNTCP] of the Government of India, pericardial TB is categorised as serious form of EPTB and new patients with TB pericarditis are treated with Category I daily treatment for six months.

Role of Adjuvant Corticosteroid Treatment

In small controlled clinical trials, the addition of predniosolone to anti-TB treatment has been shown to reduce mortality and the need for repeated pericardiocentesis in patients with TB pericarditis and effusion (5,16). The effectiveness of adjunctive corticosteroids in patients with TB pericarditis is now well justified (56).

In a double-blind study, addition of prednisolone, as an adjuvant to six months of anti-TB treatment, in patients of active TB constrictive pericarditis (5) increased the rate of clinical improvement, reduced the risk of death from pericarditis and the need of pericardiectomy was compared to placebo. It was associated with a higher proportion of patients with an overall favourable status. In a subsequent randomised controlled trial with a factorial design by the same group (16), [i] immediate, complete, open surgical drainage of pericardial fluid versus percutaneous pericardiocentesis as required; and [ii] predniosolone versus placebo, double-blind, as a supplement to six months of anti-TB treatment were compared. The authors reported that open drainage eliminated the need for repeat pericardiocentesis, though it did not reduce subsequent constriction. They also observed that prednisolone reduced the risk of death from

pericarditis and the need for repeat pericardiocentesis, and was associated with a higher propotion of patients with an overall favourable status. In both trials, the prednisolone was used for a period of 11 weeks of anti-TB treatment in a dosage of 60 mg/day for four and tapered over the next seven weeks. The authors (57), reported results of 10 years follow-up of the same cohort. In multivariate survival analysis [stratified by type of pericarditis], adjuvant prednisolone treatment reduced the overall death rate after adjusting for age and sex, and substantially reduced the risk of death from pericarditis.

In another trial (17) in HIV-seropositive patients with TB pericarditis, there was a significant reduction in all-cause mortality with use of steroids at 18 months of follow-up (17). A systematic review of all trials on adjuvant steroids concluded that while case fatality rate was markedly reduced by steroids, this did not reach statistical significance due to the small number of patients in the studies (58). A recently published international multicentre, randomised controlled clinical trial, the Investigation of the Management of Pericarditis *[IMPI]* trial (59), evaluated the effects of adjunctive glucocorticoid therapy and *Mycobacterium indicus pranii* immunotherapy in patients with TB pericarditis. In this trial (59), it was observed that there was no significant difference in the primary outcome [a composite of death, cardiac tamponade requiring pericardiocentesis, or constrictive pericarditis] between patients who received prednisolone and those who received placebo; or between those who received *M. indicus pranii* immunotherapy and those who received placebo.

As per the INDEX-TB Guidelines] (55), corticosteroids are recommended for HIV-seronegative [conditional, low quality evidence] and HIV-seropositive patients [conditional, low-quality evidence] with TB pericarditis with pericardial effusion.

Pericardiocentesis and Pericardiectomy

Pericardiocentesis is life-saving in patients with cardiac tamponade and also provides an opportunity to confirm the aetiology of the pericardial effusion. This can be performed percutaneously and by open surgical drainage. The latter method abolishes the need for repeat pericardiocentesis but does not reduce subsequent mortality or need for pericardiectomy (16). Furthermore, open surgical drainage requires general anaesthesia unlike percutaneously performed procedure, but provides an opportunity to obtain pericardial tissue for histopathological examination. Reuter *et al* (60) from South Africa studied 233 patients with TB pericardial effusion and reported that these patients responded well to closed pericardiocentesis and a six-month anti-TB treatment.

Chronic constrictive pericarditis requires pericardiectomy, which is preferably avoided in the subacute stage when a plane of cleavage has not clearly developed (61). However, pericardiectomy can be done after two to four weeks of chemotherapy and should not be unduly delayed, if indicated. Various approaches to pericardiectomy,

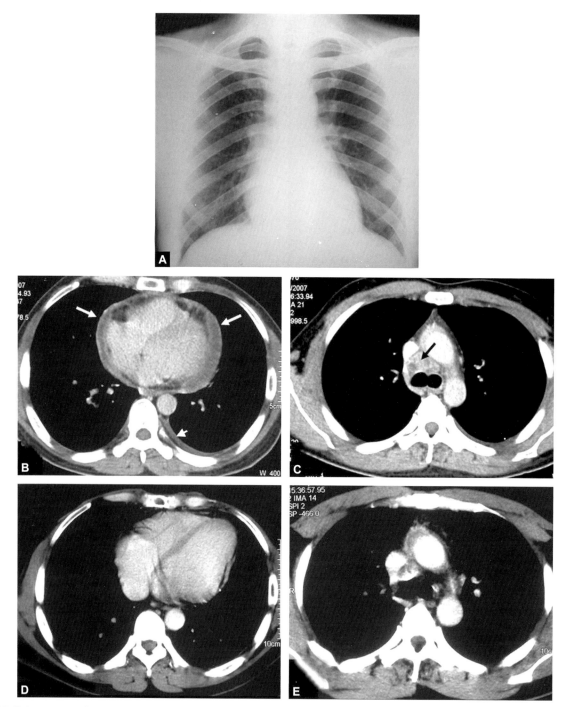

Figure 18.16: Tuberculosis effusive-constrictive pericarditis. Chest radiograph [postero-anterior view] showing cardiomegaly [A]. CT of the chest of the same patient [mediastinal window] showing pericardial effusion along with well-defined pericardial thickening [arrows], left-sided pleural effusion [arrow head] [B] and mediastinal lymphadenopathy [arrow] [C]. The lymph nodes show the characteristic peripheral rim enhancement with central attenuation. Repeat CT after completion of antituberculosis treatment showing significant regression in pericardial effusion and thickening [D] and mediastinal lymphadenopathy [E]

i.e. median sternotomy, lateral thoracotomy, bilateral thoracotomy, with or without use of cardiopulmonary bypass; and anterior or total removal of pericardium have been described depending on patient population or personal surgeon preferences. Cardiopulmonary bypass is needed for more difficult cases with extensive calcification, coronary involvement or large vessel involvement. Surgical

mortality of pericardiectomy is still high, especially in patients with calcification, in whom it was reported as 19% in a recent series (62). Other adverse predictors of outcome are long-standing disease, baseline poor functional class, low-voltage ECG complex, significantly increased atrial pressure, associated organ failure and myocardial involvement.

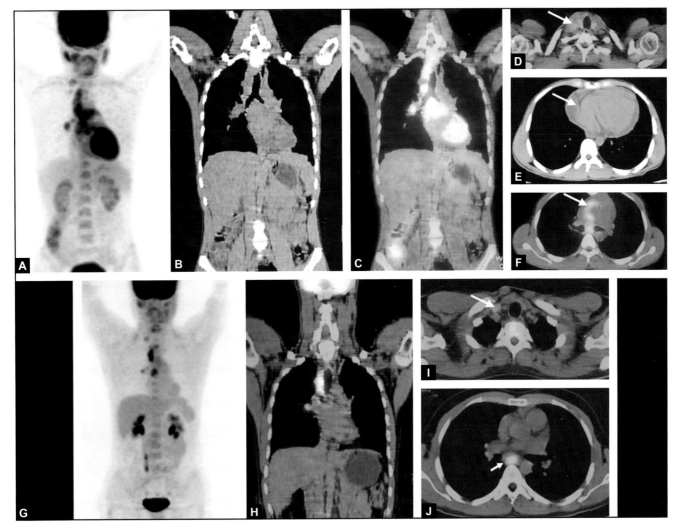

Figure 18.17: ^{18}F FDG PET-CT, maximum intensity projection image [A] showing sites of abnormal ^{18}F FDG accumulation in the mediastinum. Coronal NCCT [B] reveals multiple paratracheal, subcarinal and right hilar lymph nodes which show FDG accumulation on fused coronal PET-CT [C]. Transaxial fused PET-CT [D] showing tracer accumulation in right supraclavicular node [arrow], transaxial NCCT [E] showing pericardial effusion [arrow] and transaxial fused PET-CT [F] reveals tracer uptake in the pericardial attachment [arrow]. ^{18}F FDG PET-CT, maximum intensity projection image [G] of the same patient at six months of anti-TB treatment, showing sites of abnormal ^{18}F FDG accumulation in the mediastinum. Fused coronal PET-CT [H] showing paratracheal and right hilar lymph nodes which show FDG accumulation [C]. Transaxial fused PET-CT [I] showing tracer accumulation in right supraclavicular node [arrow], Transaxial fused PET-CT [J] showing tracer accumulation in subcarinal node [arrow]. Significant resolution of pericardial effusion is evident

PET-CT = positron emission tomography-computed tomography; FDG = fluorodeoxyglucose; TB = tuberculosis

CARDIAC TUBERCULOSIS

Myocardial TB is very rare (63,64). However with improving imaging techniques, it is being detected with increasing frequency. In patients with diffuse cardiac TB, myocardial involvement occurs but is overshadowed by the diffuse involvement. Nodular myocardial TB can, sometimes, produce a tumour-like granulomatous mass which may involve any of the cardiac chambers and multiple chambers at times (65) [Figure 18.19]. Most of these masses respond well to anti-TB treatment and may completely disappear without need for surgical excision. TB involvement with caseation necrosis of myocardium may cause aneurysm in

submitral or left ventricular anterior wall (66). Occasionally, a lymphocytic myocarditis without demonstration of *Mtb* has been described in patients with TB (63). Rare case reports of TB endocarditis have also been reported (67). Coronary arteritis from TB occurs infrequently in patients with TB pericarditis (68).

Myocardial TB is also an under-recognised aetiological cause in patients presenting with idiopathic venricular tachycardia [VT] or unexplained ventricular dysfunction (69). These patients may not have constitutional symptoms; associated intrathoracic lymphadenopathy with or without peripheral lymphadenopathy is often present.

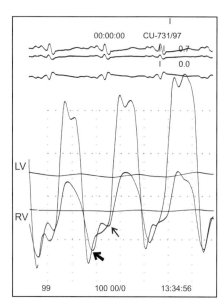

Figure 18.18: LV and RV pressure tracing at paper speed of 100 mm/s and 100 mmHg gain [each small square = 5 mmHg]. Early [thick arrow] and late [thin arrow] diastolic pressures of the two ventricles are similar [30 mmHg] and markedly elevated. Right ventricular systolic pressure is also elevated to 60 to 65 mmHg

LV = left ventricular pressure tracing; RV = right ventricular pressure tracing

Cardiac MRI and PET-CT are helpful in disease localisation. Image-guided lymph node sampling and diagnostic testing has been found to be helpful in confirming the diagnosis (69). The condition responds well to standard anti-TB treatment.

TAKAYASU'S ARTERITIS

Takayasu's arteritis, also referred to as non-specific aortoarteritis, is an inflammatory disease involving aorta and its large branches and pulmonary arteries [Figure 18.20]. The disease occurs more commonly in Asia, Africa, Mexico and South America. The role of *Mtb* in aetiopathogenesis of Takayasu's arteritis has been the subject of debate for a long time. As many as one-third of patients with Takayasu's arteritis have associated past or present TB and a large number of patients have a strongly positive tuberculin skin test. Evidence of mycobacterial involvement has also emerged from recent cytochemical and serological studies (70). There is no consensus regarding the role of anti-TB treatment in patients with Takayasu's arteritis. However, patients with evidence of active TB should be treated with anti-TB treatment and corticosteroids.

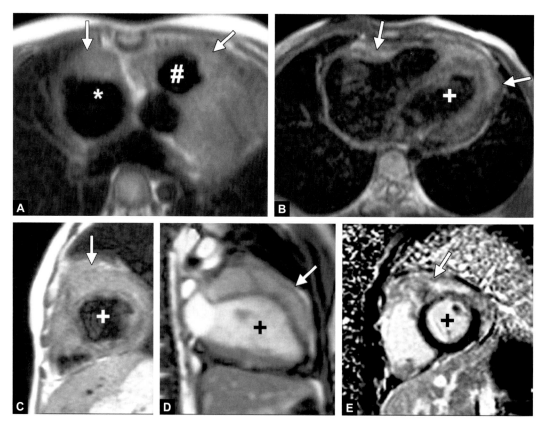

Figure 18.19: Cardiac MRI, axial T1-weighted images [A and B] showing isointense masses [arrows] along the anterior right atrium [*], right ventricular outflow tract [#], and along both ventricles [+ indicates left ventricle]. Short-axis T2-weighted image [C] showing that the lesions are mildly hyperintense. Steady state free precession image [D] revealing the infiltrative nature of the lesion along the left ventricle. The delayed enhanced short-axis image [E] shows heterogeneous enhancement of the mass

MRI = magnetic resonance imaging

Reproduced with permission from "Gulati GS, Kothari SS. Diffuse infiltrative cardiac tuberculosis. Ann Pediatr Cardiol 2011;4:87-9" (reference 65)

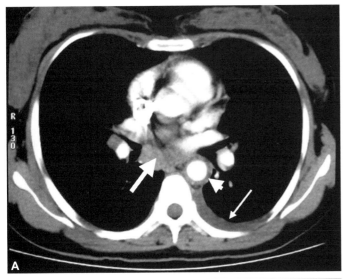

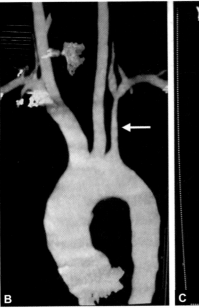
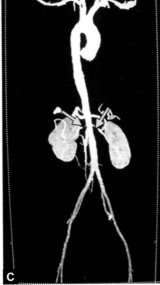

Figure 18.20: Non-specific aortoarteritis. CECT chest, axial view [A] showing aortic wall involvement [arrow head], subcarinal lympha-denopathy [thick arrow] and left sided pleural effusion [thin arrow]. Volume rendered CT angiography image showing irregular aortic wall and left subclavian artery [arrow] [B], bilateral renal artery stenosis [yellow arrows] [C]
CECT = contrast-enhanced computed tomography

ACKNOWLEDGEMENTS

Kind help rendered by Dr C Narasimhan, CARE Hospital, Hyderabad and Dr Madhavi Tripathi, Department of Nuclear Medicine, All India Institute of Medical Sciences, New Delhi, in providing Figures is thankfully acknowledged.

REFERENCES

1. Fowler NO. Tuberculous pericarditis. JAMA 1991;266:99-103.
2. Palmer JA, Watanakunakorn C. Mycobacterium kansasii pericaditis. Thorax 1984;39:876-7.
3. Bashi VV, John S, Ravikumar E, Sukumar IP, Shyamsunder K, Krishnaswamy S. Early and late results of pericardiectomy in 118 cases of constrictive pericarditis. Thorax 1988;43:637-41.
4. Das PB, Gupta, Sukumar IP, Cherian G, John S. Pericardiectomy: indications and results. J Thoracic Cardiovasc Surg 1973;66:58-70.
5. Strang JI, Kakaz HH, Gibson DG, Girling DJ, Nunn AJ, Fox W. Controlled trial of prednisolone as adjuvant in treatment of tuberculous constrictive pericarditis in Transkei. Lancet 1987;2: 1418-22.
6. Bruch C, Schmermund A, Dagres N, Bartel T, Caspari G, Sack S, et al. Changes in QRS voltage in cardiac tamponade and pericardial effusion: reversibility after pericardiocentesis and after anti-inflammatory drug treatment. J Am Coll Cardiol 2001; 38:219-26.
7. Zayas R, Anguita M, Torres F, Gimenez D, Bergillos F, Ruiz M, et al. Incidence of specific etiology and role of methods for specific etiologic diagnosis of primary acute pericarditis. Am J Cardiol 1995;75:378-82.
8. Oliver Navarrete C, Marin Ortuno F, Pineda Rocamora J, Lujan Martinez J, Garcia Fernandez A, Climent Paya VE, et al. Should we try to determine the specific cause of cardiac tamponade? Rev Esp Cardiol 2002;55:493-8.
9. Ling LH, Oh JK, Schaff HV, Danielson GK, Mahoney DW, Seward JB, et al. Constrictive pericarditis in the modern era: evolving clinical spectrum and impact on outcome after pericardiectomy. Circulation 1999;100:1380-6.
10. Oh KY, Shimizu M, Edwards WD, Tazelaar HD, Danielson GK. Surgical pathology of the parietal pericardium: a study of 344 cases [1993-1999]. Cardiovasc Pathol 2001;10:157-68.
11. Larrieu AJ, Tyers GF, Williams EH, Derrick JR. Recent experience with tuberculous pericarditis. Ann Thorac Surg 1980;29:464-8.
12. Meguire J, Kotte JH, Helm RA. Acute pericarditis. Medicine 1937; 9:425-42.
13. Harvey AM, Whitehill MR. Tubercular pericarditis. Medicine 1937;16:45-94.
14. Myers TM, Hamburger M. Tubercular pericarditis; its treatment with streptomycin and some observation on natural history of disease. Am J Med 1952;12:302-10.
15. Desai HN. Tubercular pericarditis. A review of 100 cases. S Afr Med J 1979;55:877-80.
16. Strang JI, Kakaza HH, Gibson DG, Allen BW, Mitchison DA, Evans DJ, et al. Controlled clinical trial of complete open surgical drainage and of prednisolone in treatment of tuberculous pericardial effusion in Transkei. Lancet 1988;332:759-64.
17. Hakim J, Ternouth I, Mushangi E, Siziyha S, Robertson V, Malin A. Double blind randomised placebo controlled trial of adjuvant prednisolone in the treatment of effusive tuberculous pericarditis in HIV seropositive patients. Heart 2000;84:183-8.
18. Fewell JW, Cohen RV, Miller. Tubercular pericarditis. In: Cortes FM, editor. The pericardium and its disorders. Springfield: Charles C Thomas; 1971.p.140.
19. Suwan PK, Potjalongsilp S. Predictors of constrictive pericarditis after tubercuous pericarditis. Br. Heart J 1995;73:187-9.
20. Sheffield EA. The pathology of tuberculosis. In: Davis PDO, editor. Clinical tuberculous. London: Chapman and Hall Medical; 1994:p.44-54.
21. Delacroix I, Thomas F, Godart J, Ravaud Y. Purulent tuberculous pericarditis with cardiac tamponade. Am J Med 1992;93:105.
22. Oribals DW, Avioli LV. Tuberculous pericarditis. Arch Intern Med 1979;139:231-4.
23. Talwar JR, Bhatia ML. Constrictive pericarditis. In Ahuja MMS, editor. Progress in clinical medicine in India. New Delhi: Arnold-Heinemann; 1981.p.177-89.
24. Hageman JH, D'esopo ND, Glenn WW. Tuberculosis of the pericardium. A long-term analysis of forty-four proved cases. N. Engl J Med 1964;270:327-32.
25. Rooney JJ, Crocco JA, Lyons HA. Tuberculous Pericarditis. Ann Intern Med 1970;72:73-81.
26. Spodick DH. Acute, clinically noneffusive ["dry"] pericarditis. In: Spodick DH, editor. The pericardium: a comprehensive textbook. New York: Marcel Dekker; 1977.p.94-113.

27. Komsuoglu B, Goldeli O, Kulan K, Komsuoglu SS. The diagnostic and prognostic value of adenosine deaminase in tubercular pericarditis. Eur Heart J 1995;16:1126-30.

28. Yang CC, Lee MH, Liu JW, Leu HS. Diasgnosis of tuberculous pericarditis and treatment without corticosteroids at a tertiary teaching hospital in Taiwan: a 14-year experience. J Microbiol Immunol Infect 2005;38:47-52.

29. Reuter H, Burgess L, van Vuuren W, Doubell A. Diagnosing tuberculous pericarditis. QJM 2006;99:827-39.

30. Hancock EW. On the elastic and rigid forms of constrictive pericarditis. Am Heart J 1980;100:917-23.

31. Myers RB, Spodick DH. Constrictive pericarditis: Clinical and pathophysiologic characteristics. Am Heart J 1999;138:219-32.

32. Mantri RR, Radhakrishnan S, Sinha N, Goel PK, Bajaj R, Bidwai PS. Atrio-ventricular regurgitations in constrictive pericarditis: incidence and postoperative outcome. Int J Cardiol 1993;38:273-9.

33. Permanyer-Miralda G, Sagrista-Sauleda J, Soler-Soler J. Primary acute pericardial disease; a prospective series of 231 consecutive patients. Am J Cardiol 1985;56:623-30.

34. Humphries MJ, Lam WK, Teoh R. Non-respiratory tuberculosis. In: Davis PDO, editor. Clinical tuberculosis. London: Chapman and Hall Medical;1994.p.111-9.

35. Marshall A, Ring N, Lweis T. Constrictive pericarditis: lessons from the part five years' experience in the South West Cardiothoracic Centre. Clin Med 2006;6:592-7.

36. Smedema JP, Katjitae I, Reuter H, Burgess L, Louw V, Pretorius M, et al. Twelve-lead electrocardiography in tuberculous pericarditis. Cardiovasc JS Afr 2001;12:31-4.

37. Nelson CT, Taber LH. Diagnosis of tuberculous pericarditis with a fluorochrome stain. Pediatr Infect Dis J 1995;14:1004-7.

38. Sharma SK, Kohli M, Chaubey J, Yadav RN, Sharma R, Singh BK, et al. Evaluation of Xpert MTB/RIF assay performance in diagnosing extrapulmonary tuberculosis among adults in a tertiary care centre in India. Eur Respir J 2014;44:1090-3.

39. Kohli M, Schiller I, Dendukuri N, Dheda K, Denkinger CM, Schumacher SG, et al. Xpert[®] MTB/RIF assay for extrapulmonary tuberculosis and rifampicin resistance. Cochrane Database Syst Rev 2018;8:CD012768.

40. Aggeli C, Pitsavos C, Brili S, Hasapis D, Frogoudaki A, Stefanadis C, et al. Relevance of adenosine deaminase and lysozyme measurements in the diagnosis of tuberculous pericarditis. Cardiology 2000;94:81-5.

41. Endrys J, Simo M, Shafie MZ, Uthaman B, Kiwan Y, Chugh T, et al. New nonsurgical technique for multiple pericardial biopsies. Cathet Cardiovasc Diagn 1988;15:92-4.

42. Uthaman B, Endrys J, Abushaban L, Khan S, Anim JT. Percutaneous pericardial biopsy:efficacy, safety, and value in the management of pericardial effusion in children and adolescents. Pediatr Cardiol 1997;18:414-8.

43. Feigenbaum H, Armstrong WF, Ryan T. Feigenbaum's echocardiography. 6th edition. Philadelphia: Lippincott Williams and Wilkins; 2005.p.250.

44. Agrawal S, Radhakrishnan S, Sinha N. Echocardiographic demonstration of resolving intrapericardial mass in tuberculous pericardial effusion. Int J Cardiol 1990;26:240-1.

45. Hutchison SJ, Smalling RG, Albornoz M, Colletti P, Tak T, Chandraratna PA. Comparison of transthoracic and transesophageal echocardiography in clinically overt or suspected pericardial heart disease. Am J Cardiol 1994;74:962-5.

46. Ling LH, Oh JK, Tei C, Click RL, Breen JF, Seward JB, et al. Pericardial thickness measured with transesophageal echocardiography: Feasibility and potential clinical usefulness. J Am Coll Cardiol 1997;29:1317-23.

47. Engel PJ, Fowler NO, Tei CW, Shah PM, Driedger HJ, Shabetai R, et al. M-mode echocardiography in constrictive pericarditis. J Am Coll Cardiol 1985;6:471-4.

48. Voelkel AG, Pietro DA, Folland ED, Fisher ML, Parisi AF. Echocardiographic features of constrictive pericarditis. Circulation 1978;58:871-5.

49. Hatle LK, Appleton CP, Popp RL. Differentiation of constrictive pericarditis from restrictive cardiomyopathy by Doppler echocardiography. Circulation 1989;79:357-70.

50. Glockner JF. Imaging of pericardial disease. Magn Reson Imaging Clin North Am 2003;11:149-62.

51. Masui T, Finck S, Higgins CB. Constrictive pericarditis and restrictive cardiomyopathy: evaluation with MR imaging. Radiology 1992;182:369-73.

52. Vaikus PT, Kussmaul WG. Constrictive pericarditis versus restrictive cardiomyopathy: a reappraisal and update of diagnostic criteria. Am Heart J 1991;122:1431-41.

53. Hurrell DG, Nishimura RA, Higano ST, Appleton CP, Danielson GK, Holmes DR Jr, et al. Value of dynamic respiratory changes in left and right ventricular pressures for the diagnosis of constrictive pericarditis. Circulation 1996;93:2007-13.

54. Mayosi BM, Ntsekhe M, Smieja M. Immunotherapy for tuberculous pericarditis. N Engl J Med 2014; 371:2534.

55. Sharma SK, Ryan H, Khaparde S, Sachdeva KS, Singh AD, Mohan A, et al. Index-TB guidelines: Guidelines on extrapulmonary tuberculosis for India. Indian J Med Res 2017;145:448-63.

56. Wiysonge CS, Ntsekhe M, Gumedze F, Silwa K, Blackett KN, Commerford PJ, et al. Contemporary use of adjunctive corticosteroids in tuberculous pericarditis. Int J Cardiol 2008;124:388-90.

57. Strang JI, Nunn AJ, Johnson DA, Casbard A, Gibson DG, Girling DJ. Management of tuberculous constrictive pericarditis and tuberculous pericardial effusion in Transkei: results at 10 years follow-up. QJM 2004;97:525-35.

58. Ntsekhe M, Wiysonge C, Volmink JA, Commerford PJ, Mayosi BM. Adjuvant corticosteroids for tuberculous pericarditis: promising, but not proven. QJM 2003;96:593-9.

59. Mayosi BM, Ntsekhe M, Bosch J, Pandie S, Jung H, Gumedze F, et al. IMPI Trial Investigators. Prednisolone and Mycobacterium indicus pranii in tuberculous pericarditis. N Engl J Med 2014; 371:1121-30.

60. Reuter H, Burgess LJ, Louw VJ, Doubell AF. The management of tuberculous pericardial effusion: experience in 233 consecutive paitients. Cardiovasc J S Afr 2007;18:20-5.

61. BGibson DG. Pericardial disease.In: Weatherall DJ, Ledingham JGG, Warell DA, editors. Oxford textbook of medicine. Oxford: Oxford University Press; 1989; p.13,304-12.

62. Ling LH, Oh JK, Breen JF, Schaff HV, Danielson GK, Mahoney DW, et al. Calcific constrictive pericarditis: is it still with us? Ann Intern Med 2000;132:444-50.

63. Rose AG. Cardiac tuberculosis. A study of 19 patients. Arch Pathol Lab Med 1987;111:422-6.

64. Kinare SG. Interesting facets of cardiovascular tuberculosis. Indian J Surg 1975;37:145-51.

65. Gulati GS, Kothari SS. Diffuse infiltrative cardiac tuberculosis. Ann Pediatr Cardiol 2011;4:87-9.

66. Baretti R, Eckel L, Beyersdorf F. Submitral left ventricular tuberculoma. Ann Thorac Surg 1995;60:181-2.

67. Sultan FA, Fatimi S, Jamil B, Moustafa SE, Mookadam F. Tuberculous endocarditis: valvular and right atrial involvement. Eur J Echocardiogr 2010;11:E13.

68. Daxini BV, Mandke JV, Sharma S. Echocardiographic recognition of tubercular submitral left ventricular aneurysm extending into left atrium. Am Heart J 1990;119:970-2.

69. Mohan A, Thachil A, Sundar G, Sastry BK, Hasan A, Sridevi C, et al. Ventricular tachycardia and tuberculous lymphadenopathy: sign of myocardial tuberculosis? J Am Coll Cardiol 2015;65:218-20.

70. Kothari SS. Aetiopathogenesis of Takayasu's arteritis and BCG vaccination: the missing link? Med Hypotheses 1995;45:227-30.

19

Skeletal Tuberculosis

S Bhan, HL Nag

INTRODUCTION

Existence of "tuberculosis [TB]-like" disease has been known since time immemorial. Evidence of osteoarticular TB has been found in pre-historic humans (1). In immunocompetent individuals, the osteoarticular involvement occurs in 10% of patients with extra-pulmonary TB [EPTB] (2). Commonly, TB affects the spine and the hip joint; other sites of involvement include knee joint, foot bones, elbow joint and hand bones; rarely, it also affects shoulder joint (3-5).

SKELETAL TUBERCULOSIS

Skeletal TB occurs due to haematogenous spread and affects almost all bones. The disease process can start either in the bone or in the synovial membrane. Thereafter, it spreads to other structures in a short time. Typically, an active focus forms in the metaphysis [in children] or epiphysis [in adults] and the inflammation extends peripherally along the shaft to reach the sub-periosteal space. The inflammatory exudate may extend outwards through the soft tissues to form cold abscess and sinuses. Frequently, secondary infection occurs through the sinus tract. The epiphyseal plate is not destroyed as the cartilage is resistant to destruction by the TB inflammatory process. The granulation tissue can, however, invade the area of calcified cartilage and interfere with longitudinal growth. Metaphyseal infection reaches the joint through sub-periosteal space by penetrating the capsular attachment. In adults, the inflammation can spread up to the subchondral area and enter the joint at the periphery where synovium joins the cartilage. Destruction of the subchondral bone loosens the attachments of the articular cartilage which may become displaced in the joint.

Sometimes the synovium may be infected first and the bone becomes infected secondarily. Usually, there is a low-grade synovial infection with moderate increase in joint fluid and formation of tubercles and fibrin deposits. Caseation necrosis of the synovium and the joint capsule is rare. When a destructive caseating lesion of the bone penetrates into the joint, the synovium too gets affected. Two classical forms of the disease have been described: granular and exudative [caseous]. Though both the patterns have been observed in patients with skeletal TB, one form may predominate.

Osseous Granular Type

In the osseous granular type, the bone involvement occurs at metaphysis or epiphysis often following trauma. The onset is insidious. Hydrarthrosis of the adjacent joint is non-specific and appears following exertion. Constitutional symptoms are rare. Overlying soft tissues are slightly warm and tender. Muscle atrophy appears rapidly.

Osseous Exudative [Caseating] Type

Onset of the osseous exudative [caseating] type is more rapid. Constitutional symptoms, muscle pain and spasm are more marked. The overlying soft tissues are warm, swollen, indurated and tender. When the caseous material penetrates into the joint, a severe destructive arthritis ensues.

Synovial Granular Type

The synovial granular type is characterised by intermittent joint effusion with little or no pain. Later, joint effusion occurs more frequently and becomes persistent. Constitutional symptoms are mild and muscle atrophy gradually sets in. This form of synovitis can continue for a long time without involving the bone. Rarely, the synovial granular form may get converted into caseous form and the patient may experience increase in the local and constitutional symptoms.

Synovial Exudative [Caseous] Type

The synovial exudative [caseous] type has an acute onset with marked local and constitutional symptoms. Overlying soft tissues are very tender. The joint movements are painful and regional lymph nodes are enlarged. Abscess and sinus formation are common.

Prognosis

The availability of modern anti-TB drugs has changed the outlook of patients with bone and joint TB. In the granular form of disease, healing is possible without residual joint scarring and ankylosis. Effective anti-TB treatment combined with resection of large caseous destructive foci ensures early healing and prevents the spread of infection into joint and soft tissues. In recent years, the occurrence of multidrug-resistant and extensively drug-resistant TB have, however, become a matter of concern.

SPINAL TUBERCULOSIS

Spinal TB is the most common form of skeletal involvement.

Pathology of Spinal Tuberculosis

Infection of Bone

Lower thoracic and lumbar vertebrae are the most common sites for spinal TB followed by middle thoracic and cervical vertebrae. Usually, two contiguous vertebrae are involved, but several vertebrae can be affected and skip lesions may also be seen. The infection begins in the cancellous area of vertebral body commonly in epiphyseal location and less commonly in the central or anterior area of vertebral body. TB infection produces an exudative reaction with marked hyperaemia. The infection spreads and destroys the epiphyseal cortex, the intervertebral disc and the adjacent vertebrae. It may spread beneath the anterior longitudinal ligament to reach neighbouring vertebrae. The vertebral body becomes soft and gets easily compressed to produce either wedging or total collapse. Anterior wedging is commonly seen in the thoracic spine where the normal kyphotic curve accentuates the pressure on the anterior part of vertebrae. In the cervical and lumbar spine, the centre of gravity is posteriorly located due to lordotic curve, and therefore, wedging is minimal.

A single large caseating lesion of the vertebral body is rare. This type of lesion remains isolated and calcifies centrally, appearing as a sequestrum. In this form, mechanical strength of vertebral body is reduced to lesser extent and deformity may not occur. Adjacent intervertebral disc is affected gradually.

TB infection starting in the posterior bony arch and transverse processes is uncommon. With healing, exudate is resorbed, osteoporosis decreases and density of body gradually increases to normal. When the intervertebral discs have been completely destroyed, the adjacent bodies fuse with each other.

Formation of Cold Abscess

Vertebral TB develops as an exudative lesion due to hypersensitivity reaction to *Mycobacterium tuberculosis [Mtb]*. The exudate consists of serum, leucocytes, caseous material, bone fragments and tubercle bacilli. It penetrates ligaments and follows the path of least resistance along fascial planes, blood vessels and nerves, to distant sites from the original bony lesion and forms a swelling commonly called as "cold abscess".

In the cervical region, the exudate collects behind prevertebral fascia and may protrude forward as a retropharyngeal abscess. The abscess may track down in mediastinum to enter into the trachea, oesophagus or the pleural cavity. It may spread laterally into the sternomastoid muscle and form an abscess in the neck.

In the thoracic spine, the exudate may remain confined locally for a long time and may appear in the radiographs as a fusiform or bulbous paravertebral abscess. Tension may force the exudate to enter into the spinal canal and compress the spinal cord. Rarely, a thoracic cold abscess may follow the intercostal nerve to appear anywhere along the course of nerve. It can also penetrate the anterior longitudinal ligament to form a mediastinal abscess or pass downwards through medial arcuate ligament to form a lumbar abscess.

The exudate formed at lumbar vertebrae most commonly enters the psoas sheath to manifest radiologically as a psoas abscess or clinically as a palpable abscess in the iliac fossa. Abscess can gravitate beneath the inguinal ligament to appear on the medial aspect of thigh. It can spread laterally beneath the iliac fascia to emerge at the iliac crest near the anterior superior iliac spine. Sometimes an abscess forms above the iliac crest posteriorly. Collection can follow the vessels to form an abscess in Scarpa's triangle or gluteal region if it follows femoral or gluteal vessels, respectively.

Paraplegia

While neurological complications of spinal TB are rarely encountered in developed countries, their incidence remains quite high in the developing world. Paraplegia is the most serious complication of spinal TB and its occurrence is reported to be as high as 30% in patients with spinal TB (6,7). Neurological involvement is common when the dorsal spine is involved because [i] diameter and space of the spinal canal are smallest in the dorsal region; [ii] the abscess remains confined under tension and is thereby forced into the spinal canal; [iii] TB infection is common in this area; and [iv] the spinal cord terminates below the first lumbar vertebra.

Paraplegia due to spinal TB has been known for a very long time. It is also known as *Pott's paraplegia*. It can be of early or late onset (8-11). Early onset paraplegia develops during the active phase of infection. Paraplegia of late onset can appear many years after the disease has become quiescent even without any evidence of reactivation. Most commonly paraplegia develops due to mechanical pressure on the cord, but in a small number of patients, it may occur due to non-mechanical causes as well. The mechanisms

Table 19.1: Mechanisms underlying the development of Pott's paraplegia

Extrinsic or mechanical causes
  During active disease
    Cold abscess [fluid or caseous material]
    Granulation tissue
    Sequestrated bone and disc fragments
    Pathological subluxation or dislocation of vertebra
  Following healing of lesions
    Pressure of ridge of bone anterior to cord
    Fibrosis of dura mater
    Gliosis of cord
Intrinsic or non-mechanical causes
    Spread of tuberculosis inflammation through the dura to
    meninges and eventually to the spinal cord
Rare causes
    Spinal tumour syndrome
    Thrombosis of anterior spinal artery

Adapted from reference 11

underlying the development of Pott's paraplegia are listed in Table 19.1. Frequently, more than one of these mechanisms may be operative in a given patient.

The fact that paraplegia can sometimes recover even after many years suggests that the inflammatory exudate and the resultant oedema may temporarily inhibit the nerve cell function (12). In most cases, early onset paraplegia results from cord compression due to multiple causes and these include inflammatory oedema, caseous material, TB pus and the granulation tissue. Recovery in these cases is favourable. Late onset paraplegia occurs due to long-standing persistent mechanical causes. These include internal gibbus, severe kyphotic deformity, dural fibrosis and stenosis of spinal canal. Prognosis in these cases is much less favourable (13).

Clinical Features

Spinal TB, once a disease of children and adolescents, is now often seen in the adults. Majority of patients are under 30 years of age at the time of diagnosis. Constitutional symptoms, such as, weakness, loss of appetite and weight, evening rise of temperature and night sweats generally occur before the symptoms related to the spine manifest.

Vertebral Disease

A young child may be disinclined to play and may not complain of anything else. Localised pain over the site of involvement is the most common early symptom and the pain may worsen with activity or unguarded movements. Pain may be referred along the spinal nerves to be misdiagnosed as neuralgia, sciatica or intra-abdominal pathology. As the infection progresses, pain increases and paraspinal muscle spasm occurs. Relaxation of muscles during sleep permits painful movements which may cause the child to cry during night [*night cries*].

Patient walks carefully to avoid sudden jerks which can exacerbate the pain. With the involvement of cervical spine,

head may be held with hands. Muscle spasm obliterates normal spinal curves and all spinal movements become restricted and painful. Careful palpation, percussion or pressure will reveal tenderness over the affected vertebrae. Sometimes a boggy, dusky thickening of skin may be seen over the affected area. In patients presenting late, when vertebral wedging and collapse have occurred, a localised knuckle kyphosis becomes quite obvious especially in the dorsal spine. Occasionally, patients with dorsal spine involvement present very late with an extensive destruction of multiple vertebrae. These patients have deformity of thoracic cage with a large gibbus.

Cold Abscess

Local pressure effects such as dysphagia, dyspnoea, or hoarseness of voice may occur due to a retropharyngeal abscess. Further, dysphagia may also occur due to a mediastinal abscess. Flexion deformity of the hip develops due to a psoas abscess. The abscesses may be visible and palpable if they are superficially located. Therefore, in addition to the physical examination of the bony lesion, a careful search for the presence of cold abscess in the neck, chest wall, groin, inguinal areas and thighs can be rewarding.

Paraplegia

Rarely, paraplegia may be the presenting symptom. But, in a majority of cases, the diagnosis of TB of the spine is already established when paraplegia develops. Spontaneous twitching of muscles in lower limbs and clumsiness in walking due to muscle weakness and spasticity are the earliest signs of neurological involvement. With passage of time, paralysis progresses through various stages. These include muscle weakness, spasticity, incoordination, difficulty in walking and paraplegia in extension. Subsequently, paraplegia in flexion, sensory loss and loss of sphincteric control occur. Exaggerated deep tendon reflexes, clonus, and extensor plantar reflex can be elicited. Anteriorly located motor tracts in the spinal cord are in close proximity to the disease process and are sensitive to pressure effect. Therefore, the motor functions are affected first due to the cord compression. Increasing compression of cord produces uncontrolled flexor spasms. In later stages, limbs remain in flexion [paraplegia in flexion] with complete loss of conduction in pyramidal and extra-pyramidal tracts. In very advanced cases of cord compression, varying degrees of sensory deficit and loss of bladder and sphincter control occur. The sense of position and vibration is the last to disappear. In severe cases, spasticity disappears and flaccid paralysis, sensory loss and loss of sphincter control [areflexic paraplegia] can develop.

Rarely, the cord compression may be so sudden and complete that the patient presents with sudden onset of flaccid paralysis simulating the picture of spinal shock. This may occur due to rapid accumulation of TB pus and caseation, pathological dislocation of vertebra and ischaemia of cord due to thromboembolic phenomenon. Rarely, presenting features may simulate the features of spinal tumour syndrome. These features occur due to localised tuberculoma, granuloma or peridural fibrosis producing partial or complete block without any pathology being visible on radiographs. Such cases should be differentiated from lathyrism in endemic areas since lathyrism also presents as pure motor paraplegia of insidious onset. However, patients with lathyrism will not reveal block to cerebrospinal fluid flow on lumbar puncture, myelography and magnetic resonance imaging [MRI].

Clinically, the severity of paraplegia has been classified into four grades (14-16).

Grade I Negligible paraplegia The patient is unaware of the neurological deficit but examination reveals clonus and extensor plantar response.

Grade II Mild paraplegia The patient is aware of weakness and difficulty in walking but manages to walk with or without support.

Grade III Moderate paraplegia The patient is bedridden and cannot walk due to severe weakness. Examination reveals paraplegia in extension and sensory deficit if present is less than 50%.

Grade IV Severe paraplegia Features of grade III with flexor spasm/paralysis in flexion/flaccid paralysis and sensory deficit of more than 50%.

The higher the grade of paralysis, more severe is the compression of cord and poorer is the prognosis for recovery of neurological deficit.

Radiographic Features

On an average, involvement of 2.5 to 3.8 vertebrae has been described (14-19). There are mainly four sites of infection in the vertebra: paradiscal, central, anterior and appendicial. The most common site of vertebral involvement is paradiscal. The appendicial type includes the involvement of pedicle, lamina, spinous process and transverse process. Nearly 7% of patients may show skipped lesions (17-19). Some of the vertebral bodies may become eroded not necessarily due to

the disease process *per se*, but due to the pressure effect of the paravertebral cold abscess.

Radiologically, paradiscal infection first appears as demineralisation with indistinct bony margins adjoining the disc [Figure 19.1]. Gradually, the disc space narrows signifying either atrophy of disc tissue due to lack of nutrition, or, prolapse of nucleus into the soft necrotic vertebral body. The disc space may eventually disappear and vertebral bodies reveal an enlarging area of destruction and wedging. Rarely, disc space may remain intact for a long time. It takes about three to five months for the bony destruction to become visible on a radiograph. More than 30% of mineral must be removed from the bone for a radiolucent lesion to be discernable on the plain radiograph. Computed tomography [CT] and MRI allow identification of bony lesions including prevertebral and paravertebral abscess shadows at an early stage [Figures 19.2, 19.3, and 19.4]. Abscess in the cervical region presents as a soft

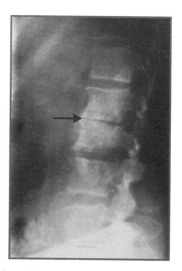

Figure 19.1: Plain radiograph of the lumbosacral spine [lateral view] showing early changes of paradiscal involvement of L2 and L3 vertebrae, indistinct bony margins of adjacent vertebrae along with loss of disc space [arrow]

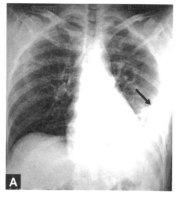
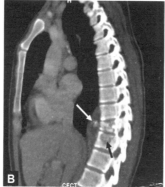
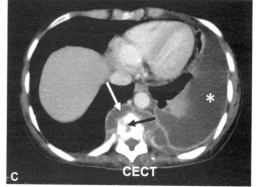

Figure 19.2: Chest radiograph [postero-anterior view] [A] showing left-sided empyema [arrow]. CECT of the chest [sagittal reconstruction] [B] and [C] showing destruction of vertebral body [black arrow], paraspinal cold abscess [white arrow] and left-sided empyema [asterisk]
CECT = contrast-enhanced computed tomography

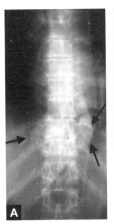
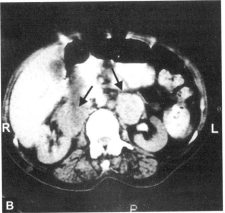

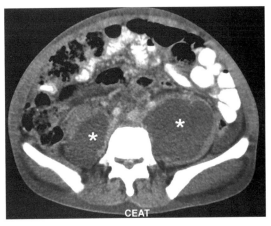

Figure 19.3: Plain radiograph of the dorsolumbar spine [antero-posterior view] [A] showing the involvement of D10 and D11 vertebrae, narrowing of intervening disc and paravertebral abscess [arrows]. CT of the dorsal spine [B] showing bilateral psoas abscesses [arrows]
CT = computed tomography

Figure 19.4: CECT of the lower abdomen showing hypodense collections [asterisks] in bilateral psoas muscles [bigger on the left side] in a patient with disseminated tuberculosis. The adjacent vertebral body appears normal
CECT = contrast-enhanced computed tomography

tissue shadow between the vertebral bodies, pharynx and trachea. Early detection of an abscess in the area of seventh cervical to fourth dorsal vertebrae requires a good quality radiograph. Abscess in the dorsal spine area produces a typical fusiform shape [*bird-nest appearance*] and a large abscess in this region may appear as mediastinal widening. An abscess arising below the attachment of diaphragm forms a psoas abscess and in a good quality radiograph appears as a bulge of the lateral border of the psoas muscle shadow. A long-standing, tense paravertebral abscess [usually in the dorsal spine] may produce concave erosions along the margin of vertebral bodies [*aneurysmal phenomenon*]. Canal compromise and cord status are best demonstrated by CT or MRI [Figures 19.5 and 19.6].

Central type lesion starts in the centre of the vertebral body. Infection at this site probably reaches through Batson's venous plexus or through branches of posterior vertebral artery. A lytic area develops in the centre of the vertebral body and may gradually enlarge resulting in the ballooning out of the vertebral body mimicking a tumour. In the later stages of advanced destruction, a concentric collapse occurs almost resembling vertebra plana. In this type of lesion, the disc space is either not affected or affected minimally and paravertebral shadow is also usually not well-marked. Therefore, this type of lesion should be differentiated from a tumour or Calve's disease.

Anterior type lesion occurs when the infection starts in front or on sides of the vertebral body beneath the anterior longitudinal ligament and periosteum. Radiologically, it is seen as a shallow excavation on anterior or lateral surface of vertebral body. Similar excavations will also appear due to the aneurysmal phenomenon in patients with paradiscal type of lesion and a long-standing, tense, paravertebral abscess.

TB of the posterior elements of vertebra is not detected in its early stage in the plain radiographs. In the late stage

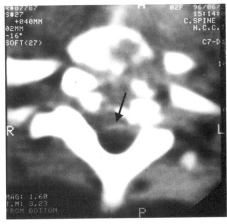

Figure 19.5: CT [transverse section through the body of C7 vertebra] showing its destruction and anterior compromise of canal by bony fragments [arrow]
CT = computed tomography

of disease, the erosive bony lesions of posterior elements can be seen in the radiographs. However, CT or MRI is invaluable in detecting these lesions at an early stage. Paravertebral abscess shadow may be present but the disc space remains intact. Sometimes more than one lesion may be present in vertebral column with one or more healthy vertebrae intervening between the diseased vertebrae [called "skip lesions"].

In late stages, anterior wedging or vertebral collapse results in the development of kyphotic deformity. Sometimes this deformity can be very severe. Destruction of vertebral body on one side can produce lateral deviation and rotation similar to that seen in patients with hemivertebra, especially when the disease affects the lower dorsal and lumbar spine [Figure 19.7]. On very rare occasions, a vertebral body may dislocate anteriorly due to destruction of the pedicles.

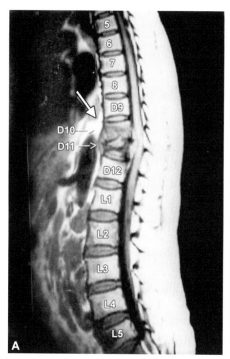
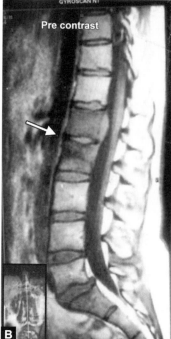
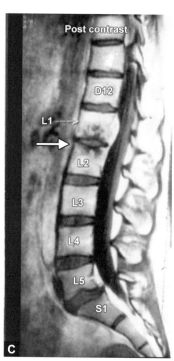

Figure 19.6: MRI of the dorsolumbar spine. Sagittal view showing profound destruction of D10 and D11 vertebrae with anterior compression of the cord [arrow] [A]. Sagittal spin-echo T1-weighted image showing hypointense L1 and L2 vertebral bodies, intervening disc and an epidural soft tissue component at L1 level [arrow] [B]. The bodies of L1 and L2 vertebrae and epidural soft tissues are brightly enhanced in T2-weighted image [arrow] [C]

MRI = magnetic resonance imaging

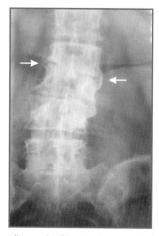

Figure 19.7: Plain radiograph of the lumbosacral spine [antero-posterior view] showing mild scoliotic chage due to the relative destruction of one side of vertebra involving L2 and L3 levels [arrows]

The severity of a gibbus can be predicted with 90% accuracy using the following formula (20a):

$y = a + bx$ where:

y = final angle of gibbus

a = constant with a value of 5.5

b = constant with a value of 30.5

x = amount of initial loss of height of vertebral body

Amount of initial loss of height of vertebral body is calculated as follows. Height of vertebral body on lateral radiograph is divided into 10 equal parts. Loss of height of

all contiguous affected vertebrae is then added together to get the value of 'x'.

Differential Diagnosis

Usually, clinical presentation and radiological findings of spinal TB are characteristic. However, in doubtful cases, clinical examination and radiological investigations including CT or MRI will help in making an accurate diagnosis. In a very small percentage of cases, biopsy of the diseased vertebra for histopathological and microbiological examinations may be required to confirm the diagnosis. Cartridge-based nucleic acid amplification tests [CBNAAT] are increasingly being used for the diagnosis of bone and joint TB (20b). In a recently published systematic review (20b) Xpert MTB/RIF was found to have a high pooled sensitivity [97.2%] and specificity [90.2%] in bone and joint fluid. The sensitivity and specificity of Xpert MTB/RIF in bone and joint tissue were found to be 94.6% and 85.3% respectively. However, some conditions [Table 19.2] may mimic TB of the spine and these conditions need to be differentiated from spinal TB, especially in patients with atypical clinical presentation.

Management

Anti-TB Treatment

Anti-TB treatment for skeletal TB is essentially the same as for TB elsewhere in the body. However, there is a difference

Table 19.2: Conditions resembling spinal tuberculosis

Developmental defects like hemivertebra, Calve's disease, Schmorl's nodes and Scheuermann's disease

Infections like pyogenic osteomyelitis, enteric fever, brucellosis, mycotic infections and syphilis

Benign neoplasms like haemangioma, aneurysmal bone cyst, giant cell tumour

Primary malignant tumours like Ewing's tumour, chordoma, osteosarcoma, fibrosarcoma, chondrosarcoma, multiple myeloma and lymphoma

Secondary neoplastic deposits

Langerhan's cell histiocytosis

Paget's disease

Traumatic fracture

Hydatid disease

Table 19.3: Indications for surgery in patients with spinal tuberculosis regardless of paraplegia

Doubtful diagnosis where open biopsy is necessary

Failure to respond to antituberculosis drugs

Radiological evidence of progression of bony lesion and/or paraspinal abscess shadow

Imminent vertebral collapse

Prevention of severe kyphosis

Instability of spine and subluxation or dislocation of vertebral body

of opinion regarding the duration of drug therapy. Though many orthpaedicians favour 18-24 months of anti-TB treatment, short-course treatment for nine months has also been shown to be equally effective in patients with disease caused by drug-susceptible microorganisms in whom the diagnosis has been established early (21,22). As per the recently published evidence-based Guidelines for Extrapulmonary TB for India [INDEX-TB Guidelines] (23), extended course of anti-TB treatment with a two-month intensive phase consisting of four drugs [isoniazid, rifampicin, pyrazinamide, ethambutol], followed by a continuation phase consisting of isoniazid, rifampicin and ethambutol lasting 10-16 months, depending on the site of disease and the patient's clinical course has been advocated.

Direct observation of treatment, an integral component of DOTS provided by the Revised National Tuberculosis Control Programme [RNTCP] of Government of India, will ensure compliance. Community DOT providers facilitate administration of drugs in non-ambulatory patients. The reader is referred to the chapters *"Treatment of tuberculosis"* [Chapter 44] and *"Revised National Tuberculosis Control Programme"* [Chapter 53] for details.

Antibiotics

Persistently draining sinuses are often secondarily infected and therefore appropriate antibiotic[s] should be administered along with anti-TB treatment after culture and drug-susceptibility testing.

Surgery

Efficacy of anti-TB treatment has significantly reduced the need for operative intervention. Indications for adjunct surgery in patients with spinal TB lesions *per se* [regardless of paraplegia] are listed in Table 19.3.

Common operative procedures include anterolateral decompression with interbody bone grafting or costotransversectomy with decompression. If a large gap is left behind after debridement, adequate bone grafting must always

be done. Anteriorly placed grafts provide good stability and heal well. An additional use of metallic implants and titanium cage filled with cancellous bone grafts may be required when nearly whole of the vertebral body has been removed during debridement.

Surgical prevention of severe kyphotic deformity requires extensive panvertebral operative procedures. These consist of anterior debridement, anterior interbody fusion and posterior fusion of affected vertebrae (15,24). It has also been suggested that, a severe deformity in the presence of active disease should be an absolute indication for debridement, correction and stabilisation since late correction of TB kyphosis is difficult and dangerous. Correction of a fixed spinal curve and severe kyphosis is a formidable surgical undertaking and should only be done in selected patients by a specially trained surgeon (25).

Formerly, posterior spinal fusion by the methods of Hibbs [fusion between laminae, articular facets and spinous processes] and Albee [fusion between spinous processes with tibial cortical graft] were frequently used. Fusion was successful because posterior elements were seldom involved in disease process. However, by these interventions, progression of lesion in body was not affected. Posterior spinal fusion is now rarely used, except to reinforce an anterior spinal fusion in regions of greatest stress at junctional areas like cervicothoracic and dorsolumbar junctions; and for panvertebral fusion in children who are at risk of developing severe kyphosis.

Cold Abscess

With anti-TB treatment, a small cold abscess will heal along with the bony lesion. Tense and large cold abscesses are usually located in the neck, chest wall, iliac fossa, lumbar triangle, inguinal region and thigh. These abscesses are frequently painful and tend to burst and form sinuses. Therefore, these abscesses must be drained as early as possible by the standard surgical approach which depends on the location of the abscess. Most surgeons do not use a drain after evacuation of abscess for fear of sinus formation. Paravertebral abscess need not be drained on its own but should be evacuated at the time of debridement of bony lesion when indicated.

Paraplegia

Three schools of thought exist in the treatment of Pott's paraplegia. One of the views is that immediate operative decompression of the cord by extensive anterior debridement results in maximum improvement in the shortest possible time (26). According to these workers, operation should be performed at an earliest because they feel that the TB infection can penetrate into the dura mater and infect the cord making recovery impossible. This view recommends early radical anterior debridement, decompression and arthrodesis in all patients with Pott's paraplegia except in patients with spinal tumour syndrome and those with paraplegia resulting from posterior spinal disease.

The second view favours initial treatment with immobilisation or complete bedrest. If this does not produce improvement and recovery within a specified time period, then the surgical decompression of the spinal cord is performed (9,10,27-29). The widely accepted indications for surgical treatment are listed in Table 19.4.

The third view, proposes the "middle path regimen" (6) and advocates rest and anti-TB treatment for four weeks and surgical decompression if there is no improvement in the neurological deficit by this time. This regimen is useful for developing countries with limited resources.

Treatment of paraplegia in severe kyphosis is by excising internal gibbus through antero-lateral approach or by anterior transposition of cord through laminectomy. Antero-lateral decompression is a surgery of lesser magnitude compared to anterior decompression and is preferred in resource limited settings. Details of surgical techniques are beyond the scope of this chapter. However, it must be pointed out that obtaining adequate surgical exposure of junctional areas of spine is difficult and this type of surgery must be undertaken only by experienced and well-trained surgeons.

Laminectomy and intraspinal exposure must be deferred if the neurological deficit is non-progressive or if the radiographs are normal. Following decompression with or without bone grafting, bedrest for a period of 10-12 weeks is indicated. Thereafter, the patient is gradually mobilised with a suitable brace.

Reactivation or reinfection may result in a relapse in a small percentage of cases and may be complicated by neurological involvement. In such situations, early operation and administration of appropriate anti-TB treatment are indicated.

TUBERCULOSIS OF HIP JOINT

TB of the hip joint occurs in about 15%-20% of all cases of osteoarticular TB and is the next common form after spinal TB.

Pathology

TB of the hip joint almost always starts in bone and the initial focus is in the acetabular roof [Figures 19.8 and 19.9], femoral epiphysis, proximal femoral metaphysis or greater trochanter. Rarely, the initial focus may be in the synovial membrane and the disease may remain as synovitis for a few months. In these patients, the diagnosis may be considerably delayed. TB of the greater trochanter may involve the overlying trochanteric bursa. Since the head and neck of

Table 19.4: Indications for surgical treatment in patients with spinal tuberculosis and paraplegia
Absolute indications
Onset of paraplegia during conservative treatment
Surgery is not performed for pyramidal tract signs but delayed till motor weakness is evident
Paraplegia getting worse or remaining stationary despite adequate conservative treatment
Persistence or complete loss of motor power for one month despite sufficient conservative treatment
Paraplegia accompanied by uncontrolled spasticity of such severity that reasonable rest and immobilisation are impossible or there is a risk of pressure necrosis of skin
Severe paraplegia of rapid onset. This usually indicates severe mechanical pressure but may also be due to vascular thrombosis. Surgery is not helpful when thrombosis causes paraplegia
Severe paraplegia, paraplegia in flexion, flaccid paraplegia, complete sensory loss or complete loss of motor power for more than six months. All these are indications for immediate surgery without trial of conservative treatment
Relative indications
Recurrent paraplegia even with paraplegia that would cause no concern in the first attack
Paraplegia with onset in old age to avoid hazards of immobilisation
Painful paraplegia. Pain may be due to spasm or root compression
Complications, such as, urinary tract infection and stones
Rare indications
Posterior spinal disease
Spinal tumour syndrome
Severe paralysis from cervical disease
Severe cauda equina paralysis
Adapted from references 28 and 29

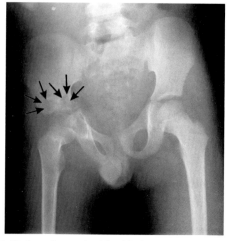

Figure 19.8: Plain radiograph of the hip joint showing lesions [arrows] at the acetabulum in a six-year-old boy at the beginning of treatment

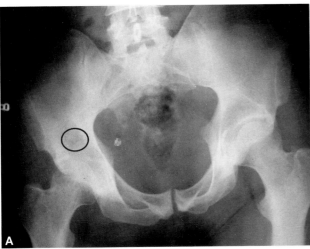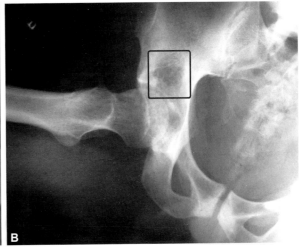

Figure 19.9: Plain radiograph of the hip joint showing early TB lesion at the acetabulum [circle] in a 34-year-old man which was missed initially [A]. Same lesion, three months after starting anti-TB treatment [rectangle] [B]
TB = tuberculosis

femur are intracapsular, a bony lesion here invades the joint early and later spreads to involve the acetabulum as well. When the disease starts in the acetabulum, symptoms related to joint involvement appear late [Figure 19.10]. Extensive destruction may result in pathological dislocation of the hip joint. A cold abscess forms in the joint, may perforate the capsule and extend anywhere around the hip joint. It may perforate the thinned acetabular floor to form an intra-pelvic abscess.

Clinical Features

TB of the hip frequently affects the children. Constitutional symptoms may precede the joint symptoms. Pain around the hip joint or along the thigh or inner aspect of the knee joint. particularly on weight bearing, is usually the first symptom. The patient limps while walking and avoids weight bearing on the affected side. During the acute stage, muscle spasm is severe. At night, relaxation of muscle spasm and unguarded movements produce *"night cries"*. All movements of the hip joint are painful and limited to a variable degree. As the acute stage subsides, pain and muscle spasm become less severe and muscle atrophy develops.

Classical untreated TB of the hip joint passes through the following three clinico-pathological stages and each stage has a definite pattern of clinical deformity.

Stage I: Stage of Synovitis

The stage of synovitis is the earliest manifestation of disease. Intra-synovial effusion and exudate distend the joint capsule. The hip joint assumes a position of flexion, abduction and external rotation. During this stage, capacity of the hip joint is maximum. Limb appears lengthened but there is no real lengthening. This is the stage when the disease is seldom diagnosed since similar physical findings are seen in traumatic synovitis, non-specific transient synovitis,

rheumatic disease, low-grade pyogenic infection, Perthes' disease and spasm of iliopsoas muscle due to an abscess in its sheath or nearby inflamed lymph nodes. In such situations, clinical and radiological examinations must be repeated at two to three weeks intervals till a definitive diagnosis has been made.

Stage II: Stage of Early Arthritis

As the capsule thickens by fibrosis and contracts, and damage to the articular surface progresses, the hip joint assumes a position of flexion, adduction and internal rotation. Limb appears short but true shortening may not be present and, if present, is not more than one centimetre. All movements of the hip joint remain painful and limited.

Stage III: Stage of Advanced Arthritis

The capsule becomes further destroyed, thickened and contracted along with advanced bony destruction producing true shortening of the limb. The joint movements become more restricted and the flexion, adduction, internal rotation deformity may become severe. With further destruction of the acetabulum, femoral head, capsule and ligaments, the joint dislocates with the destroyed head coming to lie proximally and posteriorly in wandering or migrating acetabulum. Instead of proximal migration sometimes *protrusio acetabuli* can develop with destruction of medial wall of acetabulum.

Radiographic Features

In the earliest stage, radiographs may reveal diffuse decalcification of upper end of femur. Osteolytic bony focus of infection may be visible in the acetabulum or femur a little later and this lesion may be seen to be enlarging on sequential radiographs. Soft tissue swelling may be evident on the radiograph, but ultrasonography is useful at this stage

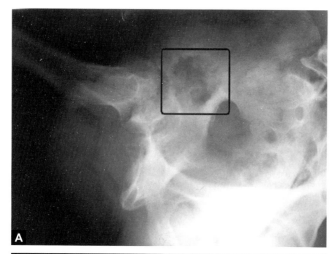

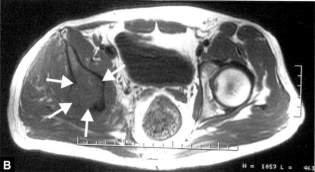

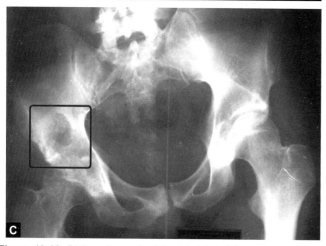

Figure 19.10: Plain radiograph of the hip joint of the patient shown in Figure 19.9 showing increase in the size of the lesion [square] despite five months of anti-TB treatment [A]. Destruction of acetabulum and granulation tissues [arrows] are seen better in transverse section in MRI [B]. Biopsy confirmed the diagnosis of TB. Radiograph at 13 months of treatment showing regression of lesion with extension into the hip joint [square] limiting the movements [C]
TB = tuberculosis

to confirm soft tissue swelling. Late stages of the disease will reveal increasing destruction of acetabulum, wandering acetabulum, small atrophic femoral head, subluxation or dislocation. Seven different types of radiological appearances have been described in advanced stage of TB arthritis of hip joint (30) and are described below [Figure 19.11].

Normal Type

The disease is mainly synovial. There may be cysts in the femoral neck, head or acetabulum, but there is no gross destruction of subchondral bone and the joint space is normal.

Perthes' Type

Most patients are under five years of age. The whole femoral head is sclerotic and differentiation from Perthes' disease can be difficult though metaphyseal changes seen in the classical Perthes' disease are not seen.

Dislocating Type

Subluxation or dislocation of the femoral head occurs. This is mainly due to capsular laxity and synovial hypertrophy and not due to accumulation of pus. Results are better after open relocation of the hip joint.

Wandering Acetabulum, Protrusio Acetabuli, Mortar and Pestle Type

These appearances occur due to the erosion of subchondral bone [Figure 19.12]. Results of surgery are generally poor in these types of TB of the hip joint.

Atrophic Type

The femoral head is irregular and the joint space is narrow. It is seen almost exclusively in adults and the results of treatment are poor and the condition almost always progresses to fibrous ankylosis [Figure 19.13].

These radiographic appearances in general also correspond to the duration of the disease before diagnosis. In the normal Perthes' dislocating and atrophic types, the mean duration of symptoms varies from four to seven months. In wandering acetabulum, protrusio acetabuli and mortar and pestle types, the mean duration of symptoms is usually longer, ranging from 10-14 months.

Management

In patients with TB of the hip joint, the prognosis depends on the stage of disease when treatment is initiated. Anti-TB treatment started at stages I and II of disease may allow an almost or near normal hip joint at the end [Figures 19.14 and 19.15]. The deformities should also be corrected as early as possible, or else fibrous ankylosis in the position of deformity will occur. Neglected cases will eventually have a markedly deformed hip joint and a short limb. The shortening is partly due to gross bony destruction and partly due to growth arrest at proximal femoral epiphysis. Occasionally, if the limb has been immobilised for more than one year, premature fusion of distal femoral epiphyseal plate can result in shortening.

Anti-TB drugs should be administered in adequate dosages for a sufficient length of time along with supportive measures to improve the general health. Skin traction is

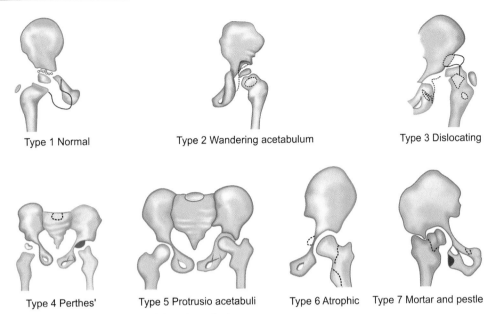

Type 1 Normal   Type 2 Wandering acetabulum   Type 3 Dislocating

Type 4 Perthes'   Type 5 Protrusio acetabuli   Type 6 Atrophic   Type 7 Mortar and pestle

Figure 19.11: Different radiological types of the hip joint tuberculosis

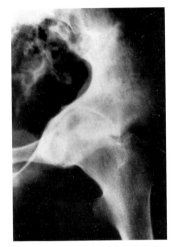

Figure 19.12: Plain radiograph of the hip joint showing the "protrusio acetabuli" type of hip involvement

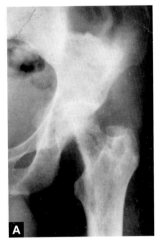
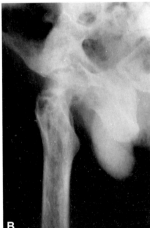

Figure 19.13: Plain radiograph of the hip joint [antero-posterior view] showing marked atrophy of head and neck of femur [A]. Radiograph of the hip joint [lateral view] of the same patient showing extensive involvement of upper shaft of the femur [B]

usually required initially in all cases. Traction corrects deformity, relieves muscle spasm and pain. It also maintains joint space, minimises chances of development of migrating acetabulum and prevents dislocation. In the presence of abduction deformity, traction should be applied to both limbs to stabilise the pelvis. Otherwise, traction to the deformed limb alone would further increase the abduction deformity. In stages I and II, a prolonged period of traction [up to 12 weeks] may be required. Traction should be continued till disease activity is well-controlled, hip movements improve and become pain free and muscle spasm does not recur. Gentle hip mobilisation and sitting in bed for short periods are started during the period of traction. For next 12 weeks, non-weight bearing walking is allowed with crutches followed by another 12 weeks period of partial weight bearing. Unprotected weight bearing should not be

permitted early, since chances of collapse and deformity of acetabulum and femoral head may persist till bones have become fully calcified after control of infection. However, currently, early weight bearing is recommended depending on the pain tolerance by the patient, since this boosts the patients' confidence and activity level (31). Drainage of cold abscess should be done without undue delay to prevent the sinus formation.

In patient with stage II disease, partial synovectomy and curettage of large or enlarging osteolytic lesions in the acetabulum [Figure 19.10] and femoral head should be done. At operation, the hip joint should not be dislocated in order to remove all TB tissue. After curettage, large lesions may be filled with cancellous grafts. Curettage of extra-articular lesions prevents spread of infection in the joint if done early enough. Post-operatively, the regimen of traction,

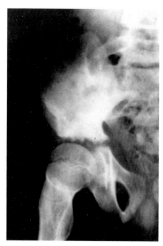

Figure 19.14: Plain radiograph of the hip joint [antero-posterior view] showing good healing of the lesion involving superior portion of acetabulum following antituberculosis treatment

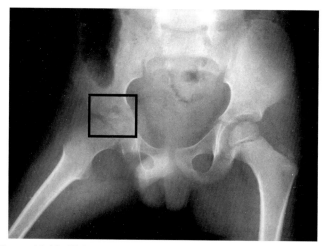

Figure 19.15: Plain radiograph the hip joint [antero-posterior view] of the patient shown in Figure 19.8, showing healed lesion [square] at completion of treatment. The patient recovered with a good function of the hip joint

non-weight bearing mobilisation, partial weight bearing and then unprotected weight bearing are followed as described above.

In patients presenting with advanced arthritis, or stage III disease, the aim is to achieve fibrous ankylosis in a functional position. Traction is applied first and, if indicated, limited operative procedure of partial synovectomy and curettage of extra-articular lesions and joint debridement are done. Once the deformities are corrected and operative wound has healed well, a plaster spica is applied. Immobilisation in the plaster is continued for six to nine months followed by partial weight bearing for another six months. Unprotected weight bearing is usually possible after about 12-18 months from the beginning of treatment.

Corrective osteotomy of proximal femur at a level just above the lesser trochanter is required in patients presenting with ankylosis in an unacceptable position. Further, with corrective femoral osteotomy, a painful, fibrous ankylosis may be converted into a painless, bony ankylosis.

Arthrodesis to achieve bony ankylosis and painless hip joint is done after about 20 years of age when proximal femur has no more potential for longitudinal growth. In the era prior to the availability of anti-TB drugs, extra-articular arthrodesis was done due to fear of reactivation of infection if the joint was opened. Two popular methods of arthrodesis were iliofemoral arthrodesis [Hibb's arthrodesis] (32) and ischiofemoral arthrodesis [Britain's arthrodesis] (33). With the availability of effective anti-TB treatment, a direct intra-articular fusion between the raw surfaces of femoral head and acetabulum is performed when arthrodesis is indicated.

Excision arthroplasty of the hip joint (34) [Girdlestone arthroplasty] consists of excision of head and neck of femur along with debridement. Post-operatively, 10-12 weeks of traction is required and this is followed by gradual weight bearing. The limb becomes shorter by about two centimeters in addition to the pre-operative shortening and the joint also becomes unstable. But this procedure offers the advantage

of retaining a good range of movements; the patient can even squat and sit cross-legged Total hip arthroplasty [THA], which has been so successful in osteoarthritis and rheumatoid arthritis [RA], is also now being performed in selected patients. For this procedure the disease must be clinically healed for over five years. At present, THA is also performed with success for active TB, though controversial, along with anti-TB treatment (35,36).

TUBERCULOSIS OF KNEE JOINT

Knee joint is the third common site for osteoarticular TB. It accounts for more than 10% of cases of osteoarticular TB.

Pathology

In the past, the knee joint involvement was mainly a disease of children presenting as "synovial type". Presently, it is increasingly being seen in adults and presents as an osseous metaphyseal lesion which spreads to the joint. The synovial type of infection is a low-grade inflammation. The synovial membrane becomes congested, oedematous and is studded with tubercles. The synovial fluid is increased. It is thin, watery, opalescent and contains flakes of fibrin and an increased number of mononuclear cells. Healing at this stage leaves the synovial membrane thickened with fibrosis and the articular surfaces remain largely intact. If healing does not occur and the infection persists, the granulation tissue forms and the synovial space is obliterated by fibrous adhesions. The granulation tissue erodes the cartilage, invades the subchondral bone, capsule and cruciate ligaments. When initial infection starts in metaphysis, it produces an acute exudative infection with caseation necrosis. This lesion can invade the joint to produce granulation tissue and extensive destruction of the articular cartilage [Figure 19.16]. Sinus formation can occur [Figure 19.17]. Wasting of thigh and calf muscles occurs early in this type of infection [Figure 19.18].

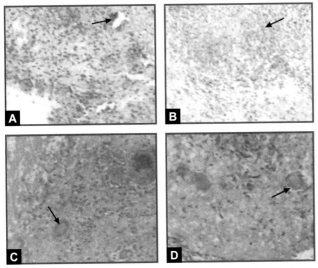

Figure 19.16: Tuberculosis synovitis with osteomyelitis. Photomicrograph showing synovial lining, chronic inflammatory changes and small necrotic bone spicules [arrow] [*Haematoxylin and eosin* × 100] [A], epithelioid granuloma with lymphocytic infiltration [arrow] [*Haematoxylin and eosin* x 200] [B], caseation necrosis, Langhans' giant cells [arrow], foreign body giant cells [*Haematoxylin and eosin* × 400] [C] and caseation necrosis, giant cells [arrow] and lymphocytes [*Haematoxylin and eosin* × 400] [D]

A low-grade synovial infection stimulates osteogenesis and ossification centers in adjoining tibia and femur. These bones may become longer than on the opposite side. If infection is not controlled early, a premature closure of neighbouring growth plate can occur and in this situation, the limb becomes shorter.

Clinical Features

The synovial type of infection is insidious in onset and starts as intermittent episodes of synovial effusion. The affected joint remains normal in appearance and function during each remission. Excessive activity and strain tend to precipitate effusion. Aspirated joint fluid is not abnormal except for the presence of some mononuclear cells. At this stage, other causes must be considered in the differential diagnosis. These include meniscal tear and synovitis due to trauma, rheumatic fever, RA and pyogenic arthritis, osteochondritis dessicans, chondromalacia patellae, haemarthrosis, villonodular synovitis and synovial chondromatosis. In doubtful cases, synovial biopsy for histopathological and microbiological investigations are necessary. When a patient presents with recurrent or persistent knee joint swelling of insidious onset, a possibility of TB must be considered. Caution must be exercised while administering intra-articular corticosteroids in such patients as a flare-up of TB can occur.

Gradually, the attacks of synovitis become more intense and presistent. The synovium and capsule become palpably thickened and tender. This feel of swelling of the knee joint in synovial TB is classically described as "doughy swelling" [Figure 19.18]. At first, the muscles, particularly, hamstrings develop spasm, atrophy and contractures may develop later. The biceps femoris muscle pulls the leg in deformity of flexion [Figure 19.19], abduction and external rotation. If this deformity persists, capsular contracture occurs and tibia gradually subluxates posteriorly. The synovial fluid is thin, opalescent and contains a large number of mononuclear cells and flakes of fibrin. When healing takes place in the early stage of intermittent synovial effusion, the knee joint

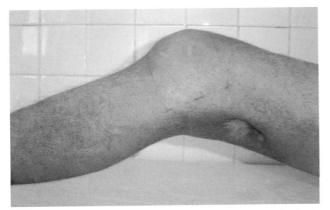

Figure 19.17: Clinical photograph showing healed tuberculosis sinus and flexion deformity of the left knee joint at eight months of treatment

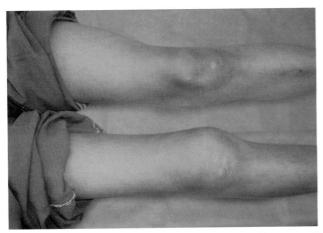

Figure 19.18: Clinical photograph showing early quadriceps wasting due to tuberculosis synovitis in the right knee joint

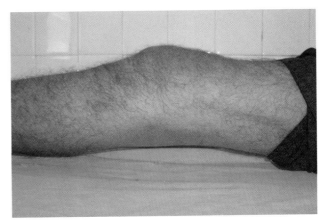

Figure 19.19: Clinical photograph showing hamstrings spasm due to tuberculosis synovitis leading to early flexion deformity of the left knee joint

may almost remain near normal. Healing in the later stages leaves behind thickened and fibrotic synovial membrane and capsule. Intra-articular adhesions lead to a fibrous ankylosis.

In the form commonly seen in adults, metaphyseal focus of infection spreads to the joint. Inflammatory signs develop suddenly and include severe pain, muscle spasm, local warmth, tenderness and restriction of movements. Constitutional symptoms are present and include fever, anorexia and night sweats. Destruction is greater and abscess and sinus formation are frequent. Stimulation of ossification may result in bony enlargement most notably in the medial femoral condyle and valgus deformity of the knee joint. A premature epiphyseal fusion results in retardation of longitudinal growth. In advanced cases, characteristic "triple deformity" of flexion, abduction, external rotation and posterior subluxation of tibia, painful fibrous ankylosis, abscess and sinus formation become evident.

Radiographic Features

In the first stage of intermittent synovitis, radiographs are normal [Figure 19.20]. In next stage of persistent synovitis, radiographs show generalised osteoporosis, loss of definition of articular margins [Figure 19.21]. Occasionally, marginal erosions are also seen. Thickened synovium and capsule may cast soft tissue shadow. In patients with advanced disease, radiographs may reveal marked narrowing of the joint space and the joint appears grossly disorganised. Osteolytic cavities and TB sequestra in bones may also be evident in an advanced stage of the disease, the classical triple deformity [Figure 19.22] is seen. When the clinical presentation is atypical, and the findings on the plain radiograph do not support the clinical features, an MRI of the knee joint can be helpful [Figure 19.23].

Management

In the early stages of synovial disease, a synovial biopsy and histopathological and microbiological examination of the material obtained may facilitate confirmation of the diagnosis.

In the stage of intermittent effusion, administration of standard anti-TB treatment alone may be sufficient. Traction is useful in all stages of the disease in children and only in the stage of persistent synovitis in adults. Pre-operative traction is used in the acute fulminating form and surgery is deferred till the acute stage of disease has been controlled. Traction is also necessary in the post-operative period following synovectomy and debridement. Simple skin traction is adequate in patients with minimal flexion deformity. But, in cases where triple deformity has developed, the double traction technique should be used. It consists of applying both horizontal and vertical tractions from a pin passed in proximal tibia. But traction has its limitations in correction of deformity of patients with advanced stage TB of the knee [Figure 19.21E]. Double traction helps in correction of deformity and prevents posterior subluxation of tibia. With quiescence of acute local signs, intermittent, gentle active and passive knee bending exercises are started. Gradual mobilisation and weight bearing are started with clinical and

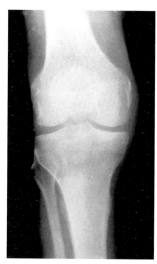

Figure 19.20: Plain radiograph of the knee joint [antero-posterior view] in a patient with tuberculosis synovitis showing normal bones

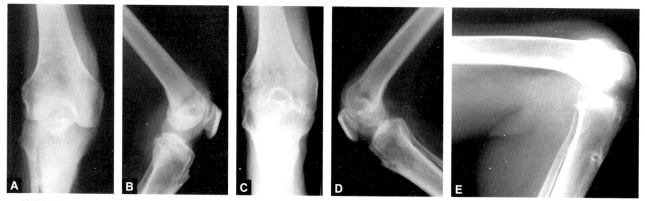

Figure 19.21: Sequentially taken plain radiographs of the left knee joint in a 54-year-old man, showing stage of synovitis with the knee in flexion before initiation of treatment [A and B]. Three months later, while on treatment, juxta-articular rarefaction of bones in early arthritis stage is evident [C and D]. The radiograph taken at the completion of treatment showing ankylosed knee joint approximately at 100° flexion despite skeletal traction [E]

radiological improvement. Clinical improvement is indicated by improvement in local and constitutional symptoms. Re-ossification of radiolucent areas and increased density of joint margins are signs of radiological improvement. In the early period of mobilisation, a bivalved plaster cast or brace can be used to prevent recurrence of flexion deformity. If the synovitis persists in spite of adequate anti-TB treatment for three months, an open arthrotomy and subtotal synovectomy are indicated. The main objective is the removal of infected tissues to render the chemotherapy more effective.

Moderately advanced disease, in addition, requires debridement with removal of loose bodies and debris. Excision of pannus covering the articular cartilage and curettage of superficial cartilage erosions and osseous necrotic foci are also done. If large metaphyseal lesions are present, they are exposed through a window at a distance from joint, curetted and packed with cancellous bone grafts. Postoperatively, traction must be continued for at least six weeks in order to prevent or to correct flexion deformity and avoid compressive forces acting against the articular surface. Thereafter, the knee joint must be protected in a bivalved plaster cast or brace and the weight bearing is started slowly and cautiously. The range of knee joint flexion is likely to remain limited to moderate or significant extent. In patients with advanced/progressive destructive arthritis or a painful fibrous ankylosis, arthrodesis may be required. During surgery, sufficient bone is removed to overcome deformity and expose normal cancellous bone and a compression device is used to obtain rapid fusion (37).

Whenever possible, arthrodesis must be deferred till the completion of growth in distal femur and proximal tibia. With arthrodesis, the knee joint remains stable and allows long hours of standing and walking. However, arthrodesis does not allow flexion of the knee joint and the leg remains sticking out while sitting.

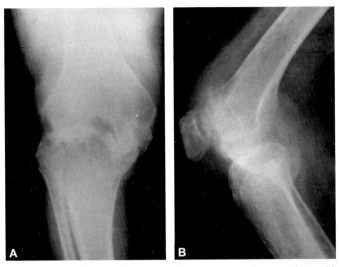

Figure 19.22: Plain radiograph of the knee joint in a patient with advanced knee joint TB. Antero-posterior view showing gross destruction of bones, lateral subluxation, flexion deformity and tricompartmental involvement can be seen [A]. Lateral view [B] of the same patient showing flexion deformity
TB = tuberculosis

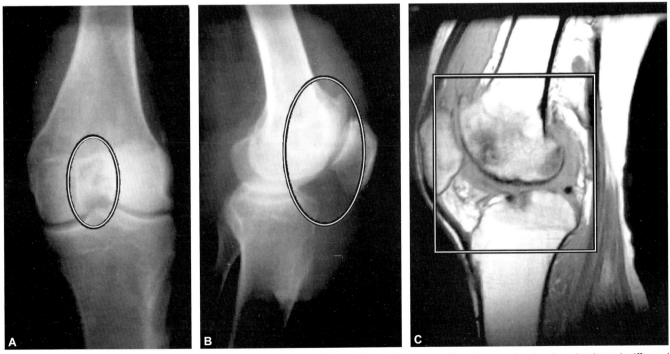

Figure 19.23: Plain radiograph of the left knee joint in an 18-year-old boy with a history of significant injury who developed pain and stiffness in the left knee joint not responding to symptomatic treatment, showing rarefaction [small oval] [A], and patellofemoral sclerosis [large oval] [B]. MRI [sagittal section] of the same patient showing infective changes affecting epiphyseal part of the femur more than tibia [C]. Biopsy confirmed the diagnosis of TB
MRI = magnetic resonance imaging; TB = tuberculosis

Healing of the wound after surgery in patients with advanced arthritis is often slow and wound dehiscence may occur. This is because, the capsule, subcutaneous tissue and the skin [that is often scarred] may also be affected by the disease process.

TUBERCULOSIS OF ANKLE AND FOOT

TB of the ankle joint and foot accounts for less than 5% of all cases of osteoarticular TB. Tarsals and the ankle joint are usually involved together in TB. This occurs due to spread of the TB infection through intercommunicating synovial channels or along soft tissue planes. The extent of bony involvement and the clinically evident swelling around the ankle joint and foot are more extensive than what is discernible on the plain radiograph.

Pathology

TB of the ankle joint and foot most commonly starts as synovitis which may be either due to infection of the synovium or less often due to inflammation in response to an adjacent focus of TB in the bone. Usually, the disease presents as synovial disease or extrasynovial soft tissue disease associated with a bony focus. The disease spreads fast to involve several joints and is clinically characterised by early occurrence of signs of inflammation. Sometimes, a central bony focus may remain clinically quiescent for some time or may produce low-grade symptoms for some weeks. Local inflammatory signs develop late, only after the cortex has been penetrated and when the adjacent soft tissues and synovium are involved.

The most commonly affected bone is calcaneum, followed in frequency by talus, first metatarsal, navicular and medial two cuneiform bones. Certain bones appear to be predisposed to TB at different ages. In infants, metatarsals are most often affected. Tarsal bones in children and bones of the ankle joint in adults are frequently involved. Talus is most often affected in old age. Multiple lesions, abscess and sinus formation are common in adults. On the other hand, fulminating synovial disease is more common in children. A metaphyseal focus in tibia can involve the growth plate and produce deformity of the ankle joint. An infective focus can develop in the epiphysis and destroy a part of it. In a child, intramedullary extension of the bony focus may precede the perforation of cortex.

Clinical Features

In the common variety of synovial disease, the onset is insidious. The clinical presentation includes pain, limp, local warmth, tenderness and a diffuse doughy swelling [Figures 19.24 and 19.25]. The soft tissue swelling is initially intermittent; subsides with rest and reappears with walking. Eventually the swelling becomes persistent, pain increases and movements of the ankle joint become restricted. The boggy and tender swelling usually starts at dorsolateral aspect of tarsal areas and with the spread of infection it extends towards tarsometatarsal joints.

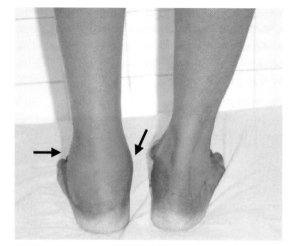

Figure 19.24: Clinical photograph of the left ankle joint showing doughy swelling [arrows] due to TB arthritis
TB = tuberculosis

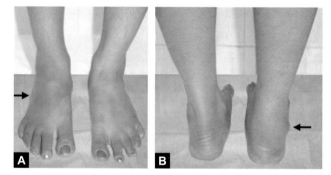

Figure 19.25: Clinical photograph of a young girl showing mid-foot swelling [A] [arrow] extending up to ankle [arrow] [B] due to TB arthritis involving right foot and ankle joint
TB = tuberculosis

In the less common type of disease, which starts as a central bony focus, usual clinical features include dull aching pain of a few weeks duration. The foot may appear deceptively normal. A careful clinical examination may reveal minimal swelling, tenderness and warmth. Sometimes, a sinus may form adjacent to the bony lesion [Figure 19.26].

Radiographic Features

An isolated destructive lesion may be seen in tarsal bones, commonly in calcaneum and talus [Figure 19.27]. In small tarsal and metatarsal bones and phalanges, single intraosseous lesion usually first produces expansion of bone. Early diffuse osteoporosis is a prominent feature. Early radiological signs, before bony destruction becomes evident, are narrowing of joint space, cortical irregularities and minimal destruction of cortical margins. In late stages of the disease, radiographs show complete obliteration and disorganisation of joint, large bony lesions and soft tissue swelling.

In selected clinical situations where either the diagnosis is not clear or radiological features are inconclusive, an MRI

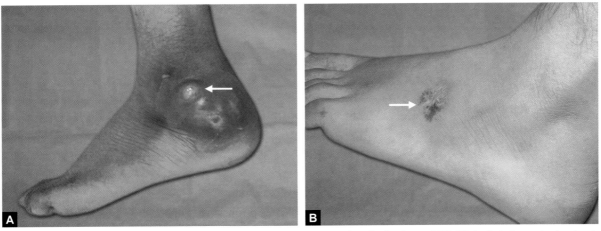

Figure 19.26: Clinical photograph of the left foot showing TB sinus over the lateral malleolus [arrow] [A]. Clinical photograph showing healed TB sinus [arrow] overlying the bony lesion in another patient [B]
TB = tuberculosis

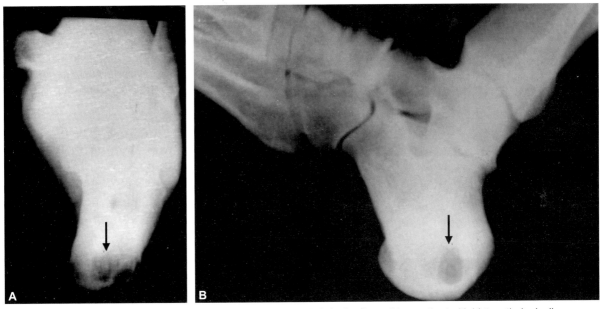

Figure 19.27: Plain radiograph of the calcaneum [axial view] [A] showing lytic lesion [arrow] in a patient with histopathologically proven calcaneal TB. The lytic lesion [arrow] is evident in the posterior part of the calcaneum in the lateral view [B]
TB = tuberculosis

is helpful. This will show the extent of the bony as well as soft tissue lesions [Figures 19.28 and 19.29].

Management

Synovial biopsy may be needed at times for confirmation of diagnosis. Anti-TB treatment is the mainstay of therapy. Plaster of paris cast is used to give rest to the affected area. The ankle joint should be immobilised in 10° equinus position. This allows ankylosis, if at all it occurs, to develop in functional position. Immobilisation and non-weight bearing should be continued till the disease becomes quiescent as evidenced by improvement in local signs. When treatment is started early, this conservative treatment will produce either completely normal or functionally normal ankle joint in over 80% of the cases.

An extensive, long-standing synovial disease requires arthrotomy and synovectomy. Along with synovectomy, pannus should be carefully peeled off the articular cartilage. The articular cartilage tends to survive for long periods and destroyed articular cartilage heals by formation of fibrocartilage.

An isolated bony lesion should be curetted and large cavities should be packed with bone grafts. This ensures early healing and prevents spread of disease into the joint and adjoining bones. An extensive destruction of one or multiple tarsal bones requires complete excision of the affected bone. Any portion of tarsus can be excised from

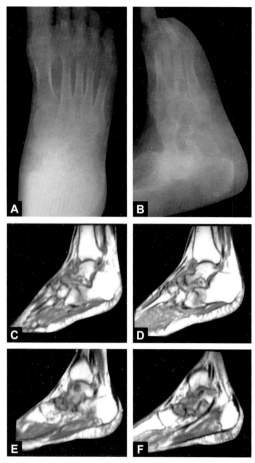

Figure 19.28: Plain radiograph of the right foot of the patient shown in Figure 19.25 antero-posterior [A] and oblique [B] views showing loss of outline of individual tarsal bones. An MRI [sagittal section] of the right foot shows involvement of talus, navicular, calcaneum, and cuboid by tuberculosis [C, D, E, and F]

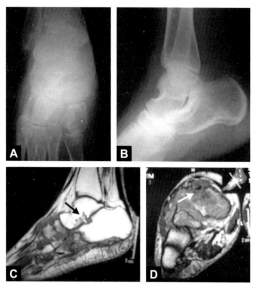

Figure 19.29: Plain radiograph of the foot showing no lesions in antero-posterior [A] and lateral [B] views. But MRI reveals extensive tuberculosis involvement of the mid-tarsal bone in the sagittal [arrow] [C] and transverse [arrow] [D] sections

the level of neck of talus proximally to metatarsal bases distally by two transverse saw cuts. The cut bone surfaces are approximated and cast applied. This results in a shortened but a well-functioning foot.

When the joint destruction is so extensive that a functional joint cannot be expected, arthrodesis of ankle or subtalar joint alone or together can result in a painless albeit stiff foot. The technique of arthrodesis is beyond the scope of this chapter.

TUBERCULOSIS OF THE SHOULDER JOINT

TB of the shoulder joint is relatively rare. It accounts for only 1%-2% of all cases of osteoarticular TB. In contrast to TB at other skeletal sites, involvement of shoulder joint by TB occurs more frequently in adults than children (38-40).

Pathology

TB of the shoulder joint seldom begins in the synovium and the clinical presentation as synovitis is rare. Commonly, the disease starts as an osseous lesion in the humeral head or glenoid. The joint is involved early and is filled with granulation tissue. Capsular contracture and fibrous ankylosis occur early and, therefore, stiffness and limitation of movements also appear early. Small osseous foci gradually enlarge and become confluent. Subsequently, a large fibro-caseous cavity forms which may lead to deformity of humeral head and glenoid. This common variety of TB of the shoulder joint is considered to be a dry and atrophic type, and hence the name *"caries sicca"*. Swelling, abscess and sinus formation occur rarely. In children, osseous lesion may start in metaphyseal region of humerus and interfere with the longitudinal growth.

Clinical Features

The onset is insidious, the early symptoms are non-specific and include sensation of heaviness or muscle weakness. Pain on movements of the shoulder joint appears next and progressively worsens. Muscle spasm fixes the shoulder joint in adduction. Examination reveals painful limitation of all movements of the shoulder joint especially external rotation and abduction. In early stages of the disease, some swelling, thickening and tenderness in soft tissues around the shoulder joint may be present. A marked wasting of deltoid supraspinatus and infraspinatus muscles may occur [Figure 19.30]. Axillary lymph nodes may be enlarged and rarely a cold abscess may be present.

In early stages, TB of the shoulder joint has to be differentiated from periarthritis of the shoulder joint. In the advanced stage, RA must be considered in the differential diagnosis. In RA, the marked soft tissue swelling and synovial effusion occur. In doubtful cases, synovial biopsy should be submitted for microbiological and histopatho-logical examinations.

Radiographic Features

Diffuse osteoporosis is an important radiological feature in early stages. Later, some soft tissue swelling occurs

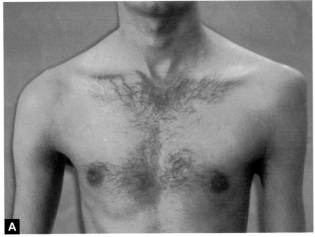

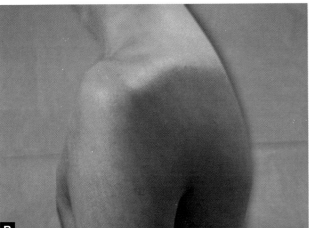

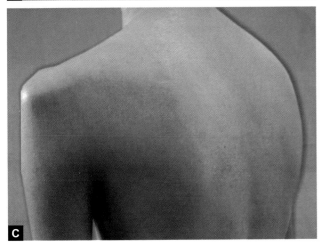

Figure 19.30: Clinical photograph showing front [A], side [B], and posterior view [C] of left shoulder joint. Gross muscle wasting involving deltoid, supraspinatus and infraspinatus can be seen.

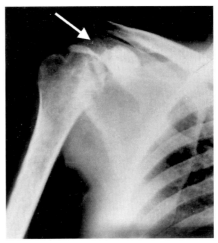

Figure 19.31: Plain radiograph of the right shoulder joint [antero-posterior view] showing late tuberculosis arthritis with destruction of the glenohumeral joint

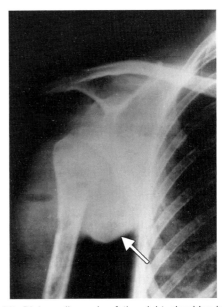

Figure 19.32: Plain radiograph of the right shoulder joint [antero-posterior view] showing pathological dislocation and a large cold abscess in axilla [arrow]. Patient had multiple sinuses located posteriorly

Management

In patients with a doubtful diagnosis, a synovial biopsy should be performed early to confirm the diagnosis. In addition to the general measures, the affected shoulder joint should be immobilised in plaster spica for three months. Currently, removable polythene brace is commonly used for this purpose. The immobilisation should be in functional position in the event of eventual healing with ankylosis. The optimum position for immobilisation is 80° abduction, 30° forward flexion and 30° of internal rotation. Usually, fibrous ankylosis occurs. Patient can perform routine activities due to compensatory movements at scapulothoracic level.

and cortical margins become indistinct. Osteolytic osseous lesions, narrowing of the joint space and deformity of the humeral head and glenoid develop in the late stages of disease [Figures 19.31 and 19.32]. Rarely, pathological subluxation or dislocation of the shoulder joint may develop [Figure 19.33].

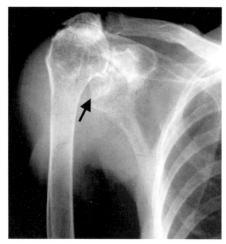

Figure 19.33: Plain radiograph of the right shoulder joint [antero-posterior view] showing pathological superior migration and osteo-porosis of the right humeral head [arrow] in treated tuberculosis arthritis of the right shoulder joint

TB of the shoulder joint responds well to anti-TB treatment. Occasionally, despite adequate anti-TB treatment, fibrous ankylosis of the shoulder joint remains painful and has to be distinguished from a relapse. In selected cases with fibrous ankylosis, surgical arthrodesis of the glenohumeral joint in the optimum functional position is helpful. This relieves pain and provides a stable joint. A shoulder spica or internal fixation with metallic implants is necessary for the success of arthrodesis. Shoulder spica is to be continued for two to three months till the radiological confirmation of arthrodesis. Subsequently, limb is supported on a sling after removal of the spica. Gradual physiotherapy is started to encourage the scapulo-thoracic movement.

An alternative to arthrodesis is available for patients with a painful shoulder joint due to TB. In the procedure known as excision arthroplasty of the shoulder joint, the diseased tissues are removed by thorough debridement, and the affected bony parts are removed from proximal humerus and glenoid. The resultant pseudoarthrosis preserves the movement at the shoulder joint. However, this procedure may render the joint unstable. Possibility of development of future relapses of the disease is also another risk with this procedure. All major surgical procedures are to be undertaken under the cover of anti-TB treatment.

TUBERCULOSIS OF ELBOW JOINT

TB of the elbow joint accounts for about 2% or less of all osteoarticular TB. Children are less often affected as compared to adults.

Pathology

The disease commonly begins as an osseous focus in the olecranon, coronoid, lower end of the humerus or upper end of the radius in order of decreasing frequency. These caseous bony lesions involve the joint to produce destruction of cartilage and pannus formation. At this stage, if healing

occurs, the eventual outcome will be a fibrous ankylosis. If caseous arthritis continues for a long period, discharging sinuses also develop. TB starting as a synovial disease is uncommon in the elbow joint.

Clinical Features

Disease is generally insidious in onset and produces pain, muscle spasm and limitation of movements. Generalised joint tenderness, boggy oedema of periarticular tissues and increased synovial effusion occur [Figure 19.34]. Swelling is most easily appreciated at the back of the elbow on both sides of the olecranon and triceps tendon. Wasting of arm and forearm muscles occurs early. Supratrochlear or axillary lymph nodes are enlarged in about one-third of cases. In advanced untreated disease, discharging sinuses may be present.

Radiographic Features

In early stage of the disease, bones around the joint show generalised osteoporosis and the articular margins become fuzzy and irregular [Figure 19.35]. Osteolytic bony lesions can be seen in the olecranon, coronoid, distal humerus or radial head [Figure 19.36]. In late stages of the disease, marked joint space narrowing and destruction of articular margins appear. Rarely, due to marked destruction of ligaments and bones, the elbow joint may develop pathological posterior dislocation. As the disease heals, fibrous ankylosis develops more frequently than bony ankylosis.

Management

If the disease starts from an osseous focus or has progressed to an advanced stage of arthritis, clinical and radiological features are usually diagnostic. In the stage of synovitis and during early stages of the joint destruction, differentiating TB of the elbow joint from RA can be difficult. In doubtful cases, an open biopsy of the synovium should be done to ascertain a definitive diagnosis.

The principles underlying the management of TB of the elbow joint are similar to those applicable to TB of other synovial joints. Anti-TB treatment forms the mainstay of therapy. In cases where sinuses have formed secondary infection with pyogenic bacteria is likely. In these cases, a broad spectrum antibiotic should also be administered.

In all stages of the disease, with or without operative intervention, the elbow joint should be immobilised for about 3 months in a plaster cast or removable polythene brace. When the disease is unilateral, immobilisation of the elbow joint in 90° flexion and forearm in the midprone position is recommended to avoid the development of ankylosis in nonfunctional position. After removal of splintage, overuse of the joint should be avoided for further six to nine months. Functionally, satisfactory range of movements at the elbow joint is retained in a majority of cases. Results, however, also depend on the stage and extent of the disease and joint destruction when treatment is started. The results are much

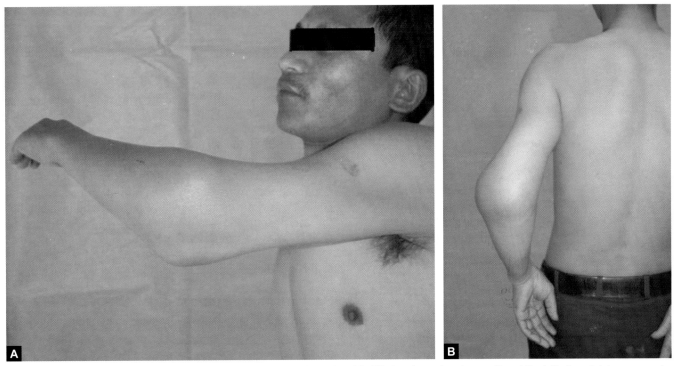

Figure 19.34: Clinical photograph with arms abducted [A] and held by the side [B] showing a doughy swelling at the left elbow joint, more marked on lateral and posterior aspects. Flexion of the elbow joint and muscle wasting in the arm are also evident

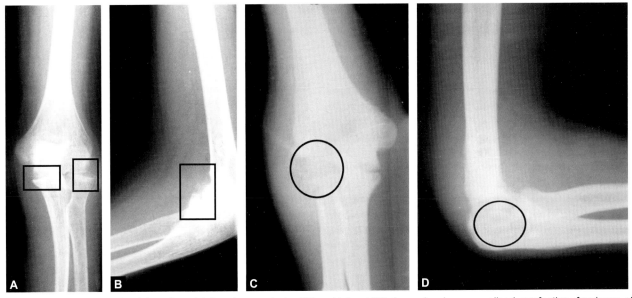

Figure 19.35: Plain radiograph of the elbow joint, antero-posterior [A] and lateral [B] views showing generalised rarefaction, fuzziness of joint surfaces [rectangles]. Plain radiograph [antero-posterior view] [C], [lateral view] [D] of the patient shown in Figure 19.34 showing soft tissue swelling and fuzziness of joint surfaces [circles] [C and D]

better in the early stage disease of synovitis and in unicompartmental disease. In advanced arthritis with involvement of all compartments of joint, the usual end result is fibrous ankylosis in a majority of patients. The bony ankylosis is uncommon.

A localised destructive lesion near the joint [usually in the olecranon or coronoid] should be curetted early to eradicate a source of future relapses and extension of disease into the joint. Synovectomy and joint debridement are indicated in patients with early arthritis when response to chemotherapy and immobilisation is not adequate.

When advanced arthritis has healed with elbow joint in tight fibrous anklylosis or anklyosis in unacceptable position, a good and functionally useful range of movements at the

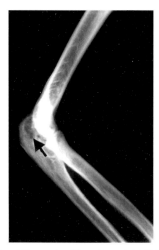

Figure 19.36: Plain radiograph of the elbow joint [lateral view] involved by tuberculosis showing lytic lesion in olecranon [arrow] and loss of joint space with flexion deformity

elbow joint can be regained with excision arthroplasty. The surgery should be deferred till growth is complete and should not be done in persons engaged in heavy manual work. The surgery consists of removing an "inverted V-shaped" segment of the lower end of humerus with the apex of "V" reaching the olecranon fossa. Supracondylar ridges, epicondyles and collateral ligaments should be carefully preserved. Upper end of the ulna [rarely along with upper end of the radius] should be sparingly trimmed and allowed to slide in the "inverted V-gap" in the humerus. After seven to ten days of operation, movements of active and assisted active flexion, extension, supination and pronation are started. Night splint should be used for three months. Light work without splint is allowed three months after the surgery (19).

In heavy manual workers, arthrodesis of the elbow joint is indicated when the joint has become extensively disorganised. For unilateral disease, a position of 90° of flexion is desirable. For bilateral cases, one elbow joint should be placed in 110° flexion to enable the hand to reach mouth and face and the other in 65° flexion to attend to personal hygiene. The optimum position is best decided after a trial immobilisation of the elbow joint in plaster cast for few weeks before operation. The surgical technique of arthrodesis of the elbow joint is beyond the scope of this chapter.

TUBERCULOSIS OF WRIST JOINT

TB of the wrist joint is rare and is seen mainly in adults.

Pathology

The most common site of initial focus of TB in the wrist joint is in the distal radius and capitate. The disease spreads to involve the wrist and intercarpal joints. Less often, the disease starts from a primary focus in the synovium and infection soon gets disseminated to intercarpal and wrist joints. Infection then spreads to involve both flexor and extensor tendon sheaths. Still less commonly, the infection may spread to wrist joint from the infected tenosynovitis (41,42). Abscess and sinus formation are common.

Clinical Features

The onset of the disease is insidious. Exacerbation of pain by movements is the early symptom. Soft tissue swelling, tenderness and limitation of flexion and extension movements at the wrist joint occur later. In progressive disease with destruction of bones and ligaments, subluxation or dislocation of radiocarpal joints occurs. This gives rise to a marked deformity and further limitation of movements. Abscess and sinus formation are frequent in advanced disease. Extension of disease to flexor and extensor tendon sheaths produces a localised boggy swelling and difficulty in movements of fingers. A monoarticular RA may be difficult to differentiate from TB.

Radiographic Features

In the early stages, radiographs show demineralisation of bones, bony erosions and some reduction of the joint space. Osteolytic bony lesions in the radius and carpal bones may be seen. In advanced stages of the disease, joint spaces of both wrist and intercarpal joints become obliterated. Bony destruction and even subluxation or dislocation of the wrist joint may occur [Figures 19.37 and 19.38].

Management

TB of the wrist joint is quite likely to be misdiagnosed as monoarticular RA and, therefore, it is essential to confirm the diagnosis with synovial biopsy.

An early diagnosis and early institution of anti-TB treatment are indicated. Periodic follow up with imaging is required. If indicated, the continuation phase may be extended and this practice of extension of treatment should be individualised. More clinical trials are required to say definitely about the efficacy as well as duration of anti-TB treatment. A prolonged splintage in plaster cast or polythene splint with wrist in 10° dorsiflexion and in midprone position is always required. Splintage should be gradually discarded during daytime but night splint is used for nearly one year. The heavy physical work should be avoided for 18-24 months in order to avoid collapse of the bones and minimising the risk of development of deformity. The combination of modern anti-TB treatment and proper splintage are adequate in nearly two-thirds of patients. Good functional range of movements can be regained with these if the treatment is started at the early stage of the disease. Gross fibrous ankylosis occurs in one-third of patients.

Synovectomy of the joint or tendon sheaths [if involved] and curettage of bony lesions are indicated in patients not responding to treatment or whenever there is doubt regarding the diagnosis. With the availability of better imaging modalities for an early diagnosis, effective drugs, use of better orthopaedic splintage and surgical intervention is rarely required (41,42).

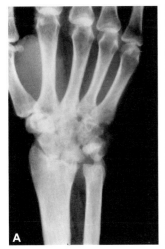
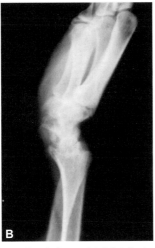

Figure 19.37: Post-treatment radiograph of the wrist joint [antero-posterior view] [A] showing ankylosed wrist, gross destruction of carpals, loss of intercarpal and radiocarpal joints. Mild volar subluxation of carpals with loss of radiocarpal joints can be seen in the lateral view [B]

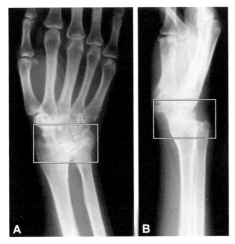

Figure 19.38: Plain radiograph of the right wrist, antero-posterior [A] and lateral [B] views of a patient who has received a full course of anti-TB treatment showing bony ankylosis [rectangles] of distal radioulnar, radiocarpal and intercarpal joints
TB = tuberculosis

Arthrodesis of the wrist joint is the treatment of choice to minimise the disability in patients where wrist joint has dislocated due to the advanced destruction, in patients with painful fibrous ankylosis or ankylosis in non-functional position [e.g., flexion]. Thorough debridement and arthrodesis are also useful for painful wrist joint with a history of recurrence of infection. Arthrodesis of both wrist and intercarpal joints is performed together from a dorsal approach. The diseased tissue, synovium and articular cartilage are removed as far as possible and joint spaces are packed with cancellous grafts. In the *Darrach's procedure*, a large cortico-cancellous graft is placed in a trough made in distal radius, lunate, capitate and proximal part of the third metacarpal. Along with this, the distal end of ulna should be excised to provide useful range of pronation and

supination. Optimum position of the wrist joint arthrodesis is in 10°–15° of dorsiflexion.

TUBERCULOSIS OF SACROILIAC JOINT

Sacroiliac joint is a true synovial joint. This joint is involved in 2%-5% cases with osteoarticular TB (43).

Pathology

TB of the sacroiliac joint may start in the synovium, in lateral masses of sacrum or ilium. Infection can either start at these sites or occur as an extension of TB from ipsilateral hip joint and lumbosacral area of spine. Destructive caseous lesions form and destroy the joint. Abscess formation is common and the abscess may present dorsally or inside the pelvis. Intrapelvic extension can lead to severe visceral lesions making the prognosis quite serious. Dorsal abscess or its extension along the iliac crest is likely to result in sinus formation. These sinuses heal with difficulty. Superadded bacterial infection through the sinuses is common.

Clinical Features

Sacroiliac TB is rare in infancy and childhood and affects adults more frequently. Females are affected more frequently than males [male: female = 2:5]. Concomitant TB at some other site is present in about half the patients. In patients with a poor general health and nutritional status, bilateral sacroiliac joint involvement is common.

The onset of the disease is insidious and it may follow trauma or pregnancy. Pain over the affected joint is the main symptom. It is referred to groin and less commonly in the sciatic nerve distribution. Pain worsens on lying either supine or on affected side. Prolonged standing and walking also aggravate pain. Sitting on the buttock on affected side is painful, whereas sitting on opposite buttock relieves pain. Bending forwards with the knee joints in extension produces tension on the hamstrings and exacerbates the pain, but, bending forwards with the knee joints in flexion is less painful as this manoeuvre relaxes the hamstrings. Sudden jerks, coughing and sneezing also worsen the pain. Localised tenderness and some boggy swelling or abscesses are present. Stressing the involved sacroiliac joints by any one of the following three manoeuvres increases pain: [i] distraction of both sacroiliac joints by simultaneous pressure on both anterior superior iliac spines; [ii] stressing the sacroiliac joint with forced flexion, abduction and external rotation of ipsilateral hip joint [*Faber's test*]; and [iii] by performing the *Gaenslen's test* of rotating the ilium on sacrum. In the *Gaenslen's test*, the hip on the unaffected side is first firmly flexed to fix the pelvis and lumbosarcal junction. The affected hip is then hyperextended, thereby rotating the corresponding ilium forwards. This stresses the inflamed ligamentous structures about the sacroiliac joint and produces pain.

Rectal examination is important to detect intraplevic abscess. In advanced disease, large cold abscesses and sinuses may be present.

Radiographic Features

In the early stages, the plain radiographs are normal. The earliest radiographic evidence is in the form of haziness or loss of definition of joint margins. Thereafter, an irregularity of the articular surface with areas of erosions may become evident. If the disease is controlled at this early stage, the joint space narrowing and sclerosis of the joint margins occur. Progressive destruction causes marked cavitation in the bone and narrowing of the joint space. Healing of advanced disease occurs by bony ankylosis and increased density of the joint margins. Ankylosing spondylitis, RA, pyogenic infection and juxta-articular bony lesions should be considered in the differential diagnosis. The CT and MRI are of great value in detecting early joint erosions, cavitation and abscess.

Management

TB of the sacroiliac joint is difficult to diagnose in the early stages as the clinical manifestations are atypical. Also, it responds slowly and less favourably to anti-TB treatment and surgical treatment becomes necessary quite often. In the pre-chemotherapeutic era, TB of the sacroiliac joint was commonly encountered in patients with generalised severe infection and the mortality was high in these patients.

Standard anti-TB treatment and general supportive therapy are initiated. Surgical intervention is indicated in patients not responding to drugs and in those with recurrence of infection or when the diagnosis is in doubt. It consists of debridement of joint, freshening of joint margins and packing the area with adequate bone grafts to achieve arthrodesis. Postoperative bedrest is required for about three months followed by gradual mobilisation in a lumbosacral belt or plaster jacket till clear bony fusion of joint is evident radiologically.

TUBERCULOSIS AT RARE SITES

Sternoclavicular Joint

TB of the sternoclavicular joint is rare. Often, the disease may be misdiagnosed to be low-grade pyogenic infection, RA, multiple myeloma or metastases. The disease usually starts in the bone at the medial end of clavicle and presents with a painful swelling of an insidious onset. The swelling may be warm, tender and boggy. A cold abscess and a sinus can form in late stages of the disease. Radiographic examination of this joint is very difficult and MRI is useful to detect early erosion and soft tissue swelling. Biopsy is necessary if the diagnosis is in doubt. Response to anti-TB treatment is usually good.

Acromioclavicular Joint

Acromioclavicular joint is also a rare site for TB and the disease may start from the lateral end of clavicle or acromion and spreads to the joint. Clinical features include pain and swelling of an insidious onset. The diagnosis is often missed. Anti-TB treatment often yields satisfactory results.

Symphysis Pubis

TB of symphysis pubis is rare. The disease usually begins in pubic bone and spreads to symphysis. Localised pain and sometimes abscess and sinuses are presenting features. Radiological assessment of this area reveals osteolytic areas in pubic bones and destruction of margins of pubic symphysis. Concomitant TB lesions in sacroiliac joint are not uncommon and some of these patients may develop displacement of symphysis. Treatment is essentially with anti-TB drugs. Cold abscess may require antigravity aspiration.

Ilium, Ischium and Ischiopubic Ramus

Isolated TB lesions are rarely seen in one of these bones. Usual presenting features include pain, swelling, tenderness, cold abscess and discharging sinuses. Radiologically, these lesions show varying number of lytic areas and some of these lesions may contain sequestra. Superimposed pyogenic infection will produce sclerosis around lytic areas. One must be aware of these conditions in order to diagnose them at an early stage. Treatment is with anti-TB drugs. Exploration and debridement of bony lesions is indicated in the following situations: [i] patients with doubtful diagnosis; [ii] disease not responding to anti-TB treatment; and [iii] recurrent disease.

Sternum and Ribs

TB very rarely involves the sternum and ribs. Often, the disease is not diagnosed till sinuses have formed. Nearly one-third of patients will have detectable TB lesion in lungs or other parts of the skeleton. Radiographic assessment of both these sites is very difficult and may reveal irregular destruction and cavities. The diseased ribs may be thickened very much or expanded with "punched out" erosions. Surgery is not required routinely in these patients. However, it may be done to establish the diagnosis or for the removal of sequestrum. Response to anti-TB treatment is good.

Scapula

The scapula is another rare site for TB. Infection may start in the angle of acromion, spine, neck of scapula and inferior or superior angle of scapula. Pain and occasionally swelling are the presenting clinical features. This is another bone where radiological evaluation is difficult. CT or MRI can be helpful to detect early lesion of the disease in scapula. Treatment is with anti-TB drugs.

Clavicle

Occurrence of TB of the clavicle without involvement of acromioclavicular or sternoclavicular joint is rare. Children are most often affected. Presenting clinical features include painful swelling of clavicle with or without cold abscess or sinuses. Radiograph shows any one of the following types of appearances: diffuse thickening and honeycombing, multiple cystic cavities and sequestra formation similar to pyogenic infection. The mainstay of therapy is anti-TB treatment. The role of surgery is limited. Biopsy may be done to confirm the diagnosis. Debridement may be helpful in patients with slow or no response to drugs. Large sequestrum should be removed surgically. If necessary, a part of clavicle can be excised without loss of function (44).

TUBERCULOSIS TENOSYNOVITIS AND BURSITIS

TB of the tendon sheaths and bursa is rare. Any synovial sheath or bursa can be affected but tendon sheaths around hand are more commonly affected as compared to other sites.

Tuberculosis Tenosynovitis

Hand is the most common site of involvement. People who work with cattle are predisposed to disease caused by *Mycobacterium bovis*. Infection can also reach the tendon sheath by haematogenous route or from neighbouring affected bone and joint. The disease usually starts as a simple inflammation of the tendon sheath with serous exudate and fibrinous deposits covering the inner surface. Gradually, the tendon sheath thickens and the exudate becomes seropurulent. With movement and friction the broken villi and fibrinous exudate get moulded to resemble *"rice bodies"* closely resembling similar looking *rice bodies* sometimes seen in RA. The tendon sheath may undergo caseation necrosis and the exudate penetrates the soft tissues to form sinuses. Rarely, necrosis of underlying tendons may occur. With healing, the sheath becomes fibrotic. The infection spreads in the sheath to involve all areas from muscle to tendinous insertion. Paratendon and fascial structures are involved by the spread of disease. TB tenosynovitis of the common sheath of forearm flexor tendons distends the sheath both proximally and distally up to flexor retinaculum. This produces a dumb-bell shaped swelling, classically known as *"compound palmar ganglion"*. Cross fluctuation can be demonstrated between the swelling proximal and distal to flexor retinaculum.

The clinical course of TB tenosynovitis is slow and insidious. Presenting features include pain, swelling, tenderness, weakness of grip and limitation of movements. The latter is minimal to start with but progressively worsens with adherence of tendons. Spontaneous tendon rupture and sinus formation are uncommon and occur as late complications. Fever and general constitutional symptoms are unusual until neighbouring bone and joint have been involved.

Treatment in early stage consists of anti-TB treatment and immobilisation. In extensive and long-standing disease, surgical resection of the diseased tissue followed by immobilisation should be done. Function becomes better after radical excision. If tendon has become necrotic, it should be excised and tendon grafting should be done. When infection has spread to bone and joint, especially the wrist joint, wide excision, debridement and arthrodesis will give best functional results.

Tuberculosis Bursitis

Bursa over greater trochanter, subdeltoid bursa and pes anserinus bursa are known to develop TB. All are rare lesions. Clinical presentation includes mild pain, localised swelling and tenderness. Differentiation from RA, ganglion and synovial tumours can be difficult and biopsy may be required for an accurate diagnosis.

TB bursitis responds well to anti-TB treatment. Large swellings may require aspiration.

TUBERCULOSIS OSTEOMYELITIS

TB of the bone alone can occur without involvement of joint (45). Any bone can be affected but long tubular bones are rarely involved. These are often diagnosed and treated like bacterial chronic osteomyelitis (40). Usually, adults are affected. The common presenting features include pain, swelling of bone with warmth, tenderness, boggy soft tissue swelling and regional lymphadenopathy. In late cases, abscess and sinus formation occurs. A high index of suspicion is required for the diagnosis. Radiographs show irregular cavities and areas of destruction with little surrounding sclerosis [Figures 19.39 and 19.40].

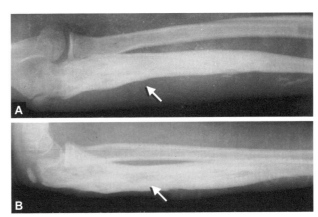

Figure 19.39: Plain radiograph of the forearm antero-posterior [A] and lateral [B] views showing TB osteomyelitis of entire ulna at the beginning of treatment [arrows]
TB = tuberculosis

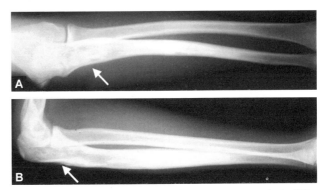

Figure 19.40: Plain radiograph of the forearm antero-posterior [A] and lateral [B] views of the patient shown in Figures 19.39A and 19.39B showing healed TB osteomyelitis of ulna at completion of treatment [arrows]
TB = tuberculosis

This commonly produces a honeycomb appearance. Some of the cavities may contain feathery sequestra. After sinus formation, superadded bacterial infection produces marked sclerosis and occasionally sequestration of cortical bone resembling pyogenic chronic osteomyelitis. Differential diagnosis includes chronic pyogenic osteomyelitis, Brodie's abscess and tumours. Biopsy for histopathological and microbiological investigations may help in the diagnosis. Occasionally, a presumptive diagnosis can be confirmed on the basis of favourable response to anti-TB treatment.

TB osteomyelitis of short tubular bones like phalanges, metacarpals and metatarsals is more often seen and is predominantly a disease of children. The disease process starts in the medullary cavity causing patchy destruction. The entire diaphysis sequestrates due to a combination of two interrelated pathological processes. Firstly, the periosteum becomes lifted up due to granulation tissue. This results in the formation of involucrum and consequently sequestration of diaphysis occurs. Secondly, because of deficient anastomosis of the osseous arteries in childhood, the thrombosis caused by TB pathology leads to sequestration of diaphysis. Rarely, the sequestrated diaphysis may be extruded before involucrum formation. As a result, gross shortening of the bone occurs. The bone becomes thickened and spindle shaped. Usually, these patients present with gradual and almost painless swelling of one of the phalanges of hand and foot. Constitutional symptoms are usually absent and the bone may be minimally tender. Radiological features of sequestration of diaphysis and subperiosteal new bone formation are diagnostic. [18]Fluorine fluorodeoxyglucose positron emission tomography [[18]FDG-PET] [Figure 19.41] has been found to be useful in localising TB disease in inaccessible or obscure sites. It also facilitates differentiating soft tissue infection as being separate from the osseous infection and monitoring response to treatment (46,47). Response to anti-TB treatment is favourable. With early treatment, sequestra may revascularise and get incorporated like a graft and nearly complete restoration of osseous structure occurs.

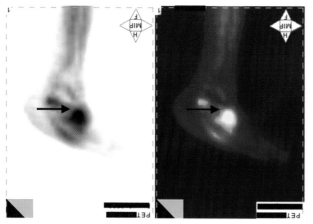

Figure 19.41: [18]FDG-PET scan showing increased FDG uptake [arrow] in small bones of foot
FDG = fluorodeoxy glucose; PET = positron emission tomography

In refractory cases involving long and short tubular bones or in the presence of abscess around the involved bone, excision of the granulation tissue and infected bone should be done. Concomitant presence of bacterial infection in the same osseous lesion, usually through sinuses, causes a delay in healing. A short-course of additional antibiotic should be given to control bacterial infection.

TUBERCULOSIS OF PROSTHETIC JOINT

As the prosthetic joint replacement is increasingly being done globally, several reports documenting TB of the prosthetic joint have been published (48-51). Prosthetic joint TB may develop due to the reactivation of the TB arthritis for which prosthetic replacement was performed. These patients present with slowly progressive joint pain. Diagnosis requires a high index of suspicion. Arthrocentesis must be done and specimens must be obtained from multiple sites for mycobacteriological studies. Eradication of TB focus is not possible without removing the prosthesis. Treatment consists of removal of the prosthesis followed by appropriate anti-TB treatment.

REFERENCES

1. Lichtor J, Lichtor A. Paleo-pathological evidence suggesting precolambian tuberculosis of spine. J Bone Joint Surg Am 1958; 39-A:1938-9.
2. Sharma SK, Mohan A. Extrapulmonary tuberculosis. Indian J Med Res 2004;120:316-53.
3. Tuli SM. Tuberculosis of the spine: an historical review. Clin Orthop Relat Res 2007;460:29-38.
4. Jain AK, Dhammi IK. Tuberculosis of the spine: a review. Clin Orthop Relat Res 2007;460:39-49.
5. Oguz E, Sehirlioglu A, Altinmakas M, Ozturk C, Komurcu M, Solakoglu C, et al. A new classification and guide for surgical treatment of spinal tuberculosis. Int Orthop 2008;32:127-33.
6. Tuli SM. Treatment of neurological complications in tuberculosis of the spine. J Bone Joint Surg Am 1969;51-A:680-92.
7. Bailey HL, Gabriel M, Hodgson AR, Shin JS. Tuberculosis of the spine in children. Operative findings and results in one hundred consecutive patients treated by removal of the lesion and anterior grafting. J Bone Joint Surg 1972;54:1633-57.
8. Butler RW. Paraplegia in Pott's disease with special reference to the pathology and etiology. Br J Surg 1935;22:738-68.
9. Seddon HJ. Pott's paraplegia, prognosis and treatment. Br J Surg 1935;22:769-99.
10. Griffiths DL, Seddon HL, Roaf R. Pott's paraplegia. London: Oxford University Press; 1956.
11. Hodgson AR, Skinsnes OK, Leong CY. The pathogenesis of Pott's paraplegia. J Bone Joint Surg 1967;49:1147-56.
12. Bosworth DM, Della Pietra A, Rahilly G. Paraplegia resulting from tuberculosis of the spine. J Bone Joint Surg 1953;35-A: 735-40.
13. Choksey MS, Powell M, Gibb WR, Casey AT, Geddes JF. A conus tuberculoma mimicking an intramedullary tumour: a case report and review of literature. Br J Neurosurg 1989;31:117-21.
14. Goel MK. Treatment of Pott's paraplegia by operation. J Bone Joint Surg 1967;49:674-81.
15. Tuli SM. Judicious management of tuberculosis of bones, joints and spine. Indian J Orthop 1985;19:147-66.
16. Kumar K. Tuberculosis of spine: natural history of disease and its judicious management. West Pac Orthop Assoc 1988;25:1-18.

17. Mukopadhaya B, Mishra NK. Tuberculosis of the spine. J Bone Joint Surg Br 1957;39-B:326-33.

18. Martin NS. Tuberculosis of the spine. A study of the results of treatment during the last twenty-five years. J Bone Joint Surg Br 1970;52:613-28.

19. Tuli SM. Tuberculosis of the skeletal system [Bones, joints, spine and bursal sheaths]. New Delhi: Jaypee Brothers Medical Publishers; 1993.

20a. Rajasekaran S, Shanmugasundaram TK. Prediction of angle of gibbus deformity in tuberculosis of spine. J Bone Joint Surg Br 1987;69:503-9.

20b. Kohli M, Schiller I, Dendukuri N, Dheda K, Denkinger CM, Schumacher SG, et al. Xpert[®] MTB/RIF assay for extrapulmonary tuberculosis and rifampicin resistance. Cochrane Database Syst Rev 2018;8:CD012768.

21. Hodgson AR, Stock FE. Anterior spinal fusion for the treatment of tuberculosis of the spine. J Bone Joint Surg 1960;42-A:295-310.

22. Dutt AK, Moers D, Stead WW. Short-course chemotherapy for extrapulmonary tuberculosis. Nine-year experience. Ann Intern Med 1986;104:7-12.

23. Sharma SK, Ryan H, Khaparde S, Sachdeva KS, Singh AD, Mohan A, et al. Index-TB guidelines: Guidelines on extrapulmonary tuberculosis for India. Indian J Med Res 2017;145:448-63.

24. Rajasekaran S, Soundarapandian S. Progression of kyphosis in tuberculosis of the spine treated by anterior arthrodesis. J Bone Joint Surg Am 1989;71:1314-23.

25. Yau AC, Hsu LCS, O'Brien JP, Hodgson AR. Tuberculous kyphosis: correction with spinal osteotomy, halopelvic distraction, and anterior and posterior fusion. J Bone Joint Surg 1947;56:1419-34.

26. Hodgson AR, Yau A, Kwon JS, Kim D. A clinical study of 100 consecutive cases of Pott's paraplegia. Clin Orthop 1964;36:128-50.

27. Bodapati PC, Vemula RCV, Mohammad AA, Mohan A. Outcome and management of spinal tuberculosis according to severity at a tertiary referral center. Asian J Neurosurg 2017;12:441-6.

28. Griffiths DL. Tuberculosis of the spine: a review. Adv Tuberc Res 1980;20:92-110.

29. Seddon HJ. The choice of treatment in Pott's disease. J Bone Joint Surg Br 1976;58-B:395-7.

30. Shanmugasundaram TK. A clinicoradiological classification of tuberculosis of hip. In: Shanmugasundaram TK, editor. Current concepts in bone joint tuberculosis. Madras; 1983.

31. Moon MS, Kim SS, Lee SR, Moon YW, Moon JL, Moon SI. Tuberculosis of hip in children: a retrospective analysis. Indian J Orthop 2012;46:191-9.

32. Hibbs RA. A Preliminary report of 20 cases of hip joint tuberculosis treated by operation fixing the joint. J Bone Joint Surg 1926;8:422.

33. Brittain HA. Ischiofemoral arthrodesis. Br J Surg 1941;29:93.

34. Girdlestone GR. Tuberculosis of bones and joints. Modern trends in orthopaedics. Series I. London: Butterworth and Company; 1950.p.35.

35. Wang Y, Wang J, Xu Z, Li Y, Wang H. Total hip arthroplasty for active tuberculosis of the hip. Int Orthop 2010;34:1111-4.

36. Neogi DS, Yadav CS, Ashok Kumar, Khan SA, Rastogi S. Total hip arthroplasty in patients with active tuberculosis of the hip with advanced arthritis. Clin Orthop Relat Res 2010;468:605-12.

37. Charnley J. Compression arthrodesis. London: E and S Livingstone; 1953.

38. Tang SC, Chow SP. Tuberculosis of the shoulder. Report of 5 cases treated conservatively. JR Coll Surg Edinb 1983;28:188-90.

39. Srivastava TP, Singh S. Osteo-articular tuberculosis in children. MS Thesis. Varanasi: Banaras Hindu University; 1987.

40. Martini M. Tuberculosis of the bones and joints. Heidelberg: Springer-Verlag; 1988.

41. Leung PC. Tuberculosis of hand. Hand 1978;10:285-91.

42. Hodgson AR, Smith TK, Gabriel Sister. Tuberculosis of the wrist. With a note on chemotherapy. Clin Orthop Relat Res 1972;83:73-83.

43. Tuli SM, Sinha GP. Skeletal tuberculosis-"unusual" lesions. Indian J Orthop 1969;3:5-18.

44. Srivastava KK, Garg LD, Kocchar VL. Tuberculous osteomyelitis of the clavicle. Acta Orthop Scand 1974;45:668-72.

45. Gardam M, Lim S. Mycobacterial osteomyelitis and arthritis. Infect Dis Clin North Am 2005;19:819-30.

46. Yago Y, Yukihiro M, Kuroki H, Katsuragawa Y, Kubota K. Cold tuberculous abscess identified by FDG-PET. Ann Nucl Med 2005;19:515-8.

47. Hu N, Tan Y, Cheng Z, Hao Z, Wang Y. FDG PET/CT in monitoring antituberculosis therapy in patient with widespread skeletal tuberculosis. Clin Nucl Med 2015;40:919-21.

48. Berbari EF, Hanssen AD, Duffy MC, Steckelberg JM, Osmon DR. Prosthetic joint infection due to Mycobacterium tuberculosis: a case series and review of the literature. Am J Orthop 1998;27:219-27.

49. Shanbhag V, Kotwal R, Gaitonde A, Singhal K. Total hip replacement infected with Mycobacterium tuberculosis. A case report with review of literature. Acta Orthop Belg 2007;73:268-74.

50. Khater FJ, Samnani IQ, Mehta JB, Moorman JP, Myers JW. Prosthetic joint infection by Mycobacterium tuberculosis: an unusual case report with literature review. South Med J 2007;100:66-9.

51. Kaya M, Nagoya S, Yamashita T, Niiro N, Fujita M. Peri-prosthetic tuberculous infection of the hip in a patient with no previous history of tuberculosis. J Bone Joint Surg Br 2006;88:394-5.

20

Musculoskeletal Manifestations of Tuberculosis

Aman Sharma, Kusum Sharma

INTRODUCTION

Extra-pulmonary tuberculosis [EPTB] has become a significant public health problem, especially in the human immuno-deficiency virus [HIV] era. Musculoskeletal tuberculosis [MSK-TB] is one of the important forms of EPTB (1). Unlike various other immunoinflammatory diseases affecting MSK system, such as, rheumatoid arthritis [RA] where achieving a cure is a dream, MSK-TB is potentially curable. Therefore, it is important to diagnose these musculoskeletal manifestations of TB early, so that anti-TB treatment can be initiated and the tissue damage can be prevented.

EPIDEMIOLOGY

There has been a surge in the number of EPTB cases in recent times (2). Share of EPTB as a proportion of total number of TB cases in USA has increased from 7.6% in 1962 to 15.7% in 1993, and to 21% in 2006 (3-5). Bone and joint TB accounted for 5337 [11%] out of a total of 47293 cases of EPTB reported in the USA from 1993–2006 (6). In the absence of a reliable epidemiological data and sparse published literature, it is not possible to give an exact figure on the relative contribution of EPTB to the total number of TB cases in India (1,7). Bone and joint TB constitutes 10%–11% of total EPTB cases which would be approximately 1%–3% of all TB cases (8,9).

Musculoskeletal TB is usually classified into spinal TB and TB of peripheral joints (10). Spinal TB constitutes nearly 50% of all MSK-TB (11). The other relatively uncommon forms of MSK-TB are Poncet's disease [parainfectious TB arthritis], TB soft tissue rheumatism, iatrogenic rheumatism and TB osteomyelitis (10). The main focus of present chapter will be on TB arthritis, Poncet's disease and TB soft tissue rheumatism. TB of the spine and peripheral joints has been covered in the chapter *"Skeletal tuberculosis" [Chapter 19].*

AETIOPATHOGENESIS AND PATHOLOGY

The causative agent of MSK-TB almost always is *Mycobacterium tuberculosis [Mtb]* (11). MSK-TB due to other mycobacteria is very rare. Anti-tumour necrosis factor-alpha [anti-TNF-α] agents are being increasingly used to treat various rheumatic diseases like RA, spondyloarthropathies, etc. There is a risk of reactivation of TB while using these agents. It might lead to disruption of tumour necrosis factor [TNF] dependent cellular migration necessary for maintaining the integrity of the granuloma (12).

The MSK-TB infection is mostly secondary to haematogenous spread from a primary focus, which may be in the lungs, lymph nodes or other organs and that the source can be demonstrated in up to 40% of these patients with the help of sensitive imaging modalities like magnetic resonance imaging [MRI] (13). The joint infection is usually a result of either spread from a TB osteomyelitis or seeding of the synovium from haematogenous spread. There is synovitis in the initial stage of infection, followed by formation of granulation tissue and pannus in the later stages, which eventually results in cartilage destruction (13). This is followed by demineralisation and necrosis resulting in severe bone damage. There may be formation of para-articular cold abscess without signs of inflammation and external fistulae (11).

Risk Factors

Host genetic factors do play a role in susceptibility to TB (14). Various studies have shown associations of different genetic polymorphisms with either increased or less risk of development of TB (15,16). EPTB like MSK-TB is predominantly a disease of children and young adults in endemic areas. In the non-endemic areas, it affects older individuals and immunocompromised patients (2,17). People with HIV infection, diabetes mellitus, and those receiving immunosuppressive and cytotoxic therapies are at increased risk of TB (18-22). Patients on treatment for underlying rheumatologic diseases, such as, systemic lupus erythematosus [SLE], RA or gout may also develop MSK-TB (23-26). There may be TB involvement of the prosthetic joints also (27).

CLINICAL MANIFESTATIONS

The clinical manifestations of MSK-TB can be divided into four major categories (28): [i] direct MSK involvement; [ii] development of TB during treatment of rheumatic disease; [iii] effects of anti-TB drugs; and [iv] reactive phenomenon.

Direct Involvement

Typical TB infection presents as a slow, smouldering localised infection of the bones [osteomyelitis], spine, peripheral joints and soft tissue. TB osteomyelitis is seen both in children and adults, but is more common in children, and may involve any bone. Femur and tibia are the most commonly involved bones, though ribs, skull, phalanx and other bones may also be involved (12). In children, TB involvement of the phalanx may cause dactylitis and present as a diffuse 'spindle-like swelling of the finger' (11). The overlying skin is shiny and stretched. Radioisotope bone scan may show 'hot spots' in the metaphysis of a short bone of the hands and feet (11).

Joint involvement is usually in the form of chronic monoarthritis of the large and medium weight-bearing joints, like hip and knee (29). Clinical manifestations are in the form of pain and swelling of the involved joint along with restriction of movements. Constitutional symptoms in the form of fever and weight loss may also be present. Other joints like sacroiliac, shoulder, elbow, ankle, carpel and tarsal joints are less commonly involved. Polyarticular or oligoarticular involvement is uncommon. There may be a polyarticular involvement in a debilitated child or adult with a past history of TB or exposure to a TB patient (11). The presentation mimicking juvenile idiopathic arthritis has also been reported rarely (30). The soft tissue TB can present as tenosynovitis, bursitis, myositis or fasciitis. There may be a delay in diagnosis of these conditions when there is a resemblance to focal soft tissue inflammatory conditions (31).

Myositis is uncommon condition and the usual causative organism is *Staphylococcus aureus* (32). TB myositis is even rarer. Most of these patients have predisposing conditions for TB (33). The proposed mechanism of involvement is thought to be due to either a 'haematogenous' spread, 'contiguous' spread from the adjoining bone and soft tissue or 'iatrogenic' due to direct inoculation through contaminated instruments (33). Abnormalities on chest radiographs have been noted in up to half of these patients. Though rare, this has been reported to have significant mortality of around 14% with even higher mortality [30%] in patients with possible haematogenous route of infection (33).

Development of Tuberculosis during Treatment of Rheumatological Diseases

Many patients with active inflammatory rheumatological disorders receive various immunosuppressive drugs, making them susceptible to reactivation of TB. Though anti-TNF therapy and corticosteroids are most commonly incriminated agents, all patients who receive any immunosuppressive therapy affecting the cellular immunity should be considered at risk of reactivation of TB (34-36). Data from a large patient registry reported a TB incidence of more than 1000 per 100,000 patient years of exposure to TNF blockers. This rate was reported to be 6 cases per 100,000 in patients with RA before the widespread use of TNF blockers (35). Etanercept has been observed to be associated with relatively lower risk (34). Reactivation TB occurs most frequently 6-12 months after initiating the TNF blockers, and is usually in form of EPTB. Proper screening for latent TB infection [LTBI] in these patients results in decrease in active TB (37). Glucocorticoids also increase the risk of reactivation in patients with LTBI. Though the risk appears to be dose related, it occurs even in patients on low physiological dose of prednisolone 7.5 mg/day.

Effects of Anti-tuberculosis Drugs

Drugs used in TB treatment can produce various clinical conditions. Isoniazid and rifampicin may produce drug-induced lupus. These patients have anti-nuclear antibody [ANA] and anti-histone antibody positivity. The disease is generally mild and reverses after stopping the offending drug. Fluoroquinolones, especially ciprofloxacin and levofloxacin, have been associated with tendon rupture (36). This risk is higher in older individuals, and those on corticosteroids. Pyrazinamide can cause hyperuricaemia due to interference with renal tubular excretion but rarely results in gout (36).

Reactive Phenomenon [Poncet's Disease]

Poncet's disease is a form of inflammatory arthritis without any evidence of direct TB involvement of the joint in the presence of TB elsewhere in the body. This was described by Poncet in 1887 in patients with current or past history of EPTB (38). In the absence of any diagnostic criteria, other disease conditions have been included in this diagnosis, and this has led to controversy over this terminology. In the recently proposed diagnostic criteria (39), there are two essential, two major and three minor criteria. Based on these criteria, the diagnosis can be either definite, probable or possible [Table 20.1] (39).

The definite pathogenesis of Poncet's is uncertain but is similar to 'reactive arthritis' as a result of molecular mimicry between *Mtb* which is arthretogenic and the articular cartilage. A CD4+ T-cell response to mycobacterial antigens has been shown to play a role (40). Chronic synovitis resembling RA can be produced by injection of complete Freund's adjuvant [heat killed and desiccated *Mtb* in oil]. Arthritis has also been reported as a side-effect

Table 20.1: Diagnostic criteria for Poncet's arthritis*

Essential criteria
  Inflammatory, non-erosive, non-deforming arthritis
  Exclusion of other causes of inflammatory arthritis
Major criteria
  Concurrent diagnosis of extra-articular TB
  Complete response to anti-TB therapy
Minor criteria
Mantoux positivity
  Presence of associated hypersensitivity phenomenon, such as,
  erythema nodosum, tuberculids or
Phlyctenular keratoconjuctivitis
Absence of sacroiliac and axial involvement

* When both essential and two major criteria are present, the diagnosis is "definite". In addition to both the essential criteria if one major and two minor criteria are present, the diagnosis is "probable". In addition to both the essential criteria, if either one major criterion and two minor criteria are present or three minor criteria are present, the diagnosis is "possible"
TB = tuberculosis
Source: reference 39

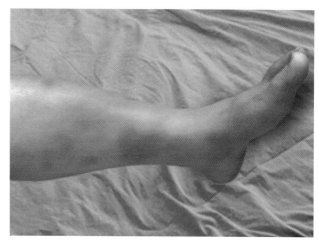

Figure 20.1: Clinical photograph showing erythema nodosum on the left shin

of the bacille Calmette-Guérin [BCG] immunotherapy in patients with urinary bladder carcinoma. The description of clinical presentations of Poncet's disease in the literature is derived from small case series and case reports (41-48). Poncet's disease is more common in juvenile and young adults. Female predilection has been osberved. Fever and constitutional symptoms may be observed in some patients. The pattern of joint involvement commonly described includes an acute or subacute symmetrical polyarthritis predominantly involving the large joints, like knees and ankles. Symmetrical small joint involvement resembling RA has also been reported occasionally. The most common site of TB in Poncet's disease is pulmonary TB; among extrapulmonary sites, lymph node TB is the most frequent site (11). Erythema nodosum [EN] was present in 6% of patients in one series (42). TB may sometimes develop during the course of Poncet's disease (47). Tuberculin skin test is usually strongly positive except in disseminated TB. Poncet's disease is a diagnosis of exclusion and there is no evidence of active TB of the joint. It resolves completely with anti-TB treatment.

Panniculitis Associated with Tuberculosis

Panniculitis is a non-suppurative inflammation of the subcutaneous fat without vasculitis. EN, a form of septal panniculitis, is the most common type of panniculitis seen in TB (49,50). EN is due to delayed type of hypersensitivity reaction to variety of antigens. These several known causes of EN like infections [bacterial, mycobacterial and fungal], drugs [especially sulphonamides and oral contraceptive pills], inflammatory bowel disease and various rheumatological conditions like Behcet's disease and sarcoidosis. This may be associated with fever and constitutional symptoms in the eruptive stage. Arthralgias or arthritis may be seen in up to half of these patients. The characteristic presentation is in the form of erythematous tender nodules over the shins [Figure 20.1], which are palpable and often tender. There is

induration of the overlying skin. Occasionally, it may be in the form of a sheet-like indurated, hyper-pigmented swelling over the ankles and shin. Though any joint may be involved, but ankle, knee and wrist are the most commonly involved joints (49,50).

Erythema induratum [EI] of Bazin type is a lobular panniculitis and has a similar presentation in the form of tender erythematous nodules (51-53). EI has clinicopathological similarity to nodular vasculitis. However, while EI occurs exclusively due to TB, nodular vasculitis can occur due to causes other than TB also. These are more commonly seen on the calves of young or middle-aged females; shin can also be involved occasionally. The other sites of involvement are trunk, buttocks, thighs and arms. Unlike EN, which heals without scarring, EI heals with ulceration or depressed scars. This can also be associated with ankle arthritis. Tuberculids are result of immunologic reactions to antigenic components of *Mtb* (51). Histopathology and polymerase chain reaction [PCR] may confirm TB in some of these patients and these respond to anti-TB treatment.

The reader is referred to the chapter *"Cutaneous tuberculosis"* [Chapter 21] for details.

UNUSUAL MANIFESTATIONS OF MUSCULOSKELETAL TUBERCULOSIS

Various types of very unusual manifestations of MSK-TB have been reported. Some of these include [i] non-healing ulcerated mass resembling a synovial sarcoma due to TB synovitis; [ii] trochanteric bursitis due to TB presenting with hip pain; [iii] sternoclavicular mass; [iv] bilateral sternoclavicular involvement; [v] involvement of great toe, lower end of fibula, midtarsal joints, and sternum [after sternotomy following bypass surgery] (54-59). Baker's cyst has also been reported due to TB (60).

MUSCULOSKELETAL DISEASES ASSOCIATED WITH NONTUBERCULOUS MYCOBACTERIA

Musculoskeletal involvement due to nontuberculous mycobacteria [NTM] is uncommon. *Mycobacterium kansasii* is the most common NTM species to cause MSK involvement, though involvement due to other species like *Mycobacterium xenopi, Mycobacterium avium intracellulare, Mycobacterium chelonei, Mycobacterium fortuitum* has also been reported (61-66). Synovial sheath infection is more common than infection of the osseous tissue (13). Most of these patients have some predisposing conditions though it has been reported in an immunocompetent patient also (67). These infections have also been reported in a patient with a rheumatic disease, like SLE or Still's disease (68). Arthritis due to NTM has also been reported after exposure to contaminated marine life (69,70). The reader is referred to the chapter *"Nontuberculous mycobacterial infections" [Chapter 41]* for details.

DIAGNOSIS OF MUSCULOSKELETAL TUBERCULOSIS

A high index of suspicion is required for making the diagnosis of MSK-TB. Common MSK manifestations are spondylitis or chronic monoarthritis. The cornerstone of diagnosis is the microbiological or histopathological evidence of TB. Patients with risk factors for TB such as immunocompromised individuals, elderly, children, those on immunosuppressive drugs must undergo these investigations in an appropriate clinical setting.

Laboratory Investigations

Laboratory abnormalities like elevated erythrocyte sedimentation rate [ESR], C-reactive protein [CRP] level have been described in patients with MSK-TB. However, these changes are not specific to TB and are found in several other inflammatory conditions.

Imaging Studies

Imaging in patients with skeletal TB is covered in detail in the chapter *"Skeletal tuberculosis" [Chapter 19]*. Certain additional features related to imaging in MSK-TB are described here. The plain radiograph of knee joint and pelvis may reveal bone destruction [Figures 20.2, 20.3 and 20.4] suggestive of MSK-TB. Among the various available imaging techniques, computed tomography [CT] is superior in depicting the degree of bony destruction and facilitating image-guided biopsy for spinal TB. On the other hand, for detailed anatomical evaluation and for distinguishing different densities of tissues [fibrous tissue, abscess, meninges, spinal cord etc.], magnetic resonance imaging [MRI] with contrast [Figures 20.5 and 20.6] is considered superior (71). The characteristic *Phemister's triad* is considered to be typical of TB. Three components of the *Phemister's triad* are [i] juxta-articular osteoporosis; [ii] peripherally located osseous erosions; and [iii] gradual narrowing of the joint space (72-75). On the other hand, in the course of RA and pyogenic arthritis, the joint space narrowing occurs early. For soft tissue TB, the ultrasonography is the method of choice as it shows the extent and degree of involvement. On the other hand, the MRI shows the extent of soft tissue, osseous and joint involvement (74). One of the other typical features

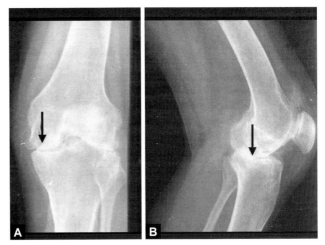

Figure 20.2: Radiograph of the knee joint [antero-posterior view] [A], [lateral view] [B], showing symmetrical decreased joint space in tibio-femoral joint with erosions [arrow]

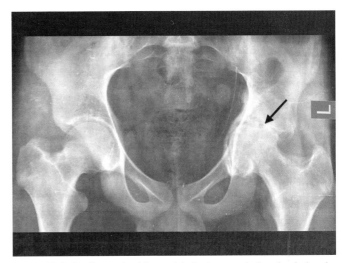

Figure 20.3: Radiograph of the pelvis [antero-posterior view] showing erosions in femoral head and acetabulum with decreased joint space in the left hip joint [arrow]

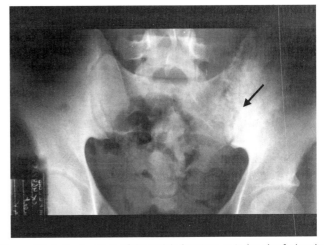

Figure 20.4: Radiograph of the pelvis [postero-anterior view] showing decreased joint space with irregularity of left sacroiliac joint with minimal subchondral sclerosis [arrow]

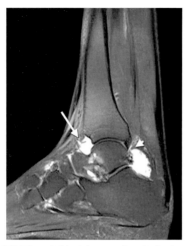

Figure 20.5: MRI T2-weighted image, [sagittal view] of ankle joint showing nodular synovitis in tibio-talar joint [arrow] with marrow oedema in talus [arrow-head]
MRI = magnetic resonance imaging

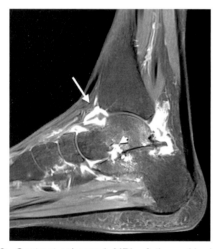

Figure 20.6: Contrast-enhanced MRI of the ankle joint showing thickening and enhancement of synovium in tibio-talar and subtalar joints [arrow] with irregularity of articular surface [arrow-head]
MRI = magnetic resonance imaging

of TB of the bones that have a relatively superficial cortical surface [e.g., metacarpals, metatarsals, phalanges, tibia and ulna] is the presence of lytic lesions surrounded by reactive subperiosteal new bone formation (13). Positron emission tomography-computed tomography [PET-CT] has been used in the diagnosis of joint involvement in TB (76). With PET-CT, an increased [18]fluorodeoxyglucose [FDG] uptake in regions of active granulomatous inflammation and cold areas in necrosed tissue containing pus has been reported (76). It needs to be emphasised that despite these advances, the 'gold standard' for the diagnosis of TB of the MSK system requires histopathological, microbiological and/or molecular confirmation.

Tuberculin Skin Test

Tuberculin skin test [TST] detects infection with *Mtb* and is a marker of LTBI. Since the purified protein derivative

[PPD] used for TST contains various *Mtb* antigens which are similar to antigens of BCG and NTM, TST may also be positive in BCG-vaccinated or NTM infected individuals. Interferon-gamma release assays [IGRAs] like QuantiFERON TB gold® and T-SPOT.TB® are also used to diagnose LTBI. The reader is referred to the chapter *"Laboratory diagnosis"* [Chapter 8] for details.

Arthrocentesis, Synovial Biopsy

Synovial fluid aspiration and synovial biopsy are required for establishing diagnosis of TB arthritis. The issues concerning procurement of adequate tissue for histopathological diagnosis of skeletal TB are discussed in the chapter *"Skeletal tuberculosis"[Chapter 19]*. The indications for a synovial biopsy in patients with MSK-TB from a rheumatologist's perspective is discussed below.

When clinical evaluation and routine investigations fail to provide a diagnosis synovial biopsy is the logical next step. It is usually the only definitive method of diagnosing infection with fastidious organisms including TB. An absolute indication for synovial biopsy is a chronic inflammatory monoarthritis where synovial fluid examination including microbiological studies may have failed to give a definitive diagnosis. Another strong indication for synovial biopsy would be a patient with persistent disease activity in a single joint.

Mycobacterial Culture, Molecular Diagnostic Methods

Conventional culture of fluid/tissue specimens on Lowenstein-Jensen [LJ] medium takes a longer time [4-8 weeks]. Newer liquid culture methods like BACTEC have reduced the isolation time to two weeks. Molecular diagnostic techniques yield faster results. Polymerase chain reaction [PCR] has been shown used for the diagnosis of various EPTB conditions including osteoarticular TB; and even for diagnosis of NTM infections like *Mycobacterium avium* (77). The recently available molecular diagnostic method, Xpert MTB/RIF® is an automated cartridge-based nucleic acid amplification test [CBNAAT] which is helpful in detecting *Mtb* and identifying rifampicin resistance in 90 minutes. It has enormously contributed to the diagnosis of EPTB (78). A recently published systemic review reported good specificity for Xpert MTB/RIF® in the diagnosis of various forms of EPTB (79). The recent World Health Organization [WHO] policy recommendation states that "Xpert MTB/RIF may be used as a replacement test for usual practice [including conventional microscopy, culture or histopathology] for testing specific non-respiratory specimens [lymph nodes and other tissues] from patients suspected of having EPTB [conditional recommendation, very low-quality evidence]" (80).

TREATMENT

Treatment of MSK-TB consists of administration of standard anti-TB treatment (81-84). The reader is referred to the chapters *"Treatment of tuberculosis"* [Chapter 44], *Revised National Tuberculosis Control Programme"* [Chapter 53] for details.

As per the recently published evidence-based Guidelines for Extrapulmonary TB for India [INDEX-TB Guidelines] (84), extended course of anti-TB treatment with a two-month intensive phase consisting of four drugs [isoniazid, rifampicin, pyrazinamide, ethambutol], followed by a continuation phase consisting of isoniazid, rifampicin and ethambutol lasting 10-16 months, depending on the site of disease and the patient's clinical course has been advocated for patients with skeletal TB.

REFERENCES

1. Sharma SK, Mohan A. Extrapulmonary tuberculosis. Indian J Med Res 2004;120:316-53.
2. Huebner RE, Castro KG. The changing face of tuberculosis. Annu Rev Med 1995;46:47–55.
3. US Department of Health and Human Services. Centers for Disease Control and Prevention. Reported tuberculosis in the United States, 2006. Atlanta: US Department of Health and Human Services. Centers for Disease Control and Prevention; 2007.
4. Iseman MD. A clinician's guide to tuberculosis. Philadelphia: Lippincott Williams & Wilkins; 2000.
5. Communicable Disease Center. Reported tuberculosis data, 1962. Atlanta: US Department of Health, Education, and Welfare; 1962.p.638.
6. Petror HR, Pratt HR, Herrington TA, LoBue PA, Armtrong LA. Epidemiology of extrapulmonary tuberculosis in the United States, 1993-2006. Clin Infect Dis 2009;49:1350-7.
7. Chakraborty AK. Epidemiology. In: Sharma SK, Mohan A, editors. Tuberculosis. New Delhi: Jaypee Brothers Medical Publishers; 2001.p.16-54.
8. Tuli SM. Tuberculosis of the skeletal system. New Delhi: Jaypee Brothers Medical Publishers; 1997.
9. Mahowald ML. Arthritis due to mycobacteria, fungi and parasites. In: Koopman WJ, editor. Arthritis and allied conditions. Fourteenth edition. Philadelphia: Lippincott Williams & Wilkins; 2000.
10. Kumar A, Malaviya AN. Musculoskeletal manifestations of tuberculosis. In: Sharma SK, Mohan A. New Delhi: Jaypee Brothers Medical Publishers; 2001.p.372-82.
11. Malaviya AN, Kotwal PP. Arthritis associated with tuberculosis. Best Pract Res Clin Rheumatol 2003;17:319-43.
12. Marquez J, Espinoza LR. Mycobacterial, brucella, fungal and parasitic arthritis. In: Hochberg MC, Silman AJ, Smolen JS, Weinblatt ME, Weisman MH, editors. Rheumatology. Philadelphia: Mosby Elsevier; 2011.p.1067-78.
13. Tuli SM. General principles of joint and bone tuberculosis. Clin Orthop Relat Res 2002;398:11-9.
14. Stein CM. Genetic epidemiology of tuberculosis susceptibility: impact of study design. PLoS Pathogens 2011;7:e1001189.
15. Li X, Yang Y, Zhou F, Zhang Y, Lu H, Jin Q, et al. SLC11A1 [NRAMP1] polymorphisms and tuberculosis susceptibility: updated systematic review and meta-analysis. PLoS One 2011;6:e15831.
16. Davies P, Grange J. The genetics of host resistance and susceptibility to tuberculosis. Ann NY Acad Sci 2001;953:151-6.
17. Puttick MP, Stein HB, Chan RM, Elwood RK, How AR, Reid GD. Soft tissue tuberculosis: a series of 11cases. J Rheumatol 1995;22:1321-5.
18. Jellis JE. Human immunodeficiency virus and joint and bone tuberculosis. Clin Orthop Relat Res 2002;398:27-31.
19. Courtman NH, Weighill FJ. Systemic tuberculosis in association with intra-articular steroid therapy. JR Coll Surg Edinb 1992;37:425.
20. Fukasawa H, Suzuki H, Kato A, Yamamoto T, Fujigaki Y, Yonemura K, et al. Tuberculous arthritis mimicking neoplasm in a hemodialysis patient. Am J Med Sci 2001;322:373-5.
21. Binymin K, Cooper RG. Late reactivation of spinal tuberculosis by low-dose methotrexate therapy in a patient with rheumatoid arthritis. Rheumatology [Oxford)] 2001;40:341-2.
22. Keane J, Gershon S, Wise RP, Mirabile-Levens E, Kasznica J, Schwieterman WD, et al. Tuberculosis associated with infliximab, a tumor necrosis factor alpha-neutralizing agent. New Engl J Med 2001;345:1098-104.
23. Hernández-Cruz B, Sifuentes-Osornio J, Ponce-de-León Rosales S, Ponce-de-León Garduño A, Díaz-Jouanen E. Mycobacterium tuberculosis infection in patients with systemic rheumatic diseases. A case-series. Clin Exp Rheumatol 1999;17:289-96.
24. Yun JE, Lee SW, Kim TH, Jun JB, Jung S, Bae SC, et al. The incidence and clinical characteristics of Mycobacterium tuberculosis infection among systemic lupus erythematosus and rheumatoid arthritis patients in Korea. Clin Exp Rheumatol 2002;20:127-32.
25. Chen YC, Hsu SW. Tuberculous arthritis mimics arthritis of the Sjogren's syndrome: findings from sonography, computed tomography and magnetic resonance images. Eur J Radiol 2001;40:232-5.
26. Lorenzo JP, Csuka ME, Derfus BA, Gotoff RA, McCarthy GM. Concurrent gout and Mycobacterium tuberculosis arthritis. J Rheumatol 1997;24:184-6.
27. Berbari EF, Hanssen AD, Duffy MC, Steckelberg JM, Osmon DR. Prosthetic joint infection due to Mycobacterium tuberculosis: a case series and review of the literature. Am J Orthop [Belle Mead NJ]. 1998;27:219-27.
28. Franco-Pardes C, Diaz-Borjon A, Senger M, Barragan L, Leonard M. The ever-expanding association of rheumatologic diseases and tuberculosis. Am J Med 2006;119:470-7.
29. Kosinski MA, Smith LC. Osteoarticular tuberculosis. Clin Podiatr Med Surg 1996;13:725-39.
30. Sawhney S, Murray KJ. Isolated tuberculosis monoarthritis mimicking juvenile rheumatoid arthritis. J Rheumatol 2002;29:857-9.
31. Chen WS, Eng HL. Tuberculous tenosynovitis of the wrist mimicking de Quervains's disease. J Rheumatol 1994;21:763-5.
32. Sharma A, Kumar S, Wanchu A, Sharma K, Sharma N, Singh R, et al. Clinical characteristics and predictors of mortality in 67 patients with primary pyomyositis: a study from North India. Clin Rheumatol 2010;29:45-51.
33. Wang JY, Lee LN, Hsueh PR, Shih JY, Chang YL, Yang PC, et al. Tuberculous myositis: a rare but existing clinical entity. Rheumatology 2003;42:836-40.
34. Mohan AK, Coté TR, Block JA, Manadan AM, Siegel JN, Braun MM. Tuberculosis following use of etanercept, a tumour necrosis factor inhibitor. Clin Infect Dis 2004;39:295.
35. Gómez-Reino JJ, Carmona L, Valverde VR, Mola EM, Montero MD; BIOBADASER Group. Treatment of rheumatoid arthritis with tumor necrosis factor inhibitors may predispose to significant increase in tuberculosis risk: a multicenter active-surveillance report. Arthritis Rheum 2003;48:2122-7.
36. Ruderman EM, Flaherty JP. Mycobacterial infections of bone and joints. In: Firestein G, Budd RC, Gabriel SE, McInnes IB, O'Dell JR, editors. Kelley's textbook of rheumatology. Ninth edition. Philadelphia: WB Saunders; 2013.p.1829-40.
37. Malaviya AN, Kapoor S, Garg S, Rawat R, Shankar S, Nagpal S, et al. Preventing tuberculosis flare in patients with inflammatory rheumatic diseases receiving tumor necrosis factor-α inhibitors in India—an audit report. J Rheumatol 2009;36:1414-20.
38. Poncet A. De La polyarthrite tuberculeuse deformante ou pseudorheumatisme chronique tuberculeux. Congres Francaise de Chirurgie 1887;1:732-9.

39. Sharma A, Pinto B, Dogra S, Sharma K, Goyal P, Sagar V, et al. A case series and review of Poncet's disease, and the utility of current diagnostic criteria. Int J Rheum Dis 2016;19:1010-7.

40. Smith-Rohrberg D, Sharma SK. Tuberculin skin test among pulmonary sarcoidosis patients with and without tuberculosis: its utility for the screening of the two conditions in tuberculosis-endemic regions. Sarcoidosis Vasc Diffuse Lung Dis 2006;23: 130-4.

41. Bhargava AD, Malaviya AN, Kumar A. Tuberculous rheumatism [Poncet's disease]: a case series. Indian J Tuberc 1998;45:215-9.

42. Kroot EJ, Hazes JM, Colin EM, Dolhain RJ. Poncet's disease: reactive arthritis accompanying tuberculosis. Two case reports and a review of the literature. Rheumatology [Oxford] 2007;46: 484-9.

43. Hansen SE, Wallenquist A. A case of chronic polyarthritis with debut in 1771: rheumatoid arthritis or Poncet's disease? Scand J Rheumatol 2007;36:322-4.

44. Ozgul A, Baylan O, Taskaynatan MA, Kalyon TA. Poncet's disease [tuberculous rheumatism]: two case reports and review of the literature. Int J Tuberc Lung Dis 2005;9:822-4.

45. Kawsar M, D'Cruz D, Nathan M, Murphy M. Poncet's disease in a patient with AIDS. Rheumatology [Oxford] 2001;40:346-7.

46. Kumar A. Rheumatic manifestations of tuberculosis. In: Sharma SK, editor. Tuberculosis. First edition. New Delhi: Jaypee Brothers Medical Publishers; 2001.p.593-6.

47. Sood R, Wali JP, Handa R. Poncet's disease in a north Indian hospital. Trop Doct 1999;29:33-6.

48. Garg S, Malaviya AN, Kapoor S, Rawat R, Agarwal D, Sharma A. Acute inflammatory ankle arthritis in northern India—Löfgren's syndrome or Poncet's disease? J Assoc Physicians India 2011;59:87-90.

49. Truong LN, O'Connell R, Oren A. A 49-year-old man with fever, erythema nodosum, and ankle swelling. final diagnosis: extrapulmonary tuberculosis with hepatic and bone marrow involvement. Ann Am Thorac Soc 2015;12:1575-7.

50. Chen S, Chen J, Chen L, Zhang Q, Luo X, Zhang W. Mycobacterium tuberculosis infection is associated with the development of erythema nodosum and nodular vasculitis. PLoS One 2013;8:e62653.

51. Hallensleben ND, de Vries HJ, Lettinga KD, Scherpbier HJ. Tuberculids: cutaneous indicator diseases of Mycobacterium tuberculosis infection in young patients. J Eur Acad Dermatol Venereol 2016;30:1590-3.

52. von Huth S, Øvrehus AL, Lindahl KH, Johansen IS. Two cases of erythema induratum of Bazin—a rare cutaneous manifestation of tuberculosis. Int J Infect Dis 2015;38:121-4.

53. Ribeiro R, Patrício C, Silva FP, Silva PE. Erythema induratum of Bazin and Ponçet's arthropathy as epiphenomena of hepatic tuberculosis. BMJ Case Rep 2016;2016. pii: bcr2015213585.

54. Ayhan S, Ozmen S, Uluoğlu O, Demirtaş Y, Boyacioglu M, Latifoğlu O, et al. Nonhealing ulcerative mass of the elbow: do not forget tuberculosis. Ann Plast Surg 2002;48:557-61.

55. Perez C, Rojas A, Baudrand R, Gonzalez S, Fontbote C. Tuberculosis bursitis: report of case. Rev Med Chil 2002;130: 319-21.

56. Dhillon MS, Gupta R, Rao KS, Nagi ON. Bilateral sternoclavicular joint tuberculosis. Arch Orthop Trauma Surg 2000;120:363-5.

57. Garcia-Porrua C, Gonzalez-Gay MA, Sanchez-Andrade A, Vazquez-Caruncho M. Arthritis in the right great toe as the clinical presentation of tuberculosis. Arthritis Rheum 1998;41: 374-5.

58. Malhan K, Kumar A, Sherman KP. Use of polymerase chain reaction in diagnosis of occult tuberculosis of the fibula. Acta Orthop Belg 2001;67:510-2.

59. Ong Y, Cheong PY, Low YP, Chong PY. Delayed diagnosis of tuberculosis presenting as small joint arthritis - a case report. Singapore Med J 1998;39:177-9.

60. Bianco G, Paris A, Venditti M, Calderini C, Anzivino C, Serra P. Popliteal [Baker's] cyst in a patient with tubercular arthritis. Report of a case and review of the literature. Recenti Prog Med 2001;92:663-6.

61. Libbrecht E, Bressieux JM, Chelius P, Roger M, Eloy C, Rezzouk L, et al. Mycobacterium xenopi osteoarthritis of the ankle in a patient followed for psoriatic rheumatism. Presse Med 2000;29:539-40.

62. Yuen K, Fam AG, Simor A. Mycobacterium xenopi arthritis. J Rheumatol 1998;25:1016-8.

63. Thariat J, Leveque L, Tavernier C, Maillefert JF. Mycobacterium marinum tenosynovitis in a patient with Still's disease. Rheumatology [Oxford] 2001;40:1419-20.

64. Ekerot L, Jacobsson L, Forsgren A. Mycobacterium marinum wrist arthritis: local and systematic dissemination caused by concomitant immunosuppressive therapy. Scand J Infect Dis 1998;30:84-7.

65. Toussirot E, Chevrolet A, Wendling D. Tenosynovitis due to Mycobacterium avium intracellulare and Mycobacterium chelonei: report of two cases with review of the literature. Clin Rheumatol 1998;17:152-6.

66. Badelon O, David H, Meyer L, Radault A, Zucman J. Mycobacterium fortuitum infection after total hip prosthesis. A report of 3 cases. Rev Chir Orthop Reparatrice Appar Mot 1979;65:39-43.

67. Frosch M, Roth J, Ullrich K, Harms E. Successful treatment of Mycobacterium avium osteomyelitis and arthritis in a non-immunocompromised child. Scand J Infect Dis 2000;32: 328-9.

68. Nakamura T, Yamamura Y, Tsuruta T, Tomoda K, Sakaguchi M, Tsukano M, et al. Mycobacterium kansasii arthritis of the foot in a patient with systemic lupus erythematosus. Intern Med 2001;40:1045-9.

69. Barton A, Bernstein RM, Struthers JK, O'Neill TW. Mycobacterium marinum infection causing septic arthritis and osteomyelitis. Br J Rheumatol 1997;36:1207-9.

70. Alloway JA, Evangelisti SM, Sartin JS. Mycobacterium marinum arthritis. Semin Arthritis Rheum 1995;24:382-90.

71. De Backer AI, Mortele KJ, Vanhoenacker FM, Parizel PM. Imaging of extraspinal musculoskeletal tuberculosis. Eur J Radiol 2006;57:119-30.

72. Prakash M, Gupta P, Sen RK, Sharma A, Khandelwal N. Magnetic resonance imaging evaluation of tubercular arthritis of the ankle and foot. Acta Radiol 2015;56:1236-41.

73. Engin G, Acunas B, Acunas G, Tunaci M. Imaging of extrapulmonary tuberculosis. Radiographics 2000;20:471-88.

74. Harisinghani MG, McLoud TC, Shepard JA, Ko JP, Shroff MM, Mueller PR. Tuberculosis from head to toe. Radiographics 2000; 20:449-70.

75. Sequeira W, Co H, Block JA. Osteoarticular tuberculosis: current diagnosis and treatment. Am J Ther 2000;7:393-8.

76. D'Souza MM, Sharma R, Tripathi M, Mondalpus A. F-18 Fluorodeoxyglucose positron emission tomography/computed tomography in tuberculosis of the hip: a case report and brief review of literature. Indian J Nucl Med 2011;26:31-3.

77. Sharma K, Sharma A, Sharma SK, Sen RK, Dhillon MS, Sharma M. Does multiplex polymerase chain reaction increase the diagnostic percentage in osteoarticular tuberculosis? A prospective evaluation of 80 cases. Int Orthop 2012;36:255-9.

78. Sharma SK, Kohli M, Chaubey J, Yadav RN, Sharma R, Singh BK, et al. Evaluation of Xpert MTB/RIF assay performance

in diagnosing extrapulmonary tuberculosis among adults in a tertiary care centre in India. Eur Respir J 2014;44: 1090-3.

79. Kohli M, Schiller I, Dendukuri N, Dheda K, Denkinger CM, Schumacher SG, Steingart KR. Xpert[®] MTB/RIF assay for extrapulmonary tuberculosis and rifampicin resistance. Cochrane Database Syst Rev 2018;8:CD012768.

80. World Health Organization. Automated real-time nucleic acid amplification technology for rapid and simultaneous detection of tuberculosis and rifampicin resistance: Xpert MTB/RIF assay for the diagnosis of pulmonary and extrapulmonary TB in adults and children: policy update. Geneva: World Health Organization; 2013.

81. Blumberg HM, Burman WJ, Chaisson RE, Daley CL, Etkind 216. SC, Friedman LN, et al. American Thoracic Society, Centers for Disease Control and Prevention and the Infectious Diseases Society. American Thoracic Society/Centers for Disease Control and Prevention/Infectious Diseases Society of America. Treatment of tuberculosis. Am J Respir Crit Care Med 2003;167:603-62.

82. World Health Organization. Treatment of tuberculosis. Guidelines. Fourth edition. WHO/HTM/TB/2009.420. Geneva: World Health Organization; 2010.

83. Central TB Division, Directorate General of Health Services, Government of India. Technical and Operational Guidelines for TB Control in India 2016. Available at URL: http://tbcindia. nic.in/index1.php?lang=1&level=2&sublinkid=4573&lid=3177. Accessed on May 20, 2018.

84. Sharma SK, Ryan H, Khaparde S, Sachdeva KS, Singh AD, Mohan A, et al. Index-TB guidelines: Guidelines on extra-pulmonary tuberculosis for India. Indian J Med Res 2017;145: 448-63.

21

Cutaneous Tuberculosis

M Ramam

INTRODUCTION

Cutaneous tuberculosis [TB] is an ancient disease. Cutaneous lesions of TB were described long before Robert Koch identified *Mycobacterium tuberculosis* [*Mtb*]. The first description of cutaneous TB is attributed to Laennec (1) in 1826 who described his own *Prosector's wart* that followed an injury sustained while performing an autopsy on a patient with spinal TB. *Mtb* was first demonstrated in tissue sections of lupus vulgaris by Demme (2) in 1883. In 1886, Reihl and Paltauf (3) established that the Prosector's wart was a TB lesion. *Apple-jelly nodules* in lupus vulgaris were first described in 1888 (4) and *tuberculids* in 1896 (5).

EPIDEMIOLOGY

World Scenario

Cutaneous TB appears to have been frequently encountered by dermatologists all around the world during the early part of this century and comprised 0.1%-2.6% of the total number of dermatology patients in various hospitals at different periods of time (6-22). Some workers had suggested that cutaneous TB was uncommon in the tropics and ascribed this difference to the abundant sunshine and consequent high levels of vitamin D in the skin (9,23). However, this view appears erroneous as evidenced by the numerous reports of cutaneous TB from India (24-36).

Indian Scenario

No systematic survey for the prevalence and incidence of cutaneous TB in the community appears to have been carried out in India. Information on the epidemiology of the disease is, therefore, based on hospital records and suffers from the usual drawbacks of such data. Cutaneous TB accounts for 0.11%-2.5% of all patients with skin diseases seen at hospitals located in different parts and this figure seems to be constant for all regions of the country (24-36). In a study from Vishakapatnam (24), cutaneous TB constituted 0.025% of all patients with TB and 15% of all patients with extra-pulmonary TB [EPTB]. One study (34) found that cutaneous TB was associated with TB in other organs in 22.1% of patients. The organs affected most commonly were lungs, followed by bones, the abdomen, central nervous system and the heart. Most studies reveal a male preponderance and a significant proportion of those affected are children (24-36). The disease is more common in the poor. In a study from Chandigarh (34), about 70% of the patients had developed the disease in spite of having been vaccinated with bacilli Calmette-Guérin [BCG]. Patients who had not been vaccinated were more likely to have TB in another organ than those who had received BCG vaccine (34).

CLINICAL FEATURES

Cutaneous TB presents in a variety of ways. The presentation is determined by the host immune response, the route of inoculation and the previous sensitisation of the host to the *Mtb*. The clinical varieties of cutaneous TB can be divided into three broad groups [Table 21.1].

Lupus vulgaris is the most common variety reported from India followed by scrofuloderma and TB verrucosa cutis. The other types are distinctly rare.

Tuberculosis Chancre

TB chancre develops at the site of inoculation of *Mtb* in a previously non-sensitised host. The bacillus enters the skin following minor wounds and abrasions. It may also gain entry following trauma, injections, circumcision and

Table 21.1: Clinical varieties of cutaneous TB

Lesions developing in those not previously exposed to
Mycobacterium tuberculosis
  TB chancre
  Acute miliary TB of the skin
Lesions developing in previously sensitised hosts
  Lupus vulgaris
  Scrofuloderma
  TB verrucosa cutis
Tuberculids
  Lichen scrofulosorum
  Papulonecrotic tuberculids
  Erythema induratum

TB = tuberculosis

ear piercing. A non-descript papule or nodule develops at the site followed by crusting and ulceration. Spontaneous healing may occur but lesions usually proceed to lupus vulgaris. The regional lymph nodes are enlarged and may break down to form a discharging sinus in three to six months. Acid-fast bacilli [AFB] can be demonstrated and grown from early lesions. Skin biopsy reveals necrosis, infiltration by neutrophils and numerous AFB in early lesions. Later, epithelioid cell granulomas develop, accompanied by the disappearance of bacilli from the lesion.

Acute Miliary Tuberculosis of the Skin

Miliary TB develops following the haematogenous dissemination of *Mtb* (37). It may follow measles or other viral exanthems (38). The skin lesions of miliary TB present as pustules, vesicles and papules that have a non-specific appearance and lack any diagnostic features [Figure 21.1]. Constitutional symptoms are usually severe and the patient is often gravely ill. The diagnosis may be suspected if the patient is known to have TB in another system. *Mtb* can be demonstrated in the lesions.

Lupus Vulgaris

Lupus vulgaris is probably the common manifestation of cutaneous TB. Classically, it presents as an indolent, asymptomatic, gradually progressive, firm plaque with central clearing and peripheral activity [Figure 21.2]. In some cases, the progressing border of the plaque reveals translucent, erythematous papules that show a residual yellowish brown colour when blanched with a glass slide, the so-called *"apple-jelly nodules"*. Though this term is associated with lupus vulgaris, it may be seen in other granulomatous diseases including sarcoidosis and leprosy. Further, apple-jelly nodules are often obscured by the hyperkeratosis and crusting of lupus vulgaris. Thus, this is not a particularly useful sign. As the lesion progresses, there is central healing with scarring while the periphery continues to spread [Figure 21.3]. The lesion may be atrophic or may show varying degrees of hyperkeratosis that may be severe enough to produce cutaneous horns. The lesion is usually dry but may occasionally be accompanied by a

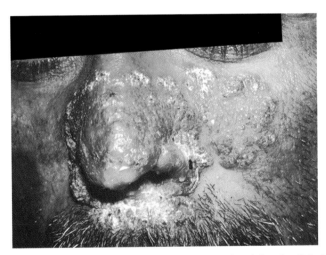

Figure 21.2: Lupus vulgaris. Central scarring and peripheral activity in a long-standing lesion

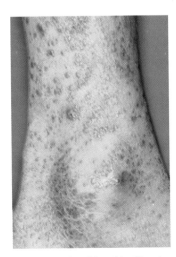

Figure 21.1: Miliary tuberculosis of the skin. Chest radiograph revelaed miliary lesions. Polymerase chain reaction from skin lesions detected mycobacterial deoxyribonucleic acid

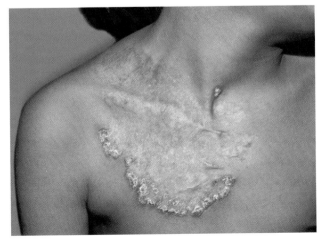

Figure 21.3: Lupus vulgaris. Annular plaque with erythematous and scaly papules at the periphery and a relatively clear centre

thin sero-purulent discharge and moist crusts. Lesions may reach enormous sizes over the years and cause considerable damage and mutilation. Squamous cell carcinoma has been described to complicate long-standing lesions (39). The classical site of lesion is the face but it is seen at least as commonly on the buttocks [Figure 21.4] and lower limbs in Indian patients. The lesion is usually single but less commonly, multiple lesions may develop in one anatomic area or may be scattered over the skin surface. Rarely, symmetrical lesions may develop. Lupus vulgaris may develop at the site of cutaneous extension of TB from an underlying focus. It has also been reported as a rare complication of BCG vaccination (40,41) [Figure 21.5]. The regional lymph nodes may be slightly enlarged but do not show any evidence of TB. In some patients, the presence of broad, atrophic scarring indicating the possibility of a previous TB infection of the regional lymph nodes may be noted [Figure 21.6]. Less commonly, the regional lymph nodes draining a lesion of lupus vulgaris may show active scrofuloderma. Most patients with lupus vulgaris are well-preserved and do not have constitutional symptoms even when lesions are extensive and multiple. The tuberculin skin test [TST] is positive in many but not all patients. Skin biopsy reveals epithelioid cell granulomas in the upper dermis abutting the epidermis which is usually thickened and hyperkeratotic. The granulomas may show necrosis though this is not a common finding. AFB cannot, as a rule, be demonstrated on sections. Culture of the biopsy material is not rewarding.

Tuberculosis Verrucosa Cutis

TB verrucosa cutis, probably a variant of lupus vulgaris, is characterised by a striking degree of hyperkeratosis in the lesions. The lesion usually develops over the acral parts of the extremities as a gradually progressive indurated plaque with a rough, horny surface but may also develop at non-acral sites [Figures 21.7 and 21.8]. With time, the lesions become progressively larger and hyperkeratotic and may involve the entire foot [Figure 21.9]. Multiple lesions are

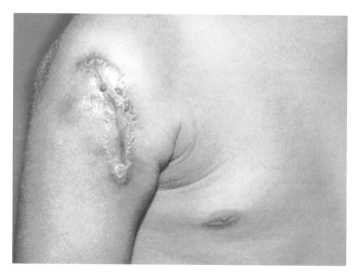

Figure 21.5: Lupus vulgaris following vaccination with BCG
BCG = bacille Calmette-Guérin

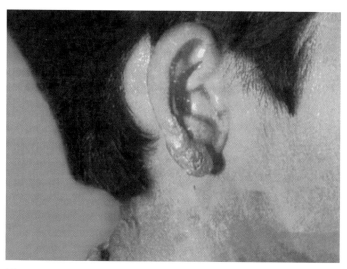

Figure 21.6: Lupus vulgaris of the ear lobe. Note scars of healed scrofuloderma on the neck

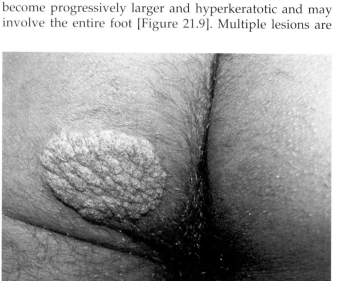

Figure 21.4: Lupus vulgaris. The buttocks are a common site

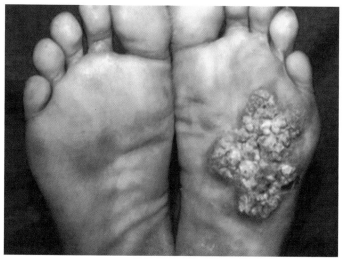

Figure 21.7: Tuberculosis verrucosa cutis. The sole is often affected

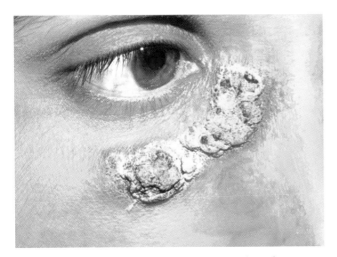

Figure 21.8: Indurated plaque with a horny, keratotic surface

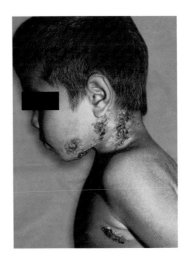

Figure 21.10: Scrofuloderma overlying tuberculosis of the cervical and axillary lymph nodes

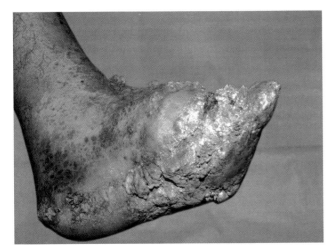

Figure 21.9: Tuberculosis verrucosa cutis. Advanced disease with the entire foot appearing to be encased in a keratotic boot

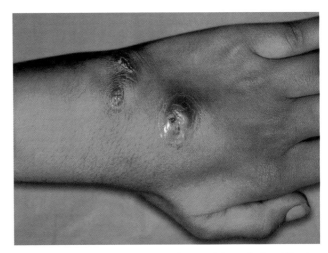

Figure 21.11: Scrofuloderma secondary to tuberculosis of the bone. Note the thickened metacarpals underlying the sinus on the dorsum of the hand

unusual and lymph nodes show changes similar to those seen in lupus vulgaris. Constitutional signs are usually absent. The TST is often positive. Skin biopsies must be taken carefully from the least keratotic area and incised deep enough to include the underlying indurated plaque, else, only thickened stratum corneum will be seen. An adequate biopsy reveals an enormously thickened epidermis with small epithelioid granulomas amidst a lichenoid infiltrate of lymphocytes and plasma cells in the upper dermis. Necrosis is absent and AFB cannot usually be demonstrated or grown from biopsy material.

Scrofuloderma

Scrofuloderma is the term applied to lesions that develop in the skin from contiguous spread or extension of TB from an underlying or adjacent structure. Most often, the primary focus is in the lymph nodes [Figure 21.10] but bones [Figure 21.11] and joints may also be the source of infection. The cutaneous lesion is a sinus or a crusted ulcer discharging thin, seropurulent material. The edge of the sinus usually shows a purple discolouration, is thinned and may be eroded. The sinus is usually attached to the underlying structure. Crusts are present and may be large. Some patients show episodic activity in lesions with the amount of discharge showing periodic variations and even drying up completely to recur after varying periods of time extending up to several months. In long-standing lesions, there are usually broad atrophic scars that represent spontaneously healed sinuses. Scarring and fibrosis of lymph nodes may lead to lymphoedema and elephantiasis [Figure 21.12]. In contrast to filariasis, the skin of the lymphoedematous area often shows lesions of cutaneous TB, usually lupus vulgaris [Figure 21.13]. AFB may be demonstrated in the discharge from lesions and *Mtb*, and rarely nontuberculous mycobacteria [NTM] such as *Mycobacterium avium complex, Mycobacterium scrofulaceum* can also be cultured. Fine needle aspiration cytology [FNAC] of the underlying structure, usually lymph node, confirms the diagnosis of TB. Biopsy from the edge of the sinus reveals a mixed cell granuloma consisting of epithelioid cells and histiocytes admixed with neutrophils and eosinophils. There are areas of necrosis and AFB may be identified in the biopsy. Culture of biopsy material grows *Mtb* or NTM in some patients.

Tuberculosis Gumma

TB gumma refers to soft, subcutaneous swellings which often break through the overlying skin to produce ulcers [Figure 21.14]. The lesions resemble scrofuloderma on clinical, histopathological and microbiological grounds and can be considered as a variant produced by haematogenous seeding of subcutaneous tissue with *Mtb*.

Tuberculosis Cutis Orificialis

TB cutis orificialis develops by the inoculation of *Mtb* derived from visceral infection into the skin around the draining

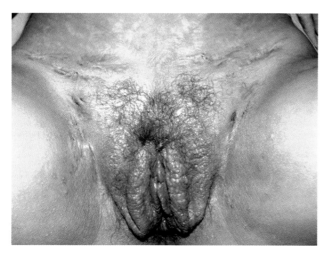

Figure 21.12: Esthiomene secondary to healed scrofuloderma of the inguinal and external iliac lymph nodes. Note the scars in the area of both inguinal ligaments

orifices. Usually lesions develop around the perianal area [Figure 21.15] or around the mouth in patients with abdominal or pulmonary TB. The lesion is a nodule that breaks down to form an indolent, deep ulcer. The diagnosis is usually suspected when the ulcer does not heal in spite of antibiotic therapy. Biopsy from the edge of the ulcer reveals epithelioid granulomas. AFB may occasionally be demonstrated or grown from the lesion.

Tuberculids

Tuberculids are skin lesions that develop as a hypersensitivity response to the presence of a TB focus elsewhere in the body. The following criteria must be fulfilled to designate a condition as tuberculid: [i] the skin lesion must show a tuberculoid histopathology; [ii] *Mtb* must not be demonstrable in the lesion; [iii] the TST must be strongly positive; and [iv] treatment of the underlying TB focus must lead to resolution of the skin lesions. In some cases, it is easy to document the focus; while in others, this may not be possible. In clinical practice, physical examination and simple imaging procedures are undertaken to look for TB elsewhere. If these tests fail to reveal a focus and clinical suspicion of a tuberculid is high, presumptive treatment for TB is administered.

Since *Mtb* cannot be demonstrated in tuberculids, there has been considerable controversy over the existence of this entity. Historically, the label was applied to all skin conditions that showed a tuberculoid granuloma on histopathology including some conditions subsequently found to be unrelated to TB. It was hypothesised that such skin lesions represented a hypersensitivity response to a manifest or occult TB focus elsewhere in the body. This led to the grouping together of a heterogeneous group of conditions that were subsequently shown to share no aetiologic or pathogenetic similarity. Presently, three conditions are unequivocally accepted as tuberculids: lichen scrofulosorum, papulonecrotic tuberculids and erythema induratum.

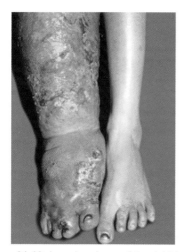

Figure 21.13: Lymphoedema of the right lower limb with gummas on the skin

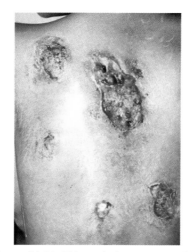

Figure 21.14: Tuberculosis gummas which have broken down to form ulcers

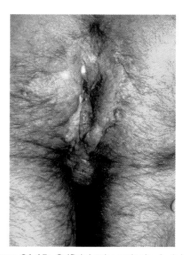

Figure 21.15: Orificial tuberculosis. Indolent, non-healing ulcer of the anus. The patient had abdominal tuberculosis

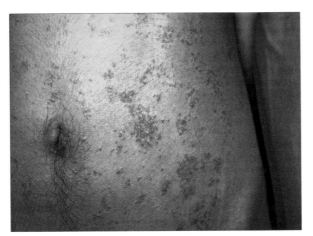

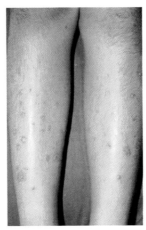

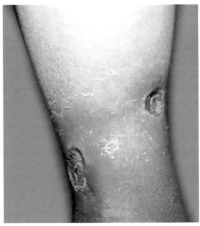

Figure 21.16: Lichen scrofulosorum. Grouped, minute erythematous papules

Figure 21.17: Papulonecrotic tuberculid. Indurated papulo-nodules with a central necrotic crust

Figure 21.18: Erythema induratum. Persistent ulcers with underlying induration on the posterior aspect of the leg

In addition, TB is an important cause of erythema nodosum in Indian patients. Recent studies employing the polymerase chain reaction [PCR] have demonstrated the presence of mycobacterial deoxyribonucleic acid [DNA] in biopsies from patients with erythema induratum (42,43) and papulonecrotic tuberculids (42,44) providing further evidence of the association between these conditions and TB.

Lichen Scrofulosorum

Lichen scrofulosorum typically presents as a crop of two to five mm erythematous papules that show a tendency to grouping [Figure 21.16]. Many papules show crusting. The eruption has a predeliction for the trunk but may occur at other sites also. Individual papules tend to resolve in about two weeks with hyperpigmentation but crops of lesions may come and go over several months. Uncommonly, the eruption may develop *after* initiation of anti-TB treatment; these lesions subsided on continuing treatment (45). The TST is strongly positive and may show ulceration. Biopsy reveals focal epithelioid cell granulomas within and around the hair follicle or the sweat duct. The underlying TB focus may be in the lymph nodes, lungs or at some other site.

Papulonecrotic Tuberculids

Papulonecrotic tuberculids present as an eruption of multiple, papulo-nodular lesions ranging in size from two to five cm occurring over the trunk and extremities. The eruption may be preceded by fever and constitutional symptoms. Individual lesions show pustulation and crusting at the centre [Figure 21.17]. Removal of the crust reveals a deep ulcer. The lesions heal gradually over four to six weeks with scarring. Crops of lesions recur at variable intervals. The TST test is strongly positive and often ulcerates. Skin biopsy reveals wedge-shaped necrosis of the epidermis and upper dermis with underlying epithelioid granulomas. A focus of active TB can usually be demonstrated in these patients.

Erythema Induratum

Erythema induratum presents as indolent, mildly tender, dull red nodules ranging in size from 5–7.5 cm that usually develop on the calves. Some nodules soften and break down to form deep persistent ulcers that gradually heal over several weeks with scarring [Figure 21.18]. New nodules may continue to develop while old lesions are resolving. The TST is positive. Skin biopsy reveals a granulomatous lobular panniculitis with vasculitis of small and/or medium vessels. A focus of TB is demonstrable in many patients. However, a significant proportion of patients who show the typical clinical and histopathological features of erythema induratum do not have TB. In these patients, the reaction pattern has presumably been triggered by some other cause.

Erythema Nodosum

Erythema nodosum presents as erythematous, tender, 2.5–5 cm nodules that usually develop on the shins [Figure 21.19] but

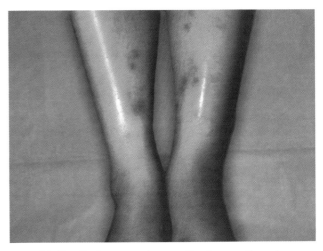

Figure 21.19: Erythema nodosum. Tender, erythematous, non-ulcerated nodules on the shins

may also involve the thighs, buttocks and forearms in severe cases. Low-grade fever and swelling of the ankle joints accompany the skin lesions in some patients. The lesions regress spontaneously becoming dull red, violaceous, finally leaving behind macular hyperpigmentation. Ulceration and scarring are not features of erythema nodosum. Recurrent crops of lesions may develop. Skin biopsy reveals a septal panniculitis with an infiltrate of lymphocytes and histiocytes. Giant cells may be seen within the thickened septum. Erythema nodosum is a reaction pattern that may be provoked by a variety of triggers, infective and non-infective. However, in India, TB is still an important cause of this condition justifying its inclusion in this section.

Others

Multiple episodes of Sweet's syndrome were recently reported during treatment of scrofuloderma and probably represent a hypersensitivity phenomenon similar to the tuberculids (46).

The reader is also referred to the chapter *"Musculoskeletal manifestations of tuberculosis" [Chapter 20]* for more details on erythema nodosum and erythema induratum.

CUTANEOUS TUBERCULOSIS IN IMMUNOCOMPROMISED HOSTS

The human immunodeficiency virus [HIV] epidemic has focused attention on the manifestations of TB in patients with acquired immunodeficiency syndrome [AIDS] (37,47-51). Similar features may, however, be seen in persons who are immunosuppressed due to other reasons as well (52,53). In patients with advanced immunodeficiency, the lesions do not fit into the above described categories and usually present as papules, nodules, vesicles or induration. Ulceration and discharge from the surface of the lesions may be a feature [Figure 21.20]. The diagnosis is usually not suspected clinically and it has been suggested that all atypical cutaneous lesions developing in immunosuppressed

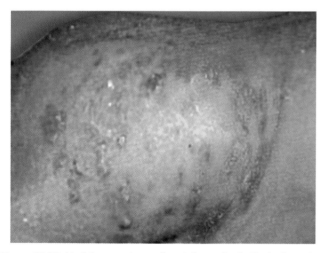

Figure 21.20: Nodules papules and pustules on the buttock of a patient with Cushing's syndrome. Numerous acid-fast bacilli were seen on biopsy

individuals should be biopsied and subjected to culture (47). Biopsy reveals a neutrophilic infiltrate which may be admixed with histiocytes. Epithelioid cells, giant cells and well-formed granulomas are uncommon; AFB are usually seen in large numbers. Culture from the lesions usually grows *Mtb* or NTM. Most patients recover with anti-TB therapy but some may die in spite of appropriate treatment. However, in those with less advanced HIV disease, the clinical manifestations are largely similar to those noted in other patients. In one study, cutaneous lesions were described to be multiple and larger with involvement of more than one underlying structure, lymph node or bone, with more common systemic involvement and less frequent tuberculin test positivity. However, histopathological findings and treatment responses were similar (54).

LABORATORY DIAGNOSIS

It is easy to obtain tissue specimens in patients with cutaneous TB; however, the diagnostic yield on direct microscopy or conventional culture methods is uniformly poor. *Mtb* has been demonstrated in 4%-9% of cases (32,33) and is hardly ever seen in lupus vulgaris and TB verrucosa cutis. AFB are found in about 35% of cases (35,36). The results of culture of biopsy material are equally disappointing. Cultures were found to be positive in less than 10% of cases (32,33,35,36). However, a much higher yield has been reported in other studies ranging from 12 of 51 cases [23.5%] (31), 29 of 51 [56.9%] cases (55), 112 of 203 cases [55.2%] (56) and 26 of 35 cases [74.3%] (57). Availability of radiometric methods has decreased the time taken for culture but is expensive and is unlikely to be of much use in cutaneous TB which is paucibacillary (58). One study has recommended the use of both conventional and liquid media to increase the isolation rate (57). Histopathological examination reveals a granulomatous dermatitis in 82–100% of cases (32-36). However, it is difficult to demonstrate *Mtb* in tissue sections.

The TST is positive in 73%-100% of patients (32-36). Increasing the cut-off for a positive test increases the specificity of the test but decreases the sensitivity (59,60). A study (61) of the utility of the TST in patients with a doubtful diagnosis of cutaneous TB revealed that the test did not perform well in differentiating TB from other diseases. In 1992, Victor *et al* (44) first described the use of PCR in cutaneous TB. Several reports have since documented the use of the test in lupus vulgaris, scrofuloderma and the tuberculids (43,62-74). Some workers (71,72) have demonstrated a high sensitivity of the technique in cutaneous TB though another group (73) did not find it useful in paucibacillary forms. In a study (74) on 66 cases and 47 controls from India, a true positive rate of 25.8% and a false positive rate of 27.7% were reported with PCR. Another study demonstrated a sensitivity of 25% and a specificity of 73.7% with DNA PCR while none of the cases or controls were positive on messenger ribonucleic acid [mRNA] PCR (75). In a recent study (76a), Xpert MTB/RIF was not found to be useful as a diagnostic test for cutaneous TB. It appears that clinical decisions about the diagnosis and treatment of patients with cutaneous TB should not be based on PCR results alone.

Finally, if the results of laboratory tests are inconclusive, a therapeutic trial with anti-TB drugs is frequently used to confirm the diagnosis in difficult cases (76b-79). Evidence is available suggesting that when a therapeutic trial is undertaken in cutaneous TB, 6 weeks of therapy with isonaizid, rifampicin, pyrazinamide and ethambutol drugs appears adequate to prove [or disprove] the diagnosis (76b-79).

If there is no improvement at all after six weeks, anti-TB treatment should be stopped and the diagnosis reconsidered. There is no benefit of continuing the trial for longer periods.

BACILLE CALMETTE-GUÉRIN AND CUTANEOUS LESIONS

Skin complications due to BCG vaccination have been classified into local and generalised forms (80,81). These details are shown in Table 21.2.

Table 21.2: Skin lesions due to BCG vaccination

Local lesions
  Keloid
  Abnormally large ulcer
  Subcutaneous abscess
  Epithelial cyst
  Eczematous reaction
  Granulomatous reaction
  Lupus vulgaris
  Warty TB
Generalised lesions
  Erythema nodosum
  Tuberculids
  Scrofuloderma
  Non-specific haemorrhagic eruptions

BCG = bacille Calmette-Guérin; TB = tuberculosis
Based on references 80,81

CUTANEOUS LESIONS DUE TO NONTUBERCULOUS MYCOBACTERIA

Skin involvement due to NTM such as, *M. marinum* and *M. ulcerans,* are clearly defined clinical entities and are considered first. This is followed by a description of miscellaneous lesions caused by a number of other NTM.

M. marinum is a pathogen of many species of fish, both fresh and salt water. Humans acquire the disease from infected fish or water through breaches in the skin, usually of the upper and the lower limb (82,83). These infections have been termed fish tank granuloma and swimming pool granuloma. A nodule, or less commonly, an ulcer, pustule or abscess develops at the site of injury about two weeks following exposure. In one-third of cases, lesions are arranged linearly along the lymphatics in a "sporotrichoid" pattern. In about a third of patients, the infection extends to the deeper tissues, usually the tenosynovium; joints and bone may also be involved. Systemic dissemination of infection

is rare. Skin biopsy reveals a range of patterns from acute neutrophilic inflammation to granulomas admixed with neutrophils. AFB are difficult to find in tissue sections (84). The organism grows best at 30 °C–33 °C on mycobacterial media. Several antibiotics have been found to be effective including rifampicin and ethambutol, doxycycline and minocycline, clarithromycin and cotrimoxazole. Treatment is recommended for two months after clinical healing; deep infections require treatment for longer periods. Surgical debridement should be considered in deep infections, immunocompromised patients or if medical therapy fails.

Buruli ulcer disease is the third most common mycobacterial disease in immunocompetent people, after TB and leprosy (85,86). It is caused by *M. ulcerans*, a mycobacteria found in soil and vegetation in many parts of the world, especially in tropical rain forests. The organism enters the skin through abrasions and injuries and is commoner on the extremities. Children are affected more frequently though no age is exempt. Three clinical stages are described: pre-ulcerative lesions may be papules, nodules or plaques. These progress to necrosis of the subcutaneous fat and undermined ulcers of the overlying skin. Untreated ulcers may extend and reach to large sizes. On skin biopsy, large number of AFB can be detected in about 60% of cases at this stage accompanied by necrosis of the dermis and subcutaneous fat with minimal inflammation (87). The final stage of scarring follows spontaneous healing of the ulcers. Scarring can lead to contractures and ankylosis and is a major cause of disability. Antibiotics are the treatment of choice with a regimen of rifampicin [10 mg/kg], orally and streptomycin [15 mg/kg], intramuscularly for 8 weeks shown to be effective in producing microbiological and clinical improvement. Alternatively, this combination can be given for 4 weeks followed by an oral regimen of rifampicin and clarithromycin [7.5 mg/kg, twice daily] for 4 weeks. Some workers have used an oral regimen of rifampicin and clarithromycin for the entire 8-week period. Moxifloxacin, 400 mg daily orally has been used instead of clarithromycin. Following antibiotic therapy, small and intermediate lesions may heal completely and surgical debridement may not be necessary. Larger lesions will require less extensive debridement and grafting if preceded by a complete course of antibiotics (88).

A large number of other NTM have been reported to cause cutaneous infections in immunocompetent and immunocompromised hosts (89-96). Most of these mycobacteria are present in the environment and gain access to the skin following an injury, including iatrogenic injuries following needle pricks and surgery. Rapid growers, *M. marinum*, *M. ulcerans* are most common species that cause skin, soft tissue infections, especially at site of skin punctures or surgery. A variety of clinical manifestations are described: papules, pustules, nodules, abscesses, cellulitis, ulcers and sinuses. The clinical features are not distinctive and the infection may be suspected from the setting. Skin biopsy reveals diverse inflammatory patterns including suppuration, granulomas, folliculitis, panniculitis and diffuse histiocytic infiltrates (61).

The histopathological features are not specific for any organism. The AFB are easily seen in immunocompromised hosts but may be difficult to find in the immunocompetent. Culture and drug-susceptibility testing [DST] testing of the causative organism is helpful for confirmation of the diagnosis and treatment.

M. chelonae also produces skin, soft tissue and bone infections. *M. chelonae* has been associated with contact lenses and laser-associated in situ keratomileusis [LASIK] surgery. Disseminated disease in immunocompromised individuals can occur with characteristic skin lesions [painless, fistulised nodules and abscesses]. Skin, soft tissue and bone infections due to *M. fortuitum* are common than pulmonary infections. Outbreaks of furunculosis have been reported following exposure to contaminated water during pedicures.

TREATMENT

The recommended therapy for cutaneous TB is the use of short-course regimens as used for pulmonary TB. As per the recently published Guidelines for Extrapulmonary TB for India [INDEX-TB Guidelines] (75), standard 6 months short-course treatment is considered adequate for cutaneous TB. The reader is referred to the chapter *"Treatment of tuberculosis"* [Chapter 45] for further details. Using these regimens, lupus vulgaris and TB verrucosa cutis were found to heal completely in 4–5 months. The skin lesions of scrofuloderma healed in 5–6 months while the lymph nodes regressed in 7–9 months. There were no relapses in the patients who were followed up for three and a-half years (73,97). Drug resistance in cutaneous TB appears to be rare though recent reports of culture-documented cases with drug resistant TB gummas and scrofuloderma are a worrisome development (98-100). Under the Revised National Tuberculosis Control Programme [RNTCP] of Government of India, daily treatment is available for patients with all forms of TB including cutaneous TB. The reader is referred to the chapter *"Revised National Tuberculosis Control Programme"* [Chapter 53] for details on this topic.

The reader is referred to the chapter *"Nontuberculous mycobacterial infections"* [Chapter 41] for details regarding treatment of cutaneous NTM disease.

REFERENCES

1. Laennec RTH. Traite de l'auscultation mediate et des maladies des peumons et du coeur. Vol.1, Paris: Asselin and Cie; 1826. p.649-50. Quoted in Marmelzat WL. Laennec and the "prosector's wart". Arch Dermatol 1962;86:122-4.
2. Demme R. Zur diagnostischen Beleutung der Tuberkelbacillen fur das Kindesalter. Berlin Klin Wschr 1883;20:217. Quoted in Michelson HE. The history of lupus vulgaris. J Invest Dermatol 1946;7:261-7.
3. Riehl G, Paltauf R. Tuberculosis verrucosa cutis. Eine bisher noch nicht beschriebene Form von Hauttuberculose. Vjschr Derm Syph 1886;13:19-19. Quoted in Marmelzat WL. Laennec and the "Prosector's wart". Arch Dermatol 1962;86:122-4.
4. Michelson HE. The history of lupus vulgaris. J Invest Dermatol 1946;7:261-7.
5. Darier J. Des tuberculides cutanees. Ann Derm Syph 1896;7:1431-6.
6. Horwitz O. Lupus vulgaris cutis in Denmark 1895-1954: its relation to the epidemiology of other forms of tuberculosis. Acta Tuberculosea Scandinavia 1960;49 Suppl:1-145.
7. Forstrom L. Frequency of other types of tuberculosis in patients with tuberculosis of the skin. Scand J Clin Lab Invest 1969; 23 Suppl:1-37.
8. Choudhury AM, Ara S. Cutaneous tuberculosis-a study of 400 cases. Bangladesh Med Res Counc Bull 2006;32:60-5.
9. Fasal P, Rhodes R. Cutaneous tuberculosis and sarcoidosis in the American Negro and in inhabitants of tropical countries. In: Simons RDGP, editor. Handbook of Tropical Dermatology and Medical Mycology, Volume 1. New York: Elsevier; 1952. p.578-603.
10. Neves H. Incidence of skin diseases 1952-65. Trans St Johns Hosp Dermatol Soc [London] 1966;52:255-70.
11. de Noronha T, de Almeida Gonclaves JC. O tratamento da tuberculose cutanea. Acrhivo Pathol 1961;33:20-45. Abstracted in Excerpta Medica [Dermatology and Venereology] 1962;16:254.
12. Ustvedt HJ, Ostensen IW. The relation between tuberculosis of the skin and primary infection. Tubercle 1951;32:36-9.
13. Amezquita R. Tuberculosis cutanea. Aspectos clinicos epidemiologicos en Mexico. Tesis recepcional. Acta Leprologica 1963; 16:1-103. Abstracted in Excerpta Medica [Dermatology and Venereology] 1965;19:674.
14. Mitchell PC. Tuberculosis verrucosa cutis among Chinese in Hong Kong. Br J Dermatol 1954;66:444-8.
15. Wong KO, Lee KP, Chiu SF. Tuberculosis of the skin in Hong Kong. Br J Dermatol 1968;80:424-9.
16. Goh YS, Ong BH, Rajan VS. Tuberculosis cutis in Singapore: a two-year experience. Sing Med J 1974;15:223-6.
17. Li HC. A preliminary study of tuberculosis of skin in Peking. Chinese J Dermatol 1957;5:13-22.
18. Lee YB, Cho BK, Houh W. Clinical and histopathological study on skin tuberculosis during 5 years [1970-74]. Korean J Dermatol 1975;13:103-8.
19. Kqn KS, Chung TA. A clinical study on skin tuberculosis. Korean J Dermatol 1977;15:181-9.
20. Kitamura K. Geographische verteilung der Haut tuberculose der lepra und der sarcoidose in Japan. Hautarzt 1967;18:524-6.
21. Takanohashi K, Yamamoto K, Ishidoya K. Statistical observations of cutaneous tuberculosis in Hirosaki University during recent 8 years [1961-1968]. Japanese J Clin Dermatol 1971;25:451-7.
22. Privat Y, Faye I, Bellossi A, Guberina I. Apropos of cutaneous tuberculosis in Senegal [presentation of 14 new cases]. Bull Soc Med Afr Noire Langue Franc 1967;12:640-4.
23. Zoon JJ. Tuberculosis of the skin. Consideration about pathogenesis. AMA Arch Dermatol 1957;75:161-70.
24. Satyanarayana BV. "Tuberculoderma" a brief review together with statistical analysis and observations. Indian J Dermatol 1963;29:25-42.
25. Ghosh LM. An analysis of 50,000 skin cases seen in the outpatient department of the School of Tropical Medicine, Calcutta, during the 5 years from 1942 to 1946. Indian Medical Gazette 1948;84:493-501.
26. Lahiri KD. Etiology and pathology of skin tuberculosis in the tropics. Indian J Dermatol 1956;2:3-7.
27. Banerjee BN. Tuberculosis of the skin and its relation with pulmonary tuberculosis. Indian J Dermatol 1957;2:69-72.
28. Singh G. Lupus vulgaris in India. Indian J Dermatol Venereol 1974;40:257-60.
29. Sobhanadri C, Gupta KG, Rao VK, Reddy DJ. Tuberculosis of the skin in Guntur [a clinico-pathological study]. Indian J Dermatol Venereol 1958;24:133-47.
30. Mammen A, Thambiah AS. Tuberculosis of the skin. Indian J Dermatol Venereol 1973;39:153-9.

31. Sharma S, Sehgal VN, Bhattacharya SN, Mahajan G, Gupta R. Clinicopathologic spectrum of cutaneous tuberculosis: a retrospective analysis of 165 Indians. Am J Dermatopathol 2015;37:444-50.

32. Pandhi RK, Bedi TR, Kanwar AJ, Bhutani LK. Cutaneous tuberculosis: a clinical and investigative study. Indian J Dermatol 1977;22:99-107.

33. Ramesh V, Misra RS, Jain RK. Secondary tuberculosis of the skin. Clinical features and problems in laboratory diagnosis. Int J Dermatol 1987;26:578-81.

34. Kumar B, Muralidhar S. Cutaneous tuberculosis: a twenty-year prospective study. Int J Tuberc Lung Dis 1999;3:494-500.

35. Sehgal VN, Srivastava G, Khurana VK, Sharma VK, Bhalla P, Beohar PC. An appraisal of epidemiologic, clinical, bacteriologic, and immunologic parameters in cutaneous tuberculosis. Int J Dermatol 1987;26:521-6.

36. Sehgal VN, Jain MK, Srivastava G. Changing patterns of cutaneous tuberculosis. A prospective study. Int J Dermatol 1989;28:231-6.

37. Rohatgi PK, Palazzolo JV, Saini NB. Acute miliary tuberculosis of the skin in acquired immunodeficiency syndrome. J Am Acad Dermatol 1992;26:356-9.

38. Kennedy C, Knowles GK. Miliary tuberculosis presenting with skin lesions. Br Med J 1975;3:356.

39. Forstrom L. Carcinomatous changes in lupus vulgaris. Ann Clin Res 1969;1:213-9.

40. Horwitz O, Meyer J. The safety record of BCG vaccination, untoward reactions observed after vaccination. Bibl Tuberc 1957;13:245-71.

41. Hartston W. Uncommon skin reactions after BCG vaccination. Tubercle 1959;40:265-70.

42. Degitz K, Steidl M, Thomas P, Plewig G, Volkenandt M. Aetiology of tuberculids. Lancet 1993;341:239-40.

43. Schneider JW, Geiger DH, Rossouw DJ, Jordaan HF, Victor T, Van Helden PD. Mycobacterium tuberculosis DNA in erythema induratum of Bazin. Lancet 1993;342:747-8.

44. Victor T, Jordaan HF, Van Niekerk DJ, Louw M, Jordaan A, Van Helden PD. Papulonecrotic tuberculid: identification of Mycobacterium tuberculosis DNA by polymerase chain reaction. Am J Dermatopathol 1992;14:491-5.

45. Thami GP, Kaur S, Kanwar AJ, Mohan H. Lichen scrofulosorum: a rare manifestation of a common disease. Pediatr Dermatol 2002;19:122-6.

46. Mahaisavariya P, Chaiprasert A, Manonukul J, Khemngern S. Scrofuloderma and Sweet's syndrome. Int J Dermatol 2002;41:28-31.

47. Freed JA, Pervez NK, Chen V, Damsker B. Cutaneous mycobacteriosis: occurrence and significance in two patients with the acquired immunodeficiency syndrome. Arch Dermatol 1987;123:1601-3.

48. Lombardo PC, Weitzman I. Isolation of Mycobacterium tuberculosis and M. avium complex from the same skin lesions in AIDS. N Engl J Med 1990;323:916-7.

49. Lanjewar DN, Bhosale A, Iyer A. Spectrum of dermatopathologic lesions associated with HIV/AIDS in India. Indian J Pathol Microbiol 2002;45:293-8.

50. Chiewchanvit S, Mahanupab P, Walker PF. Cutaneous tuberculosis in three HIV-infected patients. J Med Assoc Thai 2000;83:1550-4.

51. Daikos GL, Uttamchandani RB, Tuda C, Fischl MA, Miller N, Cleary T, et al. Disseminated miliary tuberculosis of the skin in patients with AIDS: report of four cases. Clin Infect Dis 1998;27:205-8.

52. Taylor AE, Corris PA. Cutaneous tuberculosis in an immunocompromised host: an unusual clinical presentation. Br J Dermatol 1995;132:155-6.

53. Quinibi WJ, Al-Sibai MB, Taher S, Harder EJ, deVol E, Furayh OL, et al. Mycobacterial infection after renal transplantation-report of 14 cases and review of the literature. QJM 1990;282:1039-60.

54. Varshney A, Goyal T. Incidence of various clinico-morphological variants of cutaneous tuberculosis and HIV concurrence: a study from the Indian subcontinent. Ann Saudi Med. 2011;31:134-9.

55. Gopinathan R, Pandit D, Joshi J, Jerajani H, Mathur M. Clinical and morphological variants of cutaneous tuberculosis and its relation to mycobacterium species. Indian J Med Microbiology 2001;19:193-6.

56. Umapathy KC, Begum R, Ravichandran G, Rahman F, Paramasivan CN, Ramanathan VD. Comprehensive findings on clinical, bacteriological, histopathological and therapeutic aspects of cutaneous tuberculosis. Trop Med Int Health 2006;11:1521-8.

57. Aggarwal P, Singal A, Bhattacharya SN, Mishra K. Comparison of the radiometric BACTEC 460 TB culture system and Löwenstein-Jensen medium for the isolation of mycobacteria in cutaneous tuberculosis and their drug susceptibility pattern. Int J Dermatol 2008;47:681-7.

58. Weissler JC. Tuberculosis: immunopathogenesis and therapy. Am J Med Sci 1993;305:52-65.

59. Gupta D, Saiprakash BV, Aggarwal AN, Muralidhar S, Kumar B, Jindal SK. Value of different cut-off points of tuberculin skin test to diagnose tuberculosis among patients with respiratory symptoms in a chest clinic. J Assoc Physicians India 2001;49:332-5.

60. Menzies D. What does tuberculin reactivity after bacille Calmette-Guerin vaccination tell us? Clin Infect Dis 2000;31 Suppl 3:S71-74.

61. Ramam M, Malhotra A, Tejasvi T, Manchanda Y, Sharma S, Mittal R, et al. How useful is the Mantoux test in the diagnosis of doubtful cases of cutaneous tuberculosis? Int J Dermatol. 2011;50:1379-82.

62. Schneider JW, Jordaan HF, Geiger DH, Victor T, Van Helden PD, Rossouw DJ. Erythema induratum of Bazin. A clinicopathological study of 20 cases and detection of Mycobacterium tuberculosis DNA in skin lesions by polymerase chain reaction. Am J Dermatopathol 1995;17:350-6.

63. Ban M, Kanematsu M, Ehara H, Yanagihara M, Kitajima Y. A case of acute tuberculous ulcer diagnosed rapidly by the polymerase chain reaction. Acta Derm Venereol 1995;75:245.

64. Degitz K, Messer G, Schirren H, Classen V, Meurer M. Successful treatment of erythema induratum of bazin following rapid detection of mycobacterial DNA by polymerase chain reaction. Arch Dermatol 1993;129:1619-20.

65. Taniguchi S, Chanoki M, Hamada T. Scrofuloderma: the DNA analysis of mycobacteria by the polymerase chain reaction. Arch Dermatol 1993;129:1618-9.

66. Penneys NS, Leonardi CL, Cook S, Blauvelt A, Rosenberg S, Eells LD, et al. Identification of Mycobacterium tuberculosis DNA in five different types of cutaneous lesions by the polymerase chain reaction. Arch Dermatol 1993;129:1594-8.

67. Steidl M, Neubert U, Volkenandt M, Chatelain R, Degitz K. Lupus vulgaris confirmed by polymerase-chain reaction. Br J Dermatol 1993;129:314-8.

68. Serfling U, Penneys NS, Leonardi CL. Identification of Mycobacterium tuberculosis DNA in a case of lupus vulgaris. J Am Acad Dermatol 1993;28:318-22.

69. Degitz K, Steidl M, Neubert U, Plewig G, Volkenandt M. Detection of mycobacterial DNA in paraffin-embedded specimens of lupus vulgaris by polymerase-chain reaction. Arch Dermatol Res 1993;285:168-70.

70. Welsh O, Vera-Cabrera L, Fernández-Reyes M, Gómez M, Ocampo J. Cutaneous tuberculosis confirmed by PCR in three

patients with biopsy and culture negative for Mycobacterium tuberculosis. Int J Dermatol 2007;46:734-5.

71. Quiros E, Bettinardi A, Quiros A, Piedrola G, Maroto MC. Detection of mycobacterial DNA in papulonecrotic tuberculid lesions by polymerase chain reaction. J Clin Lab Anal 2000;14:133-5.

72. Arora SK, Kumar B, Sehgal S. Development of a polymerase chain reaction dot-blotting system for detecting cutaneous tuberculosis. Br J Dermatol 2000;142:72-6.

73. Tan SH, Tan BH, Goh CL, Tan KC, Tan MF, Ng WC, et al. Detection of Mycobacterium tuberculosis DNA using polymerase chain reaction in cutaneous tuberculosis and tuberculids. Int J Dermatol 1999;38:122-7.

74. Ramam M, Ramesh V, Mittal R, Sirka CS, Achar A, Singh MK, et al. Polymerase chain reaction [PCR] for the diagnosis of cutaneous tuberculosis [Abstract]. Fourth Joint Meeting of the International Society of Dermatopathology. Washington DC; 2001.

75. Suthar C, Rana T, Singh UB, Singh M, Ramesh V, Sharma VK, Ramam M. mRNA and DNA PCR tests in cutaneous tuberculosis. Indian J Dermatol Venereol Leprol 2013;79:65-9.

76a. Sharma A. A study on clinical spectrum of cutaneous tuberculosis at a tertiary care centre in western Uttar Pradesh [MD Thesis]. Moradabad: Teerthanker Mahaveer Medical College and Research Centre; 2017.

76b. Ramam M, Mittal R, Ramesh V. How soon does cutaneous tuberculosis respond to treatment? Implications for a therapeutic test of diagnosis. Int J Dermatol 2005;44:121-4.

77. Ramam M, Tejasvi T, Manchanda Y, Sharma S, Mittal R. Six weeks is an adequate period for a therapeutic trial in cutaneous tuberculosis [Abstract]. IX International Congress of Dermatology. Beijing; 2004.

78. Ramam M, Tejasvi T, Manchanda Y, Sharma S, Mittal R. What is the appropriate duration of a therapeutic trial in cutaneous tuberculosis? Further observations. Indian J Dermatol Venereol Leprol 2007;73:243-6.

79. Sehgal VN, Sardana K, Sharma S. Inadequacy of clinical and/or laboratory criteria for the diagnosis of lupus vulgaris, re-infection cutaneous tuberculosis: fallout/implication of 6 weeks of anti-tubercular therapy [ATT] as a precise diagnostic supplement to complete the scheduled regimen. J Dermatolog Treat 2007;11:1-4.

80. Kakakhel KV, Fritsch P. Cutaneous tuberculosis. Int J Dermatol 1989;28:355-62.

81. Dostrovsky A, Sagher F. Dermatologic complications of BCG vaccination. Br J Dermatol 1963;75:181-92.

82. Aubry A, Chosidow O, Caumes E, Robert J, Cambau E. Sixty-three cases of Mycobacterium marinum infection: clinical features, treatment, and antibiotic susceptibility of causative isolates. Arch Intern Med 2002;162:1746-52.

83. Lahey T. Invasive Mycobacterium marinum infections. Emerg Infect Dis 2003;9:1496-8.

84. Travis WD, Travis LB, Roberts GD, Su DW, Weiland LW. The histopathologic spectrum in Mycobacterium marinum infection. Arch Pathol Lab Med 1985;109:1109-13.

85. van der Werf TS, van der Graaf WT, Tappero JW, Asiedu K. Mycobacterium ulcerans infection. Lancet 1999;354:1013-8.

86. Sizaire V, Nackers F, Comte E, Portaels F. Mycobacterium ulcerans infection: control, diagnosis, and treatment. Lancet Infect Dis 2006;6:288-96.

87. Guarner J, Bartlett J, Whitney EA, Raghunathan PL, Stienstra Y, Asamoa K, et al. Histopathologic features of Mycobacterium ulcerans infection. Emerg Infect Dis 2003;9:51-6.

88. World Health Organization. Treatment of Mycobacterium ulcerans disease [Buruli ulcer]: guidance for health workers. Geneva: World Health Organization; 2012.

89. Street ML, Umbert-Millet IJ, Roberts GD, Su WP. Nontuberculosis mycobacterium infection of the skin. Report of fourteen cases and review of the literature. J Am Acad Dermatol 1991;24:208-15.

90. Rotman DA, Blauvelt A, Kerdel FA. Widespread primary cutaneous infection with Mycobacterium fortuitum. Int J Dermatol 1993;32:512-4.

91. Woods GL, Washington JA 2nd. Mycobacteria other than Mycobacterium tuberculosis: review of microbiologic and clinical aspects. Rev Infect Dis 1987;9:275-99.

92. Murray-Leisure KA, Egan N, Weitekamp MR. Skin lesion caused by Mycobacterium scrofulaceum. Arch Dermatol 1897;123:369-70.

93. Hanke CW, Temofeew RK, Slama SL. Mycobacterium kansasii infection with multiple cutaneous lesions. J Am Acad Dermatol 1987;16:1122-8.

94. Cox SK, Strausbough LJ. Chronic cutaneous infection caused by Mycobacterium intracellulare. Arch Dermatol 1981;117:794-6.

95. McGovern J, Bix BC, Webster G. Mycobacterium haemophilum skin disease successfully treated with excision. J Am Acad Dermatol 1994;30:269-70.

96. Sharma SK, Ryan H, Khaparde S, Sachdeva KS, Singh AD, Mohan A, et al. Index-TB guidelines: Guidelines on extrapulmonary tuberculosis for India. Indian J Med Res 2017;145:448-63.

97. Ramesh V, Misra RS, Saxena U, Mukherjee A. Comparative efficacy of drug regimens in skin tuberculosis. Clin Exp Dermatol 1991;16:106-9.

98. Sharma N, Kumar P, Mantoo S, Patnaik S. Primary multi-drug resistant tuberculous gumma. J Commun Dis 2001;33:170-3.

99. Ramesh V, Murlidhar S, Kumar J, Srivastava L. Isolation of drug-resistant tubercle bacilli in cutaneous tuberculosis. Pediatr Dermatol 2001;18:393-5.

100. Olson DP, Day CL, Magula NP, Sahid F, Moosa MY. Cutaneous extensively drug-resistant tuberculosis. Am J Trop Med Hyg 2007;77:551-4.

22

Lymph Node Tuberculosis

Saurav Khatiwada, Arvind Kumar

INTRODUCTION

Mycobacterial lymphadenitis has plagued humanity since ancient times. It has been called as "scrofula" [a term derived from the Latin for "glandular swelling" or from the French "full necked sow"] and "King's evil". Peripheral lymph node involvement is the commonest form of extrapulmonary mycobacterial disease and the cervical region is the most frequently affected site (1-3). In the present era, *Mycobacterium tuberculosis* [*Mtb*] is the most common cause of mycobacterial lymphadenitis and lymphadenitis due to nontuberculous mycobacteria [NTM] is also being increasingly encountered. Peripheral and mediastinal lymph node tuberculosis [TB] is commonly seen in patients with human immunodeficiency virus infection [HIV] and the acquired immunodeficiency syndrome [AIDS].

EPIDEMIOLOGY

Myocobacterial lymphadenitis has shown marked geographical variation. In the developing and underdeveloped countries, TB lymphadenitis continues to be the most common and lymphadenitis due to NTM is seldom seen. In several studies from India (3-6), *Mtb* has been the most common pathogen isolated from patients with mycobacterial lymphadenitis accounting for almost all the cases (3-6). Among adults, lymph node TB is the most common form of extra-pulmonary TB [EPTB], accounting for 35% of EPTB cases (7). In a community-based, house-to-house survey of a population of 23,229 in 35 neighbouring villages with 7900 children aged 0–14 years in the rural area of Wardha district, Maharashtra State, Central India, from May 1993 to May 1994 and from March 1995 to February 1996, the prevalence of lymph node TB was reported to be 4.43/1000 children (8). On the other hand, NTM are the most frequently isolated pathogens from the lymphadenitis specimens in several

reports from the developed world (9,10). In Australia (11) and British Columbia (12), NTM have been detected 10 times more frequently than *Mtb*. In studies reported from the USA, *Mtb* accounted for 95% of all mycobacterial lymphadenitis in adults, whereas in children, 92% of the mycobacterial lymphadenitis was due to NTM (13,14).

In addition to geographical variation, there has been a changing trend in the prevalence of these organisms over a period of time at some places. In England, there has been a decline in TB lymphadenitis and a rise in NTM lymphadenitis (15). A high frequency of disease has been reported in populations hailing from areas where TB is highly endemic. In one study (2) patients from the Indian subcontinent, who otherwise constituted only 10% of the population of that region, accounted for 81% of the 61 cases of mycobacterial lymphadenitis. Similar results have been reported among Native Americans and in patients from South-East Asia and Africa (16,17). A high frequency of disease has also been reported among Asians and Hispanic patients in the San Francisco area (17). Patients of Asian origin and African-Americans also seem to have a high predilection for developing lymphadenitis due to *Mtb* (18-21).

PATHOGENESIS

TB lymphadenitis is considered to be the local manifestation of a systemic disease whereas lymphadenopathy due to NTM is truly a localised disease. *Mtb* generally enters the body via the respiratory tract and undergoes haematogenous and lymphatic dissemination. Hilar and mediastinal lymph nodes are the first lymphoid tissues encountered in the lymphatic spread from the lung parenchyma. This involvement may occur at the time of primary infection or may occur later in life due to reactivation of previous infection. Tonsil is also an important portal of entry. The infection may then spread via the lymphatics to the nearest cervical lymph nodes.

In the initial stages, the nodes may be discrete clinically. Periadenitis results in matting and fixity of the lymph nodes. The lymph nodes coalesce and break down to form caseous pus. This may perforate the deep fascia and present as a fluctuant swelling on the surface [collar-stud abscess]. Overlying skin becomes indurated, breaks down and leads to the formation of a sinus which if untreated may remain unhealed for years. Healing may occur from each of the three stages with calcification and/or scarring.

In NTM lymphadenitis, the pathogens usually enter the lymph nodes directly via oropharyngeal mucosa, salivary glands, tonsils, gingiva or conjunctiva (14,22) and lymph node involvement represents a localised disease. The reader is referred to the chapter *"Nontuberculous mycobacterial infections"* [Chapter 41] for further details.

CLINICAL PRESENTATION

Tuberculosis Lymphadenitis

Clinical presentation of TB lymphadenitis in several published studies is summarised in Tables 22.1, 22.2 and 22.3 (2-4,23,24). TB cervical lymphadenitis tends to occur more often in females and presents in young adults [Table 22.1]. Patients usually present with slowly enlarging lymph nodes and may otherwise be asymptomatic. Cervical lymph nodes are most commonly affected although axillary and inguinal lymph nodes may also be involved. Associated mediastinal lymphadenopathy may also be present sometimes.

Some patients with lymph node TB may manifest systemic symptoms. These include fever, weight loss, fatigue and occasionally night sweats [Table 22.1] (2-4,23,24). Cough may be a prominent symptom in patients with mediastinal lymphadenopathy.

Jones and Campbell (25) had classified peripheral TB lymphadenopathy into five stages [Table 22.4]. Physical examination findings depend upon the stage of the disease. The enlarged lymph nodes may be of varying size, discrete or matted. The lymph nodes may be firm or cystic inconsistency if necrosis and abscess formation has taken place [Figure 22.1]. The lymph nodes are usually not tender unless secondary bacterial infection has occurred. Physical examination may be unremarkable but for palpable lymphadenopathy. Sometimes, lymph node abscess may burst leading to a chronic non-healing TB sinus and ulcer. The typical TB sinus has thin, bluish, undermined edges with scanty watery discharge [Figure 22.2].

Various complications have also been described due to mediastinal lymph node TB. These include dysphagia due to pressure on the oesophagus (26,27), oesophago-mediastinal fistula (28-30), tracheo-oesophageal fistula (31,32). Sometimes TB tracheo-oesophageal fistula may mimick a malignant tracheo-oesophageal fistula. Occasionally, upper abdominal and mediastinal lymph nodes may cause thoracic duct obstruction and present as chylothorax, chylous ascites or chyluria (33). Rarely, jaundice occurs because of biliary obstruction due to enlarged lymph nodes (34). Cardiac

Table 22.1: Demographic characteristics and symptoms at presentation in adult patients with peripheral lymph node TB

	Studies from India		Studies from other parts of the world			
	Dandapat et al (3) [n = 80]	Subrahmanyam (4) [n = 105]	Chen et al (23) [n = 71]	Thompson et al (2) [n = 67]		Fain et al (24) [n = 59]
				Asian group* [n = 54]	White group [n = 13]	
Variable						
Place of study	Berhampur	Solapur	Taipei	Leicester	Leicester	Paris
Duration of study [years]	1	1.5	6	10	10	4
Mean age [years]	†	‡	42	41.8	46.9	37.6
Male:Female	1:12	1:1.3	1:1.5	1:1.5	1:2.3	1:1.5
History of contact with a case of TB or family history [%]	ND	5.7	ND	48	7.7	23.7
Symptoms [%]						
Fever	40	45	9.9	13	7.7	30.5
Weight loss	85	78	9.9	13	23.1	47.5
Night sweats	37	35	ND	9.3	15.4	22
Cough	10	ND	8.5	14.8	0	0
Others	ND	ND	§	‖	‖	¶

* Patients from the Indian subcontinent
† Mean age was not described. Age range = 1 to 65 years
‡ Mean age was not described. Age range = 1.5 to 68 years
§ Other symptoms included dysphagia [2.8%]; haemoptysis [2.8%]; vomiting [2.8%]
‖ Anorexia occurred in 7.4% patients in the Indian subcontinent group and 15.4% patients in the White group
¶ Asthenia occurred in 47.5% cases
TB = tuberculosis; ND = not described

Table 22.2: Physical signs at presentation observed in adult patients with peripheral lymph node tuberculosis

| | Studies from India | | Studies from other parts of the world | | | |
| | Dandapat et al (3) [n = 80] | Subrahmanyam (4) [n = 105] | Chen et al (23) [n = 71] | Thompson et al (2) [n = 67] | | Fain et al (24) [n = 59] |
Variable				Asian group* [n = 54]	White group [n = 13]	
Site of involvement [%]						
Cervical	70	93.3	91.5	85	84.5	73.1
Axillary	6	3.8	12.7	11.1	7.7	15.4
Inguinal	9	2.9	7	3.7	7.7	9.6
Multiple sites	15	ND	14.0†	ND	ND	15.3‡
Physical findings [%]						
Matting and fixity	55	68	ND	ND	ND	ND
Discrete nodes	22.5	32	ND	ND	ND	ND
Abscess formation	15	15.2	ND	ND	ND	ND
Sinuses	13	10.5	ND	ND	ND	ND
Ulcers	ND	7.6	ND	ND	ND	ND

* Patients from the Indian subcontinent
† Right elbow nodes were enlarged in 1.4% patients. Two sites were involved in 14%; three sites were involved in 7% and four sites were involved in 4.4% patients
‡ Of the 59 patients studied, 69 different lymph node sites were noted; 46 patients [78%] had exclusive lymph node disease. A superficial distribution was found in 52 cases [88.1%] and isolated superficial lymph node involvement was found in 32 patients [54.2%]. Deep lymph node involvement [mediastinal and abdominal] was observed in 17 patients [32.7%] and isolated deep lymph node involvement was found in 7 patients [11.9%]
ND = not described

Table 22.3: Evidence of associated pulmonary TB in adult patients with peripheral lymph node TB

| | Studies from India | | Studies from other parts of the world | | | |
| | Dandapat et al (3) [n = 80] | Subrahmanyam (4) [n = 105] | Chen et al (23) [n = 71] | Thompson et al (2) [n = 59]* | | Fain et al (24) [n = 59] |
Variable				Asian group† [n = 11]	White group [n = 48]	
Associated pulmonary TB [%]	5	16.2	42‡	44	18	ND

* Chest radiographs were done in 59 of the 67 patients studied
† Patients from the Indian subcontinent
‡ Among those with cervical lymph node TB, 33% of those with upper-third cervical lymph node involvement and 58.7% of patients with lower-third cervical lymph node involvement had radiological features of pulmonary TB
TB = tuberculosis; ND = not described

tamponade (35) due to TB mediastinal lymphadenitis, massive haemoptysis due to tracheo-pulmonary artery fistula and pseudoaneurysm of the pulmonary artery (36) have also been reported.

Tuberculosis Lymphadenitis in Patients with Human Immunodeficiency Virus Infection

Lymph node enlargement is a common feature in patients with HIV infection. In HIV-positive patients, lymphadenopathy can result from primary HIV-induced pathology and from diseases, such as, TB lymphadenitis, lymphadenopathy due to NTM, nodal Kaposi's sarcoma and nodal lymphoma (37,38). In HIV-negative patients, TB lymphadenitis often occurs as a focal cervical lymphadenopathy with other groups of lymph nodes being occasionally involved [Table 22.2] (2-4,23,24). The disease often presents as multifocal lymphadenopathy in HIV-positive patients. Comparison of clinical presentation of TB lymphadenitis in HIV-positive and HIV-negative patients is shown in Table 22.5 (37,38).

Nontuberculous Mycobacterial Lymphadenitis

Nontuberculous mycobacterial lymphadenitis often occurs in children. Constitutional symptoms seldom occur and the disease generally remains localised to the upper cervical area [Table 22.6]. If untreated, the nodes often progress to softening, rupture, sinus formation, healing with fibrosis

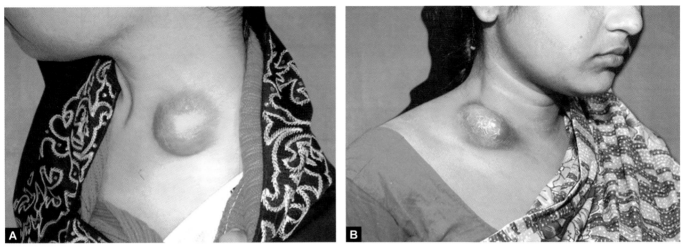

Figure 22.1: Clinical photograph showing left sided [A], right sided [B] TB cervical lymphadenitis
TB = tuberculosis

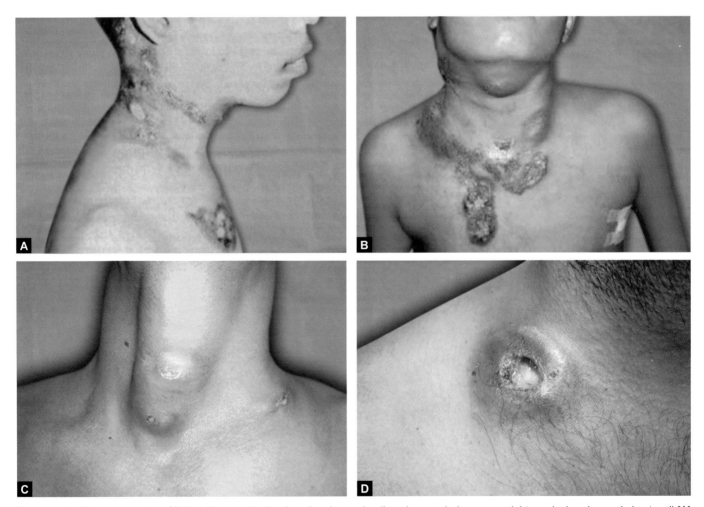

Figure 22.2: TB lymphadenitis. Clinical photograph showing chronic non-healing sinus and ulcers over right cervical region and chest wall [A]; suprahyoid, bilateral cervical and axillary lymphadenitis with chronic non-healing ulcers [B]; and suprasternal and left supraclavicular lymphadenitis with discharging sinuses [C]. Clinical photograph of another patient showing right sided cervical TB lymphadenitis with a chronic non-healing sinus and ulcer [D]
TB = tuberculosis

Table 22.4: Physical appearance of lymph node tuberculosis

Stage 1

Enlarged, firm, mobile, discrete nodes showing non-specific reactive hyperplasia

Stage 2

Larger rubbery nodes fixed to surrounding tissue owing to periadenitis

Stage 3

Central softening due to caseation necrosis and abscess formation

Stage 4

Collar-stud abscess formation

Stage 5

Sinus tract formation

Based on *"Jones PG, Campbell PE. Tuberculous lymphadenitis in childhood: the significance of anonymous mycobacteria. Br J Surg 1962;50:302-14 (reference 25)"*

and calcification (16,22,25). Appropriate laboratory tests must be performed to differentiate lymphadenitis due to NTM and *Mtb* as response to anti-TB is not good in the former. The reader is referred to the chapter *"Non-tuberculous mycobacterial infections" [Chapter 41]* for further details.

DIFFERENTIAL DIAGNOSIS

There are numerous causes of peripheral lymphadenopathy. This list includes reactive lymphadenitis [secondary to viral, bacterial infections], TB, lymphoma, sarcoidosis, secondary carcinoma and uncommon causes like fungal diseases, toxoplasmosis and diseases of the reticulo-endothelial system, among others. Multiplicity, matting and caseation are three features which help in the diagnosis of TB lymphadenitis. In patients with lymphoma, the lymph nodes are rubbery in consistency and are not matted. In patients with secondary deposits in the lymph node [from a primary somewhere in the drainage area], the lymph node is usually hard and may be fixed to surrounding structures.

Table 22.5: Comparison of clinical characteristics of lymph node TB in HIV-positive and HIV-negative patients

Variable	Bem (37)		Mohan et al (38)	
	HIV-positive [n = 157]	HIV-negative [n = 71]	HIV-positive [n = 34]	HIV-negative [n = 390]
Mean age [years]	30.6	30.6	28.4	27.8
Male:Female	1:0.9	1:1.2	1:1.3	1:1.3
Site of involvement [%]				
Cervical	99*	96	96	90
Axillary	82	43	82	37
Inguinal	84	14	71	10
Multiple sites	90	39	89	33
Physical findings [%]				
Firm and mobile	51	51	ND	ND
Matted, irregular/hard and additional local signs	49†	49	ND	ND
Histopathlogical type				
Epithelioid granulomas				
with caseation necrosis	ND	ND	18	75
without caseation necrosis	ND	ND	21	23
Suppurative variety	ND	ND	29	01
Non-reactive	ND	ND	32	01
Chest radiograph findings [%]			ND	ND
Pulmonary infiltration	46‡	60§	ND	ND
Cavitation	3‡	0§	ND	ND
Pleural effusion	17‡	13§	ND	ND
Pericardial effusion	13‡	0§	ND	ND

* Among patients with lymph node TB, lymphadenopathy was confined to the neck in 10% HIV-positive patients compared to 57% HIV-negative patients. Further, isolated unilateral TB cervical lymphadenitis was observed in only 1 of the 157 HIV-positive patients compared to 32% in HIV-negative patients

† Among HIV-positive patients with lymph node TB, local signs included sinuses [n = 2]; cold abscess [n = 3]; tender nodes [n = 3]; inflammatory mass [n = 3]. Among HIV-negative patients with lymph node TB, local signs included sinuses [n = 2]; tender nodes [n = 1]; inflammatory mass [n = 1]. None of the patients with primary HIV lymphadenopathy demonstrated local signs

‡ Tested in 110 patients

§ Tested in 15 patients

TB = tuberculosis; HIV = human immunodeficiency virus

Table 22.6: Comparison between TB lymphadenitis and NTM lymphadenitis

Variable	TB lymphadenitis	NTM lymphadenitis
Age	Any age group	Children
Sex	Female preponderance	Equal between sexes
Constitutional symptoms	Common	Rare
Lymph node involvement	Cervical lymph nodes are most commonly involved. Axillary and inguinal lymph nodes may also be involved. Bilateral involvement is common	Localised disease often involving cervical lymph nodes [jugulodigastric, submandibular, preauricular]. Unilateral involvement is common
Chest radiographic evidence of pulmonary or pleural TB	Common	Rare
Tuberculin skin test	Often reactive	Non-reactive
Response to antituberculosis treatment	Good	Poor

NTM = nontuberculous mycobacteria; TB = tuberculosis

DIAGNOSIS

Apart from a focussed history and a detailed clinical examination, several other investigations are required for confirming the diagnosis of lymph node TB. Often, one diagnostic modality might not be sufficient to make a diagnosis of TB. Hence, the concept of a composite reference standard [CRS] has been developed to make a diagnosis of EPTB including lymph node TB (39). The CRS includes yield from mycobacterial culture, histopathology, cytopathology, molecular diagnostic methods and response to treatment. In patients symptomatic for other forms of EPTB, screening with appropriate modality in such form of organ involvement should be simultaneously done. For example, in a patient with lymph node TB, presence of severe headache, evaluation for TB meningitis is warranted.

Tuberculin Skin Test and Interferon-gamma Release Assays

Tuberculin skin test [TST] is positive in about 75% immunocompetent patients with lymph node TB while it is often non-reactive in patients with NTM lymphadenitis (1,9,10). Interferon-gamma release assays [IGRAs] have also become available for the diagnosis of TB infection. However, a negative TST or IGRA does not rule out the possibility of active TB. The reader is referred to the chapter *"Laboratory diagnosis of tuberculosis: best practices and current policies"* [Chapter 8] for further details.

Imaging

Imaging modalities facilitate anatomical localisation, extent of disease. In addition, these modalities facilitate image-guided diagnostic or therapeutic aspiration from deep-seated lesions.

Chest Radiograph

A chest radiograph should be routinely performed in patients suspected to have lymph node TB. In patients with TB lymphadenitis, abnormalities are often discernible on the chest radiograph [Table 22.3] (2-4,23,24). However, there is a wide variation in the reported incidence of chest radiographic abnormalities with the figure ranging from 5%-44% [Table 22.3] (2-4,23,24). The reported incidence of paratracheal, hilar and mediastinal lymphadenopathy in patients with peripheral lymphadenopathy has varied widely from 5%-12% (2,3,14,16). In a patient with lymph node TB, presence of infiltrates in the chest radiograph will reclassify the patient to pulmonary TB as per the Revised National Tuberculosis Control Programme [RNTCP] of Government of India. From a clinician's point of view, such a patient would be considered to have disseminated TB as they have involvement of two non-contiguous sites, i.e. lymph node and lung.

Ultrasonography

Peripheral lymph node TB patients can have concomitant abdominal lymph node involvement. Although data on prevalence of abdominal lymphadenopathy in peripheral lymph node TB patients has not been studied in large cohorts, studies conducted in patients co-infected with HIV and TB have revealed a high prevalence of concomitant involvement of peripheral and abdominal lymph nodes (40). Hence, ultrasonography of the abdomen should be carried out in all patients with peripheral lymph node TB. Abdominal ultrasonography may reveal retroperitoneal, portal or mesenteric lymphadenopathy. On ultrasonography, enlarged lymph nodes or a confluent mass with central necrosis may be evident. Adrenal deposits, terminal ileal thickening, caecal fat, stranding, ascites may also be detected.

Computed Tomography

Computed tomography [CT] of the chest is required for accurate evaluation of the intrathoracic lymph nodes if the chest radiograph shows any evidence of mediastinal or hilar lymphadenopathy. CT of the abdomen is helpful in assessing the retroperitoneal, porta hepatis or mesenteric lymph

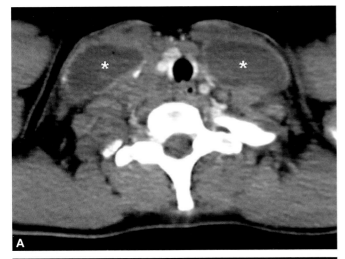

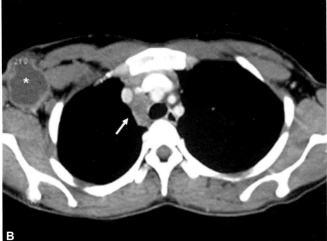

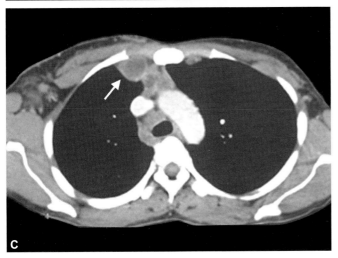

Figure 22.3: CECT of the neck and chest showing bilateral cervical [A] [asterisk]; right-sided axillary [asterisk] [B] and intrathoracic [arrow] lymphadenopathy [B,C]. Peripheral rim enhancement with central attenuation can be seen. Fine needle aspiration cytology of the cervical lymph node confirmed the diagnosis of tuberculosis

nodes. Lymph node calcification is best picked up by CT. The lymph nodes show enlargement with hypodense areas, sometimes central necrosis with peripheral rim-enhancement

or calcification [Figures 11.4, 11.5A, 11.5B, 11.5C, and 22.3]. With modern CT scanners, a simultaneous acquisition of high resolution CT [HRCT] and contrast-enhanced CT [CECT] images is possible. A simultaneous HRCT of the chest may delineate chest infiltrates that may not have been visualised on the plain chest radiograph. CT enterography which utilises administration of both oral and intravenous contrast, provides better delineation of intestinal mucosa.

Magnetic Resonance Imaging

Magnetic resonance imaging [MRI] of the chest is emerging as a useful modality to characterise and monitor mediastinal lymphadenopathy (41). MRI is useful especially when radiation hazard is considered an important concern as in children and pregnant women. The image resolution of lymph nodes and parenchymal lesions are considered slightly better than CT, although adequate studies have not been performed in this area (42). Important drawbacks of MRI include longer acquisition time, patient discomfort and high cost.

Positron Emission Tomography and Fusion Modalities

Positron emission tomography [PET] is fast emerging as a modality of choice to assess the disease extent [Figure 22.4] and monitor response to treatment. A study conducted in HIV-TB co-infected patients documented PET response in the form of change in maximum standardised uptake value [SUVmax] after 6 weeks to be highly predictive of response to anti-TB treatment (43). Similar studies in HIV-seronegative patients with lymph node TB are lacking. Also, as PET detects active inflammation, it is also being seen as a promising modality to help in deciding the end of treatment in future. As on date, PET is still an unproven yet promising investigational tool for TB. Drawbacks of PET include high cost, operational difficulty, radiation hazard to patients and operators, among others.

Fusion modalities like PET-CT, PET-MRI are fast developing imaging modalities which combine the anatomic precision of CT or MRI with the sensitivity of PET in determining active disease. These have not been adequately tested in TB. High costs and low availability may also preclude their common-place use in near future in addition to the usual drawbacks of CT, MRI or PET.

The reader is referred to the chapter *"Roentgenographic manifestations of pulmonary and extrapulmonary tuberculosis"* [*Chapter 9*] for further details.

Cytopathology/Histopathology

The definitive diagnosis of lymph node TB is established by mycobacterial culture, nucleic acid amplification tests [NAAT]. But, it is not possible to obtain microbiological diagnosis in a large proportion of cases with lymph node TB. Cytopathological and histopathological examination of lymph nodes are highly sensitive for diagnosis of TB and are, therefore, useful in such circumstances.

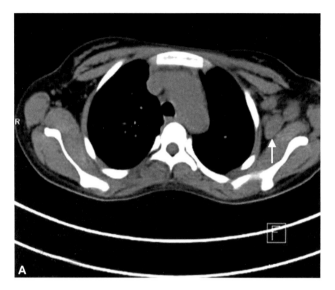

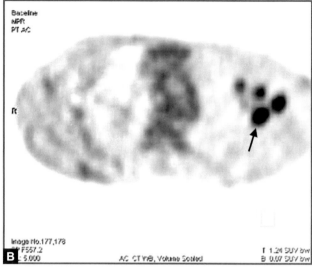

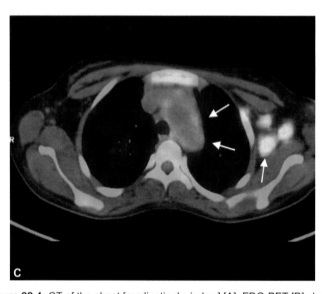

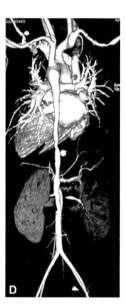

Figure 22.4: CT of the chest [mediastinal window] [A], FDG-PET [B] showing left axillary lymphadenopathy [arrows]. PET-CT image of the same patient showing increased uptake aorta [arrows] [C]. Volume rendered CT angiography image showing diffuse long segment narrowing of left subclavian artery and abdominal aorta at the renal artery origin level as well as infrarenal segment suggestive of non-specific aortoarteritis [D]. Left axillary lymph node histopathological examination confirmed the diagnosis of TB

CT = computed tomography; FDG-PET = F-18 fluorodeoxyglucose positron emission tomography; PET-CT = positron emission tomography-computed tomography; TB = tuberculosis

Fine needle aspiration cytology [FNAC], a relatively non-invasive, pain-free, out-patient procedure has established itself as a safe, cheap and reliable procedure for the diagnosis of peripheral lymphadenopathy (44-47). The characteristic cytopathological changes include epithelioid cell granulomas with or without multinucleate giant cells and caseation necrosis (44-48). Several authors have evaluated the sensitivity and specificity of FNAC in the diagnosis of peripheral lymphadenopathy by comparing it with histopathological examination and found it to be a useful technique (44-48). Lau *et al* (47) reported the sensitivity and specificity of FNAC in the diagnosis of lymph node TB to be 77% and 93%, respectively compared to histopathology. Dandapat *et al* (3) reported a true positive diagnosis in 83%, a

false negative result in 14% and equivocal results in 3%. Similar results have been documented in other studies [Table 22.7] (2-4,23,24).

In cases with suspected mediastinal lymph node TB, various techniques including transbronchial needle aspiration (49), endobronchial ultrasound [EBUS] (50) or endoscopic ultrasonography [EUS] guided FNAC or biopsy (51), ultrasonography or CT-guided transthoracic percutaneous FNAC or biopsy (52) are helpful. Cervical mediastinoscopy and video-assisted thoracoscopic surgery (53) have been used to obtain lymph node sample for diagnosis in the past, but are infrequently being used presently.

As the mycobacteria are not documented in every case, certain histopathological changes have been accepted as

Table 22.7: Method of diagnosis in adult patients with peripheral lymph node tuberculosis

	Studies from India		Studies from other parts of the world		
Variable	Dandapat et al (3) [n = 80]	Subrahmanyam (4) [n = 105]	Chen et al (23) [n = 71]	Thompson et al (2)* [n = 67]	Fain et al (24) [n = 59]
Fine needle aspiration cytology	83†	ND	ND	ND	38‡‡ [n = 26]
Lymph node biopsy Histopathology	100‡	100	100‖ [n = 64]	100** [n = 60]	100§§ [n = 39]
Microbiology	65	§	80¶ [n = 10]	100†† [n = 7]	36 [n = 39]

All values are shown as percentages
Numbers in square brackets indicate number tested
* Included 54 patients of Asian origin and 13 White patients
† False-negative results were observed in 14% and equivocal results were observed in 3% patients
‡ 80% patients had caseating granulomas; and 20% had non-caseating granulomas
§ Microbiological examination was not done in this study
‖ A total of 64 specimens were obtained for histopathological exmamination: excision biopsy [n = 32]; total excision [n = 29]; neck dissection [n = 3]. Acid-fast bacilli were found in 35 of the 64 specimens
¶ Only 10 of the 64 specimens were subjected to culture on Lowenstein-Jensen medium and eight yielded *Mycobacterium tuberculosis*.
**Histopathological examination was done in only 60 of the 67 patients. Biopsy specimens were not sent for microbiological examination in 13 of these 60 patients. Histopathology was positive in all the 60 patients. In 13 of these 60 patients, both histopathological and microbiological methods yielded the diagnosis
†† In 7 patients, histopathological exmination was not done and microbiological examination alone was done
‡‡ Of the 26 patients in whom fine needle aspiration was performed, bacteriological diagnosis was possible in 38% cases and acid-fast bacilli were positive in 2 of them
§§ Of these 39 patients, histopathological examination revealed caseating granulomas in 82%, isolated granulomata in 13% and non-specific inflammatory lesions which revealed *Mycobacterium tuberculosis* in 5%

suggestive of TB. These include granulomatous inflammation with caseation necrosis [Figure 22.5]. However, it must be clarified that, although highly suggestive, these changes are by no means specific and may sometimes be seen in other diseases also (54). Therefore, the pathological features of lymph node TB are classified as 'consistent' or 'compatible' with TB. A pattern 'consistent with TB' demonstrates acid-fast bacilli [AFB] with caseating granulomas which is almost confirmatory for *Mtb*. A pattern 'compatible with TB' has granulomas or caseation only without AFB positivity. The latter justifies treatment with anti-TB treatment if a high clinical suspicion of TB is present. In such a patient, close follow-up is necessary to monitor response as alternate diagnosis is possible.

Microbiological Methods

Microbiological tests form the backbone of investigations in lymph node TB and are summarised below.

Smear Microscopy

Smear microscopy, a fast, cheap and readily available method, is still an important diagnostic modality for the diagnosis of lymph node TB, especially in resource-limited settings (55).

Mycobacterial Culture and Drug-Susceptibility Testing

Currently, liquid culture is considered to be the "gold standard" for the diagnosis of TB while conventional solid

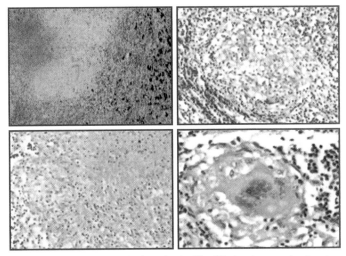

Figure 22.5: Tuberculosis lymphadenitis. Photomicrograph showing epithelioid granulomas with caseation necrosis and peripheral lympho-cyte infiltration [upper panel, left; *Haematoxylin and eosin × 100*], well-defined epithelioid granulomas with lymphocytic infiltration [upper panel, right; *Haematoxylin and eosin × 200*], epithelioid granuloma, caseation, lymphocytic infiltration [lower panel, left; *Haematoxylin and eosin × 200*] and multinucleated Langhans' giant cell and lymphocytic infiltration [lower panel, right; *Haematoxylin and eosin × 400*]

culture on Lowenstein-Jensen medium is the "gold standard" for drug-susceptibility testing [DST]. The sensitivity and specificity of TB culture is comparable to Xpert MTB/ RIF (56). Unlike the molecular methods which detect the deoxyribonucleic acid [DNA] of dead bacilli, mycobacterial culture documents the presence of live multiplying bacteria. Therefore, mycobacterial culture is also useful in assessing deciding treatment completion in patients with residual lymphadenopathy at the end of treatment. The reader is referred to the chapter *"Laboratory diagnosis of tuberculosis: best practices and current policies"* [Chapter 8] for details.

Molecular Methods

In-house polymerase chain reaction [PCR] that uses locally developed probes has been used since the 1990s for the diagnosis of lymph node TB. Though this method was highly sensitive, problems like occurrence of contamination, false positive test results, lack of reproducibility and high cost have restricted its wide applicability.

Presently, a newer diagnostic modality, Xpert MTB/RIF is increasingly being used for the diagnosis of lymph node TB. The Xpert MTB/RIF® is a cartridge-based nucleic acid amplification test [CBNAAT] which amplifies rpoB gene in the body fluid/tissue samples and uses molecular beacons to identify the resistance conferring mutations. In a systematic review (56) [598 samples, 5 studies], the pooled sensitivity and specificity of Xpert MTB/RIF in the diagnosis of lymph node TB considering CRS as the gold standard was found to be 81.2% and 99.1% respectively. Sharma *et al* (39) from New Delhi [n = 273], reported the sensitivity and specificity of Xpert MTB/RIF in the diagnosis of lymph node TB to be 78% and 91%, respectively. By detecting rifampicin resistance, Xpert MTB/RIF is also useful for rapid diagnosis of drug-resistant TB. The Xpert MTB/RIF has been approved by the World Health Organization [WHO] for use in initial diagnosis of TB in sputum, and extra-pulmonary tissue specimens, such as, lymph node aspirate, biopsy material (57). The recently published Guidelines for Extrapulmonary TB for India [INDEX-TB Guidelines] (58a), and a recent systematic review (58b), suggest that Xpert MTB/RIF may be used as additional test to conventional smear microscopy, culture and cytology in FNAC specimens for lymph node TB [*strong recommendation*].

Serodiagnostic Methods

Over 50 types of serological tests for different TB antibodies and antigen have been marketed with high claims (59). These tests have performed poorly with low sensitivity, specificity. Serological tests are discouraged by the WHO, and banned by the Government of India (60-62).

TREATMENT

Presently, it is generally agreed that anti-TB treatment alone is sufficient for majority of the cases and surgical intervention is required only in selected cases for specific situations. In India, patients with lymph node TB receive daily treatment under the RNTCP of the Government of India. The reader is referred to the chapter *"Revised National Tuberculosis Control Programme"* [Chapter 53] for details.

The number of drugs required and the ideal duration of treatment for lymph node TB have been an area of intense research. Observations from a series of randomised clinical trials conducted by the British Thoracic Society [BTS] resulted in the shortening of the duration of treatment from 18 months to 9 months initially and later to 6 months (6). In 1990, the group from Tuberculosis Research Centre [TRC], Chennai (5) reported results of their prospective trial evaluating a supervised short-course [6 months] intermittent chemotherapy regimen consisting of streptomycin, rifampicin, isoniazid and pyrazinamide three times a week for two months followed by streptomycin and isoniazid twice a week for four months on an out-patient basis in children with lymph node TB. Out of 168 patients finally analysed, favourable clinical response was noted in most patients at the end of the treatment. They concluded that in children, TB lymphadenitis can be successfully treated with a short-course chemotherapy regimen of six months. Thereafter, the British Thoracic Society's next trial (63,64) compared the following regimens: rifampicin, isoniazid, ethambutol for the initial two months, followed by rifampicin and isoniazid for the subsequent seven months; rifampicin, isoniazid, pyrazinamide for the initial two months, followed by rifampicin and isoniazid for the subsequent four months. The six months regimen was found to be equally effective in terms of response with an advantage of increased convenience and reduced cost. There was no difference in the speed of resolution of nodes, in the percentage of patients with residual nodes at the end of the treatment or in the numbers developing fluctuation or sinuses. However, seven patients in the ethambutol group and only one in the pyrazinamide group required aspiration of pus from lymph nodes. This may be because pyrazinamide, being bactericidal kills bacteria which are intracellular, making glands less likely to become fluctuant on treatment. In a study reported by Jawahar *et al* (6), patients with biopsy confirmed superficial lymph node TB were randomly allocated to receive two-drug regimens of either a daily self-administered six-month regimen [n = 136] of rifampicin and isoniazid, or a twice-weekly, directly observed, six-month regimen of rifampicin and isoniazid plus pyrazinamide for the first two months [n = 141]. Of the 277 enrolled patients, data were available for analysis in 268 patients [n = 134 from each group]. At the end of treatment, 87% patients in each treatment group had a favourable clinical response; 14 [11%] and 17 [13%] patients had a doubtful response, and 4 [3%]; and one [1%] patients had an unfavourable response among those treated with the daily and twice-weekly regimen, respectively. The authors suggested that these regimens may be considered as alternatives to the existing regimens. Experience at the Paediatric Tuberculosis Clinic at the AIIMS hospital, New Delhi (65) [n = 459], indicated that pulmonary TB was the the most common followed by lymph node TB. Of the 16 children with isolated lymph node TB who received category III treatment [thrice-weekly intermittent therapy with rifampicin, isoniazid and pyrazinamide administered for the first two months followed by rifampicin and isoniazid for the subsequent four months], 12 were cured with the primary regimen; three children achieved cure with extended primary regimen; and one child was lost to follow-up.

A multicentric study (66) conducted in 8 centres in India assessed the efficacy of the 6-month thrice-weekly intermittent directly observed treatment [DOT] and need for prolongation of treatment to 9 months for non-resolution of lymphadenopathy in patients with peripheral lymph node TB. Patients with poor resolution at the end of 6-months treatment were randomised to extended treatment up to 9 months or observation without additional treatment. At the end of 6-months of treatment, resolution of lymphadenopathy was evident in 517/551 (93.8%) patients. In the 34 patients with poor resolution at 6 months, there was no difference in response in the remaining 34 patients with [n = 16] or without [n = 18] extension of treatment to 9 months.

The evidence-based INDEX-TB guidelines (58) recommend 6 months standard first-line anti-TB treatment for peripheral lymph node TB [*strong recommendation, low quality evidence*].

However, some patients with lymph node TB invariably require longer duration of treatment. While response to anti-TB treatment may be delayed in patients with TB lymphadenitis, it is a common practice among physician and surgeons to label these patients with a diagnosis of multidrug-resistant TB [MDR-TB] lymphadentitis. But it must be understood that MDR-TB is a laboratory diagnosis and for establishing this, the organisms must be grown in the laboratory and *in vitro* resistance to rifampicin and isoniazid must be demonstrated. Since lymphadentitis is a paucibacillary disease, it is not easy to grow *Mtb* in cultures in most instances. Therefore, a label of MDR-TB lymphadenitis should be used judiciously. Where ever possible, initial phenotypic and genotypic DST should be carried out, on the lymph node tissue.

The results of various studies have shown that lymph nodes may enlarge in size during anti-TB treatment, or, new nodes may appear during or after anti-TB treatment (5,6,67). The development of new lymph node enlargement while on treatment may represent an immunological response, sometimes called the "paradoxical reaction". This phenomenon is usually transient and the nodes ultimately regress in size. Fluctuation may appear in some lymph nodes while on treatment. This cold pus should be aspirated under strict aseptic conditions. In case there is secondary bacterial infection presenting as a classical abscess, drainage and appropriate broad-spectrum antibiotics may be required in addition to anti-TB treatment.

While the term "immune reconstitution inflammatory syndrome [IRIS]" is usually used in HIV-seropositive patients who are receiving antiretroviral treatment [ART], the term "paradoxical reaction" is generally used to describe a clinical worsening of TB disease in HIV-seropositive and HIV-seronegative patients after initiation of anti-TB treatment (67). Case definitions for paradoxical TB-associated IRIS, ART-associated TB [Figure 22.6] and unmasking TB-associated IRIS [provisional] have been

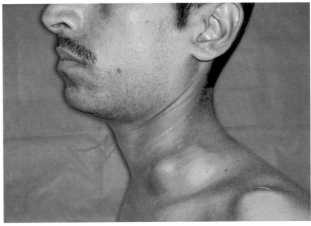

Figure 22.6: Antiretroviral treatment associated immune reconstitution inflammatory syndrome manifesting as left sided cervical lymphadenitis in a human immunodeficiency virus-seropositive patient

described (68). Symptomatic management of fever, cough, pain and other complains may be sufficient in vast majority of cases (69). Severe reactions like acute respiratory distress syndrome [ARDS], tuberculomas and pericardial effusion may require glucocorticoid therapy for few weeks (70). If DST pattern is unknown, it is usually advised to get tissue sampling done in such cases as around 10% cases of initially suspected paradoxical reactions are found to harbour drug resistance or secondary infection (69). A recent study (71a) on immunological alterations in TB-associated IRIS in people living with HIV/AIDS showed dominance of proinflammatory cells, such as, interleukin-17A cell, cytokines and chemokines, interferon-gamma [IFN-γ], IFN-γ inducible protein-10 and monokine induced by IFN-γ in TB-IRIS patients favours the development of IRIS event.

Sometimes, residual lymphadenopathy may persist at the end of the course of anti-TB treatment. These can be left as such and the patients observed under close follow-up as many of these nodes are expected to resolve over a period of time. If the nodes increase in size further or systemic features reappear, an excision biopsy of the gland for histopathology and mycobacterial culture should be done. Some workers recommend biopsy of all significant [>10 mm] residual lymph nodes and re-treatment only if cultures are positive. All culture positive isolates must be sent for DST and treatment should be tailored according to DST results. The second-line anti-TB drugs should not be added unless MDR-TB is proven in an accredited laboratory. Apart from the biopsy of the lymph nodes, surgical intervention is required only for aspiration or drainage of abcesses in a few patients or total clearance of that lymph node in some others.

Treatment of mediastinal TB poses special problems in diagnosis, monitoring as well as decision on end of therapy. A cohort study (71b) had evaluated the efficacy of anti-TB treatment in mediastinal lymph node TB. Out of 41 patients enrolled, 36 [87%] had adequate response with sub-centrimetric lymph nodes at the end of therapy, three had intercurrent paradoxical reactions and three had lymph node size greater than 1 cm at the end of therapy. The later 2 subsets were given additional treatment of 3 months and all six patients had good response. The outcomes of long-term follow-up in these patients is also unknown. These observations suggest that a standard 6 months course of anti-TB treatment is adequate in isolated mediastinal lymph node TB with an uncomplicated course.

It is generally accepted that anti-TB treatment is ineffective and complete surgical excision is recommended for lymphadenitis caused by NTM (72). Therefore, whenever a biopsy is being performed for diagnosis, especially if it happens to be from a preferred site for NTM lymphadenitis such as submandibular or pre-auricular area, a complete excision or preferably selective nodal dissection of that area should be performed. A macrolide-based regimen should be considered for patients with extensive *Mycobacterium avium-intracellulare complex* lymphadenitis or poor response to surgical therapy (72). The reader is referred to the chapter *"Nontuberculous mycobacterial infections [Chapter 41]"* for further details.

REFERENCES

1. Lazarus AA, Thilagar B. Tuberculous lymphadenitis. Dis Mon 2007; 53:10-5.
2. Thompson MM, Underwood MJ, Sayers RD, Dookeran KA, Bell PRF. Peripheral tuberculous lymphadenopathy: a review of 67 cases. Br J Surg 1992;79:763-4.
3. Dandapat MC. Mishra BM, Dash SP, Kar PK. Peripheral lymph node tuberculosis: a review of 80 cases. Br J Surg 1990;77:911-2.
4. Subrahmanyam M. Role of surgery and chemotherapy for peripheral lymph node tuberculosis. Br J Surg 1993;8: 1547-8.
5. Jawahar MS, Sivasubramaniam S, Vijayan VK, Ramakrishnan CV, Paramasivan CN, Selvakumar V, et al. Short-course chemotherapy for tuberculous lymphadenitis in children. BMJ 1990; 301:359-62.
6. Jawahar MS, Rajaram K, Sivasubramanian S, Paramasivan CN, Chandrasekar K, Kamaludeen MN, et al. Treatment of lymph node tuberculosis - a randomized clinical trial of two 6-month regimens. Trop Med Int Health 2005;10:1090-8.
7. Sharma SK, Mohan A. Extrapulmonary tuberculosis. Indian J Med Res 2004;120:316-53.
8. Narang P, Narang R, Narang R, Mendiratta DK, Sharma SM, Tyagi NK. Prevalence of tuberculous lymphadenitis in children in Wardha district, Maharashtra State, India. Int J Tuberc Lung Dis 2005;9:188-94.
9. Wright JE. Non-tuberculous mycobacterial lymphadenitis. Aust N Z J Surg 1996;66:225-8.
10. Bayazit YA, Bayazit N, Namiduru M. Mycobacterial cervical lymphadenitis. ORL J Otorhinolaryngol Relat Spec 2004;66: 275-80.
11. Llewelyn DM, Dorman D. Mycobacterial lymphadenitis. Aust Paediatr J 1971;7:97-102.
12. Roba-Kiewicz M, Grzybowski S. Epidemiologic aspects of non-tuberculous mycobacterial diseases and of tuberculosis in British Columbia. Am Rev Respir Dis 1974;109:613-20.
13. Shikhani A, Hadi UM, Mufarriz AA, Zaytoun GM. Mycobacterial cervical lymphadenitis. Ear Nose Throat J 1989; 68:660, 662-6, 668-72.
14. Manolidis S, Frenkiel S, Yoskovitch A, Black M. Mycobacterial infections of the head and neck. Otolaryngol Head Neck Surg 1993;109:427-33.
15. Yates MD, Grange JM. Bacteriological survey of tuberculous lymphadenitis in South-east England, 1981-1989. J Epidemiol Community Health 1992;46:332-5.
16. Pang SC. Mycobacterial lymphadenitis in Western Australia. Tuber Lung Dis 1992;73:362-7.
17. Lee KC, Tami TA, Lalwani AK, Schecter G. Contemporary management of cervical tuberculosis. Laryngoscope 1992;102: 60-4.
18. Cantrell R, Jensen JH, Reid D. Diagnosis and management of tuberculous cervical adenitis. Arch Otolaryngol 1975;101: 53-7.
19. Comstock GW, Edwards LB, Livesay VT. Tuberculosis morbidity in the US Navy: its distribution and decline. Am Rev Respir Dis 1974;110:571-80.
20. Rich AR. The pathogenesis of tuberculosis. Springfield: Thomas; 1950.
21. Kent DC. Tuberculous lymphadenitis: not a localized disease process. Am J Med Sci 1967;254:866.
22. Olson RN. Nontuberculous mycobacterial infections of the face and neck-practical considerations. Laryngoscope 1981;91: 1714-26.
23. Chen Y-M, Lee P-Y, Su W-J, Perng R-P. Lymph node tuberculosis: 7-year experience in Veterans GeneralHospital, Taipei, Taiwan. Tuber Lung Dis 1992;73:368-71.
24. Fain O, Lortholary O, Djouab M, Amoura I, Bainet P, Beaudreuil J, et al. Lymph node tuberculosis in the suburbs of Paris: 59 cases in adults not infected by the human immuno-deficiency virus. Int J Tuberc Lung Dis 1993;3:162-5.
25. Jones PG, Campbell PE. Tuberculous lymphadenitis in childhood: the significance of anonymous mycobacteria. Br J Surg 1962;50:302-14.
26. Singh B, Moodly M, Goga AD, Haffejee AA. Dysphagia secondary to tuberculous lymphadenitis. S Afr J Surg 1996;34:197-9.
27. Gupta SP, Arora A, Bhargava DK. An unusual presentation of oesophageal tuberculosis. Tuber Lung Dis 1992;73:174-6.
28. Ohtake M, Saito H, Okuno M, Yamamoto S, Ohgimi T. Esophago-mediastinal fistula as a complication of tuberculous mediastinal lymphadenitis. Intern Med 1996;35: 984-6.
29. Adkins MS, Raccuia JS, Acinapura AJ. Esophageal perforation in a patient with acquired immunodeficiency syndrome. Ann Thorac Surg 1990;50:299-300.
30. Im JG, Kim JH, Han MC. Computed tomography of esophago-mediastinal fistula in tuberculous mediastinal lymphadenitis. J Comput Assist Tomogr 1990;14:89-92.
31. Macchiarini P, Delamare N, Beuzeboc P, Labussiere AS, Cerrina J, Chapelier A, et al. Tracheoesophageal fistula caused by mycobacterial tuberculous adenopathy. Ann Thorac Surg 1993;55: 1561-3.
32. Lee JH, Shin DH, Kang KW, Park SS, Lee DH. The medical treatment of a tuberculous tracheo-oesophageal fistula. Tuber Lung Dis 1992;73:177-9.
33. Wilson RS, White RJ. Lymph node tuberculosis presenting as chyluria. Thorax 1976;31:617-20.
34. Kohn MD, Altman KA. Jaundice due to rare causes: tuberculous lymphadenitis. Am J Gastroenterol 1973;59:48-53.
35. Paredes C, DelCampo F, Zamarron C. Cardiac tamponade due to tuberculous mediastinal lymphadenitis. Tubercle 1990:71: 219-20.
36. Fatimi SH, Javed MA, Ahmad U, Siddiqi BI, Salahuddin N. Tuberculous hilar lymph nodes leading to tracheopulmonary artery fistula and pseudoaneurysm of pulmonary artery. Ann Thorac Surg 2006;82:e35-6.
37. Bem C. Human immunodeficiency virus-positive tuberculous lymphadenitis in Central Africa: clinical presentation of 157 cases. Int J Tuberc lung Dis 1997;1:215-9.

38. Mohan A, Reddy MK, Phaneendra BV, Chandra A. Aetiology of peripheral lymphadenopathy in adults: analysis of 1724 cases seen at a tertiary care teaching hospital in southern India. Natl Med J India 2007;20:78-80.

39. Sharma SK, Kohli M, Chaubey J, Yadav RN, Sharma R, Singh BK, et al. Evaluation of Xpert MTB/RIF assay performance in diagnosing extrapulmonary tuberculosis among adults in a tertiary care centre in India. Eur Respir J 2014;44:1090-3.

40. Patel AK, Thakrar SJ, Ghanchi FD. Clinical and laboratory profile of patients with TB/HIV coinfection: a case series of 50 patients. Lung India 2011;28:93-6.

41. Chakraborti KL, Jena A. MR evaluation of the mediastinal lymph nodes. Indian J Chest Dis Allied Sci 1997;39:19-25.

42. Rizzi EB, Schinina' V, Cristofaro M, Goletti D, Palmieri F, Bevilacqua N, et al. Detection of pulmonary tuberculosis: comparing MR imaging with HRCT. BMC Infect Dis 2011;11:243.

43. Sathekge M, Maes A, Van de Wiele C. FDG-PET imaging in HIV infection and tuberculosis. Semin Nucl Med 2013;43:349-66.

44. Gupta AK, Nayar M, Chandra M. Critical appraisal of fine needle aspiration cytology in tuberculous lymphadenitis. Acta Cytol 1992;36:391-4.

45. Finfer M, Perchik A, BursteinDE. Fine needle aspiration biopsy diagnosis of tuberculous lymphadenitis in patients with and without the acquired immunodeficiency syndrome. Acta Cytol 1991;35:325-32.

46. Gupta SK, Chugh TD, Shiekh XA, al-Rubah NA. Cytodiagnosis of tuberculous lymphadenitis. A correlative study with micro-biologic examination. Acta Cytol 1993;35:329-32.

47. Lau SK, WeiWI, Hsu C, Engzell UC. Efficacy of fine needle aspiration cytology in the diagnosis of tuberculous cervical lymphadenopathy. J Laryngol Otol 1990;104:24-7.

48. Pithie AD, Chicksen B. Fine-needle extra-thoracic lymph-node aspiration in HIV associated sputum-negative tuberculosis. Lancet 1992;340:1504-5.

49. Baron KM, Aranda CP. Diagnosis of mediastinal mycobacterial lymphadenopathy by transbronchial needle aspiration. Chest 1991;100:1723-4.

50. Eom JS, Mok JH, Lee MK, Lee K, Kim MJ, Jang SM, et al. Efficacy of TB-PCR using EBUS-TBNA samples in patients with intrathoracic granulomatous lymphadenopathy. BMC Pulm Med 2015;15:166.

51. Sharma M, Ecka RS, Somasundaram A, Shoukat A, Kirnake V. Endoscopic ultrasound in mediastinal tuberculosis. Lung India 2016;33:129-34.

52. Gulati M, Venkataramu NK, Gupta S, Sood BP, Sheena DM, Gupta SK, et al. Ultrasound guided fine needle aspiration biopsy in mediastinal tuberculosis. Int J Tuberc Lung Dis 2000;4:1164-8.

53. Kumar A, Mohan A, Sharma SK, Kaul V, Parshad R, Chatto-padhyay TK. Video assisted thoracoscopic surgery [VATS] in the diagnosis of intrathoracic pathology: initial experience. Indian J Chest Dis Allied Sci 1999;41:2-13.

54. Bharucha NE, Ramamoorthy K, Sorabjee J, Kuruvilla T. All that caseates is not tuberculosis. Lancet 1996;348:1313.

55. Abdissa K, Tadesse M, Abdella K, Bekele A, Bezabih M, Abebe G. Diagnostic performance of fluorescent light-emitting diode microscopy for tuberculous lymphadenitis in a high-burden setting. Trop Med Int Health 2015;20:1543-8.

56. Denkinger CM, Schumacher SG, Boehme CC, Dendukuri N, Pai M, Steingart KR. Xpert MTB/RIF assay for the diagnosis of extrapulmonary tuberculosis: a systematic review and meta-analysis. Eur Respir J 2014;44:435-46.

57. World Health Organization. Policy update: automated real-time nucleic acid amplification technology for rapid and simulta-neous detection of tuberculosis and rifampicin resistance: Xpert MTB/RIF system for the diagnosis of pulmonary and extrapulmonary TB in adults and children 2013. Available at URL: http://www.stoptb.org/wg/gli/assets/documents/WHO%20 Policy%20Statement%20on%20Xpert%20MTB-RIF%202013%20 pre%20publication%2022102013.pdf. Accessed on December 28, 2017.

58a. Sharma SK, Ryan H, Khaparde S, Sachdeva KS, Singh AD, Mohan A, et al. Index-TB guidelines: Guidelines on extra-pulmonary tuberculosis for India. Indian J Med Res 2017;145:448-63.

58b. Kohli M, Schiller I, Dendukuri N, Dheda K, Denkinger CM, Schumacher SG, Steingart KR. Xpert[®] MTB/RIF assay for extrapulmonary tuberculosis and rifampicin resistance. Cochrane Database Syst Rev 2018;8:CD012768.

59. Singh S, Katoch V. Commercial serological tests for the diagnosis of active tuberculosis in India: Time for introspection. Indian J Med Res 2011;134:583.

60. World Health Organization. Commercial serodiagnostic tests for diagnosis of tuberculosis: policy statement. WHO/HTM/TB/2011.5 Geneva: World Health Organization; 2011.

61. Kumar A. Directorate General of Health Services. Advisory against commercial serological tests. Central TB Division, Ministry of Health and Family Welfare. Government of India; 2011.

62. Steingart KR, Ramsay A, Dowdy DW, Pai M. Serological tests for the diagnosis of active tuberculosis: relevance for India. Indian J Med Res 2012;135:695-702.

63. British Thoracic Society Research Committee. Six months versus nine months chemotherapy for tuberculosis of lymph nodes: preliminary results. Respir Med 1992;86:15-9.

64. British Thoracic Society Research Committee. Six months versus nine months chemotherapy of tuberculosis of lymph nodes: final results. Respir Med 1993;87:621-3.

65. Kabra SK, Lodha R, Seth V. Category based treatment of tuberculosis in children. Indian Pediatr 2004;41:927-37.

66. Jindal SK, Aggarwal AN, Gupta D, Ahmed Z, Gupta KB, Janmeja AK, et al. Tuberculous lymphadenopathy: a multicentre operational study of 6-month thrice weekly directly observed treatment. Int J Tuberc Lung Dis 2013;17:234-9.

67. Cheng VC, Ho PL, Lee RA, Chan KS, Chan KK, Woo PC, et al. Clinical spectrum of paradoxical deterioration during antituberculosis therapy in non-HIV-infected patients. Eur J Clin Microbiol Infect Dis 2002;21:803-9.

68. Meintjes G, Lawn SD, Scano F, Maartens G, French MA, Worodria W, et al. International Network for the Study of HIV-associated IRIS. Tuberculosis-associated immune reconstitution inflammatory syndrome: case definitions for use in resource-limited settings. Lancet Infect Dis 2008;8:516-23.

69. Sharma SK, Soneja M. HIV and immune reconstitution inflam-matory syndrome [IRIS]. Indian J Med Res 2011;134:866-77.

70. Meintjes G, Wilkinson RJ, Morroni C, Pepper Dj, Rebe K, Rangaka MX, et al. Randomized placebo-controlled trial of prednisone for paradoxical TB-associated immune reconstitution inflammatory syndrome. AIDS Lond Engl 2010;24:2381-90.

71a. Verma C. Circulating inflammatory biomarkers as predictors of HIV-tuberculosis associated immune reconstitution inflam-matory syndrome [IRIS] [PhD Thesis]. New Delhi: All India Institute of Medical Sciences; 2016.

71b. Ayed AK, Behbehani NA. Diagnosis and treatment of isolated tuberculous mediastinal lymphadenopathy in adults. Eur J Surg Acta Chir 2001;167:334-8.

72. Griffith DE, Aksamit T, Brown-Elliott BA, Catanzaro A, Daley C, Gordin F, et al; ATS Mycobacterial Diseases Subcommittee; American Thoracic Society; Infectious Disease Society of America. An official ATS/IDSA statement: diagnosis, treatment, and prevention of nontuberculous mycobacterial diseases. Am J Respir Crit Care Med 2007;175:367-416.

23

Tuberculosis in Head and Neck

Arvind Kumar Kairo, SC Sharma

INTRODUCTION

In the pre-chemotherapeutic era, patients with active pulmonary tuberculosis [TB] often developed laryngeal, otological, nasal and paranasal sinus involvement and deteriorated progressively. The classical description of TB involving head and neck emanated from that period. With the advent of effective anti-TB treatment the incidence of otolaryngological TB has come down significantly. The resurgence of TB as a consequence of human immunodeficiency virus [HIV] infection and acquired immunodeficiency syndrome [AIDS] has brought otolaryngological TB into focus once again not only in endemic countries but also in developed countries (1-3).

TUBERCULOSIS IN HEAD AND NECK REGION

Although not as common as pulmonary TB, head and neck involvement by TB occurs in a significant proportion of cases. Head and neck TB develops due to: [i] spread of the bacilli to the upper airway by contaminated sputum from a pulmonary focus; [ii] haematogenous; and [iii] lymphatic dissemination (4). Primary involvement of the tonsil as the portal of entry with subsequent involvement of the cervical lymph nodes is also known. The site of involvement in some of the published series on head and neck TB is shown in Table 23.1 (1-3).

TUBERCULOSIS OF CERVICAL LYMPH NODES

Cervical lymph node involvement [Figures 23.1A and 23.1B] is the most frequently seen head and neck manifestation of TB (5-7). The chapter *"Lymph node tuberculosis" [Chapter 22]* covers this topic in detail. Nontuberculous mycobacterial lymphadenitis is covered in the chapter *"Nontuberculous mycobacterial infections" [Chapter 41]*.

TUBERCULOSIS OF SPINE

Patients with TB of cervical spine may occasionally present to the otorhinolaryngologist with torticollis, stiffness of neck due to spasm of the neck muscles and painful movement of the spine. Difficulty in swallowing and breathing, and a midline bulge in the posterior pharyngeal wall suggest a retropharyngeal or paravertebral abscess. Children with this condition may present with stridor. Pus from the TB lesion of the spine may track downwards and laterally along the prevertebral muscles and manifests in the neck as an abscess. Epidural sepsis in the neck can be the cause of musculoskeletal symptoms [polyradiculopathy] which can go undiagnosed before it manifests with some more obvious features (8). The reader is referred to the chapter *"Skeletal tuberculosis" [Chapter 19]* for further details on this topic.

Prevertebral Abscess

Prevertebral space extends from one transverse process to another and from the skull base superiorly to the mediastinum inferiorly. It lies directly posterior to the retropharyngeal space and posteromedial to the carotid space (9). Vertebral body destruction with associated soft tissue mass may be seen [Figures 23.2A and 23.2B]. The spinal canal and dural sac may get compromised because of vertebral body destruction and spread of abscess. The bulge and the obstruction caused by these abscesses can be so large that it may cause symptoms of paraesthesia, neck stiffness. Respiratory distress, dysphagia and paraplegia may develop depending on site and extent of infection.

TUBERCULOSIS OF ORAL CAVITY

The oral cavity is an uncommon site of involvement by TB. Infection in the oral cavity is usually acquired

Table 23.1: Site of involvement in some of the recently published series on head and neck TB

Variable	Menon et al (1) [n = 128]	Nalini and Vinayak (2) [n = 117]	Prasad et al (3) [n = 165]*
Place of study	Bradford, UK	Mumbai, India	Mangalore, India
Male:Female	68:60	41:76	108:57
Site of involvement†			
Cervical lymph nodes	111 [87]	111 [95]	121 [73.3]
Larynx	02 [1.6]	02 [1.7]	24 [14.5]
Cervical spine	0	01	03 [1.8]
Oropharynx	02 [1.6]	01	08 [5]
Nasopharynx	01	0	01
Ear	02 [1.6]	01	04 [2.4]
Eyes	02 [1.6]	0	0
Retropharyngeal abscess	01	01	0
Salivary glands	05 [3.9]	0	03 [1.8]
Thyroid	01	0	0
Temporomandibular joint	0	0	01
Skin	01	0	0
Associated pulmonary TB and TB of other organs	20	31	24.2

* Of the 65 patients who were tested, 30% were found to have co-existing HIV infection
† Values in square brackets indicate percentage
UK = United Kingdom; TB = tuberculosis; HIV = human immunodeficiency virus

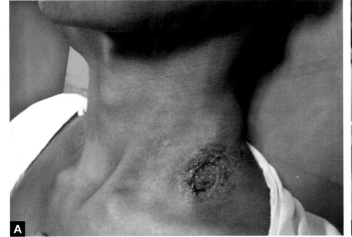 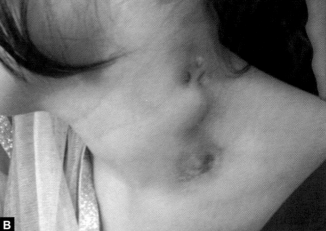

Figure 23.1: Clinical photograph showing TB cervical lymphadenitis with scrofuloderma [A]; healed TB cervical lymphadenitis with scarring and residual lymphadenopathy [B]
TB = tuberculosis

through infected sputum coughed out by a patient with open pulmonary TB. Infection may also be acquired by haematogenous spread. In general, the intact mucosa of the oral cavity is relatively resistant to invasion and saliva has inhibitory effect on the growth of mycobacteria. A breach in the mucosa due to any reason is one of the important predisposing factors for the development of TB of the oral cavity.

Tongue is the most common site of involvement and accounts for nearly half the cases. The lesions are usually found over the tip, borders, dorsum and base of the tongue. These may be single or multiple, painful or painless (10). Usually, the lesions are well-circumscribed, but, irregular ulcers may also occur [Figure 23.3]. These lesions sometimes begin as nodules, fissures or plaques (11). Initial picture may resemble a malignant process and histopathology confirms

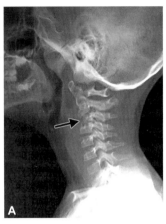
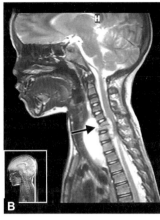

Figure 23.2: Cervial spine radiograph [lateral view] showing soft tissue shadow suggestive of prevertebral abscess. Wedging of vertebrae is also evident [arrow] [A]. Magnetic resonance imaging [T2-weighted image; saggital view] in a paediatric patient with TB of spine showing wedging of vertebrae [arrow], prevertebral abscess causing compression of trachea and oesophagus [B]

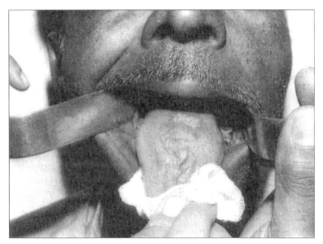

Figure 23.3: Tuberculosis of the tongue. Patient recovered completely with antituberculosis treatment

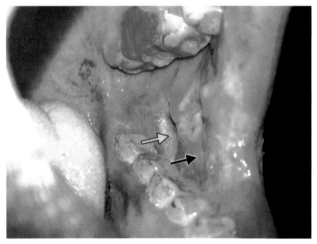

Figure 23.4: TB of buccal mucosa [black arrow]. Ulceration in posterior most part is secondary to biopsy from the lesion [yellow arrow]
TB = tuberculosis

the diagnosis of TB (12). Other sites of involvement include: floor of mouth, buccal mucosa [Figure 23.4], soft palate, anterior pillars and uvula (13). Secondary involvement of the draining lymph nodes may occur. Majority of these patients also have pulmonary TB (10-12,14-16).

TUBERCULOSIS OF LARYNX

Pathogenesis

Laryngeal TB classically develops due to direct spread to the larynx from contaminated sputum [bronchogenic spread]. This form of involvement, frequent in patients with sputum smear-positive pulmonary TB, most commonly involves the posterior glottis. It is thought to develop due to the pooling of infected sputum when the patient is in the recumbent position (17). The bronchogenic spread to the larynx results in localised oedema, granuloma or ulcerations (18). The laryngeal involvement may also occur due to lymphohaematogenous spread. Isolated laryngeal involvement may occur without any evidence of pulmonary TB. Laryngeal TB with oedematous, polypoid panlaryngitis as a consequence of lymphohaematogenous spread is not easily distinguishable from chronic laryngitis (19-23).

Epidemiology

Before the availability of anti-TB treatment, laryngeal involvement was considered a grave prognostic sign indicative of severe disease. It was seen in nearly one-third of cases with pulmonary TB (24). With the availability of effective anti-TB treatment, there has been a gradual decline in the burden of laryngeal TB. However, with the advent of the HIV infection and the AIDS, the incidence of laryngeal TB is increasing (19,21). In the present era, it has been observed that in countries where TB is highly endemic, almost all patients with laryngeal TB have been found to have radiographic evidence of pulmonary TB and many of them may be sputum smear-positive (24-26). On the contrary, most of the patients with laryngeal TB in countries with a low prevalence of TB seldom have any evidence of pulmonary TB (27,28). However, patients with a heavy bacillary load and strongly positive sputum specimens may not have laryngeal involvement. The incidence of laryngeal involvement in patients with pulmonary TB has ranged from 1.5% to 50% in published studies (25,29-32).

Pathology

The tubercle bacilli induce low-grade inflammation with the formation of typical TB granulation tissue. Coagulation necrosis occurs in large TB granulomas. Later, caseation may develop. Laryngeal lesions reveal oedema and hyperaemia, granulomas or ulceration. Vocal cord thickening and palsy can occur. Epiglottis may show irregular margins and nibbled appearance. *Mycobacterium tuberculosis* [*Mtb*] may be found in the subepithelial tissue. The process of destruction and the repair often proceeds simultaneously. The submucosa of epiglottis and aryepiglottic folds is likely to undergo fibrous infiltration resulting in pseudoedema. Described as *turban epiglottis*, this lesion is not commonly seen in the present era.

Clinical Features

Patients often present with hoarseness of voice and laryngeal TB should be considered in the differential diagnosis in any patient with unexplained hoarseness of voice. Pain is also an important feature which may radiate to one or both ears and may lead to odynophagia. In a study of laryngeal TB (25) hoarseness [98.6%], dysphagia and odynophagia or pain in throat [35.8%] and referred otalgia [28.6%] were reported to be common symptoms; in 14.3% patients, the symptoms were not referred to larynx. The physical examination findings associated with laryngeal TB include oedema, hyperaemia, nodularity, ulceration, exophytic mass, vocal cord thickening, and obliteration of anatomic landmarks. The ulcero-infiltrative lesions which predominantly affected the posterior larynx were observed frequently in the past and are rare now. Diffuse oedema or a pseudotumoural image located in any zone is often seen. Laryngeal TB should be suspected in a patient with non-specific chronic laryngitis (23). The epiglottis may be markedly oedematous [*turban epiglottis*] and the vocal cord oedema can resemble polypoid corditis. The epiglottis may show irregular margins or nibbled appearance. Subglottic oedema or granulation in the true vocal cord can result in stridor. Stridor may also result from vocal cord paralysis secondary to mediastinal lymphadenopathy (32). Any laryngeal structure can be affected by TB [Figure 23.5] and the common sites include true vocal cord, the epiglottis, the false vocal cord, the aryepiglottic fold, the arytenoids, the interarytenoid area and the subglottis (22,33,34).

Occasionally, patients may present with rapid onset of hoarseness of voice similar to that encountered in acute viral laryngitis. Because of the acute onset, TB is rarely suspected as the cause. When these patients fail to respond to conservative management, microlaryngo-scopic examination, biopsy and histopathological examination may confirm the diagnosis of vocal cord TB. Coexistence of laryngeal TB and carcinoma is well-known. Clinical features of these conditions may overlap and the lesions may look similar (26,27). The incidence of this coexistent TB and cancer of larynx has been reported to be 1.4% (35). Anti-TB treatment should be administered for at least two to three weeks before the treatment of laryngeal carcinoma is initiated. When TB develops after antineoplastic therapy, the infection is more severe with a higher mortality (26-28,35,36).

TUBERCULOSIS OF THE SALIVARY GLANDS

TB of the salivary glands is usually secondary to TB of the oral cavity or primary pulmonary TB. Primary infection of the salivary glands is also known, but, is rare. Parotid is the most common salivary gland involved [Figures 23.6A and 23.6B]. TB of the submandibular gland is also known (37). Parotid gland involvement is much more common because of its intraparotid lymph nodes. Clinical presentation can be acute or chronic. Acute presentation may resemble acute non-TB sialitis and clinical differentiation may be difficult. Occasionally, the diagnosis of TB may be a surprise following surgery performed for a suspected salivary gland tumour (38). Unsuspected TB parotid abscess may be wrongly drained mistaking it to be a pyogenic [non-TB] abscess. This may lead to the formation of a persistent sinus. In one such case (39), the diagnosis of TB was made when superficial parotidectomy was performed as part of the treatment for fistula. In patients with suspected TB sialitis, chest radiograph and fine needle aspiration cytology are useful in confirming the diagnosis.

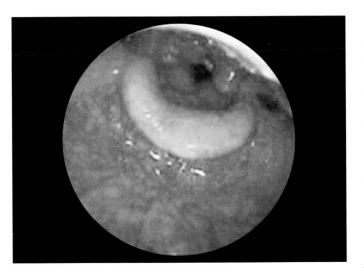

Figure 23.5: Endoscopic view of the laryngeal TB
TB = tuberculosis

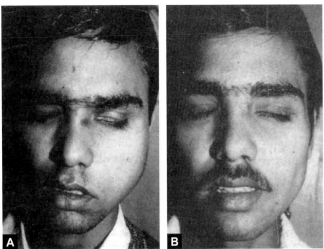

Figure 23.6: TB parotitis with facial nerve palsy before anti-TB treatment [A]. Following anti-TB treatment, facial nerve palsy recovered and parotid gland swelling subsided [B]
TB = tuberculosis

TUBERCULOSIS OF PHARYNX

TB involvement of the tonsils and pharynx is uncommon at present. These cases may be confused with pharyngeal carcinoma at the time of presentation (40). The presenting features include: [i] ulcer on the tonsil or oropharyngeal wall; [ii] granuloma of the nasopharynx; and [iii] neck abscess. Co-existence of TB (41) and cancer of pharynx could be: [i] a mere coincidence; [ii] metastatic carcinoma developing secondarily in a recent or old TB lesion; [iii] TB infection engrafted on cancer in full evolution; and [iv] chronic progressive TB in which cancer develops (42). Lymphoreticular malignancy may be associated with TB abscess and sinus of the neck. Rarely, malignancy and TB may involve two different organs (41).

TUBERCULOSIS OF THE EAR

While the association between pulmonary TB and TB of the middle ear cleft is known since early nineteenth century, primary infection of ear is rare (43-45).

Pathogenesis

Ear can become infected with *Mtb* by the bacilli invading the Eustachian tube while the infant is being fed, or, by haematogenous spread to the mastoid process.

Clinical Manifestations

Patients with aural TB present with painless otorrhoea and hearing loss. However, patients with TB mastoiditis may complain of otalgia. Pale granulation tissue may be present in the middle ear with dilatation of vessels in the anterior part of the tympanic membrane (46-49). Multiple perforations of tympanic membrane may occur as a result of caseation necrosis [Figure 23.7]. These perforations may coalesce

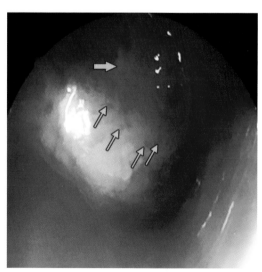

Figure 23.7: Otoscopic view in a patient with aural TB showing multiple pin-point size granulomas over the tympanic membrane [thin arrows]. These granulomas coalesce to form multiple perforations [thick arrow] TB = tuberculosis

to form a large perforation which may involve annulus as well. *Pars flaccida* is usually not involved by TB. Facial nerve palsy may occur in patients with TB of the ear with or without a sequestrum. Persistent non-healing granulations in a post-mastoidectomy patient may occasionally be the result of TB. Pre-auricular lymphadenopathy with post-auricular fistula has been considered to be pathognomonic of TB otitis media (48). TB of the external ear is uncommon. However, lupus vulgaris of the external ear has been reported (50). Very rarely it may present as *turkey ear*.

TUBERCULOSIS OF NASOPHARYNX

TB of the nasopharynx is uncommon. The most common complaint is nasal obstruction and rhinorrhoea. Physical examination may show adenoid hypertrophy without any distinguishing features. In a study [n = 40] (51), young females in the age range of 20 to 40 years were frequently affected by nasopharyngeal TB. The most common clinical manifestation was cervical lymphadenopathy [53%], followed by hearing loss [12%], tinnitus, otalgia, nasal obstruction and postnasal drip [6% each]. Systemic symptoms, such as fever, weight loss and night sweats were evident in 12% patients. Direct endoscopic examination showed nasopharyngeal mucosal irregularity or mass in the nasopharynx in a majority [70%] of the patients. Primary infection of nasopharynx by TB is very rare (52). Nasal obstruction or middle ear effusion is the common presenting features.

TUBERCULOSIS OF THE PARANASAL SINUSES

Paranasal sinus TB is a rare entity and is nearly always secondary to pulmonary or extra-pulmonary TB [EPTB] (53-55). The sinuses most frequently affected are maxillary and ethmoid though any sinus may be affected. The infection reaches the sinus either via the bloodstream or by a direct extension from TB of the skull base (56). In sinonasal TB, infection may be limited to the submucosa only. Here, the sinus mucosa may be thickened or filled with a polyp, which has a pale and boggy appearance with minimal purulent discharge. This form is more common than the second type, which is characterised by the bony involvement [osteomyelitis] with a sequestrum and fistula formation. The latter form is more difficult to treat. Like any other pyogenic infection, the sinonasal TB can also spread to the brain or orbit resulting in brain abscess, epiphora and deterioration of vision. Rarely, TB of the maxillary sinus may be associated with a carcinoma (57).

TB of the sphenoid sinus can present with blindness and features of cavernous sinus thrombosis which is of gradual onset and slow progression (55). Computed tomography [CT] may show a heterogeneous soft tissue mass lesion in a sinus with bone erosion and extension to the surrounding tissue. Magnetic resonance imaging [MRI] may delineate the soft tissue extension better.

NASAL TUBERCULOSIS

TB of nasal cavity usually manifests as nasal obstruction and catarrh. Physical examination may reveal pallor of the nasal mucosa with minute apple-jelly nodules that do not blanch with nasal decongestants. Other sites which can be involved include inferior turbinate, septal mucosa and the vestibular skin. These nodules may coalesce to form a granular lesion with subsequent perforation of the septal cartilage (19). Involvement of nasolacrimal duct can rarely occur. TB of the nose can cause complications like septal perforation, atrophic rhinitis and scarring of nasal vestibule.

DIFFERENTIAL DIAGNOSIS

Laryngeal TB must be differentiated from squamous cell carcinoma and other granulomatous inflammatory diseases, such as, fungal infections, syphilis, leprosy, Wegener's granulomatosis, and sarcoidosis. Multiple biopsies may be required to confirm the diagnosis.

TB of the nose and paranasal sinuses results in ulceration, granuloma formation and pain in the nose and the infected sinus cavity. Usually, other granulomatous disorders of the paranasal sinuses are painless. TB of the oral cavity should be differentiated from primary syphilis, fungal infections, chronic traumatic ulcers and squamous cell carcinoma.

DIAGNOSIS

Diagnosis of laryngeal TB involves demonstration of *Mtb* in sputum, laryngeal swab by smear and culture methods and histopathological examination of the biopsy material (45). Co-existent pulmonary TB should be carefully looked for by sputum smear microscopy and the chest radiography (19,50,58). A high index of suspicion is required to diagnose TB of the ear. Tissue biopsy should be done to confirm the diagnosis. However, due to the atypical nature of the clinical presentation, TB is not suspected initially and the patient may frequently undergo middle ear exploration. The diagnosis may become evident subsequently when the histopathology reveals the classical changes.

Diagnosis of TB otitis media is ascertained by smear and mycobacterial culture examination of the ear discharge and histopathologic study of the affected tissue. Smear and culture examination of the nasal discharge, nasopharyngeal secretions collected by nasal endoscopy along with histo-pathological examination of biopsy material are useful in the diagnosis of TB of the nose, paranasal sinuses and pharynx. Histopathological and microbiological examination of biopsy material is useful in confirming the diagnosis of TB of the tongue, oral cavity and salivary glands.

Diagnosis of cervical lymph node TB is covered in the chapter *"Lymph node tuberculosis"*. Molecular methods of diagnosis such as Xpert MTB/RIF seem to be useful in the diagnosis of otolaryngological TB (59a,59b).

IMAGING IN HEAD AND NECK TUBERCULOSIS

Although CT and MRI can accurately demonstrate the site, pattern and extent of the disease, however, both these modalities have limitations in the evaluation of head and neck TB (52). The radiographic features are variable and non-specific. However, CT and MRI have a definitive role in the diagnosis of TB of spine. TB lymphadenitis is often characterised by areas of low attenuation or low signal intensity with peripheral rim enhancement or calcification on CT. The CT findings in laryngeal TB are also non-specific. There may be a diffuse thickening of the epiglottis or vocal cords. Deep submucosal infiltration to pre-epiglottic space or paraglottic space and cartilage destruction is usually not seen unlike laryngeal carcinoma. In a study [n = 12] (60), CT findings in 12 patients with laryngeal TB were reported. Bilateral involvement was noted in nine patients [75%], while unilateral involvement was seen in three [25%]. Diffuse thickening of free margin of the epiglottis was a characteristic and frequent finding in TB [50%]. No deep submucosal infiltration of the pre-epiglottic and paralaryngeal fat spaces was seen even when there was extensive involvement of the laryngeal mucosa. Cartilage destruction was not found in any case. By comparison, laryngeal carcinoma presented with unilateral involvement, infiltration of the pre-epiglottic and paralaryngeal fat spaces by a submucosal mass, cartilage destruction, and extralaryngeal invasion.

In patients with TB mastoiditis, the plain radiograph or CT may reveal the presence of a sequestrum. Further, in patients with aural TB, CT of temporal bone may demonstrate destruction of the osseous chain, sclerosis of the mastoid cortex, and opacification of the middle ear and mastoid air cells. CT evidence of widespread bone destruction without clinical signs of aggressive infection, should suggest TB mastoiditis (61). MRI may show thickened seventh and eighth nerve complex in the internal auditory meatus. This finding is frequently seen in the post-contrast scans in patients with sensory neural hearing loss and facial nerve paralysis [Figure 23.8].

Positron emission tomography-computed tomography/magnetic resonance imaging [PET-CT/MRI] has been found

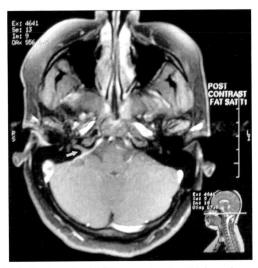

Figure 23.8: Post-contrast MRI scan showing thickened seventh and eighth nerve complex in the internal auditory meatus and arachnoiditis [arrow]

to be useful in defining the extent of disease and monitoring response to treatment.

IMPACT OF HUMAN IMMUNODEFICIENCY VIRUS INFECTION

Sparse literature is available on otorhinolaryngological TB in patients with HIV infection and AIDS (58,62-64). Singh *et al* (64) reviewed the clinical presentation of laryngeal TB in HIV-positive patients. In this study (64), eight of the 146 patients with head and neck TB had laryngeal involvement and two of these patients were HIV-positive. The most common symptoms were hoarseness, odynophagia and shortness of breath. The majority of the patients had white exophytic lesions involving any area of the larynx and these lesions resembled carcinoma or chronic laryngitis. Systemic symptoms, such as, fever, night sweats, and weight loss were very common in patients with AIDS and coupled with other illnesses masked the possibility of laryngeal disease and resulted in a delay in the diagnosis. In another recent retrospective study (58) the characteristics of TB confined to the head and neck region in 38 patients infected with HIV were reported. These patients were divided into two groups on the basis of the HIV status at presentation. Group 1 included 11 patients [29%] with AIDS at presentation. Group 2 included 27 patients [71%] with HIV infection but without AIDS. The authors reported that the cervical lymphatics were the most common site for isolated head and neck TB [89%], with the supraclavicular lymph nodes most often involved [53%]. Extralymphatic involvement was less common [11%], but involved a variety of anatomic locations [skin, spinal cord, larynx, parotid salivary gland]. The presenting history and physical examination had a low sensitivity for TB in patients with HIV infection, mainly because of the presence of multiple confounding factors. Purified protein derivative [PPD] testing was highly sensitive for TB in patients with HIV infection alone [61%]; however, its usefulness was diminished in patients with AIDS [14%]. Fine-needle aspiration biopsy was 94% sensitive for diagnosing TB and was not affected by the status of HIV infection. Surgical biopsy was the gold standard for diagnosing TB but was associated with chronically draining fistulas in a significant number of cases [14%]. These data suggest that TB should be considered in the differential diagnosis of all head and neck lesions in patients infected with HIV, even in the absence of pulmonary involvement. Six of the fourteen children with HIV-1 infection described by Schaaf *et al* (63) presented with otorrhoea. Ear swabs were the source of *Mtb* culture in three of them. Chest radiographs were abnormal in all of them.

TREATMENT OF TUBERCULOSIS IN THE HEAD AND NECK

Anti-TB treatment is the mainstay of treatment for patients with TB of head and neck region. The reader is referred to the chapter *"Treatment of tuberculosis"* [Chapter 44] for details. The recently published Guidelines for Extrapulmonary TB

for India [INDEX-TB Guidelines] (59a) suggest that patients with otorhinolaryngological TB should be treated for six to nine months; patients with bone involvement, including those with TB otitis media, should receive 9 months treatment. These guidelines (59a) also suggest that corticosteroids have no role in the treatment of otorhinolaryngological TB. As the larynx heals, fibrosis of laryngeal tissue can occur resulting in the following sequelae: cricoarytenoid joint fixation, posterior glottis stenosis and anterior glottic web, subglottic stenosis, vocal cord scarring. These specific complications are to be treated accordingly (26,28).

Indications for surgery in patients with head and neck TB are outlined in Table 23.2. Superior laryngeal nerve block has been advocated for odynophagia (27), but, is rarely required at present as effective anti-TB drugs are available. In patients with TB of the cervical spine and cold abscess, repeated aspirations may be required to decompress the abscess and relieve the difficulty in breathing and swallowing. Usually, open drainage is avoided. However, if required, external approach rather than peroral drainage is recommended to avoid sinus formation and prevent the abscess from draining into the oropharynx. Prevertebral abscess can be drained either transorally or through transcervical approach. In the transoral approach, airway is secured with a cuffed endotracheal or tracheostomy tube to prevent aspiration and drained through transoral incision through the posterior pharyngeal mucosa. For transcervical drainage an incision along the anterior border of the sternocleidomastoid muscle is employed. The space is explored by blunt dissection between the carotid sheath and pharyngeal constrictor muscle with placement of drains. Occasionally, debridement of the diseased bone and bone grafting may be required. Paraplegia may develop in patients with severe and advanced involvement of the cervical spine. To prevent this, prophylactic neck collar support is helpful. Neck collar support also relieves the pain when there is severe spasm of the muscles of the neck.

As per the INDEX-TB guidelines (59a) surgery may be indicated in some circumstances to treat complications or

---

Table 23.2: Indications for surgery in patients with head and neck TB

Diagnostic

    Biopsy of mucosal lesions

    Lymph node biopsy where the fine needle aspiration cytopathology fails to give conclusive result

Therapeutic

    Excision of a sinus or fistula which fails to heal even after adequate anti-TB therapy

    Drainage of neck abscess

    Repeated drainage or external drainage of retropharyngeal abscess

    Presence of sequestrum in the mastoid region

    Revision of cosmetically bad scars left after TB has healed

TB = tuberculosis

for reconstruction of the ear or nose. Where facial nerve palsy complicates TB otitis media, surgical decompression should be considered if there is no improvement after three to four weeks of anti-TB treatment. Surgical drainage of retropharyngeal abscess complicating TB of the cervical spine may be considered, but requires specialist judgement. Surgery should be avoided in TB of the salivary glands or thyroid as medical treatment is usually considered to be adequate. Second-line anti-TB drugs may be required in patients with drug-resistant TB [DR-TB]. Therefore, diligent efforts should be made to procure and subject the tissue specimens to mycobacterial culture and susceptibility testing in an accredited laboratory whenever nontuberculous mycobacterial infections or DR-TB is suspected.

REFERENCES

1. Menon K, Bem C, Gouldesbrough D, Strachan DR. A clinical review of 128 cases of head and neck tuberculosis presenting over a 10-year period in Bradford, UK. J Laryngol Otol 2007;121: 362-8.
2. Nalini B, Vinayak S. Tuberculosis in ear, nose, and throat practice: its presentation and diagnosis. Am J Otolaryngol 2006; 27:39-45.
3. Prasad KC, Sreedharan S, Chakravarthy Y, Prasad SC. Tuberculosis in the head and neck: experience in India. J Laryngol Otol 2007;121:979-85.
4. Kumar S, Roy BC, Sharma SC. Tuberculosis in otohinolaryngology. In: Sharma SK, Mohan A, editors. Tuberculosis. Second edition. New Delhi: Jaypee Brothers Medical Publishers; 2009.p.410-9.
5. Das S, Das D, Bhuyan UT, Saikia N. Head and neck tuberculosis: scenario in a tertiary care hospital of North Eastern India. J Clin Diagn Res 2016;10:MC04-7.
6. Bruzgielewicz A, Rzepakowska A, Osuch-Wójcikewicz E, Niemczyk K, Chmielewski R. Tuberculosis of the head and neck - epidemiological and clinical presentation. Arch Med Sci 2014;10:1160-6.
7. Yashveer JK, Kirti YK. Presentations and challenges in tuberculosis of head and neck region. Indian J Otolaryngol Head Neck Surg 2016;68:270-4.
8. Smith DF, Smith FW, Douglas JG. Tuberculous polyradiculopathy: the value of magnetic resonance imaging of the neck. Tubercle 1989;70:213-6.
9. Stäbler A, Reiser MF. Imaging of spinal infection. Radiol Clin North Am 2001;39:115-35.
10. Soni NK, Chatterji P, Chhimpa I. Lingual tuberculosis. Indian J Otolaryngol 1979;31:92-2.
11. Tyldesley WR. Oral tuberculosis–an unusual presentation. Br Med J 1978;2:928.
12. Brennan TF, Vrabec DP. Tuberculosis of the oral mucosa. Ann Otol Rhinol Laryngol 1970;79:601-5.
13. Komet H, Schaefer RF, Mahoney PL, Antonio S. Bilateral tuberculosis granulomas of the tongue. Arch Otolaryngol 1965;82:649-51.
14. Fujibayashi T, Takahashi Y, Yoneda T, Tagani Y, Kusama M. Tuberculosis of the tongue. Oral Surg 1979;47:427-35.
15. Mcandrew PG, Adekeye EO, Ajdukiewicz AB. Miliary tuberculosis presenting with multifocal oral lesions. Br Med J 1976;1:1320.
16. Weaver RA. Tuberculosis of the tongue. JAMA 1976;235: 2418.
17. Houghton DJ, Bennett JD, Rapado F, Small M. Laryngeal tuberculosis: an unsuspected danger. Br J Clin Pract 1997;51:61-2.
18. Bull TR. Tuberculosis of the larynx. Br Med J 1966;2:991-2.
19. Williams RG, Douglas-Jones T. Mycobacterium marches back. J Laryngol Otol 1995;109:5-13.
20. Soda A, Rubio H, Salazar M, Genem J, Berlanga D, Sanchez A. Tuberculosis of the larynx: clinical aspects in 19 patients. Laryngoscope 1989;99:1147-50.
21. Lazarus AA, Thilagar B. Tuberculosis of pericardium, larynx, and other uncommon sites. Dis Mon 2007;53:46-54.
22. Levenson MJ, Ingerman M, Grimes C, Robbett WF. Laryngeal tuberculosis: review of twenty cases. Laryngoscope 1984;94: 1094-7.
23. Porras AE, Martin MA, Perez RJ, Avalos SE. Laryngeal tuberculosis. Rev Laryngol Otol Rhinol 2002;123:47-8.
24. Looper EA, Lyon IB. Laryngeal tuberculosis. Ann Otol Rhinol Laryngol 1948;57:754-68.
25. Soni NK, Chatterjee P. Laryngeal tuberculosis. Indian J Otolaryngol 1978;30:115-7.
26. Rupa V, Bhanu TS. Laryngeal tuberculosis in the eighties–an Indian experience. J Laryngol Otol 1989;103:864-8.
27. Thaller SR, Gross JR, Pilch BZ, Goodman M. Laryngeal tuberculosis as manifested in the decades 1963-1983. Laryngoscope 1987;97:848-50.
28. Street I, Gillett D, Sawyer A, Weighill J. Laryngeal tuberculosis: not the usual suspect. Br J Hosp Med [Lond] 2006;67:212-3.
29. Topak M, Oysu C, Yelken K, Sahin-Yilmaz A, Kulekci M. Laryngeal involvement in patients with active pulmonary tuberculosis. Eur Arch Otorhinolaryngol 2008;265:327-30.
30. Iqbal K, Udaipurwala IH, Khan SA, Jan AA, Jalisi M. Laryngeal involvement in pulmonary tuberculosis. J Pak Med Assoc 1996;46:274-6.
31. Lim JY, Kim KM, Choi EC, Kim YH, Kim HS, Choi HS. Current clinical propensity of laryngeal tuberculosis: review of 60 cases. Eur Arch Otorhinolaryngol 2006;263:838-42.
32. Shin JE, Nam SY, Yoo SJ, Kim SY. Changing trends in clinical manifestations of laryngeal tuberculosis. Laryngoscope 2000; 110:1950-3.
33. Smallman LA, Clark DR, Raine CH, Proops DW, Shenoi PM. The presentation of laryngeal tuberculosis. Clin Otolaryngol 1987;12:221-5.
34. Galietti F, Giorgis GE, Gandolfi G, Astesiano A, Miravalle C, Ardizzi A, et al. Examination of 41 cases of laryngeal tuberculosis observed between 1975-1985. Eur Respir J 1989;2:731-2.
35. Feld R, Bodey GP, Groschell D. Mycobacteriosis in patients with malignant disease. Arch Intern Med 1976;136:67-70.
36. Kaplan MH, Armstrong D, Rosen P. Tuberculosis complicating neoplastic disease. A review of 201 cases. Cancer 1974;33: 850-8.
37. Kumar S, Dev A. Primary tuberculosis of bilateral submandibular salivary glands. Indian J Otolaryngol 1990;42:69-70.
38. El Hakim IE, Langdon JD. Unusual presentation of tuberculosis of the head and neck region. Report of three cases. Int J Oral Maxillofacial Surg 1989;18:194-6.
39. Kant R, Sahi RP, Mahendra NN, Agarwal PK, Shankhdhar R. Primary tuberculosis of the parotid gland. J Indian Med Assoc 1977;68:212.
40. Srirompotong S, Yimtae K, Srirompotong S. Clinical aspects of tonsillar tuberculosis. Southeast Asian J Trop Med Public Health 2002;33:147-50.
41. Raman R, Bakthavizian A. Tuberculosis associated with malignancy of the nasopharynx. Indian J Otolaryngol 1981;33: 149-50.
42. Broders AC. Tuberculosis associated with malignant neoplasia. JAMA 1919;72:390-4.
43. Hasan SA, Malik A. Tuberculosis otitis media. Indian J Otolaryngol 1981;33:145-6.

44. Skolink PR, Nadol JR Jr, Baker AS. Tuberculosis of the middle ear: review of literature with an instructive case report. Rev Infect Dis 1986;8:403-10.

45. Mittal OP, Singh RP, Katiyar SK, Nath N, Gupta SC. Tubercular osteomyelitis of the mastoid temporal bone. Int J Otolaryngol 1977;29:20.

46. Awan MS, Salahuddin I. Tuberculous otitis media: two case reports and literature review. Ear Nose Throat J 2002;81:792-4.

47. Di Rienzo L, Tirelli GC, D'Ottavi LR, Cerqua N. Primary tuberculosis of the middle ear: description of 2 cases and review of literature. Acta Otorhinolaryngol Ital 2001;21:365-70.

48. Greenfield BJ, Selesnick AH, Fisher L, Ward RF, Kimmelman CP, Harrison WG. Aural tuberculosis. Am J Otol 1995;16:175-82.

49. Vital V, Printza A, Zaraboukas T. Tuberculous otitis media: a difficult diagnosis and report of four cases. Pathol Res Pract 2002;198:31-5.

50. Sachdeva OP, Kukreja SM, Mohan C. Lupus vulgaris of external ear. Indian J Otolaryngol 1978;30:136-7.

51. Tse GM, Ma TK, Chan AB, Ho FN, King AD, Fung KS, et al. Tuberculosis of the nasopharynx: a rare entity revisited. Laryngoscope 2003;113:737-40.

52. Mair IWS, Johannessen TA. Nasopharyngeal tuberculosis. Arch Otolaryngol 1970;92:392-3.

53. Kukreja HK, Sacha BS, Joshi KC. Tuberculosis of maxillary sinus. Indian J Otolaryngol 1977;29:27-8.

54. Krishnan E, Rudraksha MR. Paranasal sinus tuberculosis. India J Otolaryngol 1978;3:125-6.

55. Sharma SC, Baruah P. Sphenoid sinus tuberculosis in children–a rare entity. Int J Pediatr Otorhinolaryngol 2003;67:399-401.

56. Page JR, Jash DK. Tuberculosis of the nose and paranasal sinuses. J Laryngol Otol 1974;88:579-83.

57. Vrat V, Saharia PS, Nayyer M. Co-existing tuberculosis and malignancy in the maxillary sinus. J Laryngol Otol 1985;99:397-8.

58. Singh B, Balwally N, Har-El G, Lucente FE. Isolated cervical tuberculosis in patients with HIV infection. Otolaryngol Head Neck Surg 1998;118:766-70.

59a. Sharma SK, Ryan H, Khaparde S, Sachdeva KS, Singh AD, Mohan A, et al. Index-TB guidelines: Guidelines on extra-pulmonary tuberculosis for India. Indian J Med Res 2017;145:448-63.

59b. Kohli M, Schiller I, Dendukuri N, Dheda K, Denkinger CM, Schumacher SG, Steingart KR. Xpert[®] MTB/RIF assay for extra-pulmonary tuberculosis and rifampicin resistance. Cochrane Database Syst Rev 2018;8:CD012768.

60. Kim MD, Kim DI, Yune HY, Lee BH, Sung KJ, Chung TS, et al. CT findings of laryngeal tuberculosis: comparison to laryngeal carcinoma. J Comput Assist Tomogr 1997;21:29-34.

61. Mandpe AH, Lee KC. Tuberculous infections of the head and neck. Curr Opin Otolaryngol Head Neck Surg 1998;6:190-6.

62. Srirompotong S, Yimtae K, Srirompotong S. Tuberculosis in the upper aerodigestive tract and human immunodeficiency virus coinfections. J Otolaryngol 2003;32:230-3.

63. Schaaf HS, Geldenduys A, Gie RP, Cotton MF. Culture positive tuberculosis in human immunodeficiency virus type 1-infected children. Pediatr Infect Dis J 1998;17:599-604.

64. Singh B, Balwally AN, Nash M, Har-El G, Lucente FE. Laryngeal tuberculosis in HIV-infected patients: a difficult diagnosis. Laryngoscope 1996;106:1238-40.

24

Ocular Tuberculosis

Pradeep Venkatesh, Rohan Chawla, SP Garg

INTRODUCTION

Tuberculosis [TB] is a serious public health problem. Even in the developed countries, it has re-emerged as an issue of serious health concern (1). The incidence of ocular TB in a population is difficult to estimate (2). Estimates of incidence and prevalence of ocular TB have usually been drawn from reports of histopathological- proven ocular TB, studies on experimental ocular TB, and surveys of ocular disease in patients with proven systemic TB (3). In one report from a sanatorium in the USA, 1.4% of 10,524 patients were treated for ocular TB between 1940 and 1966 (4). Of these, 14 patients had interstitial keratitis, 23 had sclerokeratitis and 3 had corneal ulcers. The incidence of TB uveitis in India has varied from 2%-30% (5,6). The large variation in the incidence rates in different reports possibly stems from differences in the diagnostic criteria. In the studies reporting higher incidence rates, the diagnosis of TB uveitis was often based on a positive tuberculin skin test [TST].

While TB can affect all areas of the visual system, the choroid is probably the most commonly infected intraocular structure. Intraocular TB is unique amongst all forms of TB in that it is paucibacillary in nature and displays multiple clinical manifestations (7). Woods (8) estimated that the choroid is involved in about 1% of patients with pulmonary TB. Primary TB of the eyelid, conjunctival sac and optic nerve is rare. TB periphlebitis has been reported to probably account for a large number of cases of Eale's disease (9,10). Further, ocular TB is usually not associated with manifestations of systemic TB (11).

The impact of acquired immunodeficiency syndrome [AIDS] epidemic on the rates of ocular TB remains unclear. Shafer and associates (12) did not report a single case of ocular TB in a study of 199 consecutive patients with human immunodeficiency virus [HIV] infection and extra-pulmonary TB [EPTB]. Small *et al* (13) reviewed 132 patients with AIDS and TB. In this study TB was entirely extrapulmonary in 30% and both pulmonary and extrapulmonary in 32% of patients and no ocular involvement was reported. However, there are a few published case reports of ocular TB in HIV-infected patients (14,15). In a study (16) from Africa in patients with TB, choroidal granulomas were seen in 2.8% cases and these patients had both AIDS and mycobacteraemia. In a study (17) from India on ocular findings in HIV-seropositive individuals, 3.8% patients were found to have evidence of intraocular TB. Interestingly, all these patients also had pulmonary TB. In a series on ophthalmic manifestations in paediatric cases with HIV co-infection, choroidal tubercles were seen in about 2.5% cases (18). In a recent study (19), it was found that amongst 980 patients with uveitis, studied over a two-year period at a tertiary care centre, only 54 patients gave a positive history of being treated in the past for proven pulmonary TB or EPTB.

PRIMARY AND SECONDARY OCULAR TUBERCULOSIS

Two different definitions have been given to "primary" ocular TB. The term *"primary ocular TB"*, has been used when the TB lesions are confined to the eyes and no systemic lesions are clinically evident. The term has also been used to describe the cases where the eye has been the initial portal of entry (20-23). *"Secondary ocular TB"* has been defined as ocular infection resulting from contiguous spread from adjacent structures or haematogenous spread from the lungs (24).

Although rare, well-documented cases of primary ocular TB do exist in the literature (21,25,26). In many of these patients, pulmonary disease could have been clinically and radiographically inapparent and perhaps would have been evident only on autopsy examination (27). It has been suggested that it is extremely unusual for a primary ocular infection to result in disseminated TB (28). Intraocular and orbital TB are considered to represent secondary infections (29,30).

Studies to detect the ability of *Mycobacterium tuberculosis* [*Mtb*] to penetrate only intact conjunctival or corneal epithelium have revealed conflicting results. Finoff (30) reported that a breach in the epithelium was necessary to initiate an infection. Therefore, epithelial injury to the cornea may lead to primary ocular TB (31,32). However, Bruckner (33), experimenting on guinea pigs, observed that *Mtb* could be carried into the subepithelial tissue by phagocytosis with chronic conjunctivitis even when the epithelium is intact. Besides *Mtb*, nontuberculous mycobacteria [NTM] can also cause ocular TB.

EYELID TUBERCULOSIS

TB affects the eyelids infrequently. The disease occurs as a result of spread of infection from the face and lymph nodes or by the haematogenous route. Primary eyelid involvement is extremely rare. TB eyelid abscess has been reported in the literature in conjunction with lung infection or sinus disease (34-36).

Eyelid lesion begins as a red papule that becomes indurated. Eventually, it enlarges to form a nodule or plaque that ulcerates. The ulcer is chronic and painless. In most cases, regional lymphadenopathy also occurs. Rarely the skin lesion is hyperkeratotic and papular.

Lupus vulgaris of the face may spread to involve the eyelid. The disease progresses slowly leading to the characteristic soft "apple-jelly" nodule appearance. This feature is said to be best appreciated on diascopy. Atrophic scars, ectropion and destruction of the lid, may develop. TB of the tarsal plate can simulate recurrent chalazion and finally causes its destruction (37).

When lid involvement occurs by spread from the underlying bone, lacrimal sac or lymph node, the initial manifestation is a red, fluctuant nodule with induration. This lesion ulcerates in several cases and a fistula surrounded by granulation tissue develops in the ulcer crater. Tuberculids of the eyelid present as small, multiple papular and chronic lesions. It is not clear whether these are a non-specific form of granuloma or a hypersensitivity reaction to tuberculoprotein. The reader is referred to the chapter *"Cutaneous tuberculosis"* [Chapter 21] for further details.

CONJUNCTIVAL TUBERCULOSIS

TB can involve the conjunctiva primarily or secondarily. Conjunctival TB and lupus vulgaris are manifestations of primary infection while tuberculids and phlyctenulosis are manifestations of secondary conjunctival infection. Primary lesions present as unilateral nodular or ulcerative conjuctivitis (38,39) associated with regional lymphadenopathy. Children are most commonly affected (20,38). Secondary lesions due to spread from contiguous disease or haematogenous dissemination are more common in older patients. The disease may be bilateral and may cause regional lymphadenopathy (38,39).

Conjunctival tuberculomas start insidiously and 3-4 weeks later lead to regional lymphadenopathy. The enlarged preauricular and rarely the submandibular lymph nodes may suppurate and drain forming a sinus. Thus, conjunctival TB is one of the causes of *Parinaud's oculoglandular* syndrome of an infectious conjunctivitis accompanied by regional lymph node enlargement. Very rarely, the disease may start as an acute purulent or muco-purulent conjunctivitis with symptoms of fever and malaise.

Several types of conjunctival granulomas have been described (40,41) and include ulcerative, nodular, polypoid or hyperplastic lesions. These lesions may be solitary or multiple. Solitary tuberculomas involving the bulbar conjunctiva are observed in 2%-30% of cases (42). The nodular prototype may simulate a trachomatous lesion. It has a propensity to involve the bulbar and upper fornix of conjunctiva (21). Associated follicles and corneal infiltration may be present. The nodule may enlarge to assume a cauliflower-like lesion with central ulceration. The ulcerative form has a propensity to involve the inferior *cul-de-sac*. It can also involve the bulbar conjunctiva and tarsus and may also spread to involve the cornea, lid or sclera. *Mtb* can often be found in the ulcer crater (40,41). The hyperplastic variety develops most commonly in the fornix and rarely on the tarsus. This form is associated with severe conjunctival chemosis and lid oedema. It may assume a pedunculated appearance like the polypoid form.

Conjunctival tuberculids are a manifestation of hypersensitivity reaction. These appear as small conjunctival nodules. These could be evanescent or remain localised. They are associated with TB involvement of the uveal tract, sclera, skin or other regions of the body. TB of the bulbar conjunctiva is usually associated with an interstitial keratitis.

Phlyctenulosis can involve the lid margin, cornea or conjunctiva. A *phlycten* [from the Greek word for blister] is a hypersensitivity reaction to tuberculoprotein. In the conjunctiva, it can affect the bulbar, conjunctival or limbal region. However, the most common site is the limbal region. It usually appears as a small nodule with surrounding hyperaemia. It gradually ulcerates and heals without scarring. This is in contrast to the corneal phlyctenulosis which leaves a scar on healing. Limbal phlyctenules leave a characteristic triangular scar because the conjunctival portion, unlike the corneal portion, heals without scar formation. TB phlctenular keratoconjunctivitis also occurs. *Mtb* has been demonstrated in only one-fourth of patients with conjunctival TB (21).

In the west, staphylococcal infection has replaced TB as the leading cause of phlyctenular keratoconjunctivitis. TB phlyctenular keratoconjunctivitis usually occurs in malnourished older children and is more common in girls. Symptoms usually last 1-2 weeks and consist of excessive lacrimation, pain, photophobia and blepharospasm. The severity of symptoms depends on the site of involvement. Corneal involvement indicates a much more severe form of the disease. Recurrence is frequent and may occur at a different site.

CORNEAL TUBERCULOSIS

The corneal manifestations in TB are phlyctenulosis, interstitial keratitis, ulceration and infiltrations (43-46). Rarely, these patients may also have active pulmonary TB (47,48). Phlyctens of the cornea usually arise from limbus. Corneal involvement is characterised by intense photophobia, pain and blepharospasm. Marginal, miliary and fasicular phlyctenular patterns have been described. Corneal phlyctenules heal with a variable degree of scarring and vascularisation.

Interstitial keratitis is uncommon in TB. However, as compared to syphilitic interstitial keratitis, TB interstitial keratitis is associated with more intense scarring and vascularisation in the deeper layers (49). Apart from being usually unilateral, TB often has selective propensity to involve the lower part of the cornea. Sclerosing keratitis may evolve as sequelae to TB involvement of the sclera. Clinically, sclerosing keratitis appears as peripheral corneal scleralisation. On resolution, it leaves behind a triangular or tongue shaped opacity with the base directed towards the limbus.

Corneal ulceration due to TB usually develops due to the contiguous spread of infection from the conjunctiva or uveal tract. These ulcers are indolent and refractory to treatment.

SCLERAL TUBERCULOSIS

Although TB was reported as a frequent cause of scleritis earlier, it was considered rare by 1926 (50). Watson and Hayreh (51) found TB of the sclera in only one of the 217 cases with episcleritis.

TB of sclera is characterised by scleral and conjunctival ulceration. Focal necrotising anterior scleritis is the most common presentation, but a diffuse presentation is also known (52,53). Physical examination may reveal preauricular and submandibular lymphadenopathy. The scleritis develops due to direct scleral infection or, by spread from the conjunctiva, uveal tract or by haematogenous route and produces a nodular lesion [Figure 24.1]. Peripheral cornea is often secondarily affected and granulomatous uveitis may also develop. The scleral nodules may undergo caseation necrosis and ulceration. Subsequently, perforation may develop.

TUBERCULOSIS OF LACRIMAL SYSTEM

TB involvement of the lacrimal gland, lacrimal canaliculi and lacrimal sac is unusual. TB dacryoadenitis usually develops during the haematogenous dissemination, occasionally due to spread from conjunctival or corneal disease and still infrequently due to an injury. It appears as a gradually enlarging painless swelling. When eyelid is involved, lid oedema and pseudoproptosis are prominent features. If the orbit is involved, proptosis and restriction of upward gaze are evident. Abscess formation with a chronic draining fistula in the upper lid can also occur. Regional lymphadenopathy is a prominent manifestation in patients with TB of lacrimal system.

ORBITAL TUBERCULOSIS

Abadie (54), in 1881, was the first to describe orbital TB. Since then, several cases of orbital TB have been reported. Orbital TB can take several forms, notably, periostitis, tuberculomas and myositis. A case of TB osteomyelitis involving the orbit and masquerading as post-traumatic haematoma has also been reported (55).

Orbital TB occurs by haematogenous spread or by extension of infection from adjacent structures such as the paranasal sinuses. It is usually unilateral and typically occurs in the first two decades of life. It usually has a protracted course. TB periostitis has an insidious onset and presents as a chronic, painless inflammation, most commonly of the malar bone. Over months, oedema and discolouration of the overlying skin can progress to cold abscess, fistula formation, cicatrisation and regional lymphadenitis. Tuberculomas, firm masses of chronic granulomatous inflammation, can occur anywhere in the orbit. These lesions can occur at any age. These cause gradual painless proptosis and sclerosis and thus mimic benign and malignant tumours, orbital pseudotumours and fungal infections. Occasionally, they involve extraocular muscles and are bilateral in location. Tuberculomas may also start in the maxillary or ethmoid sinuses, erode into the orbit and form fistula in the skin. Overt signs of chronic sinusitis accompany this presentation. Epiphora and epistaxis are also common symptoms.

TUBERCULOSIS OF THE UVEAL TRACT

Mycobacterium tuberculosis [Mtb] can involve the two principal internal layers of the eye: the uveal and the retinal layers. TB involving the uvea commonly presents as choroidal tubercles or disseminated choroiditis, choroidal mass/abscess, chronic granulomatous iridocyclitis, intermediate and panuveitis. It can rarely present as panophthalmitis (56). The authors have seen a child with pulmonary TB presenting with a

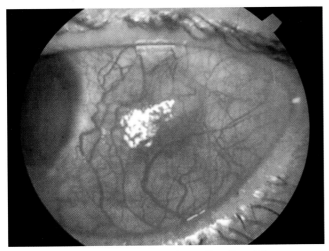

Figure 24.1: Nodular scleritis in a patient with miliary TB
TB = tuberculosis

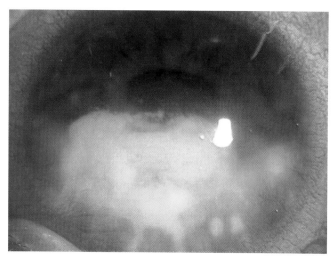

Figure 24.2A: Pre-treatment photograph of a patient with tuberculosis anterior diffuse endophthalmitis

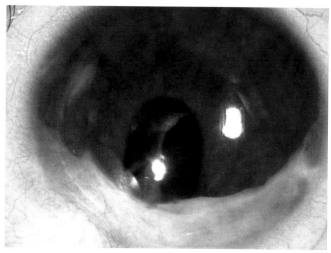

Figure 24.2B: Post-treatment photograph of the same patient showing considerable resolution of the lesion

diffuse anterior endogeneous endophthalmitis-like picture. The patient responded well to standard anti-TB treatment [Figures 24.2A and 24.2B]. TB involves the choroid more frequently than the iris and ciliary body. In a series of 40 patients with histopathological evidence of TB affecting the internal layers of the eye (3), the mean age at diagnosis was 32 years. Male and female genders were equally affected and the disease was mostly unilateral.

CHOROIDAL TUBERCULOSIS

Choroidal tubercles and tuberculomata [large, solitary masses] are the most common ocular manifestations of TB [Figures 24.3, 24.4, 24.5A, 24.5B and 24.6]. Choroid is a highly vascular structure and choroidal TB usually results from haematogenous dissemination. The presence of choroidal tubercles or choroidal masses is not diagnostic of miliary TB (57-60), although investigation for the same in a patient may be rewarding. The finding of choroidal tubercles in TB meningitis is still rarer. In one study, 28%-60% of patients with miliary TB were reported to have choroidal tubercles on ophthalmoscopic examination (60). However, in the same study, only one of the 18 patients with TB meningitis without miliary disease had choroidal tubercles. Sharma *et al* (61) found choroidal tubercles in only 4 of the 88 patients with miliary TB who were HIV-seronegative. Massaro *et al* (59) found choroidal tubercles in 30% of patients with pulmonary TB. In patients with choroidal TB, blurred vision may be the only symptom. Some patients may be asymptomatic and the tubercles may be detected on detailed fundus evaluation of a case of suspected miliary TB referred for fundus evaluation. In such patients, detection of choroidal tubercles helps the clinician in making a diagnosis of TB. On clinical examination, choroidal tubercles may be solitary or multiple and of varying dimensions ranging from about a quarter of the disc diameter to several disc diameters.

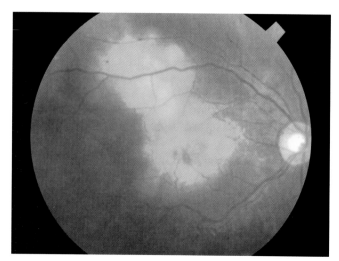

Figure 24.3: Solitary tuberculoma in miliary TB
TB = tuberculosis

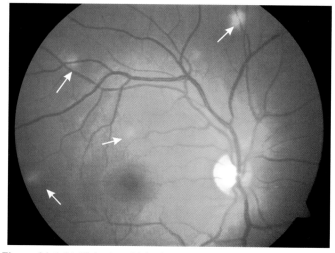

Figure 24.4: Multiple choroidal tubercles in miliary TB [arrows]
TB = tuberculosis

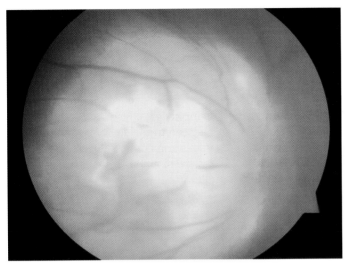

Figure 24.5A: Pre-treatment photograph in a patient with a large solitary choroidal tuberculoma

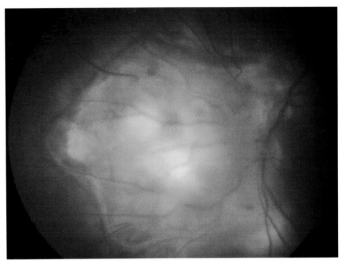

Figure 24.5B: Post-treatment photograph of the same patient showing significant resolution of the choroidal tuberculoma

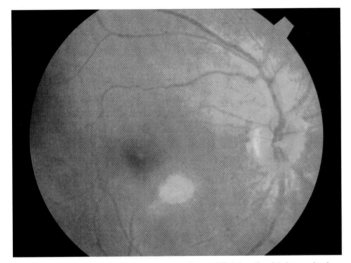

Figure 24.6: Choroidal lesion in a patient with intestinal tuberculosis

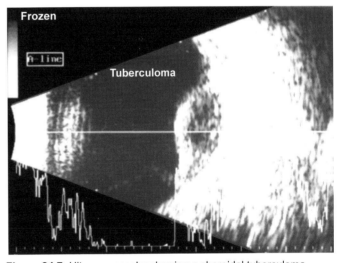

Figure 24.7: Ultrasonography showing a choroidal tuberculoma

They are most frequently situated in the posterior pole (59). Up to 60 choroidal tubercles have been described but, usually less than 5 are seen. These appear as yellowish-grey elevated nodules with overlying inflammation in the vitreous during the active stage [Figure 24.6]. The overlying and surrounding retina may be detached when the tubercles are large [tuberculoma]. Choroidal granulomas, though suggestive of TB, are not diagnostic and may occur in other conditions, such as, sarcoidosis and cryptococcosis. Most patients with miliary TB and choroidal tubercles have no anterior segment involvement (62,63) perhaps because these patients are unable to mount an effective immunologic response. Rarely, however, choroidal tubercles may co-exist with panuveitis (64,65). Brightness mode [B-mode] ultrasonography of larger choroidal masses using a 10 MHz ocular probe is considered suggestive of TB abscess if it reveals a central hypoechoic zone in a moderately reflective choroidal mass [Figure 24.7].

Some workers consider a subset of patients of serpiginous choroiditis to be of TB origin (65). A recent review on the subject provides evidence in favour and against TB as the aetiology of serpiginous choroiditis (66). The authors feel that serpiginous choroiditis is an autoimmune disorder and should be treated with corticosteroids and immunosuppressive agents (67,68).

TUBERCULOSIS IRITIS AND IRIDOCYCLITIS

Gradenigo (69), in 1869, first reported histopathological evidence of TB of the iris in a patient with miliary TB at autopsy. TB was considered an important cause of granulomatous uveitis until the early 1960s. However, there has been a dramatic decline in the number of these cases probably due to identification of other diseases, such as, sarcoidosis and toxoplasmosis. Traditionally, mutton fat keratic precipitates, early formation of dense synechiae and formation of iris nodules of Koeppe or Bussaca were considered to be characteristic of TB iridocyclitis. Such lesions must be distinguished from sarcoid nodules which are larger and more pink. Non-granulomatous anterior uveitis may also be seen in patients with systemic TB. This may be an immune reaction.

RETINAL TUBERCULOSIS

TB can affect the retina either by direct infection or because of a hypersensitivity reaction. Isolated involvement of the retina by direct infection is extremely rare. Experimental and clinical studies have revealed that *Mtb* rarely affects the retina directly (4,47,48,70). The retina is more commonly affected secondarily from adjacent choroidal lesions. Some workers have attributed retinal periphlebitis to direct infection (71,72). In an atypical presentation, Saini *et al* (73) found histopathological evidence of TB in an eye that had been enucleated for presumed retinoblastoma.

Eale's disease, an idiopathic, non-infective, inflammatory vasculitis of the retinal vasculature has been attributed the hypersensitivity to tuberculoprotein. This disease is an important cause of visual morbidity in healthy young adults, especially from the Indian subcontinent. It affects persons in their second and third decade (74). Males are more frequently involved (75). In about 90% of the patients, the disease becomes bilateral within a few years. Most patients present with painless, sudden visual loss in one eye due to vitreous haemorrhage.

Eale's disease is characterised by retinal periphlebitis and capillary non-perfusion that results in hypoxia. Retinal hypoxia leads to neovascularisation either on the retinal surface or on the optic nerve head. These new vessels being extremely fragile have a propensity to bleed into the vitreous. In some cases, this can lead to retinal detachment and an irreversible visual loss.

Ophthalmoscopically, the peripheral retinal vessels, which usually are the first to be involved, show signs of inflammation with sheathing of the vessel wall, surrounding retinal oedema and haemorrhage. New vessels may also be present on the retina or the disc. The disease can be segmental or can involve a large area. Though uncommonly used, a clinical classification and grading system has been proposed for Eale's disease (76).

The reasons for associating Eale's disease with TB include: [i] increased prevalence of tuberculoprotein hypersensitivity (28,74,76-78); [ii] presence of concurrent active or healed pulmonary TB (77,78); and [iii] response to anti-TB treatment in some patients. Further, polymerase chain reaction [PCR] positivity for TB from vitreous samples of cases of Eale's disease has been reported (80).

Histopathologically, no features typical of TB inflammation have been described (77,81,82). In most cases, a non-specific perivascular cuff of lymphocytes was the only finding. These patients may have associated neurological disease. Also most cases of Eale's vasculitis respond well to steroids alone. As of date, it is not fully established whether TB has a role to play in a subset of patients of this disease

or not. If, at all, it does have a role whether bacterial activity or secondary immunological processes are responsible for the ocular manifestations, also needs to be determined.

PATHOLOGY

Histopathologically, phlyctenules are characterised by a dense accumulation of lymphocytes, histiocytes and plasma cells. Neutrophils may be seen in the acute stage. There is a notable absence of giant cells and eosinophils. *Mtb* is seldom seen. Choroidal tubercles are similar to the tubercles found elsewhere in the body. Granulomas may be caseating or non-caseating. The characteristic giant cells may be absent. In contrast to the histopathology of choroidal tubercles, TB endophthalmitis is characterised by marked caseation necrosis and exudation.

DIAGNOSIS

Definitive diagnosis of ocular TB can be made only by demonstrating *Mtb* in the ocular tissues. However, obtaining ocular tissue for diagnostic purposes is not only difficult, but, is also associated with significant ocular morbidity. Hence, the diagnosis of TB can rarely be definitely confirmed before enucleation. Only 25% of patients with ocular TB have a history of TB and approximately 50% have normal chest radiographs (8,9,11). Orbital radiographs may reveal bony erosions. A high degree of clinical suspicion is, therefore, the key to early diagnosis. Easily accessible sites such as eyelid, conjunctiva (52), lacrimal gland and sclera (83) should preferably be biopsied to demonstrate the characteristic findings of caseating granulomas with Langhans' giant cells and *Mtb*. The emergence of multidrug-resistant TB [MDR-TB] is a compelling reason to subject ocular specimens to mycobacterial culture and sensitivity testing.

Tuberculin Skin Test

A positive TST in a patient with granulomatous uveitis is considered to be a positive evidence of ocular TB (84-87). A positive TST is indicative of infection with *Mtb* and does not necessarily reflect the disease activity. Rosenbaum and Wernik (88,89) calculated that a patient with uveitis and a positive TST has only 1% probability of having active TB. However, recent conversion of a previous non-reactor favours the diagnosis of active TB. Use of systemic corticosteroids for severe ocular inflammation can interfere with the interpretation of the TST. Therefore, though routine TST has been advocated in patients with uveitis, it is rarely diagnostic (87,90-93).

Schlaegel and Weber (87), Abrams and Schlaegel (94) have advocated the isoniazid therapeutic test for the diagnosis of suspected TB uveitis. However, therapeutic effect of isoniazid and a natural fluctuation in the course of chronic uveitis of some other aetiology needs to be distinguished. Furthermore, administration of isoniazid monotherapy can result in the development of drug resistance. Therefore, this is not widely used.

Interferon-Gamma Release Assays

Interferon-gamma release assays [IGRAs], like the TST, also cannot differentiate latent TB infection [LTBI] from active TB. In countries endemic for TB, the utility of these tests is very uncertain. Presently both the World Health Organization [WHO] and Revised National Tuberculosis Control Programme [RNTCP] of the Government of India do not encourage use of these tests to make a diagnosis of active TB (95,96).

Serological and Molecular Methods

The usefulness of enzyme-linked immunosorbent assay in the diagnosis of ocular TB is still being evaluated. The WHO and the RNTCP strongly recommend against use of serological tests for diagnosing TB (97).

Polymerase chain reaction [PCR] offers to be a promising tool to establish the definitive diagnosis of ocular TB. Kotake *et al* (98) confirm the presumptive clinical diagnosis of ocular TB using PCR in two patients. They used a sequence for the coding of MPB64 protein that is specific for *Mtb* (98,99). However just the presence of mycobacterial DNA alone does not confirm active TB (100).

More recently, detection of *Mtb* genome has been reported in vitreous samples of patients with presumed ocular TB (101b). Three methods were used in this study (101b), namely, multitargeted PCR, Gene Xpert MTB/RIF [Cepheid, Sunnyvale, CA] and line probe assay [LPA] [GenoType MTBDRplus; Hain Lifescience, GmbH, Nehren, Germany]. Of the 11 samples tested, positive results were obtained in 10, 4 and 6 subjects with multitargeted PCR, Gene Xpert MTB/RIF and LPA, respectively. This study (101b) also documented the presence of rifampicin resistance bacillus in some of the samples. In a recently published study (101b), LPA [MTBDRplus assay] testing of vitreous fluid was found to be an effective tool for the rapid diagnosis of intraocular drug-resistant TB. The utility of these molecular tests merits further study.

Imaging Studies

In cases of suspected ocular TB, a chest radiograph must be done to rule out presence of pulmonary TB. In cases where clinical suspicion based on ocular findings is very high, a high-resolution computed tomography [HRCT] of the chest can be done even if the chest radiograph is normal. Studies in miliary TB have shown computed tomography [CT] to be superior to the chest radiograph in picking up active TB lesions (102). Ultrasonography of the abdomen can help in detecting ascites, retroperitoneal lymphadenopathy and other features of abdominal TB.

Despite rapid advances in medicine, ocular TB still remains an important diagnostic challenge. The criteria for the diagnosis of ocular TB differ greatly and very often the diagnosis is based on a compatible clinical picture and good therapeutic response to anti-TB treatment rather than mycobacterial isolation.

Table 24.1: Diagnostic categories of ocular TB

Possible ocular TB

Patients with presence of the following [i], [ii] and [iii] together; or [i] and [iv] are diagnosed as having possible ocular TB:
[i]   At least one clinical sign suggestive of ocular TB,* and other aetiology excluded
[ii] Chest radiograph/CT not consistent with TB infection and no clinical evidence of extraocular TB
[iii] Presence of at least one of the following:
   • Documented exposure to TB
   • Immunological evidence of TB infection
[iv] Molecular evidence of *Mtb* infection

Clinically diagnosed ocular TB

Patients with presence of all the following [i], [ii] and [iii] together are diagnosed as having probable ocular TB:
[i]   At least one clinical sign suggestive of ocular TB,* and other aetiologies excluded
[ii] Evidence of chest radiograph consistent with TB infection or clinical evidence of extraocular TB or microbiological confirmation from sputum or extraocular sites
[iii] Documented exposure to TB and/or immunological evidence of TB infection

Bacteriologically confirmed ocular TB

A patient with at least one clinical sign of ocular TB,* along with microbiological [smear/culture] or histopathological confirmation of *Mtb* from ocular fluids/tissues

---

* A patient with one of the following clinical presentations: granulomatous anterior uveitis; non-granulomatous anterior uveitis, not associated with any other known clinical entity, e.g., HLA-B27; intermediate uveitis, with/without healed/active focal lesions; posterior uveitis, including subretinal abscess, choroidal/disc granuloma, multifocal choroiditis, retinal periphlebitis and multifocal serpiginous choroiditis; panuveitis; rarely, scleritis [anterior and posterior], interstitial and disciform keratitis has presumptive ocular TB
TB = tuberculosis; *Mtb* = *Mycobacterium tuberculosis*; HLA = human leucocyte antigen
Source: reference 104

In the past several criteria have been proposed for ocular TB (10,103). However, the diagnosis remains presumptive in most patients with suspected intraocular TB due to difficulty in obtaining the ocular tissue for histopathological examination and lack of consensus on diagnostic accuracy of molecular methods. The diagnostic categories for ocular TB defined in the recently published evidence-based Guidelines for Extrapulmonary TB for India [INDEX-TB Guidelines] (104) are shown in Table 24.1.

TREATMENT

When patients with TB elsewhere in the body develop clinical features of ocular involvement, a thorough ophthalmologic evaluation is warranted. Similarly, when patients are detected to have ocular involvement, systemic work-up to rule out active TB must be carried out. Treatment of ocular TB is on the same lines as treatment of pulmonary TB. The disease responds well to standard anti-TB treatment. The recently published Guidelines for Extrapulmonary TB for India [INDEX-TB Guidelines] (104) suggest that patients with otorhinolaryngological TB should be treated with standard anti-TB treatment with rifampicin, isoniazid, pyrazinamide and ethambutol for the first two months followed by rifampicin, isoniazid and ethambutol for the subsequent four to seven months.

Adjunctive treatment with local or systemic corticosteroids, immunosuppressants and others will also be required in specific cases. In cases of choroidal granulomas and panuveitis systemic steroids need to be started 48-72 hours after initiating anti-TB treatment. The treatment of TB phlyctenulosis involves administration of topical corticosteroids and cycloplegic agents in addition to standard anti-TB treatment. Conjunctival lesions causing only mild symptoms may respond to local astringents. Mucopurulent discharge suggests secondary bacterial infection and should be treated accordingly. Conjunctival lesions heal without scarring, but corneal phlyctenules leave superficial scars of variable severity. Adjunctive therapy with topical antibiotics such as streptomycin, amikacin or isoniazid has also been tried in the treatment of TB scleritis (59).

The INDEX-TB guidelines (104) indicate surgery in the following situations: [i] complications of retinal vasculitis, such as retinal neovascularisation, vitreous haemorrhage, tractional or combined retinal detachment, epiretinal membrane; [ii] diagnostic vitrectomy when conventional methods fail to establish diagnosis; [iii] non-resolving vitreous inflammation; [iv] visually significant vitreous floaters after completion of medical therapy; and [v] for management of complications of uveitis, such as, cataract and glaucoma.

ANTI-TUBERCULOSIS TREATMENT-INDUCED OCULAR TOXICITY

Several anti-TB drugs can cause adverse effects involving the eye, which if not recognised early, can result in an irreversible loss of vision. Often patients are referred to ophthalmologists for evaluation of ocular toxicity following prescription of drugs for TB elsewhere in the body. Sometimes patients themselves note a diminution in vision while on anti-TB drugs and get evaluated by an ophthalmologist.

Ocular toxicity due to ethambutol, isoniazid and streptomycin has been well-documented. Of these, ethambutol has the greatest potential to cause ocular toxicity. Three types of optic neuritis have been described with ethambutol (105). These include the axial, the periaxial and the mixed type. Both eyes are usually involved and the visual loss may vary from mild to severe. Colour vision is also variably affected. In the axial form of optic neuritis on visual field testing pericentral or peripheral scotoma may be evident. Quadrantic field defects have also been commonly found. Although mild disc hyperaemia and disc oedema have been reported, fundus examination may be normal in the acute phase of ethambutol toxicity (106). Peripapillary splinter haemorrhages, macular oedema and focal pigementary changes have also been described (107,108). Electophysiological studies are useful in confirming the involvement of the optic nerve and retina in patients receiving ethambutol.

Ethambutol related ocular toxicity is strongly dose related (109-118). In a study (109), 45% of patients receiving ethambutol in a dose of 60-100 mg/kg/day developed ocular toxicity. At that time the older racemic mixture of ethambutol was used (117). Another report showed the incidence of ocular toxicity to be 18.6% in patients receiving more than 53 mg/kg/day of ethambutol (111). With 25 mg/kg/day, the reported incidence of ethambutol related optic neuritis was 1.3%-15% (110). However, less than 2% patients develop this complication with doses below 15 mg/kg/day (112-117).

As the incidence of ethambutol toxicity is low with the currently favoured dose of 15-20 mg/kg/day, and also because it is reversible in most cases, sophisticated electrophysiological tests like electroretinography and visual evoked response potentials are not required in all cases. However, in all patients receiving ethambutol, a baseline best corrected visual acuity and colour vision record should be routinely obtained. Thereafter, patients should be questioned monthly about any changes in vision. Any significant alteration in vision needs to be promptly investigated. Guidelines have been proposed by the British Joint Tuberculosis Committee with respect to ethambutol-related ocular toxicity (119). These include: [i] avoiding ethambutol in patients with impaired renal function; [ii] not exceeding the recommended ethambutol dose and duration; [iii] pretreatment record of any ocular disease previously and present visual acuity must be documented; [iv] informing patients about the possibility of ethambutol affecting their vision and also the need for stopping the drugs if vision becomes impaired. That this information has been provided to the patient must also be entered in the records; [v] routine testing for visual acuity during treatment is not recommended; [vi] avoiding use of ethambutol in children and in adults in whom assessment of the visual status is difficult; and [vii] referral to a patient on ethambutol treatment, who presents with visual disturbance, to an ophthalmologist for a detailed evaluation. Treatment with ethambutol should be discontinued pending this examination. Patients receiving ethambutol in a dosage greater than 15-20 mg/kg for longer than 2 months and patients with renal insufficiency receiving ethambutol are recommended to get visual acuity and monocular color vision testing every month till completion of treatment (120).

Isoniazid has also been reported to cause optic neuritis (121-126). In these cases, the dose of isoniazid has ranged from 200-900 mg/day and symptoms have been reported as early as the tenth day. Isoniazid has to be discontinued at the first sign of ocular toxicity and pyridoxine may probably be beneficial both in the treatment as well as prophylaxis (123,124).

There have been a few reports of ocular toxicity due to streptomycin; of which, only the report by Sykowski (125) has been widely accepted.

The most common adverse effect of rifampicin in the eye is conjunctivitis. It can result in the production of tears that are orange coloured and this can stain contact lenses (126). Rifabutin has been associated with the development of an endophthalmitis-like response (127). Clofazimine has been associated with several ocular side effects; these include: a brownish discolouration of the conjunctiva, brown swirls in the cornea (128,129) and bull's eye maculopathy resulting in visual loss due to macular degeneration (130,131).

Of the newer drugs used to treat MDR-TB, optic neuritis has been reported most commonly with linezolid (132) and capreomycin (133). Linezolid-induced optic neuritis is usually reversible if diagnosed early. Following recovery, treatment can be resumed with a lower dose of linezolid. Patients receiving long-term treatment with linezolid should undergo periodic ophthalmic evaluations.

REFERENCES

1. Brudney K, Dobkin J. Resurgent tuberculosis in New York City. Am Rev Respir Dis 1991;144:745-9.
2. Dinning WJ, Starston S. Cutaneous and ocular tuberculosis: a review. J Royal Soc Med 1985;78:576-81.
3. Craig JH, Holland GN. Ocular tuberculosis. Surv Ophthalmol 1993;38:229-56.
4. Donahue HC. Ophthalmologic experience in a tuberculosis sanatorium. Am J Ophthalmol 1867;64:742-8.
5. Sen DK. Tuberculosis of the orbit and lacrimal gland. J Paed Ophthalmol 1980;17:232-8.
6. Agrwal PK, Nath J, Jain BS. Orbital involvement in tuberculosis. Indian J Ophthalmol 1977;25:12-6.
7. Basu S, Wakefield D, Biswas J, Rao NA. Pathogenesis and pathology of intraocular tuberculosis. Ocul Immunol Inflamm 2015;23:353-7.
8. Woods AC. Chronic bacterial infections: ocular tuberculosis. In: Sorsby A, editor. Modern ophthalmology. Second edition. London: Butterworths; 1973.p.2-105.
9. Mohan M, Garg SP, Kumar H. Shriniwas, Raj. SAFA test as an aid to the diagnosis of ocular tuberculosis. Indian J Ophthalmol 1990;38:57-60.
10. Goyal JL, Jain P, Arora R, Dokania P. Ocular manifestations of tuberculosis. Indian J Tuberc 2015;62:66-73.
11. Traquir HM. Manifestations of tuberculosis in ophthalmic practice. Edinburgh Med J 1940;47:57-66.
12. Shafer RW, Kim DS, Weiss JP, Quale JM. Extrapulmonary tuberculosis in patients with human immunodeficiency virus infection. Medicine 1991;70:384-97.
13. Small PM, Schecter GF, Goodman PC. Treatment of tuberculosis in patients with advanced human immunodeficiency virus infection. N Engl J Med 1991;70:384-97.
14. Blodi BA, Johnson MW, Mlash MW, Glass JDM. Presumed choroidal tuberculosis in a human immunodeficiency virus infected host. Am J Ophthalmol 1989;108:605-7.
15. Crozatto JO, Mestre C, Puente S, Gonzalez G. Non-reactive tuberculosis in a patient with acquired immunodeficiency syndrome. Am J Ophthalmol 1986;102:559-60.
16. Beare NA, Kublin JG, Lewis DK, Schijffelen MJ, Peters RP, Joaki G, et al. Ocular disease in patients with tuberculosis and HIV presenting with fever in Africa. Br J Ophthalmol 2002;86:1076-9.
17. Sudharshan S, Kaleemunnisha S, Banu AA, Shrikrishna S, George AE, Babu BR, et al. Ocular lesions in 1,000 consecutive HIV-positive patients in India: a long-term study. J Ophthalmic Inflamm Infect 2013;3:2.
18. Venkatesh P, Khanduja S, Singh S, Lodha R, Kabra SK, Garg S, et al. Prevalence and risk factors for developing ophthalmic manifestations in pediatric human immunodeficiency virus infection. Ophthalmology 2013;120:1942-3.e2.
19. Venkatesh P, Gogia V, Shah B, Gupta S, Sagar P, Garg S. Patterns of uveitis at the Apex Institute for Eye Care in India: Results from a prospectively enrolled patient data base [2011-2013]. Int Ophthalmol 2016;36:365-72.
20. Tuberculosis among foreign-born persons entering the United Sates. Recommendations of the Advisory Committee for Elimination of Tuberculosis. MMWR Morb Mortal Wkly Rep 1990;39:1-21.
21. Samuelson A. Primary tuberculosis of the conjunctiva. Arch Ophthalmol 1936;15:975-84.
22. Finoff WC. Ocular tuberculosis, experimental and clinical, Arch Ophthalmol 1924;53:130-6.
23. Gurnert C. A contribution to the subject of tuberculosis of the conjunctiva. Arch Ophthalmol 1899;28:540-6.
24. Cook CD, Hainsworth M. Tuberculosis of the conjunctiva occurring in association with a neighbouring lupus vulgaris lesion. Br J Ophthalmol 1990;74:315-6.
25. Anhatt EF, Zovell S, Chang G, Byron HM. Conjunctival tuberculosis. Am J Ophthalmol 1960;50:265-9.
26. Whitford J, Hansman D. Primary Tuberculosis of the conjunctiva. Med J Aust 1977;1:486-7.
27. Champman CB, Whorton CM. Acute generalized miliary tuberculosis in adults: clinicopathological study based on sixty-three cases diagnosed at autopsy. N Engl J Med 1946;235:239-48.
28. Licheri G. Su di un caso di tuberculosis della conjunctiva clinicomente prinotiva. Lethura Oftal 1938;15:403-17.
29. Duke-Elder S, Perkins ES. Diseases of the uveal tract. In: Duke-Elder S, editor. System of ophthalmology. Vol IX. St. Louis: CV Mosby; 1966.
30. Finoff WC. The relation of tuberculosis to chronic uveitis. Am J Ophthalmol 1931;14:1208-27.
31. Mckenzie WH. Tuberculosis of the conjunctiva. Report of a case. Am J Ophthalmol 1939;22:744-9.
32. Torres RA, Mani S, Althulz J, Bricker PW. Human immunodeficiency virus infection among homeless men in a New York City shelter: association with Mycobacterium tuberculosis infection. Arch Intern Med 1990;150:2030-6.
33. Bruckner Z. Erude histolyique de la permeability de la conjunctive aux bacilles tuberculeus. Ann Ocul 1929;166:804-24.
34. Mehta DK, Sahnikamal, Ashok P. Bilateral tubercular lid abscess-a case report. Indian J Ophthalmol 1989;37:98.
35. Mohan K, Prasad P, Benerjee AK, Dhir SP. Tubercular tarsitis. Indian J Ophthalmol 1985;33:115-6.
36. Watrin E, Mendelsohn P. Abces froid palpebral revelateur dune sinusite maxillaire tuberculeuse. Bul So Ophthalmol Fr 1967;67:1124-9.
37. Duke-Elder S, Macfaul PA. The ocular adnexa: Part I. Diseases of the eyelids. In: Duke-Elder S, editor. System of ophthalmology. Vol XIII. St. louis: CV Mosby Company; 1974.
38. Woods AC. Ocular tuberculosis. In: Sorsby A, editor. Modern ophthalmology. Philadelphia: Lippincott; 1972.p.105-40.
39. Archer D, Bird A. Primary tuberculosis of conjuctiva. Br J Ophthalmol 1967;51:679-87.
40. Eyre JWH. Tuberculosis of the conjunctiva: its etiology, pathology and diagnosis. Lancet 1912;1:1319-28.
41. Duke-Elder S. Diseases of the outer eye: part I. In: Duke-Elder S, editor. System of ophthalmology. Vol VIII. London: Henry Kimpton; 1965.
42. Boschoff PH, Grasset E. Two unusual ocular tuberculosis cases. Arch Ophthalmol 1944;32:120-2.
43. Gibson WS. The etiology of phlyctenular conjunctivitis. Am J Dis Child 1918;15:81-115.
44. Thygeson P. Phlyctenulosis. Attempts to produce an experimental model with BCG. Invest Ophthalmol Vis Sci 1962;1:262-6.

45. Aclimandos WA, Kerr-Muir M. Tuberculosis keratoconjunctivitis. Br J Ophthalmol 1992;76:175-6.

46. Ginsberg SP. Corneal problems in systemic diseases. In: Tasman W, Jaeges EA, editors. Duane's clinical ophthalmology. Philadelphia: JB Lippincott; 1982[5].p.1-23.

47. Glover LP. Some observations in tuberculosis patients at the state sanatorium, Cresson, Pennsylvania. Am J Ophthalmol 1930;13:411-2.

48. Goldenburg M, Fabricant ND. The eye in the tuberculous patient. Transact Ophthalmol Am Med Asso; 1930.p.135-65.

49. Mooney AJ. Further observations on the ocular complications of tuberculosis meningitis and their implications. Am J Ophthalmol 1959;48:297-312.

50. Weeks JE. Tuberculosis of the eye. Am J Ophthalmol 1926;9: 243-6.

51. Watson PG, Hayreh SS. Scleritis and episcleritis. Br J Ophthalmol 1976;60:163-91.

52. Nanda M, Pflugfelder SC, Holland S. Mycobacterium tuberculosis scleritis. Am J Ophthalmol 1987;108:736-7.

53. Saini JS, Sharma A, Pillai P. Scleral tuberculosis. Trop Geogr Med 1988;40:350-2.

54. Abadie C. Jumeurs Rares symebioues des paupieres. Arch Ophthalmol 1881;1:432-7.

55. Prasad N. Tubercular osteomyelitis. Bulletin of the Delhi Ophthalmological Soiety. DOS Times 1995 September.

56. Chawla R, Garg S, Venkatesh P, Kashyap S, Tewari HK. Case report of tuberculous panophthalmitis. Med Sci Monit 2004;10:CS57-9.

57. Illingworth RS, Wright T. Tuberculosis of the choroid. Br Med J 1948;365:8.

58. Jabbour NM, Faris B, Tempe CL. A case of pulmonary tuberculosis presenting with a choroidal tuberculoma Ophthalmology 1985;92: 884-7.

59. Massaro D, Katz S, Sachs M. Choroidal tuberculosis: a clue to haematogenous tuberculosis. Ann Intern Med 1964;60:231-41.

60. Olazabal Fa Jr. Choroidal tubercles a neglected sign. JAMA 1967;5:374-7.

61. Sharma SK, Mohan A, Pande JN, Prasad KL, Gupta AK, Khilnani GC. Clinical profile laboratory characteristics and outcome in miliary tuberculosis. QJM 1995;88:29-37.

62. Chung YM, Yeh TS, She SJ, Liu JH. Macular subretinal neovascularization in choroidal tuberculosis. Ann Ophthalmol 1989;21:225-9.

63. Gur S, Silverstone BZ, Zylberman R, Borson D. Chorioretinitis and extrapulmonary tuberculosis. Ann Ophthalmol 1987;19: 112-5.

64. Blodi BA, Johnson MW, McLeish NM, Gass JD. Presumed choroidal tuberculosis in a human immunodeficiency virus infected host. Am J Ophthalmol 1989;108:605-7.

65. Bansal R, Gupta A, Gupta V, Dogra MR, Sharma A, Bambery P. Tubercular serpiginous-like choroiditis presenting as multifocal serpiginoid choroiditis. Ophthalmology 2012;119:2334-42.

66. Nazari Khanamiri H, Rao NA. Serpiginous choroiditis and infectious multifocal serpiginoid choroiditis. Surv Ophthalmol 2013;58:203-32.

67. Wadhwa N, Garg SP, Mehrotra A. Prospective evaluation of intravitreal triamcinolone acetonide in serpiginous choroiditis. Ophthalmologica 2010;224:183-7.

68. Venkatesh P, Gogia V, Gupta S, Tayade A, Shilpy N, Shah B, Guleria R. Pulse cyclophosphamide therapy in the management of patients with macular serpiginous choroidopathy. Indian J Ophthalmol 2015;63:318-22.

69. Gradenigo PN. Tuberculosis of the iris. Boston Med Surg J 1869;4:285-7.

70. Ohmart WA. Experimental tuberculosis of the eye. Am J Ophthalmol 1933;16:773-8.

71. Fries JW, Patel RJ. Piesseno WF, Wirth DF, Genus and species specific DNA probes to identify mycobacteria using the polymerase chain reaction. Mol Cell Probes 1990;4:87-105.

72. Rosen PH, Spalton DJ, Gratiam EM. Intraocualr tuberculosis. Eye 1990;4:486-92.

73. Saini JS, Mukherjee AK, Nadkarni. Primary tuberculosis of the retina. Br J Ophthalmol 1986;70:533-5.

74. Gieser SC, Murphy RP. Eale's disease. In: Tasman W, Jaeger EA, editors. Duane's clinical ophthalmology. Philadelphia: JB Lippincott; 1989[3].p.1-5.

75. Elliot AJ. 30-year observation of patient with Eale's diseases. Am J Ophthalmol 1975;80:404-8.

76. Charmis J. On the classification and management of the evolutionary course of Eale's diseases. Trans Ophthalmol Soc UK 1965;85:75-160.

77. Elliot AJ. Recurrent intraoular haemorrhages in young adults [Eale's disease]: report of thirty one cases. Trans Am Ophthalmol Soc 1954;52:811-75.

78. Elliot AJ, Harris GS. The present status of the diagnosis and treatment of periphlebitis retinae [Eale's disease]. Can J Ophthalmol 1969;4:117-22.

79. Renie WA, Murphy RP, Anderson KC. The evaluation of patients with Eale's disease. Retina 1983;3:243-8.

80. Singh R, Toor P, Parchand S, Sharma K, Gupta V, Gupta A. Quantitative polymerase chain reaction for Mycobacterium tuberculosis in so-called Eales' disease. Ocul Immunol Inflamm 2012;20:153-7.

81. Ballantyne AJ, Michaelson IC. A case of perivasculitis retinae associated with symptoms of cerebral disease. Br J Ophthalmol 1937;21:22-35.

82. Finoff WC. Some impressions derived from the study of recurrent haemorrhages into the retina and vitreous of young patients. Trans Am Ophthalmol Soc 1921;19:238-58.

83. Bloomfield SE, Mondino B, Gray GF. Scleral tuberculosis. Arch Ophthalmol 1977;94:954-6.

84. Knapp A. On some forms of retinal tuberculosis. Trans Am Ophthalmol Soc 1913;13:486-9.

85. Verhoeff FH. The histologic findings in a case of tuberculous cyclitis, and a theory as to the orgin of tuberculous scleritis and keratitis. Trans Am Ophthalmol Soc 1910;12:566-86.

86. Werdenberg E. Zur Frage der Tuberkulosen Aetiologie der periphlebitis retinae: Klin Monatsbl Augenheilkd 1940;105:285-93.

87. Schlaegel TF Jr, Weber JC. Double blind therapeutic trial of isoniazid in 344 patients with uveitis. Br J Ophthalmol 1969; 53:425-7.

88. Rosenbaum JT, Wernick R. Selection and interpretation of laboratory tests for patients with uveitis. Int Ophthalmol Clin 1990;30:238-43.

89. Rosenbaum JT, Wernick R. The utility of routine screening of patients with uveitis for systemic lupus erythematosus or tuberculosis. A Bayesian analysis. Arch Ophthalmol 1990;108: 1291-3.

90. Dyorak-Theobald G. Acute tuberculous endophthalmitis. Am J Opthalmol 1958;45:403-7.

91. Mohamed MA. Tuberculous chorioretinitis: report of a florid case. Bull Ophthalmol Soc Egypt 1970;63:213-6.

92. Ni C, Papale JJ, Robinson NL, Wu BF. Uveal tuberculosis. Int Ophthalmol Clin 1982;22:103-24.

93. Smith RE. Tubrculoma of the choroid. Ophthalmology 1980;87:257-8.

94. Abrams J, Schlaegel TF Jr. The role of the isoniazed therapeutic test in tuberculous uveitis. Am J Ophthalmol 1982;94:511-5.

95. World Health Organization. Use of tuberculosis interferon-gamma release assays [IGRAs] in low- and middle-income countries: policy statement. Geneva: World Health Organization; 2011.

96. Gazette notification-G.S.R. 432[E]. Revised National Tuberculosis Control Programme, New Delhi: Ministry of Health and Family Welfare, Government of India; 2012.

97. WHO warns against the use of inaccurate blood tests for active tuberculosis. Available at URL: http://www.who.int/mediacentre/news/releases/2011/tb_20110720/en/. Accessed on October 22, 2018.

98. Kotake S, Kimura K, Yoshikawa K, Sasamoto Y, Matsuda A, Nishikawa T, et al. Polymerase chain reation for the detection of Mycobacterium tuberculosis in ocular tuberculosis. Am J Ophthalmol 1994;117:805-6.

99. Yamaguchi R, Matsuo K, Yamazaki A, Abe C, Nagai S, Terasaka K, et al. Cloning and characterization of the gene for immunogenic protein MPB 64 of Mycobacterium bovis BCG. Infect immune 1989;57:283-8.

100. Schluger NW, Kinney D, Harkin TJ, Rom WN. Clinical utility of the polymerase chain reaction in the diagnosis of infections due to Mycobacterium tuberculosis. Chest 1994;105:1116-21.

101a. Bansal R, Sharma K, Gupta A, Sharma A, Singh MP, Gupta V, et al. Detection of Mycobacterium tuberculosis genome in vitreous fluid of eyes with multifocal serpiginoid choroiditis. Ophthalmology 2015;122:840-50.

101b. Sharma K, Gupta A, Sharma M, Sharma A, Singh R, Aggarwal K, et al. MTBDRplus for the rapid diagnosis of ocular tuberculosis and screening of drug resistance. Eye [Lond] 2018;32:451-6.

102. Sharma SK, Mukhopadhyay S, Arora R, Varma K, Pande JN, Khilnani GC. Computed tomography in miliary tuberculosis: comparison with plain films, bronchoalveolar lavage, pulmonary functions and gas exchange. Australas Radiol 1996;40:113-8.

103. Gupta A, Sharma A, Bansal R, Sharma K. Classification of intraocular tuberculosis. Ocul Immunol Inflamm 2015;23:7-13.

104. Sharma SK, Ryan H, Khaparde S, Sachdeva KS, Singh AD, Mohan A, et al. Index-TB guidelines: Guidelines on extrapulmonary tuberculosis for India. Indian J Med Res 2017;145:448-63.

105. Leibold JE. Drugs having a toxic effect on the optic nerve. Int Ophthalmol Clin 1971;11:137-44.

106. Kakisu Y, adchi-Vsami E, Mizota A. Pattern electroretinogram and visual evoked cortical potential in ethambutol optic neuropathy. Doc Ophthalmol 1988;76:327-34.

107. Kuming BS, Braude L. Anterior opti neuritis caused by ethambutol toxicity. S Afr Med J 1979;55:4.

108. Rossos T, Tsolkas A. The toxicity of myambutol in the human eye. Ann Ophthalmol 1970;2:577-80.

109. Carr RE, Henkind P. Ocular manifestations of ethambutol toxicity. Arch Ophthalmol 1962;67:566-71.

110. Place VA, Perts EA, Buyske DA. Metabolic and special studies of ethambutol in normal volunteers and tuberculosis patients. Ann N Y Acad Sci 1966;135:775-95.

111. Leibold JE. The ocular toxicity of ethambutol and its relation to dose. Ann N Y Acad Sci 1966;135:904-9.

112. Citron KM. Ethambutol: a review with special reference to ocular toxicity. Tubercle 1969;50 Suppl:32-6.

113. Barron GJ. Tepper L, Lovine G. Ocular toxicity from ethambutol. Am J Ophthalmol 1974;77:256-60.

114. Donomae I, Yamamoto K. Clinical evaluation of ethambutol in primary tuberculosis. Ann N Y Acad Si 1966;135:849-81.

115. Fledelius HC, Petrera JE, Skjodt K, Trojabory W. Ocular ethambutol toxicity. Acta Ophthalmol 1987;65:251-5.

116. Gomez-Pimienta JL, Shibayama Hernandez H, Perez Fernandez LF, Perez Herrera R, Garcia Oranday O. Retreatment of pulmonary tuberculosis with ethambutol. Ann N Y Acad Sci 1966;135:882-9.

117. Pyle MM. Ethambutol in the retreatment and primary treatment of tuberculosis: four-year clinical investigation. Ann NY Acad Sci 1966;135:835-48.

118. Chaterjee VKK, Buchanan DR, Friedmann AI, Green M. Ocular toxicity following ethambutol in standard dosage. Br J Dis Chest 1986;80:288-91.

119. Citron KM, Thomas GO. Ocular toxicity from ethambutol. Thorax 1986;41:737-9.

120. Blumberg HM, Burman WJ, Chaisson RE, Daley CL, Etkind SC, Friedman LN, et al. American Thoracic Society/Centers for Disease Control and Prevention/Infectious Diseases Society of America: treatment of tuberculosis. Am J Respir Crit Care Med 2003;167:603-62.

121. Sutton PH, Beattic A. Optic atrophy after administration of isoniazid with para-aminosalicylic acid. Lancet 1955;1:650-1.

122. Kass I, Mandel W, Cohen H, Dressler SH. Isoniazid as a cause of optic neuritis and atrophy. JAMA 1957;164:1740-3.

123. Neff TA. Isoniazed toxicity: reports of lactic acidosis and keratitits. Chest 1971;59:245-8.

124. Ahmad I, Clark LA. Isoniazed hypersensitivity reaction involving the eyes: report of a case. Dis Chest 1967;52:112-3.

125. Sykowski P. Streptomycin causing retrobulbar optic neuritis: case report. Am J Ophthalmol 1951;34:1446.

126. Fraufelder FT, Meyer SM. Drug-induced ocular side effects and drug interaction. Second edition. Philadelphia: Lea and Febiger; 1982.

127. Saran BR, Maguire AM, Nichols C, Frank I, Hertle RW, Brucker AJ, et al. Hypopyon uveitis in patients with acquired immunodeficiency syndrome treated for systemic Mycobacterium avium complex infection with rifabutin. Arch Ophthalmo 1994;112:1159-65.

128. Negrel AD, Choret M, Baouillion G, Layadec R. Clofazimine and the eye: preliminary communication. Lep Rev 1981;55:349-52.

129. Walinder P, Gip L, Stempa M. Corneal changes in patients treated with cloflazimine. Br J Ophthalmol 1976;60:526-8.

130. Cunningham CA, Friedbery DN, Corr RE. Clofazimine-induced retinal degeneration. Retina 1990;10:131-4.

131. Craythorn JM, Schwartz M, Greel D. Clofazimine-induced bull's eye retinopathy. Retina 1986;6:50-2.

132. Berkovitz L, Krasnitz I, Beiran I, Blumenthal EZ, Mimouni M. Isolated reversible toxic optic neuropathy secondary to linezolid. J Clin Ophthalmol Res 2017;5:40-2.

133. Magazine R, Pal M, Chogtu B, Nayak V. Capreomycin-induced optic neuritis in a case of multidrug resistant pulmonary tuberculosis. Indian J Pharmacol 2010;42:247-8.

25

Tuberculosis in Pregnancy

Sunesh Kumar, Vatsla Dadhwal, K Aparna Sharma

INTRODUCTION

Since the days of Hippocrates, the initial presentation of tuberculosis [TB] in temporal relation to pregnancy has been a subject of concern and controversy. TB in a pregnant woman can present in several ways. Pregnant women may give a past history of TB. Occasionally, the disease may be diagnosed in a pregnant woman when she develops symptoms and signs suggestive of TB. Many a times, pregnant women may remain asymptomatic and TB may be diagnosed either incidentally or by way of a screening programme. Atypical presentation of TB in pregnant women poses difficulties in confirmation of the diagnosis. TB in pregnancy, thus, has important implications for the mother and child (1,2).

EPIDEMIOLOGY

During the year 1985, the Centres for Disease Control and Prevention [CDC], Atlanta, estimated the TB in association with pregnancy occurred at a rate of 49.6/100,000 population among the Asians and the Pacific Islanders compared to a figure of 5.7/100,000 in the American whites and 26.7/100,000 in the African-Americans (3,4). In the series reported by Schaefer *et al* (5), between 1966 and 1972, 3.2% of patients with active TB at the New York Lying-in Hospital were first diagnosed during pregnancy. Bailey *et al* (6) estimated the incidence of TB during pregnancy to be 4.8% at New Orleans. Margono *et al* (7) reported that, between 1985-1990, 12.4 cases of active TB were identified per 100000 deliveries and during 1991-1992, this number increased to 94.8 per 100,000 deliveries. In another study (8) from a district general hospital in a high prevalence area in London, UK, the incidence of active TB disease during pregnancy was reported to be 252/100,000 deliveries.

In 2011, it was estimated that more than 200,000 cases of active TB occurred among pregnant women globally; the greatest burdens were in Africa and South-East Asia (9). Various countries have been classified as high-burden [>60 cases/100,000 population per year] or low-burden [<20 cases/100,000 population per year] countries depending on the prevalence of active TB. The increasing occurrence of co-infection of human immunodeficiency virus [HIV] and TB adds an entirely new dimension to the natural history of the disease.

The epidemiology of latent TB infection [LTBI] in pregnancy is a reflection of the prevalence in general population. Small studies report prevalence of LTBI in pregnancy to be 19%-34% among HIV-negative women in India (10) and up to 49% in HIV-seropositive women in South Africa (11). In another prospective study from Pune (12), 24 of the 715 HIV infected women who were followed-up for 480 postpartum person-years developed TB, yielding a TB incidence of 5 cases per 100 person-years. A baseline CD4+ cell count less than 200 cells/mm^3, and viral load greater than 50,000 copies/mL and a positive tuberculin skin test [TST] result were found to be predictors for the development of active postpartum TB disease in HIV-seropositive women.

During pregnancy, pulmonary TB is the most common lesion and extra-pulmonary TB [EPTB] occurs less commonly. Miliary TB and TB of lymph nodes, bones and kidneys are also encountered during pregnancy (13). TB meningitis (14), TB mastitis (15), TB peritonitis (16), and perineal TB (17) have also been described.

CLINICAL PRESENTATION OF TUBERCULOSIS DURING PREGNANCY

About one-half to two-thirds of pregnant women with TB remain asymptomatic (18). Some of the symptoms,

Table 25.1: Clinical presentations of TB in pregnancy		
Variable	*Good et al (19)*	*Maurya and Sapre (20)*
Study period	1965–1974	1989–1992
Place of study	Denver	Gwalior
No. of patients		
Pulmonary TB	27*	172†
Extrapulmonary TB	0	0
Total	27	17
HIV-seropositive [%]	ND	ND
Tuberculin positive [%]	96	ND
Method of diagnosis		
Microbiological [%]	100‡	§
Histopathological [%]	0	§

* In 6 patients TB was diagnosed during pregnancy [first trimester n = 3; second trimester n = 1; third trimester n = 2]. In the remaining 11 patients, TB was diagnosed during the postpartum period [up to 12 months following delivery]
†Of the 209 patients studied, 6 patients had no evidence of TB and were tuberculin negative; 31 patients had past history of adequately treated TB
‡16 patients had drug-resistant TB
§ Detailed break up not given
TB = tuberculosis; HIV = human immunodeficiency virus; ND = not described

such as increased respiratory rate and fatigue may mimic the physiological changes that occur in pregnancy, and thus, make the diagnosis difficult. In the series reported by Schaefer *et al* (5), minimal symptoms were observed in 65% pregnant women with TB. Good *et al* (19) found 19% women to be asymptomatic among 371 women admitted to the National Jewish Hospital, Colorado. Of these, 27 patients had reactivation of TB during or within 12 months after pregnancy. They also reported cough [74%], weight loss [14%], fever [30%], malaise and fatigue [30%], and haemoptysis [19%] as the common presenting symptoms. Maurya and Sapre (20) screened 209 pregnant women for TB by TST, direct sputum examination for acid-fast bacilli and chest radiograph [done after 12 weeks of gestation with abdominal shielding]. Of these 209 patients, 12% had active TB; 70.3% were sputum smear-negative, but had chest radiographic evidence of TB and a raised erythrocyte sedimentation rate, 14% had a past history of adequately treated TB but no evidence of active disease; and 2.9% had no evidence of TB and were tuberculin negative. They found cough [75%], weight loss [23%], fever [15%] and malaise [30%] to be the common symptoms in 100 symptomatic women. Clinical presentation of TB in pregnancy as reported in some published studies is shown in Table 25.1 (19,20).

Screening for Tuberculosis in Pregnancy

In the low-burden countries, the lack of awareness towards the possibility of diagnosis of TB could be a hindrance while in the high-burden countries it is the lack of resources. Also, in women, clinical presentation with fever, night sweats and

haemoptysis has been found to be less common as compared to men (21). Presence of cough for more than 2 weeks was reported in 60% of antenatal women in a study from South Africa (22).

Co-infection with HIV further complicates the presentation and causes atypical symptoms. World Health Organization [WHO] recommends screening in symptomatic women with cough of any duration, fever or malaise (23). The Centers for Disease Control and Prevention, Atlanta, in addition recommends screening in women with a recent TB contact (24). Screening for LTBI is recommended only in high risk women in the low-burden countries. These include, those with known or suspected TB contacts, injection drug use, HIV or other immunosuppression, foreign birth, and/or residence in congregate settings (25). Pregnancy by itself is not considered high-risk. In high-burden countries, LTBI screening is not routinely done.

EFFECT OF PREGNANCY ON TUBERCULOSIS

At the start of the twentieth century it was believed that pregnancy had a deleterious effect on TB (13). In fact, therapeutic abortion was advocated for pregnant women with pulmonary TB. During this period, a number of conflicting reports evaluating the impact of pregnancy on TB appeared (13).

However, it is currently believed that pregnancy neither predisposes to the development of TB nor results in the progression of the disease. Two large studies (26,27) although somewhat old, clearly showed that pregnancy does not appear to result in the progression of the disease. One study (26) described 250 pregnant women; 189 with pulmonary and 61 with EPTB. None of them were given anti-TB treatment and the treatment largely consisted of sanatorium therapy. It was found that TB improved in 9.1% women while the disease progressed in 7% and most of the women remained stable (26). In another study, de March (27) evaluated the influence of pregnancy as a relapse factor for pulmonary TB in 215 patients who received adequate treatment and concluded that pregnancy, labour, puerperium, and lactation did not predispose to the risk of relapse of pulmonary TB when the disease was adequately treated.

Schaefer *et al* (5) compared the course and outcome of TB in pregnant women during the pre-chemotherapy and chemotherapy era; 88% women in pre-chemotherapy and 91% in the chemotherapy era remained stable during pregnancy. Eleven of the 27 cases of reactivation or relapse of pulmonary TB described by Good *et al* (17) occurred in the post-partum period. However, these and other studies highlight a small but definite of relapse and deterioration in the post-partum period (10).

EFFECT OF TUBERCULOSIS ON PREGNANCY

Contrary to old reports, following the advent of effective anti-TB treatment, current literature does not suggest that TB has much of an adverse impact either on the course of pregnancy or labour (1,2). The effects of TB on pregnancy may be influenced by many factors, including the severity of the disease, how advanced the pregnancy has progressed to at the time of diagnosis, the presence of extrapulmonary spread, HIV co-infection and the treatment instituted. The prognosis is the worst in women in whom a diagnosis of advanced disease is made in the puerperium as well as those with HIV co-infection. Failure to comply with treatment also worsens the prognosis (28).

Obstetrical complications like prematurity, foetal growth retardation, low birth weight and increased perinatal mortality have been commonly reported (29a,29b). Lymphadenitis is the most common form of EPTB reported and has no adverse effect on the maternal and foetal outcome. Other forms of EPTB, such as, intestinal, spinal, endometrial and meningeal TB are associated with an increased frequency of maternal disability, foetal growth retardation and infants with low Apgar scores (30).

However, in a prospective study from India (31), there were no statistically significant differences in pregnancy complications and pregnancy outcomes in women diagnosed with and treated for TB during pregnancy compared to matched controls who were pregnant and had no TB. The only exception was in women who started TB treatment late in pregnancy; neonatal mortality and extreme prematurity were significantly higher in this group.

Abortions

Selikoff and Dorfmann (32) reported seven early spontaneous abortions and nine antepartum or intrapartum foetal deaths in 616 pregnant women with TB, where 600 pregnancies resulted in the birth of 602 normal live infants. Maurya and Sapre (20) reported four spontaneous abortions in the group previously treated for TB.

Preterm Delivery

Schaefer *et al* (5) did not find any evidence of increased risk of prematurity in their series. Maurya and Sapre (20) reported only two premature deliveries among 31 pregnant women with a past history of TB. Bjerkedal *et al* from Norway (33) described the course and outcome of pregnancy in 542 women with TB [study group] and 112,530 women with TB [control subjects]. Study group had increased frequency of pregnancy induced hypertension [7.4% *versus* 4.7%] and vaginal bleeding [4.1% *versus* 2.2%]. Labour was induced more often in the study group than among the control subjects [14.6% *versus* 9.6%]. Labour was also reported to be more often complicated in the study group than in control subjects [15.1% *versus* 9.6] and interventions during labour were required more often in the study group [12.6% *versus* 7.7%]. Intrauterine foetal death rate between 16 and 28 weeks was nine-fold higher in the study group [20.1/1000 in cases *versus* 2.3/1000 control subjects]. However, no difference was found in the number of congenital anomalies or subsequent conception rate. There was no difference in mean gestational age, preterm births or mean birth weight among live births.

Maurya and Sapre (20) reported two preterm deliveries and on intrauterine foetal death in the subgroup with active TB. Maternal mortality and foetal complications were more frequent in pregnant women with drug-resistant TB compared to those with drug-sensitive disease in the study by Good *et al* (19).

In another study (30), 33 patients with EPTB [12 with TB lymphadenitis, 9 with intestinal, 7 with skeletal, 2 with renal, 2 with meningeal, and 1 with endometrial TB] were followed through their deliveries. Of the 33 patients, 29 received anti-TB treatment during pregnancy. The antenatal complications, intrapartum events, and perinatal outcomes were compared with those among 132 healthy pregnant women without TB who were matched for age, parity and socio-economic status. It was observed that TB lymphadenitis did not affect the course of pregnancy or labour or the perinatal outcome. However, as compared with the control subjects, 21 women with involvement of other extrapulmonary sites had significantly higher rates of antenatal hospitalisation [24% *versus* 2%], infants with low Apgar scores [<6] soon after birth [19% *versus* 3%], and low birth-weight [less than 2.5 kg] infants [33% *versus* 11%]. The authors concluded that EPTB that is confined to the lymph-nodes has no effect on obstetrical outcomes; but TB at other extrapulmonary sites does adversely affect the outcome of pregnancy (23).

TRANSPLACENTAL TRANSMISSION OF TUBERCULOSIS

Transplacental transmission of TB infection has now been conclusively proven by a number of case reports (34-36). In the literature, cases where newborn babies were found to have acquired TB from the diseased endometrium have been described. Nemir and O'Hare (34) described one female child carefully investigated and treated for congenital TB in neonatal period. This child had positive subumbilical lymph nodes indicating umbilical vein as the route of transmission.

Mycobacterium tuberculosis [*Mtb*] has also been demonstrated in placental specimens and tissues from stillborn infants (37,38). Kalpan *et al* (39) reported two interesting cases. In the first case, 25-year-old pregnant woman had been treated with multiple drugs for cavitary pulmonary TB. She desired an elective abortion of six weeks of gestation. Endometrial curettage smear revealed *Mtb*. In the second case, a 24-year-old pregnant woman presented at 34 weeks of gestation with premature rupture of membranes. An emergency caesarean section performed 24 hours later revealed fibrinous exudates on peritoneal surface and a placenta densely adherent to the uterus. Both exudates and tissue from the endometrium grew *Mtb*. These findings suggest that subclinical endometrial infections can be an important source for transplacental transmission of disease in patients with congenital TB.

CONGENITAL TUBERCULOSIS

Congenital TB (40-43) is a relatively uncommon but an important entity. The reader is referred to the chapters

"Pathology of tuberculosis" [Chapter 3] and *"Tuberculosis in children"* [Chapter 36] for more details.

DIAGNOSIS

It is important to identify pregnant women suffering from TB as it may help to prevent transmission of disease to the newborn and close contacts.

Chest Radiograph

In the past, a routine chest radiograph was advocated during pregnancy in order to detect active and inactive TB (44,45). Bonebrake *et al* (46) advised against such a policy as most patients with significant findings on chest radiograph also had positive findings on physical examination and a positive TST result. Concern about radiation exposure to foetus does not justify the policy of routine chest radiograph examination during pregnancy [34-36 weeks]. However, if a chest radiograph is indicated, pregnancy should not be considered as an absolute contraindication. A chest radiograph should be taken with abdominal shielding, preferably after the first trimester of pregnancy.

Estimated radiation from a chest radiograph is approximately 50 mrad to the chest and 2.5 to 5 mrad to the gonads (47-49). Prenatal radiation exposure has been correlated with subsequent risk of malformations and cancer. Mole (49), in a detailed analysis estimated such a risk to be zero to one case per 1000 patients of irradiated by one rad in utero during the first four months of pregnancy. Therefore, a chest radiograph carried out during pregnancy does not seem to carry a measurable risk to the foetus since radiation exposure from a chest radiograph is much less.

In symptomatic women and asymptomatic women with a recent TB contact, a shielded chest radiograph, which poses minimal risk to the foetus, sputum smear microscopy, mycobacterial culture are recommended (50,51).

Detection of Tuberculosis Infection

The TST identifies persons infected by *Mtb* but does not define the activity or extent of disease. Generally, the TST becomes positive two to ten weeks after initial exposure (52). In the past, a concern had been expressed regarding the effect of pregnancy on TST positivity (53). However, subsequent studies have not found pregnancy to affect the TST reactivity (54,55). Present and Comstock (55) evaluated 25,000 patients over a one-year period and reported that pregnancy did not affect the TST results. There appears to be no risk either to the pregnant woman or her foetus from the TST (56).

Carter and Mates (57) while reviewing cases of TB during pregnancy over a four-year span in Rhode Island found that most patients with TB infection remain asymptomatic. They concluded that the TST screening in pregnancy may prevent risk to the foetus, new born and the obstetric ward workers.

However, usefulness of such a policy in areas where TB is highly endemic remains doubtful. Although, the recently available interferon-gamma release assays [IGRAs], offer several advantages over the TST however, they should not replace TST in low-income and other middle-income countries. The reader is referred to the Chapter *"Laboratory diagnosis of tuberculosis: best practices and current policies"* [Chapter 8] for more details.

Microbiological, Molecular Methods

Demonstration of *Mtb* in sputum, body fluids or material by Ziehl-Neelsen staining and Lowenstein-Jensen culture confirms the diagnosis of TB disease. However, low yield in these specimens remains a practical problem. The utility of liquid culture, cartridge based nucleic amplification tests [CBNAAT] in the early diagnosis of TB and drug-susceptibility testing in pregnancy (58) merits further study.

TREATMENT OF ACTIVE TUBERCULOSIS DURING PREGNANCY

Pregnant women with active TB should be immediately started on ATT as untreated TB is far more hazardous to a pregnant woman and her foetus than the adverse effects related to the treatment of the disease (59). Though first-line drugs, such as isoniazid, rifampicin, streptomycin and ethambutol cross the placenta, with exception of streptomycin induced ototoxicity, none of these drugs appear to be teratogenic or toxic to the foetus (60).

Isoniazid

Even though isoniazid crosses the placenta, no significant teratogenic effects have been noted even when used during the first four months of pregnancy (61). However, one report mentioned about two-fold increase in risk of malformations when mothers were exposed to isoniazid (62).

Hepatitis is a frequently observed side-effect of isoniazid. Pregnancy and postpartum women may be particularly at higher risk for isoniazid induced hepatitis. An addition of pyridoxine in a dose of 50 mg/day has been recommended during pregnancy to prevent neurotoxicity in the mother and the foetus (59). This regimen has been shown to prevent seizures in neonates born to mothers treated with isoniazid during pregnancy (1). The reader is referred to the chapter *"Hepatotoxicity associated with anti-tuberculosis treatment"* [Chapter 45] for further details.

Rifampicin

Snider *et al* (60) failed to detect increased incidence of teratogenicity among mothers taking rifampicin during pregnancy. Presently, rifampicin is considered to be an essential component of anti-TB treatment during pregnancy (1,63).

Ethambutol

Although ethambutol is known to be teratogenic in experimental animals, there are no reports of maldevelopment including ocular injury in human foetuses (64-66).

Streptomycin

Use of streptomycin during pregnancy has been reported to be associated with vestibular and auditory impairment in the new born (67,68). Streptomycin induced ototoxicity has been reported irrespective of period of gestation. Therefore, streptomycin should not be used during pregnancy.

Pyrazinamide

Due to faster sputum conversion rate, this drug is commonly used in the short-course treatment regimens. The WHO guidelines suggest that pyrazinamide can be safely used in pregnancy (69). If pyrazinamide is not included in the initial treatment regimen, the minimum duration of treatment is nine months. Benefits of the use of pyrazinamide in HIV-seropositive pregnant women outweigh the undetermined potential risks to the foetus.

Principles of Treatment

Active disease discovered in antenatal period should be promptly treated. Daily treatment with isoniazid, rifampicin, pyrazinamide and ethambutol during the first two months followed by isoniazid, rifampicin and ethambutol for the subsequent four months should be used. The reader is referred to the *"Treatment of tuberculosis" [Chapter 44]* for more details. Duration of anti-TB treatment need not modified because of pregnancy. Active TB disease discovered close to the time of delivery should also be actively treated. Neonate should be carefully examined and kept under surveillance for development of TB. Placenta should be examined for possible infection by *Mtb*. If patients receiving anti-TB treatment conceive, pregnancy should be allowed to continue while the patient continues anti-TB treatment. Appropriate steps should be taken to prevent TB infection in the newborn.

Second-line Drugs

Little is known about the teratogenic effects of the second-line anti-TB drugs. Due to high incidence off side-effects, their usefulness is limited. Teratogenic effect has been attributed to ethionamide (70). Kanamycin and capreomycin theoretically share the potential for producing ototoxicity with streptomycin. The potential hazard of such treatment must be considered by the parents and the treating physician.

Treatment of Drug-resistant Tuberculosis During Pregnancy

Women who are being treated for drug-resistant TB should receive counselling concerning the risk to the foetus because of the known and unknown risks of second-line anti-TB drugs. There have been occasional case reports and case series in the published literature regarding the management of multidrug-resistant TB [MDR-TB] during pregnancy using second-line drugs (71-75). These data suggest that treatment of MDR-TB during pregnancy is beneficial both to the mother and the child. In a recent study (74), exposure to second-line anti-TB drugs was associated with delivery of healthy term infants. However, studies involving large sample size with a long-term follow-up are awaited.

As the majority of teratogenic effects occur in the first trimester, treatment should be delayed until the second trimester. The decision to postpone the treatment should be based on the analysis of the risks and benefits and should be acceptable to both the doctor and patient. Injectable agents, aminoglycosides and capreomycin should be avoided during pregnancy and if possible ethionamide should also be avoided (74,75). The decision should also take into consideration the severity of illness. Treatment should consist of combination of three or four drugs with demonstrated efficacy against the infecting strain.

Treatment of Human Immunodeficiency Virus-Tuberculosis Co-infection During Pregnancy

With increasing incidence of HIV and TB co-infection, the management of such cases present newer challenges especially in the pregnant women. Standard treatment guidelines (76,77) should be followed.

TREATMENT OF LATENT TUBERCULOSIS INFECTION

Evidence-based guidelines are available from the WHO for a public health approach to the management of LTBI in high risk individuals in countries with high or middle upper income and low TB incidence (78). However, efficacy and safety of isoniazid chemoprophylaxis during pregnancy, in areas where TB is highly endemic, like India, are unclear (79). A recently published systematic review (80) suggested that pregnant women benefit from screening for LTBI. The systematic review (80) also suggested that IGRAs and TST were comparable in screening for LTBI during pregnancy. The question whether the treatment should be started in pregnancy needs to be answered. For HIV-seronegative women, the Centers for Disease Control [CDC] recommends delaying treatment of LTBI until two to three months postpartum, unless the patient has had a recent known TB contact. Both the CDC and the WHO recommend early treatment of LTBI in HIV-seropositive pregnant women (81,82), but these women are at an increased risk of hepatotoxicity due to anti-TB drugs (83,84). An ongoing study (85), International Maternal Pediatric Adolescent AIDS Clinical Trials Network [IMPAACT] P1078, assessing the safety of antepartum *versus* postpartum initiation of isoniazid preventive treatment in HIV-infected women residing in TB-endemic settings is expected to provide more.

MANAGEMENT OF TUBERCULOSIS IN INFANTS BORN TO MOTHERS WITH TUBERCULOSIS

If the mother had been receiving treatment for TB during pregnancy, the newborn should be assessed for symptoms and signs of congenital TB. Infant should undergo the TST at birth. Chest radiograph and smear and culture examination of the gastric aspirate should be performed. If active TB is ruled out, the child should be treated with isoniazid for two to three months, or till such time the mother, known to be complying with treatment, becomes smear and culture negative (13).

The child should be carefully followed up thereafter. If active disease is detected, the child should receive a full course of anti-TB treatment with rifampicin, isoniazid and pyrazinamide. Ethambutol should be preferable be avoided in neonate as it is difficult to monitor the ocular toxicity.

Breast Feeding

Breast feeding should not be discouraged in nursing mothers receiving ATT as the concentrations of these drugs secreted in the breast milk seldom attain toxic levels (13). However, drugs in breast milk should not be considered to serve as effective treatment for the disease or as chemoprophylaxis in a nursing infant (86,87) Pyridoxine supplementation should be given to breast feeding women taking isoniazid.

ANTI-TUBERCULOSIS TREATMENT AND CONTRACEPTION

Rifampicin induces the P-450 mixed function oxidase system that metabolises oral contraceptives and other drugs (13). Reliability of oral contraceptives is diminished in women taking rifampicin (88,89). Alternative contraceptive measures should be considered for post-partum women who require anti-TB treatment.

REFERENCES

1. Efferen LS. Tuberculosis and pregnancy. Cur Opin Pulm Med 2007; 13:205-11.
2. Laibl VR, Sheffield JS. Tuberculosis in pregnancy. Clin Perinatol 2005;32:739-48.
3. Centers for Disease Control. Leads from the MMWR. Tuberculosis in minorities-United States. JAMA 1987;257:1291-2.
4. Centers for Disease Control. Lead from the MMWR. Tuberculosis in blacks-United States. JAMA 1987;257:2407-8.
5. Schaefer G, Zervoudakis IA, Fuchs FF, David S. Pregnancy and tuberculosis. Obstet Gynecol 1975;46:706-15.
6. Bailey WC, Thompson DH, Greenberg HB. Indigent pregnant women of New Orleans require tuberculosis control measures. Health Serv Rep 1972;87:737-42.
7. Margono F, Mroueh J, Garely A, White D, Duerr A, Minkoff HL. Resurgence of active tuberculosis among pregnant women. Obstet Gynecol 1994;83:11-4.
8. Kothari A, Mahadevan N, Girling J. Tuberculosis and pregnancy-results of a study in a high prevalence area in London. Eur J Obstet Gynecol Reprod Biol 2006;126:48-55.
9. Sugarman J, Colvin C, Moran AC, Oxlade O. Tuberculosis in pregnancy: an estimate of the global burden of disease. Lancet Glob Health 2014;2:710-6.
10. Mathad JS, Bhosale R, Sangar V, Mave V, Gupte N, Kanade S, et al. Screening for latent tuberculosis in pregnant women: a comparison of an interferon-gamma release assay with tuberculin skin testing in Pune, India. In: Programs and abstracts of the 49th Infectious Diseases Society of America, Boston, MA, 2011.
11. Nachega J, Coetzee J, Adendorff T, Msandiwa R, Gray GE, McIntyre JA, et al. Tuberculosis active case finding in a mother-to-child HIV transmission prevention programme in Soweto, South Africa. AIDS 2003;17:1398-400.
12. Gupta A, Nayak U, Ram M, Bhosale R, Patil S, Basavraj A, et al. Byrampjee Jeejeebhoy Medical College-Johns Hopkins University Study Group. Postpartum tuberculosis incidence and mortality among HIV-infected women and their infants in Pune, India, 2002-2005. Clin Infect Dis 2007;45:241-9.
13. Hamadeh MA, Glassroth J. Tuberculosis and pregnancy. Chest 1992;101:1114-20.
14. Stands JW, Jowers RG, Bryan CS. Miliary-meningeal tuberculosis during pregnancy: case report and brief survey of the problem of extra-pulmonary tuberculosis. JSC Med Assoc 1977;73:282-5.
15. Banerjee SN, Ananthakrishnan N, Mehta RB, Prakash S. Tuberculosis mastitis: a continuing problem. World J Surg 1987;11:105-9.
16. Lee GS, Kim SJ, Park IY, Shin JC, Kim SP. Tuberculous peritonitis in pregnancy. J Obstet Gynecol Res 2005;31:436-8.
17. Pal A, Mahadevan N. Perineal tuberculosis diagnosed in pregnancy: 1 case report. J Obstet Gynecol 2005;25:307-8.
18. Wilson EA, Thelin TJ, Dilts PV Jr. Tuberculosis complicated by pregnancy. Am J Obstet Gynecol 1973;115:526-9.
19. Good JT Jr, Iseman MD, Davidson PT, Lakshminarayan S, Sahn SA. Tuberculosis in association with pregnancy. Am J Obstet Gynecol 1981;140:492-8.
20. Maurya U, Sapre S. Tuberculosis and pregnancy. J Obstet Gynecol India 1996;46:460-3.
21. Long NH, Diwan VK, Winkvist A. Difference in symptoms suggesting pulmonary tuberculosis among men and women. J Clin Epidemiol 2002;55:115-20.
22. Gounder CR, Wada NI, Kensler C, Violari A, McIntyre J, Chaisson RE, et al. Active tuberculosis case finding among pregnant women presenting to antenatal clinics in Soweto, South Africa. J Acquir Immune Defic Syndr 2011;57:77-84.
23. World Health Organization. Guidelines for intensified tuberculosis case-finding and isoniazid preventive therapy for people living with HIV in resource-constrained settings. Geneva: World Health Organization; 2011.
24. Bloch AB. Screening for tuberculosis and tuberculosis infection in high-risk populations: recommendations of the Advisory Council for the Elimination of Tuberculosis. MMWR Recomm Rep 1995;44[RR-11]:18-34.
25. Geiter LJ, Gordin FM, Hershfield E, Horsburgh CR Jr, Jereb JA, Jordan TJ, et al. Targeted tuberculin testing and treatment of latent tuberculosis. MMWR Recomm Rep 2000;49:1-54.
26. Hedvell E. Pregnancy and tuberculosis. Acta Med Scand Supp 1963;286:1-101.
27. de March P. Tuberculosis and pregnancy. Five-to ten-year review of 215 patients in their fertile age. Chest 1975;68:800-4.
28. Ormerod P. Tuberculosis in pregnancy and the puerperium. Thorax 2001;56:494-9.
29a. Jana N, Vasista K, Jindal SK, Khunnu B, Ghosh K. Perinatal outcome in pregnancies complicated by pulmonary tuberculosis. Int J Gynaecol Obstet 1994;44:119-24.
29b. Sobhy S, Babiker Z, Zamora J, Khan KS, Kunst H. Maternal and perinatal mortality and morbidity associated with tuberculosis during pregnancy and the postpartum period: a systematic review and meta-analysis. BJOG 2017;124:727-33.
30. Jana N, Vasishta K, Saha SC, Ghosh K. Obstetrical outcomes among women with extra pulmonary tuberculosis. N Engl J Med 1999;341:645-9.
31. Tripathy SN. Tuberculosis and pregnancy. Int J Gynaecol Obstet 2003;80:247-53.
32. Selikoff IJ, Dorfmann HL. Management of tuberculosis. In: Rovinskey JJ, Gulmatcher AF, editors. Medical, surgical and

gynaecologic complications of pregnancy. Baltimore: Williams and Wilkins;1965:p.111.

33. Bjerkedal T, Bahna SL, Lehmann EH. Course and outcome of pregnancy in women with pulmonary tuberculosis. Scand J Respir Dis 1975;56:245-50.

34. Nemir RL, O'Hare D. Congenital tuberculosis. Review and diagnostic guidelines. Am J Dis Child 1985;139:284-7.

35. Myers JP, Perlstein PH, Light IJ, Towbin, Dincsoy HP, Dincsoy MY. Tuberculosis in pregnancy with fatal congenital infection. Pediatrics 1981;67:89-94.

36. Niles RA. Puerpal tuberculosis with death of infant. Am J Obstet Gynecol 1982;144:131-2.

37. Snider D. Pregnancy and tuberculosis. Chest 1984;86:10S-13S.

38. Siegal M. Pathological findings and pathogenesis of congenital tuberculosis. Am Rev Tuberc 1834;29:297-309.

39. Kaplan C, Benirschke K, Tarzy B. Placental tuberculosis in early and late pregnancy. Am J Obstet Gynecol 1980;137:858-60.

40. Cantwell MF, Snider DE Jr, Cauthen GM, Onorato IM. Epidemiology of tuberculosis in the United States,1985 through 1992. JAMA 1994;272:535-9.

41. American Thoracic Society, CDC, Infectious Diseases Society of America. Treatment of tuberculosis. MMWR Recomm Rep 2003; 52:1.

42. Cantwell MF, Shehab ZM, Costello AM, Sands L, Green WF, Ewing EP Jr, et al. Brief report: congenital tuberculosis. N Engl J Med 1994; 330:1051-4.

43. Biddulph J. Short course chemotherapy for childhood tuberculosis. Pediatr Infect Dis J 1990;9:793-801.

44. Freeth A. Routine X-ray examination of the chest at an antenatal clinic. Lancet 1953;1:287-8.

45. Stanton SL. Routine radiology of the chest in antenatal care. J Obstet Gynecol Br Commonw 1968;75:1161-4.

46. Bonebrake CR, Noller KL, Loehnen CP, Muhm JR, Fish CR. Routine chest roentgenography in pregnancy. JAMA 1978;240: 2747-8.

47. Mattox JH. The value of a routine prenatal chest X-ray. Obstet Gynecol 1973;41:243-5.

48. Swartz HM, Reichling BA. Hazards of radiation exposure for pregnant woman. JAMA 1978;239:1907-8.

49. Mole RH. Radiation effects on prenatal development and their radiological significance. Br J Radiol 1979;52:89-101.

50. McCarthy FP, Rowlands S, Giles M. Tuberculosis in pregnancy-case studies and a review of Australia's screening process. Aust N Z J Obstet Gynaecol 2006;46:451-5.

51. Joint Statement of the American Thoracic Society [ATS] and the Centers for Disease Control and Prevention [CDC]. Targeted tuberculin testing and treatment of latent tuberculosis infection. Am J Respir Crit Care Med 2000;161:S221-47.

52. American Thoracic Society and Centers for disease Control. The tuberculin skin test. Am Rev Respir Dis 1971;104:769-75.

53. Finn R, St Hill CA, Govan AJ, Ralfs IG, Gurney FJ, Denye V. Immunological responses in pregnancy and survival of foetal homograft. BMJ 1972;3:150-2.

54. Montgomery WP, Young RC Jr, Allen MP, Harden KA. The tuberculin test in pregnancy. Am J Obstet Gynecol 1968; 100:829-31.

55. Present PA, Comstock GW. Tuberculin sensitivity in pregnancy. Am Rev Respir Dis 1975;112:413-6.

56. Snider DE Jr, Farer LS. Package inserts of antituberculosis drugs and tuberculin. Am Rev Respir Dis 1985;131:809-10.

57. Carter EJ, Mates S. Tuberculosis during pregnancy. The Rhode Island experience, 1987 to 1991. Chest 1994;106:1466-70.

58. Bates M, Ahmed Y, Chilukutu L, Tembo J, Cheelo B, Sinyangwe S, et al. Use of the Xpert[®] MTB/RIF assay for diagnosing pulmonary tuberculosis comorbidity and multidrug-resistant TB

in obstetrics and gynaecology inpatient wards at the University Teaching Hospital, Lusaka, Zambia. Trop Med Int Health 2013;18:1134-40.

59. Warkany J. Antituberculosis drugs. Teratology 1979;20:133-7.

60. Snider DE Jr, Layde PM, Johnson MW, Lyle MA. Treatment of tuberculosis during pregnancy. Am Rev Respir Dis 1980;145: 494-8.

61. Scheinhorn DJ, Angelillo VA. Antituberculosis therapy in pregnancy. Risks to fetus. West Med J 1977;127:195-8.

62. Brost BC, Newman RB. The maternal and fetal effects of tuberculosis therapy. Obstet Gynecol Clin North Am 1997;24: 659-73.

63. Vallejo JG, Starke JR. Tuberculosis and pregnancy. Clin Chest Med 1992;13:693-707.

64. Bothamley G. Drug treatment for tuberculosis during pregnancy: safety considerations. Drug Saf 2001;24:553-65.

65. Bobrowitz ID. Ethambutol in pregnancy. Chest 1974:66:20-4.

66. Lewit T, Nebel L, Terracina S, Karman S. Ethambutol in pregnancy: observation on embryogenesis. Chest 1974;66:25-6.

67. Conway N, Birt BD. Streptomycin in pregnancy. Effects of foetal ear. BMJ 1965;2:260-3.

68. Robinson GC, Cambon KG. Hearing loss in infants of tuberculous mothers treated with streptomycin during pregnancy. N Engl J Med 1964;271:949-51.

69. World Health Organization. Treatment of tuberculosis guidelines. Fourth edition. WHO/HTM/ TB/2009.420. Geneva: World Health Organization; 2010.

70. Potworowska M, Sianozecke E, Szufladowicz. Ethionamide treatment and pregnancy. Pol Med J 1966;5:1152-8.

71. Khan M, Pillay T, Moodley J, Ramjee A, Padayatchi N. Pregnancies complicated by multidrug-resistant tuberculosis and HIV co-infection in Durban, South Africa. Int J Tuberc Lung Dis 2007;11:706-8.

72. Tabarsi P, Moradi A, Baghaei P, Marjani M, Shamaei M, Mansouri N, et al. Standardised second-line treatment of multidrug-resistant tuberculosis during pregnancy. Int J Tuberc Lung Dis 2011;15:547-50.

73. Palacios E, Dallman R, Muñoz M, Hurtado R, Chalco K, Guerra D, et al. Drug-resistant tuberculosis and pregnancy: treatment out-comes of 38 cases in Lima, Peru. Clin Infect Dis 2009;48:1413-9.

74. Dudnyk A, Pavel'chuk O. Multidrug-resistant tuberculosis in pregnant women: treatment and birth outcomes. Eur Respir J 2016;48: PA1912.

75. World Health Organization. Companion handbook to the WHO guidelines for the programmatic management of drug-resistant tuberculosis. WHO/HTM/TB/2014.11. Geneva: World Health Organization; 2014.

76. Hitti J, Frenkel LM, Stek AM, Nachman SA, Baker D, Gonzalez-Garcia A, et al. Maternal toxicity with continuous nevirapine in pregnancy: results from PACTG 1022. J Acquir Immune Defic Syndr 2004;36:772-6.

77. McIlleron H, Martinson N, Denti P, Mashabela F, Hunt J, Shembe S, et al. Efavirenz concentrations in pregnant women taking EFV-based antiretroviral therapy with and without rifampin-containing tuberculosis treatment: the TSHEPISO Study Team. In: AIDS 2012- XIX International AIDS Conference. Abstract no. MOAB0303.

78. Getahun H, Matteelli A, Abubakar I, Aziz MA, Baddeley A, Barreira D, et al. Management of latent Mycobacterium tuberculosis infection: WHO guidelines for low tuberculosis burden countries. Eur Respir J 2015;46:1563-76.

79. Sharma SK, Mohanan S, Sharma A. Relevance of latent TB infection in areas of high TB prevalence. Chest 2012;142:761-73.

80. Malhamé I, Cormier M, Sugarman J, Schwartzman K. Latent tuberculosis in pregnancy: a systematic review. PLoS One 2016;11:e0154825.

81. Centers for Disease Control and Prevention. Latent tuberculosis infection: a guide for primary health care providers. Available at URL: http://www.cdc.gov/tb/publications/LTBI/treatment.htm. Accessed on October 22, 2018.

82. World Health Organization. Guidelines for intensified tuberculosis case-finding and isoniazid preventive therapy for people living with HIV in resource-constrained settings. Geneva: World Health Organization; 2011.

83. Ouyang DW, Shapiro DE, Lu M, Brogly SB, French AL, Leighty RM, et al. Increased risk of hepatotoxicity in HIV-infected pregnant women receiving antiretroviral therapy independent of nevirapine exposure. AIDS 2009;23:2425-30.

84. Lyons F, Hopkins S, Kelleher B, McGeary A, Sheehan G, Geoghegan J, et al. Maternal hepatotoxicity with nevirapine as part of combination antiretroviral therapy in pregnancy. HIV Med 2006;7:255-60.

85. P1078 [DAIDS ID 10732]: A randomized double-blind placebo-controlled trial to evaluate the safety [hepatotoxicity] of immediate [antepartum-initiated] vs. deferred [postpartum-initiated] isoniazid preventive therapy among HIV-infected women in high TB incidence settings. Available at URL: http://www.impaactnetwork.org/studies/P1078.asp. Accessed on October 23, 2017.

86. Snider DE Jr, Powell KE. Should women taking antituberculosis drugs breast feed? Arch Int Med 1984;144:494-8.

87. Tran JH, Montakanikul P. The safety of antituberculosis medications during breast feeding. J Hum Lact 1998;14:337-40.

88. Skolnick II, Stoler BS, Katz DB, Anderson WH. Rifampin, oral contraceptives and pregnancy. JAMA 1976;236:1382.

89. Finch CK, Chrisman CR, Baciewicz AM, Self TH. Rifampin and rifabutin drug interactions: an update. Arch Intern Med 2002;162:985-92.

26

Female Genital Tuberculosis

Sunesh Kumar, JB Sharma

INTRODUCTION

Female genital tuberculosis [TB], though known to have existed for centuries, was first described by Morgagni in 1744 during an autopsy on a 20-year-old girl known to have died of TB peritonitis (1). Infertility, menstrual irregularities and chronic pelvic or lower abdominal pain are the most common manifestations of female genital TB [FGTB] (2-4). It is almost always secondary to a focus elsewhere in the body. Fallopian tubes are the first and the most commonly affected genital organs, followed by endometrium, ovary and cervix (5). Occasionally, other sites may also be affected. A number of patients may remain asymptomatic and the disease may also be discovered incidentally (6). The last century has witnessed changing trends in incidence of FGTB, initially due to improvement in economic standards in developed countries and subsequently by the global pandemic of the human immunodeficiency virus [HIV] infection (6). More liberal immigration from high to low risk areas due to globalisation has increased risk in all countries (7). Emergence of multidrug-resistant TB [MDR-TB] and extensively drug-resistant TB [XDR-TB] is a cause of serious concern (7,8).

EPIDEMIOLOGY

Genital tract TB has been reported in patients presenting with infertility, chronic pelvic pain and menstrual irregularities, in autopsy series, and recently in laparoscopy series of infertility cases and pelvic pain (5,9). Twentieth century witnessed dramatic reduction of FGTB cases in the developed world. However, a similar trend has not been observed in the developing countries. Incidence of genital TB varies greatly depending upon the geographical location ranging from less than 1% in the USA and Sweden to about 10% in infertile women in India with incidence being higher [up to 26.7%] in tertiary referral centres and in assisted reproduction (24.5%) and even higher in tubal factor infertility [up to 48.5%] and in repeated *in vitro* fertilisation [IVF] failures (6,10-16). In a study from Islamabad, Pakistan, 2.43% of the 543 women with infertility were found to have FGTB (17). FGTB can also cause abnormal uterine bleeding and postmenopausal bleeding and involves genital organs as observed on laparoscopy in pulmonary TB cases (18-21). FGTB affects older women in western countries with most women being between 40–50 years (22,23). However, in most large series from India, 68%–89% cases of genital TB were between 20 and 30 years of age [Table 26.1] (11,24-27). It may be due to younger age at marriage and child bearing in developing countries as compared to the western world. Female genital TB is less common in postmenopausal women as the atrophic endometrium in them offers a poor milieu for the growth of the bacillus (4,22-23).

PATHOGENESIS

Genital tract TB is almost always secondary to TB infection elsewhere in the body. Although pulmonary TB is most common, extrapulmonary organs, such as, kidneys, gastrointestinal tract, bone or joints may also be the primary source of infection (11,24-27). In patients with miliary TB, genital organs may be one of the many organs involved. Primary genital TB, though extremely rare, has been described in the female partners of males affected by active genitourinary TB through their semen (28,29). In patients with primary genital TB, cervix or vulva may be the site of involvement.

Haematogenous or lymphatic route is the usual mode of spread. However, direct contiguous spread from other intra-peritoneal organs may occur in a minority of patients (10,30). Simultaneous occurrence of peritoneal TB in patients with genital TB increases the possibility of ruptured caseous

Table 26.1: Age distribution of patients with female genital TB

Study (reference)	No. of patients	Age group [years]			
		<20	*20-30*	*30-40*	*>40*
Gupta (11)	47	13.0	68.0	19.0	0
Devi (24)	144	12.0	70.0	14.0	4.0
Hafeez and Tandon (25)	120	3.3	89.0	6.0	1.7
Chhabra (26)	58	1.7	74.2	8.6	15.5
Rattan *et al* (27)	50	0	76.0	24.0	0

Distribution of patients in various age groups is shown as percentage
All values are corrected to first decimal place.
TB = tuberculosis

lymph nodes or involvement of genital organs during the haematogenous spread.

Fallopian tube is usually the initial site of focus, with subsequent spread to other genital organs (6,31).

Fallopian Tube Tuberculosis

Fallopian tubes are involved in almost all patients [90%-100%] with genital TB (5,10). Ampullary portion of the fallopian tube is the most common site of the disease. Isthmus is less commonly involved and involvement of the interstitial portion is unusual. Generally, the disease tends to be bilateral. Disease may start on the peritoneal surface or in the muscularis, mucosa of the tube; however, involvement of the mucosal layer is almost universal. Gross appearance of the fallopian tube may vary depending upon the severity of disease and stage at which it is encountered. In early cases, congestion of tubes and other pelvic organs with flimsy adhesions and fine miliary tubercles on the surface of the tube and other pelvic organs may be seen. In severe disease, dense plastic adhesions between the fallopian tubes and surrounding organs are seen. In old healed cases, hydrosalpinx or pyosalpinx may be present. Failure to visualise pelvic organs at laparoscopy or laparotomy may be due to dense adhesions in patients with pelvic TB. In 25%-50% cases, the fallopian tubes remain patent with everted fimbriae giving rise to so called "tobacco pouch appearance" (32).

Microscopically, presence of chronic inflammatory cells, with or without caseation, granulomas with Langhans' giant cells may be evident. However, microscopic appearance may be variable depending upon the severity of disease and whether the disease is in active or healing phase. The tubal mucosa may be totally destroyed or may have hyperplastic or adenomatous appearance which may be confused with adenocarcinoma (33). Papillae in the endosalpinx are usually fused, and may lead to implantation of embryo in the fallopian tubes resulting in ectopic pregnancy.

Endometrial Tuberculosis

Endometrial involvement in genital TB is secondary to tubal involvement (31,32). Schaefer (31) reported endometrial involvement in 50%-80% cases of genital TB. In a large series of 1,436 cases of genital TB, Nogales-Ortiz *et al* (32) reported endometrial involvement in 79% of cases. Oosthuizen *et al* (34), in a study of 109 patients with infertility, found evidence of genital TB in the form of positive culture in menstrual blood in 16 and positive endometrial tissue for *Mycobacterium tuberculosis [Mtb]* in four patients.

Gross appearance of endometrium is mostly unremarkable. However, in advanced cases, ulcerative or atrophic endometrium or an obliterated endometrial cavity due to extensive intrauterine adhesions may be seen. Total destruction of endometrium by the disease process with resultant secondary amenorrhoea has been reported in a few cases (32).

Microscopically [Figure 26.1], diagnosis is based upon the presence of chronic inflammatory cells with or without

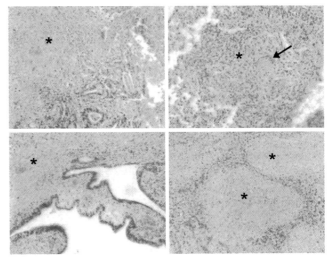

Figure 26.1: Endometrial TB. Photomicrograph showing endometrial glands with clusters of epithelioid cells and lymphocytic infiltration [asterisk] [upper panel, left; *Haematoxylin and eosin × 60]*, stroma of endometrium, epithelioid granulomas [asterisk], Langhans' giant cell [arrow] and lymphocytic infiltration [upper panel, right; *Haematoxylin and eosin × 200]*. Fallopian tube TB. Photomicrograph showing congested tubal plicae with epithelioid clusters and lymphocytic infiltration [asterisk] [lower panel, left; *Haematoxylin and eosin × 60]*, epithelioid granulomas in the fallopian tube [asterisk] [lower panel, right; *Haematoxylin and eosin × 60]*
TB = tuberculosis

caseation, granulomas with lymphocytes, Langhans' giant cells and epithelioid cells. Such lesions may be focal or generalised. Due to cyclical shedding of endometrium, such lesions may be seen close to the surface of endometrium. Granulomas may be better seen in premenstrual phase or within 12 hours after onset of menstruation (35).

However, typical granulomas may not be seen in all cases (36). Bazaz-Malik *et al* (2) in a series of 1000 cases of TB endometritis noted discrete granulomas and caseation in 60% cases only. They suggested presence of dilated glands, destruction of epithelium, inflammatory exudates in the lumen as additional criteria for diagnosis of TB endometritis. Bourno and Williams (37), suggest that focal collection of lymphocytes in the endometrium should be considered to be of TB origin unless proved otherwise.

Ovarian Tuberculosis

Ovarian involvement occurs in 15%-25% cases (5,9) and most often results from direct extension of the disease from fallopian tubes (10). In such cases, ovary may be surrounded by adhesions or may be the site of tubo-ovarian cyst formation or tubo-ovarian mass with adhesions surrounding them. In patients with haematogenous spread caseating granulomas may be seen in the parenchyma of ovary (10,32).

Tuberculosis of Cervix

TB of the cervix may be seen in 5%-15% cases of genital TB (5,9). Cervix mostly gets affected by downward spread of the disease from the endometrium. However, rarely cervical disease may occur secondary to deposition of infected semen by the male partner (28,29). Mostly, cervical lesions tend to be hypertrophic resembling cervical carcinoma (38) and less often an ulcerative lesion may be seen (32).

Microscopic examination reveals granulomatous inflammation. Inflammatory atypia with frequent hyperplastic mucosal changes may be seen along with caseation (1). The endocervical involvement is common (32) and may explain increased mucus production.

Cervical TB has been diagnosed cytologically by various workers (39-40). Multinucleated giant cells, histiocytes, epithelioid cells arranged in clusters simulating the appearance of granulomas are characteristic of the disease in Papanicolaou smear examination. Cytological diagnosis of genital TB in association with carcinoma *in situ* and *Trichomonas vaginalis* has been described (40).

Tuberculosis of the Vagina, Vulva and Bartholin Gland

TB of the vulva and vagina occurs in 1% of cases (5,9). TB of Bartholin gland and vesicovaginal fistula due to genital TB have been described (41,42). Involvement of the vagina or vulva is usually secondary to the involvement of other parts of genital tract. However, transmission of the disease by a male partner due to involvement of epididymis or seminal vesicles has been reported (28).

Lesions on vulva and vagina may present as hypertrophic lesions resembling malignancy, less often non-healing ulcers in the vulva may be seen. Histopathological examination of the lesion is useful in confirming the diagnosis.

CLINICAL PRESENTATION

Symptoms

The most frequent presenting symptoms in patients with FGTB include infertility, pelvic pain, menstrual disturbances, vaginal discharge and poor general condition [Table 26.2] (2,3,10,12,13,15,18,22,26,36,43,44). However, none of these are specific for FGTB.

Table 26.2: Clinical presentation of patients with genital TB

Study (reference)	No. of patients	Infertility	Amenorrhoea	Menorrhagia/ oligomenorrhoea	Postmenopausal bleeding	Chronic pelvic pain
Sutherland (18)	250	40	10	18	20	ND
Malkani and Rajani (13)	106	ND	43.4	43	ND	ND
Mukherjee *et al* (43)	138	100	60	19.7	ND	ND
Munjal *et al* (36)	140	37.1	42.8	41.4	1.4	ND
Klein *et al* (3)	20	70	20	ND	ND	30
Falk *et al* (10)	187	12.8	41.2	ND	ND	ND
Bazaz-Malik *et al* (2)	1000	47	26	15	1.0	2.4
Bobhate *et al* (12)*	337	58.6	26.4	ND	ND	ND
Chhabra (26)	58	29.3	18.9	15.5	3.4	43.1
Sfar *et al* (44)	118	81	ND	ND	ND	ND
Saracoglu *et al* (22)	72	47	11	ND	ND	32
Gupta *et al* (15)	40	40	10	40	ND	20

All values are shown as percentages
* These series included patients with TB endometritis only
TB = tuberculosis; ND = Not described

Infertility

Primary and secondary infertility are the most common presenting symptom in patients with FGTB. All reported series have identified this association [Table 26.2].

Chronic Lower Abdominal or Pelvic Pain

Chronic lower abdominal or pelvic pain is the second most common symptom in patients with FGTB [Table 26.2]. Pain is non-characteristic and is usually localised in the lower abdomen or pelvis. Pain tends to be chronic and is usually dull aching. Occasionally, acute pain may occur similar to that of acute pelvic inflammatory disease or a twisted pelvic organ. Episodes of acute pain, as a result of superadded bacterial infection, can occur and require administration of antibiotics. Acute episodes of pain may occur after diagnostic procedures, such as, endometrial biopsy, dilatation and curettage or hysterosalpingography [HSG]. Patients with chronic pain are more likely to have abnormal findings on pelvic examination.

Alterations in Menstrual Pattern

All types of menstrual irregularities, such as, amenorrhoea, menorrhagia, oligomenorrhoea or even postmenopausal bleeding can occur [Table 26.2].

Persistent/Abnormal Vaginal Discharge

Occasionally, patients with persistent vaginal discharge may be found to have genital TB affecting cervix or vagina (38-40). Such a symptom is more likely to occur in women with endocervical TB or in patients with TB of the cervix or vagina.

Unusual Symptoms

Several unusual symptoms as presentation of FGTB have been described from time to time. These include vulval lesions, Bartholin gland swelling (41), vesicovaginal fistula (42), pelvic masses (45), uterocutaneous fistula (46), and retention of urine due to pelvic masses of TB origin (47). Female genital TB may manifest and masquerade as ovarian cancer with rise in CA 125 levels as has been the experience of us and others (48,49).

Physical Signs

No physical sign on abdominal or pelvic examination is characteristic of genital TB. A high index of suspicion is, therefore, required to make an early diagnosis. The various signs of FGTB depend on the site of involvement of genital organs and are shown in Table 26.3 (5,23,50).

DIFFERENTIAL DIAGNOSIS

As FGTB can present in different ways with no definitive symptoms and signs, the differential diagnosis varies as per presentation [Table 26.4].

Table 26.3: Signs in female genital TB

No physical sign [common]
Systemic examination
    Fever
    Lymphadenopathy
    Chest signs [PTB]
    Other signs as per site of EPTB
Abdominal examination
    Ascites
    Doughy feel of abdomen
    Abdominal lump/vague or definite
Vaginal examination
    Enlarged uterus [pyometra]
    Induration and tenderness in adnexa
    Tubo-ovarian and adnexal masses
    Fullness and tenderness in pouch of Douglas
Unusual signs
    Ulcerative lesions on vagina, vulva, cervix [may mimic venereal diseases or cancer]
    Hypertrophic lesions on vagina, vulva, cervix [may mimic cancer]
    Uterocutaneous fistula
    Tubo-intestinal fistula
    Tubo-peritoneal fistula
    Tubo-vesical fistula
    Rectovaginal fistula
    Vesicovaginal fistula
    Bartholin swelling

TB = tuberculosis; PTB = pulmonary tuberculosis; EPTB = extra-pulmonary tuberculosis

---

Table 26.4: Differential diagnosis of female genital TB

For women presenting with pain and adnexal mass, following possibilities should be considered
    Ectopic gestation
    Acute and chronic pelvic infections
    Appendicular lump
    Endometriosis
    Ovarian malignancy
For granulomatous lesions in the pelvis
    Actinomycosis
    Brucellosis
    Crohn's disease
    Filariasis
    Granuloma inguinale
    Histoplasmosis
    Leprosy
    Schistosomiasis
    Silicosis
    Syphilis
Ulcerative or hypertrophic lesions
    Vaginal cancer
    Cervical cancer
    Bartholin abscess
    Vulval cancer
    Condyloma lata
    Condyloma acuminata
    Vaginal cyst
    Vulval and vaginal warts

TB = tuberculosis

DIAGNOSIS

As genital TB is a paucibacillary disease, it is not possible to demonstrate *Mtb* in every case. Therefore, one has to rely on imaging and histopathology. Endometrial biopsy for histopathological examination and mycobacterial culture remains the most commonly used procedure for the diagnosis of FGTB (51-54). Guinea pig inoculation is presently not being used for the diagnosis of FGTB (53,55). Laparoscopy, HSG, ultrasonography of pelvic organs, computed tomography [CT] and magnetic resonance imaging [MRI] are other investigative procedures which are carried out if the endometrial biopsy is not conclusive. Recently, a number of newer investigations such as polymerase chain reaction [PCR] have been applied for the diagnosis of genital TB [Table 26.5] with variable results. However, diagnostic hysteroscopy and laparoscopy have emerged as the most useful investigations. These investigations not only facilitate the visual examination of the lesions and confirmation of the diagnosis, but also help in picking up unsuspected pathology, such as, endometriosis or malignancy in a number of cases.

Endometrial Biopsy

Endometrial tissue obtained by endometrial biopsy curette or by aspiration with a plastic disposable cannula or by dilatation of the cervix and curettage of the endometrium [D and C] is useful for the diagnosis of TB [Figure 26.1]. Best time to perform such a procedure is shortly before the menstruation (5,9) as lesions are likely to be close to surface of endometrium during this phase of the menstrual cycle.

Histopathologically proven TB is present in 50%-76% patients with genital TB [Table 26.6] (3,10,13,15,19,32,44,51,52). In the absence of granulomas, and caseation necrosis, other features such as dilatation of glands, destruction of epithelium and inflammatory cells are seen on histopathology (3). Malkani and Rajani (13) suggested that the focal collection of chronic inflammatory cells or presence of proliferative endometrium in the premenstrual week in a patient with past history of TB in other parts of the body or a family history of TB would favour a diagnosis of FGTB.

A negative endometrial biopsy does not rule out the pelvic involvement since sampling errors are common and disease may have involved other pelvic organs without associated TB endometritis (1).

Mycobacterial Isolation

Endometrial biopsy specimen, menstrual blood, cervical and vaginal secretions, tubal biopsy material or peritoneal fluid

Table 26.5: Diagnostic modalities for female genital TB

Site	Diagnostic procedures
Fallopian tube	Laparoscopy, hysterosalpingography, peritoneal fluid smear for AFB and mycobacterial culture, tubal biopsy
Endometrium	Endometrial histology Endometrial aspirate smear for AFB and mycobacterial culture Hysteroscopy Menstrual blood culture for *Mycobacterium tuberculosis*
Cervix	Biopsy Exfoliative cytology
Vagina and vulva	Biopsy

TB = tuberculosis; AFB = acid-fast bacilli

Table 26.6: Comparison of the mycobacterial culture and histopathological examination of endometrium in the diagnosis of female genital TB

Study (reference)	No. of patients	Culture positive	HPE positive	Both culture and HPE positive
Malkani and Rajani (13)	57	17.5	100.0	*
Halbrecht and Petah Tiqua (51)	103	36.9	10.6	52.5
Klien *et al* (3)	20	37.5†	62.5†	ND
Nogales-Ortiz *et al* (32)	1436	100.0‡	76.1§	ND
Falk *et al* (10)	187	29.4	69.5	ND
Chhabra *et al* (52)	150	6.0	6.7	1.3
Sfar *et al* (44)	118	7.0	46.0	ND
Roy *et al* (19)	800	10.9	9.8	11.8
Gupta *et al* (15)	40	2.5	25	2.5

Positive yield is shown as percentage
All values have been corrected to first decimal place
* 57 endometrial biopsy-proven patients were included in the study
† Culture and histopathology yield available for 16 patients
‡ Culture yield available for 30 patients
§ Histopathology yield available for 201 patients
TB = tuberculosis; HPE = histopathological examination; ND = not described

obtained during diagnostic laparoscopy have been subjected to *Mtb* smear and culture examination (6,11,23).

Endometrial Culture *versus* Histopathology

A number of studies have evaluated histopathology and mycobacterial culture for the diagnosis of endometrial TB [Table 26.6]. Most studies have found a higher diagnostic yield with histopathological examination of endometrium than culture of biopsy material (6,11,23,44,51,52).

Hysterosalpingography

The HSG visualisation of uterine cavity and fallopian tubes by injecting a radio-opaque contrast medium into the uterus through cervix, is routinely performed for investigation of infertility [Figure 26.2]. A number of findings on HSG may suggest genital tract TB (56,57). The HSG performed during the acute stage of the disease, may however, result in exacerbation of the disease and is, therefore, contraindicated. Winifred (57) noted such an event in four of the fourteen cases subjected to HSG. Seigler (58) reported fever as the most common complication following HSG. Serious pelvic infections have been reported in 0.3%-1.3% of cases.

Magnusson (59) described two typical forms of the disease based upon HSG findings: [i] ragged and jagged tubal contour with small lumen defects [Figure 26.3]; [ii] straight rigid contour of the lumen with stem pipe-like configuration of the tube. Seigler (58) described rigid tubes, irregular tubal outline, calcification of the tubes and ovary, filling defects in the line of tubal shadow and fistulous tracts on HSG as suggestive of TB.

Rozin (60) has described several radiographic signs that were presumptive of TB. These include: [i] *golf club appearance*, when only isthmus and proximal ampulla are visualised, isthmic segment has a rigid stove pipe appearance [Figure 26.4]; [ii] a *beaded appearance* due to alternate areas of tube filled with and without radiographic contrast [Figure 26.5]; [iii] maltese cross appearance, completely filled tube with rigid, irregular

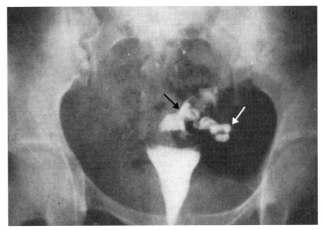

Figure 26.3: Hysterosalpingogram showing ragged and jagged contour of the tube. Only one tube could be visualised in this case [black arrow]. Terminal end of the tube presents leopard skin-like speckled appearance [white arrow]

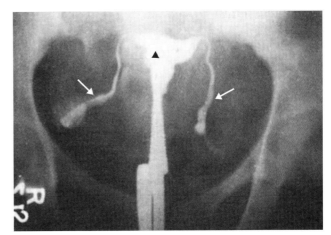

Figure 26.4: Hysterosalpingogram showing rigid stove pipe-like appearance of the fallopian tubes [arrows]. There is a small area of irregularity along the right uterine wall [arrow head]

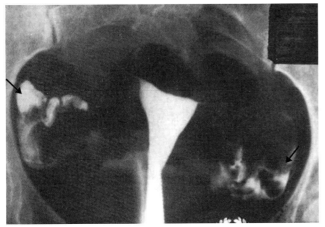

Figure 26.2: Hysterosalpingogram with normal findings. The uterine cavity has a normal outline. Both the fallopian tubes are outlined with free peritoneal spill of radio-opaque contrast [arrows]

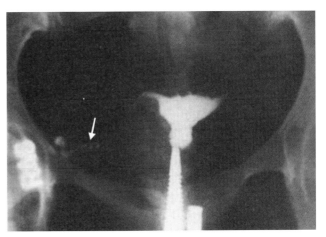

Figure 26.5: Hysterosalpingogram showing irregular uterine outline and patchy filling of the dye in the right fallopian tube resulting in beaded appearance [arrow]

outline [Figure 26.6]; [iv] rosette appearance where the distal end of tube is filled with dye [Figure 26.7]; [v] numerous diverticula in isthmic area; and [vi] leopard skin-like speckled appearance of the ampulla due to tube being partially filled with the contrast [Figure 26.3].

The presence of calcified tubes, ovary or pelvic lymph nodes is considered as the most significant finding. In addition, uterine cavity may be shrivelled and deformed. There can be extensive extravasation of radio-opaque contrast in pelvic vessels in FGTB [Figure 26.8]. The tubes may be patent in 37% of cases of TB endometritis (61). We found tubal calcification, irregularity of tubal wall, unilateral or bilateral cornual block, unilateral or bilateral hydrosalpinx, venous and lymphatic intravasation of dye in cases of genital TB in our study (62). Chauhan *et al* (63) observed synechiae formation, a distorted, and obliterated or T-shaped cavity and venous and lymphatic intravasation in their study on HSG in FGTB (63).

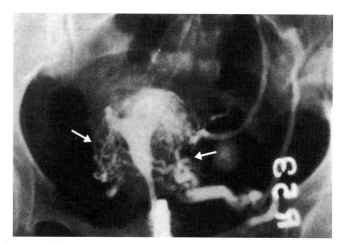

Figure 26.8: Hysterosalpingogram showing extensive extravasation of radio-opaque contrast in pelvic vessels [arrows]. Fallopian tubes are not visualised indicating bilateral cornual occlusion

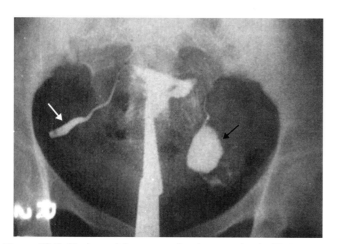

Figure 26.6: Hysterosalpingogram showing completely filled tube on the right side with a rigid outline [white arrow]. Dilatation of the distal half of the left tube with doubtful spill of the contrast is seen [black arrow]. A small filling defect is also seen in the uterine cavity

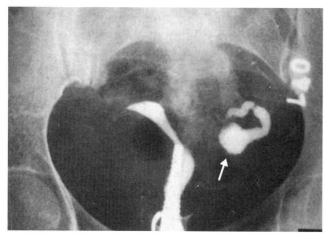

Figure 26.7: Hysterosalpingogram showing dilated portion of the left fallopian tube without any spill of dye [arrow]. Only proximal part of the right fallopian tube is seen

Laparoscopy

Laparoscopy is an important procedure in the diagnostic work-up of patients with infertility (64-73). Laparoscopy provides direct visualisation of the pelvic organs and peritoneal surfaces. In addition, it helps in confirming tubal patency. A number of observations may be made during laparoscopy in these cases. These include endometriosis, pelvic inflammatory disease or fibroids. It is important to carefully visualise whole of abdominal cavity including intestines, peritoneum, liver and gallbladder during laparoscopy to observe any TB lesion there. We have observed change in position of gallbladder [Sharma's hanging gallbladder sign] in patients with abdomino-pelvic TB (64). Despite normal physical examination, several abnormalities can be detected in about 60% of the cases during laparoscopy (65) [Figures 26.9A, 26.9B and 26.9C]. Diagnostic yield of laparoscopy in patients with infertility due to suspected FGTB has been documented in several studies (64-70) [Table 26.7] (15,65,69,70). Based upon various laparoscopic findings and guided biopsy, Palmer and Olivera (66) have described subacute and chronic stages in the natural history of pelvic TB.

Subacute Stage

The subacute stage of FGTB is characterised by the presence of whitish-yellow and opaque miliary granulations, surrounded by hyperaemic areas over the fallopian tubes and uterus. The pelvic organs may be congested, red and oedematous with adhesions. Multiple fluid filled pockets may also be seen.

Chronic Stage

The chronic stage of FGTB is recognised by the presence of the following findings.

Nodular salpingitis A series of yellow coloured small nodes may be seen on a normal looking tube.

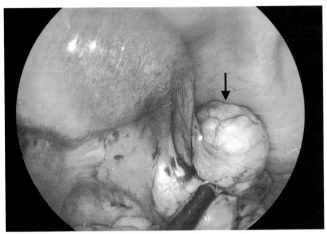

Figure 26.9A: Laparoscopy view in a patient with pelvic TB showing a large [5 × 4 cm] caseous nodule near right fallopian tube [arrow]. Biopsy from the nodule confirmed the diagnosis of TB
TB = tuberculosis

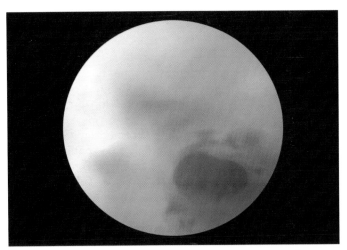

Figure 26.9D: Hysteroscopy image showing pale looking cavity

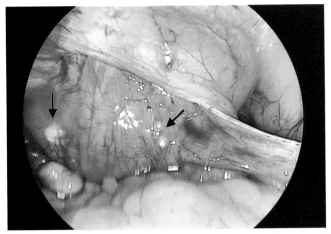

Figure 26.9B: Laparoscopy view of pelvis in a patient with pelvic TB showing surface tubercles on uterus [arrows]. Biopsy from the tubercle confirmed the diagnosis of TB
TB = tuberculosis

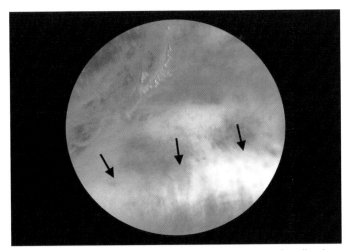

Figure 26.9E: Hysteroscopy image showing grade 3 adhesions [arrows]

Figure 26.9C: Laparoscopy view of pelvis in a patient with confirmed FGTB showing caseous nodules on the surface of right fallopian tube [white arrow] and in the Pouch of Douglas [black arrow]. Both fallopian tubes are dilated and blocked

Table 26.7: Incidence of genital TB at laparoscopy

Study (reference)	No. of patients	Incidence [%]
Krishna *et al* (70)	697	10.3
Deshmukh *et al* (69)	500	9.0
Merchant (65)	687	14.1
Gupta *et al* (15)	150	26.7
TB = tuberculosis		

Patchy salpingitis Short and swollen tubes with agglutinated fimbriae may be seen.

Hydrosalpinx Fallopian tubes are distended at their terminal end due to agglutination of fimbriae. These tubes tend to be "retort shaped". Bilateral involvement of the tubes is almost always seen.

Caseosalpinx Ampulla of the tube is deformed by an ovoid dilatation which is whitish-yellow with poor vascularisation.

The tube is distended with caseous material. This finding also tends to be bilateral.

Adhesions Bands of adhesions may be seen between loops of intestine and the omentum. Sometimes broad bands may mask the whole adnexae. Laminar adhesions covering the tubes and ovary and fixing them are occasionally seen in the chronic phase of genital TB.

Tripathy and Tripathy (20) performed laparoscopy in 62 sputum smear-positive pulmonary TB patients. They found bands of adhesion, tubercles and hyperaemia in 59.6% and intestinal adhesions in 24.2% patients. Tubercles were observed on the fallopian tubes in 22.6% and adhesions in the pouch of Douglas were evident in 11.3% patients.

Bhide et al (67), in a laparoscopy study of 71 patients with genital TB reported pelvic adhesions in 48%, tubercles in 33.8%, unilateral adnexal mass in 11.3% and bilateral adnexal masses in 21.1% patients. Further, encysted effusion [8.45%] and lesions on the bowel and/or omentum [25.4%] were also observed. Marana et al (68), in a laparoscopy study of 254 patients with primary or secondary infertility from Italy, found tubal factor to be responsible in 101 patients. Of these, only two patients had histopathological and culture positive endometrial TB. In a third patient with laparoscopic findings suggestive of TB, the organisms were cultured from urine. Deshmukh et al (69) and Krishna et al (70) also found laparoscopy useful in diagnosis of FGTB [Table 26.7]. In a study on FGTB in infertile women from New Delhi [n = 40] (15), laparoscopic examination revealed abnormally dilated, tortuous, and blocked fallopian tubes [n = 13]; peritubal and periovarian adhesions [n = 18]; Fitz-Hugh-Curtis syndrome [n = 15]; omental adhesions [n = 18]; and bowel adhesions [n = 15]. In a laparoscopic study on 85 women with FGTB, we observed tubercles on peritoneum [15.9% cases], tubo-ovarian masses [26%], caseous nodules [7.2%], encysted ascites [8.7%], various grades of pelvic adhesions [65.8%], hydrosalpinx [21.7%], pyosalpinx [2.9%], beaded tubes [10%], tobacco pouch appearance [2.9%] and inability to see tubes due to adhesions [14.2%] (71). The authors have observed a new laparoscopic sign [python sign] in tubal involvement of FGTB in which fallopian tubes become distended like a blue python with alternate constriction and dilatation on injection of methylene blue dye (72). We also observed a very high prevalence of perihepatic adhesions [Fitz-Hugh-Curtis syndrome] on laparoscopy in FGTB (73). However, we observed increased complications on laparoscopy for FGTB as compared to laparoscopy performed for non-TB patients [31% versus 4%] like inability to see pelvis [10.3% versus 1.3%], excessive bleeding [2.3% versus 0%], peritonitis [8% versus 1.8%] (74). The adhesions are typically vascular and adhesiolysis can increase the risk of bleeding and flare up of the disease (6,74).

Hysteroscopy Endoscopic visualisation of the uterine cavity in genital TB may show a normal cavity [if no endometrial TB or early stage TB] with bilateral open ostia. More often, however, the endometrium is pale looking [Figure 26.9D], the cavity is partially or completely obliterated by adhesions

of varying grade [grade 1 to grade 4] often involving ostia as observed by us (75,76) [Figure 26.9E]. Hence, FGTB is an important cause of Asherman's syndrome in India (76). There may be a small shrunken cavity. One has to be careful while performing hysteroscopy in genital TB as the procedure is associated with increased difficulty to distend the cavity and to do the procedure and increased chances of complications like excessive bleeding, perforation and flare up of genital TB as observed in our study (77). Hence, hysteroscopy in a patient of genital TB should be done by an experienced person preferably under laparoscopic guidance to avoid false passage formation and injury to the pelvic organs.

The frequent use of laparoscopy and hysteroscopy has made it possible to diagnose a number of cases of genital TB among women with infertility and chronic pelvic pain.

Ultrasonography

Ultrasonography, being non-invasive with no radiation hazard, has been increasingly used in evaluating pelvic and other abdominal masses. Lee et al (78) described sonographic features of TB endometritis in a 59-year-old female. Demonstration of bilateral, predominantly solid, adnexal masses containing scattered small calcifications is highly suggestive of TB (78).

The authors have encountered a number of patients with infertility or chronic pelvic pain with adnexal masses and free fluid in the pelvis on ultrasonography that were found to have genital TB on subsequent investigations [Figure 26.10].

Computed Tomography

A number of findings have been described on CT as suggestive of abdominal and pelvic TB. These include low density ascites, uncommon patterns of adenopathy, presence of multiple pelvic lesions, and hepatic, adrenal

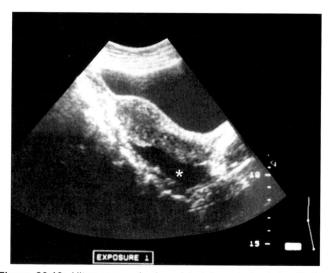

Figure 26.10: Ultrasonography in pelvic tuberculosis. A longitudinal scan in a 33-year-old parous woman with a history of oligomenorrhoea. The scan shows fluid collection in the Pouch of Douglas [asterisk]. Investigations confirmed the diagnosis of genital tuberculosis

and splenic lesions. Though these lesions may mimic malignancy, these should raise a suspicion of TB, especially if encountered in young patients suffering from infertility (79).

Magnetic Resonance Imaging

Magnetic resonance imaging [MRI] is being increasingly used for evaluating pelvic and other abdominal masses [Figures 26.11A and 26.11B] and has been found to be useful in localising soft tissue abnormalities in patients with FGTB (80). The presence of hypodense masses with rim enhancement abutting the pelvic walls is suggestive of TB [Figures 26.11A and 26.11B]. Unilateral or bilateral tubo-ovarian masses, unilateral or bilateral hydrosalpinx, adnexal cysts or TB deposits on peritoneum or liver have been described in the study of MRI in tubo-ovarian masses due to TB (80).

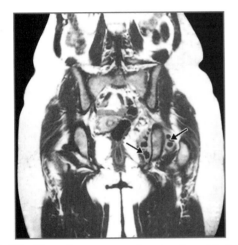

Figure 26.11A: Magnetic resonance imaging in pelvic tuberculosis. Post-gadolinium T1-weighted coronal scan in a 26-year-old nullipara with history of chronic pelvic pain unresponsive to usual treatment. Hypointense masses with rim enhancement [arrows] abutting the left pelvic wall and tracking to subgluteal region suggestive of abscesses

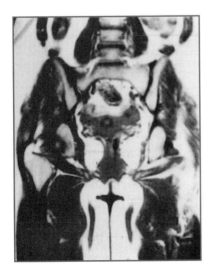

Figure 26.11B: Magnetic resonance imaging T1-weighted coronal scan of the same patient one year after antituberculosis treatment. Scan shows complete resolution of abscesses

Positron Emission Tomography

Positron emission tomography [PET] demonstrates glucose uptake by TB lesions [Figure 26.12] and is particularly useful to know whether the lesion is active or not. An active lesion shows increased glucose uptake (81). The reader is referred to the chapter *"Roentgenographic manifestations of pulmonary and extrapulmonary tuberculosis"* [Chapter 9] for details.

Serological Tests

Serological tests have been banned by Government of India and are not to be used for the diagnosis of TB presently.

Polymerase Chain Reaction

The polymerase chain reaction [PCR] is a useful supporting test for the diagnosis of FGTB (82-84). Used judiciously, the PCR can help in the diagnosis of TB in certain clinical situations. However, some authors have doubted the value of PCR in the diagnosis of TB (85). Further, false positivity of PCR, especially in-house PCR, has been observed to be high. Anti-TB treatment should not be started just on the basis of a positive PCR test result unless there is some other evidence of FGTB on clinical examination or on investigations like presence of tubercles or other stigmata of TB on laparoscopy (5).

Cartridge-based Nucleic Acid Amplification Tests

Cartridge-based nucleic acid amplification tests [CBNAAT] are increasingly being used for the diagnosis of FGTB. The Xpert MTB/RIF® is a new fully automated diagnostic molecular test with an analytic sensitivity of five genome copies of purified deoxyribonucleic acid [DNA] and 131 colony-forming units [cfu]/mL of *Mtb* in sputum. The Xpert MBT/RIF is also able to detect more than 99.5% rifampicin resistance mutations, an indicator of multidrug-resistant TB in less than two hours time (86a). Recent evidence (86b,86c) is available suggesting that in women with female genital TB with tubo-ovarian masses who are not responding to first-line anti-TB drugs, Xpert MTB/RIF is useful in early diagnosis of MDR-TB.

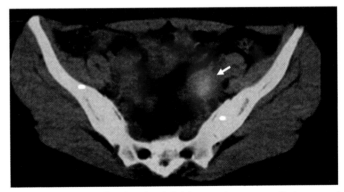

Figure 26.12: PET-CT showing left tubo-ovarian mass with increased uptake suggestive of active disease [arrow]
PET-CT = positron emission tomography-computed tomography

Diagnostic Algorithm

The diagnosis of FGTB is made based on good history, careful systemic and gynaecological examination; and judicious use of diagnostic modalities like endometrial biopsy in conjunction with imaging methods and endoscopic visualization, especially with laparoscopy. Algorithm for accurate diagnosis of FGTB by combining history taking, examination and investigations, has been reported (87). A diagnostic algorithm for FGTB is shown in Figure 26.13.

TREATMENT

Treatment of FGTB is similar to treatment of the disease as elsewhere in the body. Availability of effective anti-TB treatment has significantly decreased the requirement for surgical treatment in patients with FGTB. In India, patients with FGTB receive DOTS under the Revised National Tuberculosis Control Programme of Government of India (8). The reader is referred to the chapters *"Treatment of tuberculosis" [Chapter 44]*, and *"Revised National Tuberculosis Control Programme" [Chapter 53]* for details. The recently published evidence-based INDEX-TB guidelines (88)

recommend 6 months standard first-line anti-TB treatment regimen for FGTB. Prior to the availability of effective drug therapy, surgery produced a significant degree of morbidity and complications. These included bowel fistula [14%] and an operative mortality rate of 2.2% (31). These complications are rarely seen now. Indications for surgical intervention in patients with FGTB are shown in Table 26.8.

Minimal Genital Tuberculosis

Minimal disease is usually asymptomatic, except for infertility and is diagnosed by finding TB endometritis on curettage or biopsy or tubercle bacilli on culture of the curettings of menstrual blood. The patient is started on standard anti-TB treatment and is examined at monthly intervals. After six months, a procedure of dilatation and curettage is done and the endometrial curettings are examined histologically and bacteriologically.

Wherever feasible, the patient should be followed up annually for an indefinite period of time as exacerbations have been reported up to 10 years after apparent cure before the advent of modern short-course treatment. This is highly unlikely with current therapy.

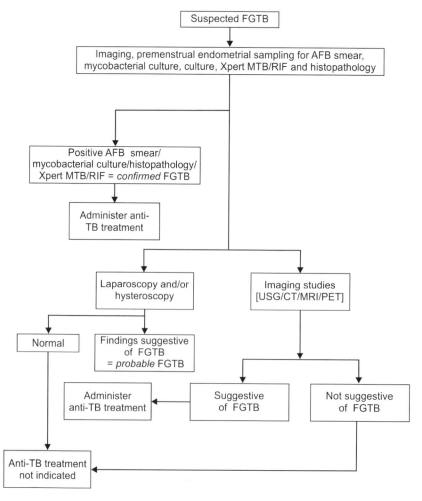

Figure 26.13: Algorithm for diagnostic work-up of FGTB

FGTB = female genital tuberculosis; RIF = rifampicin; AFB = acid-fast bacilli; TB = tuberculosis; USG = ultrasonography; CT = computed tomography; MRI = magnetic resonance imaging; PET = positron emission tomography

> **Table 26.8: Indications for surgical intervention in female genital TB**
>
> Persistence or increase of pelvic masses after a six-month course of anti-TB treatment
>
> Recurrence of positive endometrial culture or histology after six months course of anti-TB treatment
>
> Persistence or recurrence of pain or bleeding after six months of anti-TB treatment
>
> Postmenopausal patient with a recurrent pyometra due to TB
>
> TB = tuberculosis
> *Adapted from reference 9*

Advanced Genital Tuberculosis

Advanced genital TB is diagnosed by the presence of palpable tubo-ovarian masses and histopathologic or bacteriologic evidence of TB. The patient is started on standard anti-TB treatment and is examined at monthly intervals.

Schaefer (9) has suggested that, if palpable adnexal masses persist after six months, total abdominal hysterectomy and bilateral salpingo-oophorectomy are performed (9). However, there is no consensus regarding this view (9) as a number of these patients suffer from infertility and are also young. Modern short-course anti-TB treatment is highly effective for the treatment of FGTB with rare need of surgery.

There are much higher chances of complications during surgery in women with genital TB in hysteroscopy, laparoscopy, vaginal hysterectomy and laparotomy (74,77,89,90). There is excessive haemorrhage and non-availability of surgical planes at time of laparotomy with a higher risk of injury to the bowel and other pelvic and abdominal organs. In case of abdomino-pelvic TB, bowel loops may be matted together with no plane between them and uterus and adnexa may be buried underneath the plastic adhesions and bowel loops and may be inapproachable. Even trying to perform a diagnostic laparoscopy or laparotomy in such cases can cause injury to bowel necessitating resection of injured bowel. It is better to obtain biopsies from the representative areas, close the abdomen without pelvic clearance and start standard anti-TB treatment, awaiting biopsy report in cases where laparotomy is done for suspected pelvic tumours but the appearances are suggestive of TB. However, limited surgery like drainage from residual large pelvis or tubo-ovarian abscesses, pyosalpinx can be performed followed by administration of anti-TB treatment (91).

Pregnancy Following Treatment of Female Genital Tuberculosis

Full-term pregnancy is uncommon after treatment of histopathologically proven genital TB (92-98). From time to time, occasional case reports have appeared about successful term pregnancies in patients with genital TB who have undergone treatment (95,96).

If pregnancy takes place in a treated patient with FGTB, it is more likely to result in ectopic pregnancy or abortion (97). FGTB is an important cause of ectopic pregnancy in India (98).

Of the 206 patients with FGTB treated by Sutherland (99), 45 pregnancies were reported in 26 women. Of these, 11 were ectopic pregnancies and 11 pregnancies ended in abortions. Fourteen women had 23 live births (99). Merchant (65) in a study of 101 patients with FGTB, diagnosed on laparoscopy, reported 3 ectopic pregnancies, 11 intrauterine pregnancies and 9 term pregnancies. In two patients, abortion was induced for medical reasons. Jindal *et al* (95) reported three pregnancies among 14 women with histopathologically proven endometrial TB. Falk *et al* (10) in a study of 187 patients from 47 Swedish hospitals reported four ectopic pregnancies and no intrauterine pregnancy after anti-TB treatment. Saracoglu *et al* (22), in a series of 72 patients with pelvic TB from Turkey, reported one intrauterine pregnancy without any surgical or medical treatment of pelvic TB.

Tuboplasty

Since infertility is the most common symptom in patients with genital TB, reconstructive tubal surgery is often performed after adequate medical treatment. Reactivation of silent pelvic TB following tuboplasty procedure has been reported by Ballon *et al* (100). Schaefer (9) advocates against such procedures in patients with FGTB.

In Vitro Fertilisation and Embryo Transfer

Most women with genital TB present with infertility and have poor prognosis for fertility in spite of anti-TB treatment. The conception rate is low [19.2%] with live birth rate being still low [7%] (93). Parikh *et al* (101) found IVF with embryo transfer [ET] to be the only hope for some of these women whose endometrium was not damaged and reported a pregnancy rate of 16.6% per transfer. Jindal (95) observed IVF-ET to be most successful of all the assisted reproductive technology modalities in FGTB patients with 17.3% conception rate in contrast to only 4.3% observed with fertility enhancing surgery. Dam *et al* (14) found latent genital TB responsible for repeated IVF failure in young patients presenting with unexplained infertility with apparently normal pelvis and non-endometrial tubal factors. If after anti-TB treatment their tubes are still damaged but their endometrium is receptive [no adhesions or mild adhesions which can be hysteroscopically resected], IVF-ET is recommended (6). However, if they have endometrial TB causing damage to the endometrium with shrunken small uterine cavity with Asherman's syndrome, adoption or gestational surrogacy may be considered (5,6).

REFERENCES

1. Sutherland AM. The changing pattern of tuberculosis of the female genital tract. A thirty-year survey. Arch Gynaecol 1983;234:95-101.
2. Bazaz-Malik G, Maheshwari B, Lal N. Tuberculous endometritis: a clinicopathological study of 1000 cases. Br J Obstet Gynecol 1983;90:84-6.
3. Klein TA, Richmond JA, Mishell DR Jr. Pelvic tuberculosis. Obstet Gynecol 1976;48:99-104.
4. Sharma JB. Current diagnosis and management of female genital tuberculosis. J Obstet Gynaecol India 2015;65:362-71.

5. Sharma JB, Dharmendra S, Agarwal S, Sharma E. Genital tuberculosis and infertility. Fertil Sci Res 2016;3:6-18.
6. Tripathi SN. Tuberculosis manual for obstetricians and gynecologists. First edition. New Delhi: Jaypee Brothers Medical Publishers; 2015.
7. World Health Organization. Global tuberculosis report 2018. WHO/CDS/TB/2018.20. Geneva: World Health Organization; 2018.
8. Central TB Division, Government of India. TB India 2015. Revised National TB Control Programme. Annual Status Report. New Delhi: Central TB Division, Directorate General of Health Services, Ministry of Health and Family Welfare; 2018.
9. Schaefer G. Female genital tuberculosis. Clin Obstet Gynecol 1976;19:223-39.
10. Falk V, Ludviksson K, Agren G. Genital tuberculosis in women. Analysis of 187 newly diagnosed cases from 47 Swedish hospitals during the ten-year period, 1968 to 1977. Am J Obstet Gynecol 1980;138:974-7.
11. Gupta S. Pelvic tuberculosis in women. J Obstet Gynecol India 1956;7:181-98.
12. Bobhate SK, Kadar GP, Khan A, Grover S. Female genital tuberculosis. A pathological appraisal. J Obstet Gynecol India 1986;36:676-80.
13. Malkani PK, Rajani CK. Endometrial tuberculosis. Indian J Med Sci 1954;8:684-97.
14. Dam P, Shirazee HH, Goswami SK, Ghosh S, Ganesh A, Chaudhury K, et al. Role of latent genital tuberculosis in repeated IVF failure in the Indian clinical setting. Gynecol Obstet Invest 2006;61:223-7.
15. Gupta N, Sharma JB, Mittal S, Singh N, Misra R, Kukreja M. Genital tuberculosis in Indian infertility patients. Int J Gynaecol Obstet 2007;97:135-8.
16. Singh N, Sumana G, Mittal S. Genital tuberculosis: a leading cause for infertility in women seeking assisted conception in North India. Arch Gynecol Obstet 2008;278:325-7.
17. Shaheen R, Subhan F, Tahir F. Epidemiology of genital tuberculosis in infertile population. J Pak Med Assoc 2006;56:306-9.
18. Sutherland AM. Functional uterine hemorrhage. A critical review of literature since 1938. Glasgow Med J 1949;30:1-28.
19. Roy A, Mukherjee S, Bhattacharya S, Adhya S, Chakraborty P. Tuberculous endometritis in hills of Darjeeling: a clinicopathological and bacteriological study. Indian J Pathol Microbiol 1993; 36:361-9.
20. Tripathy SN, Tripathy S. Laparoscopic observation of pelvic organs in pulmonary tuberculosis. Int J Gynecol Obstet 1990;32: 129-31.
21. Gungorduk K, Ulker V, Sahbaz A, Ark C, Tekirdag AI. Postmenopausal tuberculosis endometritis. Infect Dis Obstet Gynecol 2007;2007:27028. Epub 2007 May 8.
22. Saracoglu OF, Mungan T, Tanzer F. Pelvic tuberculosis. Int J Gynecol Obstet 1992;37:115-20.
23. Neonakis IK, Spandidos DA, Petinaki E.Female genital tuberculosis: a review. Scand J Infect Dis 2011;43:564-72.
24. Devi PK. Genital tuberculosis in the female. J Indian Med Assoc 1962;38:164-6.
25. Hafeez MA, Tandon PL. Tubercular endometritits – a clinicopathologic study of 120 cases. J Indian Med Assoc 1966;46:610-16.
26. Chhabra S. Genital tuberculosis-a baffing disease. J Obstet Gynaecol India 1990;40:569-73.
27. Rattan A, Gupta SK, Singh S, Takkar D, Kumar S, Bai P, et al. Detection of antigens of Mycobacterium tuberculosis in patients of infertility by monoclonal antibody based sandwiched ELISA assay. Tuber Lung Dis 1993;74:200-3.
28. Lattimer JK, Colmore HP, Sanger G, Robertson DH, McLellan FC. Transmission of genital tuberculosis from husband to wife via the semen. Am Rev Tuberc 1954;69:618-24.
29. Sutherland AM, Glean ES, MacFarlane JR. Transmission of genitourinary tuberculosis. Health Bull 1982;40:87-91.
30. Siegler AM, Kontopoulos V. Female genital tuberculosis and the role of hysterosalpingography. Semin Roentgenol 1979;14: 295-304.
31. Schaefer G. Tuberculosis of the genital organs. Am J Obstet Gynecol 1965;14:295-304.
32. Nogales-Ortiz F, Tarancon I, Nogales FF Jr. The pathology of female genital tuberculosis – a 31-year study of 1436 cases. Obstet Gynecol 1979;53:422-8.
33. Daly JW, Monif GRG. Mycobacteria. In: Monif GRG, editor. Infectious diseases in obstetrics and gynaecology. 2nd edition. Philadelphia: Harper and Row; 1982.p.301.
34. Oosthuizen AP, Wessels PH, Hefer JN. Tuberculosis of the female genital tract in patients attending an infertility clinic. S Afr Med J 1990;77:562-4.
35. Czernobilsky B. Endometritis and infertility. Fertil Steril 1978;30:119-30.
36. Munjal S, Tandon PL, Hafeez MA. Tuberculous endometritis [clinicopathological study of 140 cases]. J Obstet Gynaecol India 1970;20:106-11.
37. Bourno AW, Williams LH [editors]. Recent advances in obstetrics and gynaecology. 10th edition. London: J and AA Churchill, 1962.p.285-318.
38. Chahtane A, Rhrab B, Jirari A, Ferhati D, Kharbach A, Chaoui A Hypertrophic tuberculosis of the cervix. Three cases. J Gynecol Obstet Biol Reprod Paris 1992;21:424-7.
39. Angrish K, Verma K. Cytologic detection of tuberculosis of the uterine cervix. Acta Cytol 1981;25:160-2.
40. Bhambani S, Das DK, Singh V, Luthra UK. Cervical tuberculosis with carcinoma in situ: a cytodiagnosis. Acta Cytol 1985;29:87-8.
41. Dhall K, Das SS, Dey P. Tuberculosis of Bartholin's gland. Int J Gynecol Obstet 1995;48:223-4.
42. Ba-Thike K, Than-Aye, Nan OO. Tuberculous vesicovaginal fistula. Int J Gynecol Obstet 1992;37:127-30.
43. Mukherjee K, Wagh KV, Agarwal S. Tubercular endometritis in primary infertility. J Obstet Gynaecol India 1967;17:619-24.
44. Sfar E, Ourada C, Kharouf M. Female genital tuberculosis in Tunisia. Apropos of 118 cases at the Rabta Neonatology and Maternity Center in Tunis [January 1984-December 1988]. Rev Fr Gynecol Obstet 1990;85:359-63.
45. Jones NC, Savage EW, Salem F, Yeager C, Davidson EC Jr. Tuberculosis presenting as a pelvic mass. J Natl Med Assoc 1981;73:758-61.
46. Malhotra D, Vasisht K, Srinivasan R, Singh G. Tuberculous uterocutaneous fistula – a rare postcaesarean complication. Aust NZ J Obstet Gynecol 1995;35:342-4.
47. Yanagizawa R, Inoue S, Itakura H, Kishi H, Fujimaaru J, Wada Y. A case of urinary retention due to tuberculous pyometra. Nippon Hinyokika Gakkai Zasshi 1992;83:690-3.
48. Sharma JB, Jain SK, Pushpraj M, Roy KK, Malhotra N, Zutshi V, et al. Abdomino-peritoneal tuberculosis masquerading as ovarian cancer: a retrospective study of 26 cases. Arch Gynecol Obstet 2010;282:643-8.
49. Koc S, Beydilli G, Tulunay G, Ocalan R, Boran N, Ozgul N, et al. Peritoneal tuberculosis mimicking advanced ovarian cancer: a retrospective review of 22 cases. Gynecol Oncol 2006;103:565-9.
50. Schaefer G, Marcus RS, Kramer EE. Postmenopausal endometrial tuberculosis. Am J Obstet Gynecol 1972;112:681-7.
51. Halbrecht I, Petah Tiqua I. The relative value of culture and endometrial biopsy in the diagnosis of genital tuberculosis. Am J Obstet Gynecol 1958;75:899-903.
52. Chhabra S, Narang P, Gupte N. A study of 150 cases of endometrial cultures for Mycobacterium tuberculosis. J Obstet Gynecol India 1986;36:146-9.
53. Seward PGR, Mitchel RW. Guinea pig inoculatin and culture for mycobacteria in tuberculosis in infertile women. A study of cost effectiveness. S Afr Med J 1985;67:126-7.
54. Morris CA, Norma Boxall F, Cayton HR. Genital tract tuberculosis in subfertile women. J Med Microbiol 1970;3:85-90.

55. Sheth SS. Lack of diagnostic value of guinea pig test for tuberculosis [letter]. Lancet 1990;336:1440.

56. Robinson SA, Shapira AA. The value of hysterosalpingography. N Engl J Med 1931;205:380.

57. Winifred JAF. Female genital tuberculosis. J Obstet Gynecol Br Common 1964;71:418-28.

58. Seigler AM. Hysterosalpingography. Fertil Steril 1983;40:139-58.

59. Magnusson WP. Liber das rant genbild ber tuberculoser slpingitus. Acta Radiol 1945;25:263.

60. Rozin S. The X-ray diagnosis of genital tuberculosis. J Obstet Gynecol Br Empire 1952;59:59-63.

61. Sharman A. Genital tuberculosis in the female. J Obstet Gynecol B Empire 1952;59:740-2.

62. Sharma JB, Pushparaj M, Roy KK, Neyaz Z, Gupta N, Jain SK, et al. Hysterosalpingographic findings in infertile women with genital tuberculosis. Int J Gynecol Obstet 2008;101:150-5.

63. Chauhan GB, Hira P, Rathod K, Zacharia TT, Chawla A, Badhe P, et al. Female genital tuberculosis: hysterosalpingographic appearances. Br J Radiol 2004;77:164-9.

64. Sharma JB. Sharma's hanging gall bladder sign: A new sign for abdominopelvic tuberculosis: An observational study, J IVF lite 2015;2:94-8.

65. Merchant R. Endoscopy in the diagnosis of genital tuberculosis. J Reprod Med 1989;34:468-74.

66. Palmar R, Olivera EM. Coelioscopy and per-coelioscopic biopsies in latent genital tuberculosis. Rippmann ET, Wenner R, editors. Latent female genital tuberculosis. Basel: Karger; 1966.p.143-51.

67. Bhide AG, Parulekar SV, Bhattacharya MS. Genital tuberculosis in females. J Obstet Gynecol India 1987;37:576-8.

68. Marana R, Muzii L, Lucisano A, Ardito F, Muscatello P, Bilancioni E, et al. Incidence of genital tuberculosis in infertile patients submitted to diagnostic laparoscopy: recent experience in an Italian University Hospital. Int J Fertil 1991;36:104-7.

69. Deshmukh KK, Lopez JA, Naidu TAK, Gaurkhede MD, Kashbhawala MV. Place of laparoscopy in pelvic tuberculosis in infertile women. Arch Gynecol 1985;237:197.

70. Krishna UR, Saathe AV, Mehta H, Wagle S, Purandare VN. Tubal factors in sterility. J Obstet Gynecol India 1979;29:663-7.

71. Sharma JB, Roy KK, Pushparaj M, Kumar S, Malhotra N, Mittal S. Laparoscopic finding in female genital tuberculosis Arch Gynecol Obstet 2008;278:359-64.

72. Sharma JB, Sharma's Python sign: A new sign in female genital tuberculosis. J Lab Physicians 2016;8:120-2.

73. Sharma JB, Roy KK, Gupta N, Jain SK, Malhotra N, Mittal S. High prevalence of Fitz-Hugh-Curtis syndrome in genital tuberculosis. Int J Gynecol Obstet 2007;99:62-3.

74. Sharma JB, Mohanraj P, Roy KK, Jain SK. Increased complication rates associated with laparoscopic surgery among patients with genital tuberculosis. Int J Gynecol Obstet 2010;109:242-4.

75. Sharma JB, Roy KK, Pushparaj M, Kumar S. Hysteroscopic findings in women with primary and secondary infertility due to genital tuberculosis. Int J Gynecol Obstet 2009;104:49-52.

76. Sharma JB, Roy KK, Pushparaj M, Gupta N, Jain SK, Malhotra N, et al. Genital tuberculosis: an important cause of Asherman's syndrome in India. Arch Gynecol Obstet 2008;277:37-41.

77. Sharma JB, Roy KK, Pushparaj M, Karmakar D, Kumar S, Singh NJ. Increased difficulties and complications encountered during hysteroscopy in women with genital tuberculosis. J Minim Inv Gynecol 2011;18:660-5.

78. Lee J, Warner L, Khalleghian R. Sonographic features of tuberculous endometritis. J Clin Ultrasound 1983;11:331-3.

79. Bankier AA, Fleischmann D, Wiesmayr MN, Putzd, Konstrus M, Hubsch P, et al. Update: abdominal tuberculosis-unusual findings on CT. Clin Radiol 1995;50:223-8.

80. Sharma JB, Karmakar D, Hari S, Singh N, Singh SP, Kumar S, et al. Magnetic resonance imaging findings among women with tubercular tubo-ovarian masses. Int J Gynecol Obstet 2011;113:76-80.

81. Sharma JB, Karmakar D, Kumar R, Shamim AS, Kumar S, Singh N, et al. Comparison of PET/CT with other imaging modalities in female genital tuberculosis in a high prevalence, tertiary care setting. Int J Gynecol Obstet 2012;118:123-8.

82. Manjunath N, Shankar P, Rajan L, Bhargava A, Saluja S, Shriniwas. Evaluation of a polymerase chain reaction for the diagnosis of tuberculosis. Tubercle 1991;72:21-7.

83. Bhanu NV, Singh UB, Chakraborty M, Suresh N, Arora J, Rana T, et al. Improved diagnostic value of PCR in the diagnosis of female genital tuberculosis leading to infertility. J Med Microbiol 2005;54:927-31.

84. Jindal UN, Bala Y, Sodhi S, Verma S, Jindal S. Female genital tuberculosis: early diagnosis by laparoscopy and endometrial polymerase chain reaction. Int J Tuberc Lung Dis 2010;14:1629-34.

85. Grosset J, Mouton Y. Is PCR a useful tool for the diagnosis of tuberculosis in 1995 Tubercl Lung Dis 1995;76:183-4.

86a. Sharma SK, Kohli M, Chaubey J, Yadav RN, Sharma R, Singh BK, et al. Evaluation of Xpert MTB/RIF assay performance in diagnosing extrapulmonary tuberculosis among adults in a tertiary care centre in India. Euro Respira J 2014;44:1090-3.

86b. Sharma JB, Kriplani A, Dharmendra S, Chaubey J, Kumar S, Sharma SK. Role of Gene Xpert in diagnosis of female genital tuberculosis: a preliminary report. Eur J Obstet Gynecol Reprod Biol 2016;207:237-8.

86c. Sharma JB, Kriplani A, Sharma E, Sharma S, Dharmendra S, Kumar S, et al. Multi drug resistant female genital tuberculosis: A preliminary report. Eur J Obstet Gynecol Reprod Biol 2017; 210:108-15.

87. Jindal UN. An algorithmic approach to female genital tuberculosis causing infertility. Int J Tuberc Lung Dis 2006;10:1045-50.

88. Sharma SK, Ryan H, Khaparde S, Sachdeva KS, Singh AD, Mohan A, et al. Index-TB guidelines: Guidelines on extrapulmonary tuberculosis for India. Indian J Med Res 2017;145: 448-63.

89. Sharma JB, Mohanraj P, Jain SK, Roy KK. Increased complication rates in vaginal hysterectomy in genital tuberculosis. Arch Gynecol Obstet 2011;283:831-5.

90. Sharma JB, Mohanraj P, Jain SK, Roy KK. Surgical complications during laparotomy in patients with abdominopelvic tuberculosis. Int J Gynecol Obstet 2010;110:157-8.

91. American Thoracic Society, Centers for Disease Control and Prevention, Prevention/Infectious Diseases Society of America. Controlling tuberculosis in the United States. Am J Respir Crit Care Med 2005;172:1169-227.

92. Jodberg H. A study on genital tuberculosis in women. Acta Obstet Gynecol Scand 1950;31:7-176.

93. Gurgan T, Urman B, Yarali H. Results of in vitro fertilization and embryo transfer in women with infertility due to genital tuberculosis. Fertil Steril 1996;65:367-70.

94. Tripathy SN, Tripathy S. Infertility and pregnancy outcome in female genital tuberculosis. Int J Gynaecol Obstet 2002;76:159-63.

95. Jindal UN, Jindal SK, Dhall GI. Short–course chemotherapy for endometrial tuberculosis in infertile women. Int J Gynecol Obstet 1990;32:75-6.

96. Schaefer G. Full-term pregnancy following genital tuberculosis. Obstet Gynecol Surv 1964;19:81-124.

97. Varma TR. Genital tuberculosis and subsequent fertility. Int J Gynecol Obstet 1991;35:1-11.

98. Sharma JB, Naha M, Kumar S, Roy KK, Singh N, Arora R. Genital tuberculosis: an important cause of ectopic pregnancy in India. Indian J Tuberc 2014;61:312-7.

99. Sutherland AM. The treatment of tuberculosis of the female genital tract with streptomycin, PAS and isoniazid. Tubercle 1976;57:137-44.

100. Ballon SC, Clewell WH, Lamb EJ. Reactivation of silent pelvic tuberculosis by reconstructive tubal surgery. Am J Obstet Gynecol 1975;122:991.

101. Parikh FR, Nandkarni SG, Kamat SA, Naik S, Soonawala SB, Parkh RM. Genital tuberculosis – a major pelvic factor causing infertility in Indian women. Fertil Steril 1997;67:497-500.

27

Genitourinary Tuberculosis

Rajeev Kumar, AK Hemal

INTRODUCTION

Genitourinary tuberculosis [GUTB] is a common term used for tuberculosis [TB] infection affecting either the urinary or genital systems. It is one of the most common forms of extra-pulmonary tuberculosis [EPTB] and, depending upon the endemicity of TB in a country, may account for up to 27% of all EPTB; making it the second or third most common form of EPTB (1-3). The common term, GUTB, is used because the pathology frequently involves both systems due to their anatomical and functional proximity, and it is usually not possible to separate affliction of one part from the other. The disease often affects individuals in the reproductive age group of 20-40 years with significant morbidity in both the renal and reproductive functions, which could include renal failure and infertility.

EPIDEMIOLOGY AND PATHOGENESIS

The GUTB complicates three to four per cent of all cases of pulmonary TB. Colabawalla (4), in a multicentric study from India, reported a prevalence of 10%-34% among patients with various urological diseases. While this may be an over-estimate of current prevalence, a meta-analysis of world-wide epidemiologic trends of GUTB found the incidence in men to be twice that in women with the mean age of involvement being 40 years (5). Overall, only about a third of these cases had evidence of previous pulmonary TB but this was almost 50% in patients from the developing world. Another important finding of this analysis was that patients in the developing world presented late and consequently had a higher incidence of severe disease and renal failure and were also more likely to have a bacteriological diagnosis than patients from the developed world. TB occurs in approximately 10% of patients with acquired immunodeficiency syndrome [AIDS] and involves

at least one extrapulmonary site in nearly 50% of the cases (6), with the kidney being the most common genitourinary site of involvement (7).

Mycobacterium tuberculosis [Mtb] is the usual cause of GUTB. Genitourinary involvement is often secondary to haematogenous dissemination from a pulmonary focus. Spread to the kidney often occurs to multiple foci which may heal with no evidence of disease or may form microscopic granulomas (8). The intensity of infection depends upon the infecting dose, virulence of the organism and the resistance of the host. Macroscopic progression of the disease is mostly unilateral (9). Usually, these multiple tubercles heal either spontaneously or as a result of anti-TB treatment administered for the primary focus. Involvement of the remaining urinary system is by contiguous spread of the infection down from the kidney. Similar haematogenous spread occurs to the epididymis which may be involved in up to 78% of all cases (10). The globus minor of the epididymis is the preferred site of involvement, possibly due to its high vascularity. Another route of involvement of the genital tract is *via* retrograde spread from the urinary bladder. Infection may travel along the ejaculatory ducts and vas deferens to involve the prostate, seminal vesicles, epididymis and testis, highlighting the common involvement of the urinary and genital systems (11).

The pathophysiologic manifestations of TB occur through a number of mechanisms; infective destruction of tissue, distortion due to formation of space-occupying lesions, and fibrosis resulting in strictures, contractures and architectural deformity. Reactivation of the renal focus may take place any time after the initial event and a latent period of up to 46 years has been reported (12). This reactivation is usually unilateral and one or more tubercles may enlarge after years of inactivity and rupture into the collecting system, producing bacilluria without a radiographically visible renal lesion (8). The bacilli descend along the nephrons and form more granulomas within the medulla and papilla. These granulomas may coalesce and form cavities which may communicate with the pelvicalyceal system [PCS] following rupture. These may also result in necrosis and sloughing. These cavities are visible on radiologic studies, often giving a 'moth eaten' appearance to the kidneys. Tuberculomas in the renal parenchyma occupy space and displace calyces with obstruction to their drainage. These may appear as dilated 'hydrocalyces'. Further, hydrocalyces may also arise as a consequence of scarring of the infundibular necks. On an intravenous contrast study, these calyces do not fill with contrast which is a characteristic feature in GUTB. Similar cicatrisation may affect the renal pelvis. Parenchymal lesions may undergo calcification and an extensively involved kidney may have extensive caseous necrosis and calcification, resulting in a 'putty' kidney. The combination of obstruction and parenchymal damage leads to a non-functioning, calcified kidney in a process called 'autonephrectomy' [Table 27.1, Figures 27.1A and 27.1B].

Gross pathological examination of the kidney may reveal destroyed papillae, ulcerated calyces, caseous masses, and cavities of varying sizes with ragged edges and containing creamy, sterile pus in the cortex. Renal calcification is often found though its aetiology is unclear. These calcific shadows tend to be ill defined and irregular, neither as dense nor as well defined as renal calculi. These lie in the cortex and strongly suggest the presence of TB. Calcification is an unfavourable prognostic sign with a high likelihood of surgical intervention as medical management will rarely cure the infection.

Ureteric pathology is typically manifest in the form of strictures (13). Downstream infection from the kidney causes mucosal and wall ulceration and fibrosis with strictures. Strictures may develop at multiple sites, giving a radiologically beaded appearance. The ureter often fails

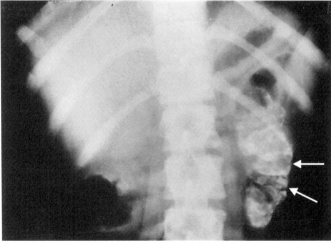

Figure 27.1A: Plain X-ray of the kidney, ureter and bladder [KUB] showing calcified kidney [arrows] on the left side resulting in autonephrectomy

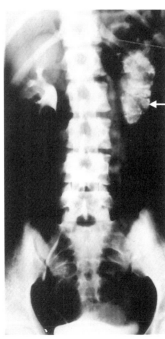

Figure 27.1B: Intravenous urogram of same patient showing normally functioning kidney on the right side and calcified nonfunctioning kidney [arrow] on the left side

Table 27.1: Pathologic changes in renal TB

Early changes
    Papillary necrosis/papillitis
Cavity formation
    From sloughed off papilla
    From rupture of abscess into the pelvi-calyceal system
Strictures
    Caliectasis
    Calyx cut-off
    Infundibular stenosis
Hydronephrosis
    Cicatrised pelvi-ureteric junction
    Ureteric strictures, reflux
    Small capacity bladder
Perinephric abscess
    Rupture of TB abscess into the perinephric space
Pseudocalculi
    Due to calcification in lesions
Caseous masses
'Putty' kidney
Dystrophic calcification

TB = tuberculosis

to dilate on the contrast studies, appearing like a fixed pipe-stem. The infection frequently occurs at the vesico-ureteric junction and causes progressive changes in the ureteric orifice within the bladder (14). The orifice may take a 'golf-hole' appearance, cause obstruction, reflux or both. Involvement of the urinary bladder begins around one or the other ureteric orifice which becomes red, inflamed and oedematous. Later, bullous granulations appear and completely obscure the ureteric orifice. TB ulcers may be present, but these are rare and are a late finding. Progressive inflammation of the mucosa leads to contractures such that results in a bladder with negligible capacity or 'thimble bladder' [Figure 27.2].

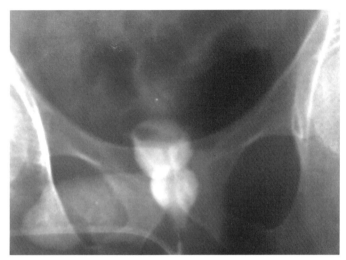

Figure 27.2: Cicatrised, small [thimble] bladder

Genital involvement may occur through haematogenous dissemination from an extragenital source (8,15), downstream involvement from the bladder or contiguous spread from an affected organ. In men, the epididymis is the most common site; while in women, the principal site of involvement is the fallopian tube. Spread from the fallopian tube to the uterus can occur in up to 50% of patients with tubal infection (16). Involvement of the testis is uncommon but may occur contiguously from the epididymis. Similar spread may involve the vas deferens, seminal vesicles and the prostate (11).

CLINICAL PRESENTATION

The clinical presentation of genitourinary TB is summarised in Table 27.2. Irritative voiding symptoms are the most common manifestation of GUTB (17). Over a half of all patients present with urinary storage symptoms, haematuria and flank pain each of which occurs in about a third of all cases. Scrotal abnormality seems to be the most common physical finding, present in almost half of all cases (5). In the study from the All India Institute of Medical Sciences

[AIIMS], New Delhi [n=241], the mean age at presentation in patients with GUTB was 34.6 years and nearly one in four had azotemia. The most common involved organ was the kidney in 130 [53.9%] cases (18).

Kidney, Ureter and Bladder

Isolated renal TB may have no symptoms initially. Progressive lesions may result in hematuria if there is cavitation into the pelvicalyceal system, back or flank pain and constitutional symptoms of fever, fatigue and malaise. Occasionally, advanced cases may present with renal, perirenal or psoas abscess. Some of these abscesses may rupture externally, resulting in a chronic sinus or fistula (18,19). Ureteric strictures may be present at the time of diagnosis. However, these often develop or progress during treatment with anti-TB drugs. Obstruction may lead to hydronephrosis which may manifest as pain and progress to a non-functioning renal unit. Typical symptoms of dysuria, haematuria, frequent voiding and nocturia usually signify a concomitant cystitis due to involvement of the bladder. These are the most common presenting symptoms and could be associated with GUTB involving any organ. As the bladder capacity progressively decreases, the patient develops incapacitating frequency to the extent of voiding every few minutes. Obstruction or reflux in the ureter and primary renal involvement result in renal impairment and may progress to end-stage renal failure. Occasionally, calcifications may be detected in the renal area.

Genital Tuberculosis

TB epididymitis may present as an acute infection with pain and swelling or with abscesses and sinuses [Figure 27.3] (11). The acute involvement may not be significant and the patient may present with chronic epididymitis or infertility if the disease involves both sides. Occasionally, this may be manifest as scrotal masses (20,21).

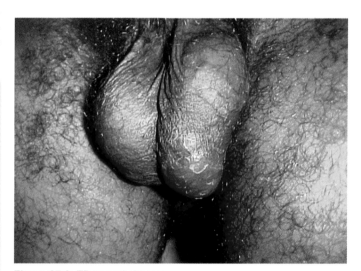

Figure 27.3: TB scrotal abscess
TB = tuberculosis
Reproduced with permission from "Kumar R. Reproductive tract tuberculosis and male infertility. Indian J Urol 2008;24:392-5" (reference 11)

Table 27.2: Clinical presentation of genitourinary TB

Common
    Irritative voiding symptoms
    Haematuria
    Flank pain
    Renal mass
    Sterile pyuria
    Recurrent urinary tract infection
    Azotemia
    Urinary calculi
    Acute presentation mimicking pyelonephritis
Uncommon
    Non-healing wound/sinuses/fistula
    Haemospermia
    Urinary fistula
Scrotal abscess

TB = tuberculosis

Involvement of the vas deferens results in infertility and clinically may be evident as a 'beaded' vas. Testicular involvement is always secondary to infection of the epididymis and orchitis without epididymal involvement is very rare. During the early phase, the testicular lesion rapidly responds to anti-TB treatment after the epididymis has been surgically removed if the destruction of the testicular tissue is not extensive.

Involvement of the prostate is rare and difficult to document. It may be diagnosed, most often, on prostate biopsy or pathological examination of a prostatectomy specimen. Very rarely, the disease spreads rapidly and cavitation may lead to a perineal sinus (22). Prostatic involvement may lead to a fibrotic obstruction of the ejaculatory ducts that pass through it. This can lead to a reduction in the semen volume which may be a presenting symptom. Obstruction of the ejaculatory ducts may also result in infertility. Some patients may develop haematospermia or blood in the ejaculate as a sign of TB. On palpation, the gland may have a nodule or feel firm. Chronic granulomatous inflammation of the prostate may result in caseation necrosis followed by fibrosis or sloughing, resulting in "autoprostatectomy" (23).

TB of the penis is very rare. Historically, it has been reported as a complication of ritual circumcision, when it was the usual practice for the operators, many of whom had open pulmonary TB, to suck the penis (24). TB lesions of the penile shaft are still occasionally seen although their aetiology is unclear. The lesion appears as a superficial ulcer of the glans penis. It may be indistinguishable from malignant disease and may progress to involve the urethra [Figure 27.4]. The diagnosis is confirmed by biopsy. The transmission of genital TB from male to female is rare and poorly documented, even though *Mtb* may be present in the semen of men with genital TB. There have been documented cases of primary urethral TB, but, despite the frequent contact of the urethra with organisms in the urine, this is anecdotal (25).

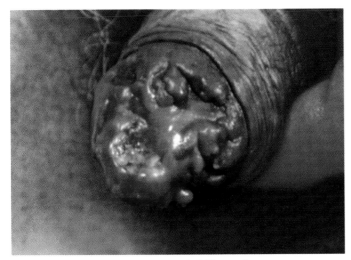

Figure 27.4: TB of the glans penis mimicking malignancy
TB = tuberculosis

DIAGNOSIS

Undiagnosed and untreated urinary tract TB can cause renal failure and death. Diagnostic difficulties in GUTB are due to the often insidious nature of disease onset, lack of bacteriological confirmation and failure to consider the diagnosis on the basis of the symptoms. The combination of a high index of suspicion and use of bacteriologic, radiologic and endourologic tools can frequently lead to the appropriate diagnosis.

The typical symptoms and features on history have been described in the segment on clinical presentation. A full blood count, erythrocyte sedimentation rate [ESR], renal function tests and serum electrolytes should be obtained. In addition, if calcification is present, a complete biochemical assessment of calcium metabolism is performed. In cases with elevated ESR, measurement at monthly intervals may give some indication regarding response to treatment. Tuberculin skin test is usually positive in most patients with GUTB.

Urine Examination

Microscopic haematuria or pyuria may be found on urine examination. Urine culture and sensitivity testing should be performed. 'Sterile pyuria' refers to the presence of leucocytes in the absence of any bacterial growth on culture. Secondary bacterial infection is found in about 20% of patients with TB and the culture may not be sterile. The usual organism is *Escherichia coli*. Persistent sterile pyuria and haematuria in the absence of recent antibiotic treatment supports a clinical suspicion of TB. Figueiredo *et al* (5) observed that detection of *Mtb* in urine was the most common method of diagnosing GUTB. This included a combination of smear and culture tests. However, in a number of cases, there may be no bacteriological evidence of TB and the diagnosis is made on the basis of a clinical and radiological picture.

Microbiological Methods

Urinary excretion of bacilli is intermittent and in order to maximise the probability of a positive growth, at least three but preferably five consecutive early morning specimen should be used for both smear examination and culture. In addition, secretions from a discharging sinus or material procured by fine-needle aspiration may be similarly investigated. In patients who have a nephrostomy placed for bypassing obstruction, urine from both the nephrostomy tube and the bladder should be examined.

Smears are stained with the Ziehl-Neelsen stain to look for acid-fast bacilli [AFB]. Bacterial cultures are performed on two slopes; Lowenstein-Jensen culture medium and a pyruvate egg medium containing penicillin to identify *M. bovis*, which is partially anaerobic and grows on the surface of the culture medium. If the cultures are positive, sensitivity tests are always conducted, in order to determine the most effective course of chemotherapy. The low sensitivity and time intensiveness of these tests means that additional tests are often required.

Molecular Methods

Polymerase chain reaction [PCR] has been used in the early diagnosis of GUTB with mixed results. However, caution must be exercised before starting anti-TB treatment on the basis of a positive PCR test alone as false-positive PCR test results can also occur in a significant number of cases and the specificity may be as low as 57% (26-29). The use of PCR testing for TB in the setting of infertility is also an area of concern. Since TB is a known cause for infertility and may often be asymptomatic, screening infertile men for TB with semen PCR tests is often performed. However, these screening tests are rarely positive and, even when the test is positive, it does not add to the management since the patient is frequently diagnosed to have GUTB based on other clinical and diagnostic tests (30,31). Similarly, the male partner of an infertile couple where the woman is diagnosed to have TB is often subjected to a screening semen TB-PCR test. Such screening does not yield any positive outcomes and should be avoided (30,31).

Considering the low yield on most bacteriological tests and the time taken for culture, newer cartridge-based nucleic acid amplification tests [CBNAAT] based on the PCR technology are now available, particularly for pulmonary TB. One of these is the Xpert MTB/RIF® [Cepheid, Sunnyvale, CA, USA] which allows detection within a two-hour period. While the test has been studied extensively for pulmonary TB, its use in GUTB is not clear. A study (32a) evaluated 55 urine samples in men with suspected GUTB TB and found 33% sensitivity and 100% specificity using cultures as the reference standard, suggesting a possible role for this test. Unlike PCR, if a sample tests positive by Xpert MTB/RIF, the case is more likely to be a true case of TB (32a). In a recently published systematic review (32b), pooled sensitivity and specificity of Xpert MTB/RIF testing in urine in the diagnosis of GUTB was reported to be 82.7% and 98.7% respectively.

Serological Tests, Interferon Gamma Release Assays

Currently serodiagnostic tests are not recommended for the diagnosis of active TB. Interferon gamma release assays [IGRAs] are useful in detecting latent TB infection [LTBI], but should not be used in the diagnosis of active TB (33). The reader is referred to the chapter *"Laboratory diagnosis"* [Chapter 8] for details.

Imaging Studies

Plain Radiograph

Plain radiographs of the urinary tract may show calcification in the renal areas [Figures 27.5A and 27.5B] and in the lower genitourinary tract. Ureteric calcification is rare in the absence of extensive renal calcification. Renal calcification is parenchymal and may be patchy or extensive. Occasionally, patients may form secondary stones following calyceal

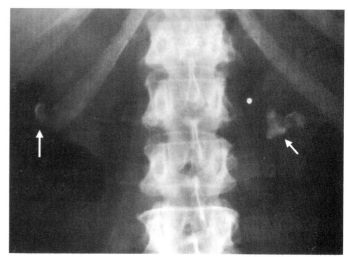

Figure 27.5A: Plain radiograph of the abdomen showing bilateral calyceal calcification [arrows]

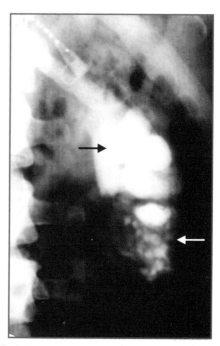

Figure 27.5B: Intravenous urogram showing lobar calcification of the inferior pole [white arrow] and dilated upper and middle calyces in the left kidney [black arrow]

infundibular stenosis and the radio-opacity seen is due to the stone and not renal parenchymal calcification.

Ultrasonography

Ultrasonography is often the first imaging investigation performed in patients presenting with complaints of abdominal pain and haematuria. However, it often fails to contribute to the diagnosis of GUTB. Its principal role is in monitoring hydronephrosis and bladder capacity during the course of disease progression and response to treatment. It is also used to guide aspiration and biopsy of renal, prostatic, epididymal and testicular lesions and for placement of nephrostomy tubes for drainage.

Contrast Imaging

Despite major advances in radiology, intravenous urography [IVU] is the principal imaging modality in suspected GUTB (34). This investigation helps in localising the disease, assessing renal function and helps in planning intervention and follow-up strategies. The renal lesion may appear as distortion of a calyx or a calyx that is fibrosed and completely occluded [lost calyx]. The renal pelvis or infundibulum of a calyx may appear cicatrised with proximal dilatation. There may be hydroureteronephrosis, a poorly functioning or a non-visualised kidney. TB ureteritis is manifested by dilatation above a ureterovesical stricture, or if the disease is more advanced, by a rigid fibrotic ureter with multiple strictures [Figures 27.6 and 27.7].

The cystographic phase of the urogram often provides significant supportive evidence of TB. Similarly, a voiding cystourethrogram is very useful in delineating bladder pathology. There is progressive decrease in bladder capacity which appears small and contracted or irregular. The bladder outline may be irregular due to localised deformity from cicatrisation or due to a hyperplastic inflammatory lesion (14). Fibrosis in the region of the trigone produces gaping ureteric orifices, which may show vesico-ureteric reflux on voiding cystourethrogram [Figure 27.8].

Computed tomography [CT] urography provides a less detailed image than conventional IVU and is not routinely indicated in evaluating GUTB. CT may, however, be useful in delineating parenchymal lesions, granulomatous masses in the kidney [Figure 27.9] and seminal vesicles (35). Magnetic resonance urography [MRU] has a role in patients with renal failure where iodinated contrast medium cannot be used. MRU can provide anatomical images of the urinary

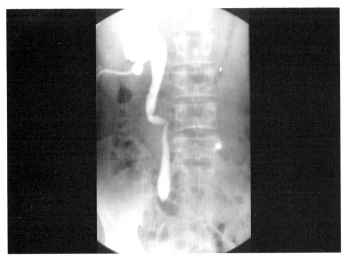

Figure 27.6: Intravenous urogram showing no excretion of contrast on the left side, hydroureteronephrosis on the right side with a lower ureteric stricture and a nephrostomy tube in the right kidney

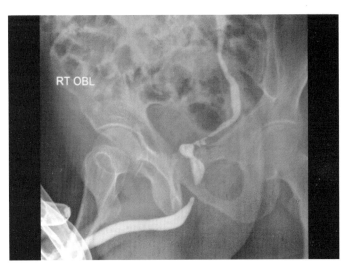

Figure 27.8: Retrograde urethrocystogram showing a thimble bladder with reflux into the left ureter

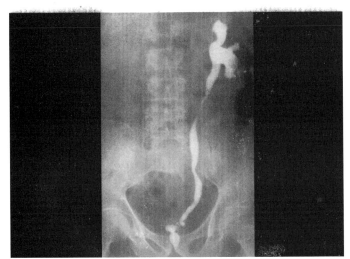

Figure 27.7: Intravenous urogram showing non-functioning kidney on the right side, hydroureteronephrosis on the left side and thimble bladder

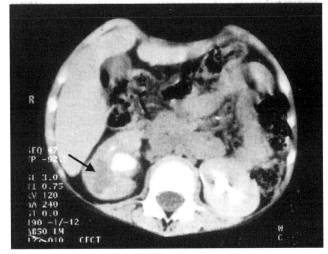

Figure 27.9: CECT of the abdomen showing an irregular hypodense lesion in the right kidney [arrow]
CECT = contrast-enhanced computed tomography

system and needs supplementation with functional studies such as a radioisotope renal scan in planning intervention.

Retrograde pyelography involves cystoscopic placement of a catheter into the ureteric orifice and injection of radiographic contrast through it under fluoroscopic control. This investigation is useful in patients with a poorly functioning kidney where the kidney does not concentrate intravenous contrast. It is also used to collect urine samples separately from each kidney. However, the procedure is invasive with attendant risks of infection. It is usually performed in conjunction with retrograde stent placement for ureteric obstruction.

Percutaneous antegrade pyelography is an alternative to retrograde ureterography in patients with hydronephrotic, obstructed kidneys. Antegrade puncture allows both instillation of contrast to visualise the system and placement of either a ureteric stent or a nephrostomy tube to drain the obstructed system. It also allows aspiration of the collected urine for examination and culture and estimation of split renal function from the two kidneys. This procedure becomes particularly relevant in advanced cases, where, following cystitis, the bladder becomes inflamed and small and visualisation of the ureteric orifice and placement of a retrograde ureteric stent becomes almost impossible. Occasionally, it may demonstrate additional pathologies and fistulous communications [Figure 27.10].

Cystoscopy

Cystoscopy serves both diagnostic and therapeutic roles in a patient suspected to have GUTB. In the absence of bacteriological confirmation, a cystoscopic examination for appearance of the bladder and ureteric orifices and taking

a biopsy may be performed. In addition, sampling urine from each kidney and stent placement as described in the section on retrograde pyelography may also be performed. Cystoscopic findings which suggest TB include a small, inflamed bladder, dilated, retracted ureteric orifices, ulcers and granulations.

TREATMENT

The recently published Guidelines for Extrapulmonary TB for India [INDEX-TB Guidelines] (36) suggest that a short-course [6 months] standard anti-TB treatment is considered adequate for GUTB. All patients, irrespective of the sequelae at presentation, are started on anti-TB treatment before further intervention (37). Several patients with GUTB will require surgical intervention at some point in time during the course of their disease. A list of the potential interventions is listed in Table 27.3.

The manifestations of GUTB continue to evolve even during the treatment phase and pathologic changes may develop due to the fibrosis and cicatrisation that occur during healing. Imaging of the kidneys and ureter is performed, mandatorily in all patients of GUTB. In patients with genital TB with no involvement of the kidney, ureter or bladder, if the initial screening ultrasound shows no abnormality, an IVU may be avoided. However, in all other patients of urinary TB, an IVU should be obtained at baseline. Another imaging study should be obtained after starting treatment with anti-TB drugs. The timing and nature of this imaging depend on the initial findings. If the first

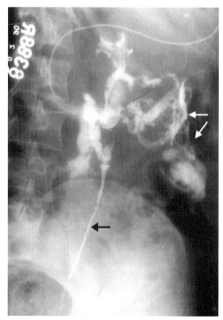

Figure 27.10: Retrograde ureteropyelogram showing reno-colo-cutaneous fistula, narrow ureter [black arrow], colon, extravasation of the contrast through the sinus tract [white arrows]

Table 27.3: Surgical interventions in genitourinary TB
Renal TB
Nephrostomy or ureteral stenting
Nephrectomy or nephroureterectomy
Partial nephrectomy
Pyeloplasty
Ureterocalicostomy
Ureteric stricture
Dilatation/endoureterotomy and stenting
Ureteroneocystostomy
Percutaneous nephrostomy
Ileal replacement
Urinary bladder: small capacity
Hydraulic dilatation
Augmentation cystoplasty
Cystectomy + orthotopic neobladder
Urinary diversion
TB of urethra
Endoscopic dilatation
Urethroplasty
Genital TB
Epididymectomy
Orchiectomy
Excision of fistula
Partial penectomy
De-roofing of prostatic abscess
Excision of seminal vesicles
TB = tuberculosis

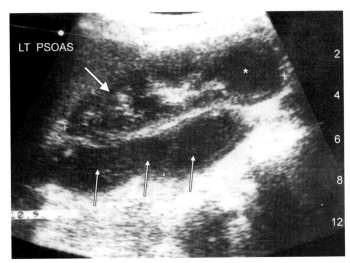

Figure 27.11: Ultrasonography showing an enlarged hypoechoic left kidney [thick arrow] with an anechoic cavity in the lower pole [asterisk] due to TB. A large psoas abscess [thin arrows] is also seen
TB = tuberculosis

imaging was normal, the repeat may be performed at three to four weeks. If there is evidence of renal, ureteric or bladder involvement on the first imaging, there is a likelihood of rapidly increasing obstruction and renal function loss and the repeat imaging may be performed as early as two weeks after starting the treatment.

In GUTB, surgical interventions aim at preventing renal damage, preserving renal function, improving drainage of the kidney and symptomatic relief. The initial intervention, which may be done concurrent with starting anti-TB treatment, involves placement of either a ureteric stent or a nephrostomy to drain an obstructed kidney or calyx (38). Renal abscesses not resolving within two weeks of the treatment can be drained under ultrasonography guidance [Figure 27.11]. Definitive treatment usually is delayed till at least four to six weeks of drug therapy are completed when no further change in the lesions is expected.

In a study from the AIIMS, New Delhi 248 surgical procedures including 33 endoscopic, 87 ablative and 128 reconstructive surgeries were conducted (18). Early complications occurred in 8% and primarily involved the bowel; 54 patients had azotemia and 81% of them had functional stabilisation or improvement.

Nephrectomy, Nephroureterectomy

Nephrectomy is indicated in patients where the kidney is either non-functioning or harbours disease that cannot be eradicated with anti-TB treatment alone (39). The disease and inflammation tend to result in extensive peri-renal fibrosis and surgery is often very difficult in these cases. On occasions, segmental or subcapsular nephrectomy may have to be performed due to the adhesions. There may be contiguous involvement of the bowel, spleen and pancreas, primarily in the inflammatory process, which may require extended resection. A peri-renal abscess may have burst onto the skin surface and all such tracts and fistulae are excised *en masse*. Laparoscopy is traditionally contraindicated in TB non-functioning kidneys due to these adhesions. However, in patients where the disease is not as extensive, laparoscopy may be successfully used (40). In patients where the ureter is also involved with strictures, the ureter is resected in continuity with the kidney [nephroureterectomy] till below the lowest stricture or the vesicoureteric junction.

Partial Nephrectomy

In patients with a localised polar lesion, partial nephrectomy may be contemplated after at least six weeks of anti-TB treatment. Renal calcification may indicate regions harbouring viable mycobacteria in up to 28% cases (41). If the remaining kidney looks normal, these may be candidates for partial nephrectomy. Small lesions can be kept under review on an annual basis. Larger areas of calcification should be excised and non-functioning kidneys with extensive calcification should be removed.

Pyeloplasty, Ureterocalicostomy

Involvement of the renal pelvis, calyceal infundibulum and upper ureter may result in stricture formation. Short segment obstructions can be managed endoscopically with incision and stenting. However, the involvement is usually extensive and fibrotic and required surgical reconstruction. If there is sufficient pelvis available, a ureteropyelostomy or pyeloplasty can be performed. Often the pelvis is completely cicatrised, precluding anastomosis. In such cases, the upper patent ureter is anastomosed to the lower calyx in ureterocalicostomy may be required.

Stricture of the Ureter

Ureteric strictures are initially managed with internal stents or nephrostomy tubes to preserve renal function. Definitive intervention is planned usually after six weeks of anti-TB treatment. Short segment strictures may be balloon dilated or endoscopically incised. For longer strictures, reconstruction is required and depends on the site and length of stricture (42). Upper ureteric strictures may require a pyeloplasty or ureterocalicostomy if the kidney is functioning. In the middle ureter, Davis' intubated ureterostomy technique over a silastic stent may be attempted. Other options include interposition of appendix or creation of a Boari's flap if the bladder capacity is still good. In the lower ureter, if strictures are identified early in the disease process, some workers have proposed that addition of corticosteroids to anti-TB treatment may limit their extent. However, there is no convincing evidence from the published literature for the use of corticosteroids as of now. Surgical reconstruction usually involves reimplantation into the bladder or creation of a Boari's flap. If the bladder is also of a small capacity, the bladder is augmented and a ureteroneocystostomy is performed. If a cystectomy is being contemplated, the ureters are reimplantation in the neobladder [Figure 27.12].

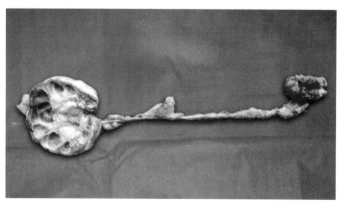

Figure 27.12: Resected surgical specimen of nephroureterectomy and cystectomy with thimble bladder

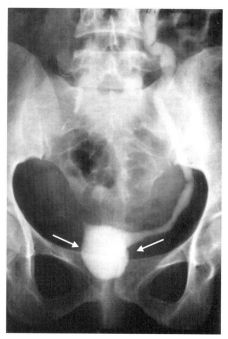

Figure 27.14A: Intravenous urogram showing small capacity thimble bladder [arrows]. The kidney is not visualised on the right side

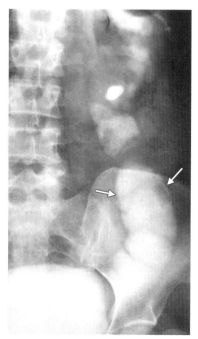

Figure 27.13: Intravenous urogram showing ileal replacement of ureter [arrows]

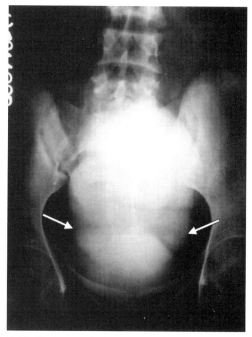

Figure 27.14B: Cystogram in the same patient following augmentation cystoplasty utilising sigmoid colon [arrows]

Patients with multiple or long segment strictures are not suitable for these interventions. If the kidney has limited function and the opposite kidney is normal, a nephro-ureterectomy may be planned. If the kidney function is good, the ureter is replaced by an ileal segment [Figure 27.13], joining a tailored or plicated ileum to the calyx of the kidney cranially, and to the urinary bladder caudally.

Surgery for Urinary Bladder Tuberculosis

Surgery for urinary bladder TB involvement aims at increasing its capacity. The procedure used depends on the residual capacity of the native bladder. If the bladder capacity is greater than 30-50 mL but small enough to incapacitate the patient [with frequency and urgency], augmentation of the native bladder is performed using a bowel segment. This can be a segment of the ileum, sigmoid or stomach (43,44). The stomach is generally reserved for patients with azotemia since it does not absorb urinary constituents as much as the other two segments. However, it is technically more difficult and has potential complication of hematuria-dysuria syndrome which can be debilitating. When the bladder capacity is less than 10-20 mL [thimble bladder], a simple cystectomy with neobladder formation is required [Figures 27.14A and 27.14B].

Surgery for Other Forms of Genitourinary Tuberculosis

Involvement of seminal vesicles, vas deferens and the prostate, can manifest as infertility. A few patients may respond to anti-TB treatment alone. Surgical intervention too has limited role in these cases. Discrete obstructions to the ejaculatory ducts within the prostate may be amenable to endoscopic resection (45,46). More extensive involvement, the fibrotic ejaculatory duct obstruction, fails to respond to surgery. Similarly, bypassing vasal obstructions with a vasoepididymostomy is possible only in a minority of cases as the involvement is multifocal. Epididymal involvement may result in chronic pain or fistulae, which would require surgical excision or an epididymectomy. Rarely, a prostatic abscess may require either trans-rectal or endoscopic drainage.

REFERENCES

1. Forssbohm M, Zwalhlen M, Loddnekemper R, Rieder HL. Demographic characteristics of patients with extrapulmonary tuberculosis in Germany. Eur Respir J 2008;1:99-105.
2. Kennedy DH. Extrapulmonary tuberculosis. In: Ratledge C, Stanford JL, Grange JM, editors. The biology of mycobacteria. New York: Academic Press; 1989.p.245-84.
3. Abbara A, Davidson RN. Etiology and management of genitourinary tuberculosis. Nat Rev Urol 2011;8:678-88.
4. Colabawalla BN. Reflections on urogenital tuberculosis. Indian J Urol 1990;6:51-9.
5. Figueiredo AA, Lucon AM, Junior RF, Srougi M. Epidemiology of urogenital tuberculosis worldwide. Int J Urol 2008;15:827-32.
6. Naidich DP, Garay SM, Leitman BS, McCauley DI. Radiographic manifestations of pulmonary disease in the acquired immuno-deficiency syndrome. Semin Roentgenol 1987;12:14-30.
7. Becker JA. Renal tuberculosis. Urol Radiol 1988;10:25-30
8. Elkin M. Urogenital tuberculosis. In: Pollack HM, editor. Clinical urography. Philadelphia: WB Saunders Company; 1990. p.1020-52.
9. Amis SE Jr, New House JH. Essentials of uroradiology. Boston: Little, Brown and Company; 1990.p.1640-66.
10. Tzvetkov D, Tzvetkova P. Tuberculosis of male genital system–myth or reality in 21st century. Arch Androl 2006;52:375-81.
11. Kumar R. Reproductive tract tuberculosis and male infertility. Indian J Urol 2008;24:392-5.
12. Figueiredo AA, LuconAM. Urogenital tuberculosis: update and review of 8961 cases from the world literature. Rev Urol 2008;10:207-17.
13. Carl P, Stark L. Indications for surgical management of genitourinary tuberculosis. World J Surg 1997;21:505-10.
14. Elkin M. Radiology of the urinary system. Boston: Little, Brown and Company; 1980.p.148-56.
15. Yoder IC. Hysterosalpingography and pelvis ultrasound imaging in infertility and gynecology. Boston: Little Brown and Company 1988.p.1166-78.
16. Greenberg JP. Tuberculous salpingitis. A clinical study of 200 cases. Johns Hopkins Hosp Rep 1991;21:97-103.
17. Gupta NP, Kumar R, Mundada OP, Aron M, Hemal AK, Dogra PN, et al. Reconstructive surgery for the management of genitourinary tuberculosis: a single center experience. J Urol 2006;175:2150-4.
18. Qureshi MA. Spontaneous nephrocutaneous fistula in tuberculous pyelonephritis. J Coll Physicians Surg Pak 2007;17:367-8.
19. Hemal AK, Gupta NP, Wadhwa SN, Songra MC, Batura D, Bhuyan UN. Primary repair of colorenocutaneous fistula in patients with genitourinary tuberculosis. Urol Int 1994;52:414.
20. Kumar R, Hemal AK. Bilateral epididymal masses with infertility. ANZ J Surg 2004;74:391.
21. Viswaroop BS, Kekre N, Gopalakrishnan G. Isolated tuberculous epididymitis: a review of forty cases. J Postgrad Med 2005;51:109-11.
22. Sporer A, Auerback MD. Tuberculosis of the prostate. Urology 1978;11:362-5
23. Hemal AK, Aron M, Nair M, Wadhwa SN. 'Autoprostatectomy': an unusual manifestation in genitourinary tuberculosis. Br J Urol 1998;82:140-1.
24. Lewis EL. Tuberculosis of the penis: a report of 5 new cases and a complete review of the literature. J Urol 1946;56:737-45.
25. Singh I, Hemal AK. Primary urethral tuberculosis masquerading as a urethral caruncle: a diagnostic curiosity! Int Urol Nephrol 2002;34:101-3.
26. Hemal AK, Gupta NP, Rajeev TP, Kumar R, Dar L, Seth P. Polymerase chain reaction in clinically suspected genitourinary tuberculosis: comparison with intravenous urography, bladder biopsy, and urine acid-fast bacilli culture. Urology 2000;56:570-4.
27. Moussa OM, Eraky I, El-Far MA, Osman HG, Ghoneim MA. Rapid diagnosis of genitourinary tuberculosis by polymerase chain reaction and non-radioactive DNA hybridization. J Urol 2000;164:584-8.
28. Chawla A, Chawla K, Reddy S, Arora N, Bairy I, Rao S, et al. Can tissue PCR augment the diagnostic accuracy in genitourinary tract tuberculosis? Urol Int 2012;88:34-8.
29. Sun L, Yuan Q, Feng JM, Yang CM, Yao L, Fan QL, et al. Rapid diagnosis in early stage renal tuberculosis by real-time polymerase chain reaction on renal biopsy specimens. Int J Tuberc Lung Dis 2010;14:341-6.
30. Gupta R, Singh P, Kumar R. Should men with idiopathic obstructive azoospermia be screened for genitourinary tuberculosis? J Hum Reprod Sci 2015;8:43-7.
31. Regmi SK, Singh UB, Sharma JB, Kumar R. Relevance of semen polymerase chain reaction positive for tuberculosis in asymptomatic men undergoing infertility evaluation. J Hum Reprod Sci 2015;8:165-9.
32a. Sharma SK, Kohli M, Chaubey J, Yadav RN, Sharma R, Singh BK, et al. Evaluation of Xpert MTB/RIF assay performance in diagnosing extrapulmonary tuberculosis among adults in a tertiary care centre in India. Eur Respir J 2014;44:1090-3.
32b. Kohli M, Schiller I, Dendukuri N, Dheda K, Denkinger CM, Schumacher SG, Steingart KR. Xpert[®] MTB/RIF assay for extra-pulmonary tuberculosis and rifampicin resistance. Cochrane Database Syst Rev 2018;8:CD012768.
33. Fan L, Chen Z, Hao XH, Hu ZY, Xiao HP. Interferon-gamma release assays for the diagnosis of extrapulmonary tuberculosis: a systematic review and meta-analysis. FEMS Immunol Med Microbiol 2012;65:456-66.
34. Valentini AL, Summaria V, Marano P. Diagnostic imaging of genitourinary tuberculosis. Rays 1998;23:126-43.
35. Premkumar A, Newhouse JH. Seminal vesicle tuberculosis: CT appearance. J Comput Assist Tomogr 1988;12:676-7.
36. Sharma SK, Ryan H, Khaparde S, Sachdeva KS, Singh AD, Mohan A, et al. Index-TB guidelines: Guidelines on extra-pulmonary tuberculosis for India. Indian J Med Res 2017;145:448-63.
37. Kadhiravan T, Sharma SK. Medical management of genitourinary tuberculosis. Indian J Urol 2008;24:362-8.

38. Krishnamoorthy S, Gopalakrishnan G. Surgical management of renal tuberculosis. Indian J Urol 2008;24:369-75.

39. Flechner SM, Gow JG. Role of nephrectomy in the treatment of nonfunctioning or poorly functioning unilateral tuberculous kidney. J Urol 1980;123:822-5.

40. Hemal AK, Gupta NP, Kumar R. Comparison of retro-peritoneoscopic nephrectomy with open surgery for tuberculous nonfunctioning kidneys. J Urol 2000;164:32-5.

41. Wong SH, Lan WY. The surgical management of non-functioning tuberculous kidneys. J Urol 1980;124:187-91.

42. Goel A, Dalela D. Options in the management of tuberculous ureteric stricture. Indian J Urol 2008;24:376-81.

43. Chan SL, Ankenman GJ, Wright JE, McLoughlin MG. Caecocysto-plasty in the surgical management of the small contracted bladder. J Urol 1980;124:338-40.

44. Hemal AK, Aron M. Orthotopic neobladder in management of tubercular thimble bladders: initial experience and long-term results. Urol 1999;53:298-301.

45. Kumar R. Surgery for azoospermia in the Indian patient: Why is it different? Indian J Urol 2011;27:98-101.

46. Yadav S, Singh P, Hemal A, Kumar R. Genital tuberculosis: current status of diagnosis and management. Transl Androl Urol 2017;6:222-33.

28

Tuberculosis in Chronic Kidney Disease

SK Agarwal

INTRODUCTION

Tuberculosis [TB] is one of the major causes of morbidity and mortality throughout the world. Susceptibility to TB has been attributed to host resistance, socioeconomic (1) and environmental factors (2). Because of the immunosuppressive effect of uraemia, use of corticosteroids and immunosuppressive drugs during renal transplantation [RT], these patients are at a high risk of developing TB. Consequently, TB has been found to occur more frequently in patients with chronic kidney disease [CKD], during maintenance haemodialysis [MHD] and following RT than in general population (3-7).

PATHOGENESIS

Uraemia is also an acquired immunodeficiency state leading to excessive morbidity and mortality related to infections. Functional abnormalities of neutrophils, T- and B-lymphocytes, monocytes and natural killer [NK] cells have been described in these patients. These abnormalities are often exacerbated by chronic haemodialysis and following RT. Bioincompatibility during haemodialysis frequently leads to immune activation and subsequent leucocyte dysfunction, thus exacerbating the underlying immune defect of uraemia. However, currently, due to change in membranes of dialysers, bioincompatibility has not remained an important issue.

Granulocyte functions such as chemotaxis, adherence and phagocytosis are marginally defective in uraemia but patients on haemodialysis have pronounced defects in these functions. Leucocyte chemotaxis has been reported to be diminished in patients with end-stage renal disease [ESRD] and MHD. In these patients, *in vitro* and *in vivo* administration of 1,25 dihydroxy vitamin D_3 has been shown to improve leucocyte adhesion and chemotaxis (8,9). Use of conventional cellulose membrane causes activation of the alternate complement pathway leading to changes in granulocyte cell adhesion molecules CD11b, CD18 [macrophage-1 antigen, MAC-1] and L-selectin. These changes correlate with development of leucopenia and its reversal (10). Similarly, phagocytosis is impaired both before and during haemodialysis. Impairment of phagocytosis during haemodialysis is more often encountered with cuprophane membrane than with newer membranes (11). Dialysis with cuprophane membrane also increases production of reactive oxygen species, thus decreasing responsiveness to an infectious challenge (12). With change of cuprophane membrane to newer more biocompatible membranes, these issues have almost eliminated.

Another major defect in lymphocyte function in uraemia and in patients on haemodialysis is decreased interleukin-2 [IL-2] production by activated T-helper cells (13). Whether the major defect is in the T-cells, antigen presentation to the T-cell or is monocyte derived, is still controversial. Altered macrophage Fc-receptor function *in vivo* and *in vitro* has been demonstrated in persons undergoing haemodialysis. This correlated very well with the incidence of severe infection during a two-year follow-up period. Defective antigen presentation by monocyte has also been demonstrated in patients on haemodialysis (14).

Following successful RT, infection remains the leading cause of morbidity and mortality, more so in high TB burden countries like India. The inflammatory response to microbial invasion in the transplant patients is attenuated by concomitant immunosuppressive therapy. The risk of infection in these patients is primarily determined by the interaction between exposure to mycobacteria and immune status of the patient. Immunosuppression is a complex state determined by the interaction of a number of factors, the most important of which are the dose, duration and temporal sequence of immunosuppressive drugs employed.

MAGNITUDE OF THE PROBLEM

There is limited information on the magnitude of the problem of TB in patients with CKD. However, a published study from China (15) reported 30 times higher prevalence of TB in patients with CKD as compared to general population of same city. The study reported inverse association between renal function and TB. Problem of TB in patients already on MHD has been more commonly studied and the incidence of TB in such patients has varied from 1%-13.3% (4-6,16-21). It has been estimated that patients undergoing dialysis have a 10- to 12-fold higher risk of developing TB compared to the general population (5,6). The incidence of TB in Indian patients receiving MHD has been reported to be 3.7%-13.3% (16,17). Majority of these patients have undergone haemodialysis for 12 to 24 months only. A report (22) also indicates transmission of TB from a healthcare worker to 29 patients and 13 employees in a dialysis centre.

The incidence of TB in RT recipients has been more systematically studied as these patients are regularly followed-up. Incidence of TB in RT patients has ranged from 1%–4% in Northern Europe (23-26); 0.5%–1% in North America (26,27) and nearly 5%–10% in several studies reported from India (28-33). Incidence of TB in RT patients has been found to be more or less similar among those who received cyclosporine and those who did not (18,30,31,33). However, few differences have been reported in these two groups. Higgins *et al* (7) reported that among RT patients who received cyclosporine-based protocols, TB developed only in those patients who were clearly at risk of developing the disease due to previous exposure. Similarly, John *et al* (33) suggested that TB developed in the early post-RT period in patients on cyclosporine, as compared to those patients who did not receive cyclosporine. At another hospital in North India, early occurrence of TB, especially miliary TB [MTB] has been observed in RT patients receiving cyclosporine compared with those who did not (34). With the use of tacrolimus and mycophenolate, it was expected that the incidence of TB in renal transplant will increase as these drugs are more potent than previously used immunosuppressive medication. In a study (35), a higher incidence of TB was found in patients receiving these drugs as compared to cyclosporine and also TB developed earlier in these patients. However, these results have not been confirmed in another study (36). A recent study (37) from the author's centre showed that with a mean follow-up of 47 [range 1-268] months, a significantly higher proportion of patients [17.3%] developed post-RT TB in cyclosporine-based triple immunosuppression as compared to 5.9% in tacrolimus-based triple immunosuppression group. TB-free survival in Kaplan-Meier analysis was significantly better in tacrolimus group as compared to cyclosporine group.

Possible transmission of TB by renal allograft has been reported (26,38,39). The most definitive report (38) was concerning a donor with culture-proven TB meningitis, whose kidneys were transplanted in two patients. Both of them developed definitive TB on days 35 and 39 respectively.

A recent meta-analysis [12 eligible studies, 71,374 ESRD patients and 560 TB cases] revealed consistent evidence suggestive of an increased risk of active TB in ESRD compared to the general population which had persisted in spite of variability in study population, design and modality of renal replacement therapy [RRT] (40).

CLINICAL PRESENTATION

Clinical Presentation of Tuberculosis during Maintenance Haemodialysis

Clinical presentation of TB in patients on MHD is summarised in [Table 28.1] (4-7,41). The age distribution of patients on MHD who developed TB was similar to that observed in general population (4). Males were nearly twice as commonly affected as compared to females (4,18). This probably reflects the gender difference observed in patients with CKD. Regular MHD usually tends to improve the general immune status of the patients with CKD. Therefore, a majority of these patients develop TB prior to initiation or within a short period from the beginning of MHD, a time when effect of uraemia on immune status is still pronounced. Sasaki *et al* (4) and Andrew *et al* (5) have reported the development of TB within six months of MHD, however, this period was much longer in other study (6). Prior exposure to TB and diabetes mellitus were found as risk factors in nearly 50% of the patients for the development of TB (6).

Constitutional symptoms attributable to TB have been reported in 30%-92% patients in various series (4-6,16) and may include low- or high-grade fever. Malhotra *et al* (17) reported that 15% of their patients on MHD, who developed TB, presented with pyrexia of unknown origin [PUO]. In other studies (6,18-21,41), this presentation has been rarely observed.

In majority of the studies (6,17-21,41), lung is the most common site of involvement in patients on MHD. In these studies (6,17-21,41), incidence of pulmonary TB ranged from 40%–92%. However, in some studies (5,6,41), isolated extra-pulmonary TB [EPTB] has been found in 56%–60% cases. Malhotra *et al* (17) have reported that pleural effusion occurred more frequently than pulmonary parenchymal lesions. However, this observation has not been corroborated by other workers who have found parenchymal lesions to be more common than pleural effusion (6,18-21). Lymph node involvement has been found to be the most common site of EPTB in patients on MHD [15%-30%] (4,6,17-19,33,41). In the series reported by Malhotra *et al* (17), lymph node TB occurred in 30% of patients; in 25% of the patients, this was the only presenting feature (17). Other sites of extrapulmonary involvement include abdomen (4-6), meninges (4), bone and joints (19,33). In a report from Taiwan, Chuang *et al* (42), while describing EPTB in dialysis patients, have reported involvement of peritoneum [35.3%], cervical lymph nodes [17.6%] and involvement of bone marrow, spine, knee joint, brain, pericardium, cutaneous tissue and genitourinary system [5.7% each]. These observations suggest that almost any organ can be affected by TB in these patients.

Table 28.1: Clinical presentation of TB in patients on maintenance haemodialysis

Variable	Sasaki et al (4) [n = 367]	Andrew et al (5) [n = 172]	Rutsky and Rostand (6) [n = 885]	Malhotra et al (17) [n = 150]	Venkata et al (41) [n = 900]
No. of TB patients [%]	12 [3.3]	10 [5.8]	9 [1]	20 [13.3]	36 [4]
Mean age [years]	45	49	48	20	52
Male:female	2:1	1.5:1	2:1	3:1	11:1
Time of diagnosis of TB in relation to duration of HD [%]	42	40	ND	0	61.1*
Prior HD					
Less than 6 months	42	50†	ND	95‡	ND
Six months to 1 year	8	0	ND	5	ND
More than 1 year	8	0	ND	0	ND
Site of TB [%]§				‖	
Pulmonary	8	60	33	10	36
Pleural	8	10	33	45	28
Lymph node	17	10	11	30¶	14
Miliary or disseminated	50	0	11	0	11
Neurological	8	10	0	0	0
Colon	8	0	0	0	0
Peritoneal	0	10	11	5	0
Bone and joints	0	0	0	5	8
Renal	0	10	0	0	0
Hepatic	0	0	0	0	0
Clinical presentation [%]					
Fever	92	**	††	‡‡	72
Appetite loss	100	**	††	‡‡	72
Weight loss	75	**	††	‡‡	25
Cough	25	**	††	‡‡	ND
Neurological deficit	50	**	††	‡‡	ND
Diagnosis [%]§§					
Microbiology ‖‖	33	50	90¶¶	20	16.6
Histopathology‖‖	17	40	20	45	30.5
Autopsy	50	10	0	5***	ND
Mortality [%]					
TB mortality	75	0	22	10	25
Overall mortality	75	20	44	60	ND

* 14 patients were on regular dialysis [13 on HD, 1 patient was on continuous ambulatory peritoneal dialysis], and 8 were on irregular dialysis. Among patients on regular dialysis, TB was identified within 1 year of dialysis in 4, and in the remaining, TB was diagnosed between 1 and 9 years of dialysis
† In 1 patient, the diagnosis of TB was made concurrent with the initiation of HD
‡ In 3 patients, the diagnosis of TB was made concurrent with the initiation of HD
§ More than one site was involved in some patients
‖ The site of TB was not clear in one patient. This patient responded well to antituberculosis treatment
¶ One patient had left hilar lymphadenopathy
** Details of clinical presentation were not described. The presenting symptoms were non-specific and constitutional in nature. Fever, malaise, anorexia and weight loss were most commonly encountered. Headache, chills, and shortness of breath were less common [<30% of the patients]
†† Of the 885 patients studied, a diagnosis of TB was made in 9 patients on HD and 8 patients who had CRF but did not require long-term dialysis. The clinical symptoms were not separately described for these 2 groups of patients
‡‡ Consolidated break-up of clinical features was not provided. Of the 20 patients in whom TB was diagnosed, 75% presented with fever, 50% with pleural effusion; 30% had lymphadenopathy, pulmonary abnormalities were found in 20% and ascites and hepatomegaly were observed in 10% patients. Other features included marked anorexia [10%], abnormal weight loss [5%] and bony swelling [5%]
§§ More than 1 method was positive in some patients
‖‖ Cumulative yield from various tissue and fluid specimens
¶¶ NTM were isolated from 3 of the 9 patients
*** A patient who had shown TB peripheral lymphadenopathy during life revealed histopathological evidence of TB in hilar and tracheobronchial lymph nodes on autopsy
TB = tuberculosis; HD = haemodialysis; ND = not described; CRF = chronic renal failure; NTM = nontuberculous mycobacteria

Disseminated TB [DTB], MTB have also been observed as the presenting feature in these patients. Nearly half of the patients studied by Sasaki *et al* (4) presented with DTB/MTB. In most of the other series, the incidence of MTB ranged between 10%-15% (6,19). None of the patients described by Malhotra *et al* (17) had MTB. Two of the 100 patients with MTB reported by Sharma *et al* (43) had CKD as a predisposing factor.

TB peritonitis has been described in patients on continuous ambulatory peritoneal dialysis [CAPD] (44,45). In these patients, the ascitic fluid may reveal predominance of polymorphonuclear leucocytes. In addition to causing morbidity, it can also cause ultrafiltration failure of CAPD and require shifting to other modality of renal replacement therapy. TB peritonitis is also one of the causes of culture-negative peritonitis in CAPD patients (44,45).

In a retrospective cohort study (46) of TB disease in 272,024 patients in the US Renal Data System initiated on dialysis therapy between April 1995 and December 1999, cumulative incidence of TB in patients undergoing either peritoneal or haemodialysis was found to be 1.2% and 1.6%, respectively. In this study (46), advanced age, unemployment, availing health insurance [Medicaid], reduced body mass index, decreased serum albumin, haemodialysis, both Asian and Native American race, ischaemic heart disease, smoking, illicit drug use and anaemia were found to be risk factors for development of TB in patients receiving peritoneal or haemodialysis. Furthermore, in patients receiving dialysis, TB was independently associated with increased mortality.

Clinical Presentation of Tuberculosis following Renal Transplantation

TB can be encountered in RT patients in two settings. First, a patient with advanced CKD suffering from TB in the pre-transplant phase may continue to suffer from TB in the post-RT phase as well. On the other hand, patients may develop TB for the first time following RT. The present description is regarding patients in the latter category.

Patients who develop TB following RT [Table 28.2] (7,30-33) are usually younger. Males are more often affected. This could be because of the fact that young males undergo RT more often in a country like India (30-32). Similar observations have been reported from the west as well as from other countries (47). Past history of TB has been reported in 5.6%–8.9% patients in studies reported from India [Table 28.2]. When TB develops, constitutional symptoms are more often encountered in RT patients than in patients on MHD (31-33). The lung is the most common site of involvement in RT patients who develop TB (29-33). Other sites of TB involvement in RT patients include abdomen (7,33); pericardium (30,33); thalamic abscess (30) and bone and joints (7,30). MTB has also been reported in 7%–36.4% of RT patients (30-33,38). Thus, RT patients develop pulmonary TB more often, and manifest constitutional symptoms more commonly compared with patients on MHD.

Comparison of presentation of TB during haemodialysis and after RT [n = 923] at the author's centre is shown in [Table 28.3] (37). Pleuropulmonary TB appears to be more common in both settings. In RT recipients, presentation with PUO and MTB is significantly more common as compared to patients on MHD. Furthermore, abdominal TB was significantly more common during dialysis and neurological TB was more common after transplantation.

Overall, patients with advanced CKD while on MHD manifest EPTB more frequently [60%] as compared to pulmonary TB [40%] [Table 28.1]. By contrast, site of involvement in RT-recipients resembles that observed in immunocompetent individuals; pulmonary TB is more frequent [60%] [Table 28.2], probably due to improvement in their immune status.

DIAGNOSIS

Definitive diagnosis of TB requires demonstration or isolation of *Mycobacterium tuberculosis [Mtb]*. In majority of studies (5-7) published from the west, diagnosis of TB was based on demonstration of the organism in the body fluids and/or tissues or on the basis of histopathological findings. In contrast, 8.6%-68% of the patients in various Indian studies (30-32) have been diagnosed to have TB only on clinical grounds. This is probably due to the low threshold for therapeutic trial with anti-TB treatment in a country like India, where TB is endemic.

Diagnosis of TB in patients with CKD is difficult. Patients with CKD can have a high erythrocyte sedimentation rate [ESR] due to anaemia and various other reasons and, therefore, ESR is not of much use in these patients. The tuberculin skin test [TST] is often negative in patients on MHD and following RT (21,48,49). A study from North India also showed that TST in patients on maintenance haemodialysis was positive only in 10.5% cases and may not be reliable test for diagnosis of TB (50). The utility of newer diagnostic methods for detecting latent TB infection [LTBI], such as, interferon-gamma release assays [IGRAs] in the diagnosis of TB infection in patients with CKD seems promising, but, needs to be explored further (51). Radiological findings in immunocompromised patients with pulmonary TB are often atypical. In these patients cavitary lesions are seldom seen and lower lung field and multiple lobar involvements are often seen. Patients on MHD can develop pleural effusion due to heart failure, uraemic pleuritis or hypoproteinaemia. Similarly, pericarditis and pericardial effusion and ascites in these patients are often due to dialysis associated pericarditis and/or ascites (52). Pleural fluid in uraemic pleuritis can also be exudative and haemorrhagic with high protein and lactate dehydrogenase levels with a predominance of lymphocytes (53,54). These findings are often encountered in TB pleural effusion and are, therefore, unreliable. Diagnostic value of adenosine deaminase activity [ADA] in pleural fluid even in RT patients is also unreliable (55). The acid-fast bacilli [AFB] can seldom be seen and mycobacteria are rarely cultured

Table 28.2: Clinical presentation of TB in renal transplant patients

Variable	Hariharan et al (32) [n = 550]	Higgins et al (7) [n = 633]	John et al (33) [n = 808]	Sakhuja et al (31) [n = 305]	Agarwal et al (30)* [n = 461]
No. of patients with TB [%]	46 [8.4]	11 [1.7]	41 [5.1]	36 [11.8]	67 [14.5]
Mean age [years]	32.5	43.9	†	33.9	14
Male:Female	4.1:1	1.8:1	4.9:1	6.2:1	3.5:1
Mean time interval between renal transplantation and detection of TB [months]	20	26.4	‡	20.7	24
Past history of TB	ND	ND	ND	5.6	8.9
Immunosuppression	D	D/T	D/T	D/T	D/T
Site of TB [%] §					
Pulmonary	39	18	49	31	37
Pleural	13	9	0	14	22
Lymph node	17	0	2	3	8
Disseminated or miliary TB	7	36	27	25	8
Neurological	4	0	0	0	5
Abdominal	4	18	7	3	5
Genitourinary	0	9	5	3	0
Skin, soft tissue	0	0	7	3	0
Pericarditis	0	0	0	0	0
Bone and joints	0	0	2	0	1.5
Diagnosis [%]‖					
Microbiology¶	52	55**	98††	14	3
Histopathology¶	26	27	10	33	12
Autopsy	4	0	0	3	11
Mortality [%]					
TB-related mortality	4	9	12	6	0
Overall mortality	9	9	46	19.4	0

Percentage values are corrected to the nearest round figures
* Figures from 1992 have been revised and updated till 1997
† Mean age of patients receiving cyclosporine immunosuppression and conventional immunosuppression was 39.9 and 37.3 years, respectively
‡ Median time [months] of diagnosis of mycobacterial infection after transplantation in patients receiving cyclosporine immunosuppression and conventional immunosuppression was 5.5 and 2.4 months, respectively
§ Some patients had involvement of more than 1 site
‖ More than 1 method was positive in some patients
¶ Cumulative yield from various tissue fluids and specimens
** 1 patient had infection with *Mycobacterium kansasii*
†† 2 patients had nontuberculous mycobacterial infection
TB = tuberculosis; ND = not described; D = double immunosuppression; T = triple immunosuppression

from the pleural fluid. Usefulness of modern diagnostic tests, such as polymerase chain reaction [PCR] has not been systematically explored in the diagnosis of TB in patients with CKD, though these are often reported as evidence of diagnosis (56). Recent evidence suggests that cartridge-based nucleic acid amplification tests [CBNAAT] like Xpert MTB/RIF have a low sensitivity and is not useful in the diagnosis of pleural TB (57). Studies with a large sample size are required to establish the usefulness of these investigations.

MANAGEMENT

Principles of anti-TB treatment during dialysis and following RT remain similar to that in other patients with TB. The choice of safe and effective anti-TB treatment for these patients depends upon the pharmacology of drugs in the setting of CKD and during MHD and their interaction with immunosuppressive drugs used in patients with RT. Pharmacological properties of anti-TB drugs that determine how the levels of these drugs are likely to be influenced by

Table 28.3: Comparison of site of TB involvement in patients with chronic kidney disease [n = 923] pre- and post-renal transplantation

Site of TB	Pre-RT No. [%]	Post-RT No. [%]
Number of cases	152	156
Pleural*	50 [32.9]	17 [10.9]
Pulmonary	44 [28.9]	45 [28.8]
Abdominal*	16 [10.5]	4 [2.6]
Nodal	14 [9.2]	13 [8.3]
Pericardial*	11 [7.2]	0
Presentation as PUO*	10 [6.6]	46 [29.5]
Genitourinary	3 [1.9]	0
Bone and joints	2 [1.3]	2 [1.3]
Miliary*	1 [0.6]	14 [8.9]
Neurological*	1 [0.6]	9 [5.8]
Miscellaneous	0	6 [3.9]
Laryngeal	0	2
Orchitis	0	1
Skin	0	1
Psoas abscess	0	1
Gluteal abscess	0	1

* Statistically significant difference
TB = tuberculosis; RT = renal transplant; PUO = pyrexia of unknown origin

renal impairment have been extensively reviewed by several workers (58-60).

Renal insufficiency complicates the management of TB because some anti-TB drugs are cleared by the kidneys. Management may be further complicated by the removal of some anti-tuberculosis agents via haemodialysis. Thus, some alteration in the dosage of anti-TB drugs is necessary in patients with CKD and ESRD receiving haemodialysis. Decreasing the dose of selected anti-tuberculosis drugs may not be the best method of treating TB because, although toxicity may be avoided, the peak serum concentrations may be too low. Therefore, increasing the dosing interval instead of decreasing the dosage of the anti-TB drugs is recommended (61).

Isoniazid

Of the administered dose of isoniazid, 96% is recoverable in the urine as unchanged drug together with its metabolites (62). All metabolites of isoniazid are devoid of anti-TB activity. These are less toxic than isoniazid and are more rapidly excreted through the kidneys (63). In anuric patients, half-life of isoniazid varies with acetylator status. Half-life is essentially unaltered in rapid acetylators; while in those who are slow acetylators, it has been observed to increase by 40%. It is, therefore, recommended that normal daily dosage of isoniazid [300 mg or 5 mg/kg body weight] should be given in patients with severe renal impairment, including anuric

patients. In slow acetylators with severe renal impairment and who are not on dialysis, 5-6 mg/kg body weight isoniazid will be equivalent to daily dose of 7-9 mg/kg body weight in normal subjects. It has been shown that isoniazid is well tolerated at this dose in these patients (64). Previous recommendation to reduce the daily dose of isoniazid to 150 mg in patients with severe CKD is, therefore, unjustified (65,66). Also, there is convincing evidence that isoniazid at a dosage less than 200 mg/day significantly decreases therapeutic response (67). Some suggestions regarding administering isoniazid eighth hourly are un-warranted (68) and there is no justification for estimation of isoniazid levels in these patients (62).

Rifampicin

Serum half-life of rifampicin and the proportion of the unchanged drug excreted in the urine increase steadily as the individual dosages are increased from 300 to 900 mg, probably as a result of biliary excretion route becoming saturated. Daily treatment with rifampicin for a period of one week or more, results in the induction of hepatic enzymes, which deacetylate the drug. Such induction significantly reduces half-life of rifampicin and probably reduces urinary excretion of the unchanged drug. About 14% of the dose is recovered in urine whether or not liver enzymes have been induced. It is thought that effect of renal impairment on rifampicin excretion is negligible at a dose of 450 mg, modest at 600 mg and substantial at 900 mg (58). Therefore, rifampicin up to a dose of 600 mg/day does not require reduction at any stage of CKD (58).

Pyrazinamide

As little as 3%-4% of ingested pyrazinamide is excreted unchanged in the urine. Its half-life is 6-10 hours and very little change is expected even in patients with severe renal failure (69,70). However, Fabre et al (70), suggested to avoid its use in severe renal failure, while Anderson et al (71), and Andrew et al (5), suggested reduction in the dose to 12-20 mg/kg/day. However, such a dosage schedule will cause suboptimal therapeutic levels (72). Controlled clinical trials have shown that thrice weekly treatment is therapeutically more effective than daily administration (73). It is, therefore, recommended that patients with renal impairment should be treated either thrice or twice weekly with 40–60 mg/kg pyrazinamide. However, in most of the published studies, patients had received daily dose of pyrazinamide (69,70).

Streptomycin

Nearly 80% of the dose of streptomycin, like other aminogly-cosides, is excreted unchanged in the urine. Aminoglycosides are excreted by glomerular filtration and not by active secretion (74,75). Line et al (74) demonstrated significant correlation between degree of renal failure and serum levels of streptomycin. Therefore, if streptomycin is to be used in the treatment of TB in presence of renal failure, its dosage must be decreased. It is preferable to give streptomycin twice or thrice weekly without decreasing the usual dose. If possible, drug through level should be measured and should not exceed 4 mg/L.

Ethambutol

About 80% of the dose of ethambutol is excreted unchanged in urine and major reduction in daily ethambutol doses are recommended in patients with renal failure. Recommended dosage in presence of renal failure varies from 5-10 mg/kg/day by various workers (6,76,77). Ethambutol can result in blindness. Moreover, measurement of streptomycin levels is much easier. Therefore, if treatment of TB in renal failure requires administration of a fourth drug, in addition to rifampicin, isoniazid and pyrazinamide, streptomycin seems to be a better choice as compared to ethambutol. However, in all the recent studies, ethambutol rather than streptomycin has been used as the fourth drug. There is report of irreversible blindness in a patient of ESRD treated with ethambutol for TB, and thus, very close watch on ophthalmic examination should be done in these patients (78).

Second-line Anti-tuberculosis Drugs

Dosages of kanamycin, amikacin, and capreomycin must be adjusted in patients with renal failure because of renal excretion of these drugs. Administration of these drugs just prior to haemodialysis, removes approximately 40% of the dosage (79). Dosing interval of these drugs should be increased. Ethionamide is not cleared by the kidneys, nor is the drug removed with haemodialysis, so no dose adjustment is necessary (80). Para-amino salicylic acid [PAS] is moderately cleared by haemodialysis [6.3%] but its metabolite, acetyl-PAS, is substantially removed by haemodialysis; twice daily dosing [4 g] should be adequate (80). Cycloserine is excreted primarily by the kidney, and is cleared by haemodialysis [56%]. Thus, an increase in the dosing interval is necessary to avoid accumulation between haemodialysis sessions, and the drug should be given after hemodialysis to avoid under-dosing (80). The fluoroquinolones undergo some degree of renal clearance that varies from drug to drug. For example, levofloxacin undergoes greater renal clearance than moxifloxacin (81). It should be noted that the fluoroquinolone dosing recommendations for ESRD provided by the manufacturers were developed for treating pyogenic bacterial infections. These recommendations may not be applicable to the treatment of TB in patients with ESRD. It is important to monitor serum drug concentrations in persons with renal insufficiency who is taking cycloserine, ethambutol, or any of the injectable agents to minimise dose-related toxicity, while providing effective doses. Currently, enough data are not available on anti-TB drug dosage modification in patients receiving peritoneal dialysis and the drug removal mechanisms differ between haemodialysis and peritoneal dialysis. Therefore, such patients may require close follow-up and therapeutic drug monitoring.

Treatment of Tuberculosis in Patients on Dialysis

Treatment of TB is imperative as soon as the diagnosis is confirmed or strongly suspected. Isoniazid and rifampicin have been used in majority of the studies (4-6,16,21). Streptomycin is not so commonly used nowadays in patients with renal failure. Isoniazid at a dosage of 200-300 mg/day does not cause significant toxicity in adult patients with renal failure. However, vitamin B6 in a dose of 10-20 mg should be administered prophylactically in all these patients. Dosage modification is not required for rifampicin but it should be administered cautiously in patients with CKD who are not on haemodialysis as it can result in acute renal failure or deterioration in the renal functions (82). Dosing recommendations for adult patients with reduced renal function [creatinine clearance <30 mL/min] and for adult patients receiving haemodialysis are shown in Table 28.4 (61). The anti-TB drugs should be administered after haemo-dialysis to avoid any loss of the drugs during the procedure, and to facilitate direct observation of treatment (61). The possibility of impaired absorption of anti-tuberculosis drugs because of comorbid clinical conditions, such as diabetes mellitus with gastroparesis that are frequently present in these patients should also be kept in mind.

Under the Revised National Tuberculosis Control Programme [RNTCP] of the Government of India, daily standard anti-TB treatment has been advocated for all patients, including those with renal failure on conservative management, MHD or following RT. Monitoring of renal or hepatic function is not done under programme conditions. As of now, there are no published data on the efficacy and safety of these regimens in patients with CKD on conservative management or MHD. There is no consensus for the duration of anti-TB treatment in these patients. These issues merit further studies.

Rifampicin is an inducer of hepatic enzymes and is known to alter the metabolism of many drugs. In this regard, rifampicin use becomes an important issue in patients before and following RT. Majority of these patients also receive anti-hypertensive drugs and with the use of rifampicin, an adequate blood pressure control may not be achieved and the dose modification may be required for the anti-hypertensive drugs. In a recently completed study on effect of rifampicin as part of anti-TB therapy on anti-hypertensive drug requirement in patients of kidney disease, it was concluded that there is a significant interaction between anti-hypertensive drugs and rifampicin, resulting in loss of blood pressure control after initiation of rifampicin-based anti-TB therapy. Most patients require an increase in their anti-hypertensive drug prescription and there is a potential risk of experiencing a hypertensive crisis. Significant decrease in serum levels of commonly prescribed anti-hypertensive drugs was observed, which correlated with the clinical findings of uncontrolled hypertension. Given the clinical impact of findings and ease of applicability, it was recommended that it would be prudent to monitor patients closely for worsening of hypertension after initiation of

Table 28.4: Dosing recommendations for adult patients with reduced renal function* and for adult patients receiving haemodialysis

Drug	Change in frequency of administration	Dosage schedule
First-line drugs		
Isoniazid	No change	5 mg/kg [maximum 300 mg] once daily, or 15 mg/kg [maximum 900 mg] per dose, three times per week
Rifampicin	No change	10 mg/kg [maximum 600 mg] once daily, or 10 mg/kg [maximum 600 mg] per dose, three times per week
Pyrazinamide	Yes	25 to 35 mg/kg per dose three times per week [not daily]
Ethambutol	Yes	15 to 25 mg/kg per dose three times per week [not daily]
Streptomycin	Yes	12 to 15 mg/kg per dose two or three times per week [not daily]
Second-line drugs		
Cycloserine	Yes	250 mg once daily, or 500 mg per dose three times per week†
Ethionamide	No change	15 to 20 mg/kg/day [maximum 1 g; usually 500 to 750 mg] in a single daily dose or two divided doses‡
Para-aminosalicylic acid	No change	8 to 12 g/day, in two or three doses
Capreomycin	Yes	12 to 15 mg/kg per dose two or three times per week [not daily]
Kanamycin	Yes	12 to 15 mg/kg per dose two or three times per week [not daily]
Amikacin	Yes	12 to 15 mg/kg per dose two or three times per week [not daily]
Levofloxacin	Yes	750 to 1000 mg per dose three times per week [not daily]

* Creatinine clearance less than 30 mL/min
† The appropriateness of 250 mg daily doses has not been established
‡ The single daily dose can be given at bed time or with the main meal. No data to support intermittent administration
The medications should be given after haemodialysis on the day of haemodialysis
Monitoring of serum drug concentrations should be considered to ensure adequate drug absorption without excessive accumulation, and to assist in avoiding toxicity
Data currently are not available for patients receiving peritoneal dialysis. Until data become available, begin with doses recommended for patients receiving haemodialysis and verify adequacy of dosing, using monitoring of serum concentration
Adapted from reference 59

rifampicin [unpublished data]. Rifampicin also decreases the efficacy of other drugs, such as, corticosteroids, cyclosporine and tacrolimus. Therefore, dosages of these drugs also need to be modified. This has led to use of non-rifampicin-based protocols for treatment of TB in RT recipients with an aim of decreasing the cost of therapy as well as avoiding frequent monitoring (83,84). However, these findings require validation in future studies. There are no published data on the efficacy and safety of the standard treatment regimens used in the RNTCP in RT recipients. Controlled trials with large sample size are required to establish the efficacy, safety, and optimum duration of these standard treatment regimens in patients with CKD.

Treatment of Latent Tuberculosis Infection in Patients with Chronic Renal Failure on Dialysis Treatment

The American Thoracic Society [ATS] guidelines (85) mention the relative risk of developing TB in patients with CKD/those on MHD to be 10-25.3 and targeted TST and treatment of LTBI is a well-accepted strategy in developed countries with low transmission of TB such as the USA (61,85). However, this approach does not seem to have much relevance in highly

endemic areas. Published data suggest that TST is not a reliable test for diagnosis of LTBI in patients with CKD (86-88). A study from India showed that TST in patients on maintenance haemodialysis is an insensitive and non-specific test for the diagnosis of LTBI and this should not be taken as criteria to prescribe prophylaxis of TB in these patients (50). The potential role of IGRAs also have been evaluated in this setting recently. It has been reported that more number of patients [35.6%] on haemodialysis test positive for QuantiFERON Gold In-Tube test [QFT-GIT] as compared to TST [17.2%]. However, there is poor agreement between the two tests. In patients on haemodialysis, Bacille-Calmette-Guérin [BCG] vaccination and history of TB in past did not seem to affect both TST and QFT-GIT test results. In the absence of a "gold standard" for the diagnosis of LTBI, the issue concerning 'true positive' test results in patients on haemodialysis needs to be resolved (89).

In a randomised, double-blind, placebo-controlled, prospective trial of isoniazid prophylaxis in patients on haemodialysis from India (90), some degree of protection was shown. This protection appeared to be insignificant when the number of cases who dropped out due to various reasons and significant number of patients developing TB in the treatment group were also taken into consideration.

Another recently published trial on isoniazid prophylaxis in patients due to undergo RT who were receiving MHD (91) documented that TB developed in 16.7% patients in the isoniazid group compared with 32.7% patients in the control group suggesting that there was a significant reduction in the incidence of TB if isoniazid was started early. These issues need further clarification.

Another issue, which is not clear, is the optimum duration of anti-TB treatment before a patient with CKD can be safely taken up for RT. Controlled trials have not been conducted to answer this question and there is no consensus. Possibly, four to six weeks treatment with an adequate anti-TB drug regimen should be enough before the surgery, especially if the patient is showing a good clinical response to treatment.

Treatment of Tuberculosis in Recipients of Renal Transplantation

Management of TB after RT is similar to the management of TB in patients on MHD with few differences. Firstly, following successful RT, renal function become normal and dosage modification done during MHD is no longer required. Secondly, anti-tuberculosis drug interaction with immunosuppressive drugs is an important issue in these patients. Three most commonly used immunosuppressive drugs in these patients are prednisolone, tacrolimus and mycophenolate mofetil. Sometimes, cyclophosphamide is also used. There have been no recommendations to decrease the dosage of immunosuppressive medication if patients develop TB after RT.

During rifampicin therapy, daily dosage of corticosteroids should be increased or maintained to nearly 1.5 times the baseline dosage, as rifampicin is known to be an inducer of the enzymes involved in the hepatic metabolism of corticosteroids (92). Azathioprine if used, sometimes, causes hepatotoxicity, which has to be differentiated from hepatotoxicity due to anti-TB treatment. The major drug interaction of anti-TB drugs is with tacrolimus. Rifampicin produces lowering of blood levels of tacrolimus by producing an increase in its hepatic metabolism (93). Ideally, tacrolimus blood levels should be monitored and its dose adjusted if the patient is also receiving rifampicin. Optimum duration of anti-TB treatment in RT recipients is again controversial. Patients who receive DOTS under the RNTCP of the Government of India are treated for six months. In individual cases, treatment duration may be prolonged by another three [e.g., EPTB] to six [e.g., TB meningitis] months. However, in some studies most patients have received treatment for 12 months or more (29-32,94). The efficacy of short-course chemotherapy has not been studied in detail in these patients.

Treatment of Latent Tuberculosis Infection in Renal Transplant Recipients

The relative risk [RR] of an RT patient developing TB has been estimated to be 37 (85). Therefore, ATS guidelines recommend treatment of LTBI in RT recipients (85).

However, it is possible for a person to develop TB in spite of chemoprophylaxis (95). In a recent study published from India (96) isoniazid prophylaxis started at the time of RT offered some protection from development of TB (96). In this study, 11.1% patients receiving isoniazid prophylaxis developed TB as compared to 25.8% in the control group [RR 0.36]. However, these differences were not statistically significant. Keeping with the END-TB strategy of the WHO, a national policy of LTBI treatment in high-risk groups, like patients with CKD, RT-recipients [after ruling our active TB] is expected to be available in near future.

Therapeutic Response and Prognosis

With the proper use of currently available anti-TB drugs, there is a potential for complete cure in a compliant patient. Major factors which determine the response to anti-TB treatment are extent of disease at the time of diagnosis, treatment regimen given to the patients, sensitivity of the mycobacteria to given drugs and compliance with drug treatment.

In the studies, where the response to anti-TB treatment was clearly reported, the cure rate varied from 50%-80% (5-6,17). Mortality varied from 7.7%-75% but TB was seldom the cause of death in these patients. Mortality due to TB occurs in nearly 10% of the RT patients (29,32,33). In RT patients, anti-TB drug-induced hepatotoxicity has been estimated to be nearly 20% in two major studies (31,32). The magnitude of the problem of multidrug-resistant TB [MDR-TB] in patients with CRF and following RT needs to be studied in detail.

NONTUBERCULOUS MYCOBACTERIAL DISEASE IN CHRONIC KIDNEY DISEASE

Nontuberculous mycobacterial disease [NTM] is uncommon in patients with CKD and following RT. In a study (6), 17.6% of mycobacterial infections in dialysis patients were caused by *M. avium-intracellulare* and *M. fortuitum*.

NTM disease has been reported more frequently in RT recipients than in patients on MHD. Among these patients, about 10% of mycobacterial infections are due to NTM, of which *M. kansasii* and *M. chelonae* are frequent (26,27,96-101). Usually these organisms cause chronic infection of bone and soft tissues. In India, mycobacterial culture and drug-susceptibility testing facilities in reliable, accredited, quality assured laboratories are seldom available and it is, therefore, possible that NTM infections are being missed. The reader is referred to the chapter *"Nontuberculous mycobacterial infections"* [Chapter 41] for details.

REFERENCES

1. Ogg CS, Toseland PA, Cameson JS. Pulmonary tuberculosis in a patient on intermittent haemodialysis. BMJ 1968;2:283-4.
2. Comstock GW. Frost revisited: the modern epidemiology of tuberculosis. Am J Epidemiol 1975;101:363-82.
3. Papadimitriou M, Memmos D, Metaxas P. Tuberculosis in patients on regular haemodialysis. Nephron 1979;24:53-7.

4. Sasaki S, Akiba T, Suenaga M, Tomura S, Yoshiyama N, Nakagawa S, et al. Ten years survey of dialysis associated tuberculosis. Nephron 1979;24:141-5.

5. Andrew OT, Schoenfeld PY, Hopewell PC, Humphreys MH. Tuberculosis in patients with end-stage renal disease. Am J Med 1980;68:59-65.

6. Rutsky EA, Rostand SG. Mycobacteriosis in patients with chronic renal failure. Arch Intern Med 1980;140:57-61.

7. Higgins RM, Cahn AP, Porter D, Richardson AJ, Mitchell RG, Hopkin JM, et al. Mycobacterial infection after renal transplantation. QJM 1991;78:145-53.

8. Tabata T, Suzuki R, Kikunami K, Matsushita Y, Inoue T, Inove T, et al. The effect of 1 alpha hydroxy-vitamin D3 on cell mediated immunity in hemodialysed patients. J Clin Endocrinol Metabol 1986;63:1218-21.

9. Venezio FR, Koseny FA, Divincenzo CA, Hano JE. Effect of 1,25 dihydroxy vitamin D3 on leukocyte functions in patients receiving chronic hemodialysis. J Infect Dis 1988;158:1102-5.

10. Himmelfarb J, Zaoui P, Hakim RM. Modulation of granulocyte LAM-1 and MAC-1 during dialysis: a prospective randomised, controlled trial. Kidney Int 1992;41:388-95.

11. Descamps-Latscha B, Goldfarb B, Nguygen AT, Landais P, London G, Cavaillon NH, et al. Establishing the relationship between complement activation and stimulation of phagocyte oxidation metabolism in randomised study. Nephron 1991;59: 279-85.

12. Himmelfarb J, Ault KA, Holbrook D, Leeber DA, Hakim RM. Intradialysis granulocyte reactive oxygen species production: a prospective crossover trial. J Am Soc Nephrol 1993;4:178-86.

13. Beaurain G, Naret C, Marcon L, Grateau G, Drueke T, Urena P, et al. In vivo T-cell reactivation in chronic uremic haemodialysed and non-haemodialysed patients. Kidney Int 1989;36:636-44.

14. Gibbons RA, Martinez OM, Garovoy MR. Altered monocyte function in uraemia. Clin Immunol Immunopathol 1990;56:66-71.

15. Yuan FH, Guang LX, Zhao SJ. Clinical comparison of 1498 chronic renal failure patients with and without tuberculosis. Ren Fail 2005;27:149-53.

16. Narula AS, Misra A, Oberoi HS, Anand AC, Chatterjee SK, Waryam S. Tuberculosis in patients of chronic renal failure on maintenance haemodialysis. Indian J Nephrol 1991;1:67.

17. Malhotra KK, Parashar MK, Sharma RK, Bhuyan UN, Dash SC, Kumar R, et al. Tuberculosis in maintenance hemodialysis patients. Postgrad Med J 1981;57:492-8.

18. Pradhan RP, Katz LA, Nidus BD, Matalon R, Eisinger RP. Tuberculosis in a dialysed patient. JAMA 1974;229:798-800.

19. Basok A, Vorobiov M, Rogachev B, Avnon L, Tovbin D, Hausmann M, et al. Spectrum of mycobacterial infections: tuberculosis and Mycobacterium other than tuberculosis in dialysis patients. Isr Med Assoc J 2007;9:448-51.

20. Christopoulos AI, Diamantopoulos AA, Dimopoulos PA, Gumenos DS, Barbalias GA. Risk of tuberculosis in dialysis patients: association of tuberculin and 2,4-dinitrochlorobenzene reactivity with risk of tuberculosis. Int Urol Nephrol 2006;38: 745-51.

21. Zyga S, Tourouki G. Tuberculosis in haemodialysis: a problem making a comeback. J Ren Care 2006;32:176-8.

22. Center for Disease Control and Prevention. Tuberculosis transmission in a renal dialysis center-Nevada, 2003. MMWR Morb Mortal Wkly Rep 2004;53:873-5.

23. Coutts II, Jegarajah S, Stark JE. Tuberculosis in renal transplant recipients. Br J Dis Chest 1979;73:141-8.

24. Riska H, Gronhagen-Riska C, Ahonen J. Tuberculosis and renal allograft transplantation. Transplant Proc 1987;19:4096-7.

25. McWhinney N, Khan O, Williams G. Tuberculosis in patients undergoing maintenance haemodialysis and renal transplantation. Br J Surg 1981;68:408-11.

26. Lichtenstein IH, Macgregor RR. Mycobacterial infection in renal transplant recipients: report of five cases and review of literature. Rev Infect Dis 1983;5:216-26.

27. Lloveras J, Peterson PK, Simmons RL, Najarian JS. Mycobac-terial infections in renal transplant patients. Arch Intern Med 1982;142: 888-92.

28. Govil S, Ojha RK, Bhatia RK, Zope JD, Shah PR, Trivedi HL. Tuberculosis and renal allograft dysfunction. Indian J Nephrol 1995;5:96-7.

29. Agarwal DK, Ammanna N, Murthy BVR, Neela P, Ratnakar KS. High incidence of post-transplant tuberculosis in India. Indian J Nephrol 1994;91.

30. Agarwal SK, Dash SC, Tiwari SC, Agarwal R, Mehta SN. Spectrum of tuberculosis in renal transplant recipients in northern India. Indian J Nephrol 1992;2:39-43.

31. Sakhuja V, Jha V, Varma PP, Joshi K, Chugh KS. The high incidence of tuberculosis among renal transplant recipients in India. Transplantation 1996;61:211-5.

32. Hariharan S, Date A, Gopalkrishnan G, Pandey AP, Jacob CK, Kirubakaran MG, et al. Tuberculosis after renal transplantation. Dialysis Transpl 1987;16:311-2.

33. John GT, Vincent L, Jeyaseelan L, Jacob CK, Shastry JCM. Cyclosporine immunosuppression and mycobacterial infections. Transplantation 1994;58:247-9.

34. Agarwal SK. Tuberculosis in chronic renal failure. In: Sharma SK, Mohan A, editors. Tuberculosis. Second edition. New Delhi: Jaypee Brothers Medical Publishers; 2009.p.479-92.

35. Atasever A, Bacakoglu F, Toz H, Basoglu OK, Duman S, Basak K, et al. Tuberculosis in renal transplant recipients on various immunosuppressive regimens. Nephrol Dial Transplant 2005; 20:797-802.

36. Vandermarliere A, Van Audenhove A, Peetermans WE, Vanrenterghem Y, Maes B. Mycobacterial infection after renal transplantation in a Western population. Transpl Infect Dis 2003;5:9-15.

37. Agarwal SK, Bhowmik D, Mahajan S, Bagchi S. Impact of type of calcineurin inhibitor on post-transplant tuberculosis: single-center study from India. Transpl Infect Dis 2017;19[1]. doi: 10.1111/tid.12626.

38. Peters TG, Reiter CG, Boswell RL. Transmission of tuberculosis by kidney transplantation. Transplantation 1984; 38:514-6.

39. Graham JC, Kearns AM, Magee JG, El-Sheikh MF, Hudson M, Manas D, et al. Tuberculosis transmitted through transplantation. J Infect 2001;43:251-4.

40. Al-Efraij K, Mota L, Lunny C, Schachter M, Cook V, Johnston J. Risk of active tuberculosis in chronic kidney disease: a systematic review and meta-analysis. Int J Tuberc Lung Dis 2015;19:1493-9.

41. Venkata RKC, Kumar S, Krishna RP, Kumar SB, Padmanabhan S, Kumar S. Tuberculosis in chronic kidney disease. Clin Nephrol 2007;67:217-20.

42. Chuang FR, Lee CH, Wang IK, Chen JB, Wu MS. Extrapulmonary tuberculosis in chronic haemodialysis patients. Ren Fail 2003; 25:739-46.

43. Sharma SK, Mohan A, Pande JN, Prasad KL, Gupta AK, Khilnani GC. Clinical profile, laboratory characteristics and outcome in miliary tuberculosis. QJM 1995;88:29-37.

44. Karayayali I, Seyrek N, Akpolat T, Ates K, Ozener C, Yilmaz ME, et al. The prevalence and clinical features of tuberculous peritonitis in CAPD patients in Turkey, report of ten cases from multicenters. Ren Fail 2003;25:819-27.

45. Gupta N, Prakash KC. Asymptomatic tuberculous peritonitis in a CAPD patient. Perit Dial Int 2001;21:416-7.

46. Klote MM, Agodoa LY, Abbott KC. Risk factors for Mycobacterium tuberculosis in US chronic dialysis patients. Nephrol Dial Transplant 2006;21:3287-92.

47. el-Agroudy AE, Refaie AF, Moussa OM, Ghoneim MA. Tuberculosis in Egyptian kidney transplant recipients: study of clinical course and outcome. J Nephrol 2003;16:404-11.

48. Amedia C, Oettinger CW. Unusual presentation of tuberculosis in chronic haemodialysed patients. Clin Nephrol 1977;8:363-6.

49. Habesoglu MA, Torun D, Demiroglu YZ, Karatasli M, Sen N, Ermis H, et al. Value of the tuberculin skin test in screening for tuberculosis in dialysis patients. Transplant Proc 2007;39:883-6.

50. Agarwal SK, Gupta S, Tiwari SC. Tuberculin skin test for the diagnosis of latent tuberculosis infection during renal replacement therapy in an endemic area: a single center study. Indian J Nephrol 2010;20:132-6.

51. Passalent L, Khan K, Richardson R, Wang J, Dedier H, Gardam M. Detecting latent tuberculosis infection in hemodialysis patients: a head-to-head comparison of the T-SPOT.TB test, tuberculin skin test, and an expert physician panel. Clin J Am Soc Nephrol 2007;2:68-73.

52. Cinque TJ, Letteri JM. Idiopathic ascites in chronic renal failure. NY State J Med 1973;73:781-4.

53. Berger HW, Rammadan G, Neff MS, Buhain WJ. Uremic pleural effusion: a study of 14 patients on chronic dialysis. Ann Intern Med 1975;82:362-4.

54. Fairshter RD, Vazin ND, Mirahmudi MK. Lung pathology in chronic hemodialysed patients. Int J Artif Organs 1982;5:97-100.

55. Chung JH, Kim YS, Kim SI, Park K, Park MS, Kim YS, et al. The diagnostic value of the adenosine deaminase activity in the pleural fluid of renal transplant patients with tuberculous pleural effusion. Yonsei Med J 2004;45:661-4.

56. Kumar S, Agarwal R, Bal A, Sharma K, Singh N, Aggarwal AN, et al. Utility of adenosine deaminase [ADA], PCR and thoracoscopy in differentiating tuberculous and non-tuberculous pleural effusion complicating chronic kidney disease. Indian J Med Res 2015;141:308-14.

57. INDEX-TB Guidelines. Guidelines on extrapulmonary tuberculosis for India. Initiative of Central TB Division, Ministry of Health and Family Welfare, Government of India; 2016. Available at URL: http://tbcindia.nic.in/showfile.php?lid=3245. Accessed on October 10, 2016.

58. Kenny MT, Strates B. Metabolism and pharmacokinetics of the antibiotic rifampicin. Drug Metab Rev 1981;12:159-218.

59. Holdiness MR. Clinical pharmacokinetics of the antitubercular drugs. Clin Pharmacokinetics 1984;9:511-44.

60. Holdiness MR. Chromatographic analysis of antitubercular drugs in biological samples. J Chromatogr 1985;340:321-59.

61. Nahid P, Dorman SE, Alipanah N, Barry PM, Brozek JL, Cattamanchi A, et al. Official American Thoracic Society/Centers for Disease Control and Prevention/Infectious Diseases Society of America Clinical Practice Guidelines: Treatment of Drug-Susceptible Tuberculosis. Clin Infect Dis 2016;63:e147-95.

62. Ellard GA, Gammon PT. Pharmacokinetics of isoniazid metabolism in man. J Pharmacokinetics Biopharma 1976;4:83-113.

63. Ellard GA. A slow release preparation of isoniazid: pharmacological aspects. Bull Int Union Tuberc 1976;51:144-54.

64. HongKong Treatment Services and East African and British Medical Research Council. First-line chemotherapy in the treatment of bacteriological relapse of pulmonary tuberculosis following a short-course regimen. Lancet 1976;1:162-3.

65. Anonymous. Tuberculosis in patients having dialysis. BMJ 1980; 280:349.

66. Whelton A. Antibacterial chemotherapy in renal insufficiency: a review. Antibiotics Chemother 1974;81:1-48.

67. East African/British Medical Research Council. Isoniazid with thiacetazone in the treatment of pulmonary tuberculosis in east Africa. Second investigation. Tubercle 1963;44:301-33.

68. Bennett WM. Guide to drug dosage in renal failure. Clin Pharmacokinetics 1988;15:326-54.

69. Stamatakis G, Montes C, Trouvin JH, Farinotti R, Fessi H, Kenouch S, et al. Pyrazinamide and pyrazanoic acid pharmacokinetics in patients with chronic renal failure. Clin Nephrol 1988;30:230-4.

70. Fabre J, Fox HM, Dayer P, Balant L. Difference in kinetic properties of drugs: implication as to the selection of a particular drug for use in patients with renal failure with special emphasis on antibiotic and beta-adrenoreceptor blocking agents. Clin Pharmacokinetics 1980;5:441-64.

71. Anderson RJ, Gambertoglio JG, Schrier RW. Drugs used in the treatment of tuberculosis and fungal infections. In: Clinical use of drugs in renal failure. Springfield: Thomas 1976.p.90-101.

72. Ellard GA. Absorption, metabolism and excretion of pyrazinamide in man. Tubercle 1969;50:144-58.

73. East African/British Medical Research Council. A controlled comparison of four regimens of streptomycin plus pyrazinamide in the retreatment of pulmonary tuberculosis. Tubercle 1969;50: 81-114.

74. Line DH, Poole GW, Waterworth PM. Serum streptomycin levels and dizziness. Tubercle 1970;51:76-81.

75. Mitchison DA, Ellard GA. Tuberculosis in patients having dialysis. BMJ 1980;280:1533.

76. Anonymous. Tuberculosis in chronic renal failure. Lancet 1980; 1:909-10.

77. Varughese A, Brater DG, Benet LZ, Lee CC. Ethambutol kinetics in patients with impaired renal function. Am Rev Respir Dis 1986;134:84-8.

78. Fang JT, Chen YC, Chang MY. Ethambutol-induced optic neuritis in patients with end-stage renal disease on haemodialysis: two case reports and literature review. Ren Fail 2004;26:189-93

79. Matzke GR, Halstenson CE, Keane WF. Hemodialysis elimination rates and clearance of gentamicin and tobramycin. Antimicrob Agents Chemother 1984;25:128-30.

80. Malone RS, Fish DN, Spiegel DM, Childs JM, Peloquin CA. The effect of hemodialysis on cycloserine, ethionamide, para-aminosalicylate, and clofazimine. Chest 1999;116:984-90.

81. Fish DN, Chow AT. The clinical pharmacokinetics of levofloxacin. Clin Pharmacokinetics 1997;32:101-19.

82. Mittal R, Saxena S, Agarwal SK, Tiwari SC, Bhuyan UN, Dash SC. Acute interstitial nephritis following first exposure to continuous rifampicin therapy. Indian J Nephrol 1993;3:54-6.

83. Vachharajani TJ, Oza UG, Phadke AG, Kirpalani AL. Tuberculosis in renal transplant recipients: Rifampicin sparing treatment protocol. Int Urol Nephrol 2002;34:551-3.

84. Jha V, Sakhuja V. Rifampicin sparing treatment protocols in post-transplant tuberculosis. Int Urol Nephrol 2004;36:287-8.

85. Joint Statement of the American Thoracic Society [ATS], and the Centers for Disease Control and Prevention [CDC], endorsed by the Council of the Infectious Diseases Society of America. [IDSA], September 1999, and the sections of this statement. Targeted tuberculin testing and treatment of latent tuberculosis infection. Am J Respir Crit Care Med 2000;161:S221-47.

86. Sester M, Sester U, Clauer P, Heine G, Mack U, Moll T, et al. Tuberculin skin testing underestimates a high prevalence of latent tuberculosis infection in haemodialysis patients. Kidney Int 2004;65:1826-34.

87. Poduval RD, Hammes MD. Tuberculosis screening in dialysis patients—is the tuberculin test effective? Clin Nephrol 2003;59:436-40.

88. Fang HC, Chou KJ, Chen CL, Lee PT, Chiou YH, Hung SY, et al. Tuberculin skin test and anergy in dialysis patients of a tuberculosis-endemic area. Nephron 2002;91:682-7.

89. Agarwal SK, Singh UB, Zaidi SH, Gupta S, Pandey RM. Comparison of interferon gamma release assay and tuberculin skin tests for diagnosis of latent tuberculosis in patients on maintenance hemodialysis in India. Indian J Med Res 2015;141:463-8.

90. John GT, Thomas PP, Thomas M, Jeyaseelan L, Jacob CK, Shastry JC. A double-blind, randomised trial of primary isoniazid prophylaxis in dialysis and transplant patients. Transplantation 1994;57:1683-4.

91. Vikrant S, Agarwal SK, Gupta S, Bhowmik D, Tiwari SC, Dash SC, et al. Prospective randomised control trial of isoniazid chemoprophylaxis during renal replacement therapy. Trans Infect Dis 2005;7:99-108.

92. Edwards OM, Courtenary Evans RJ, Galley JM, Hunter J, Tait AD. Changes in cortisol metabolism following rifampicin therapy. Lancet 1974;2:548-51.

93. Cutler RE. Cyclosporine drug interaction. Dialysis Transpl 1988;17:139-51.

94. British Thoracic and Tuberculosis Association. Short-course chemotherapy in pulmonary tuberculosis. Lancet 1976;2: 1102-4.

95. Kuruvila KC, Colabawalla BN, Joshi SS. Problem of transplantation in India. Transpl Proc 1979;2:1296.

96. Agarwal SK, Gupta S, Dash SC, Bhowmik D, Tiwari SC. Prospective randomised trial of isoniazid prophylaxis in renal transplant recipient. Int Urol Nephrol 2004;36:425-31.

97. Rosen T. Cutaneous Mycobacterium kansasii infection presenting as cellulitis. Cutis 1983;31:87-9.

98. Fraser DW, Buxton AE, Naji A, Barker C, Rudnick M, Weinstein AJ. Disseminated Mycobacterium kansasii infections presenting with cellulitis in a recipient of a renal homograft. Am Infect Dis 1975;112:125-9.

99. Spence RK, Dafoe DC, Rabin G, Grossman RA, Naji A, Barker CF, et al. Mycobacterium infections in renal allograft recipients. Arch Surg 1983;118:356-9.

100. Cruz N, Ramirex-Muxo O, Bermudez RH, Santiago-Delpin EA. Pulmonary infection with Mycobacterium kansasii in a renal transplant patient. Nephron 1980;26:187-8.

101. Sanger JR, Stampfl D, Franson T. Recurrent granulomatous synovitis due to Mycobacterium kansasii in renal transplant patient. Am J Hand Surg 1987;12:436-41.

29

Disseminated/Miliary Tuberculosis

Surendra K Sharma, Alladi Mohan

The whole surface, in front and behind, as well as within the interstitium of the major lobes, was covered with firm small white corpuscles, of the size of millet seeds…..

John Jacob Manget

INTRODUCTION

Disseminated tuberculosis [DTB] refers to concurrent involvement of at least two non-contiguous organ sites of the body, or, involvement of the blood or bone marrow by tuberculosis [TB] process (1-3). One form of DTB, miliary tuberculosis [MTB], results from a massive haematogenous dissemination of tubercle bacilli which results in tiny discrete foci usually the size of millet seeds [1 to 2 mm] more or less uniformly distributed in the lungs and the other viscera (4-9). Miliary pattern on the chest radiograph is the hallmark of MTB.

Miliary and disseminated TB continue to be a diagnostic problem even in areas endemic to TB, where clinical suspicion is very high. Mortality from MTB disease has remained high despite effective therapy being available. In patients with human immunodeficiency virus [HIV] infection acquired immunodeficiency syndrome [AIDS] DTB and MTB are particularly common (1,3,10,11).

EPIDEMIOLOGY

The epidemiology of MTB as documented in several published studies is depicted in Table 29.1 (12-36). Miliary TB accounts for less than 2% of all cases of TB and up to 20% of all TB cases in various clinical studies in immunocompetent individuals; the corresponding figures in autopsy studies have been higher [Table 29.1]. Caution must be exercised while comparing these epidemiological data as these studies are hospital based or autopsy studies.

Table 29.1: Epidemiology of miliary TB

Study (reference)	Frequency of miliary TB	
	Overall [%]	Among TB [%]
Adults, autopsy studies (12-18)	0.3 to 13.3	11.9 to 40.5
Adults, clinical studies (19-22)	1.3 to 2.0	0.64 to 20
Children, clinical studies (23-26)	0.7 to 41.3	1.3 to 3.2
All age groups, epidemiological studies, public health data (27-36)	–	0.4 to 10.7

TB = tuberculosis
Adapted from reference 4

The emergence of the HIV/AIDS pandemic and widespread use of immunosuppressive drugs have changed the epidemiology of MTB. Since its first description by John Jacob Manget, the clinical presentation of MTB has changed dramatically. Especially its occurrence as a complication of childhood infection is diminishing and the "cryptic form" [*vide infra*] in a much older group is emerging (37-39). The modulating effect of Bacille Calmette-Guérin [BCG] vaccination resulting in substantial reduction in MTB and TB meningitis among young vaccinees, increasing use of computed tomography [CT], and wider application of invasive diagnostic methods could also have contributed to the demographic shift (4).

Age and Gender Distribution

In patients with MTB, presently two additional peaks are evident—one involving adolescents and young adults and another later in life among elderly people (4-9). Sparse published data are available on DTB. In a series from northern Taiwan (2), patients with HIV/AIDS who had DTB [n = 23] were younger [mean age 37.1 years], compared with DTB patients with [n = 64; mean age 61.4 years] and without other co-morbid conditions [n = 77; mean age 58.9 years].

Male gender seems to be more frequently affected by MTB in children as well as adults (4-9). Similarly, 119 of the 164 patients with DTB reported by Wang *et al* (2) were males. However, a few recent adult series on MTB (16,20,40,41) describe a female preponderance. This shift probably reflects increased awareness and use of health services by women. Further work is required to understand the influence of other factors, such as, socio-economic and nutritional status, co-morbid illnesses, and host genetic factors other than ethnic variations in the causation of DTB/MTB.

PATHOGENESIS

Miliary TB develops due to a massive lymphohaematogenous dissemination of *Mycobacterium tuberculosis [Mtb]* from a pulmonary or extrapulmonary focus and embolisation to the vascular beds of various organs (4) [Figure 29.1]. Less commonly, simultaneous reactivation of multiple foci in various organs can result in MTB. This reactivation can occur either at the time of primary infection or later during reactivation of a dormant focus. When MTB develops during primary disease [early generalisation], the disease has an acute onset and is rapidly progressive. Late generalisation during post-primary TB can be rapidly progressive [resulting in acute MTB], episodic, or protracted, leading to chronic MTB. Re-infection also has an important role, especially in areas where TB is highly endemic. Rarely, MTB can also develop due to caseation of an extrapulmonary site, discharge of caseous material into the portal circulation and initial hepatic involvement with the classical pulmonary involvement occurring late (4-9). The reader is referred to the chapter *"Immunology" [Chapter 5]* for details regarding the molecular mechanisms underlying the pathogenesis of DTB/MTB.

Miliary TB is a common manifestation of congenital TB in neonates. Acquisition of infection during the perinatal period through aspiration and ingestion of infected maternal genital tissues and fluid may rarely lead to the development of MTB in neonates. The reader is referred to the chapter *"Pathology" [Chapter 3]* for details regarding congenital TB.

CLINICAL PRESENTATION

Most of the patients with DTB/MTB often have non-specific predisposing/associated conditions [Table 29.2]. Their pathogenetic role is unclear.

Common presenting symptoms and signs noted at presentation in patients with DTB/MTB are listed in Tables 29.3A and 29.3B (40-56). Although DTB/MTB involves almost all organs, most often the involvement is asymptomatic. Clinical manifestations of DTB/MTB are protean and can be obscure till late in the disease. Fever and inanition are relatively common. Cough and dyspnoea are often present. Chills and rigors, usually seen in patients with malaria, or, sepsis and bacteraemia, have often been described in adult

patients with MTB (2,17-23). Organomegaly is also a frequent physical finding.

Choroidal tubercles are bilateral, pale, greyish-white and oblong patches which occur less commonly in adult patients with MTB than children (4). If present, choroidal tubercles are pathognomonic of MTB and offer a valuable clue to the diagnosis [Figures 24.3, 24.4, 24.5A, 24.5B and 24.6]. Therefore, systematic ophthalmoscopic examination after mydriatic administration must be done in every suspected patient with MTB. Skin involvement in the form of erythematous macules and papules have also been described (4-9). Signs of hepatic involvement may be evident in the form of icterus and hepatomegaly. Neurological involvement in the form of meningitis or tuberculomas is common. TB meningitis has been described in 10%-30% of adult patients with MTB (14,20,40-53) Conversely, about one-third of patients presenting with TB meningitis have underlying MTB (57). Clinically significant cardiac or renal involvement is uncommon in patients with MTB (4-9). Overt adrenal insufficiency at presentation, or during treatment has also been described in MTB (58). In some studies, headache and abdominal pain when present are supposed to have specific implications in MTB, headache signifying the presence of meningitis and abdominal pain signifying abdominal involvement (4-9).

Clinical presentation of MTB in children is similar to that observed in adults, but with important differences [Tables 29.3A and 29.3B]. In children with MTB, chills, night sweats, haemoptysis, and productive cough have been reported less frequently, while peripheral lymphadenopathy and hepatosplenomegaly are more common, compared with adults. Likewise, a higher proportion of children with MTB have TB meningitis compared with adults.

Rare Manifestations

Table 29.4 (37-53,58-79) shows various atypical manifestations in patients with MTB. Atypical presentations can delay the diagnosis and DTB/MTB is often a missed diagnosis. Patients with occult DTB/MTB can present with pyrexia of unknown origin [PUO] without any focal localising clue. Clinical presentation such as absence of fever, and progressive wasting strongly mimicking a metastatic carcinoma can occur, especially in the elderly. Proudfoot *et al* (37) suggested the term "cryptic miliary TB" for this presentation. Table 29.5 (37-39) highlights the important differences between classical and cryptic forms of MTB. The reader is referred to the chapter *"Tuberculosis and acute lung injury" [Chapter 32]* for details regarding TB and acute respiratory distress syndrome [ARDS].

Disseminated/Miliary Tuberculosis in the Immunosuppressed

The clinical presentation of TB in early HIV infection [CD4+ cell counts >500/μL] is similar to that observed in immunocompetent individuals. With progression of immunosuppression in advanced HIV infection

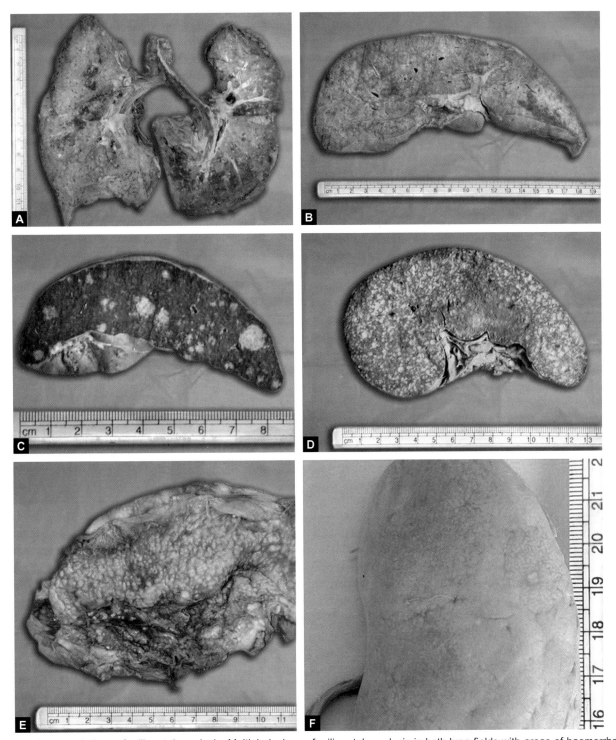

Figure 29.1: Gross pathology of miliary tuberculosis. Multiple lesions of miliary tuberculosis in both lung fields with areas of haemorrhage [A]; liver slice showing multiple confluent as well as discrete tubercles [B]; spleen showing multiple grey-white varying sized lesions [C]; cut-section of spleen showing miliary seeding [D]; omentum showing multiple tubercles, caseation is evident in larger lesions [E]; kidney with tubercles seen over the surface [F]

[CD4+ cell counts <200/μL], DTB/MTB are seen more frequently (54,80-82). Cutaneous involvement is unusual in MTB but is more commonly seen in HIV-seropositive patients with CD4+ cell counts below 100 cells/μL (83). The cutaneous lesions that have been described include

tiny papules or vesiculo-papules variously described as 'tuberculosis cutis miliaris disseminata', 'tuberculosis cutis acuta generalisita', and disseminated TB of the skin (84). Rarely, macular, pustular, or purpuric lesions, indurated ulcerating plaques, and subcutaneous abscesses have also

Table 29.2: Conditions predisposing to/associated with miliary/disseminated TB

Childhood infections
   Malnutrition
   HIV/AIDS
   Alcoholism
   Diabetes mellitus
   Chronic renal failure, dialysis
   Post-surgery [e.g., gastrectomy*]
   Organ transplantation
   Drugs

Corticosteroids

Immunosuppressive and cytotoxic drugs

Immunomodulator drugs [e.g., infliximab, etanercept]
   Connective tissue disorders
   Pregnancy, postpartum
   Underlying malignancy
   Silicosis
   Iatrogenic causes
      Ureteral catheterisation*
      Extracorporeal shockwave lithotripsy†
      Laser lithotripsy†
      Cardiac valve homograft replacement‡
      Intravesical BCG therapy for urinary bladder carcinoma

* Predisposes to TB in general
† Patient had undiagnosed genitourinary TB
‡ Contamination of homografts probably occurred at the time of harvest from cadavers
TB = tuberculosis; HIV = human immunodeficiency virus; AIDS = acquired immunodeficiency syndrome; BCG = bacille Calmette-Guerin
Adapted from reference 4

Table 29.3A: Presenting symptoms in miliary/disseminated TB

Variable	Miliary TB		Disseminated TB‡
	Adults [%]*	Children [%]†	
Fever	35-100	61-98	48
Chills	15-28	ND	ND
Anorexia	24-100	04-81	06
Weight loss	20-100	04-60	07-46
Night sweats	08-100	08-75	03
Weakness/fatigue	25-100	14-54	10-75
Cough/sputum	27-82	17-90	23-33
Chest pain	03-49	01-03	ND
Dyspnoea	08-100	07-25	11-17
Haemoptysis	03-15	01	ND
Headache	02-18	02-08	02
Altered sensorium	05-26	02-08	09
Seizures	ND	07-30	ND
Nausea	01-19	ND	ND
Abdominal pain	05-19	03-15	06
Diarrhoea	02-03	ND	ND
Urinary symptoms	02-06	ND	04

All values are expressed as percentages corrected to the nearest round figures
* Data from references 13,20,40-54
† Data from references 21,23,26,55,56
‡ Data from Wang *et al* (reference 2). In this series, 23 of the 164 patients were human immunodeficiency virus seropositive
TB = tuberculosis; ND= not described

been reported (84). In HIV/AIDS patients with DTB/MTB, intrathoracic lymphadenopathy and tuberculin anergy are more common; sputum smears are seldom positive and blood culture may grow *Mycobacterium tuberculosis,* especially in patients with profound immunosuppression (1,2,4-9,54).

Immune reconstitution inflammatory syndrome [IRIS] has been implicated as the cause of paradoxical worsening of lesions in patients with TB. Consequently, HIV-seropositive patients with MTB may develop acute renal failure (85) or ARDS (86). The reader is referred to the chapter *"Tuberculosis and human immunodeficiency virus infection" [Chapter 35]* for further details on this topic.

LABORATORY FINDINGS

Haematology and Serum Biochemistry

A number of haematological and biochemical abnormalities are known to occur in DTB/MTB but their significance is controversial [Table 29.6]. Anaemia of chronic disease, leucocytosis, leucopenia, leukaemoid reactions, thrombocytopenia and disseminated intravascular coagulation [DIC], haemophagocytic lymphohistiocytosis are all known to occur. Erythrocyte sedimentation rate is usually elevated in patients with DTB/MTB (4-9). The reader is referred to the chapter *"Haematological manifestations of tuberculosis" [Chapter 33]* for further details on this subject.

Table 29.3B: Presenting signs in miliary/disseminated TB

Variable	Miliary TB		Disseminated TB‡
	Adults [%]*	Children [%]†	
Fever	35-100	39-75	48
Pallor	36-59	31	ND
Cyanosis	01-02	ND	06
Icterus	05-09	03	07-46
Lymphadenopathy	02-30	05	03
Chest signs	29-84	34-72	10-75
Hepatomegaly	14-62	39-82	23-33
Splenomegaly	02-32	24-54	ND
Ascites	04-38	06-09	11-17
Choroidal tubercles	02-12	02-05	ND
Neurological signs	03-26	19-35	02

All values are expressed as percentages corrected to the nearest round figures
* Data from references 13,20,40-54
† Data from references 21,23,26,55,56
‡ Data from Wang *et al* (reference 2). In this series, 23 of the 164 patients were human immunodeficiency virus seropositive
TB = tuberculosis; ND = not described

Table 29.4: Atypical clinical manifestations in MTB

Cryptic miliary TB

Pyrexia of unknown origin [PUO]

Acute respiratory distress syndrome [ARDS]

"Airleak" syndrome [pneumothorax, pneumomediastinum]

Myelophthisic anaemia, myelofibrosis, pancytopenia, immune haemolytic anaemia

Acute empyema

Septic shock, multiple organ dysfunction syndrome

Thyrotoxicosis

Renal failure due to granulomatous destruction of the interstitium

Immune complex glomerulonephritis

Sudden cardiac death

Mycotic aneurysm of aorta

Massive haematemesis

Native valve and prosthetic valve endocarditis

Myocarditis, congestive heart failure, intracardiac masses

Cholestatic jaundice

Presentation as focal extrapulmonary TB

Metastatic abscess

Incidental diagnosis

Syndrome of inappropriate antidiuretic hormone secretion [SIADH]

Deep vein thrombosis

Haemophagocytic lymphohistiocytosis

Hypercalcaemia

TB = tuberculosis
Data from references 37-53,58-79

Table 29.5: Comparison of classical and cryptic miliary TB

Variable	Classical miliary TB	Cryptic miliary TB
Age at diagnosis	Majority < 40 years	Majority > 60 years
Fever	Present in >90%	Usually absent
Weight loss	Present in 60%-80%	Dominant clinical feature
Meningitis	Seen in 20%-30% adults 30%-40% children	Rare unless terminal
Lymphadenopathy	Present in 20%	Rarely present
Chest radiograph	Classical miliary pattern common	Normal
HRCT scan of the chest	Required only when classical miliary pattern is not evident	Required for diagnosis
Tuberculin skin test	Positive in 60%	Rarely positive
Confirmation of diagnosis	Invasive procedures	Usually made at autopsy

TB = tuberculosis; HRCT = high resolution computed tomography
Data from references 37-39

Table 29.6: Laboratory abnormalities in miliary/disseminated TB

Haematological
  Anaemia
  Leucocytosis
  Neutrophilia
  Lymphocytosis
  Monocytosis
  Thrombocytosis
  Leucopenia
  Lymphopenia
  Thrombocytopenia

Leukaemoid reaction
  Elevated ESR, CRP levels

Biochemical
  Hyponatraemia
  Hypoalbuminaemia
  Hyperbilirubinaemia
  Elevated transaminases
  Elevated serum alkaline phosphatase
  Hypercalcaemia

TB = tuberculosis; ESR = erythrocyte sedimentation rate; CRP = C-reactive protein

Hyponatraemia in MTB was first described in 1938 by Winkler and Crankshaw (87). Shalhoub and Antoniou (88) postulated an acquired disturbance of neurohypophyseal function resulting in unregulated antidiuretic hormone [ADH] release as the underlying mechanism. Vorherr *et al* (89) demonstrated an antidiuretic principle in the lung tissue affected by TB and suggested that it may either produce ADH or absorb an inappropriately released hormone from the posterior pituitary. Some have attributed hyponatraemia to meningeal involvement (43). Presence of hyponatraemia in patients with MTB is thought be of prognostic significance [*vide infra*]. Hypercalcaemia has been documented in MTB but is uncommon (4-9).

Tuberculin Skin Test

Majority of patients with DTB/MTB are tuberculin skin test [TST] positive. In various paediatric series (21,23,26,55,56) [Table 29.7] negative TST results were observed in 35%-74% of patients. In adult series (42-47,49-51,90) [Table 29.7] TST negativity was reported in 20%-70% of patients.

Interferon-gamma Release Assays

The reader is referred to the chapter *"Laboratory diagnosis"* [Chapter 8] for further details on this topic.

Imaging

Chest Radiograph

The radiographic hallmark of MTB is the miliary pattern on chest radiograph [Figure 9.7]. The term miliary refers to the "millet seed" size of the nodules [< 2 mm] seen on classical

Table 29.7: Results of TST in miliary TB*			
Study (reference)	No. studied	No. tested	Negative TST [%]
Paediatric series			
Kim et al (23)	84	84	51
Aderele (55)	44	26	35
Rahajoe (56)	80	80	54
Hussey et al (21)	94	94	62
Gurkan et al (26)	23	23	74
Adult series			
Biehl (42)	68	26	39
Munt (43)	69	57	48
Campbell (44)	48	30	20
Gelb et al (45)	109	72	44
Grieco and Chmel (46)	28	21	52
Onadeko et al (47)	41	23	65
Prout and Benatar (49)	62	21	62
Kim et al (50)	38	38	68
Maartens et al (51)	109	47	57
Mert (40)	38	38	62
Sharma and Mohan (90)	134	107	70

* Varying strengths and methods were employed for TST in different studies

TB = tuberculosis; TST = tuberculin skin test

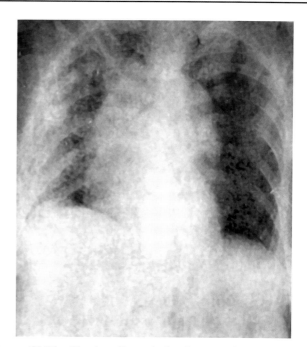

Figure 29.2A: Chest radiograph [postero-anterior view] showing confluent shadows instead of miliary mottling in a patient with miliary tuberculosis
Reproduced with permission from "Sharma SK, Mohan A, Prasad KL, Pande JN, Gupta AK, Khilnani GC. Clinical profile, laboratory characteristics and outcome in miliary tuberculosis. QJM 1995;88: 29-37 (reference 52)"

chest radiographs (4). Some patients with MTB, however, may have normal chest radiographs when they seek medical care and some have patterns that are indistinguishable from interstitial pneumonia (4,52). Some of the patients may manifest coalescent opacities [Figures 29.2A, 29.2B, 29.3, 29.4]. When patients with MTB develop ARDS, the chest radiograph may be identical to that seen in ARDS due to other causes (4,59). Majority of the patients [88%] in the study reported by Sharma *et al* (52) had chest radiographs consistent with MTB and in some, these classical radiological changes evolved over the course of the disease. The diagnosis of MTB is easier when patient presents with classical miliary shadowing on chest radiograph in an appropriate setting. However, the diagnosis may be difficult in those situations where chest radiograph does not show classical miliary shadows. This fact is highlighted by 12 patients in the series reported by Sharma *et al* (52) who had atypical chest radiographs and the case of a patient with fever of unknown origin who presented with a very subtle suggestion of miliary mottling on the chest radiograph. This chest radiograph was passed off as normal in a busy outpatient department [Figure 29.5]. High resolution computed tomography [HRCT] [*vide infra*] suggested a miliary pattern [Figure 29.6] and excision biopsy of the supraclavicular lymph node which developed over the course of the disease confirmed the diagnosis in this patient [Figure 29.7]. This re-emphasises the fact that though the clinical and laboratory parameters are indicative of the disease, these are not sensitive enough to allow an accurate provisional diagnosis. Thus, if there is a high index of suspicion of the diagnosis of MTB and the chest radiograph is atypical, it is suggested that HRCT be done to support the diagnosis.

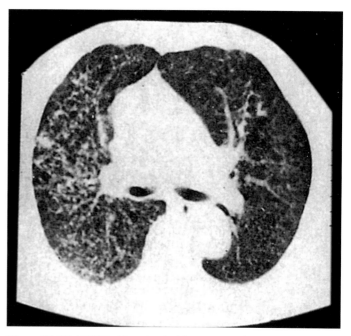

Figure 29.2B: HRCT of the chest of the same patient in Figure 29.2A, showing miliary pattern
Reproduced with permission from "Sharma SK, Mohan A, Prasad KL, Pande JN, Gupta AK, Khilnani GC. Clinical profile, laboratory characteristics and outcome in miliary tuberculosis. QJM 1995;88: 29-37 (reference 52)"
HRCT = high resolution computed tomography

Ultrasonography

In patients with DTB/MTB, ultrasonography is useful in the detection of associated lesions, such as, loculated ascites, focal hepatic and splenic lesions, adnexal masses [in women] and cold abscess. Diagnostic thoracic or abdominal paracentesis under ultrasound guidance is useful to procure fluid for diagnostic testing, especially when it is loculated. Recently, B-lines, comet-tail artifacts disseminated throughout multiple lung areas and a pattern of sub-pleural granularity have been described on ultrasonography of the chest in patients with MTB (91).

Computed Tomography and Magnetic Resonance Imaging

High-resolution computed tomography has considerably improved the ante-mortem diagnosis of DTB/MTB. The interlobular septal thickening or intralobular fine network that is evident on HRCT in MTB seems to be caused by the presence of tubercles in the interlobular septa and alveolar walls. Centrilobular nodules and branching linear structures producing a tree-in-bud appearance—a pattern seen in active post-primary pulmonary TB—may sometimes be evident in MTB. Contrast-enhanced computed tomography [CECT] is better for detecting intrathoracic lymphadenopathy, calcification, and pleural lesions (3,4).

Magnetic resonance imaging [MRI] and CECT are also useful in demonstrating miliary lesions at occult extra-pulmonary sites, an exercise that was earlier possible only at post-mortem examination. Abdominal CECT is useful in identifying lesions in the liver and spleen, intra-abdominal lymphadenopathy, and cold abscesses (3,4,92). Miliary lesions in the liver and spleen may appear as confluent or discrete hypodense lesions, sometimes with peripheral rim enhancement on the CECT scan of the abdomen (3,4,92).

Positron Emission Tomography

Recently, positron emission tomography-CT [PET-CT] and PET-MRI have been used to assess the disease activity in patients with TB (93,94). PET-CT and PET-MRI are useful in defining the disease extent in patients with DTB/MTB. The utility of these investigations in assessing the activity of lesions [Figures 29.8, 29.9] that might persist following anti-TB treatment in DTB/MTB needs to be studied further.

Ultrasonography, CECT, and MRI may help in identifying adnexal masses, ascites in women, and epididymitis and seminal vesicle lesions in men with genital tract involvement. The CECT or MRI of the brain and spine are useful in the evaluation of patients with concomitant TB meningitis or spinal TB. Interventional radiological procedures such as fine needle aspiration for cytological examination and biopsy under CT or MRI guidance are useful for procuring tissue/fluid for confirmation of diagnosis.

Imaging findings which are commonly encountered in patients with DTB are shown in [Figures 29.10. 29.11A, 29.11B, 29.12A, 29.12B, 29.13A, 29.13B, 29.14 and 29.15].

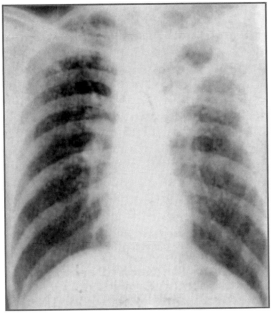

Figure 29.3: Chest radiograph [postero-anterior view] showing miliary mottling and a cavity in the left upper lobe

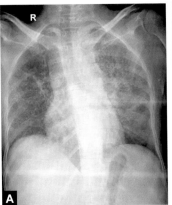
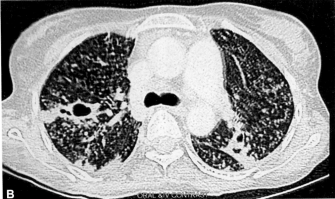
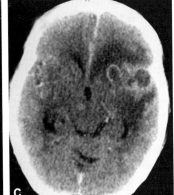

Figure 29.4: Chest radiograph [postero-anterior view] showing miliary mottling [A]. HRCT chest of the same patient showing miliary mottling and bilateral cavitary lesions [B]. CECT head of the same patient showing intracranial tuberculomas [C]
HRCT = high resolution computed tomography; CECT = contrast-enhanced computed tomography

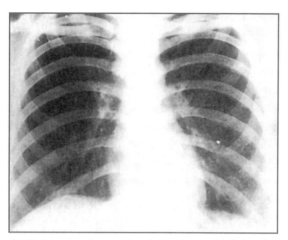

Figure 29.5: Chest radiograph [postero-anterior view] showing subtle miliary shadows
Reproduced with permission from "Sharma SK, Mohan A, Prasad KL, Pande JN, Gupta AK, Khilnani GC. Clinical profile, laboratory characteristics and outcome in miliary tuberculosis. QJM 1995;88: 29-37 (reference 52)"

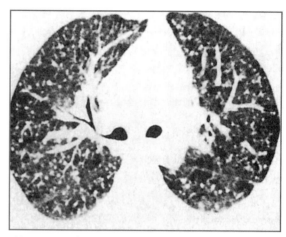

Figure 29.6: CT of the chest of the same patient in Figure 29.5 showing extensive miliary shadows
Reproduced with permission from "Sharma SK, Mohan A, Prasad KL, Pande JN, Gupta AK, Khilnani GC. Clinical profile, laboratory characteristics and outcome in miliary tuberculosis. QJM 1995;88: 29-37 (reference 52)"

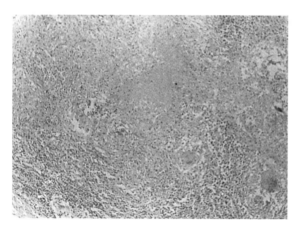

Figure 29.7: Lymph node biopsy showing confluent, caseating epithelioid cell granulomas with giant cells suggestive of tuberculosis [Haematoxylin and eosin × 80]
Reproduced with permission from "Sharma SK, Mohan A, Prasad KL, Pande JN, Gupta AK, Khilnani GC. Clinical profile, laboratory characteristics and outcome in miliary tuberculosis. QJM 1995;88:29-37 (reference 52)"

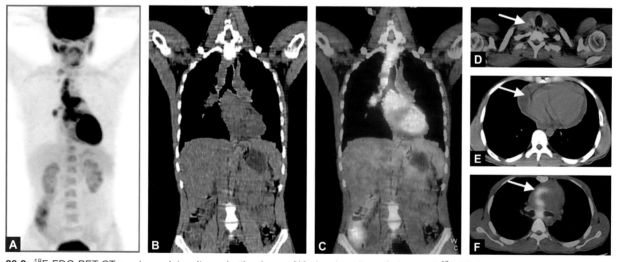

Figure 29.8: ^{18}F FDG PET-CT maximum intensity projection image [A] showing sites of abnormal ^{18}F FDG accumulation in the mediastinum. Coronal NCCT reveals multiple paratracheal, subcarinal and right hilar lymph nodes [B] which show FDG accumulation on fused coronal PET-CT [C]. Transaxial fused PET-CT showing tracer accumulation in right supraclavicular node [arrow] [D], transaxial NCCT showing pericardial effusion [arrow] [E] and transaxial fused PET-CT reveals tracer uptake in the pericardial attachment [arrow] [F]
FDG PET-CT = fluorodeoxyglucose positron emission tomography-computed tomography; NCCT = non-contrast computed tomography

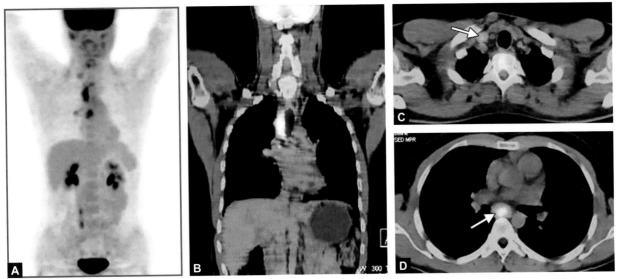

Figure 29.9: [18]F FDG PET-CT of the same patient shown in Figure 29.8, obtained at 4 months of anti-TB treatment, maximum intensity projection image showing sites of abnormal ^{18}F FDG accumulation in the mediastinum [A]. Fused coronal PET-CT reveals paratracheal and right hilar lymph nodes which show FDG accumulation [B]. Transaxial fused PET-CT showing tracer accumulation in right supraclavicular node [arrow] [C] and subcarinal node [arrow] [D]

FDG PET-CT = fluorodeoxyglucose positron emission tomography-computed tomography; TB = tuberculosis; FDG = fluorodeoxyglucose

Sharma *et al* (95) assessed the CT appearances of MTB and the CT findings were correlated with pulmonary functions and gas exchange. The effect of anti-TB treatment on various observed findings was also studied. It was found that HRCT was superior to the conventional CT in defining the parenchymal details. A significant positive correlation was observed between the visual chest radiograph and CT scores (95). Further, CT scan of the chest also revealed lymph node enlargement, calcification and pleural lesions in more patients than plain films. Curiously, Sharma *et al* (95) also described air trapping on CT scan both at presentation and during follow-up period and attributed this to TB bronchiolitis. The clinical significance of these findings is unclear at present.

Pipavath *et al* (96), in a recent report [n = 16] documented the following changes on HRCT in patients with MTB: miliary pattern [n = 16]; intrathoracic lymphadenopathy [n = 8]; alveolar lesions such as ground-glass attenuation and/or consolidation [n = 5]; pleural and pericardial effusions [2 patients each]; and peribronchovascular interstitial thickening and emphysema [one patient each].

Pulmonary Functions, Gas Exchange Abnormalities

Miliary TB is associated with abnormalities of pulmonary functions typical of diffuse interstitial disease of the lungs (4). The impairment of diffusion has been the most frequent and severe abnormality encountered (4). Sharma *et al* (97) studied the pulmonary functions [n = 31] and gas exchange abnormalities on arterial blood gas analysis [n = 13] in patients with MTB. They found a mild restrictive ventilatory defect, impairment of diffusing capacity and hypoxaemia

due to widening of alveolar-arterial oxygen gradient. A mild reduction in the flow rates suggestive of peripheral airways involvement was also observed.

With anti-TB treatment, mean arterial oxygen tension [PaO_2] showed a significant increase from the pre-treatment value. The mean post-treatment values of forced vital capacity [FVC], forced expiratory volume in the first second [FEV_1], peak expiratory flow rate [PEFR], maximal mid expiratory flow rate FEF_{25-75}, [V_{50}] and V_{25} did not show a significant increase at the end of treatment (88). The functional residual capacity [FRC] and residual volume [RV]/total lung capacity [TLC] [%] also did not decrease significantly at the end of treatment. Anti-TB treatment resulted in improvement in gas exchange.

Pipavath *et al* (96), assessed the correlation between the disease extent score as evaluated by a visual scoring system and the pulmonary functions in 16 patients with MTB. They observed a significant correlation between the disease extent score and the FVC, FEV_1, TLC, arterial oxygen saturation [SaO_2], and diffusion capacity of the lung for carbon monoxide [DLCO].

Cardiopulmonary Exercise Testing

Patients with MTB have abnormal cardiopulmonary exercise performance with lower maximum oxygen consumption, maximal work rate, anaerobic threshold, peak minute ventilation, breathing reserve, and low maximal heart rate (98,99). Other abnormalities include higher respiratory frequency, peak minute ventilation at submaximal work, and high physiological dead space/tidal volume ratio. Some of these patients manifest a demonstrable fall in oxygen saturation [to 4% or more] with exercise. Following successful

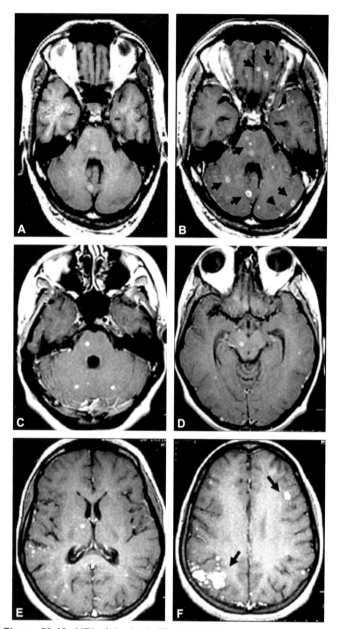

Figure 29.10: MRI of the brain [T1-weighted image, axial view] in a patient with miliary tuberculosis showing multiple hyperintense disk-like lesions [tubercles] [A] that are enhanced after the administration of contrast medium [arrows] [B]. Contrast enhanced MRI of the brain [T1-weighted image, axial section] showing multiple hyperintense enhancing disk-like lesions of varying sizes scattered within the brain [C,D, and E]. Some of them have coalesced to produce a hyperintense enhancing irregularly shaped lesions [arrows] [F]
MRI = magnetic resonance imaging

treatment, most patients reveal reversal of abnormalities. However, some of these abnormalities may persist following treatment (98,99).

Immunologic Abnormalities and Bronchoalveolar Lavage

Sharma *et al* (97) reported that patients with MTB had a significantly higher total cell count and increased proportion

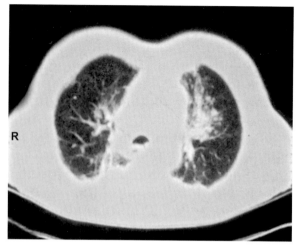

Figure 29.11A: CECT of the chest of a patient with disseminated TB showing bilateral parenchymal lesions
TB = tuberculosis; CECT = contrast-enhanced computed tomography

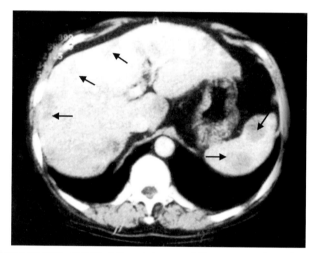

Figure 29.11B: CECT of the abdomen of the same patient showing multiple, low attenuation lesions in the liver and spleen [arrows]
CECT = contrast-enhanced computed tomography

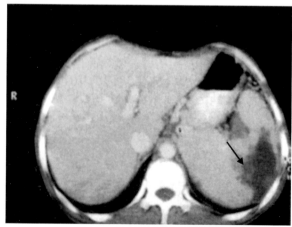

Figure 29.12A: CECT of the abdomen of a patient with disseminated tuberculosis showing a large, low attenuation lesion in the spleen [arrow]
CECT = contrast-enhanced computed tomography

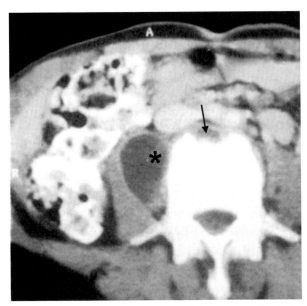

Figure 29.12B: CECT of the abdomen of the same patient showing psoas abscess [asterisk] on the right side. Erosion of the vertebral body [arrow] can also be seen
CECT = contrast-enhanced computed tomography

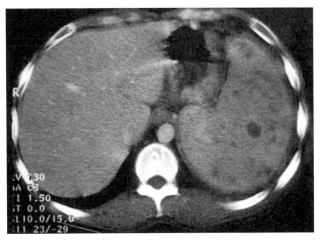

Figure 29.13A: CECT of the abdomen of a patient with disseminated tuberculosis showing multiple, low attenuation lesions in the spleen
CECT = contrast-enhanced computed tomography

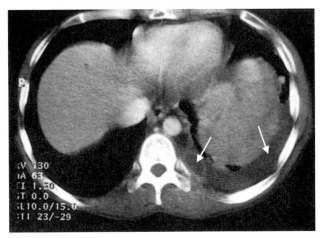

Figure 29.13B: CECT of the abdomen of the same patient showing ascites with loculations [arrows]
CECT = contrast-enhanced computed tomography

of lymphocytes, CD3+, and CD4+ T-lymphocytes in the bronchoalveolar lavage [BAL] fluid. BAL in patients with MTB showed lymphocytic alveolitis (97,100). The finding of increased helper lymphocytes in the BAL fluid and their depletion in the peripheral blood suggested compartmentalisation of lymphocytes at the site of inflammation. With anti-TB treatment, total cell count in BAL fluid decreased but continued to be higher than that in normal control subjects. The proportion of lymphocytes did not change significantly.

Sharma *et al* (97) also observed that the immunoglobulins [Ig] G, IgA, IgM were increased in the peripheral blood and BAL fluid in 18 patients suggesting polyclonal hypergammaglobulinaemia. With anti-TB treatment, serum immunoglobulins, IgG and IgA showed an insignificant increase. The decrease in serum IgM value was not statistically significant. The mean BAL fluid IgG, IgA values showed a decline following anti-TB treatment, but the difference did not attain statistical significance. Although BAL fluid IgM did not show a significant fall with anti-TB treatment, the mean post-treatment value in MTB patients was quite close to the mean in normal control subjects. Sharma *et al* (97) postulated that elevation of IgM occurred in the acute and active phase of the infection only, whereas, IgG and IgA continued to be raised even after apparent cure of infection. These increased levels were thought to be due to persistent mycobacterial antigenic stimulus. Increased BAL fluid fibronectin (97,101) and serum complement [C3] (97) have also been described in patients with MTB. The increase in serum C3 has been thought to be the result of "acute phase response" to ongoing inflammation and elevated BAL fluid fibronectin compared with peripheral blood suggested local synthesis in the lung.

DIAGNOSIS

Even in an endemic area, the diagnosis of DTB/MTB can be difficult as the clinical symptoms have been non-specific, the chest radiographs do not always reveal the classical miliary changes and atypical presentations such as ARDS, and shadows larger than miliary on chest radiograph commonly occur. In patients with suspected DTB/MTB, attempts must be made to ascertain histopathological/microbiological diagnosis. Sputum, pleural fluid, cerebrospinal fluid, urine, bronchoscopic secretions, blood and histopathological examination of tissue biopsy specimens have all been employed to confirm the diagnosis of DTB/MTB with varying results [Tables 29.8A, 29.8B and 29.8C] (42,49-53,102).

Molecular Methods

In patients with DTB/MTB, the usefulness of molecular methods like cartridge-based nucleic acid amplification tests [CBNAAT] [e.g., Xpert MTB/RIF, line probe assay] in the

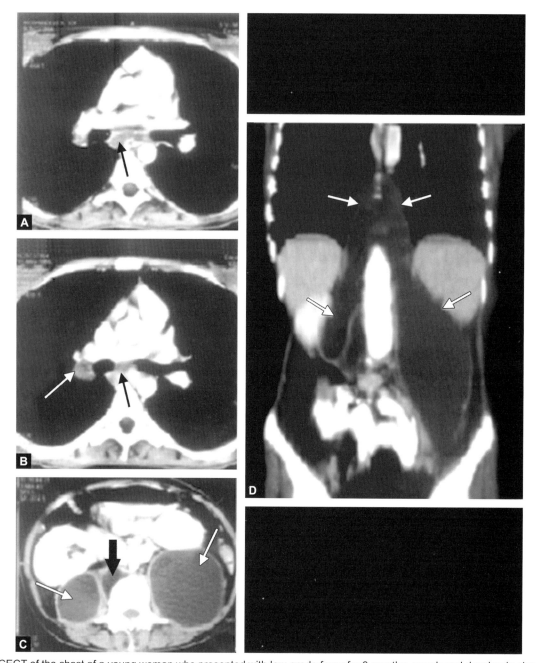

Figure 29.14: CECT of the chest of a young woman who presented with low-grade fever for 3 months, cough and dysphagia showing subcarinal [A] and right hilar [B] lymph nodes. Arrows point to hypodensities which indicate necrosis in the lymph nodes. CECT of the abdomen of the same patient showing bilateral psoas abscesses [C] [arrows]. Coronal reconstruction of the CECT of the abdomen of the same patient showing bilateral psoas abscesses [D] [arrows]. CT guided fine needle aspirate from the psoas abscess revealed numerous acid-fast bacilli
CECT = contrast-enhanced computed tomography; CT = computed tomography
Reproduced with permission from "Sharma SK, Mohan A. Extrapulmonary tuberculosis. Indian J Med Res 2004;120:316-53 (reference 3)"

field setting needs to be established. Although a positive molecular diagnostic method can support the diagnosis in the appropriate clinical setting, a negative test cannot rule out DTB/MTB and treatment should not be withheld just because of negative test[s] (3,103a).

In geographical areas where the prevalence of TB is high, when a patient presents with a compatible clinical picture and a chest radiograph suggestive of classical miliary

pattern, it is a common practice to start the anti-TB treatment straight-away keeping in mind the potential lethality of the condition. Measures to confirm the diagnosis are initiated simultaneously.

Sharma *et al* (52) suggest the following criteria for the diagnosis of MTB: [i] clinical presentation consistent with a diagnosis of TB such as, pyrexia with evening rise of temperature, weight loss, anorexia, tachycardia and night

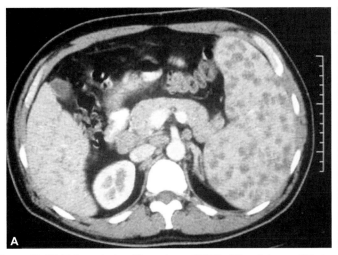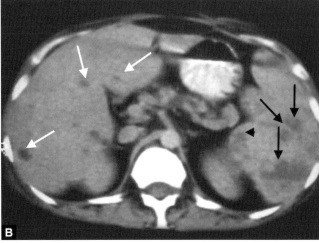

Figure 29.15: Tuberculosis of the spleen. CECT of the abdomen [A] showing multiple hypodense lesions in the spleen. CECT of the abdomen [B] showing multiple hypodense lesions in the spleen [black arrows] and liver [white arrows]

sweats of greater than six weeks duration responding to anti-tuberculosis treatment; [ii] classical miliary pattern on chest radiograph; [iii] bilateral diffuse reticulonodular lung lesions on a background of miliary shadows demonstrable either on plain radiograph or HRCT; and [iv] microbiological or histopathological evidence of TB.

The following criteria (1) have been suggested for the diagnosis of DTB: [i] clinical features suggestive of TB; [ii] concurrent involvement of at least two non-contiguous organ sites; or demonstration of *Mtb* in the blood, or, bone marrow; [iii] microbiological and/or histopathological evidence of TB; [iv] marked improvement on anti-TB therapy.

Differential Diagnosis

Many conditions that can present with a miliary pattern on the chest radiograph [Figure 29.16] are shown in Table 29.9.

TREATMENT

Untreated, DTB/MTB is uniformly fatal within one year (1,5,103,104,105a,105b). Delay in confirmation of the diagnosis often leads to delay in the institution of specific anti-TB treatment and significantly contributes to the mortality. A high clinical suspicion and efforts towards confirming the diagnosis by demonstrating *Mtb* early in the disease are imperative.

There is no consensus regarding the optimum duration of treatment in patients with DTB/MTB [Table 29.10] (105-108). According to the World Health Organization [WHO] guidelines (105a) patients with MTB receive six months of standard anti-TB treatment. The WHO guidelines (105a) mention that some experts recommend 9-12 months of treatment for TB meningitis and indicate 9 months of treatment when bone and joint TB is also present. The recently published American Thoracic Society [ATS], the Centers for Disease Control and Prevention [CDC],

Table 29.8A: Body fluids and tissues commonly tested for diagnostic confirmation in miliary/disseminated TB

Fluids
  Sputum {spontaneously expectorated, induced with hypertonic [3% or 5% saline]}

Bronchoscopic specimens
  Aspirate
  Washings
  Brush smear
  Bronchoalveolar lavage [BAL] fluid
  Transbronchial lung biopsy [TBLB]

Cerebrospinal fluid

Pleural fluid

Pericardial fluid

Peritoneal fluid

Gastric lavage*
  Pus from cold abscess

Tissues
  Lymph node
  Peripheral†
  Intrathoracic‡§
  Intra-abdominal‡||
  Peritoneum, omentum||
  Liver
  Bone marrow/bone
  Skin lesions
  Lung§
  Operative specimens

Peripheral blood¶

* Often used in children
† FNAC/excision biopsy
‡ Radiologically guided FNAC/biopsy
§ Mediastinoscopic/video-assisted thoracoscopic surgery, biopsy
|| Laparoscopic biopsy
¶ Useful in advanced HIV infection
TB = tuberculosis; FNAC = fine needle aspiration cytology;
HIV = human immunodeficiency virus

Table 29.8B: Confirmation of diagnosis by conventional methods in adults with MTB*

Variable	Biehl (42)	Prout and Benatar (49)	Kim et al (50)	Willcox et al (102)	Maartens et al (51)	Sharma et al (52)	Al-Jahdali et al (53)	Cumulative yield [%]
Sputum†	13/26	31/39	25/33	ND	29/75	10/88	6/22	41.4
Bronchoscopy‡†	ND	3/3	12/19	34/41	38/95	2/37	7/10	46.8
Gastric lavage†	20/35	ND	6/8	ND	7/11	ND	ND	61.1
CSF†	15/45	1/31	0/26	ND	14/44	ND	ND	21.2
Urine†	7/29	3/17	18/27	ND	5/28	ND	ND	32.7
Bone marrow§†	ND	20/21	9/22	ND	18/22	3/11	8/11	66.7
Liver biopsy	ND	12/13	11/12	ND	11/11	6/9	ND	88.9
Lymph node biopsy	3/3	ND	ND	ND	9/9	16/19	2/2	90.9

* Data are shown as number positive/number tested. Criteria for subjecting the patients to these tests not clearly defined in any of the studies. Often, more than one test has been performed for confirming the diagnosis. For histopathological diagnosis, presence of granulomas, caseation and demonstration of acid-fast bacilli have been variously used to define a positive test
† Yield from smear and culture
‡ Includes yield from bronchoscopic aspirate, washings, brushings, bronchoalveolar lavage and transbronchial lung biopsy
§ Yield from aspiration and/or trephine biopsy
MTB = miliary tuberculosis; CSF = cerebrospinal fluid; ND = not described

Table 29.8C: Characteristic body fluid findings in DTB/MTB

Variable	Pleural fluid	Ascitic fluid	Pericardial fluid	Cerebrospinal fluid
Appearance	Straw coloured	Straw coloured	Straw coloured or serosanguineous	Clear early; Turbid with chronicity cob web formation
Cell count				
Total count [/mm^3]	1000-5000	150-4000	Not well described. Leucocyte count is usually increased	100-500 Rarely >1000
Differential count	50% - 90% lymphocytes, eosinophils <5%	Predominantly lymphocytes	PMN preponderant early. Later mononuclear cells predominate	PMN preponderant early. Later, up to 95% mononuclear cells
Protein	Usually high [>2.5g/dL]	Usually high [>2.5 g/dL] Serum-ascitic fluid albumin gradient [SAAG] <1.1	Usually high	Usually high [100-500 mg/dL] Can be very high with blockage or chronicity
Glucose	Usually less than simultaneously collected peripheral blood value	Low	Low	Usually 40-50 mg/dL [about 50% of blood glucose]
Smear microscopy	< 10%	<3%	<1%	5%-37%
Mycobacterial culture	12%-70%	<20%	25%-60%	40%-80%

DTB = disseminated tuberculosis; MTB = miliary tuberculosis; PMN = polymorphonuclear leucocytes
Adapted from reference 38

the Infectious Disease Society of America [IDSA] (106) guidelines state that six months of treatment is adequate in MTB. These guidelines (108) also suggest that, when associated TB meningitis is also present, treatment needs to be given for at least 12 months [2-month intensive phase with isoniazid, rifampicin, pyrazinamide, and ethambutol, followed by a 7-10 month continuation phase with isoniazid and rifampicin] [Table 29.10]. In the absence of associated meningeal involvement, the 2015 Report of the Committee on Infectious Diseases, American Academy of Pediatrics [AAP] (107) advocates the use of the standard six-month treatment regimen for DTB/MTB as for pulmonary TB. When TB meningitis is present, the AAP Committee on Infectious Diseases (107) recommends an initial intensive phase with isoniazid, rifampicin, pyrazinamide and ethionamide or an aminoglycoside [in place of ethambutol] for 2 months, followed by 7-10 months of isoniazid and rifampicin. The National Institute for Health and Clinical Excellence [NICE] (108) guidelines from UK recommend 6 months of treatment for MTB.

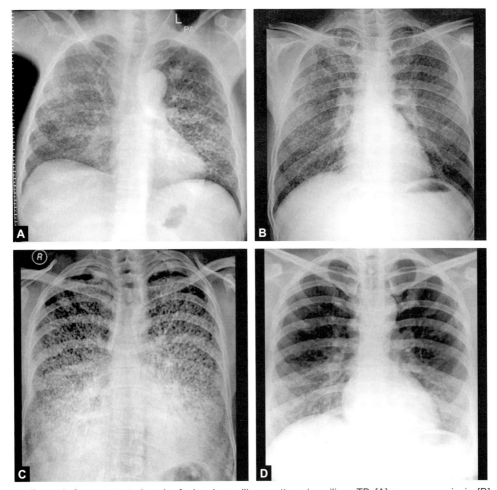

Figure 29.16: Chest radiograph [postero-anterior view] showing miliary pattern in miliary TB [A], pneumoconiosis [B], pulmonary alveolar microlithiasis [C], and sarcoidosis [D]

TB = tuberculosis

When TB meningitis is present, the evidence-based INDEX TB guidelines (109) advocate treatment for at least 9 months. The evidence-based INDEX TB guidelines (109) also suggest that when spinal TB and other forms of bone and joint TB are present, a total treatment duration of 12 months [extendable to 18 months on a case-by-case basis] is indicated.

There are no published data from randomised controlled trials assessing the efficacy of the standard WHO treatment regimens (105a) that are widely used in national TB control programmes worldwide. Furthermore, there are sparse data regarding the efficacy of standard treatment regimens in the treatment of DTB/MTB in HIV co-infected patients.

Under the Revised National Tuberculosis Control Programme [RNTCP] of Government of India, patients with DTB/MTB get treated with the DOTS. Though this duration of treatment is adequate in a majority of the patients, each patient needs to be assessed individually, and wherever indicated, treatment duration may have to be extended.

The reader is referred to the chapter *"Treatment of tuberculosis" [Chapter 44]*, for further details regarding treatment of DTB/MTB.

Corticosteroids

Sparse published data are available regarding the usefulness of adjunct corticosteroid treatment in patients with MTB with conflicting results. A beneficial response was observed in some studies (110) although such benefit could not be documented in others (111). Presence of associated adrenal insufficiency is an absolute indication for their administration. Adjunctive corticosteroid treatment may be beneficial in MTB with adrenal insufficiency, TB meningitis, large pericardial effusion, dyspnoea and/or disabling chest pain, IRIS, ARDS, immune complex nephritis, and histiocytic phagocytosis syndrome (4,103,104).

Anti-retroviral Drugs

The reader is referred to the chapter *"Tuberculosis and human immunodeficiency virus infection" [Chapter 35]* for details regarding this topic.

COMPLICATIONS

Complications are often self-limited and improve with antituberculosis treatment alone. However, at times these

Table 29.9: Common causes of fever with a miliary pattern on chest radiograph

Infections
  Mycobacteria
  Tuberculosis
  Fungal infections
    Histoplasmosis
  Blastomycosis
  Coccidioidomycosis
  Cryptococcosis
  Bacteria
  Legionellosis
  Staphylococcus aureus bacteraemia
  Mycoplasma pneumonia
  Nocardiosis
  Melioidosis
  Tularaemia
  Psittacosis
  Brucellosis
  Parasites
  Toxoplasmosis
  Strongyloides stercoralis hyperinfection
  Schistosomiasis

Immunoinflammatory disorders
  Sarcoidosis

Pneumoconiosis

Malignant
  Bronchoalveolar carcinoma
  Carcinoma lung with lymphangitis carcinomatosa
  Bronchial carcinoid
  Metastatic carcinoma
  Lymphoproliferative disorders
  Lymphoma
  Lymphomatoid granulomatosis

can be life-threatening, necessitating prompt recognition and treatment. Important complications in patients with MTB include airleak syndromes [e.g., pneumothorax, pneumopericardium], ARDS, anti-TB drug induced hepatotoxicity, and fulminant hepatic failure. Rarely, cardiovascular complications such as myocarditis, congestive

Table 29.10: Anti-TB drug regimens for drug-susceptible miliary/disseminated TB

Guideline [year] (reference)	Anti-TB drug regimen
WHO [2010] (105a)	2 months of RHZE + 4 months of RH* 2 months of RHZE + 7-10 months of RH* if TBM is also present 2 months of RHZE + 7 months of RH* if bone and joint TB is also present
ATS/CDC/IDSA [2016] (106)	2 months of RHZE + 4 months of RH 2 months of RHZE + 7-10 months of RH if TBM is also present
NICE [2016] (108)	2 months of RHZE + 4 months of RH 2 months of RHZE + 10 months of RH if TBM is also present

TB = tuberculosis; WHO = World Health Organization; ATS = American Thoracic Society; CDC = Centers for Disease Control; IDSA = Infectious Disease Society of America; NICE = National Institute for Health and Clinical Excellence; TBM = tuberculosis meningitis; TB = tuberculosis; Cy = cycloserine; E = ethambutol; Eth = ethionamide; H = isoniazid; K = kanamycin; P = para-aminosalicylic acid; R = rifampicin; S = streptomycin; Z = pyrazinamide
* Continuation phase consists of RHE in countries with high levels of H resistance in new TB patients, and where H drug-susceptibility testing in new patients is not done [or results are unavailable] before the continuation phase begins

Table 29.11: Predictors of poor outcome in patients with DTB/MTB

Study (reference)	Year of publication	Predictors of poor outcome
Gelb et al (45)*	1973	Stupor, meningismus, increasing age, cirrhosis of liver, leucopenia, leucocytosis
Grieco and Chmel (46)	1974	Increasing age, presence of underlying disease, history of cough, night sweats
Kim (50)	1990	Female gender, altered mental status
Maartens (51)	1990	Age > 60 years, lymphopaenia, thrombocytopaenia, hypoalbuminaemia, elevated transaminase levels, treatment delay
Sharma (52)	1995	Dyspnoea, chills, temperature >39.3 °C, icterus, hepatomegaly, hypoalbuminaemia, hyponatraemia, elevated serum alkaline phosphatase
Long (20)	1997	Presence of one or more risk factors†
Mert (40)	2001	Male gender, presence of atypical chest radiographic pattern, delay in instituting anti-TB treatment
Hussain (41)	2004	Presence of altered mental status, lung crackles, leucocytosis, thrombocytopaenia and the need for ventilation
Wang (2)‡	2007	Hypoalbuminaemia, hyperbilirubinaemia, renal insufficiency, and delay in instituting anti-TB treatment
Lee (112)	2014	Extent of ground-glass opacity >50%§

* No statistical analysis was performed
† Listed in Table 29.2
‡ DTB
§ Significantly associated with a delay in diagnosis, longer hospital stay, acute respiratory failure; but there was no difference in mortality
DTB = disseminated tuberculosis; MTB = miliary tuberculosis

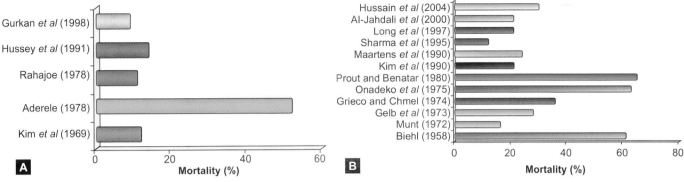

Figure 29.17: Mortality in children with miliary tuberculosis [A]. Data derived from Kim et al (23), Aderele (55), Rahajoe (56), Hussey et al (21), Gurkan et al (26). Mortality in adults with miliary tuberculosis [B]. Data derived from Biehl (42), Munt (43), Gelb et al (45), Grieco and Chmel (46), Onadeko et al (47), Prout and Benatar (49), Kim et al (50), Maartens et al (51), Sharma et al (52), Long et al (20), Al-Jahdali et al (53), Hussain et al (41)

heart failure, infective endocarditis, pericarditis, intracardiac mass, mycotic aneurysm, and sudden cardiac death have been described in MTB and should be carefully examined for (4,103,104).

PROGNOSIS

Predictors of poor outcome in DTB/MTB are shown in Table 29.11. The mortality related to MTB [Figure 29.17] is about 15%-20% in children (21,23,26,55,56) and is slightly higher [25%-30%] in adults (14,20,40-53). Delay in diagnosis and initiation of specific anti-TB treatment appears to be the most important factor responsible for mortality.

Several studies have attempted to identify predictors of poor outcome in patients with DTB/MTB. These details are shown in Table 29.11 (2,20,40,41,45,46,50-52,112,113). They may be helpful in guiding the clinicians caring for patients with DTB/MTB.

REFERENCES

1. Sharma SK, Mohan A, Sharma A. Challenges in the diagnosis & treatment of miliary tuberculosis. Indian J Med Res 2012;135: 703-30.
2. Wang JY, Hsueh PR, Wang SK, Jan IS, Lee LN, Liaw YS, et al. Disseminated tuberculosis: a 10-year experience in a medical center. Medicine [Baltimore] 2007;86:39-46.
3. Sharma SK, Mohan A. Extrapulmonary tuberculosis. Indian J Med Res 2004;120:316-53.
4. Sharma SK, Mohan A, Sharma A, Mitra DK. Miliary tuberculosis: new insights into an old disease. Lancet Infect Dis 2005;5:415-30.
5. Sahn SA, Neff TA. Miliary tuberculosis. Am J Med 1974;56: 494-505.
6. Sharma SK, Mohan A. Disseminated/miliary tuberculosis. In: Sharma SK, Mohan A, editors. Tuberculosis. New Delhi: Jaypee Brothers Medical Publishers; 2001.p.348-61.
7. Baker SK, Glassroth J. Miliary tuberculosis. In: Rom WN, Garay SM, editors. Tuberculosis. Philadelphia: Lippincott Williams & Wilkins; 2004.p.427-44.
8. Divinagracia R, Harris HW. Miliary tuberculosis. In: Schlossberg D, editor. Tuberculosis and nontuberculous myco-bacterial infection. Philadelphia: WB Saunders Company; 1999. p.271-84.
9. Sharma SK, Mohan A. Miliary tuberculosis. In: Agarwal AK, editor. Clinical medicine update – 2006. New Delhi: Indian Academy of Clinical Medicine; 2006.p.353-60.
10. Hill AR, Premkumar S, Brustein S, Vaidya K, Powell S, Li P-W, et al. Disseminated tuberculosis in the acquired immuno-deficiency syndrome era. Am Rev Respir Dis 1991;144:1164-70.
11. Sharma SK, Mohan A, Kadhiravan T. HIV-TB co-infection: epidemiology, diagnosis & management. Indian J Med Res 2005;121:550-67.
12. Lewison M, Frelich EB, Ragins OB. Correlation of clinical diagnosis and pathological diagnosis with special reference to tuberculosis: analysis of autopsy findings in 893 cases. Am Rev Tuberc 1931;24:152-71.
13. Chapman CB, Whorton CM. Acute generalised miliary tuberculosis in adults. A clinicopathological study based on sixty three cases diagnosed at autopsy. N Engl J Med 1946;235: 239-48.
14. Slavin RE, Walsh TJ, Pollack AD. Late generalized tuberculosis: a clinical pathologic analysis and comparison of 100 cases in the preantibiotic and antibiotic eras. Medicine [Baltimore] 1980;59:352-66.
15. Jacques J, Sloan JM. The changing pattern of miliary tuberculosis. Thorax 1970;25:237-40.
16. Vasankari T, Liippo K, Tala E. Overt and cryptic miliary tuberculosis misdiagnosed until autopsy. Scand J Infect Dis 2003;35:794-6.
17. Savic I, Trifunovic-Skodric V, Mitrovic D. Clinically unrecognized miliary tuberculosis: an autopsy study. Ann Saudi Med 2016;36:42-50.
18. Ansari NA, Kombe AH, Kenyon TA, Hone NM, Tappero JW, Nyirenda ST, et al. Pathology and causes of death in a group of 128 predominantly HIV-positive patients in Botswana, 1997-1998. Int J Tuberc Lung Dis 2002;6:55-63.
19. Alvarez S, McCabe WR. Extrapulmonary tuberculosis revisited: a review of experience at Boston City and other hospitals. Medicine [Baltimore] 1984;63:25-55.
20. Long R, O'Connor R, Palayew M, Hershfield E, Manfreda J. Disseminated tuberculosis with and without a miliary pattern on chest radiograph: a clinical-pathologic-radiologic correlation. Int J Tuberc Lung Dis 1997;1:52-8.
21. Hussey G, Chisholm T, Kibel M. Miliary tuberculosis in children: a review of 94 cases. Pediatr Infect Dis J 1991;10:832-6.
22. Noertjojo K, Tam CM, Chan SL, Chan-Yeung MM. Extrapulmonary and pulmonary tuberculosis in Hong Kong. Int J Tuberc Lung Dis 2002;6:879-86.

23. Kim PK, Lee JS, Yun DJ. Clinical review of miliary tuberculosis in Korean children: 84 cases and review of the literature. Yonsei Med J 1969;10:146-52.

24. Udani PM, Bhat US, Bhave SK, Ezuthachan SG, Shetty VV. Problem of tuberculosis in children in India: epidemiology, morbidity, mortality and control programme. Indian Pediatr 1976;13:881-90.

25. Somu N, Vijayasekaran D, Ravikumar T, Balachandran A, Subramanyam L, Chandrabhushanam A. Tuberculous disease in a pediatric referral centre: 16 years experience. Indian Pediatr 1994;31:1245-9.

26. Gurkan F, Bosnak M, Dikici B, Bosnak V, Yaramis A, Tas MA, et al. Miliary tuberculosis in children: a clinical review. Scand J Infect Dis 1998;30:359-62.

27. Centers for Disease Control. Tuberculosis statistics in the United States, 1990. Atlanta: US Department of Health and Human Services, Centers for Disease Control: 1992.

28. Farer LS, Lowell AM, Meador MP. Extrapulmonary tuberculosis in the United States. Am J Epidemiol 1979;109:205-17.

29. Rieder HL, Snider DE Jr, Cauthen GM. Extrapulmonary tuberculosis in the United States. Am Rev Respir Dis 1990;141: 347-51.

30. Centers for Disease Control. Reported tuberculosis in the United States, 1997. Tuberculosis cases by form of disease: States, 1997. Available at URL: http://www.cdc.gov/nchstp/tb/ surv/surv97/surv97pdf/table12.pdf. Accessed on 05 February 2008.

31. Centers for Disease Control. Reported tuberculosis in the United States, 1998. Tuberculosis cases by form of disease: States, 1998. Available at URL: http://www.cdc.gov/nchstp/ tb/surv/surv98/surv98pdf/table12.pdf. Accessed on 05 February 2008.

32. Centers for Disease Control. Reported tuberculosis in the United States, 1999. Tuberculosis cases by form of disease: States, 1999. Available at URL: http://www.cdc.gov/nchstp/tb/surv/surv99/pdfs/table21.pdf. Accessed on 05 February 2008.

33. Centers for Disease Control. Reported tuberculosis in the United States, 2000. Tuberculosis cases by form of disease: States, 2000. Available at URL: http://www.cdc.gov/nchstp/ tb/surv/surv2000/pdfs/t21.pdf. Accessed on 05 February 2008.

34. Centers for Disease Control. Reported tuberculosis in the United States, 2001. Tuberculosis cases by form of disease: States, 2001. Available at URL: http://www.cdc.gov/nchstp/tb/ surv/surv2001/pdf/t23.pdf. Accessed on 05 February 2008.

35. Centers for Disease Control Reported tuberculosis in the United States, 2002. Tuberculosis cases by form of disease: States, 2002. Available at URL: http://www.cdc.gov/nchstp/tb/ surv/surv2002/PDF/T23.pdf. Accessed on 05 February 2008.

36. Wares F, Balasubramanian R, Mohan A, Sharma SK. Extrapulmonary tuberculosis: management and control. In: Agarwal SP, Chauhan LS, editors. Tuberculosis control in India. New Delhi: Central TB Division. Directorate General of Health Services, Ministry of Health and Family Welfare, Government of India; 2005.p.95-114.

37. Proudfoot AT, Akhtar AJ, Douglas AC, Horne NW. Miliary tuberculosis in adults. BMJ 1969;2:273-6.

38. Yu YL, Chow WH, Humphries MJ, Wong RW, Gabriel M. Cryptic miliary tuberculosis. QJM 1986;59:421-8.

39. Ormerod LP. Respiratory tuberculosis. In: Davies PDO, editor. Clinical tuberculosis. London: Chapman & Hall Medical; 1997.p.76.

40. Mert A, Bilir M, Tabak F, Ozaras R, Ozturk R, Senturk H, et al. Miliary tuberculosis: clinical manifestations, diagnosis and outcome in 38 adults. Respirology 2001;6:217-24.

41. Hussain SF, Irfan M, Abbasi M, Anwer SS, Davidson S, Haqqee R, et al. Clinical characteristics of 110 miliary tuberculosis patients from a low HIV prevalence country. Int J Tuberc Lung Dis 2004;8:493-9.

42. Biehl JP. Miliary tuberculosis; a review of sixty-eight adult patients admitted to a municipal general hospital. Am Rev Tuberc 1958;77:605-22.

43. Munt PW. Miliary tuberculosis in the chemotherapy era: with a clinical review in 69 American adults. Medicine [Baltimore] 1972;51:139-55.

44. Campbell IG. Miliary tuberculosis in British Columbia. Can Med Assoc J 1973;108: 1517-9.

45. Gelb AF, Leffler C, Brewin A, Mascatello V, Lyons HA. Miliary tuberculosis. Am Rev Respir Dis 1973;108:1327-33.

46. Grieco MH, Chmel H. Acute disseminated tuberculosis as a diagnostic problem. A clinical study based on twenty-eight cases. Am Rev Respir Dis 1974;109:554-60.

47. Onadeko BO, Dickinson R, Sofowora EO. Miliary tuberculosis of the lung in Nigerian adults. East Afr Med J 1975;52:390-5.

48. Teklu B, Butler J, Ostrow JH. Miliary tuberculosis. A review of 83 cases treated between 1950 and 1968. Ethiop Med J 1977;15:39-48.

49. Prout S, Benatar SR. Disseminated tuberculosis. A study of 62 cases. S Afr Med J 1980;58:835-42.

50. Kim JH, Langston AA, Gallis HA. Miliary tuberculosis: epidemiology, clinical manifestations, diagnosis, and outcome. Rev Infect Dis 1990;12:583-90.

51. Maartens G, Willcox PA, Benatar SR. Miliary tuberculosis: rapid diagnosis, hematologic abnormalities, and outcome in 109 treated adults. Am J Med 1990;89:291-6.

52. Sharma SK, Mohan A, Pande JN, Prasad KL, Gupta AK, Khilnani GC. Clinical profile, laboratory characteristics and outcome in miliary tuberculosis. Q J Med 1995;88:29-37.

53. Al-Jahdali H, Al-Zahrani K, Amene P, Memish Z, Al-Shimemeri A, Moamary M, et al. Clinical aspects of miliary tuberculosis in Saudi adults. Int J Tuberc Lung Dis 2000;4:252-5.

54. Swaminathan S, Padmapriyadarsini C, Ponnuraja C, Sumathi CH, Rajasekaran S, Amerandran VA, et al. Miliary tuberculosis in human immunodeficiency virus infected patients not on antiretroviral therapy: clinical profile and response to short course chemotherapy. J Postgrad Med 2007;53:228-31.

55. Aderele WI. Miliary tuberculosis in Nigerian children. East Afr Med J 1978;55:166-71.

56. Rahajoe NN. Miliary tuberculosis in children. A clinical review. Paediatr Indones 1990;30:233-40.

57. Thwaites GE, Nguyen DB, Nguyen HD, Hoang TQ, Do TT, Nguyen TC, et al. Dexamethasone for the treatment of tuberculous meningitis in adolescents and adults. N Engl J Med 2004;351:1741-51.

58. Braidy J, Pothel C, Amra S. Miliary tuberculosis presenting as adrenal failure. J Can Med Assoc 1981;82:254-6.

59. Sharma SK, Mohan A, Banga A, Saha PK, Guntupalli KK. Predictors of development and outcome in patients with acute respiratory distress syndrome due to tuberculosis. Int J Tuberc Lung Dis 2006;10:429-35.

60. Penner C, Roberts D, Kunimoto D, Manfreda J, Long R. Tuberculosis as a primary cause of respiratory failure requiring mechanical ventilation. Am J Respir Crit Care Med 1995;151: 867-72.

61. Mohan A, Sharma SK, Pande JN. Acute respiratory distress syndrome in miliary tuberculosis: a 12-year experience. Indian J Chest Dis Allied Sci 1996;38:147-52.

62. Sharma N, Kumar P. Miliary tuberculosis with bilateral pneumothorax: a rare complication. Indian J Chest Dis Allied Sci 2002;44:125-7.

63. Das M, Chandra U, Natchu M, Lodha R, Kabra SK. Pneumomediastinum and subcutaneous emphysema in acute miliary tuberculosis. Indian J Pediatr 2004;71:553-4.

64. Singh KJ, Ahluwalia G, Sharma SK, Saxena R, Chaudhary VP, Anant M. Significance of haematological manifestations in

patients with tuberculosis. J Assoc Physicians India 2001;49: 790-4.

65. Kuo PH, Yang PC, Kuo SS, Luh KT. Severe immune hemolytic anemia in disseminated tuberculosis with response to antituberculosis therapy. Chest 2001;119:1961-3.

66. Runo JR, Welch DC, Ness EM, Robbins IM, Milstone AP. Miliary tuberculosis as a cause of acute empyema. Respiration 2003;70:529-32.

67. Sydow M, Schauer A, Crozier TA, Burchardi H. Multiple organ failure in generalized disseminated tuberculosis. Respir Med 1992;86:517-9.

68. Nieuwland Y, Tan KY, Elte JW. Miliary tuberculosis presenting with thyrotoxicosis. Postgrad Med J 1992;68:677-9.

69. Mallinson WJ, Fuller RW, Levison DA, Baker LR, Cattell WR. Diffuse interstitial renal tuberculosis—an unusual cause of renal failure. Q J Med 1981;50:137-48.

70. Shribman JH, Eastwood JB, Uff J. Immune complex nephritis complicating miliary tuberculosis. Br Med J [Clin Res Ed] 1983;287: 1593-4.

71. Wallis PJ, Branfoot AC, Emerson PA. Sudden death due to myocardial tuberculosis. Thorax 1984;39:155-6.

72. Cope AP, Heber M, Wilkins EG. Valvular tuberculous endocarditis: a case report and review of the literature. J Infect 1990;21:293-6.

73. Wainwright J. Tuberculous endocarditis: A report of 2 cases. S Afr Med J 1979;56:731-3.

74. Rose AG. Cardiac tuberculosis. A study of 19 patients. Pathol Lab Med 1987;111:422-6.

75. Lee SW, Wang CY, Lee BJ, Kuo CY, Kuo CL. Hemophagocytic syndrome in miliary tuberculosis presenting with noncaseating granulomas in bone marrow and liver. J Formos Med Assoc 2008;107:495-9.

76. Rathnayake PV, Kularathne WK, De Silva GC, Athauda BM, Nanayakkara SN, Siribaddana A, et al. Disseminated tuberculosis presenting as hemophagocytic lymphohistiocytosis in an immunocompetent adult patient: a case report. J Med Case Rep 2015;9:294.

77. Kato M, Shimizu A, Ishikawa O. Metastatic tuberculous abscess as a manifestation of miliary tuberculosis. J Dermatol 2014;41: 1117-8.

78. Yeow Y, Fong SS, Rao J, Sim R. Aorto-oesophageal fistula from miliary tuberculosis: a rare cause of massive haematemesis. Ann Acad Med Singapore 2014;43:559-60.

79. So E, Bolger DT Jr. Hypercalcaemia: atypical presentation of miliary tuberculosis. BMJ Case Rep 2014;2014.

80. Haas DW, Des Prez RM. Tuberculosis and acquired immuno-deficiency syndrome: a historical perspective on recent develop-ments. Am J Med 1994;96:439-50.

81. Jones BE, Young SM, Antoniskis D, Davidson PT, Kramer F, Barnes PF. Relationship of the manifestations of tuberculosis to CD4 cell counts in patients with human immunodeficiency virus infection. Am Rev Respir Dis 1993;148:1292-7.

82. Lado Lado FL, Barrio Gomez E, Carballo Arceo E, Cabarcos Ortiz de Barron A. Clinical presentation of tuberculosis and the degree of immunodeficiency in patients with HIV infection. Scand J Infect Dis 1999;31:387-91.

83. Daikos GL, Uttamchandani RB, Tuda C, Fischl MA, Miller N, Cleary T, et al. Disseminated miliary tuberculosis of the skin in patients with AIDS: report of four cases. Clin Infect Dis 1998;27:205-8.

84. del Giudice P, Bernard E, Perrin C, Bernardin G, Fouché R, Boissy C, et al. Unusual cutaneous manifestations of miliary tuberculosis. Clin Infect Dis 2000;30:201-4.

85. Jehle AW, Khanna N, Sigle JP, Glatz-Krieger K, Battegay M, Steiger J, et al. Acute renal failure on immune reconstitution in

an HIV-positive patient with miliary tuberculosis. Clin Infect Dis 2004;38:e32-5.

86. Goldsack NR, Allen S, Lipman MC. Adult respiratory distress syndrome as a severe immune reconstitution disease following the commencement of highly active antiretroviral therapy. Sex Transm Infect 2003;79:337-8.

87. Winkler AW, Crankshaw DF. Chloride depletion in conditions other than Addison's disease. J Clin Invest 1938;17:1-6.

88. Shalhoub RJ, Antoniou LD. The mechanism of hyponatremia in pulmonary tuberculosis. Ann Intern Med 1969;70:943-62.

89. Vorherr H, Massry SG, Fallet R, Kaplan L, Kleeman CR. Antidiuretic principle in tuberculous lung tissue of a patient with pulmonary tuberculosis and hyponatremia. Ann Intern Med 1970;72:383-7.

90. Sharma SK, Mohan A. Disseminated/miliary tuberculosis. In: Sharma SK, Mohan A, editors. Tuberculosis, Second edition. New Delhi: Jaypee Brothers Medical Publishers; 2009.p.493-518.

91. Hunter L, Bélard S, Janssen S, van Hoving DJ, Heller T. Miliary tuberculosis: sonographic pattern in chest ultrasound. Infection 2016;44:243-6.

92. Yu RS, Zhang SZ, Wu JJ, Li RF. Imaging diagnosis of 12 patients with hepatic tuberculosis. World J Gastroenterol 2004;10:1639-42.

93. Goo JM, Im JG, Do KH, Yeo JS, Seo JB, Kim HY, et al. Pulmonary tuberculoma evaluated by means of FDG PET: findings in 10 cases. Radiology 2000;216:117-21.

94. Ichiya Y, Kuwabara Y, Sasaki M, Yoshida T, Akashi Y, Murayama S, et al. FDG-PET in infectious lesions: the detection and assessment of lesion activity. Ann Nucl Med 1996;10:185-91.

95. Sharma SK, Mukhopadhyay S, Arora R, Varma K, Pande JN, Khilnani GC. Computed tomography in miliary tuberculosis: comparison with plain films, bronchoalveolar lavage, pulmonary functions and gas exchange. Australasian Radiol 1996;40:113-8.

96. Pipavath SN, Sharma SK, Sinha S, Mukhopadhyay S, Gulati MS. High resolution CT [HRCT] in miliary tuberculosis [MTB] of the lung: correlation with pulmonary function tests & gas exchange parameters in north Indian patients. Indian J Med Res 2007;126: 193-8.

97. Sharma SK, Pande JN, Singh YN, Verma K, Kathait SS, Khare SD, et al. Pulmonary function and immunologic abnormalities in miliary tuberculosis. Am Rev Respir Dis 1992;145:1167-71.

98. Sharma SK, Ahluwalia G. Exercise testing in miliary tuberculosis—some facts. Indian J Med Res 2007;125:182-3.

99. Sharma SK, Ahluwalia G. Effect of antituberculosis treatment on cardiopulmonary responses to exercise in miliary tuberculosis. Indian J Med Res 2006;124:411-8.

100. Sharma SK, Pande JN, Verma K. Bronchoalveolar lavage [BAL] in miliary tuberculosis. Tubercle 1988;69:175-8.

101. Prabhakaran D, Sharma SK, Verma K, Pande JN. Estimation of fibronectin in bronchoalveolar lavage fluid in various diffuse interstitial lung diseases. Am Rev Respir Dis 1990;141:A51.

102. Willcox PA, Potgieter PD, Bateman ED, Benatar SR. Rapid diagnosis of sputum negative miliary tuberculosis using the flexible fibreoptic bronchoscope. Thorax 1986;41:681-4.

103. Sharma SK, Mohan A. Tuberculosis: From an incurable scourge to a curable disease—journey over a millennium. Indian J Med Res 2013;137:455-93.

104. Sharma SK, Mohan A, Sharma A. Miliary tuberculosis: a new look at an old foe. J Clin Tuberc Other Mycobact Dis 2016;3: 13-27.

105a. World Health Organization. Treatment of tuberculosis. Guidelines, Fourth edition. WHO/HTM/TB/2009.420. Geneva: World Health Organization; 2010.

105b. World Health Organization. Guidelines for treatment of drug-susceptible tuberculosis and patient care 2017 update. WHO/HTM/TB/2017.05. Geneva: World Health Organization; 2017.

106. Nahid P, Dorman SE, Alipanah N, Barry PM, Brozek JL, Cattamanchi A, et al. Official American Thoracic Society/ Centers for Disease Control and Prevention/Infectious Diseases Society of America Clinical Practice Guidelines: Treatment of drug-susceptible tuberculosis. Clin Infect Dis 2016;63: e147-95.

107. American Academy of Pediatrics. Committee on Infectious Diseases. 2015 Red Book: Report of the Committee on Infectious Diseases. 30th edition. Elk Grove Village: American Academy of Pediatrics; 2015.

108. National Institute for Health and Clinical Excellence, National Collaborating Centre for Chronic Conditions. 2016. NICE guideline [NG33] Published date: January 2016 Last updated: May 2016. https://www.nice.org.uk/guidance/ng33/ resources/tuberculosis-1837390683589. Accessed on September 20, 2018.

109. Sharma SK, Ryan H, Khaparde S, Sachdeva KS, Singh AD, Mohan A, et al. Index-TB guidelines: Guidelines on extra-pulmonary tuberculosis for India. Indian J Med Res 2017;145: 448-63.

110. Sun TN, Yang JY, Zheng LY, Deng WW, Sui ZY. Chemotherapy and its combination with corticosteroids in acute miliary tuberculosis in adolescents and adults: analysis of 55 cases. Chin Med J [Engl] 1981;94:309-14.

111. Massaro D, Katz S, Sachs M. Choroidal tubercles. A clue to hematogenous tuberculosis. Ann Intern Med 1964;60:231-41.

112. Lee J, Lim JK, Seo H, Lee SY, Choi KJ, Yoo SS, et al. Clinical relevance of ground glass opacity in 105 patients with miliary tuberculosis. Respir Med 2014;108:924-30.

113. Sharma SK, Mohan A. Miliary tuberculosis. In: Schlossberg D, editor. Tuberculosis and nontuberculous mycobacterial infections. Sixth edition. Washington: ASM Press; 2017.p.491-513.

30

Tuberculosis at Uncommon Body Sites

Y Mutheeswaraiah, J Harikrishna

TUBERCULOSIS OF THE BREAST

Introduction

Primary tuberculosis [TB] of the breast is uncommon (1). As the clinical presentation and radiological manifestations are non-specific, TB of the breast is a diagnostic problem faced by clinicians (2-8).

Pathogenesis

Breast TB could be the only manifestation of TB, or it can occur secondary to TB elsewhere in the body (9-11). The postulated mechanisms for the development of breast TB are shown in Table 30.1. Of these, centripetal lymphatic spread from lungs to breast tissue appears to be the most likely mechanism for the development of breast TB (2,9,12). Retrograde lymphatic spread from axillary, cervical, paratracheal and internal mammary lymph nodes can also cause breast TB (10,11). Direct extension of infection from adjacent ribs, sternum, costal cartilages pleura, chest wall and direct inoculation from abrasions in skin are other postulated mechanisms (2,9-11).

Table 30.1: Pathogenetic mechanisms for development of breast TB

Haematogenous spread

Spread via the lymphatics
   Centripetal spread via lymphatics from the lung
   Retrograde lymphatic spread from axillary, paratracheal and internal mammary lymph nodes

Direct extension from contiguous structures

Direct inoculation

Ductal infection

TB = tuberculosis

EPIDEMIOLOGY

TB of the breast is thought to be rare because the environment in the breast does not favour survival and multiplication of *Mycobacterium tuberculosis* [*Mtb*] (2). The first case of breast TB was reported by Sir Astley Cooper in 1829 who called it "scrofulous swelling of the bosom" (13). Since the report of the first case of TB mastitis from India in 1957 (14), there have been occasional reports on breast TB from India (2,10-11,15-22). In developing countries, the incidence of breast TB in surgically resected specimens was found to be 3%-4.5% (23). The prevalence of breast TB in India has varied between 0.6%-3.6% (2,11,22). A high prevalence of breast TB [5.2% of all breast diseases; 32% of all infective conditions] has been reported from India (24). In low TB burden countries, the prevalence of breast TB is less than 0.1% among breast lesions examined histopathologically (25,26).

Clinical Presentation

TB of the breast is commonly seen in young women in the reproductive age group; it is rarely seen in the prepubertal age group and in older women (1,2,24). Breast TB is more common in pregnant and lactating women because of high vascularity, dilated ducts and higher likelihood of occurrence trauma (2,10,24). Spread of infection from the tonsils of the suckling infant to the mother's nipple, and from there to the lactating breast *via* lactiferous ducts has also been postulated (27). Breast TB is rare in males (28,29).

Breast TB commonly presents as a unilateral disease [Figure 30.1]. Bilateral involvement is very rare being reported in less than 3% of the cases [Figure 30.2] (10). The symptom duration varies from a few months to several years (1,2,7,8,24). TB of the breast frequently presents as a lump in the central or upper outer quadrant of the breast [Figure 30.1]. The lump may be tender, mobile or fixed to

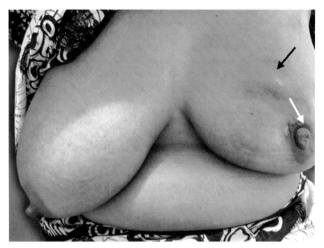

Figure 30.1: Clinical photograph showing left breast lump [arrow] and nipple retraction. Histopathological examination and mycobacterial culture confirmed the diagnosis of breast TB
TB = tuberculosis

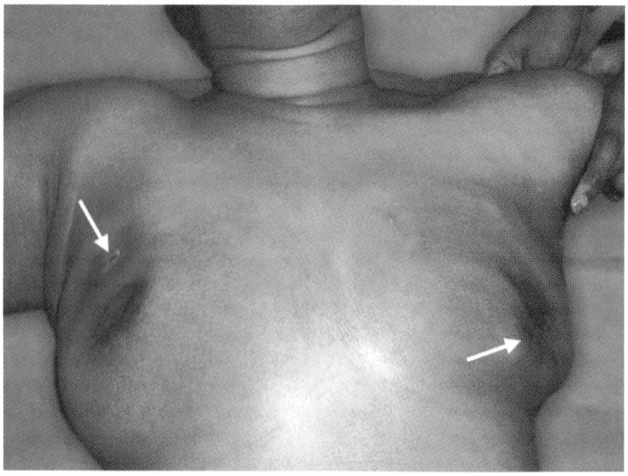

Figure 30.2: Bilateral breast TB. Clinical photograph showing ulcerating lesions in both the breasts [arrows]. Histopathological examination confirmed the diagnosis of breast TB
TB = tuberculosis

skin, muscle or the chest wall. Clinically, the lump of breast TB is irregular, ill-defined, hard in consistency mimicking breast carcinoma (1,2,7,8,24). Sometimes, nipple retraction and peau d'orange appearance may also be seen [Figure 30.3]. An ulcer in the skin overlying the breast and breast abscess have also been described [Figures 30.4, 30.5 and 30.6]. In patients with axillary lymphadenitis, breast oedema may be evident (1,2,7,8,24).

When a patient presents with a breast abscess which fails to heal in spite of adequate surgical drainage and antibiotic therapy, especially when persistent discharging sinuses are present underlying TB should be suspected.

Breast TB has been classified into different types (9). The most common form of breast TB is nodular TB mastitis. This

condition presents as a well-circumscribed, slowly growing, usually painless mass mimicking a fibroadenoma of the breast. The disease progresses to involve the overlying skin; ulceration, sinus formation, may develop and the condition may resemble breast carcinoma (30-33).

Disseminated or confluent TB mastitis is rare. It presents with multiple foci throughout the breast that may later undergo caseation necrosis resulting in sinus formation. The breast may be tense and tender, overlying skin appears thickened and stretched; painful ulcers may sometimes be seen. Matted axillary lymph nodes are often evident (33).

Sclerosing TB mastitis characterised by excessive fibrosis affects involuting breasts of older women. This condition presents as a hard painless slowly growing lump with nipple

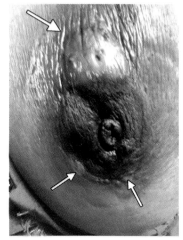

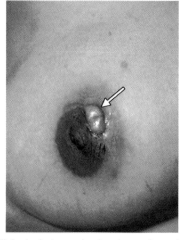

Figure 30.3: Clinical photograph showing a breast lump with shiny overlying skin and *peau de orange* appearance mimicking breast carcinoma [thick white arrow] and multiple ulcers [thin white arrows] and nipple retraction. Histopathological examination and mycobacterial culture confirmed the diagnosis of breast TB
TB = tuberculosis

Figure 30.4: Clinical photograph showing a breast lump, overlying ulceration [arrow] and nipple retraction. Histopathological examination confirmed the diagnosis of breast TB
TB = tuberculosis

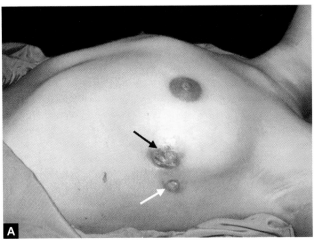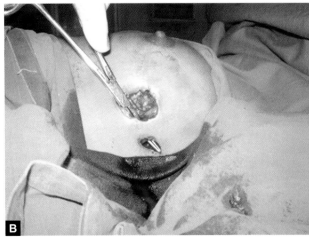

Figure 30.5: Clinical photograph showing an ulcer [black arrow] in the left breast and a sinus in the chest wall [white arrow] [A]. Operative photograph of the same patient [B] showing the sinus tract. Histopathological examination confirmed the diagnosis of TB

TB = tuberculosis

retraction resembling a schirrotic carcinoma (33). TB mastitis obliterans is characterised proliferation of lining epithelium of the ducts, marked epithelial and periductal fibrosis. Occlusion of ducts results in formation of cystic spaces and the condition mimics cystic mastitis. Rarely, breast TB may develop in patients with miliary TB.

Diagnosis

Diagnostic work-up is aimed at establishing TB as the aetiological diagnosis and ruling out other conditions, especially breast cancer.

Tuberculin Skin Test

A positive tuberculin skin test [TST] is frequently evident. However, a positive TST indicates infection with *Mtb* and is not considered to be a marker for active TB.

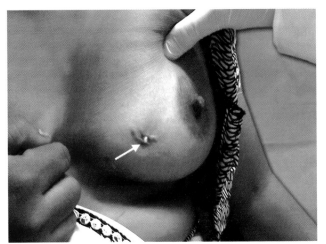

Figure 30.6: Clinical photograph showing a discharging sinus in the left breast [arrow]. Histopathological examination confirmed the diagnosis of breast TB

TB = tuberculosis

Chest Radiograph

The chest radiograph may show evidence of active or old healed pulmonary TB or miliary TB (22). Calcified axillary lymph nodes may sometimes be evident on the chest radiograph (34).

Mammography

In breast TB, various mammographic findings, such as, mass, coarse calcification, asymmetric density with spiculated margin, skin thickening, nipple retraction and axillary lymphadenopathy have been described (35). When TB abscess is present, a dense tract connecting an ill-defined breast mass to a localised skin thickening and bulge may be seen (36). The mammographic features of nodular breast TB closely resembles breast carcinoma. Disseminated TB mastitis mimics inflammatory carcinoma. In sclerosing TB mastitis, a homogeneous dense mass with fibrous septae and nipple retraction is seen (10,33). However, mammography alone cannot distinguish breast TB from breast cancer (35-38).

Ultrasonography

On breast ultrasonography, the features of breast TB are non-specific (39). Ultrasonography is useful in differentiating cystic from solid breast masses. It may also show a fistulous connection between retromammary abscess and chest wall (36,40,41). Ultrasonography-guided fine needle aspiration can be done for procuring tissue for cytopathological, microbiological and molecular studies (37).

Computed Tomography

Computed tomography [CT] is helpful in defining the extent of thoracic wall involvement especially in patients presenting with a deeply adherent breast lump (42,43). On CT, TB abscess appears as smoothly marginated, inhomogeneous, hypodense lesions; surrounding rim-enhancement may be seen on contrast-enhanced CT. Underlying rib osetomyelitis, fistulous connection with the pleura may also be seen on CT (41). Further, involvement of pleural disease, pulmonary parenchyma, intrathoracic and axillary lymph nodes may also be detected on CT (43,44).

Magnetic Resonance Imaging

Some investigators have described the magnetic resonance imaging [MRI] findings in breast TB (39,44-47). On T2-weighted gadolinium diethylenetriaminepentaacetic acid [Gd-DTPA] enhanced MRI images, breast abscess appears as a smooth or irregular ring like bright signal intensity. Further, MRI is useful in delineating the extramammary involvement as well. However, these findings are not specific to TB and may also be seen in bacterial and fungal abscesses and breast carcinoma (39,44-47).

Positron Emission Tomography

There are a few reports of the utility of positron emission tomography [PET]-CT in the diagnosis of breast TB. Intense focal fluorodeoxy glucose [FDG] uptake mimicking breast cancer has been described (48-50). However, PET-CT or PET-MRI findings alone cannot distinguish breast TB from breast cancer. Procurement of breast tissue for further diagnostic testing is required to ascertain the diagnosis of TB as the aetiological cause.

Fine Needle Aspiration Cytology

Fine needle aspiration cytology [FNAC] from the breast lump has been used to diagnose breast TB (51-54). On FNAC, features of granulomatous mastitis like epithelioid cell granulomas, necrosis are present (1); acid-fast bacilli [AFB] may also be seen sometimes (51-54). In TB breast abscess, the FNAC picture may be dominated by an acute inflammatory exudate. In this situation presence of AFB or histopathological evidence of TB is considered to be evidence of breast TB (51).

Open Biopsy

When the FNAC examination is inconclusive open [incision or excision] biopsy, or biopsy from the wall of the abscess is helpful (1). Histopathological examination reveals granulomatous inflammation and must be distinguished from other granulomaotus disorders like fungal infection and sarcoidosis.

Microbiological, Molecular Methods

Breast tissue procured for diagnostic testing should be subjected to smear and mycobacterial culture examination, as well as molecular diagnostic testing (55). The conventional diagnostic testing methods like smear for AFB and mycobacterial culture, have a low yield in breast TB. The scope of using cartridge-based nucleic acid amplification tests [CBNAAT] like Xpert MTB/RIF in the diagnosis of breast TB merits further study (56).

Differential Diagnosis

Clinical examination, imaging findings cannot reliably distinguish breast TB from breast cancer. Sometimes, co-incidental occurrence of TB and carcinoma of the breast is known; granulomatous lymphadenitis in the axillary has been reported in patients with breast cancer (31,32).

Treatment

The management of breast TB consists of administration of standard anti-TB treatment and surgery in certain situations. Anti-TB treatment is the mainstay of therapy. The standard six-month anti-TB treatment is considered adequate for most of the patients; in some patients, the treatment may have to be extended by further three months (1,2,24,15,57). In a recent retrospective study (58) 33 of the 46 [72%] patients responded to the standard six-month therapy while treatment extension to 9-12 months was required in 13 [28%] cases. The reader is referred to the chapter *"Treatment of tuberculosis" [Chapter 44]* for more details.

Surgical Treatment

Surgery may be required for excisional biopsy, drainage of abscess, procuring biopsy from abscess wall, management of sinuses in the breast; segmentectomy and occasionally simple mastectomy (1,2) have been employed. For large ulcerating masses involving the entire breast and the draining axillary lymph nodes, simple mastectomy with or without axillary clearance is required. Modified radical mastectomy is considered only if is a co-existing malignancy is present.

FEVER OF UNKNOWN ORIGIN

Since the initial classical description by Petersdorf and Beeson (59), fever of unknown origin [FUO] is a common diagnostic problem faced by clinicians. As defined by Durack and Street (60), FUO is diagnosed based on the presence of *all* of the following criteria: [i] temperature of greater than 38.3°C [>101°F] on several occasions; [ii] duration of fever more than 3 weeks; and [iii] a failure to reach a diagnosis despite three outpatient visits or three days in the hospital without elucidation of a cause or one week of "intelligent and invasive" ambulatory investigation.

Epidemiology

TB is an important cause of FUO especially in areas where TB is highly endemic. In patients presenting with FUO, atypical clinical presentation of TB is common. Focal extrapulmonary TB, disseminated TB and miliary TB that is not evident initially, but, becomes evident during the course of evaluation are common.

In studies conducted at Kolkata (61,62), New Delhi (63) and Tirupati (64) from India documented that TB was the most common cause for FUO. Kejriwal *et al* (61) in their study of FUO [n=100] reported that TB was the aetiological cause in 24% of patients. Bandyopadhyay *et al* (62) studied

164 patients with FUO and documented that in 46 [28%] patients, TB was the aetiological cause. In the study from New Delhi [n = 121], Handa *et al* (63) reported that extra-pulmonary TB [n = 26; 21.5%] was a common cause of FUO. In the recent study from Tirupati (64), TB was found to be aetiological cause in 19 of the 45 [42%] patients with FUO.

Diagnosis

A careful physical examination, and daily re-examination, may reveal valuable clues to TB as the aetiology [Figures 30.7, 30.8, 30.9, 30.10, 30.11, 30.12 and 30.13]. Imaging modalities, such as ultrasonography, CT, MRI and especially, PET-CT are useful to localise the disease site. Diagnosis is confirmed by procuring appropriate tissue/body fluids for diagnostic testing under image-guidance.

Molecular testing with CBNAAT like Xpert MTB/RIF is helpful in early confirmation of diagnosis. In patients

with FUO in whom laboratory diagnostic testing is non-contributory, aspiration and trephine biopsy of the bone marrow, cytopathological and histopathological examination [Figure 30.13] and molecular diagnostic testing of the obtained material with Xpert MTB/RIF can be helpful in confirming TB as the aetiological diagnosis.

Treatment

In resource limited, TB endemic areas, when all FUO diagnostic work-up including bone marrow examination is inconclusive, clinicians often resort to a therapeutic trial with anti-TB treatment as many clinicians consider the therapeutic benefits outweigh the risk of adverse events (65,66). In patients in whom the diagnosis of TB has been established, depending on the site and extent of involvement, standard anti-TB treatment, that may have to be extended in the individual patient yields good results.

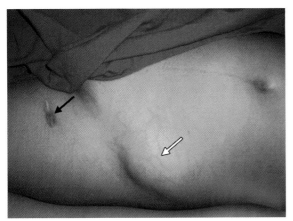

Figure 30.7: Clinical photograph of a patient who presented with fever of unknown origin showing a sinus in the left upper inner thigh [black arrow] and left sided external iliac lymphadenopathy. Histopathological examination confirmed the diagnosis of TB
TB = tuberculosis

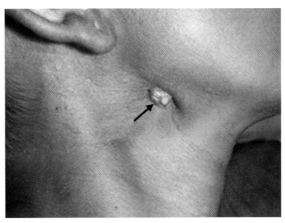

Figure 30.8: Clinical photograph of a patient who presented with prolonged low grade fever showing a discharing sinus in the right side of the neck [arrow]. Histopathological examination was suggestive of granulomatous inflammation; pus on Xpert MTB/RIF testing showed *Mycobacterium tuberculosis* sensitive to rifampicin

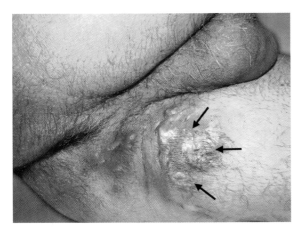

Figure 30.9: Clinical photograph of a patient who presented with prolonged low grade fever showing multiple discharing sinuses in the upper left thigh [arrows]. Histopathological examination confirmed the diagnosis of TB
TB = tuberculosis

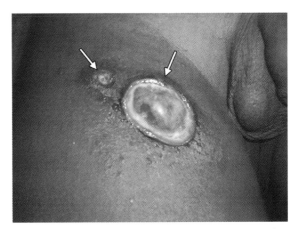

Figure 30.10: Clinical photograph of a patient presenting with prolonged fever showing ulcers with undermined margins [arrows] in the upper inner thigh. Histopathological examination confirmed the diagnosis of TB
TB = tuberculosis

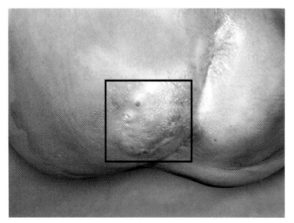

Figure 30.11: Clinical photograph showing multiple sinuses [square] in the gluteal region. Xpert MTB/RIF examination of material discharging from the sinuses detected *Mycobacterium tuberculosis* sensitive to rifampicin
TB = tuberculosis

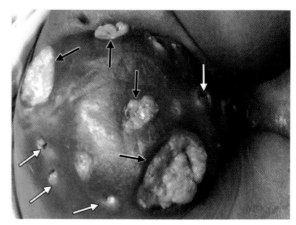

Figure 30.12: Clinical photograph showing multiple ulcers with undermined margins [black arrows] and sinuses [white arrows] in the gluteal region. Histopathological examination confirmed the diagnosis of TB
TB = tuberculosis

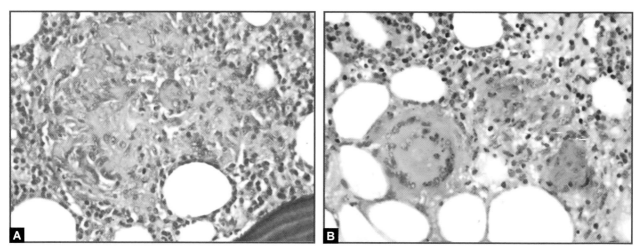

Figure 30.13: Photomicrograph of trephine biopsy of bone marrow in a patient presenting with fever of unknown origin in whom all laboratory and imaging testing was inconclusive showing ill-defined epithelioid granuloma with fatty spaces and bony trabeculae [Haematoxylin and eosin, × 200] [A]; and Langhans' giant cells amidst fatty spaces [Haematoxylin and eosin, × 200] [B] suggestive of disseminated TB. Mycobacterial culture grew *Mycobacterium tuberculosis*
TB = tuberculosis

TUBERCULOSIS PYOMYOSITIS

TB pyomyositis is an extremely rare form of extrapulmonary TB. It has been documented in immunocompromised individuals (67-69). There are occasional reports of TB pyomyositis in immunocompetent individuals also (70-72). In human immunodeficiency virus-seropositive individuals, occurrence of TB pyomyositis as a component of immune reconstitution inflammatory syndrome has also been documented (73). The disease is characterised by the formation of an abscess in the skeletal muscle. The rare occurrence of intramuscular TB nodules at multiple muscular sites has also been described (74).

Insidious onset, slow progression of symptoms, non-responsiveness to antibiotic treatment raises the possibility to TB pyomyositis. Imaging modalities like ultrasonography,

CT and MRI are helpful in localising the disease. TB pyomyositis must be distinguished from pyogenic bacterial, or fungal abscesses, haematoma and neoplasms. Diagnosis is established by microbiological and molecular testing of the aspirated pus. Treatment consists of standard anti-TB treatment that may have to be extended in the individual patient. Effective drainage of the abscess is done by anti-gravity aspiration. When these measures fail, surgical exploration may be required (72).

REFERENCES

1. Hiremath BV, Subramaniam N. Primary breast tuberculosis: diagnostic and therapeutic dilemmas. Breast Dis 2015;35:187-93.
2. Tewari M, Shukla HS. Breast tuberculosis: diagnosis, clinical features and management. Indian J Med Res 2005;122:103-10.

3. Mirsaeidi SM, Masjedi MR, Mansouri SD, Velayati AA. Tuberculosis of the breast: report of 4 clinical cases and literature review. East Mediterr Health J 2007;13:670-6.

4. Morino GF, Rizzardi G, Gobbi F, Baldan M. Breast tuberculosis mimicking other diseases. Trop Doct 2007;37:177-8.

5. Bahadur P, Aurora AL, Sibbal RM, Prabhu SS. Tuberculosis of the mammary gland. J Indian Med Assoc 1983;21:67-80.

6. Rangabashyam N, Gnanaprakasm D, Krishnaraj B, Manohar V, Vijayalakshmi SR. Spectrum of benign breast lesions in Madras. J R Coll Surg Edinb 1983;28:369-73.

7. da Silva BB, Lopes-Costa PV, Pires CG, Pereira-Filho JD, dos Santos AR. Tuberculosis of the breast: analysis of 20 cases and a literature review. Trans R Soc Trop Med Hyg 2009;103:559-63.

8. Khodabakhshi B, Mehravar F. Breast tuberculosis in northeast Iran: review of 22 cases. BMC Womens Health 2014;14:72.

9. McKeown KC, Wilkinson KW. Tuberculous diseases of the breast. Br J Surg 1952;39:420-9.

10. Banerjee SN, Ananthakrishnan N, Mehta RB, Prakash S. Tuberculous mastitis: a continuing problem. World J Surg 1987;11:105-9.

11. Dharkar RS, Kanhere MH, Vaishya ND, Bisarya AK. Tuberculosis of the breast. J Indian Med Assoc 1968;50:207-9.

12. Domingo C, Ruiz J, Roig J, Texido A, Aguilar X, Morera J. Tuberculosis of the breast: a rare modern disease. Tubercle 1990;71:221-3.

13. Cooper A. Illustrations of the diseases of the breast. Part I. London: Longman, Rees, Orme, Brown and Green; 1829.p.73.

14. Chaudhary M. Tuberculosis of the breast. Br J Dis Chest 1957;23:195-9.

15. Thimmappa D, Mallikarjuna MN, Vijayakumar A. Breast Tuberculosis. Indian J Surg 2015;77 Suppl 3:1378-84.

16. Mallick D, Saha M, Chakrabarti S, Chakrabarty J. Tubercular breast abscess—a diagnostic dilemma. J Nepal Health Res Counc 2014;12:144-6.

17. Pal P, Patra SK, Ray S. An unusual cause of breast lump: isolated tuberculosis of the breast. Am J Trop Med Hyg 2014;90:788-9.

18. Gupta S, Singh VJ, Bhatia G, Dhuria K. Primary tuberculosis of the breast manifested as abscess: a rare case report. Acta Med Indones 2014;46:51-3.

19. Singal R, Dalal AK, Dalal U, Attri AK. Primary tuberculosis of the breast presented as multiple discharge sinuses. Indian J Surg 2013;75:66-7.

20. Tandon M, Chintamani, Panwar P. Breast tuberculosis at a tertiary care centre: a retrospective analysis of 22 cases. Breast Dis 2014;34: 127-30.

21. Singal R, Bala J, Gupta S, Goyal S, Mahajan N, Chawla A. Primary breast tuberculosis presenting as a lump: a rare modern disease. Ann Med Health Sci Res 2013;3:110-2.

22. Mukherjee P, George M, Maheshwari HB, Rao CP. Tuberculosis of the breast. J Indian Med Assoc 1974;62:410-2.

23. Hamit HF, Ragsdale TH. Mammary tuberculosis. JR Soc Med 1982;75:764-5.

24. Shukla HS, Kumar S. Benign breast disorders in nonwestern populations. Part II. Benign breast disorders in India. World J Surg 1989;13:746-9.

25. O'Reilly M, Patel KR, Cummins R. Tuberculosis of the breast presenting as carcinoma. Mil Med 2000;165:800-2.

26. Al-Marri MR, Almosleh A, Almoslmani Y. Primary tuberculosis of the breast in Qatar: ten year experience and review of literature. Eur J Surg 2000;166:687-90.

27. Wilson TS, MacGregor JW. The diagnosis and treatment of tuberculosis of the breast. Can Med Assoc J 1963;89:1118-24.

28. Brown S, Thekkinkattil DK. Tuberculous cold abscess of breast: an unusual presentation in a male patient. Gland Surg 2016;5:361-5.

29. Cantisani C, Lazic T, Salvi M, Richetta AG, Frascani F, De Gado F, et al. Male tuberculous mastitis: a rare entity. Clin Ter 2013;164: e293-5.

30. Khandelwal R, Jain I. Breast tuberculosis mimicking a malignancy: a rare case report with review of literature. Breast Dis 2013;34: 53-5.

31. Siddiqui B, Akhter K, Faridi SH, Maheshwari V. A case of coexisting carcinoma and tuberculosis in one breast. J Transl Int Med 2015;3:32-4.

32. Bansal A, Sipayya V, Chintamani C, Saxena S. Carcinoma and tuberculosis of the breast coexisting in same breast with axillary lymphadenopathy: A rare association. Indian J Cancer 2015;52: 229-30.

33. Shinde SR, Chandawarkar RY, Deshmukh SP. Tuberculosis of the breast masquerading as carcinoma: a study of 100 patients. World J Surg 1995;19:379-81.

34. Fujii T, Kimura M, Yanagita Y, Koida T, Kuwano H. Tuberculosis of axillary lymph nodes with primary breast cancer. Breast Cancer 2003;10:175-8.

35. Longman CF, Campion T, Butler B, Suaris TD, Khanam A, Kunst H, et al. Imaging features and diagnosis of tuberculosis of the breast. Clin Radiol 2017; pii: S0009-9260[16]30502-5.

36. Makanjuola D, Murshid K, Al Sulaimani S, Al Saleh M. Mammographic features of breast tuberculosis: the skin bulge and sinus tract sign. Clin Radiol 1996;51:354-8.

37. Schnarkowski P, Schmidt D, Kessler M, Reiser MF. Tuberculosis of the breast: US, mammographic, and CT findings. J Comput Assist Tomogr 1994;18:970-1.

38. Muttarak M, Pojchamarnwiputh S, Chaiwun B. Mammographic features of tuberculous axillary lymphadenitis. Australas Radiol 2002;46:260-3.

39. Oh KK, Kim JH, Kook SH. Imaging of tuberculous disease involving breast. Eur Radiol 1998;8:1475-80.

40. Bassett LW, Kimme-Smith C. Breast sonography. Am J Roentgenol 1991;156:449-55.

41. Chung SY, Yang I, Bae SH, Lee Y, Park HJ, Kim HH, et al. Tuberculous abscess in retromammary region: CT findings. J Comput Assist Tomogr 1996;20:766-9.

42. Shojaku H, Noguchi K, Kamei T, Tanada Y, Yoshida K, Adachi Y, Matsui K. CT findings of axillary tuberculosis lymphadenitis: a case detected by breast cancer screening examination. Case Rep Radiol 2016;2016:9016517.

43. Romero C, Carrerira C, Cereceda C, Pinto J, Lopez R, Bolanos F. Mammary tuberculosis: percutaneous treatment of mammary tuberculous abscess. Eur Radiol 2000;10:531-3.

44. Bhatt GM, Austin HM. CT demonstration of empyema necessitates. J Comput Assist Tomogr 1985;9:1108-9.

45. Heywang SH. Contrast-enhanced MRI of the breast. Basel: Karger; 1990.

46. Fellah L, Leconte I, Weynand B, Donnez J, Berlière M. Breast tuberculosis imaging. Fertil Steril 2006;86:460-1.

47. Al-Khawari HA, Al-Manfouhi HA, Madda JP, Kovacs A, Sheikh M, Roberts O. Radiologic features of granulomatous mastitis. Breast J 2011;17:645-50.

48. Das CJ, Kumar R, Balakrishnan VB, Chawla M, Malhotra A. Disseminated tuberculosis masquerading as metastatic breast carcinoma on PET-CT. Clin Nucl Med 2008;33:359-61.

49. Bakheet SM, Powe J, Kandil A, Ezzat A, Rostom A, Amartey J. F-18 FDG uptake in breast infection and inflammation. Clin Nucl Med 2000;25:100-3.

50. Lee JW, Lee SM, Choi JH. ^{18}F-FDG PET/CT findings in a breast cancer patient with concomitant tuberculous axillary lymphadenitis. Nucl Med Mol Imaging 2011;45:152-5.

51. Kakkar S, Kapila K, Singh MK, Verma K. Tuberculosis of the breast. A cytomorphologic study. Acta Cytol 2000;44:292-6.

52. Chandanwale SS, Buch AC, Gore CR, Ramanpreet KC, Jadhav P. Fine needle aspiration cytology in breast tuberculosis: diagnostic difficulties—study of eleven cases. Indian J Tuberc 2012;59:162-7.

53. Mittal P, Handa U, Mohan H, Gupta V. Comparative evaluation of fine needle aspiration cytology, culture, and PCR in diagnosis of tuberculous lymphadenitis. Diagn Cytopathol 2011;39:822-6.

54. Bezabih M, Mariam DW, Selassie SG. Fine needle aspiration cytology of suspected tuberculous lymphadenitis. Cytopathology 2002;13:284-90.

55. Kumar P, Sharma N. Primary MDR-TB of the breast. Indian J Chest Dis Allied Sci 2003;45:63-5.

56. Polepole P, Kabwe M, Kasonde M, Tembo J, Shibemba A, O'Grady J, et al. Performance of the Xpert MTB/RIF assay in the diagnosis of tuberculosis in formalin-fixed, paraffin-embedded tissues. Int J Mycobacteriol 2017;6:87-93.

57. Kilic MO, Sağlam C, Ağca FD, Terzioğlu SG. Clinical, diagnostic and therapeutic management of patients with breast tuberculosis: analysis of 46 Cases. Kaohsiung J Med Sci 2016;32:27-31.

58. Kilic MO, Sağlam C, Ağca FD, Terzioğlu SG. Clinical, diagnostic and therapeutic management of patients with breast tuberculosis: analysis of 46 Cases. Kaohsiung J Med Sci 2016;32:27-31.

59. Petersdorf R, Beeson P. Fever of unexplained origin: report on 100 cases. Medicine [Baltimore] 1961;40:1-30.

60. Durack DT, Street AC. Fever of unknown origin—reexamined and redefined. Curr Clin Trop Infect Dis 1991;11:35-51.

61. Kejariwal D, Sarkar N, Chakraborti SK, Agarwal V, Roy S. Pyrexia of unknown origin: a prospective study of 100 cases. J Postgrad Med 2001;47:104-7.

62. Bandyopadhyay D, Bandyopadhyay R, Paul R, Roy D. Etiological study of fever of unknown origin in patients admitted to medicine ward of a teaching hospital of eastern India. J Glob Infect Dis 2011;3:329-33.

63. Handa R, Singh S, Singh N, Wali JP. Fever of unknown origin: a prospective study. Trop Doct 1996;26:169-70.

64. Arun Kumar D. Epidemiology and aetiology of pyrexia of unknown origin: a prospective study [MD Thesis]. Tirupati: Sri Venkateswara Institute of Medical Sciences; 2016.

65. Tariq SM, Tariq S. Empirical treatment for tuberculosis: survey of cases treated over 2 years in a London area. J Pak Med Assoc 2004;54:88-95.

66. Anglaret X, Saba J, Perronne C, Lacassin F, Longuet P, Leport C, et al. Empiric antituberculosis treatment: benefits for earlier diagnosis and treatment of tuberculosis. Tuber Lung Dis 1994;75:334-40.

67. Lupatkin H, Bräu N, Flomenberg P, Simberkoff MS. Tuberculous abscesses in patients with AIDS. Clin Infect Dis 1992;14:1040-4.

68. Osorio J, Barreto J, Benavides J, López Ó, Cuenca Á, García E. Tuberculous pyomyositis in an immunosuppressed patient. Biomedica 2016;36:23-8.

69. Indudhara R, Singh SK, Minz M, Yadav RV, Chugh KS. Tuberculous pyomyositis in a renal transplant recipient. Tuber Lung Dis 1992;73:239-41.

70. Sen RK, Tripathy SK, Dhatt S, Saini R, Aggarwal S, Agarwal A. Primary tuberculous pyomyositis of forearm muscles. Indian J Tuberc 2010;57:34-40.

71. Baylan O, Demiralp B, Cicek EI, Albay A, Komurcu M, Kisa O, et al. A case of tuberculous pyomyositis that caused a recurrent soft tissue lesion localized at the forearm. Jpn J Infect Dis 2005;58:376-9.

72. Narang S. Tuberculous pyomyositis of forearm muscles. Hand [N Y] 2009;4:88-91.

73. Chen WL, Lin YF, Tsai WC, Tsao YT. Unveiling tuberculous pyomyositis: an emerging role of immune reconstitution inflammatory syndrome. Am J Emerg Med 2009;27:251.e1-2.

74. Dhakal AK, Shah SC, Shrestha D, Banepali N, Geetika KC. Tuberculosis presenting as multiple intramuscular nodules in a child: a case report. J Med Case Rep 2015;9:72.

31

Complications of Pulmonary Tuberculosis

D Behera

INTRODUCTION

Complications of pulmonary tuberculosis [TB] significantly contribute to morbidity and mortality of patients and are listed in Table 31.1.

HAEMOPTYSIS

Haemoptysis is a common and potentially serious complication of pulmonary TB (1-4). The incidence of haemoptysis in patients with pulmonary TB is reported to range from 30%-35% (1-3). Occurrence of haemoptysis does not imply that the TB is active. Haemoptysis may occur as the initial manifestation of active TB, during the course of treatment, or, even after the disease is apparently cured. Haemoptysis can be streaky or massive and life-threatening. Massive haemoptysis may be associated with atelectasis [Figure 31.1]. Important causes of haemoptysis in patients with pulmonary TB are listed in Table 31.2.

Walls of a TB cavity may be affected by inflammation and necrosis and may become atrophic. Increased pressure can lead to weakening of the walls, dilatation of blood vessels and formation of Rasmussen's aneurysms (5,6) [Figure 31.2]. Further, these blood vessels rupture due to increased pressure during strenuous exercise or coughing

Table 31.1: Complications of pulmonary TB
Local
Pulmonary
Haemoptysis
Post-TB bronchiectasis
Fungal ball [aspergilloma]
TB endobronchitis and tracheitis
Scar carcinoma
Disseminated calcification of the lungs
Pulmonary function changes, obstructive airways disease
Secondary pyogenic infections
Nontuberculous mycobacterial disease
Pleural
Spontaneous pneumothorax
Pleural thickening [fibrothorax]
Acute and chronic empyema
Systemic
Secondary amyloidosis
Chronic respiratory failure [Type I and Type II]
Pulmonary hypertension
Chronic cor-pulmonale
TB = tuberculosis

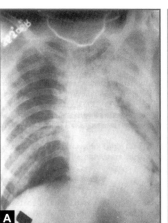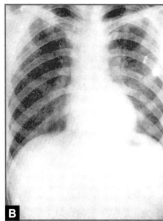

Figure 31.1: Chest radiograph [postero-anterior view] of a patient who presented with massive haemoptysis showing collapse of the left lung [A]. Chest radiograph [postero-anterior view] of the same patient following vigorous chest physiotherapy and suction showing bilateral clearance of both the lung fields. Sputum smear revealed *Mycobacterium tuberculosis* [B]
Reproduced with permission from "Sharma SK, Mohan A. Pulmonary tuberculosis: typical and atypical cases. Case track series 1. Mumbai: Merind; 1997 (reference 3)"

and can result in haemoptysis [Figure 31.3]. The vessel walls can also be eroded directly either because of endarteritis, or, vasculitis secondary to TB. Sometimes intense allergic response to antigen[s] of *Mycobacterium tuberculosis* [*Mtb*] damages the vessel wall and gives rise to haemoptysis. Bleeding from TB granulomas in the bronchi can result in haemoptysis. Blood vessels with aneurysmal dilatation and accentuated bronchopulmonary communications are present surrounding these granulomas. In this setting, the bronchial blood vessels which are under systemic pressure can be the source of bleeding. All these factors should be taken into consideration while managing haemoptysis in patients with TB.

In most instances bed rest, sedation, and resuscitative measures aimed at restoring fluid balance and haemodynamic status control the bleeding. Patients presenting with massive haemoptysis [> 600 mL of blood in 24 hours] may become haemodynamically unstable and require blood transfusion. Broad spectrum antibiotics are administered to treat super-added bacterial infection. Anti-TB treatment is indicated in patients with active TB. However, if the bleeding is massive, and repetitive, fibreoptic bronchoscopy [to localise the site of bleeding] and high resolution computed tomography [HRCT] are performed. Angiography along with bronchial artery embolisation is done in patients with massive haemoptysis [Figure 31.4] (7-9). Bronchial artery embolisation [BAE] is a good and relatively safe procedure in the management of haemoptysis due to pulmonary TB. The risk of re-bleeding after BAE in active or inactive pulmonary TB is high, particularly in patients with destroyed lung, chronic liver disease, the use of anticoagulant agents and/or antiplatelet agents, elevated pre-BAE C-reactive protein [CRP], and the existence of fungal ball (10). Rarely, resection of the site of bleeding may be indicated (11-13).

ASPERGILLOMA [MYCETOMA; "FUNGUS BALL"]

Mycetoma is a mass of fungal hyphal material that grows in a lung cavity. Although other fungi like *Zygomycetes* [mucor] and *Fusarium* may cause the formation of a fungal ball, *Aspergillus* species, particularly, *Aspergillus fumigatus*, are by far the most common aetiological agents. The overall incidence of aspergilloma in general population has been estimated to be between 0.01% in Great Britain to 0.017% in the USA (14,15). In a large multicentric study by the British Tuberculosis Association (14), which surveyed 544 patients with healed TB cavities on chest films, measuring 2.5 cm or greater in diameter, 25% had precipitins to *Aspergillus* in serum and radiographic evidence of aspergilloma was present in 11% patients. Aspergilloma occurred as frequently in patients with recently healed TB as in those with inactive disease for long periods (14). A follow-up study (15) of this group, 3 years after the first survey, revealed an increase in incidence of aspergilloma to 17%.

Table 31.2: Causes of haemoptysis in pulmonary TB
Bleeding from cavity wall
Rupture of Rasmussen's aneurysm
Direct erosion of capillaries or arteries by granulomatous inflammation
TB endobronchitis
Post-TB bronchiectasis
Aspergilloma
Broncholith, cavernolith
Scar carcinoma
TB = tuberculosis

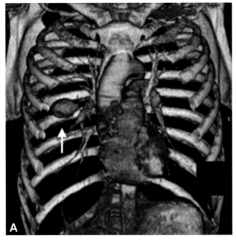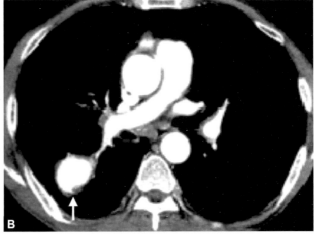

Figure 31.2: Rasmussen's aneurysm. Dynamic and three-dimensional views of the pulmonary and bronchial vasculature on computed tomography obtained after the injection of contrast material demonstrated a large pulmonary aneurysm [A and B, arrows] obtained from a 54-year-old man who presented with a 3-month history of haemoptysis. The patient underwent successful embolisation of the pulmonary artery aneurysm and its feeding vessel. However, the haemoptysis resolved only after subsequent embolisation of the bronchial artery
Reproduced with permission from "van den Heuvel MM, van Rensburg JJ. Images in clinical medicine. Rasmussen's aneurysm. N Engl J Med 2006;355:e17 (reference 5)" Copyright [2006] Massachusetts Medical Society. All rights reserved

The new aspergilloma cases were generally patients who had only serum precipitins during the first survey (14,15). Aspergillomas have been identified in cavities associated with TB, histoplasmosis, sarcoidosis, bronchial cysts, bullae, neoplasms, pulmonary infarctions, asbestosis, ankylosing spondylitis, bronchiectasis, and malignant diseases (16,17). Of these, TB is the most frequently associated condition (18). Occasionally, these are described in cavities due to other fungal infections (19,20).

The natural history of an aspergilloma is highly variable and it may remain stable, increase in size or spontaneously resolve. In the early phase of its development, the fungus ball grows inside a lung cavity consisting of both living and dead fungus. The future course depends upon the predominance of these living or dead fungi. If local conditions favour death, the fungus ball liquefies and the secretions are expectorated out. Calcification occurs less frequently.

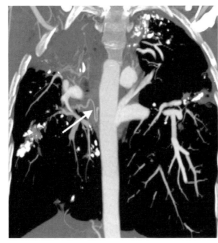

Figure 31.3: Coronal maximum intensity projection of pulmonary angiographic image showing hypertrophic and tortous right bronchial artery [arrow], branches from subclavian artery along with extensive fibrocalcific changes in both upper lobes

Clinical Features

The fungus ball may be present for long periods without any clinical symptoms and may be an incidental finding in majority of cases and the lesion remains stable. In approximately 10% of cases, it may increase in size or resolve spontaneously without treatment (21). Rarely, the aspergilloma increases in size (14). But eventually, most of these will manifest with some symptoms. The most common presentation in such cases is haemoptysis and the estimated frequency varies from 5%-90%. The amount may be very minimal to severe particularly in patients with associated TB (22). Bleeding usually occurs from the bronchial blood vessels. The exact cause of haemoptysis associated with aspergilloma is not certain, but has been ascribed to [i] mechanical friction of mycetoma; [ii] an endotoxin with haemolytic properties; [iii] an anticoagulant factor derived from *Aspergillus;* [iv] local vasculitis; and [v] direct vascular invasion in cavity wall vessels (23-26). The mortality rate varies between 2%-14%. Other features include chronic cough, weight loss, and rarely fever and dyspnoea (23-26).

Risk factors associated with poor prognosis of aspergilloma include severe underlying disease, increasing size or number of lesions as seen on chest radiograph, immunocompromised state including corticosteroid therapy, increasing *Aspergillus*-specific immunoglobulin G [IgG] titres, recurrent large volume haemoptysis, and underlying sarcoidosis or human immunodeficiency virus [HIV] infection (27).

Diagnosis

Aspergilloma usually comes to clinical attention as an incidental finding on a routine chest radiographic examination or during an evaluation of haemoptysis. The typical radiographic appearance of aspergilloma is described as a bell-like image, with the fungus ball appearing as a clapper inside a bell. A semi-circular crescentic air shadow

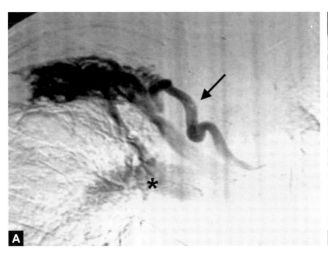
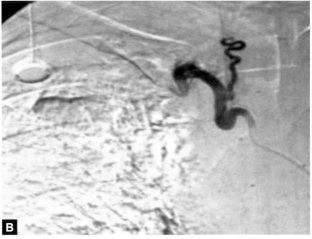

Figure 31.4: Intra-arterial digital subtraction angiography [IA-DSA] in a patient with right upper lobe pulmonary tuberculosis showing a hypertrophied intercosto-bronchial trunk [arrow] producing contrast extravasation [asterisk] and pulmonary artery filling in the region of fibrocavitary lesion [A]. The IA-DSA after embolisation with polyvinyl alcohol particles showing obliteration of the angiographic abnormality with patent parent artery [B]

appears around the radio-opaque fungus ball located in an upper lobe lung cavity (28). The fungus ball is mobile and changes its position as the patient moves, which is best seen on fluoroscopy or by taking chest radiographs or computed tomography [CT] [Figure 31.5] at different positions. A change in position of the aspergilloma with the change in position of the patient is an interesting but a variable sign (29). Occasionally, it may be difficult to recognise the mass on a routine chest radiograph, and tomography or chest CT may be necessary to visualise the aspergilloma. The adjacent pleura may be thickened. The radiographic differential diagnosis includes organised haematoma or pus inside a cavity, neoplasm, abscess, Wegener's granulomatosis and a ruptured hydatid cyst. An aspergilloma may co-exist with any of these conditions also.

The initial suspicion of a fungus ball is raised from the chest radiograph. Sputum culture may confirm the presence of fungus, but may be negative in about 50% of cases (30). The serum precipitins [IgG antibodies] to *Aspergillus* are positive in almost 100% of cases except in cases of

aspergilloma due to other *Aspergillus* species or if the patient is on corticosteroid therapy (31). Skin tests are less helpful and may be positive only in a minority of patients (30). In some cases bronchoscopy may be helpful in identifying the site of bleeding and sometimes one may see the fungus ball in direct continuity with the bronchial lumen. Bronchial washings, brushings and forceps biopsy may be carried out to isolate *Aspergillus*.

Treatment

The treatment of aspergilloma is controversial because of variability in its natural history. No therapy is warranted in asymptomatic cases. Systemic antifungal therapy is ineffective in treating these lesions. The antifungal drugs cannot penetrate into the intracavitary fungi (32). Attempts are made to instil local intrabronchial intracavitary or inhalational antifungal agents [amphotericin B, nystatin, sodium iodide] with varying success (33-35). Systemic antifungal therapy using intravenous amphotericin-B has no effect (36). Itraconazole therapy has been tried with varying

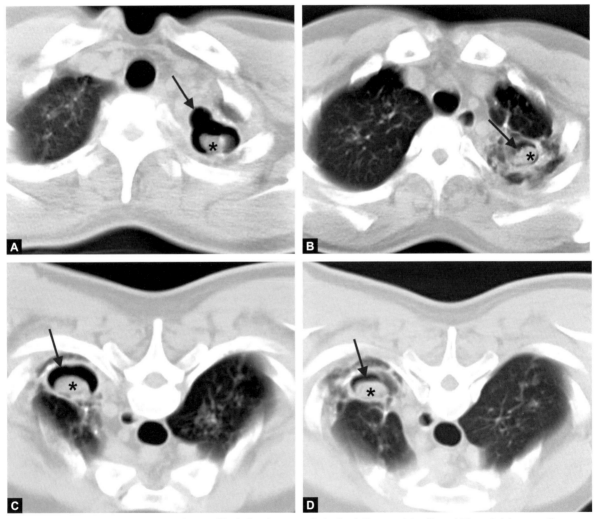

Figure 31.5: CT of the chest [lung window, supine position] showing a cavity in the left upper lobe [A and B] containing a radio-opaque shadow with a semicircular air crescent around it [arrow] suggestive of a fungal ball [asterisk]. When the CT is repeated with the patient in the prone position [C and D], the fungal ball can be seen to have changed its position

success (37). Bronchial artery embolisation rarely controls haemoptysis because of extensive collateral blood vessels. This procedure may, however, be used as a temporary measure to control massive, life-threatening haemoptysis (38).

Some advocate routine surgery because of the fear of haemoptysis in future. However, the clinical approach should be individualised. In some cases the severity of the underlying lung disease will not allow surgical resection, even in the presence of life-threatening haemoptysis. The surgical treatment of aspergilloma is associated with a relatively high mortality rate that ranges between 7% and 23% (39,40). The most common causes of death following surgery are severe underlying lung disease, pneumonia, acute myocardial infarction, and invasive pulmonary aspergillosis. In addition, there is a significant post-operative morbidity, including bleeding, residual pleural space, bronchopleural fistula, empyema, and respiratory failure. In younger patients with adequate lung reserve the morbidity and mortality are lower (41,42).

The best approach seems to wait and watch and surgery is indicated only when there is repeated and severe haemoptysis. Patients with mild infrequent haemoptysis or without symptoms may be observed carefully. Surgical approach needs to be considered in patients with massive haemoptysis and adequate pulmonary reserve (39-43).

In a recent reported series (44) of aspergilloma [n = 35; median age 43.4 years; 28 males] the average time to consultation was 19.4 [range 1-120] months. All patients had a history of pulmonary TB. Haemoptysis was the most commonly observed symptom [54.3%]. *Aspergillus* serology was positive in 22 patients. Various surgical procedures performed including 14 lobectomies, 1 bilobectomy, 1 segmentectomy, 1 bisegmentectomy, 3 lobectomies with segmentectomies, 1 bilobectomy with segmentectomy, and 14 pleuropneumonectomies. One patient with pulmonary artery damage required repair. Complications were: empyema [n = 3], a large air-leak [n = 1], parietal suppuration [n = 5], and pleural effusion [n = 3]. There was no immediate post-operative mortality. On follow-up [median duration 35 months], recurrence of haemoptysis was seen in one patient; three patients died of respiratory failure [one at 6 months and the other two at 1 year after the surgery] (44). Cavernostomy has been found to be useful in complicated cases (45).

Mycetoma and Human Immunodeficiency Virus Infection

Pulmonary mycetomas have also been documented in HIV-seropositive individuals (24,46-48). Although life-threatening haemoptysis has occasionally been documented (46), it appears to be a relatively rare manifestation in HIV-seropositive patients with pulmonary mycetoma. In a study (24) comparing the clinical presentation, disease progression, treatment, and outcome of pulmonary mycetoma in patients with [n = 10], and without [n = 15] HIV infection, the following observations were documented.

Although TB and sarcoidosis were the most prevalent predisposing diseases, a history of *Pneumocystis jirovecii* pneumonia and the consequent cavitation was found to be a risk factor for pulmonary aspergilloma in HIV-infected individuals. In HIV-seropositive patients with a CD4+ count of less than or equal to 100 cells/µL, the disease progressed despite treatment. Compared with HIV-seropositive patients, significant haemoptysis requiring intervention was more likely in HIV-seronegative individuals.

In another study (48), *Pneumocystis jirovecii* pneumonia was found to be a risk factor for pulmonary mycetoma in the HIV-infected individuals. These workers (48) also reported that though the disease progressed rapidly, life-threatening haemoptysis rarely occurred in HIV-infected patients with mycetoma. A combination of anti-fungal and antiretroviral therapy [ART] may improve the clinical outcome in HIV-infected patients with pulmonary mycetoma.

POST-TUBERCULOSIS BRONCHIECTASIS

The pathogenesis of bronchiectasis in TB is multi-factorial (49). Caseation necrosis and granulomatous inflammation in the wall of the dilated and destroyed bronchi suggest that this may represent an extension of the TB process. Scarring that follows TB inflammation produces bronchial stenosis. This, when followed by mixed bacterial infection and retention of purulent bacterial secretions, leads to destruction and dilatation of the bronchi as is the case with other types of bronchiectasis.

The ongoing pathological changes may be perpetuated by products of inflammation. Compression of the bronchial lumen by enlarged lymph nodes produces consequences similar to those of an intraluminal obstruction. This is more so in the case of young children and adolescents in whom TB hilar lymphadenitis is more common. In both these situations, inflammatory destruction of the bronchial wall is by and large the sequelae of secondary bacterial infection rather than the direct effect of *Mtb*. Another rare, but important cause of bronchial obstruction is penetration of the airway by a calcified TB lymph node and the formation of broncholith. Some or all of the bronchiectatic cavities may represent healing or healed TB cavities that have been re-lined with ciliated columnar epithelium. Bronchiectasis structurally resembles small/large cavities in the bronchial wall. Recently, it has been reported that, *M. avium-intracellulare* infection of the lungs is associated with bronchiectasis in apparently healthy individuals, or, in persons with emphysema. It seems that such an association may either be due to a primary infection or colonisation. Post-TB bronchiectasis is commonly seen in the upper lobes, since the disease is more common at this site. It is a "dry" or "sicca" type of bronchiectasis because of the effective drainage of the upper lobes by gravity. The usual presentation is with haemoptysis or repeated episodes of secondary bacterial infection.

Although the chest radiograph is important in the evaluation of a patient with suspected post-TB bronchiectasis, the findings are often non-specific. Bronchography used to be performed earlier with a radio-opaque, iodinated lipid dye for visualisation of the dilated airways. However, in the recent years, it has been replaced by CT. As compared to the bronchography, the CT is a relatively non-invasive investigation.

TUBERCULOSIS ENDOBRONCHITIS AND TRACHEITIS

TB endobronchitis and tracheitis are observed in about one-third of the patients with pulmonary TB (50). These structures can be infected by direct implantation of *Mtb*, through submucosal lymphatics, haematogenous spread or from the lymph nodes. Clinical manifestations include cough, haemoptysis, breathlessness and soreness or constriction in the sub-sternal region. Healing can lead to bronchostenosis. The reader is referred to the chapter *"Endobronchial tuberculosis" [Chapter 12]* for more details.

SPONTANEOUS PNEUMOTHORAX

Spontaneous pneumothorax has been reported in 5%-15% of patients with pulmonary TB (51,52). In countries where TB is a common problem, it is an important cause of pneumothorax [Figure 31.6]. Spontaneous pneumothorax may result from rupture of a subpleural TB cavity into the pleural space. Infection of pleural cavity results in pyopneumothorax. Other causes of pneumothorax include rupture of an open healed cavity or rupture of a bleb or bulla [Figure 31.7] secondary to fibrosis and destruction of the lung (53).

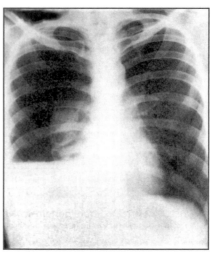

Figure 31.6: Chest radiograph [postero-anterior view] showing hydro-pneumothorax on the right side

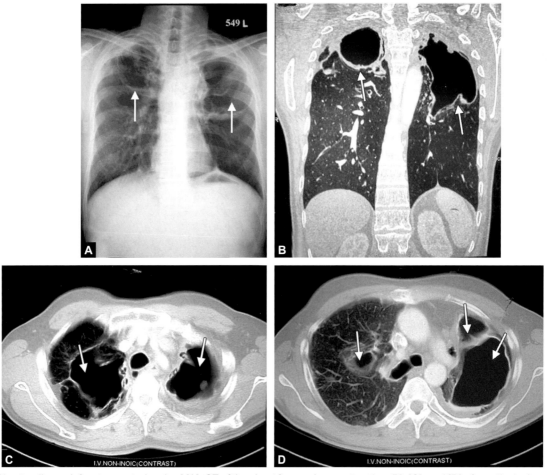

Figure 31.7: Chest radiograph [postero-anterior view] [A], CT of the chest [coronal reconstruction, B], [C], and [D] of a patient who presented with breathlessness showing bilateral bullous lung disease [arrows]. This patient had sputum smear-positive pulmonary tuberculosis a decade ago and had received adequate antituberculosis treatment

CALCIFICATION

Lung lesions of TB heal by calcification. In fact, localised or extensive calcification of the lungs is a feature of healed primary TB (52). Calcification can either be microscopic or macroscopic. Most often these calcifications are innocuous and present as discrete radio-opaque shadows in patients with parenchymal disease [Figure 31.8] and sheet-like calcification in patients with pleural disease [Figure 31.9]. Occasionally, however, these calcified concretions may get detached from the lung tissue and erode through a bronchial wall or blood vessel and result in massive haemoptysis. The patient may also give history of coughing out calcified stones in the sputum [broncholiths or pneumoliths]. Extensive calcification, may result in respiratory failure or chronic cor-pulmonale.

TUBERCULOSIS LARYNGITIS

Involvement of larynx during the course of pulmonary TB occurs in about 4%-40% of cases (54). The incidence increases with extensive involvement of lungs and presence of cavitary disease. The usual mode of infection is by direct implantation or through lymphatics and blood vessels. The symptoms include soreness or pain in the throat, dry, hacking cough and hoarseness of voice. Laryngoscopy may reveal an ulcer, granuloma, paresis or paralysis, destruction of cords, or stenosis of the vocal cords. The vocal cords, arytenoids and the inter-arytenoid space are most commonly affected. The sputum is usually positive for *Mtb*. The reader is referred to the Chapter *"Tuberculosis in head and neck" [Chapter 23]* for details.

TUBERCULOSIS ENTERITIS

TB enteritis seldom occurs as a complication of pulmonary TB in the present era. The reader is referred to the chapter *"Abdominal tuberculosis" [Chapter 15]* for further details.

"OPEN-NEGATIVE" SYNDROME

Patients with "open-negative syndrome" have thin walled cavities with epithelialisation extending from bronchioles down to the inner lining of the cavity (55-57). These are observed more frequently following the advent of chemotherapy. Although they are known as "isoniazid cavities", they can also occur due to other antituberculosis drugs. Complete epithelialisation prevents these cavities to collapse and fibrose but renders them innocuous. From a clinical point of view, they are regarded as inactive cavities. However, histopathological examination of such cavities may reveal incomplete epithelialisation and necrotic foci showing *Mtb*. These present radiologically as "ring shadows" with thin walls.

Although the cavities themselves will not produce any symptoms, they are associated with certain hazards like secondary infection, colonisation with fungi producing fungal balls, scar carcinoma, spontaneous pneumothorax, and loss of effective volume of the lungs.

SCAR CARCINOMA

Development of lung cancer in association with old scars [scar carcinoma] is common in conditions, such as progressive systemic sclerosis with lung involvement. The relationship between the scars of pulmonary TB and lung cancer has been a matter of debate for a long time. In the series reported by Auerbach *et al* (58), scar cancer was observed in 82 of the 1186 autopsied cases [1%]; 23.2% of these had originated from TB scars. A similar association between scars of TB and lung cancer has been documented in several other reports (59,60). However, other reports indicate that the association between TB and lung cancer was merely coincidental (61,62).

Impaired lung ventilation and concomitant increase in pulmonary carbon dioxide levels, which in turn causes pronounced hyperplasia of pulmonary neuroendocrine cells

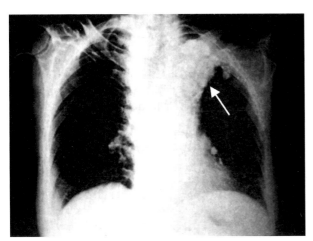

Figure 31.8: Chest radiograph [postero-anterior view] showing parenchymal calcification on the left side [arrow]

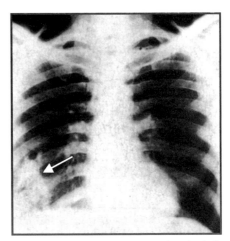

Figure 31.9: Chest radiograph [postero-anterior view] showing sheet-like pleural calcification on the right side [arrow]

have been postulated as the possible mechanisms underlying the genesis of lung cancer in patients with chronic lung diseases. A receptor with sensitivity for oxygen and carbon dioxide which produce a number of autocrine growth factors is considered to be crucial in the malignant transformation (63-65). A review (66) has discussed some of these issues including TB as a cause of lung cancer and simultaneous development of TB in lung cancer or TB developing in case of lung cancer. Various suggestions like a chance coincidence without any apparent relation, metastatic carcinoma developing in an old TB lesion, occurrence of TB in a patient with cancer, chronic progressive TB in which a carcinoma develops and simultaneous development of both TB and cancer (66). These issues merit further study.

In a population cohort study (67) of 716,872 insured subjects, incidence of lung cancer in patients with newly diagnosed TB [n=4480] and the remaining non-TB subjects was compared. Patients with TB were found to have a 11-fold higher incidence of lung cancers compared to non-TB subjects. Cox proportional hazard regression analysis showed for the TB cohort, the hazard ratio [HR] increased further with co-existing chronic obstructive pulmonary disease [COPD] or other smoking-related cancers suggesting a strong evidence of lung cancer risk among TB patients (67).

In another retrospective study (68) of 782 patients with non-small cell lung cancer [NSCLC] who had undergone surgical resection the association between lung cancer survival and the presence of old pulmonary TB lesions was assessed. The authors (68) reported that presence of an old pulmonary TB lesion was an independent predictor of poor survival [HR 1.72] in the subgroup of patients with squamous cell carcinoma.

In another surgical series (69), co-existence of TB and lung cancer in thoracic surgery was found to be fairly rare, being evident only in 46 cases [2.1%] out of 2218 operated lung cancer patients. Another study revealed that most of the patients with TB and lung cancer are smokers or former smokers, and TB is diagnosed either before or simultaneously with lung cancer. NSCLC, especially adenocarcinoma, was the most common histopathological type (70).

A systemic review and meta-analysis (71) evaluated the history of previous lung diseases as a risk factor for lung cancer. In this meta-analysis (71), it was observed that a previous history of COPD, chronic bronchitis or emphysema, pneumonia, TB had conferred an increased risk of lung cancer. The authors (71) reported that data from 30 studies suggested that a previous history of TB conferred an increased risk of lung cancer {relative risk [RR] 1.76} and this increased risk of lung cancer was independent of smoking [RR 1.90].

PULMONARY FUNCTION CHANGES

Diffuse airway obstruction has been reported in 30%-60% of cases with pulmonary TB (72,73), which is distinct from chronic bronchitis. Further, because of diffuse parenchymal fibrosis, pleural effusion and thickening, and fibrothorax, a restrictive type of pulmonary function defect is also possible. Thus, in a patient with pulmonary TB, obstructive, restrictive, or a mixed type of lung function abnormality is possible depending upon the type and extent of involvement or residual damage (74). A study (75) from New Delhi assessed the post-treatment sequelae in multidrug-resistant TB [MDR-TB] patients [n = 130] who were initiated on standardised treatment. Of these, 24 had died while on treatment. Of the remaining 106 patients, 63 [59%] patients could be traced: 51 were currently alive and 12 had died. At 24-months [range 6-63 months] of post-treatment follow-up [n = 51], 40 [78%] had persistent respiratory symptoms; 44 of the 45 tested [98%] had residual radiological sequelae with 18/45 [40%] having far advanced involvement. On pulmonary function testing [n = 47] abnormal results were observed in 45 [96%] patients. A predominantly mixed type of abnormality was seen in 31 [66%]; restrictive pattern in 9 [19%] and obstructive pattern 5 [11%] patients. None of the patients were found to be bacteriologically positive (75).

In another study (76) from Indonesia, morbidity at baseline and during treatment, and 6-month residual disability, was assessed in 200 pulmonary patients and 40 volunteers. In pulmonary TB patients, the six-minute walk test distance, quality of life and pulmonary functions were significantly lower at the baseline as well as at the end of 6 months of anti-TB treatment compared with controls. At the end of 6 months of anti-TB treatment, despite most achieving successful treatment outcomes, 57% TB patients still had respiratory symptoms and 27% had moderate to severe pulmonary function impairment. More-advanced disease at baseline and HIV-seropositivity were found to be predictors of residual disability (76). Another study (77) from Gujarat, India assessed pulmonary impairment in cured pulmonary TB patients [n = 264]. Majority of these complained of cough [n = 224, 84%] with expectoration [n = 184, 69.7%]. Physical examination revealed rhonchi, crepitations or both in 178 [67.4%] patients. The chest radiograph revealed varying degrees of lung destruction with a majority [n = 145, 38%] having involvement of two or more lobes; 223 of the 257 [87%] patients tested had obstructive airways disease. Electrocardiogram and echocardiography revealed pulmonary hypertension in 72 of the 76 patients tested (77).

CHRONIC RESPIRATORY FAILURE

Chronic respiratory failure [type I and type II] may complicate pulmonary TB, especially if the disease had been extensive and the patient survived because of adequate treatment. Respiratory failure develops due to extensive destruction of pulmonary parenchyma [Figures 31.10 and 31.11] and the resultant ventilation-perfusion [V/Q] mismatch.

Associated pleural thickening and fibrothorax result in thoracic wall malfunction and further add to the mechanical disadvantage of the lung, thus contributing to the pump failure (78-80). Atrophy or disuse of the respiratory muscles can also contribute to chronic respiratory failure. Tachypnoea, hypoxia and hypercapnia develop ultimately and the patient may die from these abnormalities.

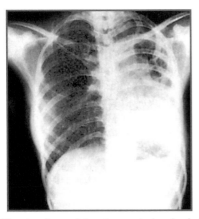

Figure 31.10: Chest radiograph [postero-anterior view] of a patient with old, healed pulmonary tuberculosis showing extensive parenchymal destruction, bronchiectatic changes and pleural thickening on the left side. On the right side, compensatory emphysema and pseudobulla formation can be seen

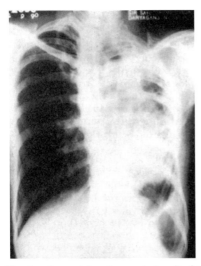

Figure 31.11: Chest radiograph [postero-anterior view] of a patient with pulmonary tuberculosis showing extensive parenchymal destruction, bronchiectatic changes and pleural thickening on the left side. On the right side, compensatory emphysema can be seen

PULMONARY HYPERTENSION AND CHRONIC COR-PULMONALE

Chronic *cor-pulmonale* is defined as enlargement [dilatation and/or hypertrophy] of the right ventricle due to increased right ventricular afterload from intrinsic pulmonary diseases including those of pulmonary circulation, inadequate function of the chest bellows or inadequate ventilatory drive from the respiratory centres; when right heart abnormalities secondary to left heart failure or congenital heart disease are excluded. Right heart failure need not be present, although this is a clinical manifestation of the overloaded right ventricle that precedes the clinically unrecognisable cor-pulmonale. Except in rare instances when the disease is complicated by massive pulmonary thromboembolism, cor-pulmonale is usually chronic.

The possible causes of chronic cor-pulmonale in pulmonary TB include abnormalities of the pulmonary parenchyma or thoracic wall. The underlying basic pathophysiology of chronic cor-pulmonale is an increase in the pulmonary artery vascular resistance and pulmonary hypertension. Mechanisms causing these changes include occlusion or destruction of vascular bed due to lung parenchymal destruction, vasculitis, and endarteritis with diminished cross-sectional area of the pulmonary circulation (81,82). Other less important causes include hypoxia, acidosis with hypercapnia, and increased blood viscosity due to polycythaemia. The latter may not be important in developing nations because of a high prevalence of malnutrition and anaemia. These causes also happen to be important in the causation of chronic cor-pulmonale in patients with COPD.

Normally, pulmonary circulation is a highly distensible, low pressure and low-resistance circulation that transmits the entire cardiac output without much change in pressure because the pulmonary arteries are thin-walled with little resting muscular tone. In adults, there is a negligible response in terms of capacity, distensibility, or resistance to flow following autonomic nervous system stimulation. Many small arterioles and capillaries are non-perfused at rest, but can be recruited when needed to expand the pulmonary vascular bed causing a decrease in pulmonary vascular resistance. There is no humoral counterpart of the renin-angiotensin system that is capable of evoking sustained pulmonary artery hypertension.

Normal mean pulmonary artery pressure is 13-14 mmHg in a young adult and is less than 18 mmHg in 80% of subjects of all ages. Pulmonary artery pressure of greater than 20 mmHg signifies pulmonary hypertension. Blood flow through the pulmonary capillaries is achieved by a pressure drop of only 5-9 mmHg [pulmonary artery to left atrial pressure] compared to 90 mmHg for the systemic circuit. Accordingly, the normal pulmonary vascular resistance is 10-20 times less than systemic vascular resistance.

It is generally agreed that the decrease in extent of the pulmonary vascular bed is insufficient to play a predominant role in the pathogenesis of pulmonary hypertension unless the reduction is extreme. The effective cross-sectional area of the pulmonary vascular bed must be reduced by more than 50% before any change in pulmonary artery pressure can be detected at rest, although exercise will increase the pressure at lower levels of increased blood flow. Experiments in dogs have shown that more than two-thirds of the lungs had to be ablated before pulmonary artery pressures approach hypertensive levels (81,82). Obliterative vascular diseases increase pulmonary vascular resistance by vascular occlusion, while diffuse interstitial and parenchymal diseases act primarily by compressing and obliterating small vessels.

The diagnosis of chronic cor-pulmonale is often not made until significant right ventricular hypertrophy or overt right ventricular failure is present. Heart failure occurs insidiously, causing further impairment of lung function and is frequently misinterpreted as worsening of the underlying lung disease. Episodes of leg oedema, atypical chest pain, exertional dyspnoea, exercise-induced cyanosis in the periphery, prior respiratory failure, and excessive daytime sleepiness are non-specific but important historical clues suggesting the possibility of cor-pulmonale.

General physical examination reveals distended neck veins, peripheral oedema, and cyanosis. Oedema in chronic cor-pulmonale may not be necessarily due to overt heart failure. Signs and symptoms suggestive of heart failure like dyspnoea, orthopnoea, oedema, hepatomegaly, and raised jugular venous pressure [JVP] can also occur due to chronic obstructive airways disease without right heart failure. However, the raised JVP is present in both phases of respiration in right heart failure.

The apical impulse and the right ventricular lift are often not palpable. The second heart sound may be palpable in the pulmonary area. The earliest sign of pulmonary hypertension is an accentuated pulmonic component of the second heart sound. A right ventricular S3 gallop is heard in the epigastrium along the sternum. With advanced pulmonary artery hypertension, characteristic diastolic murmur of pulmonary regurgitation and pansystolic murmur of tricuspid regurgitation which accentuates during inspiration can be heard along with a systolic ejection sound. Right ventricular failure is usually precipitated by some acute episode like pneumonia. Associated clinical features of the underlying basic disease will be present.

Cor-pulmonale due to restricted vascular bed is manifested by a strikingly high pulmonary arterial pressure associated with a low cardiac output. Hypoxaemia is often mild. Tachypnoea which persists even during sleep is the rule, particularly with multiple pulmonary emboli. Chest pain is common. Enlargement of right ventricle in its pure form is manifested in these disorders. Prominent "a" and "v" waves appear in the jugular veins.

The classic radiographic evidence of right ventricular enlargement [crossing the right vertebral border] will be present. This is manifested by enlargement of the outflow tract of the right ventricle, the main pulmonary arteries, and their central branches, in association with attenuated peripheral branches of the pulmonary arterial tree. Enlargement of the pulmonary artery is considered to exist when the diameter of the right descending pulmonary artery is greater than 16 mm and the left descending pulmonary artery is greater than 18 mm, although the true sensitivity and specificity of these measurements are not known.

The "suggestive" indices of pulmonary hypertension [right ventricular enlargement] in the electrocardiogram include: p pulmonale in leads II, III, aVF, S1Q3, or S1-S2-S3 patterns, right axis deviation, R:S ratio in V6 of 1.0, rSR pattern in the right precordial leads, and partial or complete right bundle branch block (83-85). Dominant R or R' in lead V1 or V3R in association with inverted T waves in the right precordial leads in combination with "suggestive" criteria, are more definite indices. Non-invasive investigations such as Doppler and 2-D transthoracic echocardiography may be used periodically to monitor pulmonary artery pressure and right ventricular function.

AMYLOIDOSIS

Secondary amyloidosis is known to occur in a wide variety of clinical situations and is characterised by the deposition of an extracellular eosinophilic substance in various organs. Although the name suggests carbohydrate deposition, in fact, the substance is predominantly, if not exclusively, protein in origin (86). Several cytokines including interleukin-1 [IL-1], interleukin-6 [IL-6] and tumour necrosis factor-α [TNF]-α stimulate hepatic synthesis of serum amyloid A precursor during TB inflammation. The incidence of renal amyloidosis in TB has been reported to range from 8%-33% (87-91). Differences in the method used to detect amyloidosis could also have contributed to this wide variation. The incidence of amyloidosis was 1.01% of 6431 postmortems and 8.4% of 1980 renal biopsies at the Postgraduate Institute of Medical Education and Research, Chandigarh (90). While 87.1% had secondary amyloidosis, 3.5% had primary amyloidosis and the remaining had multiple myeloma. TB of various organs was the most common predisposing cause accounting for 59.1% of secondary amyloidosis, followed by chronic suppurative lung diseases (90). Pulmonary TB was the leading cause in 81.6% of cases followed by glandular and abdominal TB. The interval between the onset of the predisposing disease and the first evidence of secondary renal amyloidosis varied from 1 year-30 years with a mean of 6.9 years in this study. The interval was greater than 5 years in 67% of patients. However, other reports suggest that this interval varies widely and may be as short as 6 months or as long as 43 years (91). Nonetheless, TB is still the most common cause of secondary amyloidosis in Indian patients (90). Abdominal fat pad, rectal, mucosal, liver, or kidney biopsy specimens are useful in confirming the diagnosis of secondary amyloidosis. Secondary amyloidosis can occur even in adequately treated patients with pulmonary TB (92). A study from Tunisia concluded that renal amyloidosis is an important complication of TB (93).

CHRONIC EMPYEMA, BRONCHOPLEURAL FISTULA, FIBROTHORAX/DESTROYED LUNG

Chronic empyema and bronchopleural fistula are some of the important complications of pulmonary TB, particularly if the disease is chronic. These may be due to active TB when occur for the first time or can occur as complications and persist even after the disease is inactive after full treatment and bacteriological cure. These bring about significant amount of morbidity and frequent causes of repeated infections by bacteria other than mycobacteria. The patient may require prolonged chest tubes with frozen shoulders, protein loss and respiratory and physical disability. Surgical intervention will often be required (94-104).

Destroyed lung or fibrothorax is a term which is used to denote a condition when all the three important components of the lung – the parenchyma, bronchi and pleura are often involved. The lung is grossed shrunken, fibrosed, and the mediastinum is pulled to the same side. Most often there will be features of cavity, crepitations and can complicate with repeated infections and haemoptysis. The patient can be a respiratory cripple and in advanced stages, go on to respiratory failure and *cor-pulmonale*. The reader is referred to the chapter *"Surgery for pleuropulmonary tuberculosis"* [Chapter 46] for further details.

NONTUBERCULOUS MYCOBACTERIAL DISEASE

Pulmonary disease due to nontuberculous mycobacteria [NTM] is common in persons with past history of pulmonary TB. The clinical relevance of colonisation versus active NTM disease needs to be ascertained by the treating physician. The reader is referred to the chapter *"Nontuberculous mycobacterial infections"* [Chapter 41] for details.

REFERENCES

1. Bidwell JL, Pachner RW. Hemoptysis: diagnosis and management. Am Fam Physician 2005;72:1253-60.

2. Pamra SP, Goyal SS, Raj B, Mathur GP. Epidemiology of haemoptysis. Indian J Tuberc 1970;17:111-8.

3. Sharma SK, Mohan A. Pulmonary tuberculosis: typical and atypical cases. Case track series 1. Mumbai: Merind; 1997.

4. Reechaipichitkul W, Latong S. Etiology and treatment outcomes of massive hemoptysis. Southeast Asian J Trop Med Public Health 2005;36:474-80.

5. van den Heuvel MM, van Rensburg JJ. Images in clinical medicine. Rasmussen's aneurysm. N Engl J Med 2006;355:e17.

6. Keeling AN, Costello R, Lee MJ. Rasmussen's aneurysm: a forgotten entity? Cardiovasc Intervent Radiol 2007;30:1234-7.

7. Kato A, Kudo S, Matsumoto K, Fukahori T, Shimizu T, Uchino A, et al. Bronchial artery embolization for hemoptysis due to benign diseases: immediate and long-term results. Cardiovasc Intervent Radiol 2000;23:351-7.

8. Lee JH, Kwon SY, Yoon HI, Yoon CJ, Lee KW, Kang SG, et al. Haemoptysis due to chronic tuberculosis vs. bronchiectasis: comparison of long-term outcome of arterial embolisation. Int J Tuberc Lung Dis 2007;11:781-7.

9. Ghanaati, H, Rad AS, Firouznia K, Jalali AH. Bronchial artery embolization in life-threatening massive hemoptysis. Iran Red Cres Med J 2013;15:e16618.

10. Kim SW, Lee SJ, Ryu YJ, Lee JH, Chang JH, Shim SS, et al. Prognosis and predictors of rebleeding after bronchial artery embolization in patients with active or inactive pulmonary tuberculosis. Lung 2015;193:575-81.

11. Metin M, Sayar A, Turna A, Solak O, Erkan L, Dincer SI, et al. Emergency surgery for massive haemoptysis. Acta Chir Belg 2005;105:639-43.

12. Naidoo R. Active pulmonary tuberculosis: experience with resection in 106 cases. Asian Cardiovasc Thorac Ann 2007;15:134-8.

13. Dewan RK, Moodley L. Resurgence of therapeutically destitute tuberculosis: amalgamation of old and newer techniques. J Thorac Dis 2014;6:196-201.

14. British Tuberculosis Association. Aspergillus in persistent lung cavities after tuberculosis. A report from the Research Committee of the British Tuberculosis Association. Tubercle 1968;49:1-11.

15. British Thoracic and Tuberculosis Association. Aspergilloma and residual tuberculous cavities–the results of a resurvey. Tubercle 1970;51:227-45.

16. Kauffman CA. Quandry about treatment of aspergillomas persists. Lancet 1996;347:1640.

17. Zizzo G, Castriota-Scanderbeg A, Zarrelli N, Nardella G, Daly J, Cammisa M. Pulmonary aspergillosis complicating ankylosing spondylitis. Radiol Med [Torino] 1996;91:817-8.

18. Kawamura S, Maesaki S, Tomono K, Tashiro T, Kohno S. Clinical evaluation of 61 patients with pulmonary aspergilloma. Intern Med 2000;39:209-12.

19. Rosenheim SH, Schwartz J. Cavitary pulmonary cryptococcosis complicated by aspergilloma. Am Rev Respir Dis 1975;111:549-53.

20. Sarosi GA, Silberfarb PM, Saliba NA, Huggin PM, Tosh FE. Aspergillomas occurring in blastomycotic cavities. Am Rev Respir Dis 1971;104:581-4.

21. Gefter WB. The spectrum of pulmonary aspergillosis. J Thoracic Imaging 1992;7:56-74.

22. Faulkner SL, Vernon R, Brown PP, Fisher RD, Bender HW Jr. Hemoptysis and pulmonary aspergilloma: operative versus nonoperative treatment. Ann Thorac Surg 1978;25:389-92.

23. Tomee JF, van der Werf TS, Latge JP, Koeter GH, Dubois AE, Kauffman HF. Serologic monitoring of disease and treatment in a patient with pulmonary aspergilloma. Am J Respir Crit Care Med 1995;151:199-204.

24. Addrizzo-Harris DJ, Harkin TJ, McGuinness G, Naidich DP, Rom WN. Pulmonary aspergilloma and AIDS. A comparison of HIV-infected and HIV-negative individuals. Chest 1997;111:612-8.

25. Wallace JM, Lim R, Browdy BL, Hopewell PC, Glassroth J, Rosen MJ, et al. Pulmonary Complications of HIV Infection Study Group. Risk factors and outcomes associated with identification of Aspergillus in respiratory specimens from persons with HIV disease. Chest 1998;114:131-7.

26. Aslam PA, Eastridge CE, Hughes FA Jr. Aspergillosis of the lung. An eighteen year experience. Chest 1971;59:28-32.

27. Stevens DA, Kan VL, Judson MA, Morrison VA, Dummer S, Denning DW, et al. Practice guidelines for diseases caused by Aspergillus. Infectious Diseases Society of America. Clin Infect Dis 2000;30:696-709.

28. Tuncel E. Pulmonary air meniscus sign. Respiration 1984;46:139-44.

29. Roberts CM, Citron KM, Strickland B. Intrathoracic aspergilloma. Role of CT in diagnosis and treatment. Radiology 1987;165:123-8.

30. McCarthy DS, Pepys J. Pulmonary aspergilloma: clinical immunology. Clin Allergy 1973;3:57-70.

31. Rafferty P, Biggs BA, Crompton GK, Grant IW. What happens to patients with pulmonary aspergilloma? Analysis of 23 cases. Thorax 1983;38:579-83.

32. Pennington JE. Aspergillus lung disease. Med Clin North Am 1980;64:475-90.

33. Jewkes J, Kay PH, Paneth M, Citron KM. Pulmonary aspergilloma: analysis of prognosis in relation to haemoptysis and survey of treatment. Thorax 1983;38:572-8.

34. Yamada H, Kohno S, Koga H, Maesaki S, Kaku M. Topical treatment of pulmonary aspergilloma by antifungals. Relationship between duration of the disease and efficacy of therapy. Chest 1993;103: 1421-5.

35. Munk PL, Vellet AD, Rankin RN, Muller NL, Ahmad D. Intracavitary aspergilloma: transthoracic percutaneous injection of amphotericin gelatin solution. Radiology 1993;188:821-3.

36. Hammermann KJ, Sarosi GA, Tosh FE. Amphotericin B in the treatment of saprophytic forms of pulmonary aspergillosis. Am Rev Respir Dis 1974;109:57-62.

37. Campbell JH, Winter JH, Richardson MD, Shankland GS, Banham SW. Treatment of pulmonary aspergilloma with itraconazole. Thorax 1991;46:839-41.

38. Uflacker R, Kaemmerer A, Picon PD, Rizzon CF, Neves CM, Oliveira ES, et al. Bronchial artery embolization in the management of hemoptysis: technical aspects and long-term results. Radiology 1985;157:637-44.

39. Okubo K, Kobayashi M, Morikawa H, Hayatsu E, Ueno Y. Favorable acute and long-term outcomes after the resection of pulmonary aspergillomas. Thorac Cardiovasc Surg 2007;55: 108-11.

40. Pratap H, Dewan RK, Singh L, Gill S, Vaddadi S. Surgical treatment of pulmonary aspergilloma: a series of 72 cases. Indian J Chest Dis Allied Sci 2007;49:23-7.

41. Chen JC, Chang YL, Luh SP, Lee JM, Lee YC. Surgical treatment for pulmonary aspergilloma: a 28 year experience. Thorax 1997;52: 810-3.

42. Regnard JF, Icard P, Nicolosi M, Spagiarri L, Magdeleinat P, Jauffret B, et al. Aspergilloma: a series of 89 surgical cases. Ann Thorac Surg 2000;69:898-903.

43. Glimp RA, Bayer AS. Pulmonary aspergilloma: diagnostic and therapeutic considerations. Ann Intern Med 1983;143:303-8.

44. Ba PS, Ndiaye A, Diatta S, Ciss AG, Dieng PA, Gaye M, et al. Results of surgical treatment for pulmonary aspergilloma. Med Sante Trop 2015;25:92-96.

45. Silva Pdos S, Marsico GA, Araujo MA, Braz FS, Santos HT, Loureiro GL, et al. Complex pulmonary aspergilloma treated by cavernostomy. Rev Col Bras Cir 2014;41:406-11.

46. Lombardo GT, Anandarao N, Lin CS, Abbate A, Becker WH. Fatal hemoptysis in a patient with AIDS-related complex and pulmonary aspergilloma. N Y State J Med 1987;87:306-8.

47. Hohler T, Schnutgen M, Mayet WJ, Meyer zum Buschenfelde KH. Pulmonary aspergilloma in a patient with AIDS. Thorax 1995;50: 312-3.

48. Greenberg AK, Knapp J, Rom WN, Addrizzo-Harris DJ. Clinical presentation of pulmonary mycetoma in HIV-infected patients. Chest 2002;122:886-92.

49. Rosenzweig DY, Stead WW. The role of tuberculosis and other forms of bronchopulmonary necrosis in the pathogenesis of bronchiectasis. Am Rev Respir Dis 1966;93:769-85.

50. Rikimaru T. Endobronchial tuberculosis. Expert Rev Anti Infect Ther 2004;2:245-51.

51. Kim HY, Song KS, Goo JM, Lee JS, Lee KS, Lim TH. Thoracic sequelae and complications of tuberculosis. Radiographics 2001;21: 839-58.

52. Hussain SF, Aziz A, Fatima H. Pneumothorax: a review of 146 adult cases admitted at a university teaching hospital in Pakistan. J Pak Med Assoc 1999;49:243-6.

53. Borrego Galan JC, Rivas Lopez P, Remacha Esteras MA. Recurrent tuberculous pneumothorax and tuberculous empyema: an association of two rare complications. Arch Bronconeumol 2003;39:478-9.

54. Lim JY, Kim KM, Choi EC, Kim YH, Kim HS, Choi HS. Current clinical propensity of laryngeal tuberculosis: review of 60 cases. Eur Arch Otorhinolaryngol 2006;263:838-42.

55. Elemanov MG, Kharcheva KA, Vavillin GI. Evaluation of the "open-negative" syndrome in the clinical course of tuberculosis. Probl Tuberk 1974;52:19-23.

56. Miyagi Y. "Open-negative" syndrome. Clinical course of its development and subsequent destiny. Jpn J Tuberc 1966;13:54-9.

57. Breuer J, Abeles H, Chaves AD, Robins AB. Observations on ambulatory tuberculous patients with pulmonary cavities and noninfectious sputum [the open-negative syndrome]. Am Rev Tuberc 1958;78:725-34.

58. Auerbach O, Garfinkel L, Parks VR. Scar cancer of the lung: increase over a 21 year period. Cancer 1979;43:636-42.

59. Gao YT. Risk factors for lung cancer among nonsmokers with emphasis on lifestyle factors. Lung Cancer 1996;14:S39-45.

60. Wu-Williams AH, Dai XD, Blot W, Xu ZY, Sun XW, Xiao HP, et al. Lung cancer among women in north-east China. Br J Cancer 1990;62:982-7.

61. Jindal SK, Malik SK, Bedi RS, Gupta SK. Risk of lung cancer in patients with old tuberculosis – a prospective study. Lung India 1986;4:59-61.

62. Hinds MW, Cohen HI, Kolonel LN. Tuberculosis and cancer risk in nonsmoking women. Am Rev Respir Dis 1982;125:776-8.

63. Johnson DE, Geogieff MK. Pulmonary perspective: neuro-endocrine cells in health and disease. Am Rev Respir Dis 1989;140:1807-12.

64. Youngson C, Nurse C, Yeger H, Cutz E. Oxygen sensing in airway chemoreceptors. Nature 1993;365:153-5.

65. Schuller HM, Miller MS, Park PD, Orloff MS. Promoting mechanisms of CO_2 on neuroendocrine cell proliferation mediated by nicotine receptor stimulation. Significance for lung cancer risk in individuals with chronic lung disease. Chest 1996;109: 20S-21S.

66. Harikrishna J, Sukaveni V, Kumar DP, Mohan A. Cancer and tuberculosis. J Indian Acad Clin Med 2012;13:142-4.

67. Yu YH, Liao CC, Hsu WH, Chen HJ, Liao WC, Muo CH, et al. Increased lung cancer risk among patients with pulmonary tuberculosis: a population cohort study. J Thorac Oncol 2011;6: 32-7

68. Zhou Y, Cui Z, Zhou X, Chen C, Jiang S, Hu, et al. The presence of old pulmonary tuberculosis is an independent prognostic factor for squamous cell lung cancer survival. J Cardiothorac Surg 2013; 8:123.

69. Cicėnas S, Vencevičius V. Lung cancer in patients with tuberculosis World J Surg Oncol 2007;5:22.

70. Silva DR, Valentini Jr DF, Müller AM, de Almeida CP, Dalcin Pde T. Pulmonary tuberculosis and lung cancer: simultaneous and sequential occurrence. J Bras Pneumol 2013;39:484-9.

71. Brenner DR, McLaughlin JR, Hung RJ. Previous lung diseases and lung cancer risk: a systematic review and meta-analysis. PLoS One 2011;6:e17479.

72. Hallett WY, Martin CJ. The diffuse obstructive pulmonary syndrome in a tuberculosis sanatorium. I. Etiologic factors. Ann Intern Med 1961;54:1146-55.

73. Snider GL, Doctor L, Demas TA, Shaw AR. Obstructive airway disease in patients with treated pulmonary tuberculosis. Am Rev Respir Dis 1971;103:625-40.

74. Lee JH, Chang JH. Lung function in patients with chronic airflow obstruction due to tuberculous destroyed lung. Respir Med 2003;97:1237-42.

75. Singla N, Singla R, Fernandes S, Behera D. Post treatment sequelae of multi-drug resistant tuberculosis patients. Indian J Tuberc 2009;56:206-12.

76. Ralph AP, Kenangalem E, Waramori G, Pontororing GJ, Sandjaja, Tjitra E, et al. High morbidity during treatment and residual pulmonary disability in pulmonary tuberculosis: under-recognised phenomena. PLoS One 2013;8:e80302.

77. Akkara SA, Shah AD, Adalja M, Akkara AG, Rathi A, Shah DN. Pulmonary tuberculosis: the day after. Int J Tuberc Lung Dis 2013;17:810-3.

78. Macklem PT. Respiratory muscles: the vital pump. Chest 1980;78: 753-8.

79. Park JH, Na JO, Kim EK, Lim CM, Shim TS, Lee SD, et al. The prognosis of respiratory failure in patients with tuberculous destroyed lung. Int J Tuberc Lung Dis 2001;5:963-7.

80. Bone RC. Treatment of respiratory failure due to advanced chronic obstructive lung disease. Arch Intern Med 1980;140: 1018-21.

81. Ferrer MI. Cor pulmonale [pulmonary heart disease]: present-day status. Am Heart J 1975;89:657-64.

82. Fishman AP. State of the art: chronic cor pulmonale. Am Rev Respir Dis 1976;114:775-94.

83. Kleiger RE, Senior RM. Long-term electrocardiographic monitoring of ambulatory patients with chronic airway obstruction. Chest 1974;65:483.

84. Padmavati S, Raizada V. Electrocardiogram in chronic cor pulmonale. Br Heart J 1975;34:648.

85. Prabhakar R. Laboratory aspects of tuberculosis. Indian J Tuberc 1987;34:67-80.

86. Glenner GG, Terry WD, Isersky C. Amyloidosis: its nature and pathogenesis. Semin Hematol 1973;10:65-86.

87. Shah PKD, Jain MK, Mangal HN, Singhvi NM. Kidney changes in pulmonary tuberculosis–a study by kidney biopsy. Indian J Tuberc 1975;1:23-7.

88. Mittal OP, Sharma GS, Singh SK, Agarwala MC. Renal biopsy in pulmonary tuberculosis. Indian J Chest Dis 1966;8:20-4.

89. Abdulpurkar AG, Desai MG, Shankar PS. Renal changes in pulmonary tuberculosis. Lung India 1987;5:82-5.

90. Chugh KS, Singhal PC, Sakhuja V, Datta BN, Jain SK, Dash SC. Pattern of renal amyloidosis in Indian patients. Postgrad Med J 1981;57:31-5.

91. Kennedy AC, Burton JA, Allison ME. Tuberculosis as a continuing cause of renal amyloidosis. Br Med J 1974;3:795-7.

92. Dixit R, Gupta R, Dave L, Prasad N, Sharma S. Clinical profile of patients having pulmonary tuberculosis and renal amyloidosis. Lung India 2009;26:41-5.

93. Ben Abdelghani K, Barbouch S, Ounissi M, Ounissi M, Mahfoudhi M, Ben Moussa F, et al. Etiologic profile of amyloidosis of the elderly in Tunisia. Tunis Med 2012;90:13-8.

94. Goyal VD, Gupta B, Sharma S. Intercostal muscle flap for repair of bronchopleural fistula. Lung India 2015;32:152-4.

95. Petrella F, Spaggiari L. Bronchopleural fistula treatment: from the archetype of surgery to the future of stem cell therapy. Lung India 2015;32:100-1.

96. Bagheri R, Haghi SZ, Rajabi MT, Motamedshariati M, Sheibani S. Outcomes following surgery for complicated tuberculosis: analysis of 108 patients. Thorac Cardiovasc Surg 2013;61:154-8.

97. Bai L, Hong Z, Gong C, Yan D, Liang Z. Surgical treatment efficacy in 172 cases of tuberculosis-destroyed lungs. Eur J Cardiothorac Surg 2012;41:335-40.

98. Yaldiz S, Gursoy S, Ucvet A, Kaya SO. Surgery offers high cure rates in multidrug-resistant tuberculosis. Ann Thorac Cardiovasc Surg 2011;17:143-7.

99. Acharya PR, Shah KV. Empyema thoracis: a clinical study. Ann Thorac Med 2007;2:14-7.

100. Dewan RK. Role of thoracic surgery in pulmonary tuberculosis. J Indian Med Assoc 1999;97:438-41.

101. Dewan RK, Singh S, Kumar A, Meena BK. Thoracoplasty: an obsolete procedure? Indian J Chest Dis Allied Sci 1999;41:83-8.

102. Conlan AA, Kopec SE. Indications for pneumonectomy. Pneumonectomy for benign disease. Chest Surg Clin North Am 1999;9:311-26.

103. Ashour M. Pneumonectomy for tuberculosis. Eur J Cardiothorac Surg 1997;12:209-13.

104. Iseman MD, Madsen LA. Chronic tuberculous empyema with bronchopleural fistula resulting in treatment failure and progressive drug resistance. Chest 1991;100:124-7.

32

Tuberculosis and Acute Respiratory Distress Syndrome

DR Karnad, KK Guntupalli

INTRODUCTION

Acute respiratory distress syndrome [ARDS] is a disorder characterised by inflammatory damage to the alveolar capillary membrane producing severe derangement of gas exchange, which could result from a variety of insults, ultimately resulting in severe hypoxaemia, non-cardiogenic pulmonary oedema (1). In general, abnormalities of gas exchange are uncommon in pulmonary tuberculosis [TB] because concomitant involvement of ventilation and perfusion results in maintenance of the normal ventilation-perfusion relationship (2). However, severe hypoxic respiratory failure due can sometimes complicate severe forms of pulmonary and miliary TB (3-5). This complication is associated with a very high mortality despite treatment. Hence, early recognition and appropriate management of this uncommon complication is of utmost importance.

DEFINITION

The term acute lung injury [ALI] has been loosely used until the 1994 American-European Consensus Conference [AECC] laid down a specific definition for ALI and ARDS in order to ensure uniformity in diagnosis, research and management (1,6). This definition was widely used in ARDS research for more than 15 years since then. However, issues concerning the limitations, reliability and validity of the AECC definition had emerged. Addressing these issues, recently, the Berlin definition criteria [Table 32.1] have been described for the diagnosis of ARDS (7).

PATHOGENESIS

ARDS occurs in approximately 40% of patients with sepsis and the systemic inflammatory response syndrome (6).

Table 32.1: The Berlin definition criteria for the diagnosis of ARDS

Variable	Criteria for diagnosis
Timing	Timing: within 1 week of a known clinical insult or new or worsening respiratory symptoms
Chest imaging*	Bilateral opacities—not fully explained by effusions, lobar/lung collapse, or nodules
Origin of oedema	Respiratory failure not fully explained by cardiac failure or fluid overload Need objective assessment [e.g. echocardiography] to exclude hydrostatic oedema if no risk factor present
Oxygenation†	
Mild	200 mmHg < PaO_2/FiO_2 ≤ 300 mmHg with PEEP or CPAP ≥ 5 cm H_2O‡
Moderate	100 mmHg < PaO_2/FiO_2 ≤ 200 mmHg with PEEP ≥ 5 cm H_2O
Severe	PaO_2/FiO_2 < 100 mmHg with PEEP ≥ 5 cm H_2O

* Chest radiograph or computed tomography
† If altitude is higher than 1000 m, the correction factor should be calculated as follows: {PaO_2/FiO_2 × [barometric pressure/760]}
‡ This may be delivered noninvasively in the mild acute respiratory distress syndrome group
ARDS = acute respiratory distress syndrome; PaO_2 = arterial oxygen tension; FiO_2 = fraction of inspired oxygen; PEEP = peak end-expiratory pressure; CPAP = continuous positive airway pressure
Source: reference 7

Initially, there is inflammatory damage to the pulmonary endothelial cell barrier, resulting in increased pulmonary capillary permeability. This produces leakage of protein-rich pulmonary oedema at normal pulmonary artery wedge pressure. A series of inflammatory events then damages the alveolar epithelial cells [Figures 32.1 and 32.2]. Damage to the Type I cells further worsens alveolar flooding and gas-exchange. Type II cuboidal cells, which produce surfactant, too are damaged in later stages of the disease resulting in collapse of the more severely affected

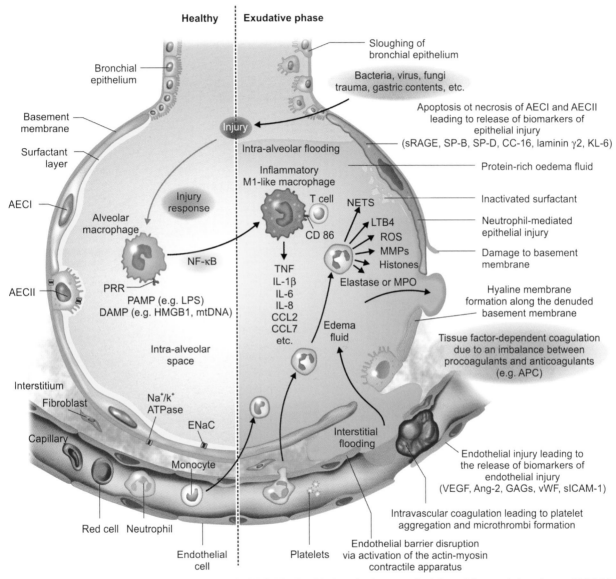

Figure 32.1: The healthy lung and the exudative phase of ARDS. The healthy lung is shown on the left, and the exudative phase of ARDS is shown on the right. Injury is initiated by either direct or indirect insults to the delicate alveolar structure of the distal lung and associated microvasculature. In the exudative phase, resident alveolar macrophages are activated, leading to the release of potent proinflammatory mediators and chemokines that promote the accumulation of neutrophils and monocytes. Activated neutrophils further contribute to injury by releasing toxic mediators. The resultant injury leads to loss of barrier function, as well as interstitial and intra-alveolar flooding. Tumour necrosis factor [TNF]–mediated expression of tissue factor promotes platelet aggregation and microthrombus formation, as well as intra-alveolar coagulation and hyaline-membrane formation ARDS = acute respiratory distress syndrome; AECI = type I alveolar epithelial cell; AECII = type II alveolar epithelial cell; Ang-2 = angiopoietin-2; APC = activated protein C; CC-16 = club cell [formerly Clara cell] secretory protein 16; CCL = chemokine [CC motif] ligand; DAMP = damage-associated molecular pattern; ENaC = epithelial sodium channel; GAG = glycosaminoglycan; HMGB1 = high-mobility group box 1 protein; KL-6 = Krebs von den Lungen 6; LPS = lipopolysaccharide; LTB4 = leukotriene B4; MMP = matrix metalloproteinase; MPO = myeloperoxidase; mtDNA = mitochondrial DNA; Na+/K+ ATPase = sodium–potassium ATPase pump; NF-κB = nuclear factor kappa light-chain enhancer of activated B-cells; NET = neutrophil extracellular trap; PAMP = pathogen-associated molecular pattern; PRR = pattern recognition receptor; ROS = reactive oxygen species; sICAM = soluble intercellular adhesion molecule; SP = surfactant protein; sRAGE = soluble receptor for advanced glycation end products; VEGF = vascular endothelial growth factor; vWF = von Willebrand factor

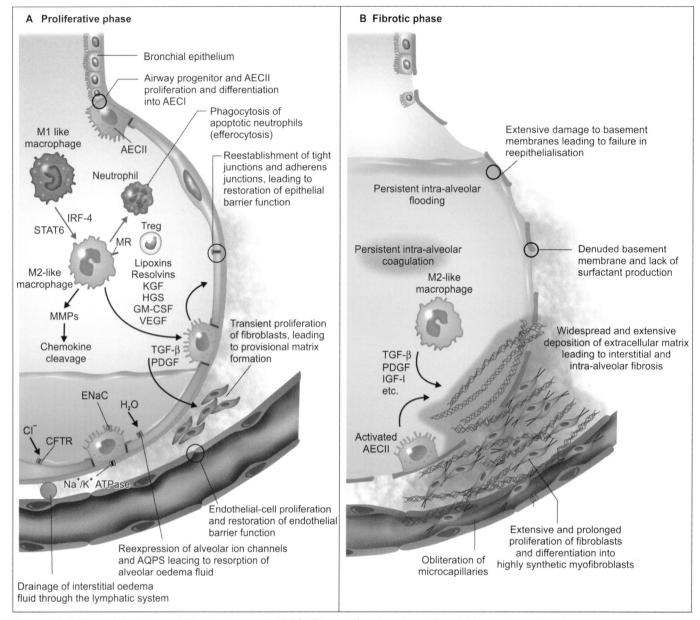

Figure 32.2: The proliferative and fibrotic phases of ARDS. The proliferative phase [Panel A] aims to restore tissue homeostasis and is characterised by the transient expansion of resident fibroblasts and the formation of a provisional matrix, as well as proliferation of airway progenitor cells and type II alveolar epithelial cells [AECII], with differentiation into type I alveolar epithelial cells [AECI]. During the fibrotic phase of ARDS [Panel B], which is strongly associated with the need for mechanical ventilation, extensive basement membrane damage and inadequate or delayed reepithelialisation lead to the development of interstitial and intra-alveolar fibrosis

ARDS = acute respiratory distress syndrome; AQP5 = aquaporin 5; CFTR = cystic fibrosis transmembrane conductance regulator; GMCSF = granulocyte–macrophage colony stimulating factor; HGF = hepatocyte growth factor; IGFI = insulin like growth factor I; IRF4 = interferon regulatory factor 4; KGF = keratinocyte growth factor; MR = mannose receptor; PDGF = platelet derived growth factor; TGFβ = transforming growth factor β

Reproduced with permission from "Thompson BT, Chambers RC, Liu KD. Acute respiratory distress syndrome. N Engl J Med 2017;377:562-72 (reference 6)." Copyright [2000] Massachusetts Medical Society. All rights reserved

alveoli during end-expiration. Pro-inflammatory cytokines interleukin-1 [IL-1], interleukin-6 [IL-6], interleukin-8 [IL-8], and tumour necrosis factor-α [TNF-α] attract and activate inflammatory cells like neutrophils, macrophages. These cells release other inflammatory substances like elastases, other proteases, oxygen free radicals, leukotrienes and platelet activating factor. Endogenous anti-inflammatory substances like soluble interleukin-1 receptor antagonist [sIL-1RA], soluble tumour necrosis factor receptor [sTNF-R] and anti-inflammatory cytokines, interleukin-10 [IL-10] and interleukin-11 [IL-11] too are present in the alveoli, but their role in the pathogenesis of ARDS is not clear (6).

The inflammatory process is not limited to the lung (8,9). Activation of coagulation is common and frank disseminated intravascular coagulation [DIC] may develop in some patients. Inflammatory mediators arising from the lung may also play a role in the development of the multiple organ dysfunction syndrome in these patients (8).

In patients with TB, ARDS is believed to result from the release of mycobacteria or their products into the pulmonary circulation (10,11). This classical situation is present in severe miliary TB where widespread distribution of the bacterial load may result in diffuse lung injury and ARDS (12). Mycobacterial cell wall component lipoarabinomannan [LAM] and mycobacterial cytosolic heat-shock protein-65kD [HSP-65] have been shown to induce release of inflammatory cytokines (13). LAM binds to CD14 receptors on human mononuclear macrophages and induces the production and release of cytokines including interleukin-1β [IL-1β], TNF-α, interleukin-1α [IL-1α], IL-6, IL-8, IL-10, and granulocyte macrophage colony-stimulating factor [GM-CSF]. Heat-shock protein-65kD too induces the release of cytokines, but to a lesser extent than LAM, and by a mechanism that does not involve the CD14 receptor (12). Mycobacteria also induce expression of the intercellular adhesion molecule-1 [ICAM-1] on endothelial cells, which facilitates adhesion of activated neutrophils to capillary walls (12). Another compound, muramyl dipeptide, stimulates chemotaxis, and enhances phagocytosis and release of inflammatory mediators (14). The subsequent series of events are probably similar to those seen in gram-negative bacterial sepsis (10,11,13).

Some authors have also suggested that ARDS may be partly due to a cell-mediated immune response to mycobacterial antigens (14). This could result either from an enhancement of the delayed hypersensitivity response or from a decrease in suppressor mechanisms (14,15). This may probably play an important role in ARDS that develops in some patients after institution of anti-TB drug therapy and in patients with human immunodeficiency virus [HIV] infection receiving antiretroviral drugs (12-16).

EPIDEMIOLOGY

Eventhough ARDS is a well recognised complication in patients with pulmonary and miliary TB, sparse epidemiological data are available on this entity. Burden of ARDS as reported in some of the clinical studies is shown in Table 32.2 (3,5,17-23). Varying denominators have been used in the published studies because of which meaningful comparison of these data is not possible. The incidence of TB-ARDS has been observed to increase with any delay in diagnosis and institution of appropriate therapy for miliary TB (24). In an autopsy study (25) from Chandigarh, 10 of the 196 cases [5.1%] with disseminated TB, 10 met the clinical criteria for ARDS; in 60% of these, histopathological evidence of diffuse alveolar damage was present.

PREDISPOSING FACTORS

Acute lung injury invariably occurs in patients with severe TB, such as miliary TB, or TB bronchopneumonia (10,11). A number of predisposing factors have been described. Malnutrition is the most common predisposing factor seen in patients with pulmonary TB developing acute respiratory failure (12,17,26). Other factors include alcoholism, diabetes mellitus, immunosuppressive therapy with corticosteroids or other drugs, HIV infection, drug addiction, chronic liver disease and pregnancy (2,12,14,26,27). Independent predictors of TB-ARDS development documented in recent studies are shown in Table 32.3 (5,20,22).

CLINICAL SYNDROMES

Acute Respiratory Distress Syndrome in Miliary Tuberculosis

In patients with miliary TB, ARDS can occur at all ages and the youngest patient reported is a seven months old child (28). Fever, non-productive cough, chest discomfort and dyspnoea are the common symptoms and the average interval between onset of symptoms and diagnosis is 14 days (17,26). In more than 50% of patients the diagnosis of TB is not known at the time of admission with respiratory failure (12). In these patients, radiological features of ARDS usually mask the typical miliary mottling (10). The interval between admission and diagnosis in a large series was one

---

Table 32.2: Burden of TB-ARDS in published clinical studies

Study [year] (reference)	Incidence of TB-ARDS
Maartens *et al* [1990] (17)	8 of the 109 patients [7.3%] with miliary TB
Sharma *et al* [1995] (3)	5 of the 100 patients [5%] with miliary TB
Choi *et al* [1999] (18)	17 of 1010 [1.7%] patients with pulmonary TB had acute respiratory failure
Parikh and Karnad [1999] (19)	1.7% of admissions to the medical intensive care unit [ICU] in Mumbai had TB-ARDS
Kim *et al* [2003] (20)	8 of the 34 patients [23.5%] patients with miliary TB developed ARDS
Agarwal *et al* [2005] (21)	9 of the 187 patients [4.8%] admitted to the respiratory ICU at a tertiary care teaching hospital in Chandigarh, had TB-ARDS
Sharma *et al* [2006] (5)	29 of the 2733 [1.06%] TB patients seen during the period 1980-2003 at two tertiary care teaching hospitals in north and south India developed TB-ARDS
Deng *et al* [2012] (22)	85 of the 466 patients with miliary TB developed TB-ARDS
Sharma *et al* [2016] (23)	5 of the 64 [7.8%] patients with ARDS admitted to a medical ICU at a tertiary care teaching hospital in north India had TB-ARDS

TB-ARDS = tuberculosis-acute respiratory distress syndrome

Table 32.3: Predictors of development of TB-ARDS in various published studies

Study [year] (reference)	Predictors of development of TB-ARDS
Kim et al [2003] (20)	Lower WBC count and platelet count, lower serum albumin, elevated serum AST, ALT and ALP levels at the time of admission*
Sharma et al [2006] (5)	Presence of miliary TB, duration of illness beyond 30 days at presentation, absolute lymphocyte count less than 1625/mm^3 and serum ALT > 100 IU/L
Deng et al [2012] (22)	Presence of diabetes mellitus, ALT [70-100U/L], AST > 94 U/L, D-dimer >1.6 mg/L, haemoglobin < 9 g/dL, serum albumin < 2.5 g/dL*

* in patients with miliary TB
TB = tuberculosis; ARDS = acute respiratory distress syndrome; WBC = white blood cell; AST = aspartate aminotransferase; ALT = alanine aminotransferase; ALP = alkaline phosphatase

to twenty days (12). In up to 10% of patients with ARDS, miliary TB may be cryptic with systemic dissemination and a normal chest radiograph (24,26,29,30). A large proportion of these patients may harbour HIV infection (24). Other clinical findings include hepatosplenomegaly, mild hepatic dysfunction and pancytopenia (26). In a patient with unexplained ARDS, a history of fever of more than 15 days duration and elevation of serum alkaline phosphatase should arouse the suspicion of disseminated TB as the underlying cause (26).

ARDS may also develop in diagnosed patients with miliary TB after anti-TB treatment is initiated (12). In patients with miliary TB, auscultation of the chest is generally normal. Tachypnoea and presence of diffuse rales while on drug therapy is are ominous signs of early ARDS.

Mortality in patients with ARDS due to miliary TB is between 40%-80%, despite use of mechanical ventilation and corticosteroids (10,12,20,31). At autopsy, alveoli may show intense perifocal inflammation, interstitial granulomas and obliterative endarteritis [Figures 32.3 and 32.4], characteristic of miliary TB (32). In addition, other changes of ARDS may be present, in the form of diffuse alveolar damage [DAD], increased vascularity, presence of dense exudates in the alveoli, and hyaline membrane formation (25,32,33).

Acute Respiratory Distress Syndrome in Tuberculosis Pneumonia

Nodular lesions resulting from air-space consolidation due to endobronchial spread to lobar or multilobar locations is termed TB pneumonia (12). The development of acute respiratory failure due to TB pneumonia was first reported in 1977 by Agarwal et al (2). They reported 16 patients with acute respiratory failure, 10 of whom required mechanical ventilation. Alcoholism and chronic liver disease were the predisposing factors in almost all cases. In a 10-year review of patients with TB requiring mechanical ventilation for ARDS, Penner et al (12) found that six of the 13 patients with respiratory failure requiring mechanical ventilation had TB pneumonia. The mean interval between the onset of symptoms of TB and treatment was 45 days. Seven of the 29 patients in the series reported by Sharma et al (5) had pulmonary TB. Chest radiographs show nodular lesions, with mixed consolidation and ground-glass opacities

[Figures 32.5 and 32.6] (3,12). High-resolution computed tomography [HRCT] shows bronchogenic dissemination with ground glass attenuation (10). The classical tree-in-bud appearance is seen on computed tomography [CT] in less than 50% of cases (18).

Acute Respiratory Distress Syndrome in Cavitary Pulmonary Tuberculosis

In a retrospective analysis of patients with TB and acute respiratory failure, Zahar et al (24) found that 11% of patients had an isolated apical cavity on chest radiograph preceding the onset of acute respiratory failure. Choi et al (18) found cavities in HRCT of 45% of patients with acute respiratory failure. Extensive endobronchial spread of TB following rupture of a cavity into the bronchus is thought to initiate ARDS (34). The initial symptoms of TB in these patients are fever and cough, which are followed after two weeks to two months by acute onset of dyspnoea and severe hypoxaemia (34). The chest radiograph shows diffuse bilateral alveolar infiltrates as in ARDS, but unlike in miliary TB complicated by ARDS, these patients tend to have unilateral preponderance of the infiltrates and physical signs (34). They may have systemic manifestations, like DIC and hypotension. Mycobacteria are easily demonstrable in tracheal aspirates in almost all cases.

Acute Respiratory Distress Syndrome after Initiation of Anti-tuberculosis Treatment

In 1986, Onwubalili et al (14) described two alcoholic, malnourished patients, with bilateral extensive sputum smear-positive pulmonary TB, who developed paradoxical worsening of the disease resulting in ARDS during the second week of anti-TB treatment. One patient had TB bronchopneumonia. Baseline tests of immune function revealed a negative tuberculin skin test [TST] with 10 tuberculin units [TU] of purified protein derivative [PPD], lymphopenia, failure of peripheral blood mononuclear cells to respond to stimulation with PPD and severely depressed natural killer cell activity. This patients experienced severe breathlessness severe hypoxaemia 11 days after starting anti-TB therapy, along with worsening of the radiological lesions. At this time, the erythrocyte sedimentation rate [ESR] had

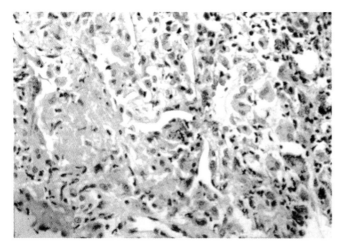

Figure 32.3: Tuberculosis pneumonia presenting as acute respiratory distress syndrome. Epithelioid cells are identified within the alveoli *[Haematoxylin and eosin, × 100]*

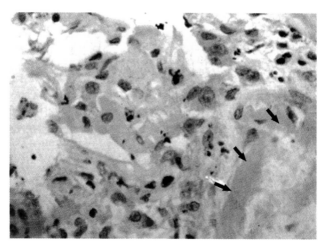

Figure 32.4: Acute respiratory distress syndrome in tuberculosis. There is an inflammatory exudate in the alveolus and fibrin deposition [arrows] along the alveoli *[Haematoxylin and eosin, × 400]*

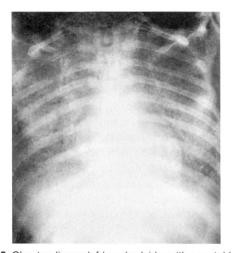

Figure 32.5: Chest radiograph [done bedside, with a portable machine] showing consolidation with air-bronchogram
Reproduced with permission from "Sharma SK, Mohan A, Pande JN, Prasad KL, Gupta AK, Khilnani GC. Clinical profile, laboratory characteristics and outcome in miliary tuberculosis. QJM 1995;88: 29-37 (reference 3)"

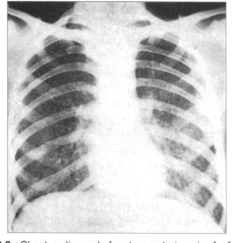

Figure 32.6: Chest radiograph [postero-anterior view] of the same patient in Figure 32.5 showing classical miliary shadows evolving after a few days
Reproduced with permission from "Sharma SK, Mohan A, Pande JN, Prasad KL, Gupta AK, Khilnani GC. Clinical profile, laboratory characteristics and outcome in miliary tuberculosis. QJM 1995;88: 29-37 (reference 3)"

increased to 110 mm at the end of first hour, TST [1 TU of PPD] revealed an induration of eight mm, and there was considerable improvement in the tests of immune function. The second patient had fibrocavitary disease and a TST [1 TU of PPD] reading of 7 mm. His condition deteriorated eight days after starting treatment; ESR increased to 100 mm at the end of first hour and there was an increase in all the parameters of immune function. He required mechanical ventilation for ARDS, and methylprednisolone was administered to reduce pulmonary inflammation. This patient died 13 days after starting treatment.

The authors (14) mention that both patients had *in vivo* and *in vitro* anergy and depression of lymphocyte function, probably due to poor nutritional status, excess alcohol consumption and the severe infection itself. On treatment, there was a progressive reversal of the immune deficiency and the acute respiratory failure may have been due to an exaggerated delayed hypersensitivity reaction to mycobacterial antigens released by the dying organisms. Tuberculoprotein and muramyl dipeptide have been implicated as possible immunogenic cell-wall components (14). Cell mediated damage to the pulmonary alveolar-capillary membrane is believed to cause ARDS in these patients (14).

Akira and Sakatani (15) have reported the radiological features in five patients who develop acute respiratory failure due to paradoxical worsening after treatment of TB. All five patients had unilateral cavitary TB restricted to one lobe. After treatment, chest radiographs revealed progression of the original lesion, and appearance of new lesions in the other lung and other regions in the same lung. HRCT revealed that in addition to the segmental or lobar cavitation in the original locations, extensive areas of ground-glass opacities were present bilaterally in all cases. However, a predominantly dependent distribution, which is characteristic of ARDS due to sepsis, was not seen. Transbronchial lung biopsy [TBLB] showed the presence of intra-alveolar and interstitial pulmonary oedema. Two of these five patients died.

Transient radiological worsening of pulmonary lesions has been reported in 3%-14% of patients receiving anti-TB treatment (35). However, the patients may remain asymptomatic in this setting. In 0.6% of cases, the process may be severe enough to cause acute respiratory failure (15). Paradoxical worsening is more frequent and also more severe in patients with HIV infection, especially those also receiving antiretroviral drugs due to the immune reconstitution inflammatory syndrome [IRIS] (16,36). However, Wendel et al (36) showed that 11% of patients with HIV infection receiving antiretroviral drugs along with anti-TB treatment developed clinically relevant paradoxical worsening compared to 7% receiving anti-TB treatment alone; the difference was not statistically significant (31).

Increase in severity of fever and a rising ESR may help identify patients who are likely to develop severe paradoxical worsening (14,15). Injectable methylprednisolone or oral prednisolone [1-2 mg/kg body weight, daily for one to two weeks which is gradually tapered] are recommended in patients with paradoxical worsening, although there are no randomised controlled studies to prove their benefit (16).

Other Manifestations

As in severe systemic sepsis, dysfunction of other organs is seen in 35% of patients with acute respiratory failure due to TB even in the absence of other bacterial infections (24,27,37). These manifestations are encountered more often in miliary TB than in TB pneumonia (12). Mycobacterial infection itself

can cause septic shock, with increased cardiac index, and low systemic vascular resistance (38). Non-mycobacterial sepsis due to secondary infection may supervene in approximately 40% of patients receiving mechanical ventilation (12). A significant number of patients also have co-existing DIC (17). Mortality in these patients is close to 100% (39). Up to 10% of patients may also have acute renal failure (24). Pancytopenia has been frequently reported in ARDS due to miliary TB (17,26). Mechanisms include bone marrow infiltration by TB granulomas and cytokine-induced bone marrow suppression. Pancytopenia responds well to anti-TB treatment, but these patients have poor survival rates (26).

DIAGNOSIS

Acute respiratory failure is suspected in patients with severe hypoxaemia, bilateral extensive rales on auscultation, presence of bilateral confluent alveolar opacities on chest radiograph in patients with proven pulmonary TB or prolonged fever (10,11,37,40). Arterial blood gas will reveal a significant alveolar-arterial oxygen gradient. Type I respiratory failure with normal or low arterial carbon dioxide tension [$PaCO_2$] is usually seen (8,11,32,37). The diagnosis is made by the Berlin definition diagnostic criteria mentioned earlier (7).

The diagnosis of TB in patients presenting with ARDS is difficult [Figure 32.7] (30), and needs a high index of suspicion. Early diagnosis is important as delay in treatment may worsen the respiratory failure and increase mortality. Radiographic changes of ARDS may mask underlying TB and alveolar infiltrates that are more organised or appear more nodular than usual should arouse suspicion (33). Choi et al (18) systematically reviewed the chest radiographic and HRCT findings in 17 patients with acute respiratory failure due to TB [Table 32.4]. During resolution, HRCT may reveal bilateral extensive thin-walled cystic lesions. Whether these represent parenchymal damage due to TB or ventilator-induced lung injury is not clear. These cysts resolve completely over several months (18).

Table 32.4: Radiological findings in patients with acute respiratory failure due to pulmonary tuberculosis

Plain radiograph		High-resolution computed tomography	
Findings	%	Findings	%
Small [<10 mm] nodular lesions	96	Nodular lesions	100
Air-space consolidation	76	Ground-glass opacities	91
Ground-glass opacities	70	Air-space consolidation	73
Reticular lesions	24	Septal thickening	73
Cavitary lesions	24	Tree-in-bud appearance	45
		Cavities	45
		Mediastinal lymphadenopathy	27
		Pleural effusion	27
		Pericardial effusion	27
		Spontaneous pneumothorax	9

Adapted from reference 16

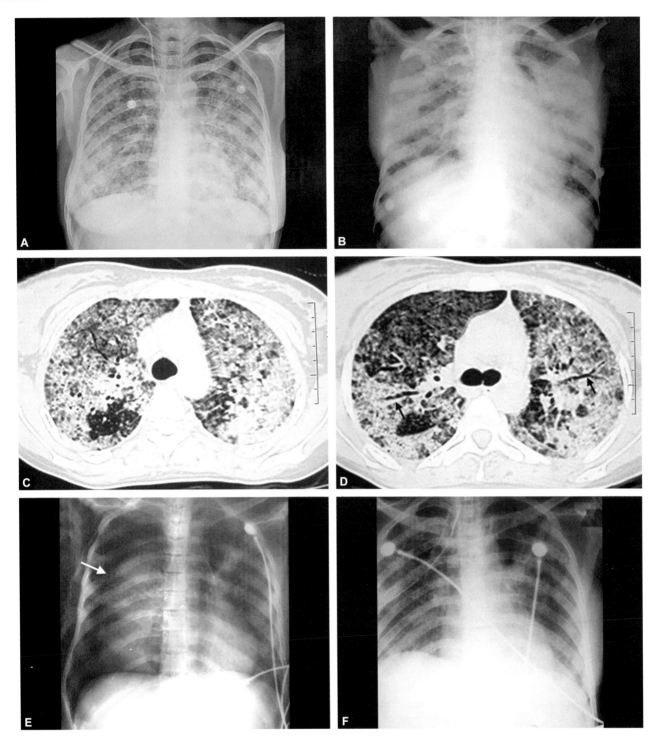

Figure 32.7: Chest radiograph [postero-anterior view] of a pregnant woman who presented with prolonged pyrexia showing a classical miliary pattern [A]. Fundus examination following mydriatic administration in both the eyes revealed choroid tubercles and had raised the suspicion of miliary TB. The patient developed ARDS during the course of her illness. Chest radiograph [antero-posterior view], obtained with a portable X-ray machine, bed-side showing bilateral frontal opacities suggestive of ARDS [B]. CT chest obtained at the same time reveals air-space consolidation [C and D]; air-bronchogram [arrows] [D]. While assisted ventilation was being administered, the patient developed pneumothorax on the right side; collapsed lung border is also evident [arrow] [E]. The patient required tube thoracostomy and underwater seal drainage. Eventually the patient was weaned off the ventilator and the intercostal tube was removed following resolution of the pneumothorax. The chest radiograph obtained thereafter shows significant improvement in the lesions [F]. The patient survived the turbulent in-hospital course, went on to complete full-term of pregnancy and was successfully delivered a live baby

TB = tuberculosis; ARDS = acute respiratory distress syndrome; CT = computed tomography

Reproduced with permission from "Sharma SK, Mohan A, Sharma A. Challenges in the diagnosis & treatment of miliary tuberculosis. Indian J Med Res 2012;135:703-30" (reference 30)

The TST is often negative (10,26). The yield of acid-fast bacilli [AFB] in the tracheal secretions depends on the type of underlying pulmonary TB lesion. In fibro-cavitary TB, TB pneumonia and endobronchial spread leading to bronchopneumonia, endotracheal aspirate will be positive for *Mycobacterium tuberculosis* [Mtb] in over 60% of cases (5,24). In miliary TB the yield is much lower at approximately 33% (17). Fiberoptic bronchoscopy with TBLB or broncho-alveolar lavage [BAL] may increase the yield to 88% (17). In many cases, especially those with cryptic miliary TB who do not have miliary mottling on chest radiograph, the diagnosis is invariably established by demonstration of TB granulomas in the liver biopsy specimen (26,29,30).

MANAGEMENT

The basic principles of management of TB-ARDS are the same as for ARDS due to other causes: treatment of basic cause, maintenance of optimum oxygen delivery, provision of adequate nutrition [preferably by the enteral route] and prevention of complications like nosocomial infections, upper gastrointestinal haemorrhage and deep vein thrombosis (6,41).

Oxygen Therapy

Initial treatment of hypocapnic acute respiratory failure consists of oxygen administration. The aim of therapy is to maintain arterial PaO_2 above 60 mmHg and arterial oxygen saturation measure by pulse oximetry [SpO_2] above 90%. Using an oxygen mask can increase fraction of inspired oxygen [FiO_2] to 50%-60%. Pulse oximetry helps in rapidly adjusting the FiO_2 to provide adequate oxygenation. If the desired SpO_2 cannot be achieved, oxygen administered by a non-rebreathing mask with a reservoir bag may help. If these measures fail, or respiratory distress is severe, or patient appears fatigued, tracheal intubation and mechanical ventilation may be needed (3,6,11,37,41).

Mechanical Ventilation

The initial ventilatory strategy in patients with ARDS is to deliver tidal volumes of 6 mL/kg of ideal body weight, using 100% FiO_2 with positive end-expiratory pressure [PEEP] (6). After PaO_2/FiO_2 ratio reaches the desired levels, the FiO_2 can be reduced gradually to less than 60%, provided SpO_2 remains above 90%. Most patients will require sedation and neuromuscular blockade to prevent discomfort (6). In patients with refractory hypoxaemia, lung recruitment manoeuvres and prone positioning of the patient may sometimes help. The possibility of barotrauma and ventilator-induced lung injury should be kept in mind when changing ventilator settings (6). The risk of developing pneumothorax due to barotrauma is particularly high in patients with TB as a cause of ARDS.

Extracorporeal Membrane Oxygenation

Extracorporeal membrane oxygenation [ECMO] has been found to be useful in the management of TB-ARDS (42).

Anti-TB Drugs

Anti-TB treatment should be instituted as soon as possible. Enteral therapy may not be possible in all patients. In these cases, parenteral therapy with streptomycin, isoniazid should be initiated. Injectable rifampicin may be added where available.

Corticosteroids

Corticosteroids have been used in TB-ARDS in various dosages (10,14,16,17,31,43). In addition to their immuno-suppressive effects, corticosteroids also inhibit synthesis of several mediators of inflammation including cytokines like, IL-1, IL-3, IL-4, IL-5, IL-6, IL-8, TNF-α and GM-CSF (43). They also prevent induction of the inducible forms of nitric oxide synthase [iNOS] and cyclo-oxygenase [COX-2] (43). Most workers recommend that corticosteroids be give to all patients with TB-ARDS along with anti-TB drugs, since up to 10% of these patients also have adrenal TB leading to adrenal insufficiency (16,17,44). The increased risk or upper gastrointestinal bleeding and secondary bacterial sepsis must be weighed before instituting corticosteroid therapy (44).

PROGNOSIS

Overall mortality in TB-ARDS is between 40%-80%. Non-survivors of ARDS, regardless of the cause, die of respiratory failure in less than 20% of cases (45). Most deaths are primarily related to the underlying disease, the severity of the acute illness, and the degree of dysfunction of other organs (45). Sharma *et al* (5) reported that acute physiology and chronic health evaluation II [APACHE II] score greater than 18; APACHE II score less than 18 in the presence of hyponatraemia and PaO_2/FiO_2 ratio less than 108.5 were predictors of death in patients with TB-ARDS. Zahar *et al* (24) have shown that patients receiving treatment more than one month after onset of symptoms have a 3.5 times higher risk of death than those in whom treatment is started early. Deng *et al* (22) have observed that in miliary TB patients with TB-ARDS, compared to non-survivors, survivors had a significantly shorter duration of time to diagnosis, time-lag from diagnosis to institution of assisted mechanical ventilation and time to anti-TB treatment.

REFERENCES

1. Bernard GR, Artigas A, Brigham KL, Carlet J, Falke K, Hudson L, et al. The American-European Consensus Conference on ARDS: definitions, mechanisms, relevant outcomes, and clinical trial coordination. Am J Respir Crit Care Med 1994;149:818-24.
2. Agarwal MK, Muthuswamy PP, Banner AS, Shah RS, Addington WW. Respiratory failure in pulmonary tuberculosis. Chest 1977;72: 605-9.
3. Sharma SK, Mohan A, Pande JN, Prasad KL, Gupta AK, Khilnani GC. Clinical profile, laboratory characteristics and outcome in miliary tuberculosis. QJM 1995;88:29-37.
4. Mohan A, Sharma SK, Pande JN. Acute respiratory distress syndrome in miliary tuberculosis: a 12-year experience. Indian J Chest Dis Allied Sci 1996;38:147-52.

5. Sharma SK, Mohan A, Banga A, Saha PK, Guntupall KK. Predictors of development and outcome in patients with acute respiratory distress syndrome due to tuberculosis. Int J Tuberc Lung Dis 2006;10:429-35.

6. Thompson BT, Chambers RC, Liu KD. Acute respiratory distress syndrome. N Engl J Med 2017;377:562-72.

7. Ranieri VM, Rubenfeld GD, Thompson BT, Ferguson ND, Caldwell E, Fan E, et al, ARDS Definition Task Force. Acute respiratory distress syndrome: the Berlin Definition. JAMA 2012;307:2526-33.

8. Ranieri VM, Suter PM, Tortorella C, De Tullio R, Dayer JM, Brienza A, et al. Effect of mechanical ventilation on inflammatory mediators in patients with acute respiratory distress syndrome: a randomized controlled trial. JAMA 1999;282:54-61.

9. Ranieri VM, Giunta F, Suter PM, Slutsky AS. Mechanical ventilation as a mediator of multisystem organ failure in acute respiratory distress syndrome. JAMA 2000;284:43-4 .

10. Jindal SK, Aggarwal AN, Gupta D. Adult respiratory distress syndrome in the tropics. Clin Chest Med 2002;23:445-55.

11. Chandana I. Tuberculosis and acute lung injury. In: Sharma SK, Mohan A, editors. Tuberculosis. New Delhi: Jaypee Brothers Medical Publishers; 2001.p.507-13.

12. Penner C, Roberts D, Kunimoto D, Manfreda J, Long R. Tuberculosis as a primary cause of respiratory failure requiring ventilation. Am J Respir Crit Care Med 1995;151:867-72.

13. Zhang Y, Doerfler M, Lee TC, Guillemin B, Rom WN. Mechanisms of stimulation of interleukin-1 beta and tumour necrosis factor alpha by Mycobacterium tuberculosis components. J Clin Invest 1993;91:2076-83.

14. Onwubalili JK, Scott GM, Smith H. Acute respiratory distress related to chemotherapy of advanced pulmonary tuberculosis: a study of two cases and a review of literature. QJM 1986;230: 599-610.

15. Akira M, Sakatani M. Clinical and high-resolution computed tomographic findings in five patients with pulmonary tuberculosis who developed respiratory failure following chemotherapy. Clin Radiol 2001;56:550-5.

16. Nahid P, Dorman SE, Alipanah N, Barry PM, Brozek JL, Cattamanchi A, et al. Official American Thoracic Society/Centers for Disease Control and Prevention/Infectious Diseases Society of America Clinical Practice Guidelines: Treatment of Drug-Susceptible Tuberculosis. Clin Infect Dis 2016;63:e147-95.

17. Maartens G, Willcox PA, Benatar SR. Miliary tuberculosis: rapid diagnosis, hematologic abnormalities, and outcome in 109 treated adults. Am J Med 1990;89:291-6.

18. Choi D, Lee KS, Suh GY, Kim TS, Kwon OJ, Rhee CH, et al. Pulmonary tuberculosis presenting as acute respiratory failure: radiologic findings. J Comput Assist Tomogr 1999;23:107-13.

19. Parikh CR, Karnad DR. Quality, cost, and outcome of intensive care in a public hospital in Bombay, India. Crit Care Med 1999;27:1754-9.

20. Kim JY, Park YB, Kim YS, Kang SB, Shin JW, Park IW, et al. Miliary tuberculosis and acute respiratory distress syndrome. Int J Tuberc Lung Dis 2003;7:359-64.

21. Agarwal R, Gupta D, Aggarwal AN, Behera D, Jindal SK. Experience with ARDS caused by tuberculosis in a respiratory intensive care unit. Intensive Care Med 2005;31:1284-7.

22. Deng W, Yu M, Ma H, Hu LA, Chen G, Wang Y, et al. Predictors and outcome of patients with acute respiratory distress syndrome caused by miliary tuberculosis: a retrospective study in Chongqing, China. BMC Infect Dis 2012;12:121.

23. Sharma SK, Gupta A, Biswas A, Sharma A, Malhotra A, Prasad KT, et al. Aetiology, outcomes & predictors of mortality in acute respiratory distress syndrome from a tertiary care centre in north India. Indian J Med Res 2016;143:782-92

24. Zahar JR, Azoulay E, Klement E, De Lassence A, Lucet JC, Regnier B, et al. Delayed treatment contributes to mortality in ICU patients with severe active pulmonary tuberculosis and acute respiratory failure. Intensive Care Med 2001;27:513-20.

25. Sharma S, Nahar U, Das A, Radotra B, Joshi K, Varma S, et al. Acute respiratory distress syndrome in disseminated tuberculosis: an uncommon association. Int J Tuberc Lung Dis 2016;20:271-5.

26. Case record of the Massachusetts General Hospital. Weekly clinicopathological exercises. Case 23-1995. A 44 year-old woman with pulmonary infiltrates, respiratory failure and pancytopenia. N Engl J Med 1995;333:241-8.

27. Gachot B, Wolff M, Clair B, Regnier B. Severe tuberculosis in patents with human immunodeficiency virus infection. Intensive Care Med 1990;16:491-3.

28. Kruger M, Woenckhaus J, Berner R, Hentschel R, Brandis M. Miliary tuberculosis and adult respiratory distress syndrome in an infant. Klin Pediatr 1998;210:425-7.

29. Sharma SK, Mohan A, Sharma A, Mitra DK. Miliary tuberculosis: new insights into an old disease. Lancet Infect Dis 2005;5:415-30.

30. Sharma SK, Mohan A, Sharma A. Challenges in the diagnosis & treatment of miliary tuberculosis. Indian J Med Res 2012;135: 703-30.

31. Tanaka G, Nagai H, Hebisawa A, Kawabe Y, Machida K, Kurashima A, et al. Acute respiratory failure caused by tuberculosis requiring mechanical ventilation. Kekkaku 2000; 75:395-401.

32. Bhalla A, Mahapatra M, Singh R, D'Cruz SD. Acute lung injury in miliary tuberculosis. Indian J Tuberc 2002;49:125-8.

33. Dee P, Teja K, Korzeniowski O, Suratt PM. Miliary tuberculosis resulting in adult respiratory distress syndrome: a surviving case. Am J Roentgenol 1980;134:569-72.

34. Dyer RA, Potgieter PD. The adult respiratory distress syndrome bronchogenic pulmonary tuberculosis. Thorax 1984;39:383-7.

35. Akira M, Sakatani M, Ishikawa H. Transient radiographic progression during initial treatment of pulmonary tuberculosis: CT findings. J Comput Assist Tomogr 2000;24:426-31.

36. Wendel KA, Alwood AS, Gachuhi R, Chaisson RE, Bishai WR, Sterling TR. Paradoxical worsening of tuberculosis in HIV-infected persons. Chest 2001;120:193-7.

37. Udwadia FE. Multiple organ dysfunction syndrome due to tropical infections. Indian J Crit Care Med 2003;7:233-6.

38. Ahuja SS, Ahuja SK, Phelps KR, Thelmo W, Hill AR. Hemodynamic confirmation of septic shock in disseminated tuberculosis. Crit Care Med 1992;20:901-3.

39. Piqueras AR, Marruecos L, Artigas A, Rodriguez C. Miliary tuberculosis and adult respiratory distress syndrome. Intensive Care Med 1987;13:175-82.

40. Befort P, Corne P, Godreuil S, Jung B, Jonquet O. Clinical review of eight patients with acute respiratory distress syndrome due to pulmonary tuberculosis. Scand J Infect Dis 2012;44:222-4.

41. Rittayamai N, Brochard L. Recent advances in mechanical ventilation in patients with acute respiratory distress syndrome. Eur Respir Rev 2015;24:132-40.

42. Nam SJ, Cho YJ. The successful treatment of refractory respiratory failure due to miliary tuberculosis: survival after prolonged extracorporeal membrane oxygenation support. Clin Respir J 2016;10:393-9.

43. Jantiz MA, Sahn SA. Corticosteroids in acute respiratory failure. Am J Respir Crit Care Med 1999;160:1079-100.

44. Sun TN, Yang JY, Zheng LY, Deng WW, Sui ZY. Chemotherapy and its combination with corticosteroids in acute miliary tuberculosis in adolescents and adults: analysis of 55 cases. Chin Med J [Engl] 1981;94:309-14.

45. Vincent JL, Sakr Y, Ranieri VM. Epidemiology and outcome of acute respiratory failure in intensive care unit patients. Crit Care Med 2003;31 Suppl 4:S296-9.

33

Haematological Manifestations of Tuberculosis

Shaji Kumar

INTRODUCTION

The interactions between the mycobacteria and the haemato-poietic system have been a major focus of interest for haematologists and mycobacteriologists alike for several decades. Patients with mycobacterial infections can present with myriad different, often puzzling, haematological abnormalities (1,2) [Table 33.1] and different mycobacterial infections often afflict patients with haematological disorders. Though haematological abnormalities associated with tuberculosis [TB] have been well recognised, few studies have carefully evaluated their prevalence and relationship with disease severity. Haematological changes have been observed with focal as well as disseminated TB and are usually reversible with anti-TB treatment. Haematological manifestations of TB can be due to direct effect of the infectious process itself or may be a consequence of anti-TB treatment. While haematological changes are also commonly seen in children with TB, a study (3) from a developing nation suggested that these may not be significantly different compared to a matched group of children without TB. In general, the reported haematological changes in TB appear to be more frequent and profound among patients with disseminated TB compared to localised disease.

ANAEMIA

Anaemia is the most common haematological manifestation of TB, and is seen in 16%-94% of patients with pulmonary or extra-pulmonary TB [EPTB]. The prevalence of anaemia is likely to be higher in the developing nations, given the high rates of nutritional deficiencies as well as other causes of iron deficiency anaemia, such as worm infestations. Morris *et al* (4) observed anaemia in 60% of patients with pulmonary TB, males being more frequently affected than females. In this study (4) there was a correlation between the degree of anaemia and the presence of acid-fast bacilli [AFB] in the sputum and failure to correct anaemia was associated with persistence of AFB in the sputum. The anaemia observed with TB is multifactorial in aetiology [Table 33.2] and tends to be mostly normocytic, normochromic and less often microcytic anaemia. The peripheral blood picture and the haematological indices usually indicate anaemia of chronic disease. The inflammatory response seen in TB leads to increased secretion of cytokines, such as, tumour necrosis factor-α [TNF-α] from the monocytes, which result in a blunted response to erythropoietin and decreased ability to utilise the marrow iron stores. Morris *et al* (4) found that 81% of patients with pulmonary TB had increased iron stores, suggesting decreased release of marrow iron stores and suppression of erythropoiesis by inflammatory response mediators. However, the bone marrow iron was found to be decreased in another study (5). Similarly, serum iron and total iron binding capacity have been observed to be decreased in patients with pulmonary TB and anaemia compared to those without anaemia. In addition, erythro-poietin level itself has been noted to be low in patients with

Table 33.1: Haematological changes in tuberculosis

Anaemia

Leucocyte changes
   Leucopenia or leucocytosis
   Lymphocytopenia
   Neutropenia or neutrophilia
   Monocytopenia or monocytosis

Thrombocytopenia or thrombocytosis

Pancytopenia

Deep vein thrombosis

Disseminated intravascular coagulation

Table 33.2: Aetiological factors for anaemia in tuberculosis

Anaemia of chronic disease

Iron deficiency
  Nutritional deficiency
  Secondary to chronic blood loss

Folate deficiency

Vitamin B_{12} deficiency

Myelophthisic anaemia

Haemolytic anaemia

Hypoplastic or aplastic anaemia

Pure red cell aplasia

Sideroblastic anaemia

Drug-induced anaemia [includes marrow aplasia and haemolysis]

Primary haematological disorder with tuberculosis disease

TB (6). Ebrahim *et al* (6) using an *in vitro* system of hepatocellular carcinoma cell lines demonstrated suppression of erythropoietin secretion by monocyte supernatants from patients with pulmonary TB. The levels of TNF-α were higher in these sera and addition of neutralising antibodies to TNF-α reversed some of these effects. Serum ferritin levels have been found to be an unreliable marker for iron deficiency in patients with TB (4,7). The inflammatory process in TB results in increased ferritin synthesis and high levels of ferritin in spite of decrease in iron stores. Ferritin acts as an acute phase reactant and the levels correlate with C-reactive protein [CRP] concentration. In patients with TB, raising the cut-off values of serum ferritin to 30 µg/L or less, correctly diagnosed 88% patients with iron deficiency compared with a figure of 61% when a cut-off value of 10 µg/L or less was used (8). A higher red blood cell volume distribution width [RDW] similar to that observed in iron deficiency anaemia has been reported in untreated anaemic patients with TB. The RDW values tended to become normal with anti-TB treatment (9). In a study (10) from Indonesia, the distribution of three polymorphisms in the solute carrier family 11 member 1 gene [SLC11A1], previously known as natural resistance-associated macrophage protein 1 [NRAMP1], including INT4, D543N and 3'UTR was examined for a possible association with susceptibility to TB. The authors (10) studied 378 patients with active pulmonary TB and 436 healthy control subjects from the same neighbourhood with the same socio-economic status. Anaemia was present in 63.2% of the patients with active pulmonary TB compared with 6.8% of the control subjects. Anaemia was more pronounced in female patients and those with extensive disease as assessed by the chest radiograph. Patients with active pulmonary TB and anaemia had lower plasma iron levels, iron binding capacity and higher ferritin levels. Even without iron supplementation, anti-TB treatment resulted in normalisation of the plasma iron, iron binding capacity and ferritin levels. However, *NRAMP1* gene polymorphisms were not associated with TB susceptibility,

TB severity or anaemia. The authors (10) concluded that anaemia in patients with active pulmonary TB was probably due to inflammation and not to iron deficiency.

Recent evidence is emerging regarding the role of hepcidin, an acute-phase reactant peptide that is the central regulator of iron homeostasis in the innate immune response to *Mycobacterium tuberculosis* [*Mtb*] infection (11-14). Hepcidin concentrations have been found to be strongly associated with mycobacterial burden and disseminated TB (15). Among patients with TB, hepcidin concentrations were also positively associated with greater anaemia severity.

Macrocytic anaemia is less frequently associated with TB and is usually unrelated to folate or vitamin B_{12} deficiency (4,16). In a study of 138 patients with megaloblastic haematopoiesis, who were also life-long vegetarians, 17 patients were found to have TB (16). However, Morris *et al* (4) found that the serum vitamin B_{12} levels were elevated in over half of the patients with pulmonary TB, while serum and red cell folate levels were normal in most of them. The vitamin B_{12} levels were higher in patients with leucocytosis possibly because of the elevated levels of R-binders which lead to increased concentration of vitamin B_{12}. In a study (17) of Nigerian patients with TB, the cobalamin status did not appear to influence the severity of anaemia seen in pulmonary or disseminated TB. Administration of vitamin B_{12} does not correct the anaemia in these patients. Low serum folate levels have been observed in a study (5), while no relationship between folate levels and megaloblastic haematopoiesis was found in another study (4). Autoimmune haemolytic anaemia has been reported in association with both pulmonary and disseminated TB and may disappear with treatment (17-19). Pure red cell aplasia [PRCA] has been seen in association with TB in children (20,21). Sideroblastic changes have been reported in the marrow of patients with localised or disseminated TB and the anaemia has been reported to respond to pyridoxine administration (22). There are only limited studies on the haematological changes in patients with disseminated and miliary TB (23-28). In a study (25) comparing patients with disseminated and miliary TB and those with pulmonary TB, normocytic, normochromic anaemia was the most common abnormality observed in both the groups. Moderate degree of anaemia has been observed in 52%-72% of the patients in most series (26,27,29). The anaemia is predominantly normocytic and normochromic (30). Autoimmune haemolytic anaemia [AIHA] and PRCA have been reported in association with disseminated TB (31-33). Anaemia can be a prominent finding in patients with gastrointestinal TB, where blood loss can complicate the anaemia of chronic disease (34).

Recent studies have shown that presence of anaemia at the time of diagnosis of TB was associated with a poor prognosis and an increased risk of death (35,36). Isanaka *et al* (37) analysed data from a randomised clinical trial of micronutrient supplementation in patients with pulmonary TB in Tanzania. The authors (37) reported that anaemia without iron deficiency was associated with an independent, four-fold increased risk of TB recurrence. Iron deficiency, anaemia with and without iron deficiency were associated with a greater than two-fold independent increase in the risk of death.

LEUCOCYTE CHANGES

Mild leucocytosis and a left shift with increased myelocytes and metamyelocytes, in the peripheral blood is the most common finding in most of the studies and has been seen in 6%-22% of patients (38). Patients with pulmonary TB more frequently have leucocytosis whereas leucopenia is rare. TB can result in increased myelopoiesis and the bone marrow and peripheral blood may show a leukaemoid reaction (39-41). Patients with advanced TB often have higher counts than those with minimal disease. Mild leucopenia with counts less than $4 \times 10^9/L$ has been documented in 1.5%-4% of patients (4). Prevalence of leucopenia in most studies is either equal to or higher than leucocytosis (38). Leucopenia and neutropenia were significantly higher in patients with disseminated TB. Neutrophilia has been observed in 20%-60% of patients while leucopenia has been documented in 10%-30% patients with miliary TB (23,24,42). Neutropenia has been observed in patients with disseminated TB (38). The mechanisms of neutropenia may include hypersplenism, increased neutrophil demand, or excessive margination of neutrophils. Cell-mediated autoimmune mechanisms may be responsible for neutropenia in some of the patients (43). Presence of Pelger-Huet anomaly [two symmetric, usually rounded nuclear lobes joined by a thin-strand formed by hypercondensation of nuclear chromatin that creates a spectacle-like appearance] has been described in TB (44).

Decrease in the peripheral blood CD4+ subset of T-lymphocytes has also been documented and may be seen in up to 15% of patients and is more common in disseminated and miliary TB (45,46). Lymphopenia appear to be more common than lymphocytosis in patients with pulmonary TB (38,46,47). The decreased count usually returns to the normal level following effective therapy (48). While the reasons behind the lymphopenia in TB are not entirely clear, it may reflect continued recruitment of CD4+ T-lymphocytes to the sites of granuloma formation (48). In a study (49) of lymphocyte populations in peripheral blood, pleural fluid, and ascites during TB infection, recent infection was associated with peripheral blood lymphocytosis involving both CD4+ and CD8+ cells compared to no changes in previously diagnosed patients. No changes were found in the numbers of B-lymphocytes or natural killer [NK] cells in either recently infected or previously diagnosed patients. The pleural effusion and ascitic fluid samples contained T-lymphocytes, the majority of which were CD4+ cells. These lymphocytes also showed an inverted CD45RA-to-CD45RO ratio, and had high-level expression of the interleukin-2 [IL-2] receptor [CD25] in some patients.

Both monocytosis and monocytopenia have been documented in patients with TB (4). Monocytopenia has been reported in as many as 50% of the patients and may correlate with the disease severity (50). Basophilia has been reported

in patients with disseminated TB (39). Hypereosinophilic syndrome with organ damage (51) as well as isolated eosinophilia (52,53) have also been reported in association with TB.

PLATELET ABNORMALITIES

Patients with pulmonary or disseminated TB usually have mild thrombocytosis, probably due to increased thrombopoiesis reflecting an acute phase reaction (38,54). The increased thrombopoiesis may be in part be driven by inflammatory cytokines, such as IL-6. The IL-6 is known to increase the megakaryocytes *in vitro* (55). In a study comparing patients with pulmonary TB with healthy volunteers, the median IL-6 concentrations were higher among those patients with thrombocytosis compared to those with normal platelet counts (56). The IL-6 concentrations were significantly correlated with acid-fast bacilli [AFB] positivity. Hence, it appears that IL-6 might play a contributory part in reactive thrombocytosis and acute phase response in TB.

Thrombocytopenia is more common in patients with disseminated TB, whereas, thrombocytosis is more common in pulmonary TB. However, isolated thrombocytopenia has occasionally been described in pulmonary TB and its pathogenesis is believed to be immune mediated (38,57-60). Anti-platelet antibodies and platelet associated immunoglobulin G [IgG] have been demonstrated in some patients. Boots *et al* (57) reported a case of immune thrombocytopenia with pulmonary TB, where additional studies showed presence of platelet bound IgG antibodies without any circulating anti-platelet anti- bodies. In contrast to antibodies in patients with idiopathic thrombocytopenic purpura, the antibodies in this patient did not react with normal donor platelets and the thrombocytopenia resolved with intravenous immunoglobulin therapy (57,58). There is an inverse correlation between platelet count and the mean platelet volume, and increased numbers of small platelets have been described in these patients which have a shortened survival (61). Thrombocytopenia is more common in patients with disseminated TB and has been reported in 23%-43% of patients (24,62,63). Majority of these patients, however, does not have any significant bleeding. Thrombotic thrombocytopenic purpura has been seen with lymph node as well as pulmonary TB and has been hypothesized to be due to an increased procoagulant activity of IL-1 on endothelial cells (64,65).

PANCYTOPENIA

Pancytopenia is infrequent and has been observed in only 3%-12% of cases (66). Pancytopenia is rare in patients with pulmonary TB and may occur occasionally as a result of drug toxicity in these patients (62,66-70). It is mostly associated with an underlying haematological disease although cases associated with severe miliary TB alone have been described. Patients with disseminated TB may have splenomegaly as a result of the disease process, underlying haematological disease or both. Splenomegaly may contribute to the haematological abnormalities including pancytopenia in some of these patients (71). The pancytopenia may resolve after splenectomy in some of these patients, suggesting that hypersplenism may be one of the mechanisms of pancytopenia in these patients. Pancytopenia in disseminated TB has also been attributed to haemophagocytosis, even though hypocellularity of the marrow has also been reported (71-73). All these haematological abnormalities including pancyto-penia often reverse with effective therapy (70).

COAGULATION ABNORMALITIES

Various coagulation abnormalities have been described in patients with pulmonary as well as disseminated TB. Disseminated intravascular coagulation [DIC] has been documented in disseminated as well as pulmonary TB and often is accompanied by a high mortality rate (68,74-79). In these patients activated partial thromboplastin time and thrombin time are increased and the antithrombin-III [AT-III] activity is often reduced. In a retrospective study of 833 culture-proven TB patients with DIC were evaluated before starting anti-TB treatment (80). Nearly 3.2% of them had TB induced DIC with a mortality rate of 63%. Seven of the 27 patients with DIC [25.9%] had disseminated TB. An early institution of anti-TB treatment significantly improved survival in this study. Acquired Factor V deficiency with variable bleeding manifestations has been described in patients with pulmonary TB. This abnormality disappears with anti-TB treatment (81). Sarode *et al* (80) reported the presence of platelet hyperaggregation in 88% patients with intestinal TB. Serum and plasma from 15 of these patients, when incubated with normal platelets caused hyperaggregation as well (80). This abnormality may be related to increased levels of CRP in these patients. Transient thrombasthenia has been reported in patients with TB (82). Transient protein S deficiency has been reported in association with TB and deep vein thrombosis [DVT]; however, a direct pathological relationship could not be established.

Deep vein thrombosis confirmed by venography has been observed in 3%-4% of patients with pulmonary TB (83). In a group of patients with active pulmonary TB, thrombo-cytosis, elevations in plasma fibrinogen, fibrin degradation products [FDP], tissue plasminogen activator [t-PA] and inhibitor [PAI-1] with depressed AT-III levels were seen (84). In another study (85) comparing 45 patients of active pulmo-nary TB with healthy volunteers, elevated levels of plasma fibrinogen, Factor VIII, PAI-1 and depressed AT-III and protein C levels were observed. Following treatment, fibrinogen and Factor VIII, protein C and AT-III levels normalized. There was no evidence of activated protein C resistance. Platelet aggregation studies demonstrated increased platelet activation. Age, gender and disease matched individuals with venographically proven DVT had higher FDP, t-PA, and functional PAI-1 activity. Fibrinogen levels in all patients rose during the first-two weeks of therapy and, together with related disturbances, corrected within 12 weeks. Bone marrow emboli have been reported in patients with miliary TB (86). Budd-Chiari syndrome has been reported in a child with hepatic TB (87). Portal vein thrombosis has been reported in association with abdominal TB (88).

BONE MARROW CHANGES IN TUBERCULOSIS

Both localised and disseminated TB, can lead to a spectrum of histopathological changes in the bone marrow [Table 33.3]. These changes include typical caseating granuloma formation, non-caseating granulomas, marrow hypoplasia, red cell aplasia, megaloblastosis, haemophago-cytosis, and necrosis of the marrow (28,89). In majority of the patients, the bone marrow shows normal to increased cellularity and myeloid hyperplasia (75). In most patients with pulmonary TB, the marrow shows "reactive changes" with increased granulocytic hyperplasia with mild to moderate plasmacytosis (4). Bone marrow plasmacytosis is seen less frequently in miliary TB and can be a helpful differentiating feature (4,28,90).

Bone marrow granulomas [Figures 33.1 and 33.2] are present in 50%-100% of patients with miliary TB and are usually absent in pulmonary TB (91). In a study (92) of 6,988 bone marrow biopsies, 6% of patients in whom granulomas were present in the bone marrow had TB as the inciting cause. Patients with peripheral blood abnormalities are

Table 33.3: Bone marrow changes in tuberculosis
Myeloid hyperplasia
Plasmacytosis
Megaloblastoid maturation
Hypoplasia or aplasia
Haemophagocytosis
Caseating and non-caseating granulomas
Bone marrow necrosis
Myelofibrosis

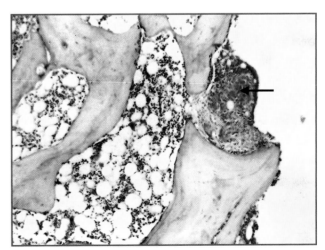

Figure 33.1: Bone biopsy showing a well-defined tuberculosis granuloma composed of epithelioid cells and Langhans' giant cells [arrow] [*Haematoxylin and eosin,* × *100*]

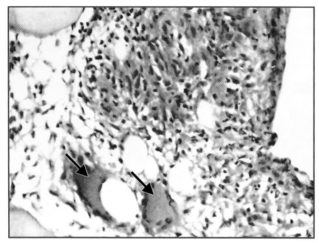

Figure 33.2: Bone biopsy showing a tuberculosis granuloma composed of epithelioid cells and Langhans' giant cells [arrows] [*Haematoxylin and eosin, × 400*]

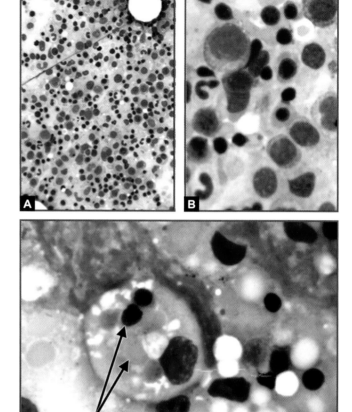

Figure 33.3: Primary HLH. A 19-year-old male who presented with fever, pancytopenia and splenomegaly. Photomicrograph of bone marrow aspirate showed increased cellularity [Giemsa, × 100] [A], [Giemsa, × 400] [B], histiocyte with ingested red blood cells and lymphocytes [arrows] [Giemsa, × 1000] [C] suggestive of HLH. Collagen vascular disease profile was negative. Further diagnostic work-up confirmed the diagnosis of primary HLH
HLH = haemophagocytic lymphohistiocytosis

more likely to have granulomas in the bone marrow (42). TB granulomas usually show the presence of Langhans' giant cells and caseation necrosis in 60%-70% of cases (24,28). Caseation necrosis and the presence of AFB in the granulomas is diagnostic of TB. It has been observed that near these granulomas the marrow cellularity is often greater or lower, and there may be an increase in reticulin fibres and in severe cases myelofibrosis may occur (93). Reticuloendothelial cells in the bone marrow may show phagocytosis of erythrocytes, leucocytes and platelets, commonly referred to as haemophagocytosis. It is more often seen in disseminated TB and disappears with treatment (94,95).

Bone marrow necrosis has been described in patients with disseminated TB (96-99). The bone marrow in patients with untreated TB may show megaloblastic changes in as many as 60% of patients with disseminated TB, but this does not reflect vitamin B_{12} or folate deficiency in these patients (28). Bone marrow aspirate iron stores are usually increased reflecting poor iron usage, though these may be decreased in some patients. Patients with poor nutritional status may have decreased iron status on bone marrow examination (31).

Bone marrow examination is often a helpful diagnostic tool in TB. The AFB may be demonstrated in the bone marrow morphologically within the granulomas or by mycobacterial culture. In a study of patients with pulmonary TB (100), AFB were detected in 55% cases in the buffy coat, and in 48.3% cases in the bone marrow. In 38.3% cases, the AFB could be demonstrated both in the buffy coat as well as the bone marrow. It is possible to use polymerase chain reaction [PCR] to detect *Mtb* in bone marrow aspirate material and this technique may be more sensitive than the conventional culture methods (53).

HAEMOPHAGOCYTIC LYMPHOHISTIOCYTOSIS, MACROPHAGE ACTIVATION SYNDROME

Haemophagocytic lymphohistiocytosis [HLH] is an under-recognised hyperinflammatory disorder characterised by haemophagocytosis, in which activated macrophages engulf blood cells or their precursors and cytokine storm (101). Primary [Figure 33.3] and secondary HLH have been described. The wrevised diagnostic criteria for HLH are shown in Table 33.4 (102). Macrophage activation syndrome [MAS] (102) is a clinical syndrome characterised by pancytopenia, elevated serum triglyceride levels, and/or hypofibrinogenaemia, evidence of haemophagocytosis in bone marrow, spleen or lymph nodes [Figure 33.4]. Other associated laboratory abnormalities include hyper-ferritinaemia and elevated blood levels of lactate dehydrogenase. Presently several workers classify MAS as a category of secondary HLH and efforts are underway to streamline the contemporary classification of histiocytic disorders.

Secondary HLH, MAS due to TB [Figure 33.4] has been described in some of the recently published reports (96,97,103-106). Shea *et al* (107) recently reported two cases and reviewed the published literature regarding

Table 33.4: Revised diagnostic guidelines for HLH*

Fever

Splenomegaly

Cytopenias in blood ≥2 cell lineages in the peripheral blood
   Haemoglobin < 9 g/dL [in infants <4 weeks < 10 g/dL]
   Platelets < 100 × 10⁹/L
   Neutrophils < 1.0 × 10⁹/L

Hypertriglyceridemia and/or hypofibrinogenemia:
   Fasting triglycerides ≥ 265 mg/dL
   Fibrinogen ≤ 1.5 g/L

Haemophagocytosis in bone marrow or spleen or lymph nodes

No evidence of malignancy

Low or absent NK-cell activity [according to local laboratory reference]

Ferritin ≥ 500 mg/L

Soluble CD25 [i.e., soluble IL-2 receptor] ≥ 2,400 U/mL

Diagnosis requires a molecular diagnosis of primary HLH or the presence of ≥ 5 of 8 diagnostic criteria
HLH = haemophagocytic lymphohistiocytosis; NK-cell = natural killer-cell; IL-2 = interleukin-2
Source: reference 102

55 cases and suggested that TB is an important treatable cause of secondary HLH which can be fatal if untreated.

NONTUBERCULOUS MYCOBACTERIAL INFECTION

Haematological abnormalities are commonly observed in patients with localised or disseminated infection caused by nontuberculous mycobacteria [NTM], but a causal relationship is often difficult to confirm given the usual immunocompromised status of the typical host and other predisposing illnesses. NTM infections are on the rise globally, especially due to the ongoing acquired immunodeficiency syndrome [AIDS] epidemic. Anaemia can be seen in almost all patients with NTM (108). Leucopenia, thrombocytopenia and pancytopenia have been observed in nearly half of the patients (109). Plasmacytosis and granulocytic hyperplasia are common findings in the bone marrow (108). Granulomas can be found in approximately half of the patients and range from small and lymphohistiocytic aggregates to larger lymphohistiocytic lesions and clusters of epithelioid cells

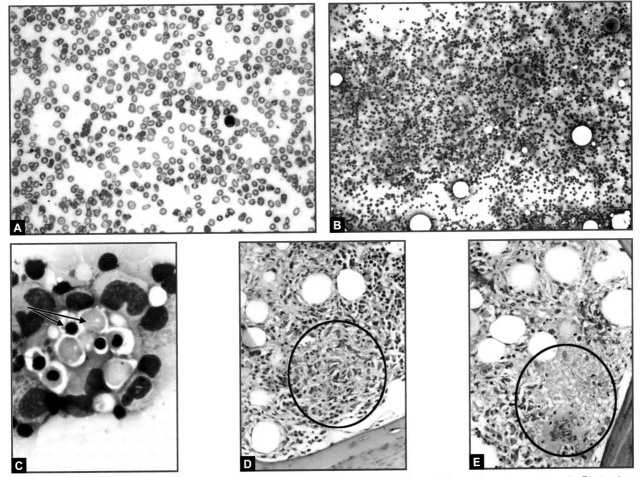

Figure 33.4: Secondary HLH due to TB. A 29-year-old male presented with fever, abdominal lymphadenopathy and pancytopenia. Photomicrograph of the peripheral blood smear showing pancytopenia [Giemsa, × 100] [A]. Photomicrograph of the bone marrow aspirate showed increased cellularity [Giemsa, × 100] [B], haemophagocytic lymphohistiocytosis [arrows] [Giemsa, × 400] [C]. Photomicrograph of the bone marrow trephine biopsy showed aggregates of epithelioid cells forming granulomas [circle] [Haematoxylin and eosin, × 400] [D], necrosis and multinucleate giant cells [circle] [Haematoxylin and eosin × 400] [E] suggestive of necrotising granulomatous inflammation. The patient responded well to anti-TB treatment
HLH = haemophagocytic lymphohistiocytosis; TB = tuberculosis

and lymphocytes (108). Unlike the granulomas associated with TB, necrosis is not commonly seen in these granulomas. Usually, few bacteria are demonstrable in the bone marrow biopsy in patients with TB, whereas numerous AFB can be seen in patients with disease due to *M. avium intracellulare* complex [MAIC]. Farhi *et al* (108) found granulomas in the bone marrow in 12 of 24 patients with disseminated MAIC infection.

DRUG-INDUCED HAEMATOLOGICAL CHANGES

Many of the abnormalities seen with TB can also be induced by the anti-TB drugs and often makes the diagnosis difficult in a patient initiated on therapy [Table 33.5]. Drug-induced AIHA can be precipitated by isoniazid, rifampicin, streptomycin as well as para- aminosalicyclic acid [PAS] (110-112). In patients receiving rifampicin, a flu-like prodrome may precede the onset of the intravascular haemolysis. In many of these patients, direct Coomb's test will become positive. Sideroblastic anaemia is a well-documented adverse effect of isoniazid therapy and usually occurs after several weeks of therapy (113,114). The bone marrow usually shows normoblastic hyperplasia with ring sideroblasts and the indices of iron metabolism are usually within normal range. The anaemia reverses on withdrawal of the drug and administration of pyridoxine. Sideroblastic anaemia has also been occasionally reported with pyrazinamide (115). Isoniazid may also produce an immune-mediated PRCA which

reverses on withdrawal of the drug (116). Aplastic anaemia has been documented with disseminated bacille Calmette-Guérin [BCG] infection (117). Treatment with PAS may cause malabsorption and result in vitamin B12 deficient megaloblastic anaemia (118).

Leucopenia, agranulocytosis and aplastic anaemia have been observed following isoniazid, rifampicin and PAS administration (86,119-123). Anti-TB treatment induced leucopenia appears to be more commonly seen in elderly patients (124). Leucopenia is rare with ethambutol use (120). Para-aminosalicylic acid can produce atypical lymphocytosis simulating infectious mononucleosis. Eosinophilia can occur with rifampicin therapy (125) and also has been reported with ethambutol (126).

The use of rifampicin may produce immune-mediated thrombocytopenia and the antibodies may be directed against the glycoprotein Ib/IX complex (127-130). Antibodies of IgG and immunoglobulin M [IgM] type have been demonstrated in many of these patients. Thrombocytopenia has been more frequently observed when twice weekly regimen of 900 mg rifampicin was used and it resolves with reduction of dose to 150-300 mg/day. Isoniazid, pyrazinamide (131), streptomycin, ethambutol (132,133), and PAS (134) may also produce thrombocytopenia. Thrombotic thrombocytopenic purpura has been reported in association with rifampicin (135).

Coagulation abnormalities are rare with anti-TB drugs. Rarely, DIC following isoniazid and rifampicin therapy has been documented (136). Acquired Factor XIII deficiency due to inhibitors has been reported with isoniazid therapy (137). In most cases, the inhibitors have been shown to be IgG antibodies and these patients may present with severe subcutaneous and retroperitoneal bleeding. The pathogenesis of isoniazid associated Factor XIII inhibitor is not fully understood. Lorand *et al* (138) have proposed that isoniazid binds to Factor XIII or one of its substrates and antigenically modifies the protein resulting in autoantibody production. PAS can produce hypothrombinemia (4). Increased incidence of DVT has been reported among patients with TB receiving rifampicin (4). This may be related to the induction of enzyme cytochrome P-450 system by rifampicin which alters the balance between anticoagulant and coagulant proteins resulting in a state of hypercoagulability. A relationship between administration of isoniazid alone or in combination with rifampicin and fibrinogen as well as AT-III blood levels has been seen in one study (139). These observations indicate a protective effect of the synchronous administration of rifampicin in the preservation of fibrinogen blood levels by enzyme induction mechanisms.

ACQUIRED IMMUNODEFICIENCY SYNDROME

Various haematological abnormalities have been described in patients with human immunodeficiency virus [HIV] infection and AIDS (140-143). In patients with AIDS, isolated thrombocytopenia has been observed during early part of the disease (144); severe degree of anaemia, leucopenia and pancytopenia are more often observed in advanced disease (145,146). Leucocytosis is more often observed in

---

Table 33.5: Haematological changes due to anti-TB treatment

Autoimmune haemolytic anaemia
    Rifampicin
    Para-aminosalicylic acid
    Isoniazid

Megaloblastic anaemia
    Para-aminosalicylic acid

Sideroblastic anaemia
    Isoniazid
    Cycloserine
    Pyrazinamide

Pure red cell aplasia
    Isoniazid

Agranulocytosis
    Streptomycin
    Thioacetazone
    Para-aminosalicylic acid

Autoimmune thrombocytopenia
    Rifampicin
    Para-aminosalicylic acid
    Isoniazid

Aplastic anaemia
    Streptomycin
    Para-aminosalicylic acid

Disseminated intravascular coagulation
    Isoniazid

TB = tuberculosis

patients with extra-pulmonary TB without HIV infection than in patients with AIDS (147). Hill *et al* (148) have observed absolute lymphocyte count of less than $1 \times 10^9/L$ in 80% of HIV-seropositive patients and in only 40% of HIV-seronegative patients.

Approximately 60% of these patients have granulomas in the bone marrow (147,148). Non-granulomatous reaction occurs in the presence of severe overwhelming infection. The granulomas may have areas of necrosis with many AFB. The surrounding inflammation when present consists mainly of polymorphonuclear cells and macrophages in contrast to usual cellular components of a granuloma seen in HIV-seronegative patients with TB (147). In a study from India (149), AFB could be demonstrated in 12.9% of the 140 bone marrow aspirates obtained from HIV-seropositive patients suggesting that in countries with a high prevalence of TB, AFB staining of the bone marrow aspirate is useful in establishing the diagnosis of TB. In a study from sub-Saharan Africa (150), low selenium concentrations, high viral load, and high IL-6 concentrations were associated with anaemia in HIV- seropositive adults with active pulmonary TB.

These manifestations could be partly secondary to anti-retroviral drug treatment or hypersplenism. Several anti-retroviral drugs, particularly zidovudine have a propensity to cause haematological manifestations, especially anaemia (151). However, a direct effect of mycobacterial infection and HIV on the haematopoietic system cannot be excluded. The underlying defect of the haematological system may also be responsible for the haematological changes and increased susceptibility to mycobacterial infection in patients with or without HIV infection. These observations merit further evaluation.

In a study (152) from Cape Town, South Africa, anaemia of chronic disease was observed to be the predominant cause of anaemia in HIV-TB patients; iron deficiency anaemia was uncommon. Another recent study (15) had shown that in patients with HIV-TB co-infection, high hepcidin concentrations were strongly associated with disseminated disease, anaemia, and poor prognosis. The authors suggested that hepcidin may be a mechanistically important mediator underlying the high prevalence of severe anaemia in HIV-TB co-infected patients.

REFERENCES

1. Dawborn JK, Cowling DC. Disseminated tuberculosis and bone marrow dyscrasias. Australas Ann Med 1961;10:230-6.
2. Corr WP Jr, Kyle RA, Bowie EJ. Hematologic changes in tuberculosis. Am J Med Sci 1964;248:709-14.
3. Wessels G, Schaaf HS, Beyers N, Gie RP, Nel E, Donald PR. Haematological abnormalities in children with tuberculosis. J Trop Pediatr 1999;45:307-10.
4. Morris CD, Bird AR, Nell H. The haematological and biochemical changes in severe pulmonary tuberculosis. QJM 1989;73:1151-9.
5. Roberts PD, Hoffbrand AV, Mollin DL. Iron and folate metabolism in tuberculosis. Br Med J 1966;2:198-202.
6. Ebrahim O, Folb PI, Robson SC, Jacobs P. Blunted erythro-poietin response to anaemia in tuberculosis. Eur J Haematol 1995;55:251-4.
7. Baynes RD, Flax H, Bothwell TH, Bezwoda WR, MacPhail AP, Atkinson P, et al. Haematological and iron-related measurements in active pulmonary tuberculosis. Scand J Haematol 1986;36:280-7.
8. Kotru M, Rusia U, Sikka M, Chaturvedi S, Jain AK. Evaluation of serum ferritin in screening for iron deficiency in tuberculosis. Ann Hematol 2004;83:95-100.
9. Baynes RD, Flax H, Bothwell TH, Bezwoda WR, Atkinson P, Mendelow B. Red blood cell distribution width in the anemia secondary to tuberculosis. Am J Clin Pathol 1986;85:226-9.
10. Sahiratmadja E, Wieringa FT, van Crevel R, de Visser AW, Adnan I, Alisjahbana B, et al. Iron deficiency and NRAMP1 polymorphisms [INT4, D543N and 3'UTR] do not contribute to severity of anaemia in tuberculosis in the Indonesian population. Br J Nutr 2007;98:684-90.
11. Shin DM, Jo EK. Antimicrobial peptides in innate immunity against mycobacteria. Immune Netw 2011;11:245-52.
12. Nemeth E, Rivera S, Gabayan V, Keller C, Taudorf S, Pedersen BK, et al. IL-6 mediates hypoferremia of inflammation by inducing the synthesis of the iron regulatory hormone hepcidin. J Clin Invest 2004;113:1271-6.
13. Ganz T. Hepcidin and iron regulation, 10 years later. Blood 2011;117:4425-33.
14. Minchella PA, Donkor S, Owolabi O, Sutherland JS, McDermid JM. Complex anemia in tuberculosis: the need to consider causes and timing when designing interventions. Clin Infect Dis 2015;60:764-72.
15. Kerkhoff AD, Meintjes G, Burton R, Vogt M, Wood R, Lawn SD. Relationship between blood concentrations of hepcidin and anemia severity, mycobacterial burden, and mortality among patients with HIV-associated tuberculosis. J Infect Dis 2016;213:61-70.
16. Chanarin I, Malkowska V, O'Hea AM, Rinsler MG, Price AB. Megaloblastic anaemia in a vegetarian Hindu community. Lancet 1985;2:1168-72.
17. Knox-Macaulay HH. Serum cobalamin concentration in tuberculosis. A study in the Guinea savanna of Nigeria. Trop Geogr Med 1990;42:146-50.
18. Siribaddana SH, Wijesundera A. Autoimmune haemolytic anaemia responding to anti-tuberculous treatment. Trop Doct 1997;27:243-4.
19. Kuo PH, Yang PC, Kuo SS, Luh KT. Severe immune haemolytic anemia in disseminated tuberculosis with response to anti-tuberculosis therapy. Chest 2001;119:1961-3.
20. Rani S, Singh T, Prakash S. Pure red cell aplasia. Indian Pediatr 1990;27:366-70.
21. Dutta S, Mohta R, Pati HP. Tuberculosis pure red cell aplasia. Int J Tuberc Lung Dis 1999;3:361-2.
22. Demiroglu H, Dundar S. Vitamin B6 responsive sideroblastic anaemia in a patient with tuberculosis. Br J Clin Pract 1997;51:51-2.
23. Sharma SK, Mohan A, Pande JN, Prasad KL, Gupta AK, Khilnani GC. Clinical profile, laboratory characteristics and outcome in miliary tuberculosis. QJM 1995;88:29-37.
24. Sharma SK, Mohan A, Sharma A, Mitra DK. Miliary tuberculosis: new insights into an old disease. Lancet Infect Dis 2005;5:415-30.
25. Singh KJ, Ahluwalia G, Sharma SK, Saxena R, Chaudhary VP, Mohan A. Significance of haematological manifestations in patients with tuberculosis. J Assoc Physicians India 2001;49:788,790-4.
26. Hussain SF, Irfan M, Abbasi M, Anwer SS, Davidson S, Haqqee R, et al. Clinical characteristics of 110 miliary tuberculosis patients from a low HIV prevalence country. Int J Tuberc Lung Dis 2004;8:493-9.

27. Yoon HJ, Song YG, Park WI, Choi JP, Chang KH, Kim JM. Clinical manifestations and diagnosis of extrapulmonary tuberculosis. Yonsei Med J 2004;45:453-61.

28. Lombard EH, Mansvelt EP. Haematological changes associated with miliary tuberculosis of the bone marrow. Tuber Lung Dis 1993;74:131-5.

29. Al-Jahdali H, Al-Zahrani K, Amene P, Memish Z, Al-Shimemeri A, Moamary M, et al. Clinical aspects of military tuberculosis in Saudi adults. Int J Tuberc Lung Dis 2000;4:252-5.

30. al-Majed SA, al-Momen AK, al-Kassimi FA, al-Zeer A, Kambal AM, Baaqil H. Tuberculosis presenting as immune thrombocytopenic purpura. Acta Haematol 1995;94:135-8.

31. Bakhshi S, Rao IS, Jain V, Arya LS. Autoimmune haemolytic anemia complicating disseminated childhood tuberculosis. Indian J Pediatr 2004;71:549-51.

32. Sinha AK, Agarwal A, Lakhey M, Ansari J, Rani S. Pure red cell aplasia–report of 11 cases from eastern Nepal. Indian J Pathol Microbiol 2003;46:405-8.

33. Blanche P, Rigolet A, Massault PP, Bouscary D, Dreyfus F, Sicard D. Autoimmune haemolytic anaemia revealing military tuberculosis. J Infect 2000;40:292.

34. Ismail Y, Muhamad A. Protean manifestations of gastro-intestinal tuberculosis. Med J Malaysia 2003;58:345-9.

35. Lee SW, Kang YA, Yoon YS, Um SW, Lee SM, Yoo CG, et al. The prevalence and evolution of anemia associated with tuberculosis. J Korean Med Sci 2006;21:1028-32.

36. Armitage AE, Moran E. HIV-associated tuberculosis: does the iron-regulatory hormone hepcidin connect anemia with poor prognosis? J Infect Dis 2016;213:3-5.

37. Isanaka S, Mugusi F, Urassa W, Willett WC, Bosch RJ, Villamor E, et al. Iron deficiency and anemia predict mortality in patients with tuberculosis. J Nutr 2012;142:350-7.

38. Olaniyi JA, Aken'Ova YA. Haematological profile of patients with pulmonary tuberculosis in Ibadan, Nigeria. Afr J Med Med Sci 2003;32:239-42.

39. Paar JA, Scheinman MM, Weaver RA. Disseminated nonreactive tuberculosis with basophilia, leukemoid reaction and terminal pancytopenia. N Engl J Med 1966;274:335.

40. Keeton GR, Naidoo G, Jacobs P. Leukaemoid reaction and disseminated tuberculosis. A case report. S Afr Med J 1975;49:1930-2.

41. Tripathi K, Prakash J, Misra KM, Srivastava PK, Dube B. Leukaemoid reaction in tuberculosis. J Indian Med Assoc 1984;82:63-4.

42. Maartens G, Willcox PA, Benatar SR. Miliary tuberculosis: rapid diagnosis, hematologic abnormalities, and outcome in 109 treated adults. Am J Med 1990;89:291-6.

43. Bagby GC Jr, Gilbert DN. Suppression of granulopoiesis by T-lymphocytes in two patients with disseminated mycobacterial infection. Ann Intern Med 1981;94:478-81.

44. Shenkenberg TD, Rice L, Waddell CC. Acquired Pelger-Huet nuclear anomaly with tuberculosis. Arch Intern Med 1982;142:153-4.

45. Kony SJ, Hane AA, Larouzé B, Samb A, Cissoko S, Sow PS, et al. Tuberculosis-associated severe CD4+ T-lymphocytopenia in HIV-seronegative patients from Dakar. SIDAK Research Group. J Infect 2000;41:167-71.

46. Sharma SK, Pande JN, Singh YN, Verma K, Kathait SS, Khare SD, et al. Pulmonary function and immunologic abnormalities in miliary tuberculosis. Am Rev Respir Dis 1992;145:1167-71.

47. Akintunde EO, Shokunbi WA, Adekunle CO. Leucocyte count, platelet count and erythrocyte sedimentation rate in pulmonary tuberculosis. Afr J Med Med Sci 1995;24:131-4.

48. Onwubalili JK, Edwards AJ, Palmer L. T4 lymphopenia in human tuberculosis. Tubercle 1987;68:195-200.

49. Gambon-Deza F, Pacheco Carracedo M, Cerda Mota T, Montes Santiago J. Lymphocyte populations during tuberculosis infection: V beta repertoires. Infect Immun 1995;63:1235-40.

50. Venter JP. Hematological, blood biochemical and certain clinical aspects of tuberculosis in the Bantu. S Afr Med J 1974;48:1559-62.

51. Farcet JP, Binaghi M, Kuentz M, Merlier JF, Mayaud C, Nebout T, et al. A hypereosinophilic syndrome with retinal arteritis and tuberculosis. Arch Intern Med 1982;142:625-7.

52. Flores M, Merino-Angulo J, Tanago JG, Aquirre C. Late generalized tuberculosis and eosinophilia. Arch Intern Med 1983;143:182.

53. Lombard EH, Victor T, Jordaan A, van Helden PD. The detection of Mycobacterium tuberculosis in bone marrow aspirate using the polymerase chain reaction. Tuber Lung Dis 1994;75:65-9.

54. Omar MA, Jogessar VB, Kamdar MC. Thrombocytosis associated with tuberculous peritonitis. Tubercle 1983;64:295-6.

55. Asano S, Okano A, Ozawa K, Nakahata T, Ishibashi T, Koike K, et al. In vivo effects of recombinant human interleukin-6 in primates: stimulated production of platelets. Blood 1990;75:1602-5.

56. Unsal E, Aksaray S, Koksal D, Sipit T. Potential role of interleukin 6 in reactive thrombocytosis and acute phase response in pulmonary tuberculosis. Postgrad Med J 2005;81:604-7.

57. Boots RJ, Roberts AW, McEvoy D. Immune thrombocytopenia complicating pulmonary tuberculosis: case report and investigation of mechanisms. Thorax 1992;47:396-7.

58. Hernandez-Maraver D, Pelaez J, Pinilla J, Navarro FH. Immune thrombocytopenic purpura due to disseminated tuberculosis. Acta Haematol 1996;96:266.

59. Surana AP, Shelgikar KM, Melinkeri S, Phadke A. Immune thrombocytopenia [ITP]: a rare association of lymph node tuberculosis. J Assoc Physicians India 2014;62:74-6.

60. Srividya G, Nikhila GP, Kaushik AV, Jayachandran K. Immune thrombocytopenia in tuberculosis: causal or coincidental? J Global infect Dis 2014;6:128-31.

61. Baynes RD, Bothwell TH, Flax H, McDonald TP, Atkinson P, Chetty N, et al. Reactive thrombocytosis in pulmonary tuberculosis. J Clin Pathol 1987;40:676-9.

62. Cockcroft DW, Donevan RE, Copland GM, Ibbott JW. Miliary tuberculosis presenting with hyponatremia and thrombocytopenia. Can Med Assoc J 1976;115:871-3.

63. Cummins D, Markham D, Ardeman S, Lubenko A. Severe thrombocytopenia in tuberculosis. Clin Lab Haematol 1993;15:150-2.

64. Pavithran K, Vijayalekshmi N. Thrombocytopenic purpura with tuberculous adenitis. Indian J Med Sci 1993;47:239-40.

65. Toscano V, Bontadini A, Falsone G, Conte R, Fois F, Fabiani A, et al. Thrombotic thrombocytopenic purpura associated with primary tuberculosis. Infection 1995;23:58-9.

66. De SRJL, Vidanapathirana NN, Rajakariar R. Pancytopenia in a paediatric unit. Ceylon Med J 1977;22:132-6.

67. Ulku B, Ilkova HM, Celikoglu SI, Aykan TB. Pancytopenia associated with disseminated tuberculosis. Haematologica 1982;67:630-5.

68. Sarma PS, Viswanathan KA, Budhiraja A, Mukherjee MM. Pancytopenia and DIC in disseminated tuberculosis. J Assoc Physicians India 1984;32:601-2.

69. Hunt BJ, Andrews V, Pettingale KW. The significance of pancytopenia in miliary tuberculosis. Postgrad Med J 1987;63:801-4.

70. Yadav TP, Mishra S, Sachdeva KJ, Gupta VK, Siddhu KK, Bakshi G, et al. Pancytopenia in disseminated tuberculosis. Indian Pediatr 1996;33:597-9.

71. Cassim KM, Gathiram V, Jogessar VB. Pancytopaenia associated with disseminated tuberculosis, reactive histiocytic

haemophagocytic syndrome and tuberculous hypersplenism. Tuber Lung Dis 1993;74:208-10.

72. Demiroglu H, Ozcebe OI, Ozdemir L, Sungur A, Dundar S. Pancytopenia with hypocellular bone marrow due to military tuberculosis: an unusual presentation. Acta Haematol 1994;91: 49-51.

73. Basu S, Mohan H, Malhotra H. Pancytopenia due to hemophagocytic syndrome as the presenting manifestation of tuberculosis. J Assoc Physicians India 2000;48:845-6.

74. Mavligit GM, Binder RA, Crosby WH. Disseminated intravascular coagulation in miliary tuberculosis. Arch Intern Med 1972;130:388-9.

75. Oluboyede OA, Onadeko BO. Observation on haematological patterns in pulmonary tuberculosis in Nigerians. J Trop Med Hyg 1978;81:91-5.

76. Stein DS, Libertin CR. Disseminated intravascular coagulation in association with cavitary tuberculosis. South Med J 1990;83:60-3.

77. Eliopoulos G, Vaiopoulos G, Kittas C, Fessas P. Tuberculosis associated hemophagocytic syndrome complicated with severe bone marrow failure and disseminated intravascular coagulation. Nouv Rev Fr Hematol 1992;34:273-6.

78. Fujita M, Kunitake R, Nagano Y, Maeda F. Disseminated intra-vascular coagulation associated with pulmonary tuberculosis. Intern Med 1997;36:218-20.

79. Wang JY, Hsueh PR, Lee LN, Liaw YS, Shau WY, Yang PC, et al. Mycobacterium tuberculosis inducing disseminated intravascular coagulation. Thromb Haemost 2005;93:729-34.

80. Sarode R, Bhasin D, Marwaha N, Roy P, Singh K, Panigrahi D, et al. Hyperaggregation of platelets in intestinal tuberculosis: role of platelets in chronic inflammation. Am J Hematol 1995;48: 52-4.

81. Aliaga JL, de Gracia J, Vidal R, Pico M, Flores P, Sampol G. Acquired factor V deficiency in a patient with pulmonary tuberculosis. Eur Respir J 1990;3:109-10.

82. Du PHA, Retief FP, Richter G, Badenhorst PN. Transient thrombasthenia in a patient with tuberculosis. S Afr Med J 1974;48:2454-6.

83. Cowie RL, Dansey RD, Hay M. Deep-vein thrombosis and pulmonary tuberculosis. Lancet 1989;2:1397.

84. Robson SC, White NW, Aronson I, Woollgar R, Goodman H, Jacobs P. Acute-phase response and the hypercoagulable state in pulmonary tuberculosis. Br J Haematol 1996;93:943-9.

85. Turken O, Kunter E, Sezer M, Solmazgul E, Cerrahoglu K, Bozkanat E, et al. Hemostatic changes in active pulmonary tuberculosis. Int J Tuberc Lung Dis 2002;6:927-32.

86. Witham RR, Burton JA. Bone marrow emboli in a patient with miliary tuberculosis. Chest 1979;75:208.

87. Gomber S, Khalil A, Vij JC, Bahl VK, Kapoor R, Saini L. Budd-Chiari syndrome in a child with hepatic tuberculosis. Indian Heart J 1986;38:226-9.

88. Ruttenberg D, Graham S, Burns D, Solomon D, Bornman P. Abdominal tuberculosis–a cause of portal vein thrombosis and portal hypertension. Dig Dis Sci 1991;36:112-5.

89. Knox-Macaulay HH. Tuberculosis and the haemopoietic system. Baillieres Clin Haematol 1992;5:101-29.

90. Kinoshita M, Ichikawa Y, Koga H, Sumita S, Oizumi K. Reevaluation of bone marrow aspiration in the diagnosis of miliary tuberculosis. Chest 1994;106:690-2.

91. Morris CD. The radiography, haematology and biochemistry of pulmonary tuberculosis in the aged. QJM 1989;71:529-36.

92. Bhargava V, Farhi DC. Bone marrow granulomas: clinico-pathologic findings in 72 cases and review of the literature. Hematol Pathol 1988;2:43-50.

93. Samuelsson SM, Killander A, Werner I, Stenkvist B. Myelofibrosis associated with tuberculous lymphadenitis. Acta Med Scand Suppl 1966;445:326-5.

94. Campo E, Condom E, Miro MJ, Cid MC, Romagosa V. Tuberculosis-associated hemophagocytic syndrome. A systemic process. Cancer 1986;58:2640-5.

95. Undar L, Karpuzoglu G, Karadogan I, Gelen T, Artvinli M. Tuberculosis-associated haemophagocytic syndrome: a report of two cases and a review of the literature. Acta Haematol 1996;96:73-8.

96. Shin BC, Kim SW, Ha SW, Sohn JW, Lee JM, Kim NS. Hemophagocytic syndrome associated with bilateral adrenal gland tuberculosis. Korean J Intern Med 2004;19:70-3.

97. Claessens YE, Pene F, Tulliez M, Cariou A, Chiche JD. Life-threatening hemophagocytic syndrome related to mycobacterium tuberculosis. Eur J Emerg Med 2006;13:172-4.

98. Katzen H, Spagnolo SV. Bone marrow necrosis from military tuberculosis. JAMA 1980;244:2438-9.

99. Paydas S, Ergin M, Baslamisli F, Yavuz S, Zorludemir S, Sahin B, et al. Bone marrow necrosis: clinicopathologic analysis of 20 cases and review of the literature. Am J Hematol 2002;70:300-5.

100. Garcia MJ, Rodriguez L, Vandervoort P. Pulmonary vein thrombosis and peripheral embolization. Chest 1996;109:846-7.

101. Brisse E, Matthys P, Wouters CH. Understanding the spectrum of haemophagocytic lymphohistiocytosis: update on diagnostic challenges and therapeutic options. Br J Haematol 2016;174: 175-87.

102. Henter JI, Horne A, Aricó M, Egeler RM, Filipovich AH, Imashuku S, et al. HLH-2004: Diagnostic and therapeutic guidelines for hemophagocytic lymphohistiocytosis. Pediatr Blood Cancer 2007;48:124-31.

103. Grom AA, Horne A, De Benedetti F. Macrophage activation syndrome in the era of biologic therapy. Nat Rev Rheumatol 2016;12:259-68.

104. Bizid S, Ben Slimane B, Msakni I, Bouali R, Ben Abdallah H, Abdelli N. Macrophage activation syndrome revealing dis-seminated Mycobacterium tuberculosis. Tunis Med 2015;93: 580-2.

105. André V, Liddell C, Guimard T, Tanguy G, Cormier G. Macro-phage activation syndrome revealing disseminated tuberculosis in a patient on infliximab. Joint Bone Spine 2013;80:109-10.

106. Le Hô H, Barbarot N, Desrues B. Pancytopenia in disseminated tuberculosis: Think of macrophage activation syndrome. Rev Mal Respir 2010;27:257-60.

107. Shea YF, Chan JF, Kwok WC, Hwang YY, Chan TC, Ni MY, et al. Haemophagocytic lymphohistiocytosis: an uncommon clinical presentation of tuberculosis. Hong Kong Med J 2012;18: 517-25.

108. Farhi DC, Mason UG 3rd, Horsburgh CR, Jr. The bone marrow in disseminated Mycobacterium avium-intracellulare infection. Am J Clin Pathol 1985;83:463-8.

109. Horsburgh CR Jr, Mason UG 3rd, Farhi DC, Iseman MD. Disseminated infection with Mycobacterium avium-intracellulare. A report of 13 cases and a review of the literature. Medicine [Baltimore] 1985;64:36-48.

110. Oguz A, Kanra T, Gokalp A, Gultekin A. Acute haemolytic anemia caused by irregular rifampicin therapy. Turk J Pediatr 1989;31:83-8.

111. Yeo CT, Wang YT, Poh SC. Mild haemolysis associated with flu-syndrome during daily rifampicin treatment–a case report. Singapore Med J 1989;30:215-6.

112. Letona JM, Barbolla L, Frieyro E, Bouza E, Gilsanz F, Fernandez MN. Immune haemolytic anaemia and renal failure induced by streptomycin. Br J Haematol 1977;35:561-71.

113. McCurdy PR, Donohoe RF. Pyridoxine-responsive anemia conditioned by isonicotinic acid hydrazide. Blood 1966;27:352-62.

114. Tomkin GH. Isoniazid as a cause of neuropathy and sideroblastic anaemia. Practitioner 1973;211:773-7.

115. McCurdy PR, Donohoe RF, Magovern M. Reversible sideroblastic anemia caused by pyrazinoic acid [pyrazinamide]. Ann Intern Med 1966;64:1280-4.

116. Claiborne RA, Dutt AK. Isoniazid-induced pure red cell aplasia. Am Rev Respir Dis 1985;131:947-9.

117. Long HJ. Aplastic anemia, a rare complication of disseminated BCG infection: case report. Mil Med 1982;147:1067-70.

118. Paaby P, Norvin E. The absorption of vitamin B12 during treatment with para-aminosalicylic acid. Acta Med Scand 1966;180:561-4.

119. Williams CK, Aderoju EA, Adenle AD, Sekoni G, Esan GJ. Aplastic anaemia associated with anti-tuberculosis chemotherapy. Acta Haematol 1982;68:329-32.

120. Mehrotra TN, Gupta SK. Agranulocytosis following isoniazid. Report of a case. Indian J Med Sci 1973;27:392-3.

121. van Assendelft AH. Leucopenia caused by two rifampicin preparations. Eur J Respir Dis 1984;65:251-8.

122. Carrington CB, Addington WW, Goff AM, Madoff IM, Marks A, Schwaber JR, et al. Chronic eosinophilic pneumonia. N Engl J Med 1969;280:787-98.

123. van Assendelft AH. Leucopenia in rifampicin chemotherapy. J Antimicrob Chemother 1985;16:407-8.

124. Umeki S. Clinical features of pulmonary tuberculosis in young and elderly men. Jpn J Med 1989;28:341-7.

125. Nigam P, Goyal BM, Saxena HN. Eosinophilia as a result of rifampicin therapy. J Indian Med Assoc 1981;77:158-9.

126. Wong PC, Yew WW, Wong CF, Choi HY. Ethambutolinduced pulmonary infiltrates with eosinophilia and skin involvement. Eur Respir J 1995;8:866-8.

127. Leggat PO. Rifampicin and thrombocytopenia. Lancet 1971;2:103-4.

128. Burnette PK, Ameer B, Hoang V, Phifer W. Rifampin-associated thrombocytopenia secondary to poor compliance. DICP 1989;23:382-4.

129. Lee CH, Lee CJ. Thrombocytopenia–a rare but potentially serious side effect of initial daily and interrupted use of rifampicin. Chest 1989;96:202-3.

130. Mehta YS, Jijina FF, Badakere SS, Pathare AV, Mohanty D. Rifampicin-induced immune thrombocytopenia. Tuber Lung Dis 1996;77:558-62.

131. Jain VK, Vardhan H, Prakash OM. Pyrazinamide induced thrombocytopenia. Tubercle 1988;69:217-8.

132. Rabinovitz M, Pitlik SD, Halevy J, Rosenfeld JB. Ethambutol induced thrombocytopenia. Chest 1982;81:765-6.

133. Prasad R, Mukerji PK. Ethambutol-induced thrombocytopaenia. Tubercle 1989;70:211-2.

134. Feigin RD, Zarkowsky HF, Shearer W, Anderson DC. Thrombocytopenia following administration of paraaminosalicylic acid. J Pediatr 1973;83:502-3.

135. Fahal IH, Williams PS, Clark RE, Bell GM. Thrombotic thrombocytopenic purpura due to rifampicin. BMJ 1992;304:882.

136. Ip M, Cheng KP, Cheung WC. Disseminated intravascular coagulopathy associated with rifampicin. Tubercle 1991;72:291-3.

137. Krumdieck R, Shaw DR, Huang ST, Poon MC, Rustagi PK. Hemorrhagic disorder due to an isoniazid-associated acquired factor XIII inhibitor in a patient with Waldenstrom's macro-globulinemia. Am J Med 1991;90:639-45.

138. Lorand L, Maldonado N, Fradera J, Atencio AC, Robertson B, Urayama T. Haemorrhagic syndrome of autoimmune origin with a specific inhibitor against fibrin stabilizing factor [factor XIII]. Br J Haematol 1972;23:17-27.

139. Farmakis M, Travlou O, Aroni S, Fertakis A. Fibrinogen and antithrombin III blood levels fluctuations during isoniazid or isoniazid plus rifampicin administration. Arzneimittel-forschung 1992;42:1041-4.

140. Evans RH, Scadden DT. Haematological aspects of HIV infection. Baillieres Best Pract Res Clin Haematol 2000;13:215-30.

141. Adias TC, Uko E, Erhabor O. Anaemia in human immuno-deficiency virus infection: a review. Niger J Med 2006;15:203-6.

142. Lee SW, Kang YA, Yoon YS, Um SW, Lee SM, Yoo CG, et al. The prevalence and evolution of anemia associated with tuberculosis. J Korean Med Sci 2006;21:1028-32.

143. Subbaraman R, Chaguturu SK, Mayer KH, Flanigan TP, Kumarasamy N. Adverse effects of highly active antiretroviral therapy in developing countries. Clin Infect Dis 2007;45:1093-101.

144. Karpatkin S. HIV-1 related thrombocytopenia. Hematol Oncol Clin North Am 1990;4:193-218.

145. Treacy M, Lai L, Costello C, Clark A. Peripheral blood and bone marrow abnormalities in patients with HIV related diseases. Br J Haematol 1987;65;289-94.

146. Zon Li, Arkin C, Groopman JE. Haematologic manifestations of human immunodeficiency virus [HIV] infection. Br J Haematol 1987;66:251-6.

147. Shafer RW, Kim DS, Weiss JP, Quale JM. Extrapulmonary tuberculosis in patients with human immunodeficiency virus infection. Medicine [Baltimore] 1991;70:384-97.

148. Hill AR, Premkumar S, Brustein S, Vaidya K, Powell S, Li PW, et al. Disseminated tuberculosis in the acquired immuno-deficiency syndrome era. Am Rev Respir Dis 1991;144:1164-70.

149. Khandekar MM, Deshmukh SD, Holla VV, Rane SR, Kakrani AL, Sangale SA, et al. Profile of bone marrow examination in HIV/AIDS patients to detect opportunistic infections, especially tuberculosis. Indian J Pathol Microbiol 2005;48:7-12.

150. van Lettow M, West CE, van der Meer JW, Wieringa FT, Semba RD. Low plasma selenium concentrations, high plasma human immunodeficiency virus load and high interleukin-6 concentrations are risk factors associated with anemia in adults presenting with pulmonary tuberculosis in Zomba district, Malawi. Eur J Clin Nutr 2005;59:526-32.

151. Antoniskis D, Easley AC, Espina BM, Davidson PT, Barnes PF. Combined toxicity of zidovudine and antituberculosis chemo-therapy. Am Rev Respir Dis 1992;145:430-4.

152. Kerkhoff AD, Meintjes G, Opie J, Vogt M, Jhilmeet N, Wood R, et al. Anaemia in patients with HIV-associated TB: relative contributions of anaemia of chronic disease and iron deficiency. Int J Tuberc Lung Dis 2016;20:193-201.

34

Endocrine Implications of Tuberculosis

CV Harinarayan, Shalini Joshi, SP Munigoti

INTRODUCTION

Tuberculosis [TB] can affect various endocrine glands in the body. Endocrine involvement has been observed in pulmonary TB, extra-pulmonary TB [EPTB], disseminated TB and miliary TB. Further, anti-TB drugs induce cytochrome P-450 oxidase enzymes which can enhance the catabolism of hormones. The present chapter provides an overview regarding the endocrine implications of TB.

TUBERCULOSIS AND HYPOTHALAMUS, PITUITARY INVOLVEMENT

Pituitary and Tuberculosis

Epidemiology

Pituitary involvement in TB remains rare. TB is responsible for 20% of the intracranial space occupying lesions in India and tuberculomas of the sellar and suprasellar region comprise 1% of all intracranial tuberculomas (1). Studies documenting hypothalamo-pituitary involvement in TB published from India are summarised in Table 34.1 (2-8). In the western countries the reported frequency of sellar tuberculomas is 0.25%-4% (4).

Pathogenesis

TB hypophysitis can occur as a localised sellar/suprasellar lesion or can be a part of a widespread disease involving the either rest of the brain parenchyma and/or meninges. Intra-sellar tuberculomas may present as apoplexy. The usual mode of spread of infection to the pituitary is *via* haematogenous route or direct spread from the paranasal sinus (9-11).

Clinical Presentation

Clinical presentation of patients with hypothalamo-pituitary involvement would depend on the extent of central nervous system [CNS] involvement. Meningeal symptoms, such as, headache are the most common amongst those reported. Sellar lesions themselves tend to be asymptomatic and get diagnosed radiologically but could manifest with endocrine abnormalities. Involvement of posterior pituitary could result in polydipsia and polyuria secondary to diabetes insipidus. A review of 54 cases (1), revealed female preponderance [females: males ratio 2:1]. Majority of patients were found to be young [< 45 years] and headache appeared to be the most common symptom [91%]. Suprasellar involvement was found in 74% of the cases while sellar enlargement was seen in 95% of the cases on neuroradiology imaging. In this study (1), non-preferential anterior pituitary involvement was described in more than half the cases and hyperprolactinaemia was observed in a quarter of the cases. Posterior pituitary involvement leading to diabetes insipidus was seen in 11% of the cases. Others reported growth hormone and gonadotropin deficiency as more common endocrine abnormalities (12-18). Less common endocrine abnormalities are those of corticotropic and thyrotropic hormones manifesting as secondary adrenocortical insufficiency or hypothyroidism. In children, the presentation could be either anterior or posterior pituitary dysfunction with compressive features. Clinical manifestations are those of short stature or hypogonadism. Isolated diabetes insipidus has been reported in a young male with supra-sellar involvement (15). Though pituitary hypofunction is more common, hormonal over activity presenting as central precocious puberty has been reported in

Table 34.1: Studies documenting hypothalamo-pituitary involvement in TB published from India

Study [year] (reference)	Clinical manifestations	Remarks
Sunil *et al* [2007] (1)	A patient with prostatic TB on treatment developed diabetes mellitus, loss of libido and headache. While on treatment for diabetes mellitus with insulin he gradually developed hypoglycaemia. Anti-diabetic medication was stopped; evaluation for hypoglycaemia revealed hypocorticism and pituitary mass, which on excision and histopathological examination revealed epithelioid granulomas, giant cell and caseation necrosis suggestive of TB	Case presentation and review of 54 previous reported cases with sellar/suprasellar TB
Ranjan *et al* [2011] (2)	Young lady presented with progressive headache, found to have with hypothyroidism, hyperprolactinaemia. She responded to anti-TB treatment and was symptom free at follow-up	Sellar abscess diagnosed after culture of purulent discharge grew *Mtb*
Mageshkumar *et al* [2011] (3)	Patient presented with sellar and suprasellar lesions with widespread CNS TB needing decompression for hydrocephalus with a shunt and also full hormone replacement therapy along with anti-TB treatment	Widespread inflammation resulted in hypopituitarism
Mittal *et al* [2010] (4)	Full resolution of a sellar mass presenting as visual loss following haemorrhage that resolved completely with surgery and anti-TB treatment	Tuberculoma with apoplexy and sellar haemorrhage causing compression of optic chiasma
Furtado *et al* [2011] (5)	Panhypopituitarism	Isolated tuberculoma presenting with hypopituitarism
Hussain *et al* [2008] (6)	Hypopituitarism	Granulomatous hypophysitis diagnosed as TB after CSF PCR tested positive
Satyarthee and Mahapatra [2003] (7)	Diabetes insipidus	Rare presentation of sellar-suprasellar tuberculoma
Dutta *et al* [2006] (8)	Patient presented with visual disturbances, diabetes insipidus with panhypopituitarism. Diagnosis of TB confirmed on histopathological examination that revealed granulomas and tested positive for acid-fast bacilli	Pituitary TB abscess presenting with compressive features and endocrine dysfunction

TB = tuberculosis; *Mtb* = *Mycobacterium tuberculosis*; CNS = central nervous system; CSF = cerebrospinal fluid; PCR = polymerase chain reaction

children with preceding history of TB meningitis in as many as 31% girls and 27% boys (16). Hyperprolactinaemia as a result of stalk compression and release of anterior pituitary from inhibiting effect of dopamine due to tuberculoma have also been recorded (14).

Diagnosis

Imaging Studies Pituitary lesions in a patient with or without background TB would be evident after neuroradiological imaging including computed tomography [CT] and magnetic resonance imaging [MRI]. Pituitary tuberculomas are isointense on T1 weighted MRI images and usually exhibit intense post-contrast enhancement on MRI and CT. Contrast MRI [Figure 34.1] demonstrates thickening of the stalk thought to be due to chronic inflammatory scarring (17). But, this thickening of the stalk is non-specific and is described in other diverse clinical conditions, such as neoplasms, sarcoidosis, syphilis, lymphocytic hypophysitis, granulomatous hypophysitis and eosinophilic granuloma. More so, suprasellar extension could make stalk evaluation difficult on neuroimaging. Peripheral ring enhancement of the mass, enhancement of the adjacent dural and basal enhancing exudates due to meningitis, isolated stalk thickening, sellar/suprasellar calcification, apoplexy and

erosion of the sellar floor (11) are some other findings described on the MRI.

Surgery

Transsphenoidal surgery is the only way to establish definitive diagnosis. Other than TB, histopathologically, the differential diagnosis of granulomatous hypophysitis includes sarcoidosis, mycotic infection, hypophysitis due to ruptured intrasellar Rathke cleft cyst, histiocytosis X and idiopathic causes (19-23). Granulomas in TB are typically described to be characterised by a central area of caseous necrosis surrounded by epithelioid cells, macrophages, lymphocytes and plasma cells. Identification of *Mycobacterium tuberculosis* [*Mtb*] itself is clearly diagnostic. Sometimes diagnosis is made after the culture results of suspected cases turn positive. In cases of further ambiguity, molecular diagnostic testing in cerebrospinal fluid could also be helpful (6).

Treatment

Standard anti-TB treatment as for other forms of EPTB is reported to result in good response. However, in some patients, full functional recovery remains uncertain in spite of adequate anti-TB treatment and patients may need hormone replacement therapy for life (1).

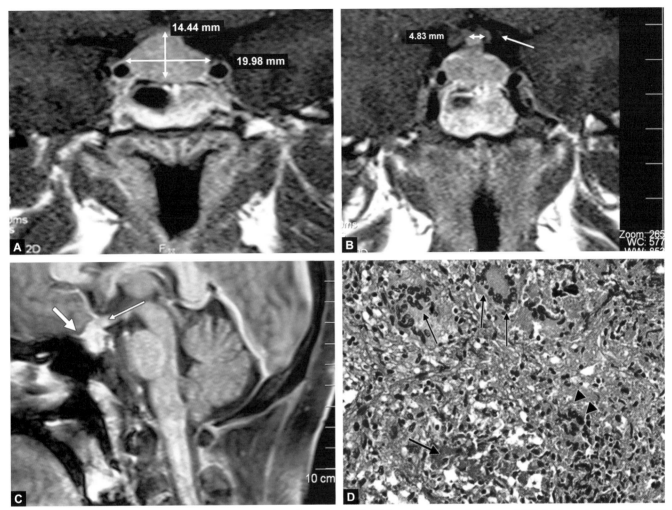

Figure 34.1: Post-contrast MRI of sella showing enlarged pituitary gland [A], thickened pituitary stalk [arrow] [B]; thickened dura [thick arrow], pituitary stalk along with enlarged pituitary gland [thin arrow] [C]. Photomicrograph [D] of the pituitary gland showing Langhans' giant cells [arrows], a small focus of caseation necrosis [thick arrow] and epithelioid cells [arrow heads]. No normal pituitary tissue is identified [Haematoxylin and eosin, × 45]

MRI = magnetic resonance imaging

Tuberculosis and Altered Water and Electrolyte Metabolism

In patients with pulmonary TB, hyponatraemia unexplained by primary renal and adrenal abnormality has been described (24). This was described as syndrome of inappropriate antidiuretic hormone [SIADH] secretion by Schwartz *et al* (25). In the presence of subnormal plasma osmolarity and no volume depletion, there is incomplete suppression of peripheral arginine vasopressin [AVP]. This syndrome presents as hyponatraemia, elevated urinary sodium concentration and urine osmolarity. This syndrome is seen mostly in EPTB such as TB meningitis (26-28), miliary TB (29) and TB epididymo-orchitis (30). Increased adsorption of the AVP in the lung tissue is one of the postulated mechanisms (31). Disturbed or down set osmoregulatory mechanisms due to active TB (32) and circulating mediators of acute phase reaction, such as, inflammatory cytokines, acting on posterior

pituitary as a stimulus for increased AVP (33-35) are some of the other postulates put forward to explain hyponatraemia.

Clinical presentation of hyponatraemia is usually mild, asymptomatic and self limiting. Water restriction as a conservative therapy should be restricted to patients with serum sodium levels less than <125 mEq/L (25,34,35). SIADH in TB meningitis carries a poor prognosis. Prompt recognition of this condition and management is important (36).

Tuberculosis and Adrenal Gland

Thomas Addison described chronic adrenocortical insufficiency in 1855. The term "Addison's Disease" refers to chronic primary adrenocortical insufficiency. Ethnic variations in the aetiology of chronic adrenal insufficiency have been described (37). While 92% of Caucasians have hypoadrenalism due to autoimmune disease, TB is the cause of hypoaderenalism 63% of Polynesians (37). TB is still the most common cause of primary hypoadrenalism in developing countries (38,39) unlike western world where autoimmune adrenalitis dominates the picture.

In up to 6% of patients with active pulmonary TB, adrenal gland involvement has been observed. Adrenal glands are a good nidus for mycobacterium not only because of rich vascular supply but also due to the fact that high levels of local corticosteroids suppress cell mediated immune response. Corticosteroid hormones have most pronounced effect on lymphocyte blast transformation with mitogens persisting even after discontinuation of their use (40). The most common sites in order of involvement are liver, spleen, kidneys and bones. Primary isolated TB adrenalitis is very rare and should be considered in any patient with fever and enlargement of adrenals (41). Similarly adrenal TB in Cushing's disease with bilateral macronodular adrenocortical hyperplasia has been documented as an incidental diagnosis on histopathological examination post-surgery (42).

Whereas release of adrenal corticosteroids is elevated in acute infections (43), adrenal reserves in chronic infections like TB is a subject of controversy. Overt adrenal insufficiency occurs when more than 80%-90% of both the adrenal glands are destroyed. But subclinical adrenal insufficiency can occur without any evidence and can manifest when there is an increased [supra] physiological requirement of adrenal hormones to meet heightened metabolic demands.

Pathogenesis

Adrenal damage caused by TB is thought to be immune mediated. Increased cortisol secretion secondary to activation of hypothalamo-pituitary axis thereby shifting Th1/Th2 balance towards Th2 T-cell dysfunction is one of the proposed mechanisms to explain TB adrenalitis and subsequent hypoadrenalism (44). Anti-TB therapy with rifampicin [a potent hepatic microsomal enzyme inducer] reduces the half-life of corticosteroids which may unmask the subclinical adrenal reserve and lead to Addisonian crisis (45). There are reports of sudden death and rapid deterioration of clinical condition with anti-TB therapy.

Clinical Presentation

Acute abdominal pain, vomiting, severe hypotension or hypovolaemic shock and fever are presenting features of acute adrenal insufficiency. Fatigue, irritability, asthenia, loss of muscle strength, weight loss, nausea, anorexia, hyperpigmentation, salt craving and failure to thrive [in children] are features of chronic adrenal insufficiency. If these symptoms appear after the initiation of anti-TB therapy, it should raise the suspicion of hypocortisolism.

Investigations

Estimation of paired sample for morning [8 AM] cortisol along with adrenocorticotrophic hormone [ACTH] differentiates primary and secondary adrenal insufficiency. Adrenal reserve is most reliably estimated by estimating serum cortisol before, 30 and 60 minutes after an intramuscular injection of 250 μg of cosyntropin (46,47).

Basal serum cortisol is either normal or increased (48,49). An autopsy series demonstrated that high basal serum cortisol was evident in patients with adrenal granulomas (50). Basal serum cortisol has been observed to be inversely proportional to duration of symptoms (51). A direct correlation between the sputum smear-positivity for acid-fast bacilli [AFB], extent of disease, pyrexia and elevated erythrocyte sedimentation rate and adrenal reserve has been documented (51). Hyperfunctioning of the adrenal glands in response to stress and infection is thought to be the cause of increased basal serum cortisol. The ACTH stimulation tests in patients with TB have shown normal or compromised to a significant extent (48,52).

Adrenal Imaging

In the active stage of the disease, TB adrenalitis shows features of enlarged adrenals associated with large, hypoattenuating necrotic areas, with or without dot like calcification [Figure 34.2], In the chronic stage the adrenal glands are typically shrunken and calcified, (44,53-55). Patients with enlarged adrenal gland have longer duration of disease.

Table 34.2 (51,56-58) summarises some of the studies from India on adrenocortical reserve in various forms of TB.

Treatment

Subjects already receiving corticosteroids need to increase the corticosteroid dose following anti-TB therapy. Reversal of adrenal function after anti-TB therapy is controversial. Reversibility has been seen as early as two weeks after the beginning of anti-TB therapy (48,59). There is a report (48) that rifampicin possibly prevents improvement of adrenal reserve with anti-TB therapy; however, observations from another study do not support this view (48,49). In a study of adrenal reserve in patients in 105 human immunodeficiency virus [HIV] seronegative patients with various forms TB [72 pulmonary TB, 33 EPTB] Sharma et al (59) reported that 49.5% of the subjects had compromised adrenal reserve at baseline. At six months of therapy the responders increased to 71% and at 24 months of therapy 97% demonstrated normal adrenal reserve. This fact has clinical relevance in acute stressful setting. Interestingly in this study (59), with anti-TB treatment the adrenal insufficiency reversed in majority of the patients.

There is sparse literature of adrenal reserve in patients co-infected with HIV and TB. The adrenal reserve was compromised in nearly 50% of patients with both HIV-seropositive and seronegative patients with active TB (60,61).

Tuberculosis and Thyroid

Epidemiology and Pathogenesis

TB affecting thyroid gland is very rare. The first case of TB of thyroid was described by Lebret, in 1862, in a patient

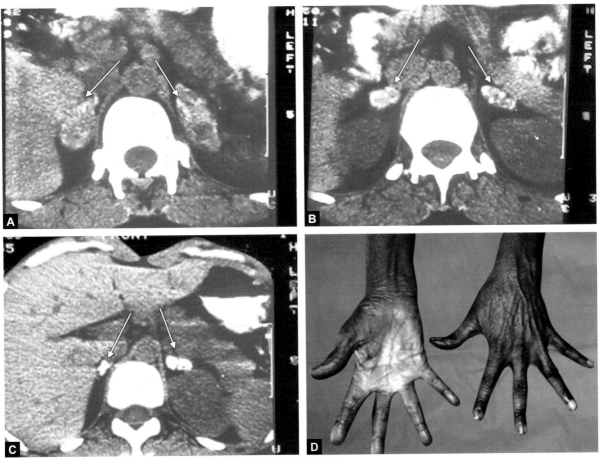

Figure 34.2: Post-contrast MRI of adrenal gland showing enlarged adrenals with calcification [arrows] [A]; shrunken adrenal with more calcification [arrows] [B]; bilateral shrunken and calcified [totally destroyed] adrenals [arrows] [C]; and clinical photograph showing hyperpigmentation of hands and palms in Addison's disease [D]
MRI = magnetic resonance imaging

Table 34.2: Studies from India on adrenocortical reserve in various forms of TB

Study [year] (reference)	No. of patients studied	Basal cortisol	Post-ACTH stimulation	Comments
Srivastava et al [1980] (51)	84 PTB	Elevated in all patients	Not described	Sputum smear-positive patients had higher cortisol. Patients with longer duration of symptoms had lower serum cortisol
Behera and Dash [1992] (56)	28 PTB 10 controls	Basal values comparable	Mean delta peak, mean and area under the response curve were significantly lower in PTB patients	There is functional impairment of adrenal cortical reserve in patients with PTB
Prasad et al [2000] (57)	30 PTB; 33 DTB/MTB 34 DR-TB	Mean cortisol lower compared to controls Difference did not attain statistical significance	Adrenal reserve compromised in 45% of TB patients	Adrenal reserve compromised in drug-sensitive TB and DR-TB
Zargar et al [2001] (58)	28 PTB,12 EPTB, 10 control subjects	Comparable among controls and patients	35% had sub-optimal cortisol reserve	Radiological severity and chronicity of PTB inversely related to adrenal reserve

TB = tuberculosis; ACTH = adrenocorticotrophic hormone; PTB = pulmonary tuberculosis; DTB = disseminated tuberculosis; MTB = miliary tuberculosis; DR-TB = drug-resistant TB; EPTB = extra-pulmonary TB

with disseminated TB (62). In 1893, Burns described primary TB of the thyroid gland even with no clinical evidence of pulmonary TB (63). Although estimates based on short case series suggests prevalence to be around 0.2% in specimens reported as chronic thyroiditis, it is reported to be as high as 14% in patients with miliary TB (64-66). There is a female preponderance with a male: female ratio of 1:2. Das *et al* (67) have reported the prevalence of TB of thyroid to be 0.6% among the 1283 thyroid lesions subjected to fine needle aspiration cytology [FNAC] (67). Association of TB of the thyroid with with papillary carcinoma thyroid has been reported (68).

The true incidence of this condition remains unknown as most cases reported in the literature are retrospectively diagnosed. Asymptomatic nature of the disease, absence of systemic TB and difficulty in demonstrating TB bacilli and/or typical lesion in histopathological examination in most of the cases are some of the reasons to explain the difficulties in estimating the true incidence. The reason for rarity of this clinical entity even in endemic areas is not known but a number of possible mechanisms, such as, rich blood flow, pattern of lymphatic drainage from the thyroid gland, excess iodine in stored form and possible anti-tubercular nature of stored thyroid hormone are proposed to explain this (64,65). The protective fibrous capsule surrounding the thyroid that separates it from other structures of the neck is thought to prevent the spread of infection to and from the gland.

Clinical Presentation

Most cases present on pre-existing multinodular goiter, solitary nodule, or even as an abscess [Figure 34.3]. Functionally, cases of patients presenting with hyperthyroidism secondary to thyroiditis and hypothyroidism secondary to total glandular destruction have been reported (69-79). It is usually a painless thyromegaly, with or without lymphadenopathy. Diagnosis of TB as a cause of clinical presentation in most cases is retrospective after histopathological demonstration of either the characteristic necrotic granuloma or TB bacilli. A cost-effective approach for diagnosis of TB of thyroid is by FNAC. If the FNAC smear is negative for AFB, molecular diagnostic methods may be helpful (80,81).

Effect of Anti-TB Treatment on Thyroid

Anti-TB drugs para-amino salicylic acid [PAS] and ethionamide are known to produce goitre (82). Usually there is complete resolution of goitre after these drugs are discontinued.

TB and Sick Euthyroid Syndrome

Serum thyroid hormones in patient with TB show low or normal serum total T4, low serum total T3, increase in reverse T3, and normal TSH, a profile consistent with sick euthyroid syndrome. Chow *et al* (83) have reported the prevalence of this syndrome in TB patients to be 63%. Low serum total T3 predicts higher mortality.

Treatment

Given the rarity of the clinical entity, prospective clinical trials evaluating the efficacy of the anti-TB therapy in treating thyroid TB are not available. The general consensus seems to favour a full course of anti-TB treatment as for other

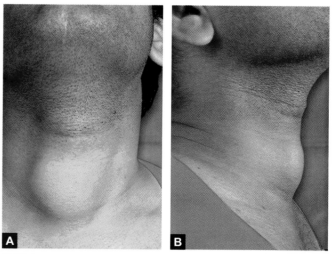

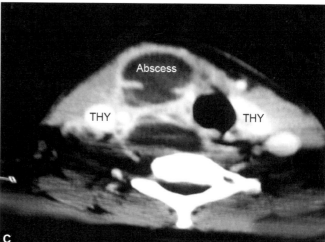

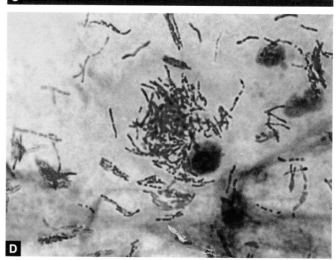

Figure 34.3: Cold abscess of the neck masquerading as a thyroid nodule. The swelling was soft, non-tender, fluctuant, and not trans-illuminant [A and B]. CT of the neck showed cold abscess of thyroid [C]. Photomicrograph of the fine-needle aspiration cytology from the swelling showing a moderate to richly cellular, mild haemorrhagic smear showing many neutrophils admixed with eosinophils, lymphocytes, and epithelioid looking cellular clusters [C]; and acid-fast bacilli [Ziehl-Neelsen, × 1000] [D]

THY = thyroid gland; CT = computed tomography

Reproduced with permission from reference 75

forms of EPTB (64,65). Thyroid binding globulin levels have been demonstrated to increase with the initiation of anti-TB treatment. Surgical intervention such as lobectomy or partial thyroidectomy may be necessary in cases where FNAC does not clarify the diagnosis of nodular presentation and also in drainage of a TB abscess. In those rare cases of hypothyroidism secondary to widespread glandular destruction, patient would need thyroid replacement therapy for life.

Diabetes Mellitus and Tuberculosis

Epidemiology

The association between diabetes mellitus [DM] and TB has been recognised for centuries. The discovery of insulin in 1920 and streptomycin in 1940 had lowered the fatality rates of individuals with TB and DM. The incidence of TB is high in countries with high rates of infection with HIV, malnutrition and crowded living conditions. It is estimated that two-thirds of the 440 million persons with DM by 2030 will be from low income countries (84). TB Co-morbid conditions like DM further complicate TB. In pulmonary TB, DM is the most common co-morbid condition.

The risk of acquiring TB in a patient with DM is 4.8% compared to 0.8% in general population (85). The relative risk of developing pulmonary TB is 3.5 times higher in DM patients compared to matched controls; in type 1 diabetes patients under 40 years of age, the risk is 24% (86). India Tuberculosis-Diabetes Study Group screened patients with DM for TB in India. Of the 7218 patients with DM screened for TB, 254 patients were identified positive for the disease and 46% were sputum smear-positive (87).

Patients with poorly controlled DM are more prone to be affected by TB. It has been shown in large studies (88,89) that DM is a moderate to strong risk for development of TB. Patients with DM who require more than 40 units of insulin per day are two-times more likely to develop TB (90). Both type 1 and type 2 DM patients with high insulin requirements are at increased risk of developing TB (91-93). The evidence for association of DM with drug-resistant TB is equivocal. While some studies have documented an increased association (94,95), no such association was evident in other studies (96,97). Interestingly, Bashar et al (95) have shown that multidrug-resistant TB was more common [36% vs 10%] in patients with DM compared with those without DM (95). DM patients have also been found to have a higher baseline mycobacterial burden; longer time for sputum conversion and higher treatment failure and relapse rate (97-100). Mortality is higher in DM patients with TB probably because of increased severity of TB or co-existing co-morbid conditions (101).

Pathogenesis

Hyperglycaemia and cellular insulinopenia directly increases the susceptibility to the disease caused by *Mtb*. Hyperglycaemia has indirect effects on the functioning of macrophages and lymphocytes, chemotaxis, phagocytosis and antigen presentation in response to mycobacterial infection. Interferon-alpha [IFN-α] production by T-cells, the growth, function and proliferation of T-cells are adversely affected by DM (102). DM patients with poor glycaemic control with TB have lower production of interleukin 1-beta [IL-1β] and tumour necrosis factor-beta [TNF-β] (103). Thickened alveolar epithelium and pulmonary basal lamina, altered diffusion capacity of the lungs and lung volume, along with reduced elastic recoil of the lungs are known to increase the susceptibility to TB in DM patients. Non-enzymatic glycosylation of tissue proteins and alteration in connective tissue in DM patients is thought to be the pathogenetic mechanism underlying these aforementioned changes in the lung causing increased susceptibility to TB (104). Further, autonomic neuropathy causing changes in the basal airway tone leading to reduced bronchial activity and dilated bronchus potentially increase the susceptibility to TB (105). The genetic predisposition towards pulmonary TB is increased in the presence of DRB[1]*09 allele, while DQB[1]*05 is observed to be protective for TB in patients with DM (106).

Clinical and Radiographic Presentation

The symptomatology and presentation of TB in patients with and without DM are similar. Radiologically, lower lung field involvement is commonly observed in DM patients with TB compared to persons without DM in whom, upper lung involvement is more common (107,108). This assumes significance as such radiological lesion could easily be misdiagnosed as community acquired pneumonia or malignancy, thereby delaying the diagnosis. Elderly patients with DM are particularly prone for this and oxygen tension variability preferably involving lower lobe is thought to be the reason for increased lower lung field predilection. Multilobar disease with multiple cavities [Figure 34.4] is also more common in patients with DM with TB (109,110).

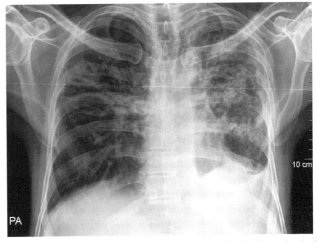

Figure 34.4: Chest radiograph [postero-anterior view] of a patient with diabetes mellitus with TB showing bilateral parenchymal infiltrates and left pleural effusion
TB = tuberculosis

Issues in Management

In the co-management of DM and TB, several issues are of concern to clinicians. TB is known to worsen diabetes control. Overlapping toxicities like peripheral neuropathy due to isoniazid treatment and poor glycaemic control must be kept in mind. Rifampicin is known to cause hyperglycaemia either by direct action by or interaction with oral antidiabetic drugs (111). Rifampicin induces cytochrome P450 enzyme which leads to accelerated metabolism of sulphonylureas, like glyburide and glipizide. The concentration of these drugs may reduced by 39% and 22% respectively (112). Netaglinide is metabolised by oxidative transformation by cytochrome CYP2C9 and CYP3A4 and has no appreciable hypoglycaemic effect when given with rifampicin. In patients with type 1 DM the insulin requirements will increase with rifampicin use. Careful monitoring of glycaemic status because of direct and indirect effect of rifampicin is a must. DM can change the effect of anti-TB drugs by decreased protein binding, renal insufficiency or fatty liver with impaired drug clearance (113).

Tuberculosis and its Influence on Glucose Metabolism

There are several studies documenting impaired glucose tolerance [IGT] in patients with TB (114-118). India Tuberculosis-Diabetes Study Group screened for DM in patients with TB [n = 8269]. Of the 8109 patients assessed, 13% were found to have DM {8% [682] were previously known to have DM and 5% were newly detected to have DM}. The prevalence of DM in patients with TB was significantly higher in tertiary care hospitals compared to a TB unit [16% vs 9%]. In south India the prevalence was significantly higher compared to north India [20% vs 10%] (119). Various postulates have been made to explain the prevalence of DM in TB. These include: [i] reciprocal relationship between both the diseases (120); [ii] occult IGT predisposing to TB infection (121); [iii] low body mass index [BMI, kg/m^2] and malnutrition in developing countries (122-126); and [iv] TB affecting the endocrine function of pancreas (118), among others. Persistent hyperglycemia in TB patients may be due to transient changes in carbohydrate metabolism (118). These abnormalities improve with commencement of anti-TB therapy. Despite well documented association between TB and diabetes, the causative link needs further scientific exploration.

Tuberculosis and Endocrine Pancreas

Pancreatic TB is a rare entity in spite of other forms of abdominal TB being common, especially in the developing countries (127). In a large autopsy study (128) which dates back to 1944, miliary TB was noted in 297 of the 1656 autopsies of patients with TB, of which only 14 had pancreatic involvement (128). In a post-mortem study from India [n = 300] spanning over a period of 12 years, none were found to have pancreatic TB (129). It is hypothesised that the pancreatic enzymes could interfere with the seeding of *Mtb*, and hence, it is biologically protected (130).

Pathogenesis

TB involvement of pancreas commonly involves the head of the pancreas because of its rich vasculature including lymphatic drainage. Haematogenous spread of the primary infection is usually the cause. Rarely, TB of the duodenum is said to be the cause of spread to pancreas due to reflux of duodenal material and bile into the pancreas due to ampulary incompetence [commonly due to submucosal fibrosis] or by lymphatic spread.

Clinical Presentation

In published literature, various clinical presentations of pancreatic TB have been documented. These include, obstructive jaundice mimicking pancreatic cancer, gastrointestinal bleeding, acute or chronic pancreatitis, pancreatic abscess, portal venous thrombosis causing portal hypertension and colonic perforation, among others (129,131). Other findings of abdominal TB like lymphadenopathy, ascites, thickening of ileoceacal region of intestines and focal hepatic and splenic lesions when present are helpful pointers to TB as the aetiological cause. Co-existence of pancreatic TB and pancreatic carcinoma is rare (132).

Miliary involvement of the pancreas may be asymptomatic initially, the caseous or nodular involvement of the pancreas may present as neoplasm. TB of pancreas presenting as pancreatic abscess is very rare.

Diagnosis

Ante-mortem diagnosis of pancreatic TB remains challenging. Liver function testing may show features suggestive of obstructive jaundice; non-specific elevation of tumour marker CA 125 is reported (129-134). Ultrasonography of the abdomen reveals a solitary hypoechoic lesion with a cystic component in the head of pancreas. CT of the abdomen reveals either a sharply delineated mass with irregular margins in the pancreatic head, diffuse enlargement of the pancreas or peripancreatic lymphadenopathy. On MRI focal involvement appears as hypointese on fat suppressed T1-weighted images and hypo/hyperintese on T2-weighted images (133). Although helpful, none of these radiological features are pathognomonic of TB of the pancreas.

Evaluation of a pancreatic mass should be done diligently keeping in mind the possibility of pancreatic TB so that unnecessary extensive surgery can be avoided. After reviewing the laboratory findings, imaging modalities and ultrasonography, CT guided biopsy, if the histopathology is consistent with malignancy standard Whipple's pancreaticoduodenectomy should be carried out. In cases where the work up is inconclusive, laparotomy with frozen section of pancreatic mass/or lymph nodes is indicated which would help in clinching the diagnosis either way. Demonstration of caseating granulomas, AFB or a positive molecular diagnostic test on specimens collected by either endoscopic ultrasonography or CT-guided biopsy is helpful in ascertaining the diagnosis.

Treatment

Standard anti-TB treatment for 6-9 months is considered adequate for pancreatic TB. Prognosis is excellent with complete clinical resolution. Radiologic regression of the pancreatic mass on follow-up is often evident. If no improvement is noted, pancreatic excision is warranted (132).

Vitamin D and Tuberculosis

Attention has now focussed on the non-classical actions of vitamin D, especially innate and adaptive immunity. In the pre-antibiotic era vitamin D was utilised as a therapy for TB (135). Williams used cod-liver oil in patients with pulmonary TB (136). Until the introduction of antimicrobial therapy in 1950s, cod liver oil was used in the treatment and prevention of TB. It is believed to be an effective treatment for TB of the skin (137,138). It was shown by Liu that with the sensing of *Mtb* by toll-like receptor 2/1[TLR2/1], the expression of vitamin D receptors [VDR] and CYP27B1 in monocytes is increased (139). Vitamin D_3 promotes VDR mediated transactivation of cathelicidin. There is direct antimicrobial function of cathelicidin which kills the intracellular *Mtb*. Vitamin D promotes phagolysosome formation playing a crucial role in immune response to *Mtb* (140).

Vitamin D deficiency is pandemic in India (141). There are studies linking development of pulmonary TB in Asian Indians (142-145). Higher levels of 25-hydroxy vitamin D_3 {$25[OH]_2D_3$} levels were associated with less extensive radiological lesions (146). In the Asian Gujarati community living in London post-primary pulmonary TB is associated with Vitamin D deficiency and single nucleotide polymorphism [SNP] in VDR (147). This study revealed association between T allele related to *Taql SNP* of *VDR* gene and vitamin D deficiency (147). In a cross-sectional study done in 897 participants in north India {MDR-TB 354, drug-susceptible pulmonary TB [DS-PTB] 338, controls 205}, $25[OH]_2D_3$, serum calcium and parathyroid hormone were measured and Genotypic and allelic frequencies of *Fok*I, *Bsm*I and *Taq*I VDR polymorphisms evaluated. MDR-TB correlated positively with *Fok*I *Ff* genotype and *Taq*I *t* allele. In both MDR-TB and DS-PTB groups *ff* genotype and *f* allele of *Fok*I frequency were higher. MDR-TB correlated inversely with *Bsm*I *Bb* genotype. MDR-TB had the lowest serum $25[OH]_2D_3$ concentrations and correlated inversely with time to sputum smear conversion. The study concluded hypovitaminosis D and VDR gene polymorphisms predispose to MDR-TB. Time to MDR-TB sputum smear negativity was increased with lower serum $25[OH]_2D_3$ levels (148). The exact mechanism liking the VDR polymorphism with TB is not known.

Tuberculosis and Hypercalcaemia

About 50% of adult patients with TB manifest hypercalcaemia (149-151). Presence of hypercalcaemia has been reported in abdominal TB too (152). Regional differences in dietary calcium intake and vitamin D status account for wide variation in the clinical presentation (150,153). Shek *et al* (150) observed it is the sixth common cause and second common cause of hypercalcaemia after malignancy. There are number of factors that are thought to be responsible for hypercalcaemia in patients with TB. Abnormal vitamin D metabolism appears to be the prime factor. The hypercalcaemia observed in these cases is not influenced by negative feedback loop involving 1α hydroxylase as the serum parathyroid hormone is suppressed and serum phosphorous tends to be on the higher side of normal (154). The main factors regulating the 1α hydroxylase in the granulomatous tissue is the locally or systemically produced lymphokines similar to sarcoidosis (155,156). The CD4+ T-lymphocytes recovered from bronchoalveolar lavage in patients with active pulmonary TB express $1,25[OH]_2D_3$. The antimycobacterial products within the granulomatous tissue could be regulating $1,25[OH]_2D_3$ production independent of parathyroid hormone and $25[OH]_2D_3$. Hypercalcaemia may be masked in initial presentation because of low serum albumin levels. Lung is the extra renal site of synthesis of $1,25[OH]_2D_3$. High concentration of $1,25[OH]_2D_3$ is detected in patients with TB pleuritis (157). Serum $1,25[OH]_2D_3$ levels are reported to be higher in TB patients compared to controls (158-161) and even in patients with end stage renal failure and TB (162). It has been shown in *in vitro* studies that $1,25[OH]_2D_3$ is produced by alveolar macrophages and lymphocytes (163,164). Studies have shown the calcium absorption is high due to high $1,25[OH]_2D_3$ levels (165-167). Anti-TB drugs are known to adversely affect the calcium and phosphate metabolism; rifampicin and isoniazid both reduce the $25[OH]_2D_3$ levels (168-170). This is further aggravated in vitamin D deficient population like in India (171).

Tuberculosis of Female Reproductive Endocrine System

The reader is referred to the chapter *"Female genital tuberculosis"* [Chapter 26] for details.

Tuberculosis of Male Reproductive Endocrine System

The reader is referred to the chapter *"Genitourinary tuberculosis"* [Chapter 27] for details.

REFERENCES

1. Sunil K, Menon R, Goel N, Sanghvi D, Bandgar T, Joshi SR, et al. Pituitary tuberculosis. J Assoc Physicians India 2007;55:453-56.
2. Ranjan R, Agarwal P, Ranjan S. Primary pituitary tubercular abscess mimicking as pituitary adenoma. Indian J Endocrinol Metab 2011;15 Suppl 3:S263-6.
3. Mageshkumar S, Patil DV, Philo AJ, Madhavan K. Hypopituitarism as an unusual sequelae to central nervous system tuberculosis. Indian J Endocrinol Metab 2011;15 Suppl 3:S259-62.
4. Mittal P, Dua S, Saggar K, Gupta K. Magnetic resonance findings in sellar and suprasellar tuberculoma with hemorrhage. Surg Neurol Int 2010;1:73.
5. Furtado SV, Venkatesh PK, Ghosal N, Hegde AS. Isolated sellar tuberculoma presenting with panhypopituitarism: clinical,

diagnostic considerations and literature review. Neurol Sci 2011;32: 301-4.

6. Husain N, Husain M, Rao P. Pituitary tuberculosis mimicking idiopathic granulomatous hypophysitis. Pituitary 2008;11:313-5.

7. Satyarthee GD, Mahapatra AK. Diabetes insipidus in sellar-suprasellar tuberculoma. J Clin Neurosci 2003;10:497-9.

8. Dutta P, Bhansali A, Singh P, Bhat MH. Suprasellar tubercular abscess presenting as panhypopituitarism: a common lesion in an uncommon site with a brief review of literature. Pituitary 2006;9: 73-7.

9. Arunkumar MJ, Rajshekhar V. Intrasellar tuberculoma presenting as pituitary apoplexy. Neurol India 2001;49:407-10.

10. Sharma MC, Vaish S, Arora R, Gaikwad S, Sarkar C. Composite pituitary adenoma and intrasellar tuberculoma: report of a rare case. Pathol Oncol Res 2001;7:74-6.

11. Sharma MC, Arora R, Mahapatra AK, Sarat-Chandra P, Gaikwad SB, Sarkar C. Intrasellar tuberculoma: an enigmatic pituitary infection: A series of 18 cases. Clin Neurol Neurosurg 2000;102: 72-7.

12. Lam KS, Sham MM, Tam SC, Ng MM, Ma HT. Hypopituitarism after tuberculous meningitis in chidhood. Ann Intern Med 1993; 118:701-6.

13. Bartsocas CS, Pantelakis SN. Human growth hormone therapy in hypopituitarism due to tuberculous meningitis. Acta Paediatr Scand 1973;62:304-6.

14. Lanigan CJ, Buckley MP. Adult panhypopituitarism with normal stature following tuberculous meningitis: a case report. Ir Med J 1983;76:353-4.

15. Nayil K, Singh S, Makhdoomi R, Ramzan A, Wani A. Sellar-suprasellar tuberculomas in children: 2 cases and literature review. Pediatr Neurol 2011;44:463-6.

16. Desai M, Colaco MP, Choksi CS, Ambadkar MC, Vaz FE, Gupte C. Isosexual precocity: the clinical and etiologic profile. Indian Pediatr 1993;30:607-23.

17. Patankar T, Patkar D, Bunting T, Catillo M, Mukherji SK. Imaging in pituitary tuberculosis. J Clin Imag 2000;24:89-92.

18. Behari S, Shinghal U, Jain M, Jaiswal AK, Wadwekar V, Das KB, et al. Clinicoradiological presentation, management options and a review of sellar and suprasellar tuberculomas. J Clin Neurosci 2009;16:1560-6.

19. Ahmad FU, Sarat Chandra P, Sanyal S, Garg A, Mehta VS. Sellar tuberculoma: an unusual infection. Indian J Tuberc 2005;52: 215-7.

20. Gazioglu N. Lymphocytic and granulomatous hypophysitis: Experience with nine cases. J Endocrinol Invest 2000;23:189-92.

21. Bullmann C, Faust M, Hoffmann A, Heppner C, Jockenhovel F, Muller-Wieland D, et al. Five cases with central diabetes insipidus and hypogonadism as first presentation of eurosarcoidosis. Eur J Endocrinol 2000;142:365-72.

22. Vasile M, Marsot-Dupuch K, Kujas M, Brunereau L, Bouchard P, Comov J, et al. Idiopathic granulomatous hypophysitis: Clinical and imaging features. Neuroradiology 1997;39:7-11.

23. Roncaroli F, Bacci A, Frank G, Calbucci F. Granulomatous hypophysitis caused by ruptured intrasellar Rathke's cleft cyst: Report of a case and review of the literature. Neurosurgery 1998;43:146-9.

24. Sims EA, Welt LG, Orloff J, Needham JW. Asymptomatic hyponatraemia in pulmonary tuberculosis. J Clin Invest 1950;29: 1545-57.

25. Schwartz WB, Bennett W, Curelop S, Bartter FC. A syndrome of renal sodium loss and hyponatremia probably resulting from inappropriate secretion of antidiuretic hormone. Am J Med 1957;23:529-42.

26. Erduran E, Mocan H, Aslan Y. Syndrome of inappropriate secretion of antidiuretic hormone in tuberculous meningits. Pediatr Nephrol 1996;10:127.

27. Cotton MF, Donald PR, Schoeman JF, Van-Zyl LE, Aalbers C, Lombard CJ. Raised intracranial pressure, the syndrome of inappropriate antidiuretic hormone secretion, and arginine vaso-pressin in tuberculous meningitis. Childs Nerv Syst 1993;9:10-5.

28. Cotton MF, Donald PR, Schoeman JF, Aalbers C, Van-Zyl LE, Lombard C. Plasma arginine vasopressin and the syndrome of inappropriate antidiuretic hormone secretion in tuberculous meningitis. Pediatr Infect Dis J 1991;10:837-42.

29. Ando T, Tanaka T, Saeki A, Ogawa K, Honda K, Sasamoto M, et al. Syndrome of inappropriate secretion of antidiuretic hormone associated with miliary tuberculosis. Kekkaku 1997;72:161-5.

30. Motiwala HG, Sanghvi NP, Barjatiya MK, Patel SM. Syndrome of inappropriate antidiuretic hormone following tuberculous epididymo-orchitis in renal transplant recipient: case report. J Urol 1991;146:1366-7.

31. Vorherr H, Massry SG, Fallet R, Kaplan L, Kleeman CR. Antidiuretic principle in tuberculous lung tissue of a patient with pulmonary tuberculosis and hyponatraemia. Ann Intern Med 1970;72:383-7.

32. DeFronzo RA, Goldberg M, Agus ZS. Normal diluting capacity in hyponatremic patients. Reset osmostat or a variant of the syndrome of inappropriate antidiuretic hormone secretion. Ann Intern Med 1976;84:538-42.

33. Silva CL, Faccioli LH. Tumour necrosis [cachectin] factor mediates induction of cachexia by cord factor from mycobacteria. Infect Immun 1988;56:3067-71.

34. Dinarello CA. Interleukin-1 and its biologically related cytokines. Adv Immunol 1989;44:153-205.

35. Hill AR, Uribarri J, Mann J, Berl T. Altered water metabolism in tuberculosis: role of vasopressin. Am J Med 1990;88:357-64.

36. Berliner S, Garfinkel D, Shoenfeld Y, Pinkhas J. Inappropriate antidiuretic hormone [ADH] secretion in a patient with extensive fibrothorax. Respiration 1980;39:283-5.

37. Eason RJ, Croxson MS, Perry MC, Somerfield SD. Addison's disease, adrenal autoantibodies and computerized adrenal tomography. N Z Med J 1982;95:569-73.

38. Keletimur F, Unlü Y, Ozesmi M, Tolu I. A hormonal and radiological evaluation of adrenal gland in patients with acute or chronic pulmonary tuberculosis. Clin Endocrinol [Oxf] 1994;41:53-6.

39. Kong MF, Jeffcoate W. Eighty-six cases of Addison's disease. Clin Endocrinol [Oxf] 1994;41:757-61.

40. Basov PV. Effect of glucocorticosteroid hormones on T lymphocytes in patients with pulmonary tuberculosis. Probl Tuberk 1989;4:30-3.

41. Del Borgo C, Urigo C, Marocco R, Belvisi V, Pisani L, Citton R, et al. Diagnostic and therapeutic approach in a rare case of primary bilateral adrenal tuberculosis. J Med Microbiol 2010;59:1527-9.

42. Kwon HS, Kim SI, Yoo SJ, Yoon KH, Lee KW, Kang MW, et al. Adrenal tuberculosis in Cushing's disease with bilateral macronodular adrenocortical hyperplasia. Endocr J 2006;53: 219-23.

43. Arlt W, Allolio B. Adrenal insufficiency. Lancet 2003;361:1881-93.

44. Kelestimur F. The endocrinology of adrenal tuberculosis: the effects of tuberculosis on the hypothalamo-pituitary-adrenal axis and adrenocortical function. J Endocrinol Invest 2004;27:380-6.

45. McAllister WA, Thompson PJ, Al-Habet SM, Rogers HJ. Rifampicin reduces effectiveness and bioavailability of prednisolone. Br Med J [Clin Res Ed] 1983;286:923-5.

46. Danowski TS, Hofmann K, Weigand FA, Sunder JH. Steroid responses to ACTH-like polypeptides. J Clin Endocrinol Metab 1968;28:1120-6.

47. Dickstein G, Shechner C, Nicholson WE, Rosner I, Shen-Orr Z, Adawi F, et al. Adrenocorticotropin stimulation test: effects of

basal cortisol level, time of day, and suggested new sensitive low dose test. J Clin Endocrinol Metab 1991;72:773-8.

48. Ellis ME, Tayoub F. Adrenal function in tuberculosis. Br J Dis Chest 1986;80:7-12.

49. Barnes DJ, Naraqi S, Temu P, Turtle JR. Adrenal function in patients with active tuberculosis. Thorax 1989;44:422-4.

50. Chan CH, Arnold M, Mak TW, Chan RC, Hoheisel GB, Chow CC, et al. Adrenocortical function and involvement in high risk cases of pulmonary tuberculosis. Tuber Lung Dis 1993;74:395-8.

51. Srivastava RML, Mukerji PK, Bhargava KP, Khanna BK. A study on plasma cortisol in pulmonary tuberculosis. Indian J Tuberc 1980;27:3-6.

52. Sarma GR, Immanuel C, Ramachandran G, Krishnamurthy PV, Kumaraswami V, Prabhakar R. Adrenocortical function in patients with pulmonary tuberculosis. Tubercle 1990;71:277-82.

53. McMurry JF Jr, Long D, McClure R, Kotchen TA. Addison's disease with adrenal enlargement on computed tomographic scanning. Report on two cases of tuberculosis and review of the literature. Am J Med 1984;77:365-8.

54. Jayakar DV, Condemi G, DeSoto-LaPaix F, Plawker M, Farag A, Ghosh BC. Adrenal tuberculosis. Eur J Surg 1998;164:975- 8.

55. Barnes DJ, Naraqi S, Temu P, Turtle JR. Adrenal function in patients with active tuberculosis. Thorax 1989;44:422-4.

56. Behera D, Dash RJ. Adreno-cortical reserve in pulmonary tuberculosis. J Assoc Physicians India 1992;40:520-1.

57. Prasad GA, Sharma SK, Mohan A, Gupta N, Bajaj S, Saha PK, et al. Adrenocortical reserve and morphology in tuberculosis. Indian J Chest Dis Allied Sci 2000;42:83-93.

58. Zargar AH, Sofi FA, Akhtar MA, Salahuddin M, Masoodi SR, Laway BA. Adrenocortical reserve in patients with active tuberculosis. J Pak Med Assoc 2001;51:427-33.

59. Sharma SK, Tandan SM, Saha PK, Gupta N, Kochupillai N Misra NK. Reversal of subclinical adrenal insufficiency through antituberculosis treatment in TB patients: a longitudinal follow up. Indian J Med Res 2005;122:127-31.

60. Prasad GA, Sharma SK, Kochupillai N. Adrenocortical reserve in patients with tuberculosis. Indian J Chest Dis Allied Sci 1996;38: 25-33.

61. Hawken MP, Ojoo JC, Morris JS, Kariuki EW, Githui WA, Juma ES, et al. No increased prevalence of adrenocortical insufficiency in human immunodeficiency virus-associated tuberculosis. Tuber Lung Dis 1996;77:444-8.

62. Lebert H. Die Kranheiten der Schilddruse und ihre Behandlung. Breslau;1862.p.264.

63. Burns P. Stuma tuberculosis. Beitr Klin Chir 1893;10:1.

64. Khan EM, Haque I, Pandey R, Mishra SK, Sharma AK. Tuberculosis of the thyroid gland: a clinicopathological profile of four cases and review of the literature. Aust N Z J Surg 1993;63:807-10.

65. Al-Mulhim AA, Zakaria HM, Abdel Hadi MS, Al-Mulhim FA, Al-Tamimi DM, Wosornu L. Thyroid tuberculosis mimicking carcinoma: report of two cases. Surg Today 2002;32:1064-7.

66. Tan KK. Tuberculosis of the thyroid gland—a review. Ann Acad Med Singapore 1993;22:580-2.

67. Das DK, Pant CS, Chachra KL, Gupta AK. Fine needle aspiration cytology diagnosis of tuberculous thyroiditis. A report of eight cases. Acta cytol 1992;36:517-22.

68. Hizawa K, Okamura K, Sato K, Kuroda T, Yoshinari M, Ikenoue H, et al. Tuberculous thyroiditis and miliary tuberculosis manifested postpartum in a patient with thyroid carcinoma. Endocrinol Jpn 1990;37:571-6.

69. Bulbuloglu E, Ciralik H, Okur E, Ozdemir G, Ezberci F, Cetinkaya A. Tuberculosis of thyroid gland. Review of literature. World J Surg 2006;30:149-55.

70. Chaudhary A, Nayak B, Guleria S, Arora R, Gupta R, Sharma MC. Tuberculosis of the thyroid presenting as multinodular goiter with hypothyroidism: a rare presentation. Indian J Pathol Microbiol 2010;53:579-81.

71. Aerts S,Gypen BJ, VanHee R, and Bomans P. Tuberculosis of the thyroid gland. A case report. Acta Chirurgica Belgica 2009;109: 805-7.

72. Sivanagamani K, Suvarna Kumari G, Aruna CA, Sikinder Hayath M. Tuberculosis of thyroid gland. Indian J Tuber 1980;27:33-4.

73. Barnes P, Weatherstone R. Tuberculosis of the thyroid: two case reports. Br J Dis Chest 1979;73:187-91.

74. Modayil PC, Leslie A, Jacob A. Tuberculous infection of thyroid gland: a case report. Case Rep Med 2009;2009:416231.

75. Harinarayan CV, Kumaraswamy Reddy M, Venkataramanappa M. Cold abscess of the neck masquerading as a thyroid nodule. Thyroid 2004;14:636.

76. Bahadur P, Bhatnagar BNS, Aurora AL, Seetharaman ML. Tuberculous abscess of thyroid gland. Indian J Tuberc 1983;30: 33-5.

77. Parmar H, Hashmi M, Rajput A, Patankar T, Castillo M. Acute tuberculous abscess of the thyroid gland. Australas Radiol 2002;46:186-8.

78. Kapoor VK, Subramani K, Das SK. Tuberculosis of the thyroid gland associated with thyrotoxicosis. Postgrad Med J 1985;61: 339-40.

79. Silva BP, Amorim EG, Pavin EJ, Martins AS, Matos PS, Zantut-Wittmann DE. Primary thyroid tuberculosis: a rare etiology of hypothyroidism and anterior cervical mass mimicking carcinoma. Arq Bras Endocrinol Metabol 2009;53:475-8.

80. Mondal A, Patra DK. Efficacy of fine needle aspiration cytology in diagnosis of tuberculosis of the thyroid gland: a study of 18 cases. J Laryngol Otol 1995;109:36-8.

81. Das DK, Pant CS, Chachra KL, Gupta AK. Fine needle aspiration cytology diagnosis of tubercular thyroiditis. A report of eight cases. Acta Cytol 1992;36:517-22.

82. Clausen KH, Kjerulf Jensen K. Artificial myxoedema during para-aminosalicylic acid. Nord Med 1951;45:475-7.

83. Chow CC, Mak TW, Chan CH, Cockram CS. Euthyroid sick syndrome in pulmonary tuberculosis before and after treatment. Ann Clin Biochem 1995;32:385-91.

84. Boutayeb A. The double burden of communicable and non-communicable diseases in developing countries. Trans R Soc Trop Med Hyg 2006;100:191-9.

85. Patel JC. Complications in 8793 cases of diabetes mellitus 14 years study in Bombay Hospital, Bombay, India. Indian J Med Sci 1989;43:177-83.

86. Kim SJ, Hong YP, Lew WJ, Yang SC, Lee EG. Incidence of pulmonary tuberculosis among diabetics. Tuber Lung Dis 1995;76:529-33.

87. India Diabetes Mellitus—Tuberculosis Study Group. Screening of patients with diabetes mellitus for tuberculosis in India. Trop Med Int Health 2013;18:646-54.

88. Dooley KE, Tang T, Golub JE, Dorman SE, Cronin W. Impact of diabetes mellitus on treatment outcomes of patients with active tuberculosis. Am J Trop Med Hyg 2009;80:634-9.

89. Dooley KE, Chaisson RE Tuberculosis and diabetes mellitus: convergence of two epidemics. Lancet Infect Dis 2009;9:737-46.

90. Stevenson CR, Forouhi NG, Roglic G, Williams BG, Lauer JA, Dye C, et al. Diabetes and tuberculosis: the impact of the diabetes epidemic on tuberculosis incidence. BMC Public Health 2007;7:234.

91. Olmos P, Donoso J, Rojas N, Landeros P, Schurmann R, Retamal G, et al. Tuberculosis and diabetes mellitus: a longitudinal-retrospective study in a teaching hospital. Rev Med Chil 1989;117:979-83.

92. Leung CC, Lam TH, Chan WM, Yew WW, Ho KS, Leung GM, et al. Diabetic control and risk of tuberculosis: a cohort study. Am J Epidemiol 2008;167:1486-94.

93. Jeon CY, Murray MB. Diabetes mellitus increases the risk of active tuberculosis: a systematic review of 13 observational studies. PLoS Med 2008;5:e152.

94. Fisher-Hoch SP, Whitney E, McCormick JB, Crespo G, Smith B, Rahbar MH, et al. Type 2 diabetes and multidrug-resistant tuberculosis. Scand J Infect Dis 2008;40:888-93.

95. Bashar M, Alcabes P, Rom WN, Condos R. Increased incidence of multidrug-resistant tuberculosis in diabetic patients on the Bellevue Chest Service, 1987 to 1997. Chest 2001;120:1514-9.

96. Subhash HS, Ashwin I, Mukundan U, Danda D, John G, Cherian AM, Thomas K. Drug resistant tuberculosis in diabetes mellitus: a retrospective study from south India. Trop Doct 2003;33:154-6.

97. Singla R, Khan N. Does diabetes predispose to the development of multidrug-resistant tuberculosis? Chest 2003;123:308-9.

98. Wang CS, Yang CJ, Chen HC, Chuang SH, Chong IW, Hwang JJ, et al. Impact of type 2 diabetes on manifestations and treatment outcome of pulmonary tuberculosis. Epidemiol Infect 2009;137:203-10.

99. Hendy M, Stableforth D. The effect of established diabetes mellitus on the presentation of infiltrative pulmonary tuberculosis in the immigrant Asian community of an inner city area of the United Kingdom. Br J Dis Chest 1983;77:87-90.

100. Al Wabel AH, Teklu B, Mahfouz AA, Al Ghamdi AS, El Amin OB, Khan AS. Symptomatology and chest roentgenographic changes of pulmonary tuberculosis among diabetics. East Afr Med J 1987;74:62-4.

101. Gómez-Gómez A, Magaña-Aquino M, López-Meza S, Aranda-Álvarez M, Díaz-Ornelas DE, Hernández-Segura MG, et al. Diabetes and other risk factors for multi-drug resistant tuberculosis in a Mexican population with pulmonary tuberculosis: case control study. Arch Med Res 2015;46:142-8.

102. Uno K, Nakano K, Maruo N, Onodera H, Mata H, Kurosu I, et al. Determination of interferon-alpha-producing capacity in whole blood cultures from patients with various diseases and from healthy persons. J Interferon Cytokine Res 1996;16:911-8.

103. Tsukaguchi K, Yoneda T, Yoshikawa M, Tokuyama T, Fu A, Tomoda K, et al. Case study of interleukin-1b, tumor necrosis factor alpha and interleukin-6 production in peripheral blood monocytes in patients with diabetes complicated by pulmonary tuberculosis. Kekkaku 1992;67:755-60.

104. Marvisi M, Marani G, Brianti M, Della Porta R. Pulmonary complications in diabetes mellitus. Recent Prog Med 1996;97:623-7.

105. Stevenson CR, Forouhi NG, Roglic G, Williams BG, Lauer JA, Dye C, et al. Diabetes and tuberculosis: the impact of the diabetes epidemic on tuberculosis incidence. BMC Public Health 2007;7:234.

106. Zhao Y, Duanmu H, Song C. Analysis of the association between HLA-DRB[1], DQB[1] gene and pulmonary tuberculosis complicated with diabetes mellitus. Zhonghua Jie He He Hu Xi Za Zhi 2001;24: 75-9.

107. Marais RM. Diabetes mellitus in black and coloured tuberculosis patients. S Afr Med J 1980;57:483-84.

108. Perez-Guzman C, Torres-Cruz A, Villarreal-Velarde H, Salazar-Lezama MA, Vargas MH. Atypical radiological images of pulmonary tuberculosis in 192 diabetic patients: a comparative study. Int J Tuberc Lung Dis 2001;5:455-61.

109. Ikezoe J, Takeuchi N, Johkoh T, Kohno N, Tomiyama N, Kozuka T, et al. CT appearance of pulmonary tuberculosis in diabetic and immunocompromised patients: comparison with patients who had no underlying disease. AJR Am J Roentgenol 1992;159:1175-9.

110. Perez-Guzman C, Torres-Cruz A, Villarreal-Velarde H, Vargas MH. Progressive age-related changes in pulmonary tuberculosis images and the effect of diabetes. Am J Respir Crit Care Med 2000;162: 1738-40.

111. Niemi M, Backman JT, Fromm MF, Neuvonen PJ, Kivisto KT. Pharmacokinetic interactions with rifampicin: clinical relevance. Clin Pharmacokinet 2003;42:819-50.

112. Niemi M, Backman JT, Neuvonen M, Neuvonen PJ, Kivisto KT. Effects of rifampin on the pharmacokinetics and pharmacodynamics of glyburide and glipizide. Clin Pharmacol Ther 2001;69:400-6.

113. Gwilt PR, Nahhas RR, Tracewell WG. The effects of diabetes mellitus on pharmacokinetics and pharmacodynamics in humans. Clin Pharmacokinet 1991;20:47-90.

114. Kishore B, Nagrath SP, Mathur KS, Hazra DK, Agarwal BD. Manifest, chemical and latent chemical diabetes in pulmonary tuberculosis. J Assoc Phycians India 1973;21:875-81.

115. Seth SC, Parmar MS, Saini AS, Lal H. Glucose tolerance in pulmonary tuberculosis. Hormone Metab Res 1982;14:50.

116. Zack MD, Fulkerson LL, Stein E. Glucose intolerance in pulmonary tuberculosis. Am Rev Respir Dis 1973;108:1164-9.

117. Singh V, Goyal RK, Mathur MN. Glucose tolerance in patients with pulmonary tuberculosis. J Indian Med Assoc 1978;70:81-3.

118. Roychowdhury AB, Sen PK. Diabetes in tuberculous patients. J Indian Med Assoc 1980;74:8-15.

119. India Tuberculosis-Diabetes Study Group. Screening of patients with tuberculosis for diabetes mellitus in India. Trop Med Int Health 2013;18:636-45.

120. Nichols GP. Diabetes among young tuberculosis patients; a review of the association of the two diseases. Am Rev Tuber 1957;76: 1016-30.

121. Bloom JD. Glucose intolerance in pulmonary tuberculosis. Am Rev Respir Dis 1969;100:38-41.

122. Samal KC, Tripathy BB, Das S. Profile of childhood onset diabetes in Orissa. Int J Diab Dev Countries 1990;10:27-34.

123. Hadden DR. Glucose free fatty acid and insulin interrelations in Kwashiorkor and marasmus. Lancet 1967;2:589-92.

124. McLarty DG, Swai ABM, Kitange HM, Masuki G, Mtinangi BL, Kilima PM, et al. Prevalence of diabetes and impaired glucose tolerance in rural Tanzania. Lancet 1989;1:871-5.

125. Broxmeyer L. Diabetes mellitus, tuberculosis and the mycobacteria: two millenia of enigma. Med Hypotheses 2005;65:433-9.

126. Martinez N, Kornfeld H. Diabetes and immunity to tuberculosis. Eur J Immunol 2014;44:617-26.

127. Weiss ES, Klein WM, Yeo CJ. Peripancreatic tuberculosis mimicking pancreatic neoplasia. J Gastrointest Surg 2005;9: 254-62.

128. Auerbach O. Acute generalized miliary tuberculosis. Am J Pathol 1944; 20:121-36.

129. Rana SS, Bhasin DK, Rao C, Singh K. Isolated pancreatic tuberculosis mimicking focal pancreatitis and causing segmental portal hypertension. JOP 2010;11:393-5.

130. Arora A, Mukund A, Garg H. Isolated pancreatic tuberculosis: a rare occurrence. Am J Trop Med Hyg 2012;87:1-2.

131. Veerabadran P, Sasnur P, Subramanian S, Marappagounder S. Pancreatic tuberculosis-abdominal tuberculosis presenting as pancreatic abscesses and colonic perforation. World J Gastroenterol 2007;13:478-9.

132. Singh DK, Haider A, Tatke M, Kumar P, Mishra PK. Primary pancreatic tuberculosis masquerading as a pancreatic tumor leading to Whipple's pancreaticoduodenectomy. A case report and review of the literature. JOP 2009;10:451-6.

133. De Backer AI, Mortele KJ, Bomans P, De Keulenaer BL, Vanschoubroeck IJ, Kockx MM. Tuberculosis of the pancreas: MRI features. AJR Am J Roentgenol 2005;184:50-4.

134. Khaniya S, Koirala R, Shakya VC, Adhikary S, Regmi R, Pandey SR, et al. Isolated pancreatic tuberculosis mimicking as carcinoma: a case report and review of the literature. Cases J 2010;3:18.

135. Ellman P, Anderson K. Calciferol in tuberculosis peritonitis with disseminated tuberculosis. BMJ 1948;1:394.

136. Williams CJB. Cod liver oil in phthisis. J Med 1849;1:1-18.

137. Dowling GB, Prosser-Thomas EW. Treatment of lupus vulgaris with calciferol. Lancet 1946;1:919-22.

138. Charpy J. Quelques traitements vitamines ou par substances fonctionnelles en dermatologie. Bull Med 1950;24:505.

139. Liu PT, Stenger S, Li H, Wenzel I, Tan BH, Krutzik SR, et al. Toll-like eceptors triggering of a vitamin D mediated anti-microbical response. Science 2006; 311:1770-3.

140. Chocano-Bedoya P, Ronnenberg AG. Vitamin D and tuberculosis. Nutr Res 2009;67:289-93.

141. Harinarayan CV, Joshi SR. Vitamin D status in India–its implications and remedial measures: a review. J Assoc Physicians India 2009; 40-8.

142. Cadranel J, Milleron B, Garabedian M, Aroun G. Serum concentrations of vitamin D metabolites in untreated tuberculosis. Thorax 1985;40:639-40.

143. Davies PD, Brown RC, Church HA, Woodhead JJ. The effect of antituberculous chemotherapy on vitamin D and calcium metabolism. Tubercle 1987;38:261-6.

144. Davies PD. A possible link between vitamin D deficiency and impaired host defense to Mycobacterial tuberculosis. Tubercle 1985;66:301-6.

145. Rook GAW. The role of vitamin D in tuberculosis. Am Rev Respir Dis 1988;138:768-70.

146. Grange JM, Davies PD, Brown RC, Woodhead JS, Kardjito T. Vitamin D levels in Indonesian patients with untreated pulmonary tuberculosis. Tubercle 1985;66:187-91.

147. Wilkinson RJ, Llewelyn M, Toossi Z, Patel P, Pasvol G, Lalvani A, et al. Influence of vitamin D deficiency and vitamin D receptor polymorphisms on tuberculosis among Gujarati Asians in west London: a case-control study. Lancet 2000;355:618-21.

148. Rathored J, Sharma SK, Singh B, Banavaliker JN, Sreenivas V, Srivastava AK, et al. Risk and outcome of multidrug-resistant tuberculosis: vitamin D receptor polymorphisms and serum 25[OH]D. Int J Tuberc Lung Dis 2012;16:1522-8.

149. Need AG, Philips PJ, Chiu F, Prisk HM. Hypercalcaemia associated with tuberculosis. Br Med J 1980;282:831.

150. Shek CC, Natkunam A, Tsang V, Cockram CS, Swaminathan R. Incidence, causes and mechanism of hypercalcaemia in a hospital population in Hong Kong. QJM 1990;284:1277-85.

151. Abbasi AA, Chemplavil JK, Farah S, Muller BF, Arnstein AR. Hypercalcaemia in active pulmonary tuberculosis. Ann Intern Med 1979;90:324-8.

152. Ramanathan M, Abdullah AD, Sivadas T. Hypercalcaemic crisis as the presenting manifestation of abdominal tuberculosis: a case report. Med J Malaysia 1998;53:432-4.

153. Chan TY. Differences in vitamin D status and calcium intake: possible explanations for the regional variation in the prevalence of hypercalcaemia in tuberculosis. Calcif Tissue Int 1997;60:91-3.

154. Singhellakis PN, Kitrou MP, Demertzi FD, Tzannes SE, Alevizaki CC, Mountokalkis TD, et al. Serum parathyroid hormone levels in active pulmonary tuberculosis. Acta Endocrinol Suppl [Copenh] 1984;265:52-4.

155. Adams JS, Gacad MA. Characterization of 1 alpha—hydroxylation of vitamin D3 sterols by cultured alveolar macrophage from patients with sarcoidosis. J Exp Med 1985;161:755-65.

156. Barnes PF, Modlin RL, Bikle DD, Adams JJ. Transpleural gradient of 1,25 dihydroxyvitamin D in tuberculosis pleuritis. J Clin Invest 1989;83:1527-32.

157. Epstein S, Stern PH, Bell NH, Dowdeswell I, Turner RT. Evidence for abnormal regulation of circulating 1 alpha, 25 dihydroxyvitamin D in patients with pulmonary tuberculosis and normal calcium metabolism. Calcif Tissue Int 1984;36:541- 4.

158. Bell NH, Shary J, Shaw S, Turner RT. Hypercalcaemia associated with increased circulating 1,25 dihydroxyvitamin D in patients with pulmonary tuberculosis. Calcif Tissue Int 1985;37:588-91.

159. Saggese G, Bertelloni S, Baroncelli GI, Fusara C, Gualtiers M. Abnormal synthesis of 1,25 dihydroxyvitamin D and hypercalcaemia in children with tuberculosis. Pediatr Med Chir 1989;11:529-32.

160. Cadranel J, Milleron B, Garabedian M, Aroun G. Serum concentrations of vitamin D metabolites in untreated tuberculosis. Thorax 1985;40:639-40.

161. Felsenfeld AJ, Drezner MK, Llacch F. Hypercalcemia and elevated calcitriol levels in a maintenance dialysis patient with tuberculosis. Arch Intern Med 1986;146:1941-5.

162. Caldranel J, Hance AJ, Milleron B, Paillard F, Akoun GM, Garabedian M. Vitamin D metabolism in tuberculosis: production of 1,25 [OH]2D3 by cells recovered by bronchoalveolar lavage and the role of this metabolite in calcium homeostasis. Am Rev Respir Dis 1988;138:984-9.

163. Reichel H, Koeffler HP, Barbers R, Norman AW. Regulation of 1,25 dihydroxyvitamin D production by cultured alveolar macrophages from normal human donors and from patients with pulmonary sarcoidosis. J Clin Endocrinol Metab 1987;65:1201-9.

164. Crowle AJ, Ross EJ, May MH. Inhibition by 1,25[OH]2 Vitamin D3 of the multiplication of virulent tubercle bacilli in cultured human macrophage. Infect Immun 1987;55:2945-50.

165. Martinez ME, Gonzalez J, Sanchez-Cabezudo MJ, Peria JM, Vazquez JJ, Felsenfeld A. Evidence of absorption hypercalciuria in tuberculosis patients. Calcif Tissue Int 1993;53:384-7.

166. Brodie MJ, Boobis AR, Hillyard CJ, Abeyasekera G, Stevenson JC, Macintyre I, et al. Effect of rifampicin and isoniazide on vitamin D metabolism. Clin Pharmacol Ther 1982;32:525-30.

167. Brodie MJ, Boobis AR, Dollery CT, Hillyard CJ, Brown DJ, Macintyre I, et al. Rifampin and vitamin D metabolism. Clin Pharmacol Ther 1980;27:810-4.

168. Davies PD, Brown RC, Church HA, Woodhead JJ. The effect of antituberculous chemotherapy on vitamin D and calcium metabolism. Tubercle 1987;38:261-6.

169. Tebben PJ, Singh RJ, Kumar R. Vitamin D-mediated hypercalcemia: mechanisms, diagnosis, and treatment. Endocr Rev 2016;37:521-47.

170. Rajendra A, Mishra AK, Francis NR, Carey RA. Severe hypercalcemia in a patient with pulmonary tuberculosis. J Family Med Prim Care 2016;5:509-11.

171. Harinarayan CV, Ramalakshmi T, Prasad UV, Sudhakar D, Srinivasarao PV, Sarma KV, et al. High prevalence of low dietary calcium, high phytate consumption, and vitamin D deficiency in healthy south Indians. Am J Clin Nutr 2007;85:1062-7.

Tuberculosis and Human Immunodeficiency Virus Infection

BB Rewari, Amitabh Kumar, Srikanth Tripathy, Jai P Narain

INTRODUCTION

Human immunodeficiency virus [HIV] infection and tuberculosis [TB] are two major public health problems in most of developing countries including India. TB is also the most common opportunistic infection [OI] seen in HIV infected patients in India (1,2). In the pre-antiretroviral therapy [ART] era, nearly one-third of HIV-acquired immunedeficiency syndrome [AIDS] related deaths have been reported to be due to TB (3). With the wider availability of ART, though the mortality of HIV-associated TB has reduced significantly; it is still higher compared to HIV-uninfected individuals (4). HIV-TB co-infection carries a high mortality risk and accounts for approximately 25% of global HIV/AIDS deaths each year (5).

In HIV-infected individuals, presentation of TB may be very different from that in a HIV-seronegative individual. Extra-pulmonary TB [EPTB] accounts for up to 20% of cases of TB in immunocompetent, HIV-seronegative persons. However, observations from India suggest that, EPTB constituted 45%-56% of all the cases of TB in persons with HIV/AIDS (6). It is not only the HIV infection that increases the incidence, dissemination and severity of TB infection but TB has also been implicated to advance the progression of the HIV disease and subsequent immunosuppression. Thus, it has been rightly called the 'deadly duet' with one disease fuelling the other.

The Central TB Division [CTD], Ministry of Health and Family Welfare, Government of India and WHO India laid down the "Standards of Care for TB in India" [SCTI] in 2014 (6). The management of active TB disease in HIV-infected persons is essentially the same as in HIV-negative persons, with a few additional considerations. In addition to anti-TB treatment, the ART must be initiated early during TB treatment for all co-infected patients to reduce the risk of death (7). Case management requires a combination of appropriate anti-TB treatment, ART, and co-trimoxazole [trimethoprim-sulphamethoxazole] preventive therapy [CPT] to prevent other OIs (8). ART reduces mortality by 64%-95% in patients with drug-susceptible TB (9), and CPT halves the mortality risk (10).

To maximise the benefits of ART and anti-TB treatment, it is essential that HIV-TB co-infected patients are identified well in time, initiated on appropriate treatments and monitored closely for better treatment outcomes. Hence, it is of utmost importance to have a close coordination between Revised National TB Control Programme [RNTCP] and National AIDS Control Programme [NACP]. Some newer initiatives taken under this initiative include innovative intensified case finding using cartridge based nucleic acid amplification test [CBNAAT], daily anti-TB treatment, single window service for anti-TB treatment and ART, isoniazid preventive therapy [IPT], pharmacovigilance of anti-TB and anti-retroviral drugs, information and communication technology [ICT] based adherence support and air borne infection control practices, among others.

This chapter provides an overview regarding the different HIV-TB coordination activities recommended globally by WHO to end TB and their implementation in India at national, state and district levels.

EPIDEMIOLOGY

As per the WHO report 2018 (2), in 2017, there were an estimated 10 million new TB cases globally. People living with HIV [PLHIV] accounted for 10% of all new TB cases. In 2017, there were an estimated 1.3 million TB deaths; an additional 0.3 million deaths resulted from TB disease in PLHIV (2). TB deaths among HIV-positive people are classified as HIV deaths in International Classification of Diseases-10 [ICD-10] (2,11).

India has the third highest number of estimated PLHIV in the world. In 2015, in India, the number of PLHIV was estimated to be 2,117,000; national adult [15-49 years] prevalence of HIV was estimated to be 0.26% [Figure 35.1] (12). An overall reduction of 66% in the annual new HIV infections over last 15 years [Figure 35.2]. As of now, around 86,000 new infections occur every year. The trend of annual AIDS deaths is showing a steady decline since roll out of the free ART programme in 2004 [Figure 35.3]. It is estimated that around 450,000 lives have been saved due to ART till 2014 (12).

In terms of numbers, India accounts for about 9% of the global burden of HIV-associated TB making it second highest globally. However, HIV prevalence among incident TB patients in India is estimated to be around 5% with a range of 0%-45% across the country. There are an estimated

110,000 HIV-associated TB patients emerging annually. In general, HIV prevalence rates are higher in southern India while TB rates are higher in northern India (13).

Occurrence of HIV-TB co-infection is a fatal combination with extremely high death rates ranging from 15%-18% reported among HIV-infected TB cases notified under the RNTCP. In terms of absolute numbers, 42,000 HIV-TB co-infected people die every year (14).

NATIONAL PROGRAMMES FOR TB AND HIV

Revised National Tuberculosis Control Programmes

The reader is referred to the Chapter *"Revised National TB Control Programme" [Chapter 53]* for details on this topic.

National AIDS Control Programme

The Government of India established National AIDS Control Organisation [NACO] and launched the NACP in 1992 with phase-wise implementation; and currently, Phase IV of the NACP is being implemented with focus on capacity building, consolidating preventive services and comprehensive care, support and treatment [Table 35.1] (13).

The Government of India launched the free ART programme on 1 April 2004, under phase II of the NACP, starting with 8 tertiary-level government hospitals in the 6 high prevalence states of Andhra Pradesh, Karnataka, Maharashtra, Tamil Nadu, Manipur and Nagaland, as well as the NCT of Delhi. As on Dec 2015, nearly 911,000 PLHIV are receiving free ART at more than 1500 ART delivery sites (12). The programme also provides second line ART to 12,500 PLHIV and is planning to introduce third line ART shortly.

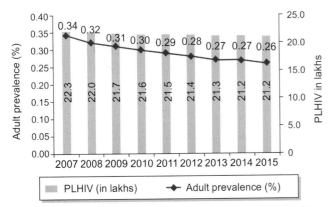

Figure 35.1: PLHIV and adult HIV prevalence in India 2007-2015
Lakh = 100,000; PLHIV = people living with HIV; HIV = human immunodeficiency virus
Source: reference 12

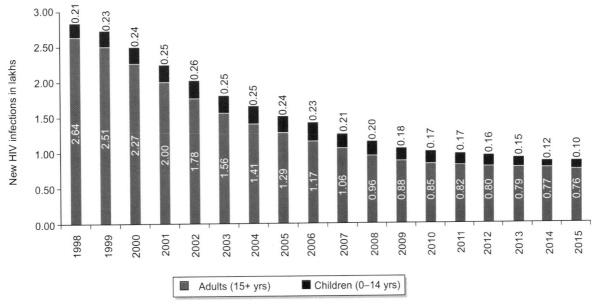

Figure 35.2: Estimated new HIV-infected persons in India, 1998-2015
Lakh = 100,000; HIV = human immunodeficiency virus
Reproduced with permission from reference 12

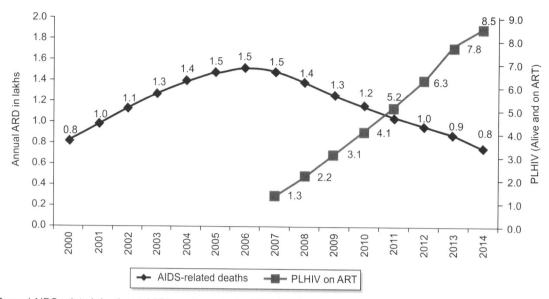

Figure 35.3: Annual AIDS-related deaths and ART scale-up, India, 2000-2014
PLHIV = people living with HIV; ARD = AIDS-related deaths; Lakh = 100,000; AIDS = acquired immunodeficiency syndrome; ART = anti-retroviral therapy
Reproduced with permission from reference 12

NACP phase	Salient features
Table 35.1: NACP: Phase-wise implementation	
Phase I [1992-1999]	Objective of slowing down the spread of HIV infections Reduce morbidity, mortality and impact of AIDS in the country NACO set up for project implementation
Phase II [1999-2007]	Focus shifted from raising awareness to changing behaviour Decentralisation of programme implementation to the state level Greater involvement of NGOs ART provision introduced in 2004
Phase III [2007-2012]	Scaling-up prevention efforts among high-risk group and general population Integrating preventive strategy with CST services Target of reducing new infections by 50% by 2012, achieved well in advance
Phase IV [2012-2017]	Aims to consolidating the gains till NACP III Accelerate the process of epidemic reversal Further strengthen the epidemic response in India through a cautious and well-defined integration process Intensifying and consolidating prevention services with a focus on high-risk groups and vulnerable population Increasing access and promoting comprehensive care, support and treatment services

NACO = National AIDS Control Organisation; NACP = National AIDS Control Programme; HIV = human immunodeficiency virus; AIDS = acquired immunodeficiency syndrome; NGOs = non-governmental organisations; ART = anti-retroviral therapy; CST = Care, Support and Treatment
Source: reference 13

HUMAN IMMUNODEFICIENCY VIRUS-TUBERCULOSIS: PATHOGENESIS

HIV is the strongest of all known risk factors for the development of TB and is known to affect Th-1 cell-mediated immune responses that are the central immune defences against *Mycobacterium tuberculosis* [*Mtb*] in the body. HIV-infected persons are at markedly increased risk for progressive disease following primary TB infection, as well as reactivation of latent TB infection [LTBI]. HIV infection increases the risk of subsequent episodes of TB from exogenous re-infection and it also increases the chance of relapse. The estimated annual risk of reactivation among those co-infected with HIV and TB is about 5%-8% with a cumulative lifetime risk of 50%-60%, which is very high when compared to a cumulative lifetime risk of 5%-10% in HIV-seronegative adult patients.

The interaction between HIV and TB infections is bi-directional. HIV infection increases the risk of both primary and reactivation TB (15), and this risk increases markedly with advancing HIV disease (15). At the time of TB diagnosis, most patients with co-infection have advanced HIV disease [Table 35.2] with low CD4+ T-cell counts and high viral loads or WHO clinical stage 3 and 4 disease [Table 35.3] (15,16). The development of active TB is also associated with increases in HIV viral load locally and systemically (16,17). There is consequently an increased risk of progression to AIDS and death (18,19).

In patients of TB there is evidence of immune activation and several studies have suggested a role of persistently activated immune system in pathogenesis of persistently elevated plasma viraemia in HIV-TB co-infection. It is proposed that immune activation leads to increased expression of chemokine receptors CXCR4 and CCR5, as well as their chemokine ligands. As CXCR4 and CCR5 being the two major co-receptors used by HIV for cell entry, increased expression leads to increased viral entry into the immune cells and subsequent high replication and viraemia. It has also been observed that there is an associated increase in plasma level of chemokines along with an increased expression of markers of immune activation (20,21).

CLINICAL PRESENTATION

The clinical presentation of HIV-associated TB is diverse and often atypical posing a diagnostic challenge. In HIV-positive cases, TB can occur at any CD4+ count (22). However, as the immunosuppression increases the likelihood of developing TB increases. In immunocompetent adult patients, pulmonary TB is the most common form of TB encountered, often with focal infiltrates and cavities. As the CD4+ count goes down, the presentation of TB becomes more atypical. While extra-pulmonary TB [EPTB] accounts for only 20% in HIV-negative persons, it accounts for 45%-56% in HIV-positive individuals (22).

Even with the pulmonary form of TB, the presentation is atypical. Patients are more likely to have diffuse pulmonary disease without cavitation often involving the lower lobes and prominent mediastinal or paratracheal adenopathies are often seen. Such patients are less likely to be sputum positive for acid-fast bacilli [AFB]. There is also a high probability of having miliary TB [Table 35.2]. TB of the lymphatic system, central nervous system, soft tissue, bone marrow, liver, spleen and other viscera may also occur. There is an increased frequency of lymph nodes involvement, pleural effusion, TB of the brain, abscesses of the chest wall, testes, spleen or elsewhere. In a study of HIV associated TB among PLHIV in New Delhi, it was observed that pulmonary TB in isolation was seen only in 38.4% patients while 39.7% patients had only EPTB and 21.9% had both pulmonary as well as EPTB at diagnosis (4).

DIAGNOSIS

Diagnosis of pulmonary TB in HIV-seronegative patient is relatively easy as sputum smear for AFB is frequently positive. There has been a huge emphasis on sputum for AFB examination in the RNTCP as the goal is also to cut the chain of transmission and halt the spread of TB. Published evidence suggests that sputum smears reveal AFB less frequently in HIV-seropositive patients with pulmonary TB, especially in late HIV disease (23). Diagnosis of such cases would, thus, require additional radiological and other relevant investigations. The reader is referred to the chapter *"Laboratory diagnosis" [Chapter 8]* for details.

Smear-negative pulmonary TB, EPTB, disseminated and miliary TB may require mycobacterial culture, nucleic acid amplification tests [NAAT] and gene probe-based tests, among others. Samples obtained from extrapulmonary sites such as bone marrow, lymph node, pleural/ascitic fluid, brain tissue, cerebrospinal fluid, urine, stool or blood should be tested by conventional and rapid molecular diagnostic tests.

Cartridge based nucleic acid amplification test [CBNAAT], Xpert MTB/RIF, has shown very high sensitivity and specificity for diagnosis of both smear-positive and smear-negative pulmonary TB cases with high rates of detection of rifampicin resistance and greater concordance with gene sequencing for rifampicin resistance when compared with mycobacterial culture (24). It is designed to extract, amplify and identify targeted rpoB nucleic acid sequences automatically with minimal specimen handling. From the patient management perspective, it provides results within 2 hours that enables same day diagnosis and prompt

Table 35.2: Clinical presentation of TB in early and late HIV infection

Features	Stage of HIV Infection	
	Early	*Late*
Clinical presentation	Often resembles post-primary TB	Often resembles primary TB
Sputum smear	Often positive	Often negative
Radiological appearance	Upper lobe involvement	Lower lung-field involvement
	Cavitatory lesions	Cavitation rare
		Intra-thoracic lymph node TB
		Disseminated/miliary TB more common
		Pleural/pericardial effusions

TB = tuberculosis; HIV = human immunodeficiency virus

treatment initiation with higher retention rates. This is the fastest turn around time as compared to 72 hours with line probe assay [LPA], nearly 2 months with liquid culture and drug-susceptibility testing [DST] and four months in solid culture and DST. Xpert MTB/RIF is now the standard of care for confirmation of TB among TB suspects, especially those who are HIV infected. This has also been proven to be of promising value in diagnosis of EPTB (25). Its usefulness in paediatric TB and drug-resistant TB has also been well documented (26). CBNAAT based testing has now been adopted by RNTCP and is being provided at 125 sites presently with plans to expand to 950 sites during the National Strategic Plan [NSP] period by 2017.

TREATMENT

Treatment of HIV-TB Co-infected Persons

TB is considered as WHO clinical stage 3 [pulmonary] or 4 [extra-pulmonary] disease [Table 35.3] (27). The estimated aggregate case fatality rate of HIV-infected TB is high at about 40%, and may be over 50% in many developing countries. While deaths in the first month of TB treatment may be due to TB, late deaths in co-infected persons are attributable to HIV disease progression (28). Immediate treatment of TB is the central priority in management of TB-HIV co-infected persons. The patient must be started on anti-TB treatment without any delay, on the diagnosis of TB. The principles of management of TB in PLHIV are essentially the same. Standards for TB Care in India lays down uniform standards for TB care for all stakeholders in the country (6). The patients should be started on RNTCP Category I or Category II regimens, as per guidelines immediately.

Several issues in the management of the two diseases together, like, pill burden, poor tolerance, poor drug absorption, poor adherence, substance abuse, drug interactions, overlapping toxicities, stigmatisation and discrimination may have a bearing on the eventual outcome of the treatment, both for TB and HIV. Outcomes of HIV-TB co-infected patients continue to be poor with less than 80% success rate amongst the new patients (29). A project has recently been launched by WHO-NACO-CTD at 30 high burden ART centres across the countries where in HIV-TB co-infected persons will be initiated on daily anti-TB regimen as well as IPT to improve their outcomes (14). A decision has now been taken by the Government of India to provide daily anti-TB treatment for all TB patients starting with HIV-TB co-infected to begin with at all ART centres across the country.

Morbidity and mortality due to TB in areas of high prevalence may not be singly contained by the current global TB control strategy using the WHO recommended DOTS (30). Good quality supervised treatment for TB under this strategy may take care of the TB, but its role in slowing or reversing HIV disease progression is doubtful. Antiretroviral treatment will reduce both the incidence of TB and mortality. The use of ART in TB-endemic areas has been associated with more than 80% reduction in the incidence of

HIV-associated TB; the protective effect of ART was seen at all stages of HIV disease, but was greatest in symptomatic patients and those with advanced disease (31,32). Concurrent use of ART during TB treatment has been found to be associated with reduced mortality (32,33).

Treatment of HIV-TB is challenging, often it is difficult to identify the optimum time to start ART for patients on TB treatment. This is associated with a complex series of competing risks that may vary between different settings and patient populations (33,34). However, it is clear that delays in ART initiation are associated with increased risk of mortality among patients with TB (34-39). WHO has revised the ART guidelines for resource-limited settings several times between 2002 and 2016, recommending progressively earlier initiation of ART during TB treatment. The revision of these guidelines, published in 2016, recommended that ART be given to all patients with TB regardless of CD4+ T-cell count, should be started as soon as possible after TB treatment is tolerated, and should definitely be initiated maximum by 8 weeks of initiating anti-TB treatment (40,41). In India, it was seen that the median time between the start of TB treatment and ART was 23 days and nearly 80% imitated ART within 8 weeks of anti-TB treatment [Table 35.4] (42). As new data emerge from trials being conducted all over the globe these guidelines may be further refined (34). In India, NACO recommends starting ART after 2 weeks of patients being put on anti-TB treatment and not later than 8 weeks of treatment. The programme is considering for simultaneous initiation of anti-TB treatment and ART for all co-infected patients with CD4+ count less than 50 cells/mm^3 in order to reduce mortality among those who are severely immune compromised.

Antiretroviral Therapy

The currently available antiretroviral drugs cannot eradicate the HIV infection as the viruses hides in 'immunological sanctuaries' in the body from where it is difficult to wipe it off. A pool of latently infected CD4+ cells is established during the earliest stages of acute HIV infection and persists within the organs/cells and fluids [e.g., liver and lymphoid tissue] despite adequate treatment. Hence, the goals of ART are to achieve suppression of viral replication for extended period with recovery of immune system and eventual prolongation of life and improving quality of life [Table 35.5] (7).

There are six major classes of drugs used to treat HIV/AIDS termed as antiretroviral drugs [ARV]. These drugs are grouped by way these interfere with steps in HIV replication [Table 35.6] (7). The current standard of care for the treatment of HIV-1 infection is "triple-drug therapy" with two nucleoside reverse transcriptase inhibitors [NRTI] or nucleotide reverse transcriptase inhibitors [NtRTI] backbones in combination with a non-nucleoside reverse transcriptase inhibitor [NNRTI] (40,41). Over the years there has been a shift towards earlier initiation of ART with simplified less toxic more robust ART regimen [Figure 35.4]. The guidelines

Table 35.3: WHO clinical staging of HIV disease in adults, adolescents and children

Adults and adolescents	Children
Clinical stage 1	*Clinical stage 1*
Asymptomatic	Asymptomatic
Persistent generalised lymphadenopathy	Persistent generalised lymphadenopathy
Clinical stage 2	*Clinical stage 2*
Moderate unexplained weight loss [<10% of presumed or measured body weight]	Unexplained persistent hepatosplenomegaly
Recurrent respiratory tract infections [sinusitis, tonsillitis, otitis media, pharyngitis]	Recurrent or chronic upper respiratory tract infections [otitis media, otorrhoea, sinusitis, tonsillitis]
Herpes zoster	Herpes zoster
Angular cheilitis	Lineal gingival erythema
Recurrent oral ulceration	Recurrent oral ulceration
Papular pruritic eruption	Papular pruritic eruption
Fungal nail infections	Fungal nail infections
Seborrhoeic dermatitis	Extensive wart virus infection
	Extensive molluscum contagiosum
Clinical stage 3	*Clinical stage 3*
Unexplained severe weight loss [>10% of presumed or measured body weight]	Unexplained moderate malnutrition not adequately responding to standard therapy
Unexplained chronic diarrhoea for longer than 1 month	Unexplained persistent diarrhoea [14 days or more]
Unexplained persistent fever [intermittent or constant for longer than 1 month]	Unexplained persistent fever [above 37.5 °C, intermittent or constant, for longer than 1 month]
Persistent oral candidiasis	Persistent oral candidiasis [after first 6 weeks of life]
Oral hairy leukoplakia	Oral hairy leukoplakia
	Lymph node TB
Pulmonary TB	Pulmonary TB
Severe bacterial infections [such as pneumonia, empyema, pyomyositis, bone or joint infection, meningitis, bacteraemia]	Severe recurrent bacterial pneumonia
Acute necrotising ulcerative stomatitis, gingivitis or periodontitis	Acute necrotising ulcerative gingivitis or periodontitis
Unexplained anaemia [<8 g/dL], neutropaenia [< 0.5 × 10^9/L] and/or chronic thrombocytopaenia [<50 × 10^9/L]	Unexplained anaemia [<8 g/dL], neutropaenia [< 0.5 × 10^9/L] and/or chronic thrombocytopaenia [<50 × 10^9/L]
	Symptomatic lymphoid interstitial pneumonitis
	Chronic HIV-associated lung disease, including bronchiectasis
Clinical stage 4	*Clinical stage 4*
HIV wasting syndrome	Unexplained severe wasting, stunting or severe malnutrition not responding to standard therapy
Pneumocystis jiroveci pneumonia	*Pneumocystis jiroveci* pneumonia
Recurrent severe bacterial pneumonia	Recurrent severe bacterial infections [such as, empyema, pyomyositis, bone or joint infection, meningitis, but excluding pneumonia]
Chronic herpes simplex infection [orolabial, genital or anorectal of more than 1 month's duration or visceral at any site]	Chronic herpes simplex infection [orolabial or cutaneous of more than 1 month's duration or visceral at any site]
Oesophageal candidiasis [or candidiasis of trachea, bronchi or lungs]	Oesophageal candidiasis [or candidiasis of trachea, bronchi or lungs]
Extra-pulmonary TB	Extra-pulmonary TB
Kaposi sarcoma	Kaposi sarcoma
Cytomegalovirus infection [retinitis or infection of other organs]	Cytomegalovirus infection [retinitis or infection of other organs with onset at age more than 1 month]
Central nervous system toxoplasmosis	Central nervous system toxoplasmosis [after the neonatal period]
HIV encephalopathy	HIV encephalopathy
Extrapulmonary cryptococcosis, including meningitis	Extrapulmonary cryptococcosis, including meningitis
Disseminated nontuberculous mycobacterial infection	Disseminated nontuberculous mycobacterial infection
Progressive multifocal leukoencephalopathy	Progressive multifocal leukoencephalopathy
Chronic cryptosporidiosis	Chronic cryptosporidiosis [with diarrhoea]
Chronic isosporiasis	Chronic isosporiasis
Disseminated mycosis [extra-pulmonary histoplasmosis, coccidioidomycosis]	Disseminated endemic mycosis [extrapulmonary histoplasmosis, coccidioidomycosis, penicilliosis]
Lymphoma [cerebral or B-cell non-Hodgkin]	Lymphoma [cerebral or B-cell non-Hodgkin]
Symptomatic HIV-associated nephropathy or cardiomyopathy	HIV-associated nephropathy or cardiomyopathy
Recurrent septicaemia [including non-typhoidal *Salmonella*]	
Invasive cervical carcinoma	
Atypical disseminated leishmaniasis	

WHO = World Health Organization; HIV = human immunodeficiency virus; TB = tuberculosis
Source: Adapted from reference 27

Table 35.4: Initiation on ART for HIV-positive TB patients in 62 facilities in India, October-November 2014

Study cohort [adults, n= 9468]	Observations
Patients diagnosed with TB [No.]	1871
Patients already on ART at the time of TB diagnosis [No.]	362
Time between start of TB treatment and ART initiation, for the 1429 HIV-positive TB patients who were not already on ART {No. [%]}	
<2 weeks	200 [14%]
2-8 weeks	933 [65%]
>8 weeks	296 [21%]
Median	23 days

ART = anti-retroviral therapy; HIV = human immunodeficiency virus; TB = tuberculosis
Source: reference 42

Table 35.5: Goals of anti-retroviral therapy

Goal	Observations
Clinical goals	Prolongation of life and improvement in quality of life
Virological goals	Maximum reduction in viral load for as long as possible
Immunological goals	Reconstitution of immunity
Therapeutic goals	Rational sequencing of drugs in a way to achieve clinical, virological and immunological goals while maintaining treatment options, limiting drug toxicity and facilitating adherence
Reduction of HIV transmission in individuals	Reduction of HIV transmission by suppression of viral load

HIV = human immunodeficiency virus
Source: reference 7

Table 35.6: Classification of anti-retroviral drugs

Drug class	Drugs
Nucleoside reverse transcriptase inhibitors [NRTI]	Zidovudine [AZT], Lamivudine [3TC], Stavudine [d4T], Didanosine [ddI], Zalcitabine [ddC], Abacavir [ABC], Tenofovir [TDF], Emtricitabine [FTC]
Non-nucleoside reverse transcriptase inhibitors [NNRTI]	Nevirapine [NVP], Efavirenz [EFV], Delavirdine [DLV]
Protease inhibitors	Indinavir [IDV], Nelfinavir [NFV], Saquinavir [SQV], Ritonavir [RTV], Atazanavir [ATV], Lopinavir [LPV], Fosamprenavir, Darunavir.[TMC114]
CCR5 co-receptor antagonist	Maraviroc
Fusion inhibitors	Enfuvirtide
Integrase inhibitors	Raltegravir, Elvitegravir

Source: reference 7

on when to initiate ART have been progressively moving from CD4+ count less than 200/mm^3 in the year 2004 to "treat all" irrespective of CD based on trials like CIPHRA HT 001, SMART trial, HPTN 052 and the recent START trial [Figure 35.5]. The current NACO guidelines now provide for a simple harmonised ART in form of a single tablet of fixed dose combination of tenofovir, lamivudine and efavirenz to all newly diagnosed PLHIV including pregnant women, those co-infected with TB or hepatitis [Table 35.7] (7). This simplification is helpful for HIV-TB patients as efavirenz has minimal drug-drug interaction with anti-TB drugs. Efavirenz which was earlier supposed to be avoided during first trimester of pregnancy is now considered safe to administer (43). The eligibility for initiation of ART in asymptomatic patients has been revised to CD4+ cut off of 500 and irrespective of CD4+ count for WHO stages 3 and 4

with HIV-TB co-infection. The first-line, second-line and proposed third-line regimen used in the programme are listed in [Table 35.8] (7).

Adverse drug reaction are a major challenge while managing HIV because of the number of drugs used. Common side effects of major drugs used in the program are enlisted in Table 35.9 (7). Drug toxicity can lead to patient often discontinuing ART (44). Some ARVs may have overlapping or additive toxicities with anti-TB treatment [Table 35.10] (45). The drugs like stavudine and didanosine which were used earlier have now been phased out due to their long-term toxicities. Once the patient is started on first-line ART, it is important to monitor the CD4+ count and viral load to identify treatment failure and switch to second line ART. The criteria for identifying treatment failure are listed in [Table 35.11] (7).

Rifampicin, the mainstay drug in treatment of TB has major interactions with NNRTIs and the PIs. The PIs and NNRTIs are metabolised mainly through the cytochrome P450 [CYP] 3A4 enzymes. Rifampicin induces the expression of CYP3A4 isoenzyme in the liver and intestines (46), decreasing the plasma concentration of PIs and the NNRTIs when co-administered (47). Rifampicin also increases the activity of the efflux multidrug transporter P-glycoprotein [P-gp], which contributes to the elimination of the PIs (48,49). Rifampicin reduces the area under the curve [AUC] of efavirenz by 22%-26% (50), and nevirapine by up to 31% (51,52); hence, rifampicin can be co-administered with efavirenz.

Rifampicin reduces the AUC of available PIs by 35%-92%, and the reduction by rifabutin is in the range of

Topic	2002	2003	2006	2010	2013	2015
When to start	CD4+ ≤200	CD4+ ≤200	CD4+ ≤200 – Consider 350 – CD4+ ≤350 for TB	CD4+ ≤350 – Regardless CD4+ for TB and HBV	CD4+ ≤500 – Regardless CD4+ for TB HBV PW and SDC –CD4+ ≤350 as priority	**Towards treatment initiation at any CD4+ cell count**
			Earlier initiation →			
1st line ART	8 options –AZT preferred	4 options –AZT preferred	8 options –AZT or TDF preferred –d4T dose reduction	6 options and FDCs –AZT or TDF preferred –d4T phase out	1 preferred option and FDCs –TDF and EFV preferred across all nops	**Continue with FDC approach and phased introduction of new options [DTG, EFV/400]**
			Simpler treatment →			
2nd line ART	Boosted and non-boosted Pls	Boosted Pls –IDV/r LPV/r. SQV/r	Boosted PI –ATV/r, DRV/r, FPV/r LPV/r, SQV/r	Boosted PI –Heat stable FDC, ATV/r. LPV/r	Boosted Pls –Heat stable FDC; ATV/r. LPV/r	**Add more heat stable PI options [DRV/r] and new strategies [NRTI sparing regimens]**
			Less toxic, more robust regimens →			
3rd line ART	None	None	None	DRV/r, RAL, ETV	DRV/r, RAL, ETV	**Encourage HIV DR to guide**
Viral load testing	No	No [Desirable]	Yes [Tertiary centers]	Yes [Phase in approach]	Yes [Preferred for monitoring use of PoC DPS]	**Support for scale up of VL using all technologies**
			Better and simpler monitoring →			

Figure 35.4: Evolution of global ARV guidelines
ARV = antiretroviral; TB = tuberculosis; HBV = hepatitis B virus; PW = pregnant women; SDC = sero-discordant couple; AZT = zidovudine; TDF = tenofovir ;d4T = stavudine; FDCs = fixed-dose combinations; EFV = efavirenz; IDV/r = indinavir/ritonavir; LPV/r = lopinavir/ritonavir; SQV/r = saquinavir/ritonavir; ATV/r = atazanavir/ritonavir; DRV/r = darunavir/ritonavir; DTV = dolutegravir; NRTI = nucleoside reverse transcriptase inhibitors; ART = anti-retroviral treatment; HIV DR = human immunodeficiency virus drug-resistance; RAL = raltegravir; ETV = etravirine; VL = viral load

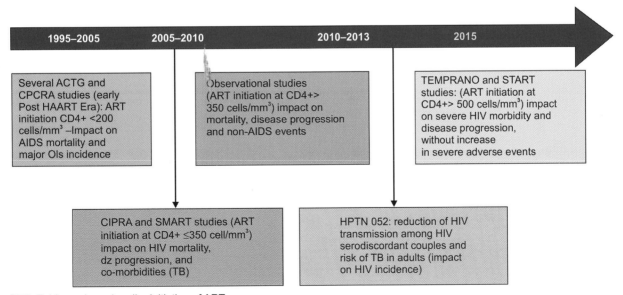

Figure 35.5: Evidence-based earlier initiation of ART
ACTG = AIDS Clinical Trials Group; CPCRA = Community Programs for Clinical Research on AIDS; HAART = highly active anti-retroviral therapy; ART = anti-retroviral therapy; AIDS = acquired immunodeficiency syndrome; TEMPRANO = A Trial of Early Antiretrovirals and Isoniazid Preventive Therapy in Africa; START = Initiation of Antiretroviral Therapy in Early Asymptomatic HIV Infection; HIV = human immunodeficiency virus; CIPRA = Comprehensive International Program of Research on AIDS; SMART = Strategies for Management of Antiretroviral Therapy; HPTN = HIV Prevention Trials Network; OIs = opportunistic infections

Table 35.7: Initiation of ART based on CD4+ count and WHO clinical staging in HIV infected persons

Situation	Recommendations	Regimen
WHO clinical stage		
Clinical stage I and II	Start ART if CD4+ <500 cells/mm^3	
Clinical stage III and IV	Start ART regardless of CD4+ count	
All pregnant and breast feeding women	Start ART regardless of CD4+ count	
All HIV infected children below 5 years of age	Start ART regardless of CD4+ count	
For HIV and TB co-infected patients		
Patients with HIV and TB co-infection [PTB or EPTB]	Start ART regardless of CD4+ count and type of TB [start ani-TB treatment first, initiate ART as early as possible between 2 weeks and 2 months when TB treatment is tolerated]	FDC of TDF 300 mg + 3TC 300 mg + EFV 600 mg [Single pill at bed time]
For HIV and hepatitis B and C co-infected patients		
HIV and HBV/HCV co-infection–without any evidence of severe/chronic liver disease	Start ART if CD4+ <500 cells/mm^3	
HIV and HBV/HCV co-infection–with documented evidence of severe/chronic liver disease	Start ART regardless of CD4+ count	

ART = anti-retroviral therapy; WHO = World Health Organization; HIV = human immunodeficiency virus; TB = tuberculosis; PTB = pulmonary TB; EPTB = extra-pulmonary TB; HBV = hepatitis B virus; HCV = hepatitis C virus; FDC = fixed-dose combination; TDF = Tenofovir; 3TC = Lamivudine; EFV = efavirenz
Source: reference 7

Table 35.8: ARV regimens used in the National AIDS Control Programme

Regimen	Dosage
First-line ARV regimen	
Tenofovir 300 mg + Lamivudine 300 mg + Efavirenz 600 mg	1 tab OD
Zidovudine 300 mg + Lamivudine 150 mg + Nevirapine 200 mg	1 tab BD
Zidovudine 300 mg + Lamivudine 150 mg/Efavirenz 600 mg	1 tab ZL BD + 1 tab EFV HS
Tenofovir 300 mg + Lamivudine 300 mg/Nevirapine 200 mg	1 tab TL OD + 1 tab NVP BD
Alternate first-line ARV regimen	
Stavudine 30 mg + Lamivudine 150 mg + Nevirapine 200 mg	1 tab BD
Stavudine 30 mg + Lamivudine 150 mg/Efavirenz 600 mg	1 tab SL BD + 1 tab EFV HS
Abacavir 600 mg + Lamivudine 300 mg/Nevirapine 200 mg	1 tab AL OD + 1 tab NVP BD
Abacavir 600 + Lamivudine 300 mg/Efavirenz 600 mg	1 tab AL OD + 1 tab EFV HS
Second-line ARV regimen	
Tenofovir 300 mg + Lamivudine 300 mg/Atazanavir 300 mg/Ritonavir 100 mg	1 tab TL OD + 1 tab ATV OD + 1 tab RTV OD
Tenofovir 300 mg + Lamivudine 300 mg/Lopinavir 200 mg + Ritonavir 50 mg	1 tab TL OD + 2 tab LPV/r BD
Zidovudine 300 mg + Lamivudine 150 mg/Atazanavir 300 mg/Ritonavir 100 mg	1 tab ZL BD + 1 tab ATV OD + 1 tab RTV OD
Zidovudine 300 mg + Lamivudine 150 mg/Lopinavir 250 mg + Ritonavir 50 mg	1 tab ZL BD + 2 tab LPV/r BD
Stavudine 30 mg + Lamivudine 150 mg/Atazanavir 300 mg/Ritonavir 100 mg	1 tab SL BD + 1 tab ATV OD + 1 tab RTV OD
Stavudine 30 mg + Lamivudine 150 mg/Lopinavir 250 mg + Ritonavir 50 mg	1 tab SL BD + 2 tab LPV/r BD
Abacavir 600 mg + Lamivudine 300 mg/Atazanavir 300 mg/Ritonavir 100 mg	1 tab AL OD + 1 tab ATV OD + 1 tab RTV OD
Abacavir 600 mg + Lamivudine 300 mg/Lopinavir 250 mg + Ritonavir 50 mg	1 tab AL OD + 2 tab LPV/r BD
Proposed third-line ARV regimen	
Raltegravir 400 mg/Darunavir 600 mg/Ritonavir 100 mg	1 tab RAL BD + 1 tab DRV BD + 1 tab RTV OD

Source: reference 7

15%-45% (42,47). In general, co-administration of rifampicin with PIs is contraindicated (47,51-53). Rifabutin is a much less potent inducer of the CYP3A4 isoenzyme and is used when using PI based second-line ART for those who have failed first-line ART and needs TB treatment as well.

IMMUNE RECONSTITUTION INFLAMMATORY SYNDROME

Starting ART in patients having HIV infection leads to rapid suppression of the virus and consequently a rapid recovery

Table 35.9: Common side effects of ARV drugs

Timing	Side effects and toxicities	Common causes
Short-term [the first few weeks]	Gastrointestinal toxicities, including nausea, vomiting, diarrhoea, anaemia and neutropenia	AZT, TDF, PIs
	Rash [most rashes occur within the first 2-3 weeks]	NVP, EFV, ABC, PIs [rarely]
	Hepatotoxicity [more common in hepatitis B or C co-infection]	NVP, EFV, PIs
	Drowsiness, dizziness, confusion and vivid dreams [normally self-resolving but can take weeks to months]	EFV
Medium-term [the first few months]	Anaemia and neutropaenia, sudden and acute bone marrow suppression can occur within the first weeks of therapy or present as a slow onset of progressive anaemia over months	AZT
	Hyperpigmentation of skin, nails and mucous membranes	AZT
	Lactic acidosis [more common after the first few months, most commonly associated with d4T]	d4T, ddI, AZT
	Peripheral neuropathy [more common after the first few months]	d4T, ddI
	Pancreatitis [can occur at any time]	ddI
Long-term [after 6-18 months]	Lipodystrophy and lipoatrophy	d4T, ddI, AZT, PIs
	Dyslipidaemia	d4T, EFV, PIs
	Diabetes mellitus	IDV
	Skin, hair and nail abnormalities	PIs especially IDV
	Renal tubular dysfunction	TDF
	Bone mineral toxicity	TDF

ARV = anti-retroviral; AZT = zidovudine; TDF = tenofovir; PIs = protease inhibitors; NVP = nevirapine; EFV = efavirenz; ABC = abacavir; d4T = stavudine; ddI = didanosine; IDV = indinavir
Source: reference 7

Table 35.10: Overlapping or additive toxicities due to ARV drugs and first-line anti-TB drugs

Toxicity	Antiretroviral agents	Anti-TB drugs
Peripheral neuropathy	Stavudine, didanosine, zalcitabine	Isoniazid, ethambutol
Gastrointestinal intolerance	All	All
Hepatotoxicity	NVP, EFV, all NRTIs and PIs	Isoniazid, rifampicin, rifabutin, pyrazinamide
Central nervous system	EFV	Isoniazid
Bone marrow suppression	AZT	Rifabutin, rifampicin
Skin rash	ABC, amprenavir, NVP, EFV and fosamprenavir	Isoniazid, rifampicin and pyrazinamide
Ocular effects	ddI	Ethambutol, rifabutin

ARV = anti-retroviral; TB = tuberculosis; NVP = nevirapine; EFV = efavirenz; NRTIs = nucleoside reverse transcriptase inhibitors; PIs = protease inhibitors; AZT = zidovudine; ABC = abacavir; ddI = didanosine
Source: reference 45

Table 35.11: Criteria for identifying treatment failure

Types of failure	Criteria
Clinical failure	New or recurrent WHO stage 4 condition after at least 6 months of ART
Immunological failure	Fall of CD4 count to pre-therapy 50% fall from the on-treatment peak value Persistent CD4 levels below 100 cells/mL
Virological failure	Plasma viral load >1,000 copies/mL after at least 6 months of ART

Source: reference 7

of the immune system. The immune reconstitution, however, can lead to an acute inflammatory reaction against infectious and non-infectious agents (54). Symptomatic disease is most common in patients starting treatment with low CD4+ T-cell counts and is attributed to poor regulation of the restored immune system (55). *Mtb* infection accounts for probably one-third of [HIV] related immune reconstitution inflammatory syndrome [IRIS] events, particularly in developing countries where HIV and TB co-infection is very common. Up to 7%-43% of patients with HIV-TB coinfection may develop IRIS (56,57). TB-associated IRIS has a wide spectrum of presentations, ranging from mild lymph node inflammation to potentially fatal disease of the central nervous system.

IRIS can be of two types [in TB]: "paradoxical" transient clinical deterioration after clinical improvement [paradoxical IRIS]; and the uncovering of active TB disease in patients with unrecognised "occult" TB ["unmasking IRIS]". In a clinical setting, TB-IRIS must be differentiated from anti-TB treatment failure. IRIS is usually accompanied by an increase in CD4+ T-cell count and/or a rapid decrease in viral load while treatment failure is associated with increasing viral load and decline in CD4+ count. TB-IRIS can occur as early as 5 days after starting ART; however, most patients develop symptoms within the first 2-6 weeks (58,59), though cases may occur even later. A low baseline CD4+ T-cell count, a shorter interval between TB diagnosis and ART initiation, and disseminated or EPTB have been proposed as risk factors for TB-IRIS (56,60).

IRIS in a TB patient may present as prolonged, high grade fever or the reappearance of fever, worsening pulmonary infiltrates, new pleural effusions, or increased or new lymphadenopathy (61). Many patients initially treated for pulmonary TB develop additional manifestations of IRIS at extrapulmonary sites (59). Hepatomegaly, lymphadenopathy [mediastinal, cervical, or abdominal], splenic abscesses, terminal ileitis leading to perforation, arthropathy, and cutaneous lesions may be manifestations of TB-IRIS, with or without exacerbation of existing TB disease (57,59,62). Neurological disease following initiation of ART may have a poor outcome (63).

Most cases of TB-IRIS are self-limiting (59), and may require no change or only minor changes in treatment. Mild cases may just require symptomatic management with non-steroidal anti-inflammatory drugs [NSAIDs]. Moderate to severe cases usually respond to corticosteroids, and occasionally interruption of ART may be needed. Rarely, needle aspiration, surgical drainage, or laparotomy may be required for severe manifestations.

Human Immunodeficiency Virus and Multidrug Resistant-Tuberculosis

Human immunodeficiency virus *per se* does not predispose a person to development of multidrug-resistant TB [MDR-TB] (64,65). However, several factors during co-treatment of HIV-TB like poor drug absorption, pill burden and overlapping toxicities leading to poor compliance, drug interactions leading to sub-therapeutic drug levels, etc. may lead to emergence of drug resistance to anti-TB drugs as well as resistance to ARVs. Second line anti-TB drugs are with more toxic and often difficult to tolerate. Combining it with ARV makes it even more difficult. Treatment of MDR-TB and HIV together is challenging and often with poor outcomes.

HIV/TB COLLABORATIVE ACTIVITIES

Considering the evidence that TB and HIV duo form the deadly synergy and the co-infected patients with these diseases more often have unfavourable treatment outcomes, WHO in 2012 released a policy document on collaborative

HIV-TB activities which outlined broad activities in the policy. The major collaborative activities recommended by WHO are listed in Table 35.12 (66,67). India has been implementing HIV/TB collaborative activities since 2001 in increasing the universal access to prevention, early diagnosis, and treatment services in combating the threat of HIV/TB. In 2008-2009, NACO and CTD jointly developed a National Framework for HIV/TB collaborative activities to address the two intersecting epidemics. The framework called "Intensified TB-HIV package" emphasised increased HIV testing of TB patients, TB screening for PLHIV and prompt treatment for persons affected with HIV/TB.

To further strengthen the HIV/TB collaborative activities in the country during 2012-2017, the 'National Framework for Joint HIV/TB Collaborative Activities' was revised in November, 2013, based on updated WHO HIV/TB policy recommendations and vision documents of both the National Programmes, NACP-IV and RNTCP National Strategic Plan (68). This document is a guidance tool for policy

Table 35.12: WHO-recommended collaborative TB/HIV activities
Establish and strengthen the mechanisms for delivering integrated TB and HIV services
Set up and strengthen a coordinating body for collaborative TB/HIV activities functional at all levels
Determine HIV prevalence among TB patients and TB prevalence among people living with HIV
Carry out joint TB/HIV planning to integrate the delivery of TB and HIV services
Monitor and evaluate collaborative TB/HIV activities
Reduce the burden the TB in people living with HIV and initiate early antiretroviral therapy [the Three I's for HIV/TB]
Intensify TB case-finding and ensure high quality antituberculosis treatment
Initiate TB prevention with isoniazid preventive therapy and early antiretroviral therapy
Ensure control of TB infection in health-care facilities and congregate settings.
Reduce the burden of HIV in patients with presumptive and diagnosed TB
Provide HIV testing and counselling to patients with presumptive and diagnosed TB
Provide HIV prevention interventions for patients with presumptive and diagnosed TB
Provide co-trimoxazole preventive therapy for TB patients living with HIV
Ensure HIV prevention interventions, treatment and care for TB patients living with HIV
Provide antiretroviral therapy for TB patients living with HIV
WHO = World Health Organization; TB = tuberculosis; HIV = human immunodeficiency virus *Source: references 66,67*

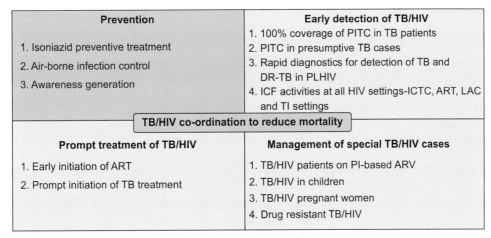

Prevention	Early detection of TB/HIV
1. Isoniazid preventive treatment 2. Air-borne infection control 3. Awareness generation	1. 100% coverage of PITC in TB patients 2. PITC in presumptive TB cases 3. Rapid diagnostics for detection of TB and DR-TB in PLHIV 4. ICF activities at all HIV settings-ICTC, ART, LAC and TI settings

TB/HIV co-ordination to reduce mortality

Prompt treatment of TB/HIV	Management of special TB/HIV cases
1. Early initiation of ART 2. Prompt initiation of TB treatment	1. TB/HIV patients on PI-based ARV 2. TB/HIV in children 3. TB/HIV pregnant women 4. Drug resistant TB/HIV

Figure 35.6: Framework of TB/HIV co-ordination activities in India to reduce mortality
TB = tuberculosis; HIV = human immunodeficiency virus; PITC = provider initiated testing and counselling; ART = anti-retroviral therapy; DR-TB = drug-resistant TB; ICTC = Integrated Counselling and Testing Centres; PLHIV = people living with HIV; PI = protease inhibitor; ICF = intensified case-finding; LAC = Link ART Centre; TI = treatment initiation
Source: reference 7

makers, programme managers, professionals at health facilities, health-care workers and partners.

The joint framework was developed to maintain close coordination between RNTCP and NACP at national, state and district levels, to decrease morbidity and mortality due to TB among persons living with HIV/AIDS, to decrease impact of HIV in TB patients and provide access to HIV-related care and support to HIV-infected TB patients, and to significantly reduce morbidity and mortality due to HIV-TB through prevention, early detection and prompt management of HIV and TB together. A four pronged strategy for strong collaboration between NACP and RNTCP has been formulated in the revised framework [Figure 35.6] (7).

National AIDS Control Programme—Revised National TB Control Programme Coordination Mechanisms at Various Levels

A National TB-HIV Coordination Committee [NTCC] has been constituted at the national level headed by the administrative heads from both the programmes. The National Technical Working Group [NTWG] comprising of key officials from NACO, CTD and other stakeholders, helps in identifying bottlenecks in policy, programme design and service delivery, explore solutions to address the bottlenecks and provides oversight for joint implementation of activities. Similarly at the state and district levels, state level coordination committees [SCC], state technical working group [SWG] and district level coordination [DCC] committees are in place to ensure smooth implementation and regular review of TB-HIV collaborative activities. There are well laid defined terms of references and meeting schedules for all these groups and joint field visits by RNTCP and NACO staff are conducted regularly for looking into implementation of collaborative activities in the facilities.

SERVICE DELIVERY

National AIDS Control Programme—Revised National TB Control Programme Coordination Activities

A 'four pronged strategy' has been formulated to ensure strong collaboration and good coordination between NACP and RNTCP. It involves early detection of TB/HIV, prevention, prompt treatment, and management of special TB/HIV cases. The Three I's used under this strategy for prevention of TB/HIV include: [i] intensified case finding [ICF]; [ii] isoniazid preventive therapy [IPT]; and [iii] infection control activities [IC].

The programme has formulated four important strategies to ensure early diagnosis of HIV and TB at all service delivery sites, namely [i] provider initiated testing and counselling [PITC] in TB patients; [ii] PITC in presumptive TB cases; [iii] rapid diagnostics for detection of TB and DR-TB in PLHIV; and [iv] ICF activities at all HIV settings, namely, Integrated Counselling and Testing Centre [ICTC], ART, Link ART Centre [LAC] settings.

Human Immunodeficiency Virus Testing of Tuberculosis Patients

PITC for HIV among TB patients is implemented across the country as a part of the intensified HIV/TB package so as to ensure early detection of HIV and linkage to care and support. HIV testing of TB patients is presently done at integrated counselling and testing centres [ICTC] which many a times leads to referral loss. It is planned that all designated microscopy centres [DMC] conducting quality assured sputum microscopy, will have a co-located HIV testing facility to minimise linkage loss. At present there are more than 13,500 DMCs of which out more than 7,500 have co-located HIV/TB testing.

Under ICF, all ICTC clients are screened by ICTC counsellors for presence of four TB symptom score [current cough, weight loss, fever, nigh sweats] at every encounter [pre-, post-, or follow-up counselling]. Further, that all patients coming to ART centres are actively screened for opportunistic infections [OIs], particularly TB. The presumptive TB cases identified at ART centres are prioritised and "fast-tracked" for evaluation by Senior Medical Officer/Medical Officer to minimise opportunities for airborne transmission of infection to other PLHIV. All TB co-infected PLHIV are initiated on ART irrespective of CD4+ count (67).

Innovative Intensified Tuberculosis Case Finding and Appropriate Treatment at High Burden Antiretroviral Treatment Centres in India

There exists a gap in early identification, screening and referral of TB among PLHIV, resulting in delayed diagnosis of TB and poor outcomes of subsequent treatment. Considering the challenges, there is a felt need to implement the comprehensive strategy to reduce the burden of TB among PLHIV. With support from WCO-India, NACO-CTD have jointly launched "Innovative, intensified TB case finding and appropriate treatment at selected 30 high burden ART centres in India" in March 2015, aimed at reducing the burden of TB among PLHIV.

The key features of this project are single window service delivery to HIV-seropositive individuals through provision of TB services at ART centres which include [i] intensified TB case finding by deployment of rapid molecular diagnostics [CBNAAT]; [ii] daily anti-TB treatment; [iii] identification and management of side

effects of drugs through pharmacovigilance programme of India [PvPI]; [iv] treatment adherence support to patient including support through use of ICT; [v] provision of IPT to HIV- infected individuals; and [vi] minimisation of risk of acquiring TB in HIV-seropositive individuals through implementation of airborne infection control measures at these ART centres.

There is the risk of transmission of TB in health care facilities including laboratories. Early diagnosis and immediate initiation and adherence to RNTCP treatment regimens will make infectious TB patients rapidly non-infectious and breaks the chain of transmission. Ensuring various administrative, environmental and personal protective measures as recommended in the airborne infection control guidelines is crucial in reducing the risk of transmission of TB at HIV-TB care settings. The assessment of these centres has been completed recently and these activities will soon be expended to all ART centres across the country.

Achievements under Human Immunodeficiency Virus/Tuberculosis Collaborative Activities in India

The NACO and RNTCP have been successful in increasing access and uptake of HIV testing and counselling for all TB patients. The trend of known HIV status among TB patients is increasing and in 2015, 78% of TB patients knew their HIV status [Figure 35.7]. The linkage of TB HIV co-infected patients to CPT and ART is showing increasing trend in India; 95% of co-infected patients received CPT in 2015 [Figure 35.8] and 31% of co-infected patients received ART in 2014 [Figure 35.9]. All these achievements have higher averages in India compared to global achievement on each indicator.

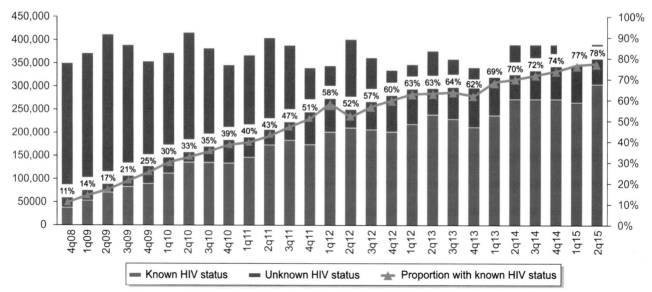

Figure 35.7: Trends in Number [%] of registered TB patients with known HIV status, 4q08- 2q15
TB = tuberculosis; HIV = human immunodeficiency virus; q = quarter
Source: Data from Basic Services Division, National AIDS Control Organisation

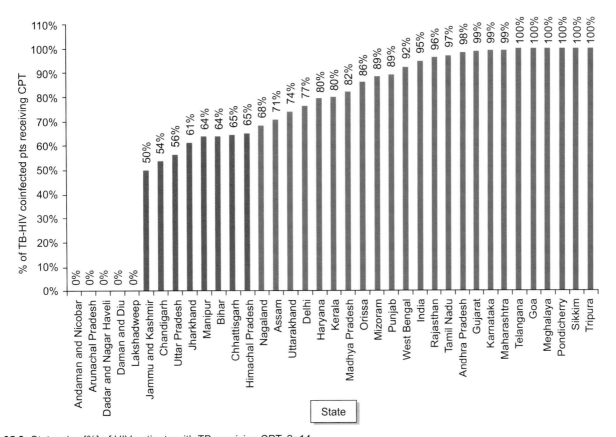

Figure 35.8: State-wise [%] of HIV patients with TB receiving CPT, 2q14
TB = tuberculosis; HIV = human immunodeficiency virus; CPT = co-trimoxazole preventive therapy; q = quarter; pts = patients
Source: Data from Basic Services Division, National AIDS Control Organisation

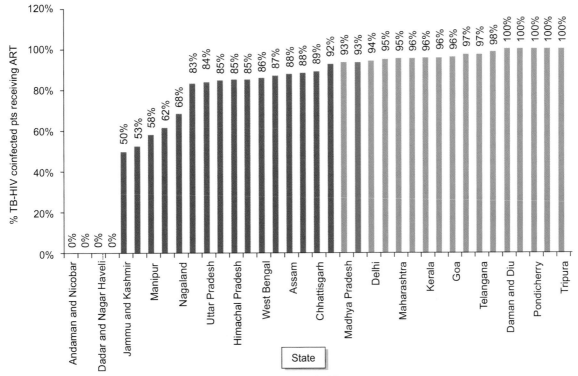

Figure 35.9: State-wise status of ART in TB-HIV co-infected patients reg. in 2q14
TB = tuberculosis; HIV = human immunodeficiency virus; ART = anti-retroviral therapy; reg. = registered in; q = quarter; pts = patients
Source: Data from Basic Services Division, National AIDS Control Organisation

The concentred efforts of Government of India have yielded results in the form of achievement of millennium development goal [MDG] 6, moving in direction of achieving high-level meeting [HLM] target 5 of UN General Assembly special session on HIV [UNGASS 2011] pertaining to reduction in TB deaths among persons living with HIV. As we move into post 2015 agenda, the achievement of Sustainable Development Goal 3 [SDG 3] pertaining to health will be on top priority of Government and HIV and TB programmes are going to be big contributor to achieving this goal. These activities will be further expanded and strengthened as India has received a specific grant now from Global Fund for HIV-TB collaborative activities.

Effective prevention strategies, early detection of HIV and TB by using newer methodologies, and prompt management of HIV and TB infections through well-coordinated efforts within RNTCP and NACP will ensure a sustainable long-term success in dealing with these dual infections.

The World Health Assembly [WHA] in May 2014 has adopted an END TB strategy with ambitious targets. The strategy aims to end the global TB epidemic, with targets to reduce TB deaths by 95% and to cut new cases by 90% between 2015 and 2035, and to ensure that no family is burdened with catastrophic expenses due to TB. In order to achieve the global End TB strategy and end AIDS epidemic as a public health threat by 2030, India needs to further enhance its HIV-TB collaborative activities.

REFERENCES

1. National AIDS Control Organization. Guidelines for prevention and management of common opportunistic infections/malignancies among HIV-infected adults and adolescents. New Delhi: National AIDS Control Organization, Ministry of Health and Family Welfare, Government of India; 2013.
2. World Health Organization. Global Tuberculosis Report 2018. Geneva: World Health Organization; 2018.
3. Sharma SK, Mohan A. Tuberculosis: From an incurable scourge to a curable disease - journey over a millennium. Indian J Med Res 2013;137:455-93.
4. Agarwal U, Kumar A, Behera D. Profile of HIV associated tuberculosis at a tertiary institute in setting of free anti-retroviral therapy. J Assoc Physicians India 2009;57:685-90.
5. Lawn SD, Churchyard G. Epidemiology of HIV-associated tuberculosis. Curr Opin HIV AIDS 2009;4:325-33.
6. WHO Country Office for India, Central TB Division. Standards for TB care in India. New Delhi: WHO Country Office for India & Central TB Division, Ministry of Health and Family Welfare, Government of India; 2014.
7. National AIDS Control Organization. Anti-retroviral therapy guidelines for HIV infected adult and adolescents including post exposure prophylaxis. New Delhi: National AIDS Control Organization, Ministry of Health and Family Welfare, Government of India; 2013.
8. Harries AD, Zachariah R, Corbett EL, Lawn SD, Santos-Filho ET, Chimzizi R, et al. The HIV-associated tuberculosis epidemic—when will we act? Lancet 2010;375:1906-19.
9. Lawn SD, Kranzer K, Wood R. Antiretroviral therapy for control of the HIV-associated tuberculosis epidemic in resource-limited settings. Clin Chest Med 2009;30:685-99.
10. Harries AD, Zachariah R, Lawn SD. Providing HIV care for co-infected tuberculosis patients: a perspective from sub-Saharan Africa. Int J Tuberc Lung Dis 2009;13:6-16.
11. International statistical classification of diseases and related health problems, 10th revision [ICD-10]. Second edition. Geneva: World Health Organization; 2007.
12. Ministry of Health and Family Welfare, Government of India. India HIV Estimations 2015. Technical report. New Delhi: Ministry of Health and Family Welfare. Government of India; 2015.
13. National AIDS Control Organization. Annual Report 2013-14. New Delhi: National AIDS Control Organization, Department of AIDS Control, Ministry of Health & Family Welfare. Government of India.
14. Central TB Division. RNTCP Annual Status Report 2016. New Delhi: Central TB Division, Ministry of Health & Family Welfare, Government of India; 2016.
15. Wolday D, Hailu B, Girma M, Hailu E, Sanders E, Fontanet AL. Low CD41 T-cell count and high HIV viral load precede the development of tuberculosis disease in a cohort of HIV positive Ethiopians. Int J Tuberc Lung Dis 2003;7:110-6.
16. Morris L, Martin DJ, Bredell H, Nyoka SN, Sacks L, Pendle S, et al. Human immunodeficiency virus-1 RNA levels and CD4 lymphocyte counts, during treatment for active tuberculosis, in South African patients. J Infect Dis 2003;187:1967-71.
17. Toossi Z. Virological and immunological impact of tuberculosis on human immunodeficiency virus type 1 disease. J Infect Dis 2003;188:1146-55.
18. Whalen CC, Nsubuga P, Okwera A, Johnson JL, Hom DL, Michael NL, et al. Impact of pulmonary tuberculosis on survival of HIV-infected adults: a prospective epidemiologic study in Uganda. AIDS 2000;14:1219-28.
19. Badri M, Ehrlich R, Wood R, Pulerwitz T, Maartens G. Association between tuberculosis and HIV disease progression in a high tuberculosis prevalence area. Int J Tuberc Lung Dis 2001;5:225-32.
20. Hoshino Y, Tse DB, Rochford G, Prabhakar S, Hoshino S, Chitkara N, et al. Mycobacterium tuberculosis-induced CXCR4 and chemokine expression leads to preferential X4 HIV-1 replication in human macrophages. J Immunol 2004;172:6251-8.
21. Wolday D, Tegbaru B, Kassu A, Messele T, Coutinho R, van Baarle D, et al. Expression of chemokine receptors CCR5 and CXCR4 on CD4+ T cells and plasma chemokine levels during treatment of active tuberculosis in HIV-1-coinfected patients. J Acquir Immune Defic Syndr 2005;39:265-71.
22. Sharma SK, Mohan A, Kadhiravan T. HIV-TB co-infection: epidemiology, diagnosis and management. Indian J Med Res 2005;121:550-67.
23. Havlir DV, Barnes PF. Tuberculosis in patients with human immunodeficiency virus infection. N Engl J Med 1999;340:367-73.
24. Sharma SK, Kohli M, Yadav RN, Chaubey J, Bhasin D, Sreenivas V, et al. Evaluating the diagnostic accuracy of Xpert MTB/RIF assay in pulmonary tuberculosis. PLoS One 2015;10:e0141011.
25. Sharma SK, Kohli M, Chaubey J, Yadav RN, Sharma R, Singh BK, et al. Evaluation of Xpert MTB/RIF assay performance in diagnosing extrapulmonary tuberculosis among adults in a tertiary care centre in India. Eur Respir J 2014;44:1090-3.
26. Raizada N, Sachdeva KS, Nair SA, Kulsange S, Gupta RS, Thakur R, et al. Enhancing TB case detection: experience in offering upfront Xpert MTB/RIF testing to pediatric presumptive TB and DR TB cases for early rapid diagnosis of drug sensitive and drug resistant TB. PLoS One 2014;9:e105346.
27. World Health Organization. WHO case definitions of HIV for surveillance and revised clinical staging and immunological classification of HIV-related disease in adults and children. Geneva: World Health Organization; 2007.

28. Corbett EL, Watt CJ, Walker N, Maher D, Williams BG, Raviglione MC, et al. The growing burden of tuberculosis: global trends and interactions with the HIV epidemic. Arch Intern Med 2003;163: 1009-21.

29. Vashishtha R, Mohan K, Singh B, Devarapu SK, Sreenivas V, Ranjan S, et al. Efficacy and safety of thrice weekly DOTS in tuberculosis patients with and without HIV co-infection: an observational study. BMC Infect Dis 2013;13:468.

30. De Cock KM, Chaisson RE. Will DOTS do it? A reappraisal of tuberculosis control in countries with high rates of HIV infection. Int J Tuberc Lung Dis 1999;3:457-65.

31. Badri M, Wilson D, Wood R. Effect of highly active antiretroviral therapy on incidence on tuberculosis in South Africa: a cohort study. Lancet 2002;359:2059-64.

32. Santoro-Lopes G, Felix de Pinho AM, Harrison LH, Schechter M. Reduced risk of tuberculosis among Brazilian patients with advanced human immunodeficiency virus infection treated with highly active antiretroviral therapy. Clin Infect Dis 2002;34: 543-6.

33. García de Olalla P, Martínez-González MA, Caylà JA, Jansà JM, Iglesias B, Guerrero R, et al. Influence of highly active anti-retroviral therapy [HAART] on the natural history of extra-pulmonary tuberculosis in HIV patients. Int J Tuberc Lung Dis 2002;6:1051-7.

34. Lawn SD, Torok ME, Wood R. Optimum time to start antiretroviral therapy during HIV-associated opportunistic infections. Curr Opin Infect Dis 2011;24:34-42.

35. Lawn SD, Wood R. Optimum time to initiate antiretroviral therapy in patients with HIV-associated tuberculosis: there may be more than one right answer. J Acquir Immune Defic Syndr 2007;46:121-3.

36. Manosuthi W, Chottanapand S, Thongyen S, Chaovavanich A, Sungkanuparph S. Survival rate and risk factors of mortality among HIV/tuberculosis-coinfected patients with and without antiretroviral therapy. J Acquir Immune Defic Syndr 2006;43: 42-6.

37. Velasco M, Castilla V, Sanz J, Gaspar G, Condes E, Barros C, et al. Effect of simultaneous use of highly active antiretroviral therapy on survival of HIV patients with tuberculosis. J Acquir Immune Defic Syndr 2009;50:148-52.

38. Blanc FX, Sok T, Laureillard D, Borand L, Rekacewicz C, Nerrienet E, et al. Earlier versus later start of antiretroviral therapy in HIV-infected adults with tuberculosis. N Engl J Med 2011;365:1471-81.

39. Abdool Karim SS, Naidoo K, Grobler A, Padayatchi N, Baxter C, Gray A, et al. Timing of initiation of antiretroviral drugs during tuberculosis therapy. N Engl J Med 2010;362:697-706.

40. World Health Organization. Consolidated guidelines on the use of antiretroviral drugs for treating and preventing HIV infection: recommendations for a public health approach. Second edition. Geneva: World Health Organization; 2016.

41. World Health Organization. Antiretroviral therapy for HIV infection in adults and adolescents. Recommendations for a publc health approach [2010 revision]. Geneva: Switzerland: World Health Organization; 2010.

42. World Health Organization. Global tuberculosis report 2015. Geneva: World Health Organization; 2015.

43. Ford N, Mofenson L, Shubber Z, Calmy A, Andrieux-Meyer I, Victoria M, et al. Safety of efavirenz in the first trimester of pregnancy: an updated systematic review and meta-analysis. AIDS 2014;28: S123-31.

44. d'Arminio Monforte A, Lepri AC, Rezza G, Pezzotti P, Antinori A, Phillips AN, et al. Insights into the reasons for discontinuation of first highly active antiretroviral therapy [HAART] regimen in a cohort of antiretroviral naïve patients. AIDS 2000;14:499-507.

45. Kwara A, Flanigan TP, Carter EJ. Highly active antiretroviral therapy [HAART] in adults with tuberculosis: current status. Int J Tuberc Lung Dis 2005;9:248-57.

46. Kolars JC, Schmiedlin-Ren P, Schuetz JD, Fang C, Watkins PB. Identification of rifampin-inducible P450IIIA4 [CYP3A4] in human small bowel enterocytes. J Clin Invest 1992;90:1871-8.

47. Burman WJ, Jones BE. Treatment of HIV-related tuberculosis in the era of effective antiretroviral therapy. Am J Respir Crit Care Med 2001;164:7-12.

48. Kim RB, Fromm MF, Wandel C, Leake B, Wood AJ, Roden DM, et al. The drug transporter Pglycoprotein limits oral absorption and brain entry of HIV-1 protease inhibitors. J Clin Invest 1998;101:289-94.

49. Schuetz EG, Schinkel AH, Relling MV, Schuetz JD. P-glycoprotein: a major determinant of rifampicin–inducible expression of cytochrome P4503A in mice and humans. Proc Natl Acad Sci 1996;93:4001-5.

50. López-Cortés LF, Ruiz-Valderas R, Viciana P, Alarcón-González A, Gómez-Mateos J, León-Jimenez. Pharmacokinetic interactions between efavirenz and rifampin in HIV. HIV-infected patients with tuberculosis. Clin Pharmacokinet 2002;41:681-90.

51. Ribera E, Pou L, Lopez RM, Crespo M, Falco V, Ocaña I, et al. Pharmacokinetic interaction between nevirapine and rifampicin in HIV-infected patients with tuberculosis. AIDS 2001;28:450-3.

52. Oliva J, Moreno S, Sanz J, Ribera E, Molina JA, Rubio R, et al. Co-administration of rifampin and nevirapine in HIV-infected patients with tuberculosis. AIDS 2003;17:637-8.

53. Centers for Disease Control and Prevention. Updated guidelines for the use of rifamycins for the treatment of tuberculosis among HIV-infected patients taking protease inhibitors or nonnucleoside reverse transcriptase inhibitors. Atlanta: Centers for Disease Control; 2004.

54. Sharma SK, Soneja M. HIV & immune reconstitution inflammatory syndrome [IRIS]. Indian J Med Res 2011;134:866-77.

55. French MA, Lenzo N, John M, Mallal SA, McKinnon EJ, James IR, et al. Immune restoration disease after the treatment of immuno-deficient HIV-infected patients with highly active antiretroviral therapy. HIV Med 2000;1:107-15.

56. Breen RA, Smith CJ, Bettinson SH, Dart B, Bannister MA, Johnson, et al. Paradoxical reactions during tuberculosis treatment in patients with and without HIV co-infection. Thorax 2004;59: 704-7.

57. Breton G, Duval X, Estellat C, Poaletti X, Bonnet D, Mvondo D, et al. Determinants of immune reconstitution inflammatory syndrome in HIV type 1-infected patients with tuberculosis after initiation of antiretroviral therapy. Clin. Infect Dis 2004;39: 1709-12.

58. Kumarasamy N, Chaguturu S, Mayer KH, Solomon S, Yepthomi HT, Balakrishnan P, et al. Incidence of immune reconstitution syndrome in HIV/tuberculosis-coinfected patients after initiation of generic antiretroviral therapy in India. J. Acquir. Immune Defic Syndr 2004;37:1574-6.

59. Lawn SD, Myer L, Bekker LG, Wood RG. Tuberculosis associated immune reconstitution disease: incidence, risk factors and impact in an antiretroviral treatment service in South Africa. AIDS 2007;21:335-41.

60. Burman W, Weis A, Vernon A, Khan A, Benator D, Jones B, et al. Frequency, severity and duration of immune reconstitution events in HIV-related tuberculosis. Int J Tuberc Lung Dis 2007;11:1282-9.

61. Karmakar S, Sharma SK, Vashishtha R, Sharma A, Ranjan S, Gupta D, et al. Clinical characteristics of tuberculosis-associated immune reconstitution inflammatory syndrome in North Indian

population of HIV/AIDS patients receiving HAART. Clin Dev Immunol 2011;2011:239021.

62. Narita M, Ashkin D, Hollender ES, Pitchenik AE. Paradoxical worsening of tuberculosis following antiretroviral therapy in patients with AIDS. Am J Respir Crit Care Med 1998;158:157-61.

63. Meintjes G, Lawn SD, Scano G, Maartens F, French MA, Worodria W, et al. International Network for the Study of HIV-associated IRIS. Tuberculosis-associated immune reconstitution inflammatory syndrome: case definitions for use in resource-limited settings. Lancet Infect Dis 2008;8:516-23.

64. Asch S, Knowles L, Rai A, Jones BE, Pogoda J, Barnes PF. Relationship of isoniazid resistance to human immunodeficiency virus infection in patients with tuberculosis. Am J Respir Crit Care Med 1996;153:1708-10.

65. Spellman CW, Matty KJ, Weis SE. A survey of drug-resistant Mycobacterium tuberculosis and its relationship to HIV infection. AIDS 1998;12:191-5.

66. World Health Organization. WHO policy on collaborative TB/HIV activities: guidelines for national programmes and other stakeholders. Geneva: World Health Organization; 2012.

67. Central TB Division & Department of AIDS Control, Ministry of Health and Family Welfare, Government of India. National Framework for Joint HIV-TB Collaborative Activities. November 2013.

68. National AIDS Control Organization. Guidelines on prevention and management of TB in PLHIV at ART centres. December 2016. New Delhi: National AIDS Control Organization. Ministry of Health and Family Welfare, Government of India.

36

Tuberculosis in Children

SK Kabra, Rakesh Lodha

INTRODUCTION

Tuberculosis [TB] is one of the major infections affecting children worldwide. It causes significant morbidity and mortality, especially in infants and young children as TB infection can progress rapidly to the disease, particularly in this group. TB in children reflects the prevalence of the disease in adults as well as current transmission rates. Developing countries in Africa and South-east Asia have the largest number of TB cases and the situation there has been worsened by the human immunodeficiency virus [HIV] epidemic. Children born to HIV-infected parents, whether infected or not, are at high risk of developing TB because of the increased risk of exposure to the disease. TB is more common among the disadvantaged and vulnerable groups in each society and the impact of overcrowding, undernutrition and poverty is particularly severe on children. *Mycobacterium tuberculosis* [*Mtb*] infects millions of children worldwide every year, yet accurate information on the extent and distribution of the disease in children is not available for most of the world. In a recent meta-analysis (1), it was observed that without adequate treatment, children with TB, especially those under five years of age, are at high risk of death. HIV-coinfected children have an increased risk of mortality even when receiving anti-TB treatment (1).

EPIDEMIOLOGY

Since most children acquire the organism from adults in their surroundings, the epidemiology of childhood TB follows that in adults. The burden of childhood TB in the world is unclear. This is because of the difficulty of confirming the diagnosis of childhood TB. The other important reason is that children do not make a significant contribution to the spread of TB. Several estimates make use of an arbitrary calculation assigning 10% of the TB burden to children (2). Available data linking the incidence of TB to the proportion of the TB caseload represented by children suggest an exponential rise in the proportion of the TB caseload caused by children. With rise in the incidence of TB; children may constitute nearly 40% of the caseload in certain high incidence communities (3).

TB infection and disease among children are much more prevalent in developing countries, where resources for control are scarce (4). It is estimated that in developing countries the annual risk of TB infection in children is 2%-5%. The estimated lifetime risk of developing TB disease for a young child infected with *Mtb* as indicated by positive tuberculin test is about 10% (5). About 5% of those infected are likely to develop disease in the first year after infection and another 5% in rest of their lifetime. These rates increase in HIV-infected individuals. Nearly 8%-20% of the deaths caused by TB occur in children (6). The age of the child at acquisition of TB infection has a great effect on the occurrence of TB disease. Approximately, 40% of infected children less than 1 year of age, if left untreated, develop radiologically significant lymphadenopathy or segmental lesions compared with 24% of children between 1-10 years and 16% of children 11-15 years of age (7). As per the Global TB Report, 2017 (8), in the year 2016, 6.9% of the 10.4 million estimated new TB cases were among children.

TRANSMISSION

Transmission of *Mtb* generally is person-to-person and occurs via inhalation of mucous droplets that become airborne when an individual with pulmonary or laryngeal TB coughs, sneezes, speaks, laughs, or sings. After drying, the droplet nuclei can remain suspended in the air for hours. Only small droplets [<5 µ in diameter] can reach alveoli. Droplet nuclei also can be produced by aerosol treatments, by sputum induction, and through manipulation of lesions.

Numerous factors are associated with the risk of acquiring *Mtb* infection (9). The risk has been associated consistently with the extent of contact with the index case, the burden of organisms in the sputum, and the frequency of cough in the index case. Patients with smear-positive pulmonary TB are more likely to transmit infection. Markers of close contact such as urban living, overcrowding, and lower socioeconomic status all are correlated with the acquisition of infection. An increased risk-developing infection has been demonstrated in multiple institutional settings, including nursing homes, correctional institutions, and homeless shelters. The risk of acquiring infection increases with age from infancy to early adulthood, likely attributable to increasing contact with other persons.

NATURAL HISTORY

The natural history of TB infection is covered in detail in the chapter *"Pulmonary tuberculosis" [Chapter 10]*. Progressive primary disease is a serious complication of the pulmonary primary complex [PPC], in which the PPC instead of resolving or calcifying, enlarges steadily and develops a large caseous center. The center then liquefies; this may empty into an adjacent bronchus leading to formation of a cavity with a large numbers of tubercle bacilli (10). From this stage, the bacilli may spread to other parts of the lobe or the entire lung. This may lead to consolidation of area of lung or bronchopneumonia. Cavitary disease is relatively uncommon in children. It may be difficult to differentiate progressive primary disease from a simple TB focus with superimposed acute bacterial pneumonia. Appearance of a segmental lesion is fan shaped on a roentgenogram, representing mainly atelectasis and almost always involves that very segment occupied by the primary pulmonary focus (11,12).

Some of the events may occur because of involvement of lymph nodes (13,14). The enlarged lymph nodes may compress the neighbouring airway (15,16). Ball-valve effect due to incomplete obstruction may lead to trapping of air distal to obstruction [emphysema] (17,18). Enlarged paratracheal nodes may cause stridor and respiratory distress. Subcarinal nodes may impinge on the esophagus and may cause dysphagia. If the obstruction of bronchus is complete, atelectasis occurs.

Outcome of Bronchial Obstruction

Bronchial obstruction may resolve in several ways, including: [i] complete expansion and resolution of the chest radiograph findings; [ii] disappearance of the segmental lesions; and [iii] scarring and progressive compression of the lobe or segment leading to bronchiectasis. A caseous lymph node may erode through the wall of the bronchus, leading to TB bronchitis or endobronchial TB. Fibrosis and bronchiectatic changes may supervene. Discharge of *Mtb* into the lumen may lead to bronchial dissemination of infection.

Haematogenous disemination of *Mtb* occurs early in the course of the disease; this results when the bacilli find their way into blood stream through lymph nodes. This may result in foci of infection in various organs. If the host immune system is good, then these foci are contained and disease does not occur. Seeding of apex of lungs leads to development of *Simon's focus*. Lowering of host immunity may lead to activation of these metastatic foci and development of disease. This is especially seen in young infants, severely malnourished children, and children with immunodeficiency [including HIV infection]. Massive seeding of blood stream with *Mtb* leads to miliary TB, where all lesions are of similar size. This usually occurs within three to six months after initial infection.

Pulmonary TB resulting from endogenous reactivation of foci of infection is uncommon in children; but may be seen in adolescents. The most common site for this type of disease is the apex of the lung [*Puhl's lesion*], because the blood flow is sluggish at apex. Regional lymph nodes are usually not involved in this type of TB (19).

CLINICAL FEATURES

Childhood TB can be divided into two broad classifications: intra- and extrathoracic TB. Most children with TB will develop pulmonary TB. Nonetheless, the recognition of extrathoracic TB is equally important because of its great potential for causing morbidity.

Intrathoracic Tuberculosis

Diagnosis of TB in a child is often difficult because of absence of typical symptoms, signs and of microbiologic evidence in the majority of children with pulmonary TB. The onset of symptoms is generally insidious, but may be relatively acute in miliary TB.

Primary infection usually passes off unrecognized. Asymptomatic infection is defined as infection associated with tuberculin hypersensitivity and a positive tuberculin skin test [TST] but with no striking clinical or radiographic manifestations. Most symptoms in children with primary complex are constitutional in the form of mild fever, anorexia, weight loss, decreased activity. Cough is an inconsistent symptom and may be absent even in advanced disease. Irritating dry cough can be a symptom of bronchial and tracheal compression due to enlarged lymph nodes. In some children, the lymph nodes continue to enlarge even after resolutions of parenachymal infiltrate (20,21). This may lead to compression of neighbouring regional bronchus. The PPC is the most commonly encountered presentation in the outpatient setting. In a community setting, often primary infection occurs without sufficient constitutional symptoms to warrant medical advice. The PPC may be picked up accidentally during evaluation of intercurrent infections (22).

Progressive primary disease is the result of progression of primary disease. Children with progressive primary disease may present with high-grade fever and cough. Expectoration of sputum and haemoptysis are usually associated with advanced disease and development of cavity or ulceration of the bronchus. Physical findings of consolidation or cavitation depend on the extent of the disease. Abnormal chest signs consist mainly of dullness, decreased air entry, and crepitations. Cavitating pulmonary TB is uncommon in children. However, Maniar (23) reported a series of 75 children, less than two years of age presenting with primary cavitatory pulmonary TB suggesting variability of clinical presentation of TB in different setting.

Children with endobronchial TB may present with fever, troublesome cough [with or without expectoration]. Dyspnoea, wheezing and cyanosis may be present. Occasionally, the child may be misdiagnosed as asthma. In a wheezing child less than two years of age, the possibility of endobronchial TB should always be considered, especially if there is poor response to asthma medications. Partial compression of the airway can lead to emphysema. Features of collapse may be present if a large airway is completely compressed (21,22).

Miliary TB is an illness characterised by heavy haematogenous spread and progressive development of innumerable small foci throughout the body. The disease is most common in infants and young children. The onset of illness is often sudden. The clinical manifestations depend on the numbers of disseminated organisms and the involved organs. The child may have high-grade fever, which is quite unlike in other forms of TB. The child may also have dyspnoea and cyanosis. There are hardly any pulmonary findings but fine crepitations and rhonchi may be present. These findings may occasionally be confused with other acute respiratory infections of childhood. The illness may be severe, with the child having high fever, rigors and alteration of sensorium. In addition, these children may have lymphadenopathy and hepatosplenomegaly. The other presentation of miliary TB may be insidious with the child appearing unwell, febrile and losing weight. Choroid tubercles may be seen in about 50% children. TB meningitis may occur in 20%-30% of cases (21,22).

The rupture of a subpleural focus into the pleural cavity may result in pleural effusion. The pleura may also be involved by haematogenous spread from the primary focus. The effusion usually occurs due to hypersensitivity to tuberculoprotein[s]. If the sensitivity is high, there is significant pleural effusion along with fever and chest pain on affected side. Minor effusions associated with the rupture of primary foci are usually not detected. TB effusion is uncommon in children under five years of age, is more common in boys, and is rarely associated with segmental lesion and miliary TB (19). The onset may be insidious or acute with rise in temperature, cough, dyspnoea and pleuritic pain on the affected side. There is usually no expectoration. The pleuritic pain may disappear once the fluid separates the inflamed pleural surfaces; and a vague discomfort may then be felt. Increase in effusion may make breathing shallow and difficult. The clinical findings depend on the amount of fluid in the pleural sac. In early stages, a pleural rub may be present. Early signs include decreased chest wall movement, impairment of percussion note and diminished air entry on the affected side. As the fluid collection increases, the signs of pleural effusion become more definite.

In some instances, acute secondary bacterial infection occurs, presenting with high fever, cough and crepitations. The symptoms and signs respond partially to the conventional antibiotics, but the chest radiographic findings due to underlying TB persist. Calcification of the primary complex occurs more commonly in children.

Extrathoracic Tuberculosis

A detailed description of extrathoracic TB is beyond the scope of this chapter, but clinicians must consider this possibility when evaluating children with a history of persistent fevers. The most common forms of extrathoracic disease in children include TB of the peripheral lymph nodes and the central nervous system. Other rare forms of extrathoracic disease in children include osteoarticular, abdominal, gastrointestinal, genitourinary, cutaneous, and congenital disease.

TB of the peripheral lymph nodes involves the supra-clavicular, anterior cervical, tonsillar, and submandibular nodes. Although lymph nodes may become fixed to surrounding tissues, low-grade fever may be the only systemic symptom. A primary focus is visible radiologically only 30%-70% of the time. TST is usually positive. Although spontaneous resolution may occur, untreated lymphadenitis frequently progresses to caseating necrosis, capsular rupture, and spread to adjacent nodes and overlying skin, resulting in a draining sinus tract that may require surgical removal (24).

Central nervous system disease is the most serious complication of TB in children and arises from the formation of a caseous lesion in the cerebral cortex or meninges that results from early occult lymphohaematogenous spread. Infants and young children are more likely to experience a rapid progression to hydrocephalus, seizures, and cerebral oedema. In older children, signs and symptoms progress over the course of several weeks, beginning non-specifically with fever, headache, irritability, and drowsiness. Disease abruptly advances with symptoms of lethargy, vomiting, nuchal rigidity, seizures, hypertonia, and focal neurologic signs. The final stage of disease is marked by coma, hypertension, decerebrate and decorticate posturing, and eventually death. Rapid confirmation of tuberculous meningitis can be extremely difficult to establish because of the wide variability in cerebrospinal characteristics, negative TST in 40% of cases, and normal chest radiographs in 50% of cases. Because improved outcomes are associated with early treatment, empiric anti-TB therapy should be considered for any child with basilar meningitis and hydrocephalus or cranial nerve involvement that has no other apparent cause (25).

DIAGNOSIS

Laboratory Tests

The diagnostic tests for pulmonary TB can be broadly divided into two categories: [i] demonstration/isolation of Mtb or one of its components; and [ii] demonstration of host's response to exposure to Mtb.

Conventional Diagnostic Methods of Smear and Mycobacterial Culture

In children with suspected pulmonary TB, spontaneously expectorated or induced sputum, gastric aspirate, bronchoscopic secretions are subjected to smear examination, mycobacterial culture and molecular diagnostic testing.

Ziehl Neelsen [ZN] stain reveals acid-fast bacilli [AFB] if the number of *Mtb* is more than 10^4/mL of specimen (26). The best specimen for demonstration of AFB in children is the early morning gastric aspirate obtained by using a nasogastric tube before the child arises and peristalsis empties the stomach of the respiratory secretions swallowed overnight (27). The yield of *Mtb* on ZN stain is less than 20% and depends on extent of pulmonary disease and number of specimen tested (28). To avoid hospitalisation, an ambulatory gastric lavage specimen has been shown to yield good results. Children are asked to come on an empty stomach for six hours and nasogastric tube is inserted to aspirate the gastric contents for smear and culture examination. If gastric contents are less, gastric lavage may be done with 10-20 mL sterile saline. Samples obtained on two consecutive days may provide smear positivity between 5%-10% (29). Neutralisation of gastric aspirate by sodabicarb is not recommended as it does not improve yield and may cause contamination (30).

When adequate sputum specimen is not being produced, sputum induction is attempted. Three mL of hypertonic saline [3%] is nebulised after priming with salbutamol. Older children may directly cough out expectoration while in younger children and infants, nasopharyngeal secretions are secured by placing a small tube in nasopharynx and applying slow suction (29).

In childhood TB, the yield of gastric aspirate is superior to bronchoalveolar lavage [BAL] fluid in detecting AFB (27,31). Bronchoscopy would allow visualisation of the tracheobronchial tree and use of BAL fluid may improve the diagnostic yield over gastric aspirate by 17%-26%. Detection of external compression by lymph nodes and endobronchial spread may help in diagnosis of TB in children (32,33). Endobronchial ultrasound-guided sampling [EBUS] commonly used in adults, has also been shown to be useful in children with mediastinal nodes on imaging (34).

The yield of mycobacterial culture in gastric aspirate specimens varies from 30%-50% in children with TB (35,36). A higher yield [up to 70%] has been reported in infants and children with extensive disease (15). The long period required for isolation of *Mtb* by conventional culture techniques has led to the development of other techniques for culture such as BACTEC radiometric assay, Septichek AFB system, and mycobacterial growth indicator tube system [MGIT] (37-41).

Serodiagnostic Methods

Serodiagnostic methods have been banned and should not be used for diagnosis of TB in children.

Molecular Methods

Conventional polymerase chain reaction [PCR] is *not recommended* for diagnosis of TB in children (42). Cartridge-based nucleic acid amplification tests [CBNAAT] are a major advance in diagnosis of TB in adults. The sensitivity of the CBNAAT, Xpert MTB/RIF in identifying intrathoracic TB in children using two gastric aspirate specimens or induced sputum has been reported to be between 60% and 70% and specificity is more than 90% (43-45a,45b). The evidence-based recommendations regarding the use of Xpert MTB/RIF in the diagnosis of TB in children as described in the recently published World Health Organization [WHO] guidelines (46) are shown in Table 36.1. The recently published evidence-based guidelines for Extrapulmonary TB for India [INDEX-TB guidelines] (47) provide current evidence for use of Xpert MTB/RIF in the diagnosis of extrapulmonary TB.

For further details on the laboratory diagnostic methods, including those used for the diagnosis of latent TB infection, the reader is referred to the chapter *"Laboratory diagnosis"* [Chapter 8] for more details.

Imaging Studies

Primary TB is the most common form encountered in children. On the chest radiograph, the PPC manifests as

Table 36.1: Evidence-based recommendations for use of Xpert MTB/RIF for the diagnosis of TB in children	
Recommendation	*Evidence*

Xpert MTB/RIF should be used rather than conventional microscopy and culture as the initial diagnostic test
   in children suspected to have MDR-TB or HIV-associated TB
   in all children suspected of having TB
	Strong recommendation, very low quality of evidence
	Conditional recommendation acknowledging resource implications, very low quality of evidence

Xpert MTB/RIF may be used as a replacement test for usual practice [including conventional microscopy, culture, and/or histopathology] for testing of specific non-respiratory specimens [lymph nodes and other tissues] from children suspected to have EPTB	Conditional recommendation, very low quality of evidence
Xpert MTB/RIF should be used in preference to conventional microscopy and culture as the initial diagnostic test in testing CSF specimens from children suspected of having TBM	Strong recommendation given the urgency of rapid diagnosis, very low quality of evidence
TB = tuberculosis; MDR-TB = multidrug-resistant tuberculosis; HIV = human immunodeficiency virus; EPTB = extra-pulmonary tuberculosis; TBM = tuberculosis meningitis *Source: reference 46*	

an area of airspace consolidation of varying sizes, usually unifocal, and homogeneous [Figure 36.1]. Enlarged lymph nodes may be seen in the hilar, or right paratracheal region. Sometimes, lymphadenopathy alone may be present in children with primary TB.

Consolidation in progressive primary disease is usually heterogeneous, poorly marginated with predilection of involvement of apical or posterior segments of the upper lobe or superior segment of the lower lobe [Figure 36.2]. Features of collapse may be present as well [Figure 36.3]. Bronchiectasis may occur in a progressive primary disease because of: [i] destruction and fibrosis of lung parenchyma resulting in retraction and irreversible bronchial dilatation; and [ii] cicatricial bronchostenosis secondary to localised endobronchial infection resulting in obstructive pneumonitis and distal bronchiectasis. In children, cavitary disease is uncommon [Figure 36.4]. Pleural effusion may occur with or without lung lesions [Figure 36.5]. In miliary TB, the lesions are less than 2 mm in diameter [Figure 36.6].

Occasionally, the chest radiograph may be normal and lymphadenopathy may be evident only on computed tomography [CT]. In addition, CT features, such as, low attenuation of lymph nodes with peripheral enhancement, calcification, branching centrilobular nodules and miliary nodules are helpful in suggesting the diagnosis in cases where the radiograph is normal or equivocal. Other features such as segmental or lobar consolidation and atelectasis are non-specific (48). In a study by Kim *et al* (49), CT including high-resolution CT [HRCT] revealed lymphadenopathy, and parenchymal lesions that were not evident in 21% and 35% of the chest radiographs, respectively. The HRCT is more sensitive than chest radiograph for the detection of miliary TB and shows randomly distributed multiple, small [< 2 mm diameter] nodules (50). The nodules may be so numerous that these coalesce to form larger nodules greater than 2 mm in diameter and at times areas of consolidation with air bronchograms may be seen. Thickening of the interlobular septa may also be a feature. Mediastinal and

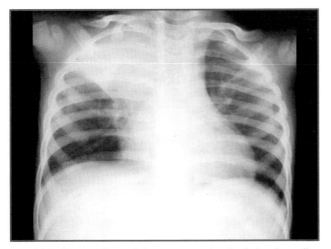

Figure 36.1: Chest radiograph [postero-anterior view] in a child with progressive primary complex showing left-sided hilar adenopathy and an ill-defined parenchymal lesion

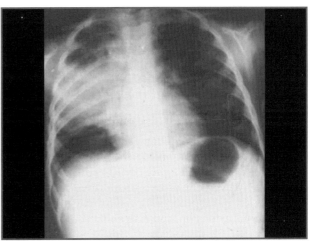

Figure 36.2: Chest radiograph [postero-anterior view] in a child with progressive primary disease showing consolidation in the right mid-zone

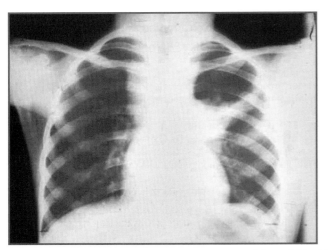

Figure 36.3: Chest radiograph [postero-anterior view] showing collapse consolidation of the right upper lobe

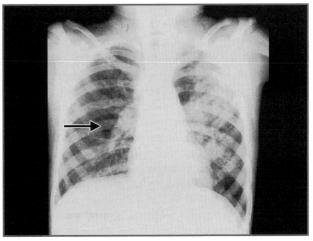

Figure 36.4: Chest radiograph [postero-anterior view] showing a cavity [arrow] in the right mid-zone

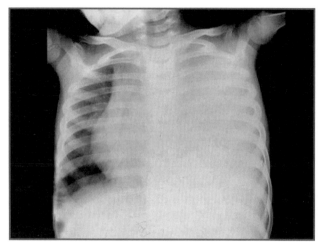

Figure 36.5: Chest radiograph [postero-anterior view] showing massive pleural effusion on the left side

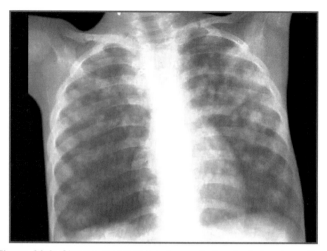

Figure 36.6: Chest radiograph [postero-anterior view] showing miliary mottling and right-sided paratracheal adenopathy

hilar lymphadenopathy may also be present. Cavitation is reported to be rare on the chest radiograph in children with TB. However, children co-infected with HIV and TB may manifest atypical radiographic features (51,52). In children co-infected with HIV and TB, CT may show areas of cavitation that are not apparent on the chest radiograph (51,52). The HRCT and colour Doppler ultrasonography have been found to be useful in the diagnosis of cervical lymphadenopathy (53).

TB of the spine is the most common site of osseous involvement and has a higher prevalence in developing nations with an increasing incidence in developed nations. Magnetic resonance imaging [MRI] findings include: contiguous involvement of two or more vertebral bodies, intraspinal or paraspinal soft tissue mass or abscess, subligamentous extension, and ring enhancement of the soft tissue mass (54). Contrast-enhanced MRI is emerging as a very useful technique for diagnosing neurological TB, as it demonstrates the localised lesions, meningeal enhancement and the brain stem lesions (55).

Scoring Systems for Predicting Childhood Tuberculosis

Diagnosis of TB in children is usually based on clinical signs and symptoms, chest radiograph, TST and history of contact with adult patients. Clinical features may be non-specific and chest radiograph and TST are difficult to interpret and do not provide conclusive evidence for the disease. Though demonstration of *Mtb* in various clinical specimens remains gold standard, this is often not possible in children due to the pauci-bacillary nature of the illness.

To overcome the problem of diagnosis in children; combination of clinical features, history of exposure to adult patient with TB, result of TST and radiological finding have been evaluated by various workers. Several scoring systems have been developed after giving different weightage to these variables (56,57). In these scoring system, more weightage is given to laboratory test, i.e. demonstration

Table 36.2: Diagnostic criteria for pulmonary tuberculosis in children in countries where mycobacterial culture facilities are not available
Gastric washings positive for AFB
or
Two or more of the following criteria
History of contact with a TB adult
Symptoms suggestive of pulmonary TB [cough for more than 2 weeks]
2 TU PPD reaction positive
> 10 mm in unvaccinated BCG patients
> 15 mm in vaccinated BCG patients
Radiological findings compatible with pulmonary TB
Response to treatment [body weight increase > 10% after 2 months of treatment, plus clinical improvement]
AFB = acid-fast bacilli; TB = tuberculosis; TU = tuberculin units; PPD = purified protein derivative; BCG = Bacille Calmette-Guérin *Source: reference 58*

of AFB, tubercles in biopsy, suggestive radiology and TST greater than 10 mm induration. These scoring systems need validation in individual countries. The criteria for diagnosis of pulmonary TB in children in countries where mycobacterial culture is not available proposed by Migliori *et al* (58) is shown in Table 36.2.

DIAGNOSTIC ALGORITHM

The new diagnostic algorithm is prepared jointly by the Indian Academy of Paediatrics and Revised National Tuberculosis Control Programme [RNTCP] of Government of India for paediatric pulmonary TB and lymph node TB (59,60) are shown in Figures 36.7A, 36.7B and 36.7C.

DRUG-RESISTANT TUBERCULOSIS

Pattern of drug resistance among children with TB tends to reflect the same found among adults in the same population. A four-year prospective study in the Western Cape province of South Africa evaluated 149-child contacts of 80-adult

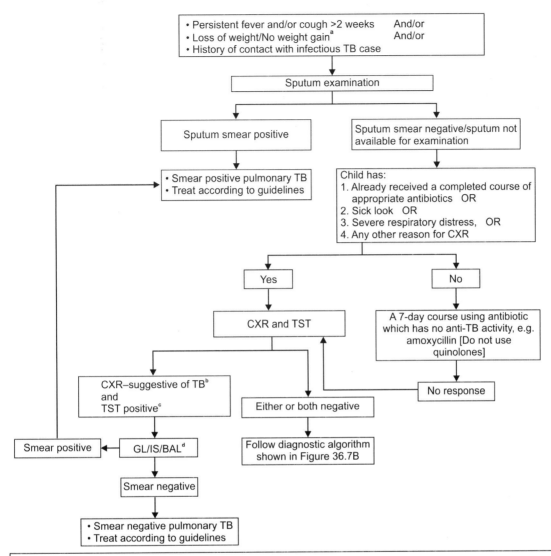

Figure 36.7A: Diagnostic algorithm for paediatric pulmonary TB
TB = tuberculosis; CXR = chest X-ray; TST = tuberculin skin test
Source: reference 59

multidrug-resistant [MDR] pulmonary TB cases (61). Culture for *Mtb* was obtained from both the adult source cases as and the child contacts. Isolates were compared by drug susceptibility testing [DST] and restriction fragment length polymorphism [RFLP] analysis. Six adult–child pairs with cultures positive for *Mtb* were identified. DST and RFLP analyses were identical for five adult-child pairs. The strain isolated from a child, in whom a source case was not evident, was different from that isolated from the source cases. However, the strain isolated from this child was prevalent in the community in which he resided. This study (61) supports the view that majority of the childhood contacts of adults with MDR-TB are likely to be infected by these source cases.

Childhood contacts of adults with MDR-TB should, therefore, be treated according to the drug susceptibility patterns of *Mtb* strains of the likely source cases unless the susceptibility pattern of the strain isolated from the child indicates otherwise. In another report from South Africa (62), of the 306 mycobacterial culture and sensitivity results available from 338 children [under 13 years of age], the prevalence of isoniazid resistance and multidrug-resistance [defined as isolates resistant to isoniazid and rifampicin

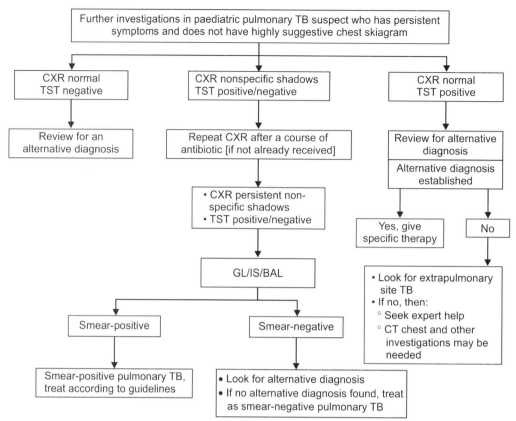

Figure 36.7B: Diagnostic algorithm for further investigations in pediatric pulmonary TB suspect who has persistent symptoms and does not have a suggestive chest radiograph

TB = tuberculosis; CXR = chest X-ray; TST = tuberculin skin test; GL = gastric lavage; IS = induced sputum; BAL = bronchoalveolar lavage
Source: reference 59

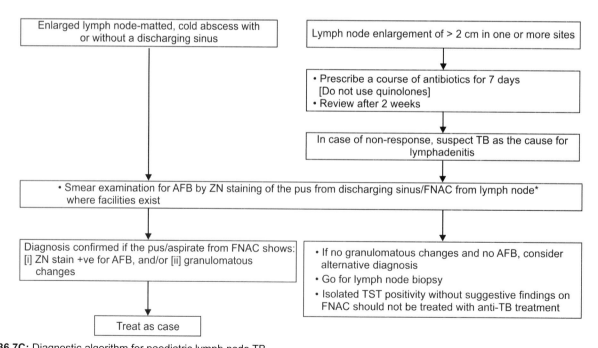

Figure 36.7C: Diagnostic algorithm for paediatric lymph node TB
*The INDEX-TB guidelines (47) recommend use of Xpert MTB/RIF for diagnosis of lymph node TB
TB = tuberculosis; AFB = acid-fast bacilli; ZN = Ziehl Neelsen; FNAC = fine needle aspiration cytology; TST = tuberculin skin test
Source: reference 59

with or without resistance to other anti-TB drugs] were 6.9% and 2.3%, respectively (62). Clinical features were similar in children with drug-susceptible and drug resistant TB (62).

TREATMENT

The principles of therapy in children with TB are similar to that of adults. Short-course anti-TB treatment is presently the standard of care for paediatric TB. It has been observed that conventional doses used in childhood TB fail to achieve serum concentrations above minimal inhibitory concentrations [MICs] (63). The recently revised anti-TB drug dosages as per the WHO guidelines are shown in Table 36.3 (46). The WHO recommended daily treatment regimens for new TB cases in children are listed in Table 36.4 (46). The WHO guidelines (46) advocate daily anti-TB treatment for paediatric TB.

In India, children with TB get treated under the RNTCP of the Government of India. The treatment categories advocated in the recently updated National Guidelines for Diagnosis and Treatment of Paediatric TB (59,60); and the treatment regimens used are described in the chapter *"Revised National Tuberculosis Control Programme"* [Chapter 53]. The reader is also referred to the chapter *"Endobronchial tuberculosis"* [Chapter 12] for details on airway stent placement.

Corticosteroids

Corticosteroids, in addition to anti-TB drugs, are useful in the treatment of children with neurological TB and in some children with pulmonary TB. These are mainly useful in settings where the host inflammatory reaction contributes significantly to tissue damage. Short-courses of corticosteroids are indicated in children with endobronchial TB that causes localised emphysema, segmental pulmonary lesions or respiratory distress. Some children with severe miliary TB may show dramatic improvement with corticosteroids, if alveolo-capillary block is present.

Management of an Infant Born to a Mother with Tuberculosis

The foetus may be infected either haematogenously through umbilical vessels or through ingestion of the infected amniotic fluid. In the former situation, there will be primary focus in liver and in the latter it will be in the lungs. It is difficult to find the route of transmission in a newborn with multiple foci of infection. It is difficult to differentiate between congenital and postnatally acquired TB (64). According to the criteria proposed by Cantwell *et al* (65) in 1994, congenital TB is diagnosed if the infant has proven TB lesion[s] and at least one of the following criteria: [i] appearance of lesions in the first week of life; [ii] a primary hepatic complex or caseating hepatic granulomas; [iii] TB infection of the placenta or the maternal genital tract; and [iv] exclusion of the possibility of postnatal transmission by a thorough investigation of contacts including the infant's hospital attendants or birth attendant.

Table 36.3: Recommended daily dosages of first-line anti-TB drugs in children

Drug	Dosage and range [mg/kg body weight]	Maximum dose [mg]
Isoniazid	10 [7-15]*	300
Rifampicin	15 [10-20]	600
Pyrazinamide	35 [30-40]	–
Ethambutol	20 [15-25]	–

*higher end of the dosage range for isoniazid applies to younger children. As the children grow older, the lower end of the dosage range becomes more appropriate
TB = tuberculosis
Source: reference 46

Table 36.4: Recommended daily treatment regimens for new TB cases in children

Diagnostic category	Anti-TB treatment regimen	
	Intensive phase	Continuation phase
HIV-negative children in low HIV prevalence and low H resistance settings		
Smear-negative pulmonary TB	2HRZ	4HR
Intrathoracic lymph node TB	2HRZ	4HR
TB peripheral lymphadenitis	2HRZ	4HR
Extensive pulmonary disease	2HRZE	4HR
Smear-positive pulmonary TB	2HRZE	4HR
Severe forms of EPTB [other than TBM/osteoarticular TB]	2HRZE	4HR
High HIV prevalence or high H resistance or both		
Smear-positive pulmonary TB	2HRZE	4HR
Smear-negative pulmonary TB with or without extensive parenchymal disease	2HRZE	4HR
Severe forms of EPTB [other than TBM/osteoarticular TB]	2HRZE	4HR
All regions		
TBM and osteoarticular TB	2HRZE	10HR
MDR-TB	Individualised treatment regimens	

The number preceding the treatment regimen indicates the duration of that phase in months; drug treatment is daily
TB = tuberculosis; H = isoniazid; R= rifampicin; Z = pyrazinamide; E = ethambutol; EPTB = extrapulmonary tuberculosis; TBM = tuberculosis meningitis; MDR-TB = multidrug-resistant tuberculosis
Source: reference 46

All infants born to mothers with active TB should be screened for evidence of disease by doing a good physical examination, TST and chest radiograph. If physical examination and investigations are negative for TB disease, the infant should be started on isoniazid prophylaxis [10 mg/kg/day] for six months.

Infants with congenital TB should be treated with four drugs [isoniazid, rifampicin, pyrazinamide, ethambutol] in the intensive phase followed by two drugs [isoniazid, rifampicin] during the continuation phase for next four months (60).

Management of a Child in Contact with an Adult with Tuberculosis

In a prospective observational study (66), nearly one-third of children [aged < 5 years] in contact with adults with active TB disease had evidence of TB infection. The infection was more commonly associated with younger age, severe malnutrition, absence of Bacilli Calmette-Guérin [BCG] vaccination, contact with an adult who was sputum-positive, and exposure to environmental tobacco smoke (66). It is suggested that children below six years of age in contact with adult patients with sputum positive TB should receive six months of isoniazid prophylaxis. It is mandatory to screen all children in the household of an adult patient with sputum-positive TB.

Monitoring of Therapy

Response to treatment can be judged by using the following criteria: clinical, radiological, bacteriological, and laboratory test results.

Clinical Criteria

Clinical improvement in a child on anti-TB treatment is the mainstay of judging response to treatment. The child should be seen once in every two to four weeks initially, and once in four to eight weeks thereafter. On each visit, improvement in fever, cough, appetite and subjective well being is assessed. The child is examined for weight gain and improvement in findings on physical examination. Compliance is assessed by talking to parents, checking medications on each visit. Majority of children show improvement in symptoms within a few weeks.

In the presence of poor response or worsening of symptoms or signs, the initial basis of diagnosis is reviewed, especially, if treatment compliance has been regular and the child should be assessed for the possibility of drug-resistant TB. After the treatment is over, follow-up every three to six months for next two years is desirable (67).

Immune reconstitution inflammatory syndrome [IRIS] has been described in 32%-36% of patients with HIV-TB, usually within days to weeks after the initiation of highly active antiretroviral therapy (68,69). Rarely, paradoxical reactions have been described in HIV-seronegative patients as well. These can be brief or prolonged with multiple recurrences. Paradoxical reactions pose a diagnostic challenge and have to be distinguished from TB treatment failure, drug resistance and other opportunistic infections that are common among HIV-infected patients (68,69).

Radiological Criteria

Clinical improvement precedes clearance of lesion on chest radiographs. The optimal frequency of radiological monitoring in children with pulmonary TB is unclear. A chest radiograph may be obtained after completing six months of treatment if the child is showing satisfactory improvement on clinical monitoring. If the child shows worsening of clinical features at any time or no improvement after two months of intensive phase, a repeat chest radiograph may be obtained (59,60). Children who show poor or no response at the end of intensive phase should be given benefit of extension of intensive phase for one more month. The child, if better, should be shifted to continuation phase; else, the child is investigated for failure of treatment and drug-resistance.

Microbiological Criteria

Most of the childhood pulmonary TB is paucibacillary. In children, where isolation of *Mtb* was possible at the time of diagnosis, every effort should be made to document disappearance of bacilli during therapy.

Other Measures

Although an elevated erythrocyte sedimentation rate [ESR] may be expected in children with TB, a recent study found that one-third of children with TB had a normal ESR at the time of diagnosis, suggesting little value in using ESR as a diagnostic and monitoring test for childhood TB (70).

REFERENCES

1. Jenkins HE, Yuen CM, Rodriguez CA, Nathavitharana RR, McLaughlin MM, Donald P, et al. Mortality in children diagnosed with tuberculosis: a systematic review and meta-analysis. Lancet Infect Dis 2016 Dec 7. pii: S1473-3099[16]30474-1.
2. Mandalakas AM, Starke JR. Current concepts of childhood tuberculosis. Semin Pediatr Infect Dis 2005;16:93-104.
3. Seddon JA, Shingadia D. Epidemiology and disease burden of tuberculosis in children: a global perspective. Infect Drug Resist 2014;7:153-65.
4. Enarson DA. The International Union Against Tuberculosis and Lung Disease Model National Tuberculosis Programmes. Tuber Lung Dis 1995;76: 95-9.
5. Comstock GW, Livesay VT, Woolpert SF. The prognosis of a positive tuberculin reaction in childhood and adolescence. Am J Epidemiol 1974;99:131-8.
6. Munoz FM, Starke JR. Tuberculosis in children. In: Reichman LB, Hershfield E, editors. Tuberculosis: a comprehensive international approach, 2nd edition. New York: Marcell-Dekker Inc; 2000. p.553-95.
7. Miller FM, Seale RME. Tuberculosis in children. Boston: Little, Brown and Company; 1963.
8. World Health Organization. Global Tuberculosis Report 2017. Geneva: World Health Organization; 2017.
9. Comstock G. Epidemiology of tuberculosis. In: Reichman LB, Hershfield E, editors. Tuberculosis: a comprehensive international approach. New York: Marcel Dekker; 2000.p.129-48.
10. Dannenberg AM, Sugimoto M. Liquefaction of caseous foci in tuberculosis. Am Rev Respir Dis 1976;113:257- 9.

11. Lamont AC, Cremin B, Pettenet B. Radiologic patterns of pulmonary tuberculosis in the pediatric age group. Pediatr Radiol 1986;16:2-7.

12. Morrison JB. Natural history of segmental lesions in primary pulmonary tuberculosis. Arch Dis Child 1973;48:90-8.

13. Lincoln EM, Harris LC, Bovornkitti S, Carretero RW. Endobronchial tuberculosis in children. Am Rev Tuberc Pulm Dis 1958;77:39-61.

14. Seale RME, Thomas SME. Endobronchial tuberculosis in children. Lancet 1956;ii:995-6.

15. Stansberry SD. Tuberculosis is infants and children. J Thorac Imag 1990;5:17-27.

16. Daly JF, Brown DS, Lincoln EM, Wilking VN. Endobronchial tuberculosis in children. Dis Chest 1952;22:380-98.

17. Matsaniotis N, Kattanis C, Economou-Mavron C, Kyriazakou M. Bullous emphysema in childhood tuberculosis. J Pediatr 1967;71:703-8.

18. Pray LG. Obstructive emphysema is infancy due to tuberculous mediastinal glands. J Pediatr 1944;25:253-6.

19. Seth V, Lodha R, Kabra SK. Pulmonary Tuberculosis. In: Seth V, Kabra SK, editors. Essentials of tuberculosis in Children. Fourth edition. New Delhi: Jaypee Brothers Medical Publishers; 2010. p.85-98.

20. Seth V, Singhal PK, Semwal OP, Kabra SK, Jain Y. Childhood tuberculosis in a referral center: clinical profile and risk factors. Indian Pediatr 1993;30:479-85.

21. Pamra S. Tuberculosis in children. Indian J Tuberc 1987;34:55-6.

22. Somu N, Vijayasekaran D, Ravikumar T, Balachandran A, Subramanyam L, Chandrabhushanam A. Tuberculous disease in a pediatric referral center: 16 years experience. Indian Pediatr 1994;31:1245-9.

23. Maniar BM. Cavitating pulmonary tuberculosis below age of 2 years. Indian Pediatr 1994;31:181-90.

24. Seth V, Donald PR. Tuberculous lymphadentis. In: Seth V, Kabra SK, editors. Essentials of tuberculosis in children. Fourth edition. New Delhi: Jaypee Brothers Medical Publishers; 2010.p.99-107.

25. Seth V, Gulati S, Udani PM. Clinical features and diagnosis of CNS tuberculosis. In: Seth V, Kabra SK, editors. Essentials of tuberculosis in children. Fourth edition. New Delhi: Jaypee Brothers Medical Publishers; 2010.p.134-61.

26. Allen BW, Mitchison DA. Counts of viable tubercle bacilli in sputum related to smear and culture gradings. Med Lab Sci 1992;49:94-8.

27. Abadco DL, Steiner P. Gastric lavage is better than bronchoalveolar lavage for isolation of Mycobacterium tuberculosis in childhood pulmonary tuberculosis. Pediatr Infect Dis J 1992;11:735-8.

28. Strumpf IJ, Tsang AY, Sayre JW. Reevaluation of sputum staining for the diagnosis of pulmonary tuberculosis. Am Rev Respir Dis 1979;119:599-602.

29. Mukherjee A, Singh S, Lodha R, Singh V, Hesseling AC, Grewal HM, et al. Ambulatory gastric lavages provide better yields of Mycobacterium tuberculosis than induced sputum in children with intrathoracic tuberculosis. Pediatr Infect Dis J 2013;32:1313-7.

30. Parashar D, Kabra SK, Lodha R, Singh V, Mukherjee A, Arya T, et al. Does neutralization of gastric aspirates from children with suspected intrathoracic tuberculosis affect mycobacterial yields on MGIT culture? J Clin Microbiol 2013;51:1753-6.

31. Somu N, Swaminathan S, Paramasivan CN, Vijayasekaran D, Chandrabhooshanam A, Vijayan VK, et al. Value of bronchoalveolar lavage and gastric lavage in the diagnosis of pulmonary tuberculosis in children. Tuberc Lung Dis 1995;76:295-9.

32. Singh M, Moosa NV, Kumar L, Sharma M. Role of gastric lavage and bronchoalveolar lavage in the bacteriological diagnosis of childhood pulmonary tuberculosis. Indian Pediatr 2000;37:947-51.

33. Menon PR, Lodha R, Singh U, Kabra SK. A prospective assessment of the role of bronchoscopy and bronchoalveolar lavage in evaluation of children with pulmonary tuberculosis. J Trop Pediatr 2011;57: 363-7.

34. Madan K, Ayub II, Mohan A, Jain D, Guleria R, Kabra SK. Endobronchial ultrasound-guided transbronchial needle aspiration [EBUS-TBNA] in mediastinal lymphadenopathy. Indian J Pediatr 2015;82:378-80.

35. Lobeto MN, Lobeto AM, Furst K, Cole B, Hopewell PC. Detection of Mycobacterium tuberculosis in gastric aspirate collected from children, hospitalization is not necessary. Pediatrics 1998;102:E40.

36. Starke JF, Tylorwalis KT. Tuberculosis in the pediatric population of Houston Texas. Pediatrics 1989;84:8-35.

37. Venkataraman P, Herbert D, Paramasivan CN. Evaluation of the BACTEC radiometric method in the early diagnosis of tuberculosis. Indian J Med Res 1998;108:120-7.

38. Roberts GD, Goodman NL, Heifets L, Larsh HW, Lindner TH, McClatchy JK, et al. Evaluation of the ACTEC radiometric method for recovery of mycobacteria and drug susceptibility testing of Mycobacterium tuberculosis from acid-fast smear-positive specimens. J Clin Microbiol 1983;18:689-96.

39. Ninan SA. Comparative study of different methods of identification of Mycobacterium tuberculosis in gastric aspirate of children suffering from pulmonary tuberculosis. MD thesis. New Delhi: All India Institute of Medical Sciences; 1997.

40. Sewell DL, Rashad AL, Rourke WJ Jr, Poor SL, McCarthy JA, Pfaller MA. Comparison of the Septi-Chek AFB and BACTEC systems and conventional culture for recovery of mycobacteria. J Clin Microbiol 1993;31: 689-91.

41. Badak FZ, Kiska DL, Setterquist S, Hartley C, O'Connell MA, Hopfer RL. Comparison of mycobacteria growth indicator tube with BACTEC 460 for detection and recovery of mycobacteria from clinical specimens. J Clin Microbiol 1996;34:2236-9.

42. Noordhoek GT, Kolk AHJ, Bjune G, Cotty D, Dale JW, Fine PEM, et al. Sensitivity and specificity of PCR or detection of Mycobacterium tuberculosis: a blind comparison study among seven laboratories. J Clin Microbiol 1994;32:277-84.

43. Walters E, Goussard P, Bosch C, Hesseling AC, Gie RP. GeneXpert MTB/RIF on bronchoalveolar lavage samples in children with suspected complicated intrathoracic tuberculosis: a pilot study. Pediatr Pulmonol 2014;49:1133-7.

44. Nicol MP, Workman L, Isaacs W, Munro J, Black F, Eley B, et al. Accuracy of the Xpert MTB/RIF test for the diagnosis of pulmonary tuberculosis in children admitted to hospital in Cape Town, South Africa: a descriptive study. Lancet Infect Dis 2011;11:819-24.

45a. Pang Y, Wang Y, Zhao S, Liu J, Zhao Y, Li H. Evaluation of the Xpert MTB/RIF assay in gastric lavage aspirates for diagnosis of smear-negative childhood pulmonary tuberculosis. Pediatr Infect Dis J 2014;33:1047-51.

45b. Memon SS, Sinha S, Sharma SK, Kabra SK, Lodha R, Soneja M. Diagnostic accuracy of Xpert Mtb/Rif assay in stool samples in intrathoracic childhood tuberculosis. J Tuberc Ther 2018;3:115.

46. World Health Organization. Guidance for national tuberculosis programmes on the management of tuberculosis in children. WHO/HTM/TB/2014.03. Second edition. Geneva: World Helath Organization; 2014.

47. Sharma SK, Ryan H, Khaparde S, Sachdeva KS, Singh AD, Mohan A, et al. Index-TB guidelines: Guidelines on extrapulmonary tuberculosis for India. Indian J Med Res 2017;145:448-63.

48. Copley SJ. Application of computed tomography in childhood respiratory infections. Br Med Bull 2002;61:263-79.

49. Kim WS, Moon WK, Kim IO, Lee HJ, Im JG, Yeon KM, et al. Pulmonary tuberculosis in children: evaluation with CT. Am J Roentgenol 1997;168:1005-9.

50. Jamieson DH, Cremin BJ. High-resolution CT of the lungs in acute disseminated tuberculosis and a pediatric radiology perspective of the term 'miliary'. Pediatr Radiol 1993;23: 380-3.

51. Haller JO, Ginsburg KJ. Tuberculosis in children with acquired immunodeficiency syndrome. Pediatr Radiol 1997;27:186-8.

52. Kornreich L, Goshen Y, Horev G, Grunebaum M. Mycobacterial respiratory infection in leukemic children. Eur J Radiol 1995;21: 44-6.

53. Papakonstantinou O, Bakantaki A, Paspalaki P, Charoulakis N, Gourtsoyiannis N. High-resolution and color Doppler ultrasono-graphy of cervical lymphadenopathy in children. Acta Radiol 2001;42:470-6.

54. Andronikou S, Jadwat S, Douis H. Patterns of disease on MRI in 53 children with tuberculous spondylitis and the role of gadolinium. Pediatr Radiol 2002;32:798-805.

55. Uysal G, Kose G, Guven A, Diren B. Magnetic resonance imaging in diagnosis of childhood central nervous system tuberculosis. Infection 2001;29:148-53.

56. Stengen G, Kenneth J, Kaplas P. Criteria for guidance in the diagnosis of tuberculosis. Pediatrics 1969;43:260-3.

57. Nair PM, Philip T. A scoring system for diagnosis of tuberculosis in children. Indian Pediatr 1981;18:299-303.

58. Migliori GB, Borghesi A, Rossanigo P, Adriko C, Neri M, Santini S, et al. Proposal of an improved score method for the diagnosis of pulmonary tuberculosis in childhood in developing countries. Tuber Lung Dis 1992;73:145-9.

59. Central TB Division, Directorate General of Health Services, Ministry of Health and Family Welfare, Indian Academy of Pediatrics. National Guidelines on Diagnosis and Treatment of Pediatric Tuberculosis. Updated January-February 2012. Available at URL: http://tbcindia.nic.in/WriteReadData/l892s/3175192227Paediatric%20guidelines_New.pdf. Accessed on December 15, 2017.

60. Kumar A, Gupta D, Nagaraja SB, Singh V, Sethi GR, Prasad J. Indian Academy of Pediatrics. Updated National Guidelines for Pediatric Tuberculosis in India, 2012. Indian Pediatr 2013;50: 301-6.

61. Schaaf HS, Van Rie A, Gie RP, Beyers N, Victor TC, Van Helden PD, et al. Transmission of multidrug-resistant tuberculosis. Pediatr Infect Dis J 2000;19:695-9.

62. Schaaf HS, Gie RP, Beyers N, Sirgel FA, de Klerk PJ, Donald PR. Primary drug-resistant tuberculosis in children. Int J Tuberc Lung Dis 2000;4:1149-55.

63. Mukherjee A, Velpandian T, Singla M, Kanhiya K, Kabra SK, Lodha R. Pharmacokinetics of isoniazid, rifampicin, pyra-zinamide and ethambutol in Indian children. BMC Infect Dis 2015;15:126.

64. Saramba MI, Zhao D. A perspective of the diagnosis and management of congenital tuberculosis. J Pathog 2016:8623825.

65. Cantwell MF, Shehab ZM, Costello AM, Sands L, Green WF, Ewing, et al. Brief report: Congenital Tuberculosis. N Engl J Med 1994;330:1051-4.

66. Singh M, Maynak ML, Kumar L, Mathew JL, Jindal SK. Prevalence and risk factors for transmission of infection among children in household contact with adults having pulmonary tuberculosis. Arch Dis Child 2005;90:624-8.

67. Kabra SK, Ratageri VH. Tuberculosis in children: Monitoring of treatment and management of side effects. Paediatr Today 1999;2:81-4.

68. Sharma SK, Mohan A, Kadhiravan T. HIV-TB co-infection: epidemiology, diagnosis and management. Indian J Med Res 2005; 121:550-67.

69. Cheng SL, Wang HC, Yang PC. Paradoxical response during antituberculosis treatment in HIV-negative patients with pulmonary tuberculosis. Int J Tuberc Lung Dis 2007;11:1290-5.

70. Al-Marri MR, Kirkpatrick MB. Erythrocyte sedimentation rate in childhood tuberculosis: is it still worthwhile? Int J Tuberc Lung Dis 2000;4:237-9.

37

Surgical Aspects of Childhood Tuberculosis

Minu Bajpai, Alisha Gupta, Manisha Jana, Arun K Gupta

INTRODUCTION

Diagnosis of tuberculosis [TB] in children poses a major problem and a high degree of suspicion is warranted to make an early diagnosis even in endemic regions. Currently, surgery has a minimal role in treatment of childhood TB, because anti-TB treatment remains the mainstay in the management. Surgery is generally performed to secure tissue for diagnosis confirmation. With the increasing application of cartridge-based nucleic acid amplification tests [CBNAAT] like Xpert MTB/RIF for the diagnosis of TB in children, surgical intervention is being resorted to more frequently for procuring tissue for confirmation of diagnosis of TB (1-3). Surgery has a role in managing sequelae or complications of TB. Sometimes, resectional surgery is carried out in children with drug-resistant active TB. In this chapter, the surgical aspects of TB in children will be discussed laying emphasis on the clinical, diagnostic and surgical principles involved.

GENITOURINARY TUBERCULOSIS

As there is a time lag of about four to twenty years between the initial infection and occurrence of genitourinary involvement, paediatric genitourinary TB presents usually in the adolescent period. The time lag noted is more than five years in two-thirds of the patients and is greater than 15 years in a quarter of the cases (4).

Clinical Presentation

TB of the genital tract is uncommon before puberty. Majority of the young children with genitourinary TB are asymptomatic. Symptoms are seen in the more advanced stages and usually after vesical involvement. Symptoms and signs commonly observed in children with genitourinary TB are listed in Table 37.1.

TB of the genitourinary tract must be suspected if a child presents with chronic or recurrent urinary tract infection [cystitis] not responding to adequate standard antibiotic therapy for recommended duration. The clinical suspicion is enhanced when pus cells are found without bacteria in an acidic urine or on methylene blue staining of the urine sediment. Gross or microscopic haematuria; an enlarged, non-tender epididymis with a thickened, beaded vas; a chronic, draining scrotal sinus in the setting of history of TB elsewhere in the body or definite history of contact, further support the diagnosis of genitourinary TB.

Urinary frequency is the earliest symptom which is diurnal and progressive in nature (5). Frequency is secondary to vesical irritation, decreased bladder capacity and rarely as a result of polyuria with tubular dysfunction. The urine may be opalescent. Occasionally, patients may present with pyuria. The child may initially complain of suprapubic pain with a moderately full bladder which gradually progresses to dysuria and strangury. Renal pain is usually absent but some patients may have a dull flank ache. Painless haematuria may result because of ulcers at the renal papilla in 5% cases (4-7).

Table 37.1: Clinical features of genitourinary tuberculosis
Symptoms
Progressive, diurnal urinary frequency
Dysuria
Macroscopic haematuria with back and flank pain
Renal colic
Systemic symptoms [fever, anorexia, night sweats, weight loss]
Hypertension
Chronic epididymitis
Other symptoms
Polyuria, hyponatraemia [with adrenal tuberculosis]
Chronic renal insufficiency

Renal and ureteric colic may occur due to passage of a blood clot, secondary calculi or debris. There is usually no renal enlargement or tenderness. Rarely, the contralateral kidney may show compensatory enlargement. Symptomatic chronic renal failure occurs rarely but subclinical impairment of renal functions may be seen more often. Hypertension may be evident in 5%-10% children with renal TB (4-7). Ocon *et al* (6) have shown that in most patients, the hypertension is not mediated by the renin-angiotensin system, and is therefore, not cured by nephrectomy. Genitourinary TB may present with other complications, such as perinephric abscess, renal calculi, secondary amyloidosis and adenocarcinoma of the renal pelvis.

TB of the genital tract most often manifests as epididymitis in boys. Fever is seldom present. Enlarged epididymis may be felt as a hard, nodular swelling. A chronic draining scrotal sinus should suggest TB aetiology unless proved otherwise. A secondary hydrocoele may accompany epididymitis. The testis may be fixed by an extension of an epididymal abscess. The prostate may be nodular or indurated and the seminal vesicle is similarly involved. In the presence of prostatitis, TB may spread via the semen. Genital TB may be a manifestation of sexual abuse and there are reports of urethral involvement and penile lesions following ritual circumcision. In girls, lower abdominal pain and amenorrhoea may be presenting symptoms of genital TB. Constitutional symptoms are rare. Free peritoneal fluid and lower abdominal mass may be evident.

Role of Surgery

Surgery is reserved for the management of local complications, such as ureteral strictures, perinephric abscesses, non-functioning kidneys and reconstruction of upper urinary tract, urinary bladder, urethra. Algorithm for the surgical management of children with genitourinary TB is shown in Figure 37.1. Surgery should be preceded by at least three weeks and preferably four months of anti-TB treatment with constant clinical and radiological monitoring. The principles of surgery for urogenital TB in children are same as those for adults. The reader is referred to the chapter *"Genitourinary tuberculosis" [Chapter 27]* for more details.

ABDOMINAL TUBERCULOSIS

The clinical manifestations of abdominal TB are protean [Figures 37.2, 37.3, 37.4, 37.5 and 37.6]. All age groups are at risk, and children between six and fourteen years of age are often affected (8,9). Clinical presentation of abdominal TB in children can be acute, sub-acute or with other manifestations. The reader is referred to the chapters *"Tuberculosis in children" [Chapter 36]* and *"Abdominal tuberculosis" [Chapter 15]* for more details regarding the clinical presentation, diagnosis and medical management of this condition.

Role of Surgery

Anti-TB treatment is the mainstay of management (4-9). Surgical intervention is helpful in procuring tissue for confirmation of aetiological diagnosis in children with peritoneal and mesenteric lymph node TB (8-12). An algorithm for assessment of suspected abdominal TB is shown in Figure 37.7 (13). Surgery is also helpful in the management of complications of intestinal TB, such as perforation of intestinal ulcer and intestinal obstruction. The possible role of surgical intervention in children with abdominal TB is shown in Figures 37.8A and 37.8B.

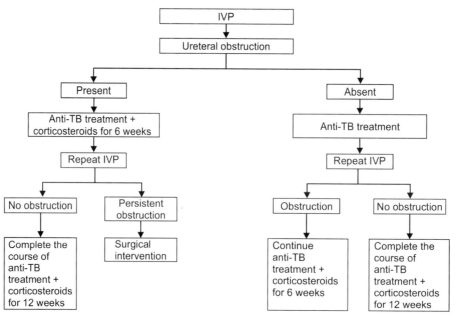

Figure 37.1: Algorithm for the surgical management of children with genitourinary TB
IVP = intravenous pyelography; TB = tuberculosis
Adapted and reproduced with permission from reference 7

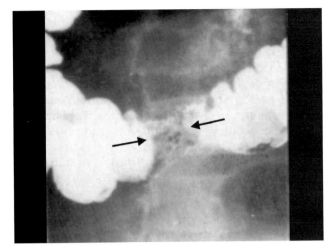

Figure 37.2: Barium meal follow through examination showing ileocaecal tuberculosis [stricture marked by arrows]

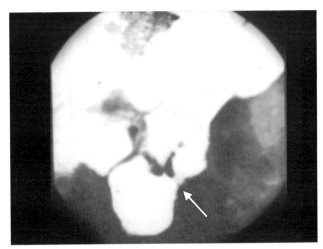

Figure 37.3: Barium meal follow through examination showing short segment tuberculosis stricture [arrow] in the small bowel with proximal dilatation

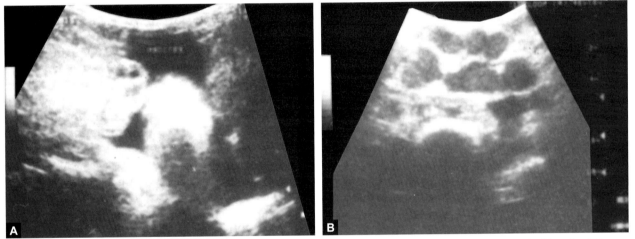

Figure 37.4: Ultrasonography of the abdomen showing ascites [A] and multiple hypoechoic masses in the prevertebral location [B] suggestive of lymphadenopathy

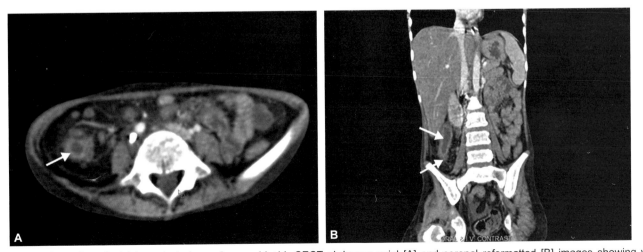

Figure 37.5: Gastrointestinal tuberculosis in an 8-year-old girl. CECT abdomen axial [A] and coronal reformatted [B] images showing wall thickening of the terminal ileum [arrow] and adjacent mesenteric lymphadenopathy
CECT = contrast-enhanced computed tomography

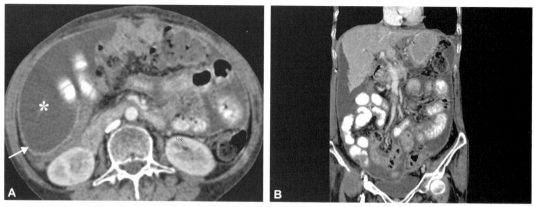

Figure 37.6: Peritoneal tuberculosis. CECT abdomen axial [A] and coronal reformatted [B] image reveal ascites [asterisk] with peritoneal thickening [arrow] and clumped bowel loops in the central abdomen
CECT = contrast-enhanced computed tomography

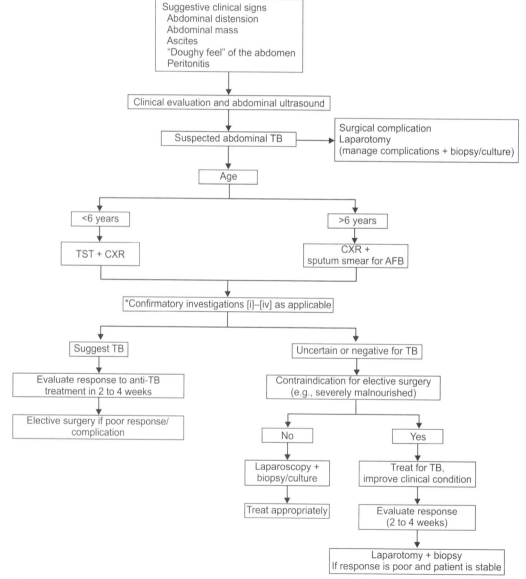

Figure 37.7: Algorithm for assessment of suspected abdominal TB
*Confirmatory investigations: [i] culture for *Mycobacterium tuberculosis* from accessible source; [ii] peripheral lymph node biopsy for histopathology and culture; [iii] adenosine deaminase levels in ascitic fluid; and [iv] CT of the abdomen if ultrasonography is inconclusive
TB = tuberculosis; AFB = acid-fast bacilli; TST = tuberculin skin test; CT = computed tomography
Adapted from reference 13

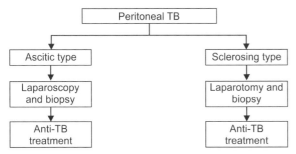

Figure 37.8A: Surgical intervention in patients with peritoneal TB
TB = tuberculosis
Adapted from reference 12

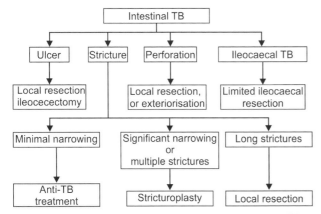

Figure 37.8B: Surgical intervention in patients with intestinal TB
TB = tuberculosis
Adapted from reference 6

The role of laparoscopy has been promising in procuring tissue for histopathological diagnosis (14). It has brought down the rate of unnecessary laparotomies in children and with experience, its role may also be extended to therapeutic purposes [stricturoplasty, adhesiolysis]. Surgery for abdominal TB must be cautious and minimal as the risk of inadvertent bowel injury with subsequent entero-cutaneous fistulae is high. Procedures commonly adopted include closure of perforation, exteriorisation of bowel, adhesiolysis and resection-anastomosis of the bowel. The choice of surgery is dependent on several factors. TB perforations carry a high mortality [30%-40%] despite surgery (15). Stricturoplasty is preferred to multiple resection anastomoses in multiple strictures as it conserves the bowel and obviates the occurrence of blind loop syndromes.

Abdominal cocoon is a rare disease in which intestinal obstruction results from the encasement of variable lengths of the bowel by a dense fibrocollagenous membrane that gives the appearance of a cocoon. Patients with tuberculous cocoon usually complain of recurrent attacks of subacute intestinal obstruction or abdominal lump, and some patients may be asymptomatic. An accurate diagnosis is difficult to make preoperatively. Surgical exploration with release of gut from the encasement membrane is the treatment of choice (16). The typical finding at surgery is a conglomeration of small bowel loops encased in a dense white membrane.

Ileum is the most common site of TB perforation and is associated with distal stricture formation. Resection and anastomosis are preferred because simple closure of the perforation is associated with a high incidence of leakage and fistula formation, and thus, higher mortality (17). Emergency surgery for intestinal obstruction is best avoided as it is associated with a high mortality (18).

PERIPHERAL LYMPH NODE TUBERCULOSIS

TB accounts for a high proportion of lymphadenopathy in children. Classically, the cervical nodes are involved in 67%-90% of cases (19,20). The exact incidence may vary in childhood but has been reported in up to 55% in a cohort of 223 children under six years of age (21). Painless enlargement, matting, fluctuant neck mass or a discharging sinus may be evident. Multifocal [> 3 sites] or generalised lymphadenopathy is uncommon without co-existent disseminated or miliary TB. Associated extralymphatic TB has been described in 5%-15% cases. Such presentation is more frequently seen in human immunodeficiency virus [HIV] infection (19-22). Isolated TB lymphadenitis at sites other than cervical region has been reported rarely.

Selective preauricular and intraparotid lymph nodal TB with or without parotid parenchymal involvement may, sometimes, be seen (23). The lower pole is usually involved presenting as a swelling antero-inferior to the ear and in front of the mastoid attachment of the sternocleidomastoid muscle. The dense parotid fascia limits the spread of infection and the resultant swelling may mimic a tumour on physical examination.

Nontuberculous Mycobacterial Lymphadenitis in Children

In lymphadenitis caused by nontuberculous mycobacteria [NTM], females are mostly affected and lymph node involvement is unilateral (24,25). High cervical lymph nodes near the mandible are characteristically involved and the enlarged lymph nodes are firm, rubbery and non-tender. These may not manifest the signs of inflammation and matting is exceedingly rare. Systemic symptoms are uncommon and history of exposure to TB is rarely obtained.

The reader is referred to the chapters *"Lymph node tuberculosis"* [Chapter 22], *"Nontuberculous mycobacterial infections"* [Chapter 41] for more details.

Role of Surgery

Anti-TB treatment is the mainstay in management of lymph node TB. The surgeon aids in obtaining tissue for the confirmation of diagnosis [e.g., in performing excision biopsy of the lymph node]. The indications for the lymph node sampling are listed in Table 37.2. NTM lymphadenitis is treated primarily by surgical excision (19). Parotid lymph nodal TB may mandate superficial extirpation of an encapsulated mass with a 1 cm margin (23). Aspiration of fluctuant lesions may also be required in some patients.

Table 37.2: Indications for lymph node sampling

Difficulty in clinical diagnosis and/or non-diagnostic fine needle aspiration cytology

Abscess formation

History of rapid increase in size

Further significant increase in size on treatment

Supraclavicular lymph nodes

Hard or matted lymph nodes

Fixation to surrounding structures

Development of new signs and symptoms [fever, weight loss, night sweats]

Significant lymph node [> 2 cm] not responding to antibiotic therapy in 4 to 6 weeks

Non-resolution of the lymphadenopathy in 8 weeks

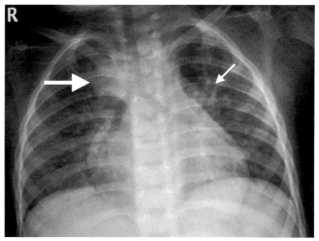

Figure 37.9: Chest radiograph [postero-anterior view] showing right paratracheal lymphadenopathy [thick arrow] and left upper zone patchy consolidation [thin arrow]

PULMONARY TUBERCULOSIS

In children with primary pulmonary TB disease [Figures 37.9 and 37.10], compression of the relatively narrow and compliant airways by the enlarged intrathoracic lymph nodes can result in atelectasis, obstructive emphysema, pulmonary infection and even asphyxia (26-28). The enlarged mediastinal lymph nodes can also cause perforation of the tracheobronchial tree. The aim of effective surgical treatment in childhood pulmonary TB includes restoring lung function to normal and managing complications. The indications for surgery are listed in Table 37.3 (26-30).

Role of Surgery

Major Airways Obstruction

When there is an obstruction of the major airways and acute respiratory distress, administration of prednisolone [2 mg/kg/day] along with anti-TB treatment and nebulised bronchodilator therapy is indicated. Lack of improvement within 48-72 hours is an indication for operative intervention. Following a pre-operative bronchoscopic assessment of the airway, usually a right thoracotomy is performed. An attempt to resect the entire nodal mass is hazardous and can lead to damage of the airway wall. Most of the nodes can be evacuated by incising the capsule and removing the caseous material or by removing the calcified contents piecemeal.

When there is chronic compromise, these patients may be asymptomatic. Superinfection by pyogenic organisms can result in an acute presentation. Also, the distal atelectatic or collapsed lung can undergo progressive damage despite effective medical therapy [Figure 37.11].

Recent evidence suggests that the early surgical decompression prevents irreversible pulmonary parenchymal damage. The risk of airway damage during evacuation of lymph nodes is higher in this group. Nodal incision and curettage of the mass is recommended.

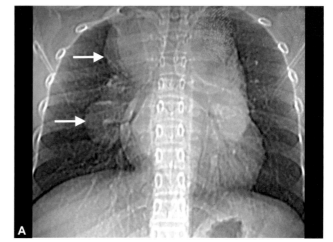

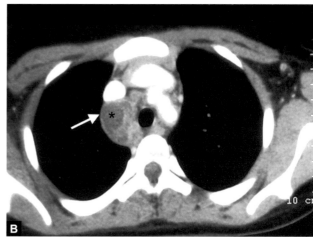

Figure 37.10: Intrathoracic lymph node involvement in TB in a child. Chest radiograph [A] shows superior mediastinal widening, lobulated soft tissue density shadows in right paratracheal and hilar regions [arrows]. CECT chest [B] shows central non-enhancing areas [asterisk] indicating caseation necrosis and peripheral thin rim enhancement [arrow] indicating inflammation in the lymph nodes
TB = tuberculosis; CECT = contrast-enhanced computed tomography

Table 37.3: Indications of surgery in childhood pulmonary TB

Major airway obstruction by extraluminal lymph node compression or intraluminal tissue

Post-TB pulmonary destruction

TB pleural disease

Other indications
  Drainage of active TB lung abscess
  Repair of broncho-oesophageal and bronchopleural fistula using vascularised muscle flaps
  Resection of persistently discharging chest wall sinuses

TB = tuberculosis

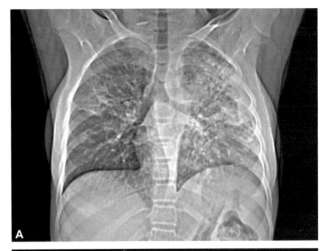

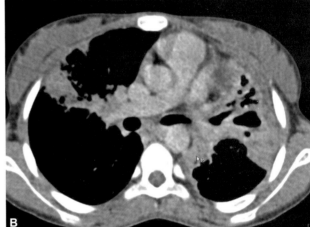

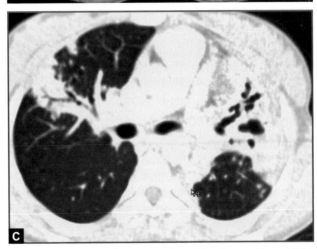

Figure 37.12: Extensive lung parenchymal involvement in a child with pulmonary TB. CT topogram [A] showing an opaque left hemithorax with areas of cavitation and bronchiectasis. CECT chest [mediastinal window] [B] and lung window [C] bilateral consolidation and areas of breakdown in left upper lobe
TB = tuberculosis; CT = computed tomography; CECT = contrast-enhanced computed tomography

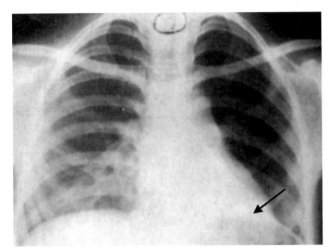

Figure 37.11: Chest radiograph [postero-anterior view] showing collapse of left lower lobe which can be seen as a triangular radiodensity [arrow] in the left retrocardiac region

When the obstruction is due to intraluminal tissue [endobronchial TB], the collapsed lung is at high risk of being permanently damaged by infection. Bronchoscopic suction and removal of granulomatous tissue with biopsy forceps results in re-inflation of the lobe or lung in more than 50% of the cases. This usually requires multiple attempts which are repeated every five to seven days. Haemorrhage during removal of the granulation tissue is a possible complication. This procedure decreases the incidence of pulmonary resection and salvages lungs or lobes which are collapsed secondary to obstruction but are otherwise normal.

Post-tuberculosis Pulmonary Destruction

Patients with post-TB pulmonary destruction present with definite evidence of extensive pulmonary damage [Figures 37.11, 37.12 and 37.13] and are usually symptomatic. Decision making regarding pulmonary resection is primarily based on symptomatology rather than the radiological findings. The risk to the remaining pulmonary tissue should be kept in mind while planning for surgery. Intensive pre-operative preparation involving physiotherapy and use of broad-spectrum antibiotic treatment is mandatory.

This regimen is continued till the sputum production is reduced to a minimum. One lung ventilation and prone position with head end lowered is recommended during surgery to avoid contamination of the normal lung.

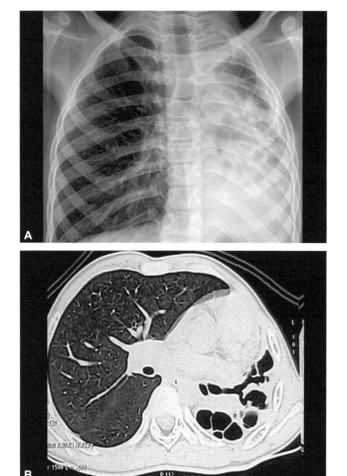

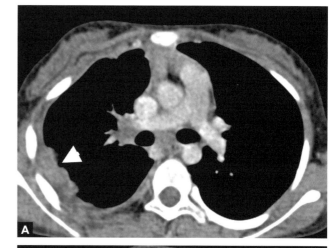

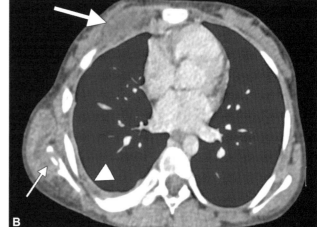

Figure 37.13: Destroyed left lung secondary to TB in an adolescent male. Chest radiograph [postero-anterior view] [A] shows opaque left hemithorax with ipsilateral mediastinal shift. CECT chest [lung window] [B] shows complete destruction of left lung parenchyma and compensatory hyperinflation of the right lung

TB = tuberculosis; CECT = contrast-enhanced computed tomography

Tuberculosis Pleural Disease

In children, TB of the pleura can, sometimes, present with associated chest wall abscess and bone involvement as well [Figure 37.14]. Late pleural fibrosis after a TB empyema requires decortication [Figures 37.15 and 37.16]. Patients with minimal or no respiratory symptoms despite radiographic evidence of pleural fibrosis do not require decortication unless there is a significant postural problem [scoliosis]. Patients with minimal symptoms cope well with pleural fibrosis which tends to regress with age and activity. It is also important to ensure that the underlying lung is not bronchiectatic and unsalvageable before undertaking decortication. Video-assisted thoracoscopic surgery [VATS] is also finding increasing use in the treatment of pleuro-pulmonary TB (31-33). VATS is a safe approach and avoids the morbidity associated with conventional thoracotomy. The current role of VATS in the management of pleuropulmonary TB is unclear but VATS has been found to be useful in the following situations (31-33): [i] VATS is safe and effective in

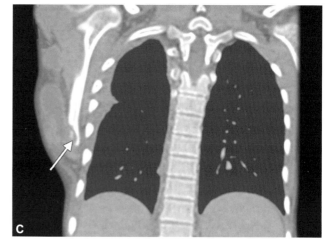

Figure 37.14: Pleural thickening and TB osteomyelitis in a 13-year-old girl. CECT chest axial images [A and B] show right-sided pleural thickening [arrow head] and anterior chest wall abscess [thick arrow], and destruction of the angle of right scapula [thin arrow]. Coronal reformatted image [bone window] [C] shows the destruction of right scapula [arrow]

TB = tuberculosis; CECT = contrast-enhanced computed tomography

achieving the diagnosis of TB through pleural biopsies or wedge lung resection of indeterminate pulmonary nodules; it is particularly useful for those patients who are debilitated,

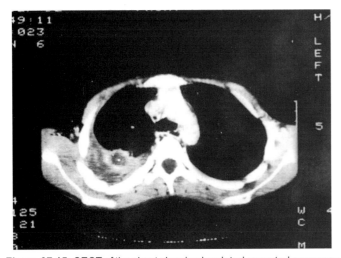

Figure 37.15: CECT of the chest showing loculated encysted empyema in right hemithorax with enhancing walls. Thickening of extrapleural soft tissues can also be seen
CECT = contrast-enhanced computed tomography

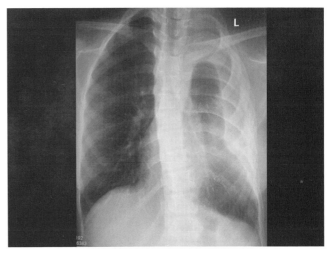

Figure 37.16: Chest radiograph [postero-anterior view] of a 12-year-old boy with left-sided TB empyema. The left hemithorax shows volume loss, rib crowding and pleural thickening
TB = tuberculosis

thus making them poor candidates for conventional open surgery; and [ii] in patients with trapped lung or TB empyema, VATS could achieve full lung re-expansion with minimal morbidity. However, therapeutic lung resection using VATS in patients with TB is technically demanding and potentially hazardous. Its role is, at present, limited. The reader is also referred to the chapter *"Surgery for pleuropulmonary tuberculosis"* [Chapter 46] for more details.

NEUROLOGICAL TUBERCULOSIS

Neurological TB constitutes almost half the cases of childhood TB. The reader is referred to the chapter *"Neurological tuberculosis"* [Chapter 17] and *"Tuberculosis in children"* [Chapter 36] for more details.

Surgical Therapy

Intrathecal hyaluronidase has been used in children with thick basal exudates. Besides clearing up meningeal adhesions hyaluronidase helps in better diffusion of drugs and reverses or reduces vasculitis. A weekly dose of 1000-1500 units for five to ten weeks has been recommended as treatment (34).

In 50% or more cases, there is established hydrocephalus [Figure 37.17] requiring treatment. Meningeal exudates not only obstruct cerebrospinal fluid [CSF] pathways but can occlude large vessels in the circle of Willis, the middle cerebral artery in the Sylvian fissure and the lenticulostriate vessels causing infarction. The aetiopathogenesis of hydrocephalus in TBM involves blockage of the basal cisterns by the TB

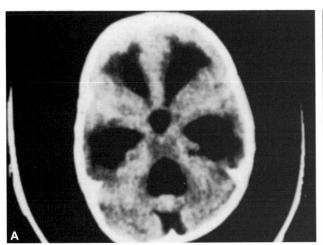
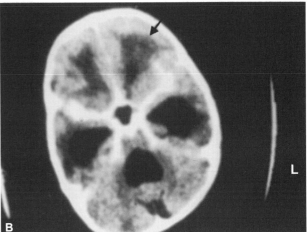

Figure 37.17: NCCT of the head showing obscured suprasellar cisterns [A] which manifest intense enhancement with intravenous contrast. Communicating hydrocephalus with periventricular ooze [arrow] is also seen [B]
NCCT = non-contrast computed tomography

exudates in the acute stage and adhesive leptomeningitis in the chronic stage resulting in communicating hydrocephalus. The aqueduct of sylvius may be blocked by circumferential compression of the brainstem by the meningeal exudates leading to non-communicating hydrocephalus. Rarely, an intraluminal subependymal tuberculoma or a plug of ependymal exudate may block the aqueduct.

In patients with hydrocephalus due to TBM, surgical management is indicated if the signs and symptoms suggestive of raised intracranial pressure persist despite adequate medical therapy. Increasing ventriculomegaly with periventricular ooze, recent onset papilloedema and signs and symptoms of raised intracranial pressure like vomiting, hypertonia, gaze palsies and bradycardia are indications for shunt surgery (35-40). Ventriculoperitoneal shunts are preferred over ventriculoatrial shunts unless the peritoneal cavity is involved in the disease. Various shunt systems are available and all of them involve a one-way pressure regulated valve. CSF examination is mandatory before shunt placement. The presence of persistent infection in the CSF can lead to a low-grade peritoneal inflammation and pseudocyst formation. Further, the high protein content of the CSF has been implicated in the higher incidence of shunt blockage seen in this setting. Intraventricular septae and ependymal adhesions complicate the picture and cause incomplete decompression of ventricles. Ventriculoscopy and adhesiolysis may be required to break the loculations and allow free CSF drainage. It must be remembered that CSF shunting has definite serious complications and, therefore, the decision to place a shunt must be individualised and based on definite indications.

Intracranial tuberculomas can be multiple [Figure 37.18]. If the tuberculoma is large or is located in the pathway of CSF circulation, surgical removal is essential [Figure 37.19]. However, in majority of the patients, tuberculomas respond well to anti-TB treatment and corticosteroids.

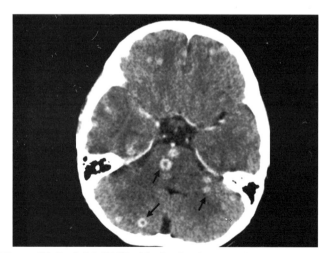

Figure 37.18: Axial CECT of brain showing multiple ring enhancing lesions in the brain suggestive of tuberculomas
CECT = contrast-enhanced computed tomography

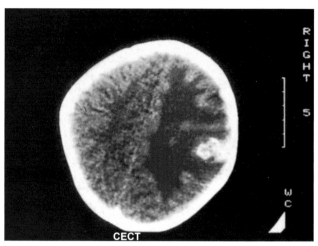

Figure 37.19: CECT of the head showing contrast-enhancing granuloma with lobulated outline and surrounding oedema. Tuberculoma is difficult to differentiate reliably from other inflammatory granulomas on the basis of CT alone
CECT = contrast-enhanced computed tomography; CT = computed tomography

COMPLICATIONS OF SURGERY FOR TUBERCULOSIS IN CHILDREN

Complications of surgery in childhood TB are shown in Table 37.4. The surgical complications or post-operative sequelae may be due to an ongoing process of cicatrisation as a result of healing. Hence, emphasis should be on initial adequate drug therapy, meticulous surgery and regular follow-up. Follow-up of at least 12 months after completion of therapy and life-long follow-up is suggested in cases with calcification.

Table 37.4: Some of the complications of surgery in childhood TB

Pulmonary TB	Contralateral spread of disease Retention of secretions Nonspecific pneumonia Symptomatic air space Infarction of middle lobe Postoperative haemorrhage Empyema
Abdominal	Inadvertent bowel injury Entero-cutaneous fistulae
Genitourinary TB	Following reconstructive surgery
TB = tuberculosis	

REFERENCES

1. Detjen AK, DiNardo AR, Leyden J, Steingart KR, Menzies D, Schiller I, et al. Xpert MTB/RIF assay for the diagnosis of pulmonary tuberculosis in children: a systematic review and meta-analysis. Lancet Respir Med 2015;3:451-61.
2. Sharma SK, Ryan H, Khaparde S, Sachdeva KS, Singh AD, Mohan A, et al. Index-TB guidelines: Guidelines on extrapulmonary tuberculosis for India. Indian J Med Res 2017;145: 448-63.

3. World Health Organization. Automated real-time nucleic acid amplification technology for rapid and simultaneous detection of tuberculosis and rifampicin resistance: Xpert MTB/RIF assay for the diagnosis of pulmonary and extrapulmonary TB in adults and children: policy update. Geneva: World Health Organization; 2013.

4. Christensen WI. Genitourinary tuberculosis. Review of 102 cases. Medicine 1974;53:377-92.

5. Wechsler H, Westfall M, Lattimer KK. The earliest signs and symptoms in male patients with genitourinary tuberculosis. J Urol 1960;83:801-3.

6. Ocon J, Novillo R, Villavicencio H, Del Rio G, Castellet R, Izquierdo F, et al. Renal tuberculosis and hypertension: value of the renal vein renin ratio. Eur Urol 1984;10:114-20.

7. Bajpai M, Dave S. Genitourinary tuberculosis. In: Seth V, editor. Essentials of tuberculosis in children. New Delhi: Jaypee Brothers Medical Publishers; 1997.p.203.

8. Millar AJW, Rode H, Cywes S. Abdominal tuberculosis in children - surgical management. A 10-year review of 95 cases. Pediatr Surg Int 1990;5:392-6.

9. Talat N, Afzal M, Ahmad S, Rasool N, Wasti AR, Saleem M. Role of diagnostic laparoscopy in evaluation and treatment of chronic abdominal pain in children. J Ayub Med Coll Abbottabad 2016;28:35-8.

10. Malik R, Srivastava A, Yachha SK, Poddar U, Lal R. Childhood abdominal tuberculosis: Disease patterns, diagnosis, and drug resistance. Indian J Gastroenterol 2015;34:418-25.

11. Sharma AK, Agarwal LD, Sharma CS, Sarin YK. Abdominal tuberculosis in children. Experience over a decade. Indian Pediatr 1993;30:1149-52.

12. Gupta DK, Bajpai M. Abdominal tuberculosis. In: Seth V, editor. Essentials of tuberculosis in children. New Delhi: Jaypee Brothers Medical Publishers; 1997.p.140.

13. Saczek KB, Schaaf HS, Voss M, Cotton MF, Moore SW. Diagnostic dilemmas in abdominal tuberculosis in children. Pediatr Surg Int 2001;17:111-5.

14. Talat N, Afzal M, Ahmad S, Rasool N, Wasti AR, Saleem M. Role of Diagnostic laparoscopy in evaluation and treatment of chronic abdominal pain in children. J Ayub Med Coll Abbottabad 2016;28:35-8.

15. Bahari HM. Perforation of tuberculous enteritis: report of a case. Med J Malays 1978;32:282-4.

16. Wani I, Ommid M, Waheed A, Asif M. Tuberculous abdominal cocoon. Ulus Travma Acil Cerrahi Derg 2010;16:508-10.

17. Ara C, Sogutlu G, Yildiz R, Kocak O, Isik B, Yilmaz S, et al. Spontaneous small bowel perforations due to intestinal tuberculosis should not be repaired by simple closure. J Gastrointest Surg 2005;9:514-7.

18. Bhansali SK. The challenge of abdominal tuberculosis in 310 cases. Indian J Surg 1978;40:65-77.

19. Venkatesh V, Everson NW, Johnstone MS. Atypical mycobacterial lymphadenopathy in children—is it underdiagnosed? J R Coll Surg Edinb 1994;39:301-3.

20. Xu JJ, Peer S, Papsin BC, Kitai I, Propst EJ. Tuberculous lymphadenitis of the head and neck in Canadian children: Experience from a low-burden region. Int J Pediatr Otorhinolaryngol 2016;91:11-4.

21. Herzog LW. Prevalence of lymphadenopathy of the head and neck in infants and children. Clin Pediatr 1983;22:485-7.

22. Dandapat MC, Mishra BM, Dash SP, Kar PK. Peripheral lymph node tuberculosis: a review of 80 cases. Br J Surg 1990;77:911-2.

23. Zheng JW, Zhang QH. Tuberculosis of the parotid gland: a report of 12 cases. J Oral Maxillofac Surg 1995;53:849-51.

24. Tebruegge M, Pantazidou A, MacGregor D, Gonis G, Leslie D, Sedda L, et al. Nontuberculous mycobacterial disease in children—epidemiology, diagnosis & management at a tertiary center. PLoS One 2016;11:e0147513.

25. López-Varela E, García-Basteiro AL, Santiago B, Wagner D, van Ingen J, Kampmann B. Non-tuberculous mycobacteria in children: muddying the waters of tuberculosis diagnosis. Lancet Respir Med 2015;3:244-56.

26. Goussard P, Gie R. Airway involvement in pulmonary tuberculosis. Paediatr Respir Rev 2007;8:118-23.

27. Freixinet J, Varela A, Lopez Rivero L, Caminero JA, Rodriguez de Castro F, Serrano A. Surgical treatment of childhood mediastinal tuberculous lymphadenitis. Ann Thorac Surg 1995;59:644-6.

28. Papagiannopoulos KA, Linegar AG, Harris DG, Rossouw GJ. Surgical management of airway obstruction in primary tuberculosis in children. Ann Thorac Surg 1999;68:1182-6.

29. Goussard P, Gie RP, Janson JT, le Roux P, Kling S, Andronikou S, et al. Decompression of enlarged mediastinal lymph nodes due to Mycobacterium tuberculosis causing severe airway obstruction in children. Ann Thorac Surg 2015;99:1157-63.

30. Pomerantz M, Brown J. The surgical management of tuberculosis. Semin Thorac Cardiovasc Surg 1995;7:108-11.

31. Yim AP, Low JM, Ng SK, Ho JK, Liu KK. Video-assisted thoracoscopic surgery in the paediatric population. J Paediatr Child Health 1995;31:192-6.

32. Yim AP. The role of video-assisted thoracoscopic surgery in the management of pulmonary tuberculosis. Chest 1996;110:829-32.

33. Chen B, Zhang J, Ye Z, Ye M, Ma D, Wang C, et al. Outcomes of video-assisted thoracic surgical decortication in 274 patients with tuberculous empyema. Ann Thorac Cardiovasc Surg 2015;21:223-8.

34. Udani PM. Management of tuberculosis meningitis. Indian J Pediatr 1985;52:171-4.

35. Bajpai M. Management of hydrocephalus. Indian J Pediatr 1997;64:48-56.

36. Harold LR. Treatment of hydrocephalus. In: Cheek WR, Marlin AE, McLone DG, Reigel DH, Walker ML, editors. Pediatric neurosurgery. Third edition. Philadelphia: WB Saunders Company; 1994.p.202-20.

37. Que S, Gao Z, Zheng J, Lu J, Qiu P, Qi X, et al. Ventricular-peritoneal shunt for an infant with post-meningitic external hydrocephalus. J Craniofac Surg 2015;26:2236-7.

38. Goyal P, Srivastava C, Ojha BK, Singh SK, Chandra A, Garg RK, et al. A randomized study of ventriculoperitoneal shunt versus endoscopic third ventriculostomy for the management of tubercular meningitis with hydrocephalus. Childs Nerv Syst 2014;30:851-7.

39. Vadivelu S, Effendi S, Starke JR, Luerssen TG, Jea A. A review of the neurological and neurosurgical implications of tuberculosis in children. Clin Pediatr [Phila] 2013;52:1135-43.

40. Savardekar A, Chatterji D, Singhi S, Mohindra S, Gupta S, Chhabra R. The role of ventriculoperitoneal shunt placement in patients of tubercular meningitis with hydrocephalus in poor neurological grade: a prospective study in the pediatric population and review of literature. Childs Nerv Syst 2013;29:719-25.

38

Tuberculosis in the Elderly

Surendran Deepanjali, Tamilarasu Kadhiravan

INTRODUCTION

The past century had witnessed an impressive improvement in human survival across the globe brought about by advances in modern medicine. Average life-expectancy at birth had improved from 48 years to 65 years over the period of 1955-1995, and is expected to improve further to 73 years by 2025 (1). This increase had been observed in all regions of the world. On the other hand, fertility rates had steadily declined all around the globe, and this secular trend continues to hold (2). As a result, the age-structure of populations is undergoing a marked change [Figure 38.1] (3). Globally, in a few years' time, elderly people will outnumber children. The elderly population [aged ≥ 65 years] is projected to grow from an estimated 524 million in 2010 to nearly 1.5 billion in 2050 (4). Notably, most of this increase would happen in the developing countries [250% *versus* 71% increase] (4). In India, the average life-expectancy improved from 56.3 years in early 1980s to 66.3 years by 2011; simultaneously, the fertility rate declined from 4.47 births

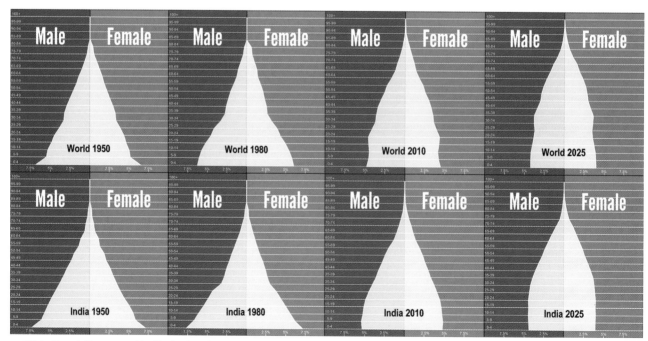

Figure 38.1: Population pyramids illustrating the age-composition of population during 1950 to 2025 [projected] in the world [top panels] and India [bottom panels]

Reproduced with permission from "http://populationpyramid.net/ Courtesy: Martin De Wulf"

in early 1980s to 2.5 births per woman in 2011 (5,6). While the elderly [aged ≥ 60 years] constituted 5.3% of Indian population in 1960, the contribution is expected to rise to 11% by 2025 (7).

Alongside this demographic transition, the relative burden of human illnesses is also witnessing a substantial change. The Global Burden of Disease Study 2010 (8) found that ageing of the world's population contributed to a 11.2% decrease in mortality due to communicable, maternal, neonatal, and nutritional disorders over the period 1990-2010; on the other hand, ageing contributed to a 39.2% increase in deaths due to non-communicable diseases. During this period, mortality due to tuberculosis [TB] saw a relative decrease of 18.7%. As a result, TB fell from 6th to 10th position among the top 25 causes of global deaths and likewise dropped to the 11th position from its previous ninth position among the top 25 causes of years of life lost globally (8). Notwithstanding this general decline in infectious diseases, TB continues to be a public health burden in developing countries (9). It has been recognised since long that ageing is a risk factor for TB, and that age is closely linked to the treatment outcome in patients with TB. The profound change in the demographic structure of populations, is thus, likely to alter the epidemiology of TB both in endemic as well as non-endemic countries.

EPIDEMIOLOGY OF TUBERCULOSIS IN THE ELDERLY

The generally accepted concept is that in low-burden, developed countries, TB is a disease of elderly native-born and the immigrant populations while it commonly affects young adults in high-burden, developing countries (10-12). However, this is a simplistic supposition since the epidemiology of TB is influenced by the interplay of multiple factors, some of which might be context specific such as the prevalence of human immunodeficiency virus [HIV] infection in the population. In the United States, persons aged 65 years and above constituted 21% of all TB cases notified in the year 2011. Interestingly, this proportion has remained fairly the same over time, despite a progressive decline in the risk of TB across all age-groups during the period 1993-2011 (13). Over this period, the incidence rates in elderly have consistently remained higher than the rest of the population [Figure 38.2]. Moreover, the higher risk among elderly was apparent in all ethnic groups such as Whites, African, Americans, Asians, Hispanics, Pacific islanders, and American Indians or Alaskans (13). In contrast, a study from Switzerland found that TB among the foreign-born most commonly affected the younger ages with less than 5% of patients aged 65 years and above, whereas among the native-born nearly 50% of patients were aged 65 years and above. Further, the native-born TB patients had a bimodal age distribution—the other peak in the younger age group was attributable to HIV infection (14). In the United Kingdom, where 74% of all cases reported in 2011 were among the foreign-born, elderly [≥ 65 years] constituted 14% of all cases (15).

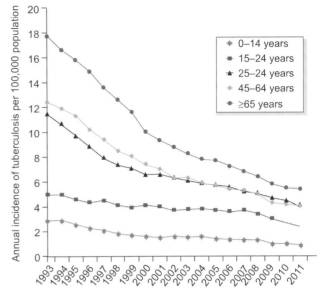

Figure 38.2: Time trends in age-specific TB incidence in the United States during 1993 to 2011
Based on data from reference 13

Population-based studies from India, a high burden country, had found increased prevalence as well as incidence of both latent TB infection [LTBI] and active TB as the age increases, especially among people aged 55 years or more. A population-based survey in southern India during 1961-1968 found that the average annual incidence of TB among those aged 55 years or more was 327 per 100,000 population while it was 153 per 100,000 among those aged 35-54 years (16). Similarly, more contemporary [1999-2006] population-based surveys from south India also confirm a substantially higher prevalence of culture-positive TB in the 55-64 and above 65 years age-groups compared to the rest of the population (17,18).

A modest over-representation of elderly is observed among TB patients in India; 8.3% of all smear-positive pulmonary TB cases notified in the year 2011 were aged 65 years or above, while they constituted only about 5.1% of the total Indian population in 2010 (7). Thus, it is reasonable to believe that the elderly are at a higher risk of TB even in high-burden settings. In fact, nearly 10% of all new smear-positive pulmonary TB notified in the year 2011 from the 22 high-burden countries was among the elderly aged 65 years or more (9). There exists a possibility that these figures might, in fact underestimate the actual burden of TB among the elderly, as sick elderly people do not always seek care and are largely dependent on others for their health care needs. On the other hand, in the World Health Organization [WHO] African region, just about 4% of smear-positive TB cases notified in 2011 were among the elderly (9). In African countries like South Africa, the major burden of TB is borne by young adults aged 20-50 years, attributable to the influence of the HIV epidemic (19).

It emerges that the contribution of elderly to the total number of TB cases depends on the relative contribution of elderly to the total population as well as the differential decline/increase in the incidence of TB in the younger age-groups. For example, a burgeoning elderly population would increase the relative contribution of elderly to the total number of TB cases. Likewise, decreasing transmission in the community brought about by effective TB control programmes with a resultant decline among the younger ages would also increase the relative contribution of elderly. It should be noted that both these factors are currently influencing the epidemiology of TB. On the other hand, any increase in the risk of TB among the younger ages and a decrease in life expectancy, as it happened in some African countries with the advent of the HIV epidemic, would attenuate the contribution of elderly to the TB burden.

Ageing and Risk of Tuberculosis

Leaving aside the issue of the relative contribution of the elderly to the total TB burden, an entirely different question that needs to be answered is, whether the elderly are intrinsically at a higher risk of TB. The absolute risk of TB in elderly is influenced mainly by two factors—prevalence of LTBI and the risk of reactivation. In light of the contribution of reinfection [detailed below], the risk of progression following a reinfection should also be considered as the third factor. In any population, irrespective of the level of endemicity, the prevalence of LTBI increases with age. The gradient in the prevalence of LTBI between the young and elderly sections of the population is more pronounced in countries with a currently low burden of TB. Historically, however, these countries had witnessed a high burden of TB several decades ago in the past. Most of the elderly people presently living in the low-burden countries were born during this era. Thus, the majority of the elderly in these countries is supposed to have got infected several decades ago when the annual risk of TB infection was high and effective anti-TB treatment was unavailable. In fact, early epidemiological studies concluded that the higher risk of TB in this population was just a reflection of a high burden of LTBI among them. This phenomenon is known as the "generation or birth cohort effect" (10,20). Frost described this as *"the peak of [tuberculosis related] mortality in late life does not represent postponement of maximum risk to a later period, but rather would seem to indicate that the present high rates in old age are the residuals of higher rates in earlier life"* (21).

Seminal epidemiological studies (21-23) have demonstrated that the apparently higher risk of TB mortality among the elderly seen in cross-sectional studies of populations is actually a fallacy. Rather when the populations were studied as birth cohorts, the risk of TB death peaked among children [0-5 years] and young adults [20-30 years] and the risk was comparatively less among the elderly (22,23). The counterintuitive finding that the risk was lower among elderly is fascinating and was attributed by Frost (21), Andord *et al* (23) to host resistance. Possibly, it represents a healthy survivor bias as a result of natural selection operating at younger ages. In fact, the phenomenon of higher incidence in the elderly compared to the young has been

described by some as a sign of successful TB control (24). However, with a substantially lesser selection pressure due to decreasing transmission and the availability of curative treatment, more and more susceptible persons might survive to old age in the future as compared to the past. As a result of this easing selection pressure, the cohort-contour that was described to be constant across generations based on data from the pre-chemotherapy era [1851-1930] might get distorted (22).

On the other hand, some authors have contested the notion that the actual risk of TB is less among the elderly, based on more contemporaneous data (25). Davies (25) reported that the decline in the risk of after adulthood has started reversing since 1978 in Hong Kong during the period 1953-1993 (26). Another study (27) from the same population covering the time period 1961-2005, employing a robust age-period-cohort modelling approach, found that after adjusting for the effects of birth cohort and time period, *"the relative risk of age began to rise in both men and women in the 5-9 year age group, peaked at 20-24 years, then quickly declined to a nadir in the 45-49 year age group, and finally showed an upturn during the eighth decade for women which was not apparent for men. Whereas both sexes [female more so than male] showed an upward inflection as they approached their 70s, this effect was only observed for people born later [1911-56] but not earlier [1876-1906]"*. It is really remarkable that the cohort-contour described by Andvord continues to hold true even today, barring the upturn in the later part of life. This upturn in the risk of TB case-notifications among the elderly is possibly an early indication of the easing selection pressure at younger ages as a result of successful TB control. While such a conclusion is entirely speculative, it is not biologically implausible given the fact that ample evidence exists to attest the fact that humans and *Mycobacterium tuberculosis* [*Mtb*] have co-evolved over a long period of time pre-dating the Neolithic period (28). Thus, at the end of this convoluted series of arguments, it emerges that the contemporary elderly are perhaps at a higher risk of TB, especially in populations where there has been a sustained improvement in control.

RE-INFECTION VERSUS RE-ACTIVATION

The higher risk of TB among the elderly is attributable to a higher risk of reactivation of LTBI. The majority of TB disease in the elderly is believed to be caused by re-activation of endogenous infection rather than by exogenous new infection/re-infection (29). In one of the earliest population-based molecular epidemiological studies from San Francisco, USA [1991-1992], clustering of isolates was seen much less frequently among the elderly compared to the rest [24% *versus* 46%], indicating that the majority of cases were not attributable to recent infection (30). A subsequent molecular epidemiological analysis of all TB cases reported over a 13-year period [1991-2003] in San Francisco also confirmed the finding that cases aged over 55 years were significantly less likely to be in a cluster (31). In Norway, 213 of 418 *Mtb* isolates during 1998-2005 from persons born before 1950 were attributed to re-activation (32).

In a population-based study from Florida, USA, HIV-seronegative persons aged over 50 years had a four-fold higher risk of re-activation (33). In another study from New York, USA, 75 [76%] of 98 TB patients aged over 60 years had a unique IS6110 deoxyribonucleic acid [DNA] fingerprint, while only 210 [47%] of 448 patients younger than 60 years had a unique isolate (34). Thus, multiple molecular epidemiological studies done in low-burden countries have shown decreased 'clustering' of cases in the elderly population, which suggests endogenous re-activation, rather than exogenous infection.

Another study from the USA which examined TB among foreign-born US residents found that the elderly immigrants with TB had a 4.5-fold higher odds of reactivation TB compared to younger immigrants [< 15 years] with TB (35). A population-based molecular epidemiologic study on a rural southern Indian population found that 38% of patients were in clusters suggesting recent transmission (36). In contrast to other studies, among patients detected by house-to-house survey, patients in clusters were significantly older than those with unique isolates [55 *versus* 43 years]. While the reason for this aberrant observation is unclear, it is possible that an elderly patient with endogenous reactivation could be the original source of infection in such clusters (36).

From the data discussed earlier, it also emerges that even in low-burden settings, at least a fourth of cases among the elderly could be the result of recent infection. Of late, an important role for exogenous re-infection has been proposed based on epidemiological and experimental evidence (37). This is particularly important in high-burden countries like India with high rates going on of TB transmission in the community (38). On the other hand, in low-burden countries like the USA, clustering of cases due to spread of infection has been reported among elderly residing in nursing homes and long-term care facilities (11,39). The risk of active TB among them is almost two- to three-fold higher compared to community-dwelling elders.

AGEING AND IMMUNOSENESCENCE

In general, the elderly are considered to be more susceptible to infectious diseases (40). 'Immunosenescence'—a decline in immunity with ageing—is characterised by defects in the haematopoietic bone marrow, impaired peripheral lymphocyte migration, maturation and function, and chronic involution of the thymus gland (41). The age-related decline in output of T-cells from thymus is compensated by an increase in the lifespan of naïve CD4+ T-cells mediated by decreased levels of the proapoptotic molecule (42,43). However, these naïve T-cells with increased lifespan are functionally defective (44,45). A robust antigen-specific CD4+ T-cell response and production of T-helper 1 [Th1]-associated cytokines, such as, interferon gamma [IFN-γ], interleukin-12 [IL-12], and tumour necrosis factor-alpha [TNF-α] are necessary for immunity against TB (46). Paradoxically, in murine experiments with aerosol delivery of *Mtb* to the lungs, old mice exhibit some early resistance to infection that is mediated by CD8+ T-cells, but they subsequently have a higher bacterial load in the lungs than the younger ones

and evidence of more haematogenous dissemination to the liver (46-48). A low antigen-specific CD4+ T-cell proliferative capacity and a decline in natural killer [NK] cell activity have also been demonstrated in the elderly (46,49). The gamut of immune system changes due to ageing is quite similar to that of HIV infection (50). Although these factors may potentially predispose to re-activation of LTBI or development of disease after exogenous infection in the elderly, conclusive evidence for the purported role of immunosenescence in humans is still not available.

RISK FACTORS

The various risk factors known to predispose otherwise healthy adults to TB, increase the risk of TB among the elderly also (51). Many studies have found a preponderance of men among the elderly TB patients. The lower prevalence of TB in women is often attributed to poor care-seeking behaviour and barriers to access healthcare. But, population-based studies from India have also found a consistently lower prevalence of TB among women of all age-groups compared to men (16,18). Diabetes mellitus is another well-recognised risk factor that increases the risk for TB by 2- to 3-fold (52,53). Globally, about 10% of TB cases are attributable to diabetes mellitus (54,55). A burgeoning elderly population in the low- and middle-income countries is set to increase the burden of diabetes in these countries, thereby posing a challenge to TB control (56,57). Likewise, tobacco smoking is another risk factor for TB whose significance is being increasingly recognised (58). Notwithstanding the fact that the prevalence of active smoking declines with ageing, a population-based study from southern India found that at least 45% of TB deaths among the urban living and at least 28% of TB deaths among the rural living elderly men aged 65 years or more were attributable to smoking (59). In addition to these risk factors, poor socio-economic conditions, such as, poverty, malnutrition, and overcrowding and other co-morbidities, like chronic renal failure, malignancy, silicosis, post-gastrectomy status, and use of immuno-suppressive drugs render the elderly population more vulnerable to TB (60).

CLINICAL FEATURES OF TUBERCULOSIS IN THE ELDERLY

Pulmonary Tuberculosis

In general, TB among the elderly is characterised by a higher frequency of atypical clinical presentations. Pulmonary TB in the elderly may also present with typical clinical and radiographic features. However, atypical presentations are often encountered in the elderly, leading to the premise whether it is a different disease altogether (61). A number of studies in the past had compared the clinical features of pulmonary TB in the elderly with younger patients, and their findings were variable and sometimes even discordant (62-66). Differences that were observed in these studies include more frequent mid- and lower-zone infiltrates, miliary shadows, post-mortem diagnosis, and concomitant comorbidities; and a comparatively infrequent occurrence of fever, weight loss, night sweats, expectoration, haemoptysis, positive tuberculin skin test [TST], cavitating lung infiltrates, and alcoholism among elderly TB patients.

In a pooled analysis of 12 studies that together had compared 859 elderly with 1,801 young pulmonary TB patients, male preponderance was similar among both younger and elderly TB patients (67). Similarly, there was no difference between young and older patients with respect to evolution time before diagnosis, frequency of cough or sputum production, weight loss, and fatigue. But, fever, night sweats, and haemoptysis were less frequent among the elderly. Interestingly, there was no significant difference in the frequency of radiographic upper lobe lesions and sputum-smear positivity, even though cavitation was significantly less common among the elderly (67). Other studies have also found that ageing does not drastically influence the frequency of upper lobe involvement in pulmonary TB; but, it definitely increases the concomitant involvement of lower lobes (68-70). The frequent involvement of lower lobes in elderly has been traditionally ascribed to poor immunity and disease caused by re-infection. However, age-related changes in lung ventilation–perfusion are thought to predominantly affect the lower lobes leading to a higher alveolar oxygen tension in the lower lobes, which favours the multiplication of *Mtb* (69).

Diabetes mellitus exhibits a complex interaction with ageing to influence the clinical and radiographic findings of pulmonary—[i] patients with diabetes and TB are comparatively older; [ii] the male preponderance of TB is not observed among patients with diabetes mellitus; [iii] in elderly diabetes mellitus increases the chances of lower lobe lesions [synergism] as well as cavitation [antagonism]; and, diabetes mellitus modestly decreases the frequency of upper lobe involvement (69,71,72). Rarely, pulmonary TB in the elderly may present as organising pneumonia. Parenchymal pseudotumoural variant of pulmonary TB does not seem to have a predilection for the elderly.

Perez-Guzman *et al* (67) also found that elderly TB patients had lower serum albumin levels, and a negative tuberculin skin test was more common. Dyspnoea was more commonly seen in the elderly, attributable to a greater prevalence of concomitant medical conditions, like cardiovascular diseases, chronic obstructive pulmonary disease, diabetes, and cancers among the elderly. On the contrary, alcoholism was more common among younger TB patients. Most of these differences could be because of the physiological changes associated with ageing (67).

After the publication of this meta-analysis, several small-sized studies from India had compared the clinical presentation of TB in the elderly, and their observations were largely similar to the findings of this meta-analysis (73-77). To date, the largest study of TB among the elderly from India is a retrospective population-based study of 1,485 TB patients aged 60 years or more who were treated under the national programme in 12 of the 32 districts of the southern state of Tamil Nadu during the second quarter of 2011 (78). However, since the study involved a review of data collected by the programme, detailed information on the differences in clinical presentation between elderly and the rest was not available. Notwithstanding, there was no excess of sputum-smear negative pulmonary cases among the newly treated elderly compared to the rest [34% *versus* 32%]. However, extra-pulmonary TB [EPTB] was much less common among the elderly [12% *versus* 23%] (78).

Fever of Unknown Origin

Sometimes, symptoms such as anorexia, fatigue, change in cognitive state, mental dullness, or simply 'failure to thrive' may be the sole manifestation of TB in an elderly patient [Figure 38.3]. As noted above, fever may not be a prominent feature. However, TB does present sometimes as fever of unknown origin [FUO] in the elderly, as it often does in the young. In two large case series from China covering the years 2000-2008, TB was the most frequent infectious cause of FUO among patients aged 60 years or more – 103 of 397 patients and 13 of 87 patients had TB in these studies (79,80). Further, contrary to the earlier assertion that extrapulmonary disease is comparatively infrequent among the elderly, a high proportion of elderly patients with presenting as FUO had EPTB (79,80). Similarly, vintage studies from developed countries also found that TB was an important cause of FUO in the elderly (81,82). In fact, 11 of the 100 cases of FUO originally studied by Petersdorf and Beeson in the 1950s were due to TB; three of their 11 TB patients were aged more than 60 years (83). However, TB is much less common in more contemporary studies from developed countries.

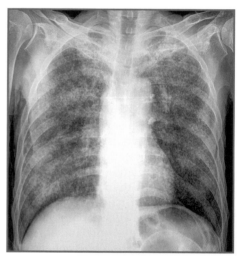

Figure 38.3: Atypical clinical presentation of TB in the elderly. Chest radiograph [postero-anterior view] of an 80-year-old man with no known comorbidities who presented with anorexia, dysphagia, and inanition since 20 days; symptoms were preceded by a low-grade fever for 2 days. Treating physician did not suspect TB; but, a routinely performed chest radiograph revealed miliary mottling, after which anti-TB treatment was started presumptively. However, patient succumbed 15 days later. TB was confirmed on post-mortem examination.
TB = tuberculosis

But, it continues to be one of the causes of FUO, and its diagnosis is often delayed (84-86). Apart from a general decline in the incidence of TB, another potential reason for a decline in TB as a cause of FUO is the widespread availability of non-invasive imaging modalities such as computed tomography and magnetic resonance imaging (86).

Cryptic Miliary Tuberculosis

A related clinical entity was described in 1969 by Proudfoot and colleagues (87) as 'cryptic military TB'. They reported a series of 16 patients that *"did not present the clinical and radiographic features associated with classical miliary TB"* (87). Most of these patients (11 of 16) were elderly that presented with malaise, weight loss, and fever that remained unexplained despite detailed investigation. Typically, these patients had a paucity of respiratory symptoms, and their chest radiographs showed no diagnostic abnormalities. In sharp contrast to other studies where the diagnosis was made only at necropsy, in this series a diagnosis of TB was suspected during life in all except two patients. Indeed, 10 patients showed a clinical response to a therapeutic trial of isoniazid and para-aminosalicylic acid (87). Proudfoot *et al* (87) concluded that, *"Cryptic miliary TB is a difficult diagnostic problem and should be suspected in any elderly patient, particularly a woman, who has an unexplained pyrexia, pancytopenia, or leukaemoid reaction"*. Such a clinical presentation was not entirely unknown before this seminal report. In 1962, several years ahead of Proudfoot's report, Bottiger *et al* (88) had described a series of 5 patients with miliary TB diagnosed at necropsy. They wrote, *"The disease resembles malignant neoplasia with weight loss, fever, and much-increased erythrocyte-sedimentation rate but without local signs"* (88). But, it was the legacy of Proudfoot *et al* (87) that popularised cryptic miliary TB as a distinct clinical entity.

When miliary TB manifests in a cryptic fashion, choroid tubercles are absent; enlargement of liver and spleen is frequently seen; and serosal cavity effusions are uncommon (89). Often, although not invariable, these patients have a non-reactive type of TB—described as *"Microscopically there is an abundance of small caseaeous [sic] necrotic lesions, especially in the liver and spleen, but characteristically no giant or epitheliod [sic] cells are found. The lesions generally contain enormous amounts of tubercle bacilli"* (88,90,91). A broad range of haematological abnormalities such as neutropenia, pancytopenia, leukaemoid reaction, and myelofibrosis have been described in such patients (91). Other laboratory abnormalities, such as, elevated alkaline phosphatase, hyponatraemia due to adrenal involvement, and hypokalaemia may also be seen (89). Nearly half the patients have associated co-morbidities such as diabetes, solid organ or haematologic cancers, and autoimmune diseases, that often distract the attention of the clinician (89,92).

As originally noted by Proudfoot *et al* (87), subsequent studies (90,92,93) also found that the age of patients with miliary TB [both overt and cryptic] had progressively increased over the years, while the number of cases actually showed a declining trend or remained stable. In a large series of 254 deaths due to miliary TB confirmed at autopsy in Finland during 1974-1993, the mean age of the patients was more than 75 years; the average age of 140 patients with cryptic form of the disease was 78 years (92). This finding is possibly attributable to a decline in childhood miliary TB as a result of improved TB control, while miliary TB in elderly increased due to re-activation in an ageing population (94). On the other hand, very few studies have been published on cryptic miliary TB during the past two decades. Presumably, the widespread availability of non-invasive imaging seems to have led to a decline in missed diagnoses. However, occasional cases of cryptic miliary TB in elderly continue to be recognised only at necropsy even in resource-replete settings (95). Hence, one must bear in mind another important observation by these studies that the cryptic variety in the elderly was as common as the overt classical miliary TB (87,90,92,93).

Extrapulmonary Tuberculosis

As mentioned earlier, the relative frequency of extrapulmonary involvement is considerably less in elderly with TB. In Poland, extrapulmonary TB constituted 8.5% of all TB notifications in elderly aged 60 years or more during the period 1974-2010, while it was 18.6% in those aged 0-19 years (96). The most common forms among the elderly were pleural effusion [34%], peripheral lymphadenitis [20%], genitourinary [13%], and osteoarticular TB [12%]. In contrast, intrathoracic lymphadenitis [44%], pleural effusion [22%], and peripheral lymphadenitis [11%] were common in the 0-19 years age-group (96). In an analysis of TB cases reported to the Centers for Disease Control and Prevention, USA, during 1993-2008, extrapulmonary disease was slightly less common among the elderly compared to younger adults aged 21-64 years [17.5% *versus* 18.9%] (97). However, 27% of all extrapulmonary notifications were among elderly aged over 60 years (98). Particularly, elderly contributed to about 35% of osteoarticular and genitourinary TB cases. Common forms of EPTB which may present differently in elderly are discussed here.

Pleural Tuberculosis

Pleural effusion occurs early during the natural history of *Mtb* infection. Most instances of TB pleural effusion develop 3-7 months following primary infection (99). Thus, understandably, TB pleural effusion is typically a disease of adolescents and young adults in high-burden settings. In a recently published large multicentric study of TB pleural effusions from India, elderly constituted less than 5% of patients (100). Similarly, of the 254 patients with tubercular pleural effusion treated at a Spanish University Hospital during 1989-1997, just 12% of patients were aged over 60 years (101). In another study from the same setting, it was also observed that 70% of pleural effusions in patients aged under 40 years were tubercular in origin (102). Whereas, only 10% of pleural effusions in those aged over 40 years were due to TB; malignancy and congestive heart failure were the most common causes in this age-group. Understanding this pre-test probability is very important from a diagnostic point of view [detailed below].

On the other hand, pleural effusion can also occur following re-activation of remote infection, especially in the elderly. Moudgil *et al* (103) observed that most cases of TB pleural effusion notified in Edinburgh during 1980-1991 were attributable to reactivation rather than primary infection; most of the pleural effusions due to re-activation were seen in persons aged 40 years or more. Similarly, in a study of 548 TB effusions from Spain, Sahn *et al* (104) noted that the mean age of patients had increased from 34 years to 43 years over the period that spanned two decades from 1991 to 2011, possibly indicating an increasing contribution of re-activation. The annual incidence of TB had fallen from 72 cases to 28 cases per 100,000 population in the study region over the period of 1996 to 2010. In Taiwan, which has a large and fast-growing elderly population and declining TB incidence, the mean age of patients with TB pleural effusion was 62 years (105). Similarly, in a series of 106 consecutive patients from South Korea, 41% were aged 60 years or more; 74% of all patients had computed tomographic features suggestive of re-activation TB, and such patients were about two decades older than those with features of primary infection (106). Pleural effusions occurring in the setting of sputum culture-positive TB indicating parenchymal disease is more common among the elderly [23% *versus* 9%] compared to the rest (70). Chest pain might be less frequent in elderly patients with TB pleural effusion; pleural thickening and calcification might be more frequently seen (107).

Tuberculosis Meningitis

Classically, the risk of meningitis is maximal during the initial 1-3 months following the primary infection when haematogenous seeding of the central nervous system [CNS] occurs (99). Thus, the risk of meningitis is disproportionately borne by children and young adults. However, empirical data from high-incidence settings suggest that tubercular meningitis is not confined to the younger ages. In a large clinical trial on tubercular meningitis in adolescents and adults aged over 14 years from Vietnam, about 13% of patients were elderly aged over 65 years, and almost 40% of all patients had chest radiographic features of active non-miliary TB, that may suggest the possibility of reactivation rather than primary infection as the proximate cause in many of them (108). In Turkey, a moderate incidence setting, a sizeable proportion of patients with tubercular meningitis diagnosed between 1985 and 1997 at 12 university hospitals, was elderly (109). The findings from low-incidence settings were also largely similar. In a nationwide study from Denmark, 18% of all adult TB meningitis patients were over 60 years of age; 45% of the cases were ethnic Danes (110). Danish natives with TB meningitis were more likely to be elderly compared to immigrants [28% *versus* 10%]. Similarly, in Houston, Texas, USA, 5% of all CNS TB diagnosed over a 10-year period [1995-2004] was among the elderly; only 27%

of all patients were foreign-born (111). It clearly emerges that irrespective of the epidemiologic setting, elderly contribute to a considerable burden of tubercular meningitis and other forms of CNS TB. However, it is unclear whether CNS involvement in the elderly is the result of reactivation or else follows fresh infection at a later age.

TB meningitis in the elderly may just present as unexplained obtundation, confusion, or irritability (112). Typical symptoms of a meningitic illness such as fever, headache, vomiting, and nuchal rigidity are often absent. Hyponatraemia caused by inappropriate secretion of antidiuretic hormone may be present contributing to the altered sensorium. Infrequently, TB meningitis in the elderly might present with cognitive defects clinically mimicking a dementia (113). In a series of 124 elderly patients evaluated for dementia at a teaching hospital in northern India, 10 were found to have CNS TB, which is potentially reversible with prompt treatment (114).

Other Forms of Extra-pulmonary Tuberculosis

TB lymphadenitis is uncommon in the elderly population (115). But, it may be encountered in specialist practices due to referral bias (116,117). In endemic regions, TB lymphadenitis may be incidentally found in nodes suspected to have metastatic cancers (118). Rarely, TB and malignancy might be present in the same lymph node (119). On the other hand, tubercular lymph nodes may closely mimic metastatic malignancy on fluorodeoxy glucose—positron emission tomography [FDG-PET] evaluation showing very high standardised uptake values (120). Paradoxical reaction, commonly encountered during treatment of tubercular lymphadenitis in the young, has also been reported in elderly patients (121).

Typically, genitourinary and skeletal TB clinically manifest a long time after the primary infection. Thus, a considerable proportion of these forms of TB will be in the elderly population. The mean age of patients with bone/joint TB and genitourinary TB in the USA was 50 years and 52 years respectively (98). Interestingly, in low-burden settings, genitourinary TB is more common among the native-born elderly than foreign-born immigrants (122). This is attributed to confounding by age rather than a true difference. Similarly, 82% of bone/joint TB in Denmark was among the native-born; the median age at diagnosis was 72 years (123). Spine and hip are the most commonly affected sites. Isolated involvement of a peripheral joint is not uncommon in the elderly, and when it presents so, the diagnosis is often delayed (124). Apart from symptoms referable to the local site of involvement, genitourinary and bone/joint TB may also present as FUO.

Comparison of clinical presentation of TB in the young and the elderly patients is shown in Table 38.1 (125).

DIAGNOSIS

The diagnostic tools for TB in the elderly do not differ from the rest. However, a diagnosis of TB in the elderly is often delayed and sometimes totally missed. Elderly contribute

Table 38.1: Comparison of clinical presentation of TB in the young and the elderly patients

Variable	Young	Elderly
Constitutional symptoms		
Fever	+	−
Night sweats	+	−
Non-specific symptoms*	+	−
Respiratory symptoms		
Cough	+	−
Haemoptysis	+	−
Dyspnoea	−	+
Comorbid conditions†	−	+
Hypoalbuminaemia	−	+
Tuberculin positivity	+	−
Adverse drug reactions	−	+

* = dizziness, mental dullness
† = chronic obstructive pulmonary disease, diabetes mellitus, bronchiectasis, stroke
TB = tuberculosis; + = more frequent; − = less frequent
Reproduced with permission from "van Cleeff M , Gondrie PCFM, Veen J. Tuberculosis in elderly. In: Sharma SK, Mohan A, editors. Tuberculosis. Second edition. New Delhi: Jaypee Brothers Medical Publishers; 2009.p.625-33" (reference 125)

to about 50% of all such missed opportunities for TB treatment (126). In the USA during 1985-1988, about 12% of TB cases among the elderly aged 65 years or more were diagnosed only at death; the figure was much higher among those aged over 85 years (126). Similarly, 8% of elderly with pulmonary TB diagnosed in Taipei city, Taiwan during 2005-2010 died before treatment could be initiated (127).

Two factors that are responsible for a delay in diagnosis are lack of suspicion and atypical clinical presentations. TB should always figure among the differentials in elderly presenting with lung infiltrates, pleural effusion, unexplained weight loss, FUO, failure to thrive, etc. A careful physical examination to look for lymphadenopathy and choroid tubercles is often rewarding in an elderly patient with FUO. The chest radiograph should be carefully looked at for miliary nodules. Biopsy of the bone marrow or liver may be considered, especially in the presence of cytopenias, hepatosplenic focal lesions, or elevated serum alkaline phosphatase.

While the sputum smear examination remains a useful diagnostic tool for pulmonary TB in the elderly (67), sometimes patients may not expectorate sputum due to frailty. In such circumstances, sputum induction and gastric washings might obviate the need for invasive procedures such as bronchoscopic sampling (128). While a high degree of suspicion is needed, entities like cryptogenic organising pneumonia are often misdiagnosed as pulmonary TB in endemic regions (129). High-resolution computed tomography could be of help in such situations (130).

Considerable caution is warranted while diagnosing TB pleural effusion in the elderly. Even if one assumes that

the sensitivity and specificity of pleural fluid adenosine deaminase [ADA] level to detect a TB pleural effusion are 100% and 95% respectively, at a disease frequency of 10%, the corresponding positive predictive value would still be just 70%, i.e., 30% of such effusions would actually be non-TB (101,131). The implication of this observation is that, an exudate with elevated ADA cannot be considered diagnostic of tubercular aetiology in elderly patients and further investigations such as pleural fluid cytology, pleural biopsy, and a contrast-enhanced computed tomographic imaging of the chest should always be done to rule out malignancy. Lymphoma is a common condition in the elderly that closely mimics tubercular pleural effusion in its clinical, radiological, and laboratory characteristics including a high ADA level in the pleural fluid (132). Drug-induced pleural effusion caused by tyrosine kinase inhibitors such as dasatinib may resemble TB effusion in its characteristics (133). Uraemic pleurisy is another condition in which it is often difficult to rule out the possibility of TB aetiology (134). The diagnostic utility of pleural fluid ADA in elderly is further complicated by issues surrounding its sensitivity. Recently, it has been recognised that elderly patients with TB pleural effusion have significantly lower levels of ADA in the pleural fluid, necessitating a lower cut-off which would further compromise its specificity (135,136). Likewise, ageing might influence the pleural fluid protein and lactate dehydrogenase levels causing difficulty in the identification of exudative pleural effusions (137). This is important, because the pleural fluid may be classified as a transudate in about 1% of otherwise proven cases of tubercular pleural effusion (104). But, the factors responsible for these aberrant transudates in TB are unknown; advanced age might be responsible in some of them. On the same note, the proportion of patients with lymphocyte predominance [>50%] on pleural fluid analysis may be considerably less among the elderly – 17% of patients had lymphocyte count less than 50% in a study of predominantly elderly (105) as opposed to 7% in another study of predominantly younger patients (101).

It is often difficult to differentiate spinal TB from metastatic cancer and myeloma, especially in early stages. In such situations, where the diagnosis of TB warrants an invasive procedure on an elderly patient, clinicians often resort to a trial of treatment with anti-TB treatment. Such decisions are only to be made on a case-by-case basis taking into consideration the various factors, such as, availability of sampling and laboratory testing facility, safety of the diagnostic procedure in a given patient, acuity of the clinical condition, turnaround time, limitations in sensitivity, risk of adverse drug reactions, possibility of promoting drug-resistance, and the dangers of missing an alternative diagnosis.

TREATMENT

General Principles and Adverse Effects

The principles of treatment of TB in the elderly are no different from that of other patient groups. But, as noted earlier, many of these patients have other medical comorbidities that might complicate the issue. They might be on drugs like oral hypoglycaemic agents, antihypertensives, digoxin, or theophylline, some of which might have clinically significant drug–drug interactions with rifampicin (12). Problems like cognitive impairment or dementia may lead to difficulty in comprehending how to take the medicines. Poor eyesight, poor memory, and lack of determination to complete 6-month long therapy may result in default (12). Elderly often depend on others to access health care and to take the drugs regularly. In countries like India, where a considerable fraction of people aged >60 years still work for livelihood, loss of wages might adversely affect adherence with directly observed therapy.

The risk of anti-TB drug-induced hepatotoxicity is at least two-fold higher in the elderly (138,139). Malnutrition and hypoalbuminaemia prevalent among the elderly may add to the risk (140). Ethambutol can cause optic neuritis in the presence of renal failure, and hence dose adjustment is needed. Advanced age is a risk factor for both nephrotoxicity and ototoxicity with aminoglycosides. The dose of streptomycin should not exceed 500-750 mg/day. The symptoms of toxicity might be presumed by patients as age-related and may not be reported early.

Treatment Outcome in the Elderly

Despite timely diagnosis and treatment, the outcomes in elderly TB patients are often worse. Only 73% of 812 elderly patients treated at a chest clinic in Delhi, India, over the period of 2005-2010 had a favourable outcome compared to 86% in the non-elderly (141). Rates of death [7.6% *versus* 1.5%] and loss to follow-up [9.9% *versus* 6.5%] were higher among the elderly. Likewise, aggregated unfavourable outcome [death, failure, or default] was more common among the elderly [16% *versus* 11%] treated under programme conditions in south India (78). Particularly, those aged over 70 years fared much worse than those aged 60-70 years [22% *versus* 14%]. Death during treatment largely accounted for these differences. Multiple studies from disparate epidemiologic settings have consistently found that elderly patients with TB are more likely to die compared to younger patients (126,142-144). The risk of death in elderly remains elevated even after the intensive phase of treatment (126,143). Further, the standardised mortality rate [SMR] in elderly TB patients aged 60 years or more was only 2.2 compared to an SMR of 15.1 in the 15-44 years age group (145). Both these observations clearly indicate that TB *per se* does not account for a substantial part of this mortality risk in the elderly. Rather, the excess risk is largely attributable to the frailty and multiple comorbidities which are often present in these patients. Very recently, it has been found that TB is independently associated with a 40% higher risk of acute coronary syndrome (146). Apart from treating early, it remains unclear at present how to mitigate the excess mortality among elderly with TB.

Drug-resistance, Human Immunodeficiency Virus Co-infection in the Elderly

While multidrug-resistant-TB [MDR-TB] and HIV-associated TB threaten to destabilise the global TB control, the situation is better in the elderly. Since most of the TB among the elderly is caused by re-activation of infection often acquired in the pre-chemotherapy era, primary drug-resistance including MDR is believed to be uncommon among the elderly (11). In the USA, during the period 1993-2007, the frequency of MDR-TB, including extensively drug-resistant TB [XDR-TB] among the elderly was 0.8% while it was 2.5% in the 25-44 years age group (147). Similarly, in the European Union and the European Economic Area, the frequency of MDR-TB [including XDR-TB] reported in 2012 was 2.1% among the elderly, while it was 5.4% in the 25-44 years age group (148). In the update to the fourth report of the WHO/International Union Against Tuberculosis and Lung Disease [IUATLD] global project on anti-TB drug resistance surveillance, in countries reporting continuous drug-resistance surveillance data, the frequency of MDR-TB decreased linearly with age and was lowest in persons aged 65 years or over (149). Even in the central and eastern European countries with a very high the frequency of MDR, it was still lowest in persons aged 65 years or more (150). But, it needs to be appreciated that the elderly are not completely protected against drug-resistant TB, and the treatment of MDR-TB, XDR-TB in an elderly patient is challenging.

As with MDR-TB, the problem of HIV-associated TB is largely confined to the younger ages even in high HIV prevalence settings. While 6.5% of all TB patients tested in 2011 had HIV co-infection in India (9), in a study from southern India only 1.5% of TB patients aged 60 years or more were HIV-infected (78). Interestingly, an age cut-off of over 50 years is customarily used to denote elderly in the context of HIV infection. At present, 7% of people living with HIV in India are aged over 50 years (150). But, with the widespread availability of life-saving antiretroviral treatment, a large number of HIV-infected persons will survive into their 60s and beyond. It is estimated that by 2015, half the people living with HIV would be aged over 50 years in the USA; a similar transition is expected in African countries as well (151). Although limited data indicate that TB is not more common in elderly with HIV (152), how this transition would impact the interaction between ageing, TB, and HIV is currently unknown.

LATENT TUBERCULOSIS INFECTION IN THE ELDERLY

Despite being an important clinical issue, TB in the elderly is not considered a problem that warrants population-level prevention, for various reasons. The present thinking is that elderly age *per se* is not an indication for targeting TB prevention. But, when elderly persons reside in settings favouring transmission to others such as elderly homes, homeless shelters, nursing homes, and other long-term care facilities, testing and treatment of LTBI is recommended in some developed countries (153). In resource-limited high burden settings, understandably, this is not a priority at present.

While a robust body of evidence from randomised controlled trials supports the efficacy isoniazid for preventing TB in general, elderly were not represented in most of these trials (154). A very low risk [<1%] of hepatitis was reported in the trial population. But, the risk of serious adverse events in the real-world setting is particularly high among the elderly. In a large population-based study from Quebec, Canada, 6% of elderly patients treated during 1998-2003 for LTBI experienced at least one hospitalisation for a serious adverse event (155). Hence, the potential benefit of preventive treatment needs to be carefully weighed against the risk of substantial harm in elderly. Stead (156) had argued that the risk-benefit ratio is favourable only in documented recent tuberculin converters among the elderly and not those with unknown timing of conversion. Decision analysis models also suggest that the direct benefit to the treated individual in terms of gain in life expectancy is very minimal (157,158). Thus, a non-selective test and treat strategy of all institutionalised elderly without taking into consideration the individual risk-benefit profile may not accrue net benefit. Perhaps for this reason, the British guidelines differ from the American guidelines—the former recommends individualised decision to treat LTBI in persons aged over 35 years (159).

REFERENCES

1. World Health Organization. World Health Report. 50 Facts: Global health situation and trends 1955-2025. Available at URL: www.who.int/whr/1998/media_centre/50facts/en/. Accessed on October 24, 2018.

2. World Bank. World Development Indicators: Reproductive health. Available at URL: http://wdi.worldbank.org/table/2.17. Accessed on November 25, 2018.

3. United Nations, Department of Economic and Social Affairs. World Population Prospects: The 2012 Revision. Demographic Profiles. Available at URL: http://esa.un.org/wpp/Demographic-Profiles/index.shtm. Accessed on November 25, 2018.

4. World Health Organisation, US National Institute of Aging. Global Health and Aging. Available at URL: http://www.who.int/ageing/publications/global_health.pdf. Accessed on November 25, 2018.

5. United Nations, Department of Economic and Social Affairs. World Population Prospects: The 2012 Revision. Detailed indicators. Life expectancy at birth: India, Medium variant, 1950-2100. Available at URL: http://esa.un.org/unpd/wpp/unpp/panel_indicators.htm. Accessed on November 25, 2018.

6. United Nations, Department of Economic and Social Affairs. World Population Prospects: The 2012 Revision. Detailed indicators. Total fertility: India, Medium variant, 1950-2100. Available at URL: http://esa.un.org/unpd/wpp/unpp/panel_indicators.htm. Accessed on Novemebr 25, 2018.

7. United Nations, Department of Economic and Social Affairs. World Population Prospects: The 2012 Revision. Detailed indicators. Population aged 60+: India, Medium variant, 1950-2100. Available at URL: http://esa.un.org/unpd/wpp/unpp/panel_indicators.htm. Accessed on November 25, 2018.

8. Lozano R, Naghavi M, Foreman K, Lim S, Shibuya K, Aboyans V, et al. Global and regional mortality from 235 causes of death for 20 age groups in 1990 and 2010: a systematic analysis for the Global Burden of Disease Study 2010. Lancet 2012;380:2095-128.

9. World Health Organization. Global tuberculosis report 2012. Geneva: World Health Organization; 2012.

10. Mori T, Leung CC. Tuberculosis in the global aging population. Infect Dis Clin North Am 2010;24:751-68.

11. Azami M, Sayehmiri K, Yekta Kooshali MH, Hafezi Ahmadi MR. The prevalence of tuberculosis among Iranian elderly patients admitted to the infectious ward of hospital: A systematic review and meta-analysis. Int J Mycobacteriol 2016;5 Suppl 1:S199-S200.

12. Schaaf HS, Collins A, Bekker A, Davies PD. Tuberculosis at extremes of age. Respirology 2010;15:747-63.

13. Centers for Disease Control and Prevention. Reported Tuberculosis in the United States, 2011. Atlanta: U.S. Department of Health and Human Services; 2012.

14. Kherad O, Herrmann FR, Zellweger JP, Rochat T, Janssens JP. Clinical presentation, demographics and outcome of tuberculosis [TB] in a low incidence area: a 4-year study in Geneva, Switzerland. BMC Infect Dis 2009;9:217.

15. Health Protection Agency, UK. Tuberculosis in the UK: Annual report on tuberculosis surveillance in the UK, 2012. London: Health Protection Agency; 2012.

16. National Tuberculosis Institute. Tuberculosis in a rural population of South India: a five-year epidemiological study. Bull World Health Organ 1974;51:473-88.

17. Subramani R, Radhakrishna S, Frieden TR, Kolappan C, Gopi PG, Santha T, et al. Rapid decline in prevalence of pulmonary tuberculosis after DOTS implementation in a rural area of South India. Int J Tuberc Lung Dis 2008;12:916-20.

18. Gopi PG, Subramani R, Radhakrishna S, Kolappan C, Sadacharam K, Devi TS, et al. A baseline survey of the prevalence of tuberculosis in a community in south India at the commencement of a DOTS programme. Int J Tuberc Lung Dis 2003;7:1154-62.

19. Wood R, Lawn SD, Caldwell J, Kaplan R, Middelkoop K, Bekker LG. Burden of new and recurrent tuberculosis in a major South African city stratified by age and HIV-status. PLoS One 2011;6:e25098.

20. Davies PD. TB in the elderly in industrialised countries. Int J Tuberc Lung Dis 2007;11:1157-9.

21. Frost WH. The age selection of mortality from tuberculosis in successive decades. 1939. Am J Epidemiol 1995;141:4-9.

22. Blomberg B, Rieder HL, Enarson DA. Kristian Andvord's impact on the understanding of tuberculosis epidemiology. Int J Tuberc Lung Dis 2002;6:557-9.

23. Andvord KF, Wijsmuller G, Blomberg B. What can we learn by following the development of tuberculosis from one generation to another? 1930. Int J Tuberc Lung Dis 2002;6:562-8.

24. Powell KE, Farer LS. The rising age of the tuberculosis patient: a sign of success and failure. J Infect Dis 1980;142:946-8.

25. Davies PD. Commentary: Tuberculosis down the generations–a comment on 'Continued studies of tuberculosis as a generation illness' by Kr F Andvord. Int J Epidemiol 2008;37:934-6.

26. Tocque K, Bellis MA, Tam CM, Chan SL, Syed Q, Remmington T, et al. Long-term trends in tuberculosis. Comparison of age-cohort data between Hong Kong and England and Wales. Am J Respir Crit Care Med 1998;158:484-8.

27. Wu P, Cowling BJ, Schooling CM, Wong IO, Johnston JM, Leung CC, et al. Age-period-cohort analysis of tuberculosis notifications in Hong Kong from 1961 to 2005. Thorax 2008;63:312-6.

28. Gagneux S. Host-pathogen coevolution in human tuberculosis. Philos Trans R Soc Lond B Biol Sci 2012;367:850-9.

29. Vynnycky E, Fine PE. The natural history of tuberculosis: the implications of age-dependent risks of disease and the role of reinfection. Epidemiol Infect 1997;119:183-201.

30. Small PM, Hopewell PC, Singh SP, Paz A, Parsonnet J, Ruston DC, et al. The epidemiology of tuberculosis in San Francisco. A population-based study using conventional and molecular methods. N Engl J Med 1994;330:1703-9.

31. Cattamanchi A, Hopewell PC, Gonzalez LC, Osmond DH, Masae Kawamura L, Daley CL, et al. A 13-year molecular epidemiological analysis of tuberculosis in San Francisco. Int J Tuberc Lung Dis 2006;10:297-304.

32. Kinander W, Bruvik T, Dahle UR. Dominant Mycobacterium tuberculosis lineages in elderly patients born in Norway. PLoS One 200918;4:e8373.

33. Horsburgh CR Jr, O'Donnell M, Chamblee S, Moreland JL, Johnson J, Marsh BJ, et al. Revisiting rates of reactivation tuberculosis: a population-based approach. Am J Respir Crit Care Med 20101;182:420-5.

34. Geng E, Kreiswirth B, Driver C, Li J, Burzynski J, DellaLatta P, et al. Changes in the transmission of tuberculosis in New York City from 1990 to 1999. N Engl J Med 2002;346:1453-8.

35. Ricks PM, Cain KP, Oeltmann JE, Kammerer JS, Moonan PK. Estimating the burden of tuberculosis among foreign-born persons acquired prior to entering the U.S., 2005-2009. PLoS One 2011;6:e27405.

36. Narayanan S, Das S, Garg R, Hari L, Rao VB, Frieden TR, et al. Molecular epidemiology of tuberculosis in a rural area of high prevalence in South India: implications for disease control and prevention. J Clin Microbiol 2002;40:4785-8.

37. Chiang CY, Riley LW. Exogenous reinfection in tuberculosis. Lancet Infect Dis 2005;5:629-36.

38. Chadha VK, Sarin R, Narang P, John KR, Chopra KK, Jitendra R, et al. Trends in the annual risk of tuberculous infection in India. Int J Tuberc Lung Dis 2013;17:312-9.

39. Stead WW, To T. The significance of the tuberculin skin test in elderly persons. Ann Intern Med 1987;107:837-42.

40. Crossley KB, Peterson PK. Infections in the elderly. Clin Infect Dis 1996;22:209-15.

41. Gruver AL, Hudson LL, Sempowski GD. Immunosenescence of ageing. J Pathol 2007;211:144-56.

42. Eaton SM, Burns EM, Kusser K, Randall TD, Haynes L. Age-related defects in CD4 T cell cognate helper function lead to reductions in humoral responses. J Exp Med 2004;200:1613-22.

43. Haynes L, Eaton SM, Burns EM, Randall TD, Swain SL. Newly generated CD4 T cells in aged animals do not exhibit age-related defects in response to antigen. J Exp Med 2005;201:845-51.

44. Tsukamoto H, Clise-Dwyer K, Huston GE, Duso DK, Buck AL, Johnson LL, et al. Age-associated increase in lifespan of naive CD4 T cells contributes to T-cell homeostasis but facilitates development of functional defects. Proc Natl Acad Sci USA 2009;106:18333-8.

45. Tsukamoto H, Huston GE, Dibble J, Duso DK, Swain SL. Bim dictates naive CD4 T cell lifespan and the development of age-associated functional defects. J Immunol 2010;185:4535-44.

46. Vesosky B, Turner J. The influence of age on immunity to infection with Mycobacterium tuberculosis. Immunol Rev 2005;205:229-43.

47. Cooper AM, Callahan JE, Griffin JP, Roberts AD, Orme IM. Old mice are able to control low-dose aerogenic infections with Mycobacterium tuberculosis. Infect Immun 1995;63:3259-65.

48. Turner J, Frank AA, Orme IM. Old mice express a transient early resistance to pulmonary tuberculosis that is mediated by CD8 T cells. Infect Immun 2002;70:4628-37.

49. Hazeldine J, Lord JM. The impact of ageing on natural killer cell function and potential consequences for health in older adults. Ageing Res Rev 2013;12:1069-78.

50. Effros RB, Fletcher CV, Gebo K, Halter JB, Hazzard WR, Horne FM, et al. Aging and infectious diseases: workshop on HIV infection and aging: what is known and future research directions. Clin Infect Dis 2008;47:542-53.

51. Reider HL. Epidemiologic basis of tuberculosis control. Paris: International Union Against Tuberculosis and Lung Disease; 1999.

52. Jeon CY, Murray MB. Diabetes mellitus increases the risk of active tuberculosis: a systematic review of 13 observational studies. PLoS Med 2008;5:e152.

53. World Health Organization, International Union Against Tuberculosis and Lung Disease. Collaborative framework for care and control of tuberculosis and diabetes. Geneva: WHO; 2011.

54. India Tuberculosis-Diabetes Study Group. Screening of patients with tuberculosis for diabetes mellitus in India. Trop Med Int Health 2013;18:636-45.

55. Creswell J, Raviglione M, Ottmani S, Migliori GB, Uplekar M, Blanc L, et al. Tuberculosis and noncommunicable diseases: neglected links and missed opportunities. Eur Respir J 2011;37:1269-82.

56. Wild S, Roglic G, Green A, Sicree R, King H. Global prevalence of diabetes: estimates for the year 2000 and projections for 2030. Diabetes Care 2004;27:1047-53.

57. Ruslami R, Aarnoutse RE, Alisjahbana B, van der Ven AJ, van Crevel R. Implications of the global increase of diabetes for tuberculosis control and patient care. Trop Med Int Health 2010;15:1289-99.

58. van Zyl, Smit RN, Pai M, Yew WW, Leung CC, Zumla A, Bateman ED, et al. Global lung health: the colliding epidemics of tuberculosis, tobacco smoking, HIV and COPD. Eur Respir J 2010;35:27-33.

59. Gajalakshmi V, Peto R, Kanaka TS, Jha P. Smoking and mortality from tuberculosis and other diseases in India: retrospective study of 43000 adult male deaths and 35000 controls. Lancet 2003;362:507-15.

60. Ministry of Statistics & Programme Implementation. Situation analysis of the elderly in India. New Delhi: Government of India; 2011.

61. Morris CD. Pulmonary tuberculosis in the elderly: a different disease? Thorax 1990;45:912-3.

62. Teale C, Goldman JM, Pearson SB. The association of age with the presentation and outcome of tuberculosis: a five-year survey. Age Ageing 1993;22:289-93.

63. Korzeniewska-Kosela M, Krysl J, Müller N, Black W, Allen E, FitzGerald JM. Tuberculosis in young adults and the elderly. A prospective comparison study. Chest 1994;106:28-32.

64. Dai DL, Tang AW, Chan VK, Leung AC. A study on tuberculosis in elderly patients. J Hongkong Geriatr Soc 1994;5:40-4.

65. Alvarez S, Shell C, Berk SL. Pulmonary tuberculosis in elderly men. Am J Med 1987;82:602-6.

66. Umeki S. Comparison of younger and elderly patients with pulmonary tuberculosis. Respiration 1989;55:75-83.

67. Pérez-Guzmán C, Vargas MH, Torres-Cruz A, Villarreal-Velarde H. Does aging modify pulmonary tuberculosis? A meta-analytical review. Chest 1999;116:961-7.

68. Geng E, Kreiswirth B, Burzynski J, Schluger NW. Clinical and radiographic correlates of primary and reactivation tuberculosis: a molecular epidemiology study. JAMA 2005;293:2740-5.

69. Perez-Guzman C, Torres-Cruz A, Villarreal-Velarde H, Vargas MH. Progressive age-related changes in pulmonary tuberculosis images and the effect of diabetes. Am J Respir Crit Care Med 2000;162:1738-40.

70. Wang CS, Chen HC, Yang CJ, Wang WY, Chong IW, Hwang JJ, et al. The impact of age on the demographic, clinical, radiographic characteristics and treatment outcomes of pulmonary tuberculosis patients in Taiwan. Infection 2008;36:335-40.

71. Pérez-Guzmán C, Vargas MH, Torres-Cruz A, Pérez-Padilla JR, Furuya ME, Villarreal-Velarde H. Diabetes modifies the male:female ratio in pulmonary tuberculosis. Int J Tuberc Lung Dis 2003;7:354-8.

72. Pérez-Guzman C, Torres-Cruz A, Villarreal-Velarde H, Salazar-Lezama MA, Vargas MH. Atypical radiological images of pulmonary tuberculosis in 192 diabetic patients: a comparative study. Int J Tuberc Lung Dis 2001;5:455-61.

73. Bhushan B, Kajal NC, Maske A, Singh SP. Manifestations of tuberculosis in elderly versus young hospitalised patients in Amritsar, India. Int J Tuberc Lung Dis 2012;16:1210-3.

74. Das SK, Mukherjee RS, Ghosh IN, Halder AK, Saha SK. A study of pulmonary tuberculosis in the elderly. J Indian Med Assoc 2007;105:432, 436, 438-9.

75. Chand N, Bhushan B, Singh D, Pandhi N, Thakur S, Bhullar SS, et al. Tuberculosis in the elderly [aged 50 years and above] and their treatment outcome under DOTS. Chest 2007;132[4_Meeting Abstracts]:640b.

76. Rawat J, Sindhwani G, Juyal R. Clinico-radiological profile of new smear positive pulmonary tuberculosis cases among young adult and elderly people in a tertiary care hospital at Deheradun [Uttarakhand]. Indian J Tuberc 2008;55:84-90.

77. Gupta D, Singh N, Kumar R, Jindal SK. Manifestations of pulmonary tuberculosis in the elderly: a prospective observational study from north India. Indian J Chest Dis Allied Sci 2008;50:263-7.

78. Ananthakrishnan R, Kumar K, Ganesh M, Kumar AM, Krishnan N, Swaminathan S, et al. The profile and treatment outcomes of the older [aged 60 years and above] tuberculosis patients in Tamil Nadu, South India. PLoS One 2013;8:e67288.

79. Ma J, Shi X, Zhao S, Meng Q, Qian Y. Fever of unknown origin in an older Chinese population. J Am Geriatr Soc 2012;60:169-70.

80. Chen Y, Zheng M, Hu X, Li Y, Zeng Y, Gu D, et al. Fever of unknown origin in elderly people: a retrospective study of 87 patients in China. J Am Geriatr Soc 2008;56:182-4.

81. Knockaert DC, Vanneste LJ, Bobbaers HJ. Fever of unknown origin in elderly patients. J Am Geriatr Soc 1993;41:1187-92.

82. Tal S, Guller V, Gurevich A, Levi S. Fever of unknown origin in the elderly. J Intern Med 2002;252:295-304.

83. Petersdorf RG, Beeson PB. Fever of unexplained origin: report on 100 cases. Medicine [Baltimore] 1961;40:1-30.

84. Vanderschueren S, Knockaert D, Adriaenssens T, Demey W, Durnez A, Blockmans D, et al. From prolonged febrile illness to fever of unknown origin: the challenge continues. Arch Intern Med 2003;163:1033-41.

85. Bleeker-Rovers CP, Vos FJ, de Kleijn EM, Mudde AH, Dofferhoff TS, Richter C, et al. A prospective multicenter study on fever of unknown origin: the yield of a structured diagnostic protocol. Medicine [Baltimore] 2007;86:26-38.

86. Naito T, Mizooka M, Mitsumoto F, Kanazawa K, Torikai K, Ohno S, et al. Diagnostic workup for fever of unknown origin: a multicenter collaborative retrospective study. BMJ Open 2013;3:e003971.

87. Proudfoot AT, Akhtar AJ, Douglas AC, Horne NW. Miliary tuberculosis in adults. Br Med J 1969;2:273-6.

88. Bottiger LE, Nordenstam HH, Wester PO. Disseminated tuberculosis as a cause of fever of obscure origin. Lancet 1962;1:19-20.

89. Yu YL, Chow WH, Humphries MJ, Wong RW, Gabriel M. Cryptic miliary tuberculosis. Q J Med 1986;59:421-8.

90. Jacques J, Sloan JM. The changing pattern of miliary tuberculosis. Thorax 1970;25:237-40.

91. O'Brien Jr. Non-reactive tuberculosis. J Clin Pathol 1954;7:216-25.

92. Vasankari T, Liippo K, Tala E. Overt and cryptic miliary tuberculosis misdiagnosed until autopsy. Scand J Infect Dis 2003;35:794-6.

93. Sime PJ, Chilvers ER, Leitch AG. Miliary tuberculosis in Edinburgh—a comparison between 1984-1992 and 1954-1967. Respir Med 1994;88:609-11.

94. Sahn SA, Neff TA. Miliary tuberculosis. Am J Med 1974;56:494-505.

95. Bourbonnais JM, Sirithanakul K, Guzman JA. Fulminant miliary tuberculosis with adult respiratory distress syndrome undiagnosed until autopsy: a report of 2 cases and review of the literature. J Intensive Care Med 2005;20:306-11.

96. Rowińska-Zakrzewska E, Korzeniewska-Koseła M, Roszkowski-Śliż K. Extrapulmonary tuberculosis in Poland in the years 1974-2010. Pneumonol Alergol Pol 2013;81:121-9.

97. Pratt RH, Winston CA, Kammerer JS, Armstrong LR. Tuberculosis in older adults in the United States, 1993-2008. J Am Geriatr Soc 2011;59:851-7.

98. Peto HM, Pratt RH, Harrington TA, LoBue PA, Armstrong LR. Epidemiology of extrapulmonary tuberculosis in the United States, 1993-2006. Clin Infect Dis 2009;49:1350-7.

99. Wallgren A. The time-table of tuberculosis. Tubercle 1948;29:245-51.

100. Sharma SK, Solanki R, Mohan A, Jain NK, Chauhan LS. Pleural Effusion Study Group. Outcomes of Category III DOTS treatment in immunocompetent patients with tuberculosis pleural effusion. Int J Tuberc Lung Dis 2012;16:1505-9.

101. Valdés L, Alvarez D, San José E, Penela P, Valle JM, García-Pazos JM, et al. Tuberculous pleurisy: a study of 254 patients. Arch Intern Med 1998;158:2017-21.

102. Valdés L, Alvarez D, Valle JM, Pose A, San José E. The etiology of pleural effusions in an area with high incidence of tuberculosis. Chest 1996;109:158-62.

103. Moudgil H, Sridhar G, Leitch AG. Reactivation disease: the commonest form of tuberculous pleural effusion in Edinburgh, 1980-1991. Respir Med 1994;88:301-4.

104. Sahn SA, Huggins JT, San José ME, Álvarez-Dobaño JM, Valdés L. Can tuberculous pleural effusions be diagnosed by pleural fluid analysis alone? Int J Tuberc Lung Dis 2013;17:787-93.

105. Ruan SY, Chuang YC, Wang JY, Lin JW, Chien JY, Huang CT, et al. Revisiting tuberculous pleurisy: pleural fluid characteristics and diagnostic yield of mycobacterial culture in an endemic area. Thorax 2012;67:822-7.

106. Kim HJ, Lee HJ, Kwon SY, Yoon HI, Chung HS, Lee CT, et al. The prevalence of pulmonary parenchymal tuberculosis in patients with tuberculous pleuritis. Chest 2006;129:1253-8.

107. Lai Y, Chang S, Yuan M, Lai J, Lin P, Kuo L, et al. Tuberculous pleural effusion in the elderly. Int J Gerontol 2012;6:224-8.

108. Thwaites GE, Nguyen DB, Nguyen HD, Hoang TQ, Do TT, Nguyen TC, et al. Dexamethasone for the treatment of tuberculous meningitis in adolescents and adults. N Engl J Med 2004;351:1741-51.

109. Hosoglu S, Geyik MF, Balik I, Aygen B, Erol S, Aygencel TG, et al. Predictors of outcome in patients with tuberculous meningitis. Int J Tuberc Lung Dis 2002;6:64-70.

110. Christensen AS, Roed C, Omland LH, Andersen PH, Obel N, Andersen ÅB. Long-term mortality in patients with tuberculous meningitis: a Danish nationwide cohort study. PLoS One 2011;6:e27900.

111. El Sahly HM, Teeter LD, Pan X, Musser JM, Graviss EA. Mortality associated with central nervous system tuberculosis. J Infect 2007;55:502-9.

112. Dixon PE, Hoey C, Cayley AC. Tuberculous meningitis in the elderly. Postgrad Med J 1984;60:586-8.

113. Sethi NK , Sethi PK, Torgovnick J, Arsura E. Central nervous system tuberculosis masquerading as primary dementia: a case report. Neurol Neurochir Pol 2011;45:510-3.

114. Jha S, Patel R. Some observations on the spectrum of dementia. Neurol India 2004;52:213-4.

115. Jindal SK, Aggarwal AN, Gupta D, Ahmed Z, Gupta KB, Janmeja AK, et al. Tuberculous lymphadenopathy: a multicentre operational study of 6-month thrice weekly directly observed treatment. Int J Tuberc Lung Dis 2013;17:234-9.

116. Prasad KC, Sreedharan S, Chakravarthy Y, Prasad SC. Tuberculosis in the head and neck: experience in India. J Laryngol Otol 2007;121:979-85.

117. Kato T, Kimura Y, Sawabe M, Masuda Y, Kitamura K. Cervical tuberculous lymphadenitis in the elderly: comparative diagnostic findings. J Laryngol Otol 2009;123:1343-7.

118. Karthikeyan VS, Manikandan R, Jacob SE, Murugan PP. Metastatic squamous cell carcinoma urinary bladder coexisting with tuberculosis in pelvic lymph nodes 2013;2013. pii: bcr2013202173.

119. Akbulut S, Sogutcu N, Yagmur Y. Coexistence of breast cancer and tuberculosis in axillary lymph nodes: a case report and literature review. Breast Cancer Res Treat 2011;130:1037-42.

120. Harkirat S, Anand SS, Indrajit IK, Dash AK. Pictorial essay: PET/CT in tuberculosis. Indian J Radiol Imaging 2008;18: 141-7.

121. Roubaud-Baudron C, Godard M, Greffard S, Boddaert J, Verny M. Lymph node tuberculosis and paradoxical evolution. J Am Geriatr Soc 2010;58:192-3.

122. Grange JM, Yates MD, Ormerod LP. Factors determining ethnic differences in the incidence of bacteriologically confirmed genitourinary tuberculosis in south-east England. J Infect 1995; 30:37-40.

123. Autzen B, Elberg JJ. Bone and joint tuberculosis in Denmark. Acta Orthop Scand 1988;59:50-2.

124. Evanchick CC, Davis DE, Harrington TM. Tuberculosis of peripheral joints: an often missed diagnosis. J Rheumatol 1986;13:187-9.

125. van Cleeff M , Gondrie PCFM, Veen J. Tuberculosis in elderly. In: Sharma SK, Mohan A, editors. Tuberculosis. Second edition. New Delhi: Jaypee Brothers Medical Publishers; 2009.p.625-33.

126. Rieder HL, Kelly GD, Bloch AB, Cauthen GM, Snider DE Jr. Tuberculosis diagnosed at death in the United States. Chest 1991;100:678-81.

127. Yen YF, Yen MY, Shih HC, Hu BS, Ho BL, Li LH, et al. Prognostic factors associated with mortality before and during anti-tuberculosis treatment. Int J Tuberc Lung Dis 2013;17:1310-6.

128. Brown M, Varia H, Bassett P, Davidson RN, Wall R, Pasvol G. Prospective study of sputum induction, gastric washing, and bronchoalveolar lavage for the diagnosis of pulmonary tuberculosis in patients who are unable to expectorate. Clin Infect Dis 2007;44:1415-20.

129. Sen T, Udwadia ZF. Cryptogenic organizing pneumonia: clinical profile in a series of 34 admitted patients in a hospital in India. J Assoc Physicians India 2008;56:229-32.

130. Marchiori E, Zanetti G, Irion KL, Nobre LF, Hochhegger B, Mançano AD, et al. Reversed halo sign in active pulmonary tuberculosis: criteria for differentiation from cryptogenic organizing pneumonia. AJR Am J Roentgenol 2011;197:1324-7.

131. Valdés L, San José E, Alvarez D, Sarandeses A, Pose A, Chomón B, et al. Diagnosis of tuberculous pleurisy using the biologic parameters adenosine deaminase, lysozyme, and interferon gamma. Chest 1993;103:458-65.

132. Yao CW, Wu BR, Huang KY, Chen HJ. Adenosine deaminase activity in pleural effusions of lymphoma patients. QJM 2014;107:887-93.

133. Bergeron A, Réa D, Levy V, Picard C, Meignin V, Tamburini J, et al. Lung abnormalities after dasatinib treatment for chronic myeloid leukemia: a case series. Am J Respir Crit Care Med 2007;176:814-8.

134. Jarratt MJ, Sahn SA. Pleural effusions in hospitalized patients receiving long-term hemodialysis. Chest 1995;108:470-4.

135. Tay TR, Tee A. Factors affecting pleural fluid adenosine deaminase level and the implication on the diagnosis of tuberculous pleural effusion: a retrospective cohort study. BMC Infect Dis 2013;13:546.

136. Lee SJ, Kim HS, Lee SH, Lee TW, Lee HR, Cho YJ, et al. Factors Influencing pleural adenosine deaminase level in patients with tuberculous pleurisy. Am J Med Sci 2014;348:362-5.

137. Zarogiannis SG, Tsilioni I, Hatzoglou C, Molyvdas PA, Gourgoulianis KI. Pleural fluid protein is inversely correlated with age in uncomplicated parapneumonic pleural effusions. Clin Biochem 2013;46:378-80.

138. Schaberg T, Rebhan K, Lode H. Risk factors for side-effects of isoniazid, rifampin and pyrazinamide in patients hospitalized for pulmonary tuberculosis. Eur Respir J 1996;9: 2026-30.

139. Hosford JD, von Fricken ME, Lauzardo M, Chang M, Dai Y, Lyon JA. Hepatotoxicity from antituberculous therapy in the elderly: a systematic review. Tuberculosis 2015;95:112-22.

140. Sharma SK, Balamurugan A, Saha PK, Pandey RM, Mehra NK. Evaluation of clinical and immunogenetic risk factors for the development of hepatotoxicity during antituberculosis treatment. Am J Respir Crit Care Med 2002;166:916-9.

141. Patra S, Lukhmana S, Tayler Smith K, Kannan AT, Satyanarayana S, Enarson DA, et al. Profile and treatment outcomes of elderly patients with tuberculosis in Delhi, India: implications for their management. Trans R Soc Trop Med Hyg 2013;107:763-8.

142. Lefebvre N, Falzon D. Risk factors for death among tuberculosis cases: analysis of European surveillance data. Eur Respir J 2008;31:1256-60.

143. Nguyen LT, Hamilton CD, Xia Q, Stout JE. Mortality before or during treatment among tuberculosis patients in North Carolina, 1993-2003. Int J Tuberc Lung Dis 2011;15:257-62.

144. Salvadó M, Garcia-Vidal C, Vázquez P, Riera M, Rodríguez-Carballeira M, Martínez-Lacasa J, et al. Mortality of tuberculosis in very old people. J Am Geriatr Soc 2010;58:18-22.

145. Kolappan C, Subramani R, Karunakaran K, Narayanan PR. Mortality of tuberculosis patients in Chennai, India. Bull World Health Organ 2006;84:555-60.

146. Chung WS, Lin CL, Hung CT, Chu YH, Sung FC, Kao CH, et al. Tuberculosis increases the subsequent risk of acute coronary syndrome: a nationwide population-based cohort study. Int J Tuberc Lung Dis 2014;18:79-83.

147. Shah NS, Pratt R, Armstrong L, Robison V, Castro KG, Cegielski JP. Extensively drug-resistant tuberculosis in the United States, 1993-2007. JAMA 2008;300:2153-60.

148. van der Werf MJ, Ködmön C, Hollo V, Sandgren A, Zucs P. Drug resistance among tuberculosis cases in the European Union and European Economic Area, 2007 to 2012. Euro Surveill 2014;19:20733.

149. World Health Organization. Multidrug and extensively drug-resistant TB [M/XDR-TB]. 2010 Global report on surveillance and response. Geneva: WHO; 2010.

150. Department of AIDS Control, Ministry of Health & Family Welfare. Annual Report 2012-13. New Delhi: Government of India; 2013.

151. Mills EJ, Bärnighausen T, Negin J. HIV and aging–preparing for the challenges ahead. N Engl J Med 2012;366:1270-3.

152. Fatti G, Mothibi E, Meintjes G, Grimwood A. Antiretroviral treatment outcomes amongst older adults in a large multicentre cohort in South Africa. PLoS One 2014;9:e100273.

153. Centers for Disease Control and Prevention. Targeted tuberculin testing and treatment of latent tuberculosis infection. MMWR Recomm Rep 2000;49:1-51.

154. Smieja MJ, Marchetti CA, Cook DJ, Smaill FM. Isoniazid for preventing tuberculosis in non-HIV infected persons. Cochrane Database Syst Rev 2000;2:CD001363.

155. Smith BM, Schwartzman K, Bartlett G, Menzies D. Adverse events associated with treatment of latent tuberculosis in the general population. CMAJ 2011;183:E173-9.

156. Stead WW, To T, Harrison RW, Abraham JH 3rd. Benefit-risk considerations in preventive treatment for tuberculosis in elderly persons. Ann Intern Med 1987;107:843-5.

157. Tsevat J, Taylor WC, Wong JB, Pauker SG. Isoniazid for the tuberculin reactor: take it or leave it. Am Rev Respir Dis 1988;137:215-20.

158. Sarasin FP, Perrier A, Rochat T. Isoniazid preventive therapy for pulmonary tuberculosis sequelae: which patients up to which age? Tuber Lung Dis 1995;76:394-400.

159. National Institute for Health and Care Excellence. Clinical diagnosis and management of tuberculosis, and measures for its prevention and control. Available at URL: http://www.nice.org.uk/guidance/cg117. Accessed on November 25, 2018.

39

Tuberculosis in Health Care Workers

SK Jindal

INTRODUCTION

The contagious nature of tuberculosis [TB] was recognised long before the bacteriological aetiology was identified (1). Historically, there are innumerable examples of relatives and close contacts of patients with TB themselves developing the disease. Similarly, the risk of TB is high in health care workers [HCWs] looking after patients suffering from an active infectious disease. This is particularly so since the infection is air-borne and the presentation of the disease after acquisition of infection is generally delayed. It seems quite appropriate to consider TB as an occupational disease as suggested in the recent medical literature (2).

TUBERCULOSIS CARE AS AN OCCUPATIONAL HAZARD

There is a large body of data to suggest that looking after patients of TB is an occupational hazard. This belief was traced to the 1950s in an elegant historical review of the

medical literature of the past 100 years (3). It was perhaps in 1938 when a high incidence of TB among nurses was demonstrated for the first time (4). Several other reports had appeared thereafter (5-8). Quite aptly, it had been termed as "the battle of a century" (9).

There is a paucity of data on this subject from this country in spite of the fact that India accounts for about one-third of the total global TB burden and that most disease indices are alarmingly high (10). A study from a teaching hospital in Chandigarh (11) revealed that, among resident doctors, the overall risk of developing TB was estimated as 11.2 cases per 1000 person-years of exposure; the overall incidence of TB was found to be 17.3 per 1000. Several of the recent reports corroborate the observation of an increased risk in HCW [Table 39.1] (12-16). In a systematic review of published studies, the median prevalence of latent TB infection [LTBI] in HCWs was reported as 63% on an average with median annual risk of 5.8% in lower and middle income countries (17). In another recent systematic review the pooled

Table 39.1: Some of the recent reports from different countries showing a higher risk of TB among HCWs				
Study [year] (reference)	*Place*	*Type of study*	*Study population*	*TB risk*
Naidoo and Jinabhai [2006] (12)	South Africa	Retrospective study	HCWs [n = 583]	TB incidence 1133/100,000 HCWs
Lopes *et al* [2008] (13)	Central Brazil	Prospective cohort study	Nurses [n = 128]	11.5 new TST conversions/100 person years
Christopher *et al* [2010] (14)	India	Prospective cohort study	Nursing trainees [n = 436]	50.2% tested TST positive
He *et al* [2010] (15)	China	Cross-sectional survey	HCWs [n = 3746]	TB prevalence 6.7 TB/1000 medical staff; 2.5/1000 administrative/ logistic staff
Claasens *et al* [2010] (16)	South Africa	Retrospective study	Community-based health care researchers [n = 180]	TB incidence 4.39 TB/100 person years of follow-up
TB = tuberculosis; HCWs = health care workers; TST = tuberculin skin test				

prevalence of LTBI in HCWs in high TB burden countries was reported to be 47% (18).

RECOGNITION OF TRANSMISSION OF TUBERCULOSIS

Diagnosis of clinical TB is made on the basis of clinical picture and microbiological positivity of sputum or other biological specimens. The presence of infection, however, is established long before the onset of disease symptoms. Based on the circumstantial evidence, it is somewhat easy to attribute the occurrence of new clinical symptoms and aetiology in an HCW to their exposure to TB. This, however, cannot be definitely said unless the mycobacterial transmission can be traced to the specific source in a health care setting. This can be done with the help of molecular techniques, such as, the deoxyribonucleic acid [DNA] fingerprinting.

Tuberculin Skin Test

A positive tuberculin skin test [TST] result is the most frequently used marker of TB infection. There are several difficulties in interpreting TST results and estimating TST conversion rates. This is generally attributed to factors such as the prior Bacille Calmette-Guérin [BCG] vaccination and/or previous exposure to environmental mycobacteria. It is difficult to attribute the presence of TB infection in HCWs to occupational exposure merely from the presence of TST positivity unless the pre-exposure status is known to be TST negative. In a study (19) from Chandigarh, a cut-off of 10 mm was found to be useful in supporting the diagnosis in patients with strong clinical suspicion of TB; in other patients, the 15 mm cut-off was more suitable. From retrospective analyses, it is perhaps more pertinent to compare the number of TB patients among HCWs *versus* general population in these areas, provided reliable data are available.

Interferon-gamma Release Assays

The interferon-gamma release assays [IGRAs] are now being extensively used for diagnosis of LTBI in HCWs (20-29). The test has been employed in both low and high TB prevalence settings. However, there is no distinct advantage of IGRAs over TST. Therefore, in view of the higher costs as well as the requirement of a blood sample for IGRAs, the TST is a preferred method for contact screening in high TB burden settings.

RISK OF INFECTION

The annual risk of TB infection [ARI] assessed using TST in HCW had varied from 0.09% to 10% in different populations in various studies published in the 1980s and 1990s (7-9,30-32). This was up to a hundred times higher than the estimated ARI in the general population of the Western Europe and the United States during this period. The calculated risk for the home staff and the pulmonary fellows *versus* general population was probably highest. Similarly, the annual incidence of TB disease was considerably more

in the HCWs. The incidence seems to have declined in the developed countries in the recent studies (23,29,33-36). Studies from the developing countries, however, continue to report a high transmission risk (12-17). Both the TB infection and the disease are reported to be significantly higher in most studies among HCWs. The criteria used for assessment of TB risk are diverse in different studies. In the Western European countries, USA, Canada and Australia where the TB prevalence is rather low, the positive TST and/or TST conversion are the most frequently employed tests to detect the presence of infection. In a large study (37) involving 4070 HCWs and 4298 non-HCWs, a positive TST was observed in 19.3% HCWs compared with 13.7% in non- HCWs; the significant differences were not explained by the employees characteristics, such as, age, country of birth and the past BCG status (37).

Besides the transmission of TB infection, there are several reports on occurrence of active TB disease amongst physicians and other HCWs from India (38,39). In a short report, TB was diagnosed to develop in 4 of 23 resident doctors during their residency period at the author's institute (11). A 10-year review of hospital records from Vellore reported the incidence of TB among HCWs to be 0.3-1.57 per 1000 pulmonary TB and 0.34-1.57 per 1000 extra-pulmonary tuberculosis [EPTB] cases (40).

DETERMINANTS OF RISK OF INFECTION

The risk of infection amongst HCWs depends upon a large number of factors. Some of the important risk factors [Table 39.2] are discussed below.

Category of HCW

Higher infection rates are reported in almost all categories of HCWs including the doctors, nurses and other ancillary

---

Table 39.2: Factors influencing nosocomial transmission of TB among HCWs

Related to HCW type

Related to the health facility

Level of exposure
  High *versus* low exposure areas
  Inadequate isolation of infected patients

Environmental
  Inadequate sanitation
  Inappropriate disposal of excreta
  Crowding in the wards
  Poor ventilation

Host factors related to HCWs
  Immune status of an individual
  Comorbidities
  BCG vaccination status

General clinical factors
  Delayed suspicion and diagnosis
  Delayed initiation of treatment
  Self-administration of drug

TB = tuberculosis; HCWs = health care workers; BCG = bacille Calmette-Guérin

staff (11,13,17,41-44). Those HCWs who are in direct care with the patients [such as nurses and doctors] are at higher risk of contacting infection. The risk is also high amongst nursing trainees who spend a significant amount of time in patient-care (14). A higher risk has also been reported in the community setting in health care researchers working in an area with high prevalence of TB and human immunodeficiency virus [HIV] infections in South Africa (16).

Level of Exposure

The risk of transmission of infection is greater when the level of exposure is high. Patients with pulmonary TB, especially those who are sputum smear positive are more likely to infect HCWs. Data from several studies indicate that medical and nursing personnel [especially chest physicians and HCWs working in chest diseases wards] have higher risk ratios of TST conversion and development of active TB (2,42,45-47). On the other hand, smear-negative TB appears to be less contagious to HCWs (34).

Nosocomial transmission, however, is also known to occur from non-pulmonary sites (48). Twelve [13%] of 95 HCWs who were initial non-reactive to tuberculin developed a positive TST after exposure to an index patient with TB prostatic abscess who had undergone abscess drainage and bilateral orchiectomy and had died after 27 days of hospitalisation (48). Such transmission is more likely to happen in the presence of other risk factors, such as altered host immunity, environmental conditions and inadequate infection control measures. The level of exposure is also high in medical wards and microbiology laboratories. In a case-control study from India, the risk was over five times higher among laboratory workers and over 12 times higher for HCWs in the medical wards (49).

High TST positivity has been recorded among physicians [45.9%] than the general Canadian population (41). Similarly, physicians in USA had a high rate of tuberculin reactivity [7%] although the TST conversion rate was low (42). A TST conversion rate of 1.7% over a 12 months period was also seen in dental HCWs (43).

A strong association has also been shown with type and duration of work; for example people working in respiratory therapy, physiotherapy and housekeeping have greater risks (9).

Environmental Factors

Environment of hospital wards and the methods employed for sanitation and disposal of waste materials and excreta affect the disease transmission. The TST conversion rate has been shown to be strongly associated with inadequate ventilation of the general patient rooms (50). Room size was the major determinant in a report from Italy where 8% of HCWs developed TST conversion after a workplace exposure to a highly infectious multidrug-resistant TB [MDR-TB] patient (51). Some of these factors are of particular importance in this country where the wards are rather overcrowded and poorly ventilated.

Immune Status and Comorbidities

The presence of diseases, which predispose to TB and the status of immunity are important factors which determine the prevalence of TB in HCWs. Prevalence of diseases such as diabetes mellitus, as well as many other conditions requiring use of corticosteroids or other immunosuppressive drugs, among HCWs, is at least similar to their prevalence in the community. Their presence in HCW is likely to augment their predisposition to TB.

Intrinsic immune status of an individual HCW is a particular point of interest. Immunodeficiency is an independent risk factor for TB. In a study on occupational transmission in a haemodialysis unit, the TB isolates from different sources showed the strains to be unrelated when tested with restriction fragment length polymorphism [RFLP] (52). Presence of HIV infection in HCWs is an important risk factor for TB (12,53-56). The impact of HIV infection on increase in number of TB patients was demonstrated in a South African district hospital where the incidence rate of TB among HCWs and ancillary staff was not significantly different from the age-specific rate in the community. But there was a five-fold increase in annualised incidence rate from 1991 to 1992 and 1993 to 1996 which was directly attributable to HIV infection (57). In another study, strains of TB bacilli infecting eight of nine HIV-seropositive HCWs had a clustered RFLP pattern, implying a common source, i.e., an unrecognised occupational transmission (58). The HIV-seropositive HCWs who developed TB following a hospital outbreak of MDR-TB had more severe disease and had died (59).

Overall 14% of 1627 HCWs with TB were found to be co-infected with HIV infection in an analysis of surveillance data on HIV-TB co-infection in England and Wales (60). This had increased from 8% in 1999 to 14% in 2005, mostly amongst non-UK born HCWs. The authors (60) had also recommended voluntary HIV testing for new HCWs for an early diagnosis.

Bacille Calmette-Guérin Vaccination

BCG vaccination is administered at birth or in early childhood as a general vaccination policy in countries with high TB prevalence, including in India. It is unclear if the BCG vaccination in childhood affects the incidence of risk in HCWs.

Clinical Factors

Besides factors related to the host, i.e., the type of HCWs and the environment in which HCWs work, factors related to awareness of occupational transmission, preventive steps being used, clinical suspicion and diagnosis of an early disease are important in influencing the occurrence of disease. There was an inadequacy of knowledge on TB transmission and infection control measures among HCWs in the USA in a questionnaire survey (61). The situation is likely to be worse in most hospitals of the developing world.

Many HCWs are likely to be more negligent in adopting routine measures while working in the hospitals and tend to ignore precautionary practices generally recommended for attendants and care providers of patients. Attitudinal desensitisation to follow guidelines is common unless repeatedly enforced.

RISK ASSESSMENT

It is known that an untreated patient with active TB transmits acid-fast bacilli [AFB] and infects other individuals. This risk is likely to be significant in the hospital surroundings with a larger number of patients staying in a closed-door environment. HCW in the in-patient and out-patient facilities and history of TB exposure in the previous year were found to be significant predictors for TST conversion in a study on 624 HCWs in Thailand (62). More than the close personal contact, it is the inhalational route which is important in spreading TB. This was amply shown following a sharp outbreak of TB abroad the naval vessel "Richard E Byrd" (63). It was concluded that the rate of infection was proportional to the amount of contaminated air.

The mathematical model for quantitative assessment of air-borne infection *vis-a-vis* room ventilation developed for measles epidemic has been also used for TB (64). The probability curve of TB infection clearly showed the diminishing effectiveness of high level of ventilation. A similar curve was drawn for TB outbreak from a brief but intense exposure during bronchoscopy (65). It can be, therefore, concluded that TB transmission can be quantitatively assessed fairly well from the amount of room ventilation (66).

CONTROLLING OCCUPATIONAL TUBERCULOSIS

An increased occurrence of TB in HCWs has more serious ramifications than a mere addition to the total pool of TB patients. There is the fear of spreading panic among the employees as well as the community. It is, therefore, an issue of great public and social importance. It is important to adopt strategies to prevent and control TB in HCWs. Implementation of protection guidelines has been shown to effectively reduce the TB risk in HCWs (35,67-69). Therefore, there is a clear need to implement infection control policies in all health care settings (13,33,35,67-70).

There are two important strategies to control occupational TB among HCWs: [i] early diagnosis and treatment; and [ii] prevention of infection and disease.

Early Diagnosis and Treatment

It is important to make diagnosis and institute anti-TB treatment at the earliest. Hospital employees have the advantage of an easy availability of medical advice and investigations. It is, therefore, simpler to make an early diagnosis in a symptomatic individual. In fact, early documentation of detection and notification of cases of TB among HCWs may partly account for some of the increased risk among them.

While HCWs are better placed to seek early interventions, they also tend to ignore early symptoms, more than the people in the community. It is a common observation that hospital personnel including doctors and nurses rely greatly on self-administered symptomatic treatments before seeking appropriate medical advice. This is particularly so in developing countries where medicines are relatively easily accessible and available to medical, nursing and paramedical personnel. These factors are likely to delay the early diagnosis. A careful approach to diagnosis among symptomatic individuals and routine screening programmes among HCWs are, therefore, important for success.

An early and aggressive approach is important for diagnosis and treatment considering the hospital work as a risk factor and the fact that more specialised expertise and care is available in a hospital setting. A simplified algorithm [Figure 39.1] for diagnosis and treatment of TB, may be useful in the evaluation of HCWs who are TB suspects. The suggested definition of a TB suspect among HCWs is different from that used in the Revised National TB Control Programme [RNTCP] in India. It is worthwhile to introduce a standardised symptoms questionnaire as an instrument for active case finding for screening of all HCWs on a regular basis. Any individual who reports with respiratory and/or general constitutional symptoms of even one week's duration [unless explained by a definite alternative aetiology] should be considered as a TB-suspect and investigated with the help of both sputum microscopy for AFB and a chest radiograph examination. In case sputum smear is positive for AFB, anti-TB treatment is given accordingly. In case, sputum smear is negative for AFB, and the chest radiograph findings suggest TB, treatment for smear-negative TB should be instituted and an attempt should be made to demonstrate AFB in the bronchoalveolar lavage [BAL] fluid and/or other appropriate investigations. In case the chest radiograph is clearly normal or negative for TB, other diagnoses should be considered and appropriate investigations done. Treatment regimens in HCWs do not differ from those recommended for TB in other groups.

Preventive Strategies

Different strategies are employed in different countries to prevent infection and mycobacterial transmission. The differences in approach in India reflect the difficulties due to the enormity of the burden and the inadequacy of the existing health care infrastructure. Nonetheless, the infection control measures which are recommended anywhere are generally similar [Table 39.3].

The Centers for Disease Control [CDC], "Guidelines for preventing the transmission of *Mycobacterium tuberculosis* in health care settings" uses a broader term "health care setting" to include not only the hospital-related scenario [e.g., in-patient and out-patient settings, TB clinics], but also correctional facilities in which health care is delivered, settings in which home-based health care and emergency medical services are provided, and laboratories handling clinical specimens that might contain *Mtb* (33). The recently

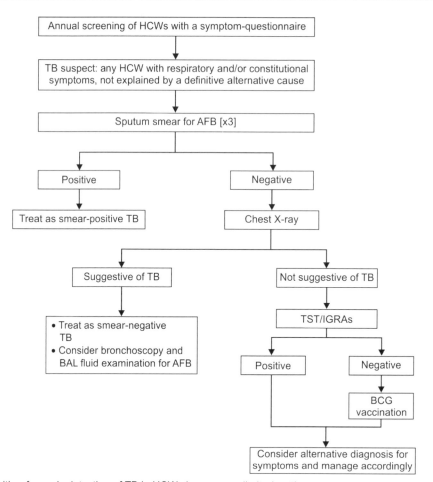

Figure 39.1: Suggested algorithm for early detection of TB in HCWs in resource-limited settings
HCWs = health care workers; TB = tuberculosis; AFB = acid-fast bacilli; TST = tuberculin skin test; IGRAs = interferon-gamma release assays; BAL = bronchoalveolar lavage; BCG = bacille Calmette-Guérin

Table 39.3: General measures used for control of tuberculosis transmission in HCWs
General Infection Control Measures
Reduction of environmental load by reducing the release of mycobacteria
Use of masks for patients
Isolation rooms
Preventing environmental spread
Negative pressure rooms
Use of HEPA filters
Use of ultra violet radiation
Individual protection measures
Inhalational prevention strategies
Use of simple masks
Use of respirators: HEPA filters/PAPR
BCG vaccination
Chemoprophylaxis
Early detection and treatment
HCWs = health care workers; HEPA = high-efficiency particulate air; PAPR = powered air-purifying respirator; BCG = bacille Calmette-Guérin

framed guidelines on "Airborne infection control in health care and other settings" published by Ministry of Health and Family Welfare, Government of India (71) provide a comprehensive framework on important preventive measures [Table 39.4]. The recommendation includes the adoption of administrative, environmental and personal protection measures (71).

Infection Control Measures

The most important source of mycobacteria in the environment is an open patient with pulmonary TB who is excreting bacilli in the sputum. Bacteria are released during coughing, laughing and talking, and transmitted to others through air-borne droplets. Infection control measures are, therefore, designed to focus on reduction of environmental load of mycobacteria by one or more of the following steps in transmission of infection.

Reducing the release of mycobacteria and preventing environmental distribution The most efficient method to prevent dispersion of infectious particles from a patient in a hospital room is to trap the particles at the patient's mouth. This can be achieved by the masks covering the mouth and nose. In resource-limited settings, simple gauze masks or a piece of cloth are commonly used for this purpose. The respiratory droplets released on coughing are impinged on the mask. A mask is fairly effective but is not convenient

Table 39.4: Recommended control measures to reduce risk of transmission of respiratory pathogens

Administrative controls
    Decompression of crowded areas
    Segregation of patients with respiratory symptoms
    Fast tracking through health care facility
    Minimise hospitalisation
    Infection control training of HCWs
    Regular assessment of TB in all HCWs

Procedures for standard precautions
    Hand hygiene
    Personal protection [gloves, gowns, masks, shields]
    Respiratory hygiene and cough etiquette
    Prevention of injury from needles or other sharp objects
    Cleaning and disinfecting medical equipments
    Cleaning the patient care environments
    Linen and waste management

Biomedical waste management protocol

Environmental controls
    Effective ventilation
    Mechanically aided means
    Natural
    Ultraviolet germicidal irradiation

Personal protection

TB = tuberculosis; HCWs = health care workers

for constant use. It gets wet very soon and cumbersome for use in a patient with persistent cough and sputum production. The use is, therefore, restricted to specific situations for limited time periods.

Adequate ventilation is useful to dilute the environmental concentration of mycobacteria. While the indoor load within a hospital is reduced, the method may prove to be counter-productive by spreading infectious, airborne droplets in the surrounding areas. This poses a risk of infection to a larger number of employees and other people in the building. Such incidents of infection in the entire building spread through mechanical ventilating systems have been reported in the literature, such as the TB outbreak through ventilation in two adjoining compartments, in the naval vessel "Richard E Byrd" and the other outbreak, where one worker with undiagnosed TB infected 27 of 67 colleagues over a four-week period (63,72). Similarly, it was shown that the exposure in the hospital building treating HIV patients with TB infection was universal and a sojourn of 40 or more hours per week was enough to get infection (73). This was attributable to recirculation of air from the infected source to the entire building. It is, therefore, more useful to contain the infection within, rather than ventilating it out. Internal containment includes the prevention of dissemination of infectious droplets in the air by entrapment procedures as well as the air disinfection.

Complete isolation of a TB patient is not feasible. As per current practice and recommendations in India, a sputum smear-positive patient need not be admitted in the hospital. If the medical indication for admission is strong, separate areas should be earmarked for such patients. The use of high-efficiency particle air [HEPA] filter is useful to prevent dispersal. Separate cubicles/booths should be made available in the wards and laboratories for performance of procedures requiring coughing, such as induced sputum induction. Similarly, bronchoscopic examination in suspected TB patients should be performed in well-equipped areas fitted with HEPA filters.

Air filtration and disinfection The air-cleaning technologies are common for prevention of all airborne infections including TB. Some of these methods include in-room air cleaners, HEPA and ultraviolet germicidal irradiation [UVGI] air technologies. No health technology assessment on air cleaning technology was found on literature review in an evidence-based analysis of studies on air (74). Cleaning technologies in Ontario, Canada (74), HEPA filters, permanently fixed for room ventilation remove droplet nuclei carrying tubercle bacilli from the air. They are capable of removing almost 100% of particles of over 0.3 mm in diameter (75). The filter units are fitted with blowers to recirculate air. The filtered air from the room or the booth can also be re-circulated through a duct to create a negative pressure within. This type of HEPA filtered self-contained booths for some specified purposes as listed earlier, are already available commercially.

Ultraviolet radiation has some advantages over HEPA air disinfection. The resistance to airflow is much less than with an HEPA filter. Therefore, the blowers used are smaller and quieter. But the main disadvantage is the possibility of causing excessive exposure to the germicidal UV causing painful superficial irritation of skin and eyes although there are no serious long-term effects (75). There is no evidence of systemic immune-suppression from UV germicidal irradiation employed for room disinfection (76). To prevent personal exposure, the germicidal UV is directed at the air in the upper part of the room. The mixing of lower air with upper air permits disinfection of all indoor air. This mixing is promoted by convection and forced air movement by supplemental fans. But when the ceilings are low, the upper air UV radiation gets deflected downwards posing a greater risk to the occupants. Ultraviolet radiation can also be used in the ventilating ducts to make the re-circulated air germ-free. Generally, the upper air disinfection in each room is more effective than central duct irradiation but it requires a more elaborate setting.

Individual Protection

Inhalational prevention strategies Protective measures which can be employed by an individual working in a health care facility include the use of devices to prevent inhalation of infectious droplet nuclei. Unfortunately, most of these methods have their fallacies and failures. The risk of infection in HCWs is minimal from paediatric patients with primary TB (77).

Historically, surgical facemasks have been employed by visitors and HCW attending upon TB patients. It is difficult to comment upon the usefulness of this method in the absence of any efficacy-study on their use. There is a complete lack of standardisation, besides the difficulties involved in wearing of a well-fitted facemask all the time.

More effective than a simple mask is a respirator which removes the infectious particles through impaction by filtration and/or electrostatic attraction. If properly worn, a respirator can prevent up to 80% of exposure. It is cumbersome to wear respirators continuously in all situations. These are generally recommended for personnel attending upon sputum-smear positive patients and during cough induction and bronchoscopic procedures (33). Leakage of droplet nuclei from a filter depends upon the filtration efficiency and facial seal. The CDC (33) recommends that a respirator should meet the following criteria: [i] it should be able to filter particles of 1 mm in size with 95% efficiency; [ii] it should have a face seal leakage of 10% or less; [iii] it should have the ability to fit the different facial sizes and characteristics of health personnel; and [iv] it should be checked for face piece fit by HCWs each time it is used.

Different types of filters which include HEPA and powered air-purifying respirator [PAPR] masks have been employed. The high cost of these gadgets is a deterrent for their use in resource-limited settings.

Bacille Calmette-Guérin vaccination Unfortunately, the role of BCG vaccination to prevent TB has remained doubtful and debatable (78). The available evidence supports a good level of protection in children (79). As per current practices in India, BCG is administered at birth. Presumably, most adults in India including the HCWs should have received BCG vaccination in childhood. There is no recommendation at present to adopt the policy of revaccinating HCWs in India. There is established practice of occupational vaccination policies in HCWs for TB in nine European countries (80). The UK Department of Health recommends that BCG vaccination should be given for all those at higher risk of TB, which includes HCWs and laboratory staff in contact with patients, clinical materials or derived isolates (81).

The subject of BCG vaccination in HCWs was addressed in a systematic review in the USA (82). All the six controlled studies included in the review, in spite of several methodological limitations, had reported a protective effect for BCG (82). It was therefore, recommended that BCG vaccinations should be offered to all the unvaccinated HCWs (83).

Treatment of Latent Tuberculosis Infection

Preventive chemotherapy for latent TB infection is recommended for people at high risk for active TB, especially those with HIV infection (84-86). There are no specific guidelines for HCWs. In an earlier study (85) in subjects with heavy TB exposure in 6 hospitals and 22 nursing homes in USA, it was concluded that healthy persons who remained nonreactive to TB after heavy exposure had escaped infection and required no chemotherapy. It was also recommended as wise to start preventive therapy if exposure was discovered immediately; treatment could be discontinued if the skin test was negative at three months.

Preventive isoniazid therapy after exposure is advisable in persons younger than 35 years of age, those with HIV infection or receiving any kind of immunosuppressive therapy. Several regimens have been used for the treatment of LTBI (87). The WHO guidelines for LTBI treatment in high income countries have recently been published (88,89). There is no consensus on these recommendations as yet in India and other resource-limited settings. It is perhaps fair to conclude that, as of today, there is sparse evidence to advocate treatment of LTBI in HCWs irrespective of their contact with sputum-smear positive patients. Personal protective measures and close supervision are important to detect an early disease and treat them immediately. The BCG vaccination policy also needs to be re-examined.

REFERENCES

1. Keers RY. Pulmonary tuberculosis: journey down the centuries. First edition. London: Bailliere Tindall; 1978.
2. Kilinc O, Ucan ES, Cakan MD, Ellidokuz MD, Ozol MD, Sayiner A, et al. Risk of tuberculosis among health care workers: can tuberculosis be considered as an occupational disease? Respir Med 2002;96:506-10.
3. Sepkowitz KA. Tuberculosis and the health care worker: a historical perspective. Ann Intern Med 1994;120:71-9.
4. Heimbeck J. Incidence of tuberculosis in young adult women with special reference to employment. Br J Tuberc 1938; 32: 154-66.
5. Badger TL, Ayvazian LF. Tuberculosis in nurses: clinical observation on its pathogenesis as seen in a fifteen-year follow up of 745 nurses. Am Rev Tuberc 1949;60:305-27.
6. Childress WG. Occupational tuberculosis in hospitals and sanatorium personnel. JAMA 1951;146:1188-90.
7. Price LE, Rutala WA, Samsa GP. Tuberculosis in hospital personnel. Infect Control 1987;8:97-101.
8. Menzies D, Fanning A, Yuan L, Fitzgerald M. Tuberculosis among health care workers. N Engl J Med 1995;332:92-8.
9. Fennelly KP, Iseman MD. Health care workers and tuberculosis: the battle of a century. Int J Tuberc Lung Dis 1999;3:363-4.
10. Chakraborty AK. Epidemiology. In: Sharma SK, Mohan A, editors. Tuberculosis. 2nd edition. New Delhi: Jaypee Brothers; 2009.p.16-54.
11. Rao KG, Aggarwal AN, Behera D. Tuberculosis among physicians in training. Int J Tuberc Lung Dis 2004;8:1392-4.
12. Naidoo S, Jinabhai CC. TB in health care workers in Kwazulu-Natal, South Africa. Int J Tuberc Lung Dis 2006;10:676-82.
13. Lopes LK, Teles SA, Souza AC, Rabahi MF, Tipple AF. Tuberculosis risk among nursing professionals from central Brazil. Am J Infect Control 2008;36:148-51.
14. Christopher DJ, Daley P, Armstrong L, James P, Gupta R, Premkumar B, et al. Tuberculosis infection among young nursing trainees in South India. PLoS One 2010;5:e10408.
15. He GX, Van denHof S, Van der Werf MJ, Wang GJ, Ma SW, Zhao DY, et al. Infection control and the burden of tuberculosis infection and disease in healthcare workers in China: a cross-sectional study. BMC Infect Dis 2010;10:313.
16. Claassens MM, Sismanidis C, Lawrence KA, Godfrey-Faussett P, Ayles H, Enarson DA, et al. Tuberculosis among community-based healthcare researchers. Int J Tuberc Lung Dis 2010;14:1576-81.
17. Menzies D, Joshi R, Pai M. Risk of tuberculosis infection and disease associated with work in healthcare settings. Int J Tuberc Lung Dis 2007;11:593-605.

18. Nasreen S, Shokoohi M, Malvankar-Mehta MS. Prevalence of latent tuberculosis among health care workers in high burden countries: a systematic review and meta-analysis. PLoS One 2016;11:e0164034.

19. Gupta D, Saiprakash BV, Aggarwal AN, Muralidhar S, Kumar B, Jindal SK. Value of different cut-off points of tuberculin skin test to diagnose tuberculosis among patients with respiratory symptoms in a chest clinic. J Assoc Physicians India 2001;49: 332-5.

20. Canadian Tuberculosis Committee. Interferon gamma release assays for latent tuberculosis infection. An Advisory Committee Statement [ACS]. Can Commun Dis Rep 2007;33:1-18.

21. Mazurek GH, Jereb J, Lobue P, Iademarco MF, Metchock B, Vernon A. Division of Tuberculosis Elimination, National Center for HIV, STD, and TB Prevention, Centers for Disease Control and Prevention [CDC]. Guidelines for using the QuantiFERON-TB Gold test for detecting Mycobacterium tuberculosis infection, United States. MMWR Recomm Rep 2005;54:49-55.

22. Pai M, Gokhale K, Joshi R, Dogra S, Kalantri S, Mendiratta DK, et al. Mycobacterium tuberculosis infection in health care workers in rural India: comparison of a whole-blood interferon gamma assay with tuberculin in skin testing. JAMA 2005;293: 2746-55.

23. Storla DG, Kristiansen I, Oftung F, Korsvold GE, Gaupset M, Gran G, et al. Use of interferon gamma-based assay to diagnose tuberculosis infection in health care workers after short-term exposure. BMC Infect Dis 2009;9:60.

24. Yoshiyama T, Harada N, Higuchi K, Nakajima Y, Ogata H. Estimation of incidence of tuberculosis infection in health care workers using repeated interferon-gamma assays. Epidemiol Infect 2009;137:1691-8.

25. Demkow U, Broniarek-Samson B, Filewska M, Lewandowska K, Maciejewski J, Zycinska K, et al. Prevalence of latent tuberculosis infection in health care workers in Poland assessed by interferon-gamma whole blood and tuberculin skin tests. J Physiol Pharmacol 2008;59:209-17.

26. De Perio MA, Tsevat J, Roselle GA, Kralovic SM, Eckman MH. Cost-effectiveness of interferon-gamma release assays vs tuberculin skin tests in health care workers. Arch Intern Med 2009;169:179-87.

27. Schablon A, Beckmann G, Harling M, Diel R, Nienhaus A. Prevalence of latent tuberculosis infection among health care workers in a hospital for pulmonary diseases. J Occup Med Toxicol 2009;9:1.

28. He GX, Wang LX, Chai SJ, Klena JD, Cheng SM, Ren YL, et al. Risk factors associated with tuberculosis infection among health care workers in inner Mongolia, China. Int J Tuberc Lung Dis 2012;16:1485-91.

29. Zwerling A, Cojocariu M, McIntosh F, Pietrangelo F, Behr MA, et al. TB screening in Canadian health care workers using interferon-gamma release assays. PLoS One 2012; 7:e43014.

30. Berman J, Levin ML, Orr ST, Desi L. Tuberculosis risk for hospital employees: analysis of a five-year tuberculin skin testing program. Am J Public Health 1981;71:1217-22.

31. Raad I, Cusick J, Sherertz RJ, Sabbagh M, Howell N. Annual tuberculin skin testing of employees at a university hospital: a cost-benefit analysis. Infect Control Hosp Epidemiol 1989;10: 465-9.

32. Ramirez AJ, Anderson P, Herp S, Raff MJ. Increased rate of tuberculi skin test conversion among workers at a university hospital. Infect Control Hosp Epidemiol 1992;13:579-81.

33. Jensen PA, Lambert LA, Iademarco MF, Ridzon R. CDC. Guidelines for preventing the transmission of Mycobacterium tuberculosis in health-care settings, 2005. MMWR Recomm Rep 2005;54:1-141.

34. Ringshausen FC, Schlosser S, Nienhaus A, Schablon A, Schultze-Werninghaus G, Rohde G. In-hospital contact investigation among healthcare workers after exposure to smear-negative tuberculosis. J Occup Med Toxicol 2009;8:11.

35. Welbel SF, French AL, Bush P, DeGuzman D, Weinstein RA. Protecting health care workers from tuberculosis: a 10-year experience. Am J Infect Control 2009;37:668-73.

36. Driver CR, Stricof RL, Granville K, Munsiff SS, Savranskaya G, Kearns C, et al. Tuberculosis in health care workers during declining tuberculosis incidence in New York State. Am J Infect Control 2005;33:519-26.

37. Stuart RL, Bennett NJ, Forbes AB, Grayson ML. Assessing the risk of tuberculosis infection among healthcare workers: the Melbourne Mantoux Study. Med J Aust 2001;174:569-73.

38. Aggarwal AN. Tuberculosis transmission at healthcare facilities in India. Lung India 2009;24:33-34.

39. Pai M, Kalantri S, Aggarwal AN, Menzies D, Blumberg HM. Nosocomial tuberculosis in India. Emerg Infect Dis 2006;12: 1311-8.

40. Gopinath KG, Siddique S, Kirubakaran H, Shanmugam A, Mathai E, Chandy GM. Tuberculosis among health care workers in a tertiary-care hospital in South India. J Hosp Infect 2004;57:339-42.

41. Plitt SS, Soskolne CL, Fanning EA, Newman SC. Prevalence and determinants of tuberculin reactivity among physicians in Edmonton, Canada 1996-1997. Int J Epidemiol 2001;30:1022-8.

42. Warren DK, Foley KM, Polish LB, Seiler SM, Fraser VJ. Tuberculin skin testing of physicians at a mid-western teaching hospital: a 6-year prospective study. Clin Infect Dis 2001;32:1331-7.

43. Porteous NB, Brown JP. Tuberculin skin test conversion rate in dental health care workers—results of a prospective study. Am J Infect Control 1999;27:385-7.

44. Louther J, Rivera P, Feldman J, Villa N, DeHovitz J, Sepkowitz KA. Risk of tuberculin conversion according to occupation among health care workers at a New York City Hospital. Am J Respir Crit Care Med 1997;156:201-5.

45. Cuhadaroglu C, Erelel M, Tabak L, Kilicaslan Z. Increased risk of tuberculosis in health care workers: a retrospective survey at a teaching hospital in Istanbul, Turkey. BMC Infect Dis 2002;2:14.

46. Kruuner A, Danilovitsh M, Pehme L, Laisaar T, Hoffner SE, Katila ML. Tuberculosis as an occupational hazard for health care workers in Estonia. Int J Tuberc Lung Dis 2001;5:170-6.

47. Tokars JI, McKinley GF, Otten J, Woodley C, Sordillo EM, Caldwell J, et al. Use and efficacy of tuberculosis infection control practices at hospitals with previous outbreaks of multi-drug resistant tuberculosis. Infect Control Hosp Epidemiol 2001;22:449-55.

48. D'Agata EM, Wise S, Stewart A, Lefkowitz LB Jr. Nosocomial transmission of Mycobacterium tuberculosis from an extra-pulmonary site. Infect Control Hosp Epidemiol 2001;22:10-2.

49. Mathew A, David T, Thomas K, Kuruvilla PJ, Balaji V, Jesudason MV, et al. Risk factors for tuberculosis among health care workers in South India: a nested case-control study. J Clin Epidemiol 2013;66:67-74.

50. Menzies D, Fanning A, Yuan L, FitzGerald JM. Hospital ventilation and risk for tuberculous infection in Canadian health care workers. Canadian Collaborative Group in Nosocomial Transmission of TB. Ann Intern Med 2000;133:779-89.

51. Franchi A, Richeldi L, Parrinello G, Franco G. Room size is the major determinant for tuberculin conversion in health care workers exposed to a multidrug resistant tuberculosis patient. Int Arch Occup Environ Health 2007;80:533-8.

52. Linquist JA, Rosaia CM, Riemer B, Heckman K, Alvarez F. Tuberculosis exposure of patients and staff in an outpatient hemodialysis unit. Am J Infect Control 2002;5:307-10.

53. Salami AK, Oluboyo PO. Health care workers and risk of hospital-related tuberculosis. Niger J Clin Pract 2008;11:32-6.

54. Casas EC, Decroo T, Mahoudo JA, Baltazar JM, Dores CD, Cumba L, et al. Burden and outcome of HIV infection and other morbidities in health care workers attending an Occupational Health Program at the Provincial Hospital of Tete, Mozambique. Trop Med Int Health 2011;16:1450-6.

55. Sacks LV, Pendle S, Orlovic D, Blumberg L, Constantinou C. A comparison of outbreak- and nonoutbreak-related multidrug-resistant tuberculosis among human immunodeficiency virus-infected patients in a South African hospital. Clin Infect Dis 1999;29:96-101.

56. Beck-Sagué C, Dooley SW, Hutton MD, Otten J, Breeden A, Crawford JT, et al. Hospital outbreak of multidrug-resistant Mycobacterium tuberculosis infections. Factors in transmission to staff and HIV-infected patients. JAMA 1992;268:1280-6.

57. Wilkinson D, Gilks CF. Increasing frequency of tuberculosis among staff in a South African district hospital: impact of the HIV epidemic on the supply side of health care. Trans R Soc Trop Med Hyg 1998;92:500-2.

58. Sepkowitz KA, Friedman CR, Hafner A, Kwok D, Manoach S, Floris M, et al. Tuberculosis among urban health care workers: a study using restriction fragment length polymorphism typing. Clin Infect Dis 1995;21:1098-101.

59. Jereb JA, Klevens RM, Privett TD, Smith PJ, Crawford JT, Sharp VL, et al. Tuberculosis in health care workers at a hospital with an outbreak of multi-drug resistant Mycobacterium tuberculosis. Arch Intern Med 1995;155:854-9.

60. Crofts JP, Kruijshaar ME, Delpech V, Ncube F, Abubakar I. Tuberculosis and HIV co-infection in healthcare workers in England and Wales, 1999-2005. Epidemiol Infact 2012;140:1873-9.

61. Lai KK, Fontecchio SA, Kelley AL, Melvin ZS. Knowledge of the transmission of tuberculosis and infection control measures for tuberculosis among health care workers. Infect Control Hosp Epidemiol 1996;17:168-70.

62. Sawanyawisuth K, Chaiear N, Sawanywisuth K, Limpawattana P, Bourpoern J, Reechaipichitkul W, et al. Can work places be predictors for recent onset latent tuberculosis in health care workers? J Occup Med Toxicol 2009;24:20.

63. Houk VN, Kent DC, Baker JH, Sorensen K. The epidemiology of tuberculosis infection in a closed environment. Arch Environ Health 1968;16:26-35.

64. Nardell EA. Nosocomial tuberculosis in the AIDS era: strategies for interrupting transmission in developed countries. Bull Int Union Tuberc Lung Dis 1991;66:107-11.

65. Catanzaro A. Nosocomial tuberculosis. Am Rev Respir Dis 1982;123: 559-62.

66. Riley RL. Transmission and environmental control of tuberculosis. In: Reichman LB, Hershfield ES, editors. Tuberculosis: acomprehensive international approach. First edition. New York: Marcel Dekker Inc; 1993.p.123-36.

67. Brotherton JM, Bartlett MJ, Muscatello DJ, Campbell-Lloyd S, Stewart K, McAnulty JM. Do we practice what we preach? Health care worker screening and vaccination. Am J Infect Control 2003;31:144-50.

68. Yanai H, Limpakarnjanarat K, Uthaivoravit W, Mastro TD, Mori T, Tappero JW. Risk of Mycobacterium tuberculosis infection and disease among health care workers, Chiang Rai, Thailand. Int J Tuberc Lung Dis 2003;7:36-45.

69. Cookson ST, Jarvis WR. Prevention of nosocomial transmission of Mycobacterium tuberculosis. Infect Dis Clin North Am 1997;11:385-409.

70. Farley JE, Tudor C, Mphahlele M, Franz K, Perrin NA, Dorman S, et al. A National infection control evaluation of drug-resistant tuberculosis hospitals in South Africa. Int J Tuberc Lung Dis 2012;16:82-9.

71. Guidelines on Airborne Infection Control in Healthcare and other settings. Central TB Division, Ministry of Health and Family Welfare, Government of India (2010). Available at URL: http://www.tbcindia.nic.in. Accessed on October 20, 2017.

72. Nardell EA, Keegan J, Cheney SA, Etkind SC. Airborne infection: theoretical limits of protection achievable by building ventilation. Am Rev Respir Dis 1991;144:302-6.

73. Centers for Disease Control. Mycobacterium tuberculosis transmission in a health clinic – Florida 1988. MMWR 1989;38: 256-64.

74. Health Quality Ontario. Air Cleaning technologies: an evidence-based analysis. Ont Health Technol Assess Ser 2005;17:1-52.

75. American College of Chest Physicians [ACCP] Consensus Statement. Institutional control measures for tuberculosis in the era of multiple drug resistance. Chest 1995;108:1690-710.

76. Riley RL, Nardell EA. Clearing the air: the theory and application of ultraviolet air disinfection. Am Rev Respir Dis 1989;139: 1286-94.

77. Munoz FM, Ong LT, Seavy D, Medina D, Correa A, Starke JR. Tuberculosis among adult visitors of children with suspected tuberculosis and employees at a children's hospital. Infect Control Hosp Epidemiol 2002;23:568-72.

78. Fine PE, Rodrigues LC. Modern vaccines: Mycobacterial diseases. Lancet 1990;335:1016-20.

79. Hershfield ES. BCG vaccination: Theoretical and practical applications. Bull Int Union Tuberc Lung Dis 1990;66:29-30.

80. Maltezou HC, Wicker S, Borg M, Heininger U, Puro V, Theodoridou M, et al. Vaccination policies for health care workers in acute health care facilities in Europe. Vaccine 2011; 29:9557-62.

81. Department of Health. Immunization against infectious disease–the 'Green Book'. London: DOH; 2006.

82. Brewer TF, Colditz GA. Bacille Calmette-Guerin vaccination for the prevention of tuberculosis in health care workers. Clin Infect Dis 1995;20:136-42.

83. National Collaborating Centre for Chronic Conditions [UK]. Tuberculosis: Clinical Diagnosis and Management of Tuberculosis, and Measures for its Prevention and Control; NICE Clinical Guidelines No. 33. London: Royal College of Physicians [UK]; 2006.

84. Guidelines for intensified tuberculosis care-finding and isoniazid preventive therapy for people living with HIV in resource-constrained settings. Geneva: World Health Organization; 2011.

85. Stead WW. Management of health care workers after inadvertent exposure to tuberculosis: a guide for the use of preventive therapy. Ann Intern Med 1995;122:906-12.

86. Zumla A, Raviglione M, Hafner R, Reyn FV. Tuberculosis – current concepts. New Engl J Med 2013;368:745-55.

87. Sharma SK, Sharma A, Kadhiravan T, Tharyan P. Rifamycins [rifampicin, rifabutin and rifapentine] compared to isoniazid for preventing tuberculosis in HIV-negative people at risk of active TB. Cochrane Database Syst Rev 2013;7:CD007545.

88. World Health Organization. Guidelines on the management of latent tuberculosis infection. WHO/HTM/TB/2015.01. Geneva: World Health Organization; 2015.

89. Getahun H, Matteelli A, Abubakar I, Aziz MA, Baddeley A, Barreira D, et al. Management of latent Mycobacterium tuberculosis infection: WHO guidelines for low tuberculosis burden countries Eur Respir J 2015;46:1563-76.

40

Nutrition and Tuberculosis

Ramnath Subbaraman, Jason Andrews

INTRODUCTION

Research has established clear connections between malnutrition and impairment of immune defense, including decreased cell-mediated protection, abnormal phagocytic function, and reduced immunoglobulin production (1). Among infectious diseases, tuberculosis [TB] has a particularly powerful historical association with malnutrition: its name has been linked to its wasting effect on the body since at least the time of Hippocrates in the 5th Century BC.

Despite this millenia-old association, several issues complicate our understanding of the relationship between TB and malnutrition. These include the probable bi-directional influence of one on the other [in which malnutrition predisposes to active TB even as TB causes wasting], the co-occurrence of malnutrition with other poverty-associated risk factors for TB, and the high incidence of TB in patients co-infected with the human immunodeficiency virus [HIV], which itself causes wasting. In this chapter, we discuss the relationship between nutrition and TB from a scientific, epidemiologic, and clinical perspective, including a review of recent trials of various forms of nutritional supplementation for patients with active TB.

IMPACT OF NUTRITION ON THE RISK OF ACTIVE TUBERCULOSIS

Like HIV, severe malnutrition can cause profound immunosuppression, compromising the body's ability to control mycobacterial infection. The mechanisms of immunological dysfunction that predispose to TB have been elucidated mostly in animal models, while the impact of malnutrition on the risk of TB at the population level has been demonstrated in epidemiological studies.

Evidence from Animal Models

Animal models have helped to characterised connections between malnutrition, immunosuppression, and the risk of active TB disease. In these models, protein malnutrition plays a more significant role in modulating TB risk than do micronutrient deficiencies. In a guinea pig model, vitamin D and zinc deficiencies were not associated with increased TB risk (2,3). In contrast, protein-malnourished guinea pigs exhibited absolute and relative deficiencies in a variety of T-lymphocyte subsets, including CD2+, CD4+, and CD8+ cells (4-6). After bacille Calmette-Guérin [BCG] vaccination, these protein-deficient guinea pigs had markedly decreased tuberculin skin test and interferon-γ assay responses, as compared to protein-replete animals (7,8).

Lymphocyte transfer experiments in both guinea pig and mouse models have helped to shed further light on the role protein malnutrition plays in blunting the immune response to TB. Lymphocytes transferred from TB-infected, protein-deficient animals to syngeneic, well-nourished animals did not protect the well-nourished animals from subsequent TB infection. However, the reverse was true: lymphocytes from TB-infected, well-nourished animals transferred into protein-deficient animals protected the protein-deficient animals against TB infection, suggesting that protein-related nutritional status has a major impact on the lymphocytic immune response to TB (9,10). Moreover, these animal models showed a significant reduction in the risk of active TB infection with improvement in protein-related nutritional status, suggesting that some recovery of the TB-specific immune response is possible with reversal of malnutrition.

Epidemiological Evidence

While several studies describe the diverse macro- and micro-nutrient deficiencies present in TB patients (11-17), most of these cross-sectional studies are unable to differentiate whether these nutritional deficits are an underlying *cause* of TB disease or an *effect* of nutritional wasting resulting from TB. Other prevalent poverty-associated risk factors—including living environments with high population density, poor sanitation, and concurrent social crises—also confound these analyses.

A couple of classic studies from the mid-20th century provide unique insight into the role of malnutrition as a risk factor for the development of TB. One study was performed while the author himself was a British prisoner-of-war in a German camp during World War II (18). Two groups of prisoners-of-war [Russian and British] were held in the camp in very similar living conditions. The Germans provided both groups the same meager rations, vividly described by the author as meat "with high percentage of bone," potatoes "largely frost-bitten and inedible," and a stew "full of small particles of grit and often containing large stones." The British soldiers, however, also received extra food rations from the Red Cross, adding 1300 extra calories to their daily diet and nearly doubling their protein intake. The Russians, by contrast, underwent a process of slow starvation on the German rations, as was evident by their higher rate of anemia and lower plasma protein levels.

Nineteen per cent of the Russian soldiers developed pulmonary TB, as compared to only 1.2% of the relatively well-fed British soldiers. This suggested a 16 times increased relative risk of developing TB that was largely attributable to undernourishment. Moreover, the character of the disease was different in the two populations. The Russians had rapidly progressive, highly fatal infection with massive tissue breakdown but little granuloma formation, while infection in the British soldiers followed a normal chronic course with good granuloma formation. Furthermore, the prevalence of malaria, dysentery, and other infections was similar between the two groups, suggesting that TB had the strongest association with malnutrition of any of the common infectious diseases affecting soldiers in the prisoner-of-war camp.

Another classic study was carried out in Norway in the 1940s, where the high rate of TB among naval recruits was initially believed to result from the young men's overcrowded and unhygienic living conditions (19). However, improvements in hygiene and housing failed to reduce TB rates, however. Authorities then heavily supplemented the recruits' diets with milk, cod liver oil, fruits, and vegetables, after which TB rates quickly declined. A similar conclusion was reached from a recent re-evaluation of the incidence of active TB among children in the classic 1918-1943 Papworth Village Settlement experiment in England (20). Children born outside of the settlement [who presumably experienced very poor nutrition and housing conditions] had a much higher incidence of TB than children born inside the settlement [where adequate nutrition and housing conditions were ensured].

The most compelling evidence from India regarding the influence of malnutrition on TB risk comes from a recent prospective cohort study in Mumbai of 148,173 adults followed for six years, with 13,261 deaths recorded during the study period (21). After controlling for other risk factors, for severely underweight individuals with a body mass index [BMI] of less than 16, the adjusted relative risks of death from TB compared to individuals with normal BMI were 7 and 14 in men and women, respectively. Mildly and moderately underweight individuals also had a markedly increased risk of death from TB, and overweight and obese individuals had a significantly decreased risk of death from TB. In a subsequent analysis, the authors found tobacco use to be a major effect modifier of the role malnutrition plays in increasing TB risk (22). Of the TB-related deaths in the cohort study, among non-tobacco users, 9% and 12% were attributable to being underweight [BMI <18.5] for men and women respectively. However, among tobacco users, 27% and 37% of TB deaths were attributable to being underweight in men and women, respectively.

A similar analysis of the prospective National Health and Nutrition Examination Survey [NHANES] collected from 1971-1992 in the US found that underweight individuals [BMI <18.5] had an adjusted hazard ratio for developing TB of 12.4, when compared to normal weight individuals (23). Being overweight or obese was protective against developing TB. A systematic review of six prospective cohort studies found a consistent inverse log-linear relationship between TB incidence and BMI, in which each unit increase in BMI is associated with a 13.8% average reduction in TB incidence (24).

A few studies have attempted to identify specific diets and micronutrient deficiencies that may increase TB risk. Two studies examining Hindu vegetarian *versus* Muslim omnivore South Asian immigrants in Britain found that vegetarianism correlated with a three- to four-fold increased risk of developing active TB (25,26). There was a notable dose-response relationship, in which decreasing meat consumption correlated with increasing TB risk (26). Another study found that increased fruit, vegetable, and berry intake decreases the risk of developing active TB (27).

While the data showing that malnutrition at the population level predisposes to active TB is persuasive, these findings have yet to be translated into public health interventions aimed at curbing the epidemic. Given TB's position as a major cause of morbidity and mortality in India, our knowledge regarding malnutrition as a central TB risk factor should be a consideration when designing policies and interventions addressing food security.

Diabetes Mellitus and Tuberculosis

While undernutrition has historically been a primary driver of TB in India, a rise in obesity has sparked recognition of the role that diabetes mellitus may be playing in increasing TB risk. Most prospective cohort and case-control studies suggest that diabetes mellitus is associated with an approximately two times increased odds of developing active TB, (28-30) though some studies suggest as much as a five to seven times increased odds (31,32).

Despite the recent rise in the prevalence of diabetes in India, it probably remains a relatively smaller contributor to the TB epidemic in India when compared to undernutrition. A recent analysis estimated that 34% of the TB burden among the poorest one-third of the Indian population was attributable to low BMI, while only 1.3% was attributable to diabetes mellitus. Even among the richest Indians, only 4% of TB was estimated to be attributable to diabetes mellitus, while 20% was attributable to low BMI (31). However, this analysis was limited by the fact that the National Family Health Survey-3 [NFHS-3], which was the dataset used for this analysis, captured diabetes mellitus data based on self-report, which likely resulted in significant underestimation of actual diabetes prevalence. Indeed, when the analysis was repeated using a higher estimated diabetes mellitus prevalence, the authors estimated that as much as 20% of the TB burden in India may be attributable to diabetes mellitus (31).

Recent surveys of TB patients in Tamil Nadu and Kerala suggest that, at least in the South Indian context, TB and diabetes frequently occur as comorbid conditions. In two districts in Tamil Nadu, among 827 TB patients who were screened, 25% were found to have diabetes and 25% were found to have pre-diabetes by oral glucose tolerance testing (33). Notably, 37% of these diabetes cases were newly detected based on screening at these TB centers. A similar survey performed using a state-wide representative sample of TB patients in Kerala, found a remarkable 44% prevalence of diabetes, based on haemoglobin A_{1C} testing (34). Forty-seven per cent of these patients with diabetes mellitus were newly diagnosed based on testing in the TB clinic, and the majority of these patients had poorly controlled diabetes. Only four TB patients needed to be screened to identify one new case of diabetes, which suggests that universal screening of TB patients for diabetes [as is already recommended for HIV] may be a highly beneficial policy in TB clinics and hospitals in India.

IMPACT OF ACTIVE TUBERCULOSIS ON NUTRITION

TB has been understood as a disease of wasting since its earliest descriptions, and we now know that it causes significant deficiencies in nearly every nutritional marker. Body mass index [BMI, kg/m^2], skin-fold thickness, mid-upper arm circumference, grip strength, body fat percentage, calorie stores, muscle mass, serum albumin, blood haemoglobin, plasma retinol, plasma zinc, selenium, iron, and vitamins A, C, D and E have all been found to be depressed in TB patients (11-14,17,35-38).

Weight Loss and Protein–Energy Malnutrition

Weight loss has long been identified as one of the most common presenting complaints of patients with TB; even in more affluent countries such as the USA, weight loss is a presenting complaint in nearly 50% of patients (39). The little research that has compared weight changes in pulmonary *versus* extra-pulmonary TB suggest that—at least as a subjective complaint—the loss is similar (40). The bulk of weight loss in patients with TB is fat mass, though the fat-free component, which is also lost in significant amounts, has more of an effect on the physical functioning of the patient. Protein deficiency has been well described in the context of TB, and albumin and prealbumin have been found to be useful markers both for the diagnosis of deficiency as well as the monitoring of its reversal (15,36,41,42). The predominant biochemical source of wasting is believed to be an increase in tumor necrosis factor-α [TNF-α], which causes a net catabolic state (42). While some have further described an "anabolic block", or decrease in protein synthesis, in the context of TB (43), other research has failed to demonstrate this abnormal metabolism (44).

The physiologic basis of TB-associated wasting is poorly understood. Leptin, a well-known cytokine involved in energy metabolism, appears not to be involved in the wasting process (45-47). There are conflicting reports regarding the role of other hormones such as ghrelin (46,47), and a recent study suggests that plasma peptide YY may modulate appetite suppression and be associated with poor prognosis in TB patients (47).

Micronutrient Deficiencies

Several vitamin deficiencies have been found to be common in TB patients and may be a result of TB wasting; however, most of these studies are cross-sectional, making it difficult to distinguish those results from the disease from those that predispose to it. Vitamin A deficiency is perhaps the best studied micronutrient deficiency in TB, with several studies demonstrating greatly decreased serum levels in TB patients (14,15,36,38,48-50). In a study in India, serum vitamin A levels in TB patients were found to be half that of household contacts, who presumably had a similar diet, suggesting that the deficiency resulted from the disease (35). Multiple studies have also consistently described a high prevalence of vitamin D deficiency in TB patients (51-56), and a recent meta-analysis of studies that compared TB patients to healthy controls found that TB patients have a much higher probability of being vitamin D deficient (57).

Wasting in HIV/TB Co-infected Individuals

Given the significant role that HIV has played in fanning the TB epidemic globally, the impact of HIV-TB co-infection on nutrition merits special mention. Like TB, HIV often leads to clinical wasting, particularly in its later stages (58,59). "Acquired immunodeficiency syndrome [AIDS] cachexia" and "HIV wasting" are well-characterised phenomena, with the latter carrying precise clinical definitions. While untreated HIV disease is, like TB, a net catabolic state, evidence has suggested that, in regions in which it is endemic, TB is the predominant cause of severe wasting in patients with HIV (60).

The combination of these two diseases produces a profound cachexia, rapidly obliterating a patient's nutritional stores (61). The resulting deficiencies are more severe than that of usually the case for patients with either HIV or TB alone, for a wide variety of nutritional indicators—including BMI, arm circumference, waist circumference, albumin, and vitamin A levels (35,62-64). The two diseases also act synergistically to cause anemia, which can have a major impact on functional status and mortality (65,66). If untreated, data suggest that HIV infection may blunt certain aspects of nutritional recuperation that normally takes place during TB treatment (61,64).

NUTRITION AND THE NATURAL HISTORY OF TUBERCULOSIS

Disease Manifestations and Mortality

Severely malnourished patients are more likely to have atypical symptoms, signs, and radiographic presentations of pulmonary TB. They are less likely to have symptoms of haemoptysis and more likely to have dyspnoea and diarrhoea (18,67). On chest imaging, upper lobe cavitation is less common than in well-nourished patients, while atypical findings of lower lobe consolidation, miliary nodules, and mediastinal lymphadenopathy are more common (68). In general, these findings parallel the presentation of TB in patients with AIDS. T-lymphocyte-associated immunodeficiency may be a common pathway for these manifestations (68).

Malnutrition in patients with active TB has been independently associated with increased mortality, as well as higher rates of treatment failure and relapse (69-71). Poor nutritional status results in similar outcomes in patients with multidrug-resistant TB (72). Indeed, multiple studies have shown initial body weight or BMI at the time of TB diagnosis to be a good prognostic indicator, at times predicting survival better than more complicated outcome instruments such as the acute physiology and chronic health evaluation [APACHE] score (41,73). Other studies have found that measuring lean tissue mass (74), assessing for iron deficiency (75) and calculating a composite nutrition score [based on multiple indicators] can add further prognostic value for predicting mortality and other adverse outcomes, such as, respiratory failure, treatment failure, and relapse (76-79). Nutrition may also alter the effects of TB medications, as undernourished patients may be more likely to have sub-therapeutic drug levels and drug-induced hepatotoxicity (80-89).

Diabetes may also alter the natural history of TB. A meta-analysis of several studies found that diabetes increased the risk of the combined outcome of treatment failure and death, with a mildly increased pooled relative risk of 1.69 (89). Interestingly, four studies which looked at the outcome of death alone and adjusted for age and other covariates showed that diabetes was associated with a much higher five times increased pooled odds of death in TB patients (82).

Nutritional Recovery

Chemotherapeutic treatment of TB interrupts the progressive wasting that is part of the natural history of the disease. A few studies have evaluated this process of nutritional recovery. Initiation of therapy and reduction in the burden of TB bacilli was associated in one study with a decline in plasma peptide YY and ghrelin (47). Decline in these hormone levels was followed by a rise in appetite and a subsequent increase in body fat and BMI. Despite general improvement in nutritional indicators, many TB patients may never fully recover back to their baseline nutritional status. A study from Chennai found that more than 80% of HIV-TB co-infected patients remained underweight even after the completion of anti-TB therapy (63).

In addition, "nutritional partitioning" may occur, in which patients experience disproportionate recovery of fat stores as compared to protein stores. In one study, patients on an average, gained 10% in body weight during the first six months of TB treatment; however, this increase in weight was mostly attributable to recovery of body fat. There was minimal improvement in protein stores or bone mineralisation (83). Diabetes may blunt nutritional recovery further. One prospective cohort study in Tanzania found that diabetics had a significantly lower increase in body weight, mid-upper arm circumference, and hemoglobin after five months of TB treatment, compared to non-diabetic TB patients (84). All these findings suggest that, despite some nutritional recovery with TB treatment, TB-associated malnutrition may still exert a long-term toll on patients' functional status and quality-of-life.

NUTRITIONAL STATUS AND THE TUBERCULIN SKIN TEST, INTERFERON GAMMA RELEASE ASSAYS, AND BACILLE CALMETTE-GUÉRIN VACCINE

Malnutrition likely decreases the sensitivity of the TST. Studies in humans and animal models have suggested that low biometric nutritional indicators, low serum albumin, and deficiencies of vitamin D and zinc are associated with decreased size of the TST reaction, which may result in false negative tests (85-90). These findings parallel TST studies in HIV patients, suggesting that clinicians should err on the side of liberally interpreting borderline TST reactions in undernourished patients. IGRAs are increasingly being used for detection of latent TB infection, and studies suggest that the sensitivity of these tests is also decreased significantly in malnourished patients (90-93).

Malnutrition may compromise the efficacy of the BCG vaccine in two different ways. First, maintenance of good nutrition is critical for continuing vaccine-induced immune protection. Deteriorating nutritional status between serial TSTs after BCG vaccination resulted in a marked decrease in the size of induration (94). Children with even mild levels of malnutrition in this study also had fewer positive TSTs after vaccination. These results suggest that vaccine-induced immune protection may be a function of nutritional status at any given time. Similar findings in animal models support these data (6,9,95).

Second, severe malnutrition at the time of BCG administration can permanently affect vaccine-induced immune protection. Children who had kwashiorkor at the time of BCG administration had very high rates of negative TSTs, despite much better nutrition between the time of vaccine administration and TST placement (96). This implies severe protein malnutrition prevented the vaccine from "registering" with the immune system in the first place. Severely protein malnourished children may, therefore, derive greater benefit from being vaccinated with the BCG after improvement of nutrition status, if such delay is feasible.

NUTRITIONAL INTERVENTIONS FOR PATIENTS WITH TUBERCULOSIS

While it is difficult to sort out the predisposing nutrient deficiencies from those caused by TB, it is probably best to understand them as a spiraling force, with nutritional deficiencies compromising the immune system, which enables TB to strengthen its hold on the body; this proliferation of TB leads to further nutritional deterioration. The challenge for clinicians is to interrupt this cycle, with TB chemotherapy serving as the most potent tool for doing so.

It would seem intuitive that adjunctive nutritional support might also serve a key role in decreasing TB-associated malnutrition, morbidity, and mortality. The scientific consensus regarding this question is not clear, however. A recent meta-analysis of randomised trials evaluating nutritional supplementation in TB patient highlights the fact that this field is limited by poor-quality studies with small sample sizes and varied methodologies (97). Interventions have included provision of daily cooked meals, high energy macronutrient supplements, combinations micronutrient supplements, and individual vitamins. The outcomes measured in these studies have variably included mortality, sputum smear or culture conversion, weight gain, treatment adherence, functional status, and quality-of-life. Table 40.1 summarises the critical nutritional considerations in the prevention and management of TB. We review below a few of the more interesting studies that may guide more definitive research in the future on the question of nutritional supplementation for TB patients.

Macronutrient Interventions

In a classic randomised trial performed in Chennai in the late 1950s, 193 patients were randomised to treatment at home or in a TB sanatorium (98). The sanatorium provided nutritional supplementation so that these patients had significantly increased caloric, protein, carbohydrate, and micronutrient intake as compared to patients treated at home. Patients were followed for six months, after which response to therapy was assessed using time to culture-negative sputum and improvement in chest radiograph. In spite of a markedly poorer diet and substantially less weight gain in the patients who received treatment at home, the overall response to therapy was similar in the two groups. In a multivariate analysis, none of the dietary factors studied [calories, carbohydrates, proteins, fats, minerals, and vitamins] were found to influence the time to attainment of quiescent disease.

Since the time of the classic Chennai sanatorium study, a handful of studies have re-evaluated the benefits of different types of macronutrient supplements, through provision of additional cereals and lentils (99), high-calorie nuts and ghee (100), high-calorie packaged supplements (101,102), peanuts high in arginine (103), and a more comprehensive nutritional meal (104). Notably, none of the studies has

---

Table 40.1: Critical nutritional considerations in the prevention and management of TB

Prevention
    Reduction of protein-energy malnutrition is critical to controlling and reducing rates of TB
    BCG vaccine efficacy may be compromised in malnourished recipients
    Protein and nutritional repletion prior to BCG vaccine administration should be considered, if possible, in severely protein malnourished children

Diagnosis
    Borderline TST in malnourished patients should be interpreted liberally, erring on the side of a positive read
    Severe malnutrition is associated with atypical presentations of TB, paralleling patterns in AIDS patients

Treatment
    It is unclear whether macronutrient supplementation in patients with active TB decreases mortality or improves treatment outcomes, but it may help improve weight gain and quality-of-life
    Combination micronutrient (i.e., multivitamin) supplementation may help decrease recurrence rates in patients with active TB
    High-dose vitamin D supplementation may improve treatment outcomes in TB patients with certain vitamin D receptor genotypes, though further research is needed
    Supplementation with 25-50 mg of pyridoxine daily during TB treatment should be considered for malnourished individuals, the elderly, pregnant women, cancer patients, chronic liver disease patients, children, and individuals with preexisting risk factors for peripheral neuropathy
    Repletion of tissue mass in TB patients probably requires greater-than-normal levels of nutritional intake, including protein and high energy supplementation
    Improvements of serum albumin may be the earliest sign of improving nutritional status in patients being treated for TB

TB = tuberculosis; BCG = bacille Calmette-Guérin; TST = tuberculin skin test; AIDS = acquired immunodeficiency syndrome

followed patients long enough or had been adequately powered to evaluate for differences in mortality. With regard to TB treatment outcomes, the studies have been mixed, with some showing improvements in sputum smear clearance, treatment completion rates, and treatment failure rates (99,100,103); while others showed trends towards these favorable outcomes that did not reach statistical significance (104). Nearly all of the studies showed increased weight gain in the intervention group, and some also captured significant increases in lean body mass (101), grip strength (100,101), and quality-of-life scores (100,101). Given the possible long-term toll of TB-associated malnutrition, these improvements in weight gain, physical functioning, and quality-of-life may provide benefits to patients that are meaningful enough to justify provision of adjunctive nutritional supplementation on a wider scale.

In the few studies where caloric intake was measured, even with the adjunctive nutritional supplementation, the intervention groups were not able to meet the minimum caloric intake of 2500 kcal/day that is recommended for the general population. TB patients may need even higher levels of caloric intake than the general population, given the profound catabolic state and possible anabolic block induced by TB. As such, future studies might focus on providing even higher levels of nutritional supplementation, though caloric intake may ultimately be limited in these patients by the profound decrease in appetite caused by TB disease.

Vitamin D

Indirectly, vitamin D has long been used to treat TB. In the mid-1800s, cod-liver oil, which contains high levels of vitamin D, was reported to be effective in improving outcomes for patients with TB (105,106). In 1895, Niels Finsen found sunlight exposure to be effective in treating lupus vulgaris [cutaneous TB], a discovery for which he won the Nobel Prize (107). More recently, several observational studies and a meta-analysis have found vitamin D deficiency to be associated with an increased risk of TB (51-55,57).

Basic science research suggests that when *Mtb* activates toll-like receptors on macrophages [a key component of the innate immune response], this results in upregulation of the vitamin D receptor [VDR]. In turn, activation of VDR by vitamin D may enhance killing of *M. tuberculosis* [*Mtb*] by increasing the phagocytic activity of macrophages and by inducing production of the antimicrobial peptide cathelicidin (108).

Individual risk for TB infection and therapeutic responses to vitamin D administration may vary due to VDR gene polymorphisms. The *FokI*, *BsmI*, *TaqI*, and *ApaI* polymorphisms have been of particular research interest. A recent meta-analysis suggests that the effect of these polymorphisms on TB risk may be especially pronounced in Asian populations, including Indians (109). Notably, there is a high diversity of VDR gene polymorphisms within the Indian population, with major differences in the distribution of the polymorphisms among Hindus, Muslims, and tribal populations (110).

Trials of vitamin D supplementation as adjunctive therapy for patients with active TB have produced mixed results, though interpretation of these studies is limited by highly varied dosing of vitamin D. Studies evaluating lower dose daily supplementation [e.g., 5,000 IU daily] or intermittent high-dose supplementation [e.g., 100,000 IU every few months] did not show improvements in mortality or sputum smear conversion rates (111,112). In contrast, a study that administered a higher dose of 10,000 IU a day showed a statistically significant improvement in the rate of sputum smear conversion (113).

In a more recent double-blind randomised controlled trial, 100,000 IU of vitamin D was administered every two weeks for the first six weeks of TB therapy (114). While vitamin D supplementation did not significantly affect the time to sputum culture conversion for the overall study population, it did improve sputum culture conversion times in patients with the VDR *TaqI* receptor polymorphism *tt* genotype. This trial suggests the possibility that therapeutic responses to vitamin D supplementation may be modulated by VDR receptor genotype. If confirmed in future studies, this finding may have significant implications for the individualised use of high-dose vitamin D supplementation as adjunctive TB therapy based on a patient's genotype—a strategy that may be of increasing importance in the era of multidrug-resistant and extensively drug-resistant TB, where other chemotherapeutic options are limited.

Other Micronutrients

A randomised trial performed among 194 families in Harlem in New York City in the 1940s suggested that regular supplementation with a combination of micronutrients may help protect against the development of active TB (115). The micronutrient supplement, which included vitamins [niacin, thiamine, riboflavin, vitamin A, and vitamin C] and minerals [calcium and iron], was provided to families in the intervention arm for five years. There was a statistically significant lower incidence of active TB among those receiving micronutrient supplementation [0.16 cases/100 person-years] compared to those not receiving supplementation [0.91 cases/100 person-years], though notably this was not an intent-to-treat analysis. No further studies have been performed evaluating the role of combination micronutrient supplementation for TB prevention, and, to our knowledge, this intervention has never been implemented on a wider scale.

Subsequent studies have evaluated the role of combination micronutrient supplementation as an adjuvant therapy for patients with active TB. A high-quality randomised, placebo-controlled trial of combination micronutrient supplementation was performed among 887 Tanzanian TB patients, about half of whom were co-infected with HIV (116). The study found a statistically significant decreases in TB recurrence of 45% and 63% in the overall intervention group and the subset of HIV-infected patients, respectively. Moreover, there was a 64% reduction in mortality in the HIV-negative intervention group that did not reach statistical significance. Rates of peripheral neuropathy were greatly decreased among those who received the micronutrient supplement. Other studies of combination micronutrient supplementation have not found evidence of improved TB treatment outcomes (117-121), though some of these studies did find evidence of increased grip strength (120) and weight gain (117-120) in the interventions groups.

Several other studies have evaluated provision of TB patients with vitamin A or zinc supplementation, either individually (15,117,122,123) or in combination (48,122-125). Notably, none of the studies showed improvements in mortality or treatment completion rates in the interventions groups, though one study found that patients receiving vitamin A and zinc had more rapid conversion of sputum cultures. Concerningly, two studies found a higher risk of mortality in HIV-infected patients who received vitamin A and zinc supplementation (123,125). Finally, one study from Odisha has suggested that iron supplementation may accelerate improvement of anemia during the first month of TB treatment; however, these benefits largely disappeared after the second month of treatment (126).

Isoniazid and Vitamin B6 Deficiency

Isoniazid-induced peripheral neuropathy is a well-recognised adverse effect of TB treatment mediated by nutritional deficiency of pyridoxine, or vitamin B6. Anti-TB therapy has been shown to cause significant reductions in plasma pyridoxine levels within one week of therapy (127), and isoniazid may also compete with pyridoxine in its role as a co-factor for synthesis of neurotransmitters, such as gamma-aminobutyric acid [GABA]. The result is a dose-dependent toxicity of numbness and tingling in the extremities in a glove and stocking distribution, though it can also present as ataxia or muscle weakness. Central nervous symptoms such as seizures and confusion are less frequent presentations of B6 deficiency from isoniazid.

Studies in Chennai in the 1960s first identified the role of low dose pyridoxine supplementation in protecting against isoniazid-induced peripheral neuropathy (128). Current guidelines for pyridoxine supplementation are based on the patient's risk for isoniazid toxicity. Malnourished individuals, the elderly, pregnant women, cancer patients, chronic alcoholics, chronic liver disease patients, and children [especially adolescent females] are at higher risk for pre-existing pyridoxine deficiency even before TB treatment. In addition, isoniazid peripheral neuropathy occurs more frequently in those already at risk for neuropathy from other causes such as diabetes, renal failure, and HIV. Patients co-infected with HIV and TB on antiretroviral regimens containing stavudine or didanosine are at especially high risk, as these drugs can also cause peripheral neuropathy (129). Patients with one or more risk factor should be supplemented with a pyridoxine dose of 25 to 50 mg daily. For patients presenting with active isoniazid-induced peripheral neuropathy, seizures, or mental status changes, 100 to 200 mg daily of pyridoxine is recommended for treatment.

FEAST AND FAMINE: NUTRITION'S CENTRAL ROLE IN INDIA'S TB EPIDEMIC

Contemporary India is in a unique moment in the epidemiological transition, in which the country is facing both pervasive and persistent under-nutrition, as well as rapidly rising rates of obesity—as one author puts it, a state of being both "stuffed and starved" (130). Remarkably, the Indian population is at historic lows in terms of daily calorie consumption (131). While the decline in calorie consumption may partly reflect a decline in calorie expenditure due to sedentary lifestyles resulting from increased urbanisation, it is also clear that the average BMI has actually decreased in recent years among already undernourished sub-sections of the population, such as rural men (132). A recent study estimated that, between 1998 and 2008, India likely experienced a rise in the number of TB cases that was disproportionate to population growth (132). The majority of this rise in TB incidence was attributable to nutritional factors—predominantly worsening under nourishment among rural men, but also the rising prevalence of diabetes.

Amartya Sen and Jean Dreze have argued that hunger in the modern world is a crisis of both food security and health care (133). Clinicians treating TB are in an ideal position to confront this combined entity of hunger and disease. They can do this not only by optimising nutritional status in those with active TB [thereby improving quality of life for these patients], but also by addressing malnutrition in all their patients as a method of TB prevention. Specific interventions might include encouraging increased protein intake, targeted micronutrient supplementation, and diabetes screening, as well as aggressively treating intestinal parasites and anemia.

Perhaps the most powerful way doctors can confront TB is by moving beyond the purely medical approach and stepping outside of their hospitals into the realm of public action. Even as malnutrition is a medical problem, so is TB inseparable from hunger. By advocating for public policies that ensure food security for the poor, doctors can confront TB as it needs to be confronted— at both the social and medical levels.

ACKNOWLEDGEMENTS

Ramnath Subbaraman is supported by a Harvard T32 post-doctoral HIV Clinical Research Fellowship [NIAID AI 007433].

REFERENCES

1. Chandra RK. Nutrition and the immune system from birth to old age. Eur J Clin Nutr 2002;56:S73-S76.
2. McMurray DN, Bartow RA, Mintzer CL, Hernandez-Frontera E. Micronutrient status and immune function in tuberculosis. Ann N Y Acad Sci 1990;587:59-69.
3. Hernandez-Frontera E, McMurray DN. Dietary vitamin D affects cell-mediated hypersensitivity but not resistance to experimental pulmonary tuberculosis in guinea pigs. Infect Immun 1993;61:2116-21.

4. Bartow RA, McMurray DN. Erythrocyte receptor [CD2]-bearing T lymphocytes are affected by diet in experimental pulmonary tuberculosis. Infect Immun 1990;58:1843-7.

5. Mainali ES, McMurray DN. Protein deficiency induces alterations in the distribution of T-cell subsets in experimental pulmonary tuberculosis. Infect Immun 1998;66:927-31.

6. McMurray DN, Bartow RA, Mintzer CL. Protein malnutrition alters the distribution of Fc gamma R+ [T gamma] and Fc mu R+ [T mu] T lymphocytes in experimental pulmonary tuberculosis. Infect Immun 1990;58:563-5.

7. Carlomagno M, Mintzer C, McFarland C, McMurray D. Differential effect of protein and zinc deficiencies on delayed hypersensitivity and lymphokine activity in BCG-vaccinated guinea pigs. Nutr Res 1985;5:959-68.

8. Dai G, McMurray DN. Altered cytokine production and impaired antimycobacterial immunity in protein-malnourished guinea pigs. Infect Immun 1998;66:3562-8.

9. Mainali ES, McMurray D. Adoptive transfer of resistance to pulmonary tuberculosis in guinea pigs is altered by protein deficiency. Nutr Res 1998;18:309-17.

10. Chan J, Tian Y, Tanaka KE, Tsang MS, Yu K, Salgame P, Carroll D, et al. Effects of protein calorie malnutrition on tuberculosis in mice. Proc Natl Acad Sci USA 1996;93:14857-61.

11. Kennedy N, Ramsay A, Uiso L, Gutmann J, Ngowi FI, Gillespie SH. Nutritional status and weight gain in patients with pulmonary tuberculosis in Tanzania. Trans R Soc Trop Med Hyg 1996;90:162-6.

12. Onwubalili JK. Malnutrition among tuberculosis patients in Harrow, England. Eur J Clin Nutr 1988;42:363-6.

13. Harries AD, Nkhoma WA, Thompson PJ, Nyangulu DS, Wirima JJ. Nutritional status in Malawian patients with pulmonary tuberculosis and response to chemotherapy. Eur J Clin Nutr 1988;42:445-50.

14. Karyadi E, Schultink W, Nelwan RH, Gross R, Amin Z, Dolmans WM, et al. Poor micronutrient status of active pulmonary tuberculosis patients in Indonesia. J Nutr 2000;130:2953-8.

15. Hanekom WA, Potgieter S, Hughes EJ, Malan H, Kessow G, Hussey GD. Vitamin A status and therapy in childhood pulmonary tuberculosis. J Pediatr 1997;131:925-7.

16. Wilkinson RJ, Llewelyn M, Toossi Z, Patel P, Pasvol G, Lalvani A, et al. Influence of vitamin D deficiency and vitamin D receptor polymorphisms on tuberculosis among Gujarati Asians in west London: a case-control study. Lancet 2000;355:618-21.

17. Kassu A, Yabutani T, Mahmud ZH, Mohammad A, Nguyen N, Huong BT, et al. Alterations in serum levels of trace elements in tuberculosis and HIV infections. Eur J Clin Nutr 2006;60:580-6.

18. Leyton GB. Effects of slow starvation. Lancet 1946;2:73-9.

19. Munro WT, Leitch I. Diet and tuberculosis. Proc Nutr Soc 1945;3:155-64.

20. Bhargava A, Pai M, Bhargava M, Marais BJ, Menzies D. Can social interventions prevent tuberculosis? the Papworth experiment [1918-1943] revisited. Am J Respir Crit Care Med 2012;186:442-9.

21. Pednekar MS, Hakama M, Hebert JR, Gupta PC. Association of body mass index with all-cause and cause-specific mortality: findings from a prospective cohort study in Mumbai [Bombay] India. Int J Epidemiol 2008;37:524-35.

22. Pednekar MS, Hakama M, Gupta PC. Tobacco use or body mass-do they predict tuberculosis mortality in Mumbai, India? Results from a population-based cohort study. PLoS One 2012;7:e39443.

23. Cegielski JP, Arab L, Cornoni-Huntley J. Nutritional risk factors for tuberculosis among adults in the United States, 1971-1992. Am J Epidemiol 2012;176:409-22.

24. Lonnroth K, Williams BG, Cegielski P, Dye C. A consistent log-linear relationship between tuberculosis incidence and body mass index. Int J Epidemiol 2010;39:149-55.

25. Chanarin I, Stephenson E. Vegetarian diet and cobalamin deficiency: their association with tuberculosis. J Clin Pathol 1988;41:759-62.

26. Strachan DP, Powell KJ, Thaker A, Millard FJ, Maxwell JD. Vegetarian diet as a risk factor for tuberculosis in immigrant south London Asians. Thorax 1995;50:175-80.

27. Hemila H, Kaprio J, Pietinen P, Albanes D, Heinonen OP. Vitamin C and other compounds in vitamin C-rich food in relation to risk of tuberculosis in male smokers. Am J Epidemiol 1999;150:632-41.

28. Shetty N, Shemko M, Vaz M, D'Souza G. An epidemiological evaluation of risk factors for tuberculosis in South India: a matched case control study. Int J Tuberc Lung Dis 2006;10:80-6.

29. Faurholt-Jepsen D, Range N, Praygod G, Jeremiah K, Faurholt-Jepsen M, Aabye MG, et al. Diabetes is a risk factor for pulmonary tuberculosis: a case-control study from Mwanza, Tanzania. PLoS One 2011;6:e24215.

30. Corris V, Unwin N, Critchley J. Quantifying the association between tuberculosis and diabetes in the US: a case-control analysis. Chronic Illn 2012;8:121-34.

31. Oxlade O, Murray M. Tuberculosis and poverty: why are the poor at greater risk in India? PLoS One 2012;7:e47533.

32. Ponce-De-Leon A, Garcia-Garcia Md Mde L, Garcia-Sancho MC, Gomez-Perez FJ, Valdespino-Gomez JL, Olaiz-Fernandez G, et al. Tuberculosis and diabetes in southern Mexico. Diabetes Care 2004;27:1584-90.

33. Viswanathan V, Kumpatla S, Aravindalochanan V, Rajan R, Chinnasamy C, Srinivasan R, et al. Prevalence of diabetes and pre-diabetes and associated risk factors among tuberculosis patients in India. PLoS One 2012;7:e41367.

34. Balakrishnan S, Vijayan S, Nair S, Subramoniapillai J, Mrithyunjayan S, Wilson N, et al. High diabetes prevalence among tuberculosis cases in Kerala, India. PLoS One 2012;7:e46502.

35. Ramachandran G, Santha T, Garg R, Baskaran D, Iliayas SA, Venkatesan P, et al. Vitamin A levels in sputum-positive pulmonary tuberculosis patients in comparison with household contacts and healthy 'normals'. Int J Tuberc Lung Dis 2004;8:1130-3.

36. Scalcini M, Occenac R, Manfreda J, Long R. Pulmonary tuberculosis, human immunodeficiency virus type-1 and malnutrition. Bull Int Union Tuberc Lung Dis 1991;66:37-41.

37. Ray M, Kumar L, Prasad R. Plasma zinc status in Indian childhood tuberculosis: impact of antituberculosis therapy. Int J Tuberc Lung Dis 1998;2:719-25.

38. Madebo T, Lindtjorn B, Aukrust P, Berge RK. Circulating antioxidants and lipid peroxidation products in untreated tuberculosis patients in Ethiopia. Am J Clin Nutr 2003;78:117-22.

39. Miller LG, Asch SM, Yu EI, Knowles L, Gelberg L, Davidson P. A population-based survey of tuberculosis symptoms: how atypical are atypical presentations? Clin Infect Dis 2000;30:293-9.

40. Hira SK, Dupont HL, Lanjewar DN, Dholakia YN. Severe weight loss: the predominant clinical presentation of tuberculosis in patients with HIV infection in India. Natl Med J India 1998;11:256-8.

41. Mehta JB, Fields CL, Byrd RP Jr, Roy TM. Nutritional status and mortality in respiratory failure caused by tuberculosis. Tenn Med 1996;89:369-71.

42. Adebisi SA, Oluboyo PO, Oladipo OO. The usefulness of serum albumin and urinary creatinine as biochemical indices for monitoring the nutritional status of Nigerians with pulmonary tuberculosis. Niger Postgrad Med J 2003;10:247-50.

43. Macallan DC, McNurlan MA, Kurpad AV, de Souza G, Shetty PS, Calder AG, et al. Whole body protein metabolism in human pulmonary tuberculosis and undernutrition: evidence for anabolic block in tuberculosis. Clin Sci [Lond] 1998;94:321-31.

44. Paton NI, Ng YM, Chee CB, Persaud C, Jackson AA. Effects of tuberculosis and HIV infection on whole-body protein metabolism during feeding, measured by the [15N] glycine method. Am J Clin Nutr 2003;78:319-25.

45. Schwenk A, Hodgson L, Rayner CF, Griffin GE, Macallan DC. Leptin and energy metabolism in pulmonary tuberculosis. Am J Clin Nutr 2003;77:392-8.

46. Kim JH, Lee CT, Yoon HI, Song J, Shin WG, Lee JH. Relation of ghrelin, leptin and inflammatory markers to nutritional status in active pulmonary tuberculosis. Clin Nutr 2010;29:512-8.

47. Chang SW, Pan WS, Lozano Beltran D, Oleyda Baldelomar L, Solano MA, Tuero I, et al. Gut hormones, appetite suppression and cachexia in patients with pulmonary TB. PLoS One 2013; 8:e54564.

48. Karyadi E, West CE, Schultink W, Nelwan RH, Gross R, Amin Z, et al. A double-blind, placebo-controlled study of vitamin A and zinc supplementation in persons with tuberculosis in Indonesia: effects on clinical response and nutritional status. Am J Clin Nutr 2002;75:720-7.

49. Evans DI, Attock B. Folate deficiency in pulmonary tuberculosis: relationship to treatment and to serum vitamin A and beta-carotene. Tubercle 1971;52:288-94.

50. Rwangabwoba JM, Fischman H, Semba RD. Serum vitamin A levels during tuberculosis and human immunodeficiency virus infection. Int J Tuberc Lung Dis 1998;2:771-3.

51. Gibney KB, MacGregor L, Leder K, Torresi J, Marshall C, Ebeling PR, et al. Vitamin D deficiency is associated with tuberculosis and latent tuberculosis infection in immigrants from sub-Saharan Africa. Clin Infect Dis 2008;46:443-6.

52. Williams B, Williams AJ, Anderson ST. Vitamin D deficiency and insufficiency in children with tuberculosis. Pediatr Infect Dis J 2008;27:941-2.

53. Wejse C, Olesen R, Rabna P, Kaestel P, Gustafson P, Aaby P, et al. Serum 25-hydroxyvitamin D in a West African population of tuberculosis patients and unmatched healthy controls. Am J Clin Nutr 2007;86:1376-83.

54. Ustianowski A, Shaffer R, Collin S, Wilkinson RJ, Davidson RN. Prevalence and associations of vitamin D deficiency in foreign-born persons with tuberculosis in London. J Infect 2005;50:432-7.

55. Huang SJ, Wang XH, Liu ZD, Cao WL, Han Y, Ma AG, et al. Vitamin D deficiency and the risk of tuberculosis: a meta-analysis. Drug Des Devel Ther 2016;11:91-102.

56. Mastala Y, Nyangulu P, Banda RV, Mhemedi B, White SA, Allain TJ. Vitamin D deficiency in medical patients at a central hospital in Malawi: a comparison with TB patients from a previous study. PLoS One 2013;8:e59017.

57. Nnoaham KE, Clarke A. Low serum vitamin D levels and tuberculosis: a systematic review and meta-analysis. Int J Epidemiol 2008;37:113-9.

58. Suttmann U, Ockenga J, Selberg O, Hoogestraat L, Deicher H, Muller MJ. Incidence and prognostic value of malnutrition and wasting in human immunodeficiency virus-infected outpatients. J Acquir Immune Defic Syndr Hum Retrovirol 1995;8:239-46.

59. Tang AM, Forrester J, Spiegelman D, Knox TA, Tchetgen E, Gorbach SL. Weight loss and survival in HIV-positive patients in the era of highly active antiretroviral therapy. J Acquir Immune Defic Syndr 2002;31:230-6.

60. Lucas SB, De Cock KM, Hounnou A, Peacock C, Diomande M, Hondé M, et al. Contribution of tuberculosis to slim disease in Africa. BMJ 1994;308:1531-3.

61. van Lettow M, Fawzi WW, Semba RD. Triple trouble: the role of malnutrition in tuberculosis and human immunodeficiency virus co-infection. Nutr Rev 2003;61:81-90.

62. Villamor E, Saathoff E, Mugusi F, Bosch RJ, Urassa W, Fawzi WW. Wasting and body composition of adults with pulmonary tuberculosis in relation to HIV-1 coinfection, socioeconomic status, and severity of tuberculosis. Eur J Clin Nutr 2006;60: 163-71.

63. Swaminathan S, Padmapriyadarsini C, Sukumar B, Iliayas S, Kumar SR, Triveni C, et al. Nutritional status of persons with HIV infection, persons with HIV infection and tuberculosis, and HIV-negative individuals from southern India. Clin Infect Dis 2008;46:946-9.

64. Mugusi FM, Rusizoka O, Habib N, Fawzi W. Vitamin A status of patients presenting with pulmonary tuberculosis and asymptomatic HIV-infected individuals, Dar es Salaam, Tanzania. Int J Tuberc Lung Dis 2003;7:804-7.

65. Saathoff E, Villamor E, Mugusi F, Bosch RJ, Urassa W, Fawzi WW. Anemia in adults with tuberculosis is associated with HIV and anthropometric status in Dar es Salaam, Tanzania. Int J Tuberc Lung Dis 2011;15:925-32.

66. Subbaraman R, Devaleenal B, Selvamuthu P, Yepthomi T, Solomon SS, Mayer KH, et al. Factors associated with anaemia in HIV-infected individuals in southern India. Int J STD AIDS 2009;20:489-92.

67. Madebo T, Nysaeter G, Lindtjorn B. HIV infection and malnutrition change the clinical and radiological features of pulmonary tuberculosis. Scand J Infect Dis 1997;29:355-9.

68. Okamura K, Nagata N, Kumazoe H, Ikegame S, Wakamatsu K, Kajiki A, et al. Relationship between computed tomography findings and nutritional status in elderly patients with pulmonary tuberculosis. Intern Med 2011;50:1809-14.

69. Rao VK, Iademarco EP, Fraser VJ, Kollef MH. The impact of comorbidity on mortality following in-hospital diagnosis of tuberculosis. Chest 1998;114:1244-52.

70. Zachariah R, Spielmann MP, Harries AD, Salaniponi FM. Moderate to severe malnutrition in patients with tuberculosis is a risk factor associated with early death. Trans R Soc Trop Med Hyg 2002;96:291-4.

71. Benator D, Bhattacharya M, Bozeman L, Burman W, Cantazaro A, Chaisson R, et al. Rifapentine and isoniazid once a week versus rifampicin and isoniazid twice a week for treatment of drug-susceptible pulmonary tuberculosis in HIV-negative patients: a randomised clinical trial. Lancet 2002;360:528-34.

72. Podewils LJ, Holtz T, Riekstina V, Skripconoka V, Zarovska E, Kirvelaite G, et al. Impact of malnutrition on clinical presentation, clinical course, and mortality in MDR-TB patients. Epidemiol Infect 2011;139:113-20.

73. Getahun B, Ameni G, Biadgilign S, Medhin G. Mortality and associated risk factors in a cohort of tuberculosis patients treated under DOTS programme in Addis Ababa, Ethiopia. BMC Infect Dis 2011;11:127.

74. Mupere E, Malone L, Zalwango S, Chiunda A, Okwera A, Parraga I, et al. Lean tissue mass wasting is associated with increased risk of mortality among women with pulmonary tuberculosis in urban Uganda. Ann Epidemiol 2012;22:466-73.

75. Isanaka S, Aboud S, Mugusi F, Bosch RJ, Willett WC, Spiegelman D, et al. Iron status predicts treatment failure and mortality in tuberculosis patients: a prospective cohort study from Dar es Salaam, Tanzania. PLoS One 2012;7:e37350.

76. Miyata S, Tanaka M, Ihaku D. The prognostic significance of nutritional status using malnutrition universal screening tool in patients with pulmonary tuberculosis. Nutr J 2013;12:42.

77. Kim DK, Kim HJ, Kwon SY, Yoon HI, Lee CT, Kim YW, et al. Nutritional deficit as a negative prognostic factor in patients with miliary tuberculosis. Eur Respir J 2008;32:1031-6.

78. Kim HJ, Lee CH, Shin S, Lee JH, Kim YW, Chung HS, et al. The impact of nutritional deficit on mortality of in-patients with pulmonary tuberculosis. Int J Tuberc Lung Dis 2010;14: 79-85.

79. Kim CW, Kim SH, Lee SN, Lee SJ, Lee MK, Lee JH, et al. Risk factors related with mortality in patient with pulmonary tuberculosis. Tuberc Respir Dis [Seoul] 2012;73:38-47.

80. Byrd RP, Jr, Mehta JB, Roy TM. Malnutrition and pulmonary tuberculosis. Clin Infect Dis 2002;35:634-5.

81. Warmelink I, ten Hacken NH, van der Werf TS, van Altena R. Weight loss during tuberculosis treatment is an important risk factor for drug-induced hepatotoxicity. Br J Nutr 2011;105:400-8.

82. Baker MA, Harries AD, Jeon CY, Hart JE, Kapur A, Lönnroth K, et al. The impact of diabetes on tuberculosis treatment outcomes: a systematic review. BMC Med 2011;9:81.

83. Schwenk A, Hodgson L, Wright A, Ward LC, Rayner CF, Grubnic S, et al. Nutrient partitioning during treatment of tuberculosis: gain in body fat mass but not in protein mass. Am J Clin Nutr 2004;79:1006-12.

84. Faurholt-Jepsen D, Range N, Praygod G, Kidola J, Faurholt-Jepsen M, Aabye MG, et al. The role of diabetes co-morbidity for tuberculosis treatment outcomes: a prospective cohort study from Mwanza, Tanzania. BMC Infect Dis 2012;12:165.

85. Harrison BD, Tugwell P, Fawcett IW. Tuberculin reaction in adult Nigerians with sputum-positive pulmonary tuberculosis. Lancet 1975;1:421-4.

86. Cegielski JP, McMurray DN. The relationship between malnutrition and tuberculosis: evidence from studies in humans and experimental animals. Int J Tuberc Lung Dis 2004;8:286-98.

87. Sakamoto M, Nishioka K, Shimada K. Effect of malnutrition and nutritional rehabilitation on tuberculin reactivity and complement level in rats. Immunology 1979;38:413-20.

88. Pelly TF, Santillan CF, Gilman RH, Cabrera LZ, Garcia E, Vidal C, et al. Tuberculosis skin testing, anergy and protein malnutrition in Peru. Int J Tuberc Lung Dis 2005;9:977-84.

89. Gofama MM, Garba AM, Mohammed AA. Mantoux test reactions among children managed for tuberculosis in Maiduguri, Nigeria. Scand J Infect Dis 2011;43:15-8.

90. Mandalakas AM, van Wyk S, Kirchner HL, Walzl G, Cotton M, Rabie H, et al. Detecting tuberculosis infection in HIV-infected children: a study of diagnostic accuracy, confounding and interaction. Pediatr Infect Dis J 2013;32:e111-8.

91. Thomas TA, Mondal D, Noor Z, Liu L, Alam M, Haque R, et al. Malnutrition and helminth infection affect performance of an interferon gamma-release assay. Pediatrics 2010;126:e1522-9.

92. Shu CC, Wu VC, Yang FJ, Pan SC, Lai TS, Wang JY, et al. Predictors and prevalence of latent tuberculosis infection in patients receiving long-term hemodialysis and peritoneal dialysis. PLoS One 2012;7:e42592.

93. Liebeschuetz S, Bamber S, Ewer K, Deeks J, Pathan AA, Lalvani A. Diagnosis of tuberculosis in South African children with a T-cell-based assay: a prospective cohort study. Lancet 2004;364:2196-203.

94. Kielmann AA, Uberoi IS, Chandra RK, Mehra VL. The effect of nutritional status on immune capacity and immune responses in preschool children in a rural community in India. Bull World Health Organ 1976;54:477-83.

95. McMurray DN, Mintzer CL, Tetzlaff CL, Carlomagno MA. The influence of dietary protein on the protective effect of BCG in guinea pigs. Tubercle 1986;67:31-9.

96. Satyanarayana K, Bhaskaram P, Seshu VC, Reddy V. Influence of nutrition on postvaccinial tuberculin sensitivity. Am J Clin Nutr 1980;33:2334-7.

97. Sinclair D, Abba K, Grobler L, Sudarsanam TD. Nutritional supplements for people being treated for active tuberculosis. Cochrane Database Syst Rev 2011:CD006086.

98. Ramakrishnan CV, Rajendran K, Jacob PG, Fox W, Radhakrishna S. The role of diet in the treatment of pulmonary tuberculosis. An evaluation in a controlled chemotherapy study in home and sanatorium patients in South India. Bull World Health Organ 1961; 25:339-59.

99. Sudarsanam TD, John J, Kang G, Mahendri V, Gerrior J, Franciosa M, et al. Pilot randomized trial of nutritional supplementation in patients with tuberculosis and HIV-tuberculosis coinfection receiving directly observed short-course chemotherapy for tuberculosis. Trop Med Int Health 2011;16:699-706.

100. Jahnavi G, Sudha CH. Randomised controlled trial of food supplements in patients with newly diagnosed. Singapore Med J 2010;51:957-62.

101. Paton NI, Chua YK, Earnest A, Chee CB. Randomized controlled trial of nutritional supplementation in patients with newly diagnosed tuberculosis and wasting. Am J Clin Nutr 2004;80:460-5.

102. PrayGod G, Range N, Faurholt-Jepsen D, Jeremiah K, Faurholt-Jepsen M, Aabye MG, et al. The effect of energy-protein supplementation on weight, body composition and. Br J Nutr 2012;107:263-71.

103. Schön T, Idh J, Westman A, Abate E, Diro E, Moges F, et al. Effects of a food supplement rich in arginine in patients with smear positive pulmonary tuberculosis--a randomised trial. Tuberculosis [Edinb] 2011;91:370-7.

104. Martins N, Morris P, Kelly PM. Food incentives to improve completion of tuberculosis treatment: randomised controlled trial in Dili, Timor-Leste. BMJ 2009;339:b4248.

105. Williams C. On the use and administration of cod-liver oil in pulmonary consumption. London J Med [currently British Medical Journal] 1849;2:1-18.

106. Young J. Cod-liver oil in phthisis. Boston Medical and Surgical Journal [currently the New England Journal of Medicine] 1849;39:509-12.

107. Zasloff M. Fighting infections with vitamin D. Nat Med 2006;12:388-90.

108. Liu PT, Stenger S, Li H, Wenzel L, Tan BH, Krutzik SR, et al. Toll-like receptor triggering of a vitamin D-mediated human antimicrobial response. Science 2006;311:1770-3.

109. Gao L, Tao Y, Zhang L, Jin Q. Vitamin D receptor genetic polymorphisms and tuberculosis: updated systematic review and meta-analysis. Int J Tuberc Lung Dis 2010;14:15-23.

110. Sharma PR, Singh S, Jena M, Mishra G, Prakash R, Das PK, et al. Coding and non-coding polymorphisms in VDR gene and susceptibility to pulmonary tuberculosis in tribes, castes and Muslims of Central India. Infect Genet Evol 2011;11:1456-61.

111. Gwinup G, Randazzo G, Elias A. The influence of vitamin D intake on serum calcium in tuberculosis. Acta Endocrinol [Copenh] 1981;97:114-7.

112. Wejse C, Gomes VF, Rabna P, Gustafson P, Aaby P, Lisse IM, et al. Vitamin D as supplementary treatment for tuberculosis: a double-blind, randomized, placebo-controlled trial. Am J Respir Crit Care Med 2009;179:843-50.

113. Nursyam EW, Amin Z, Rumende CM. The effect of vitamin D as supplementary treatment in patients with moderately advanced pulmonary tuberculous lesion. Acta Med Indones 2006;38:3-5.

114. Martineau AR, Timms PM, Bothamley GH, Hanifa Y, Islam K, Claxton AP, et al. High-dose vitamin D[3] during intensive-phase antimicrobial treatment of pulmonary tuberculosis: a double-blind randomised controlled trial. Lancet 2011;377:242-50.

115. Downes J. An experiment in the control of tuberculosis among Negroes. Milbank Mem Fund Q 1950;28:127-59.

116. Villamor E, Mugusi F, Urassa W, Bosch RJ, Saathoff E, Matsumoto K, et al. A trial of the effect of micronutrient supplementation on treatment outcome, T cell counts, morbidity, and mortality in adults with pulmonary tuberculosis. J Infect Dis 2008;197:1499-505.

117. Range N, Andersen AB, Magnussen P, Mugomela A, Friis H. The effect of micronutrient supplementation on treatment outcome in patients with. Trop Med Int Health 2005;10:826-32.

118. Range N, Changalucha J, Krarup H, Magnussen P, Andersen AB, Friis H. The effect of multi-vitamin/mineral supplementation on mortality during treatment. Br J Nutr 2006;95:762-70.

119. Semba RD, Kumwenda J, Zijlstra E, Ricks MO, van Lettow M, Whalen C, et al. Micronutrient supplements and mortality of HIV-infected adults with pulmonary TB. Int J Tuberc Lung Dis 2007;11:854-9.

120. PrayGod G, Range N, Faurholt-Jepsen D, Jeremiah K, Faurholt-Jepsen M, Aabye MG, et al. Daily multi-micronutrient supplementation during tuberculosis treatment increases. J Nutr 2011;141:685-91.

121. Mehta S, Mugusi FM, Bosch RJ, Aboud S, Chatterjee A, Finkelstein JL, et al. A randomized trial of multivitamin supplementation in children with tuberculosis in Tanzania. Nutr J 2011;10:120.

122. Pakasi TA, Karyadi E, Suratih NM, Salean M, Darmawidjaja N, Bor H, et al. Zinc and vitamin A supplementation fails to reduce sputum conversion time in. Nutr J 2010;9:41.

123. Lawson L, Thacher TD, Yassin MA, Onuoha NA, Usman A, Emenyonu NE, et al. Randomized controlled trial of zinc and vitamin A as co-adjuvants. Trop Med Int Health 2010;15: 1481-90.

124. Armijos RX, Weigel MM, Chacon R, Flores L, Campos A. Adjunctive micronutrient supplementation for pulmonary tuberculosis. Salud Publica Mex 2010;52:185-9.

125. Visser ME, Grewal HM, Swart EC, Dhansay MA, Walzl G, Swanevelder S, et al. The effect of vitamin A and zinc supplementation on treatment outcomes in pulmonary tuberculosis: a randomized controlled trial. Am J Clin Nutr 2011;93:93-100.

126. Das BS, Devi U, Mohan Rao C, Srivastava VK, Rath PK. Effect of iron supplementation on mild to moderate anaemia in pulmonary tuberculosis. Br J Nutr 2003;90:541-50.

127. Visser ME, Texeira-Swiegelaar C, Maartens G. The short-term effects of anti-tuberculosis therapy on plasma pyridoxine levels in patients with pulmonary tuberculosis. Int J Tuberc Lung Dis 2004;8:260-2.

128. Zilber LA, Bajdakova ZL, Gardasjan AN, Konovalov NV, Bunina TL, Barabadze EM. The prevention and treatment of isoniazid toxicity in the therapy of pulmonary tuberculosis 2. An assesmrnt of the prophylactic effect of pyridoxine in low dosage. Bull World Health Organ 1963;29:457-81.

129. Subbaraman R, Chaguturu SK, Mayer KH, Flanigan TP, Kumarasamy N. Adverse effects of highly active antiretroviral therapy in developing countries. Clin Infect Dis 2007;45:1093-101.

130. Patel R. Stuffed and starved: the hidden battle for the world food system. New York: Melville House Publishers; 2012.

131. Deaton A, Dreze J. Food and nutrition in India: facts and interpretations. Econ Polit Wkly 2009;44:42-65.

132. Dye C, Bourdin Trunz B, Lonnroth K, Roglic G, Williams BG. Nutrition, diabetes and tuberculosis in the epidemiological transition. PLoS One 2011;6:e21161.

133. Dreze J, Sen A. Hunger and public action. London: Oxford University Press; 1989.

41

Nontuberculous Mycobacterial Infections

VM Katoch, T Mohan Kumar, Babban Jee

INTRODUCTION

Nontuberculous mycobacteria [NTM] in the past were known by various names such as 'anonymous', 'environmental', 'opportunistic' mycobacteria and mycobacteria other than *Mycobacterium tuberculosis* [*Mtb*] complex [MOTT] (1-14). None of these terms has become universally acceptable and the name NTM seems to have better consensus and is also endorsed by the American Thoracic Society [ATS] and the Infectious Diseases Society of America [IDSA] statement (11,14).

These mycobacteria mainly exist in the environment as saprophytes. First such mycobacterium was recognised as a cause of human disease in 1908 (1). These organisms in the past were called "atypical mycobacteria", the term first coined by Pinner (2). Diseases caused by these organisms are uncommon compared with tuberculosis [TB], but there has been a significant increase in pulmonary and non-pulmonary infections due to these mycobacteria during the last two to three decades (3-8). This increase can be partly explained by the increase in the number of susceptible and immunocompromised individuals but can also be attributed to the availability of better technology and increased reporting worldwide. While the infections caused by *Mtb*, *M. bovis*, *M. leprae* are definite clinical entities, the diseases caused by NTM have varied manifestations, are usually not transmitted from man-to-man except *M. abscessus* in cystic fibrosis patients. Even though these mycobacteria have been present in the environment, the emergence of human immunodeficiency virus infection [HIV] and acquired immunodeficiency syndrome [AIDS] has significantly increased the risk of TB and disease due to NTM (9-11). In these individuals the NTM disease has been a major cause of morbidity and mortality in western countries (11). The NTM cause pulmonary and disseminated

infections in immunocompromised individuals and cervical lymphadenitis in children (3-8,11,12). Of the approximately 200 known species and 13 subspecies of NTM so far (13), only one-fourth is found to be associated with disease in humans. The important NTM species are listed in Tables 41.1A and 41.1B. Most of these NTM exhibit *in vitro* resistance to many drugs that are used for the treatment of *Mtb* (14,15). Some species, like *M. genavense* (16), *M. celatum* (17), *M. conspicuum* (18) and *M. colombiense* (19) were reported for the first time from people living with HIV/AIDS [PLHA]. *M. paratuberculosis* also appears to be the likely causative organism for Crohn's disease.

DISTRIBUTION IN THE ENVIRONMENT

Most of the NTM are ubiquitous in distribution and have been isolated from a wide variety of environmental sources including water (20), soil (21), swamp (22), biofilms (23), ice-machine (24), cigarette (25), biocide-treated metal-working fluid (26), gentian violet solution (27), moisture-damaged buildings (28), food stuffs (29) and protozoa (30). Generally, domestic, municipal and hospital water supply systems, swimming pools and whirlpools, coastal areas, hot tubs, aquaria, water and sewage treatment plants are considered main reservoirs of NTM (31). Further, NTM have extraordinary ability to survive in very odd physiological and environmental conditions and continue their life cycle even in extreme nutritional starvation and temperature fluctuations (32-35).

M. avium complex [MAC] organisms have been isolated from natural water sources, *M. kansasii* from tap water; and rapidly growing mycobacteria are found in soil and natural water sources as well as in tap water, water used for dialysis or even in surgical solution (3). Man-made changes in the environment may also have altered the risks from

Table 41.1A: NTM species

M. arupense	M. malmoense
M. aubaganense	M. marinum
M. avium	M. mucogenicum
M. avium intracellulare complex	M. neoaurum
M. boenickei	M. neworleansese
M. bohemicum	M. nonchromogenicum
M. bolletti	M. palustre
M. brisbanense	M. parascrofulaceum
M. canariasense [closely related to M. diernhoferi]	M. paratuberculosis
M. celatum	M. parmense
M. conspicuum	M. phocaicum
M. elephantis	M. porcinum
M. fortuitum- M. chelonae complex	M. pseudoshottii
M. fortuitum third biovariant complex	M. scrofulaceum
M. genavense	M. septicum
M. goodii	M. shottsii
M. gordonae	M. simiae
M. habana	M. smegmatis
M. haemophilum	M. szulgai
M. heckeshornense	M. terrae complex
M. houstonense	M. thermoresistibile
M. immunogenum	M. ulcerans
M. interjectum	M. vaccae
M. intracellulare	M. wolinskyi
M. kansasii	M. xenopi

Timpe and Runyon Classification (4) based on NTM growth rate and pigment production: growth rate >7 days; slowly growing mycobacteria [SGM]: Type I [photochromogens: *M. kansasii*, *M. marinum*, *M. asiaticum*, *M. simiae*]; Type II [scotochromogens: *M. scrofulaceum*, *M. szulgai*, *M. gordonae*, *M. flavescens*]; Type III [non-photochromogens: *MAC*, *M. xenopi*, *M. ulcerans*, *M. terrae*, *M. haemophilum*]; growth rate < 7 days: Type IV [rapidly growing mycobacteria: *M. fortuitum*, *M. abscessus*, *M. chelonae*]

NTM = nontuberculous mycobacteria

these mycobacteria. For example, hot water systems are growth nidus for some of these mycobacteria, such as *M. xenopi*, in the hospital environment and use of showers may result in droplet inhalation of the mycobacteria.

EPIDEMIOLOGY

The distribution of NTM, incidence and prevalence of diseases caused by them are difficult to determine since systems of notification vary from country to country. In the HIV-era, the United States and European countries appeared to be most affected regions of the world with NTM-associated infections. While MAC, *M. kansasii*, *M. abscessus*, *M. chelonae* and *M. fortuitum* were most frequently isolated NTM species in USA; *M. malmoense*, *M. xenopi*, *M. kansasii*, *M. abscessus* were predominant in Europe [particularly northern Europe]. *M. xenopi*, *M. kansasii* and *M. ulcerans* were much common in Canada, South Africa, Australia respectively (14,36). *M. marinum*, a common cause of skin and tendon infections, occurs in people living in coastal areas and those exposed to fish tanks or swimming pools. Recent data suggest that Asia is also becoming hot-spot of infections due to both slowly and rapidly growing NTM species. Like America, MAC was a common isolates in north-eastern Asia, especially in Japan and South Korea during 1971-2007. During this period in India, MAC, *M. terrae*, *M. scrofulaceum*, *M. flavescens*, *M. gordonae* were frequently encountered species. Interestingly, *M. fortuitum* was found to be common NTM isolate from pulmonary infections in India followed by *M. kansasii*, *M. triviale* and *M. szulgai* (37). There are several other important reports of NTM infections from India (38-45). Although *Mtb* has always been found as the major cause of mycobacterial infections and the proportion of NTM has varied (46-52). As the mycobacterial culture with strict criteria is still not routinely performed in most parts of India, and there is a tendency to ignore such isolates and in the absence of clear-cut guidelines followed in the country it is difficult to comment on the exact NTM disease burden. Moreover, NTM disease is not notifiable in India. *Mtb* has been observed to be the most common cause of TB especially EPTB in Indian patients with HIV/AIDS (52). It is emphasised that over-reliance on smear microscopy should be substituted with

Table 41.1B: Species of NTM causing infections in humans

M. abscessus complex	M. elephantis	M. marinum	M. septicum
M. arupense	M. fortuitum	M. neourum	M. shottsii
M. aubaganense	M. genavense	M. neworleanense	M. simiae
M. avium	M. goodii	M. nonchromogenicum	M. smegmatis
M. boenickei	M. gordonae	M. palustre	M. szulgai
M. bohemicum	M. haemophilum	M. parascrofulaceum	M. thermoresistibile
M. brisbanense	M. heckeshornense	M. paratuberculosis	M. terrae
M. canariense	M. houstonense	M. parmense	M. triviale
M. celatum	M. immunogenum	M. phocaicum	M. ulcerans
M. chelonae	M. interjectum	M. porcinum	M. vaccae
M. conspicuum	M. intracellulare	M. pseudoshottsii	M. wolinskyi
M. diernhoferi	M. kansasii	M. scrofulaceum	M. xenopi
	M. malmoense		

NTM = nontuberculous mycobacteria

identification, speciation including subspeciation of NTM isolates at the international level.

Source of NTM infections is usually from environmental reservoirs (53-56). Transmission of NTM from human-to-human is rare except outbreaks of infections due to *M. massiliense* in cystic fibrosis centres. Transmission of NTM from animal to human is also rare but, the possibility of person-to-person transmission cannot be ruled out (57). It was thought that NTM do not lead to latent infection but a study has shown that NTM can also undergo dormancy and eventually may develop latent infections similar to *Mtb* (58).

Exposure to NTM results in sensitisation which can be detected by skin test to NTM antigens and differential tuberculin testing with antigens prepared from other mycobacteria, e.g., purified protein derivative [PPD]-A [*M. avium*] or PPD-Y [*M. kansasii*] has been considered as a satisfactory method of distinguishing sensitisation due to NTM from *Mtb*.

PREDISPOSING FACTORS

It is well known that these environmental mycobacteria cause disease in individuals who offer some opportunity due to altered local or systemic immunity (3,4,11,59-63). While the reasons may be less clear in children with cervical lymphadenitis such factors may be quite obvious in patients with bronchiectasis, surgical procedures, injections, break in skin surface due to wounds and generalised immune deficiency states, like AIDS and use of immunosuppressive agents in transplant patients (11). However, mechanisms of pathogenesis of NTM infections are not very clear and have not been adequately investigated. The lipid-rich outer envelope of the organisms may be important as the first defense of these organism but specific moieties on the surface may also be important factors. Some NTM species, such as *M. avium* and *M. simiae* have been reported in patients with AIDS in India (60). Very low CD4+ T-cell counts in patients with AIDS and defective cytokine response[s] have been linked to development of severe infections due to *M. avium* from the common sources, such as potable water (64). Chronic obstructive pulmonary disease [COPD], emphysema, pneumoconiosis, bronchiectasis, cystic fibrosis, thoracic scoliosis, aspiration due to oesophageal disease, previous gastrectomy and chronic alcoholism are some of the conditions which have been linked to disease due to NTM. Table 41.2 provides a list of predisposing conditions to NTM infections.

HOST IMMUNE RESPONSE TO NTM INFECTIONS

Due to increasing number of NTM species identified to be associated with human infections, inadequate information is available on species specific host immune response. The knowledge about the immunoregulation in NTM infections is growing. From the risk point, *M. avium* is a most successful pathogen after *Mtb* causing a wide spectrum of diseases both in birds and human

subjects but little is known how host counters the attack of *M. avium* at immune level. It is assumed that *M. avium* enters macrophage using similar complement receptors CR1, CR3, CR4 and mannose receptors used by *Mtb* (65-67) and thereafter promotes recruitment of naïve monocytes to the site of infection by upregulating the expression of some prominent chemoattractants including interleukin [IL]-8, macrophage-inflammatory protein [MIP]1β, MIP1α, MIP2α, Regulated on Activation, Normal T-cell Expressed and Secreted [RANTES] protein, monocyte chemoattractant protein [MCP]-1 (68,69). Once phagocytosed, *M. avium* tries to adapt in the hostile environments of macrophage while host activates killing cascades. In this course, enhanced production of cytokines, like tumour necrosis factor-alpha [TNF-α], IL-1β, small inducible cytokine A5, trans-forming growth factor [TGF]-β2, IL-15, IL-9, IL-3, IL-6, IL-10, TGF-β1 (68,70), appearance of granuloma (71-75) and subsequent cell death (76-79) were thought to be the major steps in the control of infections. However, unaltered levels of iNOS, IL-12p40 and interferon-gamma [IFN-γ] during the exposure of *M. avium* to macrophage are intriguing (68). Cell death of *M. avium* infected macrophages has been shown to be under the control of Th1 immunity. Increasing amount of evidences suggests the central role of TNF-α in the apoptosis of *M. avium* infected macrophages (77,80) whereas IFN-γ appears to be major driving force behind granuloma necrosis (81). It has been reported that addition of exogenous hydrogen peroxide to macrophage culture also initiates apoptosis (82). Engulfment of apoptotic macrophage containing *M. avium* by healthy macrophages may be an additional strategy of host to limit the intracellular infection (77). Interestingly, *M. avium*, in some studies, has been observed to inhibit the apoptosis of infected macrophages (69,83,84).

Like *M. avium*, *M. avium* subsp. *paratuberculosis* [MAP] is also a multiple host pathogen causing deadly granulomatous enteritis [Johne's disease] in ruminants as well as possibly inflammatory bowel syndrome known as Crohn's disease in humans (85). Experimental data gathered from some *in vitro* and animal studies showed a clear shift in host immune responses during the infection of MAP. It was found that in early phase of pathogenesis, major pro-inflammatory cytokines are produced in larger quantity but this host action is not sustained for longer period. As infection progresses, the production of pro-inflammatory cytokines is replaced with abundant secretion of anti-inflammatory cytokines (86). A recent study using pan-genomic analysis of gene expression of MAP infected bovine monocyte derived macrophage provided a time-related picture of host's immune response. In this study, it was observed that just 2 hours after infection, MAP induced several-fold increase in expression of TNF-α, IL-1β, IL-1β, IL-6, *CXCL2* and *CCL20* genes and after 6 hours of infection, IL-1β, TNF-α, CXCL2, CCL4, CCL5, CCL20, CD40 and the complement factor B [CFB] genes were among the differentially expressed genes showing relatively higher level of expression as compared to those observed at two hours post-infection (87). In other

Table 41.2: Important host-related predisposing conditions

Association with host-related predisposing factors [NTM-PD]
Bronchiectasis [especially middle lobe and lingual]
Bronchiectasis due to cystic fibrosis-*CFTR* gene polymorphism
Chronic obstructive pulmonary disease
Destroyed lungs due to TB or other diseases like pneumoconiosis
Pulmonary alveolar proteinosis
Primary ciliary dyskinesia
Alpha 1 antitrypsin deficiency
Thoracic skeletal abnormalities [kyphoscoliosis]
Gastroesophageal reflux disease
Lady Windermere syndrome*

Immunodeficiency states
Primary†
Anti-interferon γ-antibodies [blocking of interferon γ–interleukin-12 pathway]
Anti-GM-CSF antibodies [impaired local immunity]
NEMO mutations [impaired signal transduction from Toll-like receptors, interleukin-1, and TNF-α]
STAT1 deficiency [weakened systemic immunity]
IL12 mutations [reduced T-cells and natural killer cells stimulation]
CYBB mutations [decreased bactericidal activity]
GATA2 gene mutations [impaired hematopoietic, lymphatic, and vascular development]

Acquired
HIV status [CD4 counts <50 cells/μ]
Use of biologics [anti-TNF agents and TNF receptor blockers]
Use of immunosuppressive agents and steroids in organ transplantation and other autoimmune diseases
Lung cancer

Environmental factors
Individual factors
Indoor swimming pool use [in past 4 months]
Swimming pool use at least once a month
Soil exposure
Climatic factors
Proportion of areas as surface water
Mean daily potential evapotranspiration
Higher copper soil levels [helps mycobacteria to form biofilms]
Higher sodium soil levels [more nutrition for mycobacteria]
Lower manganese soil levels [manganese inhibits mycobacterial growth]
Lower top soil depth [high nutrition for mycobacteria due to low vegetation]

* Non-smoking post-menopausal white women who are taller and leaner with scoliosis, pectus excavatum and mitral valve prolapse syndrome than their peers

† These mutations are rare and associated with disseminated NTM disease

NTM-PD = NTM pulmonary disease; BMI = body mass index; CFTR = cystic fibrosis transmembrane receptor; GM-CSF = granulocyte macrophage colony stimulating factor; NEMO = nuclear factor κB essential modulator; STAT1 = signal transducer and activator of transcription 1 [for disseminated infection]; IL-12 = interleukin-12; TNF = tumour necrosis factor; CYBB = cytochrome b-245 beta

study (88), a marked upregulation of anti-inflammatory cytokine IL-10 gene at all the experimental time-points [6, 24 and 72 hours] and concomitant downregulation of IFN-γ and TNF-α [at 6 hours] and IL-12 [at 72 hours] was noticed suggesting that development of true clinical form of disease is largely concerned with the dysregulation of host's effective defense mechanisms against this facultative pathogen. Not only in this but in many subsequent molecular studies carried out either with patients or animal monocytes/macrophages, higher expression of IL-10 and other important anti-inflammatory cytokine genes [IL-6 and TGF-β] six hours of post-infection emphasised the role of IL-10 in progression of disease (89-92). Interleukin-23 [IL-23] (93) and an imbalance in the ratio of Th17 cells and

regulatory T-cells [Treg] cells (94) have been implicated in the breakdown of host protective immunity. Further, polymorphism in IL-18 gene has also been associated with increased risk of Crohn's disease (95).

Studies carried out with murine model infected with *M. abscessus* [MAB] have shown that early neutrophilic response was an important factor in limiting the intracellular spread of this pathogen (96). Interaction of toll-like receptor-2 [TLR-2] with dectin-1 resulted in the enhanced production of TNF-α, IL-6 and p40 subunit of IL-12 in murine macrophages (97). Further study demonstrated that control of MAB infection in mice spleen was primarily dependent on T-cell while in liver, it was both T-cell and B-cell driven (98). It has been reported that an early influx of IFN-γ-producing CD4+ and

CD8+ T-cells into the lungs of C57BL/6 mice might play a pivotal role in clearing the invading agents from the host body (96). In an *in vitro* study carried out with MAB infected human cells, it was found that production of TNF-α was dependent on TLR-2 and mitogen-activated protein kinase [MAPK] p38 pathways and is a property shared with *M. avium* (99).

Prior to 2010, it was only a hypothesis that person having genetic defects in IFN-γ/IL-12 co-stimulatory axis may be more prone to NTM infections. But recent clinical data have provided evidence that such hypothesis is correct, it has been observed that production of anti-IFN-γ autoantibodies in patient's body, IFN-γ associated first-line defence machinery was not able to counter the attack of exogenous pathogens resulting in establishment of infections (100-103). Based on analysis of different studies during 1979 to 2015, Wu and Holland (104) have proposed mechanism[s] linking certain genetic/immunological defects with susceptibility to disseminated NTM disease [Figure 41.1] and have also suggested an algorithm to investigate these defects [Figure 41.2]. Further studies will be required to validate the same and adopt the strategy for clinical use in different geographical settings.

CLINICALLY IMPORTANT MYCOBACTERIA

Among the known 200 species and 13 subspecies of NTM, only one-fourth have been associated with localised and or disseminated diseases in humans [Tables 41.3 and 41.4].

Mycobacterium avium Complex

Members of MAC group have gained a major prominence in the west, especially after an increased frequency of infections produced by these organisms in patients with AIDS (105-108). However, in western countries these organisms were also an important cause of pulmonary and other infections in the pre-AIDS era (11,109,110) as well due to TB becoming rarer in these countries long back.

M. avium subsp. Avium

M. avium subsp. *avium* has been isolated from environment as well as clinical specimens including sputum from India (51,111). Certain specific serotypes of *M. avium* (11,62), plasmid containing *M. avium* (112) and in some European and African countries certain restriction fragment length polymorphism [RFLP] types of *M. avium* have been found to be more commonly isolated from patients with AIDS (62,108).

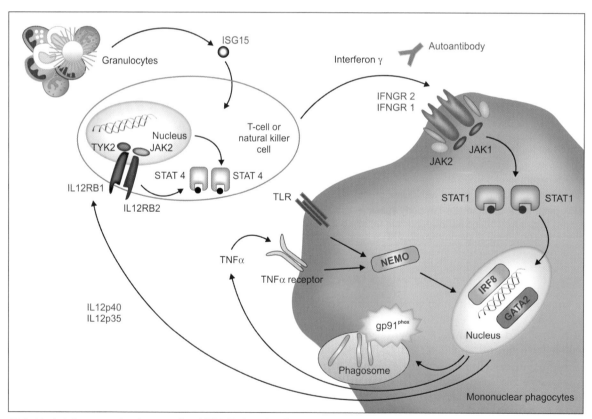

Figure 41.1: Host defence mechanisms against NTM. Defects leading to disseminated nontuberculous mycobacterial infection are shown in red ISG15 = interferon-stimulated gene 15; IFNGR = interferon-gamma receptor; TYK = tyrosine kinase; JAK = Janus kinase; STAT = signal transducer and activator of transcription; IRF = interferon regulatory factor; GATA = transcription factor implicated in early haemopoietic, lymphatic, and vascular development; NEMO = nuclear factor kappa-light-chain-enhancer of activated B cells essential modulator; IL = interleukin; TNF = tumour necrosis factor; TLR = toll-like receptors.
Reproduced with permission from "Wu UI, Holland SM. Host susceptibility to non-tuberculous mycobacterial infections. Lancet Infect Dis 2015;15:968-80 (reference 104)"

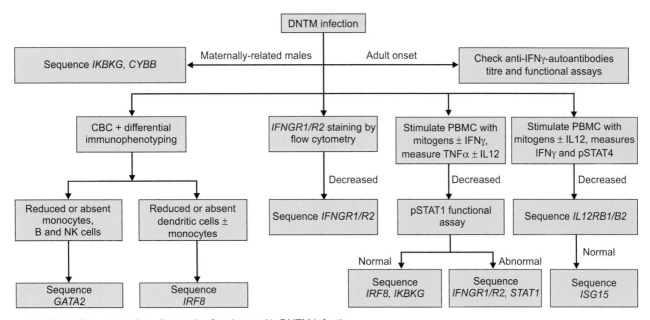

Figure 41.2: Stepwise approach to diagnosis of patients with DNTM infection

DNTM = disseminated nontuberculous mycobacterial; IFN = interferon; IL = interleukin; CBC = complete blood count; NK = natural killer; IFNGR = interferon gamma receptor; *IKBKG* = X-linked IKK-γ gene; *CYBB* = encodes the gp91[pox] submit of the phagocyte nadph oxidase; pSTAT1 = phosphorylated STAT1; NADPH = nicotinamide adenine dinucleotide phosphate; STAT = signal transducer and activator of transcription; *Reproduced with permission from "Wu UI, Holland SM. Host susceptibility to nontuberculous mycobacterial infections. Lancet Infect Dis 2015;15:968-80 (reference 104)"*

Table 41.3: Localised clinical diseases due to NTM

Type of lesion	Species
Pulmonary disease	Common: *M. avium* complex, *M. abscessus*, *M. kansasii*, *M. malmoense*, *M. xenopi* Uncommon: *M. chelonae*, *M. fortuitum*, *M. haemophilum*, *M. celatum**, *M. asiaticum**, *M. scrofulaceum*, *M. shimoidei**, *M. simiae*, *M. smegmatis*, *M. szulgai*
Lymphadenopathy	Common: *M. avium* complex, *M. scrofulaceum*, *M. malmoense* Uncommon: *M. genavense*, *M. haemophilum*, *M. chelonae*, *M. abscessus*, *M. fortuitum*, *M. kansasii*, *M. szulgai*
Skin, soft tissue, wound infections, bone disease	Common: *M. marinum*, *M. ulcerans*, *M. chelonae*, *M. fortuitum*, *M. abscessus* Uncommon: *M. avium* complex, *M. haemophilum*, *M. mucogenicum*, *M. nonchromogenicum*, *M. kansasii*, *M. malmoense*, *M. smegmatis*, *M. szulgai*, *M. terrae* complex, *M. immunogenum*
Specimen contaminant	*M. gordonae*, *M. haemophilum*, *M. mucogenicum*, *M. nonchromogenicum*, *M. terrae* complex
Crohn's disease	*M. avium* subsp. *paratuberculosis*
* Details regarding these species are available in the online supplement to reference NTM = nontuberculous mycobacteria	

Table 41.4: Disseminated disease due to NTM

Condition	Species
Disseminated disease	Common: *M. avium* complex, *M. chelonae*, *M. haemophilum*, *M. kansasii** Uncommon: *M. abscessus*, *M. celatum†*, *M. conspicuum†*, *M. fortuitum*, *M. genavense*, *M. immunogenum*, *M. malmoense*, *M. marinum*, *M. mucogenicum*, *M. scrofulaceum*, *M. simiae*, *M. szulgai*, *M. xenopi*
Without AIDS [usually transplant patients, leukaemia, etc.]	*M. avium* complex, *M. kansasii*, *M. chelonae*, *M. scrofulaceum*, *M. fortuitum* including members of *M. fortuitum* third biovariant complex-*M. boenickei*, *M. houstonense*, *M. neworleansese*, *M. brisbanense*, *M. porcinum* and *M. parascrofulaceum*, *M. septicum*, *M. canariasense* closely related to *M. diernhoferi*, *M. haemophilum*
With AIDS	*M. avium* complex, *M. haemophilum*, *M. simiae*, *M. xenopi*, *M. kansasii*, *M. fortuitum-chelonae* complex, *M. genavense*, *M. malmoense*, *M. celatum*, *M. conspicuum*
* *M. kansasii* lung disease is similar to that caused by *Mtb* and responds to rifampicin, isoniazid and ethambutol † Details regarding these species are available in the online supplement to reference NTM = nontuberculous mycobacteria; AIDS = acquired immunodeficiency syndrome; *Mtb* = *Mycobacterium tuberculosis*	

As compared to *M. intracellulare*, *M. avium* appears to have a greater predilection for causing disease in patients with AIDS (62). Further, these organisms may cause mixed infections along with other NTM, such as *M. kansasii* (106) and *M. simiae* (107), among others.

Infections caused by MAC were commonly observed in chronic bronchitis, bronchiectasis and chronic obstructive air-ways disease in the pre-AIDS era in geriatric patients. In non-HIV patients, *M. avium* has been associated with pulmonary disease, lymphadenitis and joint involvement (11). Unlike *Mtb*, the MAC strains have a low virulence and despite being commonly found in the environment rarely cause disease (64,113). These usually produce clinical disease only when the CD4+ T-cell count is very low [< 50 cells/mm^3] towards the end of natural history of disease, seen in 4%-5% of HIV/AIDS patients (61). MAC strains isolated from patients with AIDS in Africa have been shown to be different as compared with western strains (62). In AIDS patients, the portal of entry is thought to be mainly through the gut (64) and the most common presenting features include persistent high-grade fever, night sweats, anaemia and weight loss in addition to non-specific symptoms of malaise, anorexia, diarrhoea, myalgia and occasional painful adenopathy. On examination, there may be hepatomegaly and chest radiograph as well as computed tomography [CT] of the chest and abdomen may show a widespread intrathoracic and intra-abdominal lymphadenopathy. The diagnosis is generally not difficult as clinical specimens yield numerous acid–fast bacilli [AFB] which can be cultured and identified.

M. avium subsp. paratuberculosis

MAP subspecies is closely related to *M. avium* and has characteristic property of dependence on mycobactin J. This organism has been reported to be causative organisms of enteritis [Johne's disease] in cattle, goats and sheep and can be characterised rapidly with molecular techniques (114,115). With the help of gene probes, strains belonging to this subspecies have been linked to aetiology of Crohn's disease in man (115). Demonstration of specific sequences in tissue sections by *in situ* hybridisation has provided a strong evidence of an aetiological relationship of this *mycobacterium* with Crohn's disease (116).

M. avium subsp. hominissuis

M. avium subsp. *hominissuis* is a new opportunistic myco-bacterial pathogen (117) found to be associated with lympha-denitis in children (118-120), pulmonary disease (121,122) and AIDS (123). Pigs and slaughtered cattle are considered the potential sources of this NTM species in addition to human (124).

M. intracellulare

Before molecular era, the clinical disease caused by this NTM pathogen was possibly wrongly estimated due to close phenotypic similarity with *M. avium*. But, now it is possible

to determine the presence of this slowly growing pathogen in clinical samples by various molecular techniques even in a small laboratory setting. Literature suggests that like *M. avium*, this pathogen is an established aetiological agent of pulmonary disease (125-127), further its involvement in pathogenesis of cutaneous infection (128), thymoma (129) and disseminated disease (130) has been reported.

M. colombiense

M. colombiense, a slowly growing NTM species developing pigmentation over two weeks of incubation (131), is a new member of MAC which has been identified to be a human pathogen. After the first report of infection by this species in HIV-seropositive individuals in Colombia (19), it has also been isolated from an immunocompetent patient suffering with lymphadenitis (120). Recently, it was associated with the outcome of defects in IFN-γ/IL-12 costimulatory axis of a 49-year-old Canadian woman who died due to fatal pneumonia and disseminated infection. Perhaps, this was the first report that showed the role of anti-IFN-γ autoantibodies in the NTM-associated death (132).

M. chimaera

M. chimaera is another potential human pathogen recently included as a species in MAC by virtue of its greater genetic similarity with *M. avium*. It shows full resistance to ethambutol and can easily be differentiated from other members of MAC by high-performance liquid chromatography [HPLC]-mycolic acid patterns and other molecular markers (133). The clinical data revealed its greater occurrence in respiratory as well as non-respiratory samples taken from elderly people suffering with a wide range of underlying diseases including bronchiectasis, COPD, pulmonary cavitation, diabetes and non-Hodgkin's lymphoma (133-135). In addition, isolation of this slowly growing and unpigmented bacillus from respiratory tract of children with underlying cystic fibrosis highlights its expanding clinical domain (136). *M. chimaera* infection has also been reported to be the possible cause of death of patients suffering with prosthetic valve endocarditis and bloodstream infection (137). A retrospective hospital-based study (138) from Germany showed that *M. chimaera* was the most frequent isolate in MAC-positive clinical specimens analysed between the years 2002 and 2006. Overall data regarding the isolation of *M. chimaera* from environmental sources and animals are very limited.

Mycobacterium kansasii

M. kansasii are found in water and consequently in some sputum samples as non-significant commensals. Nevertheless, when repeatedly isolated from sputum they could be associated with pulmonary disease (11). Since long time, *M. kansasii* has been considered an important cause of pulmonary disease (3,11) and has become even more important in AIDS era (106,139-142). Although *in vitro* susceptibility tests suggest that members of these species are more resistant to antimicrobial agents than *Mtb*, *M. kansasii* disease frequently responds well to multiple drug therapy (6,141,142). New biotypes of *M. kansasii* have been isolated from patients with AIDS (140). As with MAC infections, these patients may present with advanced AIDS with very low CD4+ T cell count [< 50 cells/mm^3].

M. scrofulaceum

The distribution of these pigmented organisms in nature is similar to that of *M. avium* and MAC (143). The most common disease caused by these organisms is cervical lymphadenitis in children as well as chronic ulcerative and nodular lesions (11). It may cause adult pulmonary disease and disseminated infections in patients with AIDS (11,143).

M. interjectum

The first report on pathogenic behaviour of *M. interjectum* appeared in 1993 when a German group isolated this organism from an 18 months old boy with chronic lymphadenitis (144). Later on, this scotochromogenic and smooth colony-forming NTM has been found to be causative agent of disease involving lung (145,146), intestine (147), skin (148) and brain (149) of both immunocompetent and immunocompromised AIDS individuals. This microorganism has been found to be a major cause of lymphadenitis of cervical and submandibular glands mainly in children (150,151).

M. xenopi

M. xenopi is an unusual bacterium with optimal growth temperature at 45°C. It has been reported as a pathogen in patients with other underlying lung diseases (152-154). It has been isolated from hot water reservoirs of hospitals and has been found to be associated with various clinical problems (11,152,153). Clinical manifestations are similar to MAC in patients with advanced AIDS. An outbreak of pulmonary disease due to this organism from hot water supply of a hospital has been reported (11).

M. simiae Complex

M. simiae complex is a fast-expanding NTM group and so far comprises nine genetically close species *M. simiae*, *M. triplex*, *M. genavense*, *M. lentiflavum*, *M. heidelbergense*, *M. parascrofulaceum*, *M. florentinum*, *M. europaeum* and *M. stomatepiae*.

M. simiae

M. simiae, a niacin-positive *mycobacterium*, was initially isolated from a monkey in 1965 (155) and later recognised as a causative agent of pulmonary infection (156-159), lymphadenitis (160) and disseminated disease (161-163). This has been reported to be a causative agent in AIDS as well as non-AIDS patients. Like other NTM, it is less prevalent in environment and most of its isolation occurred from clinical

samples, however, not all clinical isolates had association with disease. Southwestern United States and Middle East were thought to be most affected parts of the world with this pathogen although its fatal clinical consequence was reported around the globe (164-170).

M. triplex

Before being recognised as a separate taxon, *M. triplex* was a member of "simiae-avium group"[SAV] (171). The first case of its pathologic involvement was reported in 2000 when *M. triplex* associated disseminated disease was reported in a 40-year-old HIV-seropositive individual (172). *M. triplex* has been found to be a cause of both disseminated (172,173) and pulmonary disease (174) in both immunodeficient and immunocompetent people.

M. genavense

M. genavense was isolated for the first time from patients with AIDS (16). Later, these have been emerged as major cause of disseminated infections in AIDS survivors (175-177). These organisms are grown with difficulty and need enrichment with mycobactin J. It grows in liquid media, often after prolonged incubation periods (16,178,179). Patients are usually in advanced stage of AIDS and present with weight loss, fever, abdominal pain and diarrhoea. This organism has been found to be sensitive to clarithromycin.

M. lentiflavum

M. lentiflavum was first recovered from a panel of clinical samples in 1996 (180) and later characterised as a potential human pathogen causing lung infection (181), lymphadenitis (182,183) and disseminated infections (184).

M. heidelbergense

M. heidelbergense has been recognised as an aetiological agent of cervical lymphadenitis in children (185). Its association with lung disease has also been documented (186).

M. parascrofulaceum

M. parascrofulaceum is a rare opportunistic pathogen and as of now limited information about its clinical relevance is available. It has been isolated from AIDS patients as well as some other forms of pulmonary disease in non-AIDS patients with underlying bronchiectasis, epidermoid carcinoma, COPD and emphysema (187,188). This species has also been considered as an agent of cutaneous (189) and chronic pelvic pain (190) in normal individuals. This mycobacterium was isolated for the first time from an Indian woman with a past history of TB who had immigrated to Canada in 1999 (191).

M. florentinum

M. florentinum first described in 2005, has been isolated from various clinical specimens like sputa, stool and lymph node derived from patients with known respiratory diseases and lymphadenopathy (192). There are only two recent reports which described its opportunistic nature in developing the human infections (193,194).

M. europaeum

M. europaeum is a recently discovered *mycobacterium* added to the *M. simiae* complex (195). This *mycobacterium* has been associated with pulmonary infection in people with underlying AIDS and cystic fibrosis (196).

M. terrae Complex

In classifications dating back to the 1970s, *M. terrae* complex included three species *M. terrae*, *M. nonchromogenicum* and *M. triviale*. After addition of eight new members namely *M. longobardum*, *M. engbaekii*, *M. heraklionense*, *M. algericum*, *M. senuense*, *M. arupense*, *M. kumamotonense* and *M. hiberniae* to this complex, the total number of species included in *M. terrae* complex has now reached 11.

M. terrae

M. terrae was initially considered as an environmental saprophyte (197). However, over the years, this mycobactin-dependent Runyon group III species has appeared as a significant cause of number of infections including lung infection (198,199), tenosynovitis (200,201), knee arthritis (202), knee sepsis (203), occurrence of sepsis during sickle cell disease (204), recurrent skin abscesses (205), lymphadenitis (206) and disseminated disease (207). Infection in renal transplant recipients has also been found to be associated with this organism (208). During *in vitro* testing, the organism was susceptible to rifampin (209).

M. nonchromogenicum

M. nonchromogenicum was first isolated from Japanese soil (210). The characteristic features of this NTM entity include intermediate growth on solid media and lack of pigmentation. This is usually a harmless microorganism but in some cases it was found to be pathogenic and associated with infections of intestine (211), tendons of hand and wrist (212,213), lung (214,215) and eye (216).

M. triviale

M. triviale was isolated from normal individuals in 1970s (217) and till that time this species was not reported to be associated with disease. Subsequently, this has been reported from a few clinical cases, including septic arthritis (218,219), peritonitis (220) and keratitis (216).

M. longobardum

M. longobardum is recently described NTM species isolated from clinical samples, showing rough and unpigmented colony at solid media during 7-14 days culture period and negative niacin tests (221). There is insufficient clinical data

about its pathogenic behaviour in human subjects, so far this has been found to be causative organism of chronic osteomyelitis in a 71-year-old man (222).

M. senuense

M. senuense is a new inclusion in *M. terrae* complex. It was isolated from a Korean patient with symptomatic pulmonary infections (223).

M. arupense

M. arupense is an emerging human pathogen with varied clinical manifestations. It has been reported to cause infections not only in immunocompromised AIDS patients (224) but also osteomyelitis (225), tenosynovitis (226) and lung disease (227) with or without underlying complications in immunocompetent individuals.

M. kumamotonense

M. kumamotonense was initially isolated from Japanese patients (228) but subsequently it was isolated from a Paraguayan HIV-positive patient with established extra-pulmonary disease (229).

M. marinum

M. marinum has been recognised as a causative organism of "swimming pool granuloma" or fish tank granuloma. It causes papular lesions in the extremities and may be confused with sporotrichosis (3,4,230-232). This has also been reported as a cause of infections of hands and wrist (231) and bones, joints and tendon sheaths, especially in patients with AIDS (232).

M. szulgai

M. szulgai species has been isolated on several occasions from patients with pulmonary disease. It is confused often with some of the scotochromogenic mycobacteria. This organism is also been associated with disseminated disease and also involves skin, joint and lymph nodes (233). These mycobacteria have been isolated from India also (48,49).

M. haemophilum

During the recent years this *mycobacterium* has emerged as an important human pathogen (234-238). This slowly growing organism has been recognised as a cause of life-threatening infections in immunocompromised individuals, like AIDS, bone marrow transplant recipients. The organism has been isolated from the skin lesions, lymph nodes, synovial fluid, vitreous fluid, bronchoalveolar lavage [BAL] fluid, bone marrow aspirate and blood. Recovery of this organism requires cultivation in enriched chocolate agar or haemin or ferric ammonium citrate supplement and incubation at 30°C up to eight weeks. Information about its environmental reservoirs and spread is limited. Despite aggressive therapy with multiple anti-TB drugs, the recurrence is common.

M. fortuitum Group

M. fortuitum group is a cluster of total 13 genetically close rapidly growing NTM species including members of a *M. fortuitum* third biovariant complex, *M. fortuitum*, *M. peregrinum*, *M. senegalense*, *M. mageritense* and *M. conceptionense*. *M. fortuitum* third biovariant complex consists of *M. boenickei*, *M. houstonense*, *M. neworleansense*, *M. brisbanense*, *M. porcinum* and *M. septicum*.

M. fortuitum

M. fortuitum is a widely distributed NTM species first isolated from a human abscess in 1938 by da Costa Cruz (15). With very high frequency of recovery from clinical samples studied so far, this human pathogen is ubiquitous in nature and found usually in water, soil and dust (15). This has emerged as an important cause of community acquired or health-care associated diseases and outbreaks (239-243). This has been associated with localised cutaneous and soft tissue infections (244-249), lymphadenitis (250,251), peritonitis (252), keratitis (253,254), endocarditis (255,256), meningitis/meningoencephalitis (257,258), hepatitis (259,260) and catheter-related infection (261,262) has also been reported. Disseminated infections due to this opportunistic pathogen are uncommon (263). After *M. abscessus*, it is the second most common species recovered from pulmonary infections caused due to rapidly growing mycobacteria (47,264-266). Pulmonary infection usually occurs secondary to aspiration.

M. peregrinum

M. peregrinum was first described in 1962. It is a rare cause of disseminated infections and only two cases of its kind have been reported so far (267,268). This pathogen has been associated with infections of lung (269,270), skin and soft tissue (271,272) and cervical lymph node (273) in addition to health care-related injection site and post-surgical infections (274,275).

M. fortuitum Third Biovariant Complex

M. fortuitum third biovariant complex came into existence by the work of Bönicke in 1966 (276). Members of this complex are clinically important and mainly associated with skin and soft tissues infections, traumatic injuries (277) and post-surgical infections (278). Currently, very little data regarding clinical significance of newly added members of this complex except *M. porcinum* and *M. septicum* are available.

M. porcinum

M. porcinum has been isolated from a variety of clinical samples, such as sputum, thigh and leg wound, inguinal node and lung biopsy derived from Australian and American peoples (279). This pathogen has been reported as a cause of pulmonary infections (280,281) in AIDS and non-AIDS patients with some underlying conditions, such as, prior TB and bronchiectasis. In some cases, it causes peritonitis (282),

post-mammaplasty infections (283) and postoperative sternal osteomyelitis (284).

M. septicum

This rapidly growing *mycobacterium* has been found to be associated with pulmonary disease (285), pneumonia (286) and central line sepsis (287).

M. conceptionense

M. conceptionense has been isolated for the first time from a 31-year-old woman having post-traumatic osteitis infection (288) and later this NTM has been associated with pulmonary and extrapulmonary infections (289,290), subcutaneous abscess (291) and postoperative sepsis (292).

M. mucogenicum

M. mucogenicum is a non-pigmented rapidly growing *mycobacterium* showing higher degree of susceptibility to a number of antibiotics, such as, amikacin, clarithromycin, imipenem, trimethoprim-sulfamethoxazole, linezolid, cefoxitin, ciprofloxacin and doxycycline. This *mycobacterium* has emerged as an important human pathogen and causes varied types of opportunistic infections mostly due to contaminated hospital water and health-care products. Its frequent isolation has been reported from the patients having post-organ transplantation (293), post-cosmetic surgery (294), bloodstream infections (295-298), peritonitis (299), pulmonary disease (168), cutaneous infection (300), catheter-related infection (301), central nervous system infection (302), Münchausen syndrome (303) and disseminated infection (304).

M. senegalense

M. senegalense has been associated with catheter-related sepsis (305) as well as tissue infection (306).

M. mageritense

M. mageritense, a non-pigmented mycobacterium, is an occasional cause of infections in human. There are some reports which showed the association of this pathogen to meningitis (307), bloodstream infection (308) and furunculosis (309).

M. abscessus

M. abscessus is a rapidly growing and non-chromogenic environmental mycobacteria dwelling primarily in domestic, municipal and hospital water supply systems, soil and decaying vegetations. Its initial isolation was reported from a patient's knee abscess in 1953 (310). In subsequent years, this organism has been considered as a life-threatening pathogen with worldwide occurrence. To date, this organism has been linked with a wide variety of diseases producing serious to moderate clinical consequences and many global outbreaks mainly in the United States (39,311-318). By virtue of its ability to grow at normal human body temperature, it causes deadly pulmonary disease not only in immunocompromised AIDS patients (319) but also in immunocompetent people (320,321) with underlying diseases, such as, bronchiectasis, cystic fibrosis and prior granulomatous diseases, such as TB. Clinical data showed that this pathogen is responsible for major proportion of rapidly growing mycobacterial [RGM] pulmonary disease (322) and after MAC, it is second most common NTM species isolated from pulmonary patients suffering with cystic fibrosis (323). Clinical findings also revealed that about 20% of MAB-infected people may also develop MAC diseases in their whole lifespan (322). Moreover, its frequent recovery from almost all clinical samples made this pathogen second most common NTM pathogen reported after *M. fortuitum* (15). Besides, this mycobacterial species has largely been associated with many other community acquired, health care- and hygiene-associated diseases which involve skin, soft tissue, bone, eye and heart (14,15,324,325). This species has been reported to be responsible for outbreaks mainly associated with interventions like injections (313,315,316). Studies from India (39,44,326-329) have also reported the isolation of this pathogen from a wide variety of clinical samples. It also shows complete resistance to all common anti-TB drugs.

M. chelonae

M. chelonae is an established cause of localised infections in both immunocompetent and immunosuppressed humans and has largely been associated with skin and soft tissue infections (330-335). Additionally, it has caused a wide variety of infections including disseminated disease (336), cardio-vascular infections (337,338), parotitis (339), osteomyelitis (340,341), keratitis (342), peritonitis (343), arthritis (344), nodular lymphangitis (345) and catheter-related bacter-aemia (346). This pathogen has also been recovered from patients with multiple clinical presentations (332,347,348). *M. chelonae* is occasionally associated with NTM pulmonary infection (349,350) and solitary rectal ulcer (351).

M. malmoense

M. malmoense (352-359) has emerged as another important pathogen which has not been isolated from the environ-ment (113). This *Mycobacterium* has been associated with disease in HIV (353), chronic granulocytic leukaemia (354), skin disease (355), pulmonary disease (356), cervical abscess (357), bursitis (358) and disseminated disease. Some of these infections occurred in immunocompetent individuals (355,357,359).

M. ulcerans

M. ulcerans has been established as an important skin pathogen for a long time (3,4,360-362). This pathogen was well known as a cause of Buruli ulcer in Africa (3,4), however, the skin infections caused by it are now being reported from other countries such as Japan (361).

EMERGING NEW MYCOBACTERIAL PATHOGENS

Several species of NTM have been isolated from AIDS patients over several years. Besides *M. genavense* (16), other species isolated for the first time from AIDS patients include: *M. celatum* (17), *M. conspicuum* (18) and *M. colombiense* (19). Other mycobacteria rarely associated with disease are: *M. smegmatis* (363-365), *M. thermoresistibile* (366-369), *M. neoaurum* (370,371) and *M. vaccae* (372). Due to wider use of gene sequencing using 16S ribosomal ribonucleic acid [rRNA], rpoB, these days several new species have been identified which were earlier missed as variants of known species. Within one decade (2,13) the number of identifiable distinct species has doubled. Some of them have been found to be the cause pronounced human infections. These newly identified pathogens have been isolated from a variety of conditions such as cutaneous, soft tissue and wound infections, from patients with pulmonary disease, lymphadenitis, bacteraemia, febrile conditions and disseminated disease. The exact importance of these potential pathogens in the causation of diseases will be better known with routine use of modern techniques for molecular characterisation in different parts of the world. The emerging human NTM pathogens are described in Table 41.5. Several among them, namely, *M. phlei, M. asiaticum, M. aurum, M. gordonae, M. gastri*, etc. have been taxonomically identified long back but were considered as saprophytes. Most others have been identified in recent past. It would be important to carefully analyse the pathogenic importance of all of these species in the context of emerging evidence of their association with disease. It would be appropriate to adopt and open but careful approach.

CLINICAL MANIFESTATIONS

NTM have been reported to be associated with varied clinical manifestations (3,4-8,11). In non-HIV patients, NTM has been established to be responsible for pulmonary disease usually with some local predisposing conditions, lymphadenitis, soft tissue infections, infections of joints and bones, bursae, skin ulcers and generalised disease in individuals like leukaemia, transplant patients, among others (3,4,11,373). In patients with AIDS the spectrum of clinical involvement may depend upon the degree of immune deficiency and the manifestations may range from localised pulmonary to intestinal and disseminated disease (11,374-376). Most of the NTM can be associated with both the localised and generalised disease depending upon degree of immune deficiency or local favourable conditions for their establishment and growth.

DIAGNOSIS

Diagnosis of the disease due to NTM depends upon the degree of suspicion and strict laboratory practices [Table 41.6]. The algorithm for the diagnosis of NTM infections is shown in Figure 41.3. Due to ubiquitous presence of these organisms in the environment, it is extremely important to

Table 41.5: The emerging human nontuberculous mycobacterial pathogens

M. abscessus subsp. abscessus	M. heckeshornense
M. abscessus subsp. bolletii	M. hodleri
M. abscessus subsp. massiliense	M. holsaticum
M. alvei	M. intermedium
M. arosiense	M. iranicum
M. asiaticum	M. kyorinense
M. aurum	M. llatzerense
M. austroafricanum	M. mantenii
M. bacteremicum	M. monacense
M. bohemicum	M. nebraskense
M. branderi	M. novocastrense
M. brisbanense	M. palustre
M. brumae	M. paraffinicum
M. canariasense	M. parakoreense
M. celatum	M. phlei
M. cosmeticum	M. phocaicum
M. doricum	M. poriferae
M. farcinogenes	M. rhodesiae
M. flavescens	M. riyadhense
M. fortuitum subsp. acetamidolyticum	M. saskatchewanense
M. frederiksbergense	M. setense
M. gastri	M. sherrisii
M. goodii	M. shimoidei
M. gordonae	M. shinjukuense
M. hassiacum	M. tokaiense

rule out contamination. At present, most of the experience is based on published findings from western countries and there is a general tendency of discarding these isolates as contaminants. These issues have been extensively debated and some broad guidelines have emerged (11,12,14).

Pulmonary Disease

Clinical presentation of the disease due to NTM may be like TB and pulmonary infections may present as chronic cough and infiltrates in the chest radiographs [Figures 41.4A and 41.4B]. Infection due to NTM should be suspected, especially in patients in whom initial anti-TB treatment has not produced clinical, radiographic and microbiological response. Sputum should always be sent for smear and myco-bacterial culture examination. If the cough is non-productive, bronchoscopy, and diagnostic testing of bronchial brushings, washings, aspirate, BAL and bronchoscopic biopsy material is indicated. NTM infection may be asymptomatic or may present as a subacute or chronic illness. Symptoms include cough, sputum production, weight loss, haemoptysis, shortness of breath, malaise, pleuritic chest pain, low-grade fever and night sweats. Radiographic appearances are similar to TB with cavities and infiltrates; though the upper lobes are more involved and the distribution is more variable than TB. Thin-walled cavities with lesser parenchymal infiltrates have been described as a suggestive feature (11). The changes may be unilateral or bilateral and more than one lobe may be involved. In high-resolution computed tomography [HRCT], clusters of small nodules associated with areas of bronchiectasis in the lower and middle zones

Table 41.6: Clinical and microbiological criteria for diagnosing NTM lung disease*

Clinical [both required]
i. Pulmonary symptoms, nodular or cavitary opacities on chest radiograph, or a high-resolution computed tomography scan that shows multifocal bronchiectasis with multiple small nodules [A, I]* and
ii. Appropriate exclusion of other diagnoses [A, I]*

Microbiologic
i. Positive culture results from at least two separate expectorated sputum samples [A, II]*. If the results from [i] are non-diagnostic, consider repeat sputum AFB smears and cultures [C, III]* or
ii. Positive culture result from at least one bronchial wash or lavage [C, III]* or
iii. Transbronchial or other lung biopsy with mycobacterial histopathologic features [granulomatous inflammation or AFB] and positive culture for NTM or biopsy showing mycobacterial histopathologic features [granulomatous inflammation or AFB] and one or more sputum or bronchial washings that are culture positive for NTM [A, II]*
iv. Expert consultation should be obtained when NTM are recovered that are either infrequently encountered or that usually represent environmental contamination [C, III]*
v. Patients who are suspected of having NTM lung disease but do not meet the diagnostic criteria should be followed until the diagnosis is firmly established or excluded [C, III]*
vi. Making the diagnosis of NTM lung disease does not, *per se*, necessitate the institution of therapy, which is a decision based on potential risks and benefits of therapy for individual patients [C, III]*

* Evidence quality as stated in online supplement of reference 14
NTM = nontuberculous mycobacteria; AFB = acid-fast bacilli
Reprinted with permissions of The American Thoracic Society. Copyright © 2019 American Thoracic Society, Griffith DE, Aksamit T, Brown-Elliott BA, Catanzaro A, Daley C, Gordin F, et al. An Official ATS/IDSA Statement: Diagnosis, treatment, and prevention of nontuberculous mycobacterial diseases. Am J Respir Crit Care Med 2007;175:367-416. An official Journal of The American Thoracic Society.

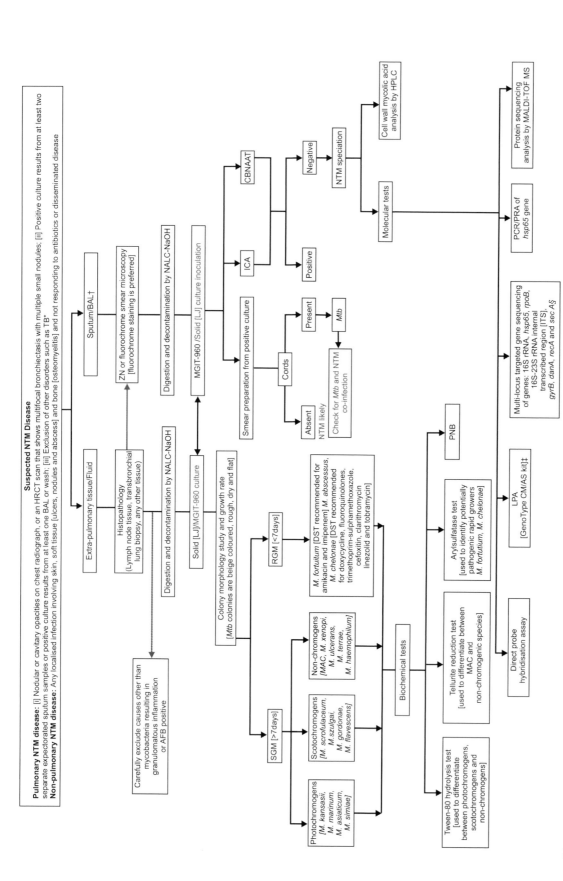

Figure 41.3: Diagnostic algorithm for NTM disease

* Three consecutive sputum samples are obtained; positive results from at least two separate expectorated sputum samples confirm the diagnosis (reference 14). They may appear as Gram-positive beaded rods [if organism burden is high]

† While sputum collection, the patient should not rinse mouth with municipal or untreated water. Spontaneous sputum should be collected or sputum should be induced if no sputum is produced by patient

‡ Common mycobacteria and additional species [CM/AS] is a strip-based reverse hybridisation technique in which 17 common mycobacterial and 17 additional mycobacterial species can be identified

§ These are target genes proposed for taxonomic identification of NTM due to their conserved nucleotide sequences. The sequencing *hsp65* and ITS genes has been widely accepted but for accurate identification multigene target approach has been recommended

NTM = nontuberculous mycobacteria; HRCT = high-resolution computed tomography; CSF = cerebrospinal fluid; ICA = immunochromatographic assay; CBNAAT = cartridge based nucleic acid amplification test; LJ = Lowenstein–Jensen media; HPLC: high performance liquid chromatography; SGM: slowly growing mycobacteria; RGM: rapidly growing mycobacteria; DST: drug susceptibility testing; LPA: line probe Assay; PNB: para-nitro benzoic acid; PCR/PRA: polymerase chain reaction/restriction endonuclease assay; MAC: *mycobacterium avium* complex; MALDI-TOF MS: matrix-assisted laser desorption ionization- time of flight mass spectrometry

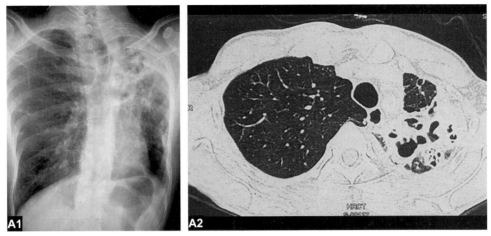

Figure 41.4A: Chest radiograph [postero-anterior view] [A1], CT chest [A2] showing destroyed left upper lobe. Sputum culture grew *M. intracellulare*
CT = computed tomography

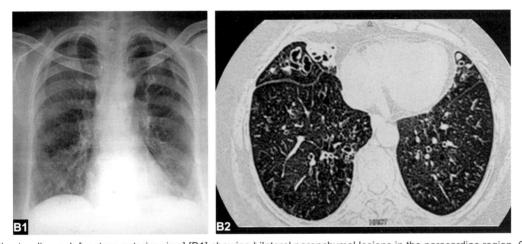

Figure 41.4B: Chest radiograph [postero-anterior view] [B1] showing bilateral parenchymal lesions in the paracardiac region. CECT chest [lung window] [B2] of the same patient showing parenchymal lesions in the medial segment of the middle lobe on the right side and lingula on the left side. Sputum culture from two separate specimens grew *Mycobacterium intracellulare*. The patient was successfully treated with drug regimen consisting of clarithromycin, rifampicin and ethambutol
CECT = contrast-enhanced computed tomography

are common. Asymptomatic solitary nodules due to MAC have been documented. Pleural thickening and effusion are not common. The gold standard for NTM disease compared to colonisation is a tissue biopsy showing granulomatous inflammation, which may or may not contain AFB and a positive culture, even if the sample is smear-negative.

Other Clinical Forms

Most of other manifestations should be considered in the differential diagnosis of any chronic infection, pyrexia of unknown origin and localised clinical disease [abscess, ulcers, nodules, infiltrates, etc.] not responding to antibiotics [Figures 41.5, 41.6, 41.7, 41.8, 41.9A, 41.9B and 41.10]. Attempts should be made to demonstrate and isolate the NTM from such lesions using most stringent criteria and precautions.

As most of the NTM are not sensitive to routine anti-TB drugs, it is imperative to correctly identify the causative

mycobacteria and, if required, determine their sensitivity profile.

Specimens

Because NTM are widely distributed in the environment and may be merely present as colonising agents on the skin and mucous membranes, proper sample collection is very important. In patients with suspicion of NTM pulmonary disease, the sputum collection should be done very carefully avoiding any environmental contamination. Prior to sputum collection, patients should not rinse mouth with municipal or untreated water and if the rinsing is required, sterilised water should be used. The specimen should be obtained directly from the lesion or organ concerned (11). It is recommended to attempt repeated isolation in significant numbers to firmly link the isolate with the aetiology. Further, the decontamination has to be gentler than *Mtb*. In case of disseminated infections, such as in patients with AIDS,

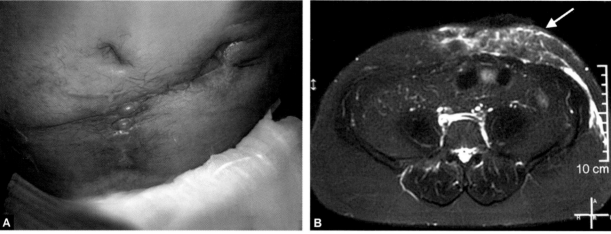

Figure 41.5: Clinical photograph [A], MRI [B] showing discharging sinus in the abdominal wall [arrow] in a patient following left inguinal hernia repair with mesh. Culture grew *M. abscessus*
MRI = magnetic resonance imaging

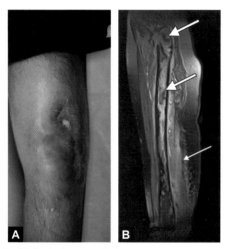

Figure 41.6: Clinical photograph [A] showing sinuses over the left knee joint and lateral aspect of upper left thigh. [B] MRI of the same patient showing intramedullary collection [thick arrows] suggestive of chronic osteomyelitis of left femur, soft tissue collection [thin arrow]. Left sided hip and knee joint involvement is also evident. Pus culture grew *M. abscessus*
MRI = magnetic resonance imaging

blood cultures have been shown to yield positive cultures. Diagnosis of MAC disease is established by growing the mycobacteria from the peripheral blood or bone marrow sample (377,378).

Histopathology

Histopathological examination of bone marrow, liver or lymph nodes [aspirates or biopsy] showing granuloma may be helpful in the diagnosis, the greatest advantage of this approach over the culture being the speed (105). It may be advisable to include some *in situ* methods [antigen detection and gene probes] to confirm the histological diagnosis straightaway.

Culture

There has been a considerable progress in developing and evaluation of methods for isolation of NTM from environment as well as clinical specimens (11,379-388). As these mycobacteria may be susceptible to decontaminating procedures like sodium hydroxide [NaOH] treatment (379), approaches like paraffin bating such as paraffin-coated slides become attractive option (380,381). Most of these mycobacteria are easy to cultivate and these can be grown on ordinary media for mycobacteria like Lowenstein-Jensen, Middle- brook and Dubos Broth, and Agar (11,380,384). Organisms like *M. haemophilum* may have special requirements like haemin for which blood containing media-chocolate agar or supplement of ferric ammonium citrate may be required. Various radiometric systems [e.g., BACTEC] (382,383,386); non-radiometric methods like mycobacteria growth inhibitor tube [MGIT] and MB/BacT (387,388) or liquid media like 13A or BACTEC 12B broth medium (60) as well as agar-based isolation systems have been described to be highly sensitive [up to 96%-98%] for MAC and other NTM (3,4,11,110,377,378,382-388). Pyruvate-containing medium may be necessary for growth of *M. bovis* or bacille Calmette-Guerin [BCG] (385). *M. genavense, M. paratuberculosis* will require supplementation with mycobactin J. Different incubation temperatures such as 30°C for *M. ulcerans* and *M. marinum*, 37°C for most pathogens, 45°C for *M. xenopi*, etc. will have to be selected depending upon the suspected organisms.

Identification of Isolates

The first scheme for identification and grouping of cultivable mycobacteria was based on growth rates and colony pigmentation. Since the days of Runyon, it is conventional to initially classify the organisms as rapid and slow growers (384).

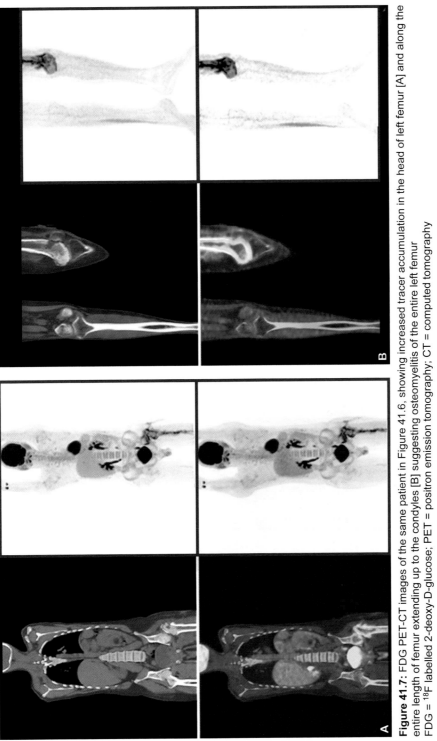

Figure 41.7: FDG PET-CT images of the same patient in Figure 41.6, showing increased tracer accumulation in the head of left femur [A] and along the entire length of femur extending up to the condyles [B] suggesting osteomyelitis of the entire left femur

FDG = [18]F labelled 2-deoxy-D-glucose; PET = positron emission tomography; CT = computed tomography

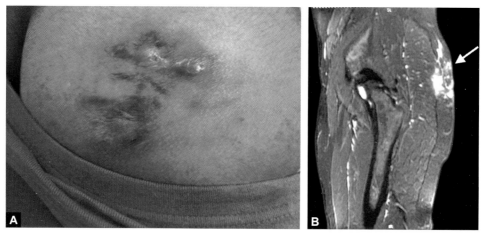

Figure 41.8: Clinical photograph [A], MRI [B] [arrow] showing right-sided post-injection gluteal abscess in a patient with NTM infection
MRI = magnetic resonance imaging; NTM = nontuberculous mycobacteria

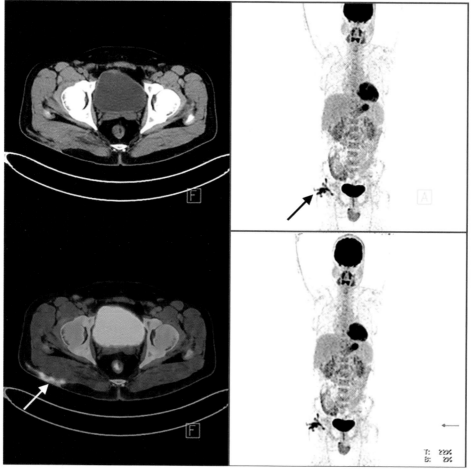

Figure 41.9A: Transaxial fused FDG PET-CT image of the same patient in Figure 41.7, at the level of acetabulum showing FDG accumulation in the subcutaneous thickening and stranding [arrow] involving the underlying right gluteus muscle superficially in right gluteal region
FDG = ^{18}F labelled 2-deoxy-D-glucose; PET = positron emission tomography; CT = computed tomography

Biochemical Tests

After classifying the mycobacteria on the basis of growth and pigmentation, most of the mycobacteria can be identified by biochemical tests (384). A few simple biochemical and culture tests can usually identify a strain to clinical satisfaction. These common tests are: niacin production, nitrate reduction, tween-80 hydrolysis, arylsulphatase, urease, and catalase [qualitative and quantitative] production, tellurite reduction, thiophene-2-carboxylic acid hydrazide sensitivity, growth on

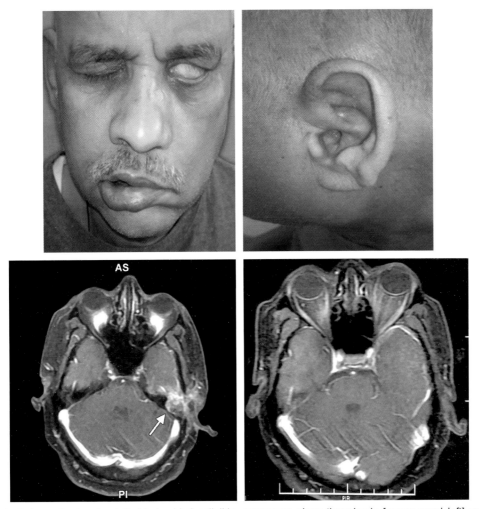

Figure 41.9B: Clinical photograph showing left-sided orbital cellulitis, cavernous sinus thrombosis [upper panel left] and pinna involvement [upper panel right]. MRI head of the same patient showing left-sided seventh nerve involvement, mastoiditis, apex of the petrous bone involvement [arrow] [lower panel left]; and meningitis [lower panel right]
MRI = magnetic resonance imaging

MacConkey agar, para-nitrobenzoic acid Lowenstein-Jensen medium [PNB-LJ] medium, sodium chloride tolerance, among others (384).

Lipid Patterns

Mycobacteria can be characterised at group and species from analysis of their cell wall lipids by thin layer chromatography and HPLC. These techniques are simple and have been developed along with easy software programmes for rapid analysis (385,386) by which isolates from liquid and solid media can be rapidly identified.

Identification Techniques for Established, Reference Laboratories

Alternative methods for identification of mycobacteria which would require special laboratories and expertise are described below:

Serotyping These methods have been well developed for the members of MAC (377,389). Based on serotype specific sera, these strains can be correctly identified and assigned to serotypes. Some serotypes (11,377) of *M. avium* have been shown to be preferentially associated with disease in patients with AIDS.

Isoenzyme and protein electropherograms Simple electrophoretic techniques and schemes based on electrophoretic mobilities of proteins and isoenzymes for the characterisation of strains of *Mtb* and NTM have been developed which can be used to confirm identity of the isolate rapidly (390-392). These patterns may be used both for rapid identification and characterisation of these mycobacteria (392).

Measurements of immunological relatedness Based on divergences in the structure of certain enzymes, such as, catalase (393) and superoxide dismutases (394), various clinically relevant mycobacterial species can be identified. This approach may also be evaluated in future studies.

New Molecular Methods for Identification and Characterisation

Recent years have witnessed many advances in the molecular genetics of various organisms including mycobacteria.

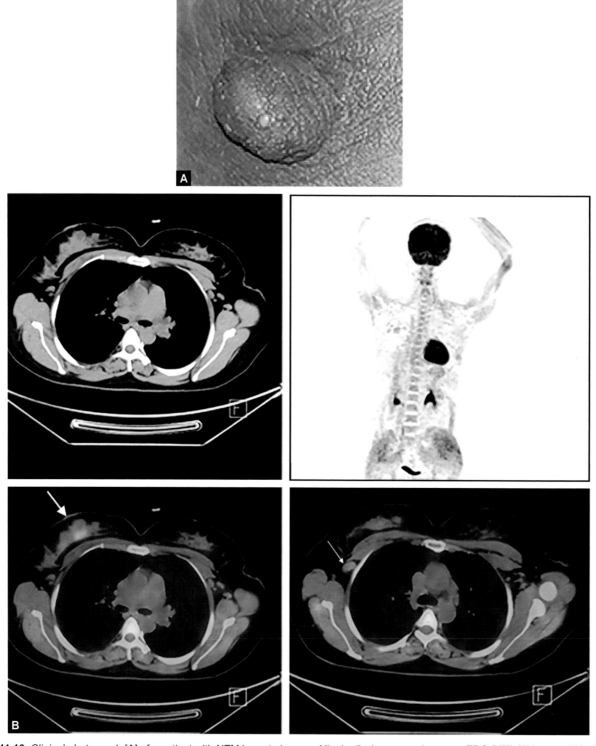

Figure 41.10: Clinical photograph [A] of a patient with NTM breast abscess. Nipple discharge can be seen. FDG PET-CT images [B] of the same patient showing FDG-avid right breast lesion [thick arrow] and right axillary lymphadenopathy [thin arrow]
FDG = 18F labelled 2-deoxy-D-glucose; PET = positron emission tomography; CT = computed tomography

As these are based on the complementarity of gene sequences, these techniques can achieve maximum sensitivity and specificity.

By hybridisation of isolated RNA, deoxyribonucleic acid [DNA] from growth or tissue with specific probes, identity of isolates is rapidly established. Based on new knowledge about the gene sequences many gene probes for the identification of isolates as well as amplification of specific gene fragments from the lesions and mycobacterial culture isolates have been developed and are described below.

Gene probes During the last 20 years, a number of gene probes for the identification of important NTM have been developed and some are also being commercially marketed (383,395-397). With the help of these probes, growth from solid slants and even liquid cultures [e.g., BACTEC] can be identified and these have been found to be fairly reliable and rapid.

Gene amplification methods Advances in gene amplification methods, especially polymerase chain reaction [PCR] technology have influenced almost every discipline of medicine. Several PCR techniques for rapid detection and identification of various clinically relevant mycobacteria have been developed (398-411). These include different types of PCR assays for detection of *M. avium, M. intracellulare* (400-402) and *M. paratuberculosis* (114,398) from the clinical specimens. The PCR assays using genus and group specific amplification followed by RFLP analysis have been developed for regions like 65 kD for *Mtb, M. avium*, etc. (399), rRNA gene region for *M. avium, M. chelonae, M. xenopi* and early secretory antigen-6 [ESAT-6] for *Mtb* and *M. kansasii*, etc. (407-412). A new PCR technique appears to be potentially useful for characterising various pathogenic NTM (411). Another PCR strategy using amplification followed by capture plate hybridisation has been reported to be useful for *M. ulcerans* (403) and *M. avium, M. chelonae, M. scrofulaceum* (404). A reverse hybridisation line probe assay [LipA][e.g., INNO-LiPA, Innogenetics, Ghent, Belgium] has been described to be quite useful for rapid identification of mycobacteria (405). The PCR targeting certain regions on rRNA has been observed to be useful for quick identification of various NTM (408). These PCR methods can be used for rapid identification of clinical isolates (399,400,402,403,407,408,411) as well direct detection of pathogens from the clinical specimens (401,406). Keeping in view the diversity of these organisms present in different geographical locations, it would be important to evaluate the usefulness of these techniques. Further, contamination from the environment will have to be carefully ruled out.

DNA fingerprinting and probes for strain differentiation Due to almost universal presence of these organisms in the environment, there has been interest in identifying the strains which would be more commonly associated with disease. Further, such identification would be important to investigate hospital infections as well other sources of such infections (413-424). The DNA fingerprinting techniques using procedures such as pulsed-field gel electrophoresis (413,422),

random amplified polymorphic DNA [RAPD]—arbitrary PCR (414), rRNA probes (415-417) and different insertion and repeat elements have been described for characterisation of NTM (237,418,420,421). Insertion elements have been described to be useful for characterisation of *M. haemophilum* (237), *M. avium* (418,419,423,424), *M. scrofulaceum* (421,423) as well as *M. kansasii* (420). Using these probes and finger-printing systems, the aetiology of Crohn's disease due to *M. paratuberculosis* has been established to a large extent (114,116). Further, some specific RFLP types of *M. avium* have been shown to be closely linked with disease in Europe and Africa (62,108). The IS1245-based RFLP analysis of Indian isolates of *M. avium* suggested birds as origin of most of human isolates (419).

Matrix associated laser desorption/ionisation-time of flight mass spectrometry [MALDI-TOF] mass spectrometry This technique has been found to be useful in identifying NTM species by analysing protein sequences.

Determination of sensitivity profiles The NTM tend to be generally resistant to low concentrations of various anti-TB drugs (11). However, at high concentrations [within the therapeutic limits], these organisms may be drug sensitive. Except for a limited number of drugs for some NTM drug susceptibility profiles have not been found to be clinically relevant (14). The media usually recommended for sensitivity screening of *Mtb* are also used for NTM. However, due to differences in the levels of sensitivity in broth (11), a caution is required. Other media, like chocolate agar supplemented with ferric ammonium salts and mycobactins, etc. will be required for sensitivity screening of other fastidious species. While newer techniques like BACTEC, MGIT and MB/BacT (387,388) have been quite promising in early detection of growth of NTM from clinical specimens, only BACTEC and E-test have been found to be useful for sensitivity determination of rapid as well as slowly growing NTM (425-427). Expert Group of American Thoracic Society [ATS] (14) has suggested that there is no use of testing of sensitivity for rifampicin and isoniazid for rapid growers as they are usually resistant to these drugs and other drugs such as sulphones, clarithromycin, cefoxitin, amikacin, etc. should be considered for the treatment of NTM disease. Likewise, higher cut-off values for determination of sensitivity should be considered for organisms, like *M. avium*. Recombinant strain of *M. avium* expressing beta galactosidase has been reported to be useful for screening of activity of antimycobacterial compounds (428a).

Laboratories with different levels of infrastructure and financial commitment can follow different strategies to deal with diagnosis and characterisation of NTM for management [Table 41.7].

A recent study from India (428b) in pulmonary and extrapulmonary specimens suggested that all mycobacterial culture positive specimens when found negative by rapid molecular testing for *Mtb* should be considered as NTM suspects and require further confirmation and NTM speciation by DNA sequencing.

Table 41.7: Recommended techniques for the diagnosis and characterisation

Low-resource settings	Moderate-resource settings	Reference laboratories
Repeated isolation on conventional media and identification by selected biochemical tests	Repeated isolation on conventional media and identification by selected biochemical tests	Repeated isolation on conventional media and identification by selected biochemical tests
Growth in any liquid medium and identification by lipid patterns	Growth in any standard liquid medium system like BACTEC/MGIT/MB-BACTEC and identification by probe hybridisation/lipid patterns	Growth in any liquid medium BACTEC/MGIT/MB-BACT and identification by probe hybridisation/lipid patterns
Histopathology	Histopathology; plus immunohistochemistry, *in situ* hybridisation, etc.	Histopathology; plus immunohistochemistry, *in situ* hybridisation, *in situ* PCR, etc.
PCR-RFLP [if PCR available]	PCR-RFLP	PCR-RFLP
	DST	DST
		DNA sequencing
		DNA fingerprinting
		MALDI-TOF mass spectrometry

Fluorochrome-staining technique is preferred for NTM. Routine DST of *M. avium* complex isolates is recommended for clarithromycin only. Routine DST of *M. kansasii* is recommended for rifampicin only. Routine DST of rapid-growing mycobacteria [*M, fortuitum, M. chelonae* and *M. abscessus*] should be with clarithromycin, cefoxitin, doxycycline, fluorinated quinolones, amikacin, a sulphonamide or trimethoprim-sulfamethoxazole, linezolid, imipenem [*M. fortuitum* only] and tobramycin [*M. chelonae* only]. For species and subspecies identification multi-locus DNA sequencing of specific target genes such as 16S rRNA, *hsp*65, *rpoB*, 16S-23S rRNA internal transcribed region, *gyrB*, *danA*, *recA* and *sec* A has been recommended and considered as a gold satndard. Recently MALDI-TOF mass spectrometry has been considered as method of choice for NTM species identification.
NTM = nontuberculous mycobacteria; PCR = polymerase chain reaction; RFLP = restriction fragment length polymorphism; MGIT = mycobacteria growth indicator tube; DST = drug-susceptibility testing; DNA = deoxyribonucleic acid; MALDI-TOF= matrix associated laser desorption/ionization-time of flight

MANAGEMENT

Prevention

NTM infections, especially those due to contamination of disinfectants, ice, wounds, injection sites, catheters, endoscopes etc. can be prevented by proper sterilisation. Avoiding the use of tap water is considered a key step to prevent hospital infections due to NTM. Further, patients undergoing cardiac surgery and transplants should receive extra attention. Besides different drug regimens, certain non-pharmacological options are available which can help in improvement of NTM disease patient. Chest physiotherapy, especially in cystic fibrosis and bronchiectasis can be helpful to improve lung functions and mucociliary clearance. Exercises including aerobic activity such as *Yoga*, are generally believed to be helpful in pulmonary rehabilitation. Apart from drugs therapy, avoidance to NTM exposure is necessary, specifically from household plumbing and water sources. Increasing hot water temperature to more than or equal to 54°C [130°F] and changing of shower heads at regular intervals can be beneficial to prevent NTM transmission. Nutrition is also important and one should maintain adequate calorie intake and BMI especially in case of surgical intervention. Monitoring pre-albumin level can be used as a marker of nutrition. In some individuals along with antibiotic regimen, probiotic therapy can be helpful.

Chemoprophylaxis with azithromycin, clarithromycin and rifabutin in HIV-AIDS cases with severe immunodeficiency [CD4+ T-lymphocyte count < 50 cells/mm^3] is recommended (14). Prevention of NTM is detailed in Table 41.8.

Treatment

Treatment of NTM disease is generally difficult. The decision for treatment of NTM patients should be based on patient's characteristic, radiographic features and species and subspecies of the isolated NTM. There are multiple potential impediments which can affect the treatment outcomes in patients and the treating clinician should keep a record of it. These impediments include [i] constitutive [innate] and additional [during treatment] antibiotic resistance of NTM; [ii] prolonged treatment for conversion; [iii] adverse events [AEs] and serious adverse events [SAEs]; [iv] co-infection with other agents like *Mtb*, fungi and other bacteria; [v] potential of permanent underlying diseases such as destroyed lungs and immunodeficiency states for their persistence.

Response to anti-TB drug regimens is poor which on many occasions serves as a lead towards diagnosis as well. As compare to *Mtb*, drug-susceptibility testing [DST] usually is not recommended as a routine except in certain situations and for certain drugs like rifampin for *M. kansasii* (429), clarithromycin and amikacin for MAC particularly when response is not good and several drugs for rapidly growing mycobacteria (14). Drug susceptibility testing for amikacin and imipenem is recommended for *M. fortuitum* and for doxycycline, sulphonamides, quinolones and tobramycin for *M. chelonae* (14). It has been suggested that routine susceptibility testing for amikacin, imipenem, doxycycline, fluroquinolones, sulphonamides [trimethoprim-sulphamethoxazole], cefoxitin, clarithromycin,

Table 41.8: Prevention of NTM disease

Health care- and hygiene-associated NTM disease
 Avoid the following:
 Exposure of injection sites, intravenous catheters and surgical wounds to tap water and tap water-derived fluids
 Cleaning of endoscopes with tap water
 Contamination of clinical specimens with tap water and ice
 Use of benzalkonium chloride as a skin disinfectant prior to local injections

Household and personal measures
 Avoid using saunas, hot tubs or any water with an aerator. Hot water usage should be done in proper ventilation
 Replacement of shower heads at regular intervals; temperature of water heater should be ≥ 54.4°C
 Sterilised water should be used in humidifiers; avoid ultrasonic humidifiers
 Household plumbing systems should be cleaned and sterilized regularly to avoid NTM biofilm formation
 Take steps to reduce gastroesophageal reflux disease [GERD]; avoid foods that may trigger it and avoid vulnerable body positions that may cause aspiration

NTM-associated hypersensitivity lung disease
 Ensure regular cleaning of indoor pools, hot tubs and hot water pipes

Chemoprophylaxis for PLHA* with CD4+ T-lymphocyte count <50 cells/µL
 Azithromycin† 1200 mg PO weekly
 or
 Clarithromycin‡ 500 mg PO twice-daily
 or
 Rifabutin 300 mg/day {dose needs to be modified based on drug-drug interaction [s]}

---

* Preventive treatment may be stopped if CD4+ T-lymphocyte count is >100/µL for more than 3 months
† First preference [in some countries where azithromycin is available as 250/500 mg preparation, the dosage is 1250 mg]
‡ Role of macrolide prophylaxis in susceptible/immunodeficient [such as, IFN-γ/IL-12 axis defect] is not clear
NTM = nontuberculous mycobacteria; PLHA = people living with human immunodeficiency virus infection/acquired immunodeficiency syndrome; PO = per orally; IFN-γ = interferon-gamma; IL = interleukin
Adapted with permissions of The American Thoracic Society. Copyright © 2019 American Thoracic Society, Griffith DE, Aksamit T, Brown-Elliott BA, Catanzaro A, Daley C, Gordin F, et al. An Official ATS/IDSA Statement: Diagnosis, treatment, and prevention of nontuberculous mycobacterial diseases. Am J Respir Crit Care Med 2007;175:367-416. An official Journal of The American Thoracic Society.

linezolid and tobramycin would be useful for taxonomic identification and also treatment of infections due to rapidly growing mycobacteria such as *M. fortuitum*, *M. chelonae* and *M. abscessus*. Rifampicin, rifabutin, ethambutol, clofazimine, amikacin, linezolid, new generation macrolides such as clarithromycin/azithromycin and quinolones like ciprofloxacin/moxifloxacin are part of regimens to treat NTM infections. Treatment of important NTM infections is summarised in Table 41.9 (14,430a). Tetracyclines [doxycycline, minocycline], sulphonamides and cephalosporins such as cefoxitin are useful against rapidly growing mycobacteria. Imipenem has been reported to be useful against *M. abscessus* and *M. chelonae* infections. Cases having significant hypersensitivity component such as hot tub disease may require additional steroid treatment (14). While macrolide clarithromycin, is considered to be the backbone of treatment of NTM disease, species and subspecies identification is important to know the presence of an active erythromycin ribosomal methylase [*erm*] 41 gene. When the organism is incubated in the presence of clarithromycin, the *erm* 41 gene is induced and the organism rapidly acquires resistance to macrolides. *M. abscessus* subsp. *abscessus*, *M. abscessus* subsp. *bolletii* and *M. fortuitum* have an inducible *erm* 41 gene while *M. abscessus* subsp. *massiliense* and *M. chelonae* have a non-functional copy of *erm* 41 gene. Therefore, patients infected with organisms having non-functional *erm* 41 gene [*M. abscessus* subsp. *massilense*, *M. chelonae*] are more likely to improve clinically than those infected with organisms that contain an inducible *erm* 41 gene, namely, *M. abscessus* subsp. *abscessus* and *M. fortuitum*. During treatment of NTM disease, treating clinicians should monitor the peak levels of drugs weekly and keep a check on conventional microbiological outcomes such as smear status, culture conversion and relapse [detailed below] for further disease management.

MAC infections are considered most important because of morbidity and mortality associated with them. Different regimens tried for the treatment of MAC infections include combinations of rifampin, isoniazid, ethambutol and streptomycin (9,430b); ansamycins, clofazimine, ethambutol and isoniazid (431), amikacin, ethambutol, rifampicin and ciprofloxacin (432), rifabutin, ethambutol, clofazimine and isoniazid (433), rifampicin, ethambutol, clofazimine and ciprofloxacin (434). Over the years, clarithromycin and azithromycin have emerged important drugs for treating these infections (14,435-438). A combination of clarithromycin or azithromycin with ethambutol and rifabutin for one year has been recommended by ATS and IDSA (14) for the treatment of nodular or bronchiectatic pulmonary infections and also disseminated forms and for severe nodular and extensive disease additional amikacin or streptomycin has been suggested (14). According to some recent studies, fluoroquinolones have been found ineffective in MAC disease and certain authors have not recommended its use. Further, it is critical to prevent the emergence of macrolide resistance as the chances of successful treatments weakens when the minimum inhibitory concentration [MIC] of macrolides for MAC is greater than 16 µg/mL. In addition, the administration of inhaled amikacin, specifically an inhaled liposomal amikacin preparation is promising in case of advanced or recalcitrant MAC pulmonary disease. Although, a recent study has shown that MAC isolates having amikacin MICs greater than 64 µg/mL were found to have amikacin resistance associated with mutated 16S rRNA gene.

M. simiae, another slowly growing NTM which is commonly isolated but rarely indicative of true infection. The clinical manifestations of *M. simiae* infection are similar to MAC pulmonary disease. But, when clinical disease occurs, *M. simiae* is very challenging to treat and requires expert consultation. With no established drug regimen, the *M. simiae* disease has been treated similar to MAC disease and multidrug DST is recommended. In few countries, *M. szulgai* is often associated with active pulmonary disease and treatment is similar to the MAC disease.

M. xenopi pulmonary disease are associated with high all-cause mortality with low overall survival rates. According to some recent literatures, severity of *M. xenopi* disease should be accounted and treated accordingly [Table 41.10] (430a). Despite unclear role in treatment, inclusion of isoniazid in drug regimen to treat *M. xenopi* is recommended. Similar approach as *M. xenopi* should be adopted to treat *M. malmoense* disease as well [Table 41.11] (430a).

For the treatment of *M. kansasii* infections, a regimen comprising rifampicin, isoniazid, ethambutol and pyridoxine

is recommended for 12 months during which time sputum culture should remain negative (439). Although, the role of isoniazid is not defined and it is not recommended by group of authors. For rifampicin-resistant disease, regimen comprising sulphonamides has been found to be effective. Any three-drug combination—clarithromycin/azithromycin, moxifloxacin, sulphonamides, streptomycin after DST is suggested for such cases (14).

Surgical debridement is of paramount importance treatment of *M. marinum* infections in addition combinations of sulphamethoxazole-trimethoprim and doxycycline (12); clarithromycin and ethambutol or ethambutol and clarithromycin have been reported to be useful (14,440-443).

The rapidly growing NTM, *M. fortuitum* and *M. chelonae* are also among frequently isolated NTM rarely cause pulmonary disease except in patients with gastrointestinal disorders, *M. fortuitium* has been found to be associated with active pulmonary disease. For the management of *M. fortuitum* and *M. chelonae* infections besides the surgical drainage/debridement, treatment with clarithromycin or azithromycin, amikacin and doxycycline is recommended (444-446).

M. abscessus Surgical resection of localised disease along with treatment with multidrug-regimens that include macrolides, especially clarithromycin is the line of management of infections due to this pathogen. Linezolid has also been found to be effective in nearly half of the infections (14). *M. abscessus* is considered as "an antibiotic nightmare" due to resistance shown towards macrolides. The *in vitro*

Table 41.9: Treatment of important/selected NTM disease conditions

Disease	Drugs and surgery	Dose and frequency	Duration
MAC pulmonary disease			
Nodular/bronchiectatic disease	Clarithromycin or	1000 mg TWI	For one year after culture conversion
	Azithromycin	500 mg TWI	
	Rifampicin	600 mg TWI	
	Ethambutol	25 mg/kg TWI	
Fibrocavitary lung disease or severe nodular/ bronchiectatic disease	Clarithromycin or	1000 mg/day [lower dose if body weight < 50 kg]	For one year after culture conversion
	Azithromycin and	250-350 mg/day	
	Rifampicin or	450-600 mg/day [lower dosage if body weight < 50 kg]	
	Rifabutin	150-300 mg/day	
	Ethambutol	15 mg/kg/day	
	Amikacin* or	15-25 mg/kg TWI during initial 3 months of therapy	
	Streptomycin†		
Recalcitrant/macrolide-resistant MAC-pulmonary disease	Rifampicin and	600 mg daily and	For one year after culture conversion
	Ethambutol and	15 mg/kg daily and	
	Isoniazid or	300 mg [*plus* pyridoxine 10 mg] daily or	
	Moxifloxacin and	400 mg daily and	
	Amikacin*	intravenous amikacin for up to 3 months	

Contd...

Contd...

Disease	Drugs and surgery	Dose and frequency	Duration
Extensive or previously treated disease	Clarithromycin or Azithromycin and Ethambutol and Rifabutin or Rifampicin and Streptomycin or amikacin*	1000 mg daily 250-300 mg daily 15 mg/kg daily 150-300 mg daily 450-600 mg daily [lower dosage if body weight < 50 kg] 15-25 mg/kg TWI during initial 3 months of therapy	
Disseminated MAC disease‡	Clarithromycin or Azithromycin [alternative] Ethambutol *plus* Rifabutin§	500 mg orally twice daily 500 mg orally daily 15 mg/kg orally daily 300-450 mg orally daily	Until resolution of symptoms and reconstitution of cell-mediated immune function
M. kansasii pulmonary disease ‖	A regimen consisting of Isoniazid Rifampicin and Ethambutol Pyridoxine	300 mg daily 450-600 mg [lower dosage if body weight < 50 kg] 15 mg/kg/day 50 mg daily	For one year following negative sputum culture
M. abscessus pulmonary disease			For one year following negative sputum culture
Clarithromycin sensitive isolates	Initial phase [≥1 month] Amikacin and Tigecycline	Intravenous 15 mg/kg/day or TIW 100 mg intravenous loading dose followed by intravenous 50 mg twice daily	
	Imipenem Clarithromycin or Azithromycin	Intravenous 1g twice daily [when tolerated] 500 mg orally twice daily 250-500 mg orally daily [when tolerated]	
	Continuation phase Nebulised amikacin¶ and Clarithromycin or Azithromycin and *1-3 of the following drugs orally as per DST and patient's tolerance*: Clofazimine Linezolid Minocycline Moxifloxacin Co-trimoxazole	500 mg nebulisation twice daily 500 mg orally twice daily or 250-500mg daily 50-100 mg daily 600 mg once daily 100 mg twice daily 400 mg once daily 960 mg twice daily	
Constitutive macrolide-resistant isolates	Initial phase [≥1 month] Amikacin and Tigecycline Imipenem	Intravenous 15 mg/kg/day or TIW 100 mg [intravenous] loading dose followed by intravenous 50 mg twice daily Intravenous 1g twice daily [when tolerated]	

Contd...

Contd...

Disease	Drugs and surgery	Dose and frequency	Duration
	Continuation phase Nebulised amikacin¶ and *2-4 of the following drugs orally as per DST and patient's tolerance:* Clofazimine Linezolid Minocycline Moxifloxacin Co-trimoxazole	 50-100 mg daily 600 mg once daily 100 mg twice daily 400 mg once daily 960 mg twice daily	
NTM cervical lymphadenitis‡	Surgical excision is the treatment of choice for single site involvement [usually in children]. Multiple sites involvement should be ruled out by appropriate imaging techniques including PET-CT or PET- MRI if available		
Patient with extensive MAC lymphadenitis or poor response to surgical treatment	Macrolide-based drug regimen Drug regimen[s] to be based on *in vitro* DST		
Non-pulmonary disease due to rapidly growing NTM	Surgical debridement is an essential component of treatment. A macrolide-based drug regimen is frequently used for *M. abscessus*		

* Liposomal amikacin is the drug of choice for nebulization, however, nebulized amikacin 500 mg twice daily may be administered in patients with macrolide resistance, fibrocavitary and treatment failure MAC pulmonary disease
† Dosage depending upon age, weight and renal function
‡ When disease is due to MAC, multiple sites involvement has to be ruled out by appropriate imaging such as CT, abdominal and pelvic ultrasonography or whole body PET-CT or PET-MRI, if available
§ Rifabutin preferred over rifampicin especially in PLHA to avoid drug–drug interactions
‖ There is no recommended prophylaxis or suppressive regimen for disseminated *M. kansasii* disease. Treatment for disseminated and pulmonary disease is similar to disease due to *Mtb*. Since MICs of isoniazid are higher as compared to *Mtb*, clarithromycin is preferred over isoniazid for treatment of *M. kansasii*. Due to resistance to pyrazinamide, the drug is not recommended for *M. kansasii* treatment. For patients with rifampicin-resistant *M. kansasii* disease, a 3-drug regimen [based on *in vitro* susceptibility] clarithromycin or azithromycin, moxifloxacin, ethambutol, sulphamethoxazole or streptomycin
¶ Amikacin for nebulisation may be re-constituted by adding injectable amikacin [250 mg/mL] to only 0.9% sodium chloride and made up to 4 mL. This should not be mixed with nebulised bronchodilator solutions or other nebulised antibiotics. Prior use of aerosolised bronchodilator [nebulised or inhaler] can be made to prevent coughing or bronchospasm
TWI = thrice-weekly intermittent; NTM = nontuberculous mycobacteria; MAC = *M. avium* complex; DST = drug-susceptibility testing; CT= computed tomography; PET = positron emission tomography; MRI = magnetic resonance imaging; PLHA = people living with human immunodeficiency virus infection/acquired immunodeficiency syndrome
Adapted from the following:
The American Thoracic Society. Copyright © 2019 American Thoracic Society, Griffith DE, Aksamit T, Brown-Elliott BA, Catanzaro A, Daley C, Gordin F, et al. An Official ATS/IDSA Statement: Diagnosis, treatment, and prevention of nontuberculous mycobacterial diseases. Am J Respir Crit Care Med 2007; 175:367-416. An Official Journal of The American Thoracic Society.
The BMJ Publishing Group Ltd., Copyright © 2015, British Medical Journal Publishing Group Haworth CS, Banks J, Capstick T, et al, British Thoracic Society guidelines for the management of non-tuberculous mycobacterial pulmonary disease [NTM-PD], Thorax 2017;72:ii1-ii64.
Philley JV, Griffith DE. Medical Management of Pulmonary Nontuberculous Mycobacterial Disease. Thorac Surg Clin 2019;29:65-76.

susceptibilities towards macrolides should be determined for *M. abscessus* [Table 41.12] and based on that the combination of drugs should be used for a successful treatment outcome (430a).

Cystic fibrosis Patients should be regularly screened for NTM infections and macrolide monotherapy for commonly occurring infections should be given only after screening for NTM. After diagnostic confirmation, NTM disease should be treated according to particular mycobacterial pathogen (14).

Lymphadenitis Surgical removal of lymph glands in case of lymphadenitis has been found to be effective in achieving full cure in majority of cases [provided imaging has ruled out multiple site involvement]. However, additional chemotherapy depending upon NTM species has also been found to be beneficial (14).

Hypersensitivity like disease The measures that are to be undertaken for the management and prevention of such cases are provided in Table 41.8 (14).

Definitions for clinical and microbiological outcomes are listed in Table 41.13 (14,430a).

Surgical Intervention

Surgical intervention is considered necessary in certain individuals with NTM pulmonary disease. These patients should have localised underlying lung disease and should have good pulmonary function reserve without having impaired gas exchange. For a successful surgical outcome, role of pulmonary and/or infectious disease specialist, respiratory therapist and nutrition expert is crucial. It is frequently reported that surgery improves the chances of success of prolonged NTM disease treatment. In extrapulmonary NTM disease, surgical intervention may be required through aggressive debridement or removal of implanted material. In patients with peripheral solitary lymph node involvement, surgical excision is the treatment of choice.

Table 41.10: Suggested antibiotic regimens for adults with *M. xenopi* pulmonary disease

M.xenopi-pulmonary disease	*Antibiotic regimen*
Non-severe *M. xenopi* pulmonary disease [i.e., AFB smear-negative respiratory tract samples, no radiological evidence of lung cavitation or severe infection, mild-moderate symptoms, no signs of systemic illness]	Treatment with a four-drug regimen consisting of: Rifampicin 600 mg daily and Ethambutol 15 mg/kg daily and either Azithromycin 250 mg/daily or clarithromycin 500 mg twice daily and Moxifloxacin 400 mg daily or isoniazid 300 mg [*plus* pyridoxine 10 mg] daily Antibiotic treatment should continue for a minimum of 12 months after culture conversion
Severe *M. xenopi* pulmonary disease [i.e., AFB smear-positive respiratory tract samples, radiological evidence or lung cavitation/severe infection, or severe symptoms/signs of systemic illness]	Rifampicin 600 mg daily and Ethambutol 15 mg/kg daily and Azithromycin 250 mg/daily or clarithromycin 500 mg twice daily Moxifloxacin 400 mg daily or isoniazid 300 mg [*plus* pyridoxine 10 mg] daily and consider intravenous or nebulised amikacin for up to 3 months Antibiotic treatment should continue for a minimum of 12 months after culture conversion

AFB = acid-fast bacilli
Reproduced with permission of the BMJ Publishing Group Ltd., Copyright © 2015, British Medical Journal Publishing Group Haworth CS, Banks J, Capstick T, et al, British Thoracic Society guidelines for the management of non-tuberculous mycobacterial pulmonary disease [NTM-PD], Thorax 2017;72:ii1-ii64.

Table 41.11: Suggested antibiotic-regimens for adults with *M. malmoense*-pulmonary disease

M.malmoense-pulmonary disease	*Antibiotic regimens*
Non-severe *M.malmoense*-pulmonary disease [i.e., AFB smear-negative respiratory tract samples, no radiological evidence of lung cavitation or severe infection, mild-moderate symptoms, no signs of systemic illness]	Treatment with a daily oral three-drug regimen consisting of: Rifampicin 600 mg daily and Ethambutol 15 mg/kg daily and Azithromycin 250 mg/daily or clarithromycin 500 mg twice daily Antibiotic treatment should continue for a minimum of 12 months after culture conversion
Severe *M.malmoense*-pulmonary disease [i.e., AFB smear-positive respiratory tract sample, radiological evidence of lung cavitation/severe infection or sever symptoms/signs of systemic illness]	Rifampicin 600 mg daily and Ethambutol 15 mg/kg daily and Azithromycin 250 mg/daily or clarithromycin 500 mg twice daily and consider intravenous amikacin for up to 3 months or nebulised amikacin Antibiotic treatment should continue for a minimum of 12 months after culture conversion

AFB = acid-fast bacilli
Reproduced with permission of the BMJ Publishing Group Ltd., Copyright © 2015, British Medical Journal Publishing Group Haworth CS, Banks J, Capstick T, et al, British Thoracic Society guidelines for the management of non-tuberculous mycobacterial pulmonary disease [NTM-PD], horax 2017;72:ii1-ii64.

Table 41.12: Interpretation of extended clarithromycin susceptibility results for *M. abscessus*

Clarithromycin susceptibility days 3-5	Clarithromycin susceptibility day 14	Genetic implication	M. abscessus subspecies	Macrolide susceptibility phenotype
Susceptible	Susceptible	Dysfunctional *erm* (41) gene	*M.a.massiliense*	Macrolide susceptible
Susceptible	Resistant	Functional *erm* (41) gene	*M.a.abscessus* *M.a.bolletii*	Inducible macrolide resistance
Resistant	Resistant	23S ribosomal RNA point mutation	Any	High-level constitutive macrolide resistance

Reproduced with permission of the BMJ Publishing Group Ltd., Copyright © 2015, British Medical Journal Publishing Group Haworth CS, Banks J, Capstick T, et al, British Thoracic Society guidelines for the management of non-tuberculous mycobacterial pulmonary disease [NTM-PD], Thorax 2017;72:ii1-ii64.

Table 41.13: Definitions for microbiological outcomes in NTM disease

Culture conversion

Three consecutive negative mycobacterial sputum cultures collected over a minimum of 3 months, with the time of conversion being the date of the first of the three negative mycobacterial cultures. In patients unable to expectorate sputum, a single negative mycobacterial culture of a CT-directed bronchial wash is indicative of culture conversion.

Recurrence

Two positive mycobacterial cultures following culture conversion. If available, genotyping may help distinguish relapse from reinfection.

Refractory disease

Failure to culture-convert after 12 months of nontuberculous mycobacterial treatment.

NTM = nontuberculous mycobacteria; CT = computed tomography
Reproduced with permission of the BMJ Publishing Group Ltd., Copyright © 2015, British Medical Journal Publishing Group, Haworth CS, Banks J, Capstick T, et al, British Thoracic Society guidelines for the management of non-tuberculous mycobacterial pulmonary disease [NTM-PD], Thorax 2017;72: ii1-ii64.

Table 41.14: Monitoring for drug toxicities and drug-drug interactions

Rifabutin + Clarithromycin	Decreases clarithromycin levels; resulting in uveitis, arthralgias neutropenia and liver function abnormalities Increases rifabutin levels
Interactions of rifampicin/rifabutin with several groups of drugs like anti-diabetic drugs, anti-coagulants, protease inhibitors	Adverse effects [side effects, altered therapeutic efficacy] to be kept in mind
Visual	Ethambutol
Central nervous system	Cycloserine, ciprofloxacin and ethambutol
Hepatic	Rifampicin/rifabutin, isoniazid and ethionamide
Auditory	Streptomycin
Haematopoietic system	Sulphonamides, cephoxitin, tetracyclines

Monitoring for Toxicity

Drugs required for management of various NTM infections have many potential adverse events [Table 41.14]. This is especially so in the elderly patients and multisystem involvement in AIDS patients. Regular clinical as well as laboratory monitoring of these systems can help in detection of side effects and permit necessary changes in the treatment.

REFERENCES

1. Duvall CW. Studies in atypical forms of tubercle bacilli isolated directly from the human tissues in cases of primary cervical adenitis. J Exp Med 1908;9:403-29.

2. Pinner M. Atypical acid-fast microorganisms. Am Rev Tuberc 1935;32:424-45.

3. Wolinsky E. Non-tuberculous mycobacteria and associated disease. Am Rev Respir Dis 1979;119:107-59.

4. Timpe A, Runyon EH. The relationship of atypical acid-fast bacteria to human disease; a preliminary report. J Lab Clin Med 1954;44:202-9.

5. Horsburgh CR Jr, Selik RM. The epidemiology of disseminated non-tuberculous mycobacterial infections in the acquired immunodeficiency syndrome [AIDS]. Am Rev Respir Dis 1989; 139:4-7.

6. Good RC. Opportunistic pathogens in the genus Mycobacterium. Annu Rev Microbiol 1985;39:347-69.

7. Smith MJ, Grange JM. Deep tissue infections due to environmental bacteria. In: Ratledge C, Stanford J, Grange MJ, editors. Biology of mycobacteria. Volume 3. London: Academic Press; 1989.p.511-64.

8. Wayne LG, Sramek HA. Agents of newly recognised or infrequently encountered mycobacterial diseases. Clin Microbiol Rev 1992;5:1-25.

9. Dolin PJ, Raviglione MC, Kochi A. Global tuberculosis incidence and mortality during 1990-2000. Bull World Health Organ 1994;72:213-20.

10. Narain JP, Raviglione MC, Kochi A. HIV-associated tuberculosis in developing countries: epidemiology and strategies for prevention. Tuber Lung Dis 1992;72:311-21.

11. Wallace RJ Jr, O'Brien R, Glassroth J, Raleigh J, Dutt A. Diagnosis and treatment of disease caused by non-tuberculous mycobacteria. Am Rev Respir Dis 1990;142:940-53.

12. Katoch VM. Infections due to non-tuberculous mycobacterial [NTM]. Indian J Med Res 2004;120:290-304.

13. Euzeby JP. List of bacterial names with standing in nomenclature - Genus Mycobacterium. Available at URL: http://www.bacterio.net/mycobacterium.html. Accessed on November 3, 2018.

14. Griffith DE, Aksamit T, Brown-Elliott BA, Catanzaro A, Daley C, Gordin F, et al. An Official ATS/IDSA Statement: Diagnosis, treatment, and prevention of nontuberculous mycobacterial diseases. Am J Respir Crit Care Med 2007;175:367-416.

15. Brown-Elliott BA, Wallace RJ Jr. Clinical and taxonomic status of pathogenic nonpigmented or late-pigmenting rapidly growing mycobacteria. Clin Microbiol Rev 2002;15:716-46.

16. Böttger EC, Teske A, Kirschner P, Bost S, Chang HR, Beer V, et al. Disseminated "Mycobacterium genavense" infection in patients with AIDS. Lancet 1992;340:76-80.

17. Butler WR, O'Connor SP, Yakrus MA, Smithwick RW, Plikaytis BB, Moss CW, et al. Mycobacterium celatum sp. nov. Int J Syst Bacteriol 1993;43:539-48.

18. Springer B, Tortoli E, Richter I, Grünewald R, Rüsch-Gerdes S, Uschmann K, et al. Mycobacterium conspicuum sp. nov. a new species isolated from patients with disseminated infections. J Clin Microbiol 1995;33:2805-11.

19. Murcia MI, Tortoli E, Menendez MC, Palenque E, Garcia MJ. Mycobacterium colombiense sp. nov., a novel member of the Mycobacterium avium complex and description of MAC-X as a new ITS genetic variant. Int J Syst Evol Microbiol 2006;56:2049-54.

20. Eilertsen E. Atypical mycobacteria and reservoir in water. Scand J Respir Dis Suppl 1969;69:85-8.

21. Davis JB, Chase HH, Raymond RL. Mycobacterium paraffinicum n. sp., a bacterium isolated from soil. Appl Microbiol 1956;4:310-5.

22. Kirschner RA Jr, Parker BC, Falkinham JO 3rd. Epidemiology of infection by nontuberculous mycobacteria. Mycobacterium avium, Mycobacterium intracellulare, and Mycobacterium scrofulaceum in acid, brown-water swamps of the southeastern United States and their association with environmental variables. Am Rev Respir Dis 1992;145:271-5.

23. Falkinham JO 3rd. Nontuberculous mycobacteria in the environment. Clin Chest Med 2002;23:529-51.

24. Covert TC, Rodgers MR, Reyes AL, Stelma GN Jr. Occurrence of nontuberculous mycobacteria in environmental samples. Appl Environ Microbiol 1999;65:2492-6.

25. Eaton T, Falkinham JO 3rd, von Reyn CF. Recovery of Mycobacterium avium from cigarettes. J Clin Microbiol 1995;33:2757-8.

26. Moore JS, Christensen M, Wilson RW, Wallace RJ Jr, Zhang Y, Nash DR, et al. Mycobacterial contamination of metal-working fluids: involvement of a possible new taxon of rapidly growing mycobacteria. AIHAJ 2000;61:205-13.

27. Safranek TJ, Jarvis WR, Carson LA, Cusick LB, Bland LA, Swenson JM, et al. Mycobacterium chelonae wound infections after plastic surgery employing contaminated gentian violet skin-marking solution. N Engl J Med 1987;317:197-201.

28. Huttunen K, Ruotsalainen M, Iivanainen E, Torkko P, Katila M, Hirvonen M. Inflammatory responses in RAW264.7 macrophages caused by mycobacteria isolated from moldy houses. Environ Toxicol Pharmacol 2000;8:237-44.

29. Dunn BL, Hodgson DJ. Atypical mycobacteria in milk. J Appl Bacteriol 1982;52:373-6.

30. Adékambi T, Ben Salah S, Khlif M, Raoult D, Drancourt M. Survival of environmental mycobacteria in Acanthamoeba polyphaga. Appl Environ Microbiol 2006;72:5974-81.

31. Primm TP, Lucero CA, Falkinham JO 3rd. Health impacts of environmental mycobacteria. Clin Microbiol Rev 2004;17:98-106.

32. Nyka W. Studies on the effect of starvation on mycobacteria. Infect Immun 1974;9:843-50.

33. Schulze-Röbbecke R, Buchholtz K. Heat susceptibility of aquatic mycobacteria. Appl Environ Microbiol 1992;58:1869-73.

34. Smeulders MJ, Keer J, Speight RA, Williams HD. Adaptation of Mycobacterium smegmatis to stationary phase. J Bacteriol 1999;181:270-83.

35. Archuleta RJ, Mullens P, Primm TP. The relationship of temperature to desiccation and starvation tolerance of the Mycobacterium avium complex. Arch Microbiol 2002;178:311-4.

36. Weiss CH, Glassroth J. Pulmonary disease caused by non-tuberculous mycobacteria. Expert Rev Respir Med 2012;6:597-612.

37. Simons S, van Ingen J, Hsueh PR, Van Hung N, Dekhuijzen PN, Boeree MJ, et al. Nontuberculous mycobacteria in respiratory tract infections, eastern Asia. Emerg Infect Dis 2011;17:343-9.

38. Kamala T, Paramasivan CN, Herbert D, Venkatesan P, Prabhakar R. Isolation and identification of environmental mycobacteria in the Mycobacterium bovis BCG trial area of south India. Appl Environ Microbiol 1994;60:2180-3.

39. Chadha R, Grover M, Sharma A, Lakshmy A, Deb M, Kumar A, et al. An outbreak of post-surgical wound infections due to Mycobacterium abscessus. Pediatr Surg Int 1998;13:406-10.

40. Rodrigues C, Mehta A, Jha U, Bharucha M, Dastur FD, Udwadia TE. Nosocomial Mycobacterium chelonae infection in laparoscopic surgery. Infect Control Hosp Epidemiol 2001;22:474-5.

41. Jesudason MV, Gladstone P. Non-tuberculous mycobacteria isolated from clinical specimens at a tertiary care hospital in South India. Indian J Med Microbiol 2005;23:172-5.

42. Reddy AK, Garg P, Babu KH, Gopinathan U, Sharma S. In vitro antibiotic susceptibility of rapidly growing nontuberculous mycobacteria isolated from patients with microbial keratitis. Curr Eye Res 2010;35:225-9.

43. Shah AK, Gambhir RP, Hazra N, Katoch R. Non-tuberculous mycobacteria in surgical wounds—a rising cause of concern? Indian J Surg 2010;72:206-10.

44. Shenai S, Rodrigues C, Mehta A. Time to identify and define nontuberculous mycobacteria in a tuberculosis-endemic region. Int J Tuberc Lung Dis 2010;14:1001-8.

45. Thomas M, D'Silva JA, Borole AJ, Chilgar RM. Periprosthetic atypical mycobacterial infection in breast implants: a new kid on the block! J Plast Reconstr Aesthet Surg 2013;66:e16-9.

46. Kaur H, Chitkara NL. A study of atypical acid-fast bacilli [culture and biochemical characteristics]. Indian J Tuberc 1964;12:16-8.

47. Katoch K, Katoch VM, Dutta AK, Sharma VD, Ramu G. Chest infection due to M. fortuitum in a case of lepromatous leprosy: a case report. Indian J Lepr 1985;57:399-403.

48. Chakrabarti A, Sharma M, Dubey ML. Isolation rates of different mycobacterial species from Chandigarh [north India]. Indian J Med Res 1990;91:111-4.

49. Singh S, Rattan A, Kumar S. Severe cutaneous Mycobacterium chelonae infection following a yellow jacket sting. Tuber Lung Dis 1992;73:305-6.

50. Sachdeva R, Gadre DV, Talwar V. Characterisation and susceptibility pattern of extrapulmonary isolates. Indian J Med Res 2002;115:102-7.

51. Bannalikar AS, Verma R. Detection of Mycobacterium avium and M. tuberculosis from human sputum culture by PCR-RFLP analysis of hsp 65 gene and pncA PCR. Indian J Med Res 2006;123:165-72.

52. Sharma SK, Kadhiravan T, Banga A, Goyal T, Bhatia I, Saha PK. Spectrum of clinical disease in a series of 135 hospitalised HIV-infected patients from north India. BMC Infect Dis 2004;4:52.

53. Meissner G, Anz W. Sources of Mycobacterium avium complex infection resulting in human diseases. Am Rev Respir Dis 1977;116:1057-64.

54. von Reyn CF, Waddell RD, Eaton T, Arbeit RD, Maslow JN, Barber TW, et al. Isolation of Mycobacterium avium complex from water in the United States, Finland, Zaire, and Kenya. J Clin Microbiol 1993;31:3227-30.

55. Tanaka E, Kimoto T, Matsumoto H, Tsuyuguchi K, Suzuki K, Nagai S, et al. Familial pulmonary Mycobacterium avium complex disease. Am J Respir Crit Care Med 2000;161:1643-7.

56. von Reyn CF, Arbeit RD, Horsburgh CR, Ristola MA, Waddell RD, Tvaroha SM, et al. Sources of disseminated Mycobacterium avium infection in AIDS. J Infect 2002;44:166-70.

57. Aitken ML, Limaye A, Pottinger P, Whimbey E, Goss CH, Tonelli MR, et al. Respiratory outbreak of Mycobacterium abscessus subspecies massiliense in a lung transplant and cystic fibrosis center. Am J Respir Crit Care Med 2012;185:231-2.

58. Benini J, Ehlers EM, Ehlers S. Different types of pulmonary granuloma necrosis in immunocompetent vs. TNFRp55-gene-deficient mice aerogenically infected with highly virulent Mycobacterium avium. J Pathol 1999;189:127-37.

59. Ramachandran R, Swaminathan S, Somasundram S, Asgar VN, Paramesh P, Paramasivan CN. Mycobacteremia in tuberculosis patients with HIV infections. Indian J Tuberc 2002;50:29-31.

60. Narang P, Narang R, Mendiratta DK, Roy D, Deotale V, Yakrus MA, et al. Isolation of Mycobacterium avium complex and M. simiae from blood of AIDS patients from Sevagram, Maharashtra, India. Indian J Tuberc 2005;52:21-6.

61. Fauci AS, Macher AM, Longo DL, Lane HC, Rook AH, Masur H, et al. Acquired immunodeficiency syndrome: epidemiologic, clinical, immunologic and therapeutic considerations. Ann Intern Med 1984;100:92-106.

62. Portaels P, Kunze ZM, McFadden JJ, Fonteyne PA, Carpels G. AIDS and mycobacterial diseases in developing and developed countries. J Chemother 1991;4:449-50.

63. Hoover DR, Graham NM, Bacellar H, Murphy R, Visscher B, Anderson R, et al. An epidemiologic analysis of Mycobacterium

avium complex disease in homosexual men infected with human immunodeficiency virus type 1. Clin Infect Dis 1995;20:1250-8.

64. von Reyn CF, Maslow JN, Barber TW, Falkinham JO, Arbeit RD. Persistent colonization of potable water as a source of Mycobacterium avium infection in patients with AIDS. Lancet 1994;343:1137-41.

65. Schlesinger LS, Bellinger-Kawahara CG, Payne NR, Horwitz MA. Phagocytosis of Mycobacterium tuberculosis is mediated by human monocyte complement receptors and complement component C3. J Immunol 1990;144:2771-80.

66. Schlesinger LS. Macrophage phagocytosis of virulent but not attenuated strains of Mycobacterium tuberculosis is mediated by mannose receptors in addition to complement receptors. J Immunol 1993;150:2920-30.

67. Bermudez LE, Young LS. Factors affecting invasion of HT-29 and HEp-2 epithelial cells by organisms of the Mycobacterium avium complex. Infect Immun 1994;62:2021-6.

68. Greenwell-Wild T, Vázquez N, Sim D, Schito M, Chatterjee D, Orenstein JM, et al. Mycobacterium avium infection and modulation of human macrophage gene expression. J Immunol 2002;169:6286-97.

69. Hale-Donze H, Greenwell-Wild T, Mizel D, Doherty TM, Chatterjee D, Orenstein JM, et al. Mycobacterium avium complex promotes recruitment of monocyte hosts for HIV-1 and bacteria. J Immunol 2002;169:3854-62.

70. Champsi J, Young LS, Bermudez LE. Production of TNF-alpha, IL-6 and TGF-beta, and expression of receptors for TNF-alpha and IL-6, during murine Mycobacterium avium infection. Immunology 1995;84:549-54.

71. Hänsch HC, Smith DA, Mielke ME, Hahn H, Bancroft GJ, Ehlers S. Mechanisms of granuloma formation in murine Mycobacterium avium infection: the contribution of CD4+ T cells. Int Immunol 1996;8:1299-310.

72. Ehlers S, Kutsch S, Ehlers EM, Benini J, Pfeffer K. Lethal granuloma disintegration in mycobacteria-infected TNFRp55-/- mice is dependent on T cells and IL-12. J Immunol 2000;165: 483-92.

73. Ehlers S, Benini J, Held HD, Roeck C, Alber G, Uhlig S. αβ T-cell receptor-positive cells and interferon-gamma, but not inducible nitric oxide synthase, are critical for granuloma necrosis in a mouse model of mycobacteria-induced pulmonary immunopathology. J Exp Med 2001;194:1847-59.

74. Yoshida YO, Umemura M, Yahagi A, O'Brien RL, Ikuta K, Kishihara K, et al. Essential role of IL-17A in the formation of a mycobacterial infection-induced granuloma in the lung. J Immunol 2010;184:4414-22.

75. Regev D, Surolia R, Karki S, Zolak J, Montes-Worboys A, Oliva O, et al. Heme oxygenase-1 promotes granuloma development and protects against dissemination of mycobacteria. Lab Invest 2012;92:1541-52.

76. Gan H, Newman GW, Remold HG. Plasminogen activator inhibitor type 2 prevents programmed cell death of human macrophages infected with Mycobacterium avium, serovar 4. J Immunol 1995;155:1304-15.

77. Fratazzi C, Arbeit RD, Carini C, Remold HG. Programmed cell death of Mycobacterium avium serovar 4-infected human macrophages prevents the mycobacteria from spreading and induces mycobacterial growth inhibition by freshly added, uninfected macrophages. J Immunol 1997;158:4320-7.

78. Flórido M, Pearl JE, Solache A, Borges M, Haynes L, Cooper AM, et al. Gamma interferon-induced T-cell loss in virulent Mycobacterium avium infection. Infect Immun 2005;73:3577-86.

79. Early J, Fischer K, Bermudez LE. Mycobacterium avium uses apoptotic macrophages as tools for spreading. Microb Pathog 2011;50:132-9.

80. Bermudez LE, Parker A, Petrofsky M. Apoptosis of Mycobacterium avium-infected macrophages is mediated by both tumour necrosis factor [TNF] and Fas, and involves the activation of caspases. Clin Exp Immunol 1999;116:94-9.

81. Aly S, Laskay T, Mages J, Malzan A, Lang R, Ehlers S. Interferon-gamma-dependent mechanisms of mycobacteria-induced pulmonary immunopathology: the role of angiostasis and CXCR3-targeted chemokines for granuloma necrosis. J Pathol 2007;212:295-305.

82. Laochumroonvorapong P, Paul S, Elkon KB, Kaplan G. H$_2$O$_2$ induces monocyte apoptosis and reduces viability of Mycobacterium avium-M. intracellulare within cultured human monocytes. Infect Immun 1996;64:452-9.

83. Lawn SD, Roberts BD, Griffin GE, Folks TM, Butera ST. Cellular compartments of human immunodeficiency virus type 1 replication in vivo: determination by presence of virion-associated host proteins and impact of opportunistic infection. J Virol 2000;74:139-45.

84. Wahl SM, Greenwell-Wild T, Hale-Donze H, Moutsopoulos N, Orenstein JM. Permissive factors for HIV-1 infection of macrophages. J Leukoc Biol 2000;68:303-10.

85. Uzoigwe JC, Khaitsa ML, Gibbs PS. Epidemiological evidence for Mycobacterium avium subspecies paratuberculosis as a cause of Crohn's disease. Epidemiol Infect 2007;135:1057-68.

86. Coussens PM. Model for immune responses to Mycobacterium avium subspecies paratuberculosis in cattle. Infect Immun 2004;72:3089-96.

87. Machugh DE, Taraktsoglou M, Killick KE, Nalpas NC, Browne JA, DE Park S, et al. Pan-genomic analysis of bovine monocyte-derived macrophage gene expression in response to in vitro infection with Mycobacterium avium subspecies paratuberculosis. Vet Res 2012;43:25.

88. Weiss DJ, Evanson OA, Moritz A, Deng MQ, Abrahamsen MS. Differential responses of bovine macrophages to Mycobacterium avium subsp. paratuberculosis and Mycobacterium avium subsp. avium. Infect Immun 2002;70:5556-61.

89. Weiss DJ, Evanson OA, Deng M, Abrahamsen MS. Gene expression and antimicrobial activity of bovine macrophages in response to Mycobacterium avium subsp. paratuberculosis. Vet Pathol 2004;41:326-37.

90. Janagama HK, Jeong Ki, Kapur V, Coussens P, Sreevatsan S. Cytokine responses of bovine macrophages to diverse clinical Mycobacterium avium subspecies paratuberculosis strains. BMC Microbiol 2006;6:10.

91. Murphy JT, Sommer S, Kabara EA, Verman N, Kuelbs MA, Saama P, et al. Gene expression profiling of monocyte-derived macrophages following infection with Mycobacterium avium subspecies avium and Mycobacterium avium subspecies paratuberculosis. Physiol Genomics 2006;28:67-75.

92. Sibartie S, Scully P, Keohane J, O'Neill S, O'Mahony J, O'Hanlon D, et al. Mycobacterium avium subsp. paratuberculosis [MAP] as a modifying factor in Crohn's disease. Inflamm Bowel Dis 2010;16:296-304.

93. Campos N, Magro F, Castro AR, Cabral J, Rodrigues P, Silva R, et al. Macrophages from IBD patients exhibit defective tumour necrosis factor-α secretion but otherwise normal or augmented pro-inflammatory responses to infection. Immunobiology 2011; 216:961-70.

94. Eastaff-Leung N, Mabarrack N, Barbour A, Cummins A, Barry S. Foxp3+ regulatory T cells, Th17 effector cells, and cytokine environment in inflammatory bowel disease. J Clin Immunol 2010;30:80-9.

95. Tamura K, Fukuda Y, Sashio H, Takeda N, Bamba H, Kosaka T, et al. IL18 polymorphism is associated with an increased risk of Crohn's disease. J Gastroenterol 2002;37:111-6.

96. Ordway D, Henao-Tamayo M, Smith E, Shanley C, Harton M, Troudt J, et al. Animal model of Mycobacterium abscessus lung infection. J Leukoc Biol 2008;83:1502-11.

97. Shin DM, Yang CS, Yuk JM, Lee JY, Kim KH, Shin SJ, et al. Mycobacterium abscessus activates the macrophage innate immune response via a physical and functional interaction between TLR2 and dectin-1. Cell Microbiol 2008;10:1608-21.

98. Rottman M, Catherinot E, Hochedez P, Emile JF, Casanova JL, Gaillard JL, et al. Importance of T cells, gamma interferon, and tumor necrosis factor in immune control of the rapid grower Mycobacterium abscessus in C57BL/6 mice. Infect Immun 2007;75:5898-907.

99. Sampaio EP, Elloumi HZ, Zelazny A, Ding L, Paulson ML, Sher A, et al. Mycobacterium abscessus and M. avium trigger toll-like receptor 2 and distinct cytokine response in human cells. Am J Respir Cell Mol Biol 2008;39:431-9.

100. Tang BS, Chan JF, Chen M, Tsang OT, Mok MY, Lai RW, et al. Disseminated penicilliosis, recurrent bacteremic nontyphoidal salmonellosis, and burkholderiosis associated with acquired immunodeficiency due to autoantibody against gamma interferon. Clin Vaccine Immunol 2010;17:1132-8.

101. Kampitak T, Suwanpimolkul G, Browne S, Suankratay C. Anti-interferon-gamma autoantibody and opportunistic infections: case series and review of the literature. Infection 2011;39:65-71.

102. Picque JB, Blot M, Binois R, Jeudy G, Simonet AL, Cagnon J, et al. Recurrent atypical mycobacterial infections in the adult: think of autoantibodies against interferon-gamma! Rev Med Interne 2012;33:103-6.

103. Browne SK, Zaman R, Sampaio EP, Jutivorakool K, Rosen LB, Ding L, et al. Anti-CD20 [rituximab] therapy for anti-IFN-gamma autoantibody-associated nontuberculous mycobacterial infection. Blood 2012;119:3933-9.

104. Wu UI, Holland SM. Host susceptibility to non-tuberculous mycobacterial infections. Lancet Infect Dis 2015;15:968-80.

105. Farhi DC, Mason UG, Horsburgh CR. Pathology of MAC infection AIDS. Human Pathol 1987;18:709-14.

106. Massenkeil G, Opravil M, Salfinger M, von Graeventz A, Luthy R. Disseminated coinfection with Mycobacterium avium complex and Mycobacterium kansasii in a patient with acquired immunodeficiency syndrome and liver abscess. Clin Infect Dis 1992;14:618-9.

107. Levy-Frebault V, Pangon B, Bure A, Katlama C, Marche C, David HL. Mycobacterium simiae, Mycobacterium avium complex—M. intracellulare mixed infection in AIDS. J Clin Microbiol 1987;25:154-7.

108. Hampson SJ, Portaels F, Thompson J, Green EP, Moss MT, Hermon-Taylor J, et al. DNA probes demonstrate single highly conserved strain of Mycobacterium avium infecting AIDS patients. Lancet 1989;1:65-8.

109. Good RC, Snider DE. Isolation of non-tuberculous mycobacteria in the United States 1980. J Infect Dis 1982;146:829-33.

110. O'Brien RJ, Geiter LJ, Snider DE. The epidemiology of non-tuberculous mycobacteria disease in the United States. Results from a national survey. Am Rev Respir Dis 1987;135:1007-14.

111. Paramasivan CN, Govindan D, Prabhakar R, Somasundaram PR, Subbammal S, Tripathy SP. Species level identification of non-tuberculous mycobacteria from south India BCG trial area during 1981. Tubercle 1985;66:9-15.

112. Meissner PS, Falkinham JO. Plasmid DNA profiles as epidemiological markers for clinical and environmental isolates of Mycobacterium avium, Mycobacterium intracellulare and Mycobacterium scrofulaceum. J Infect Dis 1986;153:325-31.

113. Kazda JF. The principles of ecology of mycobacteria. In: Stanford JL, Ratledge C, editors. Biology of mycobacteria. Volume 2. London: Academic Press; 1983.p.323-42.

114. Vary PH, Andersen PR, Green E, Hermon-Taylor J, McFadden JJ. Use of highly specific DNA probes and polymerase chain reaction for detection of Mycobacterium paratuberculosis in Johne's disease. J Clin Microbiol 1990;28:933-7.

115. McFadden JJ, Butcher PD, Chiodini R, Hermon-Taylor J. Crohn's disease-isolated related mycobacteria are identical to Mycobacterium paratuberculosis as determined by DNA probes that distinguish between mycobacterial species. J Clin Microbiol 1987;25:796-801.

116. Sechi LA, Manuela M, Francesco T, Amelia L, Antonello S, Giovanni F, et al. Identification of Mycobacterium avium subsp. paratuberculosis in biopsy specimens from patients with Crohn's disease identified by in situ hybridization. J Clin Microbiol 2001;39:4514-7.

117. Mijs W, de Haas P, Rossau R, Van der Laan T, Rigouts L, Portaels F, et al. Molecular evidence to support a proposal to reserve the designation Mycobacterium avium subsp. avium for bird-type isolates and 'M. avium subsp. hominissuis' for the human/porcine type of M. avium. Int J Syst Evol Microbiol 2002;52:1505-18.

118. Bruijnesteijn van Coppenraet LE, de Haas PE, Lindeboom JA, Kuijper EJ, van Soolingen D. Lymphadenitis in children is caused by Mycobacterium avium hominissuis and not related to 'bird tuberculosis'. Eur J Clin Microbiol Infect Dis 2008;27:293-9.

119. Kaevska M, Slana I, Kralik P, Reischl U, Orosova J, Holcikova A, et al. "Mycobacterium avium subsp. hominissuis" in neck lymph nodes of children and their environment examined by culture and triplex quantitative real-time PCR. J Clin Microbiol 2011;49:167-72.

120. Despierres L, Cohen-Bacrie S, Richet H, Drancourt M. Diversity of Mycobacterium avium subsp. hominissuis mycobacteria causing lymphadenitis, France. Eur J Clin Microbiol Infect Dis 2012;31: 1373-9.

121. Ichikawa K, Yagi T, Moriyama M, Inagaki T, Nakagawa T, Uchiya K, et al. Characterization of Mycobacterium avium clinical isolates in Japan using subspecies-specific insertion sequences, and identification of a new insertion sequence, ISMav6. J Med Microbiol 2009;58:945-50.

122. Tran QT, Han XY. Subspecies identification and significance of 257 clinical strains of Mycobacterium avium. J Clin Microbiol 2014;52:1201-6.

123. Alvarez J, García IG, Aranaz A, Bezos J, Romero B, de Juan L, et al. Genetic diversity of Mycobacterium avium isolates recovered from clinical samples and from the environment: molecular characterization for diagnostic purposes. J Clin Microbiol 2008;46:1246-51.

124. Muwonge A, Oloya J, Kankya C, Nielsen S, Godfroid J, Skjerve E, et al. Molecular characterization of Mycobacterium avium subspecies hominissuis isolated from humans, cattle and pigs in the Uganda cattle corridor using VNTR analysis. Infect Genet Evol 2014;21:184-91.

125. Thomson R, Tolson C, Carter R, Coulter C, Huygens F, Hargreaves M. Isolation of nontuberculous mycobacteria [NTM] from household water and shower aerosols in patients with pulmonary disease caused by NTM. J Clin Microbiol 2013;51:3006-11.

126. Lee G, Kim HS, Lee KS, Koh WJ, Jeon K, Jeong BH, et al. Serial CT findings of nodular bronchiectatic Mycobacterium avium complex pulmonary disease with antibiotic treatment. AJR Am J Roentgenol 2013;201:764-72.

127. Kim HS, Lee Y, Lee S, Kim YA, Sun YK. Recent trends in clinically significant nontuberculous mycobacteria isolates at a Korean general hospital. Ann Lab Med 2014;34:56-9.

128. Zhou L, Wang HS, Feng SY, Wang QL. Cutaneous Mycobacterium intracellulare infection in an immunocompetent person. Acta Derm Venereol 2013;93:711-4.

129. Satoh H, Kagohashi K, Ohara G, Miyazaki Z, Kawaguchi M, Kurishima K, et al. A case of thymoma and Mycobacterium intracellulare infection. Kekkaku 2012;87:701-5.

130. Kim WY, Jang SJ, Ok T, Kim GU, Park HS, Leem J, et al. Disseminated Mycobacterium intracellulare infection in an immunocompetent host. Tuberc Respir Dis [Seoul] 2012;72:452-6.

131. Ben Salah I, Cayrou C, Raoult D, Drancourt M. Mycobacterium marseillense sp. nov., Mycobacterium timonense sp. nov. and Mycobacterium bouchedurhonense sp. nov., members of the Mycobacterium avium complex. Int J Syst Evol Microbiol 2009;59:2803-8.

132. Poulin S, Corbeil C, Nguyen M, St-Denis A, Côté L, Le Deist F, et al. Fatal Mycobacterium colombiense/cytomegalovirus coinfection associated with acquired immunodeficiency due to autoantibodies against interferon gamma: a case report. BMC Infect Dis 2013;13:24.

133. Tortoli E, Rindi L, Garcia MJ, Chiaradonna P, Dei R, Garzelli C, et al. Proposal to elevate the genetic variant MAC-A, included in the Mycobacterium avium complex, to species rank as Mycobacterium chimaera sp. nov. Int J Syst Evol Microbiol 2004;54:1277-85.

134. Bills ND, Hinrichs SH, Aden TA, Wickert RS, Iwen PC. Molecular identification of Mycobacterium chimaera as a cause of infection in a patient with chronic obstructive pulmonary disease. Diagn Microbiol Infect Dis 2009;63:292-5.

135. van Ingen J, Hoefsloot W, Buijtels PC, Tortoli E, Supply P, Dekhuijzen PN, et al. Characterization of a novel variant of Mycobacterium chimaera. J Med Microbiol 2012;61:1234-9.

136. Cohen-Bacrie S, David M, Stremler N, Dubus JC, Rolain JM, Drancourt M. Mycobacterium chimaera pulmonary infection complicating cystic fibrosis: a case report. J Med Case Rep 2011;5:473.

137. Achermann Y, Rössle M, Hoffmann M, Deggim V, Kuster S, Zimmermann DR, et al. Prosthetic valve endocarditis and bloodstream infection due to Mycobacterium chimaera. J Clin Microbiol 2013;51:1769-73.

138. Schweickert B, Goldenberg O, Richter E, Göbel UB, Petrich A, Buchholz P, et al. Occurrence and clinical relevance of Mycobacterium chimaera sp. nov., Germany. Emerg Infect Dis 2008;14:1443-6.

139. Echevarría MP, Martín G, Pérez J, Urkijo JC. Pulmonary infection by Mycobacterium kansasii. Presentation of 27 cases [1988-1992]. Enferm Infecc Microbiol Clin 1994;12:280-4.

140. Tortoli E, Simonetti MT, Lacchini C, Penati V, Urbano P. Tentative evidence of AIDS-associated biotype of Mycobacterium kansasii. J Clin Microbiol 1994;32:1779-82.

141. Levine B, Chaisson RE. Mycobacterium kansasii: a cause of treatable pulmonary disease associated with advanced human immunodeficiency virus [HIV] infection. Ann Intern Med 1991;114:861-8.

142. Witzig RS, Fazal BA, Mera RM, Mushatt DM, Dejace PM, Greer DL, et al. Clinical manifestations and implications of coinfection with Mycobacterium kansasii and human immunodeficiency virus type 1. Clin Infect Dis 1995;21:77-85.

143. Sanders JW, Walsh AD, Snider RL, Sahn EE. Disseminated Mycobacterium scrofulaceum infection: a potentially treatable complication of AIDS. Clin Infect Dis 1995;20:549.

144. Springer B, Kirschner P, Rost-Meyer G, Schröder KH, Kroppenstedt RM, Böttger EC. Mycobacterium interjectum, a new species isolated from a patient with chronic lymphadenitis. J Clin Microbiol 1993;31:3083-9.

145. Martínez Lacasa J, Cuchi E, Font R. Mycobacterium interjectum as a cause of lung disease mimicking tuberculosis. Int J Tuberc Lung Dis 2009;13:1048.

146. Mirant-Borde MC, Alvarez S, Johnson MM. Mycobacterium interjectum lung infection. Case Rep Pulmonol 2013;2013:193830.

147. Green BA, Afessa B. Isolation of Mycobacterium interjectum in an AIDS patient with diarrhea. AIDS 2000;14:1282-4.

148. Fukuoka M, Matsumura Y, Kore-eda S, Iinuma Y, Miyachi Y. Cutaneous infection due to Mycobacterium interjectum in an immunosuppressed patient with microscopic polyangiitis. Br J Dermatol 2008;159:1382-4.

149. O'Dwyer JP, O'Connor JG, McDermott H, Sheehan S, Fanning NF, Corcoran GD, et al. Meningoencephalitis associated with non-tuberculous mycobacteria. BMJ Case Rep 2009;2009. pii: bcr03.2009.1696.

150. Tortoli E, Kirschner P, Springer B, Bartoloni A, Burrini C, Mantella A, et al. Cervical lymphadenitis due to an unusual mycobacterium. Eur J Clin Microbiol Infect Dis 1997;16:308-11.

151. Tuerlinckx D, Fauville-Dufaux M, Bodart E, Bogaerts P, Dupont B, Glupczynski Y. Submandibular lymphadenitis caused by Mycobacterium interjectum: contribution of new diagnostic tools. Eur J Pediatr 2010;169:505-8

152. Banks J, Hunter AM, Campbell IA, Jenkins PA, Smith AP. Pulmonary infection with Mycobacterium xenopi; review of treatment and response. Thorax 1984;39:376-82.

153. Ausina V, Barrio J, Luquin M, Sambeat MA, Gurgui M, Verger G, et al. Mycobacterium xenopi infections in the acquired immunodeficiency syndrome. Ann Intern Med 1988;109:927-8.

154. Shafer RW, Sierra MF. Mycobacterium xenopi, Mycobacterium fortuitum, Mycobacterium kansasii, and other nontuberculous mycobacteria in an area of endemicity for AIDS. Clin Infect Dis 1992;15:161-2.

155. Karassova V, Weissfeiler J, Krasznay E. Occurrence of atypical mycobacteria in Macacus rhesus. Acta Microbiol Acad Sci Hung 1965;12:275-82.

156. Ménard O, Tanguy B, Ahmed Z, Caligaris P, Desnanot J. Severe pulmonary mycobacteriosis caused by Mycobacterium simiae. Rev Mal Respir 1987;4:327-9.

157. Maoz C, Shitrit D, Samra Z, Peled N, Kaufman L, Kramer MR, et al. Pulmonary Mycobacterium simiae infection: comparison with pulmonary tuberculosis. Eur J Clin Microbiol Infect Dis 2008;27: 945-50.

158. Shitrit D, Peled N, Bishara J, Priess R, Pitlik S, Samra Z, et al. Clinical and radiological features of Mycobacterium kansasii infection and Mycobacterium simiae infection. Respir Med 2008;102:1598-603.

159. Qvist T, Katzenstein TL, Lillebaek T, Iversen M, Mared L, Andersen AB. First report of lung transplantation in a patient with active pulmonary Mycobacterium simiae infection. Transplant Proc 2013;45:803-5.

160. Patel NC, Minifee PK, Dishop MK, Munoz FM. Mycobacterium simiae cervical lymphadenitis. Pediatr Infect Dis J 2007;26:362-3.

161. Vandercam B, Gala J, Vandeweghe B, Degraux J, Wauters G, Larsson L, et al. Mycobacterium simiae disseminated infection in a patient with acquired immunodeficiency syndrome. Infection 1996;24:49-51.

162. Balkis MM, Kattar MM, Araj GF, Kanj SS. Fatal disseminated Mycobacterium simiae infection in a non-HIV patient. Int J Infect Dis 2009;13:e286-7.

163. Narang R, Narang P, Jain AP, Mendiratta DK, Joshi R, Lavania M, et al. Disseminated disease caused by Mycobacterium simiae in AIDS patients: a report of three cases. Clin Microbiol Infect 2010;16:912-4.

164. Krümmel A, Schröder KH, von Kirchbach G, Hirtzel F, Hövener B. Mycobacterium simiae in Germany. Zentralbl Bakteriol 1989; 271:543-9.

165. Huminer D, Dux S, Samra Z, Kaufman L, Lavy A, Block CS, et al. Mycobacterium simiae infection in Israeli patients with AIDS. Clin Infect Dis 1993;17:508-9.

166. Valero G, Peters J, Jorgensen JH, Graybill JR. Clinical isolates of Mycobacterium simiae in San Antonio, Texas. An 11-yr review. Am J Respir Crit Care Med 1995;152:1555-7.

167. Ssali FN, Kamya MR, Wabwire-Mangen F, Kasasa S, Joloba M, Williams D, et al. A prospective study of community-acquired bloodstream infections among febrile adults admitted to Mulago Hospital in Kampala, Uganda. J Acquir Immune Defic Syndr Hum Retrovirol 1998;19:484-9.

168. Amorim A, Macedo R, Lopes A, Rodrigues I, Pereira E. Non-tuberculous mycobacteria in HIV-negative patients with pulmonary disease in Lisbon, Portugal. Scand J Infect Dis 2010;42:626-8.

169. Onen ZP, Karahan ZC, Akkoca Yıldız O, Karabıyıkoğlu G. Mycobacterium simiae infection in an immunocompetent patient, with DNA analyses verification. Tuberk Toraks 2010;58:306-10.

170. Varghese B, Memish Z, Abuljadayel N, Al-Hakeem R, Alrabiah F, Al-Hajoj SA. Emergence of clinically relevant Non-tuberculous mycobacterial infections in Saudi Arabia. PLoS Negl Trop Dis 2013;7:e2234.

171. Floyd MM, Guthertz LS, Silcox VA, Duffey PS, Jang Y, Desmond EP, et al. Characterization of an SAV organism and proposal of Mycobacterium triplex sp. nov. J Clin Microbiol 1996;34:2963-7.

172. Cingolani A, Sanguinetti M, Antinori A, Larocca LM, Ardito F, Posteraro B, et al. Brief report: disseminated mycobacteriosis caused by drug-resistant Mycobacterium triplex in a human immunodeficiency virus-infected patient during highly active antiretroviral therapy. Clin Infect Dis 2000;31:177-9.

173. Zeller V, Nardi AL, Truffot-Pernot C, Sougakoff W, Stankoff B, Katlama C, et al. Disseminated infection with a mycobacterium related to Mycobacterium triplex with central nervous system involvement associated with AIDS. J Clin Microbiol 2003;41:2785-7.

174. Suomalainen S, Koukila-Kähkölä P, Brander E, Katila ML, Piilonen A, Paulin L, et al. Pulmonary infection caused by an unusual, slowly growing nontuberculous Mycobacterium. J Clin Microbiol 2001;39:2668-71.

175. Kyrilli A, Payen MC, Antoine-Moussiaux T, Dewit S, Clumeck N. Meningitis and splenic infarction due to disseminated Mycobacterium genavense infection in an HIV patient. Case report and review of the literature. Acta Clin Belg 2013;68:220-2.

176. Borde JP, Offensperger WB, Kern WV, Wagner D. Mycobacterium genavense specific mesenteritic syndrome in HIV-infected patients: a new entity of retractile mesenteritis? AIDS 2013;27:2819-22.

177. Abe K, Yamamoto T, Ishii T, Kuyama Y, Koga I, Ota Y. Duodenal Mycobacterium genavense infection in a patient with acquired immunodeficiency syndrome. Endoscopy 2013;45 Suppl 2 UCTN:E27-8.

178. Coyle MB, Carlson LC, Wallis CK, Leonard RB, Raisys VA, Kilburn JO, et al. Laboratory aspects of "Mycobacterium genavense", a proposed species isolated from AIDS patients. J Clin Microbiol 1992;30:3206-12.

179. Bessesen MT, Shlay J, Stone-Venohr B, Cohn DL, Reves RR. Disseminated Mycobacterium genavense infection; clinical and microbiological features and response to therapy. AIDS 1993;7:1357-61.

180. Springer B, Wu WK, Bodmer T, Haase G, Pfyffer GE, Kroppenstedt RM, et al. Isolation and characterization of a unique group of slowly growing mycobacteria: description of Mycobacterium lentiflavum sp. nov. J Clin Microbiol 1996;34:1100-7.

181. Molteni C, Gazzola L, Cesari M, Lombardi A, Salerno F, Tortoli E, et al. Mycobacterium lentiflavum infection in immunocompetent patient. Emerg Infect Dis 2005;11:119-22.

182. Cabria F, Torres MV, García-Cía JI, Dominguez-Garrido MN, Esteban J, Jimenez MS. Cervical lymphadenitis caused by Mycobacterium lentiflavum. Pediatr Infect Dis J 2002;21:574-5.

183. Jiménez-Montero B, Baquero-Artigao F, Saavedra-Lozano J, Tagarro-García A, Blázquez-Gamero D, Cilleruelo-Ortega MJ, et al. Comparison of Mycobacterium lentiflavum and Myco-bacterium avium-intracellulare complex lymphadenitis. Pediatr Infect Dis J 2014;33:28-34.

184. Niobe SN, Bebear CM, Clerc M, Pellegrin JL, Bebear C, Maugein J. Disseminated Mycobacterium lentiflavum infection in a human immunodeficiency virus-infected patient. J Clin Microbiol 2001;39:2030-2.

185. Haas WH, Butler WR, Kirschner P, Plikaytis BB, Coyle MB, Amthor B, et al. A new agent of mycobacterial lymphadenitis in children: Mycobacterium heidelbergense sp. nov. J Clin Microbiol 1997;35:3203-9.

186. Pfyffer GE, Weder W, Strässle A, Russi EW. Mycobacterium heidelbergense species nov. infection mimicking a lung tumor. Clin Infect Dis 1998;27:649-50.

187. Tortoli E, Chianura L, Fabbro L, Mariottini A, Martín-Casabona N, Mazzarelli G, et al. Infections due to the newly described species Mycobacterium parascrofulaceum. J Clin Microbiol 2005;43:4286-7.

188. Hibiya K, Tateyama M, Teruya H, Nakamura H, Tasato D, Kazumi Y, et al. Immunopathological characteristics of immune reconstitution inflammatory syndrome caused by Mycobacterium parascrofulaceum infection in a patient with AIDS. Pathol Res Pract 2011;207:262-70.

189. Zong W, Zhang X, Wang H, Xu XL, Wang Q, Tian W, et al. The first case of cutaneous infection with Mycobacterium parascrofulaceum.Ther Clin Risk Manag 2012;8:353-8.

190. Shojaei H, Hashemi A, Heidarieh P, Daei-Naser A. Chronic pelvic pain due to Mycobacterium parascrofulaceum in an Iranian patient: first report of isolation and molecular characterization from Asia. Braz J Infect Dis 2011;15:186-7.

191. Turenne CY, Cook VJ, Burdz TV, Pauls RJ, Thibert L, Wolfe JN, et al. Mycobacterium parascrofulaceum sp. nov., novel slowly growing, scotochromogenic clinical isolates related to Mycobacterium simiae. Int J Syst Evol Microbiol 2004;54:1543-51.

192. Tortoli E, Rindi L, Goh KS, Katila ML, Mariottini A, Mattei R, et al. Mycobacterium florentinum sp. nov., isolated from humans. Int J Syst Evol Microbiol 2005;55:1101-6.

193. Syed SS, Aderinboye O, Hanson KE, Spitzer ED. Acute cervical lymphadenitis caused by Mycobacterium florentinum. Emerg Infect Dis 2010;16:1486-7.

194. Nukui Y, Nakamura H, Ishioka H, Miyamoto H, Okamoto A, Kazumi Y, et al. Synovitis of the wrist caused by Mycobacterium florentinum. Infection 2014;42:437-40.

195. Tortoli E, Böttger EC, Fabio A, Falsen E, Gitti Z, Grottola A, et al. Mycobacterium europaeum sp. nov., a scotochromogenic species related to the Mycobacterium simiae complex. Int J Syst Evol Microbiol 2011;61:1606-11.

196. Pourahmad F, Shojaei H, Heidarieh P, Khosravi A, Hashemi A. Report of two cases of Mycobacterium europaeum from Iran. Jpn J Infect Dis 2012;65:539-41.

197. Wayne LG. Classification and identification of mycobacteria. 3. Species within group 3. Am Rev Respir Dis 1966;93:919-28.

198. Krisher KK, Kallay MC, Nolte FS. Primary pulmonary infection caused by Mycobacterium terrae complex. Diagn Microbiol Infect Dis 1988;11:171-5.

199. Hojo M, Iikura M, Hirano S, Sugiyama H, Kobayashi N, Kudo K. Increased risk of nontuberculous mycobacterial infection in asthmatic patients using long-term inhaled corticosteroid therapy. Respirology 2012;17:185-90.

200. Halla JT, Gould JS, Hardin JG. Chronic tenosynovial hand infection from Mycobacterium terrae. Arthritis Rheum 1979;22:1386-90.

201. Smith DS, Lindholm-Levy P, Huitt GA, Heifets LB, Cook JL. Mycobacterium terrae: case reports, literature review, and in vitro antibiotic susceptibility testing. Clin Infect Dis 2000;30:444-53.

202. Chen HW, Lai CC, Tan CK. Arthritis caused by Mycobacterium terrae in a patient with rheumatoid arthritis. Int J Infect Dis 2009;13:e145-7.

203. Lembo G, Goldstein EJ, Troum O, Mandelbaum B. Successful treatment of Mycobacterium terrae complex infection of the knee. J Clin Rheumatol 2012;18:359-62.

204. Esnakula AK, Mummidi SK, Oneal PA, Naab TJ. Sepsis caused by Mycobacterium terrae complex in a patient with sickle cell disease. BMJ Case Rep 2013.pii: bcr2013009159.

205. Castell P, Collet E, Chauffert B, Cuny C, Morlevat F, Lambert D, et al. Recurrent skin abscesses: pathogenic role of Mycobacterium terrae. Rev Med Interne 1993;14:1119-20.

206. Shimizu T, Furumoto H, Takahashi T, Yasuno H, Muto M. Lymphadenitis due to Mycobacterium terrae in an immunocompetent patient. Dermatology 1999;198:97-8.

207. Carbonara S, Tortoli E, Costa D, Monno L, Fiorentino G, Grimaldi A, et al. Disseminated Mycobacterium terrae infection in a patient with advanced human immunodeficiency virus disease. Clin Infect Dis 2000;30:831-5.

208. Alexander S, John GT, Jesudason M, Jacob CK. Infections with atypical mycobacteria in renal transplant recipients. Indian J Pathol Microbiol 2007;50:482-4.

209. Molavi A, Weinstein L. In vitro susceptibility of atypical mycobacteria to rifampin. Appl Microbiol 1971;22:23-5.

210. Tsukamura M. A group of mycobacteria from soil sources resembling nonphotochromogens [group 3]. A description of Mycobacterium nonchromogenicum. Igaku To Seibutsugaku 1965;71:110-3.

211. Fujisawa K, Watanabe H, Yamamoto K, Nasu T, Kitahara Y, Nakano M. Primary atypical mycobacteriosis of the intestine: a report of three cases. Gut 1989;30:541-5.

212. Ridderhof JC, Wallace RJ Jr, Kilburn JO, Butler WR, Warren NG, Tsukamura M, et al. Chronic tenosynovitis of the hand due to Mycobacterium nonchromogenicum: use of high-performance liquid chromatography for identification of isolates. Rev Infect Dis 1991;13:857-64.

213. Krusche-Mandl I, Decramer A, Boltuch-Sherif J, Vlieghe E, Brands C, Vandenberghe D. [Non-tuberculous mycobacterial infections of the hand and wrist: a retrospective review of five cases from a single centre]. Handchir Mikrochir Plast Chir 2009;41:283-7.

214. Tsukamura M, Kita N, Otsuka W, Shimoide H. A study of the taxonomy of the Mycobacterium nonchromogenicum complex and report of six cases of lung infection due to Mycobacterium nonchromogenicum. Microbiol Immunol 1983;27:219-36.

215. Sawai T, Inoue Y, Doi S, Izumikawa K, Ohno H, Yanagihara K, et al. A case of Mycobacterium nonchromogenicum pulmonary infection showing multiple nodular shadows in an immunocompetent patient. Diagn Microbiol Infect Dis 2006;54:311-4.

216. Ford JG, Huang AJ, Pflugfelder SC, Alfonso EC, Forster RK, Miller D. Nontuberculous mycobacterial keratitis in south Florida. Ophthalmology 1998;105:1652-8.

217. Kubica GP, Silcox VA, Kilburn JO, Smithwick RW, Beam RE, Jones WD, et al. Differential identification of mycobacteria. VI. Mycobacterium triviale kubica sp. nov. Int J Syst Bacteriol 1970;20:161-74.

218. Dechairo DC, Kittredge D, Meyers A, Corrales J. Septic arthritis due to Mycobacterium triviale. Am Rev Respir Dis 1973;108:1224-6.

219. Elting JJ, Southwick WO. Acute infantile septic arthritis of the hip due to Mycobacterium triviale. A case report. J Bone Joint Surg Am 1974;56:184-6.

220. Janakiraman H, Abraham G, Mathew M, Lalitha MK, Bhaskar S. Relapsing peritonitis due to co-infection with Mycobacterium triviale and Candida albicans in a CAPD patient. Perit Dial Int 2007;27:311-3.

221. Tortoli E, Gitti Z, Klenk HP, Lauria S, Mannino R, Mantegani P, et al. Survey of 150 strains belonging to the Mycobacterium terrae complex and description of Mycobacterium engbaekii sp. nov., Mycobacterium heraklionense sp. nov. and Mycobacterium longobardum sp. nov. Int J Syst Evol Microbiol 2013;63:401-11.

222. Hong SK, Sung JY, Lee HJ, Oh MD, Park SS, Kim EC. First case of Mycobacterium longobardum infection. Ann Lab Med 2013;33:356-9.

223. Mun HS, Park JH, Kim H, Yu HK, Park YG, Cha CY, et al. Mycobacterium senuense sp. nov., a slowly growing, non-chromogenic species closely related to the Mycobacterium terrae complex. Int J Syst Evol Microbiol 2008;58:641-6.

224. Heidarieh P, Hashemi-Shahraki A, Khosravi AD, Zaker-Boustanabad S, Shojaei H, Feizabadi MM. Mycobacterium arupense infection in HIV-infected patients from Iran. Int J STD AIDS 2013;24:485-7.

225. Legout L, Ettahar N, Massongo M, Veziris N, Ajana F, Beltrand E, et al. Osteomyelitis of the wrist caused by Mycobacterium arupense in an immunocompetent patient: a unique case. Int J Infect Dis 2012;16:e761-2.

226. Senda H, Muro H, Terada S. Flexor tenosynovitis caused by Mycobacterium arupense. J Hand Surg Eur Vol 2011;36:72-3.

227. Neonakis IK, Gitti Z, Kontos F, Baritaki S, Petinaki E, Baritaki M, et al. Mycobacterium arupense pulmonary infection: antibiotic resistance and restriction fragment length polymorphism analysis. Indian J Med Microbiol 2010;28:173-6.

228. Masaki T, Ohkusu K, Hata H, Fujiwara N, Iihara H, Yamada-Noda M, et al. Mycobacterium kumamotonense sp. nov. recovered from clinical specimen and the first isolation report of Mycobacterium arupense in Japan: novel slowly growing, nonchromogenic clinical isolates related to Mycobacterium terrae complex. Microbiol Immunol 2006;50:889-97.

229. Rodríguez-Aranda A, Jimenez MS, Yubero J, Chaves F, Rubio-Garcia R, Palenque E, et al. Misidentification of Mycobacterium kumamotonense as M. tuberculosis. Emerg Infect Dis 2010;16:1178-80.

230. Collins CH, Grange JM, Noble WC, Yates MD. Mycobacterium marinum infections in man. J Hyg [Lond] 1985;94:135-49.

231. Chow SP, Ip FK, Lau JH, Collins RJ, Luk KD, So YC, et al. Mycobacterium marinum infection of the hand and wrist. Results of conservative treatment in twenty four cases. J Bone Joint Surg Am 1987;69:1161-8.

232. Lambertus MW, Mathiesen GE. Mycobacterium marinum infection in a patient with cryptosporidiosis and the acquired immunodeficiency syndrome. Cutis 1988;42:38-40.

233. Maloney JM, Gregg CR, Stephens DS, Manian FA, Rimland D. Infections caused by Mycobacterium szulgai in humans. Rev Infect Dis 1987;9:1120-6.

234. Dawson DJ, Blacklock ZM, Kane DW. Mycobacterium haemophilum causing lymphadenitis in otherwise healthy child. Med J Aust 1981;2:289-90.

235. Males BM, West TE, Bartholomew WR. Mycobacterium haemophilum infection in a patient with AIDS. J Clin Microbiol 1987;25:186-90.

236. Kiehn TE, White M, Pursell KJ, Boone N, Tsivitis M, Brown AE, et al. A cluster of four cases of Mycobacterium haemophilum infection. Eur J Clin Microbiol Infect Dis 1993;12:114-8.

237. Kikuchi K, Bernard E, Kiehn TE, Armstrong D, Riley LW. Restriction fragment length polymorphism analysis of clinical isolates of Mycobacterium haemophilum. J Clin Microbiol 1994; 32:1763-7.

238. Dever LL, Martin JW, Seaworth B, Jorgensen JH. Varied presentations and responses to treatment of infections caused by Mycobacterium haemophilum in patients with AIDS. Clin Infect Dis 1992;14:1195-200.

239. Hoy JF, Rolston KV, Hopfer RL, Bodey GP. Mycobacterium fortuitum bacteremia in patients with cancer and long-term venous catheters. Am J Med 1987;83:213-7.

240. Nolan CM, Hashisaki PA, Dundas DF. An outbreak of soft-tissue infections due to Mycobacterium fortuitum associated with electromyography. J Infect Dis 1991;163:1150-3.

241. Muthusami JC, Vyas FL, Mukundan U, Jesudason MR, Govil S, Jesudason SR. Mycobacterium fortuitum: an iatrogenic cause of soft tissue infection in surgery. ANZ J Surg 2004;74:662-6.

242. Kupeli E, Bozkurt E, Azap O, Eyuboglu FO. Mycobacterium fortuitum infection presenting as community-acquired pneumonia in an immunocompetent host. J Bronchology Interv Pulmonol 2010;17:356-8.

243. Callen EC, Kessler TL. Mycobacterium fortuitum infections associated with laparoscopic gastric banding. Obes Surg 2011;21: 404-6.

244. Westmoreland D, Woodwards RT, Holden PE, James PA. Soft tissue abscess caused by Mycobacterium fortuitum. J Infect 1990;20:223-5.

245. Coney PM, Thrush S. Cutaneous Mycobacterium fortuitum complicating breast reconstruction. J Plast Reconstr Aesthet Surg 2007;60:1162-3.

246. Sarma S, Thakur R. Cutaneous infection with Mycobacterium fortuitum: an unusual presentation. Indian J Med Microbiol 2008;26:388-90.

247. Quiñones C, Ramalle-Gómara E, Perucha M, Lezaun ME, Fernández-Vilariño E, García-Morrás P, et al. An outbreak of Mycobacterium fortuitum cutaneous infection associated with mesotherapy. J Eur Acad Dermatol Venereol 2010;24:604-6.

248. Nguyen DQ, Righini C, Darouassi Y, Schmerber S. Nasal infection due to Mycobacterium fortuitum. Eur Ann Otorhinolaryngol Head Neck Dis 2011;128:197-9.

249. López Aventín D, Rubio González B, Petiti Martín G, Segura S, Rodríguez-Peralto JL, Riveiro-Falkenbach E, et al. Mycobacterium fortuitum infection in continuous subcutaneous insulin infusion sites. Br J Dermatol 2014;171:418-20.

250. Mederos LM, González D, Banderas F, Montoro EH. Ulcerative lymphadenitis due to Mycobacterium fortuitum in an AIDS patient. Enferm Infecc Microbiol Clin 2005;23:573-4.

251. Luz KG, Britto MH, Farias DC, Almeida MV, Figueirêdo NM, Silva Pde M. Mycobacterium fortuitum-related lymphadenitis associated with the varicella-zoster virus. Rev Soc Bras Med Trop 2014;47:119-21.

252. Sangwan J, Lathwal S, Kumar S, Juyal D. Mycobacterium fortuitum peritonitis in a patient on continuous ambulatory peritoneal dialysis [CAPD]: a case report. J Clin Diagn Res 2013;7:2950-1.

253. Fogla R, Rao SK, Padmanabhan P. Interface keratitis due to Mycobacterium fortuitum following laser in situ keratomileusis. Indian J Ophthalmol 2003;51:263-5.

254. Sanghvi C. Mycobacterium fortuitum keratitis. Indian J Med Microbiol 2007;25:422-4.

255. Collison SP, Trehan N. Native double-valve endocarditis by Mycobacterium fortuitum following percutaneous coronary intervention. J Heart Valve Dis 2006;15:836-8.

256. Vuković D, Parezanović V, Savić B, Dakić I, Laban-Nestorović S, Ilić S, et al. Mycobacterium fortuitum endocarditis associated with cardiac surgery, Serbia. Emerg Infect Dis 2013;19:517-9.

257. Kuruvila MT, Mathews P, Jesudason M, Ganesh A. Mycobacterium fortuitum endocarditis and meningitis after balloon mitral valvotomy. J Assoc Physicians India 1999;47: 1022-3.

258. Kell CA, Hunfeld KP, Wagner S, Nern C, Seifert V, Brodt HR, et al. Chronic meningoencephalomyelitis due to Mycobacterium fortuitum in an immunocompetent patient. J Neurol 2008; 255:1847-9.

259. Brannan DP, DuBois RE, Ramirez MJ, Ravry MJ, Harrison EO. Cefoxitin therapy for Mycobacterium fortuitum bacteremia with associated granulomatous hepatitis. South Med J 1984;77:381-4.

260. Montoliu J, Gatell JM, Bonal J, Miró JM, López-Pedret J, Revert L. Disseminated visceral infection with Mycobacterium fortuitum in a hemodialysis patient. Am J Nephrol 1985;5:205-11.

261. Brady MT, Marcon MJ, Maddux H. Broviac catheter-related infection due to Mycobacterium fortuitum in a patient with acquired immunodeficiency syndrome. Pediatr Infect Dis J 1987;6:492-4.

262. Artacho-Reinoso MJ, Olbrich P, Solano-Paéz P, Ybot-Gonzalez P, Lepe JA, Neth O, et al. Catheter-related Mycobacterium fortuitum bloodstream infection: rapid identification using MALDI-TOF mass spectrometry. Klin Padiatr 2014;226:68-71.

263. Corti M, Soto I, Villafañe F, Esquivel P, Di Lonardo M. Disseminated infection due to Mycobacterium fortuitum in an AIDS patient. Medicina [B Aires] 1999;59:274-6.

264. Glatstein M, Scolnik D, Bensira L, Domany KA, Shah M, Vala S. Lung abscess due to non-tuberculous, non-Mycobacterium fortuitum in a neonate. Pediatr Pulmonol 2012;47:1034-7.

265. de Mello KG, Mello FC, Borga L, Rolla V, Duarte RS, Sampaio EP, et al. Clinical and therapeutic features of pulmonary nontuberculous mycobacterial disease, Brazil, 1993-2011. Emerg Infect Dis 2013;19:393-9.

266. Yano Y, Kitada S, Mori M, Kagami S, Taguri T, Uenami T, et al. Pulmonary disease caused by rapidly growing mycobacteria: a retrospective study of 44 cases in Japan. Respiration 2013;85: 305-11.

267. Koscielniak E, de Boer T, Dupuis S, Naumann L, Casanova JL, Ottenhoff TH. Disseminated Mycobacterium peregrinum infection in a child with complete interferon-gamma receptor-1 deficiency. Pediatr Infect Dis J 2003;22:378-80.

268. Torres-Duque CA, Díaz C, Vargas L, Serpa EM, Mosquera W, Garzón MC, et al. Disseminated mycobacteriosis affecting a prosthetic aortic valve: first case of Mycobacterium peregrinum type III reported in Colombia. Biomedica 2010;30:332-7.

269. Marie I, Heliot P, Roussel F, Hervé F, Muir JF, Levesque H. Fatal Mycobacterium peregrinum pneumonia in refractory polymyositis treated with infliximab. Rheumatology [Oxford] 2005;44:1201-2.

270. Sawahata M, Hagiwara E, Ogura T, Komatsu S, Sekine A, Tsuchiya N, et al. [Pulmonary mycobacteriosis caused by Mycobacterium peregrinum in a young, healthy man]. Nihon Kokyuki Gakkai Zasshi 2010;48:866-70.

271. Appelgren P, Farnebo F, Dotevall L, Studahl M, Jönsson B, Petrini B. Late-onset post-traumatic skin and soft-tissue infections caused by rapid-growing mycobacteria in tsunami survivors. Clin Infect Dis 2008;47:e11-6.

272. Kamijo F, Uhara H, Kubo H, Nakanaga K, Hoshino Y, Ishii N, et al. A case of mycobacterial skin disease caused by mycobacterium peregrinum, and a review of cutaneous infection. Case Rep Dermatol 2012;4:76-9.

273. Sakai T, Kobayashi C, Shinohara M. Mycobacterium peregrinum infection in a patient with AIDS. Intern Med 2005;44:266-9.

274. Pagnoux C, Nassif X, Boitard C, Timsit J. Infection of continuous subcutaneous insulin infusion site with Mycobacterium peregrinum. Diabetes Care 1998;21:191-2.

275. Nagao M, Sonobe M, Bando T, Saito T, Shirano M, Matsushima A, et al. Surgical site infection due to Mycobacterium peregrinum: a case report and literature review. Int J Infect Dis 2009;13: 209-11.

276. Bönicke R. The occurrence of atypical mycobacteria in the environment of man and animal. Bull Int Union Tuberc Lung Dis 1966;37:361-8.

277. Wallace RJ Jr, Brown BA, Silcox VA, Tsukamura M, Nash DR, Steele LC, et al. Clinical disease, drug susceptibility, and biochemical patterns of the unnamed third biovariant complex of Mycobacterium fortuitum. J Infect Dis 1991;163:598-603.

278. Wallace RJ Jr, Musser JM, Hull SI, Silcox VA, Steele LC, Forrester GD, et al. Diversity and sources of rapidly growing mycobacteria associated with infections following cardiac surgery. J Infect Dis 1989;159:708-16.

279. Schinsky MF, Morey RE, Steigerwalt AG, Douglas MP, Wilson RW, Floyd MM, et al. Taxonomic variation in the Mycobacterium fortuitum third biovariant complex: description of Mycobacterium boenickei sp. nov., Mycobacterium houstonense sp. nov., Mycobacterium neworleansense sp. nov. and Mycobacterium brisbanense sp. nov. and recognition of Mycobacterium porcinum from human clinical isolates. Int J Syst Evol Microbiol 2004;54:1653-67.

280. Bonura C, Di Carlo P, Spicola D, Cal C, Mammina C, Fasciana T, et al. Rapidly growing mycobacteria in TB/HIV co-infection: a report of two cases focusing on difficulties in diagnosis and management. New Microbiol 2012;35:239-43.

281. de Lima CA, Gomes HM, Oelemann MA, Ramos JP, Caldas PC, Campos CE, et al. Nontuberculous mycobacteria in respiratory samples from patients with pulmonary tuberculosis in the state of Rondônia, Brazil. Mem Inst Oswaldo Cruz 2013;108:457-62.

282. Patil R, Patil T, Schenfeld L, Massoud S. Mycobacterium porcinum peritonitis in a patient on continuous ambulatory peritoneal dialysis. J Gen Intern Med 2011;26:346-8.

283. Sampaio JL, Chimara E, Ferrazoli L, da Silva Telles MA, Del Guercio VM, Jericó ZV, et al. Application of four molecular typing methods for analysis of Mycobacterium fortuitum group strains causing post-mammaplasty infections. Clin Microbiol Infect 2006;12:142-9.

284. Idigoras P, Jiménez-Alfaro JA, Mendiola J. Postoperative sternal osteomyelitis due to Mycobacterium porcinum. Enferm Infecc Microbiol Clin 2007;25:68-9.

285. Lian L, Deng J, Zhao X, Dong H, Zhang J, Li G, et al. The first case of pulmonary disease caused by Mycobacterium septicum in China. Int J Infect Dis 2013;17:e352-4.

286. Adékambi T, Drancourt M. Isolation of Mycobacterium septicum from the sputum of a patient suffering from hemoptoic pneumonia. Res Microbiol 2006;157:466-70.

287. Schinsky MF, McNeil MM, Whitney AM, Steigerwalt AG, Lasker BA, Floyd MM, et al. Mycobacterium septicum sp. nov., a new rapidly growing species associated with catheter-related bacteraemia. Int J Syst Evol Microbiol 2000;50:575-81.

288. Adékambi T, Stein A, Carvajal J, Raoult D, Drancourt M. Description of Mycobacterium conceptionense sp. nov., a Mycobacterium fortuitum group organism isolated from a post-traumatic osteitis inflammation. J Clin Microbiol 2006;44:1268-73.

289. Shojaei H, Hashemi A, Heidarieh P, Ataei B, Naser AD. Pulmonary and extrapulmonary infection caused by Mycobacterium conceptionense: the first report from Iran. JRSM Short Rep 2011;2:31.

290. Kim SY, Kim MS, Chang HE, Yim JJ, Lee JH, Song SH, et al. Pulmonary infection caused by Mycobacterium conceptionense. Emerg Infect Dis 2012;18:174-6.

291. Liao CH, Lai CC, Huang YT, Chou CH, Hsu HL, Hsueh PR. Subcutaneous abscess caused by Mycobacterium conceptionense in an immunocompetent patient. J Infect 2009;58:308-9.

292. Thibeaut S, Levy PY, Pelletier ML, Drancourt M. Mycobacterium conceptionense infection after breast implant surgery, France. Emerg Infect Dis 2010;16:1180-1.

293. Maybrook RJ, Campsen J, Wachs ME, Levi ME. A case of Mycobacterium mucogenicum infection in a liver transplant recipient and a review of the literature. Transpl Infect Dis 2013; 15:E260-3.

294. Fiore R 2nd, Miller R, Coffman SM. Mycobacterium mucogenicum infection following a cosmetic procedure with poly-L-lactic acid. J Drugs Dermatol 2013;12:353-7.

295. Cooksey RC, Jhung MA, Yakrus MA, Butler WR, Adékambi T, Morlock GP, et al. Multiphasic approach reveals genetic diversity of environmental and patient isolates of Mycobacterium mucogenicum and Mycobacterium phocaicum associated with an outbreak of bacteremias at a Texas hospital. Appl Environ Microbiol 2008;74:2480-7.

296. Shachor-Meyouhas Y, Sprecher H, Eluk O, Ben-Barak A, Kassis I. An outbreak of Mycobacterium mucogenicum bacteremia in pediatric hematology-oncology patients. Pediatr Infect Dis J 2011;30:30-2.

297. Ashraf MS, Swinker M, Augustino KL, Nobles D, Knupp C, Liles D, et al. Outbreak of Mycobacterium mucogenicum bloodstream infections among patients with sickle cell disease in an outpatient setting. Infect Control Hosp Epidemiol 2012;33:1132-6.

298. El Helou G, Hachem R, Viola GM, El Zakhem A, Chaftari AM, Jiang Y, et al. Management of rapidly growing mycobacterial bacteremia in cancer patients. Clin Infect Dis 2013;56:843-6.

299. Reddy YN, Reddy YN, Balasubramaniam L, Mathew M, Abraham G. Mycobacterium mucogenicum peritonitis in a continuous ambulatory peritoneal dialysis patient. Perit Dial Int 2012;32:226-7.

300. Shehan JM, Sarma DP. Mycobacterium mucogenicum: report of a skin infection associated with etanercept. Dermatol Online J 2008;14:5.

301. Hawkins C, Qi C, Warren J, Stosor V. Catheter-related bloodstream infections caused by rapidly growing nontuberculous mycobacteria: a case series including rare species. Diagn Microbiol Infect Dis 2008;61:187-91.

302. Adékambi T, Foucault C, La Scola B, Drancourt M. Report of two fatal cases of Mycobacterium mucogenicum central nervous system infection in immunocompetent patients. J Clin Microbiol 2006;44:837-40.

303. Fonteyn N, Wauters G, Vandercam B, Degraux J, Avesani V, Vincent V, et al. Mycobacterium mucogenicum sepsis in an immunocompetent patient. J Infect 2006;53:e143-6.

304. Vargas J, Gamboa C, Negrin D, Correa M, Sandoval C, Aguiar A, et al. Disseminated Mycobacterium mucogenicum infection in a patient with idiopathic CD4+ T lymphocytopenia manifesting as fever of unknown origin. Clin Infect Dis 2005;41:759-60.

305. Oh WS, Ko KS, Song JH, Lee MY, Ryu SY, Taek S, et al. Catheter-associated bacteremia by Mycobacterium senegalense in Korea. BMC Infect Dis 2005;5:107.

306. Talavlikar R, Carson J, Meatherill B, Desai S, Sharma M, Shandro C, et al. Mycobacterium senegalense tissue infection in a child after fish tank exposure. Can J Infect Dis Med Microbiol 2011;22:101-3.

307. Muñoz-Sanz A, Rodríguez-Vidigal FF, Vera-Tomé A, Jiménez MS. Mycobacterium mageritense meningitis in an immunocompetent patient with an intrathecal catheter. Enferm Infecc Microbiol Clin 2013;31:59-60.

308. Ali S, Khan FA, Fisher M. Catheter-related bloodstream infection caused by Mycobacterium mageritense. J Clin Microbiol 2007; 45:273.

309. Gira AK, Reisenauer AH, Hammock L, Nadiminti U, Macy JT, Reeves A, et al. Furunculosis due to Mycobacterium mageritense

associated with footbaths at a nail salon. J Clin Microbiol 2004;42:1813-7.

310. Moore M, Frerichs JB. An unusual acid-fast infection of the knee with subcutaneous, abscess-like lesions of the gluteal region; report of a case with a study of the organism, Mycobacterium abscessus, n. sp. J Invest Dermatol 1953;20:133-69.

311. Inman PM, Beck A, Brown AE, Stanford JL. Outbreak of injection abscesses due to Mycobacterium abscessus. Arch Dermatol 1969;100:141-7.

312. Villanueva A, Calderon RV, Vargas BA, Ruiz F, Aguero S, Zhang Y, et al. Report on an outbreak of postinjection abscesses due to Mycobacterium abscessus, including management with surgery and clarithromycin therapy and comparison of strains by random amplified polymorphic DNA polymerase chain reaction. Clin Infect Dis 1997;24:1147-53.

313. Zhibang Y, BiXia Z, Qishan L, Lihao C, Xiangquan L, Huaping L. Large-scale outbreak of infection with Mycobacterium chelonae subsp. abscessus after penicillin injection. J Clin Microbiol 2002; 40:2626-8.

314. Toy BR, Frank PJ. Outbreak of Mycobacterium abscessus infection after soft tissue augmentation. Dermatol Surg 2003; 29:971-3.

315. Newman MI, Camberos AE, Ascherman J. Mycobacteria abscessus outbreak in US patients linked to offshore surgicenter. Ann Plast Surg 2005;55:107-10.

316. Furuya EY, Paez A, Srinivasan A, Cooksey R, Augenbraun M, Baron M, et al. Outbreak of Mycobacterium abscessus wound infections among "lipotourists" from the United States who underwent abdominoplasty in the Dominican Republic. Clin Infect Dis 2008;46:1181-8.

317. Koh SJ, Song T, Kang YA, Choi JW, Chang KJ, Chu CS, et al. An outbreak of skin and soft tissue infection caused by Mycobacterium abscessus following acupuncture. Clin Microbiol Infect 2010;16:895-901.

318. Jamal W, Salama MF, Al Hashem G, Rifaei M, Eldeen H, Husain EH, et al. An outbreak of Mycobacterium abscessus infection in a pediatric intensive care unit in Kuwait. Pediatr Infect Dis J 2014;33:e67-70.

319. Benwill J, Babineaux M, Sarria JC. Pulmonary Mycobacterium abscessus in an AIDS patient. Am J Med Sci 2010;339:495-6.

320. Jeong YJ, Lee KS, Koh WJ, Han J, Kim TS, Kwon OJ. Nontuberculous mycobacterial pulmonary infection in immuno-competent patients: comparison of thin-section CT and histo-pathologic findings. Radiology 2004;231:880-6.

321. Varghese B, Shajan SE, Al MO, Al-Hajoj SA. First case report of chronic pulmonary lung disease caused by Mycobacterium abscessus in two immunocompetent patients in Saudi Arabia. Ann Saudi Med 2012;32:312-4.

322. Griffith DE, Girard WM, Wallace RJ Jr. Clinical features of pulmonary disease caused by rapidly growing mycobacteria. An analysis of 154 patients. Am Rev Respir Dis 1993;147:1271-8.

323. Sanguinetti M, Ardito F, Fiscarelli E, La Sorda M, D'Argenio P, Ricciotti G, et al. Fatal pulmonary infection due to multidrug-resistant Mycobacterium abscessus in a patient with cystic fibrosis. J Clin Microbiol 2001;39:816-9.

324. Petrini B. Mycobacterium abscessus: an emerging rapid-growing potential pathogen. APMIS 2006;114:319-28.

325. Medjahed H, Gaillard JL, Reyrat JM. Mycobacterium abscessus: a new player in the mycobacterial field. Trends Microbiol 2010;18:117-23.

326. Palani D, Kulandai LT, Naraharirao MH, Guruswami S, Ramendra B. Application of polymerase chain reaction-based restriction fragment length polymorphism in typing ocular rapid-growing nontuberculous mycobacterial isolates from three patients with postoperative endophthalmitis. Cornea 2007;26:729-35.

327. Gandhi V, Nagral A, Nagral S, Das S, Rodrigues C. An unusual surgical site infection in a liver transplant recipient. BMJ Case Rep 2010;2010.

328. Sarma S, Sharma S, Baweja UK, Mehta Y. Mycobacterium abscessus bacteremia in an immunocompetent patient following a coronary artery bypass graft. J Cardiovasc Dis Res 2011;2:80-2.

329. Haider M, Banerjee P, Jaggi T, Husain J, Mishra B, Thakur A, et al. Post-operative sinus formation due to Mycobacterium abscessus: a case report. Indian J Tuberc 2013;60:177-9.

330. Swetter SM, Kindel SE, Smoller BR. Cutaneous nodules of Mycobacterium chelonae in an immunosuppressed patient with preexisting pulmonary colonization. J Am Acad Dermatol 1993;28:352-5.

331. Bartralot R, Pujol RM, García-Patos V, Sitjas D, Martín-Casabona N, Coll P, et al. Cutaneous infections due to nontuberculous mycobacteria: histopathological review of 28 cases. Comparative study between lesions observed in immunosuppressed patients and normal hosts. J Cutan Pathol 2000;27:124-9.

332. Jankovic M, Zmak L, Krajinovic V, Viskovic K, Crnek SS, Obrovac M, et al. A fatal Mycobacterium chelonae infection in an immunosuppressed patient with systemic lupus erythematosus and concomitant Fahr's syndrome. J Infect Chemother 2011;17: 264-7.

333. Steyaert S, Stappaerts G, Mareen P, Dierick J. Soft tissue infections with atypical mycobacteria in two patients with inflammatory rheumatic diseases using TNF-inhibitors and/or leflunomide. Acta Clin Belg 2011;66:144-7.

334. Kennedy BS, Bedard B, Younge M, Tuttle D, Ammerman E, Ricci J, et al. Outbreak of Mycobacterium chelonae infection associated with tattoo ink. N Engl J Med 2012;367:1020-4.

335. Scott-Lang VE, Sergeant A, Sinclair CG, Laurenson IF, Biswas A, Tidman MJ, et al. Cutaneous Mycobacterium chelonae infection in Edinburgh and the Lothians, south-east Scotland, UK. Br J Dermatol 2014;171:79-89.

336. Patnaik S, Mohanty I, Panda P, Sahu S, Dash M. Disseminated Mycobacterium chelonae infection: complicating a case of hidradenitis suppurativa. Indian Dermatol Online J 2013;4: 336-9.

337. Unai S, Miessau J, Karbowski P, Bajwa G, Hirose H. Sternal wound infection caused by Mycobacterium chelonae. J Card Surg 2013;28:687-92.

338. Takekoshi D, Al-Heeti O, Belvitch P, Schraufnagel DE. Native-valve endocarditis caused by Mycobacterium chelonae, misidentified as polymicrobial Gram-positive bacillus infection. J Infect Chemother 2013;19:754-6.

339. Shaaban HS, Bishop SL, Menon L, Slim J. Mycobacterium chelonae infection of the parotid gland. J Glob Infect Dis 2012;4:79-81.

340. Rahman I, Bhatt H, Chillag S, Duffus W. Mycobacterium chelonae vertebral osteomyelitis. South Med J 2009;102:1167-9.

341. Talanow R, Vieweg H, Andresen R. Atypical osteomyelitis caused by Mycobacterium chelonae—a multimodal imaging approach. Case Rep Infect Dis 2013;2013:528795.

342. Dolz-Marco R, Udaondo P, Gallego-Pinazo R, Millán JM, Díaz-Llopis M. Topical linezolid for refractory bilateral Mycobacterium chelonae post-laser-assisted in situ keratomileusis keratitis. Arch Ophthalmol 2012;130:1475-6.

343. Lee KF, Chen HH, Wu CJ. Mycobacterium chelonae peritonitis in a patient on peritoneal dialysis. Ren Fail 2008;30:335-8.

344. Dubey M, Kalantri Y, Hemvani N, Chitnis DS. Chronic knee monoarthritis caused by Mycobacterium chelonae. Natl Med J India 2007;20:240-1.

345. Schneider P, Monsel G, Veziris N, Roujeau JC, Bricaire F, Caumes E. Successful treatment of nodular lymphangitis due to Mycobacterium chelonae in two immunosuppressed patients. Dermatol Online J 2011;17:8.

346. Jain S, Singh S, Sankar MM, Saha R, Rangaraju RR, Chugh TD. Catheter-related bacteremia due to M. chelonae in an immuno-compromised patient: an emerging nosocomial pathogen. Indian J Med Microbiol 2012;30:489-91.

347. Lin YH, Liu TC. Mycobacterium chelonae infection involving the auricle. QJM 2012;105:1021-2.

348. Iyengar KP, Nadkarni JB, Gupta R, Beeching NJ, Ullah I, Loh WY. Mycobacterium chelonae hand infection following ferret bite. Infection 2013;41:237-41.

349. van Ingen J, de Zwaan R, Dekhuijzen RP, Boeree MJ, van Soolingen D. Clinical relevance of Mycobacterium chelonae-abscessus group isolation in 95 patients. J Infect 2009;59:324-31.

350. Goto T, Hamaguchi R, Maeshima A, Oyamada Y, Kato R. Pulmonary resection for Mycobacterium chelonae infection. Ann Thorac Cardiovasc Surg 2012;18:128-31.

351. Rodríguez JC, Reyes DM, Royo G, Andrada E, Sillero C. [Mycobacterium chelonae and solitary rectal ulcer]. Gastroenterol Hepatol 2000;23:474-6.

352. Banks J, Jenkins PA, Smith AP. Pulmonary infections in Mycobacterium malmoense—a review of treatment and response. Tubercle 1985;66:197-203.

353. Claydon EJ, Coker RJ, Harris JR. Mycobacterium malmoense infection in HIV positive patients. J Infect 1991;23:191-4.

354. Engervall P, Björkholm M, Petrini B, Heurlin N, Henriques B, Källenius G. Disseminated Mycobacterium malmoense infection in a patient with chronic granulocytic leukaemia. J Intern Med 1993;234:231-3.

355. Schmoor P, Descamps V, Lebrun-Vignes B, Crickx B, Grossin M, Nouhouayi A, et al. Mycobacterium malmoense cutaneous infection in an immunocompetent patient. Ann Dermatol Venereol 2001;128:139-40.

356. Cowan CD, Hawboldt JJ, Bader M. Pulmonary infection due to Mycobacterium malmoense in a patient with Crohn disease. Can J Hosp Pharm 2009;62:496-9.

357. Duarte JN, Marques N, Barroso L, Ramos I, Sá R, Sanz D, et al. Cervical abscess in an immunocompetent patient with Myco-bacterium malmoense pulmonary disease. Oral Maxillofac Surg 2012;16:321-5.

358. Leth S, Jensen-Fangel S. Infrapatellar bursitis with Mycobacterium malmoense related to immune reconstitution inflammatory syndrome in an HIV-positive patient. BMJ Case Rep 2012;2012. pii: bcr2012007459.

359. Pigem R, Cairó M, Martínez-Lacasa X, Irigoyen D, Miró JM, Acevedo J, et al. Disseminated infection with cutaneous involvement caused by Mycobacterium malmoense in an immunocompromised patient. J Am Acad Dermatol 2013;69: e192-3.

360. Converse PJ, Nuermberger EL, Almeida DV, Grosset JH. Treating Mycobacterium ulcerans disease [Buruli ulcer]: from surgery to antibiotics, is the pill mightier than the knife? Future Microbiol 2011;6:1185-98.

361. Yotsu RR, Nakanaga K, Hoshino Y, Suzuki K, Ishii N. Buruli ulcer and current situation in Japan: a new emerging cutaneous Mycobacterium infection. J Dermatol 2012;39:587-93.

362. Chany AC, Tresse C, Casarotto V, Blanchard N. History, biology and chemistry of Mycobacterium ulcerans infections [Buruli ulcer disease]. Nat Prod Rep 2013;30:1527-67.

363. Wallace RJ, Nash DR, Tsukamura M, Blacklock ZM, Silcox VA. Human disease due to Mycobacterium smegmatis. J Infect Dis 1988;158:52-9.

364. Best CA, Best TJ. Mycobacterium smegmatis infection of the hand. Hand [NY] 2009;4:165-6.

365. Driks M, Weinhold F, Cokingtin Q. Pneumonia caused by Mycobacterium smegmatis in a patient with a previous gastrectomy. BMJ Case Rep 2011;2011:3281.

366. Weitzman I, Osadezyl D, Corrado NL, Karp D. Mycobacterium thermoresistibile; a new pathogen for humans. J Clin Microbiol 1981;14:593-5.

367. Neeley SP, Denning DW. Cutaneous Mycobacterium thermo-resistibile infection in a heart transplant recipient. Rev Infect Dis 1989;11:608-11.

368. Neonakis IK, Gitti Z, Kontos F, Baritaki S, Petinaki E, Baritaki M, et al. Mycobacterium thermoresistibile: case report of a rarely isolated mycobacterium from Europe and review of literature. Indian J Med Microbiol 2009;27:264-7.

369. Suy F, Carricajo A, Grattard F, Cazorla C, Denis C, Girardin P, et al. Infection due to Mycobacterium thermoresistibile: a case associated with an orthopedic device. J Clin Microbiol 2013;51:3154-6.

370. Davison MR, McCormack JG, Blacklock AM, Dawson DJ, Tilse MH, Crimmins PB. Bacteremia caused by Mycobacterium neoaurum. J Clin Microbiol 1988;26:62-4.

371. Jiang SH, Roberts DM, Clayton PA, Jardine M. Non-tuberculous mycobacterial PD peritonitis in Australia. Int Urol Nephrol 2013;45:1423-8.

372. Hachem R, Raad I, Rolston KV, Whimbey E, Katz R, Tarrand J, et al. Cutaneous and pulmonary infections caused by Mycobacterium vaccae. Clin Infect Dis 1996;23:173-5.

373. Lai KK, Stottmeier KD, Sherman IH, McCabe WR. Mycobacterial cervical lymphadenopathy. Relation of etiologic agents to age. JAMA 1984;251:1286-8.

374. Ahn CH, McLarty JW, Ahn SS, Ahn SI, Hurst GA. Diagnostic criteria for pulmonary disease caused by M. kansasii and M. intracellulare. Am Rev Respir Dis 1982;125:388-91.

375. Wallace RJ, Swenson JM, Silcox VA, Good RC, Tschen JA, Stone MS. Spectrum of disease due to rapidly growing mycobacteria. Rev Infect Dis 1983;5:657-79.

376. Horsburgh DR, Mason UG, Farhi DC, Iseman MD. Disseminated infection with Mycobacterium avium-intracellulare. Medicine [Baltimore] 1985;64:36-48.

377. Kiehn TE, Edwards FF, Brannon P, Tsang AY, Mary M, Jonathan WH. Infections caused by MAC in immunocompro-mised patients; diagnosis by blood culture and fecal examina-tion antimicrobial susceptibility tests, and morphological and seroagglutination characteristics. J Clin Microbiol 1985;21:168-73.

378. Gopinath K, Kumar S, Singh S. Prevalence of mycobacteremia in HIV-infected Indian patients detected by MB-BACT auto-mated culture system. Eur J Clin Microbiol Infect Dis 2008;27: 423-31.

379. Parashar D, Chauhan DS, Sharma VD, Chauhan A, Chauhan SV, Katoch VM. Optimization of procedures for isolation of mycobacteria from soil and water samples obtained in northern India. Appl Environ Microbiol 2004;70:3751-3.

380. Ollar RA, Dale JW, Feddar MS, Favate A. The use of paraffin wax metabolism in the speciation of Mycobacterium avium intracellulare. Tubercle 1990;71:23-8.

381. Narang P, Narang R, Bhattacharya S, Mendiratta DK. Paraffin slide culture technique for isolating nontuberculous mycobacteria from stool and sputum of HIV seropositive patients. Indian J Tuberc 2004;51:23-6.

382. Anargyros P, Astill DS, Lim IS. Comparison of improved BACTEC and Lowenstein-Jensen media for culture of bacteria from clinical specimens. J Clin Microbiol 1990;28:1288-91.

383. Evans KD, Nakasone AS, Sutherland PA, de la Maza LM, Peterson EM. Identification of Mycobacterium tuberculosis and Mycobacterium avium-M. intracellulare directly from primary BACTEC cultures by using acridinium ester labelled DNA probes. J Clin Microbiol 1992;30:2427-31.

384. Vestal AL. Procedure for isolation of mycobacteria. Atlanta: US Department of Health, Education and Welfare; 1977.

385. Katoch VM, Sharma VD. Advances in the diagnosis of mycobacterial infections. Indian J Med Microbiol 1997;15: 49-55.

386. Duffey PS, Guthertz LS, Evans GC. Improved rapid identification of mycobacteria by combining solid phase high performance liquid chromatography analysis of BACTEC cultures. J Clin Microbiol 1996;34:1939-43.

387. Piersimoni C, Scarparo C, Callegaro A, Tosi CP, Nista D, Bornigia S, et al. Comparison of MB/ Bact alert 3D system with radiometric BACTEC system and Lowenstein-Jensen medium for recovery and identification of mycobacteria from clinical specimens: a multicentre study. J Clin Microbiol 2001;39:651-7.

388. Leitritz L, Schubert S, Bucherl B, Masch A, Heesemann J, Roggenkamp A. Evaluation of BACTEC MGIT 960 and BACTEC 460 TB systems for recovery of mycobacteria from clinical specimens of a university hospital with low incidence of tuberculosis. J Clin Microbiol 2001;39:3764-7.

389. Schaefer WB. Serologic identification and classification of atypical mycobacteria by their agglutination. Am Rev Respir Dis 1965;92:85-93.

390. Sharma VD, Katoch VM, Shivannavar CT, Gupta UD, Sharma RK, Patil MA, et al. Protein and isoenzyme patterns of mycobacteria. I. Their role in identification of rapidly growing mycobacteria. Indian J Med Microbiol 1995;13:115-8.

391. Sharma VD, Katoch VM, Shivannavar CT, Gupta UD, Sharma RK, Patil MA, et al. Protein and isoenzyme patterns of mycobacteria. II. Their role in identification of slowly growing mycobacteria. Indian J Med Microbiol 1995;13:119-23.

392. Gupta P, Katoch VM, Gupta UD, Chauhan DS, Das R, Singh D, et al. A preliminary report on characterization and identification of non-tuberculous mycobacteria [NTM] on the basis of biochemical tests and protein/isoenzyme electrophoresis patterns. Indian J Med Microbiol 2002;20:137-40.

393. Wayne LG, Diaz GA. Reciprocal immunological distances of catalase derived from strains of M. avium, M. tuberculosis and closely related species. Int J Syst Bacteriol 1979;29:19-24.

394. Shivannavar CT, Katoch VM, Sharma VD, Patil MA, Katoch K, Bharadwaj VP, et al. Development of SOD ELISA to determine immunological relatedness among mycobacteria. Int J Lepr Other Mycobact Dis 1996;64:58-65.

395. McFadden JJ, Kunze Z, Seechurn P. DNA probes for detection and identification of non-tuberculosis mycobacteria. In: McFadden J, editor. Molecular biology of mycobacteria. Surrey: Surrey University Press; 1990.p.139-72.

396. Katoch VM, Kanaujia GV, Shivannavar CT, Katoch K, Sharma VD, Patil MA, et al. Progress in developing ribosomal RNA and rRNA gene[s]probes for diagnosis and epidemiology of infectious disease specially leprosy. In: Kumar S, Sen AK, Dutta GP, Sharma RN, editors. Molecular biology and control strategies. New Delhi: Council for Scientific and Industrial Research; 1994.p.581-7.

397. Kaminski DA, Hardy DJ. Selective utilization of DNA probes for identification of Mycobacterium species on the basis of cord formation in primary BACTEC 12B cultures. J Clin Microbiol 1995;33:1548-50.

398. Stratmann J, Strommenger B, Stevenson K, Gerlach GF. Development of peptide mediated capture of PCR for detection of Mycobacterium avium subsp paratuberculosis in milk. J Clin Microbiol 2002;40:4244-50.

399. Rodrigo G, Kallenius G, Hoffmann E, Svenson SB. Diagnosis of mycobacterial infection by PCR and restriction enzyme digestion. Lett Appl Microbiol 1992;15:41-4.

400. Chen ZH, Butler WR, Baumstark BR, Ahearn DG. Identification and differentiation of Mycobacterium avium and M. intracellulare by PCR. J Clin Microbiol 1996;34:1267-9.

401. Kulski JK, Khinsoe C, Pryce T, Christiansen K. Use of a multiplex PCR to detect and identify Mycobacterium avium and M. intracellulare in blood culture of AIDS patients J Clin Microbiol 1995;33:668-74.

402. De Beenhouwer H, Liang Z, de Rizk P, van Eekeren C, Portaels F.. Detection and identification of mycobacteria by DNA amplification and oligonucleotide specific capture plate hybridization. J Clin Microbiol 1995;33:2994-8.

403. Portaels F, Agular J, Fissetle K, Fonteyne PA, de Beenhouwer H, de Rijk P, et al. Direct detection and identification of Mycobacterium ulcerans in clinical specimens by PCR and oligonucleotide-specific capture plate hybridization. J Clin Microbiol 1997;35:1091-1100.

404. Ruiz P, Gutierrez J, Zerolo FJ, Casal M. Genotype Mycobacterium assay for identification of mycobacterial species isolated from human clinical samples by using liquid medium. J Clin Microbiol 2002;40:3076-8.

405. Suffys PN, da Silva Rocha A, de Oliveira M, Dias Campos CE, Werneck Barreto AM, Portaels F, et al. Rapid identification of mycobacterium to the species level using INNO-LiPA mycobacterium, a reverse hybridization assay. J Clin Microbiol 2001;39:4477-82.

406. Li Z, Bai GH, von Reyn CF, Marino P, Brennan MJ, Gine N, et al. Rapid detection of Mycobacterium avium in stool samples from AIDS patients by immunomagnetic PCR. J Clin Microbiol 1996;34:1903-7.

407. Vaneechoutte M, Beenhouwer HD, Claeys G, Vershraegen G, De Rouck A, Paepe N, et al. Identification of Mycobacterium species by using amplified ribosomal DNA restriction analysis. J Clin Microbiol 1993;31:2061-5.

408. Avanis Saghnjani E, Jones K, Holtzman A, Aronson T, Glover N, Boian M, et al. Molecular techniques for rapid identification of mycobacteria. J Clin Microbiol 1996;34:98-102.

409. Dobner P, Feldmann K, Rifai M, Loscher T, Rinder H. Rapid identification of mycobacterial species by PCR amplification of hypervariable 16S rRNA gene promoter region. J Clin Microbiol 1996;34:866-9.

410. Roth A, Reischl U, Streubel A, Naumann L, Kroppenstedt M, Habicht M, et al. Novel diagnostic algorithm for identification of mycobacteria using genus-specific amplification of 16S-23S rRNA gene spacer and restriction endonucleases. J Clin Microbiol 2000;38:1094-104.

411. Katoch VM, Parashar D, Chauhan DS, Singh D, Sharma VD, Ghosh D. Rapid identification of mycobacteria by gene amplification restriction analysis technique targeting 16S-23S ribosomal DNA spacer and flanking regions. Indian J Med Res 2007;125:155-62.

412. Singh S, Gopinath K, Shahdad S, Kaur M, Singh B, Sharma P. Nontuberculous mycobacterial infections in Indian AIDS patients detected by a novel set of ESAT-6 polymerase chain reaction primers. Jpn J Infect Dis 2007;60:14-8.

413. Slutsky AM, Arbeit RD, Barber TW, Rich J, von Reyn CF, Pieciak W, et al. Polyclonal infections due to Mycobacterium avium complex in patients with AIDS decided by pulsed- field gel electrophoresis of sequential clinical isolates. J Clin Microbiol 1994;32:1773-8.

414. Kauppinen J, Mantyjarvi R, Katila ML. Random amplified polymorphic genotyping of Mycobacterium malmoense. J Clin Microbiol 1994;32:1827-9.

415. Katoch VM, Shivannavar CT, Datta AK. Studies on ribosomal RNA genes of mycobacteria including M. leprae. Acta Leprol 1989;7 Suppl 1:231-3.

416. Kanaujia, Katoch VM, Shivannavar CT, Sharma VD, Patil MA. Rapid characterization of Mycobacterium fortuitum-chelonei complex by restriction fragment length polymorphism of ribosomal RNA genes. FEMS Microbiol Lett 1991;77:205-8.

417. Chiodini RJ. Characterization of Mycobacterium paratuberculosis and organisation of Mycobacterium avium complex by restriction polymorphism of rRNA gene region. J Clin Microbiol 1990;28: 489-94.

418. Picardeau M, Vincent V. Typing of Mycobacterium avium isolates by PCR. J Clin Microbiol 1996;34:389-92.

419. Kumar S, Bose M, Isa M. Genotype analysis of human Mycobacterium avium isolates from India. Indian J Med Res 2006;123:139-44.

420. Yang M, Ross BC, Dwyer B. Identification of an insertion sequence like element in subspecies of M. kansasii. J Clin Microbiol 1993;31:2074-9.

421. Falkinham JO. Molecular epidemiology: other mycobacteria. In: Ratledge C, Dale J, editors. Mycobacteria: molecular biology and virulence. Oxford: Blackwell Science Publishers Ltd; 1999. p.136-60.

422. Vanitha JD, Venkatasubramani R, Dharmalingam, Paramasivan CN. Large-restriction fragment polymorphism of Mycobacterium chelonae and Mycobacterium terrae isolates. Appl Environ Microbiol 2003;69:4337-41.

423. Jucker MT, Falkinham JO. Epidemiology of infections by nontuberculous mycobacteria. IX. Evidence for two DNA homology groups among small plasmids in Mycobacterium avium, Mycobacterium intracellulare, Mycobacterium scrofulaceum. Am Rev Respir Dis 1990;142:858-62.

424. Soini H, Eerola E, Viljanen MK. Genetic diversity among Mycobacterium avium complex Accu Probe positive isolates. J Clin Microbiol 1996;34:55-7.

425. Steadham JE, Stall SK, Simmank JL. Use of the BACTEC system for drug susceptibility testing of Mycobacterium tuberculosis, M. kansasii, and M. avium complex. Diagn Microbiol Infect Dis 1985;3:33-40.

426. Biehle JR, Cavalieri SJ, Saubolle MA, Getsinger LJ. Evaluation of E test for susceptibility testing of rapidly growing mycobacteria. J Clin Microbiol 1995;33:1760-4.

427. Fabry W, Schmid EN, Ansorg R. Comparison of the E test and a proportion dilution method for susceptibility testing of Mycobacterium kansasii. Chemotherapy 1995;41:247-52.

428a. Maisetta G, Batoni G, Pardini M, Boschi A, Bottai D, Esin S, et al. Use of recombinant strain of Mycobacterium avium expressing beta-galactosidase to evaluate the activities of the antimycobacterial agents inside macrophages. Antimicro Agents Chemother 2001;45: 356-8.

428b. Sharma SK, Sharma R, Singh BK, Upadhyay V, Mani I. A study of non-tuberculous mycobacterial [NTM] disease among tuberculosis suspects at a tertiary care center in North India. Am J Respir Crit Care Med 2019 [in press].

429. National Committee for Clinical Laboratory Standards: Susceptibility testing of mycobacteria, nocardae and other actinomycetes. Approved standard. Document number M24A. Payne: National Committee for Clinical Laboratory Standards; 2003.

430a. Haworth CS, Banks J, Capstick T, Fisher AJ, Gorsuch T, Laurenson IF, et al. British Thoracic Society Guideline for the management of non-tuberculous mycobacterial pulmonary disease [NTM-PD]. Thorax 2017;72:ii1–ii64.

430b. Ahn OH, Ahn SS, Anderson RA, Murphy DL, Mamo A. A four drug regimen for initial treatment of cavitary disease caused by Mycobacterium avium complex. Am Rev Respire Dis 1986;34: 438-41.

431. Agnes BD, Berman DS, Spicehandler D, Elsadar W, Simberkoff MS, Rahal JJ. Effect of combined therapy with ansamycin, clofazimine, ethambutol and isoniazid on Mycobacterium avium infections in patients with AIDS. J Infect Dis 1989;159:784-7.

432. Chiu J, Nussbaum J, Bozzette S, Tilles JG, Young LS, Leedom JM et al. Treatment of disseminated Mycobacterium avium complex infections in AIDS with amikacin, ethambutol, rifampin and ciprofloxacin. Ann Intern Med 1990;113:358-61.

433. Hoy J, Mijoch A, Sandland M, Grayson L, Lucas R, Dwyer S. Quadruple drug therapy in Mycobacterium avium intracellulare bacteremia in AIDS patients. J Infect Dis 1990;161:801-5.

434. Kemper CA, Meng TC, Nussbum J, Chiu J, Fiegel DF, Bartok AE, et al. Eifamin, ethambutol, clofazimine and ciprofloxacin. The California Collaborative Group. Treatment of Mycobacterium avium complex bacteremia with a four-drug oral regimen. Ann Inter Med 1992;116: 466-72.

435. Dautzenberg B, Trauffot O, Legris B, Meyohas MC, Barlie HC, Mercat AC, et al. Activity of clarithromycin against M. avium infection in acquired immune deficiency syndrome: a controlled clinical trial. Amer Rev Res Dis 1991;144:564-9.

436. Young LS, Wiviott L, Wu M, Kolonoski P, Bolan R, Inderlied CB, et al. Azithromycin for the treatment of M.avium complex infections in patients with AIDS. Lancet 1991;338:1107-9.

437. Griffith DE, Brown BA, Giard WH, Wallace RJ. Adverse events association with high dose rifabutin and macrolide containing regimens for the treatment of M. avium lung disease. Clin Infect Dis 1995;21:594-8

438. Griffith DE, Brown BA, Giard WH, Wallace RJ. Azithromycin activity against Mycobacterium avium complex lung disease in patients who were not infected with human immune deficiency virus. Clin Infect Dis 1996;23:983-9.

439. Ahn DJ, Towell JR, Ahn SS, Ahn SI, Hurst GA. Short course therapy for the pulmonary disease caused by Mycobacterium kansasii. Am Rev Res Dis 1983;128:1048-50.

440. Ahn CH, Wallace RJ Jr, Steel LC, Murphy DF. Sulphonamide containing regimen for the treatment of rifampin resistant Mycobacterium kansasii. Am Rev Res Dis 1987;135:10-6.

441. Chow SP, Ip FK, Iau JHK, Collins RJ, Luck KDK, So YC, et al. Mycobacterium marinum infection of the hand and wrist. Results of conservative management of twenty four cases. J Bone Joint Surg 1987;69A:1161-8.

442. Wolinsky E, Gomez, Zimfper F. Sporotrichoid Mycobacterium marinum infection treated with rifampin-ethambutol. Am Rev Resp Dis 1972;105:964-7.

443. Aubry A, Chosidow O, Caumes E, Robert J, Cambau E. Sixty three cases of Mycobacterium marinum infection. Arch Intern Med 2002;162:1746-52.

444. Wallace RJ, Tanvor D, Brennan PJ, Brown BA. Clinical trial of clarithromycin in cutaneous [disseminated] infections due to Mycobacterium chelonae. Ann Intern Med 1993;119:482-6.

445. Dalovisio JR, Pankey GA, Wallace RJ, Jones DB. Clinical usefulness of amikacin and doxycycline in the treatment of infection due to Mycobacterium fortuitum and Mycobacterium chelonei. Rev Infect Dis 1981;3:1968-79.

446. Kang YA, Koh WJ. Antibiotic treatment for nontuberculous mycobacterial lung disease. Expert Rev Respir Med 2016;10: 557-68.

42

Drug-resistant Tuberculosis

*Keertan Dheda, Grant Theron, Gregory Calligaro, Jason Limberis,
Malika Davids, Alisgar Esmail, Rodney Dawson*

INTRODUCTION

Although the global incidence of tuberculosis [TB] has been slowly declining, TB remains out of control in many parts of the world (1). Some of the early gains made in several parts of the world, including in Africa and Asia, are now being threatened by the emergence of drug-resistant TB [DR-TB]. Although multidrug-resistant TB [MDR-TB] defined as resistance to rifampicin and isoniazid comprises only 6%-7% of the total burden of TB it deserves public health prioritisation and is important for several reasons. First, DR-TB is associated with longer time to diagnosis and considerable pulmonary morbidity including chronic lung fibrosis, bronchiectasis, *Aspergillus*-associated a lung disease, etc. Secondly, DR-TB is associated with considerable mortality and substantial a global reduction in TB mortality will not be achievable unless the problem of DR-TB is addressed. MDR-TB and extensively drug-resistant TB [XDR-TB] [defined as MDR-TB plus resistance to at least one drug in the following classes of medicines used in the treatment of MDR-TB, namely, fluoroquinolones and second-line injectable agents] is also associated with substantial cost. For example, in South Africa, despite X/MDR-TB comprising less than 4% of the total TB burden, it is already consuming close to 40% of all TB-related healthcare resources, a situation that is unsustainable. Therefore, DR-TB has a capacity to destabilise well-functioning national TB programmes [NTPs] (2). X/MDR-TB and resistance beyond XDR-TB has become a burgeoning problem in many countries. Several issues are critical to the control of DR-TB including reducing global levels of poverty and overcrowding, and addressing drivers like human immunodeficiency virus [HIV], cigarette smoking, alcohol and substance abuse, biomass fuel exposure and diabetes. Indeed, reduction in the total burden of TB will also reduce the prevalence of DR-TB. Whilst capacity development and strengthening of NTP are of paramount importance, further research and understanding into the underlying genesis of drug resistance is critical if the development of drug resistance in the future is to be minimised.

CLINICAL EPIDEMIOLOGY

The causes of DR-TB are complex. While programmatic conditions are often responsible for promulgating MDR-TB epidemics [through, for example, frequent drug shortages and poor drug quality, inadequate drug-susceptibility testing [DST], poor training, and non-standardised treatment regimens] (3,4) certain patient-specific factors are associated with an increased likelihood of MDR-TB. Traditionally, previous TB treatment [including number of episodes, irregular treatment, and frequency of default] (5-10) has been considered the single biggest risk factor for MDR-TB. However, other factors, such as age, male sex, alcohol abuse, poverty, HIV infection (7), smoking (8), substance abuse (11), a history of imprisonment (8), hospitalisation (5,12) or recent immigration (13), or infection with certain strains [such as, atypical Beijing] (14-16) all increase the probability of DR-TB. For XDR-TB, the previous use of second-line drugs [SLDs] is the single biggest risk factor (5,6,17). However, although there are several risk factors for MDR-TB it should be noted that almost two-thirds of MDR-TB cases have never been previously been treated for TB or have none of these associated risk factors. Thus, it is not practical nor useful to risk stratify patients to guide DST, and every case of TB should, therefore undergo DST for at least rifampicin resistance.

As per the Global TB Report 2018 (1), in 2017, there were approximately 558,000 estimated new cases of MDR-TB/rifampicin resistant-TB [RR-TB] globally (1), and MDR-TB was found in approximately 3.6% of new cases and approximately 17% of retreated cases [Figures 42.1A and 42.1B] (1). More than half the MDR-TB burden lies in India, China and

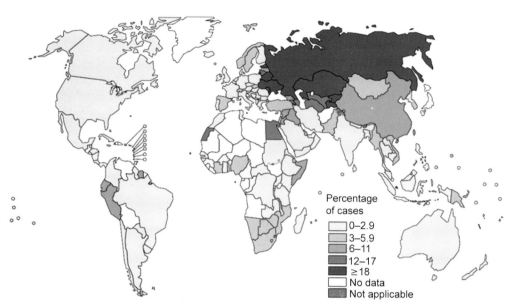

Figure 42.1A: Percentage of new TB cases with MDR/RR-TB

TB = tuberculosis; MDR = multidrug-resistant; RR = rifampicin resistant

Reproduced with permission from "World Health Organization. Global tuberculosis report. Geneva: World Health Organization; 2018" (reference 1)

The World Health Organization updates these data annually. The reader can access the updated information from the WHO report of the current year available at the URL: http://www.who.int/topics/tuberculosis/en/

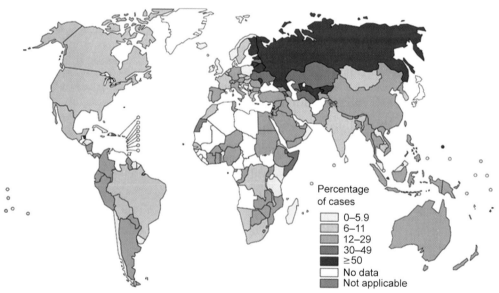

Figure 42.1B: Percentage of previously TB cases with MDR/RR-TB

TB = tuberculosis; MDR = multidrug-resistant; RR = rifampicin resistant

Reproduced with permission from "World Health Organization. Global tuberculosis report. Geneva: World Health Organization; 2018" (reference 1)

The World Health Organization updates these data annually. The reader can access the updated information from the WHO report of the current year available at the URL: http://www.who.int/topics/tuberculosis/en/

the Russian Federation. In sub-Saharan Africa and about half of the MDR-TB patients are HIV co-infected. MDR-TB is also prevalent in children roughly mirroring the MDR-TB prevalence in adults (1).

There are several worrying trends with regard to DR-TB. The global average isoniazid mono-resistance rate was 7.1% in new and 7.9% in previously treated TB (1). Although, the global burden of MDR-TB remained unchanged over

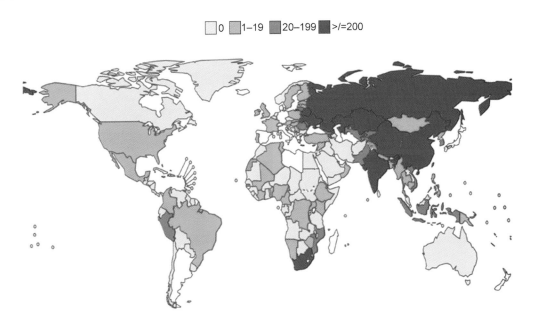

Figure 42.2: Number of patients with laboratory confirmed XDR-TB started on treatment in 2016
XDR-TB = extensively drug-resistant tuberculosis
Reproduced with permission from "World Health Organization. Multidrug-/rifampicin-resistant TB[MDR/RR-TB]: Update 2017. Available at URL:
http://www.who.int/tb/areas-of-work/drug-resistant-tb/MDR_TB_2017.pdf?ua=1. Accessed on August 29, 2018." (reference 18a)
The World Health Organization updates these data annually. The reader can access the updated information from the WHO report of the current
year available at the URL: http://www.who.int/topics/tuberculosis/en/

the period 2008 to 2017, in several countries [China, India, Pakistan, Nigeria, South Africa, Indonesia, Bangladesh, and the Democratic Republic of Congo, amongst others] the number of RR-TB cases over the period 2009 to 2017 has increased substantially. Worryingly, in 2017 the proportion of MDR-TB cases with any fluoroquinolone resistance was 22%, and disturbingly 51% of MDR-TB patients had resistance to either a fluoroquinolone, or a second-line injectable drugs [SLIDs], or both. The average proportion of MDR-TB cases with XDR-TB was 8.5% [Figure 42.2] an increase from 6.2% in 2016 (1,18a).

In India, the estimated percentage of new and retreatment cases with MDR/RR-TB was 2.2% and 18%, respectively (1). It has been estimated that, in 2017 there were an estimated 135,000 incident MDR/RR-TB cases in India. Data from different parts of India are variable. Recent studies have reported alarmingly high levels of MDR-TB in several wards of Mumbai [24% in previously untreated cases] (18b) and in Lucknow [20% of isolates] (19). A report from Mumbai documented a 11% prevalence of XDR-TB in 326 patients with MDR-TB (20). Other studies from India reported an XDR-TB prevalence ranging between 1.5% and 7.4% (21,22). One study (23) reported that 4 out of 12 HIV, MDR-TB co-infected patients had XDR-TB. In a study from New Delhi, Sharma and colleagues (24) reported that approximately 2.4% of MDR-TB cases had XDR-TB. An alarming report from Udwadia and co-workers drew attention to the problem of resistance beyond XDR-TB, i.e., totally drug-resistant TB [TDR-TB] in India (25).

Sparse published data are available on drug-resistance in extra-pulmonary tuberculosis [EPTB]. In a study (26) from New Delhi, 2553 extra-pulmonary specimens from 2468 patients, mycobacterial culture was positive in 18.9%. MDR-TB was evident in 8.1% of the specimens; pre-XDR-TB and XDR-TB were evident in 17.9% and 2.6% extra-pulmonary specimens respectively. The sensitivity and specificity of genotypic DST using both Xpert MTB/RIF and line probe assay [LPA] for detection of rifampicin resistance was 92.7% and 99.3% with 100% concordance between the two tests (26).

MOLECULAR EPIDEMIOLOGY AND TRANSMISSION DYNAMICS OF DRUG-RESISTANT TUBERCULOSIS

A basic understanding of the molecular epidemiology of DR-TB is crucial for clinicians and scientists, because not only does it enable them to identify patients at a high risk of DR-TB, but it also permits them to identify potential out-breaks of DR-TB. Drug-resistant TB may be acquired endo-genously during the course of treatment or by primary [person-to-person] spread (27). DR-TB is increasingly being seen in patients who have no history of previous TB, suggesting that these cases are mostly caused by primary transmission (1,27). Although some DR strains may be less fit [and hence may be less transmissible] (28), the fact that many patients with MDR-TB are not detected or started on treatment, and that the duration of infectiousness is longer for MDR-TB than drug-susceptible TB [DS-TB] once treatment is started (29), means that there is a large pool of infectious DR-TB cases in many high burden TB countries.

Evidence of this ongoing transmission is provided by molecular tools, such as, spoligotyping (30), IS6110 deoxyribonucleic acid [DNA] fingerprinting (31) or Mycobacterial interspersed repetitive unit-variable number tandem repeat [MIRU-VNTR] typing (32)] that identify clusters of genotypically similar strains, which can be used to trace an epidemic or determine whether a patient's DR-TB is acquired [genetically similar to earlier episode] or transmitted [genetically similar to other strains in the community]. Using these techniques, researchers have shown that 80%–90% of MDR-TB cases in settings, such as, South Africa (33) and China (9) are likely caused by primary spread (34a), and that primary transmission is likely responsible for outbreaks of XDR-TB, such as that seen in Tugela Ferry (34b). Whole genome sequencing, where all the DNA in the *Mtb* cell is sequenced, has recently started to move beyond being just a useful research tool to one where, for example, it can be used to simultaneously detect DR mutations, investigate and track outbreaks with more resolution than traditional molecular techniques (35-37), and discriminate between relapse or reinfection more accurately (38,39).

Whole genome sequencing [WGS] has recently been successfully used to trace epidemics of XDR-TB in South Africa, showing that most transmission events occur due to casual contacts in the community and that patients who are highly drug-resistant and on inadequate treatment still transmit the disease (34a,34b,40a).

Importantly, epidemics of DR-TB driven by primary transmission appear to largely be caused by a highly infectious minority of patients [the "super-spreading" phenomenon] (40b-43). Although we currently have a limited understanding of why only some patients with DR-TB are highly infectious and others are not (44,45) [which is likely a result of different bacterial, behavioural, and environmental factors], research on this phenomenon is needed to facilitate clinical interventions [e.g., inhaled antibiotics, triage for specialised infection control] that can target this minority of patients in order to halt transmission.

PATHOGENESIS

Traditional Understanding of how Drug-resistance Develops

The underlying pathogenesis of DR-TB has been summarised in Figure 42.3 (27). It is known that acquisition of resistance in *Mtb* is characterised by a low rate of spontaneous mutation, and not by horizontal gene transfer [for example ~2.6 isoniazid-specific mutations per 10^8 *Mtb* bacteria per generation occurs] (46). Thus, *Mtb* resistance arises spontaneously but at a low and predictable *de novo* rate, and in a patient with a large bacterial burden of up to 10^9 organisms, a small number of bacteria may be resistant to a single drug. However, the probability of pre-existing resistance to two or three drugs [calculated by multiplying the mutation rates for the specific drugs] is infinitesimally small. The traditional view holds that erratic therapy either due to programme-related or patient-related factors results in the killing off of susceptible bacterial sub-populations but allows the pre-existing DR populations to continue to replicate, thus eventually resulting in a predominant population of DR organisms. Thus, the traditional view holds that DR mutants are selected out because of a lack of adherence due to several factors. However, newer findings have challenged this traditional understanding.

Pharmacokinetic Variability at Population Level and Induction of Efflux Pumps

It is now well-appreciated that drug resistance can develop even when adherence to treatment is excellent (47). In some cases, pharmacokinetic [PK] mismatch occurs where a drug with a long half-life [e.g., bedaquiline or clofazimine] effectively is available to act as monotherapy. Studies using the hollowing fibre system have shown that a acquired drug resistance is strongly associated with the area under the curve and peak drug concentrations indexed to minimum inhibitory concentration [MIC], and there is, therefore facilitated at concentrations below which drug resistance is amplified and microbial killing fails. The acquired drug resistance is often accompanied or preceded by very early induction of many low-level resistance efflux pumps, which confers resistance or tolerance (48,49). These efflux pumps are thought to protect bacilli during several rounds of replication and act as a gateway for the eventual generation of chromosomal mutations associated with high level acquired resistance. This process is termed the antibiotic resistance arrow of time (50). Several studies report the co-existence of genetic mutations and multi-drug efflux pumps (51,52). However, WGS-related studies may not show this effect because efflux pumps are already encoded by the TB genome and induction is epigenetic. Furthermore, conventional susceptibility testing using breakpoints will not detect low-level resistance. Other low level mutations have been described that may act as a gateway for resistance amplification (53). The clinical relevance of such mutations require further study.

The *hollow fibre model* further showed that although therapeutic failure occurred when more than 60% of the doses were missed there was no generation of MDR-TB. More importantly, however, is the PK variability occurring in individuals and populations. In a population simulation model using PK data, it is estimated that MDR-TB would still occur in 0.68 of patients during the first 2 months of treatment despite 100% adherence because of between patient PK variability of isoniazid and rifampicin. Thus, there would effectively be monotherapy for long periods of time. A similar situation occurs in the intensive phase of short-course treatment of patients who are still culture positive but have underlying isoniazid mono-resistance. The PK variability in individuals and populations is driven mainly by genetic polymorphisms in genes coding for metabolism and drug transporters.

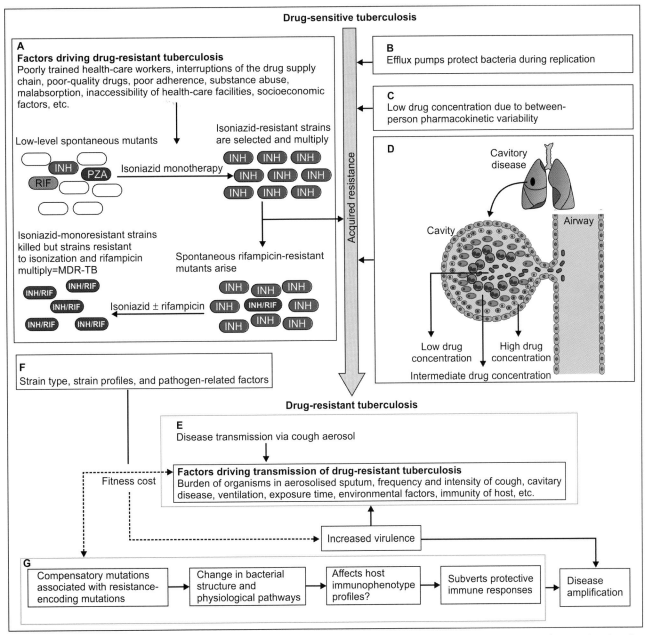

Figure 42.3: The pathogenesis of DR-TB. The traditional interpretation of resistance development is that sequential drug resistance develops through fragmented treatment [A], which can be fuelled by several programmatic and socioeconomic factors. However, resistance can develop despite excellent adherence. Several factors, including efflux pumps [B], between-person pharmacokinetic variability [C], and extensive immunopathology in the lung resulting in differential drug penetration into granulomas and cavities [D] might all drive site-specific drug concentrations below minimum inhibitory concentrations, thus probably enabling drug resistance. After acquired drug-resistance develops, person-to-person transmission might constitute the major route of spread [E]. Strain-specific genotype, newly acquired drug-encoding mutations, and compensatory mutations that can affect fitness cost [and hence transmission] might also interact [F]. Compensatory mutations could be associated with changes in structure and physiological pathways, which could affect host immune response and thereby potentially subvert protective responses and drive progressive disease [G].
DR-TB = drug-resistant tuberculosis; INH = isoniazid; RIF = rifampicin; PZA = pyrazinamide; MDR-TB = multidrug-resistant tuberculosis
Reproduced with permission from "Dheda K, Gumbo T, Gandhi NR, Murray M, Theron G, Udwadia Z, et al. Global control of tuberculosis: from extensively drug-resistant to untreatable tuberculosis. Lancet Respir Med 2014;2:321-38" (reference 27)

Differential Drug Penetration into Lung Micro Compartments

Local PK variability can also be caused by differential penetration of drugs into the lung micro compartments. The finding of different susceptibility profiles of isolates from different lesions [obtained through biopsies from the cavity wall versus the per-fibrotic margin *versus* apparently normal lung] in the same patient [also termed hetro-resistance] lend support to this hypothesis [Lenders and Dheda; unpublished observations]. The immunopathology in the lung may, therefore, drive considerable within-person PK variability, which is a key factor in the genesis of MDR-TB (27).

There are several implications of these findings. Future studies are required to: [i] evaluate the impact of therapeutic drug monitoring to minimise amplification of drug-resistance; [ii] use of a pharmaco-genomic approach where certain patient genotypes would be associated with more rapid or modulated drug metabolism, thus mandating therapeutic monitoring; and [iii] improved targeting of drugs to the disease site by dosage adjustments or targeting of drug to the lung through the inhalation route (54).

Genotype and Compensatory Mutations

Certain strains may have a higher *in vivo* mutation rates than other strains making the emergence of drug-resistance more likely (55). Mutation rates also vary between strains of the same genotype. There is limited evidence to support the hypothesis that some strains are more likely to mutate as a result of dysfunctional DNA repair mechanisms (56,57). Furthermore, the genetic background of different strains results in differing fitness costs associated with particular DR mutations (28). There may also be synergistic interaction between hyper mutable bacterial lineages and patients who rapidly metabolise first-line drugs [high PK variability], thus, accounting for the high rates of MDR-TB reported in some settings despite directly observed therapy.

Findings from WGS-related studies have shown that resistance-encoding mutations are associated with compensatory mutations elsewhere in the TB genome (58-60). It is known that compensatory mutations in *Pseudomonas* species can modulate virulence and transmissibility (27), and compensatory mutations in *Mtb* can be associated with physiological and structural changes (27). Collectively, these findings raise the possibility that drug resistance could affect mycobacterial structure and antigen specificity, and hence, perhaps even the T-cell immune responses. The underlying immunology in patients with DR-TB is poorly understood and few data are available (27). Nevertheless, several immunotherapeutic interventions have been proposed for the treatment of DR-TB, e.g., *M. vaccae*, vitamin D, and intravenous immunoglobulin [IVIG], though their effectiveness remains to be proven across different settings (60).

Fitness Cost

Transmission is driven by clinical, bacterial, behavioural, and environmental factors. However, as already outlined, transmission dynamics plays a critical role in the pathogenesis of DR-TB in terms of total case burden. For example, in South Africa, over 80% of new MDR-TB cases are due to person-to-person spread rather than by acquired resistance. Thus, over time, transmission becomes the predominant mode of acquisition of drug resistance. It is also well-recognised that a small percentage of individuals [< 10%–20%] are responsible for most of the disease transmission. The determinants of the 'super spreader' status are

poorly characterised and is currently under study by the authors' group using cough aerosol sampling [CASS] technology. The high transmissibility and virulence, characterised by high mortality and transmission of highly DR strains in South Africa and elsewhere, suggest that in many cases compensatory mutations may result in normal or possibly even enhance evolutionary fitness levels (58). Epistatic interactions may modulate fitness cost associated with drug resistance (61,62).

In summary, several newer concepts have challenged the traditional view about the pathogenesis of drug resistance. There are several clinical implications of these findings including the use of therapeutic drug monitoring, pharmacogenomics, new methods of dosing and drug delivery depending on low *versus* high level mutations, selection of drugs and regimens least likely to induce low fitness cost mutations, the potential use of immunomodulatory therapies, use of rapid diagnostic techniques to characterise super spreaders, and newer diagnostic approaches that can interrogate multiple samples and colonies for drug resistance. These aspects will need to be addressed to prevent the future emergence of TB-specific drug resistance.

DIAGNOSIS OF DRUG-RESISTANT TUBERCULOSIS

Improving the diagnosis of DR-TB is potentially the single most effective intervention that can enhance the clinical outcome of patients and limit the emergence of new cases. However, only two-thirds of the estimated 9 million cases of TB are diagnosed each year, and less than half of these undergo DST. The net effect of this phenomenon, which is due in part to the limited availability of DST methods [which themselves are often slow], is that the majority of DR-TB cases remain untreated and continue to transmit disease. If we are to enhance the diagnosis of DR-TB, which we know results in improved treatment initiation (63,64), clinical outcomes (65-67), and long-term TB incidence (41,68), we need to not only ensure that every patient diagnosed with TB also undergoes DST, but also understand the strengths and limitations of different diagnostic technologies. Current state-of-the-art methods for diagnosing DR-TB are described in Figure 42.4 and Table 42.1A. Table 42.1B (69-93) provides a comprehensive list, together with their mode of operation, and commercial manufacturers.

Culture-based Tests

Phenotypic testing involves incubating a bacterial isolate [grown from a clinical specimen] in the presence of a specific drug. As this method directly measures bacterial growth [and is not reliant on proxies of resistance, such as genetic mutations], it is the most sensitive and most specific form of DST, and is often the benchmark against which other tests are measured. Although optimised, more rapid versions are available, such as, microscopic observation direct susceptibility [MODS], phenotypic testing will always be constrained by the relatively slow growth of *Mtb*. This limits

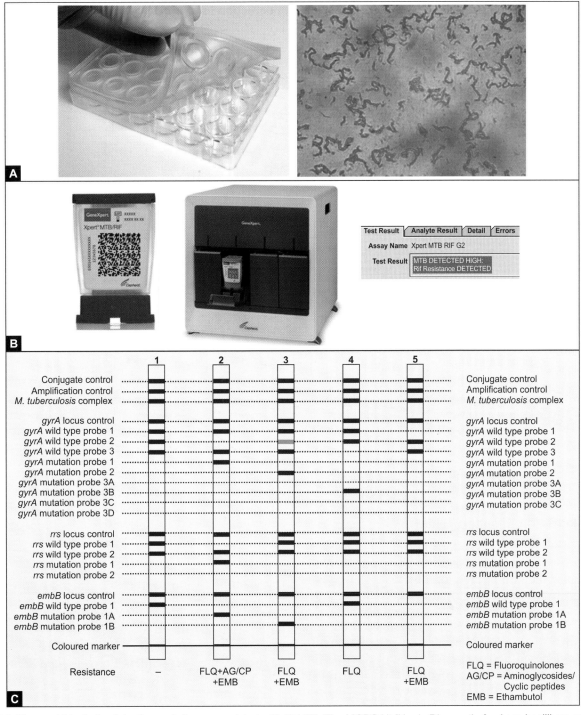

Figure 42.4: New rapid tests for detecting mutations associated with DR-TB. The MODS kit [Hardy Diagnostics], where bacilli are cultured in a micro titre well plate format, and inspected using light microscopy for distinctive cording patterns, which are indicative of *Mtb* growth. MODS is primary used for drug susceptibility testing [A]. The Xpert MTB/RIF test [Cepheid, Sunnyvale, USA], detects rifampicin resistance simultaneously with *Mtb*. The test is largely automated and endorsed by the World Health Organization. Sputum treated with sample buffer is added to a single-use MTB/RIF cartridge [left panel], prior to loading into a GeneXpert machine [middle panel; a four module GeneXpert machine is depicted], before the reading of the result about 2 hours later [right panel; information regarding the TB status, bacterial load, and rifampicin susceptibility is shown] [B]. The Genotype MTBDRsl assay, which detects mutations in the *rrs*, *gyrA* and *embB* genes [associated with resistance to the aminoglycosides, flusroquinolones, and ethambutol, respectively], shown. Nucleic acid amplification products are separated via lateral flow onto a strip containing probes corresponding to specific mutations. Upon binding to a probe, a colorimetric reaction occurs and the presence or absence of a mutation is visualised [C]. Images are courtesy of the respective manufacturers

DR-TB = drug-resistant TB; TB = tuberculosis; MODS = microscopic observation drug-susceptibility; *Mtb* = *Mycobacterium tuberculosis*

Reproduced with permission from "Dheda K, Gumbo T, Gandhi NR, Murray M, Theron G, Udwadia Z, et al. Global control of tuberculosis: from extensively drug-resistant to untreatable tuberculosis. Lancet Respir Med 2014;2:321-38" (reference 27)

Table 42.1A: Time-to-result and lower limit of bacilli detection for various diagnostic tests for TB

Diagnostic test	Time-to-result	Lower limit of bacilli detection
AFB Microscopy		
Z-N stain	45 minutes	10^4 bacilli/mL
LED-FM	30 minutes	10^4 bacilli/mL
Mycobacterial growth detection		
Solid [L-J medium] culture	Up to 6-8 weeks [average 3-4 weeks]	10-100 bacilli/mL
Solid [L-J medium] culture DST	6 weeks after detection of growth	All positive cultures
Liquid culture [MGIT-960]	Up to 6-8 weeks [average 10-14 days]	10-100 bacilli/mL
Liquid culture DST	1-2 weeks after detection of growth	All positive cultures
ICA	15 minutes	
LPA		
FL-LPA	48 hours	10^4 bacilli/mL
SL-LPA	24-48 hours	10^4 bacilli/mL
GeneXpert		
Xpert MTB/RIF	90 minutes	131 CFU/mL
Xpert MTB/RIF Ultra	90 minutes	16 CFU/mL

TB = tuberculosis; AFB = acid-fast bacilli; Z-N = Ziehl-Neelsen; LED-FM = light emitting diode-fluorescent microscopy; L-J = Lowenstein-Jensen; DST = drug-susceptibility testing; MGIT = mycobacterial growth inhibitor tube; ICA = immunochromatographic assay; LPA = line probe assay; FL = first-line; SL = second-line

the utility of currently commercially available platforms, such as the BACTEC MGIT 960 System [Becton-Dickinson], for patient management [time to result can range from 1–4 weeks after a culture isolate has grown, which itself can take 1–6 weeks] (94-96) and result in patients with DR-TB being 'lost' by the system. This, coupled with demanding technical and infrastructural requirements, means that molecular tests, which are potentially deployable close to the patient, are better for the rapid diagnosis of drug-resistance.

Nucleic Acid Amplification Tests

Nucleic acid amplification tests [NAATs] detect DNA mutations associated with drug resistance. They are inherently rapid because they do not rely on mycobacterial growth, and can go from "specimen in" to "result out" in a few hours, meaning that patients could theoretically present to the clinic, be correctly diagnosed, and started on effective treatment in a single clinical encounter. Critically, simultaneous NAAT-based DST for at least one of the first-line drugs is increasingly being incorporated into initial diagnostic tests for TB, the best example of which is Xpert MTB/RIF [Cepheid, Sunnyvale, USA].

Xpert MTB/RIF is a quantitative real-time NAAT that diagnoses TB and rifampicin resistance in less than two hours (97). It is an automated, cartridge-based system that can be performed in well-resourced decentralised locations, outside of reference laboratories by staff with minimal laboratory training (98). It has been widely validated, endorsed by the World Health Organization [WHO] (99) and the US Federal Drug Administration [FDA], (100) for the initial diagnosis of TB and for the diagnosis of MDR-TB, and is increasingly being deployed in high burden countries. A meta-analysis has reported the sensitivity

and specificity of the assay for rifampicin resistance to be 95% and 98%, respectively (101). The Xpert MTB/RIF will not detect isoniazid mono-resistance, which is in one in seven TB cases worldwide [and in half of TB cases in Eastern Europe] (102). Another concern is Xpert MTB/RIF's suboptimal false-positivity for rifampicin resistance, for which data are conflicting. For example, in settings such as India, where the MDR-TB/RR-TB prevalence is 2.2% amongst new cases (1), it is projected that half of those with a positive Xpert MTB/RIF result will be phenotypically susceptible [only 1 in 10 will be "false-positive" amongst retreatment cases] (103). However, in settings such as Brazil, which also have a low MDR-TB prevalence [~1%], empiric evidence has suggested the false-positive rate to be low [< 1 in 10] (104). In South Africa [MDR-TB prevalence of 2% in new cases], the false-positivity rate has been shown to be very low [less than 1 in 100] (105). A new version of the Xpert MTB/RIF assay cartridge called the Xpert MTB/RIF Ultra has been released in 2016. This assay includes multicopy insertion sequence targets [IS6110 and IS1081] which allow improved sensitivity in the detection and the differentiation of the *Mtb* complex. The new cartridges have decreased run-time, improved chemistry and, improved probes which target the 81bp-rifampicin resistance "hotspot" of the *Mtb* genome. These cartridges have improved sensitivity of the assay as compared to that of the Xpert G4 version by 5% but with a loss of 3% specificity when "trace" results were considered positive (106a). In addition, a new version of the GeneXpert system, which allows for one cartridge to be run at a time has been released. This device can be battery operated and is point-of-care, allowing for the detection of *Mtb* and determination of rifampicin in remote locations. In South Africa, second-line treatment is initiated based on an Xpert MTB/RIF result; however,

Table 42.1B: Available and in-development phenotypic and molecular-based tests for detecting drug resistance in *Mycobacterium tuberculosis*

Test	Description	Advantages	Limitations	Commercial versions
Culture methods				
Solid agar [Middlebrook or Lowenstein Jensen media]	Bacilli are grown in the presence or absence of each drug. An isolate is resistant when the agar plate containing the drug has ≥1% the number of colony forming units as the media without the drug	Highly sensitive and specific [considered the 'gold standard' of DST] Relatively inexpensive	Slow time-to-result [2-4 months] requires an isolate and cannot be performed directly from the specimen Standardisation challenges [e.g., drug critical concentration, reproducibility, inoculum size, media and drug pH] Technically challenging and requires strong laboratory biosafety infrastructure Unreliable for drugs with close MICs and critical concentrations [e.g., ethambutol]	Typically done using in house methods
Automated liquid techniques	Decontaminated sputum is inoculated into a liquid-media containing tube, which is automatically and continuously monitored for growth	Highly sensitive and specific [like the solid agar method is also considered the 'gold standard' of DST] Faster than solid agar DST WHO approved (1)	Similar limitations to solid agar methods Higher rates of contamination than solid agar DST	Bactec MGIT960 system and SIRE and PZA kits [Becton–Dickinson] VersaTrek/ESP [Thermo Fisher Scientific] BacT/Alert3D [bioMerieux]
Microcolony culture techniques	Drug-free or drug-containing media is inoculated with specimens from patients and examined microscopically for growth, frequently in closed micro-well plates	Highly sensitive and specific (1) Generally rapid [mean turnaround time for MODS and TLA of 10 and 11 days, respectively] Can be performed directly on specimens Relatively inexpensive and non-proprietary MODS is approved by the WHO	Limited evidence for second-line drugs May not be suited to high NTM settings Require significant technical expertise but less infrastructure than other culture methods No commercial versions of the NRA or TLA assays exist	TB MODS Kit [Hardy Diagnostics] Sensititre system [Thermoscientific, TREK Diagnostic Systems] In development: B-SMART [Sequelae]
NAATs				
Fully or partially automated nucleic acid amplification assay	For Xpert MTB/RIF which is the only commercially available test in this category, liquefied sputum is added to a cartridge and inserted into the machine. A run is completed within 2 hours. Several fast followers are expected	Rapid [potentially same day results] Can be performed directly on specimens DST may occurs simultaneously with TB detection Closed cartridge system which minimises cross-contamination and the technical expertise required Xpert MTB/RIF is WHO and FDA approved and widely available Can provide quantitative information about bacterial load, which can predict infectiousness	Xpert MTB/RIF only detects rifampicin resistance [not isoniazid] Patients with a low pre-test probability of MDR-TB who are positive for rifampicin resistance require confirmatory testing Relatively costly and requires expensive instruments	Xpert MTB/RIF, Xpert MTB/RIF Ultra [Cepheid] In development: Xpert XDR-TB cartridge [isoniazid and second-line drugs], m2000 RealTime MTB DST reflex assay [Abbott], AlereQ relex DST test [Alere], Fluorocycler [Hain Lifescience]

Contd...

Contd...

Test	Description	Advantages	Limitations	Commercial versions
LPAs	Polymerase chain reaction amplicons are passed over a lateral flow strip containing probes for specific mutations. Bound amplicons and mutations are subsequently detected colourmetrically	Good sensitivity and high specificity and can detect multiple targets in parallel Rapid [time to result of 2 days] MTBDRplus and the next iteration of the MTBDRsl assay can be performed directly on specimens Information about specific mutations [e.g., in *inhA* and *katG*] can inform dosing Some LPAs are WHO approved Low instrumentation costs	Sensitivity generally lower when performed on smear-negative samples Phenotypic DST required in specimens or isolates with a susceptible DST result in order to rule-out second-line resistance Generally open system with manual steps that is vulnerable to cross-contamination Limited performance data [expect for the Hain Lifesciences LPAs] Performance depends on the local genetic epidemiology of drug-resistant TB strains. Mutations in drug-susceptible strains can cause false positive results in some regions (1)	MTBDRplus and MTBDRsl [Hain Lifesciences] INNO LiPA RifTB [Innogenetics] TB Resistance Module [AID] AdvanSure MDR TB GenoBlot assay [LG Life Sciences] MDR-TB, INH, PZA and FLQ LPAs [NIPRO Co.] MolecuTech REBA MTB-MDR – FQ, -KM, -XDR [YD Diagnostics]
Manual NAATs	These generally require manual DNA extraction and real-time [or isothermal] PCR instrumentation	Highly multiplexed and amenable to high throughput DST often occurs in conjunction with TB detection	Very limited performance data Can only be viably performed at high level reference laboratory due to the manual processing steps and non-automated testing procedure	Anyplex plus MTB/NTM/MDR TB and Anyplex II MTB/MDR/ XDR [Seegene] MeltPro Drug Resistant TB testing kits [Xiamen Zeesan Biotech] (1) B-SMART NASBA-based test [Sequella Inc.]
Other tests	This category includes microarray platforms and mass spectrophotometry systems. They are not widely used and have limited evidence to support their use	Highly multiplexed and amenable to high throughput Several technologies are FDA-endorsed or CE-marked [e.g., INFINITI MDR-TB assay]	Very limited performance data Only suited to well-resourced reference laboratories, however some tools currently in development show promise for POC use [e.g., HYDRA 1K] Limited availability in the high burden TB countries Expensive	INFINITI MDR-TB assay [AutoGenomics] *M. tuberculosis* Drug Resistance Detection Array Kit [CapitalBio Corp.] Ibis Mass Spectrometry platform [Abbott] In development: VerePLEX Biosystem and VEreMTB Detection Kit [Veredus Laboratories], TruArray MDR-TB assays [Akonni Biosystems, MYCO assay [iCubate], HYDRA 1K [Insilixa Inc.].

DST = drug-susceptibility testing; MIC = minimum inhibitory concentration; WHO = World Health Organization; PZA = pyrazinamide; TB = tuberculosis; MODS = microscopic observation drug-susceptibility; TLA, = thin layer agar; NRA = nitrate reductase assay; NAATs = nucleic acid amplification tests; FDA = Federal Drug Administration; MDR-TB = multidrug-resistant tuberculosis; LPAs = line probe assays; DNA = deoxyribonucleic acid; PCR = polymerase chain reaction; POC = point-of-care; NTM = nontuberculous mycobacteria

Data from references 69-93

confirmatory testing is subsequently done using a LPA, the most widely available example of which is the MTBDRplus test [Hain Lifesciences], which can be performed directly on the specimen with high sensitivity and specificity (106b,107). With a vision to offer DST at the earliest time in the diagnostic process, the Guidelines on management of DR-TB in India (108a), integrated DR-TB diagnostic algorithm has been recommended. This algorithm [Figures 42.5A and 42.5B] facilitates risk assessment for DR-TB and DST-guided treatment for at least rifampicin resistance at the time of diagnosis ["universal DST"].

NAAT are often unable to target all resistance causing mutations. For example, resistance to the SLIDs is, in addition to being caused by mutations in rrs, also caused by mutations in tlyA, the eis promoter and gibB, the frequency distribution of which differs according to geographical region (108b). Thus, confirmatory phenotypic testing is still required in patients who have a susceptible result according to, for example, the MTBDRsl [Hain Lifesciences] LPA, which only targets rrs for SLID DST (109). This also applies to new tests in development, such as the Xpert XDR assay [Cepheid, Sunnyvale, USA], which targets only rrs and eis for the SLIDs, and new molecular assays for new drugs, such as bedaquiline and delamanid, for which we have an incomplete understanding of the genetic associates of resistance.

Targeted and Whole Genome Sequencing

Next generation sequencing [which can be performed on the entire genome or pre-specified regions] offers promise for the diagnosis of DR-TB (110), as the cost of sequencing has declined dramatically. Although not as rapid as molecular DST, the turn-around-time of sequencing methods is reduced by the use of "early positive" cultures [2–7 days] (111). As sequencing provides a comprehensive genotypic DST, it permits patients to have individualised treatment regimens, which is more likely to result in cure (112). However, the clinical impact of this strategy in different settings remains to be established. Next generation sequencing also allows for the detection of minority populations and information on compensatory mutations. Furthermore, it provides information on transmission and allows for tracking of outbreaks, and it can be used to identify novel mutations to newly introduced anti-TB drugs. This is of particular importance in high burden settings, where transmission can quickly drive resistance to these new drugs.

Importance of Healthcare Systems and Linkage to Care

Lastly, it should be noted that the impact of a test for DR-TB will always be undermined by the quality of the healthcare system. Healthcare workers should do everything they can to make sure diagnostic specimens arrive at laboratories timeously, are processed quickly, the result is rapidly sent back, and that drugs are readily available to rapidly start patients on treatment. For example, a study (113) in Cape Town found that Xpert MTB/RIF reduced time to MDR-TB treatment from 25 days to 17 days, however, this is nowhere near what it should be for a test that takes two hours.

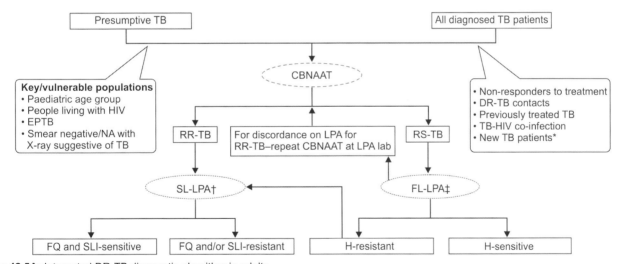

Figure 42.5A: Integrated DR-TB diagnostic algorithm in adults
*States to advance in phased manner as per PMDT scale up plan for universal DST based on lab capacity and policy on use of diagnostics
† LC DST [Mfx 2.0, Km, Cm, Lzd] will be done only for patients with any resistance on baseline SL-LPA. DST to Z, Cfz, Bdq and Dlm would be considered for policy in future, whenever available, standardised and WHO endorsed.
‡ Molecular testing is offered for H-mono/poly resistance to TB patients prioritised by risk as per the available laboratory capacity
TB = tuberculosis; DR-TB = drug-resistant TB; CBNAAT = cartridge-based nucleic acid amplification tests; HIV = human immunodeficiency virus; EPTB = extra-pulmonary TB; NA = not available; RR-TB = rifampicin resistant TB; RS-TB = rifampicin-sensitive TB; SL-LPA = second-line line probe assay; FL-LPA = first-line line probe assay; PMDT = programmatic management of drug-resistant TB; DST = drug-susceptibility testing; LC = liquid culture; Mfx 2.0 = moxifloxacin break-point concentration 2 mg/L; Km = kanamycin; Cm = capreomycin; Z = pyrazinamide; Cfz = clofazimine; Bdq = bedaquiline; Dlm = delaminid; WHO = World Health Organization
Reproduced with permission from "Revised National Tuberculosis Control Programme, Directorate General of Health Services, Ministry of Health and Family Welfare, Government of India. Guidelines on programmatic management of drug-resistant tuberculosis in India 2017. New Delhi: World Health Organization, Country Office for India; 2017" (reference 108a)

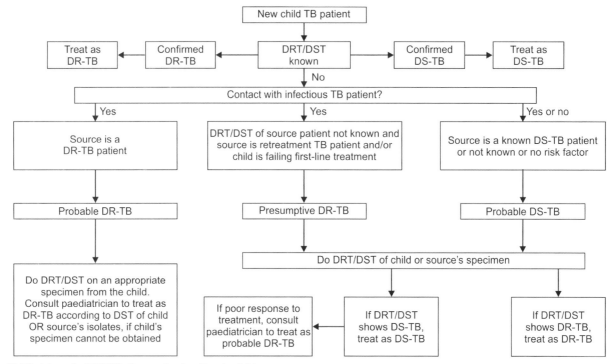

Figure 42.5B: Integrated DR-TB diagnostic algorithm in children
TB = tuberculosis; DRT = drug-resistance testing; DST = drug-susceptibility testing; DR-TB = drug-resistant TB; DS-TB = drug-sensitive TB
Reproduced with permission from "Revised National Tuberculosis Control Programme, Directorate General of Health Services, Ministry of Health and Family Welfare, Government of India. Guidelines on programmatic management of drug-resistant tuberculosis in India 2017. New Delhi: World Health Organization, Country Office for India; 2017" (reference 108a)

In summary, molecular DST is accurate and feasible in high incidence countries and should always be performed as the initial test for drug resistance; however, due to suboptimal rule-out value for drug resistance, culture-based phenotypic DST should always also be performed. Good infrastructure and training to support the use of DST results for rapid patient management are critical.

CLINICAL PRESENTATION

The clinical features of DR-TB are indistinguishable from those of DS-TB and include cough, fever, weight loss, haemoptysis and night sweats. The traditional culture-based laboratory diagnosis of DR-TB results in long delays [usually several weeks] in obtaining DST results, and as a result, DR-TB is often diagnosed late when DS-TB treatment fails or when the cultures are still positive after several months of treatment. During this delay, patients may undergo clinical worsening, and thus, are often sicker with more extensive radiological disease at the time of commencement of DR-TB. The NAATs promise to reduce the interval between sample acquisition and DST result from weeks to hours. Previous treatment for TB, local rates of drug resistance, or contact with a patient with DR-TB may raise the suspicion that the current episode is DR. Some studies have identified HIV infection, homelessness and a history of alcohol abuse as additional predictors of risk (114), but this has not been consistent across different countries. Nevertheless, almost two-thirds of patients with MDR-TB globally have not previously been treated for TB, and thus, DR-TB should always be excluded.

PRINCIPLES OF DRUG-RESISTANT TUBERCULOSIS TREATMENT

Treatment of Multidrug-resistant and Extensively Drug-resistant Tuberculosis

The updated 2016 WHO guidelines (115) recommended a standardised regimen with an intensive phase of treatment containing kanamycin [an injectable agent], moxifloxacin, prothionamide, clofazimine, isoniazid, pyrazinamide and ethambutol which are given together in an initial phase of 4 months [with the possibility to extend to 6 months if they remain sputum smear positive at the end of month 4]. This is then followed by the continuation phase of treatment for 5 months with a regimen consisting of four TB drugs: moxifloxacin, clofazimine, pyrazinamide, and ethambutol (115,116a). The suggested regimens for the programmatic management of drug-resistant TB in India are listed in Figure 42.6 (108a).

In 2018 August, December the WHO rapid communication regarding key changes to treatment of MDR/RR-TB (117a) and pre-final text ahead of a fully edited version scheduled for publication in early 2019 as part of consolidated WHO treatment guidelines on DR-TB (117b) were published.

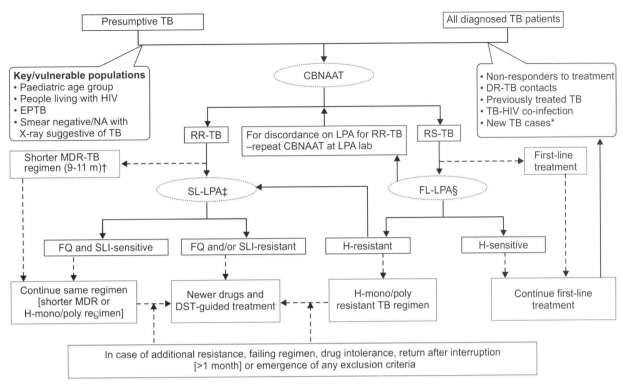

Figure 42.6: Treatment regimens for programmatic management of DR-TB in India

*States to advance in phased manner as per PMDT Scale up plan for universal DST based on lab capacity and policy on use of diagnostics

† Conventional MDR-TB regimen [24 months] for pregnant women or for EPTB patients who are not eligible for shorter regimen

‡ LC DST [Mfx 2.0, Km, Cm, Lzd] will be done only for patients with any resistance on baseline SL-LPA. DST to Z, Cfz, Bdq and Dlm would be considered for policy in future, whenever available, standardised and WHO endorsed

§ Molecular testing and treatment for H-mono/poly resistance is offered to TB patients prioritised by risk as per the available lab capacity

TB = tuberculosis; CBNAAT = cartridge-based nucleic acid amplification tests; HIV = human immunodeficiency virus; EPTB = extra-pulmonary TB; NA = not available; RR-TB = rifampicin resistant TB; RS-TB = rifampicin-sensitive TB; MDR-TB = multidrug-resistant TB; SL-LPA = second-line line probe assay; FL-LPA = first-line line probe assay; FQ = fluoroquinolones; SLI = second-line injectable drugs; H = isoniazid; PMDT = programmatic management of drug-resistant TB; DST = drug-susceptibility testing; LC = liquid culture; Mfx 2.0 = moxifloxacin break-point concentration 2 mg/L; Km = kanamycin; Cm = capreomycin; Z = pyrazinamide; Cfz = clofazimine; Bdq = bedaquiline; Dlm = delaminid; WHO = World Health Organization

Reproduced with permission from "Revised National Tuberculosis Control Programme, Directorate General of Health Services, Ministry of Health and Family Welfare, Government of India. Guidelines on programmatic management of drug-resistant tuberculosis in India 2017. New Delhi: World Health Organization, Country Office for India; 2017" (reference 108a)

Tables 42.2A, 42.2B and 42.2C (116b,117a,117b) depict the revised grouping of anti-TB medicines recommended for use in longer MDR-TB regimens. The anti-TB medicines that were grouped into *four* groups as per the WHO 2016 guidelines (115) have regrouped into *three* categories [Table 42.2C] in the WHO 2018 guidelines (117a,117b) and have been ranked based on the latest evidence as per the effectiveness and safety. As per the WHO 2018 guidelines (117a), Group A includes anti-TB medicines to be prioritized; Group B includes anti-TB medicines to be added next; and anti-TB medicines that are to be included to complete the regimens and when anti-TB medicines from Groups A and B cannot be used are listed under Group C. Kanamycin and capreomycin are no longer recommended.

Based on the currently available published evidence, the WHO 2018 rapid communication (117a) recommend implementing effective and *fully oral treatment regimens* for most patients. The guidelines (117a) also suggest the need to ensure that *drug- resistance is excluded* [at least to the fluoroquinolones and injectables] before initiating treatment,

especially in patients who are to be started on the shorter MDR-TB regimen [defined as a course of treatment for MDR/RR-TB lasting 9 to 12 months]. The WHO 2018 guidelines (117a) also address issues concerning need for close monitoring of patient safety and treatment response; a low threshold is recommended for switching non-responding patients or those experiencing drug intolerance to alternative medicines and/or new regimens. *Options for the choice of agents for the intensive and continuation phases and more detailed guidance is expected to be provided at the time of release of the final WHO guidelines later in 2019.*

In South Africa, approximately half of the MDR-TB patients receiving kanamycin develop some degree of ototoxicity and nephrotoxicity prompting substitution of kanamycin with bedaquiline. Additionally, a retrospective cohort analysis conducted by the South African Department of Health showed that, in rifampicin-resistant TB, bedaquiline resulted in a 41% increase in treatment success and a three-fold reduction in mortality, compared with those that did not receive bedaquiline (118,119). Thus, based on the superior

Table 42.2A: Characteristics of drugs* used for drug-resistant TB

Group	Dosage	Special precautions	Adverse events
Group A Include all three medicines [unless they cannot be used]			
Levofloxacin [Lfx] or	500 mg-1000 mg daily	Dose adjustment required in CKD Cr cl 30-50 mL/min = 750-1000 mg daily <30 mL/min = 750-1000 mg thrice weekly	In advanced CKD, class effect of fluoroquinolones may pose a higher risk of neuro-psychiatric adverse events and tendinopathy; QTc prolongation on ECG more with Mfx than Lfx, a combination of Bdq, Cfz and Lfx [rather Mfx] preferred
Moxifloxacin [Mfx]	400 mg daily	No dose adjustment in CKD; predominantly hepatobiliary excretion; may increase liver enzymes; has good CNS penetration; avoid concomitant administration of antacids, phosphate binders, calcium, iron, or aluminium containing medications to avoid malabsorption	
Bedaquiline [Bdq]	400 mg daily for initial 2 weeks and subsequently 200 mg thrice weekly for next 22 weeks [can be given longer]	Administration with meal increases bio-availability; no dose adjustment with renal or liver disease; ECG should be done to monitor QTc prolongation at baseline, 2, 12 and 24 weeks and stop the drug if QTc >500 ms, serum serum potassium, magnesium and calcium monitoring required for QTc prolongation; QTc monitoring required when co-administered with clarithromycin, Cfz, Lfx/Mfx	QTc prolongation, arthralgias, hepatitis, headache, anorexia, nausea
Linezolid [Lzd]	600 mg once daily; the dose can be decreased to 300 mg after 3-6 months; linezolid should be discontinued in case toxicity occurs and can be re-introduced at a lower [300 mg daily] dose following recovery	Main route of excretion is hepatic with some renal clearance. No dose adjustment is required in CKD; careful monitoring of haematological toxicity, lactic acidosis, peripheral and optic neuropathy [often reversible] required. Pyridoxine 100 mg daily can be administered to prevent haematological toxicity. Avoid concomitant use of food items rich in tyramine and medications [SSRIs and other medicines] known to increase serotonin production to prevent development of serotonin syndrome	Haematological toxicity, lactic acidosis, peripheral and optic neuropathy and serotonin syndrome. Drug toxicity is related to dose and duration of linezolid. Haematological toxicity and lactic acidosis occur in few weeks to months while neurological toxicity occurs after 3-4 months

Contd...

Contd...

Group	Dosage	Special precautions	Adverse events
Group B Add both medicines [unless they cannot be used] Clofazimine [Cfz]	100 mg daily	QTc monitoring on ECG is required when co-administered with Bdq, Lfx/Mfx; serum potassium, magnesium and calcium monitoring required for QTc prolongation. Not to be used in pregnancy and severe hepatic insufficiency. Skin problems can be prevented by application of sunscreen and lubricants	Ichthyosis and dry skin, sunburn, pink-brownish-black discoloration of skin, cornea, retina and urine; acne flare
Cycloserine [Cs] OR Terizidone [Trd]	10-15 mg/kg/day in divided doses or 250 mg morning 500 mg evening 300 mg morning 300 mg evening	Cr cl ≥ 30 mL/min: no dose adjustment required; < 30 mL/min: 250 mg daily or 500 mg on alternate days; therapeutic drug monitoring is recommended if facility is available; avoid if possible in renal disease as the main route of excretion is renal. Cs[and Trd] should be avoided in patients with a history of epilepsy, psychiatric illness or alcoholism, to prevent minor adverse reactions like insomnia administration of small dose of a tranquiliser is recommended or pyridoxine 50 mg/250 mg of administered cycloserine can be given to prevent neurotoxicity	Dizziness, slurred speech, convulsions, headache, tremor, insomnia, confusion, depression, and altered behaviour, suicidal tendency, generalised hypersensitivity reaction or hepatitis
Group C Add to complete the regimen and when medicines from Group A and B cannot be used			
Ethambutol [E]	15-25 mg/kg/day	Cr cl ≥ 30 mL/min, no dose adjustment required; < 30 mL/min: 15-25 mg/kg thrice weekly. Patients should be monitored at baseline and regularly thereafter for visual acuity and red-green colour discrimination	Dose dependent optic [retrobulbar] neuropathy [> 30 mg/kg/day or 15-25 mg/kg in CKD]; generally reverses on prompt discontinuation; hyperuricemia Uncommon: interstitial nephritis, cholestatic jaundice, neutropenia and thrombocytopenia, reversible cutaneous hypersensitivity disappearing on desensitisation
Delamanid [Dlm]	100 mg twice weekly for six months [can be administered longer]	QTc monitoring at baseline, 2, 12 and 24 weeks. Stop if > QTc 500 ms; monitor serum potassium, magnesium and calcium	QTc prolongation, nausea vomiting and abdominal pain, dizziness
Pyrazinamide [Z]	25-30 mg/kg/day [1.5 g for 50 kg, 2 g for > 50 kg]	Cr cl ≥ 30 mL/min: no dose adjustment required; < 30 mL/min: 25-30 mg/kg three times/week	GI upset, hyperuricemia, arthralgia, hepatotoxicity [not dose related]

Contd...

Contd...

Group	Dosage	Special precautions	Adverse events
Imipenem - cilastatin [Ipm-Cln] OR Meropenem	1 g IV every 12 h	Dose adjustment required in CKD	
Amoxycillin Clavulanate [Mpm/Amx/Clv]	1 g every 8-12 h IV administered with clavulanate [as amoxycillin clavulanate 250/125 mg every 8-12h]	Dose adjustment required in CKD	GI upset, transaminitis
Amikacin [Am]	15 mg/kg-maximum 1 g; five to seven times weekly or 20-25 mg/kg 2-3 times/week	Baseline audiogram and renal functions. Dose adjustment required in CKD; *prefer to avoid if possible.* Periodic monitoring of audiogram and renal functions every 2-4 weeks	Vestibular, auditory and renal toxicities
Ethionamide [Eto] or Prothionamide [Pto]	15-20 mg/kg/day in divided doses. The usual dose is 250-1000 mg/day. Most patients should be started on 250 mg doses daily or twice daily and gradually increased over several days to 750 or 1000 mg total daily dose	Should not be administered in pregnancy [teratogenicity in animals]. Careful monitoring is required if administered in patients with diabetes mellitus, liver disease, alcoholism or mental instability. No dose adjustment required in CKD. Serum TSH monitoring required periodically especially when co-administered with PAS	Pto is generally considered to be less unpleasant and better tolerated than Eto. However, profile of adverse events is similar. GI disturbances, metallic taste and sulphurous belching; psychotic reactions, hypoglycaemia [especially in diabetes mellitus patients]; hepatitis; other rare side-effects include gynaecomastia menstrual disturbance, impotence, acne, alopecia and peripheral neuropathy
p-amino salicyclic acid [PAS]	150 mg/kg or 10-12 g daily In 2-3 divided doses	Although no dose adjustment required in CKD. However, caution should be exercised, since main route of excretion is renal. Serum TSH monitoring required periodically especially when co-administered with ethionamide	GI disturbances [diarrhoea is self-limiting], hypothyroidism [more chances if given along with ethionamide], hypokalemia, hepatitis, thrombocytopenia, increased acidosis in patients with renal failure

* All are bactericidal except Cs and PAS which are bacteriostatic; Cfz and Eto are weak bactericidal
TB = tuberculosis; CKD = chronic kidney disease; Cr Cl = creatinine clearance; CKD = chronic kidney disease; ECG = electrocardiogram; SSRIs = selective serotonin reuptake inhibitors; TSH = thyroid stimulating hormone
Data from references 116b, 117a, 117b

Table 42.2B: Principles underpinning the management of drug-resistant TB

Principles underpinning the medical management of MDR-TB

A regimen is based, when possible, on proven or likely susceptibility to at least 5 drugs

A backbone of a later generation fluoroquinolone [moxifloxacin or levofloxacin], and bedaquiline and any Group C drugs* such as clofazamine, ethionamide, high dose isoniazid are recommended, such that at least 5 drugs to which the isolate is likely to be susceptible are being used is recommended. Use of an injectable in a frontline MDR-TB regimen is not recommended given the proven efficacy of bedaquiline and the toxicity of SLIDs. This proposed approach is synonymous with using bedaquiline in place of the SLID in the WHO shorter course regimen

Where toxicity, intolerance or resistance precludes use of one of the standard MDR-TB drugs, delamanid and/or linezolid may also be added to the regimen

Bedaquiline is usually used for a minimum duration of 6 months in the absence of adverse events, and longer in certain cases.

The total recommended duration of treatment using the 2016 standardised WHO shorter treatment regimen is between 9 months and 12 months [depending on culture conversion], recommend a 12 month duration of treatment if bedaquiline is included in the regimen

If the patient has previously been on treatment with a specific drug for 3 or more months, then that drug is generally avoided

Addressing psychological and social factors to ensure adherence is critical

Patients should be monitored for adverse drug reactions, which are common

A single drug should not be added to a failing regimen

Principles underpinning the medical management of pre-XDR-TB and XDR-TB

Regimens should be constructed based on prevailing DST patterns

A regimen is usually based on a backbone of bedaquiline, linezolid, PAS [and cycloserine]. Other drugs from group D such as delamanid and meropenem/clavulanate are added depending on availability.

In patients with FQ-resistant pre-XDR-TB a SLID may be considered

Given the high degree of resistance, any drug that the isolate is [potentially] susceptible to from Table 42.2A are added such that at least 4-5 effective drugs are included in the regimen

Patients should be carefully monitored for adverse drug reactions [Table 42.2A]

Attention should be given to correcting risk factors for renal failure [dehydration, nausea, vomiting and diarrhea, avoidance of other nephrotoxic drugs [cotrimoxazole and nevirapine], and early identification of underlying renal disease [diabetes and HIV-associated nephropathy]

Patients on linezolid should be monitored for the development of myelosuppression [usually develops with in 2-3 months of treatment], peripheral neuropathy [usually develops between 1 month and 4 months of treatment] and optic neuropathy [usually develops after 5 months of treatment]

Patients on bedaquiline and delamanid [especially when used with other QT prolonging drugs] should have a baseline ECG, with follow-up ECG at least 2, 6, 12, and 24 weeks after starting therapy to monitor for QT prolongation. Serum calcium, potassium, and magnesium should be measured prior to starting treatment and corrected if needed

Bedaquiline should be discontinued in patients who develop QTc interval >500 ms or a significant ventricular arrhythmia. Liver function testing should also be performed prior to initiation of treatment and repeated monthly

*Drug categories described in Table 42.2A

TB = tuberculosis; MDR-TB = multidrug-resistant tuberculosis; XDR-TB = extensively drug-resistant TB; PAS = para-amino salicylic acid; DST = drug-susceptibility testing; ECG = electrocardiogram

Table 42.2C: WHO 2018 rapid communication: grouping of medicines recommended for use in longer MDR-TB regimens

Group	Medicine [abbreviation]
Group A: Include all three medicines [unless they cannot be used]	Levofloxacin [Lfx] OR moxifloxacin [Mfx] Bedaquiline [Bdq], linezolid [Lzd]
Group B: Add both medicines [unless they cannot be used]	Clofazimine [Cfz] Cycloserine [Cs] OR terizidone [Trd]
Group C: Add to complete the regimen and when medicines from Groups A and B cannot be used	Ethambutol [E] Delamanid [Dlm] Pyrazinamide [Z] Imipenem-cilastatin [Ipm-Cln] OR meropenem [Mpm] Amikacin [Am] [OR streptomycin {S}] Ethionamide [Eto] OR prothionamide [Pto] p-amino salicylic acid [PAS]

*Longer MDR-TB regimens usually last 18-20 months and may be standardized or individualised. These regimens are usually designed to include at least 5 medicines considered to be effective

WHO = World Health Organization; MDR-TB = multidrug-resistant tuberculosis

Adapted from "World Health organization. Rapid Communication. Key changes to treatment of multidrug- and rifampicin-resistant tuberculosis [MDR/RR-TB]. WHO/CDS/TB/2018.18. Geneva: World Health organization; 2018" (reference 117a)

outcomes and better adverse event profile, the South African Department of Health has recently recommended the use of bedaquiline for all MDR-TB patients [with kanamycin being substituted for bedaqualine in the shorter course WHO regimen] (118,119). In patients who fail to respond to treatment the following must be considered: poor adherence, incorrect dosage, poor penetration of drugs in lung cavities, hetero-resistance, and malabsorption of anti-TB drugs.

The treatment regimen for XDR-TB is more complex. The current XDR-TB regimen consists of a backbone of bedaquiline, linezolid, and para-amino salicylic acid [PAS]. Other drugs [Table 42.2A] may be added depending on availability [e.g., delamanid and meropenem plus clavulanic acid] and to which susceptibility has been demonstrated, or at the discretion of the attending clinician (115,116a). Many patients with XDR-TB have been previously treated for MDR-TB (120,121), and prior exposure to drugs like ethionamide, isoniazid and clofazamine usually excludes their use in a new regimen.

Moxifloxacin has been shown to be effective against isolates phenotypically resistant to ofloxacin or ciprofloxacin (122), and may be associated with improved outcomes for patients with XDR-TB (123). In isolates where lack of isoniazid susceptibility results from mutations in the promoter region of the InhA gene (124,125), low-level resistance can likely be overcome by increased doses of the isoniazid ["high-dose isoniazid"] (126). This pattern of resistance is often accompanied with cross-resistance to other second-line anti-TB agents, specifically ethionamide, as it has a structural similarity to isoniazid (127). In recent years, linezolid has been used to treat patients with X/MDR-TB, although there have been no fully controlled trials of linezolid in a regimen for this indication. Linezolid added to the regimen of patients failing standard XDR-TB treatment has been shown to improve culture-conversion (130).

Long-term outcome data for linezolid in patients with XDR-TB, especially when combined with other effective drugs such bedaquiline, is encouraging with reported treatment success rates approaching ~70% (119,128). However, linezolid toxicity, specifically myelosuppression and peripheral neuropathy, is a major concern that prompts treatment withdrawal in up to 1/3 of patients receiving linezolid (129-134).

Adverse Effects

Treatment for DR-TB involves the use of toxic medications and drug-associated adverse effects [AEs] are common (135-137). They impact compliance, cause drug suspension and treatment interruption, and may result in serious morbidity and even death. A study (138) from South Africa in patients with XDR-TB found that 58% of patients experienced a drug-related AEs during their treatment, and culture-conversion and survival were significantly lower in those patients who had experienced severe AEs. In this study, 5% of all AEs resulted in death, and the second-line injectable drugs [in particular, capreomycin] were associated with all of these deaths. It is thus essential to monitor renal function and potassium at least monthly during the intensive phase of treatment involving an injectable. Ototoxic hearing loss is common in patients with DR-TB: another study from South Africa found that 57% of patients had developed high-frequency hearing loss after three months of aminoglycoside treatment (139), and this complication may be more common in patients with HIV infection. All patients should be screened monthly with audiometry during the intensive phase of treatment. Thyroid function should be monitored between six and nine months of treatment with ethionamide, prothionamide or PAS, and a full blood count, neurological exam and assessment of visual acuity should be checked regularly in patients taking linezolid.

Adjuvant Surgical Management

The rationale behind surgery for DR-TB is that excision of cavities [along with "debulking" of any necrotic or non-viable lung tissue] will dramatically reduce the overall organism burden in the lung while simultaneously removing the sites of high concentrations of DR bacilli. This is hoped to enhance the sterilising properties of post-surgical chemotherapy and increase the likelihood of treatment success (140,141).

Reported outcomes for surgery in DR-TB are unavoidably skewed by selection bias, as sicker patients with bilateral disease and other comorbidities are generally not considered operative candidates. However, a recent systematic review and meta-analysis of 24 comparison studies of MDR- and XDR-TB [involving more than 5000 patients] found a significant association between surgical intervention and successful outcome when compared to non-surgical treatment alone {odds ratio [OR] 2.24, 95% confidence intervals [CI] 1.68-2.97} (142). Sub-group analyses of studies involving XDR-TB patients revealed an even more pronounced treatment effect [OR 4.55, 95% CI 1.32-15.7], which would the view that surgery is a viable therapeutic option in carefully selected patients who remain culture positive despite receiving an effective regimen for drug-resistant TB, or are deemed to have a high risk of relapse. Surgery as a treatment modality for drug-resistant TB must be used in conjunction with an effective salvage regimen consisting of at least 4-5 drugs.

HUMAN IMMUNODEFICIENCY VIRUS AND DRUG-RESISTANT TUBERCULOSIS

The management of TB in HIV-infected individuals is complex. The management of DR-TB in HIV-infected persons is even more challenging, specifically due to the shared toxicity between anti-HIV and TB drugs [Table 42.3], (143-156), in addition to other factors such as greater potential for increased drug toxicity, HIV-related organ disease such as nephropathy, pharmacokinetic drug-to-drug interactions, and immune reconstitution inflammatory syndrome [IRIS]. All these factors ultimately translate into increased complexity and potentially mortality in MDR-TB-HIV co-infected patients (157).

Antiretroviral therapy [ART] improves survival in patients with MDR-TB (157-159). The WHO recommends that MDR-TB patients who are not already on ART should start ART within the first eight weeks of starting effective MDR-TB treatment irrespective of CD4 count (160). Patients with low CD4+ counts [$<50/mm^3$] should have expedited initiation of treatment with anti-retrovirals [ARVs] usually within two weeks of starting MDR-TB treatment (115,161-163), similar to the recommendation for DS-TB.

Initiating ART together with MDR-TB drugs is challenging because of overlapping adverse events, high pill burden, IRIS, and potential drug-drug interaction [Table 42.3]. In recent times introduction of new drugs such as bedaquiline, shown to be both safe and efficacious even in a high HIV prevalence settings (164), and linezolid have renewed

hope for the successful treatment of MDR-TB (130,165). It should be noted that co-administration of bedaquiline with efavirenz has the potential of reducing serum levels of bedaquiline (166). It is, therefore, recommended that bedaquiline be co-administered with two nucleoside reverse transcriptase inhibitors [NRTIs] and nevirapine or two NRTIs and a protease inhibitor [PI]. However, it should be noted that both nevirapine and certain PIs can increase bedaquiline levels by 10%–20% but the significance of this remains unclear (167). A potential alternative is an integrase inhibitor. However, this is not widely available in resource-limited settings. Other toxicity-related drug-drug interactions are described in Table 42.3.

MANAGING DRUG-RESISTANT TUBERCULOSIS IN SPECIAL SITUATIONS INCLUDING PREGNANCY, RENAL FAILURE, LIVER DISEASE AND IN THE INTENSIVE CARE UNIT

Management of DR-TB in special situations including pregnancy, renal failure, liver disease and in the intensive care unit necessitates a change in either the selection of drugs, dosage, or duration of therapy. The reader is referred to the chapters *"Tuberculosis in pregnancy"* [Chapter 25], *"Tuberculosis in chronic kidney disease"* [Chapter 28], *"Hepatotoxicity associated with anti-tuberculosis treatment"* [Chapter 45] and *"Tuberculosis and acute lung injury"* [Chapter 32] for details.

NEW DRUGS AND TREATMENT REGIMENS FOR DRUG-RESISTANT TUBERCULOSIS

It is clear that the current available treatment regimen for MDR-TB is inadequate. Issues with current treatments include multiple drug toxicities, prolonged treatment duration, development of acquired resistance, ART interactions and the on-going use of injectable agents. A promising pipeline of new drugs is emerging and at least 10 new studies are planned or underway to address this problem (168-188). Key questions that will need to be addressed are listed below.

Bedaquiline is a diarylquinoline and the first new anti-TB drug on the market in over 40 years. This orally administered agent acts via a novel mechanism that selectively inhibits mycobacterial adenosine triphosphate synthase (189). It is well tolerated (166), and has demonstrated both safety and efficacy in HIV co-infected patients (165,170). XDR-TB patients receiving a backbone of bedaquiline and linezolid had substantially better favourable outcomes compared to those not using these drugs [66.2% *versus* 13.2%; p < 0.001] (119). Bedaquiline is known to cause joint pains and prolongation of the QTc interval , which warrants regular ECG monitoring especially when using it in conjunction with fluoroquinolones [drug of choice is levofloxacin] and clofazamine.

Delamanid is an orally administered agent that acts by inhibiting mycolic acid synthesis in the mycobacterial cell wall (179). It has demonstrated increased rates of sputum culture conversion and improved clinical outcomes (181,190-192).

Table 42.3: Important drug co-toxicity and drug-drug interactions in patients with HIV/DR-TB co-infection

Description	Responsible ARV drugs	Responsible anti-TB drugs	Considerations
Renal toxicity	TDF	Aminoglycosides, Cm	TDF causes renal failure with hypophosphatemia and proteinuria Avoid TDF in patients receiving aminoglycosides and Cm Serum creatinine should be checked before switching patients onto TDF after completion of aminoglycoside Caution is advised when administering TDF or aminoglycosides in patients with underlying co-morbidities, such as, diabetes mellitus or in patients who are receiving concomitant nephrotoxic agents such as NSAIDs and amphotericin B If TDF is necessary, close monitoring of serum creatinine is required
Electrolyte derangement	TDF	Aminoglycosides, Cm	Exclude exacerbating factors, such vomiting, diarrhoea, dehydration, diuretics, etc.
Hepatitis/ hepatotoxicity	NVP, EFV, PI [especially RTV], NRTI	Z, Bdq, PAS, FQ	When severe stop both ARVs and anti-TB agents, restart TB drugs first Assess for other contributing factors such as alcohol abuse, viral aetiologies and other drugs like co-trimoxazole Avoid concomitant use of NVP and Z The risk of NVP hepatotoxicity is highest in the first 3 months of starting therapy with higher risk in patients with CD4+ >250/mm^3, the risk of NVP hepatotoxicity is lower if VL is suppressed
Myelosuppression	AZT	Lzd, H	Stop Lzd if myelosuppression occurs. Blood transfusion is indicated if haemoglobin falls below 8 g/dL Avoid co-administration of AZT and Lzd Adverse events should be managed with a combination of temporary suspension of linezolid, dose reduction and/or symptom management Reduction dose of 300 mg daily may be associated with fewer neuropathic effects but is not supported by pharmacokinetic data Consider stopping cotrimoxazole
Peripheral neuropathy	ddI, d4T	Lzd, Cs, H, Eto, E	Avoid use of D4T or ddI in combination with Cs or Lzd Use pyridoxine as prophylaxis in patients receiving Cs, H and Lzd
QT prolongation		BDQ, Mfx, Cfz Lfx, Ofx	Close monitoring of QTc is recommended when using these agents in combination
Central nervous system toxicity	EFV	Cs, H, Eto/Pto, FQ	EFV toxicity occurs in first 2–3 weeks of treatment Concurrent use of EFV with CS needs close monitoring
Headache	AZT, EFV	Cs, BDQ	Headaches may be self-limited in case of AZT, EFV and Cs Advice analgesia and hydration
Nausea and vomiting	RTV, d4T, NVP	Eto, PAS, H, BDQ, E, Z	Most drugs will cause some degree of nausea If persistent consider drug-induced pancreatitis, hepatitis
Lactic acidosis	d4T, ddI, AZT, 3TC	Lzd	High index of suspicion needed to detect hyperlactatemia to prevent overt symptoms of lactic acidosis
Pancreatitis	d4T, ddI	Lzd	Avoid co-administration where possible If pancreatitis occurs discontinue the ARVs completely
Diarrhoea	PI, ddI	PAS, FQ, Eto	For mild diarrhoea anti-motility drugs can be used May be self-limited. Exclude opportunistic infections
Optic neuritis	ddI	E, Lzd, Eto	Stop all suspected agents causing optic neuritis Screen patients using the Snellen chart and Ishihara chart
Hypothyroidism	d4T	Eto, PAS	Monitor TSH for patients receiving these agents
Joint pain	PI [Indinavir]	Z, BDQ	Mild symptoms can be managed by simple analgesia

HIV = human immunodeficiency virus; DR-TB = drug-resistant tuberculosis; TDF = tenofovir disoproxil fumarate; Cm = capreomycin; NSAIDs = nonsteroidal anti-inflammatory drugs; NVP = nevirapine; EFV = efavirenz; PI = protease inhibitor; RTV = ritonavir; NRTI = nucleoside reverse transcriptase inhibitors; ARVs = anti-retroviral drugs; Z = pyrazinamide; Bdq = bedaquiline; PAS = para-amino salicylic acid; FQ = fluoroquinolones; ARV = anti-retroviral drugs; TB = tuberculosis; VL = viral load; AZT = zidovudine; Lzd = linezolid; H = isoniazid; Lfx = levofloxacin; ddI = didanosine; d4T = stavudine; Cs = cycloserine; Eto = ethionamide; Pto = prothionamide; E = ethambutol; Mfx = moxifloxacin; Cfz = clofazimine; Gfx = gatifloxacin; Lfx = levofloxacin; Ofx = ofloxacin; TSH = thyroid stimulating hormone

Based on references 143-156

Delamanid is known to cause prolongation of the QT interval mainly via the DM-6705 metabolite which is regulated by serum albumin. Therefore, delamanid is contraindicated in patients with hypoalbuminemia, [albumin < 28 g/L], which is a frequent finding in HIV-infected individuals. This may limit its use in the HIV co-infected population despite having a safe drug-drug interaction profile with first-line antiretroviral medications (193). Additionally, delamanid is administered twice daily, 30 minutes after a standard meal (194). This dosing schedule may affect adherence (195). It seems that delamanid is potentially efficacious and well tolerated in children aged 6 years and older (196), however, data from controlled studies are scarce in the paediatric population.

How can Novel Agents Safely be Used in Combination?

The novel agents, most advanced in MDR-TB development include, the nitroimidazoles [pretonamid and delamanid] (194), the adenosine triphosphate [ATP]-synthase inhibitor bedaquiline and the oxazolidinone, sutezolid (197). Murine data and Phase II early bactericidal activity studies [EBA] inform the use of novel agents in combination. Both Bedaquiline and Delamanid have conditional regulatory approval and these two drugs may represent a feasible alternative to injectable agents, such as, the aminoglycosides. Bedaquiline, however, while promising impressive superiority to a standardised background regimen after two months of treatment for MDR-TB was associated with increased mortality, and concerns for reduced activity in combination with pretomanid will need to be addressed (197,198). Sutezolid, whilst showing activity against MDR-TB strains has not yet been clinically tested in combination with other novel agents and may be a more suitable agent than Linezolid which has been associated with bone marrow and neurotoxicity with longer term use (199).

How can Existing Agents be Effectively Integrated into Novel Regimens?

Each existing agent needs to be assessed in terms of toxicity in combination with novel agents. Fluoroquinolones and clofazimine potentially prolong the QT interval, as can novel agents bedaquiline and delamanid. While it is accepted that a FQ-containing regimens improve outcomes in MDR-TB optimal risk assessment with other novel combinations will need to be better understood.

On-going questions related to including nitroimidazoles into regimens will need to address several key factors including identification of the correct patient population [MDR-TB *versus* XDR-TB], understanding the effect of food intake on absorption, and the ideal method of constituting a regimen [individualised *versus* standardised] to prevent emergence of resistance (199).

Treatment Shortening Surrogates

There is no current consensus on endpoints that would allow easy comparability between different MDR-TB clinical trials. This step is key and harmonisation is required on definitions of treatment failure, unfavourable outcomes, and understanding loss to follow up and minimum acceptable adherence. Culture conversion should be clearly defined with uniformity on dealing with missed or contaminated samples and on documenting treatment modification across studies. Key to understanding treatment shortening is defining cure and length of follow-up particularly for agents with long half-lives such as Bedaquiline. Over all, a 6-month negative culture may be a reliable predictor of relapse-free cure in patients with drug-resistant TB (200).

Evolution to an all Oral, Injection Free, MDR-TB Regimen

South Africa is the first country to implement a standardized, all oral injection free regimen for the treatment of MDR-TB (118). This policy change is based on the observed superior treatment success rates and better adverse events profile of the bedaquiline-based shorter MDR-TB regimen when compared to the kanamycin-based regimen. However, the long-term impact of this policy change on the emergence of resistance to bedaquiline is unknown.

Several clinical trials including STREAM II, endTB, TB-Practecal and MDR-END are evaluating novel injection free regimen for M/XDR-TB. One such study is the randomised controlled trial New and Emerging Treatments for MDR-TB [NExT] (201) which is a prospective open-labelled randomised controlled trial that seeks to further reduce treatment duration by evaluating a completely new, injection-free, short-course regimen for MDR-TB. With over 100 patients randomised, this study seeks to compare a six-month five-drug regimen consisting of bedaqualine, linezolid, levofloxacin, pyrazinamide and either ethionamide, high-dose isoniazid or terizadone, depending on the presence of mutations in the *inhA* or *katG* genes [as determined by a LPA] with the conventional injection-based WHO shorter MDR-TB regimen of 12 months.

How can we Protect Novel Agents Against Developing Resistance?

It is clear that newer agents need to be introduced with a robust stewardship programme to prevent the development of acquired resistance. As MDR-TB treatment already has a high rate of treatment non-compliance there needs to be a renewed focus on psychosocial measures such as motivational interviewing and counselling for substance abuse and default. Measures such as tightened drug accountability, resistance monitoring and population PK monitoring of multiple agents needs to continue once novel regimens have attained regulatory approval.

PROGNOSIS

Globally, survival and treatment outcomes of DR-TB vary widely depending on geographical location, regimen choice, duration of treatment, and background prevalence of TB and HIV, but in general, correlate with the degree of drug resistance. The overall treatment outcomes are far from satisfactory: the WHO reports that of the estimated half a million MDR-TB patients started globally on treatment in 2009, only 48% were treated successfully (202). Treatment outcomes in XDR-TB are even worse; while the overall success rate for XDR-TB in a meta-analysis was reported to be 44% (123), additional resistance to second- and third-line TB medications beyond the minimum definition of XDR-TB was associated with further reductions in the likelihood of success. The cure rate in high-burden countries may be even lower: in South Africa, less than 20% of patients with XDR-TB, using non-bedaquiline and linezolid regimens culture-converted within six months of initiation of treatment, and this poor outcome was independent of HIV status (120). Lung function impairment and residual radiological sequelae are also more common in patients completing DR-TB treatment compared to those with DS-TB (203,204). These sequelae, together with other post-TB complications, like massive haemoptysis, aspergilloma, bronchiectasis, pneumothorax, bronchopleural fistula, tracheal or bronchial stenosis and empyema, are important contributors to chronic pulmonary disability due to TB.

PREVENTION

Active Case Finding and Contact Tracing

In countries with well performing TB programmes, it has been shown that patients with TB, even those who are smear positive, may be asymptomatic or minimally symptomatic and so do not seek medical attention (205). It, therefore, makes sense to reach out to high-risk patients to systematically look for TB. Active case finding [ACF] strives to ensure that active TB is detected as early as possible to reduce poor treatment outcomes and spread of disease.

However, there is limited or poor quality evidence that smear-microscopy-based active case finding detects earlier or less severe disease, or impacts disease burden or outcomes (206). Improved tools and approaches for active case finding are urgently required to minimise transmission and close the detection gap (207).

Several studies have suggested that mass population screening is expensive with an unfavourable risk benefit ratio and that it is much more cost effective to perform targeted screening of high-risk groups, e.g. close contacts in the home, school or workplace, HIV-infected persons, prisoners, miners especially silica-related, those with untreated fibrotic chest radiograph lesions, in high prevalence settings [>1%] those passively seeking health care, and actively in persons in shelters, slums and shanty towns where several risk factors predominate (206). The goal is to provide treatment to patients with active TB and chemoprophylaxis to those with latent TB infection [LTBI]. The main tools used for active case finding are symptom and radiographic screening (207). The predictive values of different screening algorithms have been published recently (207).

Active Case Finding for Drug-resistant Tuberculosis

Active case finding in DR-TB, when using culture, poses an added challenge in that the results of DST only become known 3–4 months after the initial sputum sample is taken. Polymerase chain reaction [PCR]-based diagnostic tests can shorten the delay and are cost effective when used in specific settings, such as, prisons in some countries (208). A strategy of screening communities at large using point of care GeneXpert MTB/RIF that is mounted in vehicles is currently being evaluated in ongoing studies. Modelling studies suggesting that point-of-care [POC] diagnostics could have transformative impact only if deployed in the context of targeted screening (209). However, little is known about the optimal strategies and utility of newer tools to screen for DR-TB.

Contact Tracing

General indications for contact tracing include sputum smear positive TB, and exposure involving persons living with HIV, and children under the age of 5 years (210). Studies have shown that contact tracing has an appreciable yield of about 4.5% [95% CI 4.3-4.8] for bacteriologically and clinically diagnosed TB in low- to middle-income countries (211). The progression to active TB among household contacts exposed to DS and MDR-TB cases have been shown to be comparable in previous studies, despite a longer duration of exposure with MDR-TB (212). Screening of household contacts of MDR and XDR-TB index cases in South Africa resulted in a MDR-TB and XDR-TB detection rate of nearly 2% in the contacts screened, in keeping with estimates for DS-TB (213). However, this is likely an under estimate since this study excluded enrollment of children who are more likely to progress to active TB. In countries with a high prevalence of HIV such as South Africa, the incidence rate of DR-TB was greater than 1700/100,000 individuals screened *versus* a community based rate of 45–65 cases/100000 (214). These high rates highlight the need to include ACF as part of the national TB control strategy as it provides an opportunity to prevent transmission. WHO recommends contact tracing for all close contacts of patients with DR-TB irrespective of smear status (210).

The general likelihood of transmission to contacts is dependent on several factors including smear positivity, cavitary disease, the closeness and intensity of the exposure, and the immune status of the host, amongst others (210). Thus, contacts should be risk stratified and screened using a combination of symptoms, chest radiograph and sputum culture/DST and/or Xpert MTB/RIF depending on local availability of these diagnostic tests. Those patients who are found to have active TB should be started on treatment based on their GeneXpert MTB/RIF or LPA results, if available. If immediate DST is unavailable and illness is severe then a case could be made for commencing the symptomatic contacts on treatment based on the DST pattern of the index patient (212). However, a study conducted in New Delhi showed that a majority of the contacts of MDR-TB actually had DS-TB (214). In settings where only conventional DST is available it is, therefore important to balance the risk of waiting for results [morbidity and mortality] to the potential toxicity from MDR-TB drugs (215,216). Symptomatic contacts whose work-up for TB is negative may be empirically treated for lower respiratory tract infection [LRTI], if indicated, with antibiotic that does not have efficacy against TB. Further investigations including bronchoscopy and/or chest computed tomography [CT] may be required.

The diagnosis of DR-TB in children can be challenging. Children under five years of age and/or children infected with HIV are at a particularly high risk of contracting TB (217). In addition to the diagnostic work up children should have a tuberculin skin test. Sputum induction and gastric aspirates are valuable tools as younger children often cannot expectorate a good sputum sample (218). It is import to remember that even if the work up for TB is negative the diagnosis of MDR-TB can be made clinically in a childhood contact if there are appropriate symptoms or radiological findings. In asymptomatic HIV-infected children or children under 5 years of age without radiological abnormalities suggestive of TB, and who are TST positive in the context of exposure to an MDR-TB index case, consideration should be given to treatment for presumed latent MDR-TB (219). Alternatively a decision may be taken to treat with isoniazid prophylaxis on the assumption that it is likely to be drug-sensitive LTBI (220). This decision should be guided by the clinical context [duration and intensity of exposure, age of the child, cavitation in the index case, HIV status, etc.], susceptibility pattern of the index case, and potential toxicity (221). If a decision is taken to administer preventative treatment for MDR-TB often two drugs are used and may include a combination selected from high-dose isoniazid, a fluoroquinolone, and ethambutol among others (219,221). Fluoroquinolone are thought to be relatively safe when used in children for TB treatment (222). The choices should reflect the local drug-susceptibility patterns and may be site or country specific. Generalised recommendations in this regards may not be appropriate (221). In older children who are HIV unin-fected preventative therapy is controversial (223) and close follow-up may be more a appropriate strategy (219,224).

INFECTION CONTROL

The reader is referred to the chapter *"Airborne infection control" [Chapter 56] for further details.*

In conclusion, although TB incidence has slowly declined in several parts of the world, DR-TB threatens to reverse the gains that have been made. Further study into the underlying pathogenesis of DR-TB will be critical in preventing the emergence of resistance with newer TB drugs, such as, bedaquiline, pretomanid and delamanid. Whilst better drug combinations and how they are delivered individual patients, together with therapeutic drug monitoring and pharmacogenomics can reduce the prevention of DR-TB and strengthening of NTP remains paramount. Without

the global reduction of the key driver of TB, including poverty, overcrowding, smoking, diabetes, exposure to biomass fuels, and HIV the problem of DR-TB will not be circumvented. Thus, like with DS-TB, control of DR-TB will only occur through global reductions in the level of poverty, overcrowding, increase funding for research and capacity development, strengthening of NTP, and political will.

REFERENCES

1. World Health Organization. Global tuberculosis report. Geneva: World Health Organisation; 2018.
2. Pooran A, Pieterson E, Davids M, Theron G, Dheda K. What is the cost of diagnosis and management of drug resistant tuberculosis in South Africa? PLoS One 2013;8:e54587.
3. Caminero JA. Multidrug-resistant tuberculosis: epidemiology, risk factors and case finding. Int J TB Lung Dis 2010;14:382-90.
4. Bateman C. Eastern Cape treatment dysfunction boosts virulent new XDR-TB strain. S Afr Med J 2015;105:165-7.
5. Andrews JR, Shah NS, Weissman D, Moll AP, Friedland G, Gandhi NR. Predictors of multidrug- and extensively drug-resistant tuberculosis in a high HIV prevalence community. PLoS One 2010;5:e15735.
6. Balaji V, Daley P, Anand AA, Sudarsanam T, Michael JS, Sahni RD, et al. Risk factors for MDR and XDR-TB in a tertiary referral hospital in India. PLoS One 2010;5:e9527.
7. Faustini A, Hall AJ, Perucci CA. Risk factors for multidrug resistant tuberculosis in Europe: a systematic review. Thorax 2006;61:158-63.
8. Skrahina A, Hurevich H, Zalutskaya A, Sahalchyk E, Astrauko A, Hoffner S, et al. Multidrug-resistant tuberculosis in Belarus: the size of the problem and associated risk factors. Bull World Health Organ 2013;91:36-45.
9. World Health Organization. Guidelines for the treatment of drug-susceptible tuberculosis and patient care, 2017 update. WHO/HTM/TB/2017.05. Geneva: World Health Organization; 2017.
10. Zhao P, Li XJ, Zhang SF, Wang XS, Liu CY. Social behaviour risk factors for drug resistant tuberculosis in mainland China: a meta-analysis. J Int Med Res 2012;40:436-45.
11. Kimerling ME, Slavuckij A, Chavers S, Peremtin GG, Tonkel T, Sirotkina O, et al. The risk of MDR-TB and polyresistant tuberculosis among the civilian population of Tomsk city, Siberia, 1999. Int J Tuberc Lung Dis 2003;7:866-72.
12. Ricks PM, Mavhunga F, Modi S, Indongo R, Zezai A, Lambert LA, et al. Characteristics of multidrug-resistant tuberculosis in Namibia. BMC Infect Dis 2012;12:385.
13. Fietta A, Cascina A, Meloni F, Morosini M, Casali L, Bono L, et al. A 10-year survey of Mycobacterium tuberculosis isolates in Pavia and their drug resistance: a comparison with other Italian reports. J Chemother 2002;14:33-40.
14. Klopper M, Warren RM, Hayes C, Gey van Pittius NC, Streicher EM, Müller B, et al. Emergence and spread of extensively and totally drug-resistant tuberculosis, South Africa. Emerg Infect Dis 2013;19:449-55.
15. Merker M, Blin C, Mona S, Duforet-Frebourg N, Lecher S, Willery E, et al. Evolutionary history and global spread of the Mycobacterium tuberculosis Beijing lineage. Nat Genet 2015;47:242-9.
16. Mokrousov I, Jiao WW, Sun GZ, Liu JW, Valcheva V, Li M, et al. Evolution of drug resistance in different sublineages of Mycobacterium tuberculosis Beijing genotype. Antimicrob Agents Chemother 2006;50:2820-3.
17. Dalton T, Cegielski P, Akksilp S, Asencios L, Campos Caoili J, Cho SN, et al. Prevalence of and risk factors for resistance to

second-line drugs in people with multidrug-resistant tuberculosis in eight countries: a prospective cohort study. Lancet 2012;380:1406-17.

18a. World Health Organization. Multidrug-/rifampicin-resistant TB [MDR/RR-TB]: Update 2017. Available at URL: http://www.who.int/tb/areas-of-work/drug-resistant-tb/MDR_TB_2017.pdf?ua=1. Accessed on August 29, 2018.

18b. D'souza DT, Mistry NF, Vira TS, Dholakia Y, Hoffner S, Pasvol G, et al. High levels of multidrug resistant tuberculosis in new and treatment-failure patients from the Revised National Tuberculosis Control Programme in an urban metropolis [Mumbai] in Western India. BMC Public Health 2009;9:211.

19. Jain A, Mondal R, Prasad R, Singh K, Ahuja RC. Prevalence of multidrug resistant Mycobacterium tuberculosis in Lucknow, Uttar Pradesh. Indian J Med Res 2008;128:300-6.

20. Jain S, Rodrigues C, Mehta A, Uwadia ZF. High Prevalence of XDR-TB from a tertiary care hospital in India. Am J Respir Crit Care Med 2007;175:A510.

21. Mondal R, Jain A. Extensively drug-resistant Mycobacterium tuberculosis, India. Emerg Infect Dis 2007;13:1429-31.

22. Thomas A, Ramachandran R, Rehaman F, Jaggarajamma K, Santha T, Selvakumar N, et al. Management of multi drug resistance tuberculosis in the field: Tuberculosis Research Centre experience. Indian J Tuberc 2007;54:117-24.

23. Singh S, Sankar MM, Gopinath K. High rate of extensively drug-resistant tuberculosis in Indian AIDS patients. AIDS 2007;21:2345-7.

24. Sharma SK, George N, Kadhiravan T, Saha PK, Mishra HK, Hanif M. Prevalence of extensively drug-resistant tuberculosis among patients with multidrug-resistant tuberculosis: a retrospective hospital-based study. Indian J Med Res 2009;130:392-5.

25. Udwadia ZF, Amale RA, Ajbani KK, Rodrigues C. Totally drug-resistant tuberculosis in India. Clin Infect Dis 2012;54:579-81.

26. Sharma SK, Chaubey J, Singh BK, Sharma R, Mittal A, Sharma A. Drug resistance pattern among extrapulmonary tuberculosis cases in a tertiary care center in North India. Int J Tuberc Lung Dis 2017;21:1112-7.

27. Dheda K, Gumbo T, Gandhi NR, Murray M, Theron G, Udwadia Z, et al. Global control of tuberculosis: from extensively drug-resistant to untreatable tuberculosis. Lancet Respir Med 2014;2:321-38.

28. Gagneux S, Long CD, Small PM, Van T, Schoolnik GK, Bohannan BJ. The competitive cost of antibiotic resistance in Mycobacterium tuberculosis. Science 2006;312:1944-6.

29. Uys PW, Warren R, van Helden PD, Murray M, Victor TC. Potential of rapid diagnosis for controlling drug-susceptible and drug-resistant tuberculosis in communities where Mycobacterium tuberculosis infections are highly prevalent. J Clin Microbiol 2009;47:1484-90.

30. Kamerbeek J. Simultaneous detection and strain differentiation of Mycobacterium tuberculosis for diagnosis and epidemiology. J Clin Microbiol 1997;35:907-14.

31. van Embden JD, Cave MD, Crawford JT, Dale JW, Eisenach KD, Gicquel B, et al. Strain identification of Mycobacterium tuberculosis by DNA fingerprinting: recommendations for a standardized methodology. J Clin Microbiol 1993;31:406-9.

32. Allix C, Supply P, Fauville-Dufaux M. Utility of fast mycobacterial interspersed repetitive unit-variable number tandem repeat genotyping in clinical mycobacteriological analysis. Clin Infect Dis 2004;39:783-9.

33. Streicher EM, Müller B, Chihota V, Mlambo C, Tait M, Pillay M, et al. Emergence and treatment of multidrug resistant [MDR] and extensively drug-resistant [XDR] tuberculosis in South Africa. Infect Gen Evol 2012;12:686-94.

34a. Dheda K, Limberis JD, Pietersen E, Phelan J, Esmail A, Lesosky M, et al. Outcomes, infectiousness, and transmission dynamics of patients with extensively drug-resistant tuberculosis and home-discharged patients with programmatically incurable tuberculosis: a prospective cohort study. Lancet Respir Med 2017;5:269-81.

34b. Gandhi NR, Moll A, Sturm AW, Pawinski R, Govender T, Lalloo U, et al. Extensively drug-resistant tuberculosis as a cause of death in patients co-infected with tuberculosis and HIV in a rural area of South Africa. Lancet 2006;368:1575-80.

35. Walker TM, Lalor MK, Broda A, Saldana Ortega L, Morgan M, Parker L, et al. Assessment of Mycobacterium tuberculosis transmission in Oxfordshire, UK, 2007-12, with whole pathogen genome sequences: an observational study. Lancet Respir Med 2014;2:285-92.

36. Walker TM, Kohl TA, Omar SV, Hedge J, Del Ojo Elias C, Bradley P, et al. Whole-genome sequencing to delineate Mycobacterium tuberculosis outbreaks: a retrospective observational study. Lancet Infect Dis 2013;13:137-46.

37. Gardy JL, Johnston JC, Ho Sui SJ, Cook VJ, Shah L, Brodkin E, et al. Whole-genome sequencing and social-network analysis of a tuberculosis outbreak. N Engl J Med 2011;364:730-9.

38. Guerra-Assunção JA, Crampin AC, Houben RM, Mzembe T, Mallard K, Coll F, et al. Large-scale whole genome sequencing of M. tuberculosis provides insights into transmission in a high prevalence area. ELife 2015;4:e05166.

39. Bryant JM, Harris SR, Parkhill J, Dawson R, Diacon AH, van Helden P, et al. Whole-genome sequencing to establish relapse or re-infection with Mycobacterium tuberculosis: a retrospective observational study. Lancet Respir Med 2013;1:786-92.

40a. Shah NS, Auld SC, Brust JCM, Mathema B, Ismail N, Moodley P, et al. Transmission of extensively drug-resistant tuberculosis in South Africa. N Engl J Med 2017;376: 243-53.

40b. Basu S, Andrews JR, Poolman EM, Gandhi NR, Shah NS, Moll A, et al. Prevention of nosocomial transmission of extensively drug-resistant tuberculosis in rural South African district hospitals: an epidemiological modelling study. Lancet 2007;370:1500-7.

41. Basu S, Friedland GH, Medlock J, Andrews JR, Shah NS, Gandhi NR, et al. Averting epidemics of extensively drug-resistant tuberculosis. Proc Natl Acad Sci USA 2009;106:7672-7.

42. Alland D, Kalkut GE, Moss AR, McAdam RA, Hahn JA, Bosworth W, et al. Transmission of tuberculosis in New York City—an analysis by DNA fingerprinting and conventional epidemiologic methods. N Engl J Med 1994;330:1710-6.

43. Small PM, Hopewell PC, Singh SP, Paz A, Parsonnet J, Ruston DC, et al. The epidemiology of tuberculosis in San Francisco—a population-based study using conventional and molecular methods. N Engl J Med 1994;330:1703-9.

44. Lloyd-Smith JO, Schreiber SJ, Kopp PE, Getz W. Superspreading and the effect of individual variation on disease emergence. Nature 2005;438:355-9.

45. Jones-López EC, Namugga O, Mumbowa F, Ssebidandi M, Mbabazi O, Moine S, et al. Cough aerosols of Mycobacterium tuberculosis predict new infection: a household contact study. Am J Respir Crit Care Med 2013;187:1007-15.

46. David HL. Probability distribution of drug-resistant mutants in unselected populations of Mycobacterium tuberculosis. Appl Microbiol 1970;20:810-4.

47. Calver AD, Falmer AA, Murray M, Strauss OJ, Streicher EM, Hanekom M, et al. Emergence of increased resistance and extensively drug-resistant tuberculosis despite treatment adherence, South Africa. Emerg Infect Dis 2010;16:264-71.

48. Pasipanodya JG, Gumbo T. A new evolutionary and pharmacokinetic-pharmacodynamic scenario for rapid emergence

of resistance to single and multiple anti-tuberculosis drugs. Curr Opin Pharmacol 2011;11:457-63.

49. Srivastava S, Musuka S, Sherman C, Meek C, Leff R, Gumbo T. Efflux-pump-derived multiple drug resistance to ethambutol monotherapy in Mycobacterium tuberculosis and the pharmacokinetics and pharmacodynamics of ethambutol. J Infect Dis 2010;201:1225-31.

50. Schmalstieg AM, Srivastava S, Belkaya S, Deshpande D, Meek C, Leff R, et al. The antibiotic resistance arrow of time: efflux pump induction is a general first step in the evolution of mycobacterial drug resistance. Antimicrob Agents Chemother 2012;56:4806-15.

51. Louw GE, Warren RM, Gey van Pittius NC, Leon R, Jimenez A, Hernandez-Pando R, et al. Rifampicin reduces susceptibility to ofloxacin in rifampicin-resistant Mycobacterium tuberculosis through efflux. Am J Respir Crit Care Med 2011;184:269-76.

52. Machado D, Couto I, Perdigão J, Rodrigues L, Portugal I, Baptista P, et al. Contribution of efflux to the emergence of isoniazid and multidrug resistance in Mycobacterium tuberculosis. PLoS One 2012;7:e34538.

53. Baquero F. Low-level antibacterial resistance: a gateway to clinical resistance. Drug Resist Updat 2001;4:93-105.

54. Dharmadhikari AS, Kabadi M, Gerety B, Hickey AJ, Fourie PB, Nardell E. Phase I, single-dose, dose-escalating study of inhaled dry powder capreomycin: a new approach to therapy of drug-resistant tuberculosis. Antimicrob Agents Chemother 2013;57:2613-9.

55. Ford CB, Shah RR, Maeda MK, Gagneux S, Murray MB, Cohen T, et al. Mycobacterium tuberculosis mutation rate estimates from different lineages predict substantial differences in the emergence of drug-resistant tuberculosis. Nature Genet 2013;45:784-90.

56. Borrell S, Gagneux S. Infectiousness, reproductive fitness and evolution of drug-resistant Mycobacterium tuberculosis. Int J Tuberc Lung Dis 2009;13:1456-66.

57. Lari N, Rindi L, Bonanni D, Tortoli E, Garzelli C. Mutations in mutT genes of Mycobacterium tuberculosis isolates of Beijing genotype. J Med Microbiol 2006;55:599-603.

58. Comas I, Borrell S, Roetzer A, Rose G, Malla B, Kato-Maeda M, et al. Whole-genome sequencing of rifampicin-resistant Mycobacterium tuberculosis strains identifies compensatory mutations in RNA polymerase genes. Nature Genet 2012;44:106-10.

59. Sun G, Luo T, Yang C, Dong X, Li J, Zhu Y, et al. Dynamic population changes in Mycobacterium tuberculosis during acquisition and fixation of drug resistance in patients. J Infect Dis 2012;206:1724-33.

60. Dheda K, Schwander SK, Zhu B, van Zyl-Smit RN, Zhang Y. The immunology of tuberculosis: from bench to bedside. Respirology 2010;15:433-50.

61. Borrell S, Gagneux S. Strain diversity, epistasis and the evolution of drug resistance in Mycobacterium tuberculosis. Clin Microbiol Infect 2011;17:815-20.

62. Müller B, Borrell S, Rose G, Gagneux S. The heterogeneous evolution of multidrug-resistant Mycobacterium tuberculosis. Trends Genet 2013;29:160-9.

63. Jacobson KR, Theron D, Kendall EA, Franke MF, Barnard M, van Helden, et al. Implementation of GenoType® MTBDRplus reduces time to multidrug-resistant tuberculosis therapy initiation in South Africa. Clin Infect Dis 2013;56:503-8.

64. Banerjee R, Allen J, Lin SY, Westenhouse J, Desmond E, Schecter GF, et al. Rapid drug susceptibility testing with a molecular beacon assay is associated with earlier diagnosis and treatment of multidrug-resistant tuberculosis in California. J Clin Microbiol 2010;48:3779-81.

65. Cox H, Hughes J, Daniels J, Azevedo V, McDermid C, Poolman M, et al. Community-based treatment of drug-resistant tuberculosis in Khayelitsha, South Africa. Int J Tuberc Lung Dis 2014;18:441-8.

66. Loveday M, Wallengren K, Voce A, Margot B, Reddy T, Master I, et al. Comparing early treatment outcomes of MDR-TB in decentralised and centralised settings in KwaZulu-Natal, South Africa. Int J Tuberc Lung Dis 2012;16:209-15.

67. Dave P, Vadera B, Kumar AM, Chinnakali P, Modi B, Solanki, et al. Has introduction of rapid drug susceptibility testing at diagnosis impacted treatment outcomes among previously treated tuberculosis patients in Gujarat, India? PLoS One 2015;10:e0121996.

68. Uys PW, Warren RM, van Helden PD. A threshold value for the time delay to TB diagnosis. PLoS One 2007;2:e757.

69. Heysell SK, Houpt ER. The future of molecular diagnostics for drug-resistant tuberculosis. Expert Rev Mol Diagn 2012;12:395-405.

70. Pfyffer G, Welscher H, Kissling P, Cieslak C, Casal MJ, Gutierrez J, et al. Comparison of the Mycobacteria Growth Indicator Tube [MGIT] with radiometric and solid culture for recovery of acid-fast bacilli. J Clin Microbiol 1997;35:364.

71. World Health Organization. Guidelines for drug susceptibility testing for second line anti-tuberculosis drugs for DOTS-PLUS. WHO/CDS/TB/2001.288. Geneva: World Health Organization; 2001.

72. Lazarus R, Kalaiselvan S, John K, Michael J. Evaluation of the microscopic observational drug susceptibility assay for rapid and efficient diagnosis of multi-drug resistant tuberculosis. Indian J Med Microbiol 2012;30:64-8.

73. Scarparo C, Ricordi P, Ruggiero G, Piccoli P. Evaluation of the fully automated BACTEC MGIT 960 system for testing susceptibility of Mycobacterium tuberculosis to pyrazinamide, streptomycin, isoniazid, rifampin, and ethambutol and comparison with the radiometric BACTEC 460TB method. J Clin Microbiol 2004;42:1109-14.

74. Rüsch-Gerdes S, Pfyffer GE, Casal M, Chadwick M, Siddiqi S. Multicenter laboratory validation of the BACTEC MGIT 960 technique for testing susceptibilities of Mycobacterium tuberculosis to classical second-line drugs and newer antimicrobials. J Clin Microbiol 2006;44:688-92.

75. Krüüner A, Yates MD, Drobniewski FA. Evaluation of MGIT 960-based antimicrobial testing and determination of critical concentrations of first-and second-line antimicrobial drugs with drug-resistant clinical strains of Mycobacterium tuberculosis. J Clin Microbiol 2006;44:811-8.

76. World Health Organization. Use of liquid TB culture and drug susceptibility testing [DST] in low- and medium-income settings. Summary report of the Expert Group Meeting on the Use of Liquid Culture Media. Geneva: World Health Organization; 2007.

77. Minion J, Leung E, Menzies D, Pai M. Microscopic-observation drug susceptibility and thin layer agar assays for the detection of drug resistant tuberculosis: a systematic review and meta-analysis. Lancet Infect Dis 2010;10:688-98.

78. Martin L, Coronel J, Faulx D, Valdez M, Metzler M, Crudder C, et al. A Field Evaluation of the Hardy TB MODS Kit™ for the Rapid Phenotypic diagnosis of tuberculosis and multi-Drug resistant tuberculosis. PLoS One 2014;9:e107258.

79. World Health Organization. Policy statement. Noncommercial culture and drug-susceptibility testing methods for screening patients at risk for multidrug-resistant tuberculosis. Geneva: World Health Organization; 2010.

80. Huang Z, Qin C, Du J, Luo Q, Wang Y, Zhang W, et al. Evaluation of the microscopic observation drug susceptibility assay for the rapid detection of MDR-TB and XDR-TB in China: a prospective multicentre study. J Antimicrob Chemother 2015;70:456-62.

81. Trollip AP, Moore D, Coronel J, Caviedes L, Klages S, Victor T, et al. Second-line drug susceptibility breakpoints for Mycobacterium tuberculosis using the MODS assay. Int J Tuberc Lung Dis 2014;18:227-32.

82. Steingart K, Sohn H, Schiller I, Kloda LA, Boehme CC, Pai M, et al. Xpert® MTB/RIF assay for pulmonary tuberculosis and rifampicin resistance in adults. Cochrane Database Syst Rev 2013;1:CD009593.

83. UNITAID. Tuberculosis diagnostic technology landscape. Available from URL: http://www.stoptb.org/wg/new_diagnostics/assets/documents/UNITAID-Tuberculosis-Landscape_2014.pdf. Accessed on September 13, 2017.

84. Theron G, Pinto L, Peter J, Mishra HM, Mishra HK, Zyl-Smit v R, et al. The use of an automated quantitative polymerase chain reaction [Xpert MTB/RIF] to predict the sputum smear status of tuberculosis patients. Clin Infect Dis 2012;54:384-8.

85. Hanrahan CF, Theron G, Bassett J, Dheda K, Scott L, Stevens W, et al. Xpert MTB/RIF as a measure of sputum bacillary burden: variation by HIV status and immunosuppression. Am J Respir Crit Care Med 2014;189:1426-34.

86. Ling DI, Zwerling AA, Pai M. GenoType MTBDR assays for the diagnosis of multidrug-resistant tuberculosis: a meta-analysis. Eur Respir J 2008;32:1165-74.

87. World Health Organization. Policy statement. Molecular line probe assays for rapid screening of patients at risk of multidrug-resistant tuberculosis [MDR-TB]. Geneva: World Health Organization; 2008.

88. Kaswa MK, Aloni M, Nkuku L, Bakoko B, Lebeke R, Nzita A, et al. Pseudo-outbreak of pre-extensively drug-resistant [Pre-XDR] tuberculosis in Kinshasa: collateral damage caused by false detection of fluoroquinolone resistance by GenoType MTBDRsl. J Clin Microbiol 2014;52:2876-80.

89. Hu S, Li G, Li H, Liu X, Niu J, Quan S, et al. Rapid detection of isoniazid resistance in Mycobacterium tuberculosis isolates by use of real-time-PCR-based melting curve analysis. J Clin Microbiol 2014;52:1644-52.

90. Liu J, Yue J, Yan Z, Han M, Han Z, Jin L, et al. Performance assessment of the Capital Bio mycobacterium identification array system for identification of mycobacteria. J Clin Microbiol 2012;50:76-80.

91. Wang F, Massire C, Li H, Cummins LL, Li F, Jin J, et al. Molecular characterization of drug-resistant Mycobacterium tuberculosis isolates circulating in China by Multilocus PCR and electrospray ionization mass spectrometry. J Clin Microbiol 2011;49:2719-21.

92. Massire C, Ivy CA, Lovari R, Kurepina N, Li H, Blyn LB, et al. Simultaneous identification of mycobacterial isolates to the species level and determination of tuberculosis drug resistance by PCR followed by electrospray ionization mass spectrometry. J Clin Microbiol 2011;49:908-17.

93. Linger Y, Kukhtin A, Golova J, Perov A, Lambarqui A, Bryant L, et al. Simplified microarray system for simultaneously detecting rifampin, isoniazid, ethambutol, and streptomycin resistance markers in Mycobacterium tuberculosis. J Clin Microbiol 2014;52:2100-7.

94. Shah NS, Moodley P, Babaria P, Moodley S, Ramtahal M, Richardson J, et al. Rapid diagnosis of tuberculosis and multidrug resistance by the microscopic-observation drug-susceptibility assay. Am J Respir Crit Care Med 2011;183:1427-33.

95. Martin A, Paasch F, Docx S, Fissette K, Imperiale B, Ribón W, et al. Multicentre laboratory validation of the colorimetric redox indicator [CRI] assay for the rapid detection of extensively drug-resistant [XDR] Mycobacterium tuberculosis. J Antimicrob Chemother 2011;66:827-33.

96. Somoskovi A, Clobridge A, Larsen SC, Sinyavskiy O, Surucuoglu S, Parsons LM, et al. Does the MGIT 960 system improve the turnaround times for growth detection and susceptibility testing of the Mycobacterium tuberculosis Complex? J Clin Microbiol 2006;44:2314-5.

97. Boehme CC, Nabeta P, Hillemann D, Nicol MP, Shenai S, Krapp F, et al. Rapid molecular detection of tuberculosis and rifampin resistance. N Engl J Med 2010;363:1005-15.

98. Theron G, Zijenah L, Chanda D, Clowes P, Rachow A, Lesosky M, et al. Feasibility, accuracy, and clinical effect of point-of-care Xpert MTB/RIF testing for tuberculosis in primary-care settings in Africa: a multicentre, randomised, controlled trial. Lancet 2013;383:424-35.

99. World Health Organization. Automated real-time nucleic acid amplification technology for rapid and simultaneous detection of tuberculosis and rifampicin resistance: Xpert MTB/RIF system for the diagnosis of pulmonary and extrapulmonary TB in adults and children. WHO/HTM/TB/2013.14. Geneva: World Health Organization; 2013.

100. Federal Drug Administration. Press statement. FDA permits marketing of first U.S. test labeled for simultaneous detection of tuberculosis bacteria and resistance to the antibiotic rifampin. Available from URL: http://www.fda.gov/NewsEvents/Newsroom/PressAnnouncements/ucm362602.htm. Accessed on January 13, 2018.

101. Steingart KR, Schiller I, Horne DJ, Pai M, Boehme CC, Dendukuri N. Xpert® MTB/RIF assay for pulmonary tuberculosis and rifampicin resistance in adults. Cochrane Database Syst Rev 2014;1:CD009593.

102. Jenkins HE, Zignol M, Cohen T. Quantifying the burden and trends of isoniazid resistant tuberculosis, 1994–2009. PLoS One 2011;6:e22927.

103. World Health Organization. Roadmap for Rolling Out Xpert MTB/RIF for Rapid Diagnosis of TB and MDR-TB Geneva: World Health Organization; 2010.

104. Trajman A, Durovni B, Saraceni V, Cordeiro-Santos M, Cobelens F, van den Hof S. High positive predictive value of Xpert in a low rifampicin resistance prevalence setting. Eur Respir J 2014;44:1711-3.

105. Osman M, Simpson JA, Caldwell J, Bosman M, Nicol MP. GeneXpert MTB/RIF version G4 for identification of rifampin-resistant tuberculosis in a programmatic setting. J Clin Microbiol 2014;52:635-7.

106a. Dorman SE, Schumacher SG, Alland D, Nabeta P, Armstrong DT, King B, et al. Xpert MTB/RIF Ultra for detection of Mycobacterium tuberculosis and rifampicin resistance: a prospective multicentre diagnostic accuracy study. Lancet Infect Dis 2018;18:76-84.

106b. Barnard M, van Pittius NCG, van Helden P, Bosman M, Coetzee G, Warren R. Diagnostic performance of Genotype® MTBDRplus Version 2 line probe assay is equivalent to the Xpert® MTB/RIF assay. J Clin Microbiol 2012;50:3712-6.

107. Crudu V, Stratan E, Romancenco E, Allerheiligen V, Hillemann A, Moraru N. First evaluation of an improved assay for molecular genetic detection of tuberculosis as well as rifampin and isoniazid resistances. J Clin Microbiol 2012;50:1264-9.

108a. Revised National Tuberculosis Control Programme, Directorate General of Health Services, Ministry of Health and Family Welfare, Government of India. Guidelines on programmatic management of drug-resistant tuberculosis in India 2017. New Delhi: World Health Organization, Country Office for India; 2017.

108b. Georghiou SB, Magana M, Garfein RS, Catanzaro DG, Catanzaro A, Rodwell TC. Evaluation of genetic mutations associated with Mycobacterium tuberculosis resistance to amikacin, kanamycin and capreomycin: a systematic review. PloS One 2012;7:e33275.

109. Theron G, Peter J, Richardson M, Barnard M, Donegan S, Warren R, et al. The diagnostic accuracy of the GenoType[®] MTBDRsl assay for the detection of resistance to second-line anti-tuberculosis drugs. Cochrane Database Syst Rev 2014;10:CD010705.

110. Witney AA, Gould KA, Arnold A, Coleman D, Delgado R, Dhillon J, et al. Clinical application of whole-genome sequencing to inform treatment for multidrug-resistant tuberculosis cases. J Clin Microbiol 2015;53:1473-83.

111. Votintseva AA, Pankhurst LJ, Anson LW, Morgan MR, Gascoyne-Binzi D, Walker TM, et al. Mycobacterial DNA extraction for whole-genome sequencing from early positive liquid [MGIT] cultures. J Clin Microbiol 2015;53:1137-43.

112. Orenstein EW, Basu S, Shah NS, Andrews JR, Friedland GH, Moll AP, et al. Treatment outcomes among patients with multidrug-resistant tuberculosis: systematic review and meta-analysis. Lancet Infect Dis 2009;9:153-61.

113. Naidoo P, du Toit E, Dunbar R, Lombard C, Caldwell J, Detjen A, et al. A comparison of multidrug-resistant tuberculosis treatment commencement times in MDRTBPlus line probe assay and Xpert® MTB/RIF-based algorithms in a routine operational setting in Cape Town. PloS One 2014;9:e103328.

114. Kliiman K, Altraja A. Predictors of extensively drug-resistant pulmonary tuberculosis. Ann Intern Med 2009;150:766-75.

115. World Health Organization. Treatment guidelines for drug-resistant tuberculosis. 2016 Update. Geneva: World Health Organization; 2016.

116a. Esmail A, Sabur NF, Okpechi I, Dheda K. Management of drug-resistant tuberculosis in special sub-populations including those with HIV co-infection, pregnancy, diabetes, organ-specific dysfunction, and in the critically ill. J Thorac Dis 2018;10:3102-18.

116b. Schecter GF, Peloquin CA. Medication fact sheets. Imipenem/cilastatin. In: Drug-Resistant tuberculosis: a survival guide for clinicians. Curry International Tuberculosis Center and California Department of Public Health, 2016, Third Edition. Available at URL: http://www.currytbcenter.ucsf.edu/sites/default/files/tb_sg3_chap5_medications.pdf. Accessed on December 24, 2018.

117a. World Health organization. Rapid Communication. Key changes to treatment of multidrug- and rifampicin-resistant tuberculosis [MDR/RR-TB]. WHO/CDS/TB/2018.18. Geneva: World Health organization; 2018.

117b. World Health Organization. WHO treatment guidelines for multidrug- and rifampicin-resistant tuberculosis 2018 update. Pre-final text. WHO/CDS/TB/2018.15. Geneva: World Health Organization; 2018. Available at URL: https://www.who.int/tb/areas-of-work/drug-resistant-tb/guideline-update2018/en/. Accessed on December 29, 2018.

118. New bedaquiline data shows reduction in TB mortality. Available at URL: http://www.tbonline.info/media/uploads/documents/new_bedaquiline_data_shows_reduction_in_tb_mortality_cases.pdf. Accessed on August 31, 2018.

119. Olayanju O, Limberis J, Esmail A, Oelofse S, Gina P, Pietersen E, et al. Long-term bedaquiline-related treatment outcomes in patients with extensively drug-resistant tuberculosis from South Africa. Eur Respir J 2018;51[5].pii:1800544.

120. Dheda K, Shean K, Zumla A, Badri M, Streicher EM, Page-Shipp L, et al. Early treatment outcomes and HIV status of patients with extensively drug-resistant tuberculosis in South Africa: a retrospective cohort study. Lancet 2010;375:1798-807.

121. Sotgiu G, Ferrara G, Matteelli A, Richardson MD, Centis R, Ruesch-Gerdes S, et al. Epidemiology and clinical management of XDR-TB: a systematic review by TBNET. Eur Respir J 2009;33: 871-81.

122. Kam KM, Yip CW, Cheung TL, Tang HS, Leung OC, Chan MY. Stepwise decrease in moxifloxacin susceptibility amongst clinical isolates of multidrug-resistant Mycobacterium tuberculosis: correlation with ofloxacin susceptibility. Microb Drug Resist 2006;12:7-11.

123. Jacobson KR, Tierney DB, Jeon CY, Mitnick CD, Murray MB. Treatment outcomes among patients with extensively drug-resistant tuberculosis: systematic review and meta-analysis. Clin Infect Dis 2010;51:6-14.

124. Sirgel FA, Donald PR, Odhiambo J, Githui W, Umapathy KC, Paramasivan CN, et al. A multicentre study of the early bactericidal activity of anti-tuberculosis drugs. J Antimicrob Chemother 2000;45:859-70.

125. Jayaram R, Shandil RK, Gaonkar S, Kaur P, Suresh BL, Mahesh BN, et al. Isoniazid pharmacokinetics-pharmacodynamics in an aerosol infection model of tuberculosis. Antimicrob Agents Chemother 2004;48:2951-7.

126. de Steenwinkel JE, de Knegt GJ, ten Kate MT, van Belkum A, Verbrugh HA, Kremer K, et al. Time-kill kinetics of anti-tuberculosis drugs, and emergence of resistance, in relation to metabolic activity of Mycobacterium tuberculosis. J Antimicrob Chemother 2010;65:2582-9.

127. Katiyar SK, Bihari S, Prakash S, Mamtani M, Kulkarni H. A randomised controlled trial of high-dose isoniazid adjuvant therapy for multidrug-resistant tuberculosis. Int J Tuberc Lung Dis 2008;12:139-45.

128. Tang S, Yao L, Hao X, Zhang X, Liu G, Liu X, et al. Efficacy, safety and tolerability of linezolid for the treatment of XDR-TB: a study in China. Eur Respir J 2015;45:161-70.

129. Zhang X, Falagas ME, Vardakas KZ, Wang R, Qin R, Wang J, Liu Y. Systematic review and meta-analysis of the efficacy and safety of therapy with linezolid containing regimens in the treatment of multidrug-resistant and extensively drug-resistant tuberculosis. J Thorac Dis 2015;7:603-15.

130. Wasserman S, Meintjes G, Maartens G. Linezolid in the treatment of drug-resistant tuberculosis: the challenge of its narrow therapeutic index. Expert Rev Anti Infect Ther 2016;14:901-15.

131. Song T, Lee M, Jeon HS, Park Y, Dodd LE, Dartois V, et al. Linezolid trough concentrations correlate with mitochondrial toxicity-related adverse events in the treatment of chronic extensively drug-resistant tuberculosis. EBioMedicine 2015;2:1627-33.

132. Srivastava S, Magombedze G, Koeuth T, Sherman C, Pasipanodya JG, Raj P, et al. Linezolid dose that maximizes sterilizing effect while minimizing toxicity and resistance emergence for tuberculosis. Antimicrob Agents Chemother 2017;61.pii: e00751-17.

133. Nuermberger E. Evolving strategies for dose optimization of linezolid for treatment of tuberculosis. Int J Tuberc Lung Dis 2016;20:48-51.

134. Ramírez-Lapausa M, Pascual Pareja JF, Carrillo Gómez R, Martínez-Prieto M, González-Ruano Pérez P, Noguerado Asensio A. Retrospective study of tolerability and efficacy of linezolid in patients with multidrug-resistant tuberculosis [1998-2014]. Enferm Infecc Microbiol Clin 2016;34:85-90.

135. Hartkoorn RC, Uplekar S, Cole ST. Cross-resistance between clofazimine and bedaquiline through upregulation of MmpL5 in Mycobacterium tuberculosis. Antimicrob Agents Chemother 2014;58:2979-81.

136. Nathanson E, Gupta R, Huamani P, Leimane V, Pasechnikov AD, Tupasi TE, et al. Adverse events in the treatment of multidrug-resistant tuberculosis: results from the DOTS-Plus initiative. Int J Tuberc Lung Dis 2004;8:1382-4.

137. Shin SS, Pasechnikov AD, Gelmanova IY, Peremitin GG, Strelis AK, Mishustin S, et al. Adverse reactions among patients being treated for MDR-TB in Tomsk, Russia. Int J Tuberc Lung Dis 2007;11:1314-20.

138. Törün T, Güngör G, Ozmen I, Bölükbaşi Y, Maden E, Biçakçi B, et al. Side effects associated with the treatment of multidrug-resistant tuberculosis. Int J Tuberc Lung Dis 2005;9:1373-7.

139. Shean K, Streicher E, Pieterson E, Symons G, van Zyl Smit R, Theron G, et al. Drug-associated adverse events and their relationship with outcomes in patients receiving treatment for extensively drug-resistant tuberculosis in South Africa. PLoS One 2013;8:e63057.

140. Harris T, Bardien S, Schaaf HS, Petersen L, De Jong G, Fagan JJ. Aminoglycoside-induced hearing loss in HIV-positive and HIV-negative multidrug-resistant tuberculosis patients. S Afr Med J 2012;102:363-6.

141. Kempker RR, Vashakidze S, Solomonia N, Dzidzikashvili N, Blumberg HM. Surgical treatment of drug-resistant tuberculosis. Lancet Infect Dis 2012;12:157-66.

142. Lalloo UG, Naidoo R, Ambaram A. Recent advances in the medical and surgical treatment of multi-drug resistant tuberculosis. Curr Opin Pulm Med 2006;12:179-85.

143. Worley MV, Estrada SJ. Bedaquiline: a novel antitubercular agent for the treatment of multidrug-resistant tuberculosis. Pharmacotherapy 2014;34:1187-97.

144. Zhang C, Wang W, Zhou M, Han Y, Xie J, Qiu Z, et al. The interaction of CD4 T-cell count and nevirapine hepatotoxicity in China: a change in national treatment guidelines may be warranted. J Acquir Immune Defic Syndr 2013;62:540-5.

145. De Lazzari E, Leon A, Arnaiz JA, Martinez E, Knobel H, Negredo E, et al. Hepatotoxicity of nevirapine in virologically suppressed patients according to gender and CD4 cell counts. HIV Med 2008;9:221-6.

146. Fortun J, Martin-Davila P, Navas E, Pérez-Elías MJ, Cobo J, Tato M, et al. Linezolid for the treatment of multidrug-resistant tuberculosis. J Antimicrob Chemother 2005;56:180-5.

147. Senneville E, Legout L, Valette M, Yazdanpanah Y, Beltrand E, Caillaux M, et al. Effectiveness and tolerability of prolonged linezolid treatment for chronic osteomyelitis: a retrospective study. Clin Therapeutics 2006;28:1155-63.

148. Gerson SL, Kaplan SL, Bruss JB, Le V, Arellano FM, Hafkin B, et al. Hematologic effects of linezolid: summary of clinical experience. Antimicrob Agents Chemother 2002;46:2723-6.

149. Anger HA, Dworkin F, Sharma S, Munsiff SS, Nilsen DM, Ahuja SD et al. Linezolid use for treatment of multidrug-resistant and extensively drug-resistant tuberculosis, New York City, 2000-06. J Antimicrob Chemother 2010;65:775-83.

150. Koh WJ, Kang YR, Jeon K, Kwon OJ, Lyu J, Kim WS et al. Daily 300 mg dose of linezolid for multidrug-resistant and extensively drug-resistant tuberculosis: updated analysis of 51 patients. The J Antimicrob Chemother 2012;67:1503-7.

151. Sotgiu G, Centis R, D'Ambrosio L, Alffenaar JW, Anger HA, Caminero JA, et al. Efficacy, safety and tolerability of linezolid containing regimens in treating MDR-TB and XDR-TB: systematic review and meta-analysis. Eur Respir J 2012;40:1430-42.

152. Centers for Disease Control and Prevention. Provisional CDC guidelines for the use and safety monitoring of bedaquiline fumarate [Sirturo] for the treatment of multidrug-resistant tuberculosis. MMWR Recomm Rep 2013;62[RR-09]:1-12.

153. Mehrzad R, Barza M. Weighing the adverse cardiac effects of fluoroquinolones: a risk perspective. J Clin Pharmacol 2015; 55:1198-206.

154. Stancampiano FF, Palmer WC, Getz TW, Serra-Valentin NA, Sears SP, Seeger KM, et al. Rare incidence of ventricular tachycardia and torsades de pointes in hospitalized patients with prolonged QT who later received levofloxacin: a retrospective study. Mayo Clin Proc 2015;90:606-12.

155. Im JH, Baek JH, Kwon HY, Lee JS. Incidence and risk factors of linezolid-induced lactic acidosis. Int J Infect Dis 2015;31:47-52.

156. Roongruangpitayakul C, Chuchottaworn C. Outcomes of MDR/XDR-TB patients treated with linezolid: experience in Thailand. J Med Assoc Thai 2013;96:1273-82.

157. Marrone MT, Venkataramanan V, Goodman M, Hill AC, Jereb JA, Mase SR. Surgical interventions for drug-resistant tuberculosis: a systematic review and meta-analysis. Int J Tuberc Lung Dis 2013;17:6-16.

158. Isaakidis P, Casas EC, Das M, Tseretopoulou X, Ntzani EE, Ford N. Treatment outcomes for HIV and MDR-TB co-infected adults and children: systematic review and meta-analysis. Int J Tuberc Lung Dis 2015;19:969-78.

159. Arentz M, Pavlinac P, Kimerling ME, Horne DJ, Falzon D, Schünemann HJ, et al. Use of anti-retroviral therapy in tuberculosis patients on second-line anti-TB regimens: a systematic review. PloS One 2012;7:e47370.

160. Padayatchi N, Abdool Karim SS, Naidoo K, Grobler A, Friedland G. Improved survival in multidrug-resistant tuberculosis patients receiving integrated tuberculosis and anti-retroviral treatment in the SAPiT Trial. Int J Tuberc Lung Dis 2014;18:147-54.

161. Dheda K, Barry CE 3rd, Maartens G. Tuberculosis. Lancet 2016;387:1211-26.

162. Abdool Karim SS, Naidoo K, Grobler A, Padayatchi N, Baxter C, Gray AL, et al. Integration of antiretroviral therapy with tuberculosis treatment. N Engl J Med 2011;365:1492-501.

163. Havlir DV, Kendall MA, Ive P, Kumwenda J, Swindells S, Qasba SS, et al. Timing of antiretroviral therapy for HIV-1 infection and tuberculosis. N Engl J Med 2011;365:1482-91.

164. Blanc FX, Sok T, Laureillard D, Borand L, Rekacewicz C, Nerrienet E, et al. Earlier versus later start of antiretroviral therapy in HIV-infected adults with tuberculosis. N Engl J Med 2011;365:1471-81.

165. Ndjeka N, Conradie F, Schnippel K, Hughes J, Bantubani N, Ferreira H, et al. Treatment of drug-resistant tuberculosis with bedaquiline in a high HIV prevalence setting: an interim cohort analysis. Int J Tuberc Lung Dis 2015;19:979-85.

166. Guglielmetti L, Le Dû D, Jachym M, Henry B, Martin D, Caumes E, et al. Compassionate use of bedaquiline for the treatment of multidrug-resistant and extensively drug-resistant tuberculosis: interim analysis of a French cohort. Clin Infect Dis 2015;60:188-94.

167. Svensson EM, Aweeka F, Park JG, Marzan F, Dooley KE, Karlsson MO. Model-based estimates of the effects of efavirenz on bedaquiline pharmacokinetics and suggested dose adjustments for patients coinfected with HIV and tuberculosis. Antimicrob Agents Chemother 2013;57:2780-7.

168. Petrella S, Cambau E, Chauffour A, Andries K, Jarlier V, Sougakoff W, et al. Genetic basis for natural and acquired resistance to the diarylquinoline R207910 in mycobacteria. Antimicrob Agents Chemother 2006;50:2853-6.

169. Huitric E, Verhasselt P, Koul A, Andries K, Hoffner S, Andersson DI, et al. Rates and mechanisms of resistance development in Mycobacterium tuberculosis to a novel diarylquinoline ATP synthase inhibitor. Antimicrob Agents Chemother 2010;54:22-8.

170. Diacon AH, Pym A, Grobusch MP, de los Rios JM, Gotuzzo E, Vasilyeva I et al. Multidrug-resistant tuberculosis and culture conversion with bedaquiline. N Engl J Med 2014;371:723-32.

171. Svensson EM, Murray S, Karlsson MO, Dooley KE. Rifampicin and rifapentine significantly reduce concentrations of bedaquiline, a new anti-TB drug. J Antimicrob Chemother 2015;70:1106-14.

172. Stover CK, Warrener P, VanDevanter DR, Sherman DR, Arain TM, Langhorne MH, et al. A small-molecule nitroimidazopyran drug candidate for the treatment of tuberculosis. Nature 2000;405:962-6.

173. Singh R, Manjunatha U, Boshoff HI, Ha YH, Niyomrattanakit P, Ledwidge R, et al. PA-824 kills nonreplicating Mycobacterium tuberculosis by intracellular NO release. Science 2008;322: 1392-5.

174. Choi KP, Kendrick N, Daniels L. Demonstration that fbiC is required by Mycobacterium bovis BCG for coenzyme F[420] and FO biosynthesis. J Bacteriol 2002;184:2420-8.

175. Choi KP, Bair TB, Bae YM, Daniels L. Use of transposon Tn5367 mutagenesis and a nitroimidazopyran-based selection system to demonstrate a requirement for fbiA and fbiB in coenzyme F[420] biosynthesis by Mycobacterium bovis BCG. J Bacteriol 2001;183:7058-66.

176. Manjunatha UH, Boshoff H, Dowd CS, Zhang L Albert TJ, Norton JE, et al. Identification of a nitroimidazo-oxazine-specific protein involved in PA-824 resistance in Mycobacterium tuberculosis. Natl Acad Sci USA 2006;103:431-6.

177. Dooley KE, Luetkemeyer AF, Park JG, Allen R, Cramer Y, Murray S, et al. Phase I safety, pharmacokinetics, and pharma-cogenetics study of the antituberculosis drug PA-824 with con-comitant lopinavir-ritonavir, efavirenz, or rifampin. Antimicrob Agents Chemother 2014;58:5245-52.

178. Sasaki H, Haraguchi Y, Itotani M, Kuroda H, Hashizume H, Tomishige T, et al. Synthesis and antituberculosis activity of a novel series of optically active 6-nitro-2,3-dihydroimidazo[2,1-b] oxazoles. J Med Chem 2006;49:7854-60.

179. Matsumoto M, Hashizume H, Tomishige T, Kawasaki M, Tsubouchi H, Sasaki H et al. OPC-67683, a nitro-dihydro-imidazo-oxazole derivative with promising action against tuberculosis in vitro and in mice. PLoS Med 2006;3:e466.

180. Wang H, Lin H, Jiang G. Pulmonary resection in the treatment of multidrug-resistant tuberculosis: a retrospective study of 56 cases. Ann Thorac Surg 2008;86:1640-5.

181. Gler MT, Skripconoka V, Sanchez-Garavito E, Xiao H, Cabrera-Rivero JL, Vargas-Vasquez DE, et al. Delamanid for multidrug-resistant pulmonary tuberculosis. N Engl J Med 2012;366:2151-60.

182. Zhang Q, Liu Y, Tang S, Sha W, Xiao H. Clinical benefit of delamanid [OPC-67683] in the treatment of multidrug-resistant tuberculosis patients in China. Cell Biochem Biophys 2013; 67:957-63.

183. Deltyba: EPAR - Product Information. European Medicines Agency. Available at URL: http://www.ema.europa.eu/docs/en_GB/document_library/EPAR—Product_Information/human/002552/WC500166232.pdf. Accessed on July 2, 2014.

184. Chen P, Gearhart J, Protopopova M, Einck L, Nacy CA. Synergistic interactions of SQ109, a new ethylene diamine, with front-line antitubercular drugs in vitro. J Antimicrob Chemother 2006;58:332-7.

185. Barbachyn MR, Hutchinson DK, Brickner SJ, Cynamon MH, Kilburn JO, Klemens SP, et al. Identification of a novel oxazolidinone [U-100480] with potent antimycobacterial activity. J Med Chem 1996;39:680-5.

186. Balasubramanian V, Solapure S, Iyer H, Ghosh A Sharma S, Kaur P, et al. Bactericidal activity and mechanism of action of AZD5847, a novel oxazolidinone for treatment of tuberculosis. Antimicrob Agents Chemother 2014;58:495-502.

187. Wallis RS, Dawson R, Friedrich SO, Venter A, Paige D, Zhu T, et al. Mycobactericidal activity of sutezolid [PNU-100480] in sputum [EBA] and blood [WBA] of patients with pulmonary tuberculosis. PloS one 2014;9:e94462.

188. Zumla A, Chakaya J, Centis R, D'Ambrosio L, Mwaba P, Bates M, et al. Tuberculosis treatment and management--an update on treatment regimens, trials, new drugs, and adjunct therapies. Lancet Respir Med 2015;3:220-34.

189. Andries K, Verhasselt P, Guillemont J, Göhlmann HW, Neefs JM, Winkler H, et al. A diarylquinoline drug active on the ATP synthase of Mycobacterium tuberculosis. Science 2005; 307:223-7.

190. Lange C, Chesov D, Heyckendorf J, Leung CC, Udwadia Z, Dheda K. Drug-resistant tuberculosis: an update on disease burden, diagnosis and treatment. Respirology 2018;23:656-73.

191. Skripconoka V, Danilovits M, Pehme L, Tomson T, Skenders G, Kummik T, et al. Delamanid improves outcomes and reduces mortality in multidrug-resistant tuberculosis. Eur Respir J 2013;41:1393-400.

192. Gupta R, Geiter LJ, Wells CD, Gao M, Cirule A, Xiao H. Delamanid for extensively drug-resistant tuberculosis. N Engl J Med 2015;373:291-2.

193. Mallikaarjun S, Wells C, Petersen C, Paccaly A, Shoaf SE, Patil S, et al. Delamanid coadministered with antiretroviral drugs or antituberculosis drugs shows no clinically relevant drug-drug interactions in healthy subjects. Antimicrob Agents Chemother 2016;60:5976-85.

194. Diacon AH, Dawson R, Hanekom M, Narunsky K, Venter A, Hittel N, et al. Early bactericidal activity of delamanid [OPC-67683] in smear-positive pulmonary tuberculosis patients. Int J Tuberc Lung Dis 2011;15:949-54.

195. Laliberté F, Bookhart BK, Nelson WW, Lefebvre P, Schein JR, Rondeau-Leclaire J, et al. Impact of once-daily versus twice-daily dosing frequency on adherence to chronic medications among patients with venous thromboembolism. Patient 2013;6:213-24.

196. Liu Y, Matsumoto M, Ishida H, Ohguro K, Yoshitake M, Gupta R, Geiter L, Hafkin J. Delamanid: From discovery to its use for pulmonary multidrug-resistant tuberculosis [MDR-TB]. Tuber-culosis [Edinb] 2018;111:20-30.

197. Sloan DJ, Davies GR, Khoo SH. Recent advances in tuberculosis: New drugs and treatment regimens. Curr Respir Med Rev 2013;9:200-10.

198. Diacon AH, Donald PR, Pym A, et al. Randomized pilot trial of eight weeks of bedaquiline [TMC207] treatment for multidrug-resistant tuberculosis: long-term outcome, tolerability, and effect on emergence of drug resistance. Antimicrob Agents Chemother 2012;56:3271-6.

199. Olaru ID, von Groote-Bidlingmaier F, Heyckendorf J, Yew WW, Lange C, Chang KC. Novel drugs against tuberculosis: a clinician's perspective. Eur Respir J 2015;45:1119-31.

200. Günther G, Lange C, Alexandru S, Altet N, Avsar K, Bang D, et al; for TBNET. Treatment outcomes in multidrug-resistant tuberculosis. N Engl J Med 2016;375:1103-5.

201. ClinicalTrials.gov. An Open-Label RCT to Evaluate a New Treatment Regimen for Patients with Multi-drug Resistant Tuberculosis [NEXT]. Available at: https://clinicaltrials.gov/ct2/show/study/NCT02454205. Accessed September 17, 2018.

202. World Health Organization. Multidrug-resistant tuberculosis [MDR-TB]: 2013 Update. Geneva: World Health Organization; 2013.

203. Collaborative Group for the Meta-Analysis of Individual Patient Data in MDR-TB treatment-2017, Ahmad N, Ahuja SD, Akkerman OW, Alffenaar JC, Anderson LF, Baghaei P, et al. Treatment correlates of successful outcomes in pulmonary multidrug-resistant tuberculosis: an individual patient data meta-analysis. Lancet 2018;392:821-34.

204. Singla N, Singla R, Fernandes S, Behera D. Post treatment sequelae of multi-drug resistant tuberculosis patients. Indian J Tuberc 2009;56:206-12.

205. Achkar JM, Jenny-Avital ER. Incipient and subclinical tuber-culosis: defining early disease states in the context of host immune response. J Infect Dis 2011;204:S1179-86.

206. Khan MS, Dar O, Sismanidis C, Shah K, Godfrey-Faussett P. Improvement of tuberculosis case detection and reduction of discrepancies between men and women by simple sputum-submission instructions: a pragmatic randomised controlled trial. Lancet 2007;369:1955-60.

207. Van't Hoog AH, Onozaki I, Lonnroth K. Choosing algorithms for TB screening: a modelling study to compare yield, predictive value and diagnostic burden. BMC Infect Dis 2014;14:532.

208. Winetsky DE, Negoescu DM, DeMarchis EH, Almukhamedova O, Dooronbekova A, Pulatov D, et al. Screening and rapid molecular diagnosis of tuberculosis in prisons in Russia and Eastern Europe: a cost-effectiveness analysis. PLoS Medicine 2012;9:e1001348.

209. Peter JG, Theron G, Pooran A, Thomas J, Pascoe M, Dheda K. Comparison of two methods for acquisition of sputum samples for diagnosis of suspected tuberculosis in smear-negative or sputum-scarce people: a randomised controlled trial. Lancet Respir Med 2013;1:471-8.

210. World Health Organization. Recommendations for investigating contacts of persons with infectious tuberculosis in low- and middle-income countries. Geneva: World Health Organization; 2012.

211. Morrison J, Pai M, Hopewell PC. Tuberculosis and latent tuberculosis infection in close contacts of people with pulmonary tuberculosis in low-income and middle-income countries: a systematic review and meta-analysis. Lancet Infect Dis 2008;8: 359-68.

212. Teixeira L, Perkins MD, Johnson JL, Keller R, Palaci M, do Valle Dettoni V, et al. Infection and disease among household contacts of patients with multidrug-resistant tuberculosis. Int J Tuberc Lung Dis 2001;5:321-8.

213. Vella V, Racalbuto V, Guerra R, Marra C, Moll A, Mhlanga Z, et al. Household contact investigation of multidrug-resistant and extensively drug-resistant tuberculosis in a high HIV prevalence setting. Int J Tuberc Lung Dis 2011;15:1170-5.

214. Singla N, Singla R, Jain G, Habib L, Behera D. Tuberculosis among household contacts of multidrug-resistant tuberculosis patients in Delhi, India. Int J Tuberc Lung Dis 2011;15: 1326-30.

215. Parr JB, Mitnick CD, Atwood SS, Chalco K, Bayona J, Becerra MC, et al. Concordance of resistance profiles in households of patients with multidrug-resistant tuberculosis. Clin Infect Dis 2014;58: 392-5.

216. Shah NS, Yuen CM, Heo M, Tolman AW, Becerra MC. Yield of contact investigations in households of patients with drug-resistant tuberculosis: systematic review and meta-analysis. Clin Infect Dis 2014;58:381-91.

217. Marais BJ, Gie RP, Schaaf HS, Hesseling AC, Obihara CC, Starke JJ, et al. The natural history of childhood intra-thoracic tuberculosis: a critical review of literature from the pre-chemotherapy era. Int J Tuberc Lung Dis 2004;8:392-402.

218. Zar HJ, Hanslo D, Apolles P, Swingler G, Hussey G. Induced sputum versus gastric lavage for microbiological confirmation of pulmonary tuberculosis in infants and young children: a prospective study. Lancet 2005;365:130-4.

219. Seddon JA, Hesseling AC, Finlayson H, Fielding K, Cox H, Hughes J, et al. Preventive therapy for child contacts of multidrug-resistant tuberculosis: a prospective cohort study. Clin Infect Dis 2013;57:1676-84.

220. Stop TBPCTBSWHO. Guidance for National Tuberculosis Programmes on the management of tuberculosis in children. Chapter 1: introduction and diagnosis of tuberculosis in children. Int J Tuberc Lung Dis 2006;10:1091-7.

221. Seddon JA, Godfrey-Faussett P, Hesseling AC, Gie RP, Beyers N, Schaaf HS, et al. Management of children exposed to multidrug-resistant Mycobacterium tuberculosis. Lancet Infect Dis 2012; 12:469-79.

222. Garcia-Prats AJ, Draper HR, Thee S, Dooley KE, McIlleron HM, Seddon JA, et al. The pharmacokinetics and safety of ofloxacin in children with drug-resistant tuberculosis. Antimicrob Agents Chemother 2015;59:6073-9.

223. van der Werf MJ, Langendam MW, Sandgren A, Manissero D. Lack of evidence to support policy development for management of contacts of multidrug-resistant tuberculosis patients: two systematic reviews. Int J Tuberc Lung Dis 2012;16:288-96.

224. Targeted tuberculin testing and treatment of latent tuberculosis infection. American Thoracic Society. MMWR Recomm Rep 2000;49[RR-6]:1-51.

43

Antituberculosis Drug Resistance Surveillance

CN Paramasivan, VH Balasangameshwara

INTRODUCTION

With the discovery of streptomycin in the 1940s and isoniazid in the 1950s, chemotherapy became the standard method of treatment of tuberculosis [TB]. In the early years of the chemotherapy era, it was found that treatment with a single drug resulted in the development of drug resistance in a high proportion of the patients, with a consequent loss of efficacy of treatment. Hence, combined chemotherapy with two or more drugs given together became the standard practice. At present fixed-dose combinations, where two or three drugs are incorporated in a single tablet or capsule, are also widely available. Despite all these advancements, in most of the disease endemic countries there was a dramatic increase in the level of initial drug resistance.

The response to treatment in patients with multidrug-resistant TB [MDR-TB] [defined as resistance to rifampicin and isoniazid, with or without resistance to other anti-TB drugs] is poor and the mortality rate is high. Since these patients have to be treated with several toxic and expensive second-line anti-TB drugs, and may need prolonged hospitalisation to manage drug toxicity and other complications, they account for a significant proportion of the health care resources (1).

In recent years, the incidence of human immunodeficiency virus [HIV] infection has increased enormously all over the world. Patients with HIV infection are known to have an increased risk of developing TB. The case fatality rate is high in patients with the acquired immunodeficiency syndrome [AIDS], who have associated MDR-TB (2). The level of initial drug resistance is said to provide an epidemiological indicator to assess the amount of resistant bacterial transmission in a community, as well as the success or otherwise of the National Tuberculosis Programme [NTP]. Further, this influences the design of therapeutic regimens, as well as policy decision (3). Hence, reliable data on the levels of drug resistance over the years in various parts of the country would be of great value.

Vigorous implementation of a multi-pronged approach in the treatment of TB resulted in a decline in the percentage of drug resistance in Korea (4) and New York city (5). But the information on drug resistance in India is available from well-conducted studies for only a small proportion of population; the percentages of drug resistance in these settings have remained almost static. In many of the drug resistance surveys conducted earlier in India, small or non-representative samples have been studied. Also, there has been no clear distinction between primary and acquired resistance, as the history of previous chemotherapy was not obtained. Despite such limitations, an attempt has been made to give an overview of the prevalence of drug resistance in India over the last three decades.

For the purpose of drug resistance surveillance [DRS] in TB, the definitions of primary drug resistance and acquired drug resistance have been revised by the World Health Organization [WHO] and International Union Against Tuberculosis and Lung Diseases [IUATLD; now called "The Union"] as 'resistance among new cases' and 'resistance in previously treated patients' (6). 'Resistance among new cases' is defined as 'the presence of resistant strains of *Mycobacterium tuberculosis* [*Mtb*] in a patient who, in response to direct questioning, denies having had any prior anti-TB treatment, [for more than one month], and, in countries where adequate documentation is available, for whom there is no evidence of such history'. For the purpose of surveillance, 'resistance in a previously treated patient' is defined as the presence of resistant strains of *Mtb* in a patient who, in response to direct questioning, admits having been treated for TB for one month or more, or, in countries where adequate documentation is available, in a patient for whom there is evidence of such history.

Since 1994, several countries have established National Tuberculosis DRS projects. These projects have adopted a standardised methodology for susceptibility testing with the assistance of the Supranational Reference Laboratories [SRLs]. Establishing surveillance of drug resistance at the country level requires strict adherence to three principles: [i] the sample of specimens should be representative of the TB patients in the country/geographical setting under study and the sample size should be determined to permit standard epidemiological analysis. It was recommended that anti-TB DRS should cover the entire country/geographical area and that the sample size is derived from the total number of new sputum-positive cases in that country; [ii] the patient's history should be carefully obtained and available medical records reviewed to clearly determine whether the patient has previously received anti-TB drugs. This was felt essential to distinguish between drug resistance among newly diagnosed cases and drug resistance among previously treated cases; and [iii] the laboratory methods for anti-TB drug susceptibility testing [DST] should be selected from among those that are internationally recommended. Four DST methods have been standardised and are widely used throughout the world (7). These are: [i] proportion method and its economic and standard variants; [ii] resistance ratio method; [iii] absolute concentration method; and [iv] radiometric method [e.g. BACTEC 460]. Comparability of data resulting from any of the above four methods is assured by the quality assurance [QA] and proficiency testing performed by the SRL network.

GLOBAL PREVALENCE OF DRUG-RESISTANT TUBERCULOSIS

The worldwide magnitude of the problem of resistance to anti-TB drugs is not known. The literature search suggests high levels of resistance in some areas. However, many of these studies were not based on representative samples and failed to distinguish between patients who had received anti-TB treatment in the past and those who had not. Further, there was no consensus on definitions and laboratory results were not standardised. The major limitation for the adequate assessment of drug resistance was the inadequate culture and DST facilities in many parts of the world. All these limitations prevented an exact assessment of the magnitude of the problem worldwide and meaningful comparisons among various countries.

Global project on anti-TB DRS represents a coordinated international effort (8). It serves as a model for surveillances of drug resistance in other diseases resulted in the establishment of multinational system for the surveillance of drug resistance. Yield of reliable results in this surveillance report comes from laboratory standardisation and QA.

The World Health Organization [WHO] and IUATLD Working Group on anti-TB DRS published report on the prevalence of resistance to four first-line drugs in 35 countries between 1994 and 1997 (8,9). As per this report (8,9) resistance to anti-TB drugs was found in all 35 countries and

regions surveyed and resistance to isoniazid or streptomycin was most common.

Despite high rates of HIV co-infection in African countries, the prevalence of drug resistance was generally low (8,9). The low level of MDR may be attributed to the unavailability of control programmes and the relatively late introduction of rifampicin.

In Western European countries, where TB notification rates were low (10), the median prevalence of primary MDR was less than 1%. Despite 28% of patients with TB having co-infection with HIV in Barcelona, Spain, the prevalence rate of MDR was only 0.5%. Reversal of previously declining rates of TB has been observed in Eastern Europe particularly in the former Soviet Union (11,12). This has been attributed to an irregular supply of drugs, non-standardised regimens, nosocomial infections and the occurrence of outbreaks in prisons (8,9). The prevalence of MDR-TB was observed to be higher in the Baltic states than in any of the other countries surveyed.

Following the publication of the first global report on anti-TB drug resistance by the WHO in 1997 with results from surveys conducted in 35 countries (8,9), by 2010, a total of five global reports (13-16) had been published. Thereafter, surveillance data have been published annually in the WHO Global Tuberculosis Report.

These surveillance results suggest link between the quality of TB control programmes and levels of drug resistance. However, this relationship is complex (18). Immigration is considered to be an important contributor to drug resistance rates (19-21).

Extensively Drug-resistant Tuberculosis

The Centers for Disease Control and Prevention [CDC], Atlanta, in March 2006 reported the extensively drug-resistant TB [XDR-TB] (22). The XDR-TB was initially defined as cases in persons with TB whose isolates were resistant to isoniazid and rifampicin and at least three of the six main classes of second-line drugs [SLDs] such as aminoglycosides, polypeptides, fluoroquinolones, thioamides, cycloserine, and para-aminosalicyclic acid (22-24). Subsequently, this definition had been modified and XDR-TB is presently defined as isolates of *Mtb* resistant to at least rifampicin and isoniazid [which is the definition of MDR-TB], any fluoroquinolone, and at least one of the three following injectable drugs, namely, capreomycin, kanamycin and amikacin (25-27). The XDR-TB has emerged worldwide as a threat to public health and TB control, raising concerns of a future epidemic of virtually untreatable TB.

WHO surveillance of TB drug resistance over the last two decades has provided evidence on the response to the MDR-TB epidemic, and recent innovations in molecular diagnostics allow a definitive shift to routine surveillance compared to special surveys hitherto being conducted. As a pathfinder with two decades of experience to draw upon, the global project on anti-TB DRS is a model for scaling up surveillance of antimicrobial resistance [AMR] to other infectious diseases. The available data indicates that considerable progress in the global and national response to the MDR-TB epidemic is evident, particularly since 2009 when the World Health Assembly [WHA] called for universal access to diagnosis and treatment of MDR-TB. The response, however, still remains insufficient. The percentage of new TB cases that have MDR-TB globally has remained unchanged. Some countries have severe epidemics and in many settings the treatment success rate is alarmingly low. WHO has suggested five priority actions [Figure 43.1], from prevention to cure to address the global MDR-TB crisis. Health system barriers, diagnostic and treatment challenges and inadequate funding for care and research and these must be urgently addressed (17).

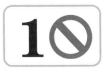

Prevent the development
of drug resistance through
high quality treatment of
drug-susceptible TB

Expand rapid testing and
detection of drug-resistant
TB cases

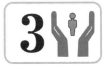

Provide immediate access
to effective treatment and
proper care

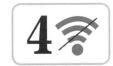

Prevent transmission
through infection control

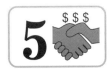

Increase political commitment with financing

Figure 43.1: Five priority actions to address the global MDR-TB crisis
Reproduced with permission from "Drug-resistant TB; surveillance and response Supplement to the Global Tuberculosis Report [2014]" (reference 28)

The global TB Supranational Reference Laboratory Network [SRLN] which included 14 laboratories in 1994 has grown to 33 laboratories in 2014, covering all six WHO regions. These laboratories are entrusted with the responsibility to conduct quality assurance, coordinate technical assistance to strengthen laboratory networks in all high TB and MDR-TB burden countries, and are the entry point for the introduction of new TB diagnostics. Since 2013, the SRLN has expanded its membership to include a new category of TB laboratory designated as 'Centres of Excellence' in large low- and middle-income countries that works specifically to build in-country laboratory capacity (28). Surveillance data compiled since 1994 has been essential to inform and guide the response to MDR-TB. The first guidance on MDR-TB treatment and care was issued in 1996. Since then updated guidance has been issued, including guidelines on laboratories, diagnostics and infection control (29).

In the earlier published previous global TB reports, estimates of the burden of DR-TB have focussed on MDR-TB. Since May 2016, the WHO issued guidance that rifampicin-resistant TB [RR-TB] with or without resistance to other anti-TB drugs, should be treated with an MDR-TB treatment regimen. This included patients with MDR-TB as well as any other patient with RR-TB. As per the global TB report 2018 (17), worldwide in 2017, an estimated 3.6% {95% confidence interval [CI] 2.6%-4.8%} of new cases and 17% [95% CI 5.6%-33%] of previously treated cases had MDR/RR-TB [Table 43.1]. In 2017, there were an estimated 58,000 [range 483,000–639,000] incident cases of MDR/RR-TB, with cases of MDR-TB accounting for 83% of the total cases. The largest numbers of MDR/RR-TB cases [47% of the global total] had occurred in China, India and the Russian Federation. There were nearly 230,000 [range 140,000-310,000] deaths from MDR/RR-TB in 2017 (17). Unpublished observations from the National Institute for Research in Tuberculosis [NIRT, earlier called Tuberculosis Research Centre], Chennai, has indicated that XDR-TB was detected in approximately 4% of 3173 isolates received during the period 2001 to 2004 from chronically ill patients with a prolonged

WHO region	Estimated % of new cases with MDR/RR-TB*	Estimated % of previously treated cases with MDR/RR-TB*	Incidence of MDR/RR-TB†
Africa	2.4 [1.4-3.7]	15 [0.81-43]	8.6 [7.2-0]
The Americas	1.9 [0.89-3.2]	14 [5.0-25]	1.1 [0.99-1.3]
Eastern Mediterranean	3.8 [2.6-5.3]	21 [4.9-4.5]	6 [4.5-7.7]
Europe	7.1 [5.9-8.4]	21 [15-29]	12 [9.4-15]
South-East Asia	3.4 [2.5-4.4]	19 [9.6-3.1]	9.7 [6.7-13]
Western Pacific	2.1 [0.99-3.6]	14 [3.9-30]	6.0 [4.7-7.5]
Global	3.6 [2.6-4.8]	17 [5.6-33]	7.4 [6.4-8.5]

Table 43.1: Estimated incidence of MDR/RR-TB in 2017 for WHO regions and globally

* Data are presented as best estimate [uncertainty level]
† Rate/100,000 population [uncertainty level]
MDR = multidrug-resistant; RR = rifampicin resistant; TB = tuberculosis; WHO = World Health Organization
Source: reference 17

and varying treatment history. As per Global TB Report 2018 (17), in 2017, XDR-TB was estimated to be present in 8.5% [95% CI 6.2%-11%] cases with MDR-TB.

Among the 40 countries with a high TB or MDR-TB burden [or both], only 20 had repeated a survey at least once. Of these, eight countries, namely, Belarus, Kazakhstan, Myanmar, Peru, Republic of Moldova, Tomsk Oblast in the Russian Federation, Thailand and Viet Nam had at least 3 years of data. There appears to be a slight trend for cases of MDR-TB to increase as a proportion of all TB cases in these countries (17).

The tripling of MDR-TB detection between 2009 and 2013 is thought to be the result of concerted efforts to strengthen laboratories and roll out rapid tests. Expanding Access to New Diagnostics for TB [EXPAND-TB], the largest multi-partner global project has focused on accelerating access to modern diagnostics for TB and MDR-TB, and is supporting 27 low- and middle-income countries. Between the start of the project in 2009 and the end of June 2014; 89,261 people with MDR-TB were detected in the 97 state-of-the-art laboratories supported by EXPAND-TB partners. Since 2010, when WHO approved the Xpert MTB/RIF assay [for the simultaneous detection of TB and rifampicin resistance], global roll out of the technology has been impressive.

An important addition to DRS is incorporation of rapid molecular tests such as the Xpert MTB/RIF assay, which provides results much faster than conventional methods [culture and phenotypic DST]. It also does not require sophisticated laboratory infrastructure, which greatly reduces and simplifies laboratory work and decrease costs. Being a molecular test, it does not suffer from some of the limitations observed in conventional methods, such as those requiring timely and refrigerated transportation of sputum samples with live bacteria, growing in laboratories prior to testing, the need to decontaminate to isolate TB bacteria and prevent the growth of other organisms, resulting in the risk of killing TB bacilli [through too harsh decontamination] or contamination from other organisms. As a result rapid molecular methods may detect TB [including drug-resistant cases] that would have been missed by conventional methods.

The Global Drug Facility [GDF] of the Stop TB Partnership has increased its supplier base for second-line anti-TB drugs from 10 to 19 between 2009 and 2014, which has resulted in an increase in the available number of second-line drugs [12-23] and also price reductions. Country progress to improve delivery of MDR-TB treatment through new approaches such as a shift away from hospitalization to ambulatory care in Central Asian countries; worldwide expansion of treatment of XDR-TB patients; and pioneering efforts of several countries in use of shorter regimens for MDR-TB under operational research conditions. However, health service capacity to treat patients has to increase with the pace of diagnosis to reduce the "waiting lists" for MDR-TB treatment in several countries. In addition, a major health service constraint is patient-centered care [including

enablers and social support] through patient follow-up and remains important activity to improve treatment outcomes.

WHO has identified TB infection control as an essential activity to minimise the risk of disease transmission which has remained one of the most neglected components of TB prevention and care". The evidence for this inference is that in 2013, more than 50% of new cases of MDR-TB were among people never before treated for TB, highlighting the importance of transmission and the lack of appropriate infection control measures, particularly at community level. MDR-TB transmission in health care facilities and in congregate settings such as prisons is a well-known public health threat. As this transmission can be effectively addressed by appropriate infection control measures, it is necessary to implement them. They are a mix of environmental, personal protection and administrative measures, rapid identification of drug resistance, and prompt, appropriate treatment of MDR-TB patients.

In view of the fact that MDR-TB is a global health security risk and carries grave consequences for those affected, WHO has called for MDR-TB to be addressed as a public health crisis in 2013. The WHO has recommended the following five actions needed on all fronts from prevention to cure; priority actions that are crucial to accelerate the response against the MDR-TB epidemic are; prevent MDR-TB as a first priority, scale up rapid testing and detection of all MDR-TB cases, ensure prompt access to appropriate MDR-TB care, including adequate supplies of quality drugs and scaled-up country capacity to deliver services, prevent transmission of MDR-TB through appropriate infection control, and underpin and sustain the MDR-TB response through high level political commitment, strong leadership across multiple governmental sectors, ever-broadening partnerships, and financing for care and research.

WHO has reiterated that adequate treatment of drug susceptible TB remains the cornerstone of efforts to prevent the emergence and spread of DR-TB. This is supported by the fact that globally, more than 95% of people who develop TB for the first time do not have rifampicin resistance or MDR-TB and can thus be treated successfully using a standard, inexpensive, six-month course of treatment. The encouraging observation is that globally in 2012, the treatment success rate for drug-susceptible TB was 86%, a level that has been maintained for several years (28). The definitions for monitoring of drug resistance-TB and MDR-TB and treatment outcomes were revised in 2013 (30) to enhance the monitoring of patients. One of the Global Plan targets is for all 27 high MDR-TB countries to manage their data on treatment of MDR-TB patients electronically by 2015. By 2013, 16 of these countries reported that national electronic databases were in place for TB patients and another five had systems for MDR-TB patients only. Guidance on the design and implementation of electronic systems for recording and reporting data was produced by WHO and technical partners in 2011 (31).

The WHO and MDR-TB global stakeholders Consultation meeting of NTP staff, donors, and all other major stakeholders during meeting recommendations of October 2013 in Paris, on indicator[s] to use and purpose were subsequently discussed and endorsed by WHO's Strategic and Technical Advisory Group for TB [STAG-TB] in June 2014 (32). Consensus was reached on the following five indicators and their application: [i] the indicator "estimated number of MDR-TB cases among notified cases of pulmonary TB" should be used for assessing programmatic performance in diagnostic and treatment coverage, at country and global levels. It is also appropriate for planning and budgeting purposes; [ii] a global estimate of MDR-TB incidence is useful for global advocacy; [iii] a global estimate of MDR-TB prevalence is also useful for advocacy; [iv] a global estimate of MDR-TB mortality is useful for global advocacy; [v] proportion of new and previously treated TB cases with MDR-TB is useful for monitoring trends in levels of drug resistance at global and country levels.

Global Surveillance of Drug Resistance: Status in 2018

Since the launch of the Global Project on Antituberculosis Drug Resistance Surveillance in 1994 (8,9,13-16), global data on anti-TB drug-resistance have been systematically collected and analysed from 82% of the 194 WHO Member States [160 countries] (17). This includes 91 countries that have continuous surveillance systems based on routine diagnostic DST of *Mtb* isolates obtained from all TB patients, and 69 countries that rely on epidemiological surveys of bacterial isolates collected from representative samples of patients. In resource limited setting, when routine diagnostic DST is not possible, surveys conducted about once in every 5 years represent the most common approach to investigating the burden of drug resistance. Of the 40 countries with a high TB burden [n = 30] and high MDR-TB burden [n = 30], 37 have data on levels of drug resistance. Of these, Congo and Liberia never conducted a drug-resistance survey and Angola has initiated a national survey in 2018. Brazil, Central African Republic, Democratic People's Republic of Korea and Papua New Guinea rely on DRS data gathered from subnational areas only.

In Eritrea, Indonesia and Lao People's Democratic Republic, the first-ever national drug-resistance surveys were completed and repeat surveys were completed in Eswatini, Sri Lanka, Togo and the United Republic of Tanzania during 2016-2017. During the period 2017-2018, drug-resistance surveys were ongoing in 12 countries [first nationwide surveys in Angola, Burundi, Haiti, Mali and Timor-Leste; and repeat surveys Bangladesh, Cambodia, Ethiopia, Malawi, the Philippines, Thailand and Turkmenistan] (17).

DRUG-RESISTANT TUBERCULOSIS IN INDIA

DR-TB has frequently been encountered in India and its presence has been known from the time anti-TB drugs were introduced.

A Historical Account of Burden of Drug-resistant Tuberculosis in India

Drug Resistance in Newly Diagnosed Cases

Though drug resistance in newly diagnosed cases is found to be low in developed countries, it is common in India and varies widely from area to area. The South-East Asia region is a major contributor, accounting for almost 40% of the global burden of MDR-TB among new cases. The data on drug resistance in newly diagnosed cases estimated by different investigators during the period 1964-1991 are listed in Table 43.2 (33-42).

In the 1960s, Indian Council of Medical Research [ICMR] conducted two nationwide surveys at nine urban chest clinics in India (33,34). The results of the first survey showed resistance level of 8.2% to isoniazid alone, 5.8% to streptomycin alone and 6.5% to both the drugs. The resistance levels among new cases seen respectively in these two surveys were 14.7% and 15.5%, respectively to isoniazid and 12.5% and 13.8%, respectively to streptomycin.

A decade later, a study was conducted to assess the prevalence of resistance among new cases in Government Chest Institute and Chest [Tuberculosis] Clinic of Government Stanley Hospital, Chennai (35). The results of this study were almost similar to the earlier ICMR surveys and the authors reported that the prevalence of resistance among new cases has not risen during the span of 10 years.

During the 1980s among five reports on primary drug resistance, while the levels of resistance among new cases to isoniazid and streptomycin were similar to that reported in earlier studies. Rifampicin resistance started appearing in North Arcot, Puducherry, Bengaluru and Jaipur but not in Gujarat (36-41). The reason for the emergence of rifampicin resistance during this period may be the introduction of short-course chemotherapy [SCC] regimens containing rifampicin.

Further, a higher level of resistance among new cases to isoniazid was observed among the rural population in Kolar (40) compared to the urban patients contradicting a Korean study where a much higher level of initial resistance was seen among urban patients giving the reason of easy access to the anti-TB drugs (4), There was also an increase in the proportion of resistance among new cases to rifampicin [4.4%] encountered in this rural population. In the early 1990s, a retrospective study done at New Delhi (42) showed a high level of resistance among new cases to isoniazid [18.5%] and a low level of rifampicin resistance.

Overall, the prevalence of resistance among new cases to isoniazid as a single agent ranged from 6% to 13% (33-38, 40-42) except among the rural population in Kolar, Karnataka (39) where a high rate has been reported. Prevalence of resistance in newly diagnosed cases to streptomycin as a single agent ranged from 1% to 5.8% and to rifampicin from 0% to 1.9% (33-42). In many of these surveys, ethambutol susceptibility was not performed. In a study conducted in Bengaluru (40), the resistance in newly detected cases was

13.7% to isoniazid, 22.5% to streptomycin; and 2.2% had MDR-TB.

For a correct evaluation of primary drug resistance, standardised methodology should have been used taking care of the following namely; eliciting patient history, adequate sample size, uniform laboratory methods, external and internal quality control, reliable drugs for setting up drug susceptibility media, standard chemicals in the preparation of media, etc. Many Indian studies may have limitations related to these methodological issues.

Resistance in Previously Treated Tuberculosis Cases

The rates of resistance in previously treated patients are invariably higher than the rates of resistance in newly diagnosed cases, though data on resistance in previously treated patients are limited. Studies on resistance in previously treated patients during the period 1980-2000 are shown in Table 43.3 (36,42-44). The longitudinal trend of drug resistance in Gujarat between 1980 and 1986 (41) showed that in treatment failure or relapsed patients, resistance to rifampicin increased from 2.8% in 1980 to 37.3% in 1986 and to isoniazid from 34.5% to 55.8%. From this study (41), it was presumed that high level of rifampicin resistance was almost entirely acquired. A study was conducted by the ICMR (43) to compare the efficacy of SCC with the conventional [non-SCC] chemotherapy in North Arcot district, Tamil Nadu. The population was examined during their follow-up period to confirm the bacterial quiescence, and in turn, the efficacy of SCC. It was found that there was an increase in the frequency of resistance in previously treated patients with 67% resistance to isoniazid, 26% to streptomycin and 12% to rifampicin. In addition, 6% of the strains tested were resistant to both isoniazid and rifampicin (43). A study from New Delhi in the 1990s (42) also showed a higher level of resistance in previously treated patients to isoniazid and rifampicin, which is almost similar to that of the Gujarat report (36). A study conducted by the Institute of Thoracic Medicine, Chennai (45) aimed at finding out the prevalence of TB resistance in four District Tuberculosis Centres of Tamil Nadu, showed that acquired resistance was 63%, out of which 23.5% were resistant to single drug and 39.5% resistant to more than one drug. In a recently conducted study in Bengaluru (44), the MDR in previously treated cases was found to be 12.8% and ranged from 8.4% to 17.2%. The proportion of 12% MDR-TB in previously treated patients appears to be similar in other DOTS implemented areas such as Hong Kong (46) and Nepal (47). The overall rates of resistance in previously treated patients to isoniazid ranged from 34.5% to 67%, for streptomycin from 26% to 26.9% and for rifampicin from 2.8% to 37.3% (33-42).

Multidrug Resistance

The rate of MDR-TB in new cases in India has been low, ranging from 0% to 3% [Table 43.2]. The drug resistance in various DRS sites in India conducted by two national reference laboratories [NRLs] of India between 1985-2003, namely Tuberculosis Research Center [TRC], Chennai and National Tuberculosis Institute [NTI], Bengaluru is shown in Figure 43.2 (40,48-50). The resistance varied from 0.5% to 3.4%. The level of MDR-TB in previously treated cases was less than 13% except in Gujarat where a high level was observed [11.4% to 18.5%] [Table 43.3]. In the report from the Institute of Thoracic Medicine, Chennai (44) on the prevalence of MDR-TB among patients undergoing treatment for varying periods of time at four District Tuberculosis Centres in Tamil Nadu, 20.3% were found to be harbouring MDR strains. Majority of these patients had irregular and interrupted treatment owing to the non-availability of drugs (44). Data documented at the TRC, Chennai (51) from 443 Category II patients from the model DOTS area in Tiruvallur district of Tamil Nadu [1999-2003] revealed that the prevalence of MDR-TB was 11.7%. In the study (52) carried out in patients co-infected with HIV-TB [n = 37], during the period 2000-2002, the incidence of MDR-TB in new and previously treated patients was 5.9%.

DRUG-RESISTANT TUBERCULOSIS IN INDIA: CURRENT SITUATION

Data documented from early 1980s during clinical trials conducted at the National Institute for Research in Tuberculosis [NIRT], Chennai [earlier called Tuberculosis Research Centre] have shown that MDR-TB has been increasing from less than 1% in the early 1990s to 2.0% in 2006 [Figure 43.3] (53). The burden of MDR-TB, MDR-TB/rifampicin-resistant TB among new and previously treated TB patients in India documented in studies between 1997 and 2016 are shown in Table 43.4 (53,54).

National Anti-TB Drug Resistance Survey 2014-2016

The Government of India conducted a National Anti-TB Drug Resistance Survey 2014-2016 [NDRS 2014-2016] (53) to know the prevalence of drug resistance among TB patients among both new and previously treated TB patients. The NDRS 2014-2016 is the largest ever conducted by any country in the world and the first ever survey having DST for 13 anti-TB drugs using the automated liquid culture system, mycobacteria growth indicator tube [MGIT] 960®. In the NDRS 2014-2016, 5280 sputum smear-positive pulmonary TB patients. This included 3240 new [DST available for 3065, 94.6%] and 2040 previously treated patients [DST available for 1893, 92.8%] diagnosed at the designated microscopy centres [DMCs] of RNTCP were enrolled. The key findings of the NDRS 2014-2016 are listed in Tables 43.5 and 43.6.

In the NDRS 2014-2016 (54) MDR-TB was evident in 2.8% new and 11.6% previously treated TB patients. Among MDR-TB patients, additional resistance to any fluoroquinolones and to any second-line injectable drugs was seen in 21.8% 3.6% respectively. Among MDR-TB patients, XDR-TB was evident in 1.3% cases.

Table 43.2: Summary of studies on resistance among new cases in *Mycobacterium tuberculosis* isolates from India

Study (reference)	Year	No. of isolates tested	Resistance to single drug [%]					Resistance to multiple drugs [%]			Total resistance [%]	Location
			H	S	R	E	T	SH	HR	SHR		
9 Urban Centres India (33)	1964-65	1838	8.2 [14.7]	5.8 [12.5]	ND	ND	–	6.5	–	–	20.4	Urban
9 Urban Centres India (34)	1965-67	851	15.5	13.8	ND	ND	–	–	–	–	22	Urban
Government Chest Institute and Stanley Hospital Chennai (35)	1976	254	10.6	9.5	ND	ND	ND	4.7	–	–	–	Urban
Gujarat* (36)	1983-86	570	7.9 [13.9]	3.2 [7.4]	0	2.5 [4]	0.5 [1.5]	3.3	0	–	20	Urban
North Arcot (37)	1985-89	2779	13	4	0.07 [2]	ND	ND	7	0.7	0.9	26	Rural
Pondicherry (37)	1985-91	2127	6	4	0.2 [0.9]	ND	ND	3	0.4	0.3	13.9	Urban
Bangalore† (38)	1980s	436	12.1 [17.4]	1.8 [5.7]	1.8 [3]	0 [0.5]	ND	3.6	0.9	0.2	21.1	Urban
Bangalore‡ (39)	1985-86	588	12.6 [17.4]	1.7 [4.8]	1.5 [2.3]	0 [0.5]	ND	2.9	1.2	0.2	20.5	Urban
Bangalore (40)	1999	271	13.7	22.5	2.6	1.8	ND	6.6	2.2	1.1	27.7	Urban
Kolar§ (39)	1987-89	292	26.7 [32.8]	1 [5.1]	1 [4.4]	0 [1.7]	ND	2.4	3.2	0.7	34.9	Rural
Jaipur¶ (41)	1988-91	1009	7.6 [10.1]	5.2 [7.6]	1.9 [3]	2 [2.6]	ND	1.6	0.7	0.1	19.9	–
New Delhi (42)	1990-91	324	18.5	–	0.6	–	–	–	–	–	–	Urban

Figures in parentheses indicate percentage of isolates resistant to a drug along with other drugs. [H] = H+SH+HR+SHR; [S] = S+SH+SR+SHR; [R] = R+SR+HR+SHR; [E] = E+HE+SE+SHE+HRE; [T] = T+HT
* Multiple resistances were also reported for HT [1.0%]; HE [0.7%]; SHE [0.9%]
† Multiple resistances were also reported for HE [0.5%]
‡ Multiple resistances were also reported for HE [0.6%]
§ Multiple resistances were also reported for HE [0.3%]; SHE [1.0%]; HRE [0.3%]
¶ Multiple resistances% were also reported for SR [0.2%]; SE [0.5%]; SHE [0.1%]
H = isoniazid; S = streptomycin; R = rifampicin; E = ethambutol; T = thiacetazone; ND = not done

Table 43.3: Summary of studies on resistance in prevviously treated patients in *Mycobacterium tuberculosis* isolates from India

Study (reference)	Year	Number of isolates	Resistance [%]							Location
			H	S	R	SH	HR	SR	SHR	
Gujarat (36)	1980-86	1574	34.5-55.8	26.3-26.9	2.8-37.3	–	–	–	–	–
Gujarat (36)	1983-86	1267	–	–	–	–	11.4-18.5	1.2-3.5	14.5-15.3	–
North Arcot (43)	1988-89	560	67.0	26.0	12.0	19.0	6.0	–	–	Rural
New Delhi (42)	1990-91	81	50.7	–	33.7	–	–	–	–	Urban
Bangalore (44)	1999-2000	226	4.7-12.1	5.4-13.2	0-3.6	0-1.3	8.4-17.2	0.2-1	0.2-4.2	Urban

H = isoniazid; S = streptomycin; R = rifampicin

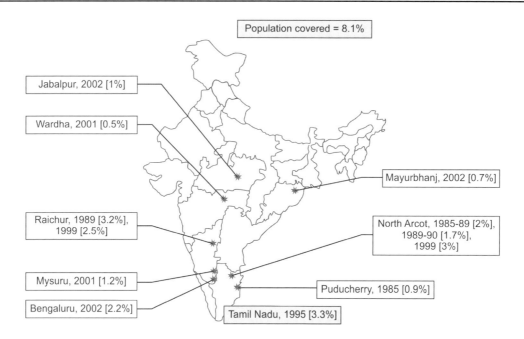

Figure 43.2: Drug-resistance data from some surveillance sites in India [1985-2003]. Figures in square brackets indicate prevalence of multidrug-resistant tuberculosis

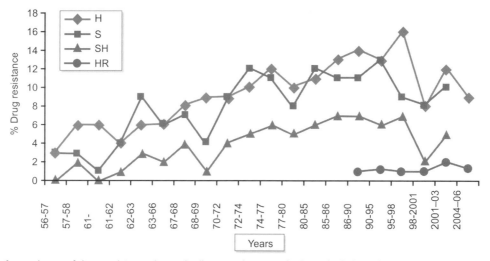

Figure 43.3: Trend of prevalence of drug resistance in newly diagnosed cases of tuberculosis in various studies conducted at National Institute for Research in Tuberculosis [NIRT, earlier called Tuberculosis Research Centre], Chennai
H = isoniazid; S = streptomycin; R = rifampcin
Reproduced with permission from reference 53

PROGRAMMATIC MANAGEMENT OF DRUG-RESISTANT TUBERCULOSIS IN INDIA: CURRENT STATUS

Following the successful national coverage of RNTCP services across the country in 2006, the Programmatic Management of Drug-resistant TB [PMDT] services were introduced in 2007 and the whole country was covered 2013. Initially, DR-TB services were offered to TB patients with the highest risk to develop drug resistance, i.e., treatment failure cases. A horizontal and vertical scale-up ensured thereafter. Definite criteria were defined to assess the risk and eligibility for DST. The DST was then offered to TB patients who remained smear-positive during follow-up; to "previously treated patients"; HIV-seropositive persons; and persons who had contact with a known DR-TB patient with a plan to achieve universal DST, to all diagnosed and notified TB patients (55,56).

Capacity building for DST then ensued from a few national reference laboratories [NRLs], and state level Intermediate reference laboratories [IRLs] with solid or liquid culture and DST facilities, a wide network of state and regional level IRLs with solid and liquid culture DST and line probe assay [LPA] facilities and district level network of laboratories capable of cartridge based

Table 43.4: MDR-TB among new and previously treated TB patients in India

Study	New TB patients %	Previously treated TB patients %
Tamil Nadu State, 1997-1998 [n = 60 million]	3.4	25
Gujarat State, 2007-2008 [n = 56 million]	2.4	17.4
Maharashtra State, 2008 [n = 108 million]	2.7	14
Undivided Andhra Pradesh State, 2009 [n = 86 million]	1.8	11.8
Tamil Nadu State, 2011 [n = 77 million]	1.8	13.2
MDR-TB/RR-TB reported under RNTCP India's routine surveillance data		
2007-2012 [n = 144,326]	NA	19
2013-2015 [n = 779,300]	5	11
2016 [n = 580,438]	4	9

n = no. studied; MDR-TB = multidrug-resistant TB; TB = tuberculosis; RR-TB = rifampicin resistant-TB; RNTCP = Revised National TB Control Programme; NA = not available
Source: references 53,54

Table 43.5: MDR-TB/XDR-TB among new and previously treated TB patients

DST results	New TB patients [n = 3065] % [95% CI]	Previously treated patients [n = 1893] % [95% CI]	All patients [n = 4958] % [95% CI]
Susceptible	77.5 [75.9-78.9]	63.2 [61-65.3]	72 [70.7-73.3]
Any drug-resistance	22.5 [21.1-24.1]	36.8 [34.6-39]	28 [26.8-29.3]
MDR-TB	2.8 [2.3-3.5]	11.6 [10.2-13.1]	6.2 [5.5-6.9]
MDR-TB + any SLI resistance	6.9 [2.6-14.4]	2.3 [0.7-5.2]	3.6 [1.8-6.3]
MDR-TB + any FQ resistance	24.1 [15.6-34.5]	20.9 [15.7-26.9]	21.8 [17.3-26.9]
XDR-TB	2.3 [0.3-8.1]	0.91 [0.1-3.3]	1.3 [0.4-3.3]

MDR-TB = multidrug-resistant TB; XDR-TB = extensively drug-resistant TB; TB = tuberculosis; CI = confidence intervals; DST = drug-susceptibility testing; SLI = second-line injectable drugs; FQ = fluoroquinolones
Source: reference 53

nucleic acid tests [CBNAAT]. Diagnostic algorithm has also undergone revision wherein CBNAAT is offered to cases who are smear-negative but have a chest X-ray suggestive of TB, as well as for new TB cases. Initially, only MDR-TB patients were offered treatment with a standard second-line regimen. Later, treatment with standard regimen was offered to XDR-TB patients and MDR-TB with additional resistance to quinolone or second-line injectables (55,56).

During 2011-12, there was a massive scale-up of procurement and supply chain management of second-line drugs with concerted efforts of multiple stakeholders, resulting in countrywide coverage by 2013. During the subsequent period, detection and management of DR-TB through RNTCP progressively increased. DR-TB case finding and treatment initiation efforts 2007-2017 are shown in Figure 43.4 (56).

In 2016, new drug bedaquiline [Bdq] was made accessible to DR-TB patients through a conditional access programme [CAP] under RNTCP. In 2017, conditional approval was accorded for use of delamanid under RNTCP. With the release of the revised Technical and Operational Guidelines in 2016, regimens to treat other forms of drug resistance, such as mono and poly resistance to first and second-line drugs were also included. This has been further updated and consolidated in the Guidelines for PMDT in India 2017 (55,56). The Guidelines for PMDT in India 2017 (55) integrates use of the shorter MDR-TB regimen and newer containing regimen under RNTCP with a DST guided regimen design. The reader is referred to the chapters *"Drug-resistant tuberculosis" [Chapter 42] and "Revised National Tuberculosis Control Programme" [Chapter 53]* for further details.

Key challenges envisaged in the MDR-TB response include; growing gaps between numbers detected and numbers started on treatment; poor treatment outcomes due to health system weaknesses; lack of effective regimens; and insufficient funding including for research. These barriers need to be urgently addressed. Further, novel drug regimens for shortened treatment of drug-susceptible and/or DR-TB, including new or re-purposed drugs, are under investigation.

Table 43.6: Individual drug resistance patterns

	New patients		Previously treated patients	
Drug	% any resistance [95% CI]	% mono-resistance [95% CI]	% any resistance [95% CI]	% mono-resistance [95% CI]
Streptomycin	6.88 [6.01-7.84]	2.22 [1.73-2.81]	13.26 [11.76-14.87]	2.48 [1.83-3.29]
Isoniazid	11.06 [9.97-12.22]	3.85 [3.20-4.60]	25.09 [23.15-27.11]	7.61 [6.45-8.89]
Rifampicin	2.84 [2.28-3.49]	0 [0.0]	11.67 [10.26-13.21]	0.05 [0.001-0.29]
Ethambutol	2.28 [1.78-2.88]	0.23 [0.092-0.47]	7.03 [5.92-8.27]	0.21 [0.06-0.54]
Pyrazinamide	6.95 [6.07-7.91]	4.11 [3.44-4.88]	8.77 [7.53-10.13]	4.07 [3.22-5.06]
Kanamycin	1.01 [0.69-1.43]	0.03 [0.0-0.18]	1.01 [0.61-1.56]	0 [0.0]
Amikacin	0.98 [0.66-1.39]	0.07 [0.01-0.24]	1.01 [0.61-1.56]	0.05 [0.001-0.29]
Capreomycin	1.04 [0.72-1.47]	0.03 [0.02-0.18]	0.85 [0.48-1.37]	0 [0.0]
Levofloxacin	2.71 [2.16-3.35]	0.1 [0.02-0.29]	3.75 [2.94-4.71]	0 [0.0]
Moxifloxacin	2.58 [2.04-3.20]	0.07 [0.01-0.24]	4.01 [3.18-4.99]	0 [0.0]
PAS	2.32 [1.81-2.91]	0.33 [0.16-0.60]	2.38 [1.74-3.17]	0.42 [0.18-0.83]
Ethionamide	2.54 [2.02-3.17]	0.33 [0.16-0.60]	3.06 [2.33-3.94]	0.26 [0.09-0.62]

CI = confidence intervals; PAS = para-amino salicylic acid
Source: reference 53

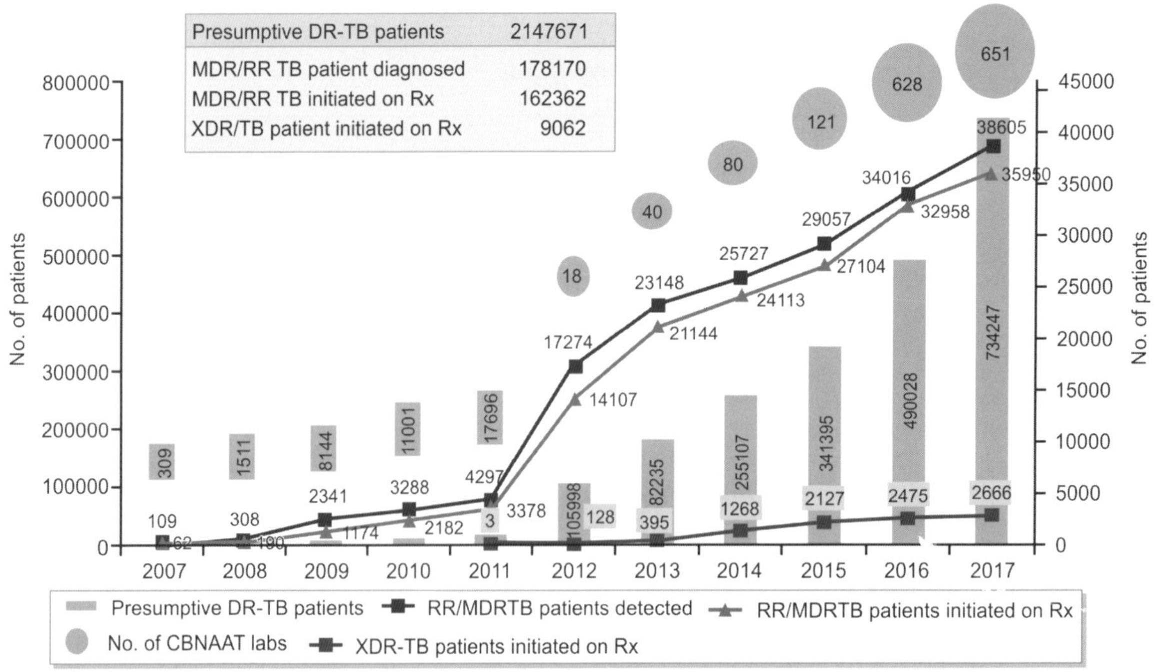

Figure 43.4: DR-TB, case-finding and treatment initiation effort, in India 2007-2017.
DR-TB = drug-resistant TB; MDR/RR TB = multidrug-resistant/rifampicin-resistant tuberculosis; Rx = treatment; XDR-TB = extensively drug-resistant tuberculosis; CBNAAT = cartridge-based nucleic acid amplification tests
Reproduced with permission from "Revised National Tuberculosis Control Programme, Directorate General of Health Services, Ministry of Health and Family Welfare, Government of India. India TB Report 2018. New Delhi: Revised National Tuberculosis Control Programme, Directorate General of Health Services, Ministry of Health and Family Welfare, Government of India; 2018" (reference 56)

ACKNOWLEDGEMENTS

The authors gratefully acknowledge Ms J Daisy Vanithai, for her painstaking help in the preparation of the first draft of the article and Mr PR Somasundaram, and Dr VK Vijayan, for their helpful comments.

REFERENCES

1. Jacobs RF. Multiple-drug-resistant tuberculosis. Clin Infect Dis 1994;19:1-8.
2. Pablos-Mendez A, Sterling TR, Frieden TR. The relationship between delayed or incomplete treatment and all-cause mortality in patients with tuberculosis. JAMA 1996;276:1223-8.
3. Bustreo F, Migliori GB, Nardini S, Raviglione MC. Anti-tuberculosis drug resistance: is it worth measuring? The WHO/IUATLD Working Group on Antituberculosis Drug Resistance Surveillance. Monaldi Arch Chest Dis 1996;51:299-302.
4. Kim SJ, Hong YP. Drug resistance of Mycobacterium tuberculosis in Korea. Tuber Lung Dis 1992;73:219-24.
5. Fujiwara PI, Cook SV, Rutherford CM, Crawford JT, Glickman SE, Kreiswirth BN, et al. A continuing survey of drug-resistant tuberculosis, New York City, April 1994. Arch Intern Med 1997;157:531-6.
6. Aziz MA, Laszlo A, Raviglione M, Rieder HL, Espinal M, Wright A, et al. Guidelines for surveillance of drug resistance in tuberculosis. Second edition. WHO/IUATLD Global Project on Anti-Tuberculosis Drug Resistance Surveillance. Geneva: World Health Organization; 2003.
7. Crofton J, Chaulet P, Mahler D. Guidelines for the management of drug resistant tuberculosis. Geneva: World Health Organization; 1997.
8. Pablos-Méndez A, Raviglione MC, Laszlo A, Binkin N, Rieder HL, Bustreo F, et al, for the WHO/IUATLD Working Group on Anti-tuberculosis Drug Resistance Surveillance. Global surveillance for antituberculosis-drug resistance: 1994-1997. N Engl J Med 1998;338:1641-9.
9. Anti-tuberculosis drug resistance in the world: the WHO/IUATLD Global Project on Anti-Tuberculosis Drug Resistance Surveillance: WHO/TB/97.229. Geneva: World Health Organization; 1997.
10. Raviglione MC, Sudre P, Rieder HL, Spinaci S, Kochi A. Secular trends of tuberculosis in western Europe. Bull World Health Organ 1993;71:297-306.
11. Raviglione MC, Rieder HL, Styblo K, Khomenko AG, Esteves K, Kochi A. Tuberculosis trends in eastern Europe and the former USSR. Tuber Lung Dis 1994;75:400-16.
12. Günther G. Multidrug-resistant and extensively drug-resistant tuberculosis: a review of current concepts and future challenges. Clin Med [Lond] 2014;14:279-85.
13. Anti-tuberculosis drug resistance in the world: the WHO/IUATLD Global Project on Anti-Tuberculosis Drug Resistance Surveillance. Report 13: Prevalence and trends: WHO/CDS/TB/2000.278. Geneva: World Health Organization; 2000.
14. Anti-tuberculosis drug resistance in the world: the WHO/IUATLD Global Project on Anti-Tuberculosis Drug Resistance Surveillance. Third global report: WHO/HTM/TB/2004.343. Geneva: World Health Organization; 2004.
15. Anti-tuberculosis drug resistance in the world: the WHO/IUATLD Global Project on Anti-Tuberculosis Drug Resistance Surveillance. Fourth global report: WHO/HTM/TB/2008.394. Geneva: World Health Organization; 2008.
16. Multidrug and extensively drug-resistant TB [M/XDR-TB]: 2010 global report on surveillance and response: WHO/HTM/TB/2010. Geneva: World Health Organization; 2010.
17. World Health Organization. Global tuberculosis report. Geneva: World Health Organization; 2018.
18. Barnes PF. The influence of epidemiologic factors on drug resistance rates in tuberculosis. Am Rev Respir Dis 1987;136:325-8.
19. Joint Tuberculosis Committee of the British Thoracic Society. Control and prevention of tuberculosis in the United Kingdom: Code of Practice 1994. Thorax 1994;49:1193-200.
20. Kennedy N, Billington O, Mackay A, Fillespie SH, Bannister B. Re-emergence of tuberculosis. BMJ 1993;306:514.
21. McKenna MT, McCray E, Onorato I. The epidemiology of tuberculosis among foreign-born persons in the United States, 1986 to 1993. N Engl J Med 1995;332:1071-6.
22. Centers for Disease Control & Prevention. Emergence of Mycobacterium tuberculosis with extensive resistance to second line drugs-worldwide, 2002-2004. MMWR 2006;55:301-5.
23. World Health Organization, XDR-TB Extensive Drug Resistant TB, September 2006. Available at URL: http://www.who.int/tb/XDR_TB_Sept_06.pdf. Accessed on September 12, 2018.
24. Masjedi MR, Farnia P, Sorooch S, Pooramiri MV, Mansoori SD, Zariffi AZ, Akbarvelayati A, Hoffner S. Extensively drug-resistant tuberculosis: 2 years of surveillance in Iran. Clin Infect Dis 2006;43:841-7.
25. Raviglione MC. The new Stop TB Strategy and the Global Plan to Stop TB, 2006-2015. Bull World Health Organ 2007;85:327.
26. Blondal K. Barriers to reaching the targets for tuberculosis control: multidrug-resistant tuberculosis. Bull World Health Organ 2007;85:387-90.
27. Migliori GB, Besozzi G, Girardi E, Kliiman K, Lange C, Toungoussova OS, et al; SMIRA/TBNET Study Group. Clinical and operational value of the extensively drug-resistant tuberculosis definition. Eur Respir J 2007;30:623-6. Epub 2007 Aug 9.
28. Supplement to the Global tuberculosis report [2014]. Drug-resistant TB—surveillance & response http://www.who.int/tb/publications/global_report/en/. Accessed on December 8, 2017.
29. Companion handbook to the WHO guidelines for the programmatic management of drug-resistant tuberculosis. WHO/HTM/TB/2014.11. Geneva: World Health Organization; 2014.
30. Definitions and reporting framework for tuberculosis – 2013 revision. WHO/ HTM/ TB/2013.2. Geneva: World Health Organization; 2013.
31. Electronic recording and reporting for TB care and control. WHO/HTM/TB/2011.22. Geneva: World Health Organization; 2012.
32. World Health Organization. Global Tuberculosis Report 2014. Geneva: World Health Organization; 2014.
33. Prevalence of drug resistance in patients with pulmonary tuberculosis presenting for the first time with symptoms at chest clinics in India. I. Findings in urban clinics among patients giving no history of previous chemotherapy. Indian J Med Res 1968;56:1617-30.
34. Prevalence of drug resistance in patients with pulmonary tuberculosis presenting for the first time with symptoms at chest clinics in India. II. Findings in urban clinics among all patients, with or without history of previous chemotherapy. Indian J Med Res 1969;57:823-35.
35. Krishnaswami KV, Rahim MA, Primary drug resistance in pulmonary tuberculosis. Indian J Chest Dis Allied Sci 1976;18:233-7.
36. Trivedi SS, Desai SC. Primary antituberculosis drug resistance and acquired rifampicin resistance in Gujarat-India. Tubercle 1988;69:37-42.

37. Paramasivan CN, Chandrasekaran V, Santha T, Sudarsanam NM, Prabhakar R. Bacteriological investigations for short-course chemotherapy under the tuberculosis programme in two districts of India. Tuber Lung Dis 1993;74:23-7.

38. Chandrasekaran S, Jagota P, Chaudhuri K. Initial drug resistance to anti-tuberculosis drugs in urban and rural district tuberculosis programme. Indian J Tuberc 1992;39:171-5.

39. Chandrasekaran S, Chauhan MM, Rajalakshmi R, Chaudhuri K, Mahadev B. Initial drug resistance to anti-tuberculosis drugs in patients attending an urban district tuberculosis centre. Indian J Tuberc 1990;37:215-6.

40. Sophia V, Balasangameshwara VH, Jagannath PS, Saorja VN, Kumar P. Initial drug resistance among tuberculosis patients under DOTS program in Bangalore city. Indian J Tuberc 2004;51:17-22.

41. Gupta PR, Singhal B, Sharma TN, Gupta RB. Prevalence of initial drug resistance in tuberculosis patients attending a chest hospital. Indian J Med Res 1993;97:102-3.

42. Jain NK, Chopra KK, Prasad G. Initial acquired isoniazid and rifampicin resistance to M. tuberculosis and its implications for treatment. Indian J Tuberc 1992; 39:121-4.

43. Datta M, Radhamani MP, Selvaraj R, Paramasivan CN, Gopalan BN, et al. Critical assessment of smear-positive pulmonary tuberculosis patients after chemotherapy under the district tuberculosis programme. Tuber Lung Dis 1993;74:180-6.

44. Sophia V, Balasangameshwara VH, Jagannatha PS, Saoja VN, Shivashankar B, Jagota P, Re-treatment outcome of smear positive tuberculosis cases under DOTS in Bangalore City. Indian J Tuber C 2002;49:195-204.

45. Vasanthakumari R, Jagannath K. Multidrug resistant tuberculosis: a Tamil Nadu study. Lung India 1997;15:178-80.

46. Kam KM, Yip CW. Surveillance of Mycobacterium tuberculosis drug resistance in Hong Kong, 1986-1999, after the implementation of directly observed treatment. Int J Tuberc Lung Dis 2001;5: 815-23.

47. Malla P, Bam DS, Shrestha B, Drug resistance surveillance of TB cases in Nepal. Int J Tuberc Lung Dis 2001;5:S 84.

48. Mahadev B, Jagota P, Srikantaramu N, Gnaneshwaran M. Surveillance of drug resistance in Mysore district, Karnataka. NTI Bulletin 2003;39:5-10.

49. Mahadev B, Kumar P, Agarwa SP, Chauhan LS, Srikantaramu N. Surveillance of Drug Resistance to Anti-tuberculosis Drugs in Districts of Hoogli in West Bengal and Mayurbhanj in Orissa. Indian J Tuber C 2005;52:5-10.

50. Paramasivan CN, Venkataraman P. Drug resistance in tuberculosis in India. Indian J Med Res 2004;120:377-86.

51. Santha T, Thomas a, Chandrasekaran V, Selvakumar N, Gopi PG, et al. Initial drug susceptibility profile of M. tuberculosis among patients under TB programme in South India. Int J tuberc Lung Dis 2006;10:52-7.

52. Swaminathan S, Paramasivan CN, Ponnuraja C, Iliayas S, Rajasekaran S, Narayanan PR. Anti-tuberculosis drug resistance in patients with HIV and tuberculosis in South India. Int J Tuberc Lung Dis 2005;9:896-900.

53. Ministry of Health and Family Welfare, Government of India. Report of the First National Anti-tuberculosis Drug Resistance Survey India 2014-16. Available at URL: https://tbcindia.gov.in/showfile.php?lid=3315. Accessed on June 26, 2018.

54. Ramachandran R, Nalini S, Chandrasekar V, Dave PV, Sanghvi AS, Wares F, et al. Surveillance of drug-resistant tuberculosis in the state of Gujarat, India. Int J Tuberc Lung Dis 2009;13:1154-60.

55. Revised National Tuberculosis Control Programme, Directorate General of Health Services, Ministry of Health and Family Welfare, Government of India. Guidelines on programmatic management of drug-resistant tuberculosis in India 2017. New Delhi: World Health Organization, Country Office for India; 2017.

56. Revised National Tuberculosis Control Programme, Directorate General of Health Services, Ministry of Health and Family Welfare, Government of India. India TB Report 2018. New Delhi: Revised National Tuberculosis Control Programme, Directorate General of Health Services, Ministry of Health and Family Welfare, Government of India; 2018.

44

Treatment of Tuberculosis

Rupak Singla, Sanjay Gupta, Amit Sharma

INTRODUCTION

Tuberculosis [TB] has been a scourge of mankind for thousands of years and remains one of the deadliest diseases in the world today. Nevertheless, TB can be cured in nearly all cases. The only way to stop the spread of disease in the community is to cure all smear-positive cases by treatment with appropriate chemotherapeutic regimens. The major landmarks in the evolution of modern anti-TB treatment are given in Table 44.1 (1-11).

ANTI-TUBERCULOSIS DRUGS

Isoniazid, rifampicin, pyrazinamide, streptomycin and ethambutol are the principal first-line anti-TB drugs used in short-course treatment. Isoniazid and rifampicin are bactericidal drugs. Pyrazinamide is bactericidal in acidic medium while streptomycin is bactericidal in alkaline medium. Ethambutol is generally considered bacteriostatic, although it is bactericidal *in vitro*. The mechanism of action and classification of anti-TB drugs are shown in Tables 44.2 and 44.3 (12,13). The reader is referred to Tables 42.2A and 42.2C for the current [year 2018] classification of anti-TB drugs.

SCIENTIFIC BASIS OF TUBERCULOSIS TREATMENT

Mycobacterium tuberculosis [*Mtb*] is a slow-growing aerobic organism with a generation doubling-time of 18 hours and can remain dormant for a long period. Therefore, prolonged treatment is required to ensure relapse-free cure.

In any drug regimen the anti-TB drugs act by three ways: [i] their bactericidal action, defined as their ability to kill rapidly large numbers of actively multiplying bacilli; [ii] their sterilising action, defined as their capacity to kill all the bacilli including semi-dormant bacilli and bacilli which show short burst of metabolic activity; [iii] their ability to prevent the emergence of acquired resistance by suppressing drug-resistant [DR] mutants which may be present in large bacterial populations [Figure 44.1, Table 44.4] (14).

The drugs with bactericidal action will lead to early sputum conversion and higher cure rates. The drugs with ability to prevent the emergence of acquired resistance will prevent failures to occur. The drugs with sterilising action will reduce the relapse rates and are very vital for reducing the treatment duration.

Bacteriological Factors

The Numerical Factor

The number of tubercle bacilli varies widely with the type of lesion. While in an encapsulated medium sized nodular lesion with no bronchial communication, the number of bacilli can be as low as 100, the number in a cavity of same size communicating with the bronchi is about 10^8 (15). Resistant mutants are likely to be present even before treatment is started if the bacterial population is larger.

The Metabolic Factor

Anti-TB drugs kill tubercle bacilli that are metabolically active and are multiplying continuously. However, in each bacterial population there are bacilli with a very low metabolic rate [Figure 44.1]. Some are inhibited due to low pH, while others remain dormant most of the time and multiply only for short periods. These bacilli are called "persisters" and "spurters". Only pyrazinamide and rifampicin are effective against them under certain conditions. This phenomenon explains to some extent why all bacilli are not killed during treatment, and why drug-susceptible bacilli are coughed up for some time thereafter. Further, endogenous reactivation and relapse

Table 44.1: Evolution of modern chemotherapy for TB

Year	Major events
1940	Bacteriostatic effect of sulphonamides and dapsone was demonstrated in guinea-pigs infected with tubercle bacilli, However, results in humans were disappointing
1944	Streptomycin showed striking therapeutic effect on experimental TB in guinea-pigs. Soon afterwards, it was used for the first time in human patients
1946	Clinical use of streptomycin, monotherapy leads to resistance
1949	PAS prevented the emergence of drug resistance if given in combination with streptomycin
1952	Anti-TB activity of isoniazid was discovered though synthesized 40 years earlier. Since then it has been an important component of all primary drug regimens as it is highly effective, inexpensive, and has low toxicity
1952-1955	Introduction of isoniazid and two drug regimens [PH and SH]
1958	Data from India suggests that supervised administration of treatment [DOT] is essential
1959	Ambulatory chemotherapy as effective as sanatorium treatment. No additional risk of disease to close contacts
1964	Intermittent regimens demonstrated to be as effective as daily regimens. Efficacy of twice weekly SH intermittent regimen [S2H2] proved
1969	Twice weekly PH as effective as daily PH
1958-1967	Emergence of daily administered 3 drug regimens [STH/TH, SPH/PH]
1970	Rifampicin introduced as the most effective medication for TB. It led to the emergence of effective short-course regimens
1970	Inclusion of rifampicin or pyrazinamide in SH regimen substantially reduced the relapse rate
1972-1974	Treatment duration shortened to 6 months by the inclusion of rifampicin and pyrazinamide in the regimen
1976	Modern SCC regimens delineated. It was shown that the sterilizing activity of pyrazinamide was confined to the first 2 months of treatment during IP, whereas the sterilising activity of rifampicin persisted throughout the CP
1977 onwards	Demonstration of the value of intermittency in short-course regimens, particularly that three times weekly treatment throughout was as effective as, and less toxic and expensive than daily regimens
1980s	6-month fully intermittent effective SCC regimens evolved
1980s	Treatment duration of less than 6 months demonstrated high relapse rates [11%-40%]
	Standardised and simplified regimens using fully intermittent, directly observed 6-month treatment shown to be effective on a mass basis

TB = tuberculosis; S = streptomycin, P = para-aminosalicylic acid; H = isoniazid; T = thiacetazone; IP = intensive Phase; CP = continuation phase; SCC = short-course chemotherapy
Source: references 1-11

Table 44.2: Mechanism of action of first-line anti-TB drugs

Drug	Mechanism of action	Genes involved in drug resistance
Streptomycin	Inhibition of protein synthesis by binding tightly to the conserved A site of 16S rRNA in the 30S ribosomal subunit	Ribosomal protein subunit 12 [rpsL] 16S ribosomal RNA [rrs]
Isoniazid	Exact mechanism of action is not known. It probably acts by its effect on nucleic acid biosynthesis, lipids and glycolysis, leading to the inhibition of the synthesis of mycolic acid of mycobacteria	Catalase-peroxidase [katG] NADH-specific enoyl acyl carrier protein [acp] reductase [inhA] Alkyl hydroperoxide reductase [ahpC] NADH dehydrogenase [ndh] Oxidative stress regulator [oxyR] Beta-ketocyl acyl carrier protein synthase [kasA]
Rifampicin	Inhibition of the beta-subunit of the enzyme DNA dependent RNA polymerase, thus suppressing the initiation of chain formation in RNA synthesis	RNA polymerase subunit B [rpoB]
Pyrazinamide	Exact mechanism of action is not known. It is postulated that the acidic pH and intracellular environment induce a component necessary for the action of pyrazinamide. However, the target is not known. Pyrazinoic acid, an active moiety of pyrazinamide has been shown to inhibit various functions at acid pH in *Mtb*	Pyrazinamidase [pncA]
Ethambutol	The exact mode of action of the drug is not known. Inhibits arabinosyl transferases involved in cell-wall biosynthesis	Arabinosyl transferase [*emb A, emb B,* and *emb C*]

TB = tuberculosis; RNA = ribonucleic acid; NADH = nicotinamide adenine dinucleotide; DNA = deoxyribonucleic acid; *Mtb = Mycobacterium tuberculosis*
Source: references 12,13

Table 44.3: Classification of anti-TB drugs

First-line drugs
 Rifampicin
 Isoniazid
 Pyrazinamide
 Ethambutol
 Streptomycin

Second-line drugs
 Broad spectrum agents
  Cycloserine
  Fluoroquinolones
   Ciprofloxacin
   Ofloxacin
   Levofloxacin
   Moxifloxacin
   Gatifloxacin
  Rifamycins [other than rifampicin]
   Rifabutin
   Rifapentene
  Macrolides
   Azithromycin
   Clarithromycin
  Narrow spectrum agents
   Capreomycin
   Kanamycin
   Amikacin
   Viomycin
   Ethionamide
   Prothionamide
   Clofazimine
   Para-aminosalicylic acid
   Thioacetazone

TB = tuberculosis
Source: reference 13

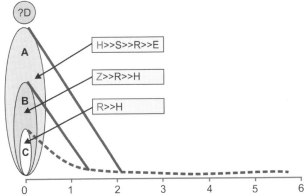

Figure 44.1: Theoretical basis of chemotherapy of tuberculosis. Three populations of *Mycobacterium tuberculosis* are postulated to exist in a tuberculosis cavity, based on their anatomic and metabolic characteristics. *Population A* refers to rapidly multiplying bacteria found in caseous debris in pulmonary cavities. Compared with streptomycin [S], rifampicin [R], and ethambutol [E], isoniazid [H] is most active against this population. Slowly multiplying bacteria because of local acidic conditions are referred to as *population B*. Pyrazinamide [Z] is the most effective antituberculosis drug active against this group followed by rifampicin [R] and isoniazid [H]. "Elimination" of populations "A" and "B" results in negative sputum cultures, typically after two months of treatment. Bacilli in the host tissue capable of sporadic bursts of metabolism, multiplication constitute population "C". This population is a potential source for relapses. Rifampicin [R] plays a major role in eliminating these organisms followed by H. Another population of bacilli designated as population "D" are dormant non-replicating bacilli that are not vulnerable to antimicrobial action and are also considered to be a potential source for relapse.
Reproduced with permission from "Balasubramanian R, Ramachandran R. Evolution of chemotherapeutic regimens in the treatment of TB and their scientific rationale. In: Sharma SK, Mohan A, editors. Tuberculosis, Second Edition. New Delhi: Jaypee Brothers Medical Publishers; 2009.p.734-50" (reference 14)

with drug-susceptible organisms after being "cured" may occur due to bacilli that have persisted in residual lesions in a dormant state for a long time.

Environmental Factors

The Anatomical Factors

All drugs are not able to penetrate into all tissues and cells or permeate biological membranes, including the normal blood-brain barrier. Isoniazid, rifampicin and pyrazinamide readily cross biological membranes, whereas streptomycin fails to enter many cells and is much less effective against intracellular bacilli (16).

The Biochemical Factors

Environmental pH and arterial oxygen tension [PaO_2] are the important biochemical factors that influence the antimicrobial effect of a drug. At a neutral pH, as in cavity walls, all the anti-TB drugs are highly effective. Streptomycin, however, is most active in a slightly alkaline [extracellular] environment, whereas pyrazinamide acts largely in acidic medium such as that found inside cells. Further, it is suggested that dormant organisms survive within cells or in necrotic areas of old encapsulated lesions [that do not communicate with a

bronchus] where pH is usually acidic and PaO_2 is decreased. Presence of small number of bacilli in closed extrapulmonary lesions also shows that the PaO_2 is an important factor.

Pharmacological Factors

Dosage

Drugs must be given in a dosage adequate enough to produce an inhibitory concentration at the site where bacilli are present, but it is not necessary to keep this concentration

Table 44.4: Grading of activities of anti-TB drugs

Extent of activity	Prevention of resistance	Early bactericidal	Sterilising
High	Isoniazid Rifampicin	Isoniazid	Rifampicin Pyrazinamide
Moderate	Ethambutol Streptomycin	Ethambutol Rifampicin	Isoniazid
Low	Pyrazinamide Thiacetazone	Streptomycin Pyrazinamide Thiacetazone	Streptomycin Thiacetazone Ethambutol

TB = tuberculosis

at a constant level. Studies on the role of dosage and serum levels of isoniazid shows that it is both, the peak level and the total exposure to the drug that are important for the response to the drug. Thus, 400 mg of isoniazid given once daily is therapeutically superior to the same dose divided into two parts and administered at 12 hours intervals (17).

Combinations of Drugs

Treatment regimens should contain a combination of three or more bactericidal drugs, particularly in the initial phase of treatment so that both the susceptible and bacilli resistant to one drug are killed rapidly. For patients who have received anti-TB drugs earlier, regimen should include at least three new drugs to which the bacilli are likely to be susceptible. Sometimes drugs are successively substituted or added, one at a time, to a failing regimen with the result that these people eventually became chronic patients with organisms resistant to all the drugs they had received. Thus, treatment of TB should never be attempted with a single drug nor should a single drug be added to a failing regimen.

The "Lag Period" Factor

In vitro experiments have shown that, when tubercle bacilli are exposed to a drug for a short-time [6-24 hours] and are transferred to a drug-free medium, the surviving bacilli start to grow again after an interval of several days. This interval, called the "lag period", varies with the type and concentration of the drug and with the length of exposure. All anti-TB drugs have been tested for their ability to produce a lag period, in order to determine whether they are suitable for intermittent regimens (18,19).

THE SCIENTIFIC BASIS OF INTERMITTENT TREATMENT

Intermittent regimens are those in which the individual drugs are given at intervals of more than one day, e.g., three or two times a week. Originally, it was believed that anti-TB drugs require daily administration to maintain drug concentrations at inhibitory levels continuously. The two main reasons why intermittent dosage was thought likely to be effective included the observation that a dose of 200 mg isoniazid given daily was more effective than the same total dosage given in divided doses twice daily, and the lag period [post-antibiotic effect] factor. Table 44.5 shows the lag period in the growth of *Mtb* after exposure to different drugs for varying times. For each bactericidal drug there is a maximum lag period that seems to indicate the practical limit beyond which the interval between two doses should not be extended. Thiacetazone is not suitable for intermittent treatment as it does not produce any lag period even after exposure for 24 hours. A series of experiments in animal models demonstrated that intermittent administration of isoniazid, rifampicin and pyrazinamide actually increased the efficacy of treatment (18,19).

Table 44.5: Lag in growth of *Mycobacterium tuberculosis* after temporary exposure to drugs

Drug	Concentration [mg/L]	Lag [days] after exposure for	
		6 hours	24 hours
Isoniazid	1	0	6-9
Rifampicin	0.2	2-3	2-3
Pyrazinamide	50	5-40	40*
Ethambutol	10	0	4-5
Streptomycin	5	8-10	8-10
Ethionamide	5	0	10
Cycloserine	100	0	4-8
Thiacetazone	10	0	0

* Depending on the pH of the medium
Source: references 17-19

Evolution of Short-course Chemotherapeutic Regimens

The monumental advances in the chemotherapy of TB in the last three decades has been the development of short course chemotherapy [SCC] regimens of six to eight months duration as against 12–24 months of conventional chemotherapy. Animal studies had shown high sterilising activities of pyrazinamide and rifampicin resulting in low relapse rates. The chances of failure due to initial drug resistance are greatly decreased because of the multiplicity and potency of the drugs used in the intensive phase [IP]. Sputum conversion occurred rapidly. This led to evolution of highly effective SCC regimens consisting of rifampicin, isoniazid, and pyrazinamide with streptomycin/ethambutol for a period of two months followed by two or three drugs like rifampicin plus isoniazid with or without ethambutol or a non-rifampicin continuation phase [CP] consisting of streptomycin or thiacetazone plus isoniazid. These regimens were found to be highly effective with no failures among patients with sensitive tubercle bacilli. The relapse rates were less than 5% during a two-year period of follow-up. In contrast, 12 months non-rifampicin conventional regimens had an overall failure [failure plus relapse] rate of maximum of 18%.

STANDARD ANTI-TUBERCULOSIS TREATMENT REGIMENS

Standardised treatment means that all patients in a defined group receive the same treatment regimen. Standard regimens have the following advantages over individualised treatment: [i] reduced errors in prescription [and thus, less risk of development of DR-TB]; [ii] facilitating the estimation of drug needs, purchasing, distribution and monitoring; [iii] staff training is facilitated; [iv] reduced costs; [v] maintaining a regular drug supply when patients move from one area to another is made easier; and [vi] outcome evaluation is convenient and results are comparable.

For assigning standard regimens, patients are grouped by the same patient registration groups used for recording and reporting, which differentiate new patients from those who have had prior treatment. Registration groups for previously treated patients are based on the outcome of their prior treatment course, i.e., failure, relapse and default.

All TB treatment regimens comprise of two phases, an initial IP of four or five bactericidal drugs and a CP of two or three drugs. The initial IP is designed to kill actively growing and semi-dormant bacilli. This means a shorter duration of infectivity with a rapid smear conversion [80%-90%] after two to three months of treatment. It usually comprises of four drugs for new patients, and five drugs for patients who had taken anti-TB treatment for more than one month in the past. Use of three drugs in the initial IP has the risk of selecting DR mutants in the smear-positive pulmonary TB patients with high bacillary loads, especially if initial DR rates are high in the area. A four-drug regimen decreases the risk of developing DR and reduces failure and relapse rates. The multiplication of susceptible organisms stops during the first few days of effective treatment, and the total number of bacilli in the sputum decreases rapidly, especially within the first two weeks of effective treatment. This will prevent early deterioration and death in the initial weeks of treatment.

The CP eliminates most residual bacilli and reduces failures and relapses. Because of a small number of bacilli at the beginning of the CP, fewer drugs are required as the chance of emergence of DR mutants is low. It usually comprises of two or three drugs given for four to five months.

World Health Organization [WHO] had revised the international guidelines for treatment of TB in 2010 (20a) in view of new evidence that became available (21-24). These guidelines (20a) were further updated in 2017 (20b). Standard treatment regimens for "new" TB patients [presumed, or known, to have drug-susceptible TB] as per the WHO guidelines (20a,20b) is shown in Table 44.6. Thrice-weekly intermittent treatment has been discontinued. Drug dosages are presented in Table 44.7. In these guidelines the emphasis has been placed on the role of drug-susceptibility testing [DST] in the management of retreatment group keeping in mind the laboratory infrastructure in a given country.

For deciding the treatment regimen, earlier, patients used to be categorised into two groups: [i] treatment naive patients [new patients or patients who have received less than 1 month of treatment]; and [ii] retreatment cases which includes treatment failure, patients returning after loss to follow-up or relapsing from their first treatment course treatment and a few other less defined groups. With availability of "universal DST", this paradigm is not in use presently.

For patients with drug-susceptible TB, treatment regimens have an initial IP for two months and a CP lasting for four months. During the initial IP of therapy four drugs, namely isoniazid, rifampicin, ethambutol and pyrazinamide, are administered which lead to rapid killing of bacilli. Majority of cases with sputum smear-positive TB will become sputum

Table 44.6: Standard treatment regimens for "new" TB patients [presumed, or known, to have drug-susceptible TB]

Intensive phase*	Continuation phase	Comment
2HRZE	4HR	Optimal regimen
2HRZE	4HRE	Applicable in countries/settings where the level of H resistance among new cases is high and H susceptibility testing is not done, or results are not available, before the continuation phase begins

* In TB meningitis, E should be replaced by S
H = isoniazid; R= rifampicin; Z = pyrazinamide; E= ethambutol; S = streptomycin
Source: references 20a,20b

Table 44.7: Recommended doses of first-line anti-TB drugs for adults

Drug	Daily	
	Dose and range [mg/kg body weight]	Maximum [mg]
Isoniazid	5 [4-6]	300
Rifampicin	10 [8-12]	600
Pyrazinamide	25 [20-30]	-
Ethambutol	15 [15-20]	-
Streptomycin*	15 [12-18]	1000

*Patients aged over 60 years may not be able to tolerate more than 500-750 mg daily, so some guidelines recommend reduction of the dose to 10 mg/kg per day in patients in this age group. Patients weighing less than 50 kg may not tolerate doses above 500-750 mg daily
TB = tuberculosis
Source: references 20a,20b

negative during this period. In the CP usually two drugs, namely isoniazid and rifampicin, are required for a period of four months. The CP should include drugs with sterilising effect so that all the bacilli including semi-dormant bacilli and bacilli which show short burst of metabolic activity are killed. This will prevent the recurrence of TB. The WHO has recommended (20a,20b) that in populations with known or suspected high levels of isoniazid resistance, new TB patients can receive ethambutol along with isoniazid and rifampicin in the CP (20a,20b).

In 2014, India Government released document for Standards for TB care in India (25). As per this document the CP should consist of three drugs [isoniazid, rifampicin and ethambutol] given for at least four months. The Standards for TB care in India (25) also states that in special situations like bone and joint TB, spinal TB with neurological involvement and neurological TB, the duration of CP may be extended by three to six months. The Presently, as per the Revised National TB Control Programme [RNTCP] Technical and Operational Guidelines for Tuberculosis Control in India (26) the CP consists of three drugs [isoniazid, rifampicin and ethambutol] given for at least four months. The reader is referred to the chapter *"Revised National Tuberculosis Control Programme" [Chapter 53]* for details.

With availability of "universal DST", molecular testing for drug resistance is done and treatment is administered as per the category of DR-TB. The new diagnostic algorithm in adults and children is shown in Figures 42.5A and 42.5B. The treatment algorithm as per the "universal DST" results is shown in Figure 42.6. The reader is referred to the chapter *"Drug-resistant tuberculosis" [Chapter 42]* for details.

Short-course Chemotherapy Regimens of less than Six Months Using First-line Drugs Only

In a study (27) conducted at Chennai, a five month regimen consisting of rifampicin, streptomycin, isoniazid and pyrazinamide daily for two months, followed by streptomycin, isoniazid and pyrazinamide twice weekly for three months was found to be effective and had a low relapse rate [7.1% of patients with organisms initially sensitive to streptomycin and isoniazid] (27). The efficacy of a three-month regimen [90 doses of RHZS] during the follow-up period of five years (28,29) has been studied in patients with pulmonary TB. Though this regimen achieved a near 100% culture conversion rate at the end of treatment, 20% of patients had bacteriologically confirmed relapse during the follow-up period of five years. In contrast, when fewer doses were administered over a longer duration [thrice-weekly for 2 months; followed by twice-weekly for 4 months, making up a total of 63 doses in 6 months], relapse rates were only 4%-6%. Thus, the duration for which the drugs are administered appears to be of prime importance and not the number of doses (30-32). Similarly, four months SCC regimens investigated in Singapore also had high relapse rates [8%-16%] (32).

Optimum Duration of Standard, Non-rifampicin Containing Regimens

There are situations where rifampicin is either not available or rifampicin and pyrazinamide cannot be given to a patient. For patients with initially sputum smear-positive TB, practically all-effective regimens reach the potential of bacteriological quiescence within six months of the start of treatment. However, relapse occurs in about one-fourth of patients treated with streptomycin, isoniazid and thiacetazone daily for six months (33). Hence, if rifampicin and pyrazinamide are not used the total duration should be at least 12 months.

With reference to study the optimum duration of initial supplement of streptomycin or the initial IP in long-term treatment, studies in East Africa had shown that two or four weeks are less effective and optimum duration of IP is eight weeks (32,34,35). There is satisfactory evidence that more than 18 months of good treatment produces little additional benefit, if any, in terms of treatment success or prevention of relapse (36).

Treatment of Smear-negative Tuberculosis

In a trial done in Hong Kong (37) the patients received daily or thrice weekly treatment with four drugs [streptomycin, isoniazid, rifampicin and pyrazinamide] for 3-4 months for smear- and culture-negative patients. The smear negative and culture positive patients received 4-6 months of treatment. The follow-up of over 60 months showed a combined relapse rate of 7% and 3% for patients who received 3 months and 4 months of treatment. The WHO guidelines (20a,20b) recommend six months treatment even for smear-negative and culture-negative patients for consistency and to allow a margin of safety.

Adverse Drug Reactions

The important adverse reactions to anti-TB drugs are listed in Table 44.8. The reader is referred to the chapter *"Hepatotoxicity associated with anti-tuberculosis treatment" [Chapter 45]* for details on this topic. Arthralgia due to pyrazinamide is due to inhibition of renal tubular secretion of uric acid by pyrazinoic acid, the main metabolite of pyrazinamide. It can be treated with non-steriodal anti-inflammatory drugs [NSAIDs]. High serum concentration of uric acid may uncommonly precipitate gout.

There are certain adverse reactions with rifampicin which occurs when it is given intermittently. These include "flu-like" syndrome, shortness of breath and shock, thrombocytopenia, acute haemolytic anaemia and acute tubular

Table 44.8: Adverse drug reactions to anti-tuberculosis drugs

Drug	Adverse drug reactions	
	Common	*Uncommon*
Isoniazid	Asymptomatic elevation of serum hepatic enzymes, cutaneous hypersensitivity, hepatitis, peripheral neuropathy	Giddiness, convulsions, psychosis, haemolytic anaemia, aplastic anaemia, lupoid reactions, arthralgias, gynaecomastia, optic neuritis
Rifampicin	Hepatitis, gastrointestinal reactions, thrombocytopenia, febrile reaction, flu syndrome, cutaneous hypersensitivity	Shortness of breath, shock, haemolytic anaemia, acute kidney injury, thrombotic thrombocytopenic purpura
Pyrazinamide	Hepatititis, arthralgia, anorexia, nausea, vomiting, flushing, photosensitivity, cutaneous reactions	Sideroblastic anaemia, gout
Ethambutol	Retrobulbar neuritis, cutaneous reactions	Peripheral neuropathy
Streptomycin	Giddiness, numbness, tinnitus, vertigo, ataxia, deafness, nephrotoxicity, cutaneous hypersensitivity	Renal failure, aplastic anaemia

necrosis (38). In last four situations the rifampicin should not be given again. With current intermittent treatment their incidence is quite low (39,40).

Isoniazid is acetylated in the liver. Europeans and southern Indians are predominantly slow acetylators; while the Japanese, Korean and Eskimo populations are predominantly rapid acetylators. The acetylator status neither affects the efficacy of isoniazid nor the risk of isoniazid induced hepatitis (41-43).

Peripheral neuropathy with isoniazid is more common in malnourished, elderly, patients with chronic liver disease, slow acetylators and in pregnancy. It can be prevented by simultaneous administration of 10 mg of pyridoxine to high risk group of patients (2). Larger doses of pyridoxine [100-200 mg per day] are needed to treat established neuropathy.

Streptomycin is toxic to eighth cranial nerve, with vestibular damage more common than auditory damage. The risk increases with the dose of drug and with age.

Management of Cutaneous Reactions

Anti-TB treatment may be associated with cutaneous reactions in the form of itching, rash etc. The rash is erythematous, macular or papular and is pruritic. In the majority of patients the treatment should be stopped until the rash has subsided to prevent the progression of reaction. Only symptomatic treatment with oral anti-histamines and local soothing lotions may be required. In serious cases exfoliative dermatitis, Stevens Johnson' syndrome and anaphylaxis may occur resulting rarely in death. Here systemic steroid therapy is required. For patients requiring desensitisation the sequence and doses of the challenged regimen to be used to identify the responsible drug is shown in Table 44.9. When other effective drugs are available one may substitute the offending drug with another effective drug rather than attempting desensitisation. Presently desensitisation is rarely required in clinical practice. Hyperpigmentation of skin and gums induced by second-line drug clofazimine used in the treatment of MDR-TB [Figure 44.2] is frequently encountered.

Management of anti-TB drug-induced hepatotoxicity is covered in *"Hepatotoxicity associated with anti-tuberculosis treatment" [Chapter 45]*. Management of TB in patients with renal impairment is covered in *"Tuberculosis in chronic kidney disease" [Chapter 28]*.

Bacteriological Monitoring of Patients during Anti-tuberculosis Treatment

In new patients, sputum smear examination for acid-fast bacilli [AFB] should be done at the end of two months, and if positive, should be repeated at the end of three months. Usually at the end of two months more than 80% of positive sputum smears would have converted to negative. By the end of three months, virtually all patients [> 90%] would be smear negative. Before the programmatic management of DR-TB was launched in India there were significant delays in diagnosis of multidrug-resistant TB [MDR-TB] as well as in the initiation of subsequent treatment of such cases (44). These delays could lead to increased defaults and deaths of MDR-TB cases.

Table 44.9: Challenge doses for detecting cutaneous or generalised hypersensitivity to anti-tuberculosis drugs

Drug	Challenge dose [mg]	
	Day 1	Day 2
Isoniazid	50	300
Rifampicin	75	300
Pyrazinamide	250	1000
Ethionamide, prothionamide	125	375
Cycloserine	125	250
Ethambutol	100	500
Para-aminosalicylic acid	1000	5000
Thiacetazone	25	50
Streptomycin or other aminoglycosides	125	500

Source: reference 20a

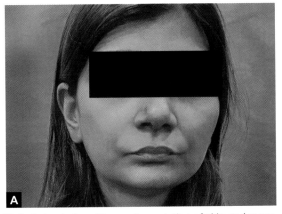
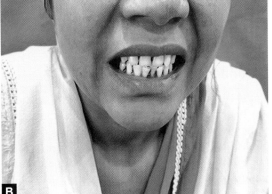

Figure 44.2: Clofazimine-induced hyperpigmentation of skin and gums

The Standards for TB Care in India (25) recommend that, if the sputum smear is positive at any time during the follow-up period, a rapid molecular DST [as the first choice] or culture-DST [at least for rifampicin and if possible for isoniazid, kanamycin and ofloxacin, if rifampicin-resistant/MDR-TB] should be performed as laboratory facilities become available.

Rapid genotypic/molecular methods can help in early detection of MDR-TB leading to early start of appropriate treatment with second line drugs. In India there has been a rapid scale up of laboratory services under programmatic management of DR-TB national programme (18) introducing use of rapid molecular methods, Xpert MTB/RIF and line probe assay [LPA] and "universal DST" is being offered to all patients presently under the RNTCP [Figures 42.5A and 42.5B].

Clinical and Radiographic Monitoring of Patients during Anti-tuberculosis Treatment

Usually after one to two months of treatment the patients start feeling better, are free from fever, cough and sputum. Chest radiograph also shows improvement. They continue to improve over next several months eventually leaving residual fibrotic/cavitary changes. Routinely monitoring of response to treatment by serial chest radiographs is not recommended as they are non-specific. However, they may be of use to look for some suspected complications such as pneumothorax, pleural effusion/empyema and in cases with haemoptysis. Also, the chest radiograph may be done at the end of treatment for future follow-up of the patient. If patients do not show clinical improvement after two or three months of treatment it should alert the clinician regarding treatment compliance and/or drug-resistant TB.

Infectivity during Treatment

Currently ambulatory treatment of TB is recommended (45-47). Hospitalisation is necessary only for some specific situations such as serious disease, compliance problems, and associated complications such as pneumothorax, empyema or haemoptysis. Usually after two weeks of treatment the patients are considered non-infectious and may return to work thereafter (48-54). Generally it is preferable to keep sputum positive patients off the work for at least four weeks.

Laboratory Monitoring during Treatment

Most of the patients complete anti-TB treatment without any significant treatment-related ADRs. Patients should be monitored clinically and counselled to inform the treating physicians in case they have any symptoms suggestive of ADRs. Except in high risk groups, such as, elderly, malnourished, patients with underlying liver disease, alcoholics, pregnant women, it is recommended that the routine laboratory monitoring is not considered necessary (20a).

Treatment of Drug-resistant Tuberculosis

MDR-TB is defined as isolates of *Mtb* resistant to at least isonizid and rifampicin. Treatment of MDR-TB is difficult and has higher failure rates and relapse rates. It requires the use of second line anti-TB drugs.

DR-TB is a man made problem. It is always preferable that national programmes should invest their resources to prevent the development of DR-TB rather than for treating it. Also it is important that the suspected MDR-TB cases are diagnosed early and are initiated on treatment as early as possible. In India programmatic management of DR-TB was launched in 2007 (18). Since then, there has been a rapid scale up of the programme and rapid genotypic laboratory methods are being used for early detection and early initiation of appropriate treatment of DR patients. The reader is also referred to the chapter "*Drug-resistant tuberculosis*" [Chapter 42] for further details.

Treatment of Extra-pulmonary Tuberculosis

Extra-pulmonary TB [EPTB] accounts for about 20% of all cases of TB in immunocompetent persons (20a). Lymph node TB, TB pleural effusion, bone or joint TB are the most common types of EPTB (55,56). Meningeal, miliary, and pericardial TB are more likely to result in a fatal outcome (55). Sparse evidence is available from controlled clinical trials regarding the treatment of EPTB. The WHO 2010 guidelines (20a) recommend that most of the EPTB should be treated with six months standard short-course regimen. Studies in India have demonstrated that six months intermittent short course chemotherapy under national programme is adequate and effective for TB pleural effusion (57) and lymph node TB (58,59).

Some authorities recommend that for miliary TB and some cases with bone and joint TB the treatment may be extended to nine months (13,60). For TB meningitis 9-12 months of treatment has been recommended (13,60). The Standards for TB Care in India (25) recommend that in bone and joint TB, spinal TB with neurological involvement and neurological TB the duration of CP may be extended by three to six months.

The evidence-based Guidelines for Extrapulmonary TB for India [INDEX-TB Guidelines] have recently been published. When TBM is present, the evidence-based INDEX-TB guidelines (61) recommend treatment for at least nine 9 months. The INDEX-TB guidelines (61) recommend that when spinal TB and other forms of bone and joint TB are present, a total treatment duration of 12 months [extendable to 18 months on a case-by-case basis] is indicated.

Details regarding treatment of various forms of EPTB have been covered in the respective chapters in the book.

Ensuring Compliance during Treatment

Many patients do not adhere to anti-TB treatment. Certain factors such as homelessness, alcohol or drug abuse, behavioural problems, mental retardation, lack of family/ social support, among others could be responsible for non-compliance (60). Directly observed treatment [DOT] was shown to be very efficacious in ensuring patients adherence by experience at Chennai and Hong Kong (62). In 1993 WHO announced the new global strategy for TB control called DOTS (63). This strategy is regarded as the most cost effective intervention in the control of TB (63). The reader is referred to the chapter *"DOTS: the strategy that ensures cure of tuberculosis"* [Chapter 47] for further details.

Fixed-dose Combination Formulations

The use of fixed-dose combination [FDC] formulations, comprising of two, three or even four drugs in the same formulation, is thought to improve the treatment compliance, lead to ease of prescription for the physician, thus, reducing in medication errors. FDCs also have the potential to simplify the drug procurement and supply under national tuberculosis programmes (64). The use of FDCs may also reduce the chances of developing DR-TB. However, the majority of clinical studies did not document the superiority of FDC formulations over the use of individual drugs regarding sputum smear-conversion, frequency of ADRs and occurrence of relapse (65,66).

While using FDCs it is important to ensure quality and bio-availability of their component drugs (67,68). Only FDC formulations of proven good quality should be used. Otherwise the bio-availability of some of the drugs, especially rifampicin, may be significantly reduced. Now FDCs are included in the list of essential drugs (69).

Surgery

The reader is referred to the chapter *"Surgery for pleuro-pulmonary tuberculosis"* [Chapter 46] for details on this topic.

Therapeutic Drug Monitoring

Measuring blood levels of anti-TB drugs during treatment is referred to as therapeutic drug monitoring [TDM].

Table 44.10 lists the clinical situations where TDM may be useful (70-73). TDM is not being used in developing countries due to high cost involved and the requirement of specialised technologies. Lack of awareness about the utility of TDM may also be a contributing factor for it's under utilisation. For accessing the peak serum concentration for most of anti-TB drugs, blood should be collected after two hours of ingestion of drug (71). For evaluating delay in absorption a second sample should be collected six hours after the drug ingestion (71). However, TDM results should always be correlated with clinical scenarios and bacteriological data (71).

NEWER ANTI-TUBERCULOSIS DRUGS

There is a need for newer anti-TB drugs which are safer, low in cost, easier to deliver and above all could reduce the duration of chemotherapy. Place of new anti-TB drugs has been extensively reviewed (74-78).

As on date, several new or repurposed anti-TB drugs are under clinical investigation. There has been progress in repurposing or redosing of known anti-TB drugs such as rifamycins [rifapentine, rifampicin], fluoroquinolones [gatifloxacin, moxifloxacin] and riminophenazines [clofazimine]. Many of the drugs have entered in advanced Phase 3 studies. Results of three major Phase 3 trials looking at treatment shortening for drug-sensitive TB are summarised in Table 44.11 (79-81).

Bedaquiline [TMC-207], linezolid, sutezolid [PNU-100480], PA-824, SQ-109 and AZD-5847, delamanid [OPC-67683] have shown encouraging results (82,83a). Bedaquiline has been found to be effective against drug-sensitive and DR strains of *Mtb* and has shown significant improvement in sputum culture conversion at two months (82). Since December 2012 bedaquiline has been approved for conditional use in USA and is the first new TB drug to be approved for use in last more than 40 years. It was recommended conditional authorisation by US-FDA for use in difficult X/MDR-TB patients in combination with other medicines when an effective treatment regimen cannot be

---

Table 44.10: Clinical situations where TDM may be useful

Patients showing unsatisfactory treatment response despite a good compliance and absence of anti-TB drug resistance to assess malabsorption of drugs

In HIV-seropositive patients with poor response [as HIV infected patients may have low levels of anti-TB drugs]

To optimise scheduling of administration and dosing of anti-tuberculous treatment in specific clinical setting such as tuberculous meningitis or some patients with MDR-TB

For evaluation and management of pharmaco-kinetic drug interaction with anti-TB drugs specially rifampicin

In presence of associated renal dysfunction, TDM to drugs such as aminoglycosides, ethambutol, ofloxacin and cyclocerine to guide optimum doses to be used without increased risk of adverse reactions and improved efficacy

For evaluation of new drug formulation such as FDC, as the bio-equivalence of individual drugs, especially rifampicin, may be affected in these

For monitoring the drug-adherence

For evaluating the influence of food or anti-ulcer medication on bio-availability of anti-TB drugs

TDM = therapeutic drug monitoring; TB = tuberculosis; HIV = human immunodeficiency virus; MDR-TB = multidrug-resistant tuberculosis; FDC = fixed-dose combination

Table 44.11: Phase 3 trials for treatment shortening in patients with drug-sensitive TB

Trial Name	Method	Result
OFLOTUB trial (79)	Trial evaluated 4-month combination regimens in which a gatifloxacin was substituted for ethambutol in test arm. In the intervention arm, 917 patients received 400 mg of gatifloxacin, six days a week, in place of ethambutol for two months, followed by two months of treatment with gatifloxacin, isoniazid and rifampicin. In the control arm patients received 6 months of conventional WHO recommended regimen	At two months and end of treatment, patients in the intervention arm fared better. However, after 24 months of completion of treatment patients in the gatifloxacin arm showed higher frequency of TB recurrence [14.6% vs 6.9%] compared to control arm
REMox TB trial (80)	Trial evaluated 4-month combination regimens in which moxifloxacin was substituted for either ethambutol or isoniazid. This was compared with standard six months conventional WHO recommended regimen	The two moxifloxacin arms had higher relapses compared to the control arm, but an earlier conversion to culture-negative sputum was observed in moxifloxacin containing arms. However, both of moxifloxacin-containing regimens were safe, with comparable incidence of grade 3 and 4 adverse events. Also there was no evidence of increased hepatic dysfunction. There was no clinical evidence of cardiac toxicity in moxifloxacin containing arms
Rifaquin Trial (81)	Trial evaluated the safety and efficacy of two regimens for patients with drug-susceptible TB. The control arm was standard 6 months WHO regimen. One study arm included 2 months of daily ethambutol, moxifloxacin, rifampicin and pyrazinamide followed by 2 months of twice weekly moxifloxacin [500 mg] and rifapentine [900 mg]. Second study arm included 2 months of daily ethambutol, moxifloxacin, rifampicin and pyrazinamide followed by 4 months of once weekly moxifloxacin [500 mg] and rifapentine [1200 mg]	The study concluded that the 6-month study regimen was non-inferior, safe and well tolerated. The 4-month study regimen was safe and well tolerated but its efficacy was inferior to the control

TB = tuberculosis; WHO = World Health Organization

devised due to resistance or tolerability. It is administered in a dosage 400 mg once daily for two weeks, followed by 200 mg thrice-weekly for 22 weeks. The drug is to be taken with food. Generally it is well tolerated. However, it can cause QT prolongation in the electrocardiogram. Therefore, one has to be careful in using it with other anti-TB drugs which can cause QT prolongation such as clofazimine, moxifloxacin, etc.

In 2013, another new drug, delamanid, was recommended conditional authorisation with similar conditions for limited. Delamanid also appears to be a promising molecule and has also been found to be effective against drug-sensitive and DR strains of *Mtb*. Delamanid has shown increased sputum culture conversion at 2 months in MDR-TB cases and also shown to reduce mortality in difficult to treat cases of DR. A Phase 3 trial [NCT01424670] is underway where delamanid with optimised background regimen for MDR-TB patients is being compared to a regimen with only background regimen with placebo. The enrolment of around 500 patients has been completed and the results of the trial are awaited (76). Bedaquiline and delamanid are available for use through conditional access under Programmatic Management of Drug-resistant Tuberculosis [PMDT] in India (83b,83c,83d). The reader is referred to chapters *"Drug-resistant tuberculosis"* [Chapter 42] and *"Revised National Tuberculosis Control Programme"* [Chapter 53] for details.

In a Phase 2b trial [TBTC trial 29X] tolerability, safety and antimicrobial activity of different doses of rifapentine [at 10, 15 and 20 mg/kg body weight] in combination with

isoniazid, pyrazinamide and ethambutol during the first-two months of treatment are being investigated. Early results demonstrated that rifapentine has good tolerability and good antimicrobial activity. A study has shown that two weeks of rifampicin up to 35 mg/kg was safe and well tolerated (84). The effects of high doses of rifampicin, 600 mg and 900 mg, in combination with other standard regimen drugs over 2 months [HIGHRIF2] are also being tried (76).

In a meta-analysis (85), linezolid, an oxazolidinone antibiotic class of drugs was found to be promising in MDR-TB. However, it has potential toxicity including anaemia, thrombocytopenia, peripheral neuropathy and optic neuritis (85). In India, linezolid has been found to be cheap, effective and relatively safe (86).

Sutezolid [PNU-100480] is an oxazolidinone and an analogue of linezolid. Sutezolid at a dosage of either 600 mg twice a day or 1200 mg once a day led to a significant reduction in log colony forming units [CFU] counts after 14 days of treatment. SQ-109, originally synthesised as derivative of ethambutol, is also being tested as part of combination regimen.

Recently there are attempts towards novel anti-TB drugs regimen which could transform therapy by shortening and simplifying the treatment of both drug-sensitive and DR-TB with the same oral regimen. NC-001, also known as new combination 1 [PaMZ], is one such regimen where drug candidate PA-824 is combined with moxifloxacin plus pyrazinamide. The early bactericidal activity of this regimen is found to be good (82). The testing of NC-001 advanced to a two months trial [called NC-002] in March, 2012 where in PaMZ was tested for drug-sensitive patients and patients with DR-TB who are sensitive to drugs included in the new regimen (87). The results showed that this combination was effective for both drug sensitive as well as for MDR-TB patients. The ADRs were similar to standard regimen (88). A second trial, NC-003 is testing the early bactericidal action of various combinations of bedaquiline, PA-824, clofazimine and pyrazinamide in drug susceptible patients (89).

There are attempts at reducing the treatment duration for MDR-TB patients also. In Bangladesh regimen, 515 MDR-TB patients were given minimum nine months of treatment regimen and followed up for 2 years. It showed 84% relapse free successful outcomes at 24 months (90). Under the umbrella of "Standardised Treatment Regimen of Anti-tuberculosis Drugs for Patients with Multi-drug-Resistant Tuberculosis [STREAM]" trials, a trial is being carried out with nine months treatment duration for MDR-TB patients with moxifloxacin replacing gatifloxacin in Bangladesh trial. The results will be compared with WHO recommended standard of care treatment for MDR-TB (91). Under the same umbrella a nine months and six months oral-only regimen using bedaquiline have been planned (91).

A recent systematic review (92) identified six drugs, which are not in the list of WHO guidelines for treatment of MDR-TB, but have potential for the management of MDR-TB. These include phenothiazines [thioridazine], co-trimoxazole, metronidazole, doxycycline, disulfiram and tigecycline. For actively replicating TB bacilli co-trimoxazole may be very effective. For dormant bacilli thioridazine appeared promising as an adjuvant drug (92).

Among new drugs some are predicted have activity against persisters populations in TB. These include clofazimine, bedaquiline and oxazolidinones [sutezolid and AZD-5847] (78). Nitroimidazopyrans [delamanid and PA-824], and benzothiazinones [BTZ-043] also have activity against persister populations.

However, despite the advancements in new drugs the search for drugs which could significantly reduce the duration of treatment for drug sensitive and DR-TB, especially avoiding the need for prolonged use of injections is still on.

Corticosteroids in Tuberculosis

Cortiosteroids should be judiciously used in the treatment of TB. The reader is referred to the chapters covering the concerned organ systems for details regarding the evidence and rationale for use and of corticosteroids in patients with active TB.

Treatment of Latent Tuberculosis Infection

The term latent TB infection [LTBI] refers to the presence of *Mtb* in the body without signs and symptoms, radiographic or bacteriologic evidence of active TB disease. Approximately one-third of the world's population is infected with *Mtb* (93). Developed countries have been successful in lowering down TB incidence by targeted testing of high risk population,

whereas poor countries, whose main objective is to cut-down TB transmission by primarily treating active cases, may have as much as 50% of the population infected, making LTBI treatment practically impossible. Yet, targeted testing of high risk populations may prove useful as shown by the successful treatment of LTBI in HIV infected individuals (94,95).

In patients with LTBI, use of potentially toxic drugs for extended intervals of time poses difficulty both to patients [mostly asymptomatic] and providers. Evidence is available demonstrating that isoniazid taken for at least six months in persons with LTBI reduced subsequent TB incidence by 25%-92%, the differences in effectiveness largely explained by differences in treatment completion (96). Use of isoniazid in LTBI treatment, however, is fraught with difficulties. Long duration of administration [6-12 months] coupled with potentially lethal albeit uncommon adverse effects, such as, drug-induced hepatotoxicity reduce its acceptability both to patients and providers alike (97,98).

The International Union Against Tuberculosis [IUAT] trial (99), conducted in Eastern Europe, showed that participants, who completed six and 12 months of isoniazid, had 69% and 93% reduction in active TB, respectively (99). However, completion of the 12 months regimen was much less than the 6 months regimen. The American Thoracic Society [ATS] in 2000 recommended 9 months isoniazid with estimated efficacy of 90% as the acceptable regimen (100). Adverse effects, especially hepatitis, may be difficult to detect and can lead to fatality which may be as high as 1% in older patients (101).

The problems with isoniazid have stimulated development and evaluation of several shorter regimens. Several randomised trials conducted to compare six to 12 months isoniazid with two months of rifampicin and pyrazinamide in HIV infected patients demonstrated equivalent efficacy (102). In 2000, ATS recommended use of rifampicin and pyrazinamide for two months along with a strong recommendation for use in HIV infected persons and a conditional recommendation for non-HIV infected persons (100). This led to widespread use of this regimen, but was quickly followed by reports of serious hepatotoxicity and death, leading to revision of recommendations that advocated cautious use in HIV infected individuals (103,104).

The WHO has published detailed guidelines for management of LTBI (105). There was consensus of the WHO Panel on the equivalence of six-month isoniazid, nine-month isoniazid, and three-month rifpentine plus isoniazid (105).

The recent 2018 WHO guidelines (106) for testing and treatment of LTBI in adults and adolescents are shown in Tables 44.12A and 44.12B.

Newer Regimens for Latent Tuberculosis Infection

One of the promising new drugs being tested for the treatment of LTBI is rifapentine, a cyclopentyl-substituted rifamycin that is as effective as rifampicin, but whose serum half-life is five times that of rifampicin, thus permitting weekly dosing. The isoniazid-rifapentine regime was investigated (107) and once-weekly, three months regimen

Table 44.12A: Treatment options for LTBI	
Risk group category	*Recommendation for treatment of LTBI*
Adults in countries with high and low TB incidence	Isoniazid monotherapy for 6 months
Adults in countries with high TB incidence	Isoniazid monotherapy for 6 months Alternative regimen: rifapentine and isoniazid weekly for 3 months
Adults in countries with a low TB incidence	Isoniazid monotherapy for 6 months Alternative regimens: Isoniazid monotherapy for 9 months; or a 3-month regimen of weekly rifapentine plus isoniazid; or 3-4 months of isoniazid plus rifampicin; or 3-4 months of rifampicin alone
Adults and adolescent PLHW who have an unknown or a positive TST and are unlikely to have active TB disease	At least 36 months of IPT, regardless of whether they are receiving ART. IPT should also be given irrespective of the degree of immunosuppression, history of previous TB treatment and pregnancy

LTBI = latent TB infection; TB = tuberculosis; PLWH = people living with HIV; HIV = human immunodeficiency virus; TST = tuberculin skin test; IPT = isoniazid preventive therapy; ART = antiretroviral treatment
Source: reference 3

Table 44.12B: Treatment regimens and dosages of drugs for LTBI	
Regimen	*Dosage*
Isoniazid alone, daily for 6 or 9 months	Adults 5 mg/kg body weight Children 10 mg/kg body weight [range 7-15 mg] Maximum dose 300 mg
Rifampicin alone, daily for 3-4 months	Adults 10 mg/kg body weight Children 15 mg/kg body weight [range 10-20 mg] Maximum dose 600 mg
Isoniazid + rifampicin daily for 3-4 months	Isoniazid Adults 5 mg/kg body weight Children 10 mg/kg body weight [range 7-15 mg] Maximum dose 300 mg Rifampicin Adults 10 mg/kg body weight Children 15 mg/kg body weight [range 10-20 mg] Maximum dose 600 mg
Rifapentine + isoniazid weekly for 3 months [12 doses]	Isoniazid Age 12 years = 15 mg/kg body weight Age 2-11 years = 5 mg/kg body weight Maximum dose = 900 mg Rifapentene 10-14 kg = 300 mg 14.1-25 kg = 450 mg 25.1-32 kg = 600 mg 32.1-50 kg = 750 mg >50 kg = 900 mg Maximum dose = 900 mg

LTBI = latent tuberculosis infection
Source: reference 106

of isoniazid-rifapentine [900 mg each] was found to be as effective as nine months of isoniazid alone in preventing TB and had a higher treatment-completion rate.

Rifabutin may be substituted for rifampicin in HIV-seropositive patients at risk for isoniazid-resistant TB owing to its lower interaction with anti-retroviral drugs as compared to RIF. The six months regimen of pyrazinamide and a fluoroquinolone, recommended for LTBI treatment of MDR-TB contacts, has been shown to have very poor completion rates due to high toxicity. This has prompted the use of monotherapy with levofloxacin or moxifloxacin, the latter showing special promise on account of published literature showing its equivalence to isoniazid (108,109).

Shorter Regimens for Treatment of Latent Tuberculosis Infection In their meta-analysis of 10 randomised controlled trials consisting of 10,717 HIV-negative adults and children, Sharma *et al* (110) concluded that shortened prophylactic regimens using rifampicin alone did not demonstrate higher rates of active TB when compared to longer regimens with isoniazid. A weekly regimen of rifapentine plus isoniazid had higher completion rates with less liver toxicity but more treatment discontinuation due to adverse events than with isoniazid (110). Further, data suggest that, treatment with four months of rifampicin had similar rates of safety and efficacy but a better adherence compared with nine months of treatment with isoniazid (111,112).

Treatment of Latent Tuberculosis Infection in India

India is home to nearly one-fourth of the global burden of TB. In India, 40% of the population are infected, the annual risk of infection being 1.5% (113,114). The priority in India has been to treat sputum smear-positive TB patients in order to interrupt the transmission in TB. Treating 40% of the population for LTBI is neither rational nor practicable, thus emphasising the need for a focussed approach. The most obvious target groups for LTBI treatment would include high-risk patients, such as, those receiving corticosteroids, immunosuppressants, HIV-infected and juvenile contacts of sputum-positive index cases, showing recent tuberculin skin test [TST] conversion.

Another major concern in LTBI treatment is development of drug-resistance. The most likely reason for development of drug-resistance with LTBI treatment is improper dosing and/or administration, which can be prevented by strict monitoring, good education and rigorous follow-up. The second reason for the development of drug-resistance could be partial treatment of active TB masquerading as LTBI. This should be avoided by a thorough clinical assessment, based on sound history and appropriate investigations such as chest radiograph and sputum testing, before starting LTBI treatment.

Finally, it is the responsibility of the health care provider team to ensure that patient complies with treatment once the decision to treat LTBI with a suitable regime on an individual basis has been taken.

REFERENCES

1. Barry V. Development of the chemotherapeutic agent for tuberculosis. In: Barry V, editor. Chemotherapy of tuberculosis. London: Butterworths; 1964.

2. Toman K, Freiden T. Toman's tuberculosis: case detection, treatment, and monitoring : questions and answers. Second edition. Geneva: World Health Organization; 2004.

3. Schatz A, Bugie E, Waksman S. Streptomycin, a substance exhibiting antibiotic activity against Gram-positive and Gram-negative bacteria. 1944 Clin Orthop Relat Res 2005;437:3-6.

4. Hinshaw H, Feldman W. Streptomycin in the treatment of clinical tuberculosis; a preliminary report. Proc Staff Meet Mayo Clin 1945;20:313-8.

5. Sense P. History of the development of rifampicin. Rev Infect Dis 1983;5:402-6.

6. East African/British Medical Research Council. Controlled clinical treatment of short course [6 months] regime of chemotherapy for treatment of pulmonary tuberculosis. Third report. Lancet 1974;2:237-48.

7. Fox W, Ellard GA, Mitchison DA. Studies on the treatment of tuberculosis undertaken by the British Medical Research Council tuberculosis units, 1946-1986, with relevant subsequent publications. Int J Tuberc Lung Dis 1999;3:S231-79.

8. Controlled trial of 2, 4, and 6 months of pyrazinamide in 6-month, three-times-weekly regimens for smear-positive pulmonary tuberculosis, including an assessment of a combined preparation of isoniazid, rifampin, and pyrazinamide. Results at 30 months. Hong Kong Chest Service/British Medical Research Council. Am Rev Respir Dis 1991;143:700-6.

9. Controlled clinical trial of five short-course [4-month] chemotherapy regimens in pulmonary tuberculosis. First report of 4th study. East African and British Medical Research Councils. Lancet 1978;2:334-8.

10. Results of directly observed short-course chemotherapy in 112,842 Chinese patients with smear-positive tuberculosis. China Tuberculosis Control Collaboration. Lancet 1996;347:358-62.

11. Khatri GR, Frieden TR. The status and prospects of tuberculosis control in India. Int J Tuberc Lung Dis 2000;4:193-200.

12. World Health Organization. Companion handbook to the WHO guidelines for the programmatic management of drug-resistant tuberculosis. Geneva: World Health Organization; 2014.

13. Blumberg HM, Burman WJ, Chaisson RE, Daley CL, Etkind SC, Friedman LN, et al. American Thoracic Society/Centers for Disease Control and Prevention/Infectious Diseases Society of America. Treatment of tuberculosis. Am J Respir Crit Care Med 2003;167:603-62.

14. Balasubramanian R, Ramachandran R. Evolution of chemotherapeutic regimens in the treatment of tuberculosis and their scientific rationale. In: Sharma SK, Mohan A, editors. Tuberculosis, Second Edition. New Delhi: Jaypee Brothers Medical Publishers; 2009.p.734-50.

15. Canetti G. The tubercle bacillus in pulmonary lesion of man; histobacteriology and its bearing on the therapy of pulmonary tuberculosis. New York: Springer; 1955.

16. Mitchison DA. Bacteriological mechanisms in recent controlled chemotherapy studies. Bull Int Union Tuberc Lung Dis 1970;43: 322-31.

17. A concurrent comparison of isoniazid plus PAS with three regimens of isoniazid alone in the domiciliary treatment of pulmonary tuberculosis in South India. Bull World Health Organ 1960;23:535-85.

18. Grumbach F, Canetti G, Grosset J, le Lirzin M. Late results of long-term intermittent chemotherapy of advanced, murine tuberculosis: limits of the murine model. Tubercle 1967;48:11-26.

19. Dickinson JM, Ellard GA, Mitchison DA. Suitability of isoniazid and ethambutol for intermittent administration in the treatment of tuberculosis. Tubercle 1968;49:351-66.

20a. World Health Organization. Treatment of tuberculosis: guidelines. Fourth Edition. Geneva: World Health Organization; 2010.

20b. World Health Organization. Treatment of tuberculosis. Guidelines for the treatment of drug-susceptible tuberculosis and patient care, 2017 update. WHO/HTM/TB/2017.05. Geneva: World Health Organization; 2017.

21. Jindani A, Nunn AJ, Enarson DA. Two 8-month regimens of chemotherapy for treatment of newly diagnosed pulmonary tuberculosis: international multicentre randomised trial. Lancet 2004;364:1244-51.

22. Mak A, Thomas A, Del Granado M, Zaleskis R, Mouzafarova N, Menzies D. Influence of multidrug resistance on tuberculosis treatment outcomes with standardized regimens. Am J Respir Crit Care Med 2008;178:306-12.

23. Menzies D, Benedetti A, Paydar A, Martin I, Royce S, Pai M, et al. Effect of duration and intermittency of rifampin on tuberculosis treatment outcomes: a systematic review and meta-analysis. PLoS Medicine 2009;6:e1000146.

24. Menzies D, Benedetti A, Paydar A, Royce S, Madhukar P, Burman W, et al. Standardized treatment of active tuberculosis in patients with previous treatment and/or with mono-resistance to isoniazid: a systematic review and meta-analysis. PLoS Medicine 2009;6:e1000150.

25. World Health Organization, Country Office for India. Standards for TB Care in India. New Delhi: World Health Organization, Country Office for India; 2014.

26. Central TB Division, Ministry of Health and family Welfare, Government of India. Revised National TB Control Programme [RNTCP] Technical and Operational Guidelines for Tuberculosis Control in India. Available at URL: http://tbcindia.nic.in/index1.php?lang=1&level=2&sublinkid=4573&lid=3177. Accessed on December 31, 2018.

27. Santha T, Nazareth O, Krishnamurthy MS, Balasubramanian R, Vijayan VK, Janardhanam B, et al. Treatment of pulmonary tuberculosis with short course chemotherapy in south India—5-year follow up. Tubercle 1989;70:229-34.

28. A controlled clinical trial of 3- and 5-month regimens in the treatment of sputum-positive pulmonary tuberculosis in South India. Tuberculosis Research Centre, Madras, and National Tuberculosis Institute, Bangalore. Am Rev Respir Dis 1986;134: 27-33.

29. Balasubramanian R, Sivasubramanian S, Vijayan VK, Ramachandran R, Jawahar MS, Paramasivan CN, et al. Five year results of a 3-month and two 5-month regimens for the treatment of sputum-positive pulmonary tuberculosis in south India. Tubercle 1990;71:253-8.

30. Clinical trial of six-month and four-month regimens of chemotherapy in the treatment of pulmonary tuberculosis. Am Rev Respir Dis 1979;119:579-85.

31. Clinical trial of six-month and four-month regimens of chemotherapy in the treatment of pulmonary tuberculosis: the results up to 30 months. Tubercle 1981;62:95-102.

32. Long-term follow-up of a clinical trial of six-month and four-month regimens of chemotherapy in the treatment of pulmonary tuberculosis. Singapore Tuberculosis Service/British Medical Research Council. Am Rev Respir Dis 1986;133:779-83.

33. Controlled clinical trial of four short-course [6-month] regimens of chemotherapy for treatment of pulmonary tuberculosis. Third report. East African-British Medical Research Councils. Lancet 1974;2:237-40.

34. Isoniazid with thiacetazone [thioacetazone] in the treatment of pulmonary tuberculosis in East Africa—fifth investigation.

A co-operative study in East African hospitals, clinics and laboratories with the collaboration of the East African and British Medical Research Councils. Tubercle 1970;51:123-51.

35. Controlled comparison of oral twice-weekly and oral daily isoniazid plus PAS in newly diagnosed pulmonary tuberculosis. Br Med J 1973;2:7-11.

36. Results at 5 years of a controlled comparison of a 6-month and a standard 18-month regimen of chemotherapy for pulmonary tuberculosis. Am Rev Respir Dis 1977;116:3-8.

37. A controlled trial of 3-month, 4-month, and 6-month regimens of chemotherapy for sputum-smear-negative pulmonary tuberculosis. Results at 5 years. Hong Kong Chest Service/Tuberculosis Research Centre, Madras/British Medical Research Council. Am Rev Respir Dis 1989;139:871-6.

38. Girling DJ, Fox W. Side effects of intermittent rifampicin. Br Med J 1971;4:231-2.

39. Dutt AK, Moers D, Stead WW. Undesirable side effects of isoniazid and rifampin in largely twice-weekly short-course chemotherapy for tuberculosis. Am Rev Respir Dis 1983;128:419-24.

40. The management of pulmonary tuberculosis in adults notified in England and Wales in 1988. The British Thoracic Society Research Committee and the Medical Research Council Cardiothoracic Epidemiology Group. Respir Med 1991;85:319-23.

41. Ellard GA, Girling DJ, Nunn AJ. The hepatotoxicity of isoniazid among the three acetylator phenotypes. Am Rev Respir Dis 1981;123:568-70.

42. Gurumurthy P, Krishnamurthy MS, Nazareth O, Parthasarathy R, Sarma GR, Somasundaram PR, et al. Lack of relationship between hepatic toxicity and acetylator phenotype in three thousand South Indian patients during treatment with isoniazid for tuberculosis. Am Rev Respir Dis 1984;129:58-61.

43. Huang YS. Recent progress in genetic variation and risk of antituberculosis drug-induced liver injury. J Chin Med Assoc 2014;77:169-73.

44. Singla R, Sarin R, Khalid UK, Mathuria K, Singla N, Jaiswal A, et al. Seven-year DOTS-Plus pilot experience in India: results, constraints and issues. Int J Tuberc Lung Dis 2009;13:976-81.

45. A concurrent comparison of home and sanatorium treatment of pulmonary tuberculosis in South India. Bull World Health Organi 1959;21:51-144.

46. Dawson JJ, Devadatta S, Fox W, Radhakrishna S, Ramakrishnan CV, Somasundaram PR, et al. A 5-year study of patients with pulmonary tuberculosis in a concurrent comparison of home and sanatorium treatment for one year with isoniazid plus PAS. Bull World Health Organ 1966;34:533-51.

47. Devadatta S, Dawson JJ, Fox W, Janardhanam B, Radhakrishna S, Ramakrishnan CV, et al. Attack rate of tuberculosis in a 5-year period among close family contacts of tuberculous patients under domiciliary treatment with isoniazid plus PAS or isoniazid alone. Bull World Health Organ 1970;42:337-51.

48. Kamat SR, Dawson JJ, Devadatta S, Fox W, Janardhanam B, Radhakrishna S, et al. A controlled study of the influence of segregation of tuberculous patients for one year on the attack rate of tuberculosis in a 5-year period in close family contacts in South India. Bull World Health Organ 1966;34:517-32.

49. Rouillon A, Perdrizet S, Parrot R. Transmission of tubercle bacilli: The effects of chemotherapy. Tubercle 1976;57:275-99.

50. Riley RL, Moodie AS. Infectivity of patients with pulmonary tuberculosis in inner city homes. Am Rev Respir Dis 1974;110:810-2.

51. Clancy LJ, Kelly P, O'Reilly L, Byrne C, Costello E. The pathogenicity of Mycobacterium tuberculosis during chemotherapy. Eur Respir J 1990;3:399-402.

52. World Health Organization. Stop TB Dept. Guidelines for the programmatic management of drug-resistant tuberculosis. Geneva: World Health Organization; 2008.

53. World Health Organization. Guidelines for the programmatic management of drug-resistant tuberculosis—2011 update. Geneva: World Health Organization; 2011.

54. Rich M. World Health Organization. Companion handbook to the WHO guidelines for the programmatic management of drug-resistant tuberculosis. WHO/HTM/TB/2014.11. Geneva: World Health Organization; 2014.

55. Sharma SK, Mohan A. Extrapulmonary tuberculosis. Indian J Med Res 2004;120:316-53.

56. Chemotherapy and management of tuberculosis in the United Kingdom: recommendations 1998. Joint Tuberculosis Committee of the British Thoracic Society. Thorax 1998;53:536-48.

57. Sharma SK, Solanki R, Mohan A, Jain NK, Chauhan LS. Outcomes of Category III DOTS treatment in immunocompetent patients with tuberculosis pleural effusion. Int J Tuberc Lung Dis 2012;16:1505-9.

58. Jindal SK, Aggarwal AN, Gupta D, Ahmed Z, Gupta KB, Janmeja AK, et al. Tuberculous lymphadenopathy: a multicentre operational study of 6-month thrice weekly directly observed treatment. Int J Tuberc Lung Dis 2013;17:234-9.

59. Kandala V, Kalagani Y, Kondapalli NR, Kandala M. Directly observed treatment short course in immunocompetent patients of tuberculous cervical lymphadenopathy treated in revised national tuberculosis control programme. Lung India 2012;29:109-13.

60. Sumartojo E. When tuberculosis treatment fails. A social behavioral account of patient adherence. Am Rev Respir Dis 1993;147:1311-20.

61. Central TB Division, Ministry of Health and Family Welfare, Government of India. INDEX-TB Guidelines. Guidelines on extra-pulmonary tuberculosis for India. Available at URL: http://tbcindia.nic.in/showfile.php?lid=3245. Accessed on October 20, 2016.

62. Short-course chemotherapy in pulmonary tuberculosis. A controlled trial by the British Thoracic and Tuberculosis Association. Lancet 1976;2:1102-4.

63. Kochi A. Tuberculosis control—is DOTS the health breakthrough of the 1990s? World Health Forum 1997;18:225-32.

64. Sbarbaro J, Blomberg B, Chaulet P. Fixed-dose combination formulations for tuberculosis treatment. Int J Tuberc Lung Dis 1999;3:S286-8.

65. Migliori GB, Raviglione MC, Schaberg T, Davies PD, Zellweger JP, Grzemska M, et al. Tuberculosis management in Europe. Task Force of the European Respiratory Society [ERS], the World Health Organization [WHO] and the International Union against Tuberculosis and Lung Disease [IUATLD] Europe Region. Eur Respir J 1999;14:978-92.

66. Monedero I, Caminero JA. Evidence for promoting fixed-dose combination drugs in tuberculosis treatment and control: a review. Bull World Health Organ 2011;15:433-9.

67. Fox W. Drug combinations and the bioavailability of rifampicin. Tubercle 1990;71:241-5.

68. Ellard GA, Fourie PB. Rifampicin bioavailability: a review of its pharmacology and the chemotherapeutic necessity for ensuring optimal absorption. Int J Tuberc Lung Dis 1999;3:S301-8.

69. Blomberg B, Spinaci S, Fourie B, Laing R. The rationale for recommending fixed-dose combination tablets for treatment of tuberculosis. Bull World Health Organ 2001;79:61-8.

70. Yew WW. Therapeutic drug monitoring in antituberculosis chemotherapy: clinical perspectives. Clinica Chemica Acta 2001;313:31-6.

71. Peloquin CA. Therapeutic drug monitoring in the treatment of tuberculosis. Drugs 2002;62:2169-83.

72. Peloquin CA, Nitta AT, Burman WJ, Brudney KF, Miranda-Massari JR, McGuinness ME, et al. Low antituberculosis drug concentrations in patients with AIDS. Ann Pharmacother 1996; 30:919-25.

73. Sahai J, Gallicano K, Swick L, Tailor S, Garber G, Seguin I, et al. Reduced plasma concentrations of antituberculosis drugs in patients with HIV infection. Ann Intern Med 1997;127: 289-93.

74. Grosset JH, Singer TG, Bishai WR. New drugs for the treatment of tuberculosis: hope and reality. Int J Tuberc Lung Dis 2012;16: 1005-14.

75. Lienhardt C, Raviglione M, Spigelman M, Hafner R, Jaramillo E, Hoelscher M, et al. New drugs for the treatment of tuberculosis: needs, challenges, promise, and prospects for the future. J Infect Dis 2012;205:S241-9.

76. Zumla A, Chakaya J, Centis R, D'Ambrosio L, Mwaba P, Bates M, et al. Tuberculosis treatment and management—an update on treatment regimens, trials, new drugs, and adjunct therapies. Lancet Respir Med 2015;3:220-34.

77. Zumla A, Nahid P, Cole ST. Advances in the development of new tuberculosis drugs and treatment regimens. Nat Rev Drug Discov 2013;12:388-404.

78. Zumla AI, Gillespie SH, Hoelscher M, Philips PP, Cole ST, Abubakar I, et al. New antituberculosis drugs, regimens, and adjunct therapies: needs, advances, and future prospects. Lancet Infect Dis 2014;14:327-40.

79. Merle CS, Fielding K, Sow OB, Gninafon M, Lo MB, Mthiyane T, et al. A four-month gatifloxacin-containing regimen for treating tuberculosis. N Engl J Med 2014;371:1588-98.

80. Gillespie SH, Crook AM, McHugh TD, Mendel CM, Meredith SK, Murray SR, et al. Four-month moxifloxacin-based regimens for drug-sensitive tuberculosis. N Engl J Med 2014;371:1577-87.

81. Jindani A, Harrison TS, Nunn AJ, Phillips PP, Churchyard GJ, Charalambous S, et al, RIFAQUIN Trial Team. N Engl J Med 2014; 371:1599-608.

82. Diacon AH, Dawson R, von Groote-Bidlingmaier F, Symons G, Venter A, Donald PR, et al. 14-day bactericidal activity of PA-824, bedaquiline, pyrazinamide, and moxifloxacin combinations: a randomised trial. Lancet 2012;380:986-93.

83a. Skripconoka V, Danilovits M, Pehme L, Tomson T, Skenders G, Kummik T, et al. Delamanid improves outcomes and reduces mortality in multidrug-resistant tuberculosis. Eur Respir J 2013; 41:1393-400.

83b. Revised National TB Control Programme. Central TB Division, Directorate General of Health Services, Ministry of Health and Family Welfare, Government of India. Guidelines for use of bedaquiline in RNTCP through conditional access under Programmatic Management of Drug-resistant Tuberculosis in India. Available at URL: https://www.tbcindia.gov.in/showfile. php?lid=3246. Accessed on December 31, 2018.

83c. Revised National TB Control Programme. Central TB Division, Directorate General of Health Services, Ministry of Health and Family Welfare, Government of India. Guidelines for use of delamanid in the treatment of drug resistant TB India 2018. Available at URL: https://tbcindia.gov.in/showfile. php?lid=3343. Accessed on December 31, 2018.

83d. Revised National Tuberculosis Control Programme, Directorate General of Health Services, Ministry of Health and Family Welfare, Government of India. Guidelines on programmatic management of drug-resistant tuberculosis in India 2017. New Delhi: World Health Organization, Country Office for India; 2017.

84. Boeree MJ, Diacon AH, Dawson R, Narunsky K, du Bois J, Venter A, et al. A dose-ranging trial to optimize the dose of rifampin in the treatment of tuberculosis. Am J Respir Crit Care Med 2015;191:1058-65.

85. Sotgiu G, Centis R, D'Ambrosio L, Alffenaar JW, Anger HA, Caminero JA, et al. Efficacy, safety and tolerability of linezolid containing regimens in treating MDR-TB and XDR-TB: systematic review and meta-analysis. Eur Respir J 2012;40:1430-42.

86. Singla R, Caminero JA, Jaiswal A, Singla N, Gupta S, Bali RK, et al. Linezolid: an effective, safe and cheap drug for patients failing multidrug-resistant tuberculosis treatment in India. Eur Respir J 2012;39:956-62.

87. Das JC, Sharma P, Singla R. A new treatment modality for phthiriasis palpebrarum. J Pediatr Ophthalmol Strabismus 2003;40:304-5.

88. Dawson R, Diacon AH, Everitt D, van Niekerk C, Donald PR, Burger DA, et al. Efficiency and safety of the combination of moxifloxacin, pretomanid [PA-824], and pyrazinamide during the first 8 weeks of antituberculosis treatment: a phase 2b, open-label, partly randomised trial in patients with drug-susceptible or drug-resistant pulmonary tuberculosis. Lancet 2015;385:1738-47.

89. Das JC, Singh K, Sharma P, Singla R. Tuberculous osteomyelitis and optic neuritis. Ophthalmic Surg Lasers Imaging 2003;34: 409-12.

90. Aung KJ, Van Deun A, Declercq E, Sarker MR, Das PK, Hossain MA, et al. Successful '9-month Bangladesh regimen' for multidrug-resistant tuberculosis among over 500 consecutive patients. Int J Tuberc Lung Dis 2014;18:1180-7.

91. Moodley R, Godec TR; STREAM Trial Team. Short-course treatment for multidrug-resistant tuberculosis: the STREAM trials. Eur Respir Rev 2016;25:29-35.

92. Alsaad N, Wilffert B, van Altena R, de Lange WC, van der Werf TS, Kosterink JG, et al. Potential antimicrobial agents for the treatment of multidrug-resistant tuberculosis. Eur Respir J 2014;43:884-97.

93. World Health Organization. Global tuberculosis report 2016. WHO/HTM/TB/2016.13. Geneva: World Health Organization; 2016.

94. Hawken MP, Meme HK, Elliott LC, Chakaya JM, Morris JS, Githui WA, et al. Isoniazid preventive therapy for tuberculosis in HIV-1-infected adults: results of a randomized controlled trial. AIDS 1997;11:875-82.

95. Akolo C AI, Shepperd S, Volmink J. Treatment of latent tuberculosis infection in HIV infected persons. Cochrane Database Syst Rev 2010;1:CD000171.

96. Ferebee SH. Controlled chemoprophylaxis trials in tuberculosis. A general review. Bibl Tuberc 1970;26:28-106.

97. Dash LA, Comstock GW, Flynn JP. Isoniazid preventive therapy: Retrospect and prospect. Am Rev Respir Dis 1980;121: 1039-44.

98. Miller B, Snider DE, Jr. Physician noncompliance with tuberculosis preventive measures. Am Rev Respir Dis 1987;135:1-2.

99. Efficacy of various durations of isoniazid preventive therapy for tuberculosis: five years of follow-up in the IUAT trial. International Union Against Tuberculosis Committee on Prophylaxis. Bull World Health Organ 1982;60:555-64.

100. Targeted tuberculin testing and treatment of latent tuberculosis infection. This official statement of the American Thoracic Society was adopted by the ATS Board of Directors, July 1999. This is a Joint Statement of the American Thoracic Society [ATS] and the Centers for Disease Control and Prevention [CDC]. This statement was endorsed by the Council of the Infectious Diseases Society of America [IDSA], September 1999, and the sections of this statement. Am J Respir Crit Care Med 2000;161:S221-47.

101. Kopanoff DE, Snider DE, Jr., Caras GJ. Isoniazid-related hepatitis: a US Public Health Service cooperative surveillance study. Am Rev Respir Dis 1978;117:991-1001.

102. Gao XF, Wang L, Liu GJ, Wen J, Sun X, Xie Y, et al. Rifampicin plus pyrazinamide versus isoniazid for treating latent tuberculosis infection: a meta-analysis. Int J Tuberc Lung Dis 2006;10:1080-90.

103. Fatal and severe hepatitis associated with rifampin and pyrazinamide for the treatment of latent tuberculosis infection—New York and Georgia, 2000. Morb Mortal Wkly Rep 2001;50:289-91.

104. Update: Fatal and severe liver injuries associated with rifampin and pyrazinamide for latent tuberculosis infection, and revisions in American Thoracic Society/CDC recommendations—United States, 2001. Morb Mortal Wkly Rep 2001;50:733-5.

105. Guidelines on the management of latent tuberculosis infection. WHO/HTM/TB/2015.01. Geneva: World Health Organization; 2015.

106. World Health Organization. Latent tuberculosis infection. Updated and consolidated guidelines for programmatic management. WHO/CDS/TB/2018.4. Geneva: World Health Organization; 2018.

107. Sterling TR, Villarino ME, Borisov AS, Shang N, Gordin F, Bliven-Sizemore E, et al. Three months of rifapentine and isoniazid for latent tuberculosis infection. N Engl J Med 2011;365:2155-66.

108. Younossian AB, Rochat T, Ketterer JP, Wacker J, Janssens JP. High hepatotoxicity of pyrazinamide and ethambutol for treatment of latent tuberculosis. Eur Respir J 2005;26:462-4.

109. Dorman SE, Johnson JL, Goldberg S, Muzanye G, Padayatchi N, Bozeman L, et al. Substitution of moxifloxacin for isoniazid during intensive phase treatment of pulmonary tuberculosis. Am J Respir Crit Care Med 2009;180:273-80.

110. Sharma SK, Sharma A, Kadhiravan T, Tharyan P. Rifamycins [rifampicin, rifabutin and rifapentine] compared to isoniazid for preventing tuberculosis in HIV-negative people at risk of active TB. Cochrane Database Syst Rev 2013;7:CD007545.

111. Menzies D, Adjobimey M, Ruslami R, Trajman A, Sow O, Kim H, et al. Four months of rifampin or nine months of isoniazid for latent tuberculosis in adults. N Engl J Med 2018;379:440-53.

112. Diallo T, Adjobimey M, Ruslami R, Trajman A, Sow O, Obeng Baah J, et al. Safety and Side Effects of Rifampin versus Isoniazid in Children. N Engl J Med 2018;379:454-63.

113. Chadha VK, Kumar P, Jagannatha PS, Vaidyanathan PS, Unnikrishnan KP. Average annual risk of tuberculous infection in India. Int J Tuberc Lung Dis 2005;9:116-8.

114. Khatri GR, Frieden TR. Controlling tuberculosis in India. N Engl J Med 2002;347:1420-5.

Hepatotoxicity Associated with Anti-tuberculosis Treatment

Divya Reddy, Jussi Saukkonen

INTRODUCTION

The treatment of both latent tuberculosis infection [LTBI] and active tuberculosis [TB] has long been challenged by effects on the liver. While isoniazid is a prototypical drug for causing hepatic dysfunction, other first and second-line antibiotics in TB treatment may also affect the liver. The extended treatment duration, the often-challenging lives, and co-morbidities of patients with TB pose unique issues of potential hepatotoxicity. There are frequent challenges in evaluating, diagnosing and determining whether observed liver abnormalities are related to TB treatment or another confounding cause. Strategies have evolved to try to prevent, evaluate, diagnose and manage hepatotoxicity related to TB medications from occurring and to such hepatotoxicity. Such strategies for preventing and monitoring drug-induced liver injury [DILI] have not been systematically developed, but have evolved from practice. Co-morbidities such as alcohol abuse, human immunodeficiency virus [HIV], and the burgeoning epidemics of viral hepatitis, complicate treatment and the potential for hepatotoxicity. The use of new regimens for latent and active TB treatment, as well as the spate of new medications is introducing both new concerns and potential opportunities for less hepatotoxicity.

MECHANISM OF ANTI-TUBERCULOSIS DRUG-INDUCED LIVER INJURY

A broad range of hepatic abnormalities may occur during anti-TB treatment, related or unrelated to the medications used. Liver dysfunction associated with anti-TB treatment ranges from asymptomatic elevation of transaminases to rare, fulminant liver failure. Low-grade transaminase elevations due to a particular medication and that do not progress to severe injury constitute hepatic adaptation to the drug. Stress on the liver, generally in the form of an administered drug or toxin, induces minor hepatocellular injury, an array of hepatic enzymes, and can be manifested as aminotransferase elevation (1). On the other hand, a progressive rise in liver transaminases, generally accompanied by hepatitis symptoms of nausea, vomiting, abdominal pain, or unexplained fatigue, and eventual jaundice are indicative of DILI (2).

The pathogenesis of anti-TB DILI is not well characterised. For isoniazid, for which the capacity for hepatotoxicity is better described and understood, DILI occurrence is idiosyncratic, and not entirely predictable, while hepatic adaptation is known to occur in up to 20% of those taking the medication. In contrast, some drugs can cause a dose-related hepatotoxicity that is at least somewhat predictable. Pyrazinamide is thought to cause both dose-related and idiosyncratic hepatotoxicity (3,4). Isoniazid can induce oxidative stress, unleashing several mechanisms of injury, including a cytokine-mediated inflammation, with a Th1 and Th2 imbalance. Covalent binding of drug or metabolites to hepatic proteins can induce potent immune and other cytotoxic responses. These oxidative and inflammatory insults lead to hepatocyte apoptosis and necrosis. Transaminase elevations signify hepatocellular injury of varying degrees. Concomitant development of jaundice or hyperbilirubinemia indicates widespread hepatocellular injury with resulting bile ductile obstruction by oedematous and necrotic tissue (2,5).

Drug metabolism, influenced by gene polymorphisms of several key enzymes, plays a role in susceptibility to potential DILI. Considerable evidence has accrued implicating specific N-acetyl transferase 2 [NAT2] genotypes associated with slow acetylation of isoniazid as a factor predisposing to varying degrees of transaminase elevation and liver injury (6-8). There are differences in prevalence of slow acetylation phenotypes that may account for reported variations in the occurrence of hepatotoxicity (9). Gene polymorphisms in cytochrome p450 2E have also been implicated in hepatotoxicity during TB treatment (10). Glutathione S-transferase [GST] gene polymorphisms at loci and alleles have also been shown to be associated with hepatotoxicity (11), likely through increased generation of free radicals. Hepatic injury is accompanied by decreased glutathione [GSH] and thiols, with increased lipid peroxidation, resulting in hepatocellular injury. N-acetylcysteine has been shown to be protective in an animal model of INH/Rif oxidative hepatic injury (12), and in one small clinical trial (13). Several other anti-oxidants appear to exert hepatoprotective effects in models of TB DILI (14,15), and curcumin when given to patients treated for TB (16). However, a recent study from India has shown that GSTM1 'null' mutation is not independently associated with DILI development in subjects receiving anti-TB treatment (17). A recent study has reported that higher concentration of plasma rifampicin is associated with subsequent development of DILI (18).

CLINICAL SIGNIFICANCE OF HEPATIC ADAPTATION

There are several essential points for the clinician regarding hepatic adaptation and true DILI. First, transaminase elevation during TB treatment should be evaluated for other causes and not immediately assumed to be related to anti-TB treatment. The serum alanine amino transferase [ALT] level is more specific for the liver then is aspartate amino transferase [AST], which may be elevated from other tissues. Thus, the former should be used for assessment for potential hepatotoxicity. Second, the association with the level of transaminase elevation for DILI has not been established. This seems to vary from drug to drug, with DILI from methotrexate appearing at ALT elevations of 3 times the upper limit of normal [ULN], on liver biopsy. Whereas with other drugs elevations of ALT that exceed even 10 the ULN, have not correlated with DILI (2). Similarly, for anti-TB treatment, the amplitude of ALT elevation that occurs during treatment has not been established. Third, the most concerning DILI is manifested by the development of jaundice or total bilirubin elevation more than twice the ULN. With this development, the risk of liver failure is escalated to about 10%, known as "Hy's law'" after the distinguished hepatologist Hyman Zimmerman (2,19).

For the TB provider the mandate is to effectively treat TB and to avoid or mitigate adverse events [AEs], especially DILI, for each patient. Simply put, the transition from transaminase elevation from hepatic adaptation to DILI is not clearly defined. The development of jaundice or hyperbilirubinemia with significant transaminase elevation is a comparatively late manifestation of liver injury with a potentially unacceptably high-risk of progression to fulminant liver failure. Thus, a strategy of interrupting treatment has evolved, using preset stopping rules for potential

manifestations of hepatotoxicity, based on expert opinion, in order to prevent those patients who might progress to severe liver injury. Unfortunately, this interrupts treatment for many patients who are experiencing either transaminase elevation unrelated to TB treatment or hepatic adaptation without progression to DILI. Evaluation of the possible causes of the hepatic event is imperative. In most cases, treatment may be resumed with the same or similar regimen, suggesting most of these cases of hepatotoxicity were those with hepatic adaption. However, the more severe the event, particularly if jaundice or hyperbilirubinemia accompanies significant transaminase elevation, more caution should be used in reintroducing some or all of the same medications.

CLINICAL MANIFESTATIONS OF HEPATOTOXICITY

Many patients found to have high-grade transaminase elevation have few or no symptoms. Constitutional symptoms may occur early, lasting often for days to weeks. In patients with severe hepatotoxicity, nausea, vomiting and abdominal pain occur in 50%-75%, while fever is noted in 10% and rash in 5%. Jaundice, dark urine and clay-coloured stools are generally late signs of severe hepatotoxicity. Coagulopathy, hypoalbuminaemia and hypoglycaemia are signs of hepatic failure. Most individuals recover with prompt discontinuation of isoniazid, but resolution usually takes weeks (20).

INCIDENCE OF HEPATOTOXICITY WITH ANTI-TUBERCULOSIS THERAPY

Among the first-line drugs used for treatment of TB, isoniazid, rifampicin and pyrazinamide can cause hepatotoxicity. Most clinical trials until more recent years were not designed to systematically capture hepatotoxicity data.

During treatment of TB with first-line therapy, hepatotoxicity has been reported to occur in 3%-25% of those treated in studies that used differing regimens and definitions of hepatotoxicity (2). Using American Thoracic Society [ATS] criteria, approximately 3% of treated individuals experience hepatotoxicity during treatment of TB (21).

For LTBI, several regimens are available with varying hepatotoxicity. These regimens include isoniazid for six to nine months, rifampicin for four months, isoniazid and rifampicin, and isoniazid with rifapentine for three months. The regimen of rifampicin and pyrazinamide given for two months is not recommended due to severe and fatal hepatotoxicity (22,23).

During treatment of LTBI, the incidence of hepatotoxicity due to isoniazid has been estimated to occur in the range from 0.1% to 0.56% of those treated with isoniazid (24-27). In a recent large multi-centre LTBI treatment trial hepatotoxicity attributed to isoniazid was 2.7% (28). Treatment of LTBI with rifampicin is associated with less hepatotoxicity, from 0.08% to 2% (29-31). A systematic review found less hepatotoxicity with rifampicin than with isoniazid in four trials, although the quality of evidence from these trials was low (32). Hepatotoxicity from the combination of isoniazid and rifampicin has been assessed in a meta-analysis and rifampicin was found to potentiate the hepatotoxicity of isoniazid (33), while another systematic review assessing two trials that yielded relatively low quality evidence (34). In a large study, isoniazid and rifapentine administered once weekly for three months was less hepatotoxic than isoniazid given daily for nine months, 0.4% *versus* 2.4%, respectively (28a). In the recent REMoxTB clinical trial (28b) patients [n = 1928] received either standard anti-TB treatment [2 months of ethambutol, isoniazid, rifampicin, pyrazinamide followed by 4 months of isoniazid and rifampicin; n = 639], or a 4-month regimen in which moxifloxacin replaced either ethambutol [isoniazid arm, 2MHRZ/2MHR; n = 654] or isoniazid [ethambutol arm, 2EMRZ/2MR; n = 635]. DILI, [defined as peak ALT more than or equal to 5 times the ULN or ALT more than or equal to 3 time the ULN with total bilirubin greater than 2 times the ULN] occurred in 58 of the 1928 [3%] at a median time of 28 days.

ASSESSMENT OF ANTI-TUBERCULOSIS TREATMENT BENEFITS, RISKS AND MITIGATION OF RISKS

A risk-benefit analysis is appropriate in all medical interventions, although for some clinical conditions the therapeutic path is clear. For patients with active disease, the benefits are clear and treatment should proceed, most commonly with a (35) standard regimen, but assessment of the risks for hepatotoxicity, other AEs and drug interactions should be done. This may, in some cases, inform the choice of regimen, monitoring strategy, and subsequent management decisions, should there be indications of DILI. For patients with LTBI, the risk/benefit analysis is less stark. In most cases, treatment of LTBI in those at high-risk for progressing to TB disease is beneficial in those whose risk of liver injury is not high. Thus, in the circumstance of LTBI the benefits of treatment are weighed more closely in relation to the risks for that individual patient. Since the patient is healthy from the standpoint of TB, i.e., does not have disease, the tragic circumstance of a healthy individual sustaining a serious or permanent liver injury is to be avoided [Table 45.1].

Risk Factors for Hepatotoxicity during Treatment for Active Tuberculosis Disease

Several risk factors for either increased incidence of or more severe liver injury include hypoalbuminemia, female gender, increasing age, pregnancy, elevated baseline transaminase (2,21). Variable data have been reported for alcohol consumption, but most consider it a risk factor. Similarly, concomitant ingestion of other potentially hepatotoxic drugs is also considered a risk factor.

Viral hepatitis co-infection often complicates treatment of patients with TB. Several studies in patients co-infected with hepatitis B indicate no increased risk, unless the baseline ALT is abnormal (36-39), with some caveats about design. However, two studies suggest increased incidence and severity risks (40,41).

Hepatitis C was reported to be associated with a higher risk of hepatotoxicity in three studies (36,42,43), but not in others (6,35,44). These viral hepatitis' are considered hepatotoxicity risk factors, particularly if transaminases are abnormal prior to TB treatment.

Assessment of cohorts of human immunodeficiency virus [HIV] infected individuals for hepatotoxicity during TB is difficult due to potential confounding factors, including concomitant hepatotoxic medications, substance abuse, and viral hepatitis. Several studies indicate a higher risk of hepatotoxicity associated with HIV infection (35,42,44), including an additive effect between hepatitis C and HIV infection (42) [Table 45.2].

Risk Factors for Hepatotoxicity during Treatment for Latent Tuberculosis Infection

Risk for hepatotoxicity during treatment for LTBI increases progressively with age (45,46). Several studies with methodologic limitations suggest that the severity of isoniazid-induced hepatotoxicity, when it does occur, may be worse in women, but incidence is not clearly increased (2). Elevated baseline transaminases are a risk factor for hepatotoxicity during treatment of LTBI (25,47). Other hepatotoxicity risk factors include alcohol consumption (48), active but not quiescent hepatitis B (49,50). Hepatitis C infection alone,

---

Table 45.1: Pre-treatment clinical evaluation and plan

A standardised history form is recommended, which includes risk factors for hepatotoxicity

The physical examination should include evaluation for signs of liver disease, such as, liver tenderness, hepatosplenomegaly, jaundice, caput medusae, spider angiomata, ascites, and oedema

Treatment indication: latent vs active TB

Consider regimen and educate patient regarding adherence and adverse effects

Decide upon and discuss monitoring plan with patient

TB = tuberculosis

Table 45.2: Potential risk factors for hepatotoxicity*

Increasing age

Malnutrition or hypoalbuminemia

Pyrazinamide in regimen

Other hepatotoxic agents

Alcohol

Elevated baseline alanine aminotransferase

Pre-existing chronic liver disease

Viral hepatitis

Human immunodeficiency virus infection

Pregnancy or post-partum

*Evidence base for each is variable

in limited data, was not associated with hepatotoxicity during treatment of LTBI (47,51). Malnutrition, prior isoniazid-related hepatotoxicity, and continued use of isoniazid while symptomatic have been described to contribute to higher-grade isoniazid hepatotoxicity (20). HIV infection alone does not appear to increase risk for hepatotoxicity (52,53), although infected patients often have other risk factors, including anti-retroviral [ARV] medications.

The risk-benefit analysis for treatment of LTBI should include the benefit at the patient's age, co-morbidities, and baseline transaminases. Concomitant medications, drug interactions, drug and alcohol use, capacity to understand instructions and communicate with staff, and ability to avoid hepatotoxic agents.

PATIENT AND REGIMEN SELECTION

Tuberculosis Treatment

Most patients with TB can be successfully treated with first-line anti-TB therapy. Treatment of patients with pre-existing significant liver disease creates substantial challenges. Serum transaminases and total bilirubin may vary as a result of the underlying liver disease, complicating monitoring for DILI. TB involving the liver may also cause elevated baseline transaminases, which improve with treatment.

For patients with significant liver disease or baseline transaminase exceed 3 times the ULN [not thought to be related to tuberculous involvement of the liver], regimens with less potentially hepatotoxic drugs should be selected. Efforts should be made to try to retain isoniazid and particularly rifampicin, if possible, due to their high efficacy. Expert consultation is recommended and adjustments during treatment are likely. Alternative regimens in the face of liver disease include treatment with first-line drugs without either pyrazinamide for a nine-month course or isoniazid [potentially with a fluoroquinolone] for at least six months. Treatment that leaves out both isoniazid and pyrazinamide entails treatment with rifampicin and ethambutol with a fluoroquinolone, injectable, or cycloserine for 12-18 months. A regimen that leaves out the first-line potentially hepatotoxic drugs for patients with severe, unstable liver disease patients includes ethambutol, a fluoroquinolone, cycloserine, and second-line injectable for 18-24 months. Some experts avoid aminoglycosides due to concerns about causing renal insufficiency or causing bleeding from injection sites due to thrombocytopenia and/or coagulopathy (2).

Latent TB Infection

The clinician and patient decide on treatment of LTBI, based on the expected benefits of treatment relative to the risks for that patient, as well as likely adherence. For patients with ALT elevation more than 2.5 to 3 times the ULN, chronic high level of alcohol consumption, or cirrhosis the risks of treatment for LTBI may outweigh benefits. If LTBI treatment is undertaken in such individuals, they should have close monitoring and a lower risk regimen should be selected, such as 3HP or rifampicin alone (54). The clinician should

evaluate for potential drug interactions if a rifamycin is being considered.

HEPATOTOXIC RISK MITIGATION AND MONITORING DURING TUBERCULOSIS TREATMENT

Steps to try to prevent and recognise early the occurrence of hepatotoxicity include patient education, discontinuation of other potentially hepatotoxic substances, modified regimens, intensive monitoring, daily directly observed therapy [DOT], and clear and prompt communication among patients and staff. Alcohol intake should be stopped, as well as any potentially hepatotoxic drugs, illicit or over the counter, such as acetaminophen or related drugs. Prescribed concomitant medications with hepatotoxic potential that cannot be replaced or discontinued are indications for close monitoring.

Patient education about hepatotoxicity should not jeopardise adherence to the regimen, but should point out that most patients do not experience hepatotoxicity. Nevertheless, patients should be educated about symptoms and signs of liver injury and to immediately notify the clinic or DOT worker. For abdominal pain, vomiting, nausea or jaundice the patient should halt ingestion of anti-TB treatment, any relevant concomitant medications and promptly communicate with TB programme staff.

A monitoring plan should be established to assess adherence, response to therapy, and for AEs. Clinical monitoring for symptoms and signs of hepatotoxicity by trained TB programme staff is complemented by biochemical monitoring, preferably of serum ALT, for those with specific risk factors for hepatotoxicity, usually every four weeks. For patients with cirrhosis, liver transplant, or who are otherwise clinically deemed at very high hepatotoxic risk, monitoring more at least every two weeks is recommended, and if the patient develops symptoms compatible with hepatitis. Adjustments of this regime based on local epidemiology and hepatotoxicity risk factors may be appropriate (2).

Hepatotoxicity tends to occur early in therapy. During treatment of TB most hepatotoxicity occurs during the four drug, intensive phase, but may occur subsequently (55). Several studies of LTBI treatment have shown that about 50%-60% of hepatotoxicity occurred in the first three months of treatment and up to about 80% in the first six months (25,26,48,56).

The benefits of scheduled as opposed to symptom-triggered biochemical monitoring have not been well studied. Rather, current monitoring practices have historically evolved to try to prevent the development of liver injury. A retrospective study suggested that scheduled monitoring reduced hospitalisations (57). An observational study of a uniform baseline and two weeks serum transaminase monitoring strategy had low sensitivity but high specificity for hepatotoxicity. Sensitivity and specificity for hepatotoxicity risk factor based strategy for monitoring were 66.7% and 65.6% (58).

TREATMENT INTERRUPTION, EVALUATION, AND SUBSEQUENT MANAGEMENT

Patients who develop symptoms of nausea, vomiting, and abdominal pain, or who develop jaundice should stop medication and be evaluated for possible hepatotoxicity as soon as possible. A careful history should be obtained for ingestion of the proper doses of TB medications, concomitant prescribed or over the counter hepatotoxic medications, alcohol and illicit drug consumption, and for risk factors for viral hepatitis. Serum transaminase and total bilirubin levels should be measured, as well as any other laboratory tests pertinent to the patient.

If the symptomatic patient has transaminases elevated beyond 3 times ULN, TB and other hepatotoxic medications should be held. For asymptomatic patients who are found through scheduled monitoring to have ALT at least 5 times ULN, TB medications should be held. The liver enzymes should be repeated and viral hepatitis serologies should be obtained to assess for coincidental infection. Other confounding hepatic insults or disease should be excluded as clinically indicated. If the transaminases are markedly elevated with or without total bilirubin elevation beyond twice the ULN or if the patient is deteriorating, tests of blood coagulation and complete blood and platelet counts should be obtained, as well. In patients with high-burden or severe TB disease in which it is felt that treatment should not be interrupted, a hepatic sparing regimen may be substituted, often temporarily.

For patients with severe liver injury thought to be TB DILI, particularly the Hy's law patient with hepatocellular injury [ALT elevation] and total bilirubin elevation or jaundice, evaluation by a hepatologist experienced in evaluating and caring for such patients is needed promptly. The role of therapeutic N-acetylcysteine in severe isoniazid DILI has not been studied. Supportive care is indicated. For patients with fulminant liver failure, evaluation for urgent liver transplant may be indicated.

The evidence base for management of hepatotoxic events is lacking. Management is often driven by the severity of the hepatic event and the patient's condition and co-morbidities. In most cases, hepatic enzymes start to improve over days to a week. Once the ALT has decreased to a level usually less than 2 times ULN, TB medication may be reinstituted. Serial single drug reintroduction is often done in an effort to determine which drug was responsible, particularly important in clinical trials. This approach may be helpful in some cases of severe DILI. However, serial drug reintroduction can be time-consuming in a high volume TB clinic, requiring multiple visits, serial transaminase measurements, staff time, and can cause delays in reaching an adequate regimen. Simultaneous reintroduction of two or more medications is also practiced. A recent study (33) assessing simultaneous versus serial introduction strategies in 175 patients who had developed hepatotoxicity found no difference in recurrent hepatotoxicity among the different strategies used, and although the sample size may not have sufficient to find small differences. Most patients can be returned to a first-line regimen. This is probably a reflection that most cases of presumed hepatotoxicity are actually experiencing hepatic adaptation or even occasionally that extraneous factors were responsible for the hepatic event.

RESEARCH ISSUES

Clearly, better approaches are needed for identifying those at risk for or progression to TB DILI with improved sensitivity and specificity. This can include better epidemiologic understanding of patients, their co-morbidities, potential co-factors for hepatotoxicity, and the biomarkers for DILI. Much work can be done with existing clinical information and technology to try to improve strategies for monitoring for adverse events. However, research into prediction, susceptibility factors, novel biomarkers, prevention strategies, hepatoprotective agents, and therapeutic drugs for hepatotoxicity are needed. Interdisciplinary collaboration between clinicians and bench researchers is needed.

Anti-TB medications commonly cause transaminase elevations that reflect hepatic adaptation. Rarely is there progression to severe TB DILI, reflected by significant transaminase elevation with jaundice or hyperbilirubinemia. Risk factors and gene polymorphisms have been associated with hepatic events during treatment of TB. A risk-benefit assessment should be employed when evaluating patients for treatment of both LTBI and TB treatment. Patient education; clinical and selective ALT monitoring; and regimen selection may help drug safety. Stopping rules have been historically implemented to allow interim evaluation of potential hepatic events and to prevent the development of severe DILI. Confounding causes of hepatic events should be excluded when such events occur. Optimal approaches for hepatotoxicity prevention, monitoring, and management are needed. The approach and rapidity of reintroducing TB treatment is likely to be guided by the severity of the hepatic event and of TB disease. Considerable research is needed to find better predictors, biomarkers, protective agents, and therapeutic drugs for DILI.

REFERENCES

1. Williams GM, Iatropoulos MJ. Alteration of liver cell function and proliferation: differentiation between adaptation and toxicity. Toxicol Pathol 2002;30:41-53.
2. Saukkonen JJ, Cohn DL, Jasmer RM, Schenker S, Jereb JA, Nolan CM, et al. An official ATS statement: hepatotoxicity of antituberculosis therapy. Am J Respir Crit Care Med 2006;174: 935-52.
3. United States Public Health Service. Hepatic toxicity of pyrazinamide used with isoniazid in tuberculous patients. Am Rev Respir Dis 1969; 59:13.
4. Centers for Disease Control and Prevention [CDC]; American Thoracic Society. Update: Fatal and severe liver injuries associated with rifampin and pyrazinamide for latent tuberculosis infection, and revisions in American Thoracic Society/CDC recommendations-United States, 2001. Morb Mortal Wkly Rep 2001;50:733-5.
5. Kaplowitz N. Biochemical and cellular mechanisms of toxic liver injury. Semin Liver Dis 2002;22:137-44.

6. Possuelo LG, Castelan JA, de Brito TC, Ribeiro AW, Cafrune PI, Picon PD, et al. Association of slow N-acetyltransferase 2 profile and anti-TB drug-induced hepatotoxicity in patients from Southern Brazil. Eur J Clin Pharmacol 2008;64:673-81.

7. Bozok Cetintaş V, Erer OF, Kosova B, Ozdemir I, Topçuoğlu N, Aktoğu S, et al. Determining the relation between N-acetyl-transferase-2 acetylator phenotype and antituberculosis drug induced hepatitis by molecular biologic tests. Tuberk Toraks 2008;56:81-6.

8. Azuma J, Ohno M, Kubota R, Yokota S, Nagai T, Tsuyuguchi K, et al. NAT2 genotype guided regimen reduces isoniazid-induced liver injury and early treatment failure in the 6-month four-drug standard treatment of tuberculosis: a randomized controlled trial for pharmacogenetics-based therapy. Eur J Clin Pharmacol 2013;69:1091-101.

9. Wilkins JJ, Langdon G, McIlleron H, Pillai G, Smith PJ, Simonsson USH. Variability in the population pharmacokinetics of isoniazid in South African tuberculosis patients. Br J Clin Pharmacol 2011; 72:51-62.

10. Huang YS, Chern HD, Su WJ, Wu JC, Chang SC, Chiang CH, et al. Cytochrome P450 2E1 genotype and the susceptibility to antituberculosis drug-induced hepatitis. Hepatology 2003;37: 924-30.

11. Roy B, Chowdhury A, Kundu S, Santra A, Dey B, Chakraborty M, et al. Increased risk of antituberculosis drug-induced hepato-toxicity in individuals with glutathione S-transferase M1 "null" mutation. J Gastroenterol Hepatol 2001;16:1033-7.

12. Attri S, Rana SV, Vaiphei K, Sodhi CP, Katyal R, Goel RC, et al. Isoniazid- and rifampicin-induced oxidative hepatic injury—protection by N-acetylcysteine. Hum Exp Toxicol 2000;19:517-22.

13. Baniasadi S, Eftekhari P, Tabarsi P, Fahimi F, Raoufy MR, Masjedi MR, et al. Protective effect of N-acetylcysteine on antituberculosis drug-induced hepatotoxicity. Eur J Gastroenterol Hepatol 2010;22:1235-8.

14. Singh M, Sasi P, Gupta VH, Rai G, Amarapurkar DN, Wangikar PP. Protective effect of curcumin, silymarin and N-acetylcysteine on antitubercular drug-induced hepatotoxicity assessed in an in vitro model. Hum Exp Toxicol 2012;31:788-97.

15. Lian Y, Zhao J, Xu P, Wang Y, Zhao J, Jia L, et al. Protective effects of metallothionein on isoniazid and rifampicin-induced hepatotoxicity in mice. PLoS ONE 2013;8:e72058.

16. Adhvaryu MR, Reddy N, Vakharia BC. Prevention of hepatotoxicity due to anti-tuberculosis treatment: a novel integrative approach. World J Gastroenterol 2008;14:4753-62.

17. Sharma SK, Jha BK, Sharma A, Sreenivas V, Upadhyay V, Jaisinghani C. Genetic polymorphisms of CYP2E1 and GSTM1 loci and susceptibility to anti-tuberculosis drug-induced hepato-toxicity. Int J Tuberc Lung Dis 2014;18:588-93.

18. Satyaraddi A, Velpandian T, Sharma SK, Vishnubhatla S, Sharma A, Sirohiwal A, et al. Correlation of plasma anti-tuberculosis drug levels with subsequent development of hepatotoxicity. Int J Tuberc Lung Dis 2014;18:188-95.

19. Zimmerman HJ. Drug-induced liver disease. In: Zimmerman HJ, editor. Hepatotoxicity: the adverse effects of drugs and other chemicals on the liver. Second edition. Philadelphia: Lippincott Williams & Wilkins; 1999.p.427-56.

20. Mitchell JR. Isoniazid liver injury: clinical spectrum, pathology, and probable pathogenesis. Ann Intern Med 1976;84:181-92.

21. Shang P, Xia Y, Liu F, Wang X, Yuan Y, Hu D, et al. Incidence, clinical features and impact on anti-tuberculosis treatment of anti-tuberculosis drug induced liver injury [ATLI] in China. PLoS ONE 2011;6:e21836.

22. Ijaz K, Jereb JA, Lambert LA, Bower WA, Spradling PR, McElroy PD, et al. Severe or fatal liver injury in 50 patients in the United States taking rifampin and pyrazinamide for latent tuberculosis infection. Clin Infect Dis 2006;42:346-55.

23. Centers for Disease Control and Prevention. Update: fatal and severe liver injuries associated with rifampin and pyrazinamide treatment for latent tuberculosis infection. JAMA 2002;288:2967.

24. Nolan CM, Goldberg SV, Buskin SE. Hepatotoxicity associated with isoniazid preventive therapy: a 7-year survey from a public health tuberculosis clinic. JAMA 1999;281:1014-8.

25. Fountain FF, Tolley E, Chrisman CR, Self TH. Isoniazid hepatotoxicity associated with treatment of latent tuberculosis infection: a 7-year evaluation from a public health tuberculosis clinic. Chest 2005;128:116-23.

26. Millard PS, Wilcosky TC, Reade-Christopher SJ, Weber DJ. Isoniazid-related fatal hepatitis. West J Med 1996;164:486.

27. LoBue PA, Moser KS. Isoniazid- and rifampin-resistant tuberculosis in San Diego County, California, United States, 1993-2002. Int J Tuberc Lung Dis 2005;9:501-6.

28a. Sterling TR, Villarino ME, Borisov AS, Shang N, Gordin F, Bliven-Sizemore E, et al. Three months of rifapentine and isoniazid for latent tuberculosis infection. N Engl J Med 2011;365:2155-66.

28b. Tweed CD, Wills GH, Crook AM, Dawson R, Diacon AH, Louw CE, et al. Liver toxicity associated with tuberculosis chemotherapy in the REMoxTB study. BMC Med 2018;16:46.

29. Page KR, Sifakis F, Montes de Oca R, Cronin WA, Doherty MC, Federline L, et al. Improved adherence and less toxicity with rifampin vs isoniazid for treatment of latent tuberculosis: a retrospective study. Arch Intern Med 2006;166:1863-70.

30. Menzies D, Long R, Trajman A, Dion MJ, Yang J, Jahdali Al H, et al. Adverse events with 4 months of rifampin therapy or 9 months of isoniazid therapy for latent tuberculosis infection. Ann Intern Med 2008;149:689-97.

31. Fresard I, Bridevaux PO, Rochat T, Janssens JP. Adverse effects and adherence to treatment of rifampicin 4 months vs isoniazid 6 months for latent tuberculosis: a retrospective analysis. Swiss Med Wkly 2011;141:w13240.

32. Sharma SK, Sharma A, Kadhiravan T. Rifamycins [rifampicin, rifabutin and rifapentine] compared to isoniazid for preventing tuberculosis in HIV-negative people at risk of active TB. Evid Based Child Health 2014;9:169-294.

33. Steele MA, Burk RF, DesPrez RM. Toxic hepatitis with isoniazid and rifampin. A meta-analysis. Chest 1991;99:465-71.

34. Sharma SK, Singla R, Sarda P, Mohan A, Makharia G, Jayaswal A, et al. Safety of 3 different reintroduction regimens of antituber-culosis drugs after development of antituberculosis treatment–induced hepatotoxicity. Clin Infect Dis 2010;50:833-9.

35. Sun HY, Chen YJ, Chen IL, Gau CS, Chang SC, Luh KT. A prospective study of hepatitis during antituberculous treatment in Taiwanese patients and a review of the literature. J Formos Med Assoc 2009;108:102-11.

36. Chien JY, Huang RM, Wang JY, Ruan SY, Chien YJ, Yu CJ, et al. Hepatitis C virus infection increases hepatitis risk during anti-tuberculosis treatment. Int J Tuberc Lung Dis 2010;14:616-21.

37. de Castro L, do Brasil PEAA, Monteiro TP, Rolla VC. Can hepatitis B virus infection predict tuberculosis treatment liver toxicity? Development of a preliminary prediction rule. Int J Tuberc Lung Dis 2010;14:332-40.

38. Hwang SJ, Wu JC, Lee CN, Yen FS, Lu CL, Lin TP, et al. A prospective clinical study of isoniazid-rifampicin-pyrazinamide-induced liver injury in an area endemic for hepatitis B. J Gastroenterol Hepatol 1997;12 :87-91.

39. Lee BH, Koh WJ, Choi MS, Suh CY, Chung MP, Kim H, et al. Inactive hepatitis B surface antigen carrier state and hepato-toxicity during antituberculosis chemotherapy. Chest 2005;127: 1304-11.

40. Wu JC, Lee SD, Yeh PF, Chan CY, Wang YJ, Huang YS, et al. Isoniazid-rifampin-induced hepatitis in hepatitis B carriers. Gastroenterology 1990;98:502-4.

41. Wong WM, Wu PC, Yuen MF, Cheng CC, Yew WW, Wong PC, et al. Antituberculosis drug-related liver dysfunction in chronic hepatitis B infection. Hepatology 2000;31:201-6.

42. Ungo JR, Jones D, Ashkin D, Hollender ES, Bernstein D, Albanese AP, et al. Antituberculosis drug-induced hepatotoxicity. The role of hepatitis C virus and the human immunodeficiency virus. Am J Respir Crit Care Med 1998;157:1871-6.

43. Lomtadze N, Kupreishvili L, Salakaia A, Vashakidze S, Sharvadze L, Kempker RR, et al. Hepatitis C virus co-infection increases the risk of anti-tuberculosis drug-induced hepatotoxicity among patients with pulmonary tuberculosis. PLoS One 2013;8:e83892.

44. Nader LA, de Mattos AA, Picon PD, Bassanesi SL. Hepatotoxicity due to rifampicin, isoniazid and pyrazinamide in patients with tuberculosis: is anti-HCV a risk factor. Ann Hepatol 2010;9:70-4.

45. Kunst H, Khan KS. Age-related risk of hepatotoxicity in the treatment of latent tuberculosis infection: a systematic review. Int J Tuberc Lung Dis 2010;14:1374-81.

46. Hosford JD, von Fricken ME, Lauzardo M, Chang M, Dai Y, Lyon JA. Hepatotoxicity from antituberculous therapy in the elderly: a systematic review. Tuberculosis 2015;95:112-22.

47. Fernández-Villar A, Sopeña B, Vázquez R, Ulloa F, Fluiters E, Mosteiro M, et al. Isoniazid hepatotoxicity among drug users: the role of hepatitis C. Clin Infect Dis 2003;36:293-8.

48. Kopanoff DE, Snider DE Jr, Caras GJ. Isoniazid-related hepatitis: a US Public Health Service cooperative surveillance study. Am Rev Respir Dis 1978;117:991-1001.

49. Patel PA, Voigt MD. Prevalence and interaction of hepatitis B and latent tuberculosis in Vietnamese immigrants to the United States. Am J Gastroenterol 2002;97:1198-203.

50. McGlynn KA, Lustbader ED, Sharrar RG, Murphy EC, London WT. Isoniazid prophylaxis in hepatitis B carriers. Am Rev Respir Dis 1986;134:666-8.

51. Sadaphal P, Astemborski J, Graham NM, Sheely L, Bonds M, Madison A, et al. Isoniazid preventive therapy, hepatitis C virus infection, and hepatotoxicity among injection drug users infected with Mycobacterium tuberculosis. Clin Infect Dis 2001;33:1687-91.

52. Cohn DL, O'Brien RJ, Geiter LJ, Gordin FM. Targeted tuberculin testing and treatment of latent tuberculosis infection. Am J Respir Crit Care Med 2000;161:S221-S247.

53. Bucher HC, Griffith LE, Guyatt GH, Sudre P, Naef M, Sendi P, et al. Isoniazid prophylaxis for tuberculosis in HIV infection: a meta-analysis of randomized controlled trials. AIDS 1999;13:501-7.

54. Sharma SK, Sharma A, Kadhiravan T, Tharyan P. Rifamycins [rifampicin, rifabutin and rifapentine] compared to isoniazid for preventing tuberculosis in HIV-negative people at risk of active TB. Cochrane Database Syst Rev 2013;7:CD007545.

55. Tostmann A, Boeree MJ, Aarnoutse RE, de lange WCM, van der Ven AJAM, Dekhuijzen R. Antituberculosis drug-induced hepatotoxicity: Concise up-to-date review. J Gastroenterol Hepatol 2008;23:192-202.

56. Efficacy of various durations of isoniazid preventive therapy for tuberculosis: five years of follow-up in the IUAT trial. International Union Against Tuberculosis Committee on Prophylaxis. Bull World Health Organ 1982;60:555-64.

57. Wu S, Xia Y, Lv X, Zhang Y, Tang S, Yang Z, et al. Effect of scheduled monitoring of liver function during anti-tuberculosis treatment in a retrospective cohort in China. BMC Public Health 2012;12:454.

58. Singanayagam A, Sridhar S, Dhariwal J, Abdel-Aziz D, Munro K, Connell DW, et al. A comparison between two strategies for monitoring hepatic function during antituberculous therapy. Am J Respir Crit Care Med 2012;185:653-9.

46

Surgery for Pleuropulmonary Tuberculosis

Abha Chandra

INTRODUCTION

Till the time effective anti-tuberculosis [anti-TB] treatment was available in the middle of the twentieth century, surgery was the only therapeutic option for pulmonary tuberculosis [TB]. Several operations were devised and practiced with the aim of controlling spread of the disease and promoting healing of the lesions. With the advent of effective anti-TB treatment, there has been a gradual decline in the need for surgical intervention in patients with pulmonary and pleural TB. The human immunodeficiency virus [HIV] infection and acquired immunodeficiency syndrome [AIDS] pandemic has resulted in the resurgence of TB worldwide. Further-more, extensively drug-resistant/multidrug-resistant TB [X/MDR-TB] have emerged as a major public health problem in several parts of the world. Because of all these factors, there has been renewed interest in surgery. Presently, there has been an increase in the number of patients with pulmo-nary and pleural TB requiring surgical intervention for diagnostic or therapeutic purposes (1).

This chapter deals with the role of surgery in the manage-ment of pleuropulmonary TB. TB of the vertebra and the oesophagus belongs to the domain of orthopaedics and gastrointestinal surgery and will not be discussed here. The reader is referred to the chapters *"Skeletal tuberculosis" [Chapter 19]* and *"Abdominal tuberculosis" [Chapter 15]* for more details.

SURGERY IN THE DIAGNOSIS OF PLEUROPULMONARY TUBERCULOSIS

Inspite of the advances in modern methods of imaging and diagnosis, a definitive diagnosis of pleural and pulmonary TB is not possible in several patients. In this setting, surgery is often performed to obtain tissue specimen to confirm the diagnosis and exclude underlying malignancy. In one study (2), pulmonary tuberculoma was confirmed as the histopathological diagnosis in 36 patients presenting with a solitary pulmonary nodule on the chest radiograph who underwent surgery for the confirmation of diagnosis. Preoperatively, lung cancer was initially suspected in 21 [58%] of these patients. In another retrospective study (3) where thoracotomy was performed to ascertain the aetio-logical diagnosis and rule out malignancy, 24 of 31 patients [77%] were found to have pulmonary TB. At the Sri Venkateswara Institute of Medical Sciences [SVIMS], Tirupati, during the period 1996 to 2000, 23 patients with a solitary lung lesion in whom TB was suspected preoperatively but diagnostic work-up did not reveal an aetiological clue underwent thoracotomy for the confirmation of diagnosis (4). Of these patients, 15 [65%] were found to have TB, five were found to have bronchogenic carcinoma and three were found to have a fungal ball [aspergilloma] and definitive treatment could be instituted in all these patients. In another retrospective study (5) from Romania, of the 144 patients who underwent pleuropulmonary surgery, TB was confirmed as the aetiological diagnosis in 21% patients with pleural effusion; 54% with empyema and pachypleuritis; 10% with pneumothorax; 11% with mediastinal lymphadenopathy; and 27% patients with pulmonary nodules.

Video-assisted Thoracoscopic Surgery

In a study reported from the All India Institute of Medical Sciences [AIIMS], New Delhi (6), video-assisted thoracoscopic surgery [VATS] was helpful in confirming the diagnosis of TB in five of the 18 patients with pulmonary pathology, three of the eight patients with mediastinal pathology and one of the five patients with pleural pathology. Importantly, VATS was helpful in providing a definitive diagnosis in all 18 patients with lung pathology, seven of the eight patients with mediastinal lesions and five of the six patients with pleural pathology who would have otherwise undergone diagnostic thoracotomy (6). In another study from Switzerland (7), VATS was useful in confirming TB as the aetiological diagnosis in 10 of the 96 patients [10.4%] in whom the pre-operative diagnoses were lung cancer [n = 4], empyema [n = 2], Pancoast tumour, pericardial effusion, pleural mesothelioma, and mediastinal lymphoma [one patient each]. Similar observations were also reported from Japan (8), and Romania (5). Thus, VATS, a minimally invasive procedure has been found to be of great assistance in confirming the diagnosis of TB in recent times.

SURGERY IN THE TREATMENT OF ACTIVE PULMONARY TUBERCULOSIS

Several surgical procedures have been used for the treatment of active pulmonary TB in the era before the advent of effective anti-TB treatment. These include cavernostomy, collapse therapy, use of phrenic nerve paralysis, artificial pneumothorax, pneumoperitoneum, extrapleural pneumonolysis and thoracoplasty. The reader is referred to the earlier editions of this textbook (4,9) for details regarding these procedures. It is likely that several of these so called "historical" procedures may have relevance in the current scenario as well.

A new modality of collapse therapy which uses percutaneous tissue expanders [the Perthes tissue expander] has been described (10). Classical thoracoplasty consists of extraperiosteal resection of seven ribs in three stages at two to three weeks intervals [Figure 46.1]. There is some deformity with thoracoplasty but not as much as might be imagined [Figure 46.2]. Compared with the classical extrapleural thoracoplasty, long-term complications such as erosion of major vessels, infection, and migration are likely to be less with this technique (10). A modified thoracoplasty with the use of a breast implant to obliterate the residual pleural space without any distortion of the chest wall has been found to be useful as an alternative to traditional thoracoplasty (11).

Current Status of Surgery

Anti-TB treatment sometimes proves ineffective or of little benefit in controlling the disease. This lack of response may vary from as low as 5% of all patients to as high as 40%-55% patients (12). This happens in patients with resistant forms of infection or in the treatment of certain forms of TB and its complications or sequelae which are associated with irreversible morphological changes in organs and tissues. Surgery is indispensable in such patients. In combination with chemotherapy, surgery can ensure sufficiently radical removal of localised lesions and save the patients life, halt progression of the disease, create better conditions for reparative processes, restore organ functions and promote complete recovery (12,13).

Although, there are conflicting views regarding the exact role of surgery in the overall management of patients with pulmonary TB, most physicians, however, consider the use of surgical methods appropriate in the situations outlined in Table 46.1 (14-18). The presence of a cavitary disease in itself is not an indication for surgery unless it is associated with one of these complications. The relative indications for resection are listed in Table 46.2.

Preoperative Work-up

The patients to be taken up for surgery for chest TB should have reasonably localised disease amenable to surgical resection and they should have adequate cardiopulmonary reserve to undergo the operation safely. The preoperative work-up apart from a chest radiograph includes computed tomography [CT] of the chest, pulmonary function tests and if possible, arterial blood gas analysis. It has been suggested that ventilation perfusion scan should also be done on all these patients as it is useful in determining the extent and the type of resection to be performed. The primary role of the ventilation perfusion scan is to confirm that the regions to be resected are physiologically inert and contributed minimally to the patient's respiratory capacity. In addition, sometimes, an area which appears normal on chest radiograph and CT may actually have no function on ventilation scan and is best removed than left inside.

These patients should also have frequent sputum analysis for smear and culture of mycobacteria. The patients should be reviewed jointly by the physician and the surgeon and they should be started on an intensive drug regimen to achieve sputum negativity or at least reduce the bacterial load to the minimum possible extent before surgery. Ideally, surgery should be performed when the smears and culture have become negative as it has a direct bearing on the incidence of bronchial stump related complications after surgery.

Pomerantz et al (14) have reported 65% success in achieving sputum conversion after an average of two and a half months of intensive anti-TB treatment. Treasure and Seaworth (18) also used intensive preoperative chemotherapeutic regimen but reported success in turning sputum negative in much higher number of patients [17 of 19 patients; 90%]. They reported that patients with persistent cavities, or disease affecting multiple segments or a lobe or with total lung destruction were candidates who benefited from surgery. Surgical removal of destroyed lung tissue harbouring a large number of bacilli protected from antibiotics by poor blood supply assists in converting the sputum negative and helps prevent relapse.

It is also recommended that bronchoscopy be performed at or before operation to exclude the presence of endobronchial disease at the proposed bronchial resection margin, as its presence will greatly increase the risk of bronchopleural fistula [BPF] after resection.

Preoperative Preparation

Nutritional Build-up

Most of the patients with chest TB would have been ill for a long time and are in a chronically debilitated condition

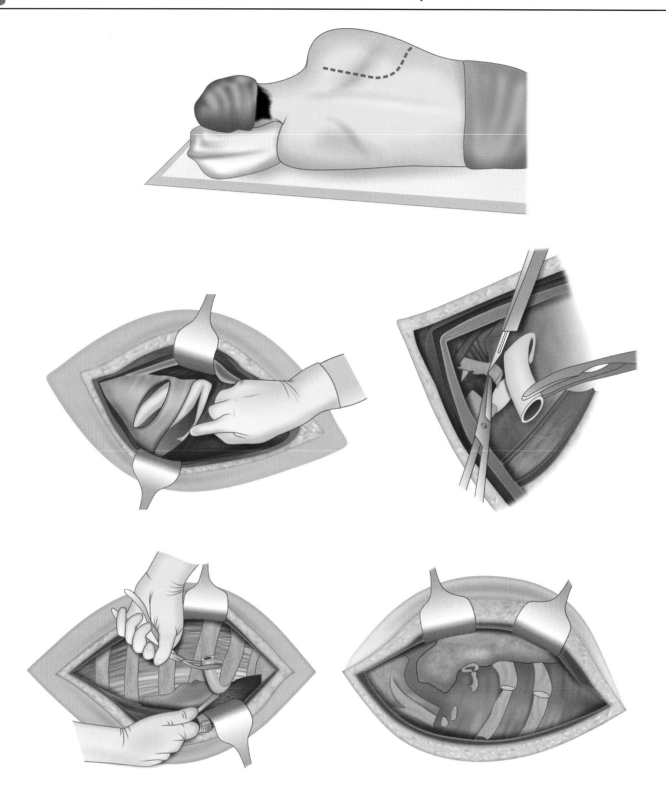

Figure 46.1: Thoracoplasty incision [upper panel centre]. Periosteum of the third, fourth and fifth ribs being peeled off [middle panel left]. Third, fourth and fifth ribs being excised [middle panel right, lower panel left]. The third, fourth and fifth ribs have been removed and the chest wall has fallen into the cavity obliterating the pleural space [lower panel right]

with poor nutritional status. Before taking up for surgery, it is important to build up nutrition of these patients. When possible this should be achieved by enteral means by encouraging high protein and calorie diet. Sometimes, patients may need hyperalimentation. The value of nutritional build up needs to be emphasised as it has a direct

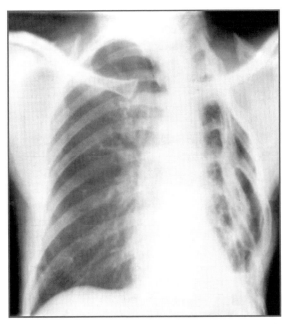

Figure 46.2: Chest radiograph [postero-anterior view] showing thoracoplasty on the left side

---

Table 46.1: Definite indications for surgery in patients with pleuropulmonary TB

To procure tissue material for confirmation of diagnosis of TB

Multidrug-resistant, extensively drug-resistant TB

Complications of TB
  Haemorrhage
  Bronchopleural fistula
  Empyema
  Bronchiectasis
  Tracheal or bronchial stenosis
  Broncholiths
  Pulmonary aspergilloma

TB = tuberculosis

Table 46.2: Relative indications for surgery in patients with pleuropulmonary TB

Destroyed lobe or lung distal to an irreversibly damaged bronchus and subject to repeated TB or, pyogenic infection

An open negative cavity of significant size [> 2 to 3 cm] in a young person

A cavity in an immunocompromised host

Demonstrable nontuberculous mycobacteria, multidrug-resistant, extensively drug-resistant organisms in a cavitary disease that can be resected clearly by lobectomy

Recurrent sputum positive infection in a given segment or lobe, even though no macroscopic cavity can be demonstrated

Asymptomatic peripheral nodule

TB = tuberculosis

Incentive Spirometry

The outcome after surgery can be improved and the incidence of complications reduced by preoperative chest exercises in the form of deep breathing and breath-holding exercises and incentive spirometry. It is important to explain the value of these simple looking exercises in improving the postoperative outcome to the patient in detail in order to achieve their maximum cooperation and compliance. Several days of such "chest training" helps tremendously in improving the outcome after surgery.

Principles of Surgery

Double lumen endotracheal tube should be used for anaesthesia in these patients to avoid cross-contamination of the contralateral lung. Patients with TB often have extensive, dense adhesions between pleura and the lung and it may be impossible to find a plane between the pleura and the lung. Additionally, dissecting through the infected material present in the pleural cavity increases the risk of postoperative empyema several folds. Due to these reasons, an extrapleural approach for pneumonectomy has been suggested (19) which decreases the morbidity as well as mortality of this operation. Dehiscence of the bronchial stump leading to BPF and empyema is the most feared and the most common complication after resectional lung surgery. Reinforcement of the bronchial stump by a vascularised tissue like intercostal muscle, pedicled extrathoracic skeletal muscle [myocutaneous flap using latissimus dorsi or serratus anterior] or omentum has been shown to significantly decrease the incidence of this complication (12,17). These should be used in all cases of resectional lung surgery for TB.

The aim of surgery in TB is to remove all the disease-bearing lung tissue at the same time preserving as much of normal lung tissue as possible. Sometimes the amount of lung tissue remaining after a resection may not be adequate to fill the entire pleural cavity and may lead to space problems post-operatively. In such cases, a concomitant tailoring thoracoplasty is recommended to reduce the chances of post-operative space problems (12). The exact procedure to be performed may vary from segmental or wedge resection to lobectomy, pneumonectomy or pleuropneumonectomy with or without myoplasty.

Extensively Drug-resistant Tuberculosis and Multidrug-resistant Tuberculosis

Indications for surgery in patients with X/MDR-TB are listed in Table 46.3. Various procedures performed for patients with MDR-TB have ranged from segmental resection to pleuropneumonectomy (14,18,20-32). In a systematic review and meta-analysis (33) that evaluated the role of pulmonary resection for MDR-TB [12 studies] and XDR-TB [3 studies] revealed substantial heterogeneity in the study characteristics. The authors (33) reported that the estimated pooled treatment success rate of pulmonary resection for

---

bearing on the outcome and the complications after surgery. Patients with anaemia and hypoproteinaemia have uniformly poor outcome after surgery.

Table 46.3: Indications for surgery in patients with X/MDR-TB

Drug resistance so extensive that there is a high probability of failure or relapse

Disease sufficiently localised so that the great preponderance of radiographically visible disease could be resected with the expectation of adequate cardiopulmonary reserve after surgery and sufficient drug activity to diminish the mycobacterial burden enough to facilitate probable healing of the bronchial stump after surgery

X/MDR-TB = extensively drug-resistant/multidrug-resistant tuberculosis

patients with MDR-TB was 84%. The rates of failure, relapse, death and default were 6%, 3%, 5% and 3%, respectively. In another published review (34) evaluating the role of surgery in the treatment of drug-resistant TB [DR-TB], the authors reviewed a total of 26 case series and cohort studies and reported that surgical resection was beneficial in the treatment of DR-TB. In another recent meta-analysis (35) that assessed the effectiveness of surgical interventions [24 comparison studies] in the treatment of DR-TB, a significant association between surgery and successful treatment compared to non-surgical interventions [Odds ratio 2.24] was observed. Meta-analysis of 23 single-arm studies showed that 92% and 87% of surgical patients achieved successful short- and long-term outcomes, respectively. The authors (35) cautioned that insufficient evidence to recommend surgery plus chemotherapy over chemotherapy alone, to evaluate the potential harm from surgery and to determine the optimal conditions for surgery.

Based on the experience reported in the literature about surgery for X/MDR-TB, it can be concluded that the operation can be performed with a low mortality. However, the complication rates are high with BPF and empyema being the major complications. Sputum positivity at the time of surgery, previous chest irradiation, prior pulmonary resection and extensive lung destruction with polymicrobial parenchymal contamination are the major factors affecting morbidity and mortality. Over 90% of the patients achieve sputum negative status postoperatively. More liberal use of muscle flaps to reinforce the bronchial stump and fill the residual space has helped significantly in reducing the rates of BPF, air leaks and residual space problems. These must be used in patients with positive sputum, when residual post-lobectomy space is anticipated, when BPF already exists pre-operatively or when extensive polymicrobial contamination is present. In patients with nontuberculous mycobacterial [NTM] infection, the outcome is poorer as compared to patients with resistant *Mycobacterium tuberculosis* infection. However, these patients should also be operated before the disease causes extensive destruction of the lung or polymicrobial infection, when the incidence of complications becomes very high.

Thus, surgery is currently recommended for patients with X/MDR-TB whose prognosis with medical treatment is poor. It should be performed after minimum of three months of intensive chemotherapeutic regimen, achieving sputum

negative status, if possible. The operative risks are acceptable and the long-term survival is much improved than that with continued medical treatment alone. However, for this to be achieved, the chemotherapeutic regimen needs to continue for prolonged periods after surgery also, probably for well over a year, otherwise recrudescence of the disease with poor survival is a real possibility.

SURGERY FOR THE COMPLICATIONS OF TUBERCULOSIS

Bronchopleural Fistula

Bronchopleural fistula may develop in TB patients following lung resections or spontaneously in association with lung lesions or empyema. Although the incidence of post-resection fistula in patients with TB has come down from as high as 28%, two or three decades ago, to 3% or less in recent years (23-25), it nevertheless, remains an important problem for the thoracic surgeon. Also, the non-surgical, spontaneously occurring BPF continues to be a problem, responsible for up to 27% of all TB-related BPF (36,37). Spontaneous BPF develops due to liquefaction necrosis and rupture of a sub-pleural TB focus. If the fistula is small and effective chemotherapy is instituted, the leak may close spontaneously and the lung re-expands as the pleural air is absorbed. Unfortunately, such is usually not the case and the leak persists with pneumothorax leading to collapse of the underlying lung and ultimately development of an empyema. It is generally believed that every patient with active pulmonary TB who develops pneumothorax has a BPF.

BPF is a serious condition with a reported mortality of 23.1%, mostly due to aspiration and its complications (36,37). In post-resection BPF, the incidence of this complication is highest during the first three months after surgery, although it can occur at any time even several years after surgery (38,39). The risk of aspiration pneumonia is highest during these first three months and its incidence decreases dramatically if BPF occurs later than three months after surgery (40).

Adequate dependent surgical drainage is the basic principle in the treatment of BPF. Drainage alone may result in closure of the fistula in some patients. In patients with non-surgical, spontaneously occurring BPF associated with pulmonary TB, intercostal tube drainage should be complemented with intensive chemotherapy as all of these patients have active, severe, often sputum positive TB infection. The pulmonary disease may vary in severity from an isolated focus to extensive disease with cavities or even bilateral disease. Continuous suction should always be applied to the tube thoracostomy and intensive antituberculosis chemotherapy continued. These patients, apart from TB infection, have associated secondary pyogenic infection also which is often polymicrobial and needs antibiotics based on the culture reports. Ihm *et al* (41) analysed 52 patients with spontaneous BPF of TB aetiology. Of these, 38 patients were treated with intercostal tube drainage with anti-TB treatment and the lung re-expanded in 28.

On analysing the factors affecting the success or failure of intercostal tube drainage, they found that the size of the BPF that gave rise to pneumothorax was the most important factor. This, in turn, was influenced by the extent of TB disease in the lung. Patients with extensive parenchymal disease, poorly controlled by drugs, had large fistulae, early development of a restrictive peel on the lung and poor outcome following tube drainage. The initial degree of collapse of the lung had no bearing on the outcome. A short time interval between the onset of pneumothorax and chest tube insertion was a favourable factor, but not dramatically so, and a long interval did not preclude success (41).

In patients failing to re-expand the lung following tube drainage, suction and chemotherapy, thoracotomy and decortication, with or without lobectomy or pneumonectomy or pleuropneumonectomy may be required depending upon the findings at surgery. The timing of this procedure is crucial. It is vital to recognise the point at which no further headway is being made with tube thoracostomy and chemotherapy and schedule the patient for definitive surgery straightaway. In the post-resection BPF, tube drainage alone may close the fistula in up to 20% patients (42), otherwise definitive surgical procedure is required. For patients with post-lobectomy or post-pneumonectomy fistula, this may involve dissection down to the lung or the mediastinum to identify the fistula site and its suture ligation. Suture ligation alone has a high failure rate. Use of pedicle muscle flaps has been recommended to fill up the empyema cavity and buttress the suture closure of the fistula site. This has been reported successful in over 75% patients (36). However, it is important that the muscle flap completely fills the empyema cavity. The muscles that have been used include intercostals, pectoralis major, serratus anterior, latissimus, dorsi and sacrospinalis. Indications for myoplasty in the treatment of BPF are listed in Table 46.4. For post-pneumonectomy fistulae, reamputation of a long bronchial stump may sometimes affect the closure especially if the BPF has been diagnosed early (42,43). Further resection of the residual lung [site of BPF] or thoracoplasty of various types have also been recommended for treating resistant post-resectional BPF but these have the disadvantage of further compromising the already compensated cardio-pulmonary reserve of these patients. On the other hand, myoplasty, can close the fistula without excision of additional lung tissue and with the removal of few, if any, additional ribs. Using the myoplasty techniques, a high rate of BPF closure with a low mortality has been reported (42-44).

Table 46.4: Indications for myoplasty in the treatment of bronchopleural fistula

A persistent bronchopleural fistula despite an adequate drainage and thoracoplasty

When thoracoplasty alone is not considered to be sufficient to close the fistula [due to a large residual cavity]

In a situation where myoplasty is likely to obviate the need for a thoracoplasty altogether

Tuberculosis Empyema

The term "TB empyema" refers to massive, frankly purulent involvement of the pleura with BPF and trapping of the lung. Some patients develop a restricting pleural peel with or without secondary pyogenic infection of the pleural fluid. It is suggested that in these patients, anti-TB treatment along with antimicrobial therapy for secondary pyogenic infection [according to culture if possible] should be continued till maximum resolution of the parenchymal disease and associated sepsis is achieved. At that point, an anatomical evaluation of the disease status by CT of the thorax should be done. In case of a residual cavity with collapsed lung, surgical intervention is indicated and decortication should be performed [Figures 46.3A and 46.3B]. If the underlying lung

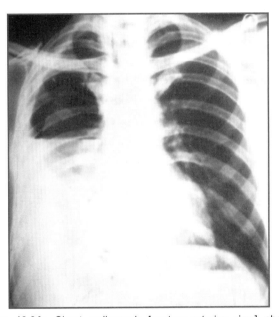

Figure 46.3A: Chest radiograph [postero-anterior view] showing hydropneumothorax on the right side

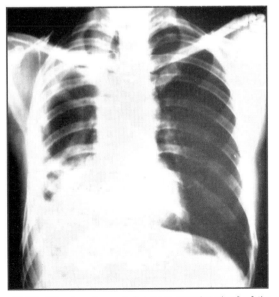

Figure 46.3B: Chest radiograph [postero-anterior view] of the same patient after decortication on the right side

is grossly diseased or destroyed or fails to expand following decortication, pulmonary resection may also be needed. In these situations also, muscle flaps should be liberally used to obliterate the residual spaces and buttress the bronchial stump to prevent the development of post-resection BPF. The use of myoplasty reduces the need for thoracoplasty in many situations or at least reduces the number of ribs that need to be resected in the thoracoplasty.

Haemoptysis

Haemoptysis is a frequent complaint in patients with pulmonary TB. Sometimes, the bleeding may be sudden and large in amount, threatening life of the patient. This topic has been dealt with in the chapter *"Complications of pulmonary tuberculosis" [Chapter 31].*

The treatment of massive or life-threatening haemoptysis has to be immediate and quick. Medical or expectant treatment is associated with an unacceptably high mortality (45,46). The first priority in treating patients with massive haemoptysis is to maintain the airway, optimise oxygenation, and stabilise the haemodynamic status. When indicated, the patient should be intubated for better gas exchange, suctioning, and protection from sudden cardiorespiratory arrest. If the bleeding site is known, the patient should be placed with the bleeding lung in the dependent position. Once stabilisation is accomplished, diagnostic and therapeutic interventions should be promptly performed because recurrent bleeding occurs unpredictably. Early bronchoscopy, preferably during active bleeding, should be performed with three goals in mind: to lateralise the bleeding side, localise the specific site, and identify the cause of the bleeding. In those patients with lateralised or localised persistent bleeding, immediate control of the airway may be obtained during the procedure with topical therapy, endobronchial tamponade, or unilateral intubation of the non-bleeding lung. If bleeding continues but the site of origin is uncertain, lung isolation or use of a double-lumen tube is reasonable, provided that the staff is skilled in this procedure. If the bleeding cannot be localised because the rate of haemorrhage makes it impossible to visualise the airway, emergent rigid bronchoscopy or urgent arteriography is indicated. Numerous reports in the recent past have outlined the value of arteriography and embolisation in the management of haemoptysis (47-55). Arteriography and embolisation should be used emergently for both diagnosis and therapy in patients who continue to bleed despite endobronchial therapy.

Mani *et al* (47) in a series of 37 patients presenting with massive or recurrent haemoptysis of TB aetiology, were able to successfully control the bleeding in all the 33 patients where embolisation with gelfoam could be performed. In two patients the bronchial artery could not be cannulated and in the remaining two embolisation was not performed because the anterior spinal artery was seen to be arising from the bronchial artery trunk. During six months of follow-up, four of these 33 patients had relapse of haemoptysis. Three were treated by re-embolisation of the abnormal bleeding vessels while one died due to aspiration. They concluded that the bronchial artery embolisation is an effective method of treatment for immediate control of life-threatening haemoptysis.

Similar experience has been reported by others (48,50,52). Sharma *et al* (50) have reported the use of an indigenous coil embolisation for controlling recurrent, massive haemoptysis secondary to post-TB bronchiectasis. This method is extremely cheap and highly effective. In patients with life-threatening haemoptysis, early operation is considered when bleeding has been localised to one side and embolisation is not available or not feasible when bleeding continues despite embolisation or it is associated with persistent haemodynamic and respiratory compromise. However, before surgery, it should be ensured that the lesion is sufficiently localised to be resectable and the patient's general condition [cardiopulmonary status] does not contraindicate thoracotomy and pulmonary resection (45,46). For patients in whom bleeding has ceased or decreased, emergent intervention may not be necessary. Surgery is the most definitive form of therapy for patients with haemoptysis because it removes the source of bleeding. Whether to proceed with elective surgery in patients with a major bleed that has stopped or one that is controlled angiographically is a difficult decision. Limited data are available to assist in this decision, even for specific diseases, such as bronchiectasis. Similarly, the long-term course of patients treated with endobronchial tamponade or topical therapy is unknown. For patients with inoperable disease, limited cardiopulmonary reserve or bilateral progressive disease, embolisation is the mainstay of treatment and should be pursued vigorously, even repeating it, if necessary. It frequently controls bleeding for prolonged periods. Majority of patients with life-threatening haemoptysis due to TB have bilateral disease, often with cavitation. Localisation of the side and the lobe from which the bleeding is originating is of para- mount importance for therapy. Bronchoscopy performed during bleeding is able to localise it in most of the cases. However, it needs to be performed quickly when the patient is actively bleeding.

In a retrospective study (56) [n = 89] of patients with massive haemoptysis caused by pulmonary TB, 36 patients [40.4%] underwent an emergency surgery and 53 [59.6%] underwent a delayed operation. The operative morbidity rate was 31.5% [28 of 89] and mortality was 2.2% [2 of 89]. Multivariate analysis showed that patients who received anti-TB treatment before surgery had a decreased risk while patients who underwent an emergency operation had an increased risk of developing postoperative complications.

Tracheal or Bronchial Stenosis, Broncholiths, Destroyed Lung, Bronchiectasis

TB is a necrotising infection, and certain patients, although cured of the infectious process, carry in their lungs the residuum of this destruction (57). Patients with a destroyed lobe or lung, bronchial stenosis with distal recurrent secondary infection and atelectasis, bronchiectasis with chronic infection and its consequences, and other similar residua may be candidates for operative intervention. These abnormalities are doubtful indications, however, unless associated with significant symptoms that cannot be controlled by current medical modalities.

In a retrospective study (58), 172 patients with destroyed lung underwent various surgical procedures, such as, total pneumonectomy [n = 110], pleuropneumonectomy [n = 37], BPF repair [n = 11], residual lobectomy [n = 10], total pneumonectomy and tracheoplasty [n = 2], lobectomy, thoracoplasty [n = 1 each], among others. The perioperative mortality was 2.9%. The surgical complication rate was 18.6%. The sputum negative conversion rate was 87.8%, and the clinical cure rate was 91.9%.

Pulmonary Aspergilloma

Pulmonary aspergilloma is often produced in residual cavities of TB origin. This topic has been covered in the chapter *"Complications of pulmonary tuberculosis" [Chapter 31]*. The surgical treatment of aspergilloma is a much debated matter. On the basis of having described its spontaneous lysis in 5%-15% of cases (59), some authors advise an expectant attitude for uncomplicated, asymptomatic cases of aspergilloma while others advise that it is preferable to treat all aspergillus lesions with respect to the future risk of complications (60). If there are accompanying clinical symptoms, and if the patient meets the conditions of operability, it is preferable to undertake surgical resection taking into account the condition of the affected lung. Lobectomy is preferred, although there may also be indications for segmental resection or pneumonectomy depending on the size of the lesion (60-62). Another surgical technique used, although only in patients with high operative risk, is simple cavernostomy and extraction of the aspergilloma as well as myoplasty in the treated zone (63). A surgical alternative in cases that precludes operation is intracavitary instillation of antifungal agents (62). In patients with massive haemoptysis, embolisation of the bronchial arteries is indicated as a primary recourse before planned surgery. Surgical treatment for aspergilloma demands individual, careful validation because it is a complex pathology with high incidence of post-resection complications.

Cold Abscess of the Chest Wall

Cold abscesses of the chest wall, though uncommonly encountered in industrialised countries, are common problems in areas where TB is highly endemic (64). Because fine needle aspiration remains an inaccurate diagnostic tool and anti-TB treatment is not always efficient, chest wall TB cold abscesses remain in most patients a surgical entity. Surgical management includes adequate debridement and a postoperative anti-TB treatment (65).

Surgery for Complications Caused by Enlarged Mediastinal Lymph Node Tuberculosis in Children

Sometimes, surgical intervention may be required in children with mediastinal lymph node TB for the management of complications caused by the enlarged lymph nodes. Surgical treatment, when performed as an adjuvant treatment for tracheobronchial complications stemming from mediastinal TB lymphadenitis, has resulted in the resolution of the lesions and has no related morbidity (66).

Surgery for Complications of Previous Surgery

Sometimes, plombage therapy can result in long-term post-operative complications. The management of these late complications is challenging and frequently requires surgical intervention (67,68).

SURGERY FOR TUBERCULOSIS: INDIAN EXPERIENCE

Indian experience regarding the role of surgery in the treatment of TB is summarised in Table 46.5 (9,69). After the advent of drug treatment for pulmonary TB, the operation of thoracoplasty became rare in the developed countries.

Table 46.5: Indications for surgery in pleuropulmonary tuberculosis: Indian experience

Variable	Lahiri et al (69) [1970-1990] [n = 1655] No. [%]	SVIMS, Tirupati (9)* [1993-2015] [n = 988] No. [%]
Tuberculosis empyema with or without bronchopleural fistula	1507 [91.0]	654 [66.1]
ICT drainage	1507 [91.0]	654 [66.1]
Thoracostoma	56 [3.4]	8 [0.8]
Decortication	45 [2.7]	293 [29.7]
Thoracoplasty	6 [0.4]	5 [0.5]
Continuous short tube drainage†	17 [1.1]	22 [2.2]
Complicated pulmonary tuberculosis	78 [4.7]	279 [28.2]
Pneumonectomy	35 [2.1]	66 [6.7]
Lobectomy	30 [1.8]	132 [13.4]
Segmental wedge resection	3 [0.2]	6 [0.6]
Thoracoplasty	10 [0.6]	2 [0.2]
Bullectomy	0 [0]	17 [1.7]
Cold abscess in the chest wall	54 [3.3]	7 [0.7]
Osteomyelitis of ribs, or sternum	16 [1.0]	16 [1.6]
Aspergilloma	0 [0]	32 [3.2]

Some patients underwent more than one procedure
* Data updated up to May 2015 from reference 9
† The intercostal tube was cut short, fixed with a safety pin and left open to atmosphere. This procedure was used in patients who were either unfit, or could not afford major surgery
ICT = intercostal tube; SVIMS = Sri Venkateswara Institute of Medical Sciences

However, this was not the case in developing countries like India. Dewan *et al* (70) reported results of thoracoplasty in 139 patients. Indications of surgery were TB empyema [n = 84], pyogenic empyema [n = 33], post-operative empyema with BPF [n = 8], drug-resistant pulmonary TB [n = 2] and recurrent haemoptysis [n = 2]. Successful outcome in the form of control of sepsis, closure of BPF, sputum conversion and control of haemoptysis was achieved in most cases. The authors concluded that with the persisting problem of pulmonary TB in the developing countries, thoracoplasty is still an operation of continued relevance. Resectional surgery (71) for pulmonary aspergilloma and its complications is also frequently used in India [Table 46.5]. In another recent study, Dewan *et al* (72) reported their experience with surgery in DR-TB. Over a period of 20 years, 107 surgical procedures [70 pneumonectomies, 20 lobectomies, 5 bilobectomies, 4 nonanatomical resections and 7 thoracoplasties] had been performed for DR-TB. The authors reported that following surgery, sputum smear-negativity could be achieved in 93 cases. At four years of follow-up, 62 patients were cured.

REFERENCES

1. Bertolaccini L, Viti A, Di Perri G, Terzi A. Surgical treatment of pulmonary tuberculosis: the phoenix of thoracic surgery? J Thorac Dis 2013;5:198-9.

2. Ishida T, Yokoyama H, Kaneko S, Sugio K, Sugimachi K, Hara N. Pulmonary tuberculoma and indications for surgery: radiographic and clinicopathological analysis. Respir Med 1992;86:431-6.

3. Whyte RI, Deegan SP, Kaplan DK, Evans CC, Donnelly RJ. Recent surgical experience for pulmonary tuberculosis. Respir Med 1989;83:357-61.

4. Kumar A, Dilip D, Chandra A. Surgery for pleuropulmonary tuberculosis. In: Sharma SK, editor. Tuberculosis, First edition. New Delhi: Jaypee Brothers Medical Publishers; 2001.p.514-9.

5. Kerti CA, Miron I, Cozma GV, Burlacu ON, Tunea CP, Voiculescu VT, et al. The role of surgery in the management of pleuropulmonary tuberculosis - seven years' experience at a single institution. Interact Cardiovasc Thorac Surg 2009;8:334-7.

6. Kumar A, Mohan A, Sharma SK, Kaul V, Parsad R, Chattopadhyay TK, et al. Video assisted thoracoscopic surgery [VATS] in the diagnosis of intrathoracic pathology: initial experience. Indian J Chest Dis Allied Sci 1999;41:5-13.

7. Beshay M, Dorn P, Kuester JR, Carboni GL, Gugger M, Schmid RA. Video thoracoscopic surgery used to manage tuberculosis in thoracic surgery. Surg Endosc 2005;19:1341-4. Epub 2005 Jun 23.

8. Hosaka N, Kameko M, Nishimura H, Hosaka S. Prevalence of tuberculosis in small pulmonary nodules obtained by video-assisted thoracoscopic surgery. Respir Med 2006;100:238-43. Epub 2005 Jun 16.

9. Kumar A, Dilip D, Chandra A. Surgery for pleuropulmonary tuberculosis. In: Sharma SK, editor. Tuberculosis. Second edition. New Delhi: Jaypee Brothers Medical Publishers; 2009.p.796-813.

10. Bertin F, Labrousse L, Gazaille V, Vincent F, Guerlin A, Laskar M. New modality of collapse therapy for pulmonary tuberculosis sequels: tissue expander. Ann Thorac Surg 2007;84:1023-5.

11. Khan H, Woo E, Alzetani A. Modified thoracoplasty using a breast implant to obliterate an infected pleural space: an alternative to traditional thoracoplasty. Ann Thorac Surg 2015;99:1418-20.

12. Perelman MI, Strelzov VP. Surgery for pulmonary tuberculosis. World J Surg 1997;21:457-67.

13. Olcmen A, Gunluoglu MZ, Demir A, Akin H, Kara HV, Dincer SI. Role and outcome of surgery for pulmonary tuberculosis. Asian Cardiovasc Thorac Ann 2006;14:363-6.

14. Pomerantz M, Madsen L, Goble M, Iseman M. Surgical management of resistant Mycobacterial tuberculosis and other mycobacterial pulmonary infections. Ann Thorac Surg 1991;52:1108-12.

15. Pomerantz M, Brown J. The surgical management of tuberculosis. Semin Thorac Cardiovasc Surg 1995;7:108-11.

16. Reed CE, Parker EF, Crawford FA. Surgical resection for complications of pulmonary tuberculosis. Ann Thorac Surg 1989;48:165.

17. Rizzi A, Rocco G, Robustellini M, Rossi G, Della-Pona S, Massera F. Results of surgical management of tuberculosis: experience in 206 patients undergoing operation. Ann Thorac Surg 1995;59:896-900.

18. Treasure RL, Seaworth BJ. Current role of surgery in Mycobacterium tuberculosis. Ann Thorac Surg 1995;59:1405-9.

19. Brown J, Pomerantz M. Extra-pleural pneumonectomy for tuberculosis chest. Surg Clin North Am 1995;5:289-96.

20. Jouveshomme S, Dautzenberg B, Bakdach H, Derenne JP. Preliminary results of collapse therapy with plombage for pulmonary disease caused by multidrug-resistant mycobacteria. Am J Respir Crit Care Med 1998;157:1609-15.

21. Kir A, Tahaoglu K, Okur E, Hatipoglu T. Role of surgery in multidrug-resistant tuberculosis: results of 27 cases. Eur J Cardiothorac Surg 1997;12:531-4.

22. van Leuven M, De Groot M, Shean KP, von Oppell UO, Willcox PA. Pulmonary resection as an adjunct in the treatment of multiple drug-resistant tuberculosis. Ann Thorac Surg 1997;63:1368-73.

23. Naidoo R, Reddi A. Lung resection for multidrug-resistant tuberculosis. Asian Cardiovasc Thorac Ann 2005;13:172-4.

24. Somocurcio JG, Sotomayor A, Shin S, Portilla S, Valcarcel M, Guerra D, et al. Surgery for patients with drug-resistant tuberculosis: report of 121 cases receiving community-based treatment in Lima, Peru. Thorax 2007;62:416-21. Epub 2006 Aug 23.

25. Mohsen T, Zeid AA, Haj-Yahia S. Lobectomy or pneumonectomy for multidrug-resistant pulmonary tuberculosis can be performed with acceptable morbidity and mortality: a seven-year review of a single institution's experience. J Thorac Cardiovasc Surg 2007;134:194-8.

26. Raymond D. Surgical intervention for thoracic infections. Surg Clin North Am 2014;94:1283-303.

27. Xie B, Yang Y, He W, Xie D, Jiang G. Pulmonary resection in the treatment of 43 patients with well-localized, cavitary pulmonary multidrug-resistant tuberculosis in Shanghai. Interact Cardiovasc Thorac Surg 2013;17:455-9.

28. Bagheri R, Haghi SZ, Rajabi MT, Motamedshariati M, Sheibani S. Outcomes following surgery for complicated tuberculosis: analysis of 108 patients. Thorac Cardiovasc Surg 2013;61:154-8.

29. Vashakidze S, Gogishvili S, Nikolaishvili K, Dzidzikashvili N, Tukvadze N, Blumberg HM, et al. Favorable outcomes for multidrug and extensively drug resistant tuberculosis patients undergoing surgery. Ann Thorac Surg 2013;95:1892-8.

30. Papiashvili M, Barmd I, Sasson L, Lidji M, Litman K, Hendler A, et al. Pulmonary resection for multidrug-resistant tuberculosis: the Israeli experience [1998-2011]. Isr Med Assoc J 2012;14:733-6.

31. Iddriss A, Padayatchi N, Reddy D, Reddi A. Pulmonary resection for extensively drug resistant tuberculosis in Kwazulu-Natal, South Africa. Ann Thorac Surg 2012;94:381-6.

32. Gegia M, Kalandadze I, Kempker RR, Magee MJ, Blumberg HM. Adjunctive surgery improves treatment outcomes among patients with multidrug-resistant and extensively drug-resistant tuberculosis. Int J Infect Dis 2012;16:e391-6.

33. Xu HB, Jiang RH, Li L. Pulmonary resection for patients with multidrug-resistant tuberculosis: systematic review and meta-analysis. J Antimicrob Chemother 2011;66:1687-95.

34. Kempker RR, Vashakidze S, Solomonia N, Dzidzikashvili N, Blumberg HM. Surgical treatment of drug-resistant tuberculosis. Lancet Infect Dis 2012;12:157-66.

35. Marrone MT, Venkataramanan V, Goodman M, Hill AC, Jereb JA, Mase SR. Surgical interventions for drug-resistant tuberculosis: a systematic review and meta-analysis. Int J Tuberc Lung Dis 2013;17:6-16.

36. Floyd RD, Hollister WF, Sealy WC. Complications in 430 consecutive resections for tuberculosis. Surg Gynecol Obstet 1959;109:467.

37. Kirsh MM, Rotman H, Behrendt DM, Orringer MB, Sloan H. Complications of pulmonary resection. Ann Thorac Surg 1975;20:215-36.

38. Malave G, Foster ED, Wilson JA, Munro DD. Bronchopleural fistula-present-day study of an old problem. A review of 52 cases. Ann Thorac Surg 1971;11:1-10.

39. Hollaus PH, Lax F, el-Nashef BB, Hauck HH, Lucciarini P, Pridun NS. Natural history of bronchopleural fistula after pneumonectomy: a review of 96 cases. Ann Thorac Surg 1997;63:1391-7.

40. Ashour M, Pandya L, Mezraqji A, Qutashat W, Desouki M, al-Sharif N, et al. Unilateral post-tuberculous lung destruction: the left bronchus syndrome. Thorax 1990;45:210-2.

41. Ihm HJ, Hankins JR, Miller JE, McLaughlin JS. Pneumothorax associated with pulmonary tuberculosis. J Thorac Cardiovasc Surg 1972;64:211-9.

42. Ali SM, Siddiqui AA, McLaughlin JS. Open drainage of massive tuberculous empyema with progressive re-expansion of the lung: an old concept revisited. Ann Thorac Surg 1996;62:218-24.

43. Hankins JR, Miller JE, Mclaughlim JS. The use of chest wall muscle flaps to close broncho-pleural fistulas: experience with 21 patients. Ann Thorac Surg 1978;25:491-9.

44. Thourani VH, Lancaster RT, Mansour KA, Miller JI Jr. Twenty-six years of experience with the modified eloesser flap. Ann Thorac Surg 2003;76:401-5; discussion 405-6.

45. Erdogan A, Yegin A, Gurses G, Demircan A. Surgical management of tuberculosis-related hemoptysis. Ann Thorac Surg 2005;79:299-302.

46. Jougon J, Ballester M, Delcambre F, Mac Bride T, Valat P, Gomez F, et al. Massive hemoptysis: what place for medical and surgical treatment. Eur J Cardiothorac Surg 2002;22:345-51.

47. Mani S, Mayekar R, Rananavare R, Maniar D, Matthews Joseph J, Doshi A. Control of tubercular haemoptysis by bronchial artery embolization. Trop Doct 1997;27:149-50.

48. Ramakantan R, Bandekar VG, Gandhi MS, Aulakh BG, Deshmukh HL. Massive haemoptysis due to pulmonary tuberculosis: control with bronchial artery embolization. Radiology 1996;200:691-4.

49. Marshall TJ, Flower CD, Jackson JE. The role of radiology in the investigation and management of patients with haemoptysis. Clin Radiol 1996;51:391-400.

50. Sharma S, Kothari SS, Bhargava AD, Dey J, Wali JP, Wasir HS. Transcatheter indigeneous coil embolization in recurrent massive hemoptysis secondary to post-tubercular bronchiectasis. J Assoc Physicians India 1995;43:127-9.

51. Wong KP, Young N, Marksen G. Bronchial artery embolization to control haemoptysis. Australasian Radiol 1994;38:256-9.

52. Sharma S, Kothari SS, Rajani M, Venugopal P. Life threatening arterial haemorrhage: results of treatment by transcatheter embolization using home-made steel coils. Clin Radiol 1994; 49:252-5.

53. Fartoukh M, Khalil A, Louis L, Carette MF, Bazelly B, Cadranel J, et al. An integrated approach to diagnosis and management of severe haemoptysis in patients admitted to the intensive care unit: a case series from a referral centre. Respir Res 2007; 8:11.

54. Lampmann LE, Tjan TG. Embolization therapy in haemoptysis. Eur J Radiol 1994;18:15-9.

55. Bin Sarwar Zubairi A, Tanveer-ul-Haq, Fatima K, Azeemuddin M, Zubairi MA, Irfan M. Bronchial artery embolization in the treatment of massive hemoptysis. Saudi Med J 2007;28:1076-9.

56. Zhang Y, Chen C, Jiang GN. Surgery of massive hemoptysis in pulmonary tuberculosis: immediate and long-term outcomes. J Thorac Cardiovasc Surg 2014;148:651-6.

57. Massard G, Olland A, Santelmo N, Falcoz PE. Surgery for the sequelae of postprimary tuberculosis. Thorac Surg Clin 2012;22:287-300.

58. Bai L, Hong Z, Gong C, Yan D, Liang Z. Surgical treatment efficacy in 172 cases of tuberculosis-destroyed lungs. Eur J Cardiothorac Surg 2012;41:335-40.

59. Wex P, Utta E, Drozdz W. Surgical treatment of pulmonary and pleuro-pulmonary Aspergillus disease. Thorac Cardiovasc Surg 1993;41:64-70.

60. Torres-Melero J, Torres AJ, Hernando F, Remezal M, Balibrea JL. Surgical treatment of pulmonary aspergilloma. Arch Bronconeumol 1995;31:68-72.

61. Zmeili OS, Soubani AO. Pulmonary aspergillosis: a clinical update. QJM 2007;100:317-34.

62. Lee KS, Kim HT, Kim YH, Choe KO. Treatment of hemoptysis in patients with cavitary aspergilloma of the lung: value of percutaneous instillation of amphotericin B. Am J Roentgenol 1993;161:727-31.

63. Rao RS, Curzon PG, Muers MF, Watson DA. Cavernoscopic evacuation of aspergilloma: an alternative method of palliation for haemoptysis in high risk patients. Thorax 984;39:394-6.

64. Kuzucu A, Soysal O, Gunen H. The role of surgery in chest wall tuberculosis. Interact Cardiovasc Thorac Surg 2004;3:99-103.

65. Faure E, Souilamas R, Riquet M, Chehab A, Le Pimpec- Barthes F, Manac'h D, et al. Cold abscess of the chest wall: a surgical entity? Ann Thorac Surg 1998;66:1174-8.

66. Freixinet J, Varela A, Lopez Rivero L, Caminero JA, Rodriguez de Castro F, Serrano A. Surgical treatment of childhood mediastinal tuberculous lymphadenitis. Ann Thorac Surg 1995;59:644-6.

67. Thomas GE, Chandrasekhar B, Grannis FW Jr. Surgical treatment of complications 45 years after extraperiosteal pneumonolysis and plombage using acrylic resin balls for cavitary pulmonary tuberculosis. Chest 1995;108:1163-4.

68. Nell H, Buxbaum A, Czedron A, Vetter N. Fatal complication of paraffin plombage after half a century. Wien Klin Wochenschr 1998;110:729-31.

69. Lahiri TK, Agrawal D, Gupta R, Kumar S. Analysis of status of surgery in thoracic tuberculosis. Indian J Chest Dis Allied Sci 1998;40:99-108.

70. Dewan RK, Singh S, Kumar A, Meena BK. Thoracoplasty: an obsolete procedure? Indian J Chest Dis Allied Sci 1999;41: 83-8.

71. Pratap H, Dewan RK, Singh L, Gill S, Vaddadi S. Surgical treatment of pulmonary aspergilloma: a series of 72 cases. Indian J Chest Dis Allied Sci 2007;49:23-7.

72. Dewan RK. Thoracic surgical interventions for DR-TB and their results. Int J Mycobacteriol 2016;5 Suppl 1:S55.

47

Stopping TB: The Role of DOTS in Global Tuberculosis Control

Deanna Tollefson, N Sarita Shah, Andrew Vernon

INTRODUCTION

In April 1993, the World Health Organization [WHO] declared tuberculosis [TB] to be a global health emergency (1). Once considered a disease of the past, TB resurged as the human immunodeficiency virus [HIV] pandemic expanded, the Soviet Union collapsed, and economies stagnated (2,3). Many countries were ill-equipped to address the expanding epidemic as general TB control practices and the structures needed to implement these practices had been neglected for decades (1,3). "The high mortality and morbidity due to TB is often the result of inadequate control measures and neglect of the disease," the WHO said in 1994 and advocated that nations adapt the directly observed therapy short-course [DOTS] strategy to quell the sudden rise in TB (1). Three years after this recommendation, the Director-General of the WHO praised the strategy, declaring, "The DOTS strategy represents the most important public health breakthrough of the decade, in terms of lives that will be saved" (4).

Since its initiation, DOTS has served as a guide for TB programmes in at least 182 countries (5). Between 1990 and 2013, the global TB mortality rate decreased 45% and global TB prevalence decreased 41%, while the global incidence of TB decreased an average of 1.5% per year from 2000-2013 (6). In raw numbers, over 56 million people were successfully treated for TB and an estimated 22 million lives saved through the programmatic implementation of DOTS between 1995 and 2012 (7). In China, the implementation and scale-up of DOTS from 1990 to 2010 corresponded to a 65% decrease in smear-positive TB prevalence; the successful DOTS scale-up is credited for China exceeding WHO's goal to reduce TB prevalence by 50% by 2015 (8). Similarly, India estimates that by embracing DOTS and by following their 2012–2017 TB Control Strategy the government can avert over 1.7 million TB cases and save 750,000 lives in the next 15 years (9).

TB incidence, prevalence, and mortality rates have decreased under DOTS, yet the burden of TB remains staggering. In 2015, the WHO estimated that TB developed in 10.4 million people and 1.4 million died from TB (6). Globally, the decline in TB incidence remains slow, and the average rate of decline in TB prevalence [3.7% per year] is insufficient to achieve the 2015 target of 50% reduction from 1990 levels, much less elimination by 2050 [≤1 active TB case per million population per year] [Figure 47.1] (10,11). Moreover, half of the world's 22 highest-burdened TB countries were not on track to meet the 2015 targets for decreases in TB incidence, prevalence, and mortality [Figure 47.2] (12). This begets the question on the role DOTS should play in the future of TB control (3,10,13-15).

In this chapter, we provide an overview on the evolution of the DOTS strategy since its global introduction and uptake, the role DOTS currently plays in TB control, and opportunities and challenges facing the control and prevention of TB in the future.

EVOLUTION OF DOTS

Original DOTS Frameworks

As TB rates increased and worries of drug resistance grew, WHO developed and began promoting DOTS as the policy package for global TB control (1). This strategy, which was published in 1994, was based on innovative practices that successful public health programmes had used since the mid twentieth-century, many of which had been first developed and tested in India [e.g., home-based, multi-drug chemotherapy] (16-19). Dr Karel Styblo, Director of Scientific Activities at the International Union Against Tuberculosis and Lung Disease [IUATLD, now called "The Union"] from 1979-1991, used the lessons learned and research on innovative practices from successful public health

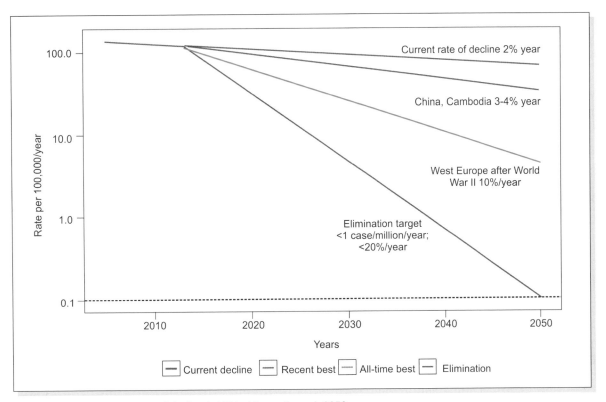

Figure 47.1: Current and potential rates of decline in TB incidence through 2050
TB = tuberculosis
Source: reference 11

Goals and targets	Global	Africa	Americas	Eastern Medi-terranean	Europe	South-East Asia	Western Pacific
TB case detection: Detect ≥70% of new sputum smear-positive TB cases	On target	On target	Met	On target	Met	On target	Met
TB treatment success: Cure at least 85% of sputum smear-positive TB cases detected	Met	On target	On target	Met	On target	Met	Met
TB incidence: Incidence rate falling	Met	Met	Met	Met	Met	Met	Met
TB prevalence: Reduce TB prevalence by 50% relative to 1990 levels by 2015	Not on target	Not on target	Met	Not on target	Not on target	On target	Met
TB mortality: Reduce TB mortality by 50% relative to 1990 levels by 2015	On target	Not on target	Met	On target	Not on target	On target	Met

Figure 47.2: Progress towards TB-related Millennium Development Goals and select stop TB targets, by WHO region
TB = tuberculosis; WHO = World Health Organization

programmes to develop the mutual assistance programme of the IUATLD, which included the core components of DOTS: the use of monitored, short-course treatment regimens to ensure TB patients complete treatment, and thus, achieve high TB cure rates (20-22). WHO adopted this strategy for TB control based on the understanding that this approach would increase cure rates, decrease transmission, and limit the development of drug resistance. The strategy became known as 'DOTS' because a shortened course of directly-observed therapy was its cornerstone. However, the DOTS framework actually consisted of five components, each necessary for TB control [Table 47.1]: political will to assure provision of adequate resources; case-finding at health facilities, primarily through microscopic examination of sputum; a short-course of anti-TB drugs provided under direct observation; adequate drug supply to ensure availability of sufficient

Table 47.1: A comparison of the original DOTS framework [1994] and the DOTS framework in the Stop TB Strategy [2006]

Original DOTS framework [1994] (1)	Updated DOTS Framework, Stop TB Strategy [2006] (5)
Government commitment	Political commitment with increased and sustained financing
Case detection through predominantly passive case finding	Case detection through quality-assured bacteriology
Short-course of anti-TB drugs given under direct observation	Standardised treatment, with supervision and patient support
Regular drug supply	An effective drug supply and management system
Monitoring system for programme supervision and evaluation	Monitoring and evaluation system and impact measurement
TB = tuberculosis	

medication to achieve cure for every patient; and a system for monitoring, with accountability for the outcome of every patient diagnosed (1).

The DOTS strategy was widely and rapidly adopted, with WHO reporting that 148 countries had embraced DOTS by 2000 (23). Despite this enthusiastic adoption, it was estimated that only 27% of people with smear-positive TB actually received treatment under DOTS and only 19% were effectively treated in 2000 (23). It became evident to public health leaders that in order to increase coverage the framework needed to expand, especially in low resource and high HIV prevalence areas (3,24).

DOTS Expansion

Expansion of the DOTS framework began when the "Stop TB Initiative" was established after the meeting of the first *Ad Hoc* Committee on the Tuberculosis Epidemic in 1998. Two years later, the "Stop TB Initiative" produced the Amsterdam Declaration to Stop TB, which called for action from ministerial delegations of 20 countries with the highest burden of TB. At this time, the World Health Assembly also endorsed the creation of a global partnership to improve TB control and achieve the Millennium Development Goals (25). The WHO Assembly recommendation led to the formation of the Stop TB Partnership, whose task was to lead efforts to extend the DOTS strategy.

Including partners from the private, public, and non-profit sectors, the Stop TB Partnership created the first *Global Plan to Stop TB [2001–2005]* which emphasised DOTS expansion (26). This re-visioning of DOTS was captured in the 2002 document, *An Expanded DOTS Framework for Effective Tuberculosis Control* (27), which described DOTS as a "comprehensive support strategy" that provided support to all persons affected by TB by placing equal emphasis on the technical, managerial, social, and political elements of TB control. This framework also led to programmatic advances in addressing the growing epidemics of HIV-associated TB [thereafter referred to as TB-HIV] and multidrug-resistant TB [MDR-TB].

By 2004, DOTS programmes had treated more than 20 million patients and cured more than 16 million (5). Nonetheless, TB control experts realised that DOTS, as designed, would not achieve the TB-related Millennium

Development Goals in all regions [i.e., halving TB mortality and prevalence by 2015], and would be insufficient to reverse the global epidemic (28). The TB epidemic had worsened in select areas in Africa, Eastern Europe, and Asia, as MDR-TB and TB-HIV increasingly hindered efforts to reduce the global burden of TB (3). Once again, it became evident that DOTS would need to expand to effectively address the evolving epidemiology and global burden of TB [Figure 47.3].

Stop TB Strategy

To further expand DOTS, in 2006 WHO and the Stop TB Partnership launched a new strategy, the *Global Plan to Stop TB 2006-2015* [commonly referred to as the "Stop TB Strategy"] (5). This plan was developed to build on the achievements of the prior decade while presenting a clear roadmap to meet the new challenges that were blocking progress towards the Millennium Development Goals and related Stop TB targets. An update to the *Global Plan to Stop TB [2011-2015]* was released in 2010 to clarify the roadmap presented in the *Global Plan to Stop TB* and to improve the plan's relevance in light of progress made towards 2015 targets (11).

In the Stop TB Strategy, DOTS is placed in the larger context of global TB control. The strategy encompasses all elements necessary for effective TB control, ranging from surveillance to programme implementation and research. In addition, the strategy was designed to frame TB control as a necessary part of poverty alleviation (5). Ultimately, the Stop TB Strategy was created to be a roadmap to enable national TB programmes and policy makers to jointly expedite TB control (29).

The Stop TB Strategy encompasses six major elements for National TB Programmes [NTPs], their local and international partners, and policy makers to pursue in order to achieve TB control (5). These elements are: [i] pursuing high-quality DOTS expansion and enhancement; [ii] addressing TB-HIV and MDR-TB and other special challenges; [iii] contributing to health system strengthening; [iv] engaging all care providers; [v] empowering people with TB and communities; and [vi] enabling and promoting research.

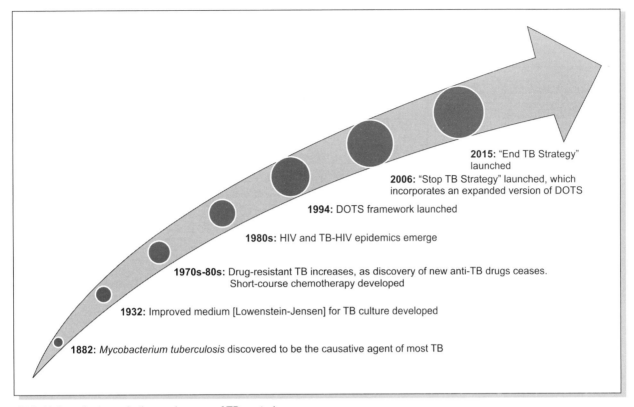

2015: "End TB Strategy" launched

2006: "Stop TB Strategy" launched, which incorporates an expanded version of DOTS

1994: DOTS framework launched

1980s: HIV and TB-HIV epidemics emerge

1970s-80s: Drug-resistant TB increases, as discovery of new anti-TB drugs ceases. Short-course chemotherapy developed

1932: Improved medium [Lowenstein-Jensen] for TB culture developed

1882: *Mycobacterium tuberculosis* discovered to be the causative agent of most TB

Figure 47.3: Major milestones in the modern era of TB control
TB = tuberculosis; HIV = human immunodeficiency virus

The pursuit of high-quality DOTS expansion is purposefully listed first among the Stop TB elements, as DOTS is the foundation upon which all elements of this framework depend (5). In other words, DOTS has an essential role in successfully addressing the other five elements of the Stop TB Strategy.

Attaining "high-quality DOTS expansion and enhancement" requires a multi-faceted and multi-sectoral approach. The following section describes in detail what comprises "high-quality" DOTS.

DOTS IN THE STOP TB STRATEGY

The DOTS strategy remains the cornerstone of the WHO and Stop TB Partnership plan for global TB control (5,11). The strategy remains based on core principles for effective public health programme implementation and continues to serve as a model for other public health programmes to emulate (29,30). The first element of the Stop TB Strategy contains the five components of DOTS, which have evolved slightly from the original 1994 DOTS framework (1,5). The original 1994 core components of DOTS, and the updated components expressed in the 2006 Stop TB Strategy, are listed in Table 47.1.

In this section we elaborate on the importance, successes, and challenges in implementation of each of the five components of DOTS in the Stop TB Strategy.

Political Commitment with Increased and Sustained Financing

Under DOTS, provision of TB services is considered a core government function, and treatment of patients with TB is a necessity to protect the public's health. TB treatment is a service not just to the individual but to all of society because treatment of infectious cases interrupts transmission of TB within the community. To ensure services are widely available, under the DOTS strategy TB programmes are encouraged to provide testing, treatment, and care *free of charge* to all people suspected of or diagnosed with TB disease. In order to do so, robust mechanisms must be in place to fund and sustain the TB control infrastructure.

While TB control is a core government function, the implementation of a successful TB control programme requires the collaborative efforts of multiple sectors in society, such as public health authorities, health facilities [public and private], academic or research institutions, non-governmental organisations, and communities [Figure 47.4]. In other words, effective TB control requires a commitment to strong partnerships. There must be both local and national partnerships, such as, the NTPs with public and private hospitals and NTP with other disease-specific programmes, and international partnerships, such as, NTP with international expert bodies, or NTP with NTPs in neighbouring countries. Domestic partnerships are necessary

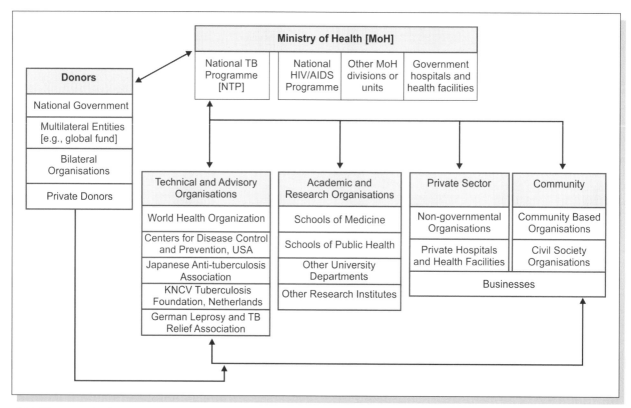

Figure 47.4: The network of partners for DOTS implementation in high TB burden settings
TB = tuberculosis; HIV = human immunodeficiency virus; AIDS = acquired immunodeficiency syndrome

to ensure uniform implementation of, and nationwide coverage with, the country's national TB guidelines. International partnerships can be used by NTP leadership to build expertise, which helps ensure that the country's TB strategy is current, efficient, and consistent with international standards.

Although DOTS is a very cost-effective public health intervention (31,32), the expanded DOTS strategy in the Stop TB framework requires significant and sustained resources to prevent, detect, treat, and report TB cases (29,33,34). This includes funding for diagnostics, drugs, and human capital to ensure that the health care system can diagnose and treat people with TB without interruption; treatment without interruption is essential to increase the likelihood of achieving cure and preventing drug-resistance. Beyond ensuring there are sufficient health care workers to treat and manage TB cases, funding must be available to train and sustain a variety of other staff, including but not limited to TB programme managers, epidemiologists, information technology [IT] specialists, community-health outreach workers, administrative and other support staff. TB programme success is dependent upon staffing to ensure strong surveillance, effective resource management, and quality patient care and management (34).

Overall, the majority of funds for global TB control come from national governments and their support for their respective NTPs. Other major funders contributing to global

TB control include multilateral entities, such as, the Global Fund to Fight AIDS, Tuberculosis and Malaria and the World Bank; bilateral organisations, such as, the US Agency for International Development [USAID], the United Kingdom's Department for International Development [DFID], or the Canadian International Development Association [CIDA], and large non-governmental organisations, such as, the Bill and Melinda Gates Foundation, the Aga Khan Foundation, and the Wellcome Trust. While there is increasing emphasis that TB funding should come from domestic sources [i.e., local governments] (5,29), the majority of high TB burden countries continue to rely heavily on non-domestic sources for TB funding [primarily the Global Fund] (35). Political commitment to global TB has been a source of contention as funding for TB has declined in recent years (13,14). Declining rates of TB [especially in donor countries], competing health priorities, and a poor fiscal environment are some of the many reasons that funding for TB control has decreased.

Case Detection through Quality-assured Bacteriology

To achieve global TB control, all countries are expected to use standardised evidence-based procedures to detect TB. To ensure quality and standardisation, WHO outlines how countries should detect cases and provides clear definitions for diagnosing TB [Table 47.2] (36). WHO guidelines specify

Table 47.2: Select WHO TB reporting definitions

Case definitions

Presumptive TB
A patient who presents with symptoms or signs suggestive of TB

Bacteriologically confirmed TB case
A case from whom a biological specimen is positive by smear microscopy, culture or WHO approved rapid diagnostic methods [such as Xpert MTB/RIF]. All cases should be notified, regardless of whether TB treatment has started

Clinically diagnosed TB case
A case that does not fulfill the criteria for bacteriological confirmation but has been diagnosed with active TB by a clinician or other medical practitioner who has decided to give the patient a full course of TB treatment. This definition includes cases diagnosed on the basis of X-ray abnormalities or suggestive histology and extrapulmonary cases without laboratory confirmation

Smear-positive pulmonary TB
A patient with one or more initial sputum smear examinations [direct smear microscopy] AFB-positive; or one sputum examination AFB positive plus radiographic abnormalities consistent with active pulmonary TB as determined by a clinician. Smear-positive cases are the most infectious, and thus, of the highest priority from a public health perspective

Smear-negative pulmonary TB
A patient with pulmonary TB who does not meet the above criteria for smear-positive disease. Diagnostic criteria should include: at least two AFB-negative sputum smear examinations; radiographic abnormalities consistent with active pulmonary TB; no response to a course of broad-spectrum antibiotics [except in a patient for whom there is laboratory confirmation or strong clinical evidence of HIV infection]; and a decision by a clinician to treat with a full course of anti-TB chemotherapy. A patient with positive culture but negative AFB sputum examination is also a smear negative case of pulmonary TB

New patient
A patient who has never been treated for TB or has taken anti-TB drugs for less than 1 month

Previously treated patient
A patient who has received 1 month or more of anti-TB drugs in the past. They are further classified by the outcome of their most recent course of treatment:

> *Relapse patient*
> A patient previously treated for TB, who was declared cured or treatment completed at the end of their most recent course of treatment, and are now diagnosed with a recurrent episode of TB [either a true relapse or a new episode of TB caused by reinfection]

> *Treatment after failure patient*
> A patient who has been previously treated for TB and whose treatment failed at the end of their most recent course of treatment

Treatment outcomes [excludes patients treated for RR-TB or MDR-TB]

Cured
A pulmonary TB patient with bacteriologically confirmed TB at the beginning of treatment who was smear- or culture-negative in the last month of treatment and on at least one previous occasion

Treatment completed
A TB patient who completed treatment without evidence of failure but with no record to show that sputum smear or culture results in the last month of treatment and on at least one previous occasion were negative, either because tests were not done or because results are unavailable

Treatment success
The sum of 'cured' and 'treatment completed'

Treatment failed
A TB patient whose sputum smear or culture is positive at month 5 or later during treatment

Died
A TB patient who dies for any reason before starting or during the course of treatment

Lost to follow-up
A TB patient who did not start treatment or whose treatment was interrupted for 2 consecutive months or more

Not evaluated
A TB patient for whom no treatment outcome is assigned. This includes cases "transferred out" to another treatment unit as well as cases for whom the treatment outcome is unknown to the reporting unit

WHO = World Health Organization; TB = tuberculosis; AFB = acid-fast bacilli; HIV = human immunodeficiency virus; RR-TB = rifampicin resistant TB; MDR-TB = multidrug-resistant TB
Source: reference 36

that bacteriological methods, including smear microscopy, culture, or approved rapid diagnostic tests, such as Xpert MTB/RIF, should be used to diagnose all persons suspected to have TB. In low-to-medium resource settings, persons suspected to have TB are first tested using smear microscopy. At least two sputum samples should be submitted [one spot and one morning sample] and local laboratories should be able to process these samples within a few hours. If a patient is smear-negative or is HIV-infected, the patient's specimens should also be tested using mycobacterial culture.

This component of DOTS highlights the importance of TB laboratories in achieving TB control (5). Successful implementation of the strategy requires that countries improve the number and quality of their TB diagnostic labs. Expanded laboratory capacity includes decentralised TB diagnostic facilities, national laboratory standards, and a functional national reference laboratory. In addition, mycobacterial culture and drug-susceptibility testing [DST] should be introduced into more laboratories and used for more patients, including all smear-negative, HIV-infected, paediatric, and possible drug-resistant cases.

In reality, the quality and availability of laboratories differs widely between and within countries. Mycobacterial culture is the gold standard for TB diagnosis, but it remains minimally available in most high-burden TB countries and is not used to confirm all smear-negative or drug-resistant TB [DR-TB]. Instead, diagnoses based on clinical and chest radiograph findings remain frequent; these diagnostic approaches have variable sensitivity and specificity for TB diagnosis, and are subject to wide variability in inter- and intra-reader agreement (37-45). Variable quality at laboratories can also lead to false-positives or false-negatives (46); inconsistent practices between labs may artificially decrease the number of cases of smear-positive TB detected and ultimately reported (47). Missed diagnoses can hamper treatment success, breed resistance, and increase both transmission and mortality. The persisting challenges in expanding access to and utilisation of appropriate TB diagnostics contributes to the WHO estimate that only 66% of people estimated to have TB and less than 25% of people estimated to have MDR-TB worldwide are actually detected and reported to NTPs (7,12).

In addition to improved laboratory services, the DOTS strategy includes an emphasis on the need for improved case detection. Active case finding, or purposeful searching to identify undiagnosed TB disease, is an essential element of the strategy. The incorporation of active case finding in the revised DOTS strategy marks a substantial change from the original framework, which focused on passive case finding (1). Today, many NTPs have procedures in place for active case finding, especially amongst persons living with HIV/AIDS where screening for TB is recommended at all clinical encounters. Select programmes even employ cough monitors or community health workers to actively seek and refer persons with TB symptoms for testing. In some places, these programmes and related efforts have been found to drastically increase the number of active cases

diagnosed (48-50). Other community-based TB programmes have not necessarily been found to be effective (51,52).

Emerging technologies provide TB programmes staff with new tools for improving case detection both within central labs and closer to the point of care for patients. GeneXpert MTB/RIF machines are a rapid diagnostic option to bacteriologically confirm TB and detect rifampicin resistance. Although culture remains the gold standard for TB diagnosis, Xpert MTB/RIF holds great promise for improving TB diagnostics in high-burden TB countries (53). Because Xpert MTB/RIF is more sensitive than sputum smear, it reduces time-to-diagnosis compared to liquid or solid culture; it is also relatively simple to use. The numbers of Xpert MTB/RIF machines are increasing in high-burden countries (54). India alone has purchased over 379,000 cartridges and dozens of machines, along with other high burden, middle-income countries [e.g., South Africa and China]. Access to this technology is greatly increasing the diagnostic capacity of TB programmes in high-TB and high-MDR-TB settings.

Molecular epidemiologic investigations rely upon another set of new tools that some countries are now using to detect TB clusters, which allows programmes to find and treat sources of transmission. If not available to NTPs, this technology is increasingly available to research institutions, even in low-resource settings; through collaboration between NTPs and research institutions, molecular technology can be used to inform the NTP's case detection efforts. The reader is referred to the chapter *"Laboratory diagnosis" [Chapter 8]* for more details.

Standardised Treatment, with Supervision and Patient Support

The DOTS strategy includes clear standards and procedures that the WHO suggests should be followed to increase cure rates, decrease transmission, and reduce development of additional drug-resistance.

Standardised Treatment

The WHO provides guidelines for standardised treatment of TB, including recommendations for the management of patients with TB and for appropriate drug regimens for each patient category (55). Recent guidelines (55) emphasise the importance of routine DST, where feasible, or to regularly evaluate the local epidemiology of DR-TB so that the best standardised treatment regimen can be prescribed. Treatment guidelines are updated as TB evolves, i.e., the development of extensively drug-resistant TB [XDR-TB] and as new TB medications become available [i.e., bedaquiline and delanamid, which were approved for use in TB therapy in 2013]. By treating patients according to the WHO guidelines, countries can be confident that their patients are receiving evidence-based therapies, maximising the chance for cure and minimising chance of patients developing anti-TB drug resistance.

Supervision during Treatment

The second aspect of this element of the strategy relates to supervision of patients while on anti-TB treatment. This includes the well-known, yet controversial, directly-observed treatment [DOT]. Note that directly-observed treatment is referred to as "DOT", while the overarching TB control strategy is referred to as "DOTS."

DOT has long been one of the cornerstones of the DOTS strategy, originating from observations and research that showed low cure rates among patients because of poor treatment adherence. Because even the "short course" of treatment for drug-susceptible TB is lengthy [i.e., six months] and far exceeds the period of time a patient feels ill, experts have long understood that it is difficult to complete a full-course of treatment. Moreover, patient characteristics are not predictive of which patients will adhere, and which will not adhere, to treatment (56,57). Failing to finish treatment is dangerous because it can lead to relapse and breed drug resistance; both of these consequences affect not only the patient, but also the community, by allowing further transmission of TB. Recognising that the consequences of incomplete treatment were dire, experts emphasised DOT for TB for all patients (34,58).

In DOT, a person trained and monitored by the health system directly observes the patient as he or she takes each dose of the prescribed TB treatment. This person could be a clinician, a community health worker, a community volunteer, a workplace associate, a community shopkeeper, a member of a non-governmental organisation, a religious leader, or another member of the community, who is trained and accountable to the health care system (57). To improve accountability, it is generally advised that this person should not be a family member (56,57), although in some settings this has been successful (59-62). Regardless of their position, the DOT provider should do more than simply watch patients as they take medications. The DOT provider should encourage the patient and teach the value of treatment success for both patients and their communities. The DOT provider also has the opportunity to inquire about TB symptoms in other family members and thus contribute to active case finding efforts. Ultimately, DOT builds bonds between the health system and patients and is intended to keep patients at the center of care, further strengthening chances for treatment success (34,56,57).

There are many approaches to DOT. Some countries ensure DOT by hospitalising all patients with TB during therapy, while others employ DOT regularly for outpatients. The most critical element for treatment success is to ensure that treatment is administered with a focus on patient-centered care (56,63,64). TB programmes have found that long-term facility-based DOT is often unsatisfactory for both patients and programmes (65,66). TB programmes in many high-burden settings are finding DOT arrangements offered in the community or a location of the patient's choosing result in equal if not higher treatment success (59,67-69). Because successful TB treatment is needed to protect the community, TB programmes must ensure treatment is convenient and accessible for patients in their jurisdiction. It is the responsibility of the public health system to ensure patients complete TB therapy, but the way in which this happens will differ from place to place, and it should be context-specific (56).

DOT continues to be recommended by WHO, but its contribution to treatment completion is controversial (56,70,71). Recent studies have found DOT to be associated with improved treatment success (21,72), decreased acquisition and transmission of DR-TB (69,70), and a decline in the prevalence of TB infection in the community (73). However, robust review of randomised trials and observational studies provide no assurance that direct observation of therapy, in comparisons to self-administered therapy [SAT], increases the rate of treatment success (71). Ethical and logistical issues make it difficult to demonstrate the effect of supervision [i.e., DOT] alone, as distinct from other, related aspects of case management (70,74). Consequently, SAT has its advocates, and it has been suggested in areas where DOT is exceptionally difficult [e.g., conflict zones, pastoralist regions] (75-78). In many high burden countries, such as India or South Africa, the volume of cases exceeds the programme capacity to provide DOT, even on an intermittent basis [e.g., thrice weekly]. Nonetheless, direct observation of each dose of therapy [i.e., DOT] currently remains the globally preferred practice for TB treatment and control.

There is intense interest in the use of mobile health [mHealth] technologies to support patients during treatment for TB. Short-message service [SMS] text messaging could be used to remind patients about appointments or track treatment, even in low resource, high burden settings (79-84), while video chatting [e.g., Skype] could be used to replace in-person DOT in areas where such infrastructure is available (85,86).

Patient Support

The third part of this strategic element is support for patients with TB. Increasingly, TB programmes are recognising the need to provide physical, social, psychological, or economic support to patients to facilitate treatment success. In part, this is because TB treatment, especially MDR-TB treatment, can cause extreme hardship socially [e.g., stigma], financially [e.g., job loss or transportation costs], and physically [e.g., illness and side effects from therapy] (87-90). Social support can be provided through establishing peer support groups (5) or dedicated community health workers who are available to patients (49). Some programmes provide nutritional support to increase treatment adherence because it can act as a behavioural incentive to continue with treatment (91). Similarly, other programmes may consider providing material incentives to bolster treatment adherence (92).

Globally, TB programmes continue to face the challenge of making TB care and treatment accessible to patients. Although the majority of TB programmes offer free treatment, per DOTS guidelines, accessing TB care costs too much money and demands too much time from patients in all parts of the world (93-97). TB programmes need policies or practices that bring TB services closer to those at high risk for TB [i.e., migrant workers, prisoners]. By improving access to TB services, an increased proportion of persons with TB disease will be able to access and complete treatment, thereby reducing transmission within the community.

An Effective Drug Supply and Management System

In order to control and reverse the TB epidemic, an effective drug supply and management system is crucial. Part of the DOTS strategy is that anti-TB drugs are to be available free of charge to patients: TB treatment is a service not just to the individual but to all of society. Furthermore, these drugs must be well-managed so that stock-outs do not occur. Lack of sustained access to effective drugs could lead to increased drug resistance, prolonged transmission within the community, and higher mortality.

The drug supply can be managed using a variety of diverse, sometimes unrelated systems. TB recording and reporting systems can be used to monitor the number of people on TB treatment, to ensure drugs can be properly planned and stocked. Drug use can also be monitored by providers. With electronic systems increasingly available, drug supplies can be monitored in real-time.

Despite the options available for managing the drug supply, maintaining a consistent supply of TB drugs, especially of second-line drugs for MDR-TB treatment, remains a challenge for many countries. There are waiting lines for MDR-TB treatment in many countries because drug shortages and difficulties in procuring drugs can lead to drug stock outs (98-100). In other countries, drugs may be plentiful but waiting lines for treatment still exist because programmes may have difficulty accessing and distributing them (101). During 2000–2009, experts estimated that fewer than 0.5% of global MDR-TB cases had received treatment with "drugs of known quality" through programmes that were competent to deliver care (98). This is problematic both because this leads to patients failing to receive the care they need and because it leads to continued transmission of MDR-TB within communities.

Strengthening the supply chain for second-line anti-TB drugs could help improve treatment and save lives (98). Indeed, countries procuring second-line drugs through the Green Light Committee Initiative—a WHO and Stop TB Partnership effort that offered reduced cost, quality assured second-line drugs, along with continuous monitoring and technical assistance—had significantly fewer MDR-TB cases develop additional second-line drug resistance during treatment, in comparison with countries not relying on the initiative (102). Efforts are underway to decentralise the work of this initiative, in an effort to expand global access to MDR-TB care (103).

Monitoring and Evaluation System, and Impact Measurement

The last component of the updated DOTS framework focuses on the development and maintenance of a strong TB surveillance system, which is vital because its data are used to understand TB epidemiology and provide the basis for estimating national, regional, and global TB trends. Strong surveillance systems also enable programmes to monitor overall programme performance and to estimate TB incidence more accurately. These types of information in turn can better inform patient management practices and improve distribution of resources.

Since the 1990s, countries have adopted WHO recommendations to use standardised recording and reporting forms and registers [e.g., registers for people suspected of having TB, treatment registers, laboratory registers, and MDR-TB registers] to systematically capture and report TB cases. These data are collected at the facility level [i.e., at points of treatment], and then transmitted up administrative levels until they reach the national programme office. Within the reformed DOTS approach, countries are advised to include an expanded number of variables on their registers. For example, registers now regularly include diagnostic information and HIV status to help guide patient care.

Today, TB surveillance is comprised of both paper-based and electronic systems. Traditionally, countries have used paper treatment cards and registers to record and report cases. However, because of expanding technology, many countries, including those traditionally considered to be low-resource countries, are converting to electronic systems. The DOTS strategy encourages countries to use electronic systems, if possible, because this facilitates individual case-based surveillance. Case-based surveillance enables more in-depth data analysis, and thus, better understanding of the TB epidemic at the local, provincial, and national levels. Some electronic, web-based surveillance systems even enable the real-time monitoring of the TB epidemic [Figure 47.5] (104). Moreover, with electronic systems, multiple TB registers can be linked on the basis of a unique identifier to further monitor and evaluate the TB programme [e.g., to identify patients not adhering to treatment or provide enhanced drug management].

In recent years, WHO has placed much emphasis on the need to strengthen the quality of TB surveillance. In 2006, it developed the WHO TB Task Force for Impact Measurement to assess global progress towards the 2015 goals and strengthen the capacity of countries to monitor and evaluate their TB control efforts. The Task Force has helped develop and implement a variety of tools and procedures to measure this progress. For example, it created the *Standards and Benchmarks for Tuberculosis Surveillance and Vital Registration Systems*, which countries can use to find possible gaps in their TB surveillance system; from this, countries can identify ways to improve the accuracy of TB case detection and notification (105). Similarly, the Task Force has promoted the use of inventory studies and capture-recapture studies to

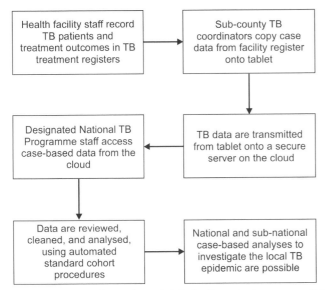

Figure 47.5: Flow of case-based data in Kenya's drug-susceptible, electronic TB surveillance system, called TIBU [meaning "to treat" in Swahili language]
TB = tuberculosis

assess the level of under-reporting of TB cases (106). Finally, there has been a renewed focus for NTPs to analyse their own surveillance data at the national and sub-national levels, so they can understand gaps in surveillance and local trends in TB, and adjust their programmes accordingly (107). This is crucial as TB cases continue to be under-diagnosed and under-reported. In both 2012 and 2013, the WHO estimated that, globally, three million TB cases were missed by national TB systems (6,12).

FUTURE OF DOTS

The Stop TB Strategy, which expanded upon the original DOTS strategy, provided the framework to make tremendous strides in TB control, but with the Stop TB Strategy continued just through 2015, a new framework, called the End TB Strategy [2015-2035], now guides TB control (6,108). The End TB Strategy includes ambitious targets for 2035, namely 95% reduction in TB mortality and 90% reduction in TB incidence compared to 2015, and no families facing catastrophic costs due to TB. It proposes three pillars building upon the achievements of the DOTS framework: integrated patient-centered care and prevention, bold policies and supportive systems, and intensified research and innovation. The End TB Strategy adds to the components of the updated DOTS strategy, calling for earlier diagnosis with universal drug susceptibility testing, collaborative TB/HIV activities, management of co-morbidities, expanded use of preventive therapy and vaccination, broader governmental and social engagement, greater attention to rational use of medications and to infection control, and a greater engagement with research and innovation. DOTS has enabled society to reach many milestones in TB control, but with this new framework

and our ever-changing world, TB control faces many new opportunities and challenges that must be considered in the quest to end TB.

Opportunities

The unceasing evolution of technology brings with it new possibilities to advance global TB control. Scale-up of access to Gene Xpert machines in high-burden countries accelerates the diagnosis of DR-TB. As internet and mobile networks grow in even the remotest corners of the world, new communications technologies [i.e., Skype or SMS] offer opportunities for TB programmes to connect to patients who would otherwise be difficult to reach because of limited human resources or high travel costs. Improved access to technology also gives traditionally resource-poor countries the possibility of real-time, electronic-based TB surveillance systems. Eventually, this technology could allow programmes to link their multiple TB data systems [i.e., NTP, laboratory, and drug-management systems], which would allow for the real-time monitoring of the TB epidemic to improve patient management, monitor patient outcomes, and prevent drug stock-outs.

In addition, the public health community is hopeful that treatment methods will advance. Although the development of new TB drugs has been a slow process, in 2013 and 2014, bedaquiline and delanamid received stringent regulatory approval, the former in the United States and the latter in Europe. Bedaquiline and delanamid are the first new drugs in decades to be successfully created for TB treatment, and there remain other drugs in the pipeline (109). These advances provide new possibilities for TB treatment and care, and thus new opportunities for DOTS. The reader is referred to the chapter *"Treatment of tuberculosis" [Chapter 44]* for further details.

Finally, TB control has the opportunity to evolve as the world reshapes its view of TB as both an international development topic and a global security threat. Rebranding TB control as an issue of international development or poverty alleviation can promote innovations in TB control that address the roots of the problem (15). Meanwhile, declaring TB as a global security issue can reinvigorate funding and resources to address TB on the global scale (110).

Challenges

Despite the opportunities that exist, TB control faces many challenges, which must be considered when envisioning the future of DOTS. First, the TB epidemic continues to evolve. Secondly, DR-TB is increasing, with the rate of MDR-TB increasing many-fold since 1990, and XDR-TB now found around the world. The majority of DR-TB globally is now the result of person-to-person transmission, not acquisition from poor adherence or poorly-designed treatment regimens. Thirdly, the co-morbidities associated with TB are also expanding. Although HIV continues to be the most serious co-morbidity, the increasing prevalence of diabetes and tobacco smoking threaten progress made in TB control, as the portion of TB attributable to diabetes or smoking grows (35,111-119). The explosion of diabetes mellitus and the high prevalence of smoking in high TB burden nations [e.g., China and India] imply that these conditions already are having a serious impact on TB (116).

In addition, TB control faces growing logistical challenges. Patients with TB have become increasingly mobile. Internal and external migration [e.g., migrant workers, students, and refugees] spread TB between cities, countries, and continents. This poses new challenges for preventing TB, linking people suspected of having TB to diagnostic services, treating cases, supervising treatment, and ensuring a stable drug supply. Another logistical challenge comes with the growth of the private health sector. More health providers offer hope for future care, but this brings logistical complications for DOTS programmes, as they strive to standardise care and ensure quality treatment among all providers. Financing DOTS in an ever globalising world will also continue to be challenging (33).

Finally, TB control faces the threat of fatigue and distraction. Although the tools needed to successfully defeat TB have been available for decades, there remains a long road toward elimination, which can cause funding to stagnate and efforts to wane. The possibilities for new approaches are enticing, but core public health principles must not be neglected in the process of utilising new technology. The fight against TB requires both perseverance and ingenuity—perseverance in implementing the basic strategies that have been consistently shown to be effective (34) and ingenuity in adapting and translating those advances that will move the world closer to the goal of eliminating TB.

The DOTS framework has been the cornerstone of TB control since the mid-1990s, but it has evolved considerably in this time. Within the Stop TB Strategy, the five core components of DOTS are political commitment with increased and sustained financing, case detection through quality-assured bacteriology, standardised treatment, with supervision and patient support, an effective drug supply and management system, and a monitoring and evaluation system, and impact measurement. TB control has made great strides with DOTS, and DOTS continues to be upheld as a model for other public health programmes to emulate. The new End TB strategy builds upon the DOTS framework, in an effort to continue progress toward the global goal of TB elimination by 2050. However, consideration of the components of DOTS reminds us that core, time-proven public health principles and practices must not be neglected in the process.

REFERENCES

1. World Health Organization. Framework for effective tuberculosis control. WHO/TB/94.179. Geneva: World Health Organization; 1994. Available from URL: http://whqlibdoc.who.int/hq/1994/WHO_TB_94.179.pdf. Accessed on December 12, 2018.
2. United Nations. World Economic Survey. UN Document E/1993/60 ST/ESA/237. Textbook Nations, 1993.
3. Lienhardt C, Glaziou P, Uplekar M, Lonnroth K, Getahun H, Raviglione M. Global tuberculosis control: lessons learnt and future prospects. Nat Rev Microbiol 2012;10:407-16.
4. World Health Organization. WHO calls for immediate use of new tuberculosis breakthrough 1997;24:1-2.
5. World Health Organization, Stop TB Partnership. The Stop TB Strategy: Building on and enhancing DOTS to meet the TB-related Millennium Development Goals. 2006. Available from URL: http://www.who.int/tb/publications/2006/who_htm_tb_2006_368.pdf. Accessed on December 12, 2018.
6. World Health Organization. Global tuberculosis report 2018. Geneva: World Health Organization.
7. World Health Organization. Countdown to 2015: Global tuberculosis report 2013 Supplement 2013. Available from URL: http://apps.who.int/iris/bitstream/10665/91542/1/WHO_HTM_TB_2013.13_eng.pdf. Accessed on December 6, 2018.
8. Wang L, Zhang H, Ruan Y, Chin DP, Xia Y, Cheng S, et al. Tuberculosis prevalence in China, 1990-2010; a longitudinal analysis of national survey data. Lancet 2014;383:2057-64.
9. Central TB Division, Ministry of Health and Family Welfare, Government of India. TB India 2013. Revised National TB Control Programme, Annual Status Report. New Delhi: Central TB Division, Ministry of Health and Family Welfare, Government of India; 2013.
10. Glaziou P, Falzon D, Floyd K, Raviglione M. Global epidemiology of tuberculosis. Semin Respir Crit Care Med 2013;34:3-16.
11. World Health Organization, Stop TB Partnership. The Global Plan to Stop TB 2011-2015: Transforming the fight towards elimination of tuberculosis. 2010. Available from URL: http://www.stoptb.org/assets/documents/global/plan/TB_Global PlanToStopTB2011-2015.pdf. Accessed on December 8, 2018.
12. World Health Organization. Global Tuberculosis Report 2013. Geneva: World Health Organization; 2013.
13. Tuberculosis—from ancient plague to modern-day nemesis. Lancet 2012;380:1359.
14. Zumla A, George A, Sharma V, Herbert N, Baroness Masham of Ilton. WHO's 2013 global report on tuberculosis: successes, threats, and opportunities. Lancet 2013;382:1765-7.
15. Ditiu L. A new era for global tuberculosis control. Lancet 2011;378:1293.
16. Tuberculosis Chemotherapy Centre. A concurrent comparison of home and sanatorium treatment of pulmonary tuberculosis in South India. Bull World Health Organ 1959;21:51-144.
17. Anonymous. A concurrent comparison of isoniazid plus PAS with three regimens of isoniazid alone in the domiciliary treatment of pulmonary tuberculosis in South India. Bull World Health Organ 1960;23:535-85.
18. Banerji D, Andersen S. A sociological study of awareness of symptoms among persons with pulmonary tuberculosis. Bull World Health Organ 1963;29:665-83.
19. Baily GV, Savic D, Gothi GD, Naidu VB, Nair SS. Potential yield of pulmonary tuberculosis cases by direct microscopy of sputum in a district of South India. Bull World Health Organ 1967;37:875-92.
20. Styblo K. Overview and epidemiologic assessment of the current global tuberculosis situation with an emphasis on control in developing countries. Rev Infect Dis 1989;11:339-46.
21. Obermeyer Z, Abbott-Klafter J, Murray CJ. Has the DOTS strategy improved case finding or treatment success? An empirical assessment. PloS One 2008;3:e1721.
22. Enarson DA. Principles of IUATLD collaborative tuberculosis progammes. Bull Int Union Tuberc Lung Dis 1991;66:195-200.
23. Dye C, Watt CJ, Bleed D. Low access to a highly effective therapy: a challenge for international tuberculosis control. Bull World Health Organ 2002;80:437-44.

24. De Cock KM, Chaisson RE. Will DOTS do it? A reappraisal of tuberculosis control in countries with high rates of HIV infection. Int J Tuberc Lung Dis 1999;3:457-65.

25. UN General Assembly. Implementation of the United Nations Millennium Declaration: Report of the Secretary-General. 2002. Fifty-seventh Session. Available from: URL: http://www.un.org/millenniumgoals/sgreport2002.pdf?OpenElement. Accessed on December 1, 2017.

26. Stop TB Partnership. Global Plan to Stop TB [2001-2005]. 2001. Available from URL: http://www.stoptb.org/assets/documents/global/plan/GLOBAL_PLAN_TO_STOP_TB_2001_2005.pdf. Accessed on December 3, 2017.

27. World Health Organization. An expanded DOTS framework for effective tuberculosis control. 2002. Available from URL: http://whqlibdoc.who.int/hq/2002/who_Cds_TB_2002.297.pdf. Accessed on December 5, 2017.

28. Dye C, Watt CJ, Bleed DM, Hosseini SM, Raviglione MC. Evolution of tuberculosis control and prospects for reducing tuberculosis incidence, prevalence, and deaths globally. JAMA 2005;293:2767-75.

29. Maher D, Dye C, Floyd K, Pantoja A, Lonnroth K, Reid A, et al. Planning to improve global health: the next decade of tuberculosis control. Bull World Health Organ 2007;85:341-7.

30. Frieden TR. Six components necessary for effective public health program implementation. Am J Public Health 2014;104: 17-22.

31. Frieden TR, Driver CR. Tuberculosis control: past 10 years and future progress. Tuberculosis [Edinburgh, Scotland] 2003;83:82-5.

32. Dye C, Floyd S. Tuberculosis. In: Jamison D, editor. Disease control priorities in developing countries. 2nd edition. Washington: World Bank; 2006.

33. Floyd K, Fitzpatrick C, Pantoja A, Raviglione M. Domestic and donor financing for tuberculosis care and control in low-income and middle-income countries: an analysis of trends, 2002-11, and requirements to meet 2015 targets. Lancet Glob Health 2013;1:e105-15.

34. Frieden TR, Brudney KF, Harries AD. Global tuberculosis: perspectives, prospects, and priorities. JAMA 2014;312:1393-4.

35. Raviglione M, Marais B, Floyd K, Lonnroth K, Getahun H, Migliori GB, et al. Scaling up interventions to achieve global tuberculosis control: progress and new developments. Lancet 2012;379:1902-13.

36. World Health Organization. Definitions and reporting framework for tuberculosis - 2013 revision. 2013. Available from URL: http://www.who.int/tb/publications/definitions/en/. Accessed on December 5, 2017.

37. Jaeger S, Karargyris A, Candemir S, Siegelman J, Folio L, Antani S, et al. Automatic screening for tuberculosis in chest radiographs: a survey. Quant Imaging Med Surg 2013;89-99.

38. Davies PD, Pai M. The diagnosis and misdiagnosis of tuberculosis. Int J Tuberc Lung Dis 2008;12:1226-34.

39. Balabanova Y, Coker R, Fedorin I, Zakharova S, Plavinskij S, Krukov N, et al. Variability in interpretation of chest radiographs among Russian clinicians and implications for screening programmes: observational study. BMJ 2005;331:379-82.

40. Muyoyeta M, Maduskar P, Moyo M, Kasese N, Milimo D, Spooner R, et al. The sensitivity and specificity of using a computer aided diagnosis program for automatically scoring chest X-rays of presumptive TB patients compared with Xpert MTB/RIF in Lusaka Zambia. PloS One 2014;9:e93757.

41. Hoog AH, Meme HK, van Deutekom H, Mithika AM, Olunga C, Onyino F, et al. High sensitivity of chest radiograph reading by clinical officers in a tuberculosis prevalence survey. Int J Tuberc Lung Dis 2011;15:1308-14.

42. Sakurada S, Hang NT, Ishizuka N, Toyota E, Hung le D, Chuc PT, et al. Inter-rater agreement in the assessment of abnormal chest X-ray findings for tuberculosis between two Asian countries. BMC Infect Dis 2012;12:31.

43. Piccazzo R, Paparo F, Garlaschi G. Diagnostic accuracy of chest radiography for the diagnosis of tuberculosis [TB] and its role in the detection of latent TB infection: a systematic review. J Rheumatol Suppl 2014 ;91:32-40.

44. Cain KP, McCarthy KD, Heilig CM, Monkongdee P, Tasaneeyapan T, Kanara N, et al. An algorithm for tuberculosis screening and diagnosis in people with HIV. N Engl J Med 2010;362:707-16.

45. Wilkinson D, Newman W, Reid A, Squire SB, Sturm AW, Gilks CF. Trial-of-antibiotic algorithm for the diagnosis of tuberculosis in a district hospital in a developing country with high HIV prevalence. Int J Tuberc Lung Dis 2000;4:513-8.

46. Colebunders R, Bastian I. A review of the diagnosis and treatment of smear-negative pulmonary tuberculosis. Int J Tuberc Lung Dis 2000;4:97-107.

47. Mekonnen A. Smear-positive pulmonary tuberculosis and AFB examination practices according to the standard checklist of WHO's tuberculosis laboratory assessment tool in three governmental hospitals, Eastern Ethiopia. BMC Res Notes 2014;7:295.

48. Yassin MA, Datiko DG, Tulloch O, Markos P, Aschalew M, Shargie EB, et al. Innovative community-based approaches doubled tuberculosis case notification and improve treatment outcome in Southern Ethiopia. PloS One 2013;8:e63174.

49. Soares EC, Vollmer WM, Cavalcante SC, Pacheco AG, Saraceni V, Silva JS, et al. Tuberculosis control in a socially vulnerable area: a community intervention beyond DOT in a Brazilian favela. Int J Tuberc Lung Dis 2013;17:1581-6.

50. Corbett EL, Bandason T, Duong T, Dauya E, Makamure B, Churchyard GJ, et al. Comparison of two active case-finding strategies for community-based diagnosis of symptomatic smear-positive tuberculosis and control of infectious tuberculosis in Harare, Zimbabwe [DETECTB]: a cluster-randomised trial. Lancet 2010;376:1244-53.

51. Ayles HM, Sismanidis C, Beyers N, Hayes RJ, Godfrey-Faussett P. ZAMSTAR, The Zambia South Africa TB and HIV Reduction Study: design of a 2 × 2 factorial community randomized trial. Trials 2008;9:63.

52. Ayles H, Muyoyeta M, Du Toit E, Schaap A, Floyd S, Simwinga M, et al. Effect of household and community interventions on the burden of tuberculosis in southern Africa: the ZAMSTAR community-randomised trial. Lancet 2013;382:1183-94.

53. Steingart KR, Schiller I, Horne DJ, Pai M, Boehme CC, Dendukuri N. Xpert[R] MTB/RIF assay for pulmonary tuberculosis and rifampicin resistance in adults. Cochrane Database Syst Rev 2014;1:CD009593.

54. World Health Organization. Tuberculosis and laboratory strengthening. 2014. Available from URL: http://www.who.int/tb/laboratory/mtbrifrollout/en/. Accessed on December 5, 2017.

55. World Health Organization. Guidelines for treatment of drug-susceptible tuberculosis and patient care, 2017 update. WHO/HTM/TB/2017.05. Geneva: World Health Organization; 2017.

56. Frieden TR, Sbarbaro JA. Promoting adherence to treatment for tuberculosis: the importance of direct observation. Bull World Health Organ 2007;85:407-9.

57. Frieden TR, Munsiff SS. The DOTS strategy for controlling the global tuberculosis epidemic. Clin Chest Med 2005;26:197-205.

58. Iseman MD, Cohn DL, Sbarbaro JA. Directly observed treatment of tuberculosis. We can't afford not to try it. N Engl J Med 1993;328: 576-8.

59. Okanurak K, Kitayaporn D, Wanarangsikul W, Koompong C. Effectiveness of DOT for tuberculosis treatment outcomes: a prospective cohort study in Bangkok, Thailand. Int J Tuberc Lung Dis 2007;11:762-8.

60. Wright J, Walley J, Philip A, Pushpananthan S, Dlamini E, Newell J, et al. Direct observation of treatment for tuberculosis: a randomized controlled trial of community health workers versus family members. Trop Med Int Health 2004;9:559-65.

61. Newell JN, Baral SC, Pande SB, Bam DS, Malla P. Family-member DOTS and community DOTS for tuberculosis control in Nepal: cluster-randomised controlled trial. Lancet 2006;367:903-9.

62. Kamolratanakul P, Sawert H, Lertmaharit S, Kasetjaroen Y, Akksilp S, Tulaporn C, et al. Randomized controlled trial of directly observed treatment [DOT] for patients with pulmonary tuberculosis in Thailand. Trans R Soc Trop Med Hyg 1999;93:552-7.

63. Scott KW, Jha AK. Putting quality on the global health agenda. N Engl J Med 2014;371:3-5.

64. Grant R. Patient-centred care: is it the key to stemming the tide? Int J Tuberc Lung Dis 2013;17:3-4.

65. Zwarenstein M, Schoeman JH, Vundule C, Lombard CJ, Tatley M. Randomised controlled trial of self-supervised and directly observed treatment of tuberculosis. Lancet 1998;352:1340-3.

66. Cavalcante SC, Soares EC, Pacheco AG, Chaisson RE, Durovni B. Community DOT for tuberculosis in a Brazilian favela: comparison with a clinic model. Int J Tuberc Lung Dis 2007;11:544-9.

67. Egwaga S, Mkopi A, Range N, Haag-Arbenz V, Baraka A, Grewal P, et al. Patient-centred tuberculosis treatment delivery under programmatic conditions in Tanzania: a cohort study. BMC Med 2009;7:80.

68. van den Boogaard J, Lyimo R, Irongo CF, Boeree MJ, Schaalma H, Aarnoutse RE, et al. Community vs. facility-based directly observed treatment for tuberculosis in Tanzania's Kilimanjaro Region. Int J Tuberc Lung Dis 2009;13:1524-9.

69. Pichenda K, Nakamura K, Morita A, Kizuki M, Seino K, Takano T. Non-hospital DOT and early diagnosis of tuberculosis reduce costs while achieving treatment success. Int J Tuberc Lung Dis 2012;16:828-34.

70. Moonan PK, Quitugua TN, Pogoda JM, Woo G, Drewyer G, Sahbazian B, et al. Does directly observed therapy [DOT] reduce drug resistant tuberculosis? BMC Public Health 2011;11:19.

71. Volmink J, Garner P. Directly observed therapy for treating tuberculosis. Cochrane Database Syst Rev 2007;[4]:CD003343.

72. Anuwatnonthakate A, Limsomboon P, Nateniyom S, Wattanaamornkiat W, Komsakorn S, Moolphate S, et al. Directly observed therapy and improved tuberculosis treatment outcomes in Thailand. PloS One 2008;3:e3089.

73. Kolappan C, Subramani R, Chandrasekaran V, Thomas A. Trend in tuberculosis infection prevalence in a rural area in South India after implementation of the DOTS strategy. Int J Tuberc Lung Dis 2012;16:1315-9.

74. Davies PD. The role of DOTS in tuberculosis treatment and control. Am J Respir Med 2003;2:203-9.

75. Das M, Isaakidis P, Armstrong E, Gundipudi NR, Babu RB, Qureshi IA, et al. Directly-observed and self-administered tuberculosis treatment in a chronic, low-intensity conflict setting in India. PloS One 2014;9:e92131.

76. Khan MA, Walley JD, Witter SN, Imran A, Safdar N. Costs and cost-effectiveness of different DOT strategies for the treatment of tuberculosis in Pakistan. Directly Observed Treatment. Health Policy Plan 2002;17:178-86.

77. Nackers F, Huerga H, Espie E, Aloo AO, Bastard M, Etard JF, et al. Adherence to self-administered tuberculosis treatment in a high HIV-prevalence setting: a cross-sectional survey in Homa Bay, Kenya. PloS One 2012;7:e32140.

78. Khogali M, Zachariah R, Reid T, Alipon SC, Zimble S, Mahama G, et al. Self-administered treatment for tuberculosis among pastoralists in rural Ethiopia: how well does it work? Int Health 2014;6:112-7.

79. Car J, Gurol-Urganci I, de Jongh T, Vodopivec-Jamsek V, Atun R. Mobile phone messaging reminders for attendance at healthcare appointments. Cochrane Database Syst Rev 2012;[7]:CD007458.

80a. Elangovan R, Arulchelvan S. A study on the role of mobile phone communication in tuberculosis DOTS treatment. Indian J Community Med 2013;38:229-33.

80b. Vivekanand K, Mohan A, Sarma KVS. Study of the structure and functioning of referral mechanism of patients receiving treatment and records linkage under Revised National Tuberculosis Control Programme [RNTCP] of Government of India. Indian J Tuberc 2017;64:77-82.

81. Gurol-Urganci I, de Jongh T, Vodopivec-Jamsek V, Atun R, Car J. Mobile phone messaging reminders for attendance at healthcare appointments. Cochrane Database Syst Rev 2013;[12]:CD007458.

82. Horvath T, Azman H, Kennedy GE, Rutherford GW. Mobile phone text messaging for promoting adherence to antiretroviral therapy in patients with HIV infection. Cochrane Database Syst Rev 2012;[3]:CD009756.

83. Iribarren S, Beck S, Pearce PF, Chirico C, Etchevarria M, Cardinale D, et al. Text TB: A mixed method pilot study evaluating acceptance, feasibility, and exploring initial efficacy of a text messaging intervention to support TB treatment adherence. Tuberc Res Treat 2013;2013:349394.

84. Lei X, Liu Q, Wang H, Tang X, Li L, Wang Y. Is the short messaging service feasible to improve adherence to tuberculosis care? A cross-sectional study. Trans R Soc Trop Med Hyg 2013;107:666-8.

85. Krueger K, Ruby D, Cooley P, Montoya B, Exarchos A, Djojonegoro BM, et al. Videophone utilization as an alternative to directly observed therapy for tuberculosis. Int J Tuberc Lung Dis 2010;14:779-81.

86. Wade VA, Karnon J, Eliott JA, Hiller JE. Home videophones improve direct observation in tuberculosis treatment: a mixed methods evaluation. PloS One 2012;7:e50155.

87. Baral SC, Aryal Y, Bhattrai R, King R, Newell JN. The importance of providing counselling and financial support to patients receiving treatment for multi-drug resistant TB: mixed method qualitative and pilot intervention studies. BMC Public Health 2014;14:46.

88. Yee D, Valiquette C, Pelletier M, Parisien I, Rocher I, Menzies D. Incidence of serious side effects from first-line antituberculosis drugs among patients treated for active tuberculosis. Am J Respir Crit Care Med 2003;167:1472-7.

89. Ralph AP, Kenangalem E, Waramori G, Pontororing GJ, Sandjaja, Tjitra E, et al. High morbidity during treatment and residual pulmonary disability in pulmonary tuberculosis: under-recognised phenomena. PloS One 2013;8:e80302.

90. Chiang CY, Schaaf HS. Management of drug-resistant tuberculosis. Int J Tuberc Lung Dis 2010;14:672-82.

91. de Pee S, Grede N, Mehra D, Bloem MW. The enabling effect of food assistance in improving adherence and/or treatment completion for antiretroviral therapy and tuberculosis treatment: a literature review. AIDS Behav 2014;18:S531-41.

92. Lutge EE, Wiysonge CS, Knight SE, Volmink J. Material incentives and enablers in the management of tuberculosis. Cochrane Database Syst Rev 2012;[1]:CD007952.

93. Pan HQ, Bele S, Feng Y, Qiu SS, Lu JQ, Tang SW, et al. Analysis of the economic burden of diagnosis and treatment of tuberculosis patients in rural China. Int J Tuberc Lung Dis 2013;17:1575-80.

94. Yen YF, Yen MY, Lin YP, Shih HC, Li LH, Chou P, et al. Directly observed therapy reduces tuberculosis-specific mortality: a population-based follow-up study in Taipei, Taiwan. PloS One 2013;8:e79644.

95. Laokri S, Drabo MK, Weil O, Kafando B, Dembele SM, Dujardin B. Patients are paying too much for tuberculosis: a direct cost-burden evaluation in Burkina Faso. PloS One 2013;8: e56752.

96. Steffen R, Menzies D, Oxlade O, Pinto M, de Castro AZ, Monteiro P, et al. Patients' costs and cost-effectiveness of tuberculosis treatment in DOTS and non-DOTS facilities in Rio de Janeiro, Brazil. PloS One 2010;5:e14014.

97. Kirwan DE, Nicholson BD, Baral SC, Newell JN. The social reality of migrant men with tuberculosis in Kathmandu: implications for DOT in practice. Trop Med Int Health 2009;14:1442-7.

98. Institute of Medicine. Developing and strengthening the global supply chain for second-line drugs for multidrug-resistant tuberculosis: workshop summary. Washington: National Academies Press; 2013.

99. D'Ambrosio L, Dara M, Tadolini M, Centis R, Sotgiu G, van der Werf MJ, et al. Tuberculosis elimination: theory and practice in Europe. Eur Respir J 2014;43:1410-20.

100. Bhaumik S. India's human rights commission seeks answers over shortage of TB drugs. BMJ 2013;347:f4301.

101. Centers for Disease Control and Prevention. Interruptions in supplies of second-line antituberculosis drugs-United States, 2005-2012. Morb Mortal Wkly Rep 2013;62:23-6.

102. Cegielski JP, Dalton T, Yagui M, Wattanaamornkiet W, Volchenkov GV, Via LE, et al. Extensive drug resistance acquired during treatment of multidrug-resistant tuberculosis. Clin Infect Dis 2014;59:1049-63.

103. World Health Organization. The new global framework to support MDR-TB management scale-up - Summary 2011 November 9, 2014. Available from URL: http://www.who. int/tb/challenges/mdr/greenlightcommittee/new_global_framework_summary.pdf?ua=1. Accesed on December 5, 2018.

104. United States Agency for International Development [USAID]. TIBU: The use of innovative technology to improve Kenya TB program management—the first in Africa! Available from URL: http://www.tbcare1.org/pdfs/download.php?file=TIBU_Factsheet.pdf. Accessed on Decemebr 2, 2018.

105. World Health Organization. Standards and benchmarks for tuberculosis surveillance and vital registration systems: checklist and user guide. Geneva: World Health Organization; 2014. Available from URL: http://www.who.int/tb/publications/standardsandbenchmarks/en/. Accessed on December 5, 2018.

106. World Health Organization. Assessing tuberculosis under-reporting through inventory studies. Geneva: World Health Organization; 2012. Available from: URL: http://www.who.int/tb/publications/inventory_studies/en/. Accessed on December 5, 2018.

107. World Health Organization. Understanding and using tuberculosis data. Geneva: World Health Organization; 2014. Available from URL: http://www.who.int/tb/publications/understanding and_using_tb_data/en/. Accessed on December 5, 2018.

108. World Health Organization. The End TB Strategy: Global strategy and targets for tuberculosis, prevention, care and control after 2015. 2014. Available from URL: http://www.who.int/tb/post2015_TBstrategy.pdf. Accessed on December 5, 2018.

109. Stop TB Partnership-Working Group on New TB Drugs. Drug pipeline 2018. Available from URL: http://www.newtbdrugs.org/pipeline.php. Accessed on September 5, 2018.

110. Global Health Security Agenda: Toward a world safe and secure from infectious disease threats. Available from URL: http://www.globalhealth.gov/global-health-topics/global-health-security/GHS%20Agenda.pdf. Accessed on December 3, 2018.

111. Chachra V, Arora VK. Study on prevalence of diabetes mellitus in patients with TB. under DOTS strategy. Indian J Tuberc 2014;61:65-71.

112. Kapur A, Harries AD. The double burden of diabetes and tuberculosis-Public health implications. Diabetes Res Clin Pract 2013;101:10-9.

113. Ruslami R, Aarnoutse RE, Alisjahbana B, van der Ven AJ, van Crevel R. Implications of the global increase of diabetes for tuberculosis control and patient care. Trop Med Int Health 2010;15:1289-99.

114. Wang HT, Zhang J, Ji LC, You SH, Bai Y, Dai W, et al. Frequency of tuberculosis among diabetic patients in the People's Republic of China. Ther Clin Risk Manag 2014;10:45-9.

115. Restrepo BI, Camerlin AJ, Rahbar MH, Wang W, Restrepo MA, Zarate I, et al. Cross-sectional assessment reveals high diabetes prevalence among newly-diagnosed tuberculosis cases. Bull World Health Organ 2011;89:352-9.

116. Marais BJ, Lonnroth K, Lawn SD, Migliori GB, Mwaba P, Glaziou P, et al. Tuberculosis comorbidity with communicable and non-communicable diseases: integrating health services and control efforts. Lancet Infect Dis 2013;13:436-48.

117. Bates MN, Khalakdina A, Pai M, Chang L, Lessa F, Smith KR. Risk of tuberculosis from exposure to tobacco smoke: a systematic review and meta-analysis. Arch Intern Med 2007;167:335-42.

118. Dooley KE, Chaisson RE. Tuberculosis and diabetes mellitus: convergence of two epidemics. Lancet Infect Dis 2009;9:737-46.

119. Jeon CY, Murray MB. Diabetes mellitus increases the risk of active tuberculosis: a systematic review of 13 observational studies. PLoS Medicine 2008;5:e152.

48

The Role of Medical Colleges in Tuberculosis Control

D Behera, MPS Kohli, Jai P Narain

INTRODUCTION

Tuberculosis [TB] continues to be a major public health problem throughout the world, more so in developing countries and India in particular. TB is a fatal infectious disease with devastating and serious socio-economic consequences. India is one of the high TB burden countries harboring the highest number of TB cases in the world (1). More adults die from TB than from any other infectious disease in India (2). With its commitment to reduce the morbidity, mortality and disability due to TB and to control and eliminate it as a public health problem, the Government of India [GoI], after piloting the DOTS strategy successfully from 1993-1996, had initiated the Revised National Tuberculosis Control Programme [RNTCP] adopting the DOTS strategy in 1997. Subsequently, the Programme expanded to cover the entire population of the country by March 2006 (3). In India, TB patients are managed by several health care providers with involvement of diverse sectors that include the government, non-governmental organisations [NGOs], the private and corporate sectors including the civil society and patients themselves. For effective TB control all stakeholders need to work together towards a common goal of Universal access.

A substantial proportion of patients with TB are managed at medical colleges across the country because of mere reputations of these colleges, public faith in their health care delivery mechanisms, availability of expertise in the field of medical sciences and infrastructure present in these medical colleges. Therefore, from the TB control point of view, medical colleges, in both the government and private sectors are recognised to occupy a key position with a unique potential for involvement with the RNTCP. To widen access and improving the quality of TB services,

involvement of medical colleges and their hospitals is of paramount importance and their importance cannot just be ignored. Being tertiary care medical centers, large numbers of patients seek care from the medical colleges. In addition, the role of medical college faculty in TB control as key opinion leaders and role models for practicing physicians and as teachers imparting knowledge, skills and shaping the attitude of medical students cannot be underestimated. There is a pressing need for all medical colleges to advocate and practice DOTS strategy and Programmatic Management of Drug Resistant TB [PMDT] guidelines which provides the best opportunity for cure of TB patients and TB control at large. In addition, medical colleges have the diagnostic facilities for extra-pulmonary TB [EPTB], human immunodeficiency virus [HIV]-TB co-infection, multidrug-resistant TB and extensively drug resistant TB [M/XDR-TB] and other forms of drug resistance like mono- or poly-resistant TB cases, associated co-morbidities like diabetes mellitus, immunosuppressed state, kidney disease and liver disease, etc.

Till the time involvement of medical colleges in the RNTCP was conceived, the interaction between the academicians in the medical colleges and the Programme managers was sparse and on many occasions discordant. The young doctors in training seldom got an opportunity to practice what was preached to them. As a result, the facilities available under the RNTCP were seldom utilised to the full extent possible. Keeping in mind the needs of the country, a future "5-Star" doctor who would take up the responsibilities as a care provider, decision maker, communicator, community leader, and a manager was visualised so that such a future doctor would not only serve the patients and the community but would also gain their respect.

EVOLUTION OF MEDICAL COLLEGE INVOLVEMENT IN THE REVISED NATIONAL TUBERCULOSIS CONTROL PROGRAMME

The involvement of medical colleges in TB control envisaged and successfully implemented by the RNTCP for more than a decade in India is an extraordinary effort. Since 1997, concerted efforts have been made to involve medical colleges and their hospitals in the Programme when the first National Consensus Conference on TB was held in New Delhi (4-7). This meeting was followed by two meetings in 2001 at the National Tuberculosis Institute [NTI], Bengaluru (8) and the All India Institute of Medical Sciences [AIIMS]-World Health Organization, South-East Asia Regional Office [WHO-SEARO], New Delhi Meeting on the Involvement of Medical Colleges in TB and Sexually Transmitted Infections [STIs]/HIV Control held at AIIMS, New Delhi (9). Professors from over 35 prestigious medical colleges/institutes participated in these meetings and accepted RNTCP as a control programme with potential for a "remarkable success" in TB control in India and expressed their commitment to the Programme. In the meeting, recommendations were made to consider medical colleges as an integral part of the RNTCP. As per these recommendations, it was envisaged that medical colleges will offer RNTCP diagnostic and treatment services, teach and carry out advocacy about RNTCP, and participate in implementation and monitoring of the Programme. The October 2002 National Level Workshop of Medical Colleges at AIIMS, New Delhi, was instrumental in developing the structure and processes required for the effective nation-wide participation of medical colleges in the Programme. Seven medical colleges located in the different zones of the country at New Delhi, Chandigarh [North], Jaipur, Mumbai [West], Kolkata [East], Vellore [South] and Guwahati [North-East] were identified as nodal centres and were requested to lead the initiative of participating in the Programme [Figures 48.1 and 48.2].

MEDICAL COLLEGE INVOLVEMENT: THE TASK FORCE MECHANISM

The Task Force mechanism has entrusted the responsibility to medical colleges to ensure their effective contribution to the efforts of GoI in TB control. A Task Force mechanism at the National, Zonal and State level [Figure 48.1] was established. Subsequently, there were consensus workshops in the States with medical colleges which further detailed the exact mechanisms for collaboration. This formed the basis for GoI's policy of involving medical colleges in TB control. The National Task Force [NTF] consisted of representatives from the zonal nodal centres, Zonal Task Forces [ZTFs], National TB Institutes, WHO-SEARO and the Central TB Division [CTD], Directorate General of Health Services, Ministry of Health and Family Welfare [MoHFW], GoI was formed. The main role of the NTF was to guide, provide leadership and advocacy for the RNTCP, develop policies regarding medical colleges' involvement in the RNTCP,

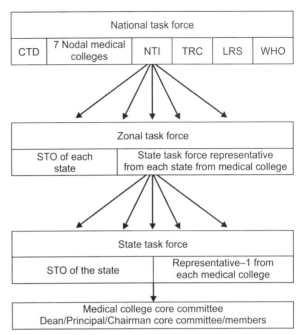

Figure 48.1: Structure of medical college involvement in RNTCP CTD = Central TB Division; NTI = National Tuberculosis Institute, Bengaluru; TRC = Tuberculosis Research Centre [presently known as National Institute for Research in Tuberculosis, NIRT], Chennai; LRS = Lala Ram Sarup Institute of Tuberculosis and Respiratory Diseases [presently known as the National Institute of Tuberculosis and Respiratory Diseases]; WHO = World Health Organization; STO = State Tuberculosis Officer; RNTCP = Revised National Tuberculosis Control Programme

coordinate with the CTD, and monitor the activities of the ZTF. The ZTF facilitated the establishment of State Task Forces [STF], coordinated between the national and STF, as well as between medical colleges and the State/District TB Centres, and monitored the activities of the STF. Because of addition and establishment of more and more Medical Colleges in the country, the south zone has been further divided in to South Zone I and South Zone II and presently there are six zones [Table 48.1].

The implementing unit is the STF, which facilitates the establishment of Designated Microscopy Centres [DMCs] and directly observed therapy [DOT] centres, as well as other activities, in all the medical colleges in the respective States. Over the years, wider interaction with medical colleges has occurred through a series of sensitisation seminars, training of medical college faculty staff at Central TB institutes, national and zonal level workshops. Steps for involvement of individual medical colleges included sensitising faculty members about RNTCP services, identifying a faculty member as a "Nodal Officer" for coordinating RNTCP activities and training of staff. Other steps included formation of a "Core committee" consisting of the heads of various departments [Table 48.2] (10-19).

Core Committees, at the level of medical colleges facilitate inter-departmental coordination for implementation of DOTS strategy. DMC and DOT Centres were established

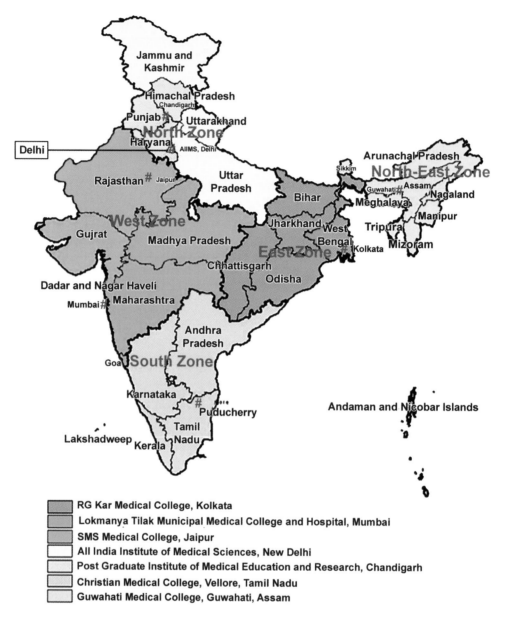

RG Kar Medical College, Kolkata
Lokmanya Tilak Municipal Medical College and Hospital, Mumbai
SMS Medical College, Jaipur
All India Institute of Medical Sciences, New Delhi
Post Graduate Institute of Medical Education and Research, Chandigarh
Christian Medical College, Vellore, Tamil Nadu
Guwahati Medical College, Guwahati, Assam

Figure 48.2: Various zones and nodal centres as per the structure of medical college involvement in RNTCP. Presently South Zone has been further sub-divided into South I and South II
RNTCP = Revised National Tuberculosis Control Programme

Table 48.1: Zonal Task Force [ZTF] in different States and Union Territories of India

Zone	States
North	Jammu and Kashmir, Himachal Pradesh, Haryana, Punjab, Chandigarh, Uttar Pradesh, Uttarakhand, Delhi
East	Bihar, Odisha, West Bengal, Jharkhand, Chhattisgarh
West	Maharashtra, Rajasthan, Gujarat, Goa, Madhya Pradesh
South 1	Andhra Pradesh, Telangana, Karnataka
South 2	Tamil Nadu, Kerala, Puducherry
North East	Assam, Meghalaya, Sikkim, Tripura, Manipur

in all government and private medical colleges and these were equipped with suitably trained additional manpower in the form of laboratory technician [LT] and TB health visitor [TBHV].

The activities of the medical colleges at the district and State level are supported through the respective Health Societies as per approved policy of RNTCP for implementation of Programme activities.

The annual ZTF and NTF meetings provided an important forum for consultation with the medical fraternity on issues or new initiatives being considered by the Programme such as external quality assurance of sputum microscopy, drug resistance surveillance, TB/HIV management and

Table 48.2: Framework for the involvement of medical colleges in RNTCP

All teaching hospitals attached to medical colleges will have a DMC and DOT centre. The following contractual staff are provided: Laboratory Technician [one] TB Health Visitor [one] Medical Officer [one; for Government Medical Colleges] with provision for providing more staff depending on workload

Medical colleges would be represented in the State/District TB Society

Constitution of the "Core Committee" consisting of at least 4 members with representatives from the department of Medicine, Chest Medicine, Microbiology, Community Medicine. Monthly conduct of Core Committee meetings

Training of medical college faculty: *STF Chairman*, who is a medical college faculty member [concise modular training at National level]; *Faculty co-ordinator of Core Committee; Trainer of trainers, Master trainers* [MO-TC modular training at National/State level]; *Heads of the departments and other senior staff* [concise modular training at State level]; other interested faculty members [MO modular training at Medical College level]; nurses, pharmacists and other paramedical staff [MPW training at Medical College level]

Recording, administration of treatment, referral for treatment, and monthly and quarterly reporting as per the format prescribed for medical colleges

Training and teaching about RNTCP
  Sensitisation of faculty members
  Posting of Interns, UGs and PGs at DOT centres
  Include questions on RNTCP in UG and PG examinations

Advocacy
  Publish articles/ newsletters, deliver radio and TB talks
  Sensitisation/ training of PPs & NGOs, IMA and other sectors
  Undertake other relevant IEC activities

Operational research
  Conducting thesis work on RNTCP [Rs 30,000 consolidated; at least one per medical college/year; more if appropriate]
  Conducting operational research on RNTCP

Mainstreaming of management of DR-TB
  Development of requisite infrastructure [e.g., microbiology laboratories in medical colleges to apply for accreditation for carrying out mycobacterial culture and drug-susceptibility testing]
  Formation of DOTS-Plus committee and DOTS-Plus site committee.
  Strengthening of the existing core committee co opting DOTS-Plus committee members

RNTCP = Revised National Tuberculosis Control Programme; TB = tuberculosis; DMC = Designated Microscopy Centre; STF = State Task Force; MO-TC = Medical Officer Tuberculosis Centre; MO = Medical Officer; MPW = Multipurpose Worker; UG = undergraduate; PG = postgraduate; PPs = private practitioners; NGOs = Non-governmental Organisations; IMA = Indian Medical Association; IEC = information, education, communication; DR-TB = drug-resistant tuberculosis

Updated and reproduced with permission from reference 18

coordination, management of M/XDR-TB and DOTS Plus (10-19).

The successful amalgamation of the public health approach and the expertise of academicians has immensely benefited the RNTCP and TB control in India and facilitated the emergence of the "future doctor" from among the medical students. Involvement of medical colleges in the RNTCP is a high priority. Continuing success of RNTCP requires involvement of all large providers of health care including medical colleges. Under RNTCP Medical Colleges play important roles in service delivery, advocacy, training and operational research.

CURRENT STATUS OF MEDICAL COLLEGE INVOLVEMENT

As on 2015-16, 382 medical colleges are involved under RNTCP with the formation of core committee, DMC and DOT Centre [Table 48.3] (4,5). STF Workshops are held once a quarter in each State to review the activities of the previous quarter and dissemination of the updates under RNTCP to all medical colleges. The annual ZTF continuing medical education [CME] lectures cum workshops are held every year. This is an opportunity for reviewing the performance of STF and medical colleges and advocating the guidelines

Table 48.3: Involvement of medical colleges under RNTCP

Variable	2009-10	2010-11	2011-12	2012-13	2013-14	2014-15	2015-16
No. of medical colleges	282	291	315	320	347	363	382
PTB cases diagnosed	141859	144303	136072	136130	156858	171627	159560
EPTB cases diagnosed	81615	83824	82067	78,200	91367	110083	101434
Total cases diagnosed	223,474	225,127	218,139	214,330	252,066	281,719	260,994

RNTCP = Revised National Tuberculosis Control Programme; PTB = pulmonary tuberculosis; EPTB = extra-pulmonary tuberculosis
Source: references 4,5

of RNTCP. In all these workshops, two representatives from each medical college in the zone, the state TB officers [STOs], STF Chairpersons, ZTF Chairpersons, Zonal operational research [OR] Committee Members and head quarter RNTCP consultants of all the states in the zone are invited to participate. NTF Workshop is the event wherein all the recommendations from the ZTF are consolidated and deliberated to enable necessary policy changes.

Impact of Medical Colleges

Medical colleges contribute about 17% of the total registered cases under the RNTCP [Table 48.3]. The main contribution is in terms of the sputum negative and extra-pulmonary TB [EPTB] where their contribution is above 30% of the overall cases diagnosed. More than 600 faculty members from Medical Colleges are trained as master trainers who support the program beyond the academics as training and facilitators for over 300 CMEs and workshops annually as part of advocacy efforts and also participating in Internal Evaluations and appraisals of the RNTCP. Currently, 382 medical colleges are involved with RNTCP. Of the total patients notified from RNTCP, medical colleges have contributed 16%-20% pulmonary TB and 50% EPTB patients (5).

Medical colleges have DMCs and DOTS Centres and referral for treatment, recording and reporting data, carrying out advocacy for RNTCP and conducting operational research relevant to RNTCP.

Majority of the medical colleges are running Integrated Counseling and Testing Centers [ICTCs] and antiretroviral treatment [ART] centres and have established standard cross referrals between TB and HIV programs (4,5). Medical colleges are contributing to diagnosis and treatment of HIV-TB co-infection and development of laboratory infrastructure for early diagnosis of MDR and/or XDR-TB and Programmatic Management of Drug-Resistant TB [PMDT].

Irrespective of which medical college in the country the patient is diagnosed to have TB, the referral mechanisms for treatment have facilitated the delivery of DOTS at the patient's place of domicile. Medical colleges, by virtue of being referral centres with more facilities for invasive procedures and histopathological and microbiological methods of diagnosis, have enhanced diagnostic yield of EPTB, such as, TB pleural effusion, lymph node TB, abdominal TB, neurological TB, among others. These have, thus, contributed to early diagnosis of EPTB cases and facilitated institution of the standard of care, i.e., DOTS for these patients. Medical college involvement has also facilitated more active involvement of pediatricians in the RNTCP and effective utilisation of RNTCP diagnostic and therapeutic services for paediatric TB.

The Medical Colleges/Institutions have settled the issue of efficacy of DOTS therapy in EPTB like, pleural effusion, lymph node TB, gastrointestinal tract TB, TB meningitis, genitourinary TB, and bone and joint TB. Currently many experts from medical colleges had contributed to the recently released INDEX-TB guidelines (19).

OR is one of the important activities of Medical Colleges. To encourage young physicians, RNTCP helps postgraduate thesis on TB with a contribution of Rs 30,000 per medical college. Besides, individual projects are supported if they have operational values for the programme. The mechanism also helps developing research capacity in medical faculty through workshops at national, zonal and state levels.

The NTF has been the voice of the collective opinion of academicians in medical colleges and has contributed in shaping key policy issues, such as, ensuring that teaching and training regarding RNTCP and provision of infrastructural facilities like DMC and DOT Centre at medical colleges are made mandatory by the Medical Council of India [MCI]; rational use of fluoroquinolone antibiotics in the treatment of respiratory tract infections; airborne infection control policy, drug regimens, ban of serological tests, rational use of anti-TB drugs, taking up drug trials among others (4,18,20). Medical College Faculty have been a part of the Joint Monitoring Mission undertaken every few years to evaluate the Programme. Some of the major contributions of NTF Workshop are shown in Table 48.4 (18).

ISSUES WITH MEDICAL COLLEGE INVOLVEMENT IN THE REVISED NATIONAL TUBERCULOSIS CONTROL PROGRAMME

Some problems have been identified in the implementation of RNTCP activities in medical colleges, especially in the new medical colleges set up in the private sector. These include delay in formation of Core Committees, establishment of DMCs in some of the medical colleges. Technical doubts about efficacy of DOTS regimens particularly in EPTB cases have lingered on. Consequently, many patients with EPTB, especially, orthopaedic and neurological TB are being treated outside the programme resulting in inadequate utilisation of the RNTCP programme. The inadequacies in staff and human resources shortage at all levels require rectification. Issues, such as, staff vacancies in medical colleges not being filled up on time, and salaries to RNTCP contractual staff not being at par with payments in the sector also need to be addressed.

In some states, delay/non-release of funds to STFs has resulted in non-performance of planned activities. There is a need to ensure financing essential for sustenance of this model. In states with a large number of medical colleges, such as Karnataka, visit by the STF Chairperson has become a practical problem. Therefore in States with large number of medical colleges there is provision of having vice chairs for every 10 medical colleges.

Poor and inadequate airborne infection control practices in most of the medical colleges, especially the overcrowded government medical colleges have been another issue of concern. There is an urgent need for advocacy regarding education on cough hygiene and etiquette. Weaknesses that are evident in supervision capacity and quality as well as in planning, monitoring and evaluation, need to be addressed.

In medical colleges, there is a need for enhanced inter-departmental sensitisation and better advocacy for

Table 48.4: The key contributions made by medical colleges in RNTCP policy formulation and programme implementation during the last decade

Defining the mechanisms for the involvement of medical colleges effectively under the programme [NTF recommendations 2002, 2003, 2004]

Management of TB cases presenting to a medical college hospital [NTF recommendations 2002, 2003, 2004]

Development of RNTCP operational research mechanisms: Identifying and addressing priority OR topics [NTF recommendations 2004, 2005, 2007]

RNTCP strategy for DRS/DOTS-Plus, role of medical colleges in the management of MDR-TB patients [NTF recommendations 2004, 2006]

Strategy for TB-HIV co-ordination at medical colleges [NTF recommendations 2004, 2006]

Recommendations for generation of evidence on effectiveness of RNTCP regimens in extra-pulmonary TB by developing generic operational research protocols on pleural effusion, lymph node [NTF recommendations 2005, 2006]

Statement on rational use of second line anti-TB drugs [NTF recommendations 2006]

Adoption and endorsement of "International Standards for Tuberculosis Care" [NTF recommendations, 2006]

Adoption and endorsement of the Chennai Consensus statement on the problem, prevention, management and control of MDR-TB and XDR-TB [NTF recommendations 2007]

Contribution to the development of RNTCP DOTS-Plus guidelines and RNTCP OR guidelines [NTF recommendations 2007]

Contribution to the development of National Airborne Infection Control Guidelines [NTF recommendations 2008]

Revision of the RNTCP Operational Research Agenda and Guidelines [NTF recommendations 2008]

Endorsed and contributed to implementation of revised diagnostic criteria of 2 weeks cough to suspect TB and 2 samples examination for diagnosis [NTF recommendations 2008]

Endorsement of proposed revision of RNTCP treatment regimen and nomenclature [2009]

Rolling out pilot of National Guidelines on Airborne Infection Control in health care and other settings in India [2009]

Promoting involvement of Medical Colleges for implementing MDR-TB diagnostic and treatment services under RNTCP [2009]

Streamlining reporting from Medical Colleges [2009]

Endorsing the RNTCP response to WHO treatment guidelines [2010]

RNTCP = Revised National Tuberculosis Control Programme; NTF = National Task Force; TB = tuberculosis; DRS = drug-resistance surveillance; MDR-TB = multidrug-resistant tuberculosis; HIV = human immunodeficiency virus; XDR-TB = extensively drug-resistant tuberculosis; WHO = World Health Organization

Updated and reproduced with permission from reference 18

RNTCP and need for more contribution in pulmonary TB [smear-positive and smear-negative cases] and EPTB cases. There is also a need for strengthening the feedback for transferred out cases. This can be facilitated by holding regular core committee meetings, more intense and sustained sensitisation regarding the Programme and enhanced inter-departmental cooperation.

Establishment of Intermediate Reference Laboratories [IRLs] and DOTS-Plus sites for M/XDR-TB in medical colleges would contribute to capacity building and strengthening of mycobacteriology laboratory services in the department of microbiology in medical colleges. Availability of quality assured accredited laboratories in medical colleges would facilitate better management of drug-resistant TB and HIV-TB co-infection.

Active medical college involvement in prior planning and efficient management of drug logistics cycle will avoid shortages and will ensure timely supply of drugs. However, in spite of all these deterrents and shortcomings, the landmark decision taken more than a decade ago to involve medical colleges in TB control appears to have extraordinary foresight. This has resulted in the establishment of DOTS as the standard of care for TB patients in all medical colleges and their hospitals. It is expected that through their own practice, senior faculty [of the rank of a professor] in medical colleges will influence the practice in the private sector as well as the future generation of physicians thus making DOTS the standard of care for TB patients in the country. This will ensure that all TB patients, irrespective of where they seek care, receive the best available care, free of cost.

Several issues need to be streamlined and improved upon in the coming years to make this partnership between the RNTCP and the medical colleges a truly effective collaboration.

THE FUTURE: THE WAY AHEAD

As the RNTCP widens the scope of services that it provides, medical colleges will have an increasingly important role to play in areas such as TB/HIV co-infection, external quality assurance of the sputum microscopy network, drug-resistance surveillance and management of MDR-TB patients. The RNTCP needs active support of medical colleges in carrying out OR in these areas to guide the development of the Programme's future policies. Recently, medical colleges have also begun participation in airborne infection control policy implementation. This will involve engineering works, renovation of existing infrastructure by involving medical college authorities.

Medical colleges also have the potential for evaluating the efficacy of isoniazid preventive treatment [IPT] in the field setting. Thus, by their active involvement in the "3Is", namely, intensified case finding, air borne infection control policy, and IPT medical colleges are active partners in the implementation of the RNTCP.

The beginning and the progress made so far seem promising. But, the need of the hour is to sustain the momentum gained and push medical college involvement forward by continuing coordination and communication. The OR relevant to the Programme needs can be further facilitated by providing attractive funding and a clear-cut *modus operandi* with a specified time-line so as to attract interested faculty members from medical colleges to take up research studies. Identifying thrust areas relevant to current needs of the Programme, and making available quality generic protocols can facilitate OR studies to be carried out in medical colleges in multicentre mode. There is also a need for visible networking to facilitate the widespread dissemination of the outcomes and results documented in the OR studies so that this will also enthuse and inspire more research relevant to the Programme needs. The experience from India in involving medical colleges in national Programme shows that tangible additional benefits can be obtained in TB control, especially by improving case detection. In view of this, involvement of medical colleges should be promoted widely and the experience replicated not only in the region but also globally. As the GoI and program is going to change or reviewing some of the strategies like 90/90 strategy, Standards for TB Care in India [STCI] in line with International Standards of TB Care [ISTC], newer and quicker diagnostics, Public Private Mix [PPM] etc., role of Medical Colleges will be more crucial. Some new initiatives have already been taken by the programme but much more need to be done.

As the Programme widens its scope, future challenges include sustenance of this contribution and facilitating universal access to quality TB care; greater involvement in operational research relevant to the Programme needs; and better co-ordination mechanisms between district, state, zonal and national level to encourage their involvement.

There is a need to integrate various National TB Institute and organisation along with medical colleges. Such linkage/lines up between RNTCP and such organisations like Indian Council of Medical Research [ICMR], National JALMA Institute for Leprosy and Other Mycobacterial Diseases, Agra; National Institute of Tuberculosis and Respiratory Diseases [NITRD], New Delhi and NTI etc. There should be active involvement of medical colleges with integrated operational and basic research. Few Medical colleges in the country are now a part of the Conditional Access Program for Bedaquiline for MDR/Pre-XDR and XDR-TB cases. New vaccines may come up in the near future which will also need trial where medical colleges will have a major role.

The efforts by the CTD and the RNTCP in organizing and developing a three-tier laboratory network consisting of DMCs, IRLs, culture and drug-susceptibility test [C-DST] laboratories and establishing Nodal DR-TB Centres [NDR-TBC] and District DR-TB Centres [DDR-TBC] in government medical colleges as a part of PMDT in India is laudable (21,22).

Although the programme has achieved a lot in TB control, there are certain lacunae still which need to be addressed. These include review of programme performance; and reorganisation, strengthening of core committees, state and zonal task force mechanisms. Teaching, training regarding RNTCP and TB control to undergraduate and postgraduate medical students, encouraging conduct of mini-projects on TB by the medical students also needs attention. There is a need for involvement of various specialties in the core committee. Medical college faculty have an important role to play regarding the operationalisation of the recently published INDEX-TB guidelines (19). Private practitioner involvement, anti-TB drug regulation, pharmacovigilance are other areas where medical colleges are expected to take a lead. Collaboration is desired from National Institutes/Medical College collaboration for capacity building in research in TB. Better co-ordination is also desired between Medical colleges/STOs/DTOs regarding fund-flow mechanism.

REFERENCES

1. World Health Organization. Global tuberculosis report 2016. Geneva: World Health Organization; 2016.
2. Central TB Division. TB India 2012. Revised National TB Control Programme. Annual Status Report. New Delhi: Central TB Division, Ministry of Health and Family Welfare, Government of India; 2012.
3. Granich R, Chauhan LS. The Revised National Tuberculosis Control Programme [RNTCP]. In: Sharma SK, Mohan A, editors. Tuberculosis. Second edition. New Delhi: Jaypee Brothers Medical Publishers; 2009.p.894-917.
4. Central TB Division. TB India 2016. Revised National TB Control Program. Annual Status Report. Central TB Division, Directorate General of Health Services, Ministry of Health and Family Welfare, Govt of India; New Delhi; 2016.
5. Central TB Division. TB India 2017. Revised National TB Control Program. Annual Status Report. Central TB Division, Directorate General of Health Services, Ministry of Health and Family Welfare, Govt of India; New Delhi; 2017.
6. Narain JP, Nath LM. The role of medical schools in tuberculosis control. In: Sharma SK, Mohan A, editors. Tuberculosis. First edition. New Delhi: Jaypee Brothers Medical Publishers; 2001. p.597-600.
7. Narain JP, Correman E, Nath LM. The role of medical colleges in tuberculosis control. In: Sharma SK, Mohan A, editors. Tuberculosis. Second edition. New Delhi: Jaypee Brothers Medical Publishers; 2009. p. 839-45.
8. Medical College Conference on RNTCP, Bangalore, September 15, 2001. Available from URL: http://www.tbcindia.nic.in/Press%20release%20Bangalore.html. Accessed on February 18, 2013.
9. AIIMS-WHO Meeting on the Involvement of Medical Schools in TB and STI/HIV Control. Report on an Informal Consultation on November 28-30, 2001 and Follow-up meeting on April 29, 2002.
10. Recommendations of the 1st NTF meeting for Involvement of Medical Colleges in the RNTCP, New Delhi, October 29-31, 2002. Available from URL: http://tbcindia.nic.in/Pdfs/NTF%20Rec%202002.pdf. Accessed on February 18, 2013.

11. Recommendations of the 2nd Meeting of the NTF for involvement of Medical Colleges in the RNTCP, New Delhi, November 22, 2003. Available at URL: http://tbcindia. nic.in/ pdfs/Recomm%202nd%20NTF%20ws%20 Nov03%20FINAL. pdf. Accessed on February 18, 2013.

12. Recommendations of the 3rd NTF Meeting for Involvement of Medical Colleges in the RNTCP, New Delhi,November 23-24, 2004. Available at URL: http://tbcindia.nic.in/pdfs/ Recomm%203rd%20NTF%20mtg%20Nov04%20Final.pdf. Accessed on February 18, 2013.

13. Recommendations of the 4th NTF Meeting for Involvement of Medical Colleges in the RNTCP, New Delhi, November 3-5, 2005. Available at URL: http://tbcindia.nic.in/Pdfs/Minutes%20 and%20Recommendations%20of%20the%20NTF%202005.pdf. Accessed on February 18, 2013.

14. Recommendations of the 5th NTF Meeting for Involvement of Medical Colleges in the RNTCP, New Delhi, November 9-11, 2006. Available at URL: http://tbcindia.nic.in/Pdfs/Minutes%20 and%20Recommendations%20of%20NTF%202006.pdf. Accessed on February 18, 2013.

15. Recommendations of the 6th NTF Meeting for Involvement of Medical Colleges in the RNTCP, New Delhi, October 29-31, 2007. Available at URL: http://tbcindia.nic.in/Pdfs/Minutes%20 and%20Recommendations%20of%20NTF%202007.pdf. Accessed on February 18, 2013.

16. Recommendations of the 7th NTF Meeting for the Involvement of Medical Colleges in the RNTCP, New Delhi, October 22-24, 2008. Available at URL: http://tbcindia.nic.in/Pdfs/NTF%20 _2008_%20recomendations.pdf. Accessed on February 18, 2013.

17. Recommendations of the 8th NTF meeting for the Involvement of Medical Colleges in the RNTCP, New Delhi, October 30-31, 2009. Available at URL: http://tbcindia.nic.in/Pdfs/NTF% 20_2009_%20recomendations.pdf. Accessed on February 18, 2013.

18. Sharma SK. Report of the NTF 2010. Presented at the NTF Meeting for involvement of Medical Colleges in the RNTCP, Hyderabad, 18-20, January2011. Available at URL: http://tbcindia.nic.in/ documents.html. Accessed on February 18, 2013.

19. Sharma SK, Mohan A, Chauhan LS, Narain JP, Kumar P, Behera D, et al. Contribution of medical colleges to tuberculosis control in India under the Revised National Tuberculosis Control Programme [RNTCP]: lessons learnt & challenges ahead. Indian J Med Res 2013;137:283-94.

20. INDEX-TB Guidelines. Guidelines on extra-pulmonary tuberculosis for India. Initiative of Central TB Division, Ministry of Health and Family Welfare, Government of India; 2016. Available at URL: http://tbcindia.nic.in/showfile.php?lid=3245. Accessed on December 10, 2016.

21. Revised National Tuberculosis Control Programme, Directorate General of Health Services, Ministry of Health and Family Welfare, Government of India. Guidelines on programmatic management of drug-resistant tuberculosis in India 2017. New Delhi: World Health Organization, Country Office for India; 2017.

22. Central TB Division. TB India 2018. Revised National TB Control Program. Annual Status Report. Central TB Division, Directorate General of Health Services, Ministry of Health and Family Welfare, Govt of India; New Delhi; 2018.

49

Public-Private Mix for TB Care

Mukund Uplekar, Sreenivas Achutan Nair

INTRODUCTION

The Mismatch of Demand and Supply

Like most public health interventions, tuberculosis [TB] control in high TB-burden countries is planned and designed by governments and implemented largely through government facilities supervised by National Tuberculosis Programmes [NTPs]. The NTPs operate through a network of public sector services with the objective of detecting and treating all people with TB. In reality, however, many people with TB, including the very poor, do not approach the network of services providing TB care under the NTP. They seek and receive care from a wide variety of public, voluntary, corporate and private health care providers (1). Public sector facilities such as hospitals and medical colleges or health facilities beyond the administrative control of health ministries such as mines and prison health services do not always follow the guidelines of the NTP. Studies have shown that in urban and rural areas alike, a private provider is often a first contact for a large proportion of TB patients especially in Asia (1,2). The uneven quality of care provided in the private sector has been widely documented (3,4). Increasing evidence from Africa also shows a rapidly growing private sector and its use by the people (1). Patient perceptions and preferences, convenience, stigma, gender are some of the factors that play a major role in determining the patient's decision to first visit a private provider (5). Inconvenient clinic timings, long waiting times, provider attitudes, direct and indirect costs and perceptions on quality of care at government health facilities are some of the reasons that drive people away from free or subsidised care at public sector health facilities (5,6).

The Need to Engage All Care Providers

The burden of TB managed outside the NTPs and roles of the diverse public and private care providers in the delivery of TB care vary greatly from country to country. Private health sector in high TB-burden countries is an unorganised and heterogeneous mix of commercial and non-commercial care providers. These may include informal and formal private practitioners, laboratories, pharmacies, non-governmental organisations [NGOs], private hospitals and academic institutions. Large and medium-sized businesses also offer health services to employees and their families. With a plethora of providers with no linkages among them, people tend to shop around for care. Government regulations on quality-assurance for laboratory services, notification of TB cases or rational prescribing and use of anti-TB drugs may exist but are rarely enforced. A study conducted based on anti-TB drug sale data revealed that enough TB drugs were sold in the private sector in India, Pakistan, the Philippines, and Indonesia to treat 65%-117% of those countries' TB burdens with a full course of regimen (7).

There are two major impediments to TB control globally and in most high TB-burden settings. First, almost every third case of TB goes undetected or unreported and secondly, among those who do get detected, there are significant delays in diagnosis leading to continued disease transmission with little impact on TB incidence in the community. On this background, there is increasing realisation that effective TB control is not possible without active engagement of all care providers in the delivery of TB care and prevention. This concern and the need to address engagement of all care providers are reflected in the Stop TB Strategy 2006-2015 and also in the End TB Strategy (8,9).

This chapter describes the evolution of public-private mix for TB care and control. The development of the concept and practice of public-private mix [PPM] is described. The current approaches and results of PPM scale up efforts underway globally and the place of PPM in the new End TB Strategy is discussed. Each country has a distinct approach in implementing and scaling up PPM and there is no "one size fits all" approach. An illustration of the progress and prospects of PPM for TB care and prevention in India, in the context of the End TB Strategy is also provided.

EVOLUTION AND EXPANSION OF PUBLIC-PRIVATE MIX FOR TB CARE

Public-Private Mix and Public-Private Partnership for TB Care

What is PPM and how it is different from public-private partnership [PPP]? PPM is nothing but PPP for delivery of TB care. The label PPM helps to differentiate partnership for care provision from all other types of partnerships that the TB community is engaged in, such as, resource mobilisation, research and new technology development, TB drugs procurement and distribution etc. PPM also conveys another meaning–a mix of mutually agreed roles for the public sector and diverse private providers to ensure TB care provision in line with national/international standards. In practising PPM, the NTP is expected always to retain the stewardship role assuming the overall responsibility of formulating policies and guidelines and managing collaborations with judicious use of incentives and disincentives.

The different types of private care providers–institutional as well as individual–play suitable roles in the mix depending upon their willingness and capacity. For example, a private non-profit or for-profit institution may take the responsibility of providing TB services in totality in a specified area and the NTP may play only supervisory role while a solo private practitioner may simply play the role of referring presumed TB cases to the NTP or managing them in his/her own clinic according to programme guidelines with or without support for free diagnosis, free drugs and supportive supervision from the NTP. Generally, collaborating with institutions, for-profit or non-profit, public or private, is much less cumbersome than working with a large number of unorganised, solo, qualified and non-qualified private practitioners. Much of the discourse on PPM is therefore centred around ways to successfully engage private practitioners in TB care and control in diverse country settings.

Global Efforts to Promote Public-Private Mix

Several PPM pilot projects were implemented successfully in many countries over the last decade and a half. These pilots were minor variations of a typical PPM model. In this model, the NTP plays the stewardship role and an intermediary agency such as a non-governmental organisation, a professional association or a franchising agency undertakes the task of mapping, enrolling, educating and engaging private practitioners and supporting them in delivering TB services. Dozens of projects linking various care providers like non-qualified village doctors, informal and formal private practitioners, private general practitioners,

---

Table 49.1: Key steps in implementing PPM and practical tools to help scale it up

Situation assessment
    Assess types of care providers and their current and potential roles
    Assess NTP capacity for PPM implementation
    Assess regulatory environment

Mobilisation of human and financial resources

Development of operational guidelines incorporating
    Objectives of implementing PPM
    Definition of task-mix for different provider types
    Description of service delivery model[s] considering incentives and enablers [based on national/International experiences] and use of digital technology
    Modules for capacity strengthening of programme staff and training and certification of private providers
    Mechanism for monitoring and periodic evaluation

Phased implementation

Generic tools presented in the PPM scale-up tool-kit
    Core Tools
        Tool to describe rationale and generic approach
        National situation assessment tool
        Operational guidelines development tool
        Tool for advocacy and communication
        International Standards for TB Care
        Monitoring and evaluation tool

Specific Tools
    Engaging solo private practitioners
    Engaging large hospitals
    Engaging non-governmental organisations
    Engaging workplaces
    Engaging social security organisations
    Engagement of TB/HIV collaborative activities
    Engagement for programmatic management of drug-resistant TB
    Engagement of pharmacies

PPM = public-private mix; TB = tuberculosis; NTP = National Tuberculosis Programme; HIV = human immunodeficiency virus
Source: references 13,14

---

specialist chest physicians, public and private hospitals, and NGOs to the NTPs have been documented (10,11). The World Health Organization [WHO]-based secretariat of the Public-Private Mix Subgroup on TB care provides a global platform for sharing of experiences of PPM implementation among countries (12). Based on available evidence, WHO and the PPM Subgroup have developed practical guidance and tools to help implement and scale up PPM. Table 49.1 lists generic implementation steps described in WHO's PPM guidance document and practical tools presented in the PPM scale up tool-kit (13,14). Evidence shows that PPM for TB care and control is a feasible, productive and a cost-effective approach to enhance TB case detection and improve treatment outcomes as well as to promote equity in access and save costs of care for the poor (15,16). The expansion of PPM over the last decade has seen two distinct development phases: the one before and the one after the application of information and communication technology in care delivery and introduction of regulatory approaches such as mandatory case notification and ensuring rational use of anti-TB drugs.

SCALING UP PUBLIC-PRIVATE MIX

Country Variations

Approaches to engage non-NTP care providers vary according to the country context. For example, in the Philippines, the national health insurance organisation has designed a special TB package for providers that collaborate with the NTP. India has diverse schemes for individual and institutional providers based on financial and non-financial incentives. China uses an internet-based system for mandatory reporting of TB cases by hospitals from where most TB patients seek care. It is also noticeable that countries have prioritised different types of care providers. These include general public hospitals [in China], private clinics and hospitals [in Nigeria and the Republic of Korea], medical colleges [in India] and health insurance organisations that also provide health services [in Egypt]. Social security organisations and prison health services are the main non-NTP providers in the Region of the Americas and in Eastern Europe, respectively (17).

Every year, countries collect and report to WHO the data on the contribution of PPM to TB case notifications. This includes contribution from the private sector through public-private mix approaches and that of the public sector providers outside the purview of NTPs through PPM initiatives. Table 49.2 gives an indication of the progress selected countries have made in scaling up PPM in 2015 (18a). In most of these countries, PPM initiatives contributed about 10%-40% of total notifications. Considering that the private medical sector in Africa is smaller than that in Asia, the contribution of private for-profit and not-for-profit providers in Ethiopia, Kenya, Nigeria and the United Republic of Tanzania is noteworthy. Progress in parts of Asia is also noticeable–almost every third or fourth case in India, Indonesia and Myanmar was notified by non-NTP care providers in 2013. Large public sector hospitals have contributed sizeable proportions of cases in China [over 50% of notified cases], Indonesia and the Philippines. In India, a large proportion of the cases notified by non-NTP providers were from medical colleges were 87% of notifications; from public non-NTP providers, 51% of notifications were from private providers, and 76% of total [public and private] notifications were from non-NTP providers. As per Global TB Report 2018 (18b), an increasing trend in the contribution of public non-NTP or private sector engagement to TB case notifications has been observed in countries,

Table 49.2: Contribution of PPM to TB case notifications in selected countries, 2015

Country	No. of TB cases notified by non-NTP public sector care providers in 2015*	Contribution of non-NTP public sector care providers to total case notifications in 2015 [%]*	No. of TB cases notified by private sector care providers in 2015†	Contribution of private sector care providers to total case notifications in 2015 [%]†
Bangladesh	ND	ND	60879	29
China	447148	56	ND	ND
Egypt	1375	17	ND	ND
Ethiopia	ND	ND	15195	ND
India	284636	16	184802	11
Indonesia	61183	18	30550	9.2
Iran	7196	69	3019	29
Iraq	2438	30	ND	ND
Kenya	ND	ND	15531	19
Malawi	ND	ND	3049	18
Myanmar	ND	ND	23513	17
Nigeria	6996	7.7	13088	14
Pakistan	ND	ND	72144	22
Philippines	79197	28	18442	6.4
Sri Lanka	4575	48	ND	ND
Swaziland	312	6.8	ND	ND
Thailand	3444	5.2	ND	ND
UR Tanzania	ND	ND	7773	13
Vietnam	6913	6.7	ND	ND

* Includes all contributions from non-NTP providers of care in the public sector, including public hospitals, public medical colleges, prisons/detention centres, military facilities, railways and public health insurance organisations
† Private sector providers include private individual and institutional providers, corporate/business sector providers, mission hospitals, NGOs and faith-based organisations
PPM = public-private mix; TB = tuberculosis; NTP = National Tuberculosis Programme; ND = not described; NGOs = non-governmental organisations
Source: reference 18

such as, Bangladesh, India, Indonesia, Kenya and Pakistan, that have prioritised PPM.

In most countries, only a small proportion of targeted care providers collaborate actively with NTPs and contribute to TB case notifications. Achieving early TB case detection to minimise disease transmission will require greater involvement of front-line care providers such as community-based traditional healers and informal practitioners, qualified general practitioners and pharmacists–who are often the first point of contact for people with symptoms of TB (17,18a).

Collaboration-Regulation Mix

Most of the country approaches to engage private care providers have been based on collaboration that involves sensitisation and training of care providers on the standards of care, support for patient care and offering financial or non-financial incentives. The result, though encouraging in terms of contribution to case notifications, has been that a large proportion of care providers do not feel obliged to contribute to national efforts to control TB. There is increasing realisation that collaborative approaches alone may not help in getting all care provider to follow the international standards of TB care or their national adaptations (19). Looking forwards, a combination of collaboration and regulation will likely elicit required actions from most private care providers. Along with introduction of information and communication technology [mHealth and eHealth] to enhance ease of collaboration, measures should also be put in place for certification and accreditation of collaborating providers, mandatory notification of TB cases by all relevant care providers, and rational use of anti-TB drugs effected through the engagement of pharmacies.

PPM IN THE 'END TB STRATEGY'

A Great Deal Remains to be Done

The End TB Strategy is presented in the chapter *"WHO's new end TB strategy" [Chapter 52]*. The PPM approach cuts across all the pillars and components of the End TB Strategy (9). A great deal remains to be done to make PPM integral to TB care and prevention in order to achieve the ambitious targets of the new Strategy. A large proportion of care providers in most high TB-burden countries still remain unengaged. Early diagnosis of TB requires understanding of patient pathways and engaging relevant informal and formal providers that people with symptoms of TB first approach. Even in countries where anti-TB drugs are not available in private pharmacies, reducing diagnostic delays requires education of and engagement with all care providers.

The PPM approach should also be employed for expansion of both–collaborative TB/human immunodeficiency virus [HIV] activities and programmatic management of multi-drug-resistant TB [MDR-TB]. Mechanisms of certification and accreditation of private providers need to be devised to ensure adherence to International Standards for TB Care [or their national adaptations]. A regulatory framework that includes mandatory TB case notification, rational use of TB drugs and infection control in health facilities should be in place and effectively enforced. Rapid and rational uptake of new diagnostics and drugs for patients in private clinics will require explicit policies and guidance. Optimising current PPM models and developing new and better ones will require operational research. New models of scaling up PPM for TB care such as social franchising and social business models have been implemented successfully in recent years with appropriate use of information and communications technology tools; their suitable application and scale up should be encouraged (20). Finally, sustainable financing of PPM interventions and ensuring social support to TB patients managed by non-NTP care providers will requires consideration under universal health coverage and social protection (21).

The Strategy-mix to Scale up Public-Private Mix

Large scale implementation of PPM to engage all care providers in TB care and prevention generally requires application of a mix of country-specific strategies based on a thorough national situation assessment and the status of PPM implementation in the country. The strategy-mix shown in Table 49.3 should be considered in scaling up PPM implementation.

Useful information and resources are available to help implement the strategy-mix [Table 49.1]. The important ones include the national situation assessment tool and the tool on inventory studies to estimate the number of TB cases treated in the private sector. Documented country experiences on engaging hospitals, engaging the business sector, setting up a certification and accreditation system and implementing mandatory case notification are also available. The PPM scale

---

Table 49.3: The strategy-mix should be considered in scaling up PPM implementation

Ensuring that the resources available–human and financial–to scale up engagement of all care providers are commensurate with [i] the magnitude of the problem of engaging all care providers; [ii] the burden of TB managed outside the NTPs; and [iii] the strengthening of capacity needed within the public sector

Optimising and expanding engagement of large hospitals, academic institutions and NGOs

Sharing the burden of engaging numerous solo private practitioners with "intermediary organisations" such as professional societies and associations; social franchising and social enterprise institutions; and NGOs with capacity and skills to work with private practitioners

Mobilising and supporting the business sector to initiate and expand TB programmes

Implementing regulatory approaches, such as mandatory case notification, rational use of TB medicines, and certification and accreditation systems to identify and support collaborating providers

Engaging communities and civil society to create demand for quality TB care from all public and private care providers

PPM = public-private mix; TB = tuberculosis; NTP = National Tuberculosis Programme; NGOs = non-governmental organisations

up tool kit provides all available guidelines and tools in a summary form along with an abstract of relevant country examples.

A COUNTRY EXAMPLE OF PUBLIC-PRIVATE MIX SCALE UP

Approaches to implementing and scaling up PPM vary according to the country contexts. With almost a quarter of global TB burden, the largest private sector and a plethora of different types of formal, informal, individual and institutional care providers, India presents a typical context to understand evolution and expansion of PPM in a country. The following paragraphs describe the progress and prospects of PPM implementation in India.

The private medical sector in India accounts for nearly 85% of the first contact of patients from all socioeconomic groups, and at least half of those treated for TB in India (22). Studies conducted since the 1990s have documented the extent to which TB is diagnosed and treated in the private sector, as well as largely inappropriate diagnostic and treatment practices.[4] The Revised National Tuberculosis Control Programme [RNTCP] has established itself as a strong and effective way to deliver TB care in the public sector providing a firm base upon which PPM efforts are being built. It is estimated that presently, private practitioners contribute just 2%-3% of case-finding and less than 1% of case management under the RNTCP. The many challenges hampering meaningful engagement of private providers include poor relationship between the private providers and the state which is often characterised by a deep mutual mistrust. Market forces are often powerful impediments to the adherence of private providers to government protocols. The state's regulatory enforcement mechanisms are too weak to control the private market, considering its size and fragmentation.

EVOLUTION

PPM had been well recognised as a requirement for effective TB control by the TB programme. As a consequence, numerous pilot projects were set up and documented. Using the experiences gained from the collaborations with NGOs and the private sector, the RNTCP published guidelines for the participation of the NGOs [2001] and private practitioners [2002] (23). These guidelines were revised in 2008 and again in 2014. In the context of engaging all care providers, involvement of public and private medical colleges in TB care and control has met with great success. By creating national, regional, state and medical college task forces, the RNTCP has managed to rope in medical colleges in expanding quality-assured TB care services. These medical colleges alone contribute about 20% of TB cases notified in the country (24). A first attempt of scaled up implementation of PPM was undertaken in 14 urban sites in India. WHO-PPM medical consultants and peripheral field supervisors were recruited and posted to these districts. An expanded version of the existing routine RNTCP

surveillance system collected disaggregated data from the different health-care providers. Providers were involved through a systematic process of situational analysis and listing of health-care facilities, sensitisation and training of practitioners on RNTCP, training of RNTCP staff on PPM-DOTS, identification of facilities for RNTCP service delivery, memoranda of understanding and RNTCP service delivery. The data from the intensified PPM sites have shown an overall increase in the number of TB cases notified under RNTCP (25).

There have been several other positive developments in the recent years. National consultations were held for better PPM engagements and a National Technical Working Group has been established. Serological testing for TB has been banned and TB has been made a notifiable disease, with a case based electronic notification [NIKSHAY] system developed for the notification of cases. Standards for TB Care in India [STCI] were developed for bringing together the right standards in diagnosis, treatment, public health and social inclusion for all (26). STCI has become the yardstick in measuring quality standards in TB care including in public and private sector. This has made the levelling of the playing field for private sector also and is helping better PPM engagement in a large way. Strategic opportunities are presented by several key developments, such as the emergence of new diagnostic technologies and advances in mobile phone penetration and applications.

CURRENT STATUS

India's national TB strategic plan aims to achieve a rapid decline in burden of TB mortality and morbidity towards ending TB in India by 2025 (27). To this effect, the RNTCP has taken steps to reach the unreached through synergising the efforts of all partners and stakeholders. This change is reflected through increased allocation of resources for partnerships, increase in manpower through sanction of dedicated positions to focus on partnership building at the state and district levels, greater flexibility to allow for innovation, capacity building through targeted training and an enabling environment to expand new approaches. The RNTCP is now engaging with private sector partners in most of the major cities of India with primary focus on notification through innovative partnership mechanisms (27-32). Some of the major PPM milestones in India include the following.

The Indian Medical Association: Revised National Tuberculosis Control Programme– Public-Private Mix Project

The Indian Medical Association [IMA]–RNTCP–PPM Project started in the year 2008 in five states and one union territory of India, covering 177 districts. Subsequently 10 more states were added. The objective of this project was to improve access to the diagnostic and treatment services of RNTCP and thereby, improve the quality of care for patients suffering from TB through the involvement of Indian Medical Association. The key activities undertaken as part of the project include state/district level workshops, publication of quarterly TB/RNTCP newsletter, publication in the Journal of Indian Medical Association, district level CME's of all the IMA branches in the target states, produce information, education and communication [IEC] materials, assist District TB Officers [DTOs] in training of private providers etc. (27).

Catholic Bishops Conference of India-Coalition for Acquired Immunodeficiency Syndrome and Related Diseases

The Catholic Bishops Conference of India-Coalition for Acquired Immunodeficiency Syndrome [AIDS] and Related Diseases [CBCI-CARD] project worked to improve access to TB diagnostic and treatment services within the Catholic Church Healthcare Facilities [CHFs]. Under this partnership, across 19 states of India, field consultants visit CHFs, conduct situational analysis, liaise with programme managers and other CHF personnel to participate in TB control and care (27).

Involvement of Pharmacists

As community pharmacies are often the first port of call for patients seeking healthcare, systematic and comprehensive engagement of pharmacists and chemists is crucial for early diagnosis and proper treatment of patients. The Central TB Division collaborated with the Indian Pharmaceutical Association [IPA], All India Organisation of Chemists and Druggists [AIOCD], Pharmacy Council of India [PCI] and South-east Asia Region [SEAR] Pharm Forum representing WHO–International Pharmaceutical Federation [FIP] Forum of National Associations in South East Asia for engaging pharmacists in TB control in India (27).

Universal Access to TB Care Project

A very important milestone for PPM in India is the Universal Access to TB Care project implemented in Mumbai in Maharashtra, Patna in Bihar and Mehesana district in Gujarat in which free anti-TB drugs for TB patients seeking care in private sector are provided to achieve universal access following Standards for TB Care in India. Once a qualified practitioner diagnose and decide to treat a TB patient outside the scope of RNTCP, s/he will notify the case using digital technology enabled mechanisms and prescription details relevant to anti-TB drugs are shared with contact centre. Based on it, a unique voucher number is generated and shared with practitioner and patient. The voucher number written on prescription is carried by patient to chemist. The voucher is validated by chemist with help of contact centre and free anti-TB drugs are given to patients. Patient is contacted telephonically for confirmation of receipt of free medicine and later at home, for extending public health services like contact screening, adherence and infection control counselling, HIV testing, drug-susceptibiliity testing services, etc. The project showed the importance of inter-mediary agencies for engagement of private practitioners

and laboratories for the required programme management activities and coordination. The project has engaged large number of private practitioners, hospitals and laboratories and have substantially increased the TB notification. There were many important factors for success of these projects such as; qualified private sector providers were allowed to manage TB patients [instead of referring them to the RNTCP], and TB patients received free services including easy digital e-vouchers for free anti-TB drugs, and laboratory tests, such as chest X-rays, sputum smears and Xpert® MTB/RIF. The field staff of intermediary agencies aggregated diverse private providers into a network, engaged, and made frequent visits to private providers, and ensured that patients were notified to the NTP and linked to care. Good adherence monitoring and support was offered to all TB patients to help them complete treatment, quality of care was monitored and targeted feedback was used to improve performance over time (30).

The National Strategic Plan 2017-2025 of RNTCP incorporated the learnings from the successful models for private sector engagement to overcome the barriers of mutual mistrust, conflicting market forces and fragmentation so that the quality of TB care is improved and encompassed within the programme (31). At the national and state levels, a technical support group [TSG], to support the programme for effective contract management and other partnership-strengthening functions Private Provider Interface Agencies [PPIAs] contracted in the states are required to manage the activities essential for engaging the private sector. An innovative strategy adapted in India that has further stimulated TB notification is the 'Nikshay Poshan Yojana' in which financial incentive to TB patients is given through direct beneficiary transfer mechanism (33). Other measures for future PPM expansion include rapid uptake of internationally approved diagnostic and treatment protocols by the RNTCP, use of mandatory TB case notification as an instrument to initiate and sustain collaboration, financial and other incentives to providers for TB notification, increased use of accreditation and contracting for further outreach to private laboratories, stronger regulations on anti TB drugs and innovative use of information and communication technologies.

The guiding principles for PPM TB are well illustrated in the following section in the National Strategic Plan for TB Elimination in India (27): "The learnings that guide the efforts to invoke support from the private sector and provide public services to its patients include the following: [i] the government will be an enabler and not see itself as the sole provider of TB care; [ii] "go where the patients go" and currently around half of the TB patients go to the private sector. This should be true of investments to address this fact as well; [iii] The cost of involving the private sector is not high. It is almost the same or marginally higher than the cost in the public sector; [iv] Investments in involving the private sector yields significant returns in case detection, with doubling or even tripling of the case notification rates; and [v] public health actions to support the private sector provides for better outcomes related to access, notifications, adherence, treatment outcomes and cost savings".

PROSPECTS

The main impediments to the successful execution of the PPM strategy include a lack of capacity within the programme in areas such as cost analysis and contract design, and protracted procurement processes. The persistent mistrust of the private sector, both in the context of the programme as well as in the broader political and administrative context, may lead to a lack of commitment to the new strategy in some states and districts. The success of the strategy is to some extent dependent on developments outside the TB programme, such as the strengthening of regulatory processes and the development of digital technology systems. Strong leadership will be of the utmost importance in tackling the possible pitfalls. A new spirit of genuine partnership will be needed, sufficient resources will have to be allocated and accountability will have to be established.

DISCLAIMER

The authors are staff members of the World Health Organization. The views expressed in this article do not necessarily represent the views or policies of the organization.

REFERENCES

1. Private sector for health. Private healthcare in developing countries. Available at URL: http://www.ps4h.org/global-healthdata.html. Accessed on December 15, 2016.
2. Mantala M. Systematic engagement of hospitals: Philippines experience 2012. Available at URL: http://www.who.int/tb/careproviders/ppm/Hospitals_Philippines_PPM_Nov12ver2.pdf. Accessed on August 15, 2018.
3. Udwadia ZF, Pinto LM, Uplekar MW. Tuberculosis management by private practitioners in Mumbai, India: has anything changed in two decades? PLoS ONE 2010;5:e12023.
4. Satyanarayana S, Subbaraman R, Shete P, Gore G, Das J, Cattamanchi A, et al. Quality of tuberculosis care in India: a systematic review. Int J Tuberc Lung Dis 2015;19:751-63.
5. Kapoor SK, Raman AV, Sachdeva KS, Satyanarayana S. How did the TB patients reach DOTS services in Delhi? A study of patient treatment seeking behavior. PLoS One 2012;7:e42458.
6. Khan MS, Salve S, Porter JD. Engaging for-profit providers in TB control: lessons learnt from initiatives in South Asia. Health Policy Plan 2015;30:1289-95.
7. Wells WA, Ge CF, Patel N Oh T, Gardiner E, Kimerling ME. Size and usage patterns of private TB drug markets in the high burden countries. PLoS One 2011;6: e18964.
8. Raviglione M, Uplekar M. WHO's new Stop TB Strategy. Lancet 2006;367:952-5.
9. Uplekar M, Weil D, Lonnroth K, Jaramillo E, Lienhardt C, Dias HM, et al. WHO's new End TB Strategy. Lancet 2015;385: 1799-1801.
10. Lönnroth K, Uplekar M, Arora VK, Juvekar S, Lan NT, Mwaniki D, et al. Public-private mix for DOTS implementation: what makes it work? Bull World Health Organ 2004;82:580-6.
11. Dewan PK, Lal SS, Lonnroth K, Wares F, Uplekar M, Sahu S, et al. Improving tuberculosis control through review public-private collaboration in India: literature review. BMJ 2006;332; 574-8.
12. Lei X, Liu Q, Escobar E, Philogene J, Zhu H, Wang Y, et al. Public-private mix for tuberculosis care and control: a systematic review. Int J Infect Dis 2015;34:20-32.
13. Subgroup on public-private mix for TB care and control. Available at URL: http://www.who.int/tb/careproviders/ppm/en/. August 14, 2018.
14. World Health Organization. Engaging all care providers in TB control: guidance on implementing public-private mix approaches. WHO/HTM/TB/2006.360. Geneva: World Health Organization; 2006.
15. World Health Organization. Stop TB partnership public-private mix for TB care and control: a toolkit 2010. http://www.who.int/tb/careproviders/ppm/PPMToolkit.pdf. Accessed on August 14, 2018.
16. Floyd K, Arora VK, Murthy KJ, Lönnroth K, Singla N, Akbar Y, et al. Cost and cost-effectiveness of PPM-DOTS for tuberculosis control: evidence from India. Bull World Health Organ 2006;84:437-45.
17. Lönnroth K, Aung T, Maung W, Kluge H, Uplekar M. Social franchising of TB care through private GPs in Myanmar: an assessment of treatment results, access, equity and financial protection. Health Policy Plan 2007;22:156-66.
18a. World Health Organization. Global tuberculosis report 2016. WHO/HTM/TB/2016.13. Geneva: World Health Organization; 2016.
18b. World Health Organization. Global tuberculosis report 2018. WHO/CDS/TB/2018.20. Geneva: World Health Organization; 2018.
19. World Health Organization. Global tuberculosis report 2014. WHO/HTM/TB/2014.08. Geneva: World Health Organization; 2014.
20. Uplekar M. Scaling up public-private mix: collaborate or regulate? Int J Tuberc Lung Dis 2013;17:1122.
21. Khan AJ, Khowaja S, Khan FS, Qazi F, Lotia I, Habib A, et al. Engaging the private sector to increase tuberculosis case detection: an impact evaluation study. Lancet Infect Dis 2012;12: 608-16.
22. USAID TB CARE II Project. Synthesis report: inclusion of TB in national insurance programs. Available at URL: http://tbcare2.org/sites/tbcare2.org/files/Synthesis%20Report%20on%20Country%20%20Assessments%20on%20TB%20Insurance%20Study%20TB%20CARE%20II%20Final.pdf. Accessed on August 14, 2018.
23. Sreeramareddy CT, Qin ZZ, Satyanarayana S, Subbaraman R, Pai M. Delays in diagnosis and treatment of pulmonary tuberculosis in India: a systematic review. Int J Tuberc Lung Dis 2014;18:255-66.
24. Sharma SK, Mohan A, Chauhan LS, Narain JP, Kumar P, Behera D, et al. Contribution of medical colleges to tuberculosis control in India under the Revised National Tuberculosis Control Programme [RNTCP]: lessons learnt & challenges ahead. Indian J Med Res 2013;137:283-94.
25. Quazi TA, Sarkar S, Borgohain G, Sreenivas A, Harries AD, Srinath S, et al. Are all patients diagnosed with tuberculosis in Indian medical colleges referred to the RNTCP? Int J Tuberc Lung Dis 2012;16:1083-5.
26. Lal SS, Sahu S, Wares F, Lönnroth K, Chauhan LS, Uplekar M. Intensified scale-up of public-private mix: a systems approach

to tuberculosis care and control in India. Int J Tuberc Lung Dis 2011;15:97-104.

27. National Strategic Plan for Tuberculosis Elimination. Central TB Division, Ministry of Health and Family Welfare, Government of India. Available at URL: https://tbcindia.gov.in/index1.php?lang=1&level=1&sublinkid=4768&lid=3266. Accessed on July 24, 2018.

28. Sachdeva KS, Kumar A, Dewan P, Satyanarayana S. New vision for Revised National Tuberculosis Control Programme [RNTCP]: universal access - "reaching the un-reached". Indian J Med Res 2012;135: 690-4.

29. Kulshrestha N, Nair SA, Rade K, Moitra A, Diwan P, Khaparde SD. Public-private mix for TB care in India: concept, evolution, progress. Indian J Tuberc 2015;62:235-8.

30. Universal access to TB care- concurrent assessment report May 2016. Available at URLL: https://tbcindia.gov.in/index1.php?lang=1&level=3&sublinkid=4711&lid=32. Accessed on July 31, 2018.

31. Uplekar M. Public-private mix for tuberculosis care and prevention. What progress? What prospects? Int J Tuberc Lung Dis 2016;20: 1424-9.

32. McDowell A, Pai M. Treatment as diagnosis and diagnosis as treatment: empirical management of presumptive tuberculosis in India. Int J Tuberc Lung Dis 2016;20:536-4.

33. Nutritional support to TB patients. Central TB Division, Ministry of Health and Family Welfare, Government of India. Available at URL: https://tbcindia.gov.in/showfile.php?lid=3318. Accessed on July 24, 2018.

50

Building Partnerships for Tuberculosis Control

Vineet Bhatia, Md Khurshid Alam Hyder

INTRODUCTION

We are in an interesting and yet challenging era of tuberculosis [TB] care and control where the goal of ending TB by 2030 has been endorsed by World Health Assembly in 2014 and yet the efforts have to gain requisite momentum. Global success of TB control efforts can be measured by the fact that the Millennium Development Goal [MDG] target to halt and reverse the TB epidemic by 2015 were achieved (1). Mortality and incidence rates are falling in all of World Health Organization [WHO] six regions and in most of the 22 high-burden countries [HBCs] that account for over 80% of the world's TB cases. However, the global burden of TB remains enormous and progress towards ending TB remains slow.

Global efforts to treat TB patients with internationally recommended, standard treatment have had a reasonable success since the year 1993, when recognising the need for enhanced response for TB control, the WHO took an unprecedented step of declaring TB a global emergency (2). To strengthen the fight against TB, WHO began to promote DOTS strategy during the same period (3). The package combined key elements from early work carried out at the Tuberculosis Research Centre [TRC] – formerly known as the Tuberculosis Chemotherapy Centre, and now renamed as National Institute of Research in Tuberculosis [NIRT], Chennai (4) and the National Tuberculosis Institute [NTI] Bengaluru (5) in India. The elements of the approach were outlined in the "Framework for effective tuberculosis control" launched by WHO in 1994 (6,7). In its report in 1993, the World Bank hailed short-course chemotherapy [SCC] with closely monitored walk-in treatment as one of the most cost-effective of health interventions (8). In 2005, a comprehensive Stop TB Strategy (9) was launched incorporating key elements that provided a long term vision for the national TB control programmes [NTPs]. In May 2014, the World Health Assembly [WHA] in its resolution WHA67.1 adopted the global strategy and targets for TB prevention, care and control after 2015 based on a bold vision of a world without TB and targets of ending the global TB epidemic, elimination of associated catastrophic costs for TB-affected households. This lays the foundation of End TB strategy (10) [Table 52.1].

OVERVIEW OF TUBERCULOSIS SITUATION AND PROGRESS IN TUBERCULOSIS CONTROL IN THE SOUTH-EAST ASIA REGION

The WHO South-East Asia Region [SEAR] consists of 11 member countries, namely, Bangladesh, Bhutan, Democratic Peoples' Republic of Korea, India, Indonesia, Maldives, Myanmar, Nepal, Sri Lanka, Thailand and Timor Leste. Six out of these 11 countries—Bangladesh, Democratic People's Republic of Korea, India, Indonesia, Myanmar and Thailand, are among the 22 global high TB burden countries. TB remains one of the major public health concerns in the SEAR of WHO (1,11).

In terms of progress in TB control, all 11 member states have sustained country-wide access to quality treatment with DOTS as one of the pillars. In 2016, more than 2.9 million TB were registered for treatment and the treatment success rate among new and relapse TB cases registered in the previous year was 78%. The TB mortality rate has decreased by 50% since 1990 and SEAR has already achieved the global target of a 50% reduction by 2015. The decline in the prevalence is observed in all member countries and in some countries it is over 50% [Figure 50.1] (12).

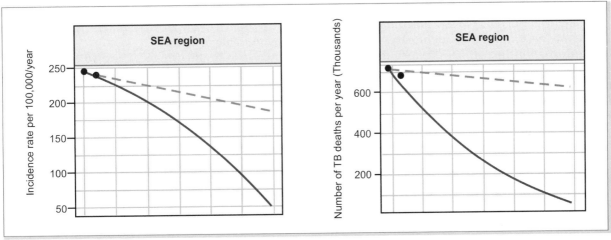

Figure 50.1: Projected regional trajectory of TB incidence and TB death 2015-2035 in South-East Asia. Dotted line representing the current trend, continuous line representing needed decline to reach targets

Table 50.1: Estimated HIV prevalence among adult populations and the number of people living with HIV infection in SEAR countries, 2013

Country	Estimated number of people newly infected with HIV	Estimated adult [15-49 years] HIV prevalence [%]	Estimated number of people living with HIV
Bangladesh	1300	<0.1	9 500
Bhutan	<200	0.1	<1000
DPR Korea	*	*	*
India	130,000	0.3	2,100,000
Indonesia	80,000	0.5	640,000
Maldives	NA	<0.1	<100
Myanmar	6700	0.6	190000
Nepal	1300	0.2	39000
Sri Lanka	<500	<0.1	2900
Thailand	8,200	1.1	440,000
Timor-Leste	NA	NA	NA
Total	230,000	0.3	3.4 million

* No reported HIV positive individual till date
HIV = human immunodeficiency virus; DPR Korea = Democratic People's Republic of Korea; NA = not available
Source: reference 14

Multidrug-resistant and Rifampicin-resistant Tuberculosis

Multidrug-resistant TB [MDR-TB] is defined as TB caused by *Mycobaterium tuberculosis* [*Mtb*] that shows *in vitro* resistance to at least isoniazid and rifampicin, the two most important first line anti-TB drugs. MDR-TB is said to be a man-made phenomenon since it is caused by inadequate, irregular or incomplete treatment with poor quality of drugs and poor adherence to treatment by the patients.

Levels of MDR-TB in WHO SEAR in terms of proportions are still low, at 2.8% among notified new TB cases [uncertainty range 2.4%-3.1%] and 13% among retreatment TB cases [uncertainty range 10%-15%]. However, given the large numbers of TB cases in the SEAR, this translates to totally 117,000 estimated RR/MDR-TB cases [uncertainty range 105,000-130,000] among notified pulmonary TB cases accounting for nearly one-third of the global burden of such cases in 2016 (1,11,12). Extensively drug-resistant TB [XDR-TB] is a subclass of MDR-TB where there is resistance to at least isoniazid, rifampicin, any fluoroquinolone, and at least one of the three injectable drugs [amikacin, kanamycin, or capreomycin]. XDR-TB has been isolated in samples from six countries in the region, namely, Bangladesh, India, Indonesia, Myanmar, Nepal and Thailand (1,11,12).

Impact of Human Immunodeficiency Virus on Tuberculosis in the Region

It is estimated that there are 3.4 million people living with human immunodeficiency virus [HIV] infection/acquired immunodeficiency syndrome [AIDS] {people living with

HIV/AIDS [PLHA]} in the WHO SEAR, accounting for nearly 10% of global PLHA. In SEAR, an estimated 210,000 cases [5.2%] of the 4 million incident cases were HIV-seropositive and an estimated 62,000 cases died of HIV-associated TB in 2014. Five countries in the region [India, Indonesia, Myanmar, Nepal and Thailand] accounted for 99% of HIV cases in the region (1,11,12). The magnitude of HIV infection differs greatly between countries of the region, and even within countries, there are marked differences [Table 50.1] (11,13).

Resources for Tuberculosis Control

In the whole Region, domestic sources continue to account for just over 62% of the funding for NTPs. Ten member countries currently benefit from funds mobilised through the Global Fund to fight AIDS, TB and Malaria [GFATM]. In addition, nine member states benefit from funds from other development partners and donor governments, the exception being Maldives, where the only external funds are WHO country budgets. Maldives is in the process of obtaining GFATM support.

There, however, remains a significant funding gap for the overall budget of TB control programmes (14). Considering the threshold of 2.28 health professionals per 1,000 population, only five of the 11 member states have sufficient human resources for health. High turnover of the staff, lack of adequate training and insufficient management of human resources is a common challenge for most of the countries in the region.

Key Challenges to Tuberculosis Control in the South-East Asia Region

Countries in the SEAR have varied socio-economic and demographic profiles, leading to diverse challenges faced by TB programmes in the respective countries. These include uncertainties regarding sustainable financial and operational resources; limited technical and management capacity; weak national laboratory networks, procurement and supply management mechanisms which in turn are slowing the planned expansion of interventions for TB-HIV and MDR-TB; case detection mainly focussed on passive case finding and lack of emphasis on management of latent TB infection.

The current laboratory capacity in the region remains inadequate to reach global and regional targets for the diagnosis of drug-resistant TB [DR-TB] and HIV-associated TB. Even in countries with a large number of laboratories, country-specific conditions such as geographically challenging situations mean that diagnostic services are currently not available to all in need.

TB prevention, care and control are heavily dependent on strong primary health care systems. Many of the constraints to effective implementation of TB prevention, care and control services in the Member States are related to underlying weak and underfinanced national health systems in general, many of which are already overstretched in terms of both infrastructure and staffing. Weak health systems are further challenged by the increasing burden of HIV/AIDS, DR-TB, as well as the growing burden and challenge of non-communicable diseases.

Access to health care including TB care in the Region is significantly funded by out-of-pocket expenditure by the patients themselves. This is direct spending by households on health services, without reimbursement of any kind and is considered the most regressive option for funding health systems – funding through general taxes, and social insurance being the most equitable forms of health financing. Of all health expenditures in countries of the SEAR, 66% are out-of-pocket, of which a substantial proportion is spent on the purchase of drugs. And, estimates suggest that as much as 30% of new poverty in some countries in the Region is caused by the catastrophic cost of accessing health care.

Low levels of community awareness also hamper the uptake of services, and there is increasing recognition that attention needs to be paid to the social, economic and behavioural determinants that impact TB, if national efforts to combat the disease are to succeed in the longer term. There is still a limited involvement of private care providers. A global study to this effect was instituted by the Global Alliance for TB drugs, which explored the private sector landscape of 10 high TB burden countries [HBCs] [that collectively account for 60% of the global TB burden] and found that the private sector treatment landscape in these countries was largely unregulated and fragmented (15). For example, the study detected 111 different first-line TB drug dosages and combinations, compared to the 14 deemed necessary by the Stop TB Partnership's Global TB Drug Facility [GDF]. Drug misuse by the private sector is likely to be responsible for many treatment failures and for escalating the emergence of MDR-TB, which is further worsening the wider TB epidemic. The impacts of these challenges are listed below.

Inadequate Access and Delayed Diagnosis of Persons with Tuberculosis, Including Children

With current notification rates, almost a third of the estimated pool of TB cases in the Region are either not detected or not notified. Factors contributing to suboptimal case detection include poor knowledge and awareness of the population; geographical, social and financial barriers; suboptimal identification by health services of persons suspected of having TB; suboptimal diagnostic procedures, referral and notification practices [public and private] including little attention paid to children; and limited screening of high-risk groups e.g. contacts, clinical risk groups and risk populations. Paediatric TB remains a neglected area as demonstrated by the very low notification rate in the age group below 15 years.

Slow Progress in Scaling up Programmatic Management of Drug-resistant Tuberculosis

In May 2009, the WHA resolution 62.15 urged the Member States "to achieve universal access to diagnosis and treatment of MDR-TB and XDR-TB" (16). However, the coverage for

MDR-TB access is far from universal access as of now with just about 20% of the estimated incidence being notified.

Slow Progress in Scaling up Tuberculosis-Human Immunodeficiency Virus Collaborative Activities

In SEAR region, 45% of all TB cases notified in SEAR knew their HIV status; of the TB patients known to be living with HIV, 85% were on anti-retroviral therapy [ART] in the region. The SEAR maintained 85% co-trimoxazole preventive therapy [CPT] enrollment of all notified HIV-seropositive TB patients since 2003 (1,11).

Addressing the Challenges through the World Health Organization South-East Asia Region Strategic Plan

The WHO SEAR Strategic Plan for TB Control was initially developed in 2006 (17) and described the future direction and focus of work for TB control in the region. The targets and strategies in the document are consistent with the global targets and strategies, but focussed on the priorities most relevant to the Region and built on past experience and successes (14).

The year 2015 has been a watershed moment in the battle against TB. It marks the deadline for global TB targets set in the context of the MDGs, and is a year of transitions: from the MDGs to a new era of Sustainable Development Goals [SDGs], and from the Stop TB Strategy to the End TB Strategy. In this transition, paradigm shifts are expected in all sectors, including health. To end the epidemic [defined as an incidence of fewer than 100 cases per million people] by 2035 will require a rapid upgrade of care and managerial standards.

Ending the TB epidemic will require an expansion of the scope and reach of interventions for TB prevention, care and control: the institution of systems and policies to promote an enabling environment, shared responsibilities with universal coverage; and aggressive pursuit of research and innovation to promote development and use of new tools for TB care and prevention.

This *Regional Strategic Plan towards Ending TB in the SEAR 2016-2020* (14) describes the future directions and focus of the work towards TB elimination aiming to support Member States in the reduction in TB mortality and incidence in line with the global targets as set in WHA resolution 67.1, guiding the countries in addressing the persisting and emerging epidemiological and demographic challenges and advancing universal health coverage and robust health systems. The plan (14) builds on and expands the existing updated Regional Strategic plan for TB Care and Control 2012-2015 (17) and focuses on the implementation of the End TB Strategy in the coming five years within the overall scope of the 20-year strategy covering the period from 2015 to 2035.

It is often beyond the capacity of NTPs alone to address these and other systemic issues. All Programmes need to work in close collaboration with other sectors within the government as well as those involved in health care outside the government. Therefore, there is a need for partnership if the problem of TB has to be adequately dealt with.

What is a Partnership?

A partnership may be defined as agreement between individuals and organisations to work towards a common goal with shared vision and responsibilities. There is generally a consensus on issues being dealt with, and motivation levels are high. In the case of TB care and control, a partnership will have a shared vision of TB elimination, and partners undertake joint activities to promote synergy of efforts.

National TB control programmes need to continue to engage a wide range of stakeholders both within the health sector and other sectors, to ensure that the distribution and coverage of quality services is equitable across all geographic locations and reach various socioeconomic groups, especially the marginalised and hard to access populations. Engaging with multiple partners requires close attention to their activities, and providing support and guidance to ensure that all activities serve their intended purpose. Partners need to be provided with relevant information, reports on achievements, a forum for regular interaction, and opportunities to share experiences and develop consensus on joint activities towards a common goal.

Relevance of Partnerships for Tuberculosis Care and Control

Partnerships are an instrument to tap diverse resources—technical, financial, human and physical infrastructure—to fill gaps in programme implementation. In resource-constrained settings, partnerships are a mechanism to induce synergies and avoid duplication. Partnerships can be viewed as a means of maximising benefits. The incentives for working in a partnership are not limited to monetary benefits; they include specific skills derived from the learning experience, greater collective capacity to respond to the problem, and increased quality of solutions.

Through partnerships, a platform is available for shared responsibility and decision making for TB care and control, where all partners feel the needs to directly or indirectly support the cause. A dialogue between the programme and other stakeholders, including the most marginalised, will lead to a common understanding and consensus for addressing challenges. This will help create an inclusive strategy and action plan for the perceived programme needs and civil society needs. This would help all partners to have a shared vision and confidence in how their individual efforts are contributing to the larger goals of the programme. Partnerships allow programmes to get diverse views and perspectives on challenges faced by the programme, creating a holistic picture. By listening to various community voices and stakeholders, the programme can gain an idea of their needs and expectations. Gaps in service delivery will also be highlighted. On the other hand, the community and stakeholders will also get a better picture of programme views on service delivery, existing constraints and efforts to improve service delivery.

Through partnerships, programmes can share information on their achievements. Partners can share their experience on a common platform. This promotes transparency and builds trust amongst stakeholders. Thus, partnerships act as an interface between programme, stakeholders and community. The partnership can carry the voice and opinion of multiple stakeholders and community members to the programme managers, and vice versa.

KEYS STEPS TO BUILDING PARTNERSHIPS

The key steps to building partnerships are listed in Table 50.2 (18).

Analysing the Potential of Various Partners

To establish a structure and align all partners for an effective response, it is important that a transparent assessment be carried out against the background of implementation of the Stop TB strategy in respective countries. Exploring options for working together and building relationships requires that this be done in a spirit of mutual respect, commitment to a common task, and sensitivity to the needs of various partners. At times, mutual trust and credibility need to be developed before partners can be expected to work together. To develop a common outlook it is useful for stakeholders to explore their expectations of tackling the ambitious task together.

Analysis of stakeholders is crucial. It will help in identifying potential partners and assessing their relevance. Questions are asked about the position, interest, influence, interrelations, networks, and other characteristics, with reference to their past and present positions as well as

to their future potential. As government determines the overall policies and outlines the framework of cooperation, government representatives are the initiators of the partnership and accept ownership and responsibility of the process.

Based on the common goals, and guided by the priorities and gaps in the Stop TB strategy implementation plan, the TB programme is responsible for assessing and grading these partners according to their value in tackling priority issues. Some examples are given in the Table 50.3.

Partner Involvement in Helping Tuberculosis Care and Control

Improving the Quality

While the national programmes strive to improve outreach, the limited availability of resources may compromise quality of services in resource constrained settings. Partners can ensure quality by pooling of resources specifically by improving access and by independent evaluation and feedback to the programme. Partners can also act as voice of community. Quality can be improved right at the stage of planning by involving communities who can help envisage implementation and access challenges for those who need it the most.

Improving Case Notification

Partners working in health and other development sectors can quickly identify chest symptomatics in community, given their proximity and close relations. Similarly industries have captive population that can be easily approached through peer support groups and through the in-house medical facilities and when available. Early recognition of symptoms will also ensure early diagnosis and hence cure.

Table 50.2: The key steps to building partnerships

Undertake a situation analysis of the programme. Identify gaps or requirements that need to be filled and list all potential partners who can contribute in these areas to fulfil the programme's goals

Identify the strengths of potential partners. Various resources available through partnerships include:
    Technical resources through technical agencies, academic institutions, professional bodies located within countries
    Public and private human resources, including NGOs and other civil society organisations, health care providers, community volunteers
    Financial resources, which can be harnessed through development partners, corporations and business houses
    Public and private physical infrastructure, including for-profit and not-for-profit organisations, health facilities, community-based groups

Shortlist the potential partners and define their roles in the programme. Share the programme goals and vision with them

Discuss the programme with them and explain why they should partner with the efforts of the programme. Address any concerns they may have in joining the programme

Obtain consensus on a common plan: targets, objectives, areas of responsibility, use of operational guidelines, procedures and timeframes. If required, help build the capacity of the partner

Implement agreed activities according to the plan

Sustain communication. Network and share information regularly with all partners on progress being made, any problems that need to be resolved and how they may maximise their contribution

Periodically and systematically monitor and evaluate progress

Document lessons learned and experiences. Share these with the partners. Appreciate and praise successes and work towards accepting failures jointly

Broaden the partnership and scope of work as the programme grows

NGOs = non-novernmental organisations

Table 50.3: Responsibility of partners in tackling priority issues

Types of organisation	Prime interest	Value for TB care and control
Human rights groups	Human rights	Awareness and legal expertise
Patient associations	Patients' rights	Advocacy and service monitoring
TB and lung associations	TB awareness	Advocacy and network
Business/corporate sectors	Benefits and profits	Service delivery
Professional associations	Education and standards	Management and training
Private practitioners, hospitals, prisons, military	Health care and medical services	Capacity building and service delivery
Ministry of Finance	Public finances	Financial resources and expertise
International and national technical agencies	Technical support	Update policies and operations research
Medical Colleges	Academic and tertiary level care	Service delivery, operations research, policy feedback and tertiary care for complicated cases and co-morbidities

TB = tuberculosis

Supporting Treatment Adherence

Treatment of TB is long-up to 9 months for susceptible TB and 20 months or more for MDR-TB. Completion of treatment is important for cure. However a long treatment may be associated with several challenges–psychological and emotional trauma, loss of job and wages, and discrimination of various kinds. Partners can provide counselling services, psychological support and rehabilitation services that may generally be outside the purview of a government run TB control programme.

Improving Communication and Community Awareness Regarding the Disease, Symptoms, Transmission and Curability

The fact that TB can be cured through a regular and compete course of treatment needs to be reinforced to reduce any associated stigma.

Illustrative List of Country Stakeholders, Possible Implementation Roles of Different Partners

The illustrative list of country stakeholders are listed in Table 50.4 (19). Possible implementation roles of different partners are shown in Table 50.5 (20).

Successful Partnerships: What Works Well

Mutual Respect and Recognition

All partners come with different strengths and varied experience. It is essential that in partnership this diversity is recognised and respected so that everyone feels included. Shared decision making leads to greater understanding and commitment. Commitment has many dimensions and is related to the extent to which participating organisations have endorsed or adopted the common mission or carried out activities in the name of partnership. The key to success is to identify bona fide partners who could also be respected leaders in the effort. Partnerships are more likely to be durable when the commitment of individual members is strong.

Information Sharing with the Partners

Communication is a binding force for the partnership. It is essential that partnership activities are regularly shared with all partners. To accomplish this task there is need to have a focal point responsible for regular communication to which all partners have a good relationship. There is also a need to share information with all partners and the programme, through newsletters, e-mails and meetings.

Frequent Discussions/Meetings with Partners and other Stakeholders

All important decisions should be consensus-based, and it is important to involve all stakeholders in discussions prior to arriving at decisions.

Clarity of Roles and Responsibilities

Partners have their own core strengths, and responsibilities within partnership can be defined accordingly. It is also important to have defined governance structures that help manage the partnership efficiently.

Forward Thinking

The partnership structure should not only be able to manage the present but also plan for the future.

Global and Regional Partnerships in Tuberculosis Care and Control

Global Partnership

In 1998, the WHO convened an "ad-hoc committee on the TB epidemic" to analyse the reasons for the slow progress and provide recommendations to the global community to support acceleration of progress (21,22). Among the recommendations made by the ad-hoc committee were

Table 50.4: Illustrative list of country stakeholders

Ministry of Health
  National TB Programme, National Public Health Laboratory, National AIDS Control Council, Joint HIV-TB Committee, National Immunisation Programme, Department of Planning, Directorate of Primary Health Care, Health Education Department, Provincial and District Health Officers, Training Department, Medicines Regulatory Authority, Pharmacy and Essential Medicines Department

Ministry of Justice
  TB control in penitentiary system/prisons

Ministry of Finance
  Directorate of health budgets
  Planning Commission

Ministry of Education
  Academic, research and training institutions
  Medical colleges, research institutes, training institutes

World Health Organization, United Nations and International technical agencies
  Interministerial groups led by WHO or the UN, such as, the HLWG on TB in the Russian Federation
  FHI 360, MSH, MSF, KNCV, PATH, The Union—specifically when agencies have a local presence

Funding agencies
  Global Fund
  World Bank
  USAID, PEPFAR, DFID, BGMF

Professional organisations
  Medical and paediatrics associations, nurses' association, pharmacists' associations, national TB/lung associations, laboratory technologists' associations

State-owned enterprises
  Manufacturers of TB-control products

Private sector health and non-health companies
  Manufacturers of TB-control products [diagnostics, medicines, vaccines], importers and wholesalers, hospitals and clinics, clinical diagnostic laboratories, faith-based organisations and NGOs, pharmacies and drug shops, traditional healers
  Local enterprises committed to corporate social responsibility

Decision-makers and opinion leaders
  National health policy-makers, academic and religious leaders, national "envoys" for TB [e.g., famous sportsmen, actors, etc.]

Community and patient advocacy groups
  Community-based organisations, patients' organisations, advocacy and community-based organisations
  Civil society organisations

Communications media
  Print media and journalists, television and radio stations

TB = tuberculosis; AIDS = acquired immunodeficiency syndrome; HIV = human immunodeficiency virus; WHO = World Health Organization; UN = United Nations; HLWG = High Level Working Group; FSI = Family Health International; MSH = Management Sciences for Health; MSF = Medicines Sans Frontieres; KNCV = Royal Netherlands Tuberculosis Association; PATH [from 1980 until 2014, PATH stood for Program for Appropriate Technology in Health. Presently it is simply referred to as PATH]; USAID = United States Agency for International Development; PEPFAR = United States President's Emergency Plan for AIDS Relief ; DFID = United Kingdom Department for International Development; BGMF = Bill and Melinda Gates Foundation; NGOs = non-governmental organisations

the creation of a global charter among all key partners and countries with the highest burdens of disease [22 countries account for 80% of global TB burden], involvement of the private sector and communities in national TB control efforts and the creation of a global drug facility.

In the same year, Dr Gro Harlem Brundtland, the then Director-General of WHO, launched the Stop TB Initiative founded on the principle of a global partnership to address the lacunae pointed out by the ad-hoc committee and to accelerate action against TB control.

As a result of the efforts of the newly launched Stop TB Initiative (23), several events with far reaching implications on global TB control followed in rapid succession. A ministerial conference on TB and sustainable health involving several global partners and ministers of health, finance and planning from HBCs was held in Amsterdam in March 2000 leading to the landmark "Amsterdam Declaration" to stop TB. In May 2000, the WHA endorsed the formation of a global partnership for TB control and, at the same time, considering that most countries had not reached the targets set in 1991, postponed these targets to 2005 (24). In 2001 a structure for a global Stop TB partnership was developed and this was endorsed at first meeting of the Stop TB Partners forum in Washington in October 2001 (25). At the first forum of the partnership, 80 partners and HBCs endorsed the Washington Commitment to Stop TB, committing themselves to the 2005 targets and to specific actions as outlined in the global plan to stop TB (26). From early 2015, the Stop TB Partnership has moved to United Nations Office for Project Services [UNOPS] with same functions as before.

Table 50.5: Possible implementation roles of different partners

Public sector departments
Education: training teachers and educating children about TB; including TB in school health campaigns; including TB awareness education in non-formal education and adult literacy programmes
Social welfare: possibly offering food subsidies and social assistance to families of TB patients
Labour: promoting treatment and prevention at the workplace; ensuring that work environments are not places in which TB is easily transmitted
Defence and police: promoting treatment and prevention within these forces; coordination and collaboration between their health facilities, where available, and those of the NTPs
Women's welfare: raising awareness through organised women's groups and ensuring supportive environments for women to seek and complete treatment more readily
Youth and sports: promoting TB awareness among young people
Media/communications: raising public awareness and helping shape public attitudes and opinions about people with TB, making the communities aware of how they may participate in control, and informing people about public policies and facilities that are in place to treat TB

NGOs
Providing community-based care
Training health care workers and volunteers to provide DOTS
Generating awareness and educating the community on prevention and treatment
Involving the community in implementing DOTS
Conducting operational research
Playing a major role in advocacy and in mobilizing community support

Private sector
Notification of diagnosed TB patients and providing DOTS services in partnership
Referring patients to the public sector from private dispensaries, clinics and hospitals when treatment is not feasible
Undertaking research and development of drugs and simpler diagnostics
Maintaining a healthy work environment to prevent the spread of TB

Academic bodies, professional associations
Influencing health policy and practices at political and decision making levels
Educating all health professionals on national guidelines for the diagnosis and treatment of TB
Assisting in setting codes of ethics and maintaining standards, especially in research for TB control

International/regional organisations and associations
Mobilizing resources and providing technical assistance to national programmes
Promoting innovative approaches, including intercountry collaboration for TB control
Co-ordinating national laws, standards and regulations on cross-border movement

Media
Disseminating evidence-based information
Educating the public and specific interest groups on TB
Influencing attitudes and behaviour with regard to TB
Advocating and communicating with policy makers to influence decisions relating to TB control

Opinion leaders [political, religious, traditional, etc.]
Influencing attitudes and behaviour of and towards people with TB
Influencing policy decisions relating to TB control

Communities
Supporting TB patients and their families by fostering positive attitudes and non-discriminatory practices
Involvement in planning, problem-solving, monitoring and reviewing TB programme initiatives
Critical feedback on availability of services

Patients and their families
Ownership of their health through active involvement to ensure that any affected member of their own family is treated properly until cured

TB = tuberculosis; NTPs = National Tuberculosis Programmes; NGOs = non-governmental organisations

Also in 2001, the G-8 at their 26th summit in Okinawa (27), committed to reducing TB deaths and prevalence by half by 2010. In January 2002, the GFATM was set up as a financial instrument to resource activities aimed at control of these three diseases (28). TB control was now firmly established on the global health agenda. TB control also features in the newly established UN SDG. Goal 3 specifically pertains to health: Ensure healthy lives and promote well-being for all at all ages. Target 3.3 states: By 2030, end the epidemics of AIDS, TB, malaria and neglected tropical diseases and combat hepatitis, water-borne diseases and other communicable diseases (29).

Partners in the South-East Asia Region

It had long been recognised in the Region that public health systems alone could not deliver health care to all. Health systems in the Region are already overstretched and countries in the Region did not have sufficient sustainable resources to meet the basic health needs of their populations. Many are also undergoing a difficult process of health sector reform in order to address these challenges.

Therefore, partnership building has been a priority for countries in the SEAR. Specifically for pooling resources and strengthen the on-going care and control activities, Programmes have collaborated with international agencies, as illustrated in Table 50.6. Joint efforts of national programmes, funding agencies, technical agencies, non-governmental organisations [NGOs] and grass roots organisations have led to considerable success in the SEAR in combatting TB. There are several examples available from the region that have been exemplified globally.

Success Stories From the Region

One deliberate and important strategy within SEAR to increase case detection and treatment success rates has been the inclusion of public health care providers operating outside the Ministry of Health, such as the railways, military, corporate sectors and prison health services, as well as private providers in TB management. In some countries, the percentage of patients seeking services through the private health sector is very high. Currently, all member countries have clear policies and strategies to involve other sectors, and their contribution to TB case notification stands at more than 25%.

A recent initiative have been the formal inclusion of the principles and practices of TB control in pre-service training and the establishment of referral mechanisms through providing lists of treatment centres [DOT centres] to teaching institutes. More than 1,000 private laboratories are now included in national diagnostic networks and undergo quality assurance mechanisms. Indonesia has intensified training of private and public hospital and laboratory staff. The country has also introduced co-ordination meetings between community health facilities and hospitals to improve transfer mechanisms between lung clinics and puskesmas. In Myanmar, TB services are provided throughout the network of Sun Quality Clinics and the NTP plans further expansion of public-private mix services through the Myanmar Medical Association.

Universities and medical schools in the region are contributing to evidence-based policies and strategies through technical advisory groups at national level.

Table 50.6: List of major donors and partners supporting TB control in South-East Asia Region

Australian Agency for International Development [AusAID]

Bangladesh Rural Advancement Committee [earlier used as an acronym. Now only the "BRAC" is used]

Centers for Disease Control and Prevention [CDC], Atlanta, USA

Clinton Health Access Initiative [CHAI]

Canadian International Development Agency [CIDA]

Challenge TB [CTB, one of the flagship projects of United States Agency for International Development]

Danish International Development Agency [DANIDA]

Damien Foundation Belgium [DFB]

UK Department for International Development [DFID]

Global TB Drug Facility/Stop TB partnership [GDF]

Global Fund to fight AIDS, TB and Malaria [GFATM, also called GF]

Japan Foundation for AIDS Prevention [JFAP]

Japan International Co-operation Agency [JICA]

Royal Netherlands Tuberculosis Association [KNCV]

Norwegian Association of Heart and Lung Patients [LHL]

Management Sciences for Health [MSH]

Norwegian Agency for International Development [NORAD]

Research Institute for Tuberculosis [Japan] [RIT]

South Asian Association for Regional Co-operation [SAARC]

International Union Against TB and Lung Disease

United Nations Development Programme [UNDP]

United Nations High Commission for Refugees [UNCHR]

United States Agency for International Development [USAID]

World Bank [WB]

World Health Organization [WHO]

TB = tuberculosis; AIDS = acquired immunodeficiency syndrome

More than 1,000 medical colleges, 25,000 private practitioners, 1,800 large public and private hospitals, 250 corporate institutions, 2,500 NGOs, nearly 100 faith-based organisations and over 900 prisons are now working with NTPs.

The International Standards of TB Care [ISTC] (30) have been endorsed by professional bodies and medical associations in Bangladesh, DPR Korea, India, Indonesia, Maldives, Myanmar, Nepal and Thailand. Intersectoral collaboration and public-private partnerships for delivery of services have been further scaled up in eight member countries [Bangladesh, India, Indonesia, Myanmar, Nepal, Sri Lanka, Thailand and Timor-Leste].

Partnership with international and national NGOs have enabled TB service delivery outreach in remote areas and among marginalised populations in several countries of the Region. Several thousand of community-based initiatives are also being incorporated into routine service delivery by national programmes. However, successful approaches should be systematically documented in order to replicate winning models in similar settings in the countries of the region.

Business alliances in the region such as the Thai Business Coalition and the Business Alliance in India are emerging as players from the non-health private sector introducing TB services into their workplaces.

Some Country Specific Examples of Successful Partnerships

Bangladesh–Community-based DOTS Implementation through Non-Governmental Organisations

Bangladesh is an outstanding example of implementing TB control in partnership with NGOs.

Community-based DOTS implemented through village doctors and the network of *shasthya shebikas* [community health volunteers] is the most common mechanism for supervising drug intake.

The Bangladesh Rural Advancement Committee [BRAC] approach for TB diagnosis and treatment focusses on community level education and engagement. The BRAC conducts orientation with different stakeholders of the community to engage them in efforts to identify patients, ensure treatment adherence, and reduce stigma. The stakeholders include: cured TB patients, local opinion and religious leaders, girls' guides and scouts, other NGO workers, village doctors, pharmacists and private practitioners.

The BRAC has created and trained a cadre of community health volunteers known as *shasthya Shebikas* to serve as front-line health care providers. *Shasthya Shebikas* educate and empower people in the community about TB control during household visits and health forums and also provide referral services. They disseminate TB messages, identify suspects, refer them for sputum examination to Upazila Health Complex [Government sub-district health complex] or BRAC laboratory services, ensure daily intake of medicine for identified TB patients through DOT and

refer for proper management of the side effects during TB treatment (31).

TB control in the Chittagong export processing zone
Chittagong is the largest industrial city in Bangladesh, and therefore, attracts a large number of people seeking work. There are over 600 garment factories in the city in the addition to industries in the Chittagong Export Processing Zone [CEPZ]. Within the CEPZ, operated by Bangladesh Export Processing Zone authority [BEPZA], there are 117 industries, employing 83,589 workers, mostly young women. These garment factories alone employ 1.8 million workers, 80% of whom are females, between the ages of 15-35 years. Recognising that health facilities at individual factory premises were inadequate, the Bangladesh garment manufacturers and exporters established two health centres with one doctor and one nurse at each. There are 43 DOT treatment centres, seven of which function also as diagnostic centres. These centres were established through collaboration between the NTP, the city corporation, local NGOs and the National Anti-TB Association of Bangladesh [NATAB]. TB cases identified at the health centres are referred to nearest NTP centre.

The Youngone Group in Bangladesh, which produces and exports sportswear including garments, shoes, nylon fabrics, quilting and luggage, operates within the CEPZ. It employs 24,000 employees of which 80% are females in the age group between 18-30 years, coming from many different districts in Bangladesh. TB was found to be common among these factory workers. The medical staff also recognised that most workers concealed their illness for fear of losing their jobs. Those with TB in the CEPZ either had to attend the CEPZ hospital, or the nearest NTP centre as a result, most workers suffering from TB preferred to consult private practitioners. This resulted in most being treated incompletely. Recognising that these workers were among the most vulnerable to TB on account of close regular contact with affected workers, the management of Youngone Industries decided to establish DOTS at Youngone Industry in the CEPZ. So far the Youngone Industries have registered 186 cases of TB among its workers, of whom a third were smear positive cases.

As a result of this initiative, the company enjoys the economic benefit accruing from increased work efficiency and better morale among its workers, national and international recognition, and a better corporate image. There is growing interest at the CEPZ hospital in establishing DOTS centre under NTP, due to the initiative by the Youngone Group. Youngone is also interested in establishing a wider partnership to address TB-HIV co-infection (32).

India–Public-Private Mix through Non-Governmental Organisation Interface

Resource Group for Education and Advocacy for Community Health [REACH] is an organisation formed in 1998 to raise awareness on issues which are critical to community health. REACH is a registered society being managed by an executive committee, with the main office based in Chennai,

Tamil Nadu, India. One of the major issues addressed by REACH is TB control. For the past 10 years REACH has been involved in creating awareness on TB in slums, schools and the community and specially caters to the lower socio-economic strata of society.

Private practitioners and private hospitals in Chennai, Tamil Nadu were actively sensitised by REACH for participation in the Revised National TB Control Program [RNTCP]. Advocacy and training of Private Physicians was carried out. The PPM project was set up as an informal non-profit collaboration initiated by REACH and Corporation of Chennai. The objectives of the PPM model were to increase access for patients to RNTCP services by involving private healthcare providers and devise innovative methods to overcome barriers to successful PPM. REACH facilitated treatment of the private patients by providing assistance to the PPM centres and the private practitioners. Since 1998-2010 the project has treated 5,264 patients with successful treatment outcomes. Advocacy, Communication and Social Mobilisation [ACSM] activities are presently being carried out in the 12 districts of Tamil Nadu as part of the GFATM supported Axshya TB Project.

As part of the initiative to increase awareness about TB among journalists and journalist students and to increase media reporting on TB, the website www.media4tb.org was launched which gives a whole range of information about TB, facts on TB, frequently raised questions on TB, some of the international agencies working towards TB control, different stakeholders in the partnership, communication materials developed by REACH (33).

Corporate sector-public sector undertaking collaborates to "Stop TB" Hindustan Copper Ltd, established in 1924 as Indian Copper Corp Ltd., is one of the oldest copper mines in India. It runs its own hospital for employees and ex-employees. The hospital has 80 beds, a fully functional lab, an operation theatre and an X-ray unit. As per the last available data, 14 doctors including four specialists, 21 nurses and 62 paramedical staff were working there. The company is also involved in community outreach programmes as part of its Corporate Social Responsibility and conducts regular health camps in the surrounding villages every month. The hospital is in a remote area and caters to a large rural population. Keeping this in mind a Designated Microscopy Centre [DMC] and a DOT centre was started in the hospital in October, 2007. Two doctors, 4 pharmacists and 3 laboratory technicians have been trained in RNTCP at the District Tuberculosis Centre, Jamshedpur. The whole programme is running under the able leadership of the Chief Medical Superintendent, whose enthusiastic response and initiative has made this programme possible in HCL. He was responsible for encouraging his staff to take active part in getting trained and following RNTCP norms (34).

Indonesia–Faith-based Organisation with Gender Sensitivities

Aisyiyah *Aisyiyah* formed in 1917 and is the first women's muslim organisation in Indonesia. Since, 2000 this organisation is involved in TB Programme. *Aisyiyah* efforts are to increase community participation in interventions like case detection and accompanying TB confirmed patients for treatment through DOTS. *Aisyiyah* also is engaged in increasing the role of non-governmental clinics to adopt counselling and treatment of TB patients through DOTS.

Activities of *Aisyiyah* include advocacy to local government, DOTS training for TB Cadres, developing DOTS curricula in Medical school, TB control in workplace and social mobilisation in the community. *Aisyiyah* managed to increase case detection rate in the working area with close co-ordination to primary health care.

To foster acceleration of hospital involvement in DOTS, 750 out of 1,645 hospitals has been trained in DOTS strategy with funding from Global Fund Round 1, Round 5 and USAID. With funding from TBCAP/USAID through KNCV, several provinces were supported by Technical Officers who specifically deal with DOTS expansion in hospital. Coordination at central level with the Directorate General of Medical Service has significantly intensified. Two guidelines have been developed, namely the Managerial Guideline for TB service provision with DOTS strategy in hospital and Guideline for TB diagnosis and treatment in hospital. In addition, the Directorate General of Medical Service has conducted assessment to several DOTS hospitals. Efforts to integrate implementation of DOTS strategy into the current hospital accreditation system are underway (35).

National movement for partnership *Gerdunas* [Gerakan Terpadu National or National Integrated Movement] is a cross sector movement formed in 1999 at central and local government levels in order to promote acceleration of TB control measures through an integrated approach, involving hospitals, private sectors, academia, NGOs, funding agencies, and other stakeholders. Following high level meetings held during 2002, *Gerdunas* provincial chapters were established in nearly all provinces. The function of partnership can be grouped into three categories: [i] planning and stewardship; [ii] financing, resource allocation and use; and [iii] service provision (36).

Nepal–Youth Organisation Involved in Human Immunodeficiency Virus Control

Bidhyarthi Jagarn Manch [BIJAM, Student Awareness Forum] is a non-profitable and non-governmental organisation focusing mainly on youth development, harm reduction, HIV, AIDS and sexually transmitted infections [STI] prevention and control and recently in TB diagnosis and treatment.

BIJAM has worked for the last 17 years to reduce HIV and AIDS related prejudice, behaviour change communication interventions, access to clean needles and syringes, condom distribution, STI treatment, HIV counselling and treatment.

Recently, BIJAM has been implementing active case finding for TB diagnosis among vulnerable groups in hard to reach populations by screening for TB symptoms, sputum collection of suspected cases, and referral of positive cases to government treatment centres.

The TB interventions are part of the Stop TB Partnership TB Reach funding with Family Health International [FHI]

Nepal managing the grant. BIJAM is one of the many FHI partners implementing the grant. Bijam works for the promotion of community initiative by strengthening existing health and education system. Focusing to increase knowledge and understanding by promoting education on health related issues (37).

Sri Lanka—Foundation as a Partner for Tuberculosis Control

Sevalanka Foundation *Sevalanka*, a registered non-profit, works with two "daughter organisations" to provide an integrated and complementary package of services. Seva Finance is a registered microfinance institution that provides financial services to community organisations and rural entrepreneurs. Seva Economic Development Company [SEDCO] is a social enterprise that focuses on fair trade, value chain investments.

Sevalanka is currently active in 22 of Sri Lanka's 25 districts. While the headquarters ensures accountability and provides specialised support services, most implementation decisions are taken at the district level by staff from that region.

Sevalanka's decentralised structure enables the organisation to respond more quickly and appropriately to local needs. Specific activities vary from district-to-district and region-to-region, but all areas follow a common strategy for facilitating a community-centred development process through social mobilisation, institutional capacity building of civil society organisations, network formation, and livelihood support services. Psychosocial well-being, environmental sustainability, gender equality, and peace-building are considered cross-cutting issues and are incorporated into all programmes (38). This has also helped incorporate TB control in their overall service provision with great success.

These success stories have led to reaffirmation of the belief that considerable success in TB care and control can be achieved by NTPs working in coordination and synergy with partners. The available strengths need to be adequately tapped to fill in the gaps of the national programmes. The need now is to identify best practices in these examples, check what interventions are replicable, adapt them to local needs and scale up, to reach out all those afflicted by TB.

REFERENCES

1. World Health Organization. Global tuberculosis control: WHO report 2018. Geneva: World Health Organization; 2018.
2. Nakajima H. Tuberculosis: a global emergency. World Health 1993;46:3.
3. Kochi A. The global tuberculosis situation and the new control strategy of the World Health Organization. Tubercle 1991;72:1-6.
4. Tuberculosis Chemotherapy Centre. A concurrent comparison of home and sanatorium treatment of pulmonary tuberculosis in south India. Bull World Health Organ 1959;21:51-144.
5. Nagpaul DR, Savic DM, Rao KP, Baily GV. Case-finding by microscopy. Bull Int Union Tuberc 1968;41:48-158.
6. World Health Organization. Global Tuberculosis Programme. Framework for effective tuberculosis control. WHO/TB/94.179. Geneva: World Health Organization; 1994.
7. World Health Organization. What is DOTS—a Guide to understanding the WHO-recommended TB control strategy known as DOTS. WHO/CDS/TB/99.270. Geneva: World Health Organization; 1999.
8. World Bank. World Development Report 1993. Investing in health. New York: Oxford University Press; 1993.
9. World Health Organization. The Stop TB Strategy: Building on and enhancing DOTS to meet the TB-related Millennium Development Goals. WHO/HTM/TB/2006.368. Geneva: World Health Organization; 2006.
10. World Health Organization. The End TB strategy. Available at URL: http://www.who.int/tb/strategy/en/. Accessed on December 18, 2017.
11. World Health Organization, Regional Office for South-East Asia. Bending the curve-ending TB: annual report 2017. Available at URL: http://apps.who.int/iris/bitstream/handle/10665/254762/978929022584-eng.pdf?sequence=1&isAllowed=y. Accessed on July 16, 2018.
12. World Health Organization, Regional Office for South-East Asia. The South-East Asia Regional Response Plan for Drug-resistant TB Care and Control 2011-2015, SEA-TB-334. New Delhi: World Health Organization, Regional Office for South-East Asia; 2011.
13. World Health Organization, Regional Office for South-East Asia. Health sector response to HIV in the South-East Asia Region 2013. New Delhi: World Health Organization, Regional Office for South-East Asia; 2013.
14. World Health Organization, Regional Office for South-East Asia. Ending TB in South East Asia-Regional Strategic Plan 2016-2020. New Delhi: World Health Organization, Regional Office for South-East Asia; 2016.
15. Wells WA, Ge CF, Patel N, Oh T, Gardiner E, Kimerling ME. Size and usage patterns of private TB drug markets in the high burden countries. PLOS One 2011;6:e18964.
16. World Health Organization. Sixty-Second World Health Assembly. WHA62/2009/REC/1. Geneva: World Health Organization; 2009.
17. World Health Organization, Regional Office for South-East Asia. Updated Regional Strategic Plan for TB Control 2012-2015. SEA-TB-345. New Delhi: World Health Organization, Regional Office for South-East Asia; 2012.
18. World Health Organization, Stop TB Partnership. A pocket guide to building partnerships: WHO/HTM/STB/2003.25. Geneva: World Health Organization; 2003.
19. World Health Organization, Stop TB Partnership. Engaging stakeholders for retooling TB control. Geneva: World Health Organization; 2008.
20. World Health Organization, Regional Office for South-East Asia. Leadership and strategic management for TB control managers. Module 8. Building Partnerships. SEA-TB-274. New Delhi: World Health Organization, Regional Office for South-East Asia.
21. Raviglione MC, Dye C, Schmidt S, Kochi A. Assessment of worldwide tuberculosis control. WHO Global Surveillance and Monitoring Project. Lancet 1997;350:624-9.
22. World Health Organization. Global Tuberculosis Programme. Report of the Ad-hoc Committee on the tuberculosis epidemic. WHO/TB/98.245. Geneva: World Health Organization; 1998.
23. World Health Organization, Stop TB Initiative. Tuberculosis and sustainable development. Report of a conference. WHO/CDS/STB/2000.6. Geneva: World Health Organization; 2000.
24. World Health Organization. Fifty-third World Health Assembly. Resolution WHA 53.1. WHA53/2000/REC. Geneva: World Health Organization; 2000.
25. Global Partnership to Stop TB. Washington Commitment to Stop TB. WHO/CDS/STB/2001.14a. Geneva: World Health Organization; 2001.

26. Global Partnership to Stop TB. Global Plan to Stop TB. WHO/CDS/STB/2001.16. Geneva: World Health Organization; 2001.

27. The Okinawa G-8 Summit. Building a global development partnership. Available at URL: http://clinton4.nara.gov/WH/EOP/nec/html/G8GlobalDevPartnership000722.html. Accessed on December 12, 2016.

28. The Global Fund to Fight AIDS, TB and Malaria. Available at URL: www.theglobalfund.org/en/. Accessed on December 22, 2018.

29. UN Sustainable Development Goals. Available at URL: https://sustainabledevelopment.un.org/sdgs. Accessed on December 22, 2016.

30. International Standards for Tuberculosis Care. Diagnosis, treatment, public health.Third edition. 2014. Available at URL: http://www.who.int/tb/publications/ISTC_3rdEd.pdf?ua=1. Accessed on December 22, 2016.

31. BRAC. Available at URL: http://www.brac.net/. Accessed on December 22, 2016.

32. World Health Organization South-East Asia Regional Office. Report of DOTS in the workplace. World Health Organization Regional Office for South-East Asia. New Delhi; 2004.

33. Resource Group for Education and Advocacy for Community Health. Available at URL: http://www.reachtbnetwork.org. Accessed on December 26, 2018.

34. Success stories. Jharkhand. Public sector undertaking collaborates to "Stop TB". Available at URL: http://www.tbcindia.nic.in/index1.php?linkid=383&level=1&lid=2749&lang=1. Accessed on December 28, 2018.

35. Muhammadiyah. Available at URL: http://www.muhammadiyah.or.id/content-199-det-aisyiyah.html. Accessed on December 18, 2018.

36. Kementerian Kesehatan Republik Indonesia. Ministry of Health Republic of Indonesia. Available at URL: http://www.depkes.go.id/. Accessed on December 22, 2018.

37. Bidhyarthi Jagarn Mancha. Available at URL: http://www.bijam.org/. Accessed on December 12, 2016.

38. Sevalanka. Available at URL: http://www.sevalanka.org/. Accessed on December 2, 2018.

51

Integrating Community-based Tuberculosis Activities into the Work of Non-governmental and other Civil Society Organisations [The ENGAGE-TB Approach]

Haileyesus Getahun, Thomas Joseph

INTRODUCTION

In 2017, an estimated 10 million people around the world became ill with tuberculosis [TB], and 1.3 million died from it (1). About 13% of TB occurs among people living with human immunodeficiency virus [HIV], and TB causes almost a quarter of acquired immunodeficiency syndrome [AIDS] deaths. One-third of people estimated to have TB are either not reached for diagnosis and treatment by the current health systems or are not being reported. Even in patients who are identified, TB is often diagnosed and treated late. In order to reach the unreached and to find TB patients early in the course of their illness, a wider range of stakeholders already involved in community-based activities needs to be engaged. These include the non-governmental organisations [NGOs] and other civil society organisations [CSOs] that are active in community-based development, particularly in primary health care, HIV infection and maternal and child health, but have not yet included TB in their priorities and activities (2).

NGOs and other CSOs are non-profit organisations that operate independently from the state and from the private for-profit sector. They include a broad spectrum of entities such as international, national and local NGOs, community-based organisations [CBOs], faith-based organisations [FBOs], patient-based organisations and professional associations. NGOs and other CSOs engage in activities that range from community mobilisation, service delivery, and technical assistance to research and advocacy (2).

The strengths of NGOs and other CSOs active in health care and other development interventions at the community level include their reach and spread and their ability to engage marginalised or remote groups. These organisations have a comparative advantage because of their understanding of the local context. Greater collaboration between NGOs and other CSOs and local and national governments could greatly enhance development outcomes (3) that will in turn benefit TB prevention, treatment and care activities.

The implementation and scaling up of community-based TB activities remains weak, despite the clear need, the documented cost-effectiveness of community-based TB activities (4) and the tremendous efforts that have been expended in recent years. Effective and mutual engagement of NGOs and other CSOs and the national TB programmes [NTPs] or their equivalents is essential to scale up community based TB activities.

The core principles for effective engagement and to improve collaboration and foster effective partnership between NGOs and other CSOs and the NTPs or their equivalents include mutual understanding and respect recognising differences and similarities in background, functions and working culture; consideration and respect for local contexts and values while establishing collaborative mechanisms and scaling-up integrated community-based TB activities; and support to a single national system for monitoring implementation of activities by all actors with standardised indicators (5). Respect for these principles will help to remove barriers and bottlenecks affecting implementation of integrated community-based TB activities.

COMMUNITY-BASED TUBERCULOSIS ACTIVITIES

Community-based TB activities cover a wide range of activities contributing to prevention, diagnosis, improved treatment adherence and care that positively influence the outcomes of drug-sensitive, drug-resistant and HIV-associated TB. While diagnostic tests for TB continue to be performed in clinical settings, for lack of simpler diagnostic methods, community-based TB activities are conducted outside the premises of formal health facilities

Table 51.1: Examples of community-based TB activities

Theme	Possible activities
Prevention	Awareness-raising, IEC, BCC, infection control, training providers
Detection	Screening, contact tracing, sputum collection, sputum transport, training providers
Referral	Linking with clinics, transport support and facilitation, accompaniment, referral forms, training providers
Treatment adherence support	Home-based DOT support, adherence counselling, stigma reduction, pill counting, training providers, home-based care and support
Social and livelihood support	Cash transfers, insurance schemes, nutrition support and supplementation, voluntary savings and loans, inclusive markets, training providers, income generation
Advocacy	Ensure availability of supplies, equipment and services, training providers, governance and policy issues, working with community leaders
Stigma reduction	Community theatre/drama groups, testimonials, patient/peer support groups, community champions, sensitising and training facility and CHWs and leaders

TB = tuberculosis; IEC = information, education, communication; BCC = behaviour change communication; DOT = directly observed therapy; CHWs = community health workers
Source: reference 6

[e.g., hospitals, health centres and clinics] in community-based structures [e.g., schools, places of worship, congregate settings] and homesteads.

Community health workers [CHWs] and community volunteers [CVs] carry out community-based TB activities, depending on national and local contexts. CHWs are people with some formal education who are given training to contribute to community-based health services, including TB prevention and patient care and support. CVs are community members who have been systematically sensitised about TB prevention and care, either through a short, specific training scheme or through repeated, regular contact sessions with professional health workers.

Community-based TB activities could and should be integrated into other community-based activities supporting primary health care services, including those for HIV infection, maternal and child health and non-communicable diseases to improve synergy and impact. Community-based TB activities utilise community structures and mechanisms through which community members, CBOs and groups interact, coordinate and deliver their responses to the challenges and needs affecting their communities (6). Some examples of community-based TB activities are shown in Table 51.1 (7).

NGOs and other CSOs could integrate TB into their community-based work in many ways, without trained medical staff. It is particularly important for them to do so when they are working with high-risk populations, [such as people living with HIV and the very poor], people living in congested environments [urban slums and prisons], people who use drugs, sex workers and migrant workers. Examples of how NGOs and other CSOs could integrate TB into their ongoing activities are shown in Table 51.2.

THE ENGAGE-TB APPROACH

The ENGAGE-TB approach seeks to shift the global perspective of TB from only a medical illness to a more comprehensive socioeconomic and community problem. It proposes six areas to facilitate the engagement of NGOs and other CSOs in community-based TB activities. These are a situation analysis; an enabling legal and policy environment; guidelines and tools; assessing the relevant TB tasks needed to be undertaken and included in action plans; monitoring and evaluation to enable learning and continuous improvement; and enhancing the capacity of organisations to scale up their work sustainably. The ENGAGE-TB approach emphasises the value of collaboration and partnership between NGOs and other CSOs and the NTPs or equivalents. It also requires close alignment of systems, especially in TB monitoring and reporting, to ensure that national data adequately capture the contributions of community-based TB activities. Each component of ENGAGE-TB is independent, and all six components are not always required to implement community-based TB activities [Figure 51.1].

Situation Analysis

A situation analysis helps to identify the specific needs and tasks for integrated community-based TB activities. It involves information-gathering to analyse and understand the existing situation. It is useful to involve and engage multiple stakeholders, including the NTP, NGOs and other CSOs, and community members, including patients and their families. An NGO or CSO should take the lead for the situational analysis of its own operational area. The situation analysis should identify and prioritise problems and needs in TB prevention and care, especially those of vulnerable groups such as prisoners, migrants, sex workers and injecting drug users who might face stigma and have difficulty in using the services of the formal health system. Information on the available TB diagnostic and treatment facilities helps in understanding how the system will work in terms of activities, such as, referral, sputum collection, diagnosis, treatment and follow-up.

Table 51.2: Examples of how NGOs and other CSOs could integrate TB into their ongoing activities

HIV programmes and projects
    TB/HIV awareness raising and stigma reduction
    TB detection through screening, contact tracing and sputum collection and transport
    TB referral by linking patients with clinics and assisting with transport
    Treatment adherence support including home-based TB and HIV care
    Social and livelihood support through nutrition supplementation, income generation and vocational training

Maternal and child health programmes and projects
    TB prevention through awareness raising, stigma reduction, infection control and improved vaccine coverage, including BCG for infants
    TB detection through screening at all ANC clinics, contact tracing and referrals to TB clinics
    Treatment adherence support through home-based DOT by CHWs and CVs
    TB advocacy on availability of supplies and drugs at facilities and on increasing access to services for women with young children who find it difficult to travel

Education programmes and projects
    TB prevention by teaching about TB, especially the signs and symptoms of TB and cough hygiene, through simple curricula in school at all levels
    TB detection by training teachers to screen for TB
    Teachers and literacy class facilitators can refer those with signs and symptoms
    Treatment adherence can be improved with teachers supporting children to take medication
    Stigma can be reduced by discussing TB in class and increasing knowledge and awareness of the disease

Livelihood development programmes and projects
    Assist in prevention by including TB education during regular visits to families and also use supervisors of such programmes to raise awareness
    Increase detection by providing training to leaders and participants on signs and symptoms to enable community-based screening
    Link village development committees and staff to health facilities to enable referrals of all those with presumptive TB
    Improve treatment outcomes through DOT support at home by staff and volunteers
    Provide extra support to TB patients in livelihood programmes, such as, special nutrition or additional stipends during their treatment period

NGO = non-governmental organisations; CSOs = civil society organisations; TB = tuberculosis; HIV = human immunodeficiency virus; BCG = bacille Calmette-Guérin; ANC = antenatal care; DOT = directly observed therapy; CHW = community health worker; CV = community volunteer

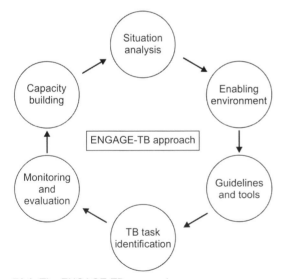

Figure 51.1: The ENGAGE-TB approach

Enabling Environment

A mutually enabling legal and policy environment will increase the engagement of NGOs and other CSOs in TB activities, particularly those who are newly engaged in TB prevention and care. A facilitated registration process of NGOs and other CSOs in accordance with local norms and needs and ensuring greater integration of processes and requirements between different government departments could be key areas for government to support the operations of NGO and other CSOs. Reducing the complexity of transactions and increasing the speed of facilitation are other factors that improve the operating environment for NGOs and other CSOs. NTPs or their equivalents have the responsibility of creating enabling national or local legal, policy and administrative environments to support the effective engagement of NGOs and other CSOs in TB activities. NGOs and other CSOs should also stimulate and support the development of an enabling legal and policy environment through constructive dialogue and engagement with the NTPs or relevant legislative structures, with the participation of the segments of society they represent. This can be best done on a sustained, continuing basis if NGOs and other CSOs form an umbrella NGO co-ordinating body [NCB] to represent their best interests and to allow systematic sharing and dissemination of lessons learnt by individual organisations. NTPs should support the formation of such NGO coalitions and make time to meet with them in order to understand their needs, constraints and the lessons learnt.

Guidelines and Tools

The NTPs or their equivalents should work with NGOs and other CSOs in the NCB to prepare national operational guidelines and standard tools based on internationally recommended, evidence-based policies and guidelines.

They should be adaptable to the mission, mandate, resources and activities of the NGOs and other CSOs. If necessary, NTPs or their equivalents should facilitate clearances and approvals of these instruments. Existing tools and instruments should be used when feasible and adapted to the needs of NGOs and other CSOs.

Task Identification

TB is linked to HIV infection and also to social determinants of health and non-communicable diseases such as poverty, crowding, malnutrition, drug and alcohol use and diabetes mellitus. Therefore, the opportunities, capacities and comparative advantages of the NGOs and other CSOs working in such areas should be considered in determining how best to address TB. Consideration must also be given to the availability of resources and expertise and ensuring synergy. Community-based TB activities could range from prevention, detection, referral and treatment adherence support to social and livelihood support, advocacy and stigma reduction. To increase synergy and effectiveness, all the parties involved [NGOs and other CSOs, NTPs or equivalents] must determine which tasks are to be carried out by each organisation.

The NTPs or their equivalents should include the implementation and scaling up of community-based TB activities through the engagement of NGOs and other CSOs in their medium- and long-term national TB strategic plans and budgets as well as in annual national and subnational operational plans.

Monitoring and Evaluation

Regular monitoring and evaluation will help in assessing the quality, effectiveness, coverage and delivery of community-based TB activities and the engagement of NGOs and other CSOs. It promotes a learning culture and serves as a foundation to ensure continuous improvement of programme implementation. NTPs or their equivalents should ensure that there is a single national monitoring and evaluation system that recognises the contribution and engagement of NGOs and other CSOs.

Quarterly reviews of progress would help to uncover issues in implementation and enable mid-stream correction to plans and budgets and to overall strategy. The NTP should help to smooth any operational difficulties that NGOs and other CSOs may face and cannot independently resolve. Quarterly meetings to discuss the review findings could be held at subnational or local levels so that there is cross-fertilisation of learning between NGOs and other CSOs and with the NTP. Annual meetings at the national level should be organised by the NCB and a broad spectrum of implementing NGOs and other CSOs invited to share their findings and report progress. The resulting national report issued by the NTP should be shared widely with all stakeholders within government, NGOs and other CSOs, patients and community members, donors and the general public.

Evaluation should be an ongoing process and include evaluation of both the activities [process evaluation] and achievement of the objectives [impact evaluation] of the action plan. Qualitative methods and periodic surveys could be used to provide an understanding of how well NGOs and other CSOs are supported and how they have engaged in community-based TB activities. One of the main challenges of monitoring the implementation of community-based TB activities has been the lack of standardised indicators. The suggested core indicators to measure the implementation of community-based activities that need to be included in the TB monitoring system of all stakeholders and linked with the national monitoring and evaluation system of the NTP or its equivalent are shown in Tables 51.3 and 51.4.

Periodic evaluation provides a qualitative view of the progress of community-based TB activities [Table 51.5]. In particular, it helps to assess the contributions of NGOs and other CSOs to new case notifications and to treatment outcomes. It also indicates whether NGO contributions are increasing or decreasing and reflects the quality of the relations between NTPs and NGOs on the basis of variables such as the frequency of meetings, the quality of such meetings, the cooperation of people involved, the factors in success and the overall interest and drive of the NTP in involving NGOs and other CSOs in TB activities.

Capacity-building

Capacity-building is necessary for strengthening and sustaining the engagement of NTPs, NGOs and other CSOs in implementing and scaling-up community-based TB activities. It requires joint actions by the NTPs or their equivalents and NGOs and other CSOs and will be of mutual benefit. Increasing financial resources is crucial for scaling-up community-based TB activities and the effective engagement of NGOs and other CSOs. Innovative resource mobilisation from internal [e.g. national governments, private donors, philanthropists] and external sources [e.g., the Global Fund to Fight AIDS, TB and Malaria, bilateral donors and charitable foundations] should be undertaken by NGOs and other CSOs and the NTPs.

In some countries, NTPs may have little prior experience of engaging with NGOs and other CSOs. Their capacities should also be built to cultivate and maintain effective relationships with the nongovernmental sector. Health sector governmental staff might require training in community mobilisation, including communication styles and methods. Health systems should be strengthened further to meet increased demand for services from affected communities.

Capacity-building interventions should also support sharing and transfer of knowledge, skills and resources between international CSOs and national CSOs, with both groups gaining from the process. Regular forums for sharing knowledge, experience and good practices should be established. Mutual learning and support can increase confidence and capability to scale-up activities.

The WHO's End TB Strategy clearly recognises the value and importance of engaging with NGOs and other

Table 51.3: Indicators for monitoring implementation. Indicator 1: referrals and new notifications

Definition	Number of new TB patients [all forms] diagnosed and notified with TB who were referred by CHWs and CVs expressed as a percentage of all new TB patients notified in the BMU during a specified period
Numerator	Number of new TB patients [all forms] referred by CHWs or CVs to a health facility for diagnosis and notified in the BMU[s] in a specified period
Denominator	Number of new TB patients [all forms] notified in the BMU[s] in the same period
Purpose	To measure the level of engagement of CHWs and CVs in increasing new notifications of TB. It can also indicate the effectiveness of the referral system in ensuring the flow of persons with presumptive TB from community-based structures to the BMU
Method	Community health worker refers to a person with some formal education who is trained to contribute to community-based health services including TB prevention and patient care and support. Community volunteer refers to a community member who has been systematically sensitised about TB prevention and care, either through a short and specific training scheme or through repeated contact with professional health workers. Both can be supported by NGOs, other CSOs and/or the government. It is important to use the definitions in this guidance in order to standardise the documentation, monitoring and evaluation of community-based activities. This will prevent confusion about what constitutes 'community engagement' in TB prevention and care. Entries on TB treatment cards, the presumptive TB register [also known as 'TB suspects' register] kept at facilities, the BMU TB register and the laboratory register should be modified to include 'Referral by community health workers and community volunteers', to allow standardised recording of the community contribution to referral. The quarterly report on TB registration in the BMU should also be adjusted to record this contribution. These forms and registers should be adapted locally and used by CHWs and CVs to ensure that data are reported to the NTP's monitoring and evaluation system. Indirect sources of data include historical data analysis of overall TB notifications and comparisons of geographical areas with and without community-based activities, time trends in TB notifications and comparisons of referrals in areas with and without community-based activities
Periodicity	Quarterly and annually
Strengths and limitations	This indicator will depend on the completeness and reliability of community-initiated referral data at clinic level, especially ensuring that referred persons with presumptive TB when confirmed with TB are tagged as having been referred by CHWs and CVs, supported either by an NGO, other CSO or the NTP
Responsibility	All stakeholders [NGOs, other CSOs or the NTP or its equivalent] implementing community-based TB activities will ensure accurate data collection at community and facility levels. NTP and their equivalents will aggregate data at district, subnational and national level, depending on the local context, to ensure that the information is included in the national TB monitoring system
Measurement tools	Presumptive TB patients should be recorded on the 'persons with presumptive TB' register [also known as 'TB suspects' register], which should specify who referred them. If confirmed with TB, they should then be recorded in the TB register as having been referred by CHWs or CVs supported by either the NTP structure or NGOs and other CSOs. Data should be aggregated quarterly for the quarterly report on TB registration and for the yearly report on programme management in districts or BMUs

TB = tuberculosis; CHWs = community health workers; CVs = community volunteers; BMU = basic management unit; NGO = non-governmental organisations; CSO = civil society organisations; NTP = National Tuberculosis Programme

Table 51.4: Indicators for monitoring implementation. Indicator 2: treatment success

Definition	New TB patients [all forms] successfully treated [cured plus completed treatment] who received support for treatment adherence from CHWs or CVs among all new TB patients [all forms] provided with treatment adherence support by CHWs or CVs [number and percentage]
Numerator	Number of new TB patients [all forms] successfully treated and provided with treatment adherence support by CHWs or CVs in the BMU[s] in a specified period
Denominator	Total number of new TB patients [all forms] given treatment adherence support by CHWs or CVs in the same period
Purpose	To measure the scope and quality of implementation of community-based TB activities particularly relating to treatment outcome of patients. It can also indicate the acceptability of CHWs or CVs to patients with TB as treatment adherence support providers
Method	Community health worker refers to a person with some formal education who is trained to contribute to community-based health services including TB prevention and patient care and support. Community volunteer refers to a community member who has been systematically sensitised about TB prevention and care, either through a short and specific training scheme, or through repeated contact with professional health workers. Both can be supported by NGOs, other CSOs and/or the government. It is important to use the definitions in this guidance in order to standardise the documentation, monitoring and evaluation of community-based activities. This will prevent confusion about what constitutes 'community engagement' in TB prevention and care
	Treatment adherence includes all efforts and services provided by CHWs and CVs to TB patients receiving treatment to help them complete their treatment successfully. These can include treatment observation, adherence counselling, pill counting and other activities to monitor both the quantity and timing of the medication taken by a patient

Contd...

Contd...

Periodicity	Quarterly and annually
Strengths and limitations	Monitors how well treatment adherence is supported by the community-based activities of NGOs, other CSOs or the government
Responsibility	All NGOs, other CSOs and the NTP or its equivalent implementing community-based TB activities will ensure that data are collected at the community and facility levels. NTP and their equivalents will ensure that data are aggregated at district, subnational and national levels, depending on the local context, to ensure that the information is included in the national TB monitoring system
Measurement tools	TB register

TB = tuberculosis; CHWs = community health workers; CVs = community volunteers; NGO = non-governmental organisation; CSO = civil society organisation; NTP = National Tuberculosis Programme

Table 51.5: Periodic evaluation

Indicators	Existence of a NCB
	    Trends in membership
	    Frequency of meetings
	    Spread to subnational levels
	    Coordination between levels
	    Mechanisms for transferring knowledge, skills and resources
	Quality of interaction with the NTP at various levels
	    Frequency of meetings
	    Quality of follow-up on agreed actions
	    Availability of TB diagnostic services and drugs
	The relative contributions of NGOs and other CSOs and of the government to new case notifications and treatment success, with trends in these variables over time
	Challenges and hurdles faced by different actors in government and civil society as well as successes and new opportunities

Method	Qualitative techniques should be used, including focus group discussions and key informant interviews. Appreciative inquiry techniques will help improve the quality of the feedback. NTP managers and district and clinic staff should be interviewed both singly and in groups. Similarly, representatives of NGOs and CBOs at national, district and local levels should be interviewed singly and jointly. The main issues emerging from the interviews should be identified, shared and discussed at a meeting between the staff of the NTP at various levels and representatives of NGOs and CSOs at various levels. The emphasis should be on sharing and learning in order to understand and improve the programme, rather than on fault finding or 'finger pointing'
Periodicity	Every 3–5 years
Strengths and limitations	Provides a periodic assessment of the contributions of NGOs and other CSOs as well as the quality of the relations with the NTPs. The value of such studies depends on the professionalism and ability of the evaluators and the biases they may bring to the process
Responsibility	All NGOs, other CSOs and the NTP or its equivalent implementing community-based TB activities must be willing to participate and share their views. The primary responsibility for organising such evaluations is with the NTP. They could coincide with the national TB reviews generally held every 5 years in each country

NCB = non-governmental oranisation co-ordinating body; NTP = National Tuberculosis Programme; TB = tuberculosis; CSO = civil society organisations; NGO = non-governmental oranisation

civil society organisations in order to achieve the goal of ending the global TB epidemic. One of the four principles of the WHO strategy is "strong coalition with CSOs and communities." The engagement of communities and CSOs is also one of the key components of the implementation strategy (8). It is clear that many marginalised and vulnerable groups are unable to access the formal health system and seek diagnosis, treatment and care. For these segments of society, it will be necessary to go outside the health facilities to reach them in their own homesteads, within their own community settings. NGOs and other CSOs are able to do so effectively and already reach them with other programmes in health, education and economic development. The remaining challenge is for NTPs to more actively seek out and engage such organisations and encourage them to integrate community-based TB activities into their work. As NGOs and other CSOs start integrating TB services into their work with communities, more and more of those previously unreached will be reached and will gain access to diagnosis, treatment and care. Community and civil society engagement must be seen as a necessary and vital component of NTP strategies to secure the vision of a world free of TB with zero deaths, disease and suffering due to TB.

REFERENCES

1. World Health Organization. Global TB report 2018. WHO/CDS/TB/2018.20. Geneva: World Health Organization; 2018.

2. Getahun H, Raviglione M. Transforming the global tuberculosis response through effective engagement of civil society organizations: the role of the World Health Organization. Bull World Health Organ 2011;89:616-8.

3. Jareg P, Kaseje DC. Growth of civil society in developing countries: implications for health. Lancet 1998;351:819-22

4. Sinanovic E, Floyd K, Dudley L, Azevedo V, Grant R, Maher D. Cost and cost-effectiveness of community-based care for tuberculosis in Cape Town, South Africa. Int J Tuberc Lung Dis 2003;7:S56-62.

5. World Health Organization. ENGAGE-TB: integrating community-based TB activities into the work of NGOs and other CSOs – operational guidance. Geneva: World Health Organization; 2012.

6. The Global Fund to Fight AIDS, Tuberculosis and Malaria. Community systems strengthening framework. Geneva; 2010.

7. World Health Organization. ENGAGE-TB: integrating community-based TB activities into the work of NGOs and other CSOs – implementation manual. Geneva: World Health Organization; 2013.

8. World Health Organization. Global strategy and targets for tuberculosis prevention, care and control after 2015. World Health Assembly resolution 67. Geneva: World Health Organization; 2014.

52

WHO's New End TB Strategy

Mukund Uplekar, Diana Weil

INTRODUCTION

A Persisting Challenge

According to the 2018 Global TB Report of the World Health Organization [WHO] (1), tuberculosis [TB] remains a persistent development challenge. TB is one of the leading causes of death worldwide and the leading cause from a single infectious agent. In 2017, there were an estimated 1.3 million TB deaths among HIV-negative people and an additional 300,000 deaths among HIV-positive people. An estimated 10 million people fell ill with TB in 2017: 90% were adults, 58% were male, 9% were people living with human immunodeficiency virus [HIV] [74% in Africa] and two-thirds were in eight countries: India, China, Indonesia, the Philippines, Pakistan, Nigeria, Bangladesh and South Africa. Drug-resistant TB [DR-TB] is a continuing threat. In 2017, there were 558,000 new cases with resistance to rifampicin [RR-TB], the most effective first-line drug, of which 82% had multidrug-resistant TB [MDR-TB]. Almost half [47%] of these cases were in India, China and the Russian Federation. Globally, the TB mortality rate is falling at about 3% per year. TB incidence is falling at about 2% per year and 16% of TB cases die from the disease. Most deaths from TB could be prevented with early diagnosis and appropriate treatment. Millions of people are diagnosed and successfully treated for TB each year, averting millions of deaths [53 million 2000-2016], but there are still large gaps in detection and treatment (1).

In 2017, 6.4 million new cases of TB were reported, equivalent to 64% of the estimated incidence of 10 million; the latest treatment outcome data show a global treatment success rate of 82%, in 2016 (1). There were 464,633 reported cases of HIV-positive TB [46% of the estimated incidence], of whom 84% were on antiretroviral therapy [ART].

A total of 139,114 people were started on treatment for drug-resistant TB, only 29.9% of the estimated incidence; treatment success remains low, at 55% globally. Making large inroads into these gaps requires progress in a particular subset of high TB burden countries. Ten countries accounted for 80% of the total gap between TB incidence and reported cases; the top three were India [26%], Indonesia [11%] and Nigeria [9%]. Ten countries accounted for 75% of the incidence-treatment enrolment gap for MDR-TB/RR-TB; India and China accounted for 39% of the global gap. Most of the gaps related to HIV-associated TB were in the WHO African Region. TB preventive treatment is expanding, especially in the two priority risk groups of people living with HIV and children under 5. However, most people eligible for TB preventive treatment are not accessing it (1).

Financing for TB care and prevention has been increasing for more than 10 years, but funding gaps still exist [US\$ 2.3 billion in 2017]. Total health spending also falls short of the resources needed to achieve universal health coverage. Closing these gaps requires more resources from both domestic sources [especially in middle-income countries] and international donors [especially in low-income countries]. Broader influences on the TB epidemic include levels of poverty, HIV infection, undernutrition and smoking. Most high TB burden countries have major challenges ahead to reach SDG targets related to these and other determinants (1).

The pipelines for new diagnostics, drugs, treatment regimens and vaccines are slowly progressing. Increased investment in research and development is needed for there to be any chance of achieving the technological breakthroughs needed by 2025. The WHO Global Ministerial Conference on ending TB in the SDG era in November 2017 and the first UN General Assembly high-level meeting on TB in 2018 have provided historic opportunities to galvanize

Table 52.1: The End TB Strategy at a glance

Vision	A world free of TB – zero deaths, disease and suffering due to TB
Goal	End the global TB epidemic
Milestones for 2025	75% reduction in TB deaths [compared with 2015] 50% reduction in TB incidence rate [less than 55 TB cases per 100,000 population] No affected families facing catastrophic costs due to TB
Targets for 2035	95% reduction in TB deaths [compared with 2015] 90% reduction in TB incidence rate [less than 10 TB cases per 100,000 population] No affected families facing catastrophic costs due to TB

Principles
1. Government stewardship and accountability, with monitoring and evaluation
2. Strong coalition with civil society organisations and communities
3. Protection and promotion of human rights, ethics and equity
4. Adaptation of the strategy and targets at country level, with global collaboration

Pillars and components

1. Integrated, patient-centred care and prevention
  A. Early diagnosis of TB including universal drug-susceptibility testing; and systematic screening of contacts and high-risk groups
  B. Treatment of all people with TB including drug-resistant TB; and patient support
  C. Collaborative TB/HIV activities; and management of co-morbidities
  D. Preventive treatment of persons at high-risk; and vaccination against TB

2. Bold policies and supportive systems
  A. Political commitment with adequate resources for TB care and prevention
  B. Engagement of communities, civil society organisations, and public and private care providers
  C. Universal health coverage policy, and regulatory frameworks for case notification, vital registration, quality and rational use of medicines, and infection control
  D. Social protection, poverty alleviation and actions on other determinants of TB

3. Intensified research and innovation
  A. Discovery, development and rapid uptake of new tools, interventions and strategies
  B. Research to optimise implementation and impact, and promote innovations

TB = tuberculosis; HIV = human immunodeficiency virus

---

the political commitment needed to step up the battle against TB and put the world and individual countries on the path to ending the TB epidemic (2,3).

On 19 May 2014, the 67th World Health Assembly adopted the "Global strategy and targets for TB prevention, care and control after 2015" labelled subsequently as the "End TB Strategy" (4). Table 52.1 presents the "End TB Strategy" at a glance and the strategy is elaborated below.

WHO'S END TB STRATEGY

Vision, Goal, Milestones and Targets

The vision for the End TB Strategy is "a world free of TB", also expressed as "zero deaths, disease and suffering due to TB". The goal is to end the global TB epidemic by 2035. Ending the TB epidemic implies bringing the levels of TB in the whole world down to those already attained by many rich countries: less than 10 new TB cases per 100,000 population per year and TB deaths reduced by 95%. An additional target is that by 2020, no TB-affected person or family should face catastrophic costs due to TB care. Milestones that need to be reached before 2035 are also proposed for 2020, 2025,

and 2030. Table 52.2 presents key global indicators, milestones and targets for the new strategy (5).

Achievements with existing tools complemented by Universal Health Coverage [UHC] and social protection may not be sufficient to obtain the rate of decline required to achieve the 2035 targets. In particular, a new vaccine that is effective pre- and post-exposure and better diagnostics as well as safer and easier treatment for TB and LTBI will be needed. For such new tools to be available by 2025, greatly enhanced and immediate investments in research and development will be required. Figure 52.1 shows the projected acceleration of the decline in global TB incidence rates with optimisation of current tools combined with progress towards UHC and social protection from 2015, and the additional impact of new tools by 2025.

The Cross-cutting Principles of the Strategy

Government Stewardship and Accountability with Monitoring and Evaluation

The success of the End TB Strategy will depend on effective enhancement of the stewardship role of governments in

Table 52.2: Key indicators, milestones and targets for the post-2015 Global TB Strategy

	Milestones		Targets	
Indicators with baseline values for 2015	*2020*	*2025*	*2030*	*2035*
Percentage reduction in deaths due to TB [projected 2015 baseline: 1.3 million deaths]	35%	75%	90%	95%
Percentage and absolute reduction in TB incidence rate [projected 2015 baseline 110/100,000]	20% [<85/100,000]	50% [<55/100,000]	80% [<20/100,000]	90% [<10/100,000]
Percentage of affected families facing catastrophic costs due to TB [projected 2015 baseline: not yet available]	Zero	Zero	Zero	Zero
TB = tuberculosis				

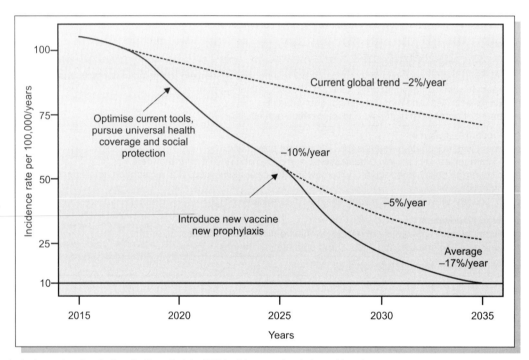

Figure 52.1: Projected acceleration in the decline of global TB incidence rates to target levels
TB = tuberculosis

engaging all stakeholders. To ensure accountability, regular monitoring and evaluation needs to be expanded to set and pursue ambitious national targets and indicators. Table 52.3 presents an illustrative list of key global indicators that should be considered and adapted for national use.

Strong Coalition with Civil Society and Communities

The affected communities must also be an integral part of the solution. Community representatives and civil society must be enabled to engage actively in expressing needs, programme planning and design, service delivery, patient support and monitoring and evaluation, and advocacy. A national coalition can also help drive greater action on the determinants of the TB epidemic.

Protection and Promotion of Human Rights, Ethics and Equity

The End TB Strategy explicitly addresses human rights, ethics and equity (6). This strategy is built on a rights-based approach that ensures protection of human rights and promotion of rights-enhancing policies and interventions. These include engagement of affected persons and communities in facilitating implementation of all pillars and components of the draft strategy with special attention to key affected populations. TB care and prevention demand clarity on ethical values and sometimes pose ethical dilemmas which need to be addressed in design and implementation of services. The strategy promotes equity through identification of the risks, needs and demands of those affected, to enable equal opportunities to prevent disease transmission, equal

Table 52.3: Illustrative list of key indicators for the draft post-2015 Global TB Strategy

Component	Illustrative indicators
Pillar one: Integrated, patient-centred care and prevention	
A. Early diagnosis	Percentage of people with suspected TB tested using WHO recommended rapid diagnostics Percentage of all TB patients for whom results of drug susceptibility testing were available Percentage of eligible index cases of TB for which contact investigations were undertaken
B. Treatment	TB treatment success rate Percentage of patients with drug-resistant TB enrolled on second-line treatment
C. TB/HIV and co-morbidities	Percentage of TB patients screened for HIV Percentage of HIV-positive TB patients on antiretroviral therapy
D. Preventive treatment	Percentage of eligible people living with HIV and children aged under-five who are contacts of TB patients being treated for latent TB infection
Pillar two: Bold policies and supportive systems	
A. Government commitment	Percentage of annual budget defined in TB national strategic plans that is funded
B. Engagement of communities and providers	Percentage of diagnosed TB cases that were notified
C. Universal health coverage and regulatory frameworks	Percentage of population without catastrophic health expenditures Percentage of countries with a certified TB surveillance system
D. Social protection, social determinants	Percentage of affected families facing catastrophic costs due to TB Percentage of population without undernutrition
Pillar three: Intensified research and innovation	
A. Discovery	Percentage of desirable number of candidates in the pipelines of new diagnostics, drugs and vaccines for TB
B. Implementation	Percentage of countries introducing and scaling-up new diagnostics, drugs or vaccines

TB = tuberculosis; HIV = human immunodeficiency virus; WHO = World Health Organization

access to diagnosis and treatment services, and equal access to means to prevent associated social and economic impacts.

Adaptation of the Strategy at Country Level, with Global Collaboration

The End TB Strategy must be adapted to diverse country settings and epidemics and requires a comprehensive national strategic plan. Prioritisation of interventions should be undertaken based on local needs and capacities. This includes mapping of people at a greater risk, understanding of socioeconomic contexts of vulnerable populations, and understanding the health system context including underserved areas. Ending the global epidemic requires recognising its global reach and enabling close collaboration among countries, including to address cross-border spread and the special needs of migrants.

Pillars and Components

Pillar One: Integrated, Patient-centred Care and Prevention

Pillar one comprises patient-centred interventions required for TB care and prevention. The national TB programme, or equivalent, needs to engage and coordinate closely with other public health programmes, social support programmes, public and private health care providers, non-governmental and civil society organisations, communities and patient associations in order to help ensure provision of high-

quality, integrated, patient-centred TB care and prevention across the health system.

Component 1A: Early diagnosis of TB including universal drug susceptibility testing, and systematic screening of contacts and high-risk groups Ensuring universal access to early and accurate diagnosis of TB and drug-resistance will require strengthening and expansion of a network of diagnostic facilities enabling easy access to new rapid molecular tests and systematic screening in selected high-risk groups. Further, additional screening tools such as a chest radiograph may facilitate referral for diagnosis of bacteriologically negative TB, extra-pulmonary TB [EPTB] and TB in children.

The burden of undetected TB is large in many settings, especially in high-risk groups. Mapping of high-risk groups and carefully planned systematic screening for active disease among them may improve early case detection (7). Contacts of people with TB, especially children aged five years or less, people living with HIV [PLHIV], and workers exposed to silica dust should always be screened for active TB (8). Other risk-groups should be considered for screening based on assessment of epidemiology, resources, system capacity and feasibility of approaches.

Component 1B: Treatment of all people with TB including drug-resistant TB, and patient support New policies incorporating molecular diagnostics will help to strengthen management of smear-negative pulmonary TB and EPTB as well as TB among children (9). Globally, about 4% of new

TB patients and about 20% of patients receiving retreatment have MDR-TB. Providing universal access to services for DR-TB will require a rapid scale up of diagnosis and treatment services. New models of delivering patient-centred treatment will need to be devised. Ambulatory, community-based services should be given preference over hospitalisation, which should be limited to severe cases (10).

The proportion of DR-TB patients successfully completing treatment remains far too low on average due to a range of factors. New safer, affordable and more effective medicines allowing treatment regimens that are shorter in duration and easier to administer are key to improving treatment outcomes. Strengthened pharmacovigilance capacity is needed. Interventions to improve quality of life for patients while enabling adherence to treatment include management of adverse drug reactions and events, access to comprehensive palliative and end-of-life care, measures to alleviate stigmatisation and discrimination, and social support and protection. Strong infection control practices need to be in place in all health services providing TB care (11).

TB is an important cause of morbidity and mortality among children. In countries with a high prevalence of TB, women of child-bearing age also carry a heavy burden of the disease. Maternal TB associated with HIV is a risk factor for transmission of TB to the infant and is associated with premature delivery, low birth-weight of neonates, and higher maternal and infant mortality. NTPs need to address systematically the challenges of caring for children with TB, and child contacts of adult TB patients. These may include, for instance, developing and using child-friendly formulation of medicines, and family-centred approaches to improve adherence. Proper management of TB among children requires development of affordable and sensitive diagnostic tests that are not based on sputum specimens. TB care should be integrated within community based maternal and child health services (12).

Patient-centred care and support, sensitive and responsive to patients' educational, emotional and material needs, is fundamental to the End TB Strategy. Treatment and support must also extend beyond cure to address any sequelae associated with TB. Examples of patient-centred support include providing treatment partners trained by health services and acceptable to the patient, access to social protection, use of eHealth technology, and patient peer groups to enable exchange information and experience.

Component 1C: Collaborative TB/HIV activities; and management of co-morbidities

HIV-associated TB accounts for about one quarter of all TB deaths and a quarter of all deaths due to acquired immunodeficiency syndrome [AIDS]. The vast majority of these cases and deaths are in the African and South-East Asia regions. All TB patients living with HIV should receive ART. Integrated TB and HIV service delivery has been shown to increase the likelihood that a TB patient will receive ART, shorten the time to treatment initiation, and reduce mortality by almost 40%. Reducing delays in diagnosis, using new diagnostic tools and instituting prompt treatment can improve textbook outcomes among PLHIV.

TB and HIV care should be further integrated with services for maternal and child health and prevention of mother-to-child transmission of HIV in high-burden settings (13).

Several non-communicable diseases and other health conditions including diabetes mellitus, undernutrition, silicosis, as well as smoking, harmful alcohol and drug use, and a range of immune-compromising disorders and treatments are risk factors for TB. Presence of co-morbidities may complicate TB management and result in poor treatment outcomes. Conversely, TB may worsen or complicate management of other diseases. Therefore, as a part of basic and coordinated clinical management, people diagnosed with TB should be routinely assessed for relevant comorbidities, based on local epidemiology (14).

Component 1D: Preventive treatment of persons at high-risk; and vaccination against TB

LTBI is diagnosed by a tuberculin skin test [TST] or interferon-γ release assay [IGRA]. However, these tests cannot predict which persons will develop active TB disease. Isoniazid preventive therapy is recommended for the treatment of LTBI among PLHIV, close contacts of patients with TB and miners exposed to silica dust. Management of LTBI in people with a high-risk of developing active TB is an essential component of TB elimination, particularly in low TB-incidence countries (15).

The bacille Calmette-Guerin [BCG] vaccination prevents disseminated disease including TB, meningitis and miliary TB, which are associated with high mortality in infants and young children. However, its preventive efficacy against pulmonary TB, which varies among populations, is only about 50%. BCG vaccination soon after birth should continue to be given to all infants except for those persons with HIV living in high TB prevalence settings.

Pillar Two: Bold Policies and Supportive Systems

The second pillar encompasses strategic actions that will enable care delivery as well as wider action to prevent TB through addressing social determinants. These include actions by and beyond NTPs, from across ministries and departments. This will require a well-resourced, organised and coordinated health system response backed up by supportive health policies. In parallel, swift progress is essential to achieve UHC and social protection while also strengthening regulatory systems. NTPs, their partners and those overseeing the programmes need to engage actively in the setting of broader social and economic development agenda that reduce poverty and vulnerability to disease. Eliciting actions from across diverse ministries will require commitment and stewardship from the highest levels of government.

Component 2A: Political commitment with adequate resources for TB care and prevention

Scaling up and sustaining interventions for TB care and prevention will require high-level political commitment along with adequate financial and human resources for central coordination and capacity across the system. This must lead to, as a first step, development of a national strategic plan embedded in a national health sector plan. A national TB strategic plan should be ambitious and comprehensive. Coordinated efforts are required to mobilise additional resources to fund truly ambitious national strategic plans with a progressive increase in domestic funding.

Component 2B: Engagement of communities, civil society organisations, and all public and private care providers

Informed communities can help identify people with suspected TB, refer them for diagnosis, provide support during treatment and help to alleviate stigmatisation and discrimination. Civil society organisations may have the key competencies required to reach out to vulnerable groups, mobilise communities, channel information, and help create demand for care. NTPs should engage with civil society organisations and communities in policy development and planning, in service delivery, as well as in programme monitoring and evaluation (16).

In many countries, TB care is delivered by diverse public, voluntary, private and corporate care providers. The private providers include pharmacists, formal and informal practitioners, non-governmental and faith-based organisations as well as private and corporate hospitals. Several public sector providers outside the purview of NTPs also provide TB care. These include large public hospitals, social security organisations, prison health services and military health services. Leaving a large proportion of care providers out of an organised response to TB has contributed to stagnating case notification, inappropriate TB management, and irrational use of TB medicines leading to the spread of DR-TB. NTPs must scale up country-specific public–private mix approaches already working well in many countries. To this effect, close collaboration with health professionals' associations will be essential (17). The *International Standards for TB Care*, other tools and guidelines developed by WHO as well as modern information and communication technology platforms can help increase effective involvement (18).

Component 2C: Universal health coverage policy, and regulatory frameworks for case notification, vital registration, quality and rational use of medicines, and infection control

UHC is defined as "the situation where all people are able to use the quality health services that they need and do not suffer financial hardship paying for them". UHC is achieved through adequate, fair and sustainable prepayment financing of health care with full geographical coverage, combined with effective service quality assurance and monitoring and evaluation. For TB specifically, this implies expanding: [i] the array of quality health services provided in line with this strategy; [ii] financing for all direct and indirect health care costs associated with diagnosis, treatment and prevention; and [iii] access for all populations, especially vulnerable groups (19).

National policy on UHC and essential regulatory frameworks are powerful levers for TB response. A comprehensive and effectively enforced infectious disease legislation, that includes compulsory notification of TB cases by all health care providers, is essential. Most countries with a high burden of TB do not have essential vital registration systems and the quality of information about the number of deaths due to TB is often inadequate. Efforts underway to broadly strengthen vital registration systems in low-income countries need to be supported (20).

Poor quality TB medicines put patients at great risk. Irrational prescription of treatment regimens leads to poor treatment outcomes and may cause drug resistance. Use of inappropriate diagnostics, such as, serological tests leads to inaccurate diagnosis. Regulation and adequate resources for enforcement are required for the registration, importation and manufacturing of medical products. Appropriate regulation is also required to ensure effective infection control in health care services and other settings where the risk of disease transmission is high (21). Calls for coherent national prevention of antimicrobial resistance can further bolster support for such measures.

Component 2D: Social protection, poverty alleviation and actions on other determinants of TB

A large proportion of households affected by TB face a catastrophic economic burden related to the direct and indirect costs of illness and health care. Its negative consequences often extend to the family of the persons ill with TB. Even when TB diagnosis and treatment is offered free of charge, social protection measures are needed to alleviate the burden of income loss and non-medical costs of seeking and staying in care.

Social protection should cover the needs associated with TB through mechanisms such as: [i] schemes for compensating the financial burden associated with illness such as sickness insurance, disability pension, social welfare payments, other cash transfers, vouchers or food packages; [ii] legislation to protect people with TB from discrimination such as expulsion from workplaces, educational or health institutions, transport systems or housing; and [iii] instruments to protect and promote human rights, including addressing stigma and discrimination, with special attention to gender, ethnicity, and protection of vulnerable groups. These instruments should include capacity-building for affected communities to be able to express their needs and protect their rights, and to call to account those who impinge on human rights, as well as those who are responsible for protecting those rights.

Actions on the determinants of ill health through approaches that ensure "health-in-all-policies" will immensely benefit TB care and prevention. Such actions include, for example: [i] pursuing overarching poverty reduction strategies and expanding social protection; [ii] improving living and working conditions and reducing food insecurity; [iii] addressing the health issues of migrants and strengthening cross-border collaboration; [iv] involving diverse stakeholders, including TB affected communities, in mapping the likely local social determinants of TB; and [v] preventing direct risk factors for TB, including smoking and harmful use of alcohol and drugs, and promoting healthy diets, as well as proper clinical care for co-morbidities such as diabetes mellitus.

Pillar Three: Intensified Research and Innovation

Ending the TB epidemic will require substantial investments in the development of novel diagnostic, treatment and prevention tools, and for ensuring their accessibility and optimal uptake in countries alongside better and wider use of existing technologies. This will be possible only through increased investments and effective engagement of the broader National Health Research Institutions, TB Programmes, civil society, funders and policy makers. An International Roadmap for TB Research has outlined priority areas for future scientific investment across the research continuum (21).

Component 3A: Discovery, development and rapid uptake of new tools, interventions and strategies Since 2007, several new tests and diagnostic approaches have been endorsed by WHO. However, an accurate and rapid point-of-care test that is usable in field conditions is still missing. This requires greater investments in biomarker research, and overcoming difficulties in transforming sophisticated laboratory technologies into robust, accurate and affordable point-of-care platforms.

The pipeline of new drugs has expanded substantially over the last decade. There are nearly a dozen new or repurposed TB drugs under clinical investigation. As mentioned above, two new TB drugs have been introduced for the treatment of MDR-TB (22). Novel regimens, including new or repurposed medicines and adjuvant and supportive therapies, are being investigated.

Globally, more than 2000 million people are estimated to be infected with *Mycobacterium tuberculosis* [*Mtb*], but only 5% to 15% of those infected will develop active disease during their lifetime. Ending the TB epidemic will require eliminating this pool of infection. Research is needed to develop new diagnostic tests to identify people with LTBI who are likely to develop TB disease. Further, treatment strategies that could be safely used to prevent development of TB in latently infected persons will also need to be identified. Moreover, research will be required to investigate the impact and safety of targeted and mass preventive strategies (21).

Currently, there are 12 vaccine candidates in clinical trials (23). A post-exposure vaccine that prevents the disease in latently infected individuals will be essential to eliminating TB in the foreseeable future.

Component 3B: Research to optimise implementation and impact; and promote innovations Research can identify bottlenecks and help devise better policies and strengthen health systems and service delivery. Research is also critical to improve the speed of roll-out of new strategies and tools. An enabling environment for performing programme-based research and translating results into policy and practice needs to be reinforced, especially in low-income countries.

ADAPTING AND IMPLEMENTING THE STRATEGY

A first recommended step in adapting and implementing the strategy is to hold inclusive national consultations with a wide range of stakeholders, including communities most affected by TB, in order to consider, adopt and prepare for adaptation of the strategy. The scope of existing TB advisory panels will need to be expanded to include a wider range of capacities from civil society and from the fields of finance and development policy, human rights, social protection, regulation, health technology assessment, the social sciences, and communications. National vision statements extending to 2030 or 2035 should be devised and medium-term plans for the next five to ten years should be drafted. Proper mapping should provide important information such as population groups most affected by the disease and most at risk of developing it; age and sex characteristics and trends; prevalence of different forms of TB and dominant comorbidities, important urban–rural variations; distribution and types of care providers; health financing, access and social protection schemes and their current and their potential implications for TB care and prevention. Where data is lacking, expert and stakeholder consultations and assessments to estimate burdens and system capacities will be needed. WHO is currently in the process of developing guidance for countries to help implement the End TB Strategy.

MEASURING PROGRESS AND IMPACT

Target setting and monitoring of progress across the components of the strategy are essential. Monitoring should be done routinely using standardised methods based on data with documented quality (20). Table 52.3 provides examples of the indicators that can be considered. Given the overarching targets of the End TB Strategy, particular attention to measurement of trends in mortality and incidence is required. WHO provides a number of tools to assist in improving routine TB reporting, conducting TB prevalence surveys and utilising vital registration data, assessing under-reporting of cases and estimating incidence. Global financing and technical partners are keen to help improve TB monitoring, evaluation and impact measurement (24-27). Such data will be critical to measure progress and drive commitment to move faster and with increased impact.

ACKNOWLEDGEMENT

This chapter is an abridged updated version of the WHO document on "Global strategy and targets for tuberculosis prevention, care and control after 2015" prepared by the Global TB Programme.

REFERENCES

1. World Health Organization. Global tuberculosis report 2018. Geneva: World Health Organization; 2018.
2. The WHO Global Ministerial Conference on ending TB in the SDG era; 2017. Available URL: http://www.who.int/conferences/tb-global-ministerial-conference/en/. Accessed on September 12, 2018.
3. UN General Assembly High-Level meeting on ending TB; 2018. Available at URL: http://www.who.int/tb/features_archive/

UNGA_HLM_ending_TB/en/. Accessed on September 12, 2018.

4. World Health Organization. Documentation for World Health Assembly 67. http://apps.who.int/gb/ebwha/pdf_files/WHA67/A67_11-en.pdf Accessed Accessed on September 12, 2018.

5. Raviglione M, Ditiu L. Setting new targets in the fight against tuberculosis. Nat Med 2013;19:263.

6. World Health Organization. Guidance on ethics of tuberculosis prevention, care and control. WHO/HTM/TB/2010.6. Geneva: World Health Organization; 2010.

7. World Health Organization. Systematic screening for active tuberculosis - principles and recommendations. WHO/HTM/TB.2013.04. Geneva: World Health Organization; 2013.

8. World Health Organization. Recommendations for investigating the contacts of persons with infectious tuberculosis in low- and middle-income countries. WHO/HTM/TB/2012.9. Geneva: World Health Organization; 2012.

9. World Health Organization. Rapid implementation of the Xpert® MTB/RIF diagnostic test: technical, operational 'how-to' and practical considerations. Geneva: World Health Organization; 2011.

10. World Health Organization. Guidelines for the programmatic management of drug-resistant tuberculosis. WHO/HTM/TB/2011.6. Geneva: World Health Organization; 2011.

11. World Health Organization. WHO policy on TB infection control in health-care facilities, congregate settings and households. WHO/HTM/TB/2009.419. Geneva: World Health Organization; 2009.

12. World Health Organization. Roadmap for childhood tuberculosis: towards zero deaths. WHO/HTM/TB/2013.12. Geneva: World Health Organization; 2013.

13. World Health Organization. WHO policy on collaborative TB/HIV activities: guidelines for national programmes and other stakeholders. WHO/HTM/TB/2012.1. Geneva: World Health Organization; 2012.

14. Marais BJ, Lönnroth K, Lawn SD, Migliori GB, Mwaba P, Glaziou P, et al. Tuberculosis co-morbidity with infectious and non-communicable diseases: integrating health services and control efforts. Lancet Infect Dis 2013;13:436-48.

15. World Health Organization. Guidelines on the management of latent tuberculosis infection. WHO/HTM/TB/2015.01. Geneva: World Health Organization; 2014.

16. World health Organization. Engage-TB: integrating community-based tuberculosis activities into the work of nongovernmental and other civil society organizations: implementation manual. WHO/HTM/TB/2013.10. Geneva: World Health Organization; 2013.

17. World Health Organization. Public-private mix for TB care and control: a toolkit. WHO/HTM/TB/2010.12. Geneva: World Health Organization; 2010.

18. Hopewell P, Fair E, Uplekar M. Updating the International Standards for Tuberculosis Care- Entering the Era of Molecular Diagnostics. Ann Am Thorac Soc 2014;11:277-85.

19. Lönnroth K, Glaziou P, Weil D, Floyd K, Uplekar M, Raviglione M. Beyond UHC: monitoring health and social protection coverage in the context of tuberculosis care and prevention. PLoS Med 2014;11:e1001693.

20. World Health Organization. Standards and benchmarks for tuberculosis surveillance and vital registration systems checklist and user guide. WHO/HTM/TB/2014.2. Geneva: World Health Organization; 2014.

21. World Health Organization. An international roadmap for tuberculosis research: towards a world free of tuberculosis. Geneva: World Health Organization; 2011.

22. Treatment Action Group, 2016. Drugs, diagnostics, vaccines, preventive technologies, research toward a cure, and immune-based and gene therapies in development. Available at URL: http://www.pipelinereport.org/2015/tb-diagnostics. Accessed on September 12, 2018.

23. World Health Organization. The use of delamanid in the treatment of multidrug-resistant tuberculosis: interim policy guidance. WHO/HTM/TB2014.23. Geneva: World Health Organization; 2014.

24. World Health Organization. WHO Global Task Force on TB impact measurement. Available at URL: http://www.who.int/tb/advisory_bodies/impact_measurement_taskforce/en/.Accessed on September 12, 2018.

25. Uplekar M. Implementing the End TB Strategy: Well begun will be half done. Indian J Tuberc 2015;62:61-3.

26. Uplekar M, Weil D, Lonnroth K, Jaramillo E, Lienhardt C, Dias HM, et al; WHO's Global TB Programme.. WHO's new end TB strategy. Lancet 2015;385:1799-801.

27. Lönnroth K, Raviglione M. The WHO's new End TB Strategy in the post-2015 era of the Sustainable Development Goals. Trans R Soc Trop Med Hyg 2016;110:148-50.

The Revised National Tuberculosis Control Programme

Jagdish Prasad, Sunil D Khaparde, KS Sachdeva

INTRODUCTION

Tuberculosis [TB] remains a serious public health problem in India, accounting for nearly one-fourth of the global burden (1). India has more people with active TB than any other country in the world. Each year, in India an estimated 2.74 million people develops TB disease and approximately 410,000 people die from TB (1).

Most TB patients are in the economically productive age group. A study of mortality in India has estimated that TB is among the top 4 causes of death between the ages of 30 and 69, with an impact similar to cancer (2). The socio-economic impact of TB in India is devastating and India continues to incur huge costs due to TB amounting to nearly US$ 350 billion between 2006 and 2015 (3). Studies indicate that around 10% of children have to leave school as a result of their parents' TB (4).

Ironically, TB persists as a major health problem in spite of the fact that many of the basic scientific precepts of the World Health Organization [WHO] recommended DOTS programme were discovered in India.

HISTORY OF TUBERCULOSIS CONTROL IN INDIA

TB control in India has a long and illustrious past (5-7). In the early 1900s, TB was recognised as a serious problem and the first open air sanitarium for treatment and isolation of TB patients was founded in 1906 in Tiluania, near Ajmer. The main line of treatment relied on good food, open air and dry climate. Without effective treatment, progress in TB control was minimal and despite an active sanatorium movement, millions of TB patients remained largely untreated. By 1920, public opinion gained a momentum for effective measures for control of TB. India became a member of the International Union against Tuberculosis [IUAT] in 1929 and the anti-TB movement grew with support from the government.

In 1946, the Bhore Committee estimated that about 2.5 million patients required treatment in the country while only 6000 beds were available (8). Work with Bacillus Calmette-Guérin [BCG] started in India as a pilot project in two centres in 1948 and in 1951 mass BCG vaccination campaigns were introduced.

In the 1950s and 1960s, research at the Tuberculosis Research Centre [TRC] in Chennai demonstrated that domiciliary treatment was as effective as and less costly than in-patient treatment for TB (9). Additionally, use of directly observed treatment [DOT], in which patients are observed taking their medications, was shown to be essential (10). These seminal findings led to a radical change in thinking regarding TB care worldwide (11). Indian researchers also pioneered the efficacy of intermittent treatment where medications were successfully given 2-3 times a week (12). Improved case-finding using microscopy among patients attending health services was also demonstrated in India (13,14).

In 1962, these and other path-breaking sociological and epidemiological studies led to the establishment of the National Tuberculosis Control Programme [NTP] in 1962. The NTP was implemented nationwide in a phased manner through the establishment of District TB Centres, urban chest clinics and in-patient beds. Short-course chemotherapy [SCC] was introduced in 1985. Despite this intervention, ensuring drug supply and adherence continued to be a problem and programme goals to control TB were not achieved.

In 1992, a comprehensive joint review of the TB programme in India by members of several organizations including the Government of India, WHO and Swedish International Development Agency found that less than half the patients with TB received an accurate diagnosis and that less than half of those were effectively treated (15). Importantly, the NTP had not made significant epidemiological impact on the prevalence of TB. Further, the human immunodeficiency virus [HIV]-acquired immunodeficiency syndrome [AIDS] epidemic and the spread of multi-drug resistance tuberculosis [MDR-TB] were threatening to worsen the situation. In order to overcome these limitations, in 1993 the Government of India [GOI] decided to reenergise the NTP, with assistance from international agencies. The Revised National TB Control Programme [RNTCP] thus formulated, adopted the internationally recommended DOTS strategy, as the most systematic and cost-effective approach for TB control in India.

The RNTCP began in October 1993 as a pilot project. Large-scale implementation of the RNTCP began in 1997 [Figure 53.1]. The systems were further strengthened and the programme was scaled up for national coverage in 2006. The RNTCP encompasses the five principles of the DOTS strategy. These five principles are: [i] political and administrative commitment; [ii] good quality diagnosis by sputum smear microscopy; [iii] uninterrupted supply of good quality drugs; [iv] directly observed treatment; and [v] systematic monitoring and accountability. The key objectives of the RNTCP were to achieve and maintain at least 85% cure rate among the new smear-positive cases initiated on treatment, and thereafter a case detection rate of at least 70% of such cases. The RNTCP was built on the infrastructure and systems built through the NTP.

The programme has made rapid strides ever since its implementation and has consistently been achieving global benchmarks of case detection and treatment success rates since 2007 [Figure 53.2]. Since inception of RNTCP in 1997 and up to December 2017, more than 20 million patients were initiated on treatment and about 3.5 million additional lives have been saved.

RNTCP has achieved Millennium Development Goals for TB and has prepared the National Strategic Plan [NSP] [2017-25] to achieve Sustainable Development Goals for TB by 2025, five years ahead of the Global Timelines. Goal of NSP is to achieve a rapid decline in burden of TB, morbidity and mortality while working towards ending TB in India by 2025. In the 12th plan period, RNTCP achieved the annual decline in new incident TB cases of around 1%-2%. Over the period of the NSP 2017-25, RNTCP aims to accelerate the decline by 10%-12% annually to achieve the goal by 2025.

STRUCTURE OF REVISED NATIONAL TUBERCULOSIS CONTROL PROGRAMME

The structure of RNTCP comprises of five levels: National level, State level, District level, Sub-district level and Peripheral health institution level [Figure 53.3].

National Level

At the central level, the RNTCP is managed by the Central TB Division [CTD] of the under the Ministry of Health and Family Welfare [MoHFW]. The respective Joint Secretary of the MoHFW looks after the financial and administrative aspects of the programme A national programme manager— Deputy Director General-TB [DDG-TB], is in-charge of RNTCP. The CTD is assisted by 6 national level institutes, namely the NTI in Bengaluru, the NIRT in Chennai, the National Institute of TB and Respiratory Diseases [NITRD] in New Delhi, National Japanese Leprosy Mission for Asia [JALMA] Institute of Leprosy and other Mycobacterial Diseases in Agra, Bhopal Memorial Hospital and Research Centre [BMHRC], Bhopal and Regional Medical Research Centre [RMRC], Bhubaneshwar.

State Level

At the State level, the State Tuberculosis Officer [STO] is responsible for the planning, training, supervising and

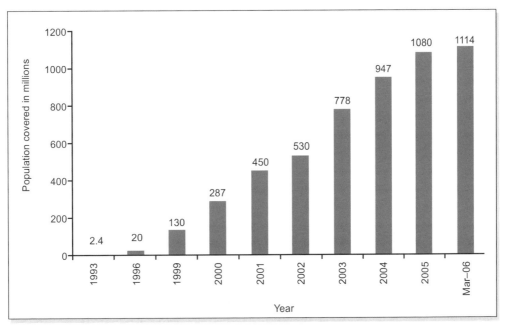

Figure 53.1: Revised National Tuberculosis Control Programme geographical coverage: India

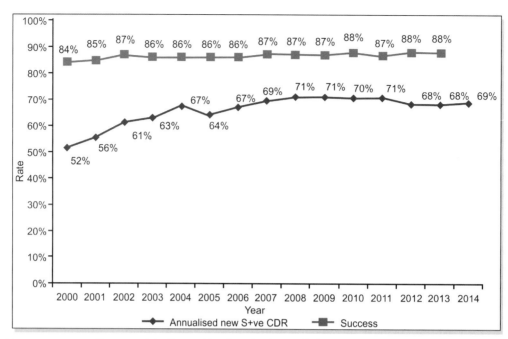

Figure 53.2: Trend in new smear-positive case detection and treatment outcome: India
S+ve = smear-positive; CDR = case-detection rate

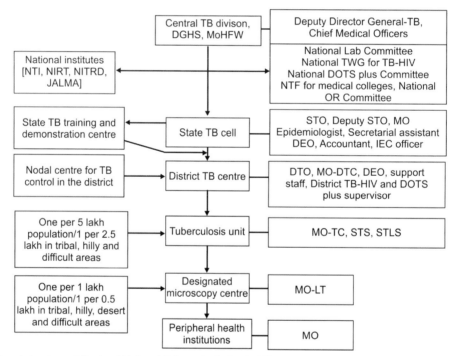

Figure 53.3: Organisational structure of Revised National Tuberculosis Control Programme
TB = tuberculosis; DGHS = Directorate General of Health Services; MoHFW = Ministry of Health and Family Welfare; NTI = National Tuberculosis Institute, Bengaluru; NIRT = National Institute for Research in Tuberculosis, Chennai; NITRD = National Institute of TB Respiratory Diseases, New Delhi; JALMA = National Japanese Leprosy Mission for Asia Institute of Leprosy and other Mycobacterial Diseases, Agra; TWG = Technical Working Group; HIV = human immunodeficiency virus; STO = State TB Officer; MO = Medical Officer; DEO = Data Entry Operator; IEC = Information, Education and Communication; DTO = District TB Officer; lakh = 100,000; MOTC = Medical Officer TB Control; STS = Senior Treatment Supervisor; STLS = Senior Tuberculosis Laboratory Supervisor; LT = Laboratory Technician.

monitoring of the programme in their respective states as per the guidelines of the State Health Society and CTD. The STO, based at the State TB Cell, is answerable to their respective State Government, whilst implementing the technical policies and guidelines issued by the CTD. The State TB Cells [STC] have been provided with equipment, infrastructure and

RNTCP contractual staff to carry out its functions. In most of the larger states, a State TB Training and Demonstration Centre [STDC] support's the State TB Cell. The STDC has 3 units: a training unit, supervision and monitoring unit and an Intermediate Reference Laboratory [IRL]. There is State Drug Store [SDS] for the effective management of anti-TB drug logistics. One SDS per 50 million populations is established in all larger states.

District Level

The District Tuberculosis Centre [DTC] is the nodal point for all TB control activities in the district. In RNTCP, the primary role of the DTC has shifted from clinical to managerial functions. The District TB Officer [DTO] at the DTC has the overall responsibility of management of RNTCP at the district level as per the programme guidelines and the guidance of the District Health Society. The DTO is also responsible for involvement of other sectors in RNTCP and is assisted by a Medical Officer, District Programme Coordinator, District PPM Coordinator, District DR-TB/HIV-TB supervisor, and other Office Operation staff.

Sub-District Level [Tuberculosis Unit Level]

The creation of a sub-district level Tuberculosis Unit [TU] is a major organizational change in RNTCP. The TU consists of a designated Medical Officer-Tuberculosis Control [MO-TC] who does RNTCP work in addition to other responsibilities. There are two full-time RNTCP contractual supervisory staff exclusively for TB work—a Senior TB Treatment Supervisor [STS] and a Senior TB Laboratory Supervisor [STLS]. These TUs cover a population of approximately 150,000-250,000 population [largely aligned with NHM Blocks]. The MO-TC at the TU has the overall responsibility of management of RNTCP at the sub-district level, assisted by the STS and STLS.

There is one RNTCP Designated Microscopy Centre [DMC] for every 100,000 population under a TU [50,000 in tribal, desert, remote and hilly regions]. DMCs are also established in Medical Colleges, Corporate hospitals, ESI and Railway health facilities, NGOs, private hospitals, etc., depending upon the requirement.

Peripheral Health Institutions

For the purpose of RNTCP, a peripheral health institution [PHI] is a health facility which is manned by at least a medical officer. At this level, there are dispensaries, peripheral health clinics, community health centres, referral hospitals, major hospitals, specialty clinics or hospitals [including other health facilities], TB hospitals, and Medical Colleges within the respective district. All health facilities in the private and non-governmental organisation [NGO] sectors participating in RNTCP are also considered as PHIs by the programme. Some of these PHIs also function as DMCs. Peripheral health institutions undertake TB case-finding and treatment activities as a part of the general health services. In this regard, they are supervised by the TU contractual paramedical staff [STS and STLS].

CASE FINDING AND DIAGNOSTICS

Once a patient is diagnosed and appropriately treated they rapidly become non-infectious. Thus, prompt case finding and treatment is the principal means of controlling transmission and reducing TB incidence.

Direct sputum smear microscopy by Ziehl-Neelsen/fluorescence staining are the primary case detection tool in RNTCP for patients with infectious TB and is also for monitoring their response to treatment. From 2018, under Programmatic Management of Drug-resistant TB [PMDT] (16), "universal DST" and molecular testing {cartridge-based nucleic acid amplification test [CBNAAT]}, is being offered to all patients as per the new diagnostic algorithm under the programme [Figures 42.5A and 42.5B]. Chest radiograph is obtained simultaneously to avoid any delay in diagnosis of TB patients with smear-negative results.

Chest radiograph is obtained simultaneously to avoid any delay in diagnosis of TB patients with smear-negative results. Extra-pulmonary TB is also diagnosed based on other tests like cytology, histopathology, CBNAAT, radio-imaging, and other supportive tests.

Enormous efforts and achievements were highlighted in case finding under the 11th Five-Year Plan [2006-2011]. In the 12th plan period, India's Revised National TB Control Programme notified about 70 lakh [lakh = 100,000] TB patients [Figure 53.4]. The programme is exploring significant new opportunities for improvement of case finding at an early stage and achieve "Universal Access". Over the period of the NSP 2017-25, RNTCP aims to notify 260 lakh [lakh = 100,000] TB patients in 8 years including public and private sector.

Strategies to Augment Case Finding

The following strategies have been adopted by RNTCP in 12th Five-Year Plan to increase notification under the programme.

Screening clinically vulnerable and socially vulnerable risk groups who are known to suffer disproportionately from TB: The clinically vulnerable population includes PLHA, household contacts of TB cases, malnourished children, diabetics, tobacco users, and those living in houses with indoor air pollution. Socially vulnerable groups include backward and tribal, migrants and urban slum dwellers, prisoners, occupational high risk groups, etc. These groups have been prioritized for systematic active TB case finding and linking with diagnostic facilities.

Ensuring use of rapid diagnostic technologies: CBNAAT provides a diagnosis of TB and rifampicin resistance within 2 hours. At present, CBNAAT laboratories are functional, covering all districts of the country.

RNTCP has successfully field tested implementation of TrueNat—an indigenous rapid molecular diagnostic technique which gives results in less than an hour, battery

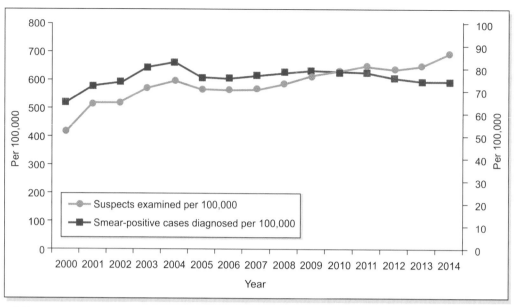

Figure 53.4: Rate of TB suspects examined per 100,000 population and smear-positive cases diagnosed, corrected for population covered under Revised National Tuberculosis Control Programme
TB = tuberculosis

operated, and with minimal infrastructure requirement. Established systems for programme-based evaluation of new TB diagnostics, and support the establishment of minimum performance standards for licensure of TB diagnostic tests. Systems developed and deployed for notifying patients at TB diagnosis from all sources.

Laboratory Network

The RNTCP laboratory network is composed of a three-tier system with National Level Reference Laboratories [NRLs], state level IRLs, and peripheral level laboratories as DMCs [Figure 53.5]. At the top of laboratory network hierarchy are six designated NRLs at national level under National institutes.

National reference laboratories assist the programme on technical issues, to develop laboratory guidelines, standard operating procedures [SOPs], conduct trainings to state level IRL, conduct annual on-site evaluation/supervisory visits to laboratories for microscopy, culture and drug-susceptibility testing [C and DST], and for providing support for overall laboratory quality improvement. National reference laboratories are quality assured through the supra-reference laboratory [SRL] coordinating laboratory at Antwerp, Belgium. All NRLs are also participating in evaluation of newer diagnostic technologies and research activities.

There is at least one IRL per major state. Each IRL conducts on-site evaluation visits to districts for panel testing of STLS at each DTC at least once a year to ensures the proficiency of staff performing smear microscopy activities by providing training to LTs and STLS. Intermediate reference laboratory also provides technical support to C and DST laboratories in medical college, private and NGO, other laboratories under RNTCP. The IRL also visit CBNAAT sites across the state, monitor performance and provide

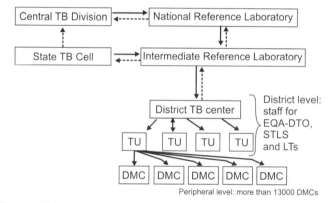

Figure 53.5: Revised National Tuberculosis Control Programme hierarchical lab network
TB = tuberculosis; TU = Tuberculosis Unit; DMC = designated microscopy centre; EQA = external quality assurance; DTO = District TB Officer; STLS = Senior TB Laboratory Supervisor; LT = laboratory technician

feedback for the same. Intermediate reference laboratory also monitors the quality assurance of DST by solid, liquid, line probe assay [LPA] and CBNAAT. There are 28 IRLs, at the State level, at least one per major state, and one additional IRL for larger states having more than 100 million population.

A network of 1135 CBNAAT laboratories have been established across the country, covering every district for access to rapid molecular diagnostic test for diagnosis of TB and DR-TB at decentralised level.

The most peripheral laboratory under the RNTCP network is the DMC. Revised national tuberculosis control programme has provided a binocular microscope for each DMC. The 200 high workload DMCs at Medical Colleges have also been provided with LED-FM. Designated microscopy centre are manned by a trained LT of the state health system. Smear Microscopy services are available through a network of more than 14,000 DMCs which are spread across the health systems and quality assured through a system of External Quality Assurance Programme [EQAP] in line with the international guidelines. Thousands of trained LTs perform sputum smear microscopy at the DMCs within general public health system.

Quality Assurance for Smear Microscopy in the Country

In order to provide high quality smear microscopy services within the programme for avoiding false results in TB case diagnosis and to achieve uniform results across the country, EQA programme has been established through national laboratory network for sputum smear microscopy. The quality assurance [QA] activities include the: on-site evaluation; panel testing; and random blinded rechecking

[RBR]. The Programme has provided a STLS, at each TU for carrying out EQA activities-on-site evaluation visits to DMCs and random blinded rechecking of routine DMC slides at the DTC level. STLS prepare staining solution for smear microscopy, check the quality through internal quality control [QC] slides and extends on-site training with trouble shooting for quality improvement. The schematic representation of the EQA reporting process is shown in Figure 53.6.

Extrapulmonary Tuberculosis

RNTCP in the recent past has prioritized the diagnosis and management of EPTB with use of CBNAAT as the first test of choice and has also developed SOPs for the IRLs and C and DSTs laboratories for processing EPTB specimens using other technologies [smear/culture and DST]. Table 53.1 describes various technologies used for diagnosis of different types of TB.

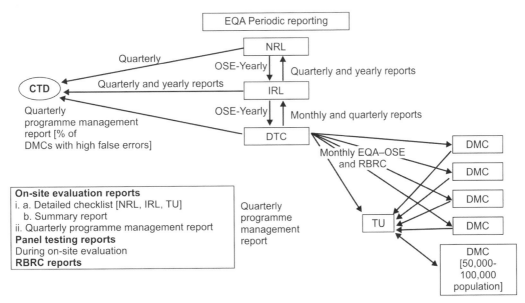

Figure 53.6: External quality assurance reporting process
CTD = Central TB Division; EQA = external quality assurance; NRL = National Reference Laboratory; OSE = on-site evaluation; RBRC = random blinded rechecking; IRL = Intermediate Reference Laboratory; DTC = District Tuberculosis Centre; TU = Tuberculosis Unit; DMC = Designated Microscopy Centre

Table 53.1: Technologies used for diagnosis of different types of TB	
Type of TB	*Technologies Used by RNTCP*
Pulmonary TB [HIV-Neg/presumed drug-sensitive]	Smear Microscopy [ZN/LED-FM]
Pulmonary TB [PLHA and paediatric age]	CBNAAT [+smear/CxR]
At risk of DR-TB [as per RNTCP]	CBNAAT / LPA / MGIT
Confirmed MDR-TB [for FL/SLD]	Automated MGIT System
Follow-up for DR-TB management	Automated MGIT System and or LJ medium
EPTB	CBNAAT, Automated MGIT System, other modalities [smear, FNAC, Biopsy, USG, CT Scan, MRI, etc.]

TB = tuberculosis; HIV = human immunodeficiency virus; ZN = Ziehl-Neelsen; LED-FM = Light-emitting diode fluorescence microscopy; PLHA = people living with HIV/ AIDS; CBNAAT = cartridge-based nucleic acid amplification test; LPA = line probe assay; DR-TB = drug resistant tuberculosis; RNTCP = Revised National Tuberculosis Control Programme; MGIT = mycobacteria growth indicating tube; MDR-TB = multidrug-resistant tuberculosis; FL = first-line; SLD = second-line drug susceptibility; LJ = Lowenstein-Jensen; FNAC = fine needle aspiration cytology; USG = ultrasonography; CT = computed tomography; MRI = magnetic resonance imaging; EPTB = extrapulmonary tuberculosis

Drug-resistant Tuberculosis

Patients at risk of DR-TB as defined by the programme [MDR-TB], are diagnosed using WHO endorsed rapid diagnostics [WRD] like CBNAAT/LPA. Response to treatment for MDR is done by follow-up culture on liquid Culture [MGIT] system [critical follow-ups requiring clinical response] and Lowenstein-Jensen [LJ] medium for [for crucial follow-ups], with identification of mycobacterial species is performed by commercial immunochromatic test.

From 2018 onwards, the programme has introduced policy of "universal DST" i.e. testing of all TB patients for at least rifampicin Sensitivity. With revision in diagnostic algorithm of PMDT, all rifampicin resistant TB patients are tested for second-line drug susceptibility testing [Figures 42.5A and 42.5B]. All rifampicin sensitive TB patients supposed to be tested for isoniazid resistance.

Culture and anti-TB DST services are provided by all States IRL as well as certified culture and DST laboratories and are currently available at 74 places. Culture and DST services are also available outside the RNTCP, in the NGO and Private sectors through provision of RNTCP certification. As on March 2018, 40 laboratory certified for SLD and it will be further expanded.

Quality Assurance

EQA for C and DST is ensured by a process of pre-assessment, on-site evaluation visit to the facility and the actual certification procedure. The process of certification was adopted from the standard international guidelines, and has been in place from 2005. This inter-laboratory culture exchange and testing process involves both NRL panel cultures testing at IRL, and re-testing of select IRL cultures by the NRL. All certified laboratories regularly participate in the Proficiency Testing programmes/rounds conducted by NRLs. The certified laboratory submits quarterly laboratory performance indicators to CTD and NRLs. The data from the performance indicators are analysed by CTD and NRLs and technical guidance provided for corrective actions.

TREATMENT SERVICES

A standardised four drug [HRZE] daily regimen is used to treat all new TB cases under RNTCP. Earlier, "previously treated" TB patients were treated using a standardised 5 drug [HRZES] regimen for 8-9 months [Table 53.2A]. Presently, the regimen for "previously treated patients" has been discontinued. Policy of Universal DST has been implemented. Under it, all diagnosed TB patients are offered DST at least for rifampicin. The non-responders and failures of first-line treatment are also offered DST. The regimens currently used for drug sensitive TB patients in RNTCP are daily regimens with fixed dose combination [FDC] medications. Patients are given drugs according to body weight [Tables 53.2B and 53.2C].

Directly observed treatment is the one of the patient support systems that creates a human bond between the provider and the patient and motivate the patient to adhere

---

Table 53.2A: Type of patients and regimens prescribed under Revised National Tuberculosis Control Programme

Treatment groups	Types of patient	Regimen	
		Intensive phase [IP]	Continuation phase [CP]
New	Sputum smear-positive Sputum smear-negative Extrapulmonary Others	2HRZE	4HRE
Previously treated*	Smear-positive relapse Smear-positive failure Smear-positive treatment after default Others	2HRZES/ 1HRZE	5HRE

* With implementation of "universal DST" this treatment category has been discontinued from December 2018

IP = intensive phase; CP = continuation phase

Table 53.2B: Drug dosage for adult TB

Weight category [kg]	Number of tablets [FDCs]		Injection streptomycin [g]*
	Intensive phase	Continuation phase	
	HRZE [75/150/400/275]	HRE [75/150/275]	
25-39	2	2	0.5
40-54	3	3	0.75
55-69	4	4	1
≥70	5	5	1

* Injection streptomycin to be added in IP phase for 2 months in the retreatment regimen of drug sensitive patients. In patients above 50 years of age, maximum dose of streptomycin should be 0.75 g Adults weighing less than 25 kg will be given loose drugs as per body weight

TB = tuberculosis; FDCs = fixed-dose combinations

Table 53.2C: Drug dosage for paediatric TB

Weight category [kg]	Number of tablets [dispersible FDCs]			Injection streptomycin [mg]
	Intensive phase		Continuation phase	
	HRZ [50/75/150]	E [100]	HRE [50/75/100]	
4-7	1	1	1	100
8-11	2	2	2	150
12-15	3	3	3	200
16-24	4	4	4	300
25-29	3 + 1A*	3	3 + 1A*	400
30-39	2 + 2A*	2	2 + 2A*	500

*A = Adult FDC [HRZE = 75/150/400/275; HRE = 75/150/275]

TB = tuberculosis; FDC = fixed-dose combinations

to and complete the treatment. Basic premises in identifying the treatment supporter [DOT providers] is that treatment supporter should be accessible and acceptable to the patient and accountable to the health system. The treatment supporter [DOT provider] can be a medical or para-medical personnel or a community volunteer or someone from the NGOs and private sector facility involved in the programme. With community treatment supporters, community-based care is ensured. Direct observation of treatment ensures that the patient consumes every dose of the treatment before a trained health worker and provides additional opportunity to support treatment.

However, the principle of direct observation is to be applied logically and judiciously. Other modalities of treatment adherence are deployed to enhance adherence to treatment. Intelligent deployment of information communication technologies [ICT] is an example of such modalities. A patient who is unable to undergo supervised treatment should not be denied treatment. Frequent on-job travellers, truck drivers, sailors, etc. may require identification of proper treatment supporter. To promote treatment adherence among these patients, ICT modalities like frequent calls, SMS reminders, interactive voice response system [IVRS], Pill Box, Pill in Hand method, etc. may be deployed.

Standards for Tuberculosis Care in India

The standards for TB care in India [STCI] (17) were released on World TB Day 2014. This is India's step towards the bold policy for Universal access to quality TB care. On one side, these standards propagate best practices in TB control in the private sector at the same time these also challenge the current policies and strategies of RNTCP to upgrade to meet these standards and provide highest quality TB care under the programme. These standards highlight improved high sensitivity diagnostic approaches and tools, daily treatment regimen with FDC, universal DST with DST guided treatment regimen to tackle the menace of DR-TB, more patient friendly treatment support systems including family DOT and ICT enabled support systems, psychosocial support systems, etc. public health responsibilities of providers and standards for social inclusion. To implement these standards across India, RNTCP has developed the draft revised technical and operational guidelines for all forms of TB in public sector as well as e-tools cum training tool kits for promoting STCI in the private sector.

PROGRAMMATIC MANAGEMENT OF DRUG-RESISTANT TB

World Health Organization Global TB Report 2018, India accounted for 24% of global MDR-TB cases (1). The RNTCP is implementing the component for DR-TB services, programmatic management of Drug resistant TB [PMDT], [erstwhile DOTS Plus] since year 2007. After a modest gradual scale up till 2010, PMDT services were systematically accelerated since 2011 to achieve complete geographical coverage in March 2013.

Strategies for controlling DR-TB include: [i] sustained high-quality DOTS implementation, daily regimen in high risk groups and patient friendly treatment to improve treatment adherence; [ii] implementing airborne infection control [AIC] measures; cut down diagnostic delays with rapid diagnostics, offer universal DST and prompt appropriate decentralized treatment; [iii] strengthening procurement, supply chain management of SLD: strengthen the procurement, supply and availability of second-line anti-TB drugs in India; [iv] nutritional assessment and supplementation: linkages with Public distribution systems, Panchayati Raj Institutions, Corporate social responsibility, etc; and [v] improving adherence through counselling support: one DR-TB counselor per DR-TB centre and district each for both institutional and home-based counselling.

The Guidelines for PMDT in India are available since 2006 and are regularly updated based on evolving evidence-based policy decisions and implementation experiences to enhance operational efficiency and ease. These guidelines were last updated in 2017 (16). The key features are as follows.

Diagnosis of M/XDR-TB

Decentralised diagnosis with WRD with specimen transport to laboratory in cold chain. Rapid Molecular DST [CBNAAT or LPA] is the first choice of DST. The subsequent choice of diagnostic technology depends on locally available laboratory capacity through an RNTCP Certified laboratory [Table 53.3]. RNTCP has been implementing "universal DST". All TB patients are tested with rapid molecular DST [CBNAAT or LPA]. All failures of first-line regimen, any patient with smear positive follow-up results, are also offered DST.

Treatment of M/XDR-TB

Under PMDT, since 2018, treatment is based on DR/DST results. Initial hospitalisation is done at DR-TB Centre followed by ambulatory care. Standardised treatment algorithm for DR-TB (16) is shown in Figure 42.6.

Status and Progress in Scaling-up of Programmatic Management of Drug-resistant Tuberculosis Services in India

The year-wise scale up of PMDT service delivery components is detailed in the Figure 53.7.

Table 53.3: Diagnosis of multidrug/extensively drug-resistant tuberculosis	
Drug susceptibility testing technology	*Choice*
Molecular DST [e.g., CBNAAT or LPA DST]	First
Liquid culture isolation and LPA DST	Second
Solid culture isolation and LPA DST	Third
Liquid culture isolation and liquid DST	Fourth
Solid culture isolation and DST	Fifth
DST = drug susceptibility testing; CBNAAT = cartridge-based nucleic acid amplification test; LPA = line probe assay	

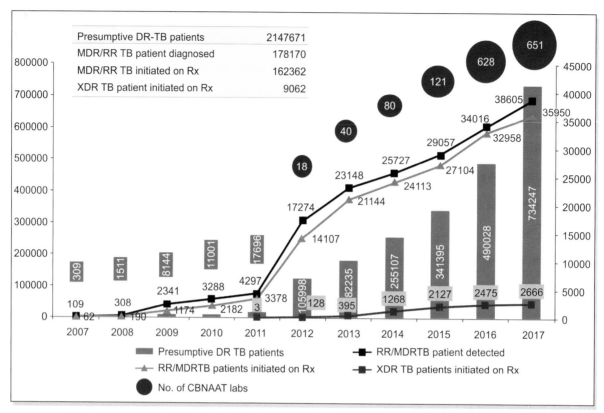

Figure 53.7: DR-TB case finding and treatment initiation effort, 2007-2017
TB = tuberculosis; DR-TB = drug-resistant TB; MDR TB = multidrug-resistant TB; RR TB = rifampicin-resistant TB; XDR TB = extensively drug-resistant TB; CBNAAT = cartridge-based nucleic acid amplification test

TUBERCULOSIS-HUMAN IMMUNODEFICIENCY VIRUS COLLABORATIVE ACTIVITIES

TB is the most common opportunistic infection in HIV-infected individuals and HIV-infection is an important risk factor for acquiring TB infection and its progression to active TB disease (18). About 87,000 HIV-associated TB patients are emerging annually in India and accounts for 8% of the global burden of HIV-associated TB. The mortality in this group is very high with nearly 12,000 people dying every year.

The interventions to reduce the burden of TB among People Living with HIV/AIDS [PLHA] include the early provision of ART for people living with HIV in line with WHO guidelines and the three I's for HIV/TB – Intensified TB case finding followed by high quality ATT, Isoniazid preventive therapy [IPT] and Infection control for TB, all of which are being implemented under the programme.

The National Framework for Joint TB-HIV Collaborative activities was developed in 2007 and has been updated based on experiential learning and scientific evidence in 2009 and 2013. The mechanism for collaboration includes coordinated service delivery at field level, and oversight and advisory groups at National, State and District level. To enable effective coordination, joint trainings, standard recording and reporting, joint monitoring and evaluation and operational research are strategically implemented. Currently, the TB/HIV package is being implemented

nationwide by both, National AIDS Control Programme [NACP] and RNTCP.

Progress so Far

The HIV testing of TB patients is now routinely offered through provider-initiated testing and counselling [PITC] implemented in all states. In 2017, 75% TB patients knew their HIV status and 36,315 were diagnosed as HIV positive [Figure 53.8]. All HIV-TB patients were provided CPT and 87% co-infected patients were put on ART. India has adopted all the recommendations suggested by the WHO for TB/HIV collaborative activities. Rapid Diagnostics are used for early diagnosis of TB among PLHIV, measures for effective implementation of AIC guidelines in HIV care settings are taken and IPT has been implemented across all ART centres in the country.

With technical support from WHO, RNTCP-NACP joined hands for the implementation of 'Innovative, Intensified TB case finding and appropriate treatment at selected 30 high burden ART centres in India' aimed at reducing the burden of TB among PLHA which was launched on 24th March 2015. The project features single window for service delivery of TB and HIV services from ART centres, diagnosis of TB by CBNAAT and treatment of TB patients with daily regimen among others. Based on the success of the project, the initiative has been scaled up across all States in 2016.

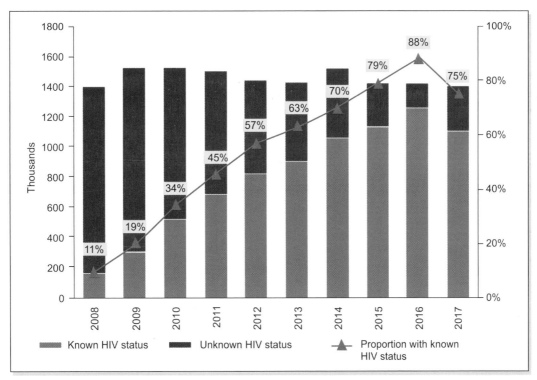

Figure 53.8: Trends in Number [%] of registered TB patients with known HIV status, 2008-2017
TB = tuberculosis; HIV = human immunodeficiency virus; q = quarter

The reader is referred to the chapter *"Tuberculosis and human immunodeficiency virus infection"* *[Chapter 35]* for details on this topic.

TUBERCULOSIS AND NON-COMMUNICABLE COMORBIDITIES [TOBACCO, DIABETE MELLITUS]

The increasing co-occurrence of TB with tobacco consumption and Diabetes Mellitus [DM] is well evident. Smoking is three times more prevalent in TB patients and is strongly associated with increased rates of TB infection. Similarly, the prevalence of DM is as high as 13% and the prevalence even goes higher in MDR-TB cases. Patients with TB may have lung damage that is aggravated by continued tobacco use. Diabetes Mellitus is supposed to depress immunity and conversely TB is supposed to impair glucose tolerance resulting in concurrence.

Feasibility of including tobacco cessation activities with RNTCP, a TB Tobacco pilot project was conducted in Gujarat by GOI in 2010. The pilot projects done by the TB-DM collaborative group has demonstrated at 8 tertiary care centres that missed opportunities can be addressed through developing routine screening system in RNTCP with no additional cost to programme.

Based on the above learning CTD, National Programme for Prevention and Control of Cardiovascular Diseases, Cancers, Diabetes and Stroke [NPCDCS] and National Tobacco Control Programme [NTCP] took a decision to develop a collaborative framework to integrate tobacco cessation advice and DM screening protocol in RNTCP; and TB screening in NPCDCS and NTCP programme. The Framework for TB-Diabetes Collaborative activities and TB-Tobacco collaborative activities has been launched on World TB Day and World No Tobacco Day respectively. Bi-directional screening for TB-DM and TB-Tobacco is being implemented in all districts wherein NPCDCS and NTCP are functional.

CHILDHOOD TUBERCULOSIS

As per the Global TB Report 2018 (1), children [under 15 years of age], accounted for more than one-fifth of the global TB burden among children. There are certain key programme features for paediatric TB. The RNTCP in association with Indian Academy of Paediatrics [IAP] has revised the paediatric TB guideline in 2012. It laid down specific algorithm diagnosis of TB among children. The treatment strategy comprises two key components. First, as in adults, children with TB are treated with standard SCC, given under direct observation and the disease status is monitored during the course of treatment. Second, patient wise boxes designed according to weight bands for complete course of anti-TB drugs (19). In order to simplify the management of paediatric TB, RNTCP has recently introduced a simplified diagnostic algorithm for paediatric TB offering upfront CBNAAT for TB diagnosis [Figure 42.5B] and introduced child-friendly dispersible FDC formulation for treatment [Table 53.2C] (16).

Considering difficulties in diagnosis of paediatric TB under field condition, the notification rates can be further strengthened. Contact screening is one of the ways for intensified case finding activity which RNTCP has implemented since its inception. Under RNTCP all children less than 6 years of age, contacts of the family member suffering with active TB are expected to be screened for TB and provided INH chemoprophylaxis once active TB has been ruled out.

The National Technical Working Group on Paediatric TB is in place to examine the policy and practices and provides suggestions to CTD for improving situation of childhood TB. To accelerate access to quality TB diagnosis for paediatric population, RNTCP had initiated a project in 10 major cities in India: RNTCP United States Agency for International Development [USAID] Foundation for Innovative New Diagnostics [FIND] Paediatric TB Xpert Project. Key hospitals and private clinics catering to paediatric populations were identified and referral network was established for sample collection and transport to facilitate early diagnosis using CBNAAT. RNTCP has incorporated the processes and learning's of the project in programme guidelines.

PUBLIC-PRIVATE MIX DOTS IN REVISED NATIONAL TUBERCULOSIS CONTROL PROGRAMME

In India, the private sector is the first point of care in many episodes of ill health (20,21). While most TB cases are ultimately treated by the RNTCP, most patients by then have already approached the private sector for TB diagnosis and treatment. Hence, engaging the private sector [both for profit and not for profit entities] effectively is an important intervention for RNTCP to achieve the overall goal of universal access and early detection.

Efforts, though isolated, have been made by RNTCP since the earlier days of its inception to widen access to quality TB care. After experiences of implementing models of private sector collaboration, CTD published guidelines for the participation of the NGOs [in 2001] and private practitioners [in 2002]. These guidelines provided opportunity to many NGOs and private practitioners to formally collaborate with RNTCP. Based on experience of implementation, the schemes are revised in 2008 (20) and in 2014 to increase its uptake. Currently, 24 partnership options for involvement of NGOs, corporates, private practitioners and research institutions are incorporated under the National Guidelines for Partnership (21).

Indian Medical Association has been engaged with the programme through Global Fund to Fight AIDS, Tuberculosis and Malaria [GFATM] supported project in 16 states and UTs. The objective of this project has been to improve the quality care for the TB patients availing services from the private sector. Similarly, civil society organisation, CBCI-CARD [Catholic Bishops Conference of India-Coalition for AIDS & Related Diseases] is working under GFATM project of RNTCP, to improve access to the diagnostic and treatment services provided by the RNTCP within the Catholic Church Healthcare Facilities [CHFs] and thereby to improve the quality of care for patients suffering from TB in India.

In addition partners like UNION, World Vision, FIND, also support the programme. These partners and national institutes work in close liaison with RNTCP and play a key role in setting national priorities, training, carrying out operational research [OR] and also in assisting the programme in its monitoring and evaluation activities.

Medical colleges have been effectively organised at a large scale through task force mechanisms at state, zonal and national levels, with RNTCP supporting with additional human resources, logistics for microscopy, funds to conduct sensitisations, trainings and research in RNTCP priority areas. RNTCP has partnered with more than 350 Medical Colleges in India and they have contributed in a major way in finding more TB cases, especially smear-negative and EPTB cases (22).

ADVOCACY COMMUNICATION AND SOCIAL MOBILISATION

Advocacy communication and social mobilisation [ACSM] is an inbuilt component of RNTCP and is recognised as an important element of all activities of TB control essential to achieve the goal of universal access. Advocacy communication and social mobilisation activities are expected to strengthen the efforts towards TB control in India by mobilising political administrative commitment resulting in availability of better resources for TB, early case detection and early complete treatment, combating stigma and discrimination, motivating and empowering community and generating awareness and demand in community.

National Advisory Committee was constituted in 2013 for a period of two years to advise and guide the CTD by infusion of newer ideas and experience. It includes experts from field of Health communication, research, National and state teaching institutes, etc.

Under RNTCP, ACSM planning and implementation has been decentralised, and helps percolate relevant messages in a language, that's best understood by the local population through the best possible medium [e.g. miking at bazaar haats or local festivals]. States develop information, education and communication [IEC] materials based on their needs and keeping in mind the local cultural context, and have budgets allocated for this purpose. Additionally, IEC materials are also developed at the national level and shared with States for use-'as is' or post-modification to suit local requirements. Several of these materials including TV spots, radio jingles and posters are available in nearly 13 regional languages. Advocacy communication and social mobilization module is incorporated in all health workers training on basic DOTS. To update the technical and operational aspects of the programme a revised training module has been prepared for the private practitioners.

TUBERCULOSIS–PATIENT SUPPORT SYSTEMS IN INDIA

In addition to better diagnostic tool and treatment regimens, other patient supportive initiatives including better nutrition,

Table 53.4: Enhanced enables and incentives under Revised National Tuberculosis Control Programme

Item	Existing norm	Proposed by MoHFW and approved by MSG
Revision of incentives to Community DOT provider providing treatment support to Category I TB patients	₹250/- for completed course of treatment	₹1000/- for the completed course of treatment
Revision of incentives to Community DOT provider providing treatment support to Category II TB patients	₹250/- for completed course of treatment	₹1500/- for the completed course of treatment
Revision of incentives to Community DOT provider providing treatment support to DR-TB patients	₹2500/- for completed course of treatment [₹1000/- at the end of IP and ₹1500/- at the end of CP]	₹5000/- for completed course of treatment. [₹2000/- at the end of IP and ₹3000/- at the end of CP]
Incentives to patient in tribal and difficult areas	₹250/patient and one attendant	₹750/patient and one attendant
Incentive to volunteers for sputum sample transport in tribal and difficult areas	₹200/month/volunteer. If less than one visit per week then ₹100/ month	₹25 per sample transported to the DMC
Travel cost to MDR-TB patient/suspect to DR-TB centre [outside district]	Actual travel cost using any public transport	Up to ₹1000/visit/patient restricted to actuals by a public transport
Travel cost to MDR-TB patient/suspect to DR-TB centre [within district]	Actual travel cost using any public transport	Up to ₹400/visit/patient restricted to actuals by a public transport
Transportation cost for co-infected TB-HIV patient travel	Nil	Up to ₹500/patient for only the first visit restricted to actuals by a public transport
Incentive related to Injection prick	Nil	₹25/injection prick

MoHFW = Ministry of Health and Family Welfare; MSG = mission-steering group; DOT = directly observed treatment; TB = tuberculosis; DR-TB = drug-resistant tuberculosis; IP = intensive phase; CP = continuation phase; MDR-TB = multidrug-resistant tuberculosis; HIV = human immunodeficiency virus

counselling and financial support are equally essential. World Health Organization 'End TB strategy' has this important target of 'no affected family face catastrophic costs due to TB'.

Revised National Tuberculosis Control Programme provides free diagnosis and treatment to all TB patients who access care from the programme. Pre-treatment investigations, ancillary drugs for managing side effects are ensured free of cost. Enhanced enables and incentives under programme are listed in Table 53.4.

However the free diagnosis and treatment is only accessible to those patients seeking care under RNTCP. Large number of patients seeking care in private sector has to bear substantial cost for TB care. Revised National Tuberculosis Control Programme under the guidelines for partnership has initiated number of schemes in which services are procured from private sector for reducing cost to the patients in the private sector. Innovative private sector engagement pilots are on in which diagnosis and treatment for TB patients in the private sector is also given free.

Though large part of cost of treatment is born by the programme, patients still have to bear expenditures such as cost for travel to the facilities, loss of wages due to sickness, etc. Apart from financial hardship, nutritional and counselling supports to TB patients are other elements the national programme was not supporting directly. In order to address these challenges, CTD had sent recommendation to state programmes to facilitate TB patients to have access to various social support programmes and systems already existing, and to actively support innovative models.

As a result of state and district programme initiatives, large number of innovative patient support activities has been implemented in the country to extend nutritional support to patient and families, financial support, vocational support, counselling support. The support activities are implemented through departments such as social welfare department, public distribution system, NGOs, CSR funding, etc. Significant role of local self-governments can be seen in many of these initiatives, where financing for these are done through their own local fund.

HUMAN RESOURCES MANAGEMENT

The goal of RNTCP's HRD strategy is to optimally utilize available health system staff to deliver quality TB services, and to strengthen the supervisory and managerial capacity of programme staff overseeing these services. TB care and control services are becoming more complex and demanding, with multiple new tasks for MDR-TB management and TB-HIV care. An adequately staffed, trained, and motivated health workforce is required to achieve the ambitious TB control objective of Universal Access.

In the 12th Five year plan of RNTCP a cadres/series of new positions have been approved under program at all level to strengthen programme management, laboratory services and PPM services.

Training institutes [national and state] play pivotal role in capacity building of all concerned. National Training institutes like NTI, Bangalore; NITRD, New Delhi and NIRT, Chennai are capacity building arms of CTD,

MoHFW-GoI. The efficient state level institutes can also come up as regional level training hubs, e.g. State TB Training & Demonstration Centres of many states.

MONITORING AND SUPERVISION

Proper supervision, modular training, and regular cross-checking of work plays a key role in maintaining quality services. Regular reviews of the programme at the state and district level are a key component of the process. In addition to the routine supervision and monitoring by the programme staff, each state conducts internal evaluation of two districts in a quarter. Central evaluations are conducted by the team from the CTD to evaluate one or two districts each month. The CIE team consists of representatives from CTD, National AIDS Control Organization [NACO], WHO, STO's from other state and also from civil society partners, etc. These activities help program managers in understanding determinants of good as well as poor performance for replication of good practices in other states/districts and take appropriate measures for improvement.

The programme is also reviewed in terms of State co-ordination committee meetings for TB HIV and review of Programmatic Management of DR-TB, both at the state and regional level. National Task Force meeting regarding the involvement and contribution of Medical colleges at the state, zonal and national level are also conducted to review their participation and also for taking suggestions for improvement of the programme. With respect to DR-TB, Coordination committee meeting of the NRL along with the annual Meeting of the National Diagnosis and Treatment Committee for RNTCP was held to formulate the future course of action.

One of the greatest strengths of the RNTCP is the recording and reporting system. Based on the patient treatment card, the laboratory registers and the TB notification register, this simple but robust system ensures accountability for each and every patient initiated on treatment.

However, the data available at district, state or national level was in aggregated form, with a lead time of >4 months, excluding private sector and neither could help much for TB burden estimation or individual case management or monitoring. To address this CTD in collaboration with National Informatics Centre [NIC] undertook the initiative to develop a Case Based Web online [cloud] application named NIKSHAY. The objectives of NIKSHAY implementation are to facilitate tracking and monitoring of individual TB patient, automated reporting, online referral/transfer mechanism, eliminate lead time in reporting, aid focused supervision, and for real-time programme management.

The notification of all TB patients in the notification register in NIKSHAY ensures monitoring and follow-up of each patient individually and real time. Reports on case finding, sputum conversion and treatment outcome then can be obtained from them for analysis of the performance indicators of the respective areas [TB unit, District, State or National].

TUBERCULOSIS NOTIFICATION AND SURVEILLANCE

The Government of India declared TB as a notifiable disease through a Government Order dated 7th May 2012. All public and private health providers are now required to notify TB cases diagnosed and/or treated by them to the District nodal officers. This is an initiative which is intended not only to improve epidemiological surveillance but also to extend the range of services available to patients regardless of whether they are registered under the public sector or treated in the private sector. These services are listed in the STCI. The RNTCP has developed a guide for notification that enables cases to be notified through email, mobile application or paper-based records.

With efforts for sensitisation of programme officials and staff and then subsequently to private sector, the number of private health facilities registered in Nikshay for TB notification further increased in 2018.

PROCUREMENT AND SUPPLY CHAIN MANAGEMENT

Procurement

Ensuring a reliable and un-interrupted supply of good quality anti-TB drugs and other commodities is the main objective of the supply chain management. The Procurement & Supply Chain Management Unit in CTD carries out procurement planning and monitoring, policy formulations, coordination with procurement agents, reporting and coordination with the donors, implementation of procurement risk mitigation plans, handling day-to-day supply related issues and monitoring of the contracts (23).

First-line and second-line Anti-TB drugs are procured under RNTCP and the logistics function ensures its seamless availability of all these essential items at the different levels of the programme to be further provided to the patients.

In addition to drugs RNTCP also procures various diagnostics and equipment's under RNTCP like LED-FM, CBNAAT kits. For diagnosis of TB patients, appropriate arrangements shall be made to ensure that X-ray facilities in the states from the RNTCP budget. States have been permitted for local procurement of purified protein derivative vials, as per their requirement, following RNTCP specifications/guidelines.

Quality Assurance of anti-TB drugs has been accorded special importance by RNTCP and measures are taken to ensure both pre- and post-dispatch inspection of all the anti-TB drugs.

Drug Logistics Management

The first-line anti-TB drugs procured are stored at the six Government Medical Store Depots [GMSDs] situated in Chennai, Guwahati, Hyderabad, Karnal, Kolkata and Mumbai which are the direct consignees. The second-line anti-TB drugs [MDR and XDR] are received directly by the

States as loose drugs and the States [i.e. State Drug Store] is the direct consignee. The States then repack these into monthly patient wise boxes which are then distributed to the districts.

Drugs are released by CTD from the GMSDs every quarter to the States considering closing stocks at the end of quarter, consumption of drugs during the quarter, with a reserve stock of 7 months using Nikshay aushadhi. The SDS subsequently releases drugs to their respective districts for one quarter's consumption, with a reserve stock of 4 months. From the districts, the drugs are released to each TB unit every quarter to maintain a reserve stock of two months, and from the TU drugs are released to the PHIs with one month stock for consumption and one month's stock as reserve after receipt at the TUs of the monthly report from the PHIs. In addition, drugs are also released any time during the month or quarter, from all levels in the instance of an increase in consumption or extra requirement of drugs due to other reasons, after submission of an "Additional Drug Request" [ADR].

Trainings on drug logistics is a regular feature in RNTCP to ensure that the capacity of the concerned staff in this important area are built adequately from time to time. SOP and manuals have been developed for Drug Management at State and District Drug Stores under RNTCP, along with a Training Manual.

FINANCE

Under the National Health Mission [NHM], which functions as an umbrella society, the erstwhile societies for most Schemes under Health including TB control have been merged into integrated "State Health Society". At present, funds for the RNTCP are maintained in a separate account within these Societies and existing Annual Action Plans have been incorporated into the NHM framework. As per the current arrangements, the Programme Implementation Plan [PIP] of the RNTCP are approved by the Government of India on year to year basis.

States receive funds for further distribution to Districts for carrying out day-to-day activities. Additionally, higher level state staff receives training from the Centre. They are also provided guidelines and modular training materials to train staff in the field.

The Government of India in line with the objective of providing adequate health care for its citizen has been steadily increasing the allocations in health sector as well as in TB Control Programme since commencement of the five year plan [Tables 53.5 and 53.6]. The RNTCP receives its funding from a World Bank credit and a Global Fund Grant. In addition, the RNTCP receives extra budgetary support from other donors including the USAID, Bill and Melinda Gates Foundation [BMGF], EXPAND TB, Centre for Disease Control [CDC]. International Union Against Tuberculosis and Lung Disease [The Union] and World Vision support the national programme with funding from The Global Fund. Technical support is provided by WHO, with a network of consultants deployed at the national, state and district levels

Table 53.5: The consistent increase in allocation in health sector in last three Five Year Plans

Five Year Plans	10th [2002-07]	11th [2007-12]	12th [2012-17]
Allocation [₹ in crore]	37,153	1,40,135	3,00,018
Crore = 10,000,000			

Table 53.6: Allocation and expenditure under Tuberculosis Control Programme in India

Five Year Plans	Plan period	Allocation	Expenditure ₹ in crore
Tenth	2002-07	743.17	757.15
Eleventh	2007-12	1447.00	1595.13
Twelfth	2012-17	4500.15	2161.14.
Crore = 10,000,000			

to provide technical support and assistance in monitoring the programme. As per analysis of the Joint TB Programme Review of 2003, RNTCP is highly economical, costing on an average less than two rupees [5 US cents] per capita per year (24). Policy direction, supervision, surveillance, drugs and microscopes are provided by the Central Government.

REFERENCES

1. World Health Organization. Global Tuberculosis Report 2018. WHO/CDS/TB/2018.20. Geneva: World Health Organization.
2. Westly E. One million deaths: what researchers are learning from an unprecedented survey of mortality in India. Nature 2013;504:22-3.
3. Laxminarayan R, Klein EY, Darley S, Adeyi O. Global investments in TB Control: economic benefits. Health Aff [Millwood] 2009;28:730-42.
4. Rajeswari R, Balasubramanian R, Muniyandi M, Geetharamani S, Theresa X, Venkatesan P. Socio-Economic impact of tuberculosis on patient and family in India. Int J Tuberc Lung Dis 1999;3: 869-77.
5. Mahadev B, Kumar P. History of tuberculosis control in India. J Indian Med Assoc 2003;101:142-3.
6. Rao KN. Textbook of tuberculosis. First edition. Bombay: Kothari Book Depot; 1972.p. 4-15.
7. Tuberculosis Association of India. India's fight against tuberculosis; New Delhi: Tuberculosis Association of India; 1956.p.7.
8. Bhore J. Report of the Health Survey and Development Committee. New Delhi: Ministry of Health, Government of India; 1946.p.157-67.
9. Tuberculosis Chemotherapy Centre. A concurrent comparison of home and sanatorium treatment of pulmonary tuberculosis in south India. Bull World Health Organ 1959;21:51-144.
10. Fox W. Self-administration of medicaments. A review of published work and a study of the problems. Bull Int Union Tuberc 1961;31:307-31.
11. Tuberculosis Research Centre, Madras. Ten year report. New Delhi: Indian Council of Medical Research; 1966.p.5-8.
12. Lotte A, Hatton F, Perdrizet S, Rouillon A. A concurrent comparison of intermittent [twice-weekly] isoniazid plus streptomycin and daily isoniazid plus PAS in the domiciliary treatment of pulmonary tuberculosis. Tuberculosis Chemotherapy Centre, Madras Bull World Health Organ 1964;31:247-71.

13. Banerji D, Anderson S. A sociological study of awareness of symptoms among persons with pulmonary tuberculosis. Bull World Health Organ 1963;29:665-83.

14. Baily GV, Savic D, Gothi GD, Naidu VB, Nair SS. Potential yield of pulmonary tuberculosis cases by direct microscopy of sputum in a district in South India. Bull World Health Organ 1967;37:875-92.

15. Khatri GR, Frieden TR. Controlling Tuberculosis in India. N Engl J Med 2002;347:1420-5.

16. Revised National Tuberculosis Control Programme, Directorate General of Health Services, Ministry of Health and Family Welfare, Government of India. Guidelines on programmatic management of drug-resistant tuberculosis in India 2017. New Delhi: World Health Organization, Country Office for India; 2017.

17. World Health Organization, Country Office for India. Standards for TB Care in India. New Delhi: World Health Organization, Country Office for India; 2014.

18. Guidelines for use of Pediatric Patient Wise boxes under the Revised National Tuberculosis Control Programme. Available at URL: http://www.tbcindia.org/pdfs/ PediatricGuidelinesFinal. pdf. Accessed on October 11, 2008.

19. The behaviour and interaction of TB patients and private for-profit health care providers in India: a review. WHO/TB/97.223. Geneva: World Health Organization; 1997.

20. Central TB Division. Revised schemes for NGOs and private providers. Available at URL: http://www.tbcindia.org/pdfs/ New%20Schemes%20NGO-PP%20140808.pdf. Accessed on October 12, 2008.

21. Central Tuberculosis Division, Ministry of Health and Family Welfare, Govt. of India. Partnerships. Technical and Operational Guidelines for TB Control in India. Available at URL: https:// tbcindia.gov.in/showfile.php?lid=3211. Accessed on December 29, 2018.

22. Sharma SK, Mohan A, Chauhan LS, Narain JP, Kumar P, Behera D, et al. Contribution of medical colleges to tuberculosis control in India under the Revised National Tuberculosis Control Programme [RNTCP]: lessons learnt & challenges ahead. Indian J Med Res 2013;137:283-94.

23. Salhotra VS. Drug procurement and management. J Indian Med Assoc 2003;101:175-6.

24. World Health Organization. Joint tuberculosis programme review: India. WHO/SEA/TB/265/. New Delhi: World Health Organization Regional Office for South-East Asia; 2003.

54

Tuberculosis Vaccine Development: A Current Perspective

AK Tyagi, B Dey, R Jain

INTRODUCTION

Tuberculosis [TB] is one of the most fatal infectious diseases, which continues to be a major global health problem (1-3). However, in spite of all the available drugs, difficulty in maintaining compliance to long treatment regimens along with complications in the diagnosis of drug-resistant pattern, there is a general perception that in the absence of an effective vaccine, the real control of TB on a worldwide basis is unlikely. A vaccine represents one of the most efficacious and potent defenses against infectious diseases, however, a perfect vaccine against TB that would be most effective in the control of this disease has eluded us all the time. Unfortunately, Bacille Calmette-Guérin [BCG], the currently used TB vaccine that was developed more than 90 years ago, has generated little protection and a great deal of controversy.

HISTORY OF THE BACILLE CALMETTE-GUÉRIN VACCINE: THE SCIENTIFIC FABLE AND THE LESSONS LEARNED

BCG is the only available and widely used vaccine against TB. It was developed by Calmette and Guérin between 1908 and 1921 by serial passaging of *Mycobacterium bovis* for 13 years (4). Based on the encouraging results in infants during the next four years, BCG was distributed around the world and its use as a preventive vaccine against TB was encouraged. By 1948, more than 10 million immunisations were carried out and in the first international BCG congress held in the same year in Paris, it was concluded that BCG vaccination was effective in preventing TB. In 1974, BCG vaccination was included in the expanded immunisation programme of the World Health Organization [WHO] to strengthen the fight against TB in children in developing countries (5). In India, the BCG vaccine laboratory was established in Chennai, Tamil Nadu, in 1948 to aid the BCG immunisation programme in the country and to supply BCG to some neighboring countries. Though Pasteur strain remains the international reference strain of BCG (6), owing to the variations in production and preservation methodologies in different countries, BCG strains with genotypic and phenotypic differences have emerged. Variations in these strains have been observed with respect to tuberculin conversion rate, frequency of adverse reactions and even vaccine efficacy ranging from 0% to 80% (7-10). Nevertheless, more than 3 billion children all over the world have been vaccinated with BCG. Despite the global use of BCG, scepticism about its safety and efficacy has persisted till date. Other than the most frequent and mild side effects of BCG vaccination like local indurations and regional suppurative adenitis (11), the only serious complication observed is disseminated BCG disease seen in some children with human immunodeficiency virus [HIV] infection (12). However, the variable efficacy of BCG in different human populations has remained the most controversial issue. Meta-analyses of several BCG efficacy trials in humans have resulted in some important observations concerning the susceptibility to infection and elicitation of immune responses (13-16). Different human populations respond differently to immunisation as well as *Mycobacterium tuberculosis* [Mtb] infection. Various host factors, variability in the BCG strains, and differences in the virulence of *Mtb* strains represent some of the multifactorial reasons for the apparent variability in the protective efficacy of BCG.

The role of host factors is well exemplified by the fact that only 10% of the exposed individuals actually develop the disease and rest 90% are efficiently able to control the infection, which may remain latent for many years (17). Several animal as well as human studies have provided strong evidence of genetic influence on immunity to

Mtb infection (18). For example, several investigations have demonstrated association of polymorphism in genes encoding interferon-γ [IFN-γ] receptor, human leucocyte antigen-D related [HLA-DR], natural resistance-associated macrophage protein [NRAMP], dendritic cell-specific intercellular adhesion molecule-3-grabbing non-integrin [DC-SIGN], nucleotide-binding oligomerisation domain-containing protein 2 [NOD2], vitamin D receptor, etc. with pulmonary TB (19). In addition, the contribution of other factors like age, nutritional status, co-existence of other diseases, immune status, etc. may play an important role in determining the risk of developing TB. While HIV infection is well known to weaken the immune system, infections, such as schistosomiasis and hookworm infections have also been found to downregulate the T-cell responses, thereby resulting in a reduced protection by BCG against TB (20-22).

Apart from the host genetic factors and differences in BCG strains, which result in enormous variability, there is emerging evidence that various *Mtb* strains may vary in their genetic composition as well as phenotype, and thus, may substantially affect the evaluation of vaccine candidates. The Beijing strain of *Mtb*, for example, which is one of the most prevalent strains in Asian countries, has been implicated in TB outbreaks in BCG-vaccinated populations and has been found to be frequently associated with drug resistance (23). This strain has also been found to be much more virulent in mice than the laboratory strain *Mtb* H37Rv, which is conventionally used in the guinea pig and mouse models of *Mtb* infection. Thus, evaluation of new vaccines against the challenge of Beijing strain requires serious consideration. Castañon-Arreola and colleagues (24) have reported that a recombinant BCG strain over-expressing the 38kDa antigen of *Mtb* was able to provide better protection against a Beijing strain of *Mtb* than BCG. The enhanced protective efficacy of recombinant BCG was not apparent when *Mtb* H37Rv was employed as the challenge organism. The mechanism of influence of various strains of *Mtb* on the final outcome of the TB pathogenesis is not yet fully understood. However, rapid characterisation of various strains of *Mtb* by robust deoxyribonucleic acid [DNA] and ribonucleic acid [RNA] sequencing technologies are improving our understanding regarding the strain variation and its effect on TB pathogenesis.

The inadequate and variable protective efficacy imparted by BCG suggests that a new vaccine may require to be tested in several populations as it may exhibit optimum effectiveness only in certain populations based on age, genetic and environmental background, immune status, nutritional status and lifestyle. Thus, a single TB vaccine may not meet the global expectations.

UNIQUE FEATURES OF THE PATHOGEN

The TB bacillus, one of the most virulent and pathogenic species of its kind, belongs to the genus *Mycobacterium*, which contains at least 100 different species; a majority of these are saprophytic, water and/or soil-borne organisms (25,26). *Mtb* is described as a slow-growing, strictly aerobic, acid-fast

bacilli, which requires special enriched media for its growth *in vitro*. The TB bacillus has characteristic thick, hydrophobic and waxy cell wall rich in mycolic acids (27,28). This unique cell wall structure imparts natural resistance to a number of antibiotics that disrupt cell wall biosynthesis. In addition, tubercle bacilli can survive long exposure to acids, alkali, detergents, oxidative agents and lysis by complement (29). The exceptionally slow growth of *Mtb* and its unique ability to enter a quiescent state on exposure to stress conditions encountered *in vitro* or *in vivo* offers survival advantage to the pathogen even in the presence of anti-bacterial agents, which act only on actively dividing bacteria (30). In addition, its ability to subvert the host immune responses and manipulate the host machinery for its own survival makes it one of the most successful human pathogens (31,32).

IMMUNOPATHOLOGY OF TUBERCULOSIS

Immune mechanisms involved in TB primarily comprise a complex series of interactions between the bacilli and various cells of the immune system resulting either in the elimination of the bacilli completely, or containment of infection for a prolonged period or immediate progression to active disease with clinical illness (33-58). Thus, a complete understanding of this disease with varying outcomes requires extensive research. Several excellent studies have addressed the role of different components of the immune system and their involvement in the containment of tubercle bacilli during infection. However, the knowledge about the specificity of immune responses required for the clearance of bacilli still remains fragmented. The reader is referred to the chapter *"Immunology of tuberculosis"* [Chapter 5] for more details.

Tuberculosis–Human Immunodeficiency Virus Co-infection and its Impact on Tuberculosis Vaccine Development

A significant proportion of HIV/acquired immunodeficiency syndrome [AIDS]-related deaths are caused by TB, which is the single largest killer of HIV/AIDS patients (1,59). Individuals living with HIV are 20-30 times more likely to develop active TB than people without HIV. In most of the cases, HIV-infected patients develop active TB due to endogenous reactivation of latent infection and not due to exogenous infection. In addition, pregnant women and children are at a high risk of death when co-infected with HIV and TB.

During HIV infection, a progressive decline in CD4+ T-cell count, especially Th1 subtype with a shift towards Th2, results in failure to control most of the invading opportunistic organisms. *Mtb*, being the robust of all, is often the earliest to break the host defense (60). Besides the potentiating effect of HIV on the progression of TB, generation of cytokines like tumour necrosis factor-alpha [TNF-α] during control of TB infection may act as a potent enhancer of HIV replication resulting in an increased viral burden (61). Furthermore, the immune response generated during active TB has been shown to prime peripheral blood cells and enhances their susceptibility to HIV infection (62).

Another important aspect is 'BCG–HIV' inter-dependence and their counter responses. While BCG vaccination in HIV-infected children may cause severe disseminated mycobacteriosis (63), it also accelerates the course of HIV infection (64). HIV infection has also been reported to reduce the efficacy of BCG against extra-pulmonary TB (65,66). Due to these reasons, the WHO has recommended to discontinue BCG vaccination in HIV-infected children (67). Taking into account the dangerous liaison between HIV–TB and the adverse events associated with BCG vaccine in the face of HIV infection, development of subunit and non-replicating viral vector-based vaccines has been proposed as a suitable option for HIV-infected individuals.

Importance of Animal Models in TB Vaccine Development

Contribution of different animal models to TB research has a long-standing history that can be traced back to the time of Robert Koch. TB being an extremely complex disease with diverse clinical outcomes, requires adequate animal models that can mimic the disease process in humans. The animal models, such as, mouse, guinea pig, rabbit and non-human primate, have vastly contributed to the understanding of TB. Each animal model has its strengths and weaknesses with varying degrees of extrapolation of their research findings to humans. Nevertheless, all these animal models resemble important facets of human TB in one way or the other. First, animals can be easily infected by pulmonary route, which precisely epitomises the way humans acquire infection. Secondly, various stages of disease progression in TB, like granuloma formation, liquefaction, cavity formation and hematogenous spread, can be easily studied in some of the animal models, especially in guinea pigs, rabbits and non-human primates [NHP]. Thirdly, distinctive signs of TB, like fever, weight loss, radiological abnormalities and respiratory distress can also be observed in these animal models. If left untreated, infected animals eventually die of pulmonary insufficiency, a fate typical of human TB patients. Hence, various animal models have been successfully used for screening new TB vaccines as well as chemotherapeutic agents. Figure 54.1 depicts the protocol used for the screening of TB vaccine candidates. For short-term evaluation, two major parameters are conventionally assessed for vaccine efficacy studies in the animal models: [i] bacillary load in lungs and spleen and [ii] pathology. In long-term studies [i] survival of animals, and [ii] clinical symptoms, such as, weight loss, radiological abnormalities, and blood parameters, are measured.

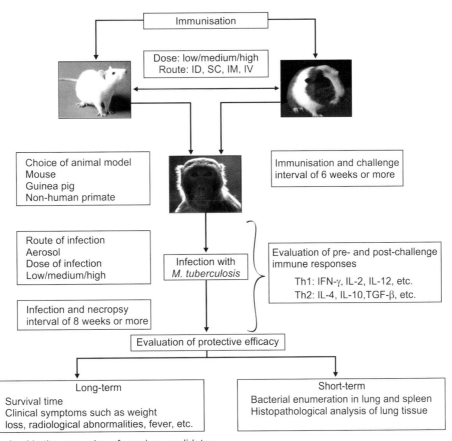

Figure 54.1: Variables involved in the screening of vaccine candidates
ID = intradermal; SC = subcutaneous; IM = intramuscular; IV = intravenous; IFN-γ = interferon-gamma; IL-2 = interleukin-2; IL-12 = interleukin-12; IL-4 = interleukin-4; IL-10 = interleukin-10; TGF-β = transforming growth factor-beta

Mouse Model of Tuberculosis

Amongst various animal models of TB, mouse model is the most popular and has provided huge wealth of information regarding the basic mechanisms of immune responses. The evidence for involvement of lymphocytes in mediating immunity to TB was successfully shown by the ability of whole blood and spleen homogenates [from an infected mice] to transfer delayed-type hypersensitivity [DTH] to a naive mice (68). It was also observed that CD4+ cells, when adoptively transferred, conferred immunity to TB and a population of CD4+ memory cells also remains in the system after clearance of the infection by chemotherapy (69,70). Further, seminal work in mouse model firmly established the importance of Th1 pathway in the expression of protective immunity (71,72). The mouse data have also shown a potential role for CD8+ (73), CD4-/CD8- (74) and γ/δ T-cells (75) in generating immune response to TB vaccines. In fact, there are several instances, where findings originally obtained in the mouse model have later been verified in humans. For example, knockout mice deficient in IFN-γ and interleukin –12[IL-12] genes were found to be highly susceptible to Mtb infection akin to patients with hereditary deficiency in IFN-γ and IL-12 signalling (76). Mice with deficient TNF-α signalling exhibited similarity with rheumatoid arthritis patients who developed reactivation TB on treatment with anti-TNF-α monoclonal antibodies. The most evident similarity is observed with dramatically increased incidence of primary and secondary TB in knockout mice devoid of CD4+ cells, thus mimicking HIV infection (76).

The usefulness of the mouse model has grown tremendously over the last two decades due to the availability of a vast array of reagents like monoclonal antibodies to T-cell surface markers, cytokines and chemokines. Moreover, advancement in the field of transgenic expression, gene knock-out, gene knock-in technologies, along with the availability of a large variety of mouse mutants with defined immune deficiencies have immensely helped the scientific investigators in dissecting the precise nature of immune response to Mtb infection. The mouse genome sequence has further helped in designing genome-based experiments to pinpoint the importance of key genes involved in innate and adaptive immunity against TB and understanding the role of downstream signaling pathways.

Although, mouse model provides a huge advantage in terms of cost effectiveness, it fails to completely mimic the entire spectrum of human TB. The mouse is innately resistant to TB and generates a strong cellular immune response against Mtb infection and controls bacterial growth and disease progression. However, mouse does not develop a strong DTH response in contrast to what is observed in humans. In addition, the cellular organisation in the granuloma in mice is characterised by aggregation of lymphocytes towards the centre, which is in striking contrast to humans and guinea pigs wherein lymphocytes form a peripheral ring with arrangements of macrophages towards

the center (77,78). Further, the event of cavity development, which is one of the hallmark events in clinical TB, does not form in mouse TB (79). Thus, despite its definite advantages in the study of immunological aspects of TB, mouse model has only been recommended for the first order screening of vaccine candidates, which needs further validation from other animal models such as guinea pig, rabbit and NHP.

Guinea Pig Model of Tuberculosis

Guinea pig is currently one of the most useful models of human TB for evaluation of new vaccines. The primary reason for this preference stems from the ability of guinea pigs to initially develop a strong immunity leading to the formation of well-organised granulomas as seen in humans. These granulomas then undergo extensive caseation and tissue necrosis eventually killing the animal. Moreover, guinea pigs are sensitive to skin testing and can be used to determine vaccination-induced DTH reaction. Further, in contrast to mouse model, guinea pigs, like human beings, have a group of CD1+ molecules that are responsible for the presentation of mycobacterial glycolipids to a specialised T-cell population. These CD1+ molecules have been shown to present mycolic acids, lipoarabinomannan and other components of the mycobacterial cell wall to human T cells in vitro.

The guinea pig model has also been employed to study the effect of malnutrition on TB, which is known to induce a state of immunodeficiency. McMurray and colleagues have documented a series of immunological abnormalities associated with protein deficiency in guinea pigs, which, when viewed in a clinical context, mimic the situation, where malnutrition in humans results in an increased susceptibility to TB (80). Malnutrition is known to impair several aspects of mycobacterial antigen-specific peripheral T-cell function, including lympho-proliferation, interleukin-2 [IL-2] production, expression of the CD2 marker and the ability to mount a DTH response (81-83). These immunological alterations, which seem to be associated with the loss of vaccine-induced and naturally acquired resistance to pulmonary TB in guinea pigs, can serve as suitable surrogate markers for protection.

Most of the vaccine candidates are first screened in mouse model of TB and only promising candidates are taken up for screening in guinea pigs. But this strategy of prioritising any vaccine candidate should be analysed very carefully as there are chances of losing those candidates, which, though may not be efficacious in mice, but may have tremendous potential in guinea pigs. For several years, paucity of immunological reagents for guinea pigs, has precluded its use as a first-order screening model. However, recent advancements in microarray (84) and RNA sequencing technology (85) as well as availability of immunological reagents, is now allowing simultaneous assessment of immune responses and vaccine efficacy in this extremely valuable animal model.

Non-human Primate Model of Tuberculosis

On comparative assessment of all the existing animal models of TB, NHP like rhesus monkey, cynomolgus monkeys, etc. were found to mimic several aspects of human TB (86). Apart from the susceptibility to natural infection with a range of mycobacterial species, NHPs are very similar to humans in terms of granuloma architecture and various stages of disease progression (87,88). In addition, NHP [rhesus monkey] and humans share the presence of similar functional major histocompatibility complex [MHC] molecules, which bind specifically to mycobacterial peptides (89,90). Further, both humans and NHP have CD1 molecules in common, those are required for presenting several non-peptide mycobacterial products to the T cells (91,92). Besides, in NHP, the course of infection can be easily followed up by chest radiograph, weight loss, as well as by performing a variety of immunological assays, which provide a detailed insight into the disease progression. It has also been further developed to study HIV and TB co-infection, which has helped in understanding the disease pathogenesis and treatment of HIV-related TB (93). Langermans and colleagues (94) using the macaque model showed that protection against a high dose of *Mtb* infection could be achieved in cynomolgus monkeys with BCG vaccination, although no such protection was observed in case of rhesus monkeys. Though rhesus and cynomolgus monkeys are closely related species, they, differ markedly in their susceptibility to *Mtb* infection and BCG-induced protection; these two species, thus-represent the two extremes of the degree of protection induced by BCG in humans. Since most of the vaccines need to be compared to BCG, cynomolgus can be very useful for the evaluation of subunit and DNA vaccines, whereas live attenuated vaccines [like recombinant BCG] may show a clear improvement over BCG in rhesus monkeys (94,95). Though the studies in macaque model have tremendously helped gaining an insight into the immune responses and pathogenesis associated with human TB, several critical disadvantages have reserved this model only for the final stage of vaccine evaluation. The disadvantages, such as, high cost, requirement of extensive biohazard containment facility, difficulty in handling, difficulty in maintaining disease-free colonies of these primates, which are extremely susceptible to mycobacterial infections, have resulted in the testing of only a few candidate vaccines in primates till date.

IDENTIFICATION OF VACCINE TARGETS IN THE POST-GENOMIC ERA

The complete genome sequencing of *Mtb* in 1998 has not only brought a paradigm shift in the cellular and biochemical dissection of the pathogen but has also tremendously accelerated the vaccine development program (96). Modern bio-informatic methods have provided means for *in silico* genome wide characterisation of immuno-dominant antigens allowing rapid discovery and development of new vaccines. Further, sequencing of the genomes of 18 *Mycobacterium* species has opened up several new vistas and has significantly helped the process of identification of vaccine candidate by interspecies comparison of the genome sequences (97,98). Moreover, it has also helped to understand the source of antigenic variation among different strains of *Mtb*. Application of microarray and RNA-sequencing technologies have revealed a repertoire of new-stage specific antigens of *Mtb*, which are expressed in different phases of infection (99,100). Unlike the conventional targeted gene knockout methodology, application of techniques like transposon mutagenesis and signature-tagged mutagenesis have made it possible to screen a large number of mutants simultaneously for their growth and virulence in experimental animal models (101,102). Two other areas namely subunit and DNA vaccines have also been significantly benefited from the genome sequencing of *Mtb*. For example, several secreted or surface-exposed proteins, which are widely used as vaccine candidates, were discovered based on the presence of specific sequences or motifs. This *in silico* analysis to identify new vaccine candidates, which is termed as 'reverse vaccinology', has tremendously boosted the entire vaccine development program (103,104). It has also provided access to the entire repertoire of *Mtb* antigens. With the application of advanced immuno-informatic tools, several antigenic secretory proteins and their potent T-cell epitopes have been identified for the development of novel protein, peptide or epitope-based vaccines.

STRATEGIES FOR THE DEVELOPMENT OF TB VACCINES

Despite the lack of a perfect understanding about protective immunity against TB, there are several reasons to believe that a better TB vaccine is biologically possible. Less than 10% of individuals infected with *Mtb* develop the disease which strongly supports the notion that most people are immunocompetent and well equipped to keep the pathogen in check. However, reactivation of persistent tubercle bacilli in asymptomatic individuals suggests that natural infection with *Mtb* does not provide complete sterility, leaving behind some bacilli in dormant state. Thus, to outperform natural *Mtb* infection, a vaccine should induce a more potent immune response than the pathogen. Figure 54.2 depicts various stages of the disease progression, where specific intervention strategies like drugs and vaccines can be used. Various vaccination strategies that have emerged in the last two decades are listed in Table 54.1.

Recombinant Bacille Calmette-Guérin

It is well acclaimed that BCG protects children against childhood TB. Hence, instead of replacing BCG with another vaccine, it is now logical to improve the current vaccine by expressing in BCG the immuno-dominant *Mtb* antigens involved in pathogenesis, persistence and immuno-modulation. Alternatively, BCG or a recombinant BCG [rBCG] can be employed in a prime boost strategy. Thus, without hampering the childhood immunisation programme, an rBCG vaccine would help in improving the protective

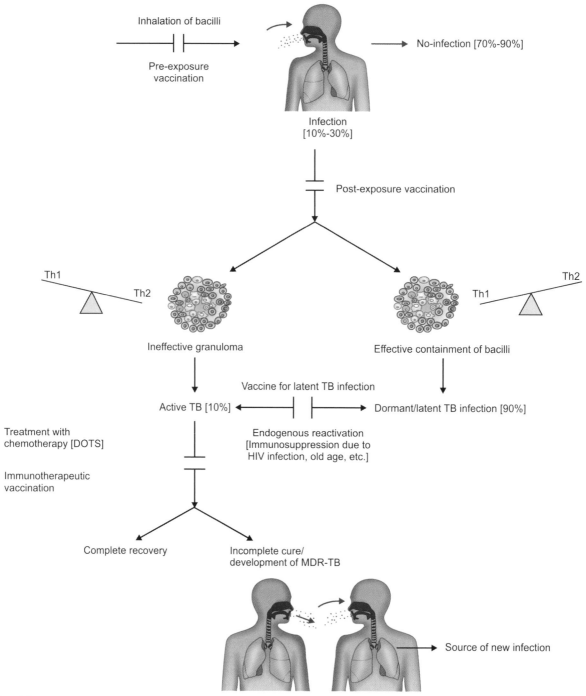

Figure 54.2: Different stages of *Mycobacterium tuberculosis* infection and intervention strategies. The figure illustrates the heterogeneity in terms of the outcome of infection in different individuals and various stages of the disease progression, where specific intervention strategies like drugs and vaccines can be used

TB = tuberculosis; HIV = human immunodeficiency virus; MDR-TB = multidrug-resistant tuberculosis

efficacy against adult pulmonary TB. Along with its potent immuno-adjuvant property, high degree of safety for human use and the availability of expression systems that provide enhanced and stable expression of genes in mycobacteria, BCG became a very attractive vehicle for the development of new rBCG vaccines. In addition, several strategies have been devised to enhance the expression and/or secretion of a protein into the extra-cellular *milieu* (105-111). Apart from the restoration of the lost genes like early secretory antigenic target-6 [ESAT-6] and MPB-64, which are absent from BCG, several other antigens like major secretory 30-32 kDa protein, 16 kDa HspX, etc. have been expressed in BCG and evaluated for their protective efficacy in mice and guinea pig models of TB (112-114). It is an excellent

Table 54.1: Various vaccination strategies that have emerged in the last two decades

Recombinant BCG

Live attenuated mutants and auxotrophs of *Mycobacterium tuberculosis*

NTM vaccines

Subunit vaccines

DNA vaccines

Epitope-based vaccines

Prime-boost immunisation strategies

BCG = bacille Calmette-Guérin; NTM = nontuberculous mycobacteria; DNA = deoxyribonucleic acid

approach and has resulted in the development of several promising new TB vaccine candidates (112-114). However, care must be exercised in the selection of genes as over-expression of the genes involved in pathogenesis may result in a BCG strain with enhanced virulence. For example, re-introduction of complete region of difference-1 [RD1] locus, although resulted in a better protection in immunocompetent mice, it was found cause virulence in immunocompromised mice (115,116). Also, over-expression of antigens like 19 kDa lipoprotein or superoxide dismutase [soda] in RBCG has resulted in an overall change in the immunomodulatory nature of BCG, resulting in loss of protective immune responses induced by BCG alone (117,118).

An efficient anti-TB immunity relies upon a Th1 immune response, which has led to the development of rBCG vaccines expressing human Th1 cytokines like IFN-γ, interferon-alpha [IFN-α], IL-2 and IL-12 (119-122). Although, all these recombinant strains exhibited improved Th1 response, their protective efficacy is not satisfactory. BCG is known to induce a detectable cytotoxic T-lymphocyte [CTL] response, however, its inability to access class I antigen-processing pathway has necessitated procedures to augment CD8+ T-cell response. An rBCG strain expressing listeriolysin of *Listeria monocytogenes*, which forms pores in the phagolysosomal membrane, has been reported to escape to the cytoplasm thereby promoting antigen processing by class I pathway resulting in a greater cytotoxic T cell response and a better protection against *Mtb* infection (123). This vaccine is now undergoing phase II clinical trial for its protective efficacy against TB.

Live Attenuated Mutants and Auxotrophs of *Mycobacterium tuberculosis*

The development of *Mtb* mutants as vaccine candidates primarily relies upon the assumption that the vaccine strain should be antigenically as identical as possible to the disease-causing organism. By comparative genomics, it has been revealed that in comparison to *Mtb* 16 defined regions [RD1-RD16] are deleted from the currently used BCG strains. These regions encode 129 open reading frames [ORFs], including several regulatory genes as well as some of the

highly immuno-dominant antigens (124). This has provided rationale for the development of live vaccines using an *Mtb* background rather than *M. bovis* BCG background. Such strains can be developed by either producing auxotrophic mutants of *Mtb* with limited replication capacity in immuno-compromised subjects or by disrupting virulence genes necessary for host–pathogen interaction (125).

A number of auxotrophic *Mtb* mutant strains developed by random transposon-mutagenesis, signature-tagged mutagenesis, illegitimate recombination and allelic exchange-homologous recombination have been assessed for their protective efficacy in experimental animal models (125-130). For example, a leucine auxotroph of *Mtb* that was severely attenuated in severe combined immunodeficiency syndrome [SCID] mice was completely cleared from mouse organs within a few weeks of immunisation. However, at least two doses were required to elicit significant protection in immunocompetent C57BL/6 mice. Due to its remarkable safety in immunocompromised mice, it is a potential candidate vaccine for use in immunodefficient individuals (130). The tryptophan and proline auxotrophs of *Mtb* have also been found to be highly attenuated and confer protection equivalent to proline or better tryptophan than BCG against *Mtb* infection in DBA/2 mice (129). A *pan*CD mutant of *Mtb* [genes required for *de novo* biosynthesis of pantothenate] was observed to be highly attenuated in immuno-compromised SCID and IFN-γ deficient mice. The *pan*CD mutant was found to be much safer than BCG and elicited long-term memory response, which persisted for several months after immunisation (131). A double auxotroph of *Mtb* [leucine and pantothenate] also provided long-term protection against *Mtb* infection in guinea pig model and was found to be safe in non-human primate model (127,132). Further, lysine *lysA* and *secA2* double mutant of *Mtb* was found to be highly efficacious and safe in mouse model compared to BCG vaccination (133).

A second approach relies on attenuation of *Mtb* genes required for virulence. Till date, several virulence genes have been identified, disrupted and the resulting mutants assessed for their growth *in vitro* and *in vivo* (134-139). These knock-out strains were found to have differences in their virulence and growth characteristics. For example, *Mtb* mutants deficient in dormancy-associated genes replicate in mice lungs in an unconstrained manner early after infection, but cease to grow at later stages due to their impaired dormancy gene program (134).

Due to highly pathogenic nature of *Mtb*, development of mutant strains for vaccine development requires careful consideration. An ideal *Mtb* mutant should have at least two or more unlinked genes deleted to reduce the probability of reversion. However, such mutants should be able to survive inside the host for sufficient time to generate an efficient immune response. Altogether, mutations should result in a fine balance between attenuation and immuno-genicity as over-attenuated bacilli may be devoid of key antigens necessary for protective immunity. In addition, these mutants need to be tested rigorously in immuno-suppressed animal models to ensure complete safety.

Atypical Mycobacterial Vaccines

Atypical and saprophytic species of mycobacteria that are closely related to *Mtb* have been evaluated for their vaccine efficacy in various animal models and human trials. The close phylogenetic relationship of these organisms with *Mtb* renders them antigenically similar to the pathogen. Apart from having an adjuvant-like property, these atypical mycobacteria are non-pathogenic even in immuno-compromised individuals. In a human trial, *M. microti,* when used in a prophylactic mode, conferred 77% protection, comparable to BCG against TB in infants (140,141). Several studies have also been carried out with killed/live or recombinant *M. vaccae* in both prophylactic and immuno-therapeutic mode resulting in protective efficacy comparable to BCG (142-144). In a separate study, *M. habana* exhibited improved protection over BCG in a mouse model (145,146). In another approach, killed *Mycobacterium indicus pranii* [previously known as *M. w*] caused reduction in the bacillary load in mice and prevented formation of granulomatous lesions in guinea pigs (147-151). A long-term human trial covering a very large population in north India revealed protective efficacy of *M. indicus pranii* against leprosy. The follow-up studies on the same population showed that *M. indicus pranii* also reduced the incidence of TB in this population by 61.5% (152,153). However, the unpublished data on *M. indicus pranii* in phase III clinical trials shows that the vaccine failed to show any protection against TB.

Subunit Vaccines

Subunit vaccines represent one of the most popular approaches for vaccine development. Subunit vaccines against *Mtb* mainly comprise secretory [culture filtrate proteins] and non-secretory proteins, lipids and carbohydrate antigens derived from *Mtb* cell wall, which have been used in adjuvanted or non-adjuvanted formulations. In addition, several subunit vaccines have been developed by using non-mycobacterial vectors, such as attenuated pox and adenoviruses.

Mtb alters its antigenic repertoire when it shifts from an active state to a dormant non-replicating state (154). Thus, it can be advocated that for a prophylactic vaccine, the candidate antigens should comprise proteins that are rapidly secreted during early infection. On the other hand, the proteins associated with dormancy-induced genes would serve better for a post-exposure vaccine. Indeed, a vaccine that includes antigens from both the classes is most likely to protect individuals from various populations with different age groups and exposure levels. The widespread use of BCG in neonates and its apparent effectiveness against paediatric TB has made it difficult to replace BCG with a new vaccine. Thus recently, the focus of TB vaccine research has shifted towards using these subunit vaccine candidates as a boosting agent in populations that have already been immunised with BCG (155-157).

The apparent inability of the subunit vaccines to mount a strong T-cell response has accelerated the process of adjuvant discovery required to induce a potent Th1 response by these subunit vaccines. New adjuvants like dimethyl dioctadecyl ammonium bromide [DDA], monophosphoryl lipid A [MPL-A] and AS02A, which are potent modulators of T-cell responses, have been shown to enhance the immunogenicity and protective efficacy of several subunit vaccines when compared with the traditional adjuvants (158-160). For instance, early secreted antigenic target 6 [ESAT 6] as a stand-alone purified protein failed to stimulate the adaptive arm of immune response, but stimulated protective immune responses equivalent to BCG, when injected along with a mixture of DDA and MPL-A (161). The fusion protein 72f, when used along with an adjuvant AS01, exhibited very promising results in several animal models and is currently in phase II clinical trials (153). In addition, fusion of antigen 85B and ESAT-6 proteins in two different adjuvant formulations [IC31 and CAF01] are currently in phase I clinical trials (153).

Deoxyribonucleic Acid Vaccines

The observation that immunisation with naked DNA could direct the immune system towards stronger and persistent cellular and humoral immune responses attracted many investigators towards this area (162,163). Intramuscular injection of a mammalian expression vector encoding a desired gene, results in the expression of corresponding protein, which subsequently induces a potent cellular immune response against the encoded antigen. This is especially advantageous in the context of TB as the protective immunity against *Mtb* is primarily dependent on the cellular fraction of the immune system (76). DNA vaccine allows continuous expression of a particular antigen, thereby exposing the immune system to the antigen for a prolonged time. The usefulness of DNA vaccines has led to the development of a variety of methods for their delivery to a desired site in the host. Direct injection, electroporation or gene–gun based delivery into muscles, delivery to the respiratory mucosa using liposome encapsulated DNA vaccines, etc., are in common use for delivery of DNA vaccines (164-168). Expression of antigens by DNA vaccines and their subsequent processing and presentation along with the MHC class I molecules mimic the antigen-processing pathway followed by an intracellular pathogen. Several DNA vaccines have been developed in the last decade and have been evaluated for their efficacy against TB in various animal models. DNA vaccination with genes encoding the members of Ag 85 complex of *Mtb* and 65 kDa heat shock protein of *M. leprae* conferred protection equal to BCG (169,170). A significant protection [equivalent to BCG] was also observed in case of ESAT-6, MPT-64 [a 24-kDa protein secreted by *Mtb*] (171), phosphate-binding protein [*PstS*] (172) and a proline-proline-glutamic acid [PPE] protein (173) when used as DNA vaccines in mouse model of experimental TB. The advancements in the field of recombinant DNA technology have facilitated simultaneous expression of more than one gene using a mammalian expression vector. DNA vaccines based on fusion of antigen Ag85B with either ESAT-6 or MPT-64 gene conferred protection better or equivalent to BCG (174). DNA vaccines expressing latency-associated antigen HspX has demonstrated remarkable protection as a booster vaccine following BCG or rBCG vaccination in animal models (113,157). Moreover, expression of co-stimulatory molecules, such as, different cytokines and chemokines and inclusion of CpG motifs in the DNA vaccine backbone has helped in enhancing the immunogenicity of DNA vaccines. Despite several promising results in animal models, issues related to antibiotic markers in the plasmid DNA backbone, concerns regarding integration of these plasmids in host genome and development of anti-DNA antibodies leading to autoimmune diseases have prevented their entry into the human clinical trials till date. However, several regulatory measures have been introduced globally to improve the safety and usefulness of DNA vaccines in humans (175-177).

Epitope-based Vaccines

Epitope-based vaccines, the latest entry in the field of vaccine development, have quickly emerged as one of the promising advancements in the field of vaccine discovery. Recently, strategies for exclusive delivery of immuno-dominant T-cell epitopes of a single or multiple proteins have emerged. One of the potential advantages of this epitope-based approach includes higher safety as it helps in getting rid of the unwanted, toxic or immunosuppressive regions from a protein. This also provides the opportunity to appropriately engineer the epitopes to elicit a desired immune response. Several immuno-dominant epitopes have been identified by employing either the bioinformatics or by screening the T-cells derived from TB patients at various stages of disease progression by *in vitro* assays employing different overlapping peptides of a protein (178-180). Moreover, comparative genomics have also helped in the identification of conserved epitopes across various pathogenic organisms, which can be incorporated along with the *Mtb* epitopes to generate a multipurpose vaccine (181). This approach can prove to be extremely beneficial, if the specificity of T-cells isolated from exposed but asymptomatic individuals is characterised against a vast array of peptides isolated from *Mtb* proteome. These peptides can be further assessed for their immunogenicity in the form of multivalent epitope-based vaccine. Till date, several epitope-based vaccines have been developed and evaluated in animal models (182-185). Some of these vaccines have shown encouraging results; however, none of the vaccines have moved to clinical trials. With the availability of an effective delivery system, a multi-epitope-based vaccine may emerge as one of the potential means of immunisation.

Prime-boost Immunisation Strategies

The concept of 'boosting' the immune responses traces its history back to the time of Louis Pasteur. The fact that

the immune system once primed with an antigen elicits a heightened response to the secondary exposure of the antigen, has been utilised to develop effective prime-boost vaccination strategies against TB. Repeated administration with the same vaccine [called homologous boosting] has proved to be relatively inefficient at boosting cellular immunity, instead it generates a very strong humoral response. This has been especially observed in case of BCG which, when administered, repeatedly offered little benefit in humans as well as in various animal models (186). Besides, these studies also demonstrated that the myco-bacterial sensitisation dramatically lowers the effectiveness of BCG (187-190). In order to circumvent this problem, 'heterologous boosting' came into being, which involves sequential administration of vaccines with appropriate intervals using different antigen-delivery system such that the immune system is primed to the antigen using one vector and is then boosted with the same antigen delivered through a different vector. The key strength of this strategy lies in the synergistic effect of vaccines on immunity, instead of the additive effect generally observed in the case of homologous boosting (191-193). This synergistic enhancement of immunity to the target antigen is reflected by an increased number of antigen-specific T cells and selective enrichment of high avidity T cells. Moreover, it also induces an elevated level of both CD4+ and CD8+ T-cell response. The tremendous power of prime-boost was highlighted in a murine model, wherein intranasal vaccination of mice with BCG, followed by a booster of a recombinant modified vaccinia virus Ankara expressing antigen 85A [MVA85A], resulted in a nearly 300-fold reduction in bacillary load in the lungs following aerosol infection with *Mtb* (194). This would mimic the situation where a gradually declining immunity of BCG can be enhanced by boosting with a candidate antigen specifically recognised by memory immunity. Under the European Union, TB vaccine screening program, 26 different strategies involving various antigens and delivery approaches were simultaneously evaluated in guinea pig model. Amongst all the strategies, the MVA85A-based prime boost vaccination described above was the only successful strategy that significantly prolonged the survival of guinea pigs in comparison to BCG vaccination (195). This vaccine became the first new generation TB vaccine to enter the human trials. Although, the vaccine was found to be safe and immunogenic in phase I and phase II human trials, however, the vaccine failed to show any protection against TB in phase III trial (196-199). Apart from the viral vectors, which have been highly recommended as boosting agents, subunit vaccines including both recombinant proteins and DNA vaccines, are now being used to boost the immunity imparted by BCG. In a study, it was observed that with age, mice vaccinated with BCG gradually lose their capacity to resist an aerosol infection with *Mtb*. However, if these mice are boosted with the Ag85A protein [with MPLA as an adjuvant] in midlife, it restored back the resistance in elderly mice to levels equivalent to young ones; with reduced pathological damage and bacillary load on lung (200).

Besides the use of BCG as the priming agent, several efforts to develop other heterologous prime-boost immunisation strategies have also been tested, wherein, subunit or DNA vaccines have been employed as priming agents (201-204). Success of heterologous prime-boost immunisation strategies has generated optimism for the development of effective anti-tubercular vaccines in future.

IMMUNOTHERAPEUTIC APPROACH TO COMBAT TUBERCULOSIS

Current strategies for TB control are based on the reduction of transmission by treatment of active cases and prevention of disease by prophylactic vaccination. The available chemotherapy comprises a very lengthy treatment schedule [6-9 months] with a combination of four drugs, namely, isoniazid, pyrazinamide, rifampicin and ethambutol. This therapy, although successful against drug sensitive TB, often fails due to non-compliance with the lengthy treatment regimens. Non-compliance with anti-TB treatment often leads to relapse and emergence of drug resistance. Thus, in order to reduce the incidence of relapse and emergence of drug resistance cases, it is imperative to develop effective means to reduce the duration of TB therapy. However, till the difficult goal of shorter chemotherapy is achieved, parallel research is underway to develop effective immuno-therapeutic agents that can serve as an adjunct to standard chemotherapy (205-207). It may not only reduce the prolonged chemotherapy period but may also eliminate dormant bacilli and consequently prevent reactivation. Additionally, a reduction in the conversion of re-infection into active disease may be another possible spin-off.

DNA vaccine immunotherapy along with chemotherapy has shown considerable promise in the treatment of TB disease in pre-clinical animal models. In a study, a combi-nation of two DNA vaccines [Ag85A and PstS-3] in mice along with chemotherapy was found to prevent exogenous re-infection as well as endogenous reactivation (208). Supplementing the chemotherapy with DNA vaccine encoding the *Mycobacterium leprae* hsp60 also resulted in a significantly reduced course of treatment (209). In an alternative approach, the use of *Mycobacterium vaccae* as an immunotherapeutic agent successfully enhanced the Th1 response, however, the expected improvement in the treatment of HIV- infected adults with pulmonary TB was not observed (210,211).

Immunotherapy can also be used to downregulate a highly exaggerated immune response in the patients with severe disease. The aggravated pathological damage in active pulmonary TB, which stems from a localised and a systemic production of high levels of Th1 cytokines such as IFN-γ or TNF-α, can be reduced by targeted suppression of these cytokines by using neutralising antibodies. Besides, the use of systemic immuno-suppressing agents like corticosteroids, etc. can also produce similar effects. However, in the use of these immuno-modulatory agents, extreme care should be taken to avoid over-suppression of the immune system, which may have unfavorable consequences. For instance, use of anti-TNF-α antibodies although reduced the pathology and inflammation associated with rheumatoid arthritis, it resulted in increased incidence of reactivation of latent infections in these patients (212,213). However, when anti-TNF-α antibodies were used as an adjunct to chemotherapy, it substantially improved the body weight, radiological scores and sputum culture conversion in patients with TB-HIV co-infection (214). Due to these dual effects, use of anti-TNF-α antibodies for the treatment of TB patients is still in the pre-clinical stage.

With growing evidence for the role of various cytokines like IFN-γ, IL-2, interleukin-4 [IL-4], IL-12, interleukin-18 [IL-18] etc., in TB pathogenesis and protection, several immuno-therapeutic strategies have been developed. For example, an aerosol delivery of IFN-γ was found to produce clini-cally encouraging response in treating multidrug-resistant TB [MDR-TB], although the effect was transient (215,216). In another study, treatment with granulocyte-macrophage colony-stimulating factor [GM-CSF] along with IFN-γ successfully treated patients with refractory central nervous system MDR-TB (217,218). Further, a cocktail of six recombi-nant proteins [six antigens: 85B, 38Kda, ESAT6, CFP21, Mtb8.4, and 16Kda] along with IFN-γ and Ribi adjuvant, monophosphoryl lipid A-trehalose dicorynomycolate [MPLA-TD] conferred a significant protection against *Mtb* infection in mouse model (218). Besides, IL-2 immunotherapy in MDR-TB patients resulted in a significant immune activation and reduced bacillary burden (219). However, in a separate study, no significant reduction in the clinical symptoms was observed when IL-2 was used as an immuno-therapeutic agent in adults suffering from drug-susceptible TB (220).

Another important class of immunotherapeutic agents are modulators of host cell signalling pathways, however, most of them are involved in regulating various cytokine pathways. One of the recent examples is the use of phospho-diesterase inhibitor, which increases the cyclic adenosine monophosphate [c-AMP] production by macrophages leading to reduced levels of TNF-α and TB-associated pathology. Phosphodiesterase inhibitors when used along with TB chemotherapy demonstrated enhanced bacterial clearance compared to treatment with the chemotherapy alone (221,222).

Poor nutrition has long been associated with the increased risk of TB (223,224). Several studies have addressed the role of vitamin D supplements and its immunotherapeutic effects in TB patients. Particularly, vitamin D supplement was found to be beneficial as an adjunct to chemotherapy in patients with severe vitamin D deficiency. The proposed mechanism behind the effect of vitamin D is the action of bioactive 1,25-dihydroxy vitamin D_3 in potentiating autophagy, phagolysosomal fusion and release of antibacterial peptide cathelicidin (225,226). Although adjunctive immunotherapy is reasonably effective, it still poses serious problems such as, high cost, occasional adverse effects and induction of tolerance during long-term application of immune adjunctive agents. Identification of newer immuno-therapeutic agents, their delivery mode and dosage may possibly help in shortening the prolonged chemotherapy period and an effective management of the disease in future.

Impact of Zoonosis on TB Vaccine Development

Zoonotic diseases in humans include all the diseases that are acquired from or transmitted to any other vertebrate animal. Among the various zoonotic diseases, TB represents one of the most common diseases transmitted to humans. Although, *Mtb* is the causative agent of human TB, a significant proportion of human infections is caused by *Mycobacterium bovis*—the aetiological agent of bovine TB. The pulmonary TB caused by *Mtb* and *Mycobacterium bovis* are clinically indistinguishable with similar radiographic and pathological features (227,228). In many African and Asian countries, where cattle are an integral part of social life, close physical contact between humans and infected animals leads to significant proportion of human TB of bovine origin. Several incidences of human TB caused by *Mycobacterium bovis* were reported from Africa (229,230), Latin America (231,232) and some of the Asian countries (227,233). In Latin America, 2% of the total pulmonary cases and 8% of extra-pulmonary TB cases were reported to be caused by *Mycobacterium bovis* (227). Analysis of the cerebrospinal fluid from patients suffering from TB meningitis in India revealed that in comparison to *Mtb* (2.8%), 17% of the samples were found to be positive for *Mycobacterium bovis* (234). In addition, 8.7% and 35.7% of the samples collected from human sources and cattle, respectively were classified as mixed infections with *Mtb* and *Mycobacterium bovis* (235). The incidences of TB due to *Mycobacterium bovis* infection have also been reported in HIV-seropositive TB patients. For example, in France, 1.6% of TB cases in HIV-positive patients were found to be caused by *Mycobacterium bovis* infection (236). On the other hand, cases of *Mtb* infection in cattle have also been reported from India as well as some of the European countries, though the incidence rate was not very high (235,237).

As the performance of BCG in preventing bovine TB is doubtful, devising an effective vaccination strategy against bovine TB would be a viable option in controlling *Mycobacterium bovis*-based human infections in addition to reducing the burden of bovine TB. Several recombinant BCG strains, subunit vaccines and DNA vaccines expressing *Mtb* antigens, have also been assessed for their efficacy in bovine model against *M. bovis* infection. Prime-boost vaccination strategies by using DNA vaccines encoding Hsp65, Hsp70 and Apa as priming agent followed by a booster of BCG have provided substantial evidence that this regimen can provide better protection in calves than either of the vaccines when used alone (202). In another strategy, Martin and colleagues reported substantial protection in cattle immunised with BCG followed by a booster of MVA85A and attenuated fowl pox strain FP9 [FP85A], expressing antigen 85A (238). Furthermore, a combination of DNA vaccines encoding Ag85B, MPT64 and MPT83 when tested for their efficacy using DDA as an adjuvant, was found to be highly effective in controlling bovine TB (239).

In some industrialised and developed countries, animal TB control and eradication programme, together with milk pasteurisation have drastically lowered the incidence of TB caused by *Mycobacterium bovis* in both animal and human population (240), however, a developing country like India, which has the largest livestock population in the world, has no effective control and eradication programme for bovine TB. Apart from developing vaccines against both human and bovine form of TB, control of zoonotic TB in India and other developing countries needs co-ordination between the human and bovine TB vaccine development programmes along with strict regulatory measures. As the degree of cattle movement in a country also enhances the incidence of TB and other zoonotic diseases, strict surveillance of animal migration may further help in bringing down the incidence rate (241). In addition, specific and effective surveillance strategies for different species of *Mycobacterium* will aid in detection of TB cases of diverse origin, which would help in developing effective prevention and treatment strategies for TB.

Tuberculosis Vaccines in Clinical Trials: Key Issues

Last decade has clearly witnessed a resurgence in the field of TB vaccine research; more than 200 new vaccine candidates have already been evaluated for their efficacy in various animal models and several promising candidates are now in various phases of human clinical trials (153). These vaccine candidates have shown encouraging results in various pre-clinical animal models, including the non-human primate model. However, success in various animal models does not always guarantee effectiveness of a vaccine in human trials. The best examples are MVA85A, one of the most promising candidate vaccines. Recent report of MVA85A phase IIb trial in infants in South Africa, showed no evidence of protection against *Mtb* infection, although, it did meet the primary objective of the trial, i.e. safety (199). TB being a chronic disease with diverse clinical and pathological outcomes in different individuals, it may be unwise to expect a single vaccine to work efficiently in all these different situations. Hence, lack of protection in one population does not negate the possibility of beneficial effects of MVA85A in other populations. This also justifies testing of new vaccine candidates in multiple target populations encompassing different age groups, immune and nutritional status as well as geographical and genetic background. Another important question that emerged from this study is regarding the existing immunological correlates of protection. Although, in animal models, induction of antigen-specific Th1 and Th17 responses were found to be associated with protection conferred by MVA85A, a similar immune response in humans did not lead to protection (199). These observations raised an alarm regarding the insufficiency of the existing immunological correlates of protection and, thus, demand identification and development of new parameters that can be employed both in animal models and humans. Recently, primary analysis of the ongoing randomised, double-blind, placebo-controlled, phase IIb trial (242) of the M72/AS01E TB vaccine in Kenya, South Africa, and Zambia, revealed that M72/AS01E provided 54.0% protection for *Mtb*-infected adults against active pulmonary TB disease. Nonetheless, the ongoing clinical trials have generated tremendous hope in the TB research community as well as in general population. These trials have not only addressed the safety issues pertaining to different types of vaccines, but also provided the opportunity to perform detailed immunological assays on multiple samples obtained from different populations. The detailed characterisation of immune responses will prove to be instrumental in selecting the most reliable set of immunological parameters for future studies.

Table 54.2 shows the current status of the pipeline for new TB vaccines (153). Presently, eight vaccines are in phase II or phase III trials. An efficient management of regulatory and operational issues is one of the major challenges while conducting a successful clinical trial for TB vaccines. This requires [i] a focused and co-ordinated effort of multi-disciplinary expertise or networks, such as mycobacteriologists, epidemiologists, clinical trial specialists, vaccine biologists, immunologists, clinicians, statisticians, social workers, etc.; [ii] selection of an appropriate trial site based on detailed epidemiological knowledge of TB, HIV and incidences of other infectious and non-infectious

diseases in the area; [iii] identification of specific inclusion and exclusion criteria of subjects for enrolment of volunteers in the clinical trial based on the type of vaccine and its target population; [iv] development of novel, cost-effective and easy-to-perform robust diagnostic assays and harmonisation of the assay procedures and data analysis are critical for comparison among various vaccine candidates tested in different trials; [v] along with adherence to the global ethical and regulatory norms, local factors at the trial sites such as, cultural perceptions, economic condition, language, education, technological advancements must be given due consideration; and [vi] finally, a continuous financial support and participation from governmental as well as non-governmental organisations is the key to the success of any clinical trial.

One of the greatest challenges of the 21st century medical research is developing an improved TB vaccine, which provides complete protection against TB. Although several key questions related to TB still need to be answered, a great deal of hope has emerged due to rapid increase in our understanding of cellular immunity, knowledge of entire genome of several *Mycobacterium* species and advent of new and improved approaches for studying global gene regulatory patterns. Besides, development in the area of proteomics and metabolomics is facilitating the identification and characterisation of new virulent determinants and immunodominant antigens, which is allowing the development of novel intervention strategies. In addition to a strict regional surveillance and international cooperation, if all the necessary resources are committed for the development of TB vaccines, we might be able to go a long way in our fight against this enormous global health problem.

ACKNOWLEDGEMENTS

A part of the work included in this chapter was supported by financial grants received from the Department of Biotechnology, Government of India. The help rendered by Rajiv Chawla in the preparation of the manuscript is also acknowledged.

Table 54.2: The development pipeline for new TB vaccines, 2018

Phase I
  Boosting vaccines
    Ad5 Ag85A [McMaster, CanSino]
    IDR93 + GLA-SE [IDRI, Aeras]
    DAR-901 [Darmouth University, Aeras]
    ChAdOx1.85A [Oxford, Birmingham]
    Crucell Ad35 – MV85A prime-boost [UOXF, Aeras, Crucell]
  Priming vaccines
    MTBVAC [Biofabri, TBVI, Zaragosa]

Phase IIa
  Boosting vaccines
    Crucell Ad35 / Aeras402 [Crucell, Aeras]
    H I + IC31 [SSI, TBVI, Intercell, EDCTP]
    H56: IC31 [SSI, Intercell, Aeras]
    H4: IC31 [SSI, SP, Aeras]
    ID93 + GLA-SE [IDRI, Wellcome Trust]
  Priming vaccines
    VPM1002 [MPIIB, VPM, TBVI, SII]
  Immunotherapeutic vaccines
    RUTI [Archivel Pharma, SL]

Phase IIb
  Boosting vaccines
    MVA85A / Aeras-485 [UOXF, Aeras]
    M72 + ASO1$_E$ [GSK, Aeras]
    DAR-90 [Dartmouth, GHIT]

Phase III
  Immunotherapeutic vaccines
    M. indicus pranii [DBT, Govt. of India, Cadila]
    M. vaccae [An Hui Longcom]

TB = tuberculosis
Source: references 153,243

REFERENCES

1. World Health Organization. Global tuberculosis report 2018. Geneva: World Health Organization; 2018.
2. Kaufmann SH, McMichael AJ. Annulling a dangerous liaison: vaccination strategies against AIDS and tuberculosis. Nat Med 2005;11:S33-44.
3. Central TB Division, Ministry of Health and Family Welfare, Government of India. TB India 2018. RNTCP annual status report. New Delhi: Central TB Division, Ministry of Health and Family Welfare, Government of India; 2018.
4. Calmette A, Guerin C. Nouvelles recherches experimentales sur la vaccination der bovides contre la tuberculose. Ann Inst Pasteur 1920;34:553-61.
5. Lugosi L. Theoretical and methodological aspects of BCG vaccine from the discovery of Calmette and Guérin to molecular biology. A review. Tuber Lung Dis 1992;73:252-61.
6. Milstien JB, Gibson JJ. Quality control of BCG vaccine by WHO: a review of factors that may influence vaccine effectiveness and safety. Bull World Health Organ 1990;68:93-108.

7. Hyge TV. The efficacy of BCG-vaccination; epidemic of tuberculosis in a State School, with an observation period of 12 years. Acta Tuberc Scand 1956;32:89-107.

8. Pönnighaus JM, Fine PE, Sterne JA, Wilson RJ, Msosa E, Gruer PJ, et al. Efficacy of BCG vaccine against leprosy and tuberculosis in northern Malawi. Lancet 1992;339:636-9.

9. Brosch R, Gordon SV, Buchrieser C, Pym AS, Garnier T, Cole ST. Comparative genomics uncovers large tandem chromosomal duplications in Mycobacterium bovis BCG Pasteur. Yeast 2000;17:111-23.

10. Brosch R, Gordon SV, Garnier T, Eiglmeier K, Frigui W, Valenti P, et al. Genome plasticity of BCG and impact on vaccine efficacy. Proc Natl Acad Sci USA 2007;104:5596-601.

11. Lotte A, Wasz-Höckert O, Poisson N, Dumitrescu N, Verron M, Couvet E. BCG complications. Estimates of the risks among vaccinated subjects and statistical analysis of their main characteristics. Adv Tuberc Res 1984;21:107-93.

12. von Reyn CF, Clements CJ, Mann JM. Human immunodeficiency virus infection and routine childhood immunisation. Lancet 1987;2:669-72.

13. Comstock GW. Simple, practical ways to assess the protective efficacy of a new tuberculosis vaccine. Clin Infect Dis 2000; 30 Suppl 3:S250-3.

14. Bloom BR, Fine PEM. The BCG experience: implications for future vaccines against tuberculosis. In: Bloom BR, editor. Tuberculosis: pathogenesis, protection and control. Washington: ASM Press; 1994.p.531-58.

15. Colditz GA, Brewer TF, Berkey CS, Wilson ME, Burdick E, Fineberg HV, et al. Efficacy of BCG vaccine in the prevention of tuberculosis. Meta-analysis of the published literature. JAMA 1994;271:698-702.

16. Clemens JD, Chuong JJ, Feinstein AR. The BCG controversy. A methodological and statistical reappraisal. JAMA 1983;249:2362-9.

17. Comstock GW. Epidemiology of tuberculosis. Am Rev Respir Dis 1982;125:8-15.

18. Skamene E. Genetic control of resistance to mycobacterial infection. Curr Top Microbiol Immunol 1986;124:49-66.

19. Wilkinson RJ. Human genetic susceptibility to tuberculosis: time for a bottom-up approach? J Infect Dis 2012;205:525-7.

20. Hotez PJ, Molyneux DH, Fenwick A, Ottesen E, Ehrlich Sachs S, Sachs JD. Incorporating a rapid-impact package for neglected tropical diseases with programs for HIV/AIDS, tuberculosis, and malaria. PLoS Med 2006;3:e102.

21. Borkow G, Weisman Z, Leng Q, Stein M, Kalinkovich A, Wolday D, et al. Helminths, human immunodeficiency virus and tuberculosis. Scand J Infect Dis 2001;33:568-71.

22. Elias D, Akuffo H, Pawlowski A, Haile M, Schön T, Britton S. Schistosoma mansoni infection reduces the protective efficacy of BCG vaccination against virulent Mycobacterium tuberculosis. Vaccine 2005;23:1326-34.

23. Kremer K, Glynn JR, Lillebaek T, Niemann S, Kurepina NE, Kreiswirth BN, et al. Definition of the Beijing/W lineage of Mycobacterium tuberculosis on the basis of genetic markers. J Clin Microbiol 2004;42:4040-9.

24. Castañon-Arreola M, López-Vidal Y, Espitia-Pinzón C, Hernández-Pando R. A new vaccine against tuberculosis shows greater protection in a mouse model with progressive pulmonary tuberculosis. Tuberculosis [Edinb] 2005;85:115-26.

25. Devulder G, Pérouse de Montclos M, Flandrois JP. A multi-gene approach to phylogenetic analysis using the genus Mycobacterium as a model. Int J Syst Evol Microbiol 2005;55:293-302.

26. List of prokaryotic names with standing in nomenclature. Genus Mycobacterium. Available from URL: http://www.bacterio.net/mycobacterium.html. Accessed on December 22, 2016.

27. Chatterjee D. The mycobacterial cell wall: structure, biosynthesis and sites of drug action. Curr Opin Chem Biol 1997;1:579-88.

28. Liu J, Barry CE 3rd, Nikaido H. Cell wall: physical structure and permeability. In: Ratledge C, Dale J, editors. Mycobacteria: molecular biology and virulence. Oxford: Blackwell Publishing Ltd; 1999.p.220-39.

29. Baulard AR, Besra GS, Brennan PJ. The cell-wall core of Mycobacterium: structure, biogenesis and genetics. In: Ratledge C, Dale J, editors. Mycobacteria: molecular biology and virulence. Oxford: Blackwell Publishing Ltd; 1999.p.240-59.

30. Baek SH, Li AH, Sassetti CM. Metabolic regulation of mycobacterial growth and antibiotic sensitivity. PLoS Biol 2011;9:e1001065.

31. Agarwal N, Lamichhane G, Gupta R, Nolan S, Bishai WR. Cyclic AMP intoxication of macrophages by a Mycobacterium tuberculosis adenylate cyclase. Nature 2009;460:98-102.

32. Singhal A, Jaiswal A, Arora VK, Prasad HK. Modulation of gamma interferon receptor 1 by Mycobacterium tuberculosis: a potential immune response evasive mechanism. Infect Immun 2007;75:2500-10.

33. Philips JA, Ernst JD. Tuberculosis pathogenesis and immunity. Annu Rev Pathol 2012;7:353-84.

34. Dannenberg AM Jr. Cellular hypersensitivity and cellular immunity in the pathogensis of tuberculosis: specificity, systemic and local nature, and associated macrophage enzymes. Bacteriol Rev 1968;32:85102.

35. Stenger S, Modlin RL. T-cell-mediated immunity to Mycobacterium tuberculosis. Curr Opin Microbiol 1999;2:89-93.

36. Vasselon T, Detmers PA. Toll receptors: a central element in innate immune responses. Infect Immun 2002;70:1033-41.

37. Goldszmid RS, Caspar P, Rivollier A, White S, Dzutsev A, Hieny S, et al. NK cell-derived interferon-γ orchestrates cellular dynamics and the differentiation of monocytes into dendritic cells at the site of infection. Immunity 2012;36:1047-59.

38. Feng CG, Kaviratne M, Rothfuchs AG, Cheever A, Hieny S, Young HA, et al. NK cell-derived IFN-γ differentially regulates innate resistance and neutrophil response in T-cell-deficient hosts infected with Mycobacterium tuberculosis. J Immunol 2006;177:7086-93.

39. Herrmann JL, Lagrange PH. Dendritic cells and Mycobacterium tuberculosis: which is the Trojan horse? Pathol Biol [Paris] 2005;53:35-40.

40. van Kooyk Y, Geijtenbeek TB. DC-SIGN: escape mechanism for pathogens. Nat Rev Immunol 2003;3:697-709.

41. Winau F, Hegasy G, Kaufmann SH, Schaible UE. No life without death—apoptosis as prerequisite for T-cell activation. Apoptosis 2005;10:707-15.

42. Roura-Mir C, Wang L, Cheng TY, Matsunaga I, Dascher CC, Peng SL, et al. Mycobacterium tuberculosis regulates CD1 antigen presentation pathways through TLR-2. J Immunol 2005;175:1758-66.

43. Shen Y, Zhou D, Qiu L, Lai X, Simon M, Shen L, et al. Adaptive immune response of Vgamma2Vdelta2+ T cells during mycobacterial infections. Science 2002;295:2255-8.

44. Fischer K, Scotet E, Niemeyer M, Koebernick H, Zerrahn J, Maillet S, et al. Mycobacterial phosphatidylinositol mannoside is a natural antigen for CD1d-restricted T cells. Proc Natl Acad Sci USA 2004;101:10685-90.

45. Kaufmann SH. Protection against tuberculosis: cytokines, T cells, and macrophages. Ann Rheum Dis 2002;61:ii54-ii58.

46. Petruccioli E, Romagnoli A, Corazzari M, Coccia EM, Butera O, Delogu G, et al. Specific T cells restore the autophagic flux inhibited by Mycobacterium tuberculosis in human primary macrophages. J Infect Dis 2012;205:1425-35.

47. Trinchieri G. Type I interferon: friend or foe? J Exp Med 2010;207:2053-63.

48. Desvignes L, Wolf AJ, Ernst JD. Dynamic roles of type I and type II IFNs in early infection with Mycobacterium tuberculosis. J Immunol 2012;188:6205-15.

49. Novikov A, Cardone M, Thompson R, Shenderov K, Kirschman KD, Mayer-Barber KD, et al. Mycobacterium tuberculosis triggers host type I IFN signaling to regulate IL-1β production in human macrophages. J Immunol 2011;187:2540-7.

50. Dannenberg AM, Dey B. Perspectives for developing new tuberculosis vaccines derived from the pathogenesis of tuberculosis: I. basic principles, II. preclinical testing, and III. clinical testing. Vaccine 2013;1:58-76.

51. Agger EM, Andersen P. Tuberculosis subunit vaccine development: on the role of interferon-gamma. Vaccine 2001;19:2298-302.

52. Ting LM, Kim AC, Cattamanchi A, Ernst JD. Mycobacterium tuberculosis inhibits IFN-gamma transcriptional responses without inhibiting activation of STAT1. J Immunol 1999;163:3898-906.

53. Dalton DK, Haynes L, Chu CQ, Swain SL, Wittmer S. Interferon γ eliminates responding CD4 T cells during mycobacterial infection by inducing apoptosis of activated CD4 T cells. J Exp Med 2000;192:117-22.

54. Hirsch CS, Toossi Z, Vanham G, Johnson JL, Peters P, Okwera A, et al. Apoptosis and T-cell hyporesponsiveness in pulmonary tuberculosis. J Infect Dis 1999;179:945-53.

55. Ottenhoff TH. New pathways of protective and pathological host defense to mycobacteria. Trends Microbiol 2012;20:419-28.

56. Ancelet L, Kirman J. Shaping the CD4+ memory immune response against tuberculosis: the role of antigen persistence, location and multi-functionality. Biomol Concepts 2012;3:13-20.

57. Seder RA, Darrah PA, Roederer M. T-cell quality in memory and protection: implications for vaccine design. Nat Rev Immunol 2008;8:247-58.

58. Scriba TJ, Tameris M, Mansoor N, Smit E, van der Merwe L, Isaacs F, et al. Modified vaccinia Ankara-expressing Ag85A, a novel tuberculosis vaccine, is safe in adolescents and children, and induces polyfunctional CD4+ T cells. Eur J Immunol 2010;40:279-90.

59. Sgaragli G, Frosini M. Human tuberculosis I. Epidemiology, diagnosis and pathogenetic mechanisms. Curr Med Chem 2016;23:2836-73.

60. Clerici M, Shearer GM. A TH1 --> TH 2 switch is a critical step in the etiology of HIV infection. Immunol Today 1993;14:107-111.

61. Del Amo J, Malin AS, Pozniak A, De Cock KM. Does tuberculosis accelerate the progression of HIV disease? Evidence from basic science and epidemiology. AIDS 1999;13:1151-8.

62. Toossi Z, Sierra-Madero JG, Blinkhorn RA, Mettler MA, Rich EA. Enhanced susceptibility of blood monocytes from patients with pulmonary tuberculosis to productive infection with human immunodeficiency virus type 1. J Exp Med 1993;177:1511-6.

63. Clements CJ, von Reyn CF, Mann JM. HIV infection and routine childhood immunization: a review. Bull World Health Organ 1987;65:905-11.

64. Quinn TC. Interactions of the human immunodeficiency virus and tuberculosis and the implications for BCG vaccination. Rev Infect Dis 1989;11:S379-84.

65. Rodrigues LC, Diwan VK, Wheeler JG. Wheeler, Protective effect of BCG against tuberculous meningitis and miliary tuberculosis: a meta-analysis. Int J Epidemiol 1993;22:1154-8.

66. Arbeláez MP, Nelson KE, Muñoz A. BCG vaccine effectiveness in preventing tuberculosis and its interaction with human immunodeficiency virus infection. Int J Epidemiol 2000;29:1085-91.

67. World Health Organization. Global Programme for vaccines and immunization. Immunization Policy. Geneva: World Health Organization; 1996.p.1-51.

68. Orme IM, Andersen P, Boom WH. T-cell response to Mycobacterium tuberculosis. J Infect Dis 1993;167:1481-97.

69. Orme IM. The dynamics of infection following BCG and Mycobacterium tuberculosis challenge in T-cell-deficient mice. Tubercle 1987;68: 277-83.

70. Orme IM. Characteristics and specificity of acquired immunologic memory to Mycobacterium tuberculosis infection. J Immunol 1988;140:3589-93.

71. Cooper AM, Flynn JL. The protective immune response to Mycobacterium tuberculosis. Curr Opin Immunol 1995;7:512-6.

72. Flynn JL, Chan J, Triebold KJ, Dalton DK, Stewart TA, Bloom BR. An essential role for interferon gamma in resistance to Mycobacterium tuberculosis infection. J Exp Med 1993;178:2249-54.

73. Kaufmann SH. CD8+ T lymphocytes in intracellular microbial infections. Immunol Today 1988;9:168-74.

74. Schaible UE, Kaufmann SH. CD1 molecules and CD1-dependent T cells in bacterial infections: a link from innate to acquired immunity? Semin Immunol 2000;12:527-35.

75. Janis EM, Kaufmann SH, Schwartz RH, Pardoll DM. Activation of gamma delta T cells in the primary immune response to Mycobacterium tuberculosis. Science 1989;244:713-6.

76. Flynn JL, Chan J. Immunology of tuberculosis. Annu Rev Immunol 2001;19:93-129.

77. Ulrichs T, Kaufmann SH. New insights into the function of granulomas in human tuberculosis. J Pathol 2006;208:261-9.

78. Turner OC, Basaraba RJ, Orme IM. Immunopathogenesis of pulmonary granulomas in the guinea pig after infection with Mycobacterium tuberculosis. Infect Immun 2003;71:864-71.

79. Kaplan G, Post FA, Moreira AL, Wainwright H, Kreiswirth BN, Tanverdi M, et al. Mycobacterium tuberculosis growth at the cavity surface: a microenvironment with failed immunity. Infect Immun 2003;71:7099-108.

80. Cohen MK, Bartow RA, Mintzer CL, McMurray DN. Effects of diet and genetics on Mycobacterium bovis BCG vaccine efficacy in inbred guinea pigs. Infect Immun 1987;55:314-9.

81. McMurray DN, Mintzer CL, Bartow RA, Parr RL. Dietary protein deficiency and Mycobacterium bovis BCG affect interleukin-2 activity in experimental pulmonary tuberculosis. Infect Immun 1989;57:2606-11.

82. Bartow RA, McMurray DN. Erythrocyte receptor [CD2]-bearing T lymphocytes are affected by diet in experimental pulmonary tuberculosis. Infect Immun 1990;58:1843-7.

83. McMurray DN, Carlomagno MA, Mintzer CL, Tetzlaff CL. Mycobacterium bovis BCG vaccine fails to protect protein-deficient guinea pigs against respiratory challenge with virulent Mycobacterium tuberculosis. Infect Immun 1985;50:555-9.

84. Jain R, Dey B, Tyagi AK. Development of the first oligonucleotide microarray for global gene expression profiling in guinea pigs: defining the transcription signature of infectious diseases. BMC Genomics 2012;13:520.

85. Wang Z, Gerstein M, Snyder M. RNA-Seq: a revolutionary tool for transcriptomics. Nat Rev Genet 2009;10:57-63.

86. Walsh GP, Tan EV, dela Cruz EC, Abalos RM, Villahermosa LG, Young LJ, et al. The Philippine cynomolgus monkey [Macaca fasicularis] provides a new nonhuman primate model of tuberculosis that resembles human disease. Nat Med 1996;2: 430-6.

87. Sharpe SA, McShane H, Dennis MJ, Basaraba RJ, Gleeson F, Hall G, et al. Establishment of an aerosol challenge model of tuberculosis in rhesus macaques and an evaluation of endpoints for vaccine testing. Clin Vaccine Immunol 2010;17:1170-82.

88. Fourie PB, Odendaal MW. Odendaal, Mycobacterium tuberculosis in a closed colony of baboons [Papio ursinus]. Lab Anim 1983;17:125-8.

89. Bontrop RE, Otting N, de Groot NG, Doxiadis GG. Major histocompatibility complex class II polymorphisms in primates. Immunol Rev 1999;167:339-50.

90. Geluk A, Elferink DG, Slierendregt BL, van Meijgaarden KE, de Vries RR, Ottenhoff TH, et al. Evolutionary conservation of major histocompatibility complex-DR/peptide/T cell interactions in primates. J Exp Med 1993;177:979-87.

91. Porcelli S, Morita CT, Brenner MB. CD1b restricts the response of human CD4-8- T lymphocytes to a microbial antigen. Nature 1992;360:593-7.

92. Shinkai K, Locksley RM. CD1, tuberculosis, and the evolution of major histocompatibility complex molecules. J Exp Med 2000;191:907-14.

93. Shen Y, Zhou D, Chalifoux L, Shen L, Simon M, Zeng X, et al. Induction of an AIDS virus-related tuberculosis-like disease in macaques: a model of simian immunodeficiency virus-mycobacterium coinfection. Infect Immun 2002;70:869-77.

94. Langermans JA, Andersen P, van Soolingen D, Vervenne RA, Frost PA, van derLaan T, et al. Divergent effect of bacillus Calmette-Guerin [BCG] vaccination on Mycobacterium tuberculosis infection in highly related macaque species: implications for primate models in tuberculosis vaccine research. Proc Natl Acad Sci USA 2001;98:11497-502.

95. Langermans JA, Doherty TM, Vervenne RA, van der Laan T, Lyashchenko K, Greenwald R, et al. Protection of macaques against Mycobacterium tuberculosis infection by a subunit vaccine based on a fusion protein of antigen 85B and ESAT-6. Vaccine 2005;23:2740-50.

96. Cole ST, Brosch R, Parkhill J, Garnier T, Churcher C, Harris D, et al. Deciphering the biology of Mycobacterium tuberculosis from the complete genome sequence. Nature 1998;393:537-44.

97. Fleischmann RD, Alland D, Eisen JA, Carpenter L, White O, Peterson J, et al. Whole-genome comparison of Mycobacterium tuberculosis clinical and laboratory strains. J Bacteriol 2002;184:5479-90.

98. Mycobacterium. Available at URL: http://www.sanger.ac.uk/resources/downloads/bacteria/mycobacterium.html. Accessed on December 19, 2017.

99. Zvi A, Ariel N, Fulkerson J, Sadoff JC, Shafferman A. Whole genome identification of Mycobacterium tuberculosis vaccine candidates by comprehensive data mining and bioinformatic analyses. BMC Med Genomics 2008;1:18.

100. He Y. Omics-Based Systems Vaccinology for vaccine target identification. Drug Development Research 2012;73:559-68.

101. Sassetti CM, Boyd DH, Rubin EJ. Genes required for mycobacterial growth defined by high density mutagenesis. Mol Microbiol 2003;48:77-84.

102. Lamichhane G, Zignol M, Blades NJ, Geiman DE, Dougherty A, Grosset J, et al. A postgenomic method for predicting essential genes at subsaturation levels of mutagenesis: application to Mycobacterium tuberculosis. Proc Natl Acad Sci USA 2003;100:7213-8.

103. Sette A, Rappuoli R. Reverse vaccinology: developing vaccines in the era of genomics. Immunity 2010;33:530-41.

104. Capecchi B, Serruto D, Adu-Bobie J, Rappuoli R, Pizza M. The genome revolution in vaccine research. Curr Issues Mol Biol 2004;6:17-27.

105. Das Gupta SK, Jain S, Kaushal D, Tyagi AK. Expression systems for study of mycobacterial gene regulation and development of recombinant BCG vaccines. Biochem Biophys Res Commun 1998;246:797-804.

106. Jain S, Kaushal D, DasGupta SK, Tyagi AK. Construction of shuttle vectors for genetic manipulation and molecular analysis of mycobacteria. Gene 1997;190:37-44.

107. Stover CK, de la Cruz VF, Fuerst TR, Burlein JE, Benson LA, Bennett LT, et al. New use of BCG for recombinant vaccines. Nature 1991;351:456-60.

108. Jacobs WR Jr, Tuckman M, Bloom BR. Introduction of foreign DNA into mycobacteria using a shuttle phasmid. Nature 1987;327:532-5.

109. Snapper SB, Lugosi L, Jekkel A, Melton RE, Kieser T, Bloom BR, et al. Lysogeny and transformation in mycobacteria: stable expression of foreign genes. Proc Natl Acad Sci USA 1988;85:6987-91.

110. Dhar N, Rao V, Tyagi AK. Recombinant BCG approach for development of vaccines: cloning and expression of immunodominant antigens of M. tuberculosis FEMS Microbiol Lett 2000;190:309-16.

111. Matsuo K, Yamaguchi R, Yamazaki A, Tasaka H, Terasaka K, Totsuka M, et al. Establishment of a foreign antigen secretion system in mycobacteria. Infect Immun 1990;58:4049-54.

112. Horwitz MA, Harth G, Dillon BJ, Maslesa-Galic' S. Recombinant Bacillus Calmette-Guérin [BCG] vaccines expressing the Mycobacterium tuberculosis 30-kDa major secretory protein induce greater protective immunity against tuberculosis than conventional BCG vaccines in a highly susceptible animal model. Proc Natl Acad Sci USA 2000;97:13853-8.

113. Dey B, Jain R, Khera A, Gupta UD, Katoch VM, Ramanathan VD, et al. Latency antigen alpha-crystallin-based vaccination imparts a robust protection against TB by modulating the dynamics of pulmonary cytokines. PLoS One 2011;6: e18773.

114. Jain R, Dey B, Dhar N, Rao V, Singh R, Gupta UD, et al. Enhanced and enduring protection against tuberculosis by recombinant BCG-Ag85C and its association with modulation of cytokine profile in lung. PLoS One 2008;3:e3869.

115. Pym AS, Brodin P, Majlessi L, Brosch R, Demangel C, Williams A, et al. Recombinant BCG exporting ESAT-6 confers enhanced protection against tuberculosis. Nat Med 2003;9:533-9.

116. Pym AS, Brodin P, Brosch R, Huerre M, Cole ST. Loss of RD1 contributed to the attenuation of the live tuberculosis vaccines Mycobacterium bovis BCG and Mycobacterium microti. Mol Microbiol 2002;46:709-17.

117. Rao V, Dhar N, Shakila H, Singh R, Khera A, Jain R, et al. Increased expression of Mycobacterium tuberculosis 19 kDa lipoprotein obliterates the protective efficacy of BCG by polarizing host immune responses to the Th2 subtype. Scand J Immunol 2005;61:410-7.

118. Jain R, Dey B, Khera A, Srivastav P, Gupta UD, Katoch VM, et al. Over-expression of superoxide dismutase obliterates the protective effect of BCG against tuberculosis by modulating innate and adaptive immune responses. Vaccine 2011;29:8118-25.

119. Luo Y, Chen X, Han R, O'Donnell MA. Recombinant bacille Calmette-Guérin [BCG] expressing human interferon-alpha 2B demonstrates enhanced immunogenicity. Clin Exp Immunol 2001;123:264-70.

120. Kong D, Kunimoto DY. Secretion of human interleukin 2 by recombinant Mycobacterium bovis BCG. Infect Immun 1995;63:799-803.

121. Murray PJ, Aldovini A, Young RA. Manipulation and potentiation of antimycobacterial immunity using recombinant bacille Calmette-Guérin strains that secrete cytokines. Proc Natl Acad Sci USA 1996;93:934-9.

122. Wangoo A, Brown IN, Marshall BG, Cook HT, Young DB, Shaw RJ. Bacille Calmette-Guérin [BCG]-associated inflammation and fibrosis: modulation by recombinant BCG expressing interferon-gamma [IFN-gamma]. Clin Exp Immunol 2000;119:92-8.

123. Hess J, Miko D, Catic A, Lehmensiek V, Russell DG, Kaufmann SH. Mycobacterium bovis Bacille Calmette-Guérin strains secreting listeriolysin of Listeria monocytogenes. Proc Natl Acad Sci USA 1998;95:5299-304.

124. Mahairas GG, Sabo PJ, Hickey MJ, Singh DC, Stover CK. Molecular analysis of genetic differences between Mycobacterium bovis BCG and virulent M. bovis. J Bacteriol 1996;178:1274-82.

125. Sambandamurthy VK, Jacobs WR Jr. Live attenuated mutants of Mycobacterium tuberculosis as candidate vaccines against tuberculosis. Microbes Infect 2005;7:955-61.

126. Ackson M, Phalen SW, Lagranderie M, Ensergueix D, Chavarot P, Marchal G, et al. Persistence and protective efficacy of a Mycobacterium tuberculosis auxotroph vaccine. Infect Immun 1999;67:2867-73.

127. Sampson SL, Dascher CC, Sambandamurthy VK, Russell RG, Jacobs WR Jr, Bloom BR, et al. Protection elicited by a double leucine and pantothenate auxotroph of Mycobacterium tuberculosis in guinea pigs. Infect Immun 2004;72:3031-7.

128. Collins DM, Kawakami RP, de Lisle GW, Pascopella L, Bloom BR, Jacobs WR Jr. Mutation of the principal sigma factor causes loss of virulence in a strain of the Mycobacterium tuberculosis complex. Proc Natl Acad Sci USA 1995;92:8036-40.

129. Smith DA, Parish T, Stoker NG, Bancroft GJ. Characterization of auxotrophic mutants of Mycobacterium tuberculosis and their potential as vaccine candidates. Infect Immun 2001;69:1142-50.

130. Hondalus MK, Bardarov S, Russell R, Chan J, Jacobs WR Jr, Bloom BR. Attenuation of and protection induced by a leucine auxotroph of Mycobacterium tuberculosis. Infect Immun 2000;68:2888-98.

131. Sambandamurthy VK, Derrick SC, Jalapathy KV, Chen B, Russell RG, Morris SL, et al. Long-term protection against tuberculosis following vaccination with a severely attenuated double lysine and pantothenate auxotroph of Mycobacterium tuberculosis. Infect Immun 2005;73:1196-203.

132. Sampson SL, Mansfield KG, Carville A, Magee DM, Quitugua T, Howerth EW, et al. Extended safety and efficacy studies of a live attenuated double leucine and pantothenate auxotroph of Mycobacterium tuberculosis as a vaccine candidate. Vaccine 2011;29:4839-47.

133. Hinchey J, Jeon BY, Alley H, Chen B, Goldberg M, Derrick S, et al. Lysine auxotrophy combined with deletion of the SecA2 gene results in a safe and highly immunogenic candidate live attenuated vaccine for tuberculosis. PLoS One 2011;6:e15857.

134. McKinney JD, Höner zu Bentrup K, Muñoz-Elías EJ, Miczak A, Chen B, Chan WT, et al. Persistence of Mycobacterium tuberculosis in macrophages and mice requires the glyoxylate shunt enzyme isocitrate lyase. Nature 2000;406:735-8.

135. Pethe K, Alonso S, Biet F, Delogu G, Brennan MJ, Locht C, et al. The heparin-binding haemagglutinin of M. tuberculosis is required for extrapulmonary dissemination. Nature 2001;412:190-4.

136. Berthet FX, Lagranderie M, Gounon P, Laurent-Winter C, Ensergueix D, Chavarot P, et al. Attenuation of virulence by disruption of the Mycobacterium tuberculosis erp gene. Science 1998;282:759-62.

137. Singh A, Gupta R, Vishwakarma RA, Narayanan PR, Paramasivan CN, Ramanathan VD, et al. Requirement of the mymA operon for appropriate cell wall ultrastructure and persistence of Mycobacterium tuberculosis in the spleens of guinea pigs. J Bacteriol 2005;187:4173-86.

138. Singh R, Rao V, Shakila H, Gupta R, Khera A, Dhar N, et al. Disruption of mptpB impairs the ability of Mycobacterium tuberculosis to survive in guinea pigs. Mol Microbiol 2003;50:751-62.

139. Reddy PV, Puri RV, Khera A, Tyagi AK. Iron storage proteins are essential for the survival and pathogenesis of Mycobacterium tuberculosis in THP-1 macrophages and the guinea pig model of infection. J Bacteriol 2012;194:567-75.

140. Hart PD, Sutherland I. BCG and vole bacillus vaccines in the prevention of tuberculosis in adolescence and early adult life. Br Med J 1977;2:293-5.

141. Manabe YC, Scott CP, Bishai WR. Naturally attenuated, orally administered Mycobacterium microti as a tuberculosis vaccine is better than subcutaneous Mycobacterium bovis BCG. Infect Immun 2002;70:1566-70.

142. Onyebujoh PC, Abdulmumini T, Robinson S, Rook GA, Stanford JL. Immunotherapy with Mycobacterium vaccae as an addition to chemotherapy for the treatment of pulmonary tuberculosis under difficult conditions in Africa. Respir Med 1995;89:199-207.

143. Skinner MA, Yuan S, Prestidge R, Chuk D, Watson JD, Tan PL. Immunization with heat-killed Mycobacterium vaccae stimulates CD8+ cytotoxic T cells specific for macrophages infected with Mycobacterium tuberculosis. Infect Immun 1997;65:4525-30.

144. Abou-Zeid C, Gares MP, Inwald J, Janssen R, Zhang Y, Young DB, et al. Induction of a type 1 immune response to a recombinant antigen from Mycobacterium tuberculosis expressed in Mycobacterium vaccae. Infect Immun 1997;65:1856-62.

145. Chaturvedi V, Srivastava A, Gupta HP, Srivastava BS. Protective antigens of Mycobacterium habana are distributed between peripheral and integral compartments of plasma membrane: a study in experimental tuberculosis of mouse. Vaccine 1999;17:2882-7.

146. Prem Raj P, Srivastava S, Jain SK, Srivastava BS, Srivastava R. Protection by live Mycobacterium habana vaccine against Mycobacterium tuberculosis H37Rv challenge in mice. Indian J Med Res 2003;117:139-45.

147. Singh IG, Mukherjee R, Talwar GP. Resistance to intravenous inoculation of Mycobacterium tuberculosis H37Rv in mice of different inbred strains following immunization with a leprosy vaccine based on Mycobacterium w. Vaccine 1991;9:10-4.

148. Gupta A, Geetha N, Mani J, Upadhyay P, Katoch VM, Natrajan M, et al. Immunogenicity and protective efficacy of "Mycobacterium w" against Mycobacterium tuberculosis in mice immunized with live versus heat-killed M. w by the aerosol or parenteral route. Infect Immun 2009;77:223-31.

149. Gupta A, Ahmad FJ, Ahmad F, Gupta UD, Natarajan M, Katoch VM, et al. Protective efficacy of Mycobacterium indicus pranii against tuberculosis and underlying local lung immune responses in guinea pig model. Vaccine 2012;30:6198-209.

150. Saini V, Raghuvanshi S, Khurana JP, Ahmed N, Hasnain SE, Tyagi AK, et al. Massive gene acquisitions in Mycobacterium indicus pranii provide a perspective on mycobacterial evolution. Nucleic Acids Res 2012;40:10832-50.

151. Saini V, Raghuvanshi S, Talwar GP, Ahmed N, Khurana JP, Hasnain SE, et al. Polyphasic taxonomic analysis establishes Mycobacterium indicus pranii as a distinct species. PLoS One 2009;4:e6263.

152. Katoch K, Katoch VM, Natrajan M, Sreevatsa, Gupta UD, Sharma VD, et al. 10-12 years follow-up of highly bacillated BL/LL leprosy patients on combined chemotherapy and immunotherapy. Vaccine 2004;22:3649-57.

153. Global TB clinical vaccine pipeline. Available at URL: http://www.newtbvaccines.org/vaccine-candidates/. Accessed on September 24, 2018.

154. Demissie A, Leyten EM, Abebe M, Wassie L, Aseffa A, Abate G, et al. Recognition of stage-specific mycobacterial antigens differentiates between acute and latent infections with Mycobacterium tuberculosis. Clin Vaccine Immunol 2006;13:179-86.

155. McShane H, Pathan AA, Sander CR, Keating SM, Gilbert SC, Huygen K, et al. Recombinant modified vaccinia virus Ankara expressing antigen 85A boosts BCG-primed and naturally acquired antimycobacterial immunity in humans. Nat Med 2004;10:1240-4.

156. Tchilian EZ, Desel C, Forbes EK, Bandermann S, Sander CR, Hill AV, et al. Immunogenicity and protective efficacy of prime-boost regimens with recombinant [delta]ureC hly+ Mycobacterium bovis BCG and modified vaccinia virus Ankara expressing M. tuberculosis antigen 85A against murine tuberculosis. Infect Immun 2009;77:622-31.

157. Dey B, Jain R, Gupta UD, Katoch VM, Ramanathan VD, Tyagi AK. A booster vaccine expressing a latency-associated antigen augments BCG-induced immunity and confers enhanced protection against tuberculosis. PLoS One 2011;6:e23360.

158. Ulrich JT, Myers KR. Monophosphoryl lipid A as an adjuvant. Past experiences and new directions. Pharm Biotechnol 1995;6: 495-524.

159. Coler RN, Bertholet S, Moutaftsi M, Guderian JA, Windish HP, Baldwin SL, et al. Development and characterization of synthetic glucopyranosyl lipid adjuvant system as a vaccine adjuvant. PLoS One 2011;6:e16333.

160. Bertholet S, Ireton GC, Ordway DJ, Windish HP, Pine SO, Kahn M, et al. A defined tuberculosis vaccine candidate boosts BCG and protects against multidrug resistant Mycobacterium tuberculosis. Sci Transl Med 2010;2:53-74.

161. Brandt L, Elhay M, Rosenkrands I, Lindblad EB, Andersen P. ESAT-6 subunit vaccination against Mycobacterium tuberculosis. Infect Immun 2000;68:791-5.

162. Fynan EF, Webster RG, Fuller DH, Haynes JR, Santoro JC, Robinson HL. DNA vaccines: protective immunizations by parenteral, mucosal, and gene-gun inoculations. Proc Natl Acad Sci USA 1993;90:11478-82.

163. Ulmer JB, Donnelly JJ, Parker SE, Rhodes GH, Felgner PL, Dwarki VJ, et al. Heterologous protection against influenza by injection of DNA encoding a viral protein. Science 1993;259: 1745-9.

164. Lin F, Shen X, McCoy JR, Mendoza JM, Yan J, Kemmerrer SV, et al. A novel prototype device for electroporation-enhanced DNA vaccine delivery simultaneously to both skin and muscle. Vaccine 2011;29: 677180.

165. Palumbo RN, Zhong X, Wang C. Polymer-mediated DNA vaccine delivery via bystander cells requires a proper balance between transfection efficiency and cytotoxicity. J Control Release 2012;157:86-93.

166. Li A, Qin L, Wang W, Zhu R, Yu Y, Liu H, et al. The use of layered double hydroxides as DNA vaccine delivery vector for enhancement of anti-melanoma immune response. Biomaterials 2011;32:469-77.

167. Yen MC, Lai MD. Biolistic DNA Delivery to Mice with the Low Pressure Gene Gun. Methods Mol Biol 2013;940:169-74.

168. Saade F, Petrovsky N. Technologies for enhanced efficacy of DNA vaccines. Expert Rev Vaccines 2012;11:189-209.

169. Lozes E, Huygen K, Content J, Denis O, Montgomery DL, Yawman AM, et al. Immunogenicity and efficacy of a tuberculosis DNA vaccine encoding the components of the secreted antigen 85 complex. Vaccine 1997;15:830-3.

170. Tascon RE, Colston MJ, Ragno S, Stavropoulos E, Gregory D, Lowrie DB. Vaccination against tuberculosis by DNA injection. Nat Med 1996;2:888-92.

171. Kamath AT, Feng CG, Macdonald M, Briscoe H, Britton WJ. Differential protective efficacy of DNA vaccines expressing secreted proteins of Mycobacterium tuberculosis. Infect Immun 1999;67:1702-7.

172. Tanghe A, Lefèvre P, Denis O, D'Souza S, Braibant M, Lozes E, et al. Immunogenicity and protective efficacy of tuberculosis DNA vaccines encoding putative phosphate transport receptors. J Immunol 1999;162:1113-9.

173. Vipond J, Vipond R, Allen-Vercoe E, Clark SO, Hatch GJ, Gooch KE, et al. Selection of novel TB vaccine candidates and their evaluation as DNA vaccines against aerosol challenge. Vaccine 2006;24:6340-50.

174. Derrick SC, Yang AL, Morris SL. A polyvalent DNA vaccine expressing an ESAT6-Ag85B fusion protein protects mice against a primary infection with Mycobacterium tuberculosis and boosts BCG-induced protective immunity. Vaccine 2004;23:780-8.

175. Jodar L, Duclos P, Milstien JB, Griffiths E, Aguado MT, Clements CJ. Ensuring vaccine safety in immunization programmes—a WHO perspective. Vaccine 2001;19:1594-1605.

176. Williams JA, Carnes AE, Hodgson CP. Plasmid DNA vaccine vector design: impact on efficacy, safety and upstream production. Biotechnol Adv 2009;27:353-70.

177. Klug B, Reinhardt J, Robertson J. Current Status of Regulations for DNA Vaccines. Gene Vaccines; 2012.p.285-95.

178. Boesen H, Jensen BN, Wilcke T, Andersen P. Human T-cell responses to secreted antigen fractions of Mycobacterium tuberculosis. Infect Immun 1995;63:1491-7.

179. Vordermeier HM, Harris DP, Friscia G, Román E, Surcel HM, Moreno C, et al. T-cell repertoire in tuberculosis: selective anergy to an immunodominant epitope of the 38-kDa antigen in patients with active disease. Eur J Immunol 1992;22:2631-7.

180. Axelsson-Robertson R, Magalhaes I, Parida SK, Zumla A, Maeurer M. The immunological footprint of Mycobacterium tuberculosis T-cell epitope recognition. J Infect Dis 2012;205: S301-S315.

181. Ardito M, Moise L, Martin W, De Groot AS. Immunoinformatic approach to a multi-pathogen genome-derived epitope-driven vaccine. In: Proceedings of the First ACM International Conference on Bioinformatics and Computational Biology. New York: Association for Computing Machinery; 2010.p.616-20.

182. Christy AJ, Dharman K, Dhandapaani G, Palaniyandi K, Gupta UD, Gupta P, et al. Epitope-based recombinant BCG vaccine elicits specific Th1 polarized immune responses in BALB/c mice. Vaccine 2012;30:1364-70.

183. De Groot AS, McMurry J, Marcon L, Franco J, Rivera D, Kutzler M, et al. Developing an epitope-driven tuberculosis [TB] vaccine. Vaccine 2005;23:2121-31.

184. Billeskov R, Grandal MV, Poulsen C, Christensen JP, Winther N, Vingsbo-Lundberg C, et al. Difference in TB10. 4 T-cell epitope recognition following immunization with recombinant TB10. 4, BCG or infection with Mycobacterium tuberculosis. Eur J Immunol 2010;40:1342-54.

185. Geluk A, van den Eeden SJ, van Meijgaarden KE, Dijkman K, Franken KL, Ottenhoff TH. A multistage-polyepitope vaccine protects against Mycobacterium tuberculosis infection in HLA-DR3 transgenic mice. Vaccine 2012;30:7513-21.

186. Karonga Prevention Trial Group. Randomised controlled trial of single BCG, repeated BCG, or combined BCG and killed Mycobacterium leprae vaccine for prevention of leprosy and tuberculosis in Malawi. Lancet 1996;348:17-24.

187. Tala-Heikkilä MM, Tuominen JE, Tala EO. Bacillus Calmette-Guérin revaccination questionable with low tuberculosis incidence. Am J Respir Crit Care Med 1998;157:1324-7.

188. Leung CC, Tam CM, Chan SL, Chan-Yeung M, Chan CK, Chang KC. Efficacy of the BCG revaccination programme in a cohort given BCG vaccination at birth in Hong Kong. Int J Tuberc Lung Dis 2001;5:717-23.

189. Buddle BM, Wedlock DN, Parlane NA, Corner LA, De Lisle GW, Skinner MA. Revaccination of neonatal calves with Myco-bacterium bovis BCG reduces the level of protection against bovine tuberculosis induced by a single vaccination. Infect Immun 2003;71:6411-9.

190. Basaraba RJ, Izzo AA, Brandt L, Orme IM. Decreased survival of guinea pigs infected with Mycobacterium tuberculosis after multiple BCG vaccinations. Vaccine 2006;24:280-6.

191. McShane H. Prime-boost immunization strategies for infectious diseases. Curr Opin Mol Ther 2002;4:23-7.

192. Estcourt MJ, Ramsay AJ, Brooks A, Thomson SA, Medveckzy CJ, Ramshaw IA. Prime-boost immunization generates a high frequency, high-avidity CD8[+] cytotoxic T lymphocyte population. Int J Immunol 2002;14:31-7.

193. Woodland DL. Jump-starting the immune system: prime-boosting comes of age. Trends Immunol 2004;25:98-104.

194. Goonetilleke NP, McShane H, Hannan CM, Anderson RJ, Brookes RH, Hill AV. Enhanced immunogenicity and protective efficacy against Mycobacterium tuberculosis of bacille Calmette-Guérin vaccine using mucosal administration and boosting with a recombinant modified vaccinia virus Ankara J Immunol 2003;171:1602-9.

195. Williams A, Hatch GJ, Clark SO, Gooch KE, Hatch KA, Hall GA, et al. Evaluation of vaccines in the EU TB Vaccine Cluster using a guinea pig aerosol infection model of tuberculosis. Tuberculosis [Edinb] 2005;85:29-38.

196. McShane H, Pathan AA, Sander CR, Goonetilleke NP, Fletcher HA, Hill AV. Boosting BCG with MVA85A: the first candidate subunit vaccine for tuberculosis in clinical trials. Tuberculosis [Edinb] 2005;85:47-52.

197. Sander CR, Pathan AA, Beveridge NE, Poulton I, Minassian A, Alder N, et al. Safety and immunogenicity of a new tuberculosis vaccine, MVA85A, in Mycobacterium tuberculosis—infected Individuals. Am J Respir Crit Care Med 2009;179:724-33.

198. Scriba TJ, Tameris M, Smit E, van der Merwe L, Hughes EJ, Kadira B, et al. A Phase IIa trial of the new tuberculosis vaccine, MVA85A, in HIV- and/or Mycobacterium tuberculosis—infected adults. Am J Respir Crit Care Med 2012;185:769-78.

199. Tameris MD, Hatherill M, Landry BS, Scriba TJ, Snowden MA, Lockhart S, et al. Safety and efficacy of MVA85A, a new tuberculosis vaccine, in infants previously vaccinated with BCG: a randomised, placebo-controlled phase 2b trial. Lancet 2013;381:1021-8.

200. Brooks JV, Frank AA, Keen MA, Bellisle JT, Orme IM. Boosting vaccine for tuberculosis. Infect Immun 2001;69:2714-7.

201. Dey B, Jain R, Khera A, Rao V, Dhar N, Gupta UD, et al. Boosting with a DNA vaccine expressing ESAT-6 [DNAE6] obliterates the protection imparted by recombinant BCG [rBCGE6] against aerosol Mycobacterium tuberculosis infection in guinea pigs. Vaccine 2009;28:63-70.

202. Skinner MA, Buddle BM, Wedlock DN, Keen D, de Lisle GW, Tascon RE, et al. A DNA prime-Mycobacterium bovis BCG boost vaccination strategy for cattle induces protection against bovine tuberculosis. Infect Immun 2003;71:4901-7.

203. Skinner MA, Wedlock DN, de Lisle GW, Cooke MM, Tascon RE, Ferraz JC, et al. The order of prime-boost vaccination of neonatal calves with Mycobacterium bovis BCG and a DNA vaccine encoding mycobacterial proteins Hsp65, Hsp70, and Apa is not critical for enhancing protection against bovine tuberculosis. Infect Immun 2005;73:4441-4.

204. Hatherill M, Mahomed H, Hanekom W. Novel vaccine prime and selective BCG boost: a new tuberculosis vaccine strategy for infants of HIV-infected mothers. Vaccine 2010;28:4550-2.

205. Tomioka H. Adjunctive immunotherapy of mycobacterial infections. Curr Pharm Des 2004;10:3297-312.

206. Coler RN, Bertholet S, Pine SO, Orr MT, Reese V, Windish HP, et al. Therapeutic immunization against Mycobacterium tuberculosis is an effective adjunct to antibiotic treatment. J Infect Dis 2012;207:1242-52.

207. Churchyard GJ, Kaplan G, Fallows D, Wallis RS, Onyebujoh P, Rook GA. Advances in immunotherapy for tuberculosis treatment. Clin Chest Med 2009;30:769-82.

208. Ha SJ, Jeon BY, Youn JI, Kim SC, Cho SN, Sung YC. Protective effect of DNA vaccine during chemotherapy on reactivation and reinfection of Mycobacterium tuberculosis. Gene Ther 2005;12:634-8.

209. Silva CL, Bonato VL, Coelho-Castelo AA, De Souza AO, Santos SA, Lima KM, et al. Immunotherapy with plasmid DNA encoding mycobacterial hsp65 in association with chemotherapy is a more rapid and efficient form of treatment for tuberculosis in mice. Gene Ther 2005;12:281-7.

210. Mwinga A, Nunn A, Ngwira B, Chintu C, Warndorff D, Fine P, et al. Mycobacterium vaccae [SRL172] immunotherapy as an adjunct to standard antituberculosis treatment in HIV-infected adults with pulmonary tuberculosis: a randomised placebo-controlled trial. Lancet 2002;360:1050-5.

211. Johnson JL, Nunn AJ, Fourie PB, Ormerod LP, Mugerwa RD, Mwinga A, et al. Effect of Mycobacterium vaccae [SRL172] immunotherapy on radiographic healing in tuberculosis. Int J Tuberc Lung Dis 2004;8:1348-54.

212. Gómez-Reino JJ, Carmona L, Valverde VR, Mola EM, Montero MD. Treatment of rheumatoid arthritis with tumor necrosis factor inhibitors may predispose to significant increase in tuberculosis risk: a multicenter active-surveillance report. Arthritis Rheum 2003;48:2122-7.

213. Wolfe F, Michaud K, Anderson J, Urbansky K. Tuberculosis infection in patients with rheumatoid arthritis and the effect of infliximab therapy. Arthritis Rheum 2004;50:372-9.

214. Wallis RS, Kyambadde P, Johnson JL, Horter L, Kittle R, Pohle M, et al. A study of the safety, immunology, virology, and microbiology of adjunctive etanercept in HIV-1-associated tuberculosis. AIDS 2004;18:257-64.

215. Condos R, Rom WN, Schluger NW. Treatment of multidrug-resistant pulmonary tuberculosis with interferon-gama via aerosol. Lancet 1997;349:1513-5.

216. Gao XF, Yang ZW, Li J. Adjunctive therapy with interferon-gamma for the treatment of pulmonary tuberculosis: a systematic review. Int J Infect Dis 2011;15:e594-e600.

217. Raad I, Hachem R, Leeds N, Sawaya R, Salem Z, Atweh S. Use of adjunctive treatment with interferon-gamma in an immunocompromised patient who had refractory multidrug-resistant tuberculosis of the brain. Clin Infect Dis 1996;22:572-4.

218. Hovav AH, Fishman Y, Bercovier H. Gamma interferon and monophosphoryl lipid A-trehalose dicorynomycolate are efficient adjuvants for Mycobacterium tuberculosis multivalent acellular vaccine. Infect Immun 2005;73:250-7.

219. Johnson BJ, Bekker LG, Rickman R, Brown S, Lesser M, Ress S, et al. rhuIL-2 adjunctive therapy in multidrug resistant tuberculosis: a comparison of two treatment regimens and placebo. Tuber Lung Dis 1997;78:195-203.

220. Johnson JL, Ssekasanvu E, Okwera A, Mayanja H, Hirsch CS, Nakibali JG, et al. Randomized trial of adjunctive interleukin-2 in adults with pulmonary tuberculosis. Am J Respir Crit Care Med 2003;168:185-91.

221. Subbian S, Tsenova L, O'Brien P, Yang G, Koo MS, Peixoto B, et al. Phosphodiesterase-4 inhibition alters gene expression and improves isoniazid–mediated clearance of Mycobacterium tuberculosis in rabbit lungs. PLoS Pathog 2011;7:e1002262.

222. Maiga M, Agarwal N, Ammerman NC, Gupta R, Guo H, Maiga MC, et al. Successful shortening of tuberculosis treatment using adjuvant host-directed therapy with FDA-approved phosphodiesterase inhibitors in the mouse model. PLoS One 2012;7: e30749.

223. Shetty P. Nutrition, HIV/AIDS and tuberculosis. In: Nutrition, immunity and infection. Oxfordshire: CABI; 2010.p.114-30.

224. Spence DP, Hotchkiss J, Williams CS, Davies PD. Tuberculosis and poverty. BMJ 1993;307:759-61.

225. Fabri M, Stenger S, Shin DM, Yuk JM, Liu PT, Realegeno S, et al. Vitamin D is required for IFN-gamma-mediated

antimicrobial activity of human macrophages. Sci Transl Med 2011;3:104ra102.

226. Realegeno S, Modlin RL. Shedding light on the vitamin D–tuberculosis–HIV connection. Proc Natl Acad Sci USA 2011;108: 18861-2.

227. Cosivi O, Grange JM, Daborn CJ, Raviglione MC, Fujikura T, Cousins D, et al. Zoonotic tuberculosis due to Mycobacterium bovis in developing countries. Emerg Infect Dis 1998;4:59-70.

228. LoBue PA, Enarson DA, Thoen CO. Tuberculosis in humans animals: an overview. Int J Tuberc Lung Dis 2010;14:1075-8.

229. Katale BZ, Mbugi EV, Kendal S, Fyumagwa RD, Kibiki GS, Godfrey-Faussett P, et al. Bovine tuberculosis at the human-livestock-wildlife interface: is it a public health problem in Tanzania? A review. Onderstepoort J Vet Res 2012;79:463.

230. Idigbe EO, Anyiwo CE, Onwujekwe DI. Human pulmonary infections with bovine and atypical mycobacteria in Lagos, Nigeria. J Trop Med Hyg 1986;89:143-8.

231. Barrera L, De Kantor IN. Nontuberculous mycobacteria and Mycobacterium bovis as a cause of human disease in Argentina. Trop Geogr Med 1987;39:222-7.

232. Pérez-Guerrero L, Milián-Suazo F, Arriaga-Díaz C, Romero-Torres C,Escartín-Chávez M. Molecular epidemiology of cattle and human tuberculosis in Mexico. Salud Pública de México 2008;50:286-91.

233. Prasad HK, Singhal A, Mishra A, Shah NP, Katoch VM, Thakral SS, et al. Bovine tuberculosis in India: potential basis for zoonosis. Tuberculosis 2005;85:421-8.

234. Shah NP, Singhal A, Jain A, Kumar P, Uppal SS, Srivatsava MV, et al. Occurrence of overlooked zoonotic tuberculosis: detection of Mycobacterium bovis in human cerebrospinal fluid. J Clin Microbiol 2006;44:1352-8.

235. Mishra A, Singhal A, Chauhan DS, Katoch VM, Srivastava K, Thakral SS, et al. Direct detection and identification of Mycobacterium tuberculosis and Mycobacterium bovis in bovine samples by a novel nested PCR assay: correlation with conventional techniques. J Clin Microbiol 2005;43:5670-8.

236. Dupon M, Ragnaud JM. Tuberculosis in patients infected with human immunodeficiency virus 1. A retrospective multicentre study of 123 cases in France. The Groupe des Infectiologues du Sud de la France. QJM 1992;85:719-30.

237. Ocepek M, Pate M, Zolnir-Dovc M, Poljak M. Transmission of Mycobacterium tuberculosis from human to cattle. J Clin Microbiol 2005;43:3555-7.

238. Vordermeier HM, Rhodes SG, Dean G, Goonetilleke N, Huygen K, Hill AV, et al. Cellular immune responses induced in cattle by heterologous prime-boost vaccination using recombinant viruses and bacille Calmette-Guérin. Immunology 2004; 112:461-70.

239. Cai H, Tian X, Hu XD, Li SX, Yu DH, Zhu YX. Combined DNA vaccines formulated either in DDA or in saline protect cattle from Mycobacterium bovis infection. Vaccine 2005;23:3887-95.

240. de la Rua-Domenech R. Human Mycobacterium bovis infection in the United Kingdom: incidence, risks, control measures and review of the zoonotic aspects of bovine tuberculosis. Tuberculosis [Edinb] 2006;86:77-109.

241. Gilbert M, Mitchell A, Bourn D, Mawdsley J, Clifton-Hadley R, Wint W. Cattle movements and bovine tuberculosis in Great Britain. Nature 2005;435:491-6.

242. Van Der Meeren O, Hatherill M, Nduba V, Wilkinson RJ, Muyoyeta M, Van Brakel E, et al. Phase 2b controlled trial of M72/AS01E vaccine to prevent tuberculosis. N Engl J Med. DOI: 10.1056/NEJMoa1803484.

243. The Global Report on Tuberculosis Vaccines 2018. Available at URL: http://www.tbvi.eu/wp-content/uploads/2018/02/Summary-SWRTV_Finalproof.pdf. Accessed on September 12, 2018.

55

Ethical and Legal Issues in Tuberculosis Control

John Porter

INTRODUCTION

Scientific thought succumbed because it violated the first law of culture, which says that the more man controls anything, the more uncontrollable both become

Tyler SA (1)

In the early years of the twenty-first century, increasing links are being made between communities, countries and continents. There are more opportunities for us to witness life in other places and to view and review our own structures and perceptions of the way we live and to learn from people of different cultures and religions. This new 'internationalism' brings with it increasing 'complexity' and an added importance for each of us to review our own beliefs and perceptions in order to allow increasing co-operation and understanding.

In the field of public health there are discussions aimed at widening the scope of health care beyond the treatment of diseases like tuberculosis [TB], to a broader concept of 'the creation of health'; that health is an entity that communities and societies have the opportunity of developing (2). This broader perception, uses biomedical health care concepts and systems, but adds to them by including other disciplines like anthropology, environmental sciences, ethics and human rights. It is anticipated that the result of this fusion, created through inter-disciplinary work, will be a change in biomedicine's perception of health and health care. Now, those of us working in TB control have an opportunity to view our control measures from different perspectives. Perhaps it is time to take note of the quotation at the beginning of the chapter and to consider whether the current, control methods for TB are violating the first law of culture, and therefore, making TB more uncontrollable. Is this why we have an increasing international problem with multi-drug-resistant TB [MDR-TB] and extensively drug-resistant TB [XDR-TB]?

The field of ethics, because it is to do with questions about 'how we ought to live' (3), provides a framework which is included in the other disciplines which address health care issues and is also a useful tool for creating a framework with which to untangle the dilemmas that occur around the treatment and 'control' of people with TB. The morality of the individual is intimately connected with the ethics of the medical and public health fraternity and both of these entities also link with the legal profession and the law [Figure 55.1]. The law and the legal system provide a framework within a society to 'assist and protect people' (4); protecting the rights of individuals but at the same time protecting the rights of institutions and organisations like professional medical bodies. The basic function of the law is to establish legal rights, and the basic purpose of the legal

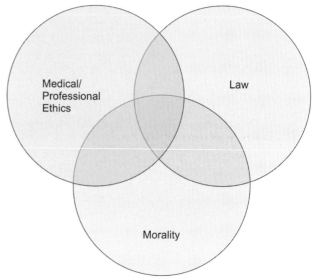

Figure 55.1: Ethics and the law

system is to define and enforce these rights (5). Ethics is not separate from the law, it is an integral part of the legal system and how laws are made and enforced.

This chapter looks at TB control from the perspectives of ethics and law. It begins with an introduction to the two disciplines and then applies them to the current international strategy for TB control. The 'ethical' issues of TB are addressed through highlighting the potential problems for a TB patient who is seeking care through the health care system [relationship with the health care worker, interaction with the health care system, etc.]. The legal issues concentrate on groups of people at high-risk for TB [e.g., alcoholics, prisoners, etc.,] to try to untangle the legal problems. Examples from India, the United States and the United Kingdom are used to provide the context for the discussion.

BACKGROUND

Public Health and Tuberculosis

The control of infectious diseases is an important part of public health policy. In most countries, TB control is the responsibility of public health departments. Public health is 'the science and art of preventing disease, prolonging life and promoting health through the organised efforts of society' (6). A more succinct definition comes from the Institute of Medicine in the United States, which says that public health is 'what we, as a society, do to assure the conditions for people to be healthy' (7). Both definitions imply an imperative to balance the needs of the individual with the needs of the population in the control of infectious diseases. Inherent in this, as in all balances, is a tension, and this tension often engenders debate and even conflict between decision makers. The framework of ethics can assist in developing a course of action to resolve these conflicts by providing clarification of the questions and a system for weighing alternatives through ethical debate (8).

During the past 150 years, scientific structure and discourse have framed the development of technological medicine which has produced sophisticated treatments and medications to treat illnesses, like TB. From the time that Koch discovered the tubercle bacillus in 1882, there has been an understanding that TB is caused by *Mycobacterium tuberculosis* [*Mtb*] and that destroying the bacillus with drugs would provide an appropriate treatment. With the development of streptomycin and the subsequent development of other anti-TB drugs, short-course chemotherapy was developed; a solution for controlling TB worldwide had been found (9). However, by the early 1990s, there were signs of increasing TB cases in all countries associated with the movement of people from high to low TB prevalence countries, the increasing spectre of human immunodeficiency virus [HIV] infection and acquired immunodeficiency syndrome [AIDS], and decreasing funds to support public health infrastructures to control TB (9). In the early 1990s, the World Health Organization [WHO] developed the DOTS strategy to try to improve the uptake of TB control measures around the world, particularly

in order to combat the increasing problem of multidrug resistance. The strategy includes: government commitment to a national programme; case detection through 'passive' case finding [sputum smear microscopy for pulmonary TB suspects]; short course chemotherapy for all smear positive pulmonary TB cases [under direct observation for at least the initial phase of treatment]; regular, uninterrupted supply of all essential anti-TB drugs; and a monitoring system for programme supervision and evaluation (10,11).

The international strategy for controlling TB, has been developed from a science base and has been created from many disciplines including medicine, epidemiology and the basic science. Now, however, with several new TB drug and vaccine candidates, who are in various stages of trials and testing, the health care fraternity has to look at the basic human behavioural issues in TB control. The issues of how individual patients interact with health care systems, and in particular, how they interact with health care workers (12,13). For a person to complete their six months of anti-TB treatment, they need to be supported and cared for and this requires strong health systems. This is a basic function of health care provision but one which has been increasingly neglected with the rise of the rapid technological approaches to treating disease. Are the current TB control methods consistent with the broad public health agenda of preventing disease and promoting health? Is there sufficient emphasis on the care of TB patients in order to promote/create health? All of these questions become increasingly difficult and complex with the increase in prevalence of HIV in communities and its link with TB (14).

Infectious Disease Control and Tuberculosis

Methods for the control of infectious diseases have been developed principally through the study of epidemiology. The perspectives of biomedical scientists have dominated thinking in this area, and the control methods currently used reflect this focus. Epidemiologists look at the interaction between the agent, host and environment, and the main strategies for control are to attack the source [e.g., the treatment or isolation of cases/carriers]; to interrupt transmission [e.g., environmental and personal hygiene, vector control]; or to protect the susceptible population [e.g., immunisation, chemoprophylaxis] [Table 55.1] (15).

The categories, attacking the source and protecting the susceptible population, both relate to the treatment of patients. Attacking the source refers to the treatment of a case of disease: the patient is treated [a benefit to him/her] and the population is protected from being infected by him [a benefit to the population]. A person with infectious pulmonary TB needs to be treated not only for his/her benefit but also for the benefit of the public health, to prevent further transmission of *Mtb* to others. Protecting the susceptible population requires the use of medication to prevent the development of a disease [treatment of latent TB infection].

The four principle methods for controlling TB are stated to be: the improvement of socioeconomic conditions, case

Table 55.1: Main strategies for control of infectious disease

Attack source	Interrupt transmission	Protect susceptible people
Treatment of cases and carriers	Environmental hygiene	Immunisation
Isolation of cases	Personal hygiene	Chemoprophylaxis
Surveillance of suspects	Vector control	Personal protection
Control of animal reservoir	Disinfection and sterilisation	Better nutrition
Notification of cases	Restrict population movements	–

Adapted from reference 12

finding and treatment, chemoprophylaxis and bacille Calmette-Guérin [BCG] vaccination (16). Although the improvement of socioeconomic conditions undoubtedly has a major impact on TB (17) in public health terms, TB control focuses on finding infectious cases [sputum positive] and treating them so that they are no longer infectious to others. This is the method for disrupting transmission; it concentrates on the individual with the aim of treating the person and protecting the community from further infection and disease. As has already been mentioned, the current international TB control strategy is DOTS. Part of the strategy is direct observation of treatment [DOT] which has been established to prevent the development of drug resistant strains of TB. The 'direct observation' component of the strategy introduces ethical issues around the right to 'control' individuals with TB, in order to protect the majority [community].

But is case finding and treatment sufficient? Although it makes scientific and logical sense to concentrate on infectious TB cases, are there no other social, environmental and economic issues that need to be considered? What about structural interventions for example?

Structural factors within the field of HIV infection have been broadly defined as physical, social, cultural, organisational, community, economic, legal or policy aspects of the environment that impede or facilitate persons' efforts to avoid infection (18). With the increasing complexity of health care, the requests for a broad perception of health, and with the increasing inter-disciplinary nature of public health work, there is an opportunity to re-evaluate the current control measures. Are these control measures for TB appropriate? Are they sensitive to the needs of people with TB? Can they be improved to ensure the rights and dignity of all patients?

ETHICS

When one speaks of ethics, one might be speaking from one or a combination of three mutually interconnected perspectives: [i] the study of ethics; [ii] the adherence to ethical guidelines laid down by governments and professional bodies; and/or [iii] the application of ethical principles in daily life (19). The ethical process is not a once-and-for-all, nor a once-in-a while pursuit. On the contrary it forms part of our day to day interactions and is an integral part of our public health interventions (19). In the study of ethics, philosophers develop theories about the interaction between moral values and the ways in which societies operate. Morals–the values and norms that frame societies' ideas about 'right' and 'wrong'–are inherently cultural constructions. All cultures and societies have moral codes, but because these are culturally and historically contingent, they shift and change over time. The work of moral philosophers both reflects and to some extent informs this process.

With the increasing co-operation and collaboration between countries in public health research, this cultural and historical contingency is important to understand. People's perceptions and understanding of TB, ethics and the law, are framed by the cultural values and historical background of the society in which they live. The moral construct used in some societies is seen as 'absolute'; for example, certain religious texts dictate the 'way the community ought to live', whereas in others, moral values are seen as 'relative' and more flexible, being seen to be different according to the context of the situation in which the ethical dilemma arises. Each community needs to be understood in terms of its history and cultural values.

Ethics in the West

In the western industrialised world, there has been a shift in moral thinking from absolute to relative values: from a *deonotological* model of ethics to a *utilitarian* model. The utilitarian theories suggest that answers to moral questions on right and wrong depend solely on the nature of the consequences of those actions or proposed actions, whereas deontology relates to moral rules not related to consequences, from the Greek word deon meaning duty (20). Although to some extent framed within the Judaic Christian religious traditions, the ethical theories and models developed in the west attempt to be ahistorical, abstract and formal.

It has been argued that the 'utilitarian' structure has emerged with the growth of technology in the North (21). If one accepts Bell's definition of technology as 'the effort to transform nature for utilitarian purposes' (21,22), one may then step back for a moment and look at the profound social and moral dilemmas inherent in this phenomenon. When applied to health one consequence of the 'utilitarian' approach is the generation of interventions which are geared towards maximising majority over individual benefit (19).

Ethics in the East

It is difficult to locate the Eastern tradition in the historical, abstract and formal theories of ethics that have been developed in the West. Ethics in the East is framed by the religions of Islam, Hinduism and Buddhism as well as many others.

In the Brahmanical-Hindu and Jaina traditions for example, it is recognised that ethics is the 'soul' of the complex spiritual and moral aspirations of the people, co-mingled with social and political structures forged over a vast period of time. This accounts for the cultures profuse literature in wisdom, legends, epics, liturgical texts, legal and political treatises. There are a variety of ethical systems within the Hindu tradition, but the tradition itself contains within it a diverse collection of social, cultural, religious and philosophical systems (23). The highest good is identified with the total harmony of the cosmic or natural order, characterised as *rita*: this is the creative purpose that circumscribes human behaviour. The social and moral order is, thus, seen as a correlate of the natural order. This is the ordered course of things, the truth of being or reality [*sat*], and hence, the 'Law' (24). The convergence of the cosmic and the moral orders is universally commended in the all-embracing category of *dharma*, which becomes more or less the Indian analogue for ethics (23). What counts as 'ethics' then although in appearance naturalistic, is largely normative; the justification usually is that this is the 'divined' ordering of things, and hence, there is a tendency also to view the moral law as absolute.

Ethics Principles and Tasks

In the development of international guidelines for the control of infectious diseases like TB the western philosophical model tends to dominate the process. There is, however, continuing research to try to develop an appropriate set of international ethical principles (25). In 1994 at the 38th Council for International Organisations of Medical Sciences [CIOMS] Conference in Ixtapa a declaration was issued describing the emergence of bioethics as a global and multi-layered enterprise and 'the need to continue to work towards an ethics of health which calls on us to consider the interconnections among all of our choices and actions that affect the health status of people anywhere' [CIOMS, Declaration of Ixtapa] (26,27).

There have been suggestions as to how ethics can be used in practice to assist with ethical dilemmas in medicine and public health. De Beaufort and Dupuis (28) have suggested that the ethical process might be used to [i] clarify concepts, [ii] analyse and structure arguments, [iii] weigh alternatives; and [iv] provide advice on an "appropriate" course of action. Another way of looking at ethical argument is that it can assist us to identify the obstacles that prevent us from acting "morally". Once these obstacles have been identified, it is easier to find ways of overcoming them.

As human beings we are moral agents: we interact daily with our family, friends, colleagues and acquaintances and these interactions are framed by the values and norms that prevail in our society. By going to our jobs, taking care of our families and talking to our neighbours, we are acting as engaged participants in our moral community. As health care workers, we are moral agents too. In this we do not stop engaging with our moral community, but we expand the boundaries of that community: at this level we also interact with our professional ethics and with the legal system of the wider society (29).

The four principles which currently dominate international bio-ethical debate are: respect for autonomy, beneficence, non-maleficence and justice (30). These principles-plus attention to their scope [i.e., how and to whom they apply] provide the basis for a rigorous consideration and resolution of ethical dilemmas. Although they do not provide "rules", these principles can help public health workers make decisions when moral issues arise. In effect they make a common set of moral commitments, a common moral language, and a common set of moral issues (20) more visible and more accessible. These principles are considered to be prima facie: they are binding unless they conflict with other moral principles. They are outlined briefly below.

Autonomy

Autonomy, "self-rule", although perceived differently in different cultures, is an attribute of all moral agents. Autonomy gives one the ability to make decisions on the basis of deliberation. Autonomy is also reciprocal: we have a moral obligation to respect the autonomy of others as long as it is compatible with equal respect for the autonomy of all those potentially affected. According to the Western philosopher Kant, respect for autonomy means 'treating others as ends in themselves and never merely as means' to some [externally defined] end (20). The person with TB is an autonomous individual, a decision maker, and the decisions that they make about their treatment should be respected not only by the health care worker with whom they are interacting but also by the health care system that is providing the treatment. The quality of the relationship between the patient and the health care provider is a key to the provision of appropriate TB treatment.

Beneficence and Non-maleficence

There is always a need to balance the effort to help and the risk of causing harm. The traditional Hippocratic moral obligation of medicine is to provide beneficence with non-maleficence: net medical benefit to patients with minimal harm. Once again, the relationship between the health care provider and the patient determines whether there is a net benefit to the TB patient. It is also important to remember, however, that the health care provider will be more able to provide support and be beneficent to the person with TB if they are appropriately supported in their job by the organisation/system that employ them. So, although the relationship between health care worker and the patient is important, the relationship of the health care worker with their employer is also part of the process of ensuring beneficent/non-maleficent care.

Justice

Justice refers to the moral obligation to act on the basis of fair adjudication between competing claims. Equality is at the heart of justice, but as Aristotle argued, justice is more than mere equality—people can be treated unjustly even if they are treated equally (31). Equity entails treating no portion of the population in a disproportionate manner. Inequity, then, is a descriptive term used to denote existing differences between groups or individuals in the distribution of or access to resources. However, inequity also denotes the reasons behind and responsibilities for underlying conditions of inequality. As such, it is inherently a statement of justice (32).

People with TB need to be treated fairly and justly. If a community wishes to prevent the spread of TB, patients need to have access to a health care structure that provides them with treatment and care. This access needs to be available to all TB patients equally.

The Application of Ethics in Public Health

Little has been written in regard to moral issues in public health (33) or the application of ethics to public health decision making. In 1980, Shindell (34) suggested that a public health intervention should: [i] relate to well-understood disease aetiology; [ii] be feasible; and [iii] entail only an appropriate trade-off of the rights of the individual against the benefits that accrue to the population. It is the third point that leads to moral debate and a tension between public health and civil liberties. In infectious disease control, interventions usually relate to diseases with a well-understood aetiology. The feasibility of a particular intervention will depend on the details of the disease outbreak [location, numbers, demographic character of people involved, etc.,] and the possibility of using standard control measures to intervene. In TB control, the aetiology of the disease is fairly well understood, the intervention [case finding and treatment] is feasible and there is an accepted [taken for granted] trade-off between the rights of the individual and the benefits of the population.

Public health interventions tend to embody an imbalance of power and capacity between the implementers and the recipients: public health professionals decide when and where to intervene, and normally what the intervention will consist of. It is presumed that whatever 'harm' the intervention may impose on individuals is outweighed by the 'good' it will bring to the population as a whole. This form of practice does not exemplify respect for the autonomy of the people at the receiving end of the intervention (35,36). Hall has argued that although individuals surrender some degree of personal freedom in exchange for membership of a society, 'individual autonomy remains to some degree'. He states that this residual autonomy is not addressed within public health and suggests that the utilitarian support for the practice of public health must be subordinated to the deontological rights of the individual (35).

Within liberal democracies it is generally accepted that the state may intervene when the exercise of one person's freedom may result in harm to another (8). This is known as the 'harm principle.' The nineteenth century philosopher John Stuart Mill defined this principle in the following way: 'The only purpose for which power can be rightfully exercised over any member of a civilised community, against his will, is to prevent harm to others. His own good, either physical or moral, is not a sufficient warrant (37). This principle provides the ethical and legal foundation for establishing public health programmes designed to require those with communicable diseases to behave in ways that are likely to reduce the risk of transmission.

THE LAW

What is it and what does it Do?

The values that are contained within a community help to define the legal statutes that are created. Ethics and the law are intimately connected [Figure 55.1]. The legal system in every country is unique, although it may use certain structures or processes, like 'common law', as a foundation (5).

It is useful to have a working definition of the law to assist with the legal issues that pertain to TB control. Wing, from the United States, states that the law is 'the sum or set or conglomerate of all the laws in all of the jurisdictions: the constitutions, the statutes and the regulations that interpret them, the traditional principles known as common law, and the judicial opinions that apply and interpret all these legal rules and principles'. Wing argues that the law is also the legal profession and the legal process–legislatures and their politics and finally 'the law is what it is interpreted to be' (5).

The basic function of the law is to establish legal rights, and the basic purpose of the legal system is to define and enforce those rights. Legal rights are the relationships that establish privileges and responsibilities among those governed by the legal system. Finally, some rights are protected, not by statute or regulation, but by an understanding and application of the prevailing ethics in an area. In general, ethics are regulated through whatever sanctions are imposed against censured behaviour by peers or colleagues. These statements underlie the essential link between ethics and the law, but 'it is normally accepted that ethics is something more than the law' (38).

Legislation for Infectious Disease Control in the United States and United Kingdom

Surveillance of infectious diseases began in the United States in 1874 in Massachusetts, when the State Board of Health instituted the first state wide voluntary plan for weekly reporting of the prevalence of diseases by physicians. By the turn of the century, the forerunners of the Public Health Service had been established, and laws in all states required that certain communicable diseases be reported to local authorities (39). During the period 1940 to 1970, states added many diseases to their mandatory lists. Even in states that did not enact legislation to require additional reporting, surveillance and reporting efforts were broadened during this period through state regulation or directives from the state health commissioners (40).

In the United Kingdom, the Infectious Disease Notification Act of 1988 amended the Infectious Disease [Notification]

Extension Act of 1899 which required compulsory nation-wide notification of certain infectious diseases [but not TB]. In England and Wales, this list was re-enacted with modifications on a number of occasions and the current 'notifiable diseases' are contained in section 10 of the Public Health [Control of Disease] Act of 1984. Notification of TB is contained in Schedule 1 of the 1988 Regulations.

The law for infectious diseases has two parts: surveillance and control, with control being further subdivided into control of the environment [in its widest sense to include premises and articles] and control of people. The control of actions by people is contained in both the 1984 Act and the 1988 Regulations, and the powers are wide ranging, from exclusion to incarceration. Section 10 of the 1984 Act allows the proper officer of any district to request any person to discontinue work 'with a view to preventing the spread' of TB and if they fail to do so, this may be an offence under section 19 of the 1984 Act. Under the powers contained in section 32[1][a]a person can be requested to leave his or her residence and under section 32[1] [b] compulsory removal can be effected, under a court order, to alternative accommodation when any infectious disease occurs in a house. In addition, provisions are included in the 1984 Act to allow compulsory removal to and incarceration in a hospital if the person is considered a serious risk (41).

Legislation for the control of diseases like TB can have a range of 'control' measures, from 'an order to complete treatment', to 'an order for detention while infectious' (42). In New York City in 1993, the health code was revised to permit 'compulsory actions to protect the public health' in relation to TB (42). The types of regulatory action included: order for examination for suspected TB as outpatient or in detention; order to complete treatment; order for DOT; written warning of possible detention; order for detention while infectious; order for detention while non-infectious; discharge from detention before cure [for non-infectious patient] (43).

Legislation in India

In India, health regulation is a responsibility of each state. The central government has some authority but the laws are created through the state legislature; each state can make and enforce its own laws. Central government can also develop health legislation but has to depend solely on each state to enforce it.

Just before independence in 1948, the Bhore Committee (44) produced recommendations on health laws including statements on the control of infectious diseases. While showing great concern for the measures required to prevent and combat the spread of diseases between provinces, it made recommendations for giving the central government some legal powers in line with those existing in the United States at the time. Public Health Acts were recommended for the central as well as state governments to bring together existing legal provisions relating to health, to modify sections of the laws which required change in the interest of promoting efficient administration and to incorporate new provisions

necessary for the health programmes recommended by the Bhore Committee. However, in keeping with the government policy of doing as little legislation in the field of health as possible, such a consolidated act was never adopted (38).

TUBERCULOSIS CONTROL—ETHICAL ISSUES

The following section looks at the ethical issues and dilemmas within the treatment and control of a person with TB. It focuses on the interaction between the patient and the health care provider, the interaction of the patient with the health care system, and on the separate stages of TB treatment from the problems of access to the systems established for monitoring and follow-up. Many of the ethical questions that arise in the control of TB are to do with relationship, particularly the relationship between the patient and the health care provider whether that person is a nurse, physician, community worker or manager, but also the broader interaction of the patient with the overall health structure.

In public health decision making, there is always the issue of balancing the rights of the individual *versus* the rights of the population. Each of us is inextricably linked to the community in which we live and what happens to us affects the wider community. Our individual morality is interlinked with the ethics of the public health system [in this case the TB control programme] and with the laws of the state [Figure 55.2].

In the case of TB control, the biomedical model has established that a person with sputum positive TB is infectious to others and is therefore capable of transmitting the infection with the risk of the development of TB disease. However, it is important to remember that the *determinants of risk* for TB are personal, societal and programmatic [Figure 55.3]. The main ethical issue therefore in TB control is the perspective on this balance between the individual and

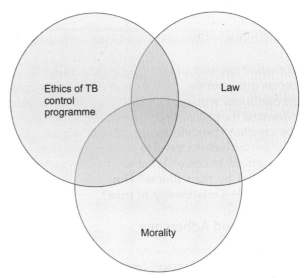

Figure 55.2: Ethics of TB control programme, law and morality
TB = tuberculosis

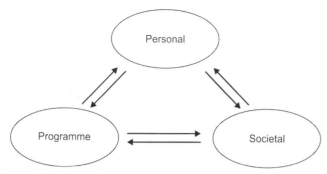

Figure 55.3: Determinants of risk of tuberculosis

the community in which she/he lives; the balance between accepting the autonomy of the individual *versus* the process of justice and equity. The official process of justice in a society is provided through the legal system which through the law courts provides a structure for people to be heard and also develops the laws to govern and protect the society. The law is there to assist and protect people (4). It can be argued that in the case of TB, the rights of the individual are justifiably sacrificed for the overall good of the population (45). As stated above, however, ethics demands a balance: while infected people have a right to be treated with dignity, worth, value and respect, they have a duty not to spread the infection to others (46).

Relationship of a Tuberculosis Patient with the Health Care Provider

A patient with TB wants both to understand what is wrong with them and to receive treatment. A person with a persistent cough will seek advice from members of their community who they know to have knowledge of health and disease. In some places this person will be the local traditional healer, in others it will be a physician practising in the private or government health system. The relationship that is developed with this person and with the health care system to which they belong will dictate how the person is treated and whether they are treated with dignity and respect.

The whole 'context' of where a person comes from, their socioeconomic conditions and level of education is essential for the health care worker to understand. Without an attempt to understand the patient's perspective, health care providers will be unable to provide an appropriate service. How far does the person have to travel to come to the health facility? Can they afford to come? What is their job and how is it being affected by their illness? How can the health care worker provide a relationship of trust?

Compliance and Adherence

Compliance can be defined as the extent to which a person's health related behaviour coincides with medical advice (47). When seeking care patients carry out their own "cost/benefit analyses", balancing out their understandings of the

severity of the illness, its impacts on their family members and their ability to obtain access to treatment, against the other conflicting priorities and demands of daily life. Patients with acute TB tend to comply with treatment because of the desire to get well and to be free from troubling symptoms of fever, cough and night sweats. Compliance after the initial phase of treatment, when the patient feels well, is more difficult to ensure—the balance of benefits and priorities has shifted from an immediate benefit to the patient, to a more abstract [from the patient's perspective] benefit to the community. From the patient's point of view the "costs" of staying on treatment once symptoms have disappeared may well outweigh the benefits, which must be difficult to assess. Thus, while the "failure" of patients to comply with maintenance therapy may appear to be irrational from the physicians' or health care workers' perspective, it is intelligible when seen from the patient's point of view (48).

Ethically, compliance relates to the interaction between the autonomy of the TB patient and the beneficence of the health care worker. Although health care workers may be trying to 'do good' and to avoid harm to the patient, however, they have difficulty acting as independent moral agents because they are participants in a health structure, and are therefore, bound to uphold the ethics of that structure [Figure 55.2]. As members of professional organisations and players in TB programmes, they are expected to conduct themselves in a particular manner, to follow the regulations of the programme, and to encourage patients to take and complete their treatment until cured. Cure is the goal, the outcome measure, which health care worker are obliged to bring about. But, there is a danger inherent in this process. At some stage the health care worker's compliance to the system may lead to coercion of patients: the end [cure] may come to justify any means taken to reach it, even if those means transgress against respect for the autonomy of patients. If patients are treated autonomously, then it must be accepted that they may choose not to follow the 'orders' of the system. The relationship between the health care worker and the patient, the trust and respect between them and the success of their communication, are vital for ensuring an ethical approach to TB treatment (12,13).

Improved adherence to TB therapy will depend on an improved understanding of the social epidemiology of TB. Wherever it occurs TB is a disease of poverty. There is strong evidence that the poorest compliance occurs in the poorest communities (49). It is, therefore, essential that the social and economic factors involved in non-compliance are understood and appreciated. Compliance will only be improved if these factors are taken into account. As Farmer has noted, "those least likely to comply are those least able to comply" with treatment (50). In the United States and other industrialised nations TB is concentrated among the elderly and people from minority ethnic groups, many of whom are poor and/or have compromised access [social, physical and economic] to care (14,51). The main TB burden, however, occurs in the developing world where TB cases occur across a wide spectrum of society (52,53).

Direct Observation of Treatment

As has already been mentioned in the background to this chapter, DOT is part of the international DOTS strategy for TB control (10). But, DOT has potential difficult ethical questions relating to coercion and control, an imbalance between the autonomy of the individual patient and the control exerted by the health care worker in the system. It can be argued that 'if a person's health related behaviour does not coincide with medical advice, then it is appropriate to ensure that it does' (19).

The ethical, legal and constitutional principles that justify efforts to control TB in the United States are broad enough to justify efforts to ensure that all patients with TB are treated until cured. Legal commentators have endorsed the goal of treatment to cure (44,54,55). There has been controversy, however, over the nature of the public health interventions that might be employed to achieve this goal and the extent to which the legal and ethical principles that guide medical and public health practice should constrain those interventions (8).

In the United States, DOT has proven effective in increasing rates of treatment completion (56,57) and in decreasing the prevalence of drug resistance and relapse in communities in which it is used (58). It was initially recommended for persons with poor records of treatment adherence and for those whose demographic or psychological profile suggested a high risk of failure. Now, however, DOT has emerged as a standard of care (57). This change has come about because of the rise of drug resistance in the United States.

In the United States, it has been argued that because DOT is standardised [is the same for all patients], the initial treatment decisions should not violate the principle of justice, and should thus, preclude acts of discrimination (59). The fact that all patients start their post-hospitalised treatment under a common programme of supervision should help to reduce the stigma of being under treatment and create an effective public health plan for the control of TB. Yet is it reasonable to assume that such a programme will be equally appropriate in all settings, no matter how socially or economically diverse? Does DOT respect the autonomy of individuals everywhere in the same way? Indeed universal DOT has been challenged as an unethical intrusion on autonomy, as 'gratuitously annoying' (60), as a violation of the Constitutional requirement that the least restrictive measure be used, and as contrary to the requirements of the Americans with Disabilities Act [That decisions involving restrictions on those with disabilities be based on an individualised assessment (61). DOT has also been criticised on the basis that it is resource and manpower intensive, and so may be wasteful of scarce resources (59,62).

It has been argued that the discourse of direct observation is one of domination and control of the health care worker over the patient (63). In ethical terms, it can be argued that the approach fails to respect the autonomy of the person with TB. The 'care relationship' between patients and providers should, in ethical terms, be characterised by a balance between the autonomy of the TB patients and the beneficence/non-maleficence of the health care worker and should lead to net benefit with minimal harm. If the health worker attempts to force the patient into a type of treatment which they do not understand or agree with, then the relationship becomes coercive.

A person goes to a medical practitioner because he is sick and wants to get well. The practitioner has access to technology and knowledge that the patient needs. It is an inherently unequal relationship. Yet this relationship is also the key relationship in health care. In TB control, the discipline of ethics helps to frame this relationship in order to ensure that this inequality is not abused. Indeed codes of conduct are an important part of ethics in medicine. The stronger this relationship the more appropriate the care provided. This relationship is destroyed if power is abused.

Those opposing direct observation may feel that it threatens this very important relationship. It is not that DOT is wrong. In fact, the DOT is a rational approach to the delivery of TB drugs. The problem comes, however, with the abuse of power that is potentially inherent in a relationship between a powerful medical worker and a sick vulnerable patient (19).

Interaction/Relationship of a Tuberculosis Patient with the Health Care Structure [Official and Unofficial]

In every country there is a health care structure whether official or unofficial. In some, it is organised and controlled by the government [regulated system], and in others it is a system established through traditional systems of medicine and health care [unregulated system]. Increasingly, the health care systems in many countries are being administered through a mixture of public and private providers.

The Health Care Structure

For a health care system to work and to provide appropriate care for people, it must be consistent with the underlying health beliefs and social norms of the community (64). If the government does not provide appropriate health care for communities, they will establish their own systems. The rise of the private sector in countries in Asia is an example. The ethical issues that relate to health care structures are to do with the rights of individuals to have a system of health care provided for them by government. In western industrialised countries, governments are considered to have a duty to provide systems of health care for the population and individuals consider that it is their right to be provided with a service.

Access

While it is important for health care to be consonant with patient belief systems, it must also be accessible to them in physical/geographic and economic terms (50,65). Not all people have equal access to health care structures and it is usually the most vulnerable groups [e.g., displaced populations, the poor, the unemployed, etc.,] that find it most difficult to use the health care services (66). In terms of ethics, it is important to look at the relative autonomy of people with TB within their community, the balance between beneficence and non-maleficence, the net gain for being enrolled in TB treatment [the DOTS strategy for example], and finally whether they are treated justly.

Social and Cultural Burden

How people use the health care system [treatment seeking] relates to cultural as well as social and economic factors. While the burden of has been well-defined from the epidemiological perspective, there have been surprisingly few attempts to define the social and economic burden of TB (52). Similarly, there are only a limited number of studies on the actual costs or economic consequences of TB borne by families, communities, and economies in the developing world (67). Nevertheless it is apparent that not all people are equally able to access health care structures (50). This is a question of equity. Ethical processes are critical in promoting equity. 'Equity-promoting action in the health sector must put the needs and interests of the poorest and most vulnerable at their heart, as the relatively worse health outcomes of this group in comparison with other groups are most often a function of circumstances beyond their control' (68).

Stigma

Another issue which needs to be highlighted when considering a patient's interaction with the health care structure as well as the ethics of the 'passive case-finding' approach [The health care system waits 'passively' for patients to present with TB rather than 'actively' looking for patients] advocated in TB control strategies, is stigma. TB carries a social stigma. It is also a disease which affects the most marginalised, most poor and most vulnerable groups in communities, the very groups who tend to have the least autonomy. Although it is clear that the effects of stigma on passive case-finding needs to be better understood, there is evidence which indicates that it will have an effect on delaying treatment-seeking and that it may substantially constrain the ability of young people and women in particular to seek and obtain care (67). Passive case finding is the method of waiting for people with TB to present to health facilities rather than actively going out to find cases.

Passive case-finding may well be sound in public health terms, and even in macro-economic terms, but the ethical implications need to be taken into consideration as well. Considered and well-informed debate should enable the development of solutions which meet the needs of the system as well as the needs of the patients and the communities in which they live.

Treatment and Drugs

Once the patient has accessed the system and been diagnosed with TB, she/he needs to be provided with a regular supply of anti-TB drugs. This requires a system to have been developed to ensure that there is a regular drug supply. For this to be achieved, questions need to be asked about the type of health care system established in a country. It asks governments to be committed to dealing with TB and to ensuring an appropriate management and distribution system for TB drugs. It is not simply the uninterrupted supply of drugs that is important, however, it is also the access to those drugs by the people who need them.

Monitoring

Monitoring and evaluation of the TB system is obviously essential and can either promote equity and efficiency or seriously detract from it (10,11). It is important, for example, that health care workers are able to perform the tasks and achieve the targets they are being evaluated on: the criteria for evaluation need to be realistic and appropriate for particular contexts and given the real constraints faced on the ground. Recent operations research in India, for example, indicate that targets set at the national and international level may be placing stresses on health workers that do not promote the care of patients (12,13,69).

Ethical questions that need to be asked in relation to monitoring and evaluation include: Is the system just and equitable? Does the system respect both the TB patients and the health care workers that care for them? Does the system encourage health care workers to identify problems or does it penalise them for 'not doing it right?' Problems need to be identified and dealt with positively. This is the art of making difficult problems soluble, a process which Medawar called the 'art of the soluble' (70). After all it is through tackling problems that we find a process of engagement and integration between people with TB, their communities, districts, states, government and the international community (71).

The international DOTS strategy makes sense scientifically, but if the emphasis is only on targets rather than the process developed to achieve these targets, then health care workers and patients may be used as 'means' to achieving a particular 'end': they may be abused. A system needs to be established in which both patients and providers are respected. The health service is, after all, there to provide a service for patients. A danger of having inappropriate targets for the health care worker is that they will focus on attaining these targets rather than on caring for the patient. This may lead to coercion by the health worker of the patient, or to the exclusion of the patient from the system. Targets need to be adapted to the local community situation and made appropriate to them.

As noted above, ethics requires people to treat each other as ends in themselves and not merely as the means to achieving a particular outcome 'end' (72). Concentrating on the moral and social aspects of a monitoring system will help to ensure that this is achieved, that people are respected and TB patients are not abused in the process. 'The provision of social services has a strong person element:

the quality of service depends heavily on the attitudes of the people undertaking it, and it is hard to monitor. Service provisioning, furthermore, often involves a position of power over users. Hence, the importance of professional ethics (73).

TUBERCULOSIS CONTROL—LEGAL ISSUES

The next section focuses on some legal issues contained within the current TB control strategy. The examples used are from a western legal perspective.

In the industrialised world the legal cases that are reported in the literature tend to relate to the loss of civil liberties. For example, in order to protect 'the majority', the legal system is used to 'control' people with TB who fail to follow public health recommendations and regulations to prevent the spread of *Mycobacterium tuberculosis [Mtb]* (8). These people are a minority of cases but affect certain groups who are themselves 'minorities'; for example, the homeless, ethnic minorities, drug users and alcoholics (19). It can be argued that these people are the 'outliers' of a community, people who live on the fringes of society and who are not seen as part of the majority, i.e. they are different from 'the norm'. If 'equality' is the only aspect of justice that is important, then it could be argued that this situation is appropriate. However, the question of equity is also important. In the section on 'ethics, principles and tasks' it has already been stated that inequity denotes the reasons behind and responsibilities for underlying conditions of inequality, and it is therefore inherently a statement of justice (32). Ethical processes are critical in promoting equity (29,68).

Legal Processes Affect the Minority of Tuberculosis Patients

A study conducted in New York City and published in 1999 indicates that between 1992 and 1997, legal action was required only for a minority of patients with TB (42). In 1993, because of the increasing rates of TB and cases of multi-drug resistance, the New York City Department of Health updated its Health Code to permit compulsory action to protect the public health. From this date, the commissioner of health could issue orders compelling a person to be examined for suspected TB, to complete treatment, to receive treatment under direct observation, or to be detained for treatment (43). The types of regulatory action ranged from 'an order for examination for suspected TB' to 'an order for detention while infectious'.

The study by Gasner evaluated legal actions in TB control and showed that regulatory orders were issued for less than 4% of the 8000 TB patients treated between 1993 and 1995 (42). The paper strikingly highlights the social and demographic characteristics of those who were detained ['the outliers']; of the 304 patients who required regulatory action, 211 [69%] were black, 68 [22%] were Hispanic, 21 [7%] were white and 4 [1%] were Asian. HIV infection was documented in 147 cases [48%]. One hundred and fifty-two [50%] had a history of homelessness, 128 [42%] had used injection drugs, 183 [60%] had used 'crack' cocaine, 191 [63%] had a history of alcohol abuse and 145 [48%] had a history of incarceration (42).

High-risk Groups

In ethics there is a dictum which states 'ought implies can' (8). It can be argued, therefore, that a person cannot be held ethically accountable for failing to adhere to moral or legal standards [e.g., TB treatment], if he or she cannot do so, or if he or she faces insuperable obstacles to adherence. This statement highlights the plight of the most vulnerable groups in our communities (52). Ethically it is important to consider the duties of the community to support these groups of vulnerable people to ensure that they are appropriately treated for TB, but perhaps more importantly, to find ways of preventing them from acquiring TB.

This ethical principle of 'ought implies can' compels us to recognise that the elimination of impediments that impinge on the capacity of an individual to cooperate in his or her own care for TB is essential and we need to look for appropriate structural interventions (18). For example, homeless persons cannot reasonably be expected to comply with their treatment unless they are provided with a secure residence, and in many cases with other social supports (8). This is echoed in social science research which indicates that those with strong community and/or familial support are more likely to adhere to a full course of TB therapy (64,67,74,75). The New York City Tuberculosis Working Group has argued that 'the government that fails to provide adequate social supports for the most vulnerable loses the legal, as well as the moral, authority to threaten with a deprivation of liberty those whose behaviour poses a health risk' (61).

Thus, the laws we develop in our communities and societies are a reflection of how we see the world, of the values we use to frame our legal system and in the case of TB control, how we perceive and deal with these vulnerable groups of TB patients. Is it not easier to develop a law which confines high-risk groups to ensure that they do not spread the disease to the larger population than to address the difficult; some may say impossible, social questions of homelessness? Is there not also the moral responsibility of the society to try to find ways of supporting these groups of people to prevent them from acquiring TB without resorting to coercion and control? Indeed is we are to believe Tyler's statement at the beginning of the chapter, our efforts to control TB patients in this way may be making the TB situation worse.

Prisons

Incarceration is the final legal action that can be taken to ensure that a person with TB takes their medication. However, prison itself is an important site for the transmission of TB as demonstrated by recent outbreaks of MDR-TB in prisons in the United States, Spain and Russia (76,77). These outbreaks have called for 'inter- national efforts to ensure effective global initiatives to control TB in these setting; strategies to screen, diagnose, and treat frequently neglected populations residing in jails and prison throughout the developing world' (78).

Prisoners have been confined to prison through the legal system in a particular country, but it is the responsibility of the government system which manages the prisons to ensure that prisoners are treated and cared for appropriately [duties]. In the case of TB, this means both 'establishing the conditions in which people can be healthy' in prisons [i.e., no overcrowding, poor nutrition, etc.] as well as providing appropriate treatment of TB cases when they arise. In many countries, the primary reason for the higher prevalence of *Mtb* infection and increased incidence of TB disease within prisons is the disproportionate number of inmates who are otherwise at high-risk for acquiring infection and developing active disease (78).

The discussion of ethical and philosophical matters in health care is not new. Over 2000 years ago the writings of Hippocrates debated the duties of doctors towards their patients and the community. However, the last three decades of the 20th century and the start of the 21st have seen a dramatic transformation in medical ethics. What has been limited in the past to codes of professional conduct became in the 1960s the new academic discipline called biomedical ethics or bioethics (27). By the 1980s bioethics had included the societal debate encompassing discussions about priority setting and health care reform. Now, in the 1990s, a new phase is evolving which transcends health care matters, encompassing the full range of health determinants. This phase has moved towards the 'bioethics of population health' with a focus on the broader ethical issues in public health such as social justice, equity, sustainable health, sustainable living, globalisation and environmentalism (79). As was stated in the introduction, the 1990s and early 2000 is witnessing increasing 'internationalism' and 'complexity' and the increasing need to address cross cultural ethical issues as well as the theoretical and practical convergence of public health and human rights (80). This is highlighted in the spectre of the HIV pandemic and the research being conducted in this area, which is driving an international agenda that is forcing individuals and governments to address broad ethical concerns about research and control.

At the 38th CIOMS [Council for International Organisations of Medical Sciences] Conference in 1994, a Declaration was issued describing the emergence of bioethics as a global and multi-layered enterprise. The following statement from that conference sums up the contemporary importance of ethics to public health; It is time to move beyond medical ethics, beyond bioethics, beyond an ethics of health care of health policy, towards an ethics of health which calls on us to consider the interconnections among all of our choices and actions that affect the health status of people anywhere. In doing so, we should acknowledge the equal moral worth of all people, and should recognise that the human condition is inherently a condition of vulnerability (26).

Ethical and legal debates provide an important focus for TB control activity. For too long, public health has been operating in an 'ethical vacuum'. It is important to ensure that the autonomy and freedom of individuals is not being inappropriately jeopardised by the government, the legal system or the public health profession. It is important to protect the population from infectious disease epidemics, but it is equally important to ensure that the rights of the infected individual are not being violated, and that these individuals are supported by their communities and by their legal systems. If we agree that 'the human condition is inherently a condition of vulnerability but that some are more vulnerable than others, then the most vulnerable groups in our populations need to be protected and supported. It can even be argued in TB control strategies that if the socially vulnerable are targeted and their issues are addressed, then the problems of the remainder [the majority] of TB patient will also be covered (81).

With increasing globalisation, it continues to be important to remember that individuals as well as communities need to be respected and treated with the dignity they deserve. TB control methods developed for one country may not be appropriate for another. If the ethical principles discussed in this chapter were to become part of the public health process, notions of autonomy, empowerment and justice would feature in public health decision-making at all levels. International, national and local decision-makers would be compelled to engage in a debate which problematised the taken-for-granted assumptions behind the principle of non-harming. Public health paternalism could no longer prevent control programmes from achieving the success they promise, and individuals and communities might come to enjoy the freedom to obtain care, and cure, for TB without having to compromise their autonomy (19).

ETHICAL ISSUES IN TUBERCULOSIS CARE AND CONTROL: RECENT DEVELOPMENTS

Recently, greater range of concerns associated with ethical issues in TB care, control and research are increasingly being recognised, especially in the context of X/MDR-TB and HIV-TB co-infection. In order to help governments and their national TB programmes and other stake-holders, the WHO had issued guidance to facilitate implementation of efforts at TB prevention, care control and research in an ethical manner (82-85). Further integration of these ethical principles in TB control programmes is expected in the ensuing years.

REFERENCES

1. Tyler SA. Post-modern ethnography: from document of the occult to occult document. In: Clifford J, Marcus GE, editors. Writing culture: the poetics and politics of ethnography. Berkeley: University of California Press; 1986.p.122-40.
2. Kickbusch A. New players for a new era: responding to the global public health challenges. J Public Health Med 1997;19:171-8.
3. Rachels J. The elements of moral philosophy. New York: McGraw-Hill; 1997.p.1.
4. Lerner BH. Temporarily detained: tuberculous alcoholics in Seattle, 1949 through 1960. Am J Public Health 1996;86:257-65.

5. Wing KR. The law and the public's health. Ann Arbor: Health Administration Press; 1990.p.1-50.

6. Acheson Report. Public health in England: The report of the committee of inquiry into the future development of the public health function. London: HMSO; 1988.

7. Institute of Medicine. Future of public health. Washington DC: National Academy Press; 1988.p.1-7.

8. Bayer R, Dupuis LJ. Tuberculosis, public health and civil liberties. Annu Rev Public Health 1995;16:307-26.

9. Snider DE. Tuberculosis: the world situation. History of the disease and efforts to combat it. In: Porter JDH, McAdam KPWJ, editors. Tuberculosis-back to the future. London: John Wiley and Sons; 1994.

10. World Health Organization. WHO TB Programme. Framework for effective TB control. Geneva: World Health Organization; 1994. WHO/TB/94.179.

11. Harries AD, Mayer D. TB/HIV: a clinical manual. WHO/TB/96.200. Geneva: World Health Organization; 1996.

12. Singh V, Jaiswal A, Porter JD, Ogden JA, Sarin R, Sharma PP, et al. TB control, poverty and vulnerability in Delhi, India. Trop Med Int Health 2002;7:693-700.

13. Jaiswal A, Singh V, Ogden JA, Porter JD, Sarin R, Sharma PP, et al. Adherence to tuberculosis treatment: lessons from the urban setting of Delhi, India. Trop Med Int Health 2003;8:625-33.

14. Brudney K, Dobkin J. Resurgent tuberculosis in New York City: human immunodeficiency virus, homelessness and the decline of tuberculosis control programs. Am Rev Respir Dis 1991;144: 745-9.

15. Vaughan JP, Morrow RH. Manual of epidemiology for district health management. Geneva: World Health Organization; 1989.

16. Rodrigues LC, Smith PG. Tuberculosis in developing countries and methods for control. Trans Royal Soc Trop Med 1990;84: 739-44.

17. McKeown T. The role of medicine: dream, mirage or nemesis? Princeton: Princeton University Press; 1979.p.45-65,92-96.

18. Sumartojo E. Structural factors in HIV prevention: concepts, examples, and implications for research. AIDS 2000;14 Suppl 1: S3-10.

19. Porter JD, Ogden JA. Ethics of directly observed therapy for the control of infectious diseases. Bull Inst Pasteur 1997;95:117-27.

20. Gillon R. Medical ethics: four principles plus attention to scope. BMJ 1994;309:184-8.

21. Hill P. The cultural and philosophical foundations of normative medical ethics. Soc Sci Med 1994;39:1149-54.

22. Bell D. Technology, nature and society. In: The winding Passage: essays and sociological journeys 1960-1980. Cambridge: ABT Books: 1980.

23. Bilimoria P. Indian ethics. In: Singer PA, editor. A companion to ethics. Blackwell Companions to Philosophy. Oxford: Blackwell; 1991.

24. Rigveda. The hymns [Translation: Menen A]. New York: Scriber's; 1954.

25. Stanley JM. The four principles in practice: facilitating international medical ethics. In: Gillon R, editor. Principles of health care ethics. London: John Wiley and Sons; 1994.

26. Declaration of Ixtapa. In: Bankowski Z, Bryant JH, Gallagher J. Ethics, equity and health for all 1994. Geneva: Council for International Organizations of Medical Sciences; 1997.

27. Wikler D. Bioethics, human rights and the renewal of health for all: an overview. Geneva: Council for International Organizations of Medical Sciences; 1997.p.23-4.

28. Beaufort ID, Dupuis HM. Handboek gezondheidsethiek. Assen/Maastricht: Van Gorcum; 1988.

29. Porter JD, Ogden JA. Public health, ethics and tuberculosis. Indian J Tuber 1999;46:3-10.

30. Beauchamp TL, Childress JF. Principles of biomedical ethics, Second edition. New York: Oxford University Press; 1983.

31. Aristotle. Nichomachean ethics. In: McKeon R. The basic works of Aristotle. Book 5. New York: Random House; 1941.

32. Stephens C. Environment, health and development: addressing complexity in the priority setting process. Geneva: World Health Organization Office of Global and Integrated Environmental Health; 1997.

33. Cole P. The moral bases for public health interventions. Epidemiology 1995;6:78-83.

34. Shindell S. Legal and ethical aspects of public health. In: Last JM, Maxcy-Rosenau, editors. Public health and preventive medicine. Eleventh edition. New York: Appleton Century Crofts; 1980. p.1834-45.

35. Skrabanek P. Why is preventative medicine exempted from ethical constraints? J Med Ethics 1990;16:187-90.

36. Hall SA. Symposium on ethics and public health: should public health respect autonomy? J Med Ethics 1992;18:97-201.

37. Mill JS. On Liberty. In: Wishy B, editor. Prefaces to liberty: selected writings of John Stuart Mill. Lanham: University Press of America; 1959.

38. Jesani A, Iyer A, Desai M, Adenwala M. Laws and health care providers. A study of legislation and legal aspects of health care delivery. Mumbai: Research Centre of Anusandhan Trust; 1996.

39. Thacker SB, Berkelman RL. Public health surveillance in the United states. Epidemiol Rev 1988;10:165.

40. Hogue LL. Public health and the law: issues and trends. Rockville: Aspen Systems Corporation; 1980.p.10.

41. Painter M, Button J. Legal aspects of communicable disease control. In: Noah N, O'Mahony M, editors. Communicable disease epidemiology and control. London: Wiley and Sons;1988.

42. Gasner MR, Maw KL, Feldman GE, Fujiwara PI, Frieden TR. The use of legal action in New York City to ensure treatment of tuberculosis. N Engl J Med 1999;340:359-66.

43. New York City Health Code. 1994. 11.47[d].

44. Bhore Committee. Report of the health survey and development committee 1946. Volume I: Survey, Volume II: Recommendations, Volume III: Appendices. New Delhi: Government of India, Manager of Publications; 1946.

45. Gittler J. Controlling resurgent tuberculosis: public health agencies, public policy, and law. J Health Polit Policy Law 1994;19:107-47.

46. Westaway MS, Wolmarans L. Cognitive and affective reactions of black urban South Africans towards tuberculosis. Tuberc Lung Dis 1994;75:47-453.

47. Snider DE. General view of problems with compliance in programme for the treatment of tuberculosis. Bull Int Union Tuberc 1982;57:255-60.

48. Donovan JL, Blake DR. Patient non-compliance: deviance or reasoned decision-making? Soc Sci Med 1992;34:507-13.

49. Yach D. Tuberculosis in the Western Cape health region of South Africa. Soc Sci Med 1988;27:683-9.

50. Farmer P. Social scientists and the new tuberculosis. Soc Sci Med 1997;44:347-58.

51. Selwyn PA. Tuberculosis and AIDS: epidemiological, clinical and social dimensions. J Law Med Ethics 1993;21:279-88.

52. Rangan S, Uplekar M, Ogden J, Porter J, Brugha R, Zwi A, et al. Shifting the paradigm in tuberculosis control: a state of the art review. Int J Tuberc Lung Dis 1999;3:855-61.

53. Porter JDH, Ogden JA. Social inequalities in the emergence of infectious disease. In: Strickland SS, Shetty PS, editors. Human biology and social inequality. Cambridge: Cambridge University Press; 1998.p.96-113.

54. Gostin LO. Controlling the resurgent tuberculosis epidemic: a 50-state survey of TB statutes and proposals for reform. JAMA 1993;269:255-61.

55. Reilly RG. Combating the tuberculosis epidemic: the legality of coercive treatment measures. Columbia J Law Social Prob 1993;27:101-49.

56. Centers for Disease Control and Prevention. Approaches to improving adherence to antituberculosis therapy-South Carolina, and New York, 1986-1991. Morb Mortal Wkly Rep 1993;42: 74-75, 81.

57. Centers for Disease Control and Prevention. Initial therapy for tuberculosis in the era of multidrug resistance: recommendations of the Advisory Council for the elimination of tuberculosis. Morb Mortal Wkly Rep 1993;42:1-8.

58. Weis SE, Slocum PC, Blais FX, King B, Nunn M, Matney GB, et al. The effect of directly observed therapy on the rates of drug resistance and relapse in tuberculosis. N Engl J Med 1994;330:1179-84.

59. Dubler NN, Bayer R, Landesman S; New York City Tuberculosis Working Group. Tuberculosis in the 1990's: ethical, legal and public policy issues in screening, treatment and the protection of those in congregate facilities. A report from the working group on TB and HIV. The tuberculosis revival: individual rights and societal obligations in a time of AIDS. New York: United Hospital Funds of New York; 1992.p.1-42.

60. Annas GJ. Control of tuberculosis–the law and the public's health. N Engl J Med 1993;328:585-8.

61. New York Working Group. Developing a system for tuberculosis prevention and care in New York City. The tuberculosis revival: individual rights and societal obligations in a time of AIDS. New York: United Hospital Fund of New York; 1992. p.51-8.

62. Hansel A. The TB and HIV epidemics: history learned and unlearned. J Law Med Ethics 1993;21:376-81.

63. Ogden JA. Compliance versus adherence: just a matter of language? The politics and poetics of public health. In: Porter JDH, Grange JM, editors. Tuberculosis – an interdisciplinary perspective. London: Imperial College Press; 1999.p.213-34.

64. Barnhoorn F, Adriaanse H. In search of factors responsible for non-compliance among tuberculosis patients in Wardha District, India. So Sci Med 1992;34:291-306.

65. Kimerling ME, Petri L. Tracing as part of tuberculosis control in a rural Cambodian district during 1992. Tuber Lung Dis 1995;76:156-9.

66. Parker RG. Empowement, community mobilization and social change in the face of HIV/AIDS. AIDS 1996;10 Suppl 3: S27-31.

67. Uplekar M, Rangan S. Tackling TB. The search for solutions. Bombay: FRCH; 1996.

68. Gilson L. Re-addressing equity: the search for the holy grail? The importance of ethics processes. In: Mills A, editor. Reforming health sectors. London: Wiley and Sons; 1998.

69. Lala Ram Swarup Institute of Tuberculosis and Allied Diseases. Final Report of the Operations Research to assess needs and persepctives of TB patients and providers of tuberculosis care in Nehru Nagar and Moti Nagar chest clinic areas of Delhi. Delhi: DFID Health and Population Office; 1998.

70. Medawar P. In Pluto's republic incorporating the 'art of the soluble'. London: Oxford University Press; 1984.

71. Pronyk P, Porter JD. Public health and human rights: the ethics of international public health interventions for tuberculosis. In: Porter JD, Grange JM, editors. Tuberculosis—an interdisiplinary perspective. London: Imperial College Press; 1999.p.99-120.

72. Gillon R. Deontological foundations for medical ethics? Chichester: John Wiley and Sons; 1994.p.14.

73. Mackintosh M. Competition and contracting in selective social provisioning. Eur J Dev Res 1995;7:26-52.

74. Sumartojo E. When tuberculosis treatment fails. A social behavioural account of patient adherence. Am Rev Resp Dis 1993;147:1311-20.

75. Rubel AJ, Garro LC. Social and cultural factors in the successful control of tuberculosis. Public Health Rep 1992;107:626-36.

76. Drobniewski F. Tuberculosis in prisons: forgotten plague. Lancet 1995;346:948-9.

77. Bureau of Justice. Prisoners in 1996, Bureau of Justice Statistics. Washington DC: US Department of Justice, Office of Justice Program; 1997.

78. Kendig N. Tuberculosis control in prisons. Int J Tuberc Lung Dis 1998;2:S57-63.

79. Lerer LB, Lopez A, Kjellstrom T, Yach D. Health for all: analyzing health status and determinants. World Health Stat Q 1998;51: 7-20.

80. Mann J. Human rights and the new public health. Health and Human Rights 1994;1:229-33.

81. Porter JDH, Ogden JA, Pronyk P. The way forward: an integrated approach to tuberculosis control. In: Porter JDH, Grange JM, editors. Tuberculosis—an interdisciplinary perspective. London: Imperial College Press; 1999.p.359-78.

82. Selgelid MJ, Reichman LB. Ethical issues in tuberculosis diagnosis and treatment. Int J Tuberc Lung Dis 2011;15 Suppl 2: S9-13.

83. Mamotte N, Wassenaar D, Koen J, Essack Z. Convergent ethical issues in HIV/AIDS, tuberculosis and malaria vaccine trials in Africa: Report from the WHO/UNAIDS African AIDS Vaccine Programme's Ethics, Law and Human Rights Collaborating Centre consultation, 10-11 February 2009, Durban, South Africa. BMC Med Ethics 2010;11:3.

84. World Health Organization. Guidance on ethics of tuberculosis prevention, care and control. WHO/HTM/TB/2010.16. Geneva: World Health Organization; 2010. Available at URL: http://apps.who.int/iris/bitstream/10665/44452/1/9789241500531_eng.pdf. Accessed on June 12, 2018.

85. World Health Organization. Ethical issues in tuberculosis prevention, care and control. Geneva: World Health Organization; 2014. Available at URL: http://www.who.int/tb/publications/ethics_in_tb_factsheet_28jan11rev.pdf. Accessed on June 12, 2018.

56

Airborne Tuberculosis Transmission and Infection Control Strategies

Kamini Walia, Jai P Narain

INTRODUCTION

Tuberculosis [TB] is transmitted through inhalation of droplet nuclei or residue from evaporated droplets containing TB bacilli. These bacilli can survive outside the body and remain suspended in the air for long periods of time. Unsuspected TB cases contribute to TB transmission as these patients are not being treated and may go unsuspected for weeks and visit number of health facilities or even may remain indoor patients also before being diagnosed as TB and put on treatment. The risk of contracting infection becomes higher in the closed settings, such as, home, health care settings, prisons, etc., where a TB patient may cough and sneeze putting others at risk of exposure. The health care workers are also at high-risk as they are continuously exposed to patients with infectious TB, and therefore, require protection from the disease at their work environment.

Recently, the international health community has set an ambitious goal to eliminate TB by 2050 and to cut the annual incidence of new cases to less than 1 per million population. These targets cannot be achieved without comprehensively addressing all aspects of disease transmission, rapid diagnosis and appropriate management (1,2). Of all the measures which are likely to bring down the TB cases, infection control strategies have been most neglected yet most important as highlighted by various studies in India and globally (3). Given that the annual risk of TB infection in high prevalence countries remains high, reducing person-to-person transmission of TB should be a top priority (4). Recognising this, India's Revised National TB Control Programme [RNTCP] issued infection control guidelines in April 2010 (5).

AIRBORNE TUBERCULOSIS TRANSMISSION DYNAMICS

Mycobacterium tuberculosis complex [*Mtb*] which principally causes TB in humans is carried in airborne particles, called droplet nuclei, of 1-5 µ in diameter, generated by persons with active pulmonary or laryngeal TB disease, when they cough, or sneeze. Droplet nuclei remain airborne lasting for several hours. Those who inhale these droplets can become infected. The infectiousness of a person with TB disease is directly related to the number of tubercle bacilli that he or she expels into the air (6). Fennelly *et al* (7) documented that cough aerosol emanating directly from TB patients contained 3-4 colony forming units [CFU] to a maximum of 633 CFU containing viable, growing, and infectious organisms.

TB transmission occurs when a healthy person inhales droplet nuclei containing *Mtb*. The probability that a person who is exposed to *Mtb* will become infected depends primarily on immune status of the exposed individual, environmental factors that affect the concentration of *Mtb* and the proximity, frequency and duration of exposure to a person with infectious TB disease (6). The closer the proximity and the longer the duration of exposure, the higher the risk is for being infected. The risk is often also associated with infectious load, although infectiousness gets reduced after initiation of an effective therapy. Persons at higher risk for exposure to and infection with *Mtb* are shown in Table 56.1. It is well recognised that TB outbreaks are facilitated in crowded living conditions with prolonged close exposure to an infectious person among close contacts.

Table 56.1: Persons at a higher risk for exposure to and infection with *Mtb*

Persons in crowded living conditions with prolonged close exposure to an infectious case of TB among close contacts
Residents and employees of congregate settings that are at high risk [e.g., correctional facilities, long-term care facilities, and homeless shelters]
Health care workers who serve patients who are at high-risk
Health care workers with unprotected exposure to a patient with TB disease before the identification and correct airborne precautions of the patient
Certain populations who are medically underserved and who have low income, as defined locally
Populations at high-risk who are defined locally as having an increased incidence of TB disease
Infants, children and adolescents exposed to adults in high-risk categories

Mtb = *Mycobacterium tuberculosis*; TB = tuberculosis

FACTORS ENHANCING TUBERCULOSIS TRANSMISSION AT VARIOUS SETTINGS

The patterns of communicable disease are influenced by the existence of pockets of high transmission (8). Outbreaks are often initiated among persons exposed to poor living conditions, characterised by poor ventilation, crowding, migration, and limited health care access (9-11). Many TB outbreaks have been documented in resource-poor hospitals in which dozens of patients share poorly ventilated rooms and waiting halls, and in crowded prison cells or mining barracks (12-17). Hence hospital wards, nursing homes for elderly, prisons and mines are also referred to as institutional amplifiers for TB transmission (18,19). In the past several years, the World Health Organization [WHO] and other major public health bodies have recognised social factors critical to influencing TB transmission risks and the risks of recurrent or resistant disease (20).

Health Care/Hospital Settings

In hospital settings, TB transmission has been associated with variety of factors like cough-generating procedures (21), and other medical examination and treatment such as broncho-scopy (22), endotracheal intubation and suctioning (23), open abscess irrigation (24), and autopsy (25). All these situations and procedures create infectious droplets and environmental factors like poor ventilation and air circulation enhance the risk of TB transmission by increasing the exposure to the source of infectious droplet nuclei thus increasing the TB transmission. Transmission of TB can have serious consequences, particularly with multidrug-resistant TB [MDR-TB]. Several outbreaks in the United States demonstrated the role that hospitals can play as focal points of MDR-TB transmission (26-29), a phenomenon also seen in Europe, South America, South Africa, and Russia (30-32). These outbreaks have been associated with high death rates as hospitalised patients are often immunocompromised (33,34).

In India, airborne transmission of TB at health care facilities is an important issue for a variety of reasons. Prevalence of TB is higher among patients attending the health care facilities than in general population, therefore the likelihood of airborne transmission is higher in health facilities. Many of these patients remain infectious for a longer period of time due to delays in diagnosis and treatment. There is general lack of awareness regarding infection control principles and practice among health care workers. The patients lack cough etiquette and patient education is sub-optimal. Many health facilities do not have policies and programmes relating to infection control, nor are there adequate infrastructure or a system in place.

Nosocomial transmission poses major threat for the health care workforce, which could adversely affect health-care services over time (35). Studies in hospitals and health care facilities have documented that poor ventilation design or construction contributes to the transmission of infection, particularly among clinical personnel in patient rooms with fewer than two air changes per hour (36). In a study of skin test conversion from Lima, Peru a 25.5% conversion risk among medical students doing their clinical training in a hospital with a room volume of 16.2 m^3/bed, compared to 12.7% for students training in a hospital with 41.4 m^3/bed (37) thus indicating efficacy of good ventilation system (38,39).

Communities and Household Settings

In communities, factors such as urban dwelling, crowding, poor housing with lack of ventilation, limited access to health services and, at individual level, smoking and alcohol use, human immunodeficiency virus [HIV] infection, exposure to indoor air pollution, diabetes mellitus, and under-nutrition have been linked to enhanced susceptibility and thus increased transmission (40-42).

Overcrowding has been identified as a risk factor for TB transmission (43,44). In communities where persons with TB disease live, crowded housing with limited air movement leads to an increased risk in terms of exposure to *Mtb* (37,43). Lienhardt (38) has summarised a number of studies showing that crowding is a risk factor for infection and for increased risk of disease after infection. Beggs *et al* (44) noted that occupancy density, room volume and air change rate are all directly correlated with the number of new TB infections among persons who share airspace (44). Inadequate air change rates, negative airflow and recirculation of air have been identified as an occupational hazard in hospitals with respect to TB transmission (36).

TB transmission in families in which there are two or more new cases [apart from the index case] of TB, within a specified time period, are identified as microepidemics (45). In communities where the prevalence of TB is high, micro-epidemics may go unnoticed simply because the pattern is not apparent. It was found that new TB cases more frequently [41%] came from families that had been characterised as having microepidemics than from families in which only a single new case had occurred [21%], and that it was a small number of families that generated the most new TB cases in the study of contacts.

Congregate Settings

The congregate settings are those where a group of people share an environment or facilities. These range from prisons and military barracks, to homeless shelters, refugee camps, and nursing homes. Of these, prison settings are considered high risk-group for TB. Infection and disease rates have been documented to be as high as 5 up to more than 80 times higher compared to national averages (45-47). The fact that prison inmates mostly come from marginalised populations with poor socioeconomic living conditions, suffer from malnutrition, co-morbidities and live in poorly ventilated prison cells explains the markedly high TB incidence and prevalence in prison populations.

TB in prison has been found to strongly influence TB and TB control in general populations by Stuckler *et al* (48) who established a clear relationship between rises in incarceration rates and increased TB incidence and MDR-TB prevalence rates in Eastern European and Central Asian countries. Prisons thus play the role of a pocket of high transmission of TB with, similarly like, mines and communal hospital wards among others.

OVERALL STRATEGIES FOR REDUCING AIRBORNE TRANSMISSION

In order to prevent airborne transmission of TB, the World Health Organization [WHO], Centers for Disease Control and Prevention [CDC] and other agencies recommend implementation of basic TB infection control programmes in all health care settings (49,50). Implementing interventions to prevent TB transmission requires action from the national policy to the institution level, and all levels in between (50). The WHO recommends developing an infection control plan, educating healthcare workers and patients, improving sputum collection practices, performing triage and evaluation of suspected TB patients in outpatient settings, and reducing exposure in the laboratory (35). Early diagnosis, triaging infected persons, and rapidly and effectively treating persons with TB are crucial for an effective TB infection control in healthcare settings (51-53). Current TB transmission control guidelines assume a prominent role for hospitals and clinics who manage MDR-TB and extensively drug resistant TB [XDR-TB] owing to substantial delays in the identification of TB patients and the diagnosis of drug-resistant cases because of the diagnostic limitations.

The standard approach to TB transmission control in health care settings includes: [i] administrative measures; [ii] environmental or engineering measures, and [iii] personal respiratory protection (50).

This approach is detailed in both the WHO TB infection control policy and the existing facility-level document, (35,50) as well as the CDC guidelines, although the latter are written primarily for low-prevalence, resource-rich settings.

Administrative Controls

The rationale for implementing administrative control measures is to minimise potential opportunities of exposure of susceptible individuals to infectious TB patients. Administrative controls are important since environmental controls and personal respiratory protection will not work in the absence of solid administrative control measures.

Administrative measures include [i] identifying rapidly persons with respiratory symptoms; [ii] separating or isolating them into appropriate environment; [iii] using simple surgical masks on patients with infectious TB, especially if they are not segregated; [iv] fast-tracking them through the health care facility to reduce exposure time to others; [v] diagnosing and treating those likely to have TB, with minimal delay; [vi] minimising hospitalisation of TB patients; and [vii] educate admitted patients for cough hygiene and have adequate sputum disposal provision.

At facility level, administrative interventions play a major role in reducing the risk of TB transmission and are essential for the implementation of other controls [i.e. environmental controls and personal protective equipment]. In the United States, administrative measures [early detection, isolation, and treatment of patients with TB] have been the most effective components of TB infection control programmes (28). In India, of all the recommended interventions, implementing administrative controls is likely to be the most feasible and effective strategy (54).

Administrative measures are often said to be the least expensive and most effective interventions such as rapid diagnosis and community-based treatment, are both administrative policy decisions. They are likely to be highly effective and cost-effective in terms of both treatment outcomes and transmission prevention. Conventional administrative strategies includes early detection of patients with infectious TB, isolating or at least segregating those with infectious pulmonary TB from other patients, and rapidly initiating anti-TB treatment, supported by measures to improve adherence [e.g., DOTS]. Depending on existing conditions, building renovations or new construction may be essential for effective airborne infection control (54).

Implementing Environmental Controls

Implementing many of the recommended environmental or engineering measures is not feasible in most health care facilities in resource-limited settings because of the high costs of such interventions [e.g., negative-pressure isolation rooms]. Studies indicate that ventilation has an important role in reducing the risk of airborne transmission of TB (36). These include mechanical as well as natural ventilation, such as, simply keeping windows open. A "Finding TB cases Actively, Separating safely, and Treating effectively" [FAST] approach is recommended (55). In fact, separation or segregation of smear-positive TB patients in private or semi-private rooms or wards with simple mechanical exhaust ventilation [e.g., window fans] could be feasible in some settings, particularly in the private sector and well-funded public hospitals. These measures have been shown to be useful in terminating an outbreak of nosocomial TB (26). This intervention is particularly necessary at centres that manage patients with MDR-TB; at such centres, patients with infectious TB must not be admitted to the same wards as patients with HIV infection.

There is a growing need for architects and engineers trained in airborne infection control owing to growing awareness on the *role of design* in limiting transmission of infections. The design process includes: [i] an in-depth study of work practices; [ii] patient volume and flow; [iii] an understanding of high-risk and lower risk areas; and [iv] an appreciation of local climate and resource limitations.

Comprehensive, evidence-based guidelines on natural ventilation to control airborne infections in health care settings have recently been issued by the WHO (56). A number of minimal hourly average ventilation rates is suggested, taking into account fluctuations in conditions and the indoor gas exchange rates are monitored using carbon dioxide as tracer gas when windows are open compared to when they are closed in some settings (57). Facilities in warm climates can take advantage of outdoor waiting areas, covered open walkways and open windows most of the time of the year. While facility planners try to take full advantage of natural ventilation, it may not be sufficient owing to different direction of airflow under various climatic conditions and at different times of day. The effect of opening and closing interior doors is also considered. When these rates and airflow direction cannot be reliably achieved by natural ventilation alone, mechanical ventilation or mixed mode systems are recommended.

Germicidal air-disinfection is also an attractive alternative as a low-cost complementary system to natural ventilation, for example at night or during cold seasons when windows may be closed (58), especially in cold climates not suitable for natural ventilation or high-volume mechanical ventilation systems (59). Germicidal irradiation is used in three different ways: [i] direct, unshielded room disinfection; [ii] disinfection in ventilation duct or room air cleaners; and [iii] upper room air disinfection.

The application of ultraviolet germicidal irradiation [UVGI] for TB transmission control is not very effective as [i] there is no evidence that *Mtb*, once settled on surfaces, can be resuspended as particles small enough to reach the alveoli of the lung where infection must begin; [ii] UV is not an ideal surface decontaminant, missing any shadowed surfaces; and [iii]air disinfection is most useful for protecting room occupants when the infectious source is present (45). UVGI in a properly designed room air cleaner will effectively disinfect the air going through it, but the overall effect in a room is limited to the number of germ-free equivalent room air changes added per hour, or 'clean air delivery rate' (46).

Small air cleaning units, sold as a quick and easy solution for TB transmission control, with very low clean air delivery rates are often mounted to the walls of corridors or placed in patient rooms. These units give a false sense of security and no meaningful risk reduction. The same limitations apply to room air cleaners using filters with or without germicidal lamps. The efficacy of UV germicidal lights is being evaluated in other low-income countries, and results of such studies are needed to determine their value in reducing nosocomial transmission.

Use of Personal Protection Measures

The first two levels of the infection control hierarchy, administrative and environmental controls, minimise the exposure to *Mtb* might occur but do not eliminate, the risk. The third level of the hierarchy is the use of respiratory protective equipment in situations that pose a high-risk for exposure. Respirators encompass a range of devices that vary in complexity from flexible masks covering only the nose and mouth, to units that cover the user's head, such as, loose-fitting or hooded powered air purifying respirators [PAPRs] and to those that have independent air supplies [e.g., airline respirators] (60).

The overall effectiveness of respiratory protection is affected by [i] the level of respiratory protection selected [e.g., the assigned protection factor]; [ii] the fit characteristics of the respirator model; [iii] the care in donning the respirator; and [iv] the adequacy of the fit-testing program. Although data on the effectiveness of respiratory protection from various hazardous airborne materials have been collected, the precise level of effectiveness in protecting health care workers from *Mtb* transmission in health care settings has not been determined.

The most widely used respirators are certified in the United States as N95 [Figure 56.1] and in Europe as FFP2. The disposable models consist of a filtering face piece in various configurations [cup, duckbill] and sizes, generally two elastic bands to achieve a tight face seal, and a malleable nose clip to prevent leaks around the nose. The US CDC provides guidance on all aspects of an effective respirator programme (61).

Besides high cost, many barriers have been identified that prevent the effective use of respirators in resource-limited

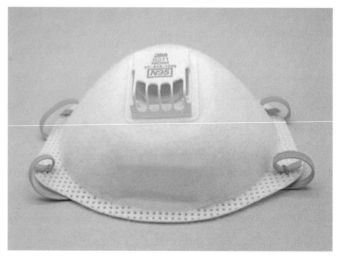

Figure 56.1: N95 respirator

settings as respirators are uncomfortable and cannot be worn continuously. For respirator to function optimally respirator models and sizes should be available since no single model or size fits everyone. All of this entails cost and training. There is a concern around the cost [ranging from US$1-$2] each in low-resource settings. The masks tend to become flaccid fairly quickly, depending on quality and how often the respirator is doffed and donned.

Better non-disposable respirator designs that have a more clinical appearance and allow better verbal communication are needed for medical use in resource-limited settings (39).

SPECIFIC STRATEGIES FOR REDUCING AIRBORNE TRANSMISSION OF TUBERCULOSIS AT HEALTH CARE FACILITIES

TB infection control requires action at national and sub-national level to provide policy and managerial direction, and at health facility level to implement TB infection control measures. The recommended set of activities for national and subnational TB infection control is necessary to facilitate implementation of TB infection control in health care facilities, congregate settings and households [Tables 56.2 and 56.3].

These activities should be integrated within existing national and sub-national management structures for general infection prevention and control.

Based upon international recommendations [WHO, CDC, etc.] following specific measures may be undertaken [Table 56.4]. For reducing transmission in the health care settings, the TB infection-control programme should be based on a three-level hierarchy of control measures that have been described earlier, namely, administrative, engineering/environmental and personal protective equipment.

Reducing Transmission in the Laboratory Facilities

TB bacteriology laboratory activities that may generate aerosols include preparing specimens for centrifugation

and mycobacterial culture, centrifugation of specimens, inoculating cultures from specimen sediment, handling unopened primary- isolation plates or tubes, staining smear of material from culture, manipulating cultures [suspension preparation, vortex, and transferring] of *Mtb* complex on solid medium, transferring large volumes of cultures or suspensions of bacilli, disposing of cultures of *Mtb* complex, inactivation of specimens for isolation of deoxyribonucleic acid [DNA] and other macromolecules on *Mtb* complex species and during shipping of cultures or specimens of *Mtb* complex.

Table 56.3: Recommendations for TB ward

TB wards should be located away from the other wards, with adequate facilities for hand washing and good maintenance and cleaning

TB wards should have adequate ventilation [natural and/or assisted] to ensure >12 ACH at all times

In TB wards there should be adequate space [at least 6 feet] between 2 adjacent beds

Cough hygiene should be promoted through signage and practice ensured through patients and staff training, ongoing reinforcement by staff

Adequate sputum disposal, with individual container with lid, containing 5% phenol, for collection of sputum should be provided

All staff should be trained on standard precautions, airborne infection control precautions, and the proper use of personal respiratory protection. A selection of different sizes of re-usable N95 particulate respirators should be made available for optional use by staff

Sputum pots in the inpatient wards should be disinfected with 5% phenol for one hour, and then emptied into the routine drain

TB = tuberculosis; ACH = air changes per hour

Table 56.4: Specific strategies for reducing airborne transmission of TB at health care facilities

Developing an infection control plan and allocation of specific budget and time line for the activity

Identifying and strengthening local coordinating bodies for TB infection control, and developing a facility plan [including human resources, and policies and procedures to ensure proper implementation of the controls listed below] for implementation

Rethinking the use of available spaces and considering renovation of existing facilities or construction of new ones to optimise implementation of controls

Conduct on-site surveillance of TB disease among health workers and assess the facility

Address ACSM for health workers, patients and visitors

Organising training of health care workers

Monitor and evaluate the set of TB infection control measures

Participate in research efforts

TB = tuberculosis; ACSM = advocacy, communication and social mobilisation

---

Table 56.2: Set of activities for national and sub-national TB infection control

Identify and strengthen a coordinating body for TB infection control, and develop a comprehensive budgeted plan that includes human resource requirements for implementation of TB infection control at all levels

Conduct surveillance of TB disease among health workers, and conduct assessment at all levels of the health system and in congregate settings

Ensure that health facility design, construction, renovation and use are appropriate

Address TB infection control advocacy, communication and social mobilisation [ACSM], including engagement of civil society

Monitor and evaluate the set of TB infection control measures

Enable and conduct operational research

TB = tuberculosis

While general principles of instituting administrative, engineering and personal protective activities [outlined above], given the greater mycobacterial burden in environment of laboratories, some of the additional important actions need to be taken. These include the following. Written TB infection control measures {standard operating procedures, [SOP]} for laboratory are available, and laboratory technologists [LTs] are trained/oriented in laboratory standard operating procedures in ensuring airborne precautions through periodic trainings. Shipping of cultures to reference laboratory needs to follow bio-safe-triple packaged containers. Laboratory is either placed at the blind-end of building and/physically isolated from the common laboratory/hospital environments. Access to the culture and drug susceptibility testing [DST] rooms is through an anteroom. The entry to lab is restricted to trained laboratory personnel. The containment room where culture and DST is carried out is sealable in case of spill and aerosolisation for decontamination. Biological safety cabinets [BSCs] class II, with 100% exhaust [i.e. ducted outside] are provided and used. BSCs ducted to outside, while switched "on", would maintain an inward air flow into the culture and DST facilities. Bio-safe centrifuges with aerosol-seal buckets is provided and used. Handwash sink is provided in the culture and DST room with effective disinfectant. Autoclave [steam sterilisation facility] is provided within the laboratory facility. Following protection measures to be followed in the laboratory by staff [Table 56.5].

Table 56.5: Protection measures to be followed in the laboratory by staff

For sputum collection and smear microscopy

Proper cough hygiene needs to be explained to the patients

Collection should be in an open area, or in a properly designed and maintained indoor sputum collection booth

Laboratory technician would maintain at least one arm length distance and upwind when a patient is collecting a sputum sample

Wear lab coats while performing the laboratory work

For culture and DST activities

All personnel working in culture laboratory need to wear separate clothing, not the common laboratory coat

Separate closed-toe foot-wear to be used at all times. *Chappals* or sandals are not appropriate

All personnel are to wear an N95 particulate respirator while performing

DST, or manipulating cultures for any reason

Decontaminate lab coat before laundering or disposal

Personal protective equipment should be worn in the following order: [i] disposable gloves; [ii] coats/suits/overalls; and [iii] respirator/mask

Personal protective equipment should be removed in the following order before leaving the laboratory: [i] respirator/mask; [ii] coats/suits/overalls; and [iii] disposable gloves

DST = drug-susceptibility testing

In laboratories where only smear microscopy is performed, personal respiratory protection [e.g., respirators] is not needed. Laboratories working with liquid suspensions of *Mtb* should be equipped with a BSC class I. Personal respiratory protection is not recommended if the BSC is functioning appropriately and all work with liquid suspensions is carried out in the cabinet.

Designated Microscopy Centres

Direct sputum microscopy is a relatively low-risk activity as long as safe work practices are implemented properly. The following work practices are recommended to ensure that microscopy laboratory technicians are not exposed to aerosols from sputum specimens.

Sputum collection Sputum must be collected in a well ventilated area with direct sunlight. It should not be collected in laboratories, toilets, waiting rooms, reception rooms, or any other enclosed space. If indoor sputum collection is required due to space constraints, it should be done in sputum collection booth.

Smear preparation Smears should be prepared in a well ventilated environment, near an open flame.

Work bench Work Benches should be cleaned daily with 70% alcohol.

Sputum container/applicator sticks/slides Sputum containers, applicator sticks and slides should be disinfected with 5% Phenol overnight before discarding. They may be discarded in deep burial pits or may be tagged for appropriate disposal via the hospital biomedical waste management system.

Acid-fast Bacilli Smear Preparation

Many laboratories which process infectious sputum in resource-limited countries perform only direct smear microscopy. Performing direct smear microscopy has not been documented to result in the transmission of *Mtb* [assuming centrifugation is not being used]. Direct smear microscopy can be safely performed on the open bench. Neither environmental controls nor personal respiratory protection are necessary during the preparation of smears.

In laboratories performing only smear preparation without the use of a centrifuge, perhaps the greatest threat to the personnel is contact with coughing patients. Administrative controls should be used to limit this exposure.

Preparation of Liquid Suspensions of Mycobacterium tuberculosis

Laboratories which process liquid preparations of suspended *Mtb* [e.g., centrifugation, cultures, and DST] should be considered at higher risk for nosocomial *Mtb* transmission. Safety can be improved by enhancing ventilation in areas where culture and susceptibility testing of *Mtb* isolates is performed; reducing the number of laboratories handling concentrated specimens containing *Mtb*; and only allowing laboratories with appropriate biosafety cabinets [BSC I or BSC II] and experienced staff to work with liquid suspensions of *Mtb*.

Reducing Transmission in Households and Communities

To reduce exposure in households, patients and their families should be educated on the importance of infection control practices to be observed at home. Houses should be adequately ventilated, particularly rooms where people with infectious TB spend considerable time [natural ventilation may be sufficient to provide adequate ventilation]. Anyone who coughs should be educated on cough etiquette and respiratory hygiene, and should follow such practices at all times while smear positive, TB patients should spend as much time as possible outdoors; sleep alone in a separate, adequately ventilated room, if possible; and spend as little time as possible in congregate settings or in public transport.

Patients with MDR-TB usually sputum convert later than those with drug-susceptible TB and remain infectious for much longer, thus prolonging the risk of transmission in the household. Additional infection control measures should, therefore, be implemented for the management of MDR-TB patients at home. Awareness of infection control in the community should be promoted. In households with culture-positive MDR-TB patients, the following guidance should be observed, in addition to the measures given above. While culture positive, MDR-TB patients who cough should always practice cough etiquette [including use of masks] and respiratory hygiene when in contact with people. Ideally, health service providers should wear particulate respirators when attending patients in enclosed spaces. Further, family members living with HIV, or family members with strong clinical evidence of HIV infection, should ideally not provide care for patients with culture-positive MDR-TB. If there is no alternative, HIV-positive family members should wear respirators, if available.

Children below five years of age should spend as little time as possible in the same living spaces as culture-positive MDR-TB patients. Such children should be followed up regularly with TB screening and, if positive, DST and treatment. While culture positive, XDR-TB patients should be isolated at all times, and any person in contact with a culture positive XDR-TB patient should wear a particulate respirator. If at all possible, HIV-positive family members, or family members with a strong clinical evidence of HIV infection, should not share a household with culture positive XDR-TB patients. If possible, potential renovation of the patient's home should be considered, to improve ventilation [e.g. building of a separate bedroom, or installation of a window or wind catcher, or both].

Reducing Transmission in Congregate Settings

Like any other health care facility, the set of TB infection control measures should be implemented in congregate settings especially prisons, as the incidence of TB infection and TB disease among individuals in congregate settings exceeds the incidence among the general population particularly among inmates of prisons. Therefore, the policy makers responsible for congregate settings should be made part of the coordinating system for planning and implementing interventions to control TB infection. In particular, the medical service of the ministry of justice and correctional facilities should be fully engaged and encouraged to implement TB infection control. Congregate settings should be part of the country surveillance activities, and should be included in facility assessment for TB infection control. Any advocacy and information, education and communication material should include a specific focus on congregate settings, as should monitoring and evaluation of TB infection control measures.

Facility-level Managerial Activities should Also Apply with Some Adaptation to Congregate Settings

To decrease TB transmission in congregate settings, cough etiquette and respiratory hygiene, and early identification, followed by separation and proper treatment of infectious cases should be implemented. All staff should be given appropriate information and encouraged to undergo TB diagnostic investigation if they have signs and symptoms suggestive of TB. People suspected of having TB should be diagnosed as quickly as possible and managed.

In congregate settings with a high prevalence of HIV [in particular in correctional services], patients living with HIV and other forms of immunosuppression should be separated from those with suspected or confirmed infectious TB. All staff and persons residing in the setting should be encouraged to undergo HIV testing and counselling. If diagnosed with HIV, they should be offered a package of prevention and care that includes regular screening for active TB. In congregate settings with patients having, or suspected of having, drug-resistant TB, such patients should be separated from other patients [including other TB patients], and referral for proper treatment should be established. Buildings in congregate settings should comply with national norms and regulations for ventilation in public buildings, and specific norms and regulations for prisons, where these exist.

India has the highest number of patients with MDR-TB globally. Given the threat of drug-resistant TB, in addition to unprecedented massive scale-up of complex, effective treatment programmes, simultaneous seismic shift in efforts to control transmission in congregate settings as well as in communities is the need of the hour. The apparent solutions to improve the current situation includes the introduction of improved diagnostic methods, rapid detection of drug resistance, newer drugs and regimes, and strengthen the infection control practices to reduce the spread of infection as well as curtail the re-infection by instituting measures to reduce transmission in hospital and community settings (62,63).

The most affordable measures which can be easily adapted are improving natural ventilation through open windows and sunlight. Educating healthcare workers about nosocomial TB and measures that can help prevent such transmission, educating patients on cough etiquette and respiratory hygiene and using simple surgical masks on patients with infectious TB [especially if they are not segregated] who are coughing is another low hanging fruit that can be utilised to break the cycle of transmission in hospital settings. Enhanced screening of health care/institutional workers followed by prompt treatment should be embedded in the institutional policy as part of administrative controls. In addition to the above measures, hospitals should make every effort to treat TB patients on an ambulatory basis. If hospitalisation is required, every effort should be made to segregate potentially infectious patients from immunocompromised patients, rapidly diagnose and initiate treatment, and discharge patients promptly with directly observed therapy [DOT] on an outpatient basis.

While international evidence-based guidelines are available, the national programmes would have to take necessary steps to ensure that this guideline is put to practice in terms of creating awareness around the benefits of reducing transmission and making sufficient resources available for supplies and infrastructure improvements.

REFERENCES

1. Dye C, Williams BG. Eliminating human tuberculosis in the twenty-first century. J R Soc Interface 2008;5:653-62.
2. Stop TB Partnership. Available at URL: http://www.stoptb.org/. Accessed on September 16, 2018.
3. World Health Organization. A ministerial meeting of high M/XDR-TB burden countries: meeting report. Geneva: World Health Organization; 2009.
4. Yates TA, Khan PY, Knight GM, Taylor JG, Mchugh TD, Lipman M, et al. The transmission of Mycobacterium tuberculosis in high burden settings. Lancet Infect Dis 2016;16:227-38.
5. Directorate General of Health Services, Ministry of Health and Family Welfare, Government of India. Guidelines on airborne infection control in healthcare and other settings. New Delhi: Directorate General of Health Services, Ministry of Health and Family Welfare, Government of India; 2010.
6. Core curriculum on tuberculosis: What the clinician should know. Available at URL: http://www.cdc.gov/tb/education/corecurr/pdf/introduction.pdf. Accessed on September 20, 2018.
7. Fennelly KP, Martyny JW, Fulton KE, Orme IM, Cave DM, Heifets LB. Cough generated aerosols of Mycobacterium tuberculosis: a new method to study infectiousness. Am J Respir Crit Care Med 2004;169:604-9.
8. Post WM, De Angelisa DL, Travis CC. Endemic disease in environments with spatially heterogeneous host populations. Math Biosci 1983; 63:289-302.
9. World Health Organization. Global tuberculosis control: surveillance, planning, financing. WHO report 2008. WHO/HTM/TB 2008.393. Geneva: World Health Organization; 2008.
10. Dormandy T. The white death: A history of tuberculosis. London: Hambledon and London; 2001.
11. Iseman MD. A clinician's guide to tuberculosis. Hagerstown: Lippincott Williams and Wilkins; 2000.
12. Gandhi NR, Moll A, Sturm AW, Pawinski R, Govender T, Lalloo U, et al. Extensively drug-resistant tuberculosis as a cause of death in patients co-infected with tuberculosis and HIV in a rural area of South Africa. Lancet 2006;368:1575-80.
13. Basu S, Friedland GH, Medlock J, Andrews JR, Shah NS, Gandhi NR, et al. Averting epidemics of extensively drug-resistant tuberculosis. Proc Natl Acad Sci USA 2009;106:7672-7.
14. Lobacheva T, Sazhin V, Vdovichenko E, Giesecke J. Pulmonary tuberculosis in two remand prisons [SIZOs] in St Petersburg, Russia. Euro Surveill 2005;10:93-6.
15. Godfrey-Faussett P, Sonnenberg P, Shearer SC, Bruce MC, Mee C, Morris L, et al. Tuberculosis control and molecular epidemiology in a South African gold-mining community. Lancet 2000;356:1066-71.
16. Moro ML, Errante I, Infuso A, Sodano L, Gori A, Orcese CA, et al. Effectiveness of infection control measures in controlling a nosocomial outbreak of multidrug-resistant tuberculosis among HIV patients in Italy. Int J Tuberc Lung Dis 2000;4:61-8.
17. Keshavjee S, Gelmanova IY, Farmer PE, Mishustin SP, Strelis AK, Andreev YG, et al. Treatment of extensively drug-resistant tuberculosis in Tomsk, Russia: a retrospective cohort study. Lancet 2008;372:1403-9.
18. Basu S, Stuckler D, McKee M. Addressing institutional amplifiers in the dynamics and control of tuberculosis epidemics. Am J Trop Med Hyg 2011;84:30-7.
19. Narain JP, Warren E, Lofgren JP, Stead WW. Epidemic tuberculosis in a nursing home: A retrospective cohort study. J Am Geriatr Soc 1985;33:258-63.
20. World Health Organization. Commission on Social Determinants of Health. Closing the gap in a generation: health equity through action on the social determinants of health. Final Report of the Commission on Social Determinants of Health. Geneva: World Health Organization; 2008.
21. Malasky C, Jordan T, Potulski F, Reichman LB. Occupational tuberculosis infections among pulmonary physicians in training. Am Rev Respir Dis 1990;142:505-7.
22. Catanzaro A. Nosocomial tuberculosis. Am Rev Respir Dis 1982;125:559-62.
23. Haley CE, McDonald RC, Rossi L, Jones Jr WD, Haley RW, Luby JP. Tuberculosis epidemic among hospital personnel. Infect Control Hosp Epidemiol 1989;10:204-10.
24. Hutton MD, Stead WW, Cauthen GM, Bloch AB, Ewing WM. Nosocomial transmission of tuberculosis associated with a draining abscess. J Infect Dis 1990;161:286-95.
25. Kanto HS, Poblete R, Pusateri SL. Nosocomial transmission of tuberculosis from unsuspected disease. Am J Med 1988;84:833-8.
26. Blumberg HM, Watkins DL, Berschling JD, Antle A, Moore P, White N, et al. Preventing the nosocomial transmission of tuberculosis. Ann Intern Med 1995;122:658-63.
27. Beck-Sague C, Dooley SW, Hutton MD, Otten J, Breeden A, Crawford JT, et al. Hospital outbreak of multidrug-resistant Mycobacterium tuberculosis infections. Factors in transmission to staff and HIV-infected patients. JAMA 1992;268:1280-6.
28. Edlin BR, Tokars JI, Grieco MH, Crawford JT, Williams J, Sordillo EM, et al. An outbreak of multidrug-resistant tuberculosis among hospitalized patients with the acquired immunodeficiency syndrome. N Engl J Med 1992;326:1514-21.
29. Zaza S, Blumberg HM, Beck-Sague C, Haas WH, Woodley CL, Pineda M, et al. Nosocomial transmission of Mycobacterium tuberculosis: role of health care workers in outbreak propagation. J Infect Dis 1995;172:1542.
30. Moro ML, Gori A, Errante I, Infuso A, Franzetti F, Sodano L, et al. An outbreak of multidrug-resistant tuberculosis involving HIV infected patients of two hospitals in Milan, Italy. Italian Multidrug-resistant Tuberculosis Outbreak Study Group. AIDS 1998;12:1095-102.

31. Ritacco V, Di Lonardo M, Reniero A, Ambroggi M, Barrera L, Dambrosi A, et al. Nosocomial spread of human immunodeficiency virus–related multidrug-resistant tuberculosis in Buenos Aires. J Infect Dis 1997;176:637-42.

32. Drobniewski F, Balabanova Y, Nikolayevsky V, Ruddy M, Kuznetzov S, Zakharova S, et al. Drug-resistant tuberculosis, clinical virulence, and the dominance of the Beijing strain family in Russia. JAMA 2005;293:2726-31.

33. Nardell EA. Indoor environmental control of tuberculosis and other airborne infections. Indoor Air 2016;26:79-87.

34. Rieder HL. Epidemiological basis of tuberculosis control. Paris: International Union Against Tuberculosis and Lung Diseases; 1999.

35. World Health Organization. Guidelines for the prevention of tuberculosis in health care facilities in resource-limited settings. Geneva: World Health Organization; 1999.

36. Menzies D, Fanning A, Yuan L, FitzGerald JM, and the Canadian Collaborative Group in Nosocomial Transmission of TB. Hospital ventilation and risk for tuberculosis infection in Canadian health care workers. Ann Intern Med 2000; 133:779-89.

37. Accinelli R, Alvarez L, Valles P. Annual risk of tuberculosis infection among medical students of Universidad Peruana Cayetano Heredia. Am J Respir Crit Care Med 2002;165:A439.

38. Lienhardt C. From exposure to disease: The role of environmental factors in susceptibility to and development of tuberculosis. Epidemiol Rev 2001;23:288-301

39. Nardell E, Dharmadhikari A. Turning off the spigot: reducing drug-resistant tuberculosis transmission in resource-limited settings. Int J Tuberc Lung Dis 2010;14:1233-43.

40. Lönnroth K, Jaramillo E, Williams BG, Dye C, Raviglione M. Drivers of tuberculosis epidemics: the role of risk factors and social determinants. Soc Sci Med 2009;68:2240-6.

41. Lönnroth K, Castro KG, Chakaya JM, Chauhan LS, Floyd K, Glaziou P, et al. Tuberculosis control and elimination 2010-50: cure, care, and social development. Lancet 2010;375:1814-29.

42. Murray M, Oxlade O, Linh HH. Modeling social, environmental and biological determinants of tuberculosis. Int J Tuberc Lung Dis 2011; 15:S64-S70.

43. Hawker JI, Bakhshi SS, Ali S, Farrington CP. Ecological analysis of ethnic differences in relation between tuberculosis and poverty. BMJ 1999; 319:1031-34.

44. Beggs CB, Noakes CJ, Sleigh PA, Fletcher LA, Siddiqi K. The transmission of tuberculosis in confined spaces: An analytical review of alternative epidemiological models. Int J Tuberc Lung Dis 2003;7:1015-26.

45. Conninx R, Eshaya-Chauvin B, Reyes H. Tuberculosis in Prisons. Lancet 1995; 346:238-39.

46. Aerts A, Hauer B, Wanlin M, Veen J. Tuberculosis and tuberculosis control in European prisons. Int J Tuber Lung Dis 2006;10:1215-23.

47. Dara M, Grzemska M, Kimerling ME, Reyes H, Zagorsky A. Guidelines for control of tuberculosis in prisons. Tuberculosis Coalition for Technical Assistance and International Committee of the Red Cross; 2009.

48. Stuckler D, Basu S, McKee M, King L. Mass incarceration can explain population increases in TB and multidrug-resistant TB in European and central Asian countries. Proc Natl Acad Sci USA 2008;105:13280-5.

49. Centers for Disease Control and Prevention. Guidelines for preventing the transmission of Mycobacterium tuberculosis in health-care settings, 2005. MMWR Recomm Rep 2005;54: 1-141.

50. World Health Organization. WHO Policy on TB infection control in health-care facilities, congregate settings, and households. Geneva: World Health Organization; 2009.

51. Blumberg HM. Tuberculosis infection control in healthcare settings. In: Lautenbach E, Woeltje K, editors. Practical handbook for healthcare epidemiologists. New Jersey: Slack Incorporated; 2004.p.259-73.

52. Menzies D, Fanning A, Yuan L, Fitzgerald M. Tuberculosis among health care workers. N Engl J Med 1995;332:92-8.

53. Blumberg HM. Tuberculosis infection control. In: Reichman LB, Hershield E, editors. Tuberculosis: a comprehensive international approach, 2nd edn. New York: Marcel-Dekker, Inc; 2000. p.609-44.

54. Joshi R, Reingold AL, Menzies D, Pai M. Tuberculosis among health-care workers in low- and middle-income countries: a systematic review. PLoS Med 2006;3:e494.

55. Nardell EA, Bucher SJ, Brickner PW, Wang C, Vincent RL, Becan-McBride K, et al. Safety of upper-room ultraviolet germicidal air disinfection for room occupants: results from the Tuberculosis Ultraviolet Shelter Study. Public Health Rep 2008;123:52-60.

56. World Health Organization. Natural ventilation for infection control in healthcare settings. Geneva: World Health Organization; 2009.

57. Escombe AR, Oeser CC, Gilman RH, Navincopa M, Ticona E, Pan W, et al. Natural ventilation for the prevention of airborne contagion. PLoS Med 2007;4:e68.

58. Nardell EA. Use and misuse of germicidal UV air disinfection for TB in high-prevalence settings. Int J Tuberc Lung Dis 2002;6: 647-8.

59. Nardell EA. Environmental infection control of tuberculosis. Semin Respir Infect 2003;18:307-19.

60. Centers for Disease Control and Prevention [CDC], National Center for HIV/AIDS, Viral Hepatitis, STD, and TB Prevention. Prevention and control of tuberculosis in correctional and detention facilities: recommendations from CDC. Endorsed by the Advisory Council for the Elimination of Tuberculosis, the National Commission on Correctional Health Care, and the American Correctional Association. MMWR Recomm Rep 2006;55[RR-9]:1-44.

61. The National Institute for Occupational Safety and Health [NIOSH]. TB Respiratory Protection Program In Health Care Facilities - Administrator's Guide. DHHS [NIOSH] Publication Number 99-143. Available at URL: https://www.cdc.gov/niosh/docs/99-143/. Accessed on December 24, 2018.

62. Parmar MM, Sachdeva KS, Rade K, Ghedia M, Bansal A, Nagaraja SB, et al. Airborne infection control in India: Baseline assessment of health facilities. Indian J Tuberc 2015;62:211-7.

63. Akshaya KM, Shewade HD, Aslesh OP, Nagaraja SB, Nirgude AS, Singarajipura A, et al. "Who has to do it at the end of the day? Programme officials or hospital authorities?" Airborne infection control at drug resistant tuberculosis [DR-TB] centres of Karnataka, India: a mixed-methods study. Antimicrob Resist Infect Control 2017;6:111.

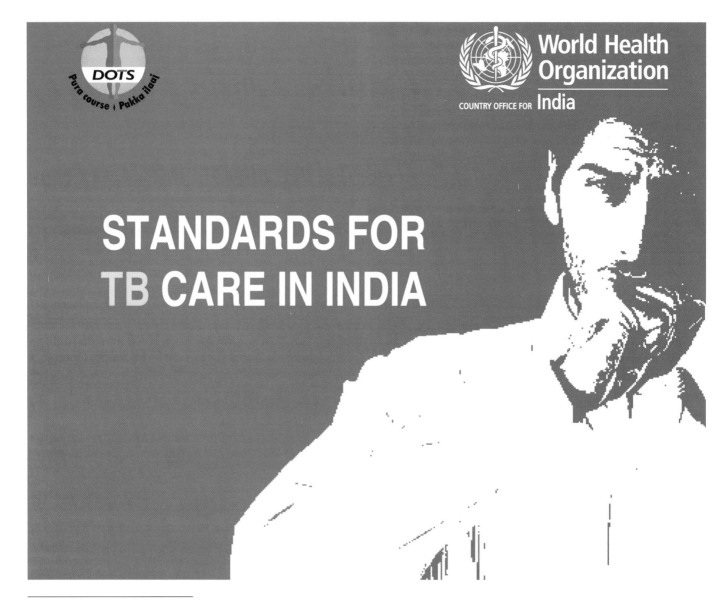

STANDARDS FOR
TB CARE IN INDIA

Table of contents

Acknowledgements

Development of the Standards for TB Care in India (STCI) is the culmination of a series of discussions involving various stakeholders and review of literature. Central TB Division, Ministry of Health & Family Welfare, Government of India and WHO Country Office for India took the lead in the process. The national TB institutions in India namely National Institute of TB and Respiratory Diseases (NITRD) New Delhi, National Institute for Research in Tuberculosis (NIRT) Chennai and National TB Institute (NTI) Bangalore contributed significantly in the development process. USAID has provided funding support to this initiative through WHO Country Office for India.

We acknowledge the contribution of all participants of the workshop and also those experts who reviewed the report and made comments for its betterment. Programme managers of Revised National Tuberculosis Control Programme (RNTCP) at central, state and district level have contributed substantially to finalize this document. Special appreciation is due for the medical consultants of WHO-RNTCP technical assistance network for their contribution in literature search and in providing necessary technical and operational support for the development of STCI. WCO-India communications team has provided crucial support in editing this document and we thank them for this.

The writing group comprised of (alphabetically) Dr A Sreenivas, Dr K Rade, Dr KS Sachdeva, Dr M Ghedia, Dr M Parmar, Dr R Ramachandran and Dr Shepherd J.

The draft guidelines have been reviewed and valuable comments have been provided by a group of experts comprising of: (alphabetically) Dr A Mohan, Dr A Joshi, Dr B John, Dr C Rodrigues, Dr GR Sethi, Dr N Kulshrestha, Dr N Wilson, Dr O George, Dr P Dewan, Dr RN Solanki, Dr R Sarin, Dr RV Ashokan, Dr S Gutta, Dr S Sahu, Dr S Swaminathan, Dr S Vijayan and Dr V Singh. These contributions are gratefully acknowledged.

Development process

The first edition of the Standards for TB Care in India was conceived by a wider community of clinicians, public health specialists, community workers and patient advocates both within and outside of the Government of India as a necessary step in requiring and monitoring a widely accepted standard of TB care for the people of India. International guidelines and standards for TB care which existed such as International Standards for TB Care 2006 and 2009 editions, American Thoracic Society Standards, European Standards 2011, WHO Guideline for Treatment of TB 2010 and WHO Guidelines for PMDT 2011 were used as a foundation for developing India's standards. However with its unique challenges, approximately one third of the world's TB burden, and long history of dealing with a TB problem that appears to be resilient to the best efforts, it was felt that India should have its own standards that could be used as a benchmark by all providers managing TB patients within India. It is hoped that a set of standards recognized as appropriate for the specific challenges of India will spur observance to these standards by all care providers of India when managing a TB patient.

The standards developed and described here are the result of a long process that culminated in a three day national workshop organized by Central TB Division at New Delhi in December 2012 with technical assistance from WHO Country Office for India. The objective of the workshop was to develop the Standards for Tuberculosis Care in India that will be applicable to providers in public, private and other settings across India. About 120 experts from national and international level including various public health administrators, programme managers, representatives from various professional associations (Indian Medical Association, Association of Physicians of India, College of Physicians Association of India, Indian Association of Paediatricians, Federation of Obstetricians and gynecologists congress of India, Family Physician Association of India etc.), academicians and specialists from public and private sectors (pulmonologists, physicians, surgeons, paediatricians, gynaecologists, orthopaedic surgeons, microbiologists, public health specialist etc.), donors, technical and implementation partners, pharmaceutical companies, pharmacists association, consultants, management experts, social science experts and civil society representatives participated at the workshop and actively worked to develop the evidence based Standards for Tuberculosis Care in India.

The methodology consisted of panel discussions and group work and the approach was to find appropriate answers to the following questions:

- What should be the standard tools and strategies for early and complete detection?
- What should be the standards of treatment in terms of drugs and regimens for best patient outcome?
- What should be the public health standards including regulations, strategies and systems for public health impact?
- What should be standards for patient support systems, both in public and private sectors and for community engagement for social inclusion?

As part of the development process, noted experts in the field of TB in India modified the international standards, following detailed review of Indiaspecific and India-relevant evidence. As an output of the workshop, 26 standards developed and the India-relevant evidence debated, and listed for each of the standards in this document. This includes a new set of standards for social inclusion that goes beyond the areas covered in the International Standards for TB Care (ISTC) 2009. After the statement of each standard a brief summary of the international and national evidence are described along with the references to the literature. The standards thus evolved, are intended to be used to enhance quality and mutually acceptable engagement with the private and other sectors in India to enhance TB care. This is thus, an important tool for achieving the goal of universal access to quality TB care.

Introduction

India, the world's second most populous country, accounts for a quarter of the world's annual incidence of TB. Every year around two million people develop TB in India and 300,000 die of TB. Over 15 million patients have been treated and three million additional lives have been saved by the Revised National TB Control Programme (RNTCP) over the last decade. Cure rates have consistently been above 85% and the TB Millennium Development Goals are reachable. However, despite a comprehensive national TB control program guiding states for implementation of TB diagnosis and treatment there is still a long way to go. The decline in TB incidence has been slow, mortality remains unacceptably high and the emergence of drug-resistant TB has become a major public health concern.

There are many challenges for TB control in India. Prompt, accurate diagnosis and effective treatment of TB are not only essential for good patient care, but they are also the key elements in the public health response to tuberculosis and the cornerstone of any initiative for tuberculosis control. The private sector holds a factual predominance of health care service delivery in India. There is very little information about the TB patient from the private sector available to the programme and little is known about their quality of treatment, including treatment outcomes. Engaging the private sector effectively is the single most important intervention required for India to achieve the overall goal of universal access to quality TB care.

The vision of India's national TB control programme is that the people suffering from TB receive the highest standards of care and support from healthcare providers of their choice. It is spelt out in the National Strategic Plan (2012-17) to extend the umbrella of quality TB care and control to include those provided by the private sector (1). The need for quality and standards for TB care is made particularly acute where a largely unregulated and unmonitored private sector accounts for almost half of the TB care delivered in India with gross challenges as far as quality of diagnosis and treatment is concerned. Thus, it was felt essential to develop and disseminate the standards of TB care that is particularly relevant in Indian context, acceptable to the medical fraternity in both the public and private sector in India.

Also, the availability of new diagnostic tools and strategies for early TB diagnosis, emerging evidences on existing regimens and newer regimens, and the need for better patient support strategies including addressing social inclusiveness necessitated the development of Standards for TB Care in India.

To paraphrase the ISTC, the standards in this document differ from existing guidelines in that the standards present what should be done whereas guidelines describe how the action is to be accomplished. There are comprehensive national guidelines from the Central TB Division, GoI [www.tbcindia.nic.in] that are regularly reviewed and updated. These standards represent the first what is expected from the Indian healthcare system. It is expected that the standards discussed in this document are clear and usable and will be accessible to all TB providers as an easy reference.

Reference:

1. Rosenblatt MB. Pulmonary tuberculosis: evolution of modern therapy. Bull NY Acad Med 1973;49:163-96.

STCI summary

Standard 1: Testing and screening for Pulmonary TB

1.1 Testing:
  - Any person with symptoms and signs suggestive of TB including cough >2 weeks, fever >2 weeks, significant weight loss, haemoptysis etc. and any abnormality in chest radiograph must be evaluated for TB.
  - Children with persistent fever and/or cough >2 weeks, loss of weight/no weight gain, and/or contact with pulmonary TB cases must be evaluated for TB.

1.2 Screening:
  - People living with HIV (PLHIV), malnourished, diabetics, cancer patients, patients on immunosuppressant or maintenance steroid therapy, should be regularly screened for signs and symptoms suggestive of TB.
  - Enhanced case finding should be undertaken in high risk populations such as health care workers, prisoners, slum dwellers, and certain occupational groups such as miners.

Standard 2: Diagnostic technology

2.1 Microbiological confirmation on sputum:
  - All patients (adults, adolescents, and children who are capable of producing sputum) with presumptive pulmonary TB should undergo quality-assured sputum test for rapid diagnosis of TB (with at least two samples, including one early morning sample for sputum smear for AFB) for microbiological confirmation.

2.2 Chest X-ray as screening tool:
  - Where available, chest X-ray should be used as a screening tool to increase the sensitivity of the diagnostic algorithm.

2.3 Serological tests:
- Serological tests are banned and not recommended for diagnosing tuberculosis.

2.4 Tuberculin Skin Test (TST) & Interferon Gamma Release Assay (IGRA)
- TST and IGRA are not recommended for the diagnosis of active tuberculosis. Standardised TST may be used as a complimentary test in children.

2.5 CB-NAAT (cartridge-based nucleic-acid amplification test) is the preferred first diagnostic test in children and PLHIV.

2.6 Validation of newer diagnostic tests:
- Effective mechanism should be developed to validate newer diagnostic tests.

Standard 3: Testing for extra-pulmonary TB

- For all patients (adults, adolescents and children) with presumptive extra-pulmonary TB, appropriate specimens from the presumed sites of involvement must be obtained for microscopy/culture and drug sensitivity testing (DST)/CB-NAAT/molecular test/histo-pathological examination.

Standard 4: Diagnosis of HIV co-infection in TB patients and Drug Resistant TB (DR-TB)

4.1 Diagnosis of HIV in TB patients:
- All diagnosed TB patients should be offered HIV counselling and testing.

4.2 Diagnosis of multi-drug resistant TB (MDR-TB):
- Prompt and appropriate evaluation should be undertaken for patients with presumptive MDR-TB or Rifampicin (R) resistance in TB patients who have failed treatment with first line drugs, paediatric non-responders, TB patients who are contacts of MDR-TB (or R resistance), TB patients who are found positive on any follow-up sputum smear examination during treatment with first line drugs, diagnosed TB patients with prior history of anti-TB treatment, TB patients with HIV co-infection and all presumptive TB cases among PLHIV. All such patients must be tested for drug resistance with available technology, a rapid molecular DST (as the first choice) or liquid/solid culture-DST (at least for R and if possible for Isoniazid (H); Ofloxacin (O) and Kanamycin (K), if R-resistant/MDR).
- Wherever available DST should be offered to all diagnosed tuberculosis patients prior to start of treatment.

4.3 Diagnosis of Extensively Drug Resistant TB (XDR-TB):
- On detection of Rifampicin resistance alone or along with isoniazid resistance, patient must be offered sputum test for second line DST using RNTCP approved phenotypic or genotypic methods, wherever available.

Standard 5: Probable TB

- Presumptive TB patients without microbiological confirmation (smear microscopy, culture and molecular diagnosis), but with strong clinical and other evidence (e.g. X-ray, Fine Needle Aspiration Cytology (FNAC, histopathology) may be diagnosed as "Probable TB" and should be treated.
- For patients with presumptive TB found to be negative on rapid molecular test, an attempt should be made to obtain culture on an appropriate specimen.

Standard 6: Paediatric TB

6.1 Diagnosis of paediatric TB patients:
- In all children with presumptive intra-thoracic TB, microbiological confirmation should be sought through examination of respiratory specimens (e.g. sputum by expectoration, gastric aspirate, gastric lavage, induced sputum, broncho-alveolar lavage or other appropriate specimens) with quality assured diagnostic test, preferably CB-NAAT, smear microscopy or culture.

6.2 Diagnosis of probable paediatric TB patients:
- In the event of negative or unavailable microbiological results, a diagnosis of probable TB in children should be based on the presence of abnormalities consistent with TB on radiography, a history of exposure to pulmonary tuberculosis case, evidence of TB infection (positive TST) and clinical findings suggestive of TB.

6.3 Diagnosis of extra-pulmonary paediatric TB patients:
  • For children with presumptive extra-pulmonary TB, appropriate specimens from the presumed sites of involvement should be obtained for rapid molecular test, microscopy, culture and DST, and histo-pathological examination.

Standard 7: Treatment with first-line regimen

7.1 Treatment of New TB patients:
  • All new patients should receive an internationally accepted first-line treatment regimen for new patients. The initial phase should consist of two months of Isoniazid (H), Rifampicin (R), Pyrazinamide (Z), and Ethambutol (E). The continuation phase should consist of three drugs (Isoniazid, Rifampicin and Ethambutol) given for at least four months.

7.2 Extension of continuation phase:
  • The duration of continuation phase may be extended by three to six months in special situations like bone & joint TB, spinal TB with neurological involvement and neuro-tuberculosis.

7.3 Drug dosages:
  • The patients should be given dosages of the drugs depending upon body weight in weight bands.

7.4 Bio-availability of drugs:
  • The bio-availability of the drug should be ensured for every batch, especially if fixed dose combinations (FDCs) are used, by procuring and prescribing from a quality-assured source.

7.5 Dosage frequency:
  • All patients should be given daily regimen under direct observation. However, the country programme may consider daily or intermittent regimen for treatment of TB depending on the available resources and operational considerations as both are effective provided all doses are directly observed.
  • All paediatric and HIV infected TB patients should be given daily regimen under direct observation.

7.6 Drug formulations:
  • Fixed dose combinations (FDCs) of four drugs (Isoniazid, Rifampicin, Pyrazinamide, and Ethambutol), and three drugs (Isoniazid, Rifampicin and Ethambutol) and two drugs (Isoniazid and Rifampicin) are recommended.

7.7 Previously treated TB patients:
  • After MDR-TB (or R resistance) is ruled out by a quality assured test, TB patients returning after lost to follow up or relapse from their first treatment course or new TB patients failing with first treatment course may receive the retreatment regimen containing first-line drugs: 2HREZS/1HREZ/5HRE.

Standard 8: Monitoring treatment response

8.1 Follow-up sputum microscopy:
  • Response to therapy in patients with pulmonary tuberculosis, new as well as retreatment cases, should be monitored by follow-up sputum microscopy (one specimen) at the time of completion of the intensive phase of treatment and at the end of treatment.

8.2 Extension of intensive phase:
  • The extension of the intensive phase is not recommended.

8.3 Offer DST in follow-up sputum positive cases:
  • If the sputum smear is positive in follow-up at any time during treatment, a rapid molecular DST (as the first choice) or culture-DST (at least for R and if possible for Isoniazid (H); Ofloxacin (O) and Kanamycin (K), if R-resistant/MDR) should be performed as laboratory facilities become available.

8.4 Response to treatment in extra-pulmonary TB:
  • In patients with extra-pulmonary tuberculosis, the treatment response is best assessed clinically. The help of radiological and other relevant investigations may also be taken.

8.5 Response to treatment in children:
  • In children, who are unable to produce sputum the response to treatment may be assessed clinically. The help of radiological and other relevant investigations may also be taken.

8.6 Long-term follow-up:
- After completion of treatment the patients should be followed up with clinical and/or sputum examination at the end of six months and 12 months.

Standard 9: Drug Resistant TB management

9.1 Treatment of M/XDR-TB (or R resistant TB):
- Patients with tuberculosis caused by drug-resistant organisms (especially M/XDR or only R resistance or with O or K resistance), microbiologically confirmed by quality assured test, should be treated with specialized regimens containing quality assured second-line anti-tuberculosis drugs.

9.2 Model of care for drug resistant TB:
- Patients with MDR-TB should be treated using mainly ambulatory care rather than models of care based principally on hospitalization. If required, a short period of initial hospitalisation is recommended.

9.3 Regimen for MDR/R-Resistant TB cases:
- The regimen chosen for MDR-TB may be standardized and/or based on microbiologically confirmed drug susceptibility patterns. At least four drugs (second line) to which the organisms are susceptible, or presumed susceptible, should be used. Most importantly the regimen should include at least a later-generation Fluoro-quinolone (such as high dose Levofloxacin) and a parenteral agent (such as Kanamycin or Amikacin), and may include Pyrazinamide, Ethambutol, Ethionamide (or Prothionamide), and either Cycloserine or PAS (P-aminosalicylic acid) if Cycloserine cannot be used.

9.4 Regimen for MDR patients with Ofloxacin and/or Kanamycin resistance detected early:
- Treatment regimen may be suitably modified in case of Ofloxacin and/or Kanamycin resistance at the initiation of MDR-TB treatment or during early intensive phase, preferably not later than four to six weeks.

9.5 Surgery in MDR/XDR TB patients:
- All patients of MDR/XDR-TB should be evaluated for surgery at the initiation of treatment and/or during follow up.

9.6 Treatment Duration in MDR TB patients:
- Till newer effective drugs are available with proven efficacy with shorter duration of MDR-TB treatment; total treatment should be given for at least 24 months in patients newly diagnosed with MDR-TB (i.e. not previously treated for MDR-TB) with recommended intensive phase of treatment being six to nine months. The total duration may be modified according to the patient's response to therapy.

9.7 Specialist consultation in M/XDR TB patients:
- Consultation with a specialist experienced in treatment of patients with MDR/XDR tuberculosis should be obtained, whenever possible.

9.8 Ensuring adherence in M/XDR TB patients:
- Patient support systems, including direct observation of treatment, are required to ensure adherence. It should be ensured that the patient consumes all the doses of the drugs.

9.9 Single sample follow-up culture in M/XDR TB patients:
- The use of sputum culture (1 sample) is recommended for monitoring of patients with MDR-TB during treatment.

9.10 Second line DST during treatment of MDR TB:
- During the course of MDR TB treatment, if the sputum culture is found to be positive at 6 months or later, the most recent culture isolate should be subjected to DST for second-line drugs (at least O and K) to decide on further course of action. DST to other drugs namely Moxifloxacin, Amikacin and Capreomycin may also be done if laboratory facilities are available to guide treatment.

9.11 Regimen for MDR patients with Ofloxacin and/or Kanamycin resistance detected later:
- The patients with MDR-TB found to be resistant to at least Ofloxacin and/or Kanamycin during the later stage of MDR TB treatment must be treated with a suitable regimen for XDR TB using second line drugs including Group 5 drugs such as Amoxicillin Clavulanate, Clarithromycin, Clofazimine, Linezolid, Thioacetazone, Imipenem to which the organisms are known or presumed to be susceptible.

9.12 New drugs:

- New drugs need to be considered for inclusion in regimens whenever scientific evidence for their efficacy and safety becomes available as per the national policy for newer antimicrobials. Appropriate regulatory mechanisms for distribution control needs to be ensured.

Standard 10: Addressing TB with HIV infection and other comorbid conditions

10.1 Treatment of HIV infected TB patients:

- TB patients living with HIV should receive the same duration of TB treatment with daily regimen as HIV negative TB patients.

10.2 Anti-retroviral & Co-trimoxazole prophylactic therapy in HIV infected TB patients:

- Antiretroviral therapy must be offered to all patients with HIV and TB as well as drug-resistant TB requiring second-line anti-tuberculosis drugs, irrespective of CD4 cell-count, as early as possible (within the first eight weeks) following initiation of anti-tuberculosis treatment. Appropriate arrangements for access to antiretroviral drugs should be made for patients. However, initiation of treatment for tuberculosis should not be delayed. Patients with TB and HIV infection should also receive Co-trimoxazole as prophylaxis for other infections.

10.3 Isoniazid preventive therapy in HIV patients without active TB:

- People living with HIV should be screened for TB using four symptom complex (current cough or, fever or weight loss or night sweats) at HIV care settings and those with any of these symptoms should be evaluated for ruling out active TB. All asymptomatic patients in whom active TB is ruled out, Isoniazid Preventive Therapy (IPT) should be offered for six months or longer.

Standard 11: Treatment adherence

11.1 Patient centered approach for adherence:

- Both to assess and foster adherence, a patient-centered approach to administration of drug treatment, based on the patient's needs and mutual respect between the patient and the provider, should be developed for all patients.

11.2 Measures for treatment adherence:

- Supervision and support should be individualized and should draw on the full range of recommended interventions and available support services, including patient counselling and education. A central element of the patient centred strategy is the use of measures to assess and promote adherence to the treatment regimen and to address poor adherence when it occurs. These measures should be tailored to the individual patient's circumstances based on details of the patient's clinical and social history and be mutually acceptable to the patient and the provider.

11.3 Trained treatment supporter for treatment adherence:

- Such measures may include identification and training of a treatment supporter (for tuberculosis and, if appropriate, for HIV, Diabetes Mellitus etc.) who is acceptable, accessible and accountable to the patient and to the health system.

11.4 Use of Information Communication Technology (ICT) to promote treatment literacy and adherence:

- Optimal use of ICT should be done to promote treatment literacy and adherence.

Standard 12: Public health responsibility

- Any practitioner treating a patient for tuberculosis is assuming an important public health responsibility to prevent on-going transmission of the infection and the development of drug resistance.
- To fulfil this responsibility the practitioner must not only prescribe an appropriate regimen, but when necessary, also utilize local public health services/community health services, and other agencies including NGOs to assess the adherence of the patient and to address poor adherence when it occurs.

Standard 13: Notification of TB cases

- All health establishments must report all TB cases and their treatment outcomes to public health authorities (District Nodal Officer for Notification).
- Proper feedback need to be ensured to all healthcare providers who refer cases to public health system on the outcome of the patients which they had referred.

Standard 14: Maintain records for all TB patients

- A written record of all medications given, bacteriologic response, adverse reactions and clinical outcome should be maintained for all patients.

Standard 15: Contact investigation

- All providers of care for patients with tuberculosis should ensure all household contacts and other persons who are in close contact with TB patients are screened for TB
- In case of pediatric TB patients, reverse contact tracing for search of any active TB case in the household of the child must be undertaken.

Standard 16: Isoniazid Prophylactic therapy

- Children <6 years of age who are close contacts of a TB patient, after excluding active TB, should be treated with isoniazid for a minimum period of 6 months and should be closely monitored for TB symptoms.

Standard 17: Airborne infection control

- Airborne infection control should be an integral part of all health care facility infection control strategy.

Standard 18: Quality assurance (QA) systems

18a   QA for diagnostic tests:
- All health care providers should ensure that all diagnostic tests used for diagnosis of TB are quality assured.

18b   QA for anti-TB drugs:
- Quality assurance system should ensure that all anti-TB drugs used in the country are subjected to stringent quality assurance mechanisms at all levels.

Standard 19: Panchayati Raj Institutions

- Panchayati Raj Institutions and elected representatives have an important role to share the public health responsibility for TB control with the healthcare providers, patients and the community.

Standard 20: Health education

- Every TB symptomatic should be properly counselled by the healthcare provider.
- TB patients and their family members should get proper counselling and health education at every contact with healthcare system

Standard 21: Death audit among TB patients

- Death among TB patients should be audited by a competent authority.

Standard 22: Information on TB prevention and care seeking

- All individuals especially women, children, elderly, differently abled, other vulnerable groups and those at increased risk should receive information related to TB prevention and care seeking.

Standard 23: Free and quality services

- All patients, especially those in vulnerable population groups, accessing a provider where TB services are available should be offered free or affordable quality assured diagnostic and treatment services which should be provided at locations and times so as to minimize workday or school disruptions and maximize access.

Standard 24: Respect, confidentiality and sensitivity

- All people seeking or receiving care for TB should be received with dignity and managed with promptness, confidentiality and gender sensitivity. Ensure that infection control procedures do not stigmatise TB patients.

Standard 25: Care and support through social welfare programmes

- Patient support system should endeavour to derive synergies between various social welfare support systems to mitigate out of pocket expenses such as transport and wage loss incurred by people affected by TB for the purpose of diagnosis and treatment.

Standard 26: Addressing counselling and other needs

- Persons affected by TB should be counselled at every opportunity, to address information gaps and to enable informed decision making. Counselling should address issues such as treatment adherence, adverse drug reactions, prognosis and physical, financial, psycho-social and nutritional needs.

Standard 1
Testing and screening for Pulmonary TB

1.1 Testing:
- Any person with symptoms and signs suggestive of TB including cough >2 weeks, fever >2 weeks, significant weight loss, haemoptysis etc. and any abnormality in chest radiograph must be evaluated for TB.
- Children with persistent fever and/or cough >2 weeks, loss of weight/no weight gain, and/or h/o contact with pulmonary TB cases must be evaluated for TB.

1.2 Screening:
- People living with HIV (PLHIV), malnourished, diabetics, cancer patients, patients on immunosuppressant or maintenance steroid therapy, should be regularly screened for signs and symptoms suggestive of TB.
- Enhanced case finding should be undertaken in high risk populations such as healthcare workers, prisoners, slum dwellers, and certain occupational groups such as miners.

The most common symptom of pulmonary TB is prolonged cough that lasts longer than the cough with most other acute lung infections. However cough is a common symptom and most coughing patients do not have TB (1). Many countries have attempted to distinguish likely TB cases from other lung infections by specifying a chronic cough lasting two to three weeks (2,3). The evidence from India suggests that cough lasting > 2 weeks is a more sensitive indicator for TB than >3 weeks cough and is thus recommended here (4,5,7,8). A high level of clinical suspicion for TB is necessary as many TB patients will not have a cough, particularly if they are infected with HIV or are otherwise immuno-suppressed. Children can present a diagnostic challenge and a high level of suspicion for TB must accompany the approach to any child with prolonged illness not otherwise explained, especially if there is a history of contact with a pulmonary TB case (5).

Enhanced case finding means maintaining a high index of suspicion for TB in all encounters, with proactive exclusion of TB using the appropriate combination of clinical queries, radiographic or microbiologic testing. For PLHIV, the WHO has developed a four-symptom screen that has proven highly sensitive for active TB (3,6). Recent evidence from surveys in southern India has pointed to the significant comorbidities of TB and type 2 diabetes (10,11) and consequently diabetics are included in the high risk categories for regular screening (12). Any other immunosuppressed patients are also at considerably heightened risk and should be enquired about symptoms of TB at every healthcare encounter. In addition, slum dwellers are a large and recognized portion of Indian urban society where the transmission of infection is high. A recent estimate of the ARTI in Delhi was 2.3-3% (9), indicating that screening for active TB may be cost-effective and sensible. Occupational groups such as miners have been reported to have high risk of tuberculosis and they could be specially targeted for active case finding. An additional group with high risk for TB is certain indigenous populations in the tribal areas of India.

References:

1. International Standards for TB Care, Second Edition (2009) Tuberculosis Coalition for Technical Assistance, The Hague, 2009.
2. Treatment of Tuberculosis: guidelines 4th Ed. (2009) World Health Organization, Geneva
3. Systematic Screening for Active Tuberculosis: Principles and Recommendations (2013) World Health Organization, Geneva
4. Revised Guidelines for Diagnosis of Pulmonary TB (2009) Revised National TB Control Programme, Delhi

5. National Guidelines on Diagnosis and Treatment of Paediatric Tuberculosis (2012) Revised National TB Control Programme, Delhi

6. Cain, KP et al; An Algorithm for TB Screening and Diagnosis in People with HIV (2010) New England Journal of Medicine 362, 707

7. Santha T et al, Comparison of cough of 2 weeks and 3 weeks to improve detection of smear-positive tuberculosis cases among out-patients in India, IJTLD, 2005, 9(1), 61-68

8. Thomas A et al., Increased yield of smear positive pulmonary TB case by screening patients with >2weeks cough compared to >3 weeks cough and adequacy of 2 sputum smear examinations for diagnosis, IJTLD 2008, 55: 77-83

9. Sarin R, Behera D et al, Annual Risk of Tuberculosis Infection (ARTI) in the slum population covered under RNTCP by LRS Institute, National OR Committee for RNTCP, meeting, 2012. (under publication)

10. Viswanathan V. et al, Prevalence of Diabetes and Pre-Diabetes and Associated Risk Factors among Tuberculosis Patients in India, PLOS ONE. 2012 7(7); e41367

11. Balakrishnan S. et al, High Diabetes Prevalence among Tuberculosis Cases in Kerala, India, PLOS ONE, 2012. 10 (7); e46502

12. Baker et al. The impact of diabetes on tuberculosis treatment outcomes–A systematic review: BMC Medicine 2011. 9 (81);1741-7015

Standard 2
Diagnostic technology

2.1 Microbiological confirmation on sputum:
   - All patients (adults, adolescents, and children who are capable of producing sputum) with presumptive pulmonary TB should undergo a quality-assured sputum test for rapid microbiological diagnosis of TB

2.2 Chest X-ray as screening tool:
   - Where available, chest X-ray should be used as a screening tool to increase the sensitivity of the diagnostic algorithm

2.3 Serological tests:
   - Serological tests are banned and not recommended for diagnosing tuberculosis.

2.4 Tuberculin Skin Test (TST) & Interferon Gamma Release Assay (IGRA):
   - TST and IGRA are not recommended for the diagnosis of active tuberculosis. Standardized TST may be used as a complimentary test in children.

2.5 Cartridge-Based Nucleic-acid Amplification Test (CB NAAT) is the preferred first diagnostic test in children and PLHIV

2.6 Validation of newer diagnostic tests:
   - Effective mechanism should be developed to validate newer diagnostic tests. One of the first responsibilities of the TB programme is to endeavour to make a bacteriological diagnosis of TB if at all possible. Currently, only sputum tests are sufficient and recommended under the programme for the microbiologic testing of TB (1). The Government of India recently issued government orders banning the manufacture, importation, distribution and use of serological tests for diagnosing TB (2). In addition Tuberculin Skin Test (TST) and Interferon-Gamma Release Assays (IGRA) are not recommended for diagnosis of TB, although in certain cases TST may be useful as an additional test for the diagnosis of children (3). Chest radiograph is an unquestionably sensitive test for the detection of pulmonary disease in adults and children, and is recommended as a screening tool for TB. Due to the non-specific nature of radiographic testing for TB, any abnormal chest radiograph should prompt further bacteriologic and clinical assessment for TB (4).

As sputum tests are the key to TB diagnosis, attention to collection of a good sputum sample is paramount; a number of studies have looked at this, including studies in India. A consensus is that two samples are almost as good as three samples and a morning sample is better than a spot sample for detection of mycobacteria (5,6,7).

Acceptable methods for bacteriologic testing of sputum include sputum smear microscopy (both conventional and fluorescent), culture (on solid or liquid media), commercial line probe assay (LPA), or CB NAAT. The most commonly-used method for bacteriologic diagnosis of TB for the last 70 years, sputum smear microscopy, has had enormous value in TB diagnosis, but has limited sensitivity, particularly in children where microscopy is less than 50% sensitive. Sputum culture remains a highly sensitive, specific, and under-utilized method for TB diagnosis, but requires weeks to yield results and hence alone does not help clinicians for early diagnosis. Nucleic acid amplification testing (NAAT) offers enormous potential for accurate rapid diagnosis, but only commercial kits have been validated and are trustworthy for replicable results (8).

While both "in-house" manual NAAT is widely available, their lack of reproducibility and quality assurance concerns means that such in-house assays cannot be recommended (9). Commercial semi-automated NAAT have been developed in India, these are yet to be validated, hence are not recommended. With the advent of CB-NAAT the sensitivity and specificity of rapid TB diagnosis from sputum has increased to approximately levels seen in solid-media sputum culture, particularly valuable for the assessment of children.

A list of RNTCP approved diagnostics tests are given in the guidelines for TB notification accessible at www.tbcindia. nic.in.

References

1. Technical and Operational Guidelines for Tuberculosis. 2005. www.tbcindia.nic.in/pdf
2. TB India 2013. Pg 53. www.tbcindia.nic.in/annual reports/pdf
3. New Paediatric TB guidelines. www.tbcindia.nic.in/documents/pdf
4. Koppaka R, Bock N. How reliable is chest radiography? In: Frieden TR, ed. Toman's tuberculosis. Case detection, treatment and monitoring, 2nd Edition. Geneva: World Health Organization, 2004:51-60.
5. Van Deun A, Salim AH, Cooreman E, et al. Optimal tuberculosis case detection by direct sputum smear microscopy: how much better is more? Int J Tuberc Lung Dis 2002; 6(3): 222–30.
6. Sarin R, Mukerjee S, Singla N, Sharma PP. Diagnosis of tuberculosis under RNTCP: examination of two or three sputum specimens. Indian J Tuberc 2001(48):13–16.
7. TB diagnostics and laboratory strengthening–WHO policy. www.stoptb/wg/gli/resources
8. WHO policy statement: automated real-time nucleic acid amplification technology for rapid and simultaneous detection of tuberculosis and rifampicin resistance: Xpert MTB/RIF assay. WHO/HTM/TB/2011.4
9. Pai M. The accuracy and reliability of nucleic acid amplification tests in the diagnosis of tuberculosis. Natl Med J India 2004;17(5): 233–6.

Standard 3
Testing for extra-pulmonary TB

3.1 Testing for extra-pulmonary TB
- For all patients (adults, adolescents and children) with presumptive extra-pulmonary TB, appropriate specimens from the presumed sites of involvement must be obtained for microscopy/culture/CB-NAAT/molecular test/histopathology examination and drug sensitivity testing (DST).

Even as pulmonary TB presents significant diagnostic challenges, extra-pulmonary TB diagnosis can be more challenging. Signs and symptoms are not specific and yield of mycobacteria are generally low from most tissue and fluid sources (1,2,3). Extra-pulmonary TB is comparatively common in PLHIV (approximately 30% of cases) and in these hosts the non-specificity of symptoms and low yield of mycobacteria present an even greater challenge. The basic principle of seeking bacteriologic diagnosis at every opportunity where TB is suspected applies to extra pulmonary TB as well. The use of unvalidated non-commercial 'in-house' NAAT on tissue specimens is not recommended; histopathology examination, smear microscopy, culture and validated commercial NAAT are the only acceptable options. Recently the use of CB-NAAT for specimens other than sputum was explored in many studies; although the test is not as sensitive on most of these samples compared with its sensitivity on sputum nevertheless it performs well and in all cases better than smear microscopy (4,5).

References:

1. Wares F et al.; Extrapulmonary Tuberculosis: Management and Control (2011) Revised National TB Control Program, Delhi
2. International Standards for TB Care, Second Edition (2009) Tuberculosis Coalition for Technical Assistance, The Hague, 2009
3. National Guidelines on Diagnosis and Treatment of Paediatric Tuberculosis (2012) Revised National TB Control Programme, Delhi. www.tbcindia.nic.in
4. Rapid Molecular Detection of Extra pulmonary Tuberculosis by the Automated GeneXpert MTB/RIF System. Journal Clin Micro. 2011; 4:1202–1205
5. Gerardo A-U, Azcona JM, Midde M, Naik P.K, Reddy S and Reddy Ret al. Hindawi Publishing Corporation Tuberculosis Research and Treatment, Volume 2012, Article ID 932862

Standard 4
Diagnosis of HIV co-infection in TB patients and diagnosis of Drug Resistant TB (DR-TB)

4.1 Diagnosis of HIV in TB patients:
- All diagnosed TB patients should be offered HIV counselling and testing.

4.2 Diagnosis of Multi-Drug Resistant TB (MDR-TB):
- Prompt and appropriate evaluation should be undertaken for patients with presumptive MDR-TB or Rifampicin (R) resistance in TB patients who have failed treatment with first line drugs, paediatric non-responders, TB patients who are contacts of MDR-TB (or R resistance), TB patients who are found positive on any follow-up sputum smear examination during treatment with first line drugs, diagnosed TB patients with prior history of anti-TB treatment, TB patients with HIV co-infection and all presumptive TB cases among PLHIV. All such patients must be tested for drug resistance with available technology, a rapid molecular DST (as the first choice) or liquid/solid culture-DST (at least for R and H; and at least for Ofloxacin (O) and Kanamycin (K), if MDR).

Wherever available DST should be considered and offered to all diagnosed tuberculosis patients prior to star of treatment.

4.3 Diagnosis of Extensively Drug Resistant TB (XDR-TB):
- On detection of Rifampicin and isoniazid resistance, patient must be offered sputum test for second line DST using quality assured phenotypic or genotypic methods, wherever available.

TB is a very clear clinical sign of possible HIV infection, and all TB patients deserve to have HIV ruled out through voluntary counselling and testing. India is considered a low HIV endemic area with high rates of TB, and the countrywide average HIV prevalence in TB patients is around 5%. In any given case of TB, at any age, HIV infection is possible. Early detection of HIV offers the opportunity for potentially life-saving additional interventions. Thus it is recommended that all patients with active TB be tested for HIV (1). If HIV infection is detected then, TB treatment and anti-retroviral therapy is as described in Standard 10.

Drug resistant TB is a growing problem worldwide including in India. Current surveillance data estimates a prevalence of MDR-TB of 2-3% in new, untreated TB patients and more than 15% in previously treated TB cases (2). The Programmatic Management of Drug Resistant TB (PMDT) has recently been expanded in order to treat DR-TB in the RNTCP and extend standards and monitoring of DR-TB treatment to the private sector. The laboratory support for this programme is in development and a growing network of accredited, quality-assured drug sensitivity testing labs will support the goal of universal DST for all TB patients. In order to provide timely information to the clinical team treating the patient and reduce primary transmission of DR-TB, rapid testing for rifampicin resistance is recommended (3).

The emergence of extensively-drug resistant TB (XDR-TB) underlines the importance of developing a laboratory infrastructure to support DST for second-line drugs. The most important tests are for resistance to the Fluoroquinolones (Ofloxacin) and the injectable agent (Kanamycin), which forms the backbone of MDR-TB treatment and resistance to these drugs defines XDR-TB (4). It is recommended that, as facilities allow, all MDR-TB isolates are further tested for Ofloxacin and Kanamycin resistance.

References:

1. WHO policy on collaborative TB/HIV activities guidelines for national programmes and other stakeholders. Updated version of a document originally published in 2004 as Interim policy on collaborative TB/HIV activities (WHO/HTM/TB/2004.330; WHO/HTM/HIV/2004.1) WHO/HTM/TB/2012.1 and 012.1 WHO/HIV/2012
2. Ramachandran R, Nalini S, Chandrasekar V, Dave PV, Sanghvi AS, Wares F, Paramasivan CN, Narayanan PR, Sahu S, Parmar M, Chadha S, Dewan P, Chauhan LS. Surveillance of drug-resistant tuberculosis in the state of Gujarat, India. Int J Tuberc Lung Dis. 2009. 13(9):1154-60
3. Guidelines for the programmatic management of drug-resistant tuberculosis, 2011 update. WHO/HTM/TB/2011.6
4. Gandhi NR, Nunn P, Dheda K, Schaaf HS, Zignol M, van Soolingen D, Jensen P, Bayona J. Multidrug-resistant and extensively drug-resistant tuberculosis: a threat to global control of tuberculosis. Lancet. 2010. 375(9728):1830-43

Standard 5
Probable TB

5.1 Probable TB
  - Patients with symptoms suggestive of TB without microbiological confirmation (sputum smear microscopy, culture and molecular diagnosis), but with strong clinical and other evidence (e.g. X-ray, Fine Needle Aspiration Cytology (FNAC), histopathology) may be diagnosed as "Probable TB" (1).

Despite the advent of new tests for TB diagnosis with greater sensitivity than smear microscopy of appropriate sputum samples, about 20-30% of TB patients will not have microbiologic confirmation. This figure may be much higher in children and patients with extra-pulmonary TB or PLHIV. Although it is recommended that any sample from a suspected TB patient that is initially negative by a rapid diagnostic test be cultured for TB growth and confirmed diagnosis, there will be a group of patients that have TB but without microbiologic confirmation. These are included in the Government of India TB case notification as "patients diagnosed clinically as a case of TB, without microbiologic confirmation, and initiated on anti-TB drugs" (2).

References:

1. WHO Case Definitions 2011 Update. http://www.stoptb.org/wg/gli/assets/documents
2. TB Notification, GO No. Z-28015/2/2012-TB, dated 7th May 2012, Ministry of Health, Government of India

Standard 6
Paediatric TB

6.1 Diagnosis of paediatric TB patients:
  - In all children with presumptive intra-thoracic TB, microbiological confirmation should be sought through examination of respiratory specimens (e.g. sputum by expectoration, gastric aspirate, gastric lavage, induced sputum, broncho-alveolar lavage or other appropriate specimens) with a quality assured diagnostic test, preferably CB-NAAT, smear microscopy or culture.

6.2 Diagnosis of probable paediatric TB patients:
  - In the event of negative or unavailable microbiological results, a diagnosis of probable TB in children should be based on the presence of abnormalities consistent with TB on radiography, a history of exposure to pulmonary TB case, evidence of TB infection (positive TST) and clinical findings suggestive of TB.

6.3 Diagnosis of extra-pulmonary paediatric TB patients:
  - For children with presumptive extra-pulmonary TB, appropriate specimens from the presumed sites of involvement should be obtained for rapid molecular test, microscopy, culture and DST, and histo-pathological examination.

Diagnosis of TB in children is particularly challenging as in small children it can be difficult to collect samples and the paucibacillary nature of TB in children reduces the sensitivity of testing. Regardless, there should be every effort to obtain bacteriologic diagnosis. Standardised TST may be used as a complimentary test in children, in combination with microbiological investigations, history of contact, radiology, and symptoms. The guidelines of the Indian Academy of Paediatrics (IAP) and paediatric TB guidelines of the RNTCP recommend obtaining specimens for mycobacteriology, the use of standardised TST with a cut-off of 10mm induration in non-immunosuppressed children, and specialist consultation. Serodiagnostic tests and IGRA have no role in paediatric TB diagnosis.

References:

1. Emily C. Pearce, A Systematic Review of Clinical Diagnostic Systems Used in the Diagnosis of Tuberculosis in Children, Hindawi Publishing Corporation AIDS Research and Treatment Volume 2012, Article ID 401896, 11 pages doi: 10.1155/2012/401896)
2. National Guidelines on diagnosis and treatment of Paediatric Tuberculosis, In consultation with Indian Academy Paediatrics during January- February 2012
3. New Paediatric TB guidelines. www.tbcindia.nic.in/documents/pdf

Standard 7
Treatment with first-line regimen

7.1 Treatment of New TB patients:
- All new patients should receive an internationally accepted first-line treatment regimen for new patients. The initial phase should consist of two months of Isoniazid (H), Rifampicin (R), Pyrazinamide (Z), and Ethambutol (E). The continuation phase should consist of three drugs (Isoniazid, Rifampicin and Ethambutol) given for at least four months.

7.2 Extension of continuation phase:
- The duration of continuation phase may be extended by three to six months in special situations like Bone & Joint TB, Spinal TB with neurological involvement and neuro-tuberculosis.

7.3 Drug dosages:
- The patients should be given dosages of the drugs depending upon body weight in weight bands.

7.4 Bio-availability of drugs:
- The bioavailability of the drug should be ensured for every batch, especially if fixed dose combinations (FDCs) are used, by procuring and prescribing from a quality-assured source.

7.5 Dosage frequency:
- All patients should be given daily regimen under direct observation. However, the country programme may consider daily or intermittent regimen for treatment of TB depending on the available resources and operational considerations as both are effective provided all doses are directly observed.
- All paediatric TB patients and HIV associated TB patients should be given daily regimen under direct observation.

7.6 Drug formulations:
- Fixed dose combinations (FDCs) of four drugs (Isoniazid, Rifampicin, Pyrazinamide, and Ethambutol), three drugs (Isoniazid, Rifampicin and Ethambutol) and two drugs (Isoniazid and Rifampicin) are recommended.

7.7 Previously treated TB patients:
- After MDR-TB (or R resistance) is ruled out by a Quality Assured test, TB patients returning after lost to follow up, relapsing from their first treatment course or new TB patients failing with first treatment course may receive the retreatment regimen containing first-line drugs: 2HREZS/1HREZ/5HRE.

Treatment of drug-susceptible pulmonary TB with RHZE for two months followed by four months of RH or RHE has been highly effective in clinical trials (1). More than 95% of patients are cured using this regimen (1,2,3). The results are so impressive and repeatable that the lower rates of cure in national TB programs highlight the operational challenges of delivering a daily regimen over an extended period of time (4,5). The concept of daily, directly observed therapy, incorporating a full six months of R has been adopted by the majority of countries worldwide as a major part of Stop TB Strategy (5). India implemented the Revised National TB Control Program (RNTCP) in 1996 as a national government run system that used a thrice weekly regimen administered by DOT (6). Cure rates in India have been comparable with countries using daily dosing, TB mortality has dropped significantly, and the prevalence of TB has declined slightly over the last two decades (6). Nevertheless, high relapse rate of 11-13% has been reported in patients treated by DOT in the RNTCP in India from several different locations over the last several years (21,23,24). In places where the background of H resistance is high and/or HIV co-infection is common and in patients with cavitary disease the daily regimen is preferred because the intermittent dosing schedules result in higher rates of treatment failure and relapse (7,8,9). In India, H resistance is 11% in untreated TB patients and 37% in previously treated cases and the prevalence of HIV co-infection is 5% (6). In countries where H resistance is prevalent a full six months course of Rifampicin is recommended with a third drug, Ethambutol, added to the four months continuation phase (2,3,18,19). Recent data indicates that this is also safe in paediatric patients (20). The extension of the continuation phase for extra-pulmonary TB to 9 or 12 months is based on expert opinion rather than evidence.

The recommendation for "category 2" treatment for previously treated cases with the addition of streptomycin to the intensive phase is currently under review and it is safe to say that a drug sensitivity test, if available, is a better guide to retreating TB than a "category 2" regimen (13,14,15,16,17,18,19,21,22,23). The addition of a single drug to a failing regimen violates one of the tenets of TB therapy so close follow up of patients on a retreatment regimen is especially important (14).

Fixed dose combinations (FDCs) are desirable as they simplify drug procurement and logistics, the delivery of DOT and may increase adherence (10). It is important that the provider prescribe only quality-assured pills of fixed drug combinations in RNTCP and WHO recommended dosing (2,3,10). Individual drug dosing should be reserved for patients with toxicities or contraindications to one or more components of the FDC (10). The RNTCP guidelines outline dosing based on weight bands. Suggested weight bands for adults are: 30-39 kg, 40-54 kg, 55-70 kg and >70 kg. Recommended weight bands for paediatric patients are: 6-8 kg, 9-12 kg, 13-16 kg, 17-20 kg, 21-24 kg and 25-30 kg.

The expert group acknowledged that the intermittent regimen used under the programme over the past decade is equally effective under direct observation as compared to the daily regimen, and choosing daily regimen does not undermine the successes of the programme (11,12). However, based on the above evidences and in the interest of having uniformity of care across all healthcare sectors to achieve the future vision of the programme for universal access to quality TB care and prevention of further drug resistance to TB; the choice for daily regimen was required. It was recommended that the programme to undertake an operational research to assess the feasibility of implementing daily therapy using FDCs under direct observation under programmatic settings.

References

1. Menzies D, Benedetti A, Paydar A, Martin I, Royce S, et al. (2009) - Effect of Duration and Intermittency of Rifampin on Tuberculosis Treatment Outcomes: A Systematic Review and Meta-Analysis. PLoS Med 2009. 6(9): e1000146. doi:10.1371

2. World Health Organisation. Treatment of Tuberculosis Guidelines. 4th edition. Geneva: World Health Organisation; 2010.

3. International Standards for TB Care, Second Edition (2009) Tuberculosis Coalition for Technical Assistance, The Hague 2009.

4. World Health Organization, Global Tuberculosis Report 2012; Geneva 2012

5. World Health Organization, Stop TB Strategy, 2013; Geneva 2013

6. Revised National TB Control Programme, 2013; tbcindia.nic.in

7. Kwok Chiu Chang et al. Dosing Schedules of 6-Month Regimens and Relapse for Pulmonary TB. Amer Journal of Respir Crit Care Medicine. 2006; 174: 1153-1158.

8. Chang KC et al. Treatment of tuberculosis and optimal dosing schedules – Downloaded from thorax.bmj.com on June 29, 2011 – Published by group.bmj.com

9. Chang K Cetal. – A Nested Case-Control Study on Treatment – related Risk Factors for Early Relapse of Tuberculosis. Amer Journal of Respir Crit Care Medicine. 2004; 170: 1124-1130.

10. MonederoI. et al. Evidence for promoting fixed-dose combination drugs in tuberculosis treatment and control: a review. Int J Tuberc Lung Dis. 2011;15(4):433–439.

11. Alvarez TA et al.Prevalence of drug-resistant Mycobacterium tuberculosis in patients under intermittent or daily treatment. J Bras Pneumol. 2009;35(6):555-560.

12. Wells AW et al. Implications of the current tuberculosis treatment landscape for future regimen change. Int J Tuberc Lung Dis. 2011; 15(6):746–753.

13. Ramachandran R, S Nalini, V. Chandrasekar, P. V. Dave, A. S. Sanghvi, F. Wares, C. N. Paramasivan, P. R. Narayanan, Sahu S, Parmar M, Chadha S, Dewan P, L. S. Chauhan.Surveillance of drug-resistant tuberculosis in the state of Gujarat, India - Int J Tuberc Lung Dis. 13(9):1154–1160.

14. Bhargava A, Pai M, et al. - Mismanagement of tuberculosis in India: Causes, consequences, and the way forward - Hypothesis 2011, 9(1): e7.

15. Mahmoudi A, Iseman MD. Pitfalls in the Care of Patients with Tuberculosis. JAMA 1993 July 7, 1993; 270:65

16. Bhargava A, Jain Y. The Revised National Tuberculosis Control Programme in India: Time for Revision of Treatment regimens and rapid up – scaling of DOTS–Plus initiative. National Medical Journal of India 2008;21(4):187–91

17. Espinal MA. Time to abandon the standard retreatment regimen with first–line drugs for failures of standard treatment. Int J Tuberc Lung Dis 2003;7:607–8.

18. Patricio E et al. – Treatment of Isoniazid-Resistant Tuberculosis in Southeastern Texas – Chest 2001; 119; 1730-1736

19. Menzies D et al. Standardized Treatment of Active Tuberculosis in Patients with Previous Treatment and/or with Mono-resistance to Isoniazid: A Systematic Review and Meta-analysis – PLoS Med 6(9): e1000150.doi: 10.1371.

20. Donald PR, Maher D, Maritz JS, Qazi S. Ethambutol dosage for the treatment of children: literature review and recommendations 2006; 10;1318-1330.

21. GS Azhar – DOTS for TB relapse in India: A Systematic Review. Lung India. 2012. 29(2).

22. Poncea M, et al. (2009) - Additional evidence to support the phasing-out of treatment category II regimen for pulmonary tuberculosis in Peru - Transactions of the Royal Society of Tropical Medicine and Hygiene 106 (2012) 508– 510

23. Thomas A et al. Predictors of relapse among pulmonary tuberculosis patients treated in a DOTS programme in a DOTS programme in South India. International Journal of Tuberculosis and Lung Diseases 2005;9(5):556-561

24. Dave P, Rade K, Modi B, Solanki R, Patel P, Shah A, Vadera B. Assessment of Long-term Outcome among New Smear Positive Pulmonary TB Patients Treated with Intermittent Regimen under RNTCP – A Retrospective Cohort Study. Natl J Community Med 2013; 4(2):189-194.

Standard 8
Monitoring treatment response

8.1 Follow-up sputum microscopy:
- Response to therapy in patients with pulmonary tuberculosis, new as well as retreatment cases, should be monitored by follow-up sputum microscopy/culture (one specimen) at the time of completion of the intensive phase of treatment and at the end of treatment.

8.2 Extension of intensive phase:
- The extension of the intensive phase is not recommended.

8.3 Offer DST in follow up sputum positive cases:
- If the sputum smear is positive in follow-up at any time during treatment, a rapid molecular DST (as the first choice) or culture-DST (at least for R and if possible for Isoniazid (H); Ofloxacin (O) and Kanamycin (K), if R-resistant/MDR) should be performed as laboratory facilities become available.

8.4 Response to treatment in extra-pulmonary TB:
- In patients with extra-pulmonary tuberculosis, the treatment response is best assessed clinically. The help of radiological and other relevant investigations may also be taken.

8.5 Response to treatment in children:
- In children, who are unable to produce sputum, the response to treatment may be assessed clinically. The help of radiological and other relevant investigations may also be taken.

8.6 Long- term follow up:
- After completion of treatment the patients should be followed up with clinical and/or sputum examination at the end of six and 12 months.

International standards recommend that a sputum sample should be collected at the end of the intensive phase (two months) and at the end of treatment (six months) to monitor the success of therapy (1,2). Recent evidence from India shows that collecting more than one sample added little to the detection of failure of treatment and therefore only one sample at two months is recommended for initial treatment monitoring (3,4,6). If the sample is positive for TB then it is recommended that a DST be done to guide further selection of therapy, either by a molecular probe for drug resistant loci or phenotypic DST in liquid culture. Consensus summarised by the WHO found little benefit for extending the intensive phase to three months if the two months smear was positive (2). It is, however, necessary to re-address adherence issues and/or other comorbid conditions that may have affected proper completion of the two months intensive phase (1).

Follow up of extra-pulmonary and smear negative TB is challenging and best done by regular clinical review. Chest X-ray has shown limited accuracy (5).

References:

1. International Standards of TB Care (2009)
2. WHO Guidelines of Treatment of TB (2010) Geneva
3. Kundu D, MV Kumar A, Satyanarayana S, Dewan PK, Achuthan Nair S, et al. (2012) Can Follow-Up Examination of Tuberculosis Patients Be Simplified? A Study in Chhattisgarh, India. PLoS ONE 7(12): e51038. doi:10.1371/journal.pone.0051038
4. Toshniwal M, MV Kumar A, Satyanarayana S, Dewan PK, Achuthan Nair S, et al. (2012) – IUATLD – Abstract Book – UNION World Conference for Lung Health, November 2012 – Kuala Lumpur, Malaysia
5. Horne et al., Lancet Infectious Diseases 2010 Gandhi MP, Kumar AMV, Toshniwal MN, Reddy RHR, Oeltmann JE, et al. (2012) Sputum Smear Microscopy at Two Months into Continuation- Phase: Should It Be Done in All Patients with Sputum Smear-Positive Tuberculosis? PLoS ONE 7(6): e39296. doi: 10.1371/journal.pone.0039296

Standard 9
Drug Resistant TB management

9.1 Treatment of M/XDR-TB(or R resistant TB):
   - Patients with TB caused by drug-resistant organisms (especially M/XDR or only R resistance or with O or K resistance), microbiologically confirmed by an accredited laboratory, should be treated with specialized regimens containing quality assured second-line anti-tuberculosis drugs.

9.2 Model of care for drug resistant TB:
   - Patients with DR-TB should be treated using mainly ambulatory care rather than models of care based principally on hospitalization. If required, a short period of initial hospitalisation is recommended.

9.3 Regimen for MDR-TB (or R resistant cases):
   - The regimen chosen for MDR-TB may be standardized and/or based on microbiologically confirmed drug susceptibility patterns. At least four drugs (second line) to which the organisms are known or presumed to be susceptible, should be used. Most importantly the regimen should include at least Pyrazinamide, Ethambutol, a later-generation Fluoroquinolone (such as high dose Levofloxacin) and a parenteral agent (such as Kanamycin or Amikacin), Ethionamide (or Prothionamide), and either Cycloserine or PAS (P-aminosalicylic acid), if Cycloserine cannot be used.

9.4 Regimen for MDR-TB patients with O and/or K resistance detected early:
   - Treatment regimen may be suitably modified in case of Ofloxacin and/or Kanamycin resistance at the initiation of MDR-TB treatment or during early intensive phase, preferably not later than four to six weeks.

9.5 Surgery in M/XDR-TB patients:
   - All patients of M/XDR-TB should be evaluated for surgery at the initiation of treatment and/or during follow up.

9.6 Treatment duration in MDR-TB patients:
   - Till newer effective drugs are available with proven efficacy with shorter duration of MDR-TB treatment; total treatment should be given for at least 24 months in patients newly diagnosed with MDR-TB (i.e. not previously treated for MDR-TB) with recommended intensive phase of treatment being six to nine months. The total duration may be modified according to the patient's response to therapy.

9.7 Specialist consultation in M/XDR-TB patients:
   - Consultation with a specialist experienced in treatment of patients with M/XDR-TB should be obtained, whenever possible.

9.8 Ensuring adherence in M/XDR-TB patients:
   - Patient support systems, including direct observation of treatment, are required to ensure adherence. It should be ensured that the patient consumes all the doses of the drugs.

9.9 Single sample follow up culture in M/XDR-TB patients:
   - The use of sputum culture (1 sample) is recommended for monitoring of patients with M/XDR-TB during treatment.

9.10 Second line DST during treatment of MDR-TB:
   - During the course of MDR-TB treatment, if the sputum culture is found to be positive at 6 months or later, the most recent culture isolate should be subjected to DST with second-line drugs (at least Ofloxacin and Kanamycin) to decide on further course of action. DST to other additional drugs may also be done if laboratory facilities are available to guide treatment.

9.11 Regimen for MDR-TB patients with Ofloxacin and/or Kanamycin resistance detected later:
   - The patients with MDR-TB found to be resistant to at least Ofloxacin and/or Kanamycin during the later stage of MDR-TB treatment must be treated with a suitable regimen for XDR-TB using second line drugs including Group 5 drugs such as Amoxicillin-Clavulanate, Clarithromycin, Clofazimine, Linezolid, Thioacetazone, Imipenem to which the organisms are known or presumed to be susceptible.

9.12 New drugs:
   - The new drugs e.g. Bedaquiline, Delaminid may be considered whenever scientific evidence for their efficacy and safety becomes available as per the national policy for newer antimicrobials. Appropriate regulatory mechanisms for distribution control needs to be ensured.

The treatment of drug resistant TB is much more complex and challenging than the treatment of drug susceptible TB and requires drugs with greater toxicities for longer periods of time with relatively less encouraging outcomes. Unfortunately the evidence for drug regimen recommendations for drug-resistant TB are based on observational studies and expert opinion and no large scale randomized controlled clinical trial data has been generated across the globe. Newer agents and newer regimens are becoming available and it is hoped the level of evidence for treatment choices increases in the next few years.

The new drugs e.g. Bedaquiline, however, may be considered whenever scientific evidence for their efficacy and safety is available as per the national policy for newer antimicrobials. Appropriate regulatory mechanisms for distribution control need to be ensured. This is of utmost importance to safeguard the new drugs from the risk of unregulated irrational use and emergence of resistance to these precious drugs.

Laboratory based microbiological confirmation of drug resistance is an important pre-requisite for deciding on an appropriate treatment regimen under consultation with a specialist experienced in management of M/XDR TB, wherever possible. Patients with tuberculosis caused by drug-resistant organisms (especially M/XDR or only Rifampicin resistance or with Ofloxacin or Kanamycin resistance), microbiologically confirmed by an accredited laboratory, should be treated with specialized regimens containing quality assured second-line anti-tuberculosis drugs. For all practical purposes, Rifampicin resistance should be considered as a surrogate of MDR-TB and treated with the same regimen for MDR-TB. While all efforts should be made for microbiological confirmation, in exceptional circumstances (e.g. paediatric and extra-pulmonary cases) the MDR treatment may be considered in absence of the microbiological confirmation. Clear guiding principles need to be laid down by the national programme to define the eligibility of patients under such exceptional circumstances for treatment with second line anti-TB drugs in absence of microbiological confirmation.

The basic principles of drug-resistant TB treatment include using at least four second line drugs that the organism has demonstrated susceptibility to through DST or that guided by the current epidemiology of drug-resistance in the relevant population. In the treatment of patients with MDR-TB, four second-line anti-TB drugs likely to be effective (including a parenteral agent), as well as Pyrazinamide and Ethambutol should be included in the intensive phase (1,2), the duration of that should be at least for six to nine months. Consider extending treatment at least 18 months beyond the last evidence of mycobacteria in a culture from the patient. Thus, the total duration of treatment should be at least 24 months up to a maximum of 27 months in patients newly diagnosed with MDR-TB (i.e. not previously treated for MDR-TB). The total duration of treatment may be modified according to the patient's response to therapy.

In the treatment of patients with MDR-TB, regimens should thus include at least Pyrazinamide, a Fluoroquinolone, a parenteral agent, Ethionamide (or Prothionamide), and either Cycloserine or PAS (P-aminosalicylic acid) if Cycloserine cannot be used (1,2). Treatment regimen may be suitably modified in case of Ofloxacin and/or Kanamycin resistance detected early at the initiation of MDR-TB treatment or during early intensive phase, preferably not later than four to six weeks. However, for patients on MDR-TB regimen that are found to be resistant to at least Ofloxacin and/or Kanamycin during the later stage of MDR-TB treatment; they must be treated with a suitable regimen for XDR-TB using second line drugs including Group 5 drugs to which the organisms are known or presumed to be susceptible.

Ambulatory care is the preferred choice for management of DR-TB patients rather than models of care based principally on hospitalization as there are convincing evidences that improving access to treatment for DR-TB through decentralization of care to centers near the patient's residence reduced the risk of default (2,3). However, if required, a short period of initial hospitalisation is recommended (2). Patient support systems, including direct observation of treatment, are required to ensure adherence. It should be ensured that the patient consumes all the doses of the drugs as missed doses for more than a week increases the odds of further augmentation of drug resistance and adversely affects treatment outcomes. Monitoring of treatment should be done by collecting a single monthly sample of sputum for culture from month three to month seven and then quarterly until the end of therapy. It has been observed in an operational research conducted under the RNTCP that there is no meaningful advantage in using two specimens and a single specimen policy could be safely implemented with negligible clinical effect on MDR-TB patients and favourable resource implications for RNTCP (4). Prompt identification of early failures of MDR-TB regimen and timely actions for initiating second line DST in culture isolates of such patients is alluded to in Standard 4. However, if the sputum culture is found to be positive at six months or later and the patient has no clinical or radiological deterioration, a repeat DST may be done to confirm sensitivity status.

Last but not the least, it must be emphasized that treatment of drug resistant TB can be complicated by drug toxicities, drug to drug interactions and emerging DST patterns and enlisting the help of an expert in DR-TB should be sought sooner rather than later through more than 100 established DR TB centers across the country.

References:

1. Guidelines for the programmatic management of drug-resistant tuberculosis (2011 update), World Health Organization, WHO/HTM/TB/2011.6. www.who.int/publications
2. Guidelines on Programmatic Management of Drug Resistant TB (PMDT) in India, Revised National Tuberculosis Control Programme, Central TB Division, Directorate General of Health Services,Ministry of Health & Family Welfare, Nirman Bhavan, New Delhi, www.tbcindia.nic.in/documents
3. M. T. Gler,* L. J. Podewils,† N. Munez,* M. Galipot,* M. I. D. Quelapio,* T.E. Tupasi* et al. (2012) - Impact of patient and program factors on default during treatment of multidrug-resistant tuberculosis-INT J TUBERC LUNG DIS 16(7):955–960 © 2012 The Union http://dx.doi.org/10.5588/ijtld.11.0502-7 May 2012
4. Nagaraja SB, Kumar AMV, Sachdeva KS, Ramachandran R, Satyanarayana S, Parmar M et al. (2012) Is One Sputum Specimen as Good as Two during Follow-Up Cultures for Monitoring Multi Drug Resistant Tuberculosis Patients in India? PLoS ONE 7(9): e45554. doi:10.1371/journal.pone.0045554

Standard 10
Addressing TB with HIV infection and other comorbid conditions

10.1 Treatment of HIV infected TB patients:
- TB patients living with HIV infection should receive the same duration of TB treatment with daily regimen as HIV-negative TB patients.

10.2 Anti-retroviral therapy and co-trimoxazole prophylactic therapy in HIV infected TB patients:
- Anti-retroviral therapy must be offered to all patients with HIV and TB as well as drug-resistant TB who require second-line anti-TB drugs, irrespective of CD4 cell-count, as early as possible (within the first eight weeks) following initiation of anti-TB treatment. Appropriate arrangements for access to anti-retroviral drugs should be made for patients. However, initiation of treatment for TB should not be delayed. Patients with TB and HIV infection should also receive Co-trimoxazole as prophylaxis for other infections.

10.3 Isoniazid preventive therapy in HIV patients without active TB:
- People living with HIV (PLHIV) should be screened for TB using four symptom complexes (current cough or fever or weight loss or night sweats) at HIV care settings and those with any of these symptoms should be evaluated for ruling out active TB. All asymptomatic patients in whom active TB is ruled out, Isoniazid Preventive Therapy (IPT) should be offered to them for six months or longer.

PLHIV are more susceptible to TB infection, more likely to develop active TB disease after infection and more likely to suffer from severe TB and disseminated, extra-pulmonary TB. In general, the treatment for TB in PLHIV is the same as treatment for patients without HIV and treatment outcomes are successful although the mortality rate of PLHIV is higher, more so with DR-TB comorbidity than the HIV uninfected (1).With growing evidences it is globally recommended, that HIV infected TB patients should be treated with daily regimen (2,3,4,5). Intermittent regimen has been proven to lead to higher risk for relapse and development of acquired Rifampicin resistance if intermittent dosing of Rifampicin was started during the intensive phase of treatment in HIV-infected patients treated with Rifampicin-based regimens (2,3,4,5).

Anti-retroviral therapy must be offered to all patients with HIV and TB as well as drug-resistant TB who require second-line anti-TB drugs, irrespective of CD4 cell-count, as early as possible (within the first eight weeks) following initiation of anti-TB treatment (2,3,5). A number of recent studies have investigated the optimal timing of TB and HIV treatment to reduce mortality and it seems clear that as soon as possible after initiating treatment for active TB in a PLHIV they should be started on antiretroviral therapy (2,5). ART reduces the risk of TB relapse and acquired drug resistance to rifampicin in HIV infected TB patients (2,3,5). Further, in settings with high Fluoroquinolone resistance and extensive prior second-line treatment, encouraging results are being achieved in an ambulatory MDR-TB programme in a slum setting in India. Rapid scale up of both Antiretroviral Therapy (ART) and second-line treatment for MDR-TB are needed to ensure survival of co-infected patients and mitigate this growing epidemic (6). Considerations such as the ability to tolerate a large pill burden, drug interactions and toxicities all have to be balanced with the life-saving treatment of both TB and HIV simultaneously.

Appropriate arrangements for access to anti-retroviral drugs should be made for patients. However, initiation of treatment for TB should not be delayed. Patients with TB and HIV infection should also receive co-trimoxazole as prophylaxis for other infections (3). In PLHIV that do not appear acutely ill and do not have one or more of the WHO recommended four symptom screens for active TB are very unlikely to be suffering from active TB and may safely be given Isoniazid Preventative Therapy (IPT) for at least six months as part of a comprehensive package of HIV care (7). IPT should be given to such individuals irrespective of the degree of immunosuppression, and also to those on ART, those who have previously been treated for TB and pregnant women (7). Recent studies have demonstrated the profound protective effect of IPT although those that derive the most benefit are TST positive. In addition, evidence from India, along with other countries, points to a prolonged course of IPT being more protective than the standard six month course.

References:

1. S. Tripathy, A. Anand, V. Inamdar et. al - Clinical response of newly diagnosed HIV seropositive &seronegative pulmonary tuberculosis patients with the RNTCP Short Course regimen in Pune, India - Indian J Med Res 133, May 2011, pp 521-528
2. Faiz Ahmad Khan, Jessica Minion, Abdullah Al-Motairi, Andrea Benedetti, Anthony D. Harries, and Dick Menzies - An Updated Systematic Review and Meta-analysis on the Treatment of Active Tuberculosis in Patients With HIV Infection - 1154 CID 2012:55 (15 October) HIV/AIDS
3. WHO Guidelines for Treatment of Tuberculosis –2010 update
4. Jiehui Li et.al. Relapse and Acquired Rifampicin Resistance in HIV-Infected Patients with Tuberculosis Treated with Rifampicin– or Rifabutin-Based Regimens in New York City, 1997-2000 – Clinical Infectious Diseases 2005;41:83-91
5. PayamNahid et.al. – Treatment outcomes of patients with HIV and Tuberculosis - American Journal of Respiratory Critical Care Medicine – Vol 175 pp 1199-1206, 2007
6. Isaakidis P, Cox HS, Varghese B, Montaldo C, Da Silva E, et al. (2011) Ambulatory Multi-Drug Resistant Tuberculosis Treatment Outcomes in a Cohort of HIV-Infected Patients in a Slum Setting in Mumbai, India. PLoS ONE 6(12): e28066. doi:10.1371/journal.pone.0028066
7. DelphineSculier and HaileyesusGetahun.Scaling up TB screening and Isoniazid preventive therapy among children and adults living with HIV: new WHO guidelines. Africa Health, November 2011, page 18-23

Standard 11
Treatment adherence

11.1 Patient-centered approach for adherence:
- To assess and foster adherence, a patient-centered approach to administration of drug treatment, based on the patient's needs and mutual respect between the patient and the provider, should be developed for all patients.

11.2 Measures for treatment adherence:
- Supervision and support should be individualized and should draw on the full range of recommended interventions and available support services, including patient counselling and education. A central element of the patient centered strategy is the use of measures to assess and promote adherence to the treatment regimen and to address poor adherence when it occurs. These measures should be tailored to the individual patient's circumstances based on details of the patient's clinical and social history and be mutually acceptable to the patient and the provider.

11.3 Trained treatment supporter for treatment adherence:
- Such measures may include identification and training of a treatment supporter (for tuberculosis and, if appropriate, for HIV, Diabetes Mellitus etc.) who is acceptable, accessible and accountable to the patient and to the health system.

11.4 Use of ICT to promote treatment literacy and adherence:
- Optimal use of ICT should be done to promote treatment literacy and adherence.

Treatment adherence is a critical determinant of treatment outcomes, prognosis and further emergence of DR-TB in patients experiencing irregular and incomplete treatment. The DOTS Strategy has been the backbone of most country's

TB programmes for the last decade. In certain places, strict healthcare worker DOTS has been cost-effective and sustainable and resulted in control of limited TB epidemics. However, accumulating evidence has pointed to the effectiveness of a wide variety of approaches including community and family-centered DOTS, which is more achievable for most developing healthcare systems and produce comparable outcomes to healthcare worker supervised DOTS (1).

However, treatment adherence goes beyond the realm of DOTS to a larger concept of treatment support system developed with mutual trust and respect between the patient, family, providers, treatment supporters and the health system at large to promptly identify and address all possible factors that could lead to treatment interruptions. This includes not only medical factors such as promptly addressing co-morbidities, adverse drug reactions and emergencies but also spans out to addressing various social, vocational, nutritional, economic, psychological stress experienced by the patient throughout the course of treatment. Periodic regular and effective supervision by the public health supervisors at various levels and close monitoring of the progress made by the patient on treatment by the treating provider are critical components to ensure high standards of care. Capacity building and engaging with local community based organizations, self-help groups and patient support groups could prove to be effective interventions to promote treatment adherence (2,3).

India is enabled with highly functional ICT systems and a population that is technology-literate. Through the use of SMS reminders and call center linkages between patients, providers and pharmacists, it is hoped that adherence to treatment will reach the necessary levels to reduce the prevalence of TB throughout India.

References:

1. International Standards of TB Care
2. Volmink J, Garner P - Directly observed therapy for treating tuberculosis (Review) - The Cochrane Library - 2009, Issue 1, http://www.thecochranelibrary.com
3. Munro SA, Lewin SA, Smith H, Engel ME, Fretheim A, et al. (2007) Patient adherence to Tuberculosis treatment: A systematic review of qualitative research. PLoS Med 4(7): e238. doi:10.1371/journal.pmed.

Standard 12
Public health responsibility

12.1 Any practitioner treating a patient for tuberculosis is assuming an important public health responsibility to prevent on-going transmission of the infection and the development of drug resistance.

12.2 To fulfil this responsibility, the practitioner must not only prescribe an appropriate regimen, but when necessary, also utilize local public health services/community health services, and other agencies including NGOs to assess the adherence of the patient and to address poor adherence when it occurs (1).

India continues to have high TB incidence and the mortality due to TB is still unacceptably high. The challenges of TB control in India are magnified by the existence of parallel systems for TB diagnosis and treatment – the public and private. Each system takes care of approximately half the TB cases (2) and methods and standards vary greatly depending on whether public or private care is accessed and furthermore what type of private care is sought, from super-speciality tertiary institutions to non-qualified providers (3). In part publishing, these standards of care attempts to standardise care so that certain responsibilities of the provider, whether public or private, are clear. In addition Standard 13, the notification of TB cases from both public and private providers, is expected to improve surveillance and quality of the care delivered and a subsequent reduction in the burden of TB in India.

References:

1. International Standards of TB Care
2. Satyanarayana S, Nair SA, Chadha SS, Shivashankar R, Sharma G, et al. (2011) From Where Are Tuberculosis Patients Accessing Treatment in India?
   Results from a Cross-Sectional Community Based Survey of 30 Districts. PLoS ONE 6(9): e24160. doi:10.1371/journal.pone.0024160
3. AnuragBhargava et al., Mismanagement of Tuberculosis in India: Causes, Consequences, and the Wayforward. Hypothesis 2011, 9(1): e7.

Standard 13
Notification of TB cases

13.1 All health establishments must report all TB cases and their treatment outcomes to public health authorities (District Nodal Officer for Notification).

13.2 Proper feedback need to be ensured to all healthcare providers who refer cases to public health system on the outcome of the patients which they had referred.

TB is a notifiable disease in India as per the government order dated 7 May, 2012 and requires that all healthcare providers who have diagnosed a case of TB through microbiological testing or clinically diagnosed and/or started treatment for TB must report to the District Nodal Officer for Notification (1). Notification is a basic public health activity common to diseases of public health importance. With notification, public health authorities can identify TB patients and offer necessary public health care, supervise and support for the quality of treatment, and monitor disease trends. Ensuring notification of all TB cases is the most important step for a comprehensive TB surveillance system, which is required for effective TB control in the country. Cases are defined as anyone who has a microbiological (smear or culture) or approved molecular test proven disease or anyone who has a clinical syndrome consistent with active TB and is started on TB treatment. The requirement for reporting applies equally to government-run facilities and to private facilities. In both settings, it is the primary TB care provider or laboratory diagnostician's responsibility to ensure that the required notification is completed (2). RNTCP has an electronic TB notification system (NIKSHAY) wherein all providers can register and notify cases -http://nikshay.gov.in

References:

1. Notification of TB in India http://www.tbcindia.nic.in/pdfs/TB%20Notification%20Govt%20%20Or der%20dated%2007%2005%202012.pdf
2. Guidance tool for TB notification http://tbcindia.nic.in/pdfs/Guidance%20tool%20for%20TB%20notificati on%20in%20India% 20-%20FINAL.pdf

Standard 14
Maintain records for all TB patients

14.1 A written record of all medications given, bacteriologic response, adverse reactions and clinical outcome should be maintained for all patients.

Patient-level recording of details of diagnosis, treatment and outcome are the foundations of any effective public health surveillance system. Use of appropriate technology such as Nikshay should improve the quality and accessibility to a primary provider initiated record that is linked at every level from a primary clinic to the State Department of Health. In turn, it is the duty of the programme to monitor outcomes, both at primary level and aggregated into larger units, on a regular basis and reports the information that allow timely actions to improve services as needed.

The Government of India through a gazette notification has made all anti-TB drugs under schedule H1. These drugs should not be dispensed without a valid prescription from a qualified practitioner. A copy of the prescription should be maintained and details of the patient to be recorded by the chemist and should be made available for verification by the responsible public health authorities.

Standard 15
Contact investigation

15.1 All care providers to patients with TB should ensure all household contacts and other persons who are in close contact with TB patients are screened for TB as per defined Diagnostic Standards.

15.2 In case of paediatric TB patients, reverse contact tracing for search of any active TB case in the household of the child must be undertaken.

The highest priority contacts for active screening are:

- Persons with symptoms suggestive of tuberculosis
- Children aged <six years
- Contacts with known or suspected immune-compromised patient, particularly HIV infection
- Contacts with Diabetes Mellitus
- Contacts with other higher risks including pregnancy, smokers and alcoholics etc.
- Contacts of patients with DR-TB. In case of contact with a DR-TB index case, close clinical monitoring should be provided, as there is no evidence that treatment of latent infection with available drugs is presently effective

A contact investigation should focus on those in close contact with the index case, most importantly family members and other members of the household who may have prolonged exposure. Among this group of contacts past studies have found 4.5% to have TB (1,2). A recent study in India found 8.7% of household contacts were diagnosed with TB (3). Particular attention should be paid to contacts with the highest susceptibility to TB infection and subsequent active disease, namely small children and immunosuppressed people.

References:

1. Recommendations for investigating contacts of persons with infectious tuberculosis in low and middle income countries. www.who.int/tb/publications/2012/en/index.html
2. Fox GJ, Barry SE, Britton WJ, Marks GB. Contact investigation of tuberculosis, a systematic review and meta-analysis. European Respiratory Journal, 2012
3. Evaluation of TB case finding through systematic contact investigation, Chhattisgarh, India – Presented at the 43rd UNION World Lung Conference, Nov 2012, Kuala Lumpur, Malaysia

Standard 16
Isoniazid Prophylactic therapy

16.1 Children <6 years of age who are close contacts of a TB patient, after excluding active TB, should be treated with isoniazid for a minimum period of six months and should be closely monitored for TB symptoms.

Because children are more susceptible to TB infection, more likely to develop active TB disease soon after infection, and more likely to develop severe forms of disseminated TB, it is widely recommended (The Union, WHO) that close contacts of index cases under the age of 6 who do not have active TB should receive IPT. Close contacts of index cases with proven or suspected DR-TB should be monitored closely for signs and symptoms of active TB as isoniazid may not be prophylactic in these cases.

Standard 17
Airborne infection control

- Airborne infection control should be an integral part of all health care facility infection control strategy.

Each healthcare facility caring for patients who have, or are suspected of having, TB should develop and implement an appropriate airborne infection control plan as per the national guidelines. Administrative, environmental and personal protective measures should be implemented in all health care facilities as per national airborne infection control guidelines. Protection of health care workers from airborne infection should be ensured through adequate preventive measures including training, personal protection measures in high risk situations and periodic screening at least once a year.

TB is an airborne bacillus spread through inhalation of droplets. Therefore, in addition to general infection control procedures recommended for all health care facilities such as regular hand-washing, attention must be paid to limiting risk from airborne transmission. Airborne infection control measures are generally grouped into three main categories; environmental, administrative and managerial. Environmental controls require safe infrastructure and involve designing buildings and systems that promote safe air exchange e.g. HVAC systems, air flow management and UV light sterilization of areas. These tend to be expensive and installation is disruptive. Managerial controls refer to management plans that promote and enable safe practices in every facility and as such every healthcare facility, whether public or private, should have clear plans for an airborne infection control strategy that are implemented and monitored for completeness. Administrative controls are the most cost-effective and should be within the reach of every facility. They include screening and timely diagnosis of TB in all clients of the facility, respectful and non-stigmatizing removal of people with active TB from the general circulation of clients for rapid assessment and care, and use of personal protective equipment by active TB patients and staff to protect both staff and other patients. Such guidelines for Indian facilities are available at www.tbcindia.nic.in

Standard 18
Quality assurance systems

18.1 Quality assurance for diagnostic tests:
- All healthcare providers should ensure that all diagnostic tests used for diagnosis of TB are quality assured.

18.2 Quality assurance for anti-TB drugs:
- Quality assurance system should ensure that all anti-TB drugs used in the country are subjected to stringent quality assurance mechanisms at all levels (from manufacturer to patients). Providers should ensure that all anti-TB drugs prescribed come from a Quality assured source.

India has banned the use of commercial serology tests for diagnosis of TB. However, any diagnostic test used for diagnosing TB should have a quality assurance system in place. India's national TB programme (RNTCP) have established a good external quality assurance system for TB diagnostics, and is available to both public and private laboratories.

The same principle applies to the use of drugs; the drugs should be from a quality assured source and should be under a standard Quality Assurance process.

Standard 19
Panchayati Raj Institutions

19.1 Panchayati Raj Institutions (PRIs) and elected representatives have an important role to share the public health responsibility for TB control with the healthcare providers, patients and the community.

Health being an important responsibility of the PRIs in India, there are many opportunities for greater involvement of the PRIs for TB control. Because the diagnosis and treatment of TB is complicated and takes long, and mistreatment of TB and emergence of drug-resistant TB affects everybody in the community, the Panchayat should be involved in all aspects of TB control. PRIs can facilitate good communication between facilities, public or private, that diagnose and treat TB and the communities, which they serve thus greatly helping in mobilizing community support for TB control. PRIs can help TB patient to link to other social welfare schemes, can help in nutritional and rehabilitation support etc.

Standard 20
Health education

20.1 Every TB symptomatic should be properly counselled by the healthcare providers

20.2 TB patients and their family members should get proper counselling and health education at every contact with healthcare system

Proper health education to the patient and family is very important for TB care. There should be systems for education and counselling as an integral part of TB treatment. Every visit of the patient to the healthcare provider and visit of the health worker to the patient's home should be utilised for health education.

Standard 21
Death audit among TB patients

21.1 Every death among TB patients should be audited by a competent authority.

Investigation into the cause of death is an important standard which needs to be followed to study the conditions that led to the death in order to initiate actions to prevent development of such conditions to other TB patients. Every TB death should be notified to the concerned authority. Competent authority at the district level should do the death audit of every TB death and provide a report to the programme to take necessary steps for preventing avoidable deaths.

Introduction to Standards for
Social Inclusion for TB

The principles for introducing Standards for Social Inclusion in TB Care are:
- To ensure all individuals presenting to the healthcare facility are treated with dignity, irrespective of their health and socio-economic status.
- To ensure universal delivery of quality assured TB diagnostic and treatment services across public and private sector.
- To ensure visibility and accessibility of the TB service programme to all, irrespective of socio-economic status.
- To find and treat women, children and the elderly within hard to reach populations (Marginalized communities in rural and urban populations).
- To eliminate out of pocket expenditure including those incurred on covering travel costs and bridging the nutrition gap.
- To address loss of income when work day is lost due to TB.
- To ensure no one is left without a plan of action to address their presenting complaint if it is not because of TB.

The Patients Charter (accompanying the ISTC) is the key operational guideline in engaging with patients in all TB care settings.

Standard 22
Information on TB prevention and care seeking

22.1 All individuals especially women, children, elderly, differently abled, other vulnerable groups and those at increased risk should receive information related to TB prevention and care seeking.

Standard 23
Free and quality services

23.1 All patients, especially those in vulnerable population groups, should be offered free or affordable quality assured diagnostic and treatment services, which should be provided at locations and times so as to minimize workday or school disruptions and maximize access.

Standard 24
Respect, confidentiality and sensitivity

24.1 All people seeking or receiving care for TB should be received with dignity and managed with promptness, confidentiality and gender sensitivity. Public health responsibilities including notification, contact tracing, chemo-prophylaxis, fast tracking, outcome monitoring etc. should be sensitive to respect and confidentiality of patients.

Standard 25
Care and support through social welfare programmes

25.1 Healthcare providers should endeavour to derive synergies between various social welfare support systems such as RSBY, nutritional support programmes, national rural employment guarantee scheme etc. to mitigate out of pocket expenses such as transport and wage loss incurred by people affected by TB.

Standard 26
Addressing counseling and other needs

26.1 Persons affected by TB and their family members should be counselled at every opportunity, to address information gaps and to enable informed decision-making. Counseling should also address issues such as healthcare, physical, financial, psycho-social and nutritional needs.

International Standards for Tuberculosis Care

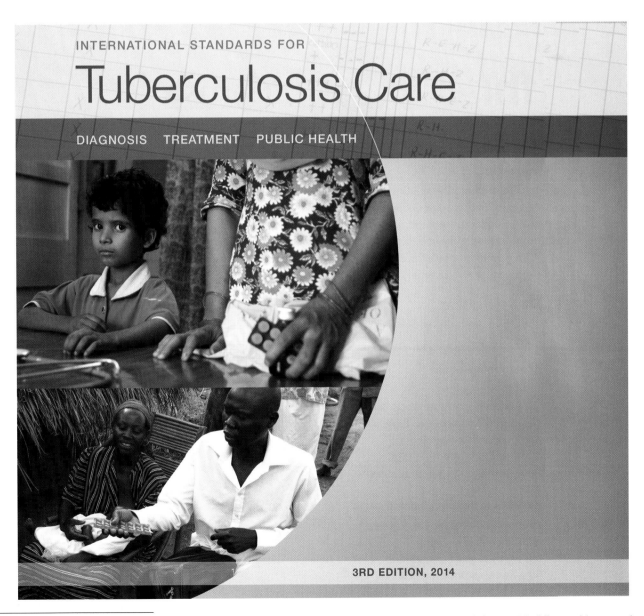

Reproduced (in part) with kind permission of Dr PC Hopewell. Full document can be accessed from URL://https://www.who.int/tb/publications/ISTC_3rdEd.pdf accessed on August 3, 2019

Developed by TB CARE I with funding by the United States Agency for International Development (USAID)

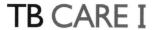 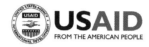

TB CARE I Organizations

 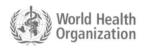

 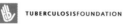 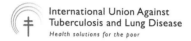

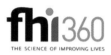 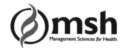

Disclaimer:

The Global Health Bureau, Office of Health, Infectious Disease and Nutrition (HIDN), US Agency for International Development, financially supports this publication through TB CARE I under the terms of Agreement No. AID-OAA-A-10-00020. This publication is made possible by the generous support of the American people through the United States Agency for International Development (USAID). The contents are the responsibility of TB CARE I and do not necessarily reflect the views of USAID or the United States Government.

Suggested citation:

TB CARE I. *International Standards for Tuberculosis Care*, Edition 3. TB CARE I, The Hague, 2014.

Contact information:

Philip C. Hopewell, MD
Curry International Tuberculosis Center
University of California, San Francisco
San Francisco General Hospital
San Francisco, CA 94110, USA
Email: phopewell@medsfgh.ucsf.edu

Available at the following web sites:

http://www.tbcare1.org/publications
http://istcweb.org
http://www.currytbcenter.ucsf.edu/international
http://www.who.int/tb/publications
To access a mobile version of ISTC, go to www.walimu.org/istc

INTERNATIONAL STANDARDS FOR

Tuberculosis Care

DIAGNOSIS   TREATMENT   PUBLIC HEALTH

3RD EDITION, 2014

Table of Contents

Acknowledgments

Development of the third edition of the *International Standards for Tuberculosis Care* was guided by a steering committee of World Health Organization Global Tuberculosis Programme staff and by an expert committee whose members were chosen to represent perspectives and areas of expertise relevant to tuberculosis care and control. Both committees are listed below. The expert committees for editions 1 and 2 are in Annex 1.

Steering Committee (WHO)

- **Haileyesus Getahun**
- **Chris Gilpin**
- **Malgosia Grzemska**
- **Ernesto Jaramillo**
- **Knut Lönnroth**
- **Mario Raviglione**
- **Mukund Uplekar**
- **Diana Weil**

Expert Committee

- **RV Asokan,** India
- **Erlina Burhan,** Indonesia
- **J.M. Chakaya,** Kenya
- **Gavin Churchyard,** South Africa
- **Marcus Conde,** Brazil
- **Charles Daley,** USA
- **Saidi Egwaga,** Tanzania
- **Elizabeth Fair,** USA
- **Paula Fujiwara,** USA
- **Haileyesus Getahun,** WHO
- **Chris Gilpin,** WHO
- **Steve Graham,** Australia
- **Malgosia Grzemska,** WHO
- **Philip Hopewell,** USA (Co-chair)
- **Ernesto Jaramillo,** WHO
- **Aamir Khan,** Pakistan
- **Knut Lönnroth,** WHO
- **G. B. Migliori,** Italy
- **Dyah Mustikawati,** Indonesia
- **Madhukar Pai,** Canada
- **Rose Pray,** USA
- **Mario Raviglione,** WHO
- **Elizabeth Soares,** Brazil
- **Mukund Uplekar,** WHO (Co-Chair)
- **Dalene Von Delft,** South Africa
- **Jan Voskens,** Netherlands
- **Diana Weil,** WHO
- **Gini Williams,** UK

Elizabeth Fair (University of California, San Francisco) in addition to being a member of the expert committee, provided scientific staffing and coordination.

Fran Du Melle (American Thoracic Society) provided administrative coordination as well as guidance on dissemination and implementation.

Cecily Miller and **Baby Djojonegoro** (University of California, San Francisco) provided assistance in organizing and preparing the document.

In addition to the committees, many individuals have provided valuable input. All comments received were given serious consideration by the co-chairs, although not all were incorporated into the document.

List of Abbreviations

AFB	Acid-fast bacilli
AIDS	Acquired immunodeficiency syndrome
ART	Antiretroviral therapy
ATS	American Thoracic Society
BCG	Bacille Calmette-Guérin
CDC	Centers for Disease Control and Prevention
CI	Confidence interval
COPD	Chronic obstructive pulmonary disease
CPT	Cotrimoxazole
CRI	Colorimetric redox-indicator
DOT	Directly observed treatment
DOTS	The internationally recommended strategy for tuberculosis control
DR	Drug-resistant
DST	Drug susceptibility testing
EMB	Ethambutol
FDA	Food and Drug Administration (US)
FDC	Fixed-dose combination
FHI 360	Formerly Family Health International
FM	Fluorescence microscopy
HAART	Highly active antiretroviral therapy
HIV	Human immunodeficiency virus
IDSA	Infectious Diseases Society of America
IGRA	Interferon-gamma release assay
INH	Isoniazid
IMAAI	Integrated Management of Adolescent and Adult Illness
IMCI	Integrated Management of Childhood Illness
IPT	Isoniazid preventive therapy
IRIS	Immune reconstitution inflammatory syndrome
ISTC	International Standards for Tuberculosis Care
IUATLD	International Union Against Tuberculosis and Lung Disease (The Union)
JATA	Japan Anti-tuberculosis Association
KNCV	KNCV Tuberculosis Foundation
LED	Light emitting diode
LPA	Line probe assay
LTBI	Latent tuberculosis infection
M&E	Monitoring and Evaluation
MDR	Multidrug-resistant
MIC	Minimal inhibitory concentration

MODS	Microscopic observation drug susceptibility
MSH	Management Sciences for Health
NAAT	Nucleic acid amplification test
NALC	N-acetyl L-cysteine
NaOH	Sodium hydroxide
NIOSH	National Institute for Occupational Services and Health
NNRTI	Non-nucleoside reverse transcriptase inhibitors
NRA	Nitrate reductase assay
NTM	Non-tuberculous mycobacteria
NTP	National tuberculosis control program
PCTC	Patients' Charter for Tuberculosis Care
PI	Protease inhibitor
PLHIV	People living with HIV
PPM	Public-private mix
PZA	Pyrazinamide
RIF	Rifampicin
RR	Risk ratio
STI	Sexually transmitted infection
TB	Tuberculosis
TBCTA	Tuberculosis Coalition for Technical Assistance
TNF	Tumor necrosis factor
TST	Tuberculin skin test (Mantoux)
USAID	United States Agency for International Development
WHO	World Health Organization
XDR	Extensively drug-resistant
ZN	Ziehl-Neelsen staining

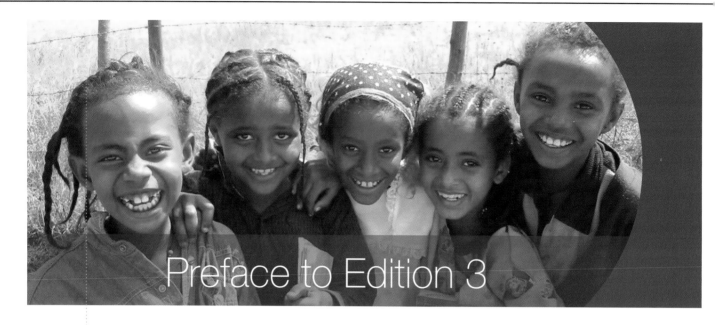

Preface to Edition 3

Development Process

The standards in the ISTC are all supported by existing WHO guidelines and policy statements, many of which had recently been developed using rigorous methodology.

Development of the first edition of the *International Standards for Tuberculosis Care* (*ISTC*) was funded by the United States Agency for International Development (USAID) via the Tuberculosis Coalition for Technical Assistance (TBCTA) and was guided by an expert committee of 28 members from 14 countries representing relevant perspectives and areas of expertise. The committee was co-chaired by Mario Raviglione of the World Health Organization (WHO) and Philip Hopewell of the American Thoracic Society (ATS). The group first agreed on a content outline and then identified areas in which systematic reviews were needed. Six reviews, largely related to approaches to diagnosis, were conducted and subsequently published in peer-reviewed publications.

Development of Edition 2 of the *ISTC* was also funded by USAID via its TB Control Assistance Program (TBCAP). A new expert committee of 56 persons from 15 countries, plus WHO, chaired by Drs. Raviglione and Hopewell guided the process. Only one systematic review, related to contact investigation (subsequently published), was identified.

Edition 3 was again funded by USAID via TB CARE I and was developed using essentially the same process. Development was led by Mukund Uplekar (WHO) and Philip Hopewell (ATS). A steering committee from the staff of the Global TB Programme at the WHO identified areas in which revisions were needed. It was felt that no new systematic reviews were needed for this edition. The standards in the *ISTC* are all supported by existing WHO guidelines and policy statements, many of which had recently been developed using rigorous methodology, including systematic reviews. The draft document was then reviewed by an expert committee of 27 members from 13 countries, co-chaired by Drs. Uplekar and Hopewell. Subsequent drafts were also reviewed and approved by the expert committee. The final draft was reviewed and approved by the TB CARE I member organizations (ATS, FHI 360, the Japan Antituberculosis Association [JATA], KNCV Tuberculosis Foundation [KNCV], Management Sciences for Health [MSH], the International Union against Tuberculosis and Lung Disease [The Union], and WHO).

Key differences between *ISTC* Edition 2 and Edition 3

Edition 1 of the *ISTC* stated, "The *Standards* should be viewed as a living document that will be revised as technology, resources, and circumstances change." It has now been five years since Edition 2 of the *ISTC* was published (2009); new information has emerged; new approaches are now feasible; and new guidelines have been written. These changes warrant an updating of the *ISTC* to be consistent with the concept of a "living document."

It was also stated in Edition 1 that, "As written, the *Standards* are presented within a context of what is generally considered to be feasible now or in the near future." There is continued recognition that not all of the standards in this edition can be met in all places at this time. However, given the rapidity of technical advances and deployment of new technologies and approaches, it is anticipated that compliance with the standards will be possible in most places in the near future. It is hoped that having standards that are higher than the minimum necessary will serve to stimulate more rapid improvements in tuberculosis care worldwide.

It must be emphasized that the basic principles that underlie the *ISTC* have not changed. Case detection and curative treatment remain the cornerstones of tuberculosis care and control and the fundamental responsibility of providers to ensure completion of treatment is unchanged. Within these basic principles, however, there have been changes that are of sufficient importance to be incorporated into the *ISTC*. The areas of change that are addressed are summarized in Table 1.

An important companion document of which the reader should be aware is *The Handbook for Utilizing the International Standards for Tuberculosis Care*. The *Handbook* is based mainly on experiences in countries that began utilizing the *ISTC* soon after it was developed and provided documentation of these experiences. The findings from these pilot countries are summarized briefly in the Introduction. The *Handbook* is available at www.istcweb.org. A set of training modules based on the third edition of the ISTC is also available on the same website. Summaries of the utilization handbook and the training materials are in Annexes 2 and 3, respectively. Revisions of the *Handbook* and training modules will be available online in October 2014.

A second companion document, the *Patients' Charter for Tuberculosis Care* (*PCTC*), was developed in tandem with the first edition of the ISTC and describes patient rights and responsibilities. The *ISTC* and the *PCTC* are mutually reinforcing documents, serving to define expectations from both the provider and the patient perspective. The *PCTC* is also available at www.istcweb.org.

TABLE 1.

Key differences between the 2009 and 2014 editions of the *ISTC*

Section	Key Differences
Overall	• Relevant WHO guidelines published since 2008 have been included. • References have been reviewed and, where necessary, replaced with new references to reflect current information. • The wording has been tightened and made more concise throughout.
Introduction	• Language has been added indicating that an additional purpose of the *ISTC* is to provide support to the integrated, patient-centered care and prevention component of WHO's global strategy for tuberculosis prevention, care, and control after 2015. Engagement of all providers is a critical component of the updated strategy and the *ISTC* will serve as a means of facilitating implementation of the strategy, especially among private providers. • Also noted is the importance of identifying individuals or groups at increased risk of tuberculosis and utilizing appropriate screening methods and preventive interventions in these persons or groups.
Standards for Diagnosis	
Standard 1	• This is a new standard emphasizing the responsibility of providers to be aware of individual and population risk factors for tuberculosis and to reduce diagnostic delay.
Standard 2	• Formerly Standard 1. The wording has been changed to include radiographic abnormalities as an indication for evaluation for tuberculosis. • The discussion of the standard emphasizes the importance of including not only cough, but also fever, night sweats, and weight loss as indications for evaluation for tuberculosis.
Standard 3	• Formerly Standard 2. The current WHO recommendations for use of rapid molecular testing as the initial microbiologic test in specified patients are now included. • The WHO recommendation against using serologic assays for diagnosing tuberculosis is emphasized.
Standard 4	• Previous Standard 4 now combined with Standard 1. • The importance of microbiological diagnosis of extrapulmonary tuberculosis is emphasized. • WHO recommendations for the use of rapid molecular testing for samples from extrapulmonary sites are included.
Standard 5	• The WHO recommendations for use of rapid molecular testing for diagnosis of tuberculosis among persons who are suspected of having the disease but have negative sputum smear microscopy are presented.
Standard 6	• The WHO recommendations for the use of rapid molecular testing for the diagnosis of tuberculosis in children are presented.

TABLE 1.

Key differences between the 2009 and 2014 editions of the *ISTC*

Section	Key Differences
Standards for Treatment	
Standard 7	• No change
Standard 8	• No change
Standard 9	• No change
Standard 10	• The role of microscopy in monitoring response in patients who had the diagnosis established by a rapid molecular test is described.
Standard 11	• This standard describes the use of Xpert® MTB/RIF in assessing for rifampicin resistance and line probe assay for detecting resistance to both isoniazid and rifampicin.
Standard 12	• The standard has been changed to reflect the revised WHO recommendations for programmatic management of drug-resistant tuberculosis.
Standard 13	• No change
Standards for Addressing HIV Infection and other Co-morbid Conditions	
Standard 14	• No change
Standard 15	• The standard has been modified to reflect the current WHO recommendations for treating HIV in PLHIV who have tuberculosis .
Standard 16	• No change
Standard 17	• No change
Standards for Public Health and Prevention	
Standard 18	• No change
Standard 19	• No change
Standard 20	• No change
Standard 21	• No change

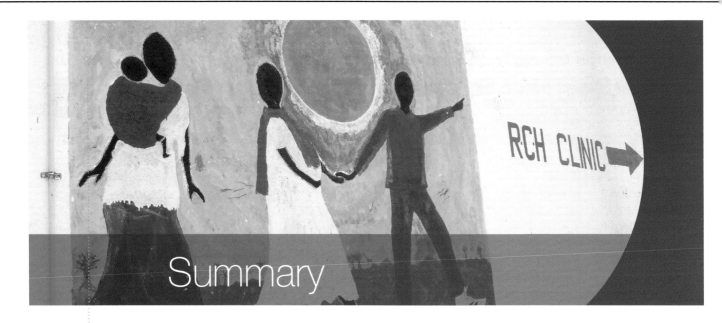

Summary

All providers who undertake evaluation and treatment of patients with tuberculosis must recognize that, not only are they delivering care to an individual, they are assuming an important public health function.

The purpose of the *International Standards for Tuberculosis Care* (*ISTC*) is to describe a widely accepted level of care that all practitioners, public and private, should seek to achieve in managing patients who have, are suspected of having, or are at increased risk of developing tuberculosis. The standards are intended to promote the effective engagement of all providers in delivering high quality care for patients of all ages, including those with sputum smear-positive and sputum smear-negative pulmonary tuberculosis, extrapulmonary tuberculosis, tuberculosis caused by drug-resistant *Mycobacterium tuberculosis* complex (*M. tuberculosis*) organisms, and tuberculosis combined with HIV infection and other co-morbidities. Moreover, there is increasing recognition of the importance for providers to employ proven approaches to screening and prevention of tuberculosis in persons at increased risk of developing the disease.

The basic principles of care for persons with, or suspected of having, tuberculosis are the same worldwide: a diagnosis should be established promptly and accurately; standardized treatment regimens of proven efficacy should be used, together with appropriate treatment support and supervision; the response to treatment should be monitored; and the essential public health responsibilities must be carried out. Prompt, accurate diagnosis and appropriate treatment are the most effective means of interrupting transmission of *M. tuberculosis*. As well as being essential for good patient care, they are the foundation of the public health response to tuberculosis. **Thus, all providers who undertake evaluation and treatment of patients with tuberculosis must recognize that, not only are they delivering care to an individual, they are assuming an important public health function that entails a high level of responsibility to the community and to the individual patient.**

Many national and international guidelines are directed toward and accessible to providers working for government tuberculosis control programs. Moreover, these providers are subject to regular monitoring and evaluation. However, private providers are generally not considered to be the main target for guidelines and recommendations and don't undergo assessments of the care they provide. Consequently, the *ISTC* is focused mainly on private and non-program public sector providers. It should be emphasized, however, that national and local tuberculosis control programs may need to develop policies and procedures that enable non-program providers to adhere to the *ISTC*. Such accommodations may be necessary, for example, to facilitate treatment supervision and contact investigations, as described in the *ISTC*.

In addition to private sector health care providers and government tuberculosis programs, both patients and communities are part of the intended audience. Patients are increasingly aware of and expect that their care will measure up to a high standard. Having generally agreed upon standards will empower patients to evaluate the quality of care they are being provided. Good care for individuals with tuberculosis is also in the best interest of the community.

The standards in the *ISTC* are intended to be complementary to local and national tuberculosis control policies that are consistent with WHO recommendations. They are not intended to replace local guidelines and were written to accommodate local differences in practice. They focus on the contribution that good clinical care of individual patients with or suspected of having tuberculosis makes to population-based tuberculosis control. A balanced approach emphasizing both individual patient care and public health principles of disease control is essential to reduce the suffering and economic losses from tuberculosis.

The *ISTC* is also intended to serve as a companion to and support for the *Patients' Charter for Tuberculosis Care*. The *Charter* specifies patients' rights and responsibilities and will serve as a set of standards from the point of view of the patient, defining what the patient should expect from the provider and what the provider should expect from the patient.

The *ISTC* should be viewed as a living document that will be revised as technology, resources, and circumstances change. As written, the standards in the *ISTC* are presented within a context of what is generally considered to be feasible now or in the near future.

The standards are as follows:

Standards for Diagnosis

Standard 1. To ensure early diagnosis, providers must be aware of individual and group risk factors for tuberculosis and perform prompt clinical evaluations and appropriate diagnostic testing for persons with symptoms and findings consistent with tuberculosis.

Standard 2. All patients, including children, with unexplained cough lasting two or more weeks or with unexplained findings suggestive of tuberculosis on chest radiographs should be evaluated for tuberculosis.

Standard 3. All patients, including children, who are suspected of having pulmonary tuberculosis and are capable of producing sputum should have at least two sputum specimens submitted for smear microscopy or a single sputum specimen for Xpert® MTB/RIF* testing in a quality-assured laboratory. Patients at risk for drug resistance, who have HIV risks, or who are seriously ill, should have Xpert MTB/RIF performed as the initial diagnostic test. Blood-based serologic tests and interferon-gamma release assays should not be used for diagnosis of active tuberculosis.

*As of this writing, Xpert®MTB/RIF (Cepheid Corp. Sunnyvale, California, USA) is the only rapid molecular test approved by WHO for initial use in diagnosing tuberculosis, thus, it is specifically referred to by its trade name throughout this document.

Standard 4. For all patients, including children, suspected of having extrapulmonary tuberculosis, appropriate specimens from the suspected sites of involvement should be obtained for microbiological and histological examination. An Xpert MTB/RIF test is recommended as the preferred initial microbiological test for suspected tuberculous meningitis because of the need for a rapid diagnosis.

Standard 5. In patients suspected of having pulmonary tuberculosis whose sputum smears are negative, Xpert MTB/RIF and/or sputum cultures should be performed. Among smear- and Xpert MTB/RIF negative persons with clinical evidence strongly suggestive of tuberculosis, antituberculosis treatment should be initiated after collection of specimens for culture examination.

Standard 6. For all children suspected of having intrathoracic (i.e., pulmonary, pleural, and mediastinal or hilar lymph node) tuberculosis, bacteriological confirmation should be sought through examination of respiratory secretions (expectorated sputum, induced sputum, gastric lavage) for smear microscopy, an Xpert MTB/RIF test, and/or culture.

Standards for Treatment

Standard 7. To fulfill her/his public health responsibility, as well as responsibility to the individual patient, the provider must prescribe an appropriate treatment regimen, monitor adherence to the regimen, and, when necessary, address factors leading to interruption or discontinuation of treatment. Fulfilling these responsibilities will likely require coordination with local public health services and/or other agencies.

Standard 8. All patients who have not been treated previously and do not have other risk factors for drug resistance should receive a WHO-approved first-line treatment regimen using quality assured drugs. The initial phase should consist of two months of isoniazid, rifampicin, pyrazinamide, and ethambutol.* The continuation phase should consist of isoniazid and rifampicin given for 4 months. The doses of antituberculosis drugs used should conform to WHO recommendations. Fixed-dose combination drugs may provide a more convenient form of drug administration.

*Ethambutol may be omitted in children who are HIV-negative and who have non-cavitary tuberculosis.

Standard 9. A patient-centered approach to treatment should be developed for all patients in order to promote adherence, improve quality of life, and relieve suffering. This approach should be based on the patient's needs and mutual respect between the patient and the provider.

Standard 10. Response to treatment in patients with pulmonary tuberculosis (including those with tuberculosis diagnosed by a rapid molecular test) should be monitored by follow up sputum smear microscopy at the time of completion of the initial phase of treatment (two months). If the sputum smear is positive at completion of the initial phase, sputum microscopy should be performed again at 3 months and, if positive, rapid molecular drug sensitivity testing (line probe assays or Xpert MTB/RIF) or culture with drug susceptibility testing should be performed. In patients with extrapulmonary tuberculosis and in children, the response to treatment is best assessed clinically.

Standard 11. An assessment of the likelihood of drug resistance, based on history of prior treatment, exposure to a possible source case having drug-resistant organisms, and the community prevalence of drug resistance (if known), should be undertaken for all patients. Drug susceptibility testing should be performed at the start of therapy for all patients at a risk of drug resistance. Patients who remain sputum smear-positive at completion of 3 months of treatment, patients in whom treatment has failed, and patients who have been lost to follow up or relapsed following one or more courses of treatment should always be assessed for drug resistance. For patients in whom drug resistance is considered to be likely an Xpert MTB/RIF test should be the initial diagnostic test. If rifampicin resistance is detected, culture and testing for susceptibility to isoniazid, fluoroquinolones, and second-line injectable drugs should be performed promptly. Patient counseling and education, as well as treatment with an empirical second-line regimen, should begin immediately to minimize the potential for transmission. Infection control measures appropriate to the setting should be applied.

Standard 12. Patients with or highly likely to have tuberculosis caused by drug-resistant (especially MDR/XDR) organisms should be treated with specialized regimens containing quality-assured second-line antituberculosis drugs. The doses of antituberculosis drugs should conform to WHO recommendations. The regimen chosen may be standardized or based on presumed or confirmed drug susceptibility patterns. At least five drugs, pyrazinamide and four drugs to which the organisms are known or presumed to be susceptible, including an injectable agent, should be used in a 6–8 month intensive phase, and at least 3 drugs to which the organisms are known or presumed to be susceptible, should be used in the continuation phase. Treatment should be given for at least 18–24 months beyond culture conversion. Patient-centered measures, including observation of treatment, are required to ensure adherence. Consultation with a specialist experienced in treatment of patients with MDR/XDR tuberculosis should be obtained.

Standard 13. An accessible, systematically maintained record of all medications given, bacteriologic response, outcomes, and adverse reactions should be maintained for all patients.

Standards for Addressing HIV Infection and other Co-morbid Conditions

Standard 14. HIV testing and counseling should be conducted for all patients with, or suspected of having, tuberculosis unless there is a confirmed negative test within the previous two months. Because of the close relationship of tuberculosis and HIV infection, integrated approaches to prevention, diagnosis, and treatment of both tuberculosis and HIV infection are recommended in areas with high HIV prevalence. HIV testing is of special importance as part of routine management of all patients in areas with a high prevalence of HIV infection in the general population, in patients with symptoms and/or signs of HIV-related conditions, and in patients having a history suggestive of high risk of HIV exposure.

Standard 15. In persons with HIV infection and tuberculosis who have profound immunosuppression (CD4 counts less than 50 cells/mm^3), ART should be initiated within 2 weeks of beginning treatment for tuberculosis unless tuberculous meningitis is present. For all other patients with HIV and tuberculosis, regardless of CD4 counts, antiretroviral therapy should be initiated within 8 weeks of beginning treatment for tuberculosis. Patients with tuberculosis and HIV infection should also receive cotrimoxazole as prophylaxis for other infections.

Standard 16. Persons with HIV infection who, after careful evaluation, do not have active tuberculosis should be treated for presumed latent tuberculosis infection with isoniazid for at least 6 months.

Standard 17. All providers should conduct a thorough assessment for co-morbid conditions and other factors that could affect tuberculosis treatment response or outcome and identify additional services that would support an optimal outcome for each patient. These services should be incorporated into an individualized plan of care that includes assessment of and referrals for treatment of other illnesses. Particular attention should be paid to diseases or conditions known to affect treatment outcome, for example, diabetes mellitus, drug and alcohol abuse, undernutrition, and tobacco smoking. Referrals to other psychosocial support services or to such services as antenatal or well-baby care should also be provided.

Standards for Public Health and Prevention

Standard 18. All providers should ensure that persons in close contact with patients who have infectious tuberculosis are evaluated and managed in line with international recommendations. The highest priority contacts for evaluation are:

- Persons with symptoms suggestive of tuberculosis
- Children aged <5 years
- Contacts with known or suspected immunocompromised states, particularly HIV infection
- Contacts of patients with MDR/XDR tuberculosis

Standard 19. Children <5 years of age and persons of any age with HIV infection who are close contacts of a person with infectious tuberculosis, and who, after careful evaluation, do not have active tuberculosis, should be treated for presumed latent tuberculosis infection with isoniazid for at least six months.

Standard 20. Each health care facility caring for patients who have, or are suspected of having, infectious tuberculosis should develop and implement an appropriate tuberculosis infection control plan to minimize possible transmission of *M. tuberculosis* to patients and health care workers.

Standard 21. All providers must report both new and re-treatment tuberculosis cases and their treatment outcomes to local public health authorities, in conformance with applicable legal requirements and policies.

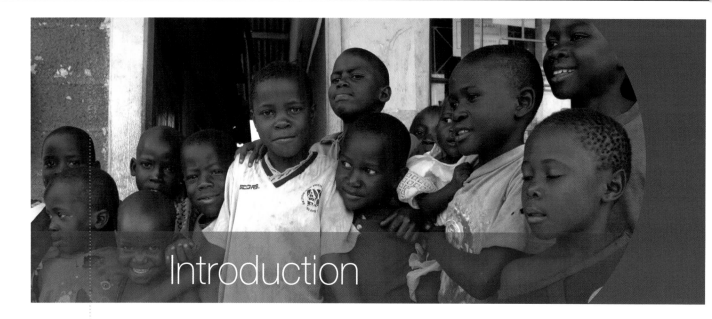

Introduction

Purpose

The ISTC is intended to facilitate the effective engagement of all care providers in delivering high quality care utilizing established best practices for patients of all ages with all forms of tuberculosis.

The fundamental purpose of the *International Standards for Tuberculosis Care* (*ISTC*) is to describe a widely accepted level of care that all practitioners, public and private, should seek to achieve in managing patients who have or are suspected of having tuberculosis, or are at increased risk of developing the disease. The *ISTC* is intended to facilitate the effective engagement of all care providers in delivering high quality care utilizing established best practices for patients of all ages with all forms of tuberculosis. In addition, providers must be aware of conditions and epidemiologic circumstances that impose an increased risk of tuberculosis and of approaches to screening for tuberculosis and applying preventive therapies in these situations.[1]

The *ISTC* is also intended to provide support to the integrated, patient-centered tuberculosis care and prevention component of WHO's proposed *Global Strategy and Targets for Tuberculosis Prevention, Care and Control after 2015*.[2] Engagement of all providers is a critical component of the updated strategy and the *ISTC* will serve as a means of facilitating implementation of the strategy especially among non-program providers.[3,4] The updated strategy presents the framework necessary for effective tuberculosis care and control and, when fully implemented, provides the elements essential for delivery of good tuberculosis care and prevention.

Much of the information presented in the *ISTC* is derived from existing WHO documents. Thus, the *ISTC* serves as a compendium of recommendations and guidelines developed by a rigorous, evidence-based process required by WHO.[5] Taken together these documents provide comprehensive guidance for best practices in tuberculosis care and control.

In addition to the fundamental purpose of the *ISTC*, an important goal is to promote unified approaches to the diagnosis, management, and prevention of tuberculosis among all care providers offering services for tuberculosis and to facilitate coordination of activities and collaboration between tuberculosis control programs and non-program providers. Given that public health authorities are responsible for normative functions, surveillance, monitoring, evaluation, and reporting, it is crucial that there is coordination between control programs and non-program providers, especially in dealing with complicated issues such as diagnosis and management of patients with drug-resistant tuberculosis. The

ISTC provides a common ground of understanding on which to build collaborations at national, regional, or local levels, or even within individual institutions.

The basic principles of care for persons with, or suspected of having, tuberculosis are the same worldwide: a diagnosis should be established promptly and accurately; standardized treatment regimens of proven efficacy should be used, together with appropriate treatment support and supervision; the response to treatment should be monitored; and the essential public health responsibilities must be carried out. Additionally, persons at increased risk of tuberculosis should be identified, evaluated, and preventive measures applied when appropriate.[1] The ways in which these principles are applied vary depending on available technology and resources. However, prompt, accurate diagnosis and effective timely treatment are not only essential for good patient care; they are the key elements in the public health response to tuberculosis and are the cornerstone of tuberculosis control. Thus, all providers who undertake evaluation and treatment of patients with tuberculosis must recognize that, not only are they delivering care to an individual, they are also assuming an important public health function that entails a high level of responsibility to the community, as well as to the individual patient.

Audience

The *ISTC* is addressed to all health care providers, private and public, who care for persons with proven tuberculosis, with symptoms and signs suggestive of tuberculosis, or with factors that place them at increased risk of developing the disease. In many instances clinicians (both private and public) who are not part of a government-coordinated tuberculosis control program lack the guidance and systematic evaluation of outcomes provided by programs and, commonly, are not in compliance with the *ISTC*. Although government program providers are not exempt from adherence to the *ISTC*, non-program providers are the main target audience. It should be emphasized, however, that public tuberculosis control programs may need to develop policies and procedures that enable non-program providers to adhere to the *ISTC*. Such accommodations may be necessary, for example, to facilitate treatment supervision and contact investigations.[6-8] In addition to health care providers and government tuberculosis programs, both patients and communities are part of the intended audience. Patients are increasingly aware of and have the right to care that measures up to a high standard, as described in the *Patients' Charter for Tuberculosis Care* (available at http://www.istcweb.org and at http://www.who.int/tb/publications/2006/istc_charter.pdf). Having generally agreed upon standards will empower patients to evaluate the quality of care they are being provided. Good care for individuals with tuberculosis is also in the best interest of the community. Community contributions to tuberculosis care and control are increasingly important in raising public awareness of the disease, providing treatment support, encouraging adherence, reducing the stigma associated with having tuberculosis, and demanding that health care providers in the community adhere to a high standard of tuberculosis care.[9] The community should expect that care for tuberculosis will be up to the accepted standard and, thus, create a demand for high quality services.

The standards focus on the contribution that good clinical care of individual patients with or suspected of having tuberculosis makes to population-based tuberculosis control.

Scope

The *ISTC* draws from a number of existing WHO guidelines and recommendations developed using modern rigorous methodology to provide its evidence base. In addition, generally we have cited summaries, meta-analyses, and systematic reviews of evidence that have examined and synthesized primary data, rather than referring to the primary data themselves. Throughout the document we have used the terminology recommended in the *Definitions and Reporting Framework for Tuberculosis, 2013 Revision.*[10]

The *ISTC* is intended to be complementary to and provide support for local and national tuberculosis control policies that are consistent with WHO recommendations. They are not intended to replace local guidelines and were written to accommodate local differences in practice while at the same time fostering a high standard of care. They focus on the contribution that good clinical care of individual patients with or suspected of having tuberculosis makes to population-based tuberculosis control. A balanced approach emphasizing both individual patient care and public health principles of disease control is essential to reduce the suffering and individual and community economic losses from tuberculosis.

To meet the requirements of the *ISTC*, approaches and strategies determined by local circumstances and practices and developed in collaboration with local and national public health authorities will be necessary. There are many situations in which local conditions, practices, and resources will support a level of care beyond what is described in the *ISTC*.

The *ISTC* should be viewed as a living document that will be revised as technology, resources, and circumstances change. As written, the standards are presented within a context of what is generally considered to be feasible now or in the near future. Within the standards priorities may be set that will foster appropriate incremental changes, such as moving in a stepwise from no, or very limited, drug susceptibility testing to universal testing.

The *ISTC* is also intended to serve as a companion to and support for the *Patients' Charter for Tuberculosis Care.* The *Charter* specifies patients' rights and responsibilities and serves as a set of standards from the point of view of the patient, defining what the patient should expect from the provider and what the provider should expect from the patient.

An additional use of the *ISTC* has been to serve as a model framework for adaptation (see below) by countries or regions as has been done, for example, for the European Union and India.[11,12]

There are several critical areas that are beyond the scope of the document. The *ISTC* does not address the issue of access to care. Obviously, if there is no care available, the quality of care is not relevant. Additionally, there are many factors that impede access even when care is available: poverty, gender, stigma, and geography are prominent among the factors that interfere with persons seeking or receiving care. Also, if the residents of a given area perceive that the quality of care provided by the local facilities is substandard, they will not seek care there. This perception of quality is a component of access that adherence to these standards will address.[3]

Also not addressed by the *ISTC* is the necessity of having a sound, effective tuberculosis control program based on established public health principles. The level of care described in the *ISTC* cannot be achieved without there being an enabling environment, generally provided by an effective public health program supported by appropriate legal and regulatory framework and financial resources. The requirements of such programs are described in publications from the WHO, the US Centers for Disease Control and Prevention (CDC), and The International Union Against Tuberculosis and Lung Disease (The Union).[13-16] Having an effective control program at the national or local level with linkages to non-program providers enables bidirectional communication of information including case notification, consultation, patient referral, provision of drugs or services such as treatment supervision/ support for private patients, and contact evaluation. In addition, the program may be the only source of quality-assured laboratory services for the private sector.

In providing care for patients with or suspected of having tuberculosis, or at risk of the disease, clinicians and persons responsible for health care facilities should take measures that reduce the potential for transmission of *M. tuberculosis* to health care workers and to other patients by following local, national, or international guidelines for infection control.[17-19] This is especially true in areas or specific populations with a high prevalence of HIV infection. Detailed recommendations are contained in the WHO document, *WHO Policy on TB Infection Control in Health-care Facilities, Congregate Settings and Households*.[18]

Rationale

Although in the past decade there has been substantial progress in the development and implementation of the strategies necessary for effective tuberculosis control, the disease remains an enormous global health problem.[20,21] It is estimated that one-third of the world's population is infected with *M. tuberculosis*, mostly in developing countries where 95% of cases occur. In 2012, there were an estimated 8.6 million new cases of tuberculosis. The number of tuberculosis cases that occur in the world each year has been declining slightly for the past few years, and the global incidence per 100,000 population is decreasing at slightly more than 2%/year.[21] Incidence, prevalence, and mortality are now decreasing in all six of the WHO regions. In Africa, the case rate has only recently begun to decrease but remains very high both because of the epidemic of HIV infection in sub-Saharan countries and the poor health systems and primary care services throughout the region. In Eastern Europe, after a decade of increases, case rates reached a plateau in the early 2000's and now have begun to decrease slightly. The increases in the 1990's are attributable to the collapse of the public health infrastructure, increased poverty, and other socio-economic factors complicated further by the high prevalence of drug-resistant tuberculosis.[22] In many countries, because of incomplete application of effective care and control measures, tuberculosis case rates are either stagnant or decreasing more slowly than should be expected. This is especially true in high-risk groups such as persons with HIV infection, the homeless, and recent immigrants. The failure to bring about a more rapid reduction in tuberculosis incidence, at least in part, relates to a failure to fully engage non-tuberculosis control program providers in the provision of high quality care, in coordination with local and national control programs. Fostering such engagement is an important purpose of the *ISTC*.[6]

It is widely recognized that many providers are involved in the diagnosis and treatment of tuberculosis.[23] Traditional healers, general and specialist physicians in private practice, nurses, clinical officers, academic physicians, unlicensed practitioners, and community organizations, among others, all play roles in tuberculosis care and, therefore, in tuberculosis control. In addition, other public providers, such as those working in prisons, army hospitals, or public hospitals and facilities, regularly evaluate persons suspected of having tuberculosis and treat patients who have the disease.

Little is known about the adequacy of care delivered by non-program providers, but evidence from studies conducted in many different parts of the world show great variability in the quality of tuberculosis care, and poor quality care continues to plague global tuberculosis control efforts even in low-prevalence, high-income settings.[24,25] A global situation assessment reported by WHO suggested that delays in diagnosis were common.[26,27] The delay was more often in receiving a diagnosis rather than in seeking care, although both elements have been shown to be important.[27,28] Even after a patient is found to have a positive sputum smear, delays are common.[29] The WHO survey and other studies also show that clinicians, in particular those who work in the private health care sector, often deviate from standard, internationally recommended, tuberculosis management practices. These deviations include under-utilization of sputum smear microscopy for diagnosis, generally associated with over-reliance on radiography; use of non-recommended drug regimens with incorrect combinations of drugs and mistakes in both drug dosage and duration of treatment; and failure to supervise and assure adherence to treatment.[25,26,30-36] Recent evidence also suggests over-reliance on poorly validated or inappropriate diagnostic tests such as serologic assays, often in preference to conventional bacteriological evaluations.[37] Because of the unreliability of these tests the WHO has taken the unusual step of specifically recommending against their use.[38]

Together, these findings highlight flaws in health care practices that lead to substandard tuberculosis care for populations that, sadly, are most vulnerable to the disease and are least able to bear the consequences of such systemic failures. Any person anywhere in the world who is unable to access quality health care should be considered vulnerable to tuberculosis and its consequences.[3] Likewise, any community with no or inadequate access to appropriate diagnostic and treatment services for tuberculosis is a vulnerable community. The *ISTC* is intended to reduce vulnerability of individuals and communities to tuberculosis by promoting high quality care for persons with, or suspected of having, tuberculosis.

There is also an ethical imperative, which applies equally to program and non-program providers, to the provision of effective, appropriate tuberculosis care.[39] Tuberculosis care (including prevention) is a public good. The disease not only threatens the health of individuals, the health of the community is also at risk. It is generally agreed that universal access to health care is a human right and governments have the ethical responsibility to ensure access, a responsibility that includes access to quality-assured tuberculosis services. In particular, tuberculosis disproportionately affects poor and marginalized people, groups that governments and health care systems have an ethical obligation to protect. Tuberculosis not only thrives on poverty, it breeds poverty by consuming often very limited personal and family resources. Poor care compounds the costs that already impoverished individuals and families cannot afford and commonly results in persons being unable to work for long periods while at the same time incurring catastrophic costs.[40,41] Substandard care, be it on the part of program or non-program providers, is unethical. The care and control measures in the *ISTC* describe approaches to tuberculosis care, control, and prevention that are consistent with the ethical standards articulated by the *Guidance on Ethics of Tuberculosis Prevention, Care, and Control* developed by the WHO.[39]

Utilization of the *ISTC*

The *ISTC* is potentially a very powerful tool to improve the quality of tuberculosis care. Because of the way in which the *ISTC* was developed and the international endorsements it has received through the two previous editions, the document is authoritative and broadly credible across categories of practitioners. This credibility is a major strength of the *ISTC* and should be capitalized upon in its utilization. A variety of possible ways in which the *ISTC* can be utilized is summarized in Annex 2.

Ideally, the *ISTC* should be used in conjunction with a set of tools developed by WHO, *Public-Private Mix for TB Care and Control: A Toolkit.*[6] The tools included in the *Toolkit* present a framework for analyzing the role of all sectors in providing tuberculosis care and control and a variety of tools to facilitate engagement of all providers. In addition, the *ISTC* should be used in conjunction with the *Patients' Charter for Tuberculosis Care,* which was developed in tandem with the *ISTC* and specifies the rights and responsibilities of patients. A third document developed by The Union, *Management of Tuberculosis: A Guide to the Essentials of Good Practice*[16], focuses on the critical roles of nurses and other health workers in providing tuberculosis services and in managing tuberculosis control programs. Taken together these documents provide a framework and guidance that can be used to develop a tailored, comprehensive multi-sectoral approach to tuberculosis care and control at the local or national level, with each component having a set of defined roles and responsibilities.

Adaptation of the *ISTC*

The *ISTC* has been developed for a global audience and it is expected and desirable that regions and countries adapt and operationalize the document to suit their own circumstances. These circumstances include consideration of the epidemiology of tuberculosis and the facilities and resources available in both the public and private sectors. The ultimate goal of these adaptations should be to improve the quality of services for tuberculosis within a more limited setting. Ideally, a consultative process involving all relevant stakeholders should be undertaken to ensure that the adaptation of the *ISTC* is appropriate for the environment and provides appropriate guidance for implementation of the practices described in the document. Moreover, broad input is necessary to ensure that the document reflects the perspectives of all sectors of the health care system and creates a sense of ownership of and commitment to the principles and practices described in the *ISTC*.

As with any set of guidelines, there should be establishment of an effective and standardized monitoring and evaluation (M&E) system. To enable global M&E it is strongly suggested that adaptations retain the title *International Standards for Tuberculosis Care* as part of the adapted document's title.

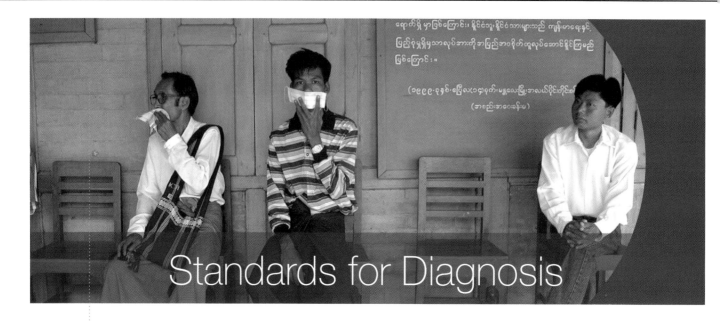

Standards for Diagnosis

STANDARD 1. To ensure early diagnosis, providers must be aware of individual and group risk factors for tuberculosis and perform prompt clinical evaluations and appropriate diagnostic testing for persons with symptoms and findings consistent with tuberculosis.

Providers must recognize that in evaluating persons who may have tuberculosis they are assuming an essential public health function that entails a high level of responsibility to the community as well as to the individual patient.

Rationale and Evidence Summary

Providers must recognize that in evaluating persons who may have tuberculosis they are assuming an essential public health function that entails a high level of responsibility to the community as well as to the individual patient. Early and accurate diagnosis is critical to tuberculosis care and control.[42] Despite dramatically improved access to high quality tuberculosis services during the past two decades[21], there is substantial evidence that failure to identify cases early is a major weakness in efforts to ensure optimal outcomes for the patient and to control the disease. Diagnostic delays result in ongoing transmission in the community and more severe, progressive disease in the affected person.

There are three main reasons for delays in diagnosing tuberculosis: the affected person either not seeking or not having access to care; the provider not suspecting the disease; and the lack of sensitivity of the most commonly available diagnostic test, sputum (or other specimen) smear microscopy.[27,28,42] Approaches to reducing these delays are, obviously, quite different. Reducing delays on the part of the affected person entails providing accessible health care facilities, enhancing community and individual awareness, and active case-finding in high risk populations—all of which are largely beyond the scope of this document.[9] Reducing provider delay is best approached by increasing provider awareness of the risks for and symptoms of tuberculosis and of the appropriate and available WHO-approved diagnostic tests in their communities. Rapid molecular tests that increase both the speed and the sensitivity for identifying *Mycobacterium tuberculosis* are increasingly available and, in some situations as described in Standards 3, 5, and 6, are the recommended initial diagnostic test.

Providers commonly fail to initiate appropriate investigations when persons with symptoms suggestive of tuberculosis, especially respiratory symptoms, seek care.[29] Of particular note, in at least one study women were less likely to receive an appropriate diagnostic evaluation than men.[43] There must be a clinical suspicion of tuberculosis before proper diagnostic tests are ordered. Clinical suspicion is prompted largely by the presence of clinical symptoms, suggestive radiographic findings, and by awareness of co-morbidities and epidemiological circumstances that increase the risk of tuberculosis in an individual patient. These risks are summarized in the WHO guidelines for screening for tuberculosis.[1] Vulnerable groups such as persons living with HIV and other co-morbidities, children, and populations at increased risk such as prisoners and persons living in high-incidence urban areas require special attention, even in the absence of typical symptoms, as noted subsequently.

STANDARD 2. **All patients, including children, with unexplained cough lasting two or more weeks or with unexplained findings suggestive of tuberculosis on chest radiographs should be evaluated for tuberculosis.**

Rationale and Evidence Summary

The most commonly reported symptom of pulmonary tuberculosis is persistent cough that generally, but not always, is productive of mucus and sometimes blood (hemoptysis). In persons with tuberculosis the cough is often accompanied by systemic symptoms such as fever, night sweats, and weight loss. In addition, findings such as lymphadenopathy consistent with concurrent extrapulmonary tuberculosis, may be noted, especially in patients with HIV infection. However, chronic cough with sputum production is not always present, even among persons having sputum smears showing acid-fast bacilli. Data from several tuberculosis prevalence surveys show that an important proportion of persons with active tuberculosis do not have cough of 2 or more weeks that conventionally has been used to define suspected tuberculosis.[44-46] In these studies 10–25% of patients with bacteriologically-confirmed tuberculosis do not report cough. These data suggest that evaluation for tuberculosis, using a symptom review that includes, in addition to cough of 2 weeks or more, cough of any duration, fever, night sweats, or weight loss, may be indicated in select risk groups, especially in areas where there is a high prevalence of the disease and in high risk populations and individuals with increased susceptibility, such as persons with HIV infection.[1] Use of this broadened set of questions in a population of PLHIV was found to have a negative predictive value of 97.7% for tuberculosis.[47]

Although many patients with pulmonary tuberculosis have cough, the symptom is not specific to tuberculosis; it can occur in a wide range of respiratory conditions, including acute respiratory tract infections, asthma, and chronic obstructive pulmonary disease.[48] Having cough of 2 weeks or more in duration serves as the criterion for defining suspected tuberculosis and is used in most national and international guidelines, particularly in areas of moderate to high prevalence of tuberculosis, as an indication to initiate an evaluation for the disease.[16,49,50] In a survey conducted in primary health care services of 9 low- and middle-income countries with a low prevalence of HIV infection, respiratory complaints, including cough, constituted on average 18.4% of symptoms that prompted a visit to a health center for persons older than 5 years of age.[51] Of this group, 5% of patients overall were categorized as possibly having tuberculosis because of the presence of an unexplained cough for more than 2–3 weeks. This percentage varies somewhat depending on whether there is pro-active questioning concerning the presence of

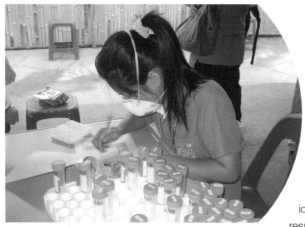

Missed opportunities for earlier detection of tuberculosis lead to increased disease severity for the patients and a greater likelihood of transmission of M. tuberculosis to family members and others in the community.

cough. Respiratory conditions, therefore, constitute a substantial proportion of the burden of diseases in patients presenting to primary health care services.

Even in patients with cough of less than 2 weeks there may be an appreciable prevalence of tuberculosis. An assessment from India demonstrated that by using a threshold of ≥2 weeks to prompt collection of sputum specimens, the number of patients with suspected tuberculosis increased by 61% but, more importantly, the number of tuberculosis cases identified increased by 46% compared with a threshold of >3 weeks.[52] The results also suggested that actively inquiring as to the presence of cough in all adult clinic attendees may increase the yield of cases; 15% of patients who, without prompting, volunteered that they had cough, had positive smears. In addition, 7% of patients who did not volunteer that they had cough but, on questioning, admitted to having cough ≥2 weeks had positive smears.

In countries with a low prevalence of tuberculosis, it is likely that chronic cough will be due to conditions other than tuberculosis. Conversely, in high prevalence countries, tuberculosis will be one of the leading diagnoses to consider, together with other conditions, such as asthma, bronchitis, and bronchiectasis that are common in many areas. Tuberculosis should also be considered in the differential diagnosis of community acquired pneumonia, especially if the pneumonia fails to resolve with appropriate antimicrobial treatment.[53,54] Several features have been identified that suggest tuberculosis in patients hospitalized for community acquired pneumonia. These are age less than 65 years, night sweats, hemoptysis, weight loss, exposure to tuberculosis, and upper lobe opacities on chest radiograph.[54]

Unfortunately, several studies suggest that not all patients with respiratory symptoms receive an adequate evaluation for tuberculosis.[26-30,32-35,43,55-58] These failures result in missed opportunities for earlier detection of tuberculosis and lead to increased disease severity for the patients and a greater likelihood of transmission of *M. tuberculosis* to family members and others in the community.

Although sputum (or other specimen) smear microscopy remains the most widely available test to establish a microbiological diagnosis, other more sensitive means of identifying *M. tuberculosis*, particularly rapid molecular tests, are rapidly gaining acceptance as their performance and applicability are increasingly understood.[59,60] Table 2 presents a succinct summary of the performance and evidence base for the various diagnostic tests for tuberculosis.

In many settings chest radiographic examination is the initial test used for persons with cough since it is a useful tool to identify persons who require further evaluation to determine the cause of radiographic abnormalities, including tuberculosis.[1] Thus, radiographic examination (film, digital imaging, or fluoroscopy) of the thorax or other suspected sites of involvement may serve as the entry point for a tuberculosis diagnostic evaluation. Also, chest radiography is useful to evaluate persons who are suspected of having tuberculosis but have negative sputum smears and/or negative Xpert MTB/RIF. The radiograph is useful to find evidence of pulmonary tuberculosis and to identify other abnormalities that may be responsible for the symptoms. However, a diagnosis of tuberculosis cannot be established by radiography alone. Although the sensitivity of chest radiography for the presence of tuberculosis is high, the specificity is low, as shown in Table 2. Reliance on the chest radiograph as the sole test for the diagnosis of tuberculosis will result in both over-diagnosis of tuberculosis and missed diagnoses of tuberculosis and other diseases. Thus, the use of radiographic examinations alone to diagnose tuberculosis is unacceptable.

Scoring systems in which the likelihood of tuberculosis is estimated based on specific radiographic criteria, each of which is given a preset value, have similar sensitivity and specificity as radiographic assessment not using a scoring system.[61] Such systems are useful in ruling-out pulmonary tuberculosis, particularly for infection control purposes in hospitals, but their low specificity precludes ruling-in tuberculosis.

TABLE 2.

WHO-approved microbiologic tests for tuberculosis

Test	Site	Major Findings/results of Systematic Reviews
Diagnosis of Active Tuberculosis		
Sputum smear microscopy	**Pulmonary**	• Fluorescence microscopy is on average 10% more sensitive than conventional microscopy. Specificity of both fluorescence and conventional microscopy is similar. Fluorescence microscopy is associated with improved time efficiency.[62] • Same-day sputum smear microscopy is as accurate as standard smear microscopy. Compared with the standard approach of examination of two smears with light microscopy over 2 days, examination of two smears taken on the same day had much the same sensitivity (64% for standard microscopy vs 63% for same-day microscopy) and specificity (98% vs 98%)[63-65]
Nucleic acid amplification tests (NAATs) [other than Xpert MTB/RIF]	**Pulmonary and extra-pulmonary TB**	• Commercial, standardized NAATs have high specificity and positive predictive value, however, they have relatively lower (and highly variable) sensitivity and negative predictive value for all forms of TB, especially in smear-negative and extrapulmonary disease.[66-73]
Xpert MTB/RIF	**Pulmonary TB and extrapulmonary TB and RIF resistance**	• Xpert MTB/RIF used as an initial diagnostic test for detection of *M. tuberculosis* and rifampicin is sensitive and specific. Xpert MTB/RIF is also valuable as an add-on test following microscopy for patients who are smear-negative. An Xpert MTB/RIF result that is positive for rifampicin resistance should be carefully interpreted and take into consideration the risk of MDR TB in a given patient and the expected prevalence of MDR TB in a given setting.[73] • When used as an initial test replacing smear microscopy Xpert MTB/RIF achieved a pooled sensitivity of 88% and pooled specificity of 98%. The pooled sensitivity was 98% for smear-positive, culture-positive cases and 68% for smear-negative cases; the pooled sensitivity was 80% in people living with HIV.[73] • For detection of rifampicin resistance Xpert MTB/RIF achieved a pooled sensitivity of 94% and pooled specificity of 98%.[73]
Automated liquid cultures and rapid MPT64-based species identification tests	**Pulmonary TB and extrapulmonary TB; speciation**	• Automated liquid cultures are more sensitive than solid cultures; time to detection is more rapid than solid cultures.[72,74] • MPT64-based rapid immunochromatographic tests (ICT) for species identification has high sensitivity and specificity.[75]

TABLE 3.

Performance of chest radiography as a diagnostic test for tuberculosis

Radiographic Finding (modified from Ref 1)	Pooled Sensitivity (%)	Pooled Specificity (%)
Any abnormality compatible with TB (active or inactive)	98 (95–100)	75 (72–79)
Abnormalities suggestive of active TB	87 (79–95)	89 (87–92)
After positive screening for symptoms (one study)	90 (81–96)	56 (54–58)
Chest radiography scoring systems[61]	96 (93–98)	46 (35–50)

STANDARD 3.   All patients, including children, who are suspected of having pulmonary tuberculosis and are capable of producing sputum should have at least two sputum specimens submitted for smear microscopy or a single sputum specimen for Xpert® MTB/RIF* testing in a quality-assured laboratory. Patients at risk for drug resistance, who have HIV risks, or who are seriously ill, should have Xpert MTB/RIF performed as the initial diagnostic test. Blood-based serologic tests and interferon-gamma release assays should not be used for diagnosis of active tuberculosis.

* As of this writing, Xpert® MTB/RIF (Cepheid Corp. Sunnyvale, California, USA) is the only rapid molecular test approved by WHO for initial use in diagnosing tuberculosis, thus, it is specifically referred to by its trade name throughout this document.

Rationale and Evidence Summary

To establish a diagnosis of tuberculosis every effort must be made to identify the causative agent of the disease.[76] A microbiological diagnosis can only be confirmed by culturing *M. tuberculosis* complex or identifying specific nucleic acid sequences in a specimen from any site of disease. Because the recommended initial microbiological approach to diagnosis varies depending on risks for drug resistance, the likelihood of HIV infection and the severity of illness, clinical assessment must address these factors. Currently, WHO recommends that the Xpert MTB/RIF assay should be used rather than conventional microscopy, culture, and DST as the initial diagnostic test in adults and children suspected of having MDR TB or HIV-associated tuberculosis.[77] Although availability of rapid molecular tests is rapidly increasing, in practice there are many resource-limited settings in which rapid molecular tests or culture are not available currently. Microscopic examination of stained sputum is feasible in nearly all settings and, in high-prevalence areas, finding acid-fast bacilli in stained sputum is the equivalent of a confirmed diagnosis. It should be noted that in persons with HIV infection sputum microscopy is less sensitive than in persons without HIV infection; however, mortality rates are greater in persons with HIV infection with clinically-diagnosed tuberculosis who have negative sputum smears than among HIV-infected patients who have positive sputum smears.[78,79]

Data suggest that a combination of sputum smear microscopy and Xpert MTB/RIF can substantially increase the diagnostic yield. Xpert MTB/RIF as an add-on test following a negative smear microscopy result has a sensitivity of 68% and specificity of 99% compared with culture. WHO recommendations also indicate that Xpert MTB/RIF may be used as the initial test in all patients if resources are available.

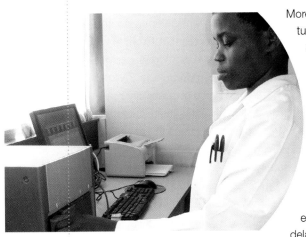

More rapid methods of identifying growth of *M. tuberculosis* such as micro culture techniques (MODS) and thin layer agar have variable performance characteristics and are not approved for general use by WHO at this time.[76]

Generally, it is the responsibility of government health systems (national tuberculosis programs [NTPs] or others) to ensure that providers and patients have convenient access to quality-assured diagnostic microbiology laboratories. As with any laboratory test it is critical that tuberculosis microbiological examinations be performed in a quality-assured laboratory.

Failure to perform a proper diagnostic evaluation before initiating treatment for tuberculosis potentially exposes the patient to the risks of unnecessary or wrong treatment with no benefit. Moreover, such an approach may delay accurate diagnosis and proper treatment. This standard applies to adults, adolescents, and children. With proper instruction and supervision many children five years of age and older can generate a specimen. Thus, age alone is not sufficient justification for failing to attempt to obtain a sputum specimen from a child or adolescent.

During the past few years Xpert MTB/RIF has been validated under field conditions and, in a systematic review, shown to have excellent performance characteristics for detecting M. tuberculosis and rifampicin resistance.

The optimum number of sputum specimens to establish a diagnosis has been examined in a number of studies that have served to support recommendations to decrease the minimum number of sputum specimens examined from 3 to 2, assuming they are examined in a quality-assured laboratory. In a systematic review of 37 studies on the yield of sputum smear microscopy, it was found that, on average, the initial specimen was positive in 85.8% of all patients ultimately found to have acid-fast bacilli detected, in an additional 11.9% with the second specimen, and a further 2.3% on the third specimen. In studies that used culture as the reference standard, the mean incremental yield in sensitivity of the second specimen was 11.1% and that of the third was 3.1%.[64]

A re-analysis of data from a study involving 42 laboratories in four high-burden countries showed that the incremental yield from a third sequential specimen ranged from 0.7% to 7.2%.[80] Thus, it appears that in a diagnostic evaluation for tuberculosis, at least two specimens should be obtained. In some settings, because of practicality and logistics, a third specimen may be useful, but examination of more than two specimens adds minimally to the number of positive specimens obtained.[64] Ideally, the results of sputum microscopy should be returned to the clinician within no more than one working day from submission of the specimen. Early detection of patients with infectious tuberculosis is an important component of infection control in health care facilities, thus, sputum specimens should be collected promptly from patients suspected of having the disease and laboratories should quickly return the results.

A variety of methods have been used to improve the performance of sputum smear microscopy.[63,64,81] However, a comprehensive systematic review of 83 studies describing the effects of various physical and/or chemical methods for concentrating and processing sputum prior to microscopy found highly variable results.[63] Moreover, processing increases complexity and may be associated with increased infection risk to laboratory personnel. For these reasons these methods are not recommended by WHO for regular use in low-resource settings.

Fluorescence microscopy (FM), in which auramine-based staining causes the acid-fast bacilli to fluoresce against a dark background, is widely used in many parts of the world. A comprehensive systematic review of 45 studies, in which the performance of direct sputum smear microscopy using fluorescence staining was compared with Ziehl-Neelsen (ZN) staining using culture as the gold standard, indicates that FM is the more sensitive method.[62] This review showed that FM is on average 10% more sensitive than conventional light microscopy. The specificity of FM was comparable to ZN microscopy. The combination of increased sensitivity with little or no loss of specificity makes FM a more accurate test, although the increased cost and complexity has restricted its use in many areas. For this reason conventional FM has best been used in centers with specifically trained and proficient microscopists, in which a large number of specimens are processed daily, and in which there is an appropriate quality control program. However, lower cost, light emitting diode (LED) fluorescence microscopes with performance characteristics superior to conventional microscopes are now endorsed by WHO and are widely available.[82]

During the past few years Xpert MTB/RIF has been validated under field conditions and, in a systematic review, shown to have excellent performance characteristics for detecting *M. tuberculosis* and rifampicin resistance. The pooled sensitivity estimate was 98% for specimens that were smear positive and 68% for smear-negative specimens.[73] The overall sensitivity when used as an initial test in place of smear microscopy was found to be 89% with a specificity of 99%. Among persons with HIV infection the overall sensitivity was 79% (61% for persons with smear-negative culture positive tuberculosis and 97% for smear-positive specimens) and the specificity 98%. For detecting rifampicin resistance the sensitivity was 95% and the specificity 99%. The obvious advantage of Xpert MTB/RIF, in addition to its performance characteristics, is the rapidity with which an answer can be obtained—about two hours if the specimen is tested upon receipt in the laboratory—and its adaptability for use in more peripheral laboratories. It must be emphasized, however, that optimum benefit from any rapid molecular test can only be realized if the response to the result is also rapid.

Assessment of the performance characteristics and the practicalities of implementation (including costs) led WHO to issue recommendations for the use of Xpert MTB/RIF.[83] The WHO evidence synthesis process confirmed a solid evidence base to support widespread use of Xpert MTB/RIF for detection of *M. tuberculosis* and rifampicin resistance.[22, 59, 73, 83] Based on the evidence WHO recommended that Xpert MTB/RIF:

- **should** be used rather than conventional microscopy, culture, and drug susceptibility testing as the initial diagnostic test in individuals presumed to have MDR or HIV-associated tuberculosis;
- **may** be used as a follow-on test to microscopy in adults where MDR and HIV is of lesser concern, especially in further testing of smear-negative specimens;

- **may** be used rather than conventional microscopy and culture as the initial diagnostic test in all adults presumed to have tuberculosis;
- **should** be used rather than conventional microscopy, culture, and drug susceptibility testing as the initial diagnostic test in children presumed to have MDR or HIV-associated tuberculosis;
- **may** be used rather than conventional microscopy and culture as the initial diagnostic test in all children presumed to have tuberculosis.

Detection of rifampicin resistance in groups with a low prevalence of MDR TB should be an uncommon finding and a second Xpert MTB/RIF test on a different sample from the patient should be performed to exclude errors in performing the test. In patients with repeated rifampicin resistance, a WHO recommended MDR TB regimen that includes isoniazid should be initiated. Patients with discordant rifampicin resistance results by Xpert MTB/RIF should be assumed to have susceptible organisms and be given a first-line regimen. Discrepancies in the determination of rifampicin resistance by Xpert MTB/RIF may require resolution by DNA sequencing.[83-85]

Using Xpert MTB/RIF does not eliminate the need for conventional microscopy, culture, and drug susceptibility testing that are required to monitor treatment and to detect resistance to drugs other than rifampicin.

Commercial line probe assay performance characteristics have been adequately validated in direct testing of sputum smear-positive specimens and on isolates of *M. tuberculosis* complex grown from smear-negative and smear-positive specimens. Direct use of line probe assays on smear-negative clinical specimens is not recommended at present.[86]

Neither the tuberculin skin test nor Interferon-gamma release assays (IGRAs) have value for diagnosing active tuberculosis in adults although the result may serve to increase or decrease the diagnostic suspicion.[38,87] Both sensitivity and specificity are generally low and variable, especially among persons living with HIV.[87] Commercial serological antibody detection tests produce inconsistent and imprecise estimates of sensitivity and specificity.[88] For this reason WHO recommends against the use of these tests and the governments of India and Cambodia have banned their use.[38]

STANDARD 4. For all patients, including children, suspected of having extrapulmonary tuberculosis, appropriate specimens from the suspected sites of involvement should be obtained for microbiological and histological examination. An Xpert MTB/RIF test on cerebrospinal fluid is recommended as the preferred initial microbiological test in persons suspected of having tuberculous meningitis because of the need for a rapid diagnosis.

Rationale and Evidence Summary

Extrapulmonary tuberculosis (without associated lung involvement) accounts for at least 15–20% of tuberculosis in populations with a low prevalence of HIV infection.[21,89] In populations with a high prevalence of HIV infection, the proportion of cases with extrapulmonary tuberculosis is higher. Because appropriate specimens may be difficult to obtain from some of these sites, bacteriological confirmation of extrapulmonary tuberculosis is often

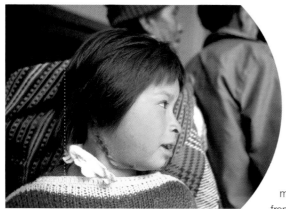

more difficult than for pulmonary tuberculosis. In spite of the difficulties, however, the basic principle that bacteriological confirmation of the diagnosis should be sought still holds.

Generally, there are fewer *M. tuberculosis* organisms present in extrapulmonary sites so identification of acid-fast bacilli by microscopy in specimens from these sites is less frequent and rapid molecular tests and/or culture are more important. Microscopic examination of pleural fluid in tuberculous pleuritis detects acid-fast bacilli in only about 5–10% of cases, and the diagnostic yield is similarly low in tuberculous meningitis although some studies have reported a higher sensitivity.[90,91] Given the low yield of microscopy, both microbiological and histological or cytological examination of tissue specimens, such as may be obtained by open or closed pleural biopsy or needle biopsy of lymph nodes, are important diagnostic tests. A systematic review showed the pooled sensitivity of Xpert MTB/RIF for the detection of TB in cerebrospinal fluid (compared with culture) was 79.5%. Although the sensitivity is not optimal, the speed with which a result is returned makes the test highly useful and, thus, is the preferred initial test (although culture should be concurrently performed if sufficient specimen is available). For lymph node tissue and aspirates the sensitivity of Xpert MTB/RIF was 84.9% compared with culture. In pleural fluid the sensitivity was only 43.7%, much greater than the sensitivity of pleural fluid microscopy, but still not sufficiently sensitive to be used as the sole test in the evaluation of pleural effusions.[77]

In view of these findings it is recommended that Xpert MTB/RIF may be used as a replacement test for conventional microscopy, culture, and/or histopathology for testing of gastric lavage fluid and specific non-respiratory specimens.[77] However, patients suspected of having extrapulmonary tuberculosis but with a single Xpert MTB/RIF-negative result should undergo further diagnostic testing, and those with high clinical suspicion for TB (especially children) should be treated even if an Xpert MTB/RIF result is negative or if the test is not available. In patients who have an illness compatible with tuberculosis (pulmonary and/or extrapulmonary) that is severe or progressing rapidly, initiation of treatment should not be delayed pending the results of microbiological examinations. Even the best test may not detect tuberculosis when there is a low bacillary load such as occurs in tuberculous meningitis, in patients with HIV infection, and in young children. In these situations, or in critically ill patients where tuberculosis is suspected, clinical judgment may justify empirical treatment while waiting for final test results, or even when test results are negative.

In addition to the collection of specimens from the sites of suspected tuberculosis, examination of sputum and a chest radiograph may also be useful, especially in patients with HIV infection, in whom asymptomatic or minimally symptomatic pulmonary tuberculosis has been noted.[92,93]

STANDARD 5. In patients suspected of having pulmonary tuberculosis whose sputum smears are negative, Xpert MTB/RIF and/or sputum cultures should be performed. Among patients with sputum that is negative by smear and Xpert MTB/RIF who have clinical evidence strongly suggestive of tuberculosis, antituberculosis treatment should be initiated after collection of specimens for culture examination.

Rationale and Evidence Summary

The designation of "sputum smear-negative tuberculosis" (now broadened to include patients with a negative Xpert MTB/RIF test) presents a difficult diagnostic dilemma. In a systematic review the sensitivity of sputum smear microscopy ranged from 31% to 69%, thus, many cases may not be identified by smear microscopy alone.[64] However, given the nonspecific nature of the symptoms of tuberculosis and the multiplicity of other diseases that could be the cause of the patient's illness, it is important that a rigorous approach be taken in diagnosing tuberculosis in a patient in whom at least two adequate sputum specimens are negative by microscopy or one specimen is negative by Xpert MTB/RIF. Because patients with HIV infection and tuberculosis frequently have negative sputum smears, and because of the broad differential diagnosis, including *Pneumocystis jiroveci* pneumonia and bacterial and fungal lower respiratory infections, a systematic approach to diagnosis is crucial. As indicated in Standard 3, persons who have HIV risks, or who are seriously ill, Xpert MTB/RIF should be performed as the initial diagnostic test.

Ideally, Xpert MTB/RIF and, if negative, culture should be included in the evaluation of patients with negative sputum smears.

It is important to balance the need for a systematic approach, in order to avoid both over- and under-diagnosis of tuberculosis, with the need for prompt treatment in a patient with an illness that is progressing rapidly. Over-diagnosis of tuberculosis when the illness has another cause will delay proper diagnosis and treatment of the true illness, whereas under-diagnosis will lead to more severe consequences of tuberculosis, including disability and possibly death, as well as ongoing transmission of *M. tuberculosis*. It should be noted that in making a diagnosis of smear-negative tuberculosis, a clinician who decides to treat with a full course of antituberculosis chemotherapy should report this as a case of sputum smear-negative pulmonary tuberculosis to local public health authorities (as described in Standard 21).

Algorithms, including a widely used approach developed by WHO,[94] may present a systematic approach to diagnosis. Performance of the WHO algorithm has been variable under field conditions, and there is little information or experience on which to base approaches to the diagnosis of smear-negative tuberculosis in persons with HIV infection when culture or Xpert MTB/RIF is not routinely available.[95-97]

There are several points of caution regarding the use of algorithms for the diagnosis of smear-negative tuberculosis. First, completion of all of the steps requires a substantial amount of time; thus, it may not be appropriate for patients with an illness that is progressing rapidly. This is especially true in patients with HIV infection in whom tuberculosis and other infections may be rapidly progressive. Second, several studies have shown that patients with tuberculosis may respond, at least transiently, to broad spectrum antimicrobial treatment.[98,99] Obviously such a response will lead one to delay a diagnosis of tuberculosis. Fluoroquinolones, in particular, are bactericidal for *M. tuberculosis* complex. Empiric fluoroquinolone monotherapy for respiratory tract infections has been associated with delays in initiation of appropriate antituberculosis therapy and acquired resistance to the fluoroquinolones.[100-102] Third, applying all the steps in an algorithm may be costly and deter the patient from continuing with the diagnostic evaluation. Given all these concerns, application of a complex sequence of diagnostic steps in patients with at least two negative sputum specimen examinations and/or one negative Xpert MTB/RIF test must be done in a flexible manner. Ideally, the evaluation of smear-negative tuberculosis should be guided by locally-validated approaches, suited to local conditions, and the needs (financial or otherwise) of the patient.

Ideally, Xpert MTB/RIF and, if negative, culture should be included in the algorithm for evaluating patients with negative sputum smears. A positive Xpert MTB/RIF will greatly reduce the time to diagnosis and initiation of appropriate treatment, possibly saving money as well as staff time. Culture adds a significant layer of complexity and cost but also increases sensitivity, which should result in case detection earlier in the course of the disease.[103,104] While, commonly, the results of culture are not be available until after a decision to begin treatment has to be made, treatment can be stopped subsequently if cultures from a reliable laboratory are negative, the patient has not responded clinically, and the clinician has sought other evidence in pursuing the differential diagnosis. It must be emphasized that, for seriously ill patients (particularly patients with HIV infection), a clinical decision to start treatment often must be made without waiting for the results of cultures. Such patients may die if appropriate treatment is not begun promptly. A rapid molecular test such as Xpert MTB/RIF, although less sensitive than culture on liquid media (but equal in sensitivity to culture on solid media), especially for smear-negative specimens, has the clear advantage of providing a result very quickly, thus, enabling appropriate treatment to be initiated promptly.[85]

The probability of finding acid-fast bacilli in sputum smears by microscopy is directly related to the concentration of bacilli in the sputum. Sputum microscopy is likely to be positive when there are at least 10,000 organisms per milliliter of sputum. At concentrations below 1,000 organisms per milliliter of sputum, the chance of observing acid-fast bacilli in a smear is less than 10%.[105,106] In contrast, a properly performed culture, especially if liquid media are used, can detect far lower numbers of acid-fast bacilli (detection limit is about 100 organisms per ml).[104] The culture, therefore, has a higher sensitivity than microscopy and, at least in theory, can increase case detection, although this potential has not been demonstrated in low-income, high-incidence areas. Further, culture makes it possible to identify the mycobacterial species and to perform full drug susceptibility testing in patients in whom there is reason to suspect drug-resistant tuberculosis.[104] The disadvantages of culture are its cost, technical complexity, infrastructure requirements, and the time required to obtain a result. In addition, ongoing quality assessment is essential for culture results to be credible.

In many countries, although culture facilities are not uniformly available, there is the capacity to perform culture or rapid molecular testing in some areas. Providers should be aware of the local capacity and use the resources appropriately, especially for the evaluation of persons suspected of having tuberculosis who have negative sputum smears and for persons with HIV infection or who are suspected of having tuberculosis caused by drug-resistant organisms.

Traditional culture methods use solid media such as Lowenstein-Jensen and Ogawa. Cultures on solid media are less technology-intensive and the media can be made locally. However, the time to identify growth is significantly longer than in liquid media systems such as the MGIT® system. Decisions to provide culture facilities for diagnosing tuberculosis depend on financial resources, infrastructure, trained personnel, and the ready availability of supplies and service for the equipment.

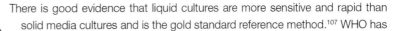

There is good evidence that liquid cultures are more sensitive and rapid than solid media cultures and is the gold standard reference method.[107] WHO has issued policy guidance on the use of liquid media for culture and drug susceptibility testing in low-resource settings.[108] This policy recommends phased implementation of liquid culture systems as a part of a country-specific comprehensive plan for laboratory capacity strengthening that addresses issues such as biosafety, training, maintenance of infrastructure, and reporting of results. However, development of the capacity to do cultures requires a well-functioning health care system, adequate laboratory infrastructure, and trained personnel.

In June 2008, WHO endorsed the use of molecular line-probe assays for rapid screening of patients at risk of MDR TB.[86] This policy statement was based in part on evidence summarized in systematic reviews,[107] expert opinion, and results of field demonstration projects. The recommended use of line probe assays is currently limited to culture isolates and direct testing of smear-positive sputum specimens. Line probe assays are not recommended as a complete replacement for conventional culture and drug susceptibility testing. Culture is still required for smear-negative specimens, and conventional drug susceptibility testing is still necessary to confirm resistance to drugs other than isoniazid and rifampicin.

Chest radiography may also play an important role in the evaluation of persons suspected of having tuberculosis but who have negative sputum smears. Cough is a nonspecific symptom; the chest radiograph can assist in determining the cause of the cough in persons with negative sputum smear microscopy. Commonly, in areas where adequate radiographic facilities are available the chest radiograph is obtained as the first test. Finding an abnormality consistent with tuberculosis should prompt the ordering of sputum specimens. Although the radiograph is a useful adjunct in diagnosing tuberculosis, as noted above, the radiograph alone cannot establish a diagnosis. However, in combination with clinical assessment, the radiograph may provide important circumstantial evidence as to the diagnosis.[109]

It is important to note that, just as with the microbiology laboratory, radiography requires quality control, both in terms of technical quality and interpretation. There are several resources that are useful both for assuring technical quality of the radiograph and for interpretation of the findings.[109-111]

STANDARD 6. For all children suspected of having intrathoracic (i.e., pulmonary, pleural, and mediastinal or hilar lymph node) tuberculosis, bacteriological confirmation should be sought through examination of respiratory secretions (expectorated sputum induced sputum, gastric lavage) for smear microscopy, an Xpert MTB/RIF test and/or culture.

Rationale and Evidence Summary

The diagnosis of tuberculosis in children relies on a thorough assessment of all the evidence derived from a careful history of exposure, clinical examination, and other relevant investigations. Although most children with tuberculosis have pulmonary involvement they commonly have paucibacillary disease without evident lung cavitation but frequently with involvement of intrathoracic lymph nodes. Consequently, compared with adults, sputum smears from children are more likely to be negative. Although bacteriological confirmation of tuberculosis in children is not always feasible, it should be sought whenever possible by sputum (or other specimen) examination with Xpert MTB/RIF, smear microscopy, and culture.[77,112-116] Because many children less than five years of age do not cough and produce sputum effectively, culture of gastric lavage obtained by naso-gastric tube or induced sputum has a higher yield than spontaneous sputum.[115,116] A trial of treatment with antituberculosis medications is not recommended as a means of diagnosing tuberculosis in children. The decision to treat a child for tuberculosis should be carefully considered and once such a decision is made, the child should be treated with a full course of therapy. The approach to diagnosing tuberculosis in children recommended by WHO is summarized in Table 4.[114]

As a component of evaluating a child for tuberculosis, the social situation and nutritional status of the child must be taken into account and the need for support services assessed The parent or responsible adult must be informed as to the importance of treatment in order to be an effective treatment supporter.

TABLE 4.

Guidance on approach to diagnose TB in children

1. Careful history (including history of TB contact and symptoms consistent with TB)
2. Clinical examination (including growth assessment)
3. Tuberculin skin testing
4. Chest X-ray if available
5. Bacteriological confirmation whenever possible
6. Investigations relevant for suspected pulmonary TB and suspected extrapulmonary TB
7. HIV testing

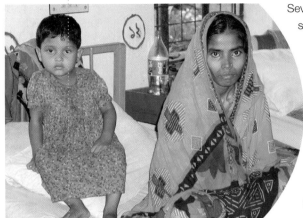

Several reviews have examined the effectiveness of various diagnostic tools, scoring systems, and algorithms to diagnose tuberculosis in children.[112-115,117-119] Many of these approaches lack standardization and validation, and, thus, are of limited applicability. Though scoring systems and diagnostic criteria remain widely used in the diagnosis of tuberculosis in children, validation has been difficult due to lack of an established and accessible gold standard.[120] Estimates of sensitivity and specificity vary widely, especially in populations with high HIV co-infection.[120]

In children the risk of tuberculosis is increased when there is an active case (infectious, smear-positive tuberculosis) in the same house, or when the child is malnourished, is HIV-infected, or has had measles in the past few months. WHO's Integrated Management of Childhood Illness (IMCI)[121] program, which is widely used in first-level facilities in low- and middle-income countries states that tuberculosis should be considered in any child with:

- Unexplained weight loss or failure to grow normally;
- Unexplained fever, especially when it continues for more than 2 weeks;
- Chronic cough;
- Exposure to an adult with probable or definite pulmonary infectious tuberculosis.

Findings on examination that suggest tuberculosis include:

- Fluid on one side of the chest (reduced air entry, dullness to percussion);
- Enlarged non-tender lymph nodes or a lymph node abscess, especially in the neck;
- Signs of meningitis, especially when these develop over several days and the spinal fluid contains mostly lymphocytes and elevated protein;
- Abdominal swelling, with or without palpable lumps;
- Progressive swelling or deformity in the bone or a joint, including the spine.

As a component of evaluating a child for tuberculosis, the social situation and nutritional status of the child must be taken into account and the need for support services assessed.

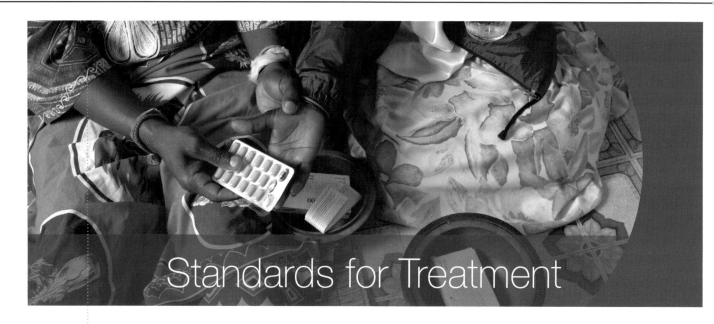

Standards for Treatment

STANDARD 7. To fulfill her/his public health responsibility, as well as responsibility to the individual patient, the provider must prescribe an appropriate treatment regimen, monitor adherence to the regimen and, when necessary, address factors leading to interruption or discontinuation of treatment. Fulfilling these responsibilities will likely require coordination with local public health services and/or other agencies.

Failure of a provider to ensure adherence could be equated with, for example, failure to ensure that a child receives the full set of immunizations.

Rationale and Evidence Summary

Effective treatment of tuberculosis prevents ongoing transmission of the infection and the development of drug resistance and restores the health of the patient. As described in the Introduction, the main interventions to prevent the spread of tuberculosis in the community are the early detection of patients with tuberculosis and provision of effective treatment to ensure a rapid and lasting cure. Consequently, treatment for tuberculosis is not only a matter of individual health, as is the case with, for example, treatment of hypertension or asthma; it is also a matter of public health. Thus, all providers, public and private, who undertake to treat a patient with tuberculosis must have the knowledge to prescribe a recommended treatment regimen and the means to assess adherence to the regimen and to address poor adherence to ensure that treatment is completed.[14,122] National and local tuberculosis programs commonly possess approaches and tools, including incentives and enablers, as well as other means of support, to ensure adherence with treatment and, when properly organized, can offer these to non-program providers. Failure of a provider to ensure adherence could be equated with, for example, failure to ensure that a child receives the full set of immunizations. Communities and patients deserve to be assured that providers treating tuberculosis are doing so in accordance with this principle and are, thereby, meeting this standard.

STANDARD 8. All patients who have not been treated previously and do not have other risk factors for drug resistance should receive a WHO recommended first-line treatment regimen using quality assured drugs. The initial phase should consist of two months of isoniazid, rifampicin, pyrazinamide, and ethambutol.* The continuation phase should consist of isoniazid and rifampicin given for 4 months. The doses of antituberculosis drugs used should conform to WHO recommendations. Fixed-dose combination drugs may provide a more convenient form of drug administration.

*Ethambutol may be omitted in children who are HIV-negative and who have non-cavitary tuberculosis.

Rationale and Evidence Summary

A large number of well-designed clinical trials have provided the evidence base for this standard and several sets of treatment recommendations based on these studies have been written in the past few years.[14,16,122] All these data indicate that with the current treatment options, a rifampicin-containing regimen is the backbone of antituberculosis chemotherapy and is highly effective in treating tuberculosis caused by drug-susceptible *M. tuberculosis*. It is also clear from these studies that the minimum duration of treatment for smear- and/or culture-positive tuberculosis is six months. Regimens of less than six months have an unacceptably high rate of relapse.[123] Thus, the current international standard duration of treatment for tuberculosis is a minimum of six months.[14,16,122] For the six-month treatment duration to be maximally effective, the regimen must include pyrazinamide during the initial two-month phase and rifampicin must be included throughout the full six months. Moreover, a systematic review of the outcome of treatment in the presence of single or poly-drug resistance (not multidrug resistance) demonstrated that failure, relapse, and acquisition of additional resistance were associated with shorter duration of rifampicin therapy.[124]

A retrospective review of the outcomes of treatment of tuberculosis in patients with HIV infection showed that relapse is minimized by the use of a regimen containing rifampicin throughout a six-month course of treatment.[125] This finding was confirmed in a more rigorous systematic review of treatment of tuberculosis in patients with HIV infection showing that better outcomes were associated with daily use of rifampicin in the initial phase of treatment and with rifampicin duration of ≥ 8 months. However, these effects of rifampicin duration were not seen in a small number of studies in which patients also received antiretroviral treatment.[126]

There are several variations in the frequency of drug administration that have been shown to produce acceptable results.[14,16,122] Intermittent administration of antituberculosis drugs enables supervision to be provided more efficiently and economically with no reduction in efficacy, although daily administration provides a greater margin of safety. The evidence on effectiveness of intermittent regimens has been reviewed.[127-128] These reviews, based on several trials, suggest that antituberculosis treatment may be given intermittently three times a week throughout the full course of therapy or twice weekly in the continuation phase without apparent loss of effectiveness except among individuals with advanced HIV infection.[128-136] However, the WHO does not recommend the use of twice-weekly intermittent regimens because of the potentially greater consequences of missing one of the two doses.

The evidence base for currently recommended antituberculosis drug dosages derives from human clinical trials, animal models, and pharmacokinetic and toxicity studies. The evidence on drug dosages and safety and the biological basis for dosage recommendations have been extensively reviewed in publications by WHO, ATS, the United States Centers for Disease Control and Prevention (CDC), and the Infectious Diseases Society of America (IDSA), The Union, and others.[14,16,122] The recommended daily and thrice weekly doses are shown in Table 5.

TABLE 5.

Doses of first-line antituberculosis drugs in adults and children

| Drug* | Recommended Dose in mg/kg Body Weight (Range) | |
	Daily	Three Times Weekly
Isoniazid**		
Children	10 (7–15), maximum 300 mg/day	——
Adults	5 (4–6), maximum 300 mg/day	10 (8–12), maximum 900 mg/dose
Rifampicin		
Children	15 (10–20), maximum 600 mg/day	——
Adults	10 (8–12), maximum 600 mg/day	10 (8–12), maximum 600 mg/dose
Pyrazinamide		
Children	35 (30–40), maximum 2,000 mg/day	——
Adults	25 (20–30), maximum 2,000 mg/day	35 (30–40), maximum 3,000 mg/dose
Ethambutol		
Children	20 (15–25), maximum 1,000 mg/day	——
Adults	15 (15–20), maximum 1,600 mg/day	30 (25–35), maximum 2,400 mg/dose

* The recommended daily doses of all 4 antituberculosis medicines are higher in children who weigh less than 25 kg than in adults, because the pharmacokinetics are different (and to achieve the same plasma concentration as in adults, the doses need to be increased)

**Same dosing for treatment of active disease and treatment of latent tuberculosis infection

Treatment of tuberculosis in special clinical situations such the presence of liver disease, renal disease, pregnancy, and HIV infection may require modification of the standard regimen or alterations in dosage or frequency of drug administration. For guidance in these situations see the WHO and ATS/CDC/IDSA treatment guidelines.[14,122]

In a clinical trial comparing a fixed-dose combination (FDC) of isoniazid, rifampicin, ethambutol, and pyrazinamide with a regimen of the same drugs given as separate pills, there was no difference in treatment outcome or adverse effects.[137] A systematic review came to the same conclusion.[138] However, because the FDC reduces the number of pills taken daily in the intensive phase of treatment from 9–16 to 3–4, patient convenience is increased and the potential for medication errors is decreased.[137,139-141]

STANDARD 9. A patient-centered approach to treatment should be developed for all patients in order to promote adherence, improve quality of life, and relieve suffering. This approach should be based on the patient's needs and mutual respect between the patient and the provider.

Rationale and Evidence Summary

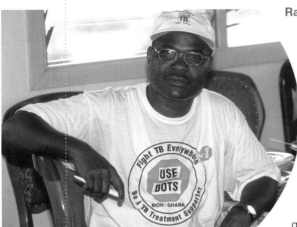

The approach described in the standard is designed to encourage and facilitate a positive partnership between providers and patients, working together to improve adherence. Adherence to treatment is the critical factor in determining treatment success.[14,122] A successful outcome of treatment for tuberculosis, assuming an appropriate drug regimen is prescribed, depends largely on patient adherence to the regimen. Achieving adherence is not an easy task, either for the patient or the provider. Anti-tuberculosis drug regimens, as described above, consist of multiple drugs given for a minimum of six months, often when the patient feels well (except, perhaps, for adverse effects of the medications). Commonly, treatments of this sort are inconsistent with the patient's cultural background, belief system, and living circumstances. Consequently, it is not surprising that, without appropriate treatment support, a significant proportion of patients with tuberculosis discontinues treatment before completion of the planned duration or is erratic in drug taking. Yet, failure to complete treatment for tuberculosis may lead to prolonged infectivity, poor outcomes, and drug resistance.

Interventions that target adherence must be tailored or customized to the particular situation and cultural context of a given patient.

Adherence is a multi-dimensional phenomenon determined by the interplay of several sets of factors.[13,142] In a systematic review of qualitative research on patient adherence to tuberculosis treatment, eight major themes were identified across the studies reviewed (Table 6).[142] These themes were then further refined into four sets of interacting factors that influence adherence: structural factors including poverty and gender discrimination, the social context, health service factors, and personal factors. From this synthesis it was concluded that a group of factors was likely to improve patient adherence. These are listed in Table 7.

Despite evidence to the contrary, there is a widespread tendency to focus on patient-related factors as the main cause of poor adherence.[13,142] Sociological and behavioral research during the past 40 years has shown that patients need to be supported, not blamed.[13] Less attention is paid to provider and health system-related factors. Several studies have evaluated various interventions to improve adherence to tuberculosis therapy (Table 7). Among the interventions evaluated, DOT has generated the most debate and controversy.[143,144] The main advantage of DOT is that treatment is carried out entirely under close, direct supervision. This provides both an accurate assessment of the degree of adherence and greater assurance that the medications have actually been ingested. When a second individual directly observes a patient swallowing medications there is greater certainty that the patient is actually receiving the prescribed medications. Also, because there is a close contact between the patient and the treatment supporter, adverse drug effects and other complications can be recognized quickly and managed appropriately and the need for additional social support can be identified. Moreover, such case management can also serve to identify and assist in addressing the myriad other problems experienced by patients with tuberculosis such as under-nutrition, poor housing, and loss of income, to name a few.

TABLE 6.

Primary themes identified in a systematic review of qualitative research on adherence to tuberculosis treatment

Organization of treatment and care for TB patients

- Access to services (urban ambulatory, distance, transport)
- Health center problems (long waiting hours, queues, physical condition of clinic)
- Treatment requirements (continuity, charging for drug, number of tablets, DOT, flexibility, and choice)
- Relationship between treatment provider and patient (poor follow up, increased contact, maltreatment of patients)

Interpretation of illness and wellness

- Individual interpretations of recovery
- Perceptions of TB
- Recognition of TB as a disease

Financial burden

- Conflict between work and treatment; costs of treatment; expenses exceeding available resources
- More pressing issues to attend to
- Increased expenditure on food

Knowledge, attitudes, and beliefs about treatment

- Limited understanding of treatment, duration, and consequences of default
- Beliefs about treatment efficacy
- Denial and difficulty accepting diagnosis
- Use of other medication, treatment requirements

Law and immigration

- Completion cards; impact on immigration status; fear of detention

Personal characteristics and adherence behavior

- Substance abuse
- Mental illness
- Ethnic characteristics
- Residential mobility
- Religion
- Personal motivation
- Gender
- Structured environment
- Personal agency

Side effects

- Real, anticipated, or culturally interpreted; insufficient information; insufficient communication; insufficient attention

Family, community, and household influence

- Peer influence
- Stigma
- Providing for family
- Family support
- Marriage

Source: Munro SA, Lewin S A, Smith H J, Engel M E, Fretjheim, A, Volmink J. Patient adherence to tuberculosis treatment: a systematic review of qualitative research. PLoS Med. 4: 2007; e238.

TABLE 7.

Factors likely to improve TB treatment adherence

- Increase the visibility of TB programs in the community, which may increase knowledge and improve attitudes towards TB
- Provide more information about the disease and treatment to patients and communities
- Increase support from family, peers, and social networks
- Minimize costs and unpleasantness related to clinic visits and increase flexibility and patient autonomy
- Increase flexibility in terms of patient choice of treatment plan and type of support

- Increase the patient-centeredness of interactions between providers and clients
- Address structural and personal factors, for example compensating high cost of treatment and income loss through cash transfers, travel vouchers, food assistance, micro-financing, and other empowerment initiatives and preventing loss of employment though addressing employment policies.
- Provide more information about the effects of medication to reduce the risk of patients becoming nonadherent when experiencing treatment side effects

Source: Modified from Munro SA, Lewin S A, Smith H J, Engel M E, Fretjheim, A, Volmink J. Patient adherence to tuberculosis treatment: a systematic review of qualitative research. PLoS Med. 4: 2007; e238.

The exclusive use of health facility-based DOT may be associated with disadvantages that must be taken into account in designing a patient-centered approach. For example, these disadvantages may include loss of income and time, stigma and discrimination, physical hardship, and travel difficulties, all factors that can have an important effect on adherence. Ideally a flexible mix of health facility- and community-based DOT, often with a family member serving as a treatment supporter, should be available.[145]

In a Cochrane systematic review that synthesized the evidence from six controlled trials comparing DOT with self-administered therapy,[143,144] the authors found that patients allocated to DOT and those allocated to self-administered therapy had similar cure rates and rates of cure plus treatment completion. They concluded that direct observation of medication ingestion did not improve outcomes. A more recent systematic review reached the same conclusion.[146] In contrast, programmatic assessments in several countries have found DOT to be associated with high cure and treatment completion rates.[147-150] It is likely that these inconsistencies are due to the fact that primary studies are often unable to separate the effect of DOT alone from the overall DOTS Strategy.[13,144] In a retrospective review of programmatic results, the highest rates of success were achieved with "enhanced DOT" which consisted of "supervised swallowing" plus social supports, incentives, and enablers as part of a larger program to encourage adherence to treatment.[147] Such complex interventions are not easily evaluated within the conventional randomized controlled trial framework.

Interventions other than DOT have also shown promise.[147-150] Incentives, peer assistance (for example, using cured patients), repeated motivation of patients, and staff training and motivation, all have been shown to improve adherence significantly.[13,142,147] In addition, adherence may be enhanced by provision of more comprehensive primary care (as described in the Integrated Management of Adolescent and Adult Illness),[151,152] as well as by provision of specialized services such as opiate substitution for injection drug users.

Providing every patient with a copy of the *PCTC* short version in their language may also serve to improve adherence.

Systematic reviews and extensive programmatic experience demonstrate that there is no single approach to case management that is effective for all patients, conditions, and settings. Consequently, interventions that target adherence must be tailored or customized to the particular situation and cultural context of a given patient.[13,142] Such an approach must be developed in concert with the patient to achieve optimum adherence. This patient-centered, individualized approach to treatment support is now a core element of all tuberculosis care and control efforts. It is important to note that treatment support measures, *and not the treatment regimen itself,* must be individualized to suit the unique needs of the patient.

Mobile technologies may provide a means of implementing a "remote DOT" form of supervision. Most health care workers and many patients in even the poorest countries are familiar with mobile phone technologies and many use them regularly in their daily lives. Voice messages, or possibly in the future video reminders, may serve both to support treatment and to monitor for adverse drug reactions.

In addition to one-on-one support for patients being treated for tuberculosis, community support is also of importance in creating a therapeutic milieu and reducing stigma.[9,153] Not only should the community expect that optimum treatment for tuberculosis is provided, but, also, the community should play a role in promoting conditions that facilitate and assist in ensuring that the patient will adhere to the prescribed regimen.

A number of studies have shown that persons with tuberculosis may incur catastrophic costs in seeking a diagnosis and appropriate treatment.[40,41] Sickness insurance, disability grants, and other social protection schemes are available in many countries, though they may not cover the entire population. Persons with tuberculosis may be eligible for financial support through such schemes, but may not be aware of them or have the capacity to access them. Health care providers should assist patients to access existing schemes, including help with administrative procedures, issuing sickness certificates, etc.

STANDARD 10. Response to treatment in patients with pulmonary tuberculosis (including those with tuberculosis diagnosed by a rapid molecular test) should be monitored by follow-up sputum smear microscopy at the time of completion of the initial phase of treatment (two months). If the sputum smear is positive at completion of the initial phase, sputum microscopy should be performed again at 3 months and, if positive, rapid molecular drug sensitivity testing (line probe assays or Xpert MTB/RIF) should be performed. In patients with extrapulmonary tuberculosis and in children, the response to treatment is best assessed clinically.

Rationale and Evidence Summary

Patient monitoring and treatment supervision are two separate functions. Patient monitoring is necessary to evaluate the response of the disease to treatment and to identify adverse drug reactions. To judge response of pulmonary tuberculosis to treatment, the most expeditious method is sputum smear microscopy. Ideally, where quality-assured

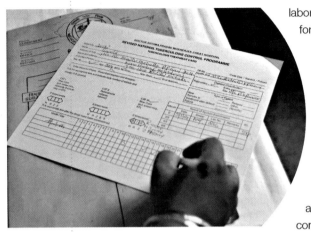

laboratories are available, sputum cultures, as well as smears, should be performed for monitoring.

Molecular tests, including Xpert MTB/RIF, are not suitable for patient monitoring because these tests detect residual DNA from non-viable bacilli.[154] However, Xpert MTB/RIF is useful for detecting rifampicin resistance in patients who remain sputum smear positive after 3 or more months of treatment. Patients whose diagnosis of tuberculosis is confirmed by Xpert MTB/RIF and who have rifampicin susceptible organisms should be monitored during treatment with sputum smear microscopy. For these patients, microscopy should be performed at completion of the intensive phase of treatment, five months into treatment and at the end of treatment as per current WHO guidelines.[14] Patients with TB and rifampicin resistance confirmed by Xpert MTB/RIF and placed on MDR TB treatment should be monitored by sputum smear and culture. If resources permit, monthly culture throughout treatment is recommended.[155,156]

A positive sputum smear at the end of the initial phase of treatment should trigger an assessment of the patient's adherence and a careful clinical re-evaluation.

Approximately 80% of patients with sputum smear-positive pulmonary tuberculosis should have negative sputum smears at the time of completion of the initial phase of treatment (2 months of therapy).[128] Patients who remain sputum smear-positive require particular attention. A positive sputum smear at the end of the initial phase of treatment should trigger an assessment of the patient's adherence and a careful re-evaluation to determine if co-morbid conditions, particularly HIV infection or other forms of immunosuppression and diabetes mellitus, are present that might interfere with response to treatment. However, a positive smear at the time of completion of the initial phase is not an indication to prolong this phase of treatment. If the sputum smear is positive at month two, sputum smear examination should be repeated at month three. Having a positive sputum smear after completion of three months of treatment raises the possibility of drug resistance and Xpert MTB/RIF, culture, and drug susceptibility testing should be performed in a quality-assured laboratory.[14]

Chest radiographs may be a useful adjunct in assessing response to treatment but are not a substitute for microbiologic evaluation. Similarly, clinical assessment can be unreliable and misleading in the monitoring of patients with pulmonary tuberculosis especially in the presence of co-morbid conditions that could confound the clinical assessment. However, in patients with extrapulmonary tuberculosis and in children, clinical evaluations may be the only available means of assessing the response to treatment.

STANDARD 11. An assessment of the likelihood of drug resistance, based on history of prior treatment, exposure to a possible source case having drug-resistant organisms, and the community prevalence of drug resistance (if known), should be undertaken for all patients. Drug susceptibility testing should be performed at the start of therapy for all patients at a risk of drug resistance. Patients who remain sputum smear-positive at completion of 3 months of treatment, patients in whom treatment has failed, and patients who have been lost to follow up or relapsed following one or more courses of treatment should always be assessed for drug resistance. For patients in whom drug resistance is considered to be likely, an Xpert MTB/RIF should be the initial diagnostic test. If rifampicin resistance is detected, culture and testing for susceptibility to isoniazid, fluoroquinolones, and second-line injectable drugs should be performed promptly. Patient counseling and education, as well as treatment with an empirical second-line regimen, should begin immediately to minimize the potential for transmission. Infection control measures appropriate to the setting should be applied.

Rationale and Evidence Summary

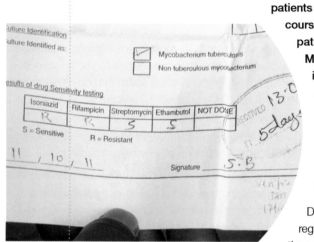

Errors that lead to drug resistance include: failure to provide effective treatment support, inadequate drug regimens, adding a single new drug to a failing regimen, and failure to recognize existing drug resistance.

Drug resistance is largely man-made and is a consequence of suboptimal regimens and treatment interruptions.[25] Clinical errors that commonly lead to the emergence of drug resistance include: failure to provide effective treatment support and assurance of adherence; inadequate drug regimens; adding a single new drug to a failing regimen; and failure to recognize existing drug resistance. In addition, co-morbid conditions associated with reduced serum levels of antituberculosis drugs (e.g., malabsorption, rapid transit diarrhea, use of antifungal agents) and interruptions caused by adverse drug reactions may also lead to the acquisition of drug resistance.[157] Programmatic causes of drug resistance include drug shortages and stock-outs, administration of poor-quality drugs and lack of appropriate supervision to prevent erratic drug intake.[155-157] Transmission of drug-resistant strains of *M. tuberculosis* has been well described in health care facilities, congregate settings, and in susceptible populations, notably HIV-infected persons.[158-162] However, multidrug-resistant (MDR) tuberculosis (tuberculosis caused by organisms that are resistant to at least isoniazid and rifampicin) may spread in the population at large as was shown in data from a number of countries, including China, the Baltic States, and countries of the former Soviet Union.[163-166]

Drug resistance surveillance data suggest that more cases of MDR tuberculosis occur among new cases of tuberculosis than among previously treated cases, although the proportion in the previously treated group is much higher.[164] In 2010, 30 countries with antituberculosis drug resistance surveillance data were each estimated to have more than 700 multidrug-resistant tuberculosis cases among their notified cases each year. Patients who had not had previous treatment comprised a median of 54% of the MDR cases. The occurrence of MDR TB in a new patient is an indication that MDR organisms are spreading in a community. Although case-finding efforts for MDR tuberculosis should first prioritize previously treated patients for drug sensitivity testing, identification of all MDR TB cases will require screening for drug resistance in a much wider group of patients.[164]

The strongest factor associated with drug resistance is previous antituberculosis treatment, as shown by the WHO/IUATLD Global Project on Anti-TB Drug Resistance Surveillance, started in 1994.[22,166] In previously treated patients, the odds of any resistance are at least 4-fold higher, and that of MDR TB at least 10-fold higher, than in new (untreated) patients.[155] Patients with chronic tuberculosis (sputum-positive after re-treatment) and those who fail treatment (sputum-positive after 5 months of treatment) are at highest risk of having MDR tuberculosis, especially if rifampicin was used throughout the course of treatment.[155] Persons who are in close contact with confirmed MDR tuberculosis patients, especially children and HIV-infected individuals, also are at high risk of being infected with MDR strains. In some closed settings prisoners, persons staying in homeless shelters and certain categories of immigrants and migrants are at increased risk of MDR tuberculosis.[155,167] These factors are summarized and presented in descending order of level of risk in Table 8.

By the mid-1990's, most countries participating in the global survey of antituberculosis drug resistance registered cases of MDR tuberculosis. Not surprisingly, in 2006, extensively drug-resistant (XDR) tuberculosis (defined as tuberculosis caused by *M. tuberculosis* resistant to at least isoniazid and rifampicin, as well as to any one of the fluoroquinolones and to at least one of three injectable second-line drugs [amikacin, capreomycin, or kanamycin]) was described and rapidly recognized as a serious emerging threat to global public health, as well as being deadly in the initial outbreak.[168] Subsequent reports have identified XDR tuberculosis in all regions of the world and, to date, treatment outcomes have been significantly worse than MDR tuberculosis outcomes.[168-171] In one cohort from KwaZulu-Natal, 98% of XDR tuberculosis patients co-infected with HIV died, with a median time of death of only 16 days from time of specimen collection.[168] The two strongest risk factors for XDR tuberculosis are:

1. Failure of a tuberculosis treatment which contains second-line drugs including an injectable agent and a fluoroquinolone.

2. Close contact with an individual with documented XDR tuberculosis or with an individual for whom treatment with a regimen including second-line drugs is failing or has failed.

More recently, strains of *M. tuberculosis* with resistance patterns beyond XDR tuberculosis have been described. The available evidence suggests that treatment outcomes are worse when resistance patterns become more complicated.[172-174]

TABLE 8.

Assessing risk for drug resistance

Risk Factors for Resistance	Comments
Failure of re-treatment regimen (a second course of treatment after failure, relapse, or default)	Patients who are still sputum smear-positive at the end of a re-treatment regimen have perhaps the highest MDR TB rates of any group, often exceeding 80%.
Close contact with a known drug-resistant case	Most studies have shown that tuberculosis occurring in close contacts of persons with MDR TB are also likely to have MDR TB.
Failure of the initial treatment regimen	Patients who fail to become sputum smear-negative while on treatment are likely to have drug-resistant organisms. However, the likelihood depends on a number of factors, including whether rifampicin was used in the continuation phase and whether DOT was used throughout treatment. Thus, a detailed history of drugs used is essential. This is especially true for patients treated by private providers, often with non-standard regimens.
Relapse after apparently successful treatment	In clinical trials most patients who relapse have fully susceptible organisms. However, under program conditions an apparent relapse, especially an early relapse, may, in fact, be an unrecognized treatment failure and thus have a higher likelihood of drug resistance.
Return after default without recent treatment failure	The likelihood of MDR TB varies substantially in this group, depending in part on the duration of treatment and the degree of adherence before default.
Exposure in institutions that have outbreaks or a high prevalence of TB with any drug resistance	Patients who frequently stay in homeless shelters, prisoners in many countries, and health care workers in clinics, laboratories, and hospitals can have high rates of TB with any drug resistance pattern.
Residence in areas with high drug-resistant TB prevalence	Drug-resistant TB rates in many areas of the world can be high enough to justify routine DST in all new cases.

[155] Modified from World Health Organization. Guidelines for the programmatic management of drug-resistant tuberculosis. WHO/HTM/TB/2008.402.

Drug susceptibility testing (DST) to the first-line antituberculosis drugs should be performed in laboratories that participate in an ongoing, rigorous quality assurance program. DST for first-line drugs is currently recommended for all patients with a history of previous antituberculosis treatment; patients who have failed treatment, especially those who have failed a standardized re-treatment regimen, are the highest priority.[156] Testing with Xpert MTB/RIF is recommended for patients judged to be at risk for having MDR tuberculosis.[85] Tests (other than Xpert MTB/RIF) for identifying drug resistance in *M. tuberculosis* are shown in Table 9. It should be noted that in some instances phenotypic DST may miss low level rifampicin resistance due to uncommon mutations in the *rpo*B gene, thus accounting for discordance between genotypic and phenotypic methods of performing DSTs.[175,176] The determination of the specificity of a molecular DST method based only on phenotypic DST as a reference may, therefore, underestimate the specificity of the molecular DST. In light of these findings, it is currently unclear whether and to what extent Xpert MTB/RIF might out-perform phenotypic DST methods for rifampicin resistance.[77]

Patients who develop tuberculosis and are known to have been in close contact with persons known to have MDR tuberculosis also should have DST performed on an initial isolate. Although HIV infection has not been conclusively shown to be an independent risk factor for drug resistance, MDR tuberculosis outbreaks in HIV settings and high mortality rates in persons with MDR tuberculosis and HIV infection justify routine DST in all HIV-infected tuberculosis patients, resources permitting.[159,160,162,168]

All patients suspected of having XDR tuberculosis should have DST to isoniazid, rifampicin, the second-line injectable agents, and a fluoroquinolone. When epidemiological or other factors suggest that there is a risk for XDR tuberculosis in a person with HIV infection, liquid media or other validated rapid techniques for DST of first- and second-line drugs is recommended. HIV-infected patients with XDR tuberculosis have been observed to have a rapidly fatal course, thus, in patients (with or without HIV infection) who have a severe or rapidly progressive illness an empirical treatment regimen, based on international recommendations, should be initiated promptly, generally prior to having drug susceptibility test results.[168]

TABLE 9.

WHO approved tests for identification of drug resistance

Tests	Purpose	Comments
Line probe assays: GenoType MTBDRplus assays	Rapid detection of rifampicin resistance	The GenoType MTBDR® assays have good sensitivity and specificity for rifampicin resistance in AFB positive sputum samples and positive cultures.[177] LPAs are approved by WHO[86]
Colorimetric redox-indicator (CRI) methods and nitrate reductase assays (NRA)	Rapid detection of rifampicin and isoniazid resistance	WHO recommends NRA and CRI as interim solutions, pending the development of capacities for genotypic DST.[178,179]
Microscopic Observation Drug Susceptibility [MODS]	Rapid detection of rifampicin and isoniazid resistance	MODS is suitable for use at reference laboratory level;[180] scaling-up and decentralization to lower level laboratories is not recommended. The WHO recommends MODS as interim solution, pending the development of capacities for genotypic DST.
Phenotypic drug susceptibility testing methods for first-line and second-line antituberculosis drugs:	Detection of resistance to first- and second-line drugs	DST for isoniazid and rifamipicin shows good reliability and reproducibility when tested in commercial liquid and solid media. WHO recommends that among Rif-resistant or MDR TB cases, phenotypic testing for all fluoroquinolones (ofloxacin, moxifloxacin, levofloxacin) and second-line injectable agents (kanamycin, amikacin, and capreomycin) available to national TB programmes should be done.[181] **Note:** Genotypic methods for detection of second-line drug susceptibility are available but not approved by WHO.[182]
Pyrosequencing for RIF resistance	Rapid detection of rifampicin resistance	Pyrosequencing is a highly sensitive and specific tool for the detection of RIF resistance in *M. tuberculosis*. Overall sensitivity and specificity were estimated at respectively 0.94 (95% CI 0.92–0.96) and 0.98 (95% CI 0.97–0.99).[183] Pyrosequencing is considered the reference method for genotypic DST methods.

STANDARD 12. Patients with or highly likely to have tuberculosis caused by drug-resistant (especially MDR/XDR) organisms should be treated with specialized regimens containing quality-assured second-line antituberculosis drugs. The doses of antituberculosis drugs should conform to WHO recommendations. The regimen chosen may be standardized or based on suspected or confirmed drug susceptibility patterns. At least five drugs—pyrazinamide and four drugs to which the organisms are known or presumed to be susceptible, including an injectable agent—should be used in a 6-8 month intensive phase and at least 3 drugs to which the organisms are known or presumed to be susceptible, should be used in the continuation phase. Treatment should be given for at least 18–24 months beyond culture conversion. Patient-centered measures, including observation of treatment, are required to ensure adherence. Consultation with a specialist experienced in treatment of patients with MDR/XDR tuberculosis should be obtained.

Rationale and Evidence Summary

Because randomized controlled treatment trials for MDR/XDR tuberculosis are difficult to design, none has been conducted to evaluate currently available regimens of second-line drugs. However, study designs similar to those used for new antiretroviral drugs in which a new drug plus an optimized regimen, based on DST, is compared to the optimized regimen are being used for studies of new drugs for MDR/XDR tuberculosis.[184] In the absence of clinical trial data, current recommendations for treating MDR/XDR tuberculosis are based on observational studies, general microbiological and therapeutic principles, extrapolation from available evidence from pilot MDR tuberculosis treatment projects, expert opinion,[155,156,169,185-193] and more recently, a carefully conducted individual patient meta-analysis.[194] The individual patient data meta-analysis examined the outcomes of treatment for MDR tuberculosis and concluded that treatment success, compared with failure/relapse or death, was associated with use of later generation fluoroquinolones, as well as ofloxacin, ethionamide or prothionamide, use of four or more likely effective drugs in the initial intensive phase, and three or more likely effective drugs in the continuation phase.[156,174,194] In addition, not surprisingly, outcomes in patients with XDR tuberculosis were worse when there was resistance to additional drugs beyond those that comprise the definition of XDR.[172]

There are three strategic options for treatment of MDR/XDR tuberculosis: standardized, empiric, and individualized regimens. The approach is dependent on having access to either reliable DST results for individual patients or population data on the prevalent resistance patterns. The choice among the three approaches should be based on availability of second-line drugs and DST for first- and second-line drugs, local drug resistance patterns, and the history of use of second-line drugs.[155,156,187,193] Basic principles involved in the design of any regimen include the use of at least four drugs with either certain or highly likely effectiveness, drug administration at least six days a week, drug dosage determined by patient weight, the use of an injectable agent (an aminoglycoside or capreomycin) for 6–8 months, treatment duration of approximately 20 months, and patient-centered DOT throughout the treatment course.

Based on their activity, efficacy, route of administration, tolerance, availability, and costs, antituberculosis drugs can be classified in five groups.[187] Group 1 consists of first-line

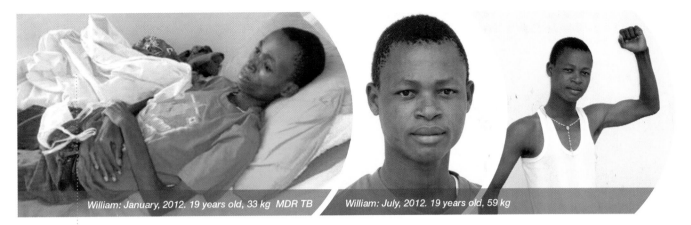

William: January, 2012. 19 years old, 33 kg MDR TB

William: July, 2012. 19 years old, 59 kg

"My grandfather lived with my family and he was very sick with cough and losing weight. He had TB and was treated several times but never got cured. He died. Then I got sick."

—William

He has now completed treatment and is working as a volunteer in the TB program in Dar es Salaam.

drugs: isoniazid, rifampicin, ethambutol, pyrazinamide, and rifabutin. Any of these drugs should be used if it is thought that susceptibility remains. Only one drug should be selected from Group 2 (injectable agents—kanamycin, amikacin, capreomycin, streptomycin) and Group 3 (fluoroquinolones), because of documented total or partial cross-resistance and similar toxicities within the groups. Group 4 consists of less potent oral agents: ethionamide, prothionamide, cycloserine, terizidone, p-aminosalicylic acid. Group 5 is composed of drugs for which antituberculosis action has not been documented in clinical trials (except for thiacetazone): clofazimine, linezolid, amoxicillin/clavulanate, thioacetazone, imipenem/cilastatin high-dose isoniazid, and clarithromycin. A drug that has been used within a failing regimen should not be counted in the total of four drugs for re-treatment, even if susceptibility is shown in the laboratory. The doses and adverse effects of second-line drugs are described in detail the ATS/CDC/IDSA Treatment of Tuberculosis.[122]

Standardized treatment regimens are based on representative drug resistance surveillance data or on the history of drug usage in the country.[155] Based on these assessments, regimens can be designed that will have a high likelihood of success. Advantages include less dependency on highly technical laboratories, less reliance on highly specialized clinical expertise required to interpret DST results, simplified drug ordering and logistics, and easier operational implementation. A standardized approach is useful in settings where second-line drugs have not been used extensively and where resistance levels to these drugs are consequently low or absent.

Empiric treatment regimens are commonly used in specific groups of patients while the DST results are pending.[155,156] Empiric regimens are strongly recommended to avoid clinical deterioration and to prevent transmission of MDR strains of *M. tuberculosis* to contacts while awaiting the DST results.[155] Once the results of DST are known, an empiric regimen may be changed to an individualized regimen. Ongoing global efforts to address the problem of MDR tuberculosis will likely result in broader access to laboratories performing DST and a faster return of results.

Individualized treatment regimens (based on DST profiles and drug history of individual patients or on local patterns of drug utilization) have the advantage of avoiding toxic and expensive drugs to which the MDR strain is resistant.[155] However, an individualized approach requires access to substantial human, financial, and technical (laboratory) capacity. DSTs for second-line drugs are notoriously difficult to perform, largely because of drug instability and the fact that critical concentrations for defining drug resistance are very close to the minimal inhibitory concentration (MIC) of individual drugs.[195] Laboratory proficiency testing results are not yet available for second-line drugs; as a result little can be said about the reliability of DST for these drugs. [195] Clinicians treating MDR tuberculosis

Often second-line drugs are the last best hope for patients with drug-resistant tuberculosis, and it is crucial that such treatment be designed with the active participation of the patient.

patients must be aware of these limitations and interpret DST results with this in mind.

A shorter course standardized regimen used in Bangladesh has been described with good results reported in a small observational study.[196] Although promising, at this point there is insufficient evidence to recommend the use of this regimen for treating MDR tuberculosis. A clinical trial is underway that should provide substantial new information on which to base recommendations. Current advice from WHO is that a short regimen for MDR tuberculosis should be used only under operational research conditions.[197]

Substantial treatment support that may include financial assistance is commonly needed to enable patients to complete a second-line regimen. MDR/XDR tuberculosis treatment is a complex health intervention and medical practitioners are strongly advised to obtain consultation with a specialist experienced in the management of these patients. Often second-line drugs are the last best hope for patients with drug-resistant tuberculosis, and it is crucial that such treatment be designed for maximal effectiveness with the active participation of the patient to overcome the challenges faced by both provider and patient with MDR/XDR tuberculosis.[198] Physicians undertaking treatment of patients with MDR TB must be committed to finding and administering a regimen using quality-assured drugs for the full recommended duration of treatment. Commonly this requires collaboration with public health tuberculosis control programs.

Two new second-line drugs, delaminanid and bedaquiline,[199-201] have been introduced, although as of this writing only bedaquiline has been approved by the US FDA. Given the paucity of data describing outcomes and adverse events, the recommendation by WHO states that bedaquiline may be added to a WHO-recommended regimen in adult patients with pulmonary tuberculosis caused by MDR organisms.[200] The recommendations also specify fairly rigid conditions under which the drug should be used. Thus, informed consent should be obtained from the patient and there should be careful monitoring for adverse drug effects.

Of great concern, tuberculosis caused by organisms resistant to all drugs tested has been described in India, but likely exists elsewhere as well.[202,203] However, because of uncertainties about the connection between second-line DST results and patient outcomes it is not clear that there are no treatment options. Nevertheless, at least at this time there are no specific recommended treatment options for such patients and symptomatic or palliative care may be required. Although the number of such cases is likely to be small providers should be attuned to the possibility of such situations and be prepared to provide appropriate palliative management to relieve suffering caused by the disease.

STANDARD 13. An accessible, systematically maintained record of all medications given, bacteriologic response, outcomes, and adverse reactions should be maintained for all patients.

Rationale and Evidence Summary

Recording and reporting of data are fundamental components of care for patients with tuberculosis and for control of the disease. Data recording and reporting are necessary to monitor trends in tuberculosis at global, national, and subnational levels; to monitor progress in the treatment and in the quality of care for individual patients and groups (cohorts) of patients; to ensure continuity when patients are referred between health care facilities; to plan, implement, and evaluate programmatic efforts; and to support advocacy for adequate funding for tuberculosis control programs.[10] When high quality data are available, successes can be documented and corrective actions taken to address problems that are identified.[204,205]

There is a sound rationale and clear benefits for individual patients of a well-maintained record keeping system. It is common for individual physicians to believe sincerely, generally without documentation, that a majority of the patients in whom they initiate antituberculosis therapy are cured. However, when systematically evaluated, it is often seen that only a minority of patients have successfully completed the full treatment regimen. The recording and reporting system enables targeted, individualized follow-up to identify patients who are failing therapy. It also helps in facilitating continuity of care, particularly in settings (e.g., large hospitals) where the same practitioner might not be seeing the patient during every visit. A good record of medications given, results of investigations such as smears, cultures, and chest radiographs, and progress notes on clinical improvement, adverse events, and adherence will provide for more uniform monitoring and ensure a high standard of care.

Records are important to provide continuity when patients move from one care provider to another and enable tracing of patients who miss appointments.

Records are important to provide continuity when patients move from one care provider to another and enable tracing of patients who miss appointments. In patients who default and then return for treatment, and patients who relapse after treatment completion, it is critical to review previous records in order to assess the likelihood of drug resistance. Lastly, management of complicated cases (e.g., MDR tuberculosis) is not possible without an adequate record of previous treatment, adverse events, and drug susceptibility results. It should be noted that, wherever patient records are concerned, care must be taken to assure confidentiality of the information, yet the records should be made available to the patient upon request.

It is anticipated that electronic data systems will play an increasing role in tuberculosis data collection and analysis.[204] Most health care workers in even the poorest countries are familiar with mobile phone technologies and many use them regularly in their daily lives. The spread of mobile and web-based technologies is dramatically reducing the barriers to implementing electronic systems that existed until the very recent past. In this context, it is not surprising that there is growing use of and interest in electronic recording and reporting of tuberculosis data.

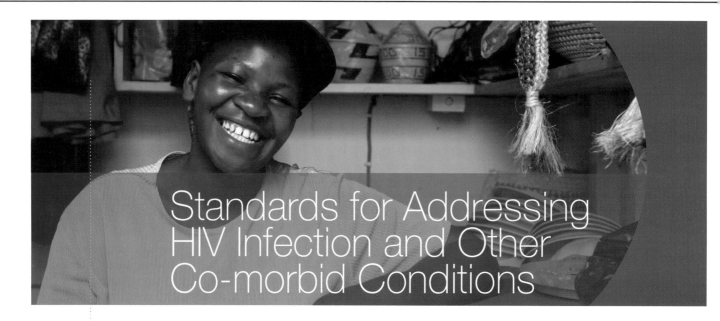

Standards for Addressing HIV Infection and Other Co-morbid Conditions

Knowledge of a person's HIV status influences the approach to a diagnostic evaluation and treatment for tuberculosis.

STANDARD 14. HIV testing and counseling should be conducted for all patients with, or suspected of having, tuberculosis unless there is a confirmed negative test within the previous two months. Because of the close relationship of tuberculosis and HIV infection, integrated approaches to prevention, diagnosis, and treatment of both tuberculosis and HIV infection are recommended in areas with high HIV prevalence. HIV testing is of special importance as part of routine management of all patients in areas with a high prevalence of HIV infection in the general population, in patients with symptoms and/or signs of HIV-related conditions, and in patients having a history suggestive of high risk of HIV exposure.

Rationale and Evidence Summary

Tuberculosis is strongly associated with HIV infection and is estimated to cause more than a quarter of deaths among persons with HIV.[21,206] An autopsy study conducted among adults with HIV infection who died at home in a South African setting found microbiological evidence of tuberculosis in 34% and active tuberculosis in 19%.[207] Similarly, an autopsy study conducted in Kenya among adults with HIV infection who died after receiving a median 10 months of antiretroviral therapy (ART) found microbiological or histological evidence of tuberculosis in 52% and tuberculosis was thought to be the cause of death in 41% of people living with HIV who died within 3 months of ART initiation.[208]

Infection with HIV increases the likelihood of progression from infection with *M. tuberculosis* to active tuberculosis. The risk of developing tuberculosis in people living with HIV is between 20 and 37 times greater than among those who do not have HIV infection.[206] Although the prevalence of HIV infection varies widely between and within countries, among persons with HIV infection there is always an increased risk of tuberculosis. The wide differences in HIV prevalence mean that a variable percentage of patients with tuberculosis will have HIV infection as well. This ranges from less than 1% in low HIV prevalence countries up to 50–77% in countries with a high HIV prevalence, mostly sub-Saharan African countries.[21] Even though in low HIV prevalence countries few tuberculosis patients are HIV-infected, the connection is sufficiently strong and the impact on the patient sufficiently great that provider-initiated HIV counseling and testing should always be conducted in managing individual patients, especially among groups in which the prevalence

Integrated care facilitates early detection and prompt treatment of tuberculosis resulting in a reduction of mortality and improved treatment success.

of HIV is higher, such as injecting drug users. In countries having a high prevalence of HIV infection, the yield of positive results will be high and, again, the impact of a positive result on the patient will be great.[209] Thus, the indication for HIV testing is strong; co-infected patients will benefit by access to antiretroviral therapy and by administration of cotrimoxazole for prevention of opportunistic infections.[209] Testing for HIV among presumptive tuberculosis cases in sub-Saharan Africa also yields high HIV-positive results.[210,211] In addition, in South Africa testing household contacts of patients with tuberculosis for both HIV and tuberculosis resulted in detection of a large number of undiagnosed tuberculosis cases and persons with HIV infection.[212] A study in Thailand also showed higher HIV prevalence among contacts of tuberculosis patients living with HIV than among contacts of HIV-negative tuberculosis patients.[213]

Infection with HIV changes the clinical manifestations of tuberculosis.[214,215] Further, in comparison with non-HIV infected patients, patients with HIV infection who have pulmonary tuberculosis have a lower likelihood of having acid-fast bacilli detected by sputum smear microscopy.[216] Moreover, data consistently show that the chest radiographic features are atypical and the proportion of extrapulmonary tuberculosis is greater in patients with advanced HIV infection compared with those who do not have HIV infection. Consequently, knowledge of a person's HIV status influences the approach to a diagnostic evaluation for tuberculosis. For this reason it is important, particularly in areas in which there is a high prevalence of HIV infection, that provider-initiated HIV testing and counseling be implemented for persons suspected of having tuberculosis and those known to have tuberculosis.[210,217] In addition, the history and physical examination should include a search for indicators that suggest the presence of HIV infection. A comprehensive list of clinical criteria/algorithms for HIV/AIDS clinical staging is available in the WHO document *WHO Case Definitions of HIV for Surveillance and Revised Clinical Staging and Immunological Classification of HIV-Related Disease in Adults and Children*.[218]

Studies of integrated tuberculosis and HIV services have demonstrated that integrated care facilitates early detection and prompt treatment of tuberculosis resulting in a reduction of mortality and improved treatment success.[219-223] The integrated model of tuberculosis and HIV services in a single health facility also improves ART enrollment and ART update, and supports early initiation of ART.[209,219-223] Thus, integrated approaches to prevention, diagnosis, and treatment of tuberculosis and HIV are strongly recommended in areas of high HIV prevalence.

STANDARD 15. In persons with HIV infection and tuberculosis who have profound immunosuppression (CD4 counts less than 50 cells/mm³), ART should be initiated within 2 weeks of beginning treatment for tuberculosis unless tuberculous meningitis is present. For all other patients with HIV and tuberculosis, regardless of CD4 counts, antiretroviral therapy should be initiated within 8 weeks of beginning treatment for tuberculosis. Patients with tuberculosis and HIV infection should also receive cotrimoxazole as prophylaxis for other infections.

Rationale and Evidence Summary

The evidence on effectiveness of treatment for tuberculosis in patients with HIV co-infection versus those who do not have HIV infection has been reviewed extensively.[14,122,125,126,224-227]

These reviews suggest that, in general, the outcome of treatment for tuberculosis is the same in HIV-infected and non-HIV-infected patients with the notable exception that death rates are greater among patients with HIV infection, presumably due in large part to complications of HIV infection. Tuberculosis treatment regimens are largely the same for HIV-infected and non-HIV-infected patients; however, the results are better if rifampicin is used throughout and treatment is given daily at least in the intensive phase.[126]

In patients with HIV-related tuberculosis, treating tuberculosis is the first priority. In the setting of advanced HIV infection, untreated tuberculosis can progress rapidly to death. As noted above, however, antiretroviral treatment may be lifesaving for patients with advanced HIV infection. Therefore, all patients with tuberculosis and HIV infection should receive antiretroviral therapy as early as possible regardless of CD4 counts.[228] Antiretroviral therapy results in remarkable reduction in mortality and AIDS-related morbidity, and greatly improves survival and quality of life of HIV-infected persons. ART is associated with reduction of mortality risk that in different studies has ranged from 54% to 95% in both resource-limited and high-income settings.[229] Recent clinical trials, STRIDE and SAPIT, showed reduction of deaths and AIDS-related events by 42% and 68%, respectively, with early ART in combination with tuberculosis treatment in persons with advanced HIV infection.[230,231] The CAMELIA trial found reduction of mortality by 34% when ART was initiated 2 weeks compared with 8 weeks following initiation of tuberculosis treatment in patients with profound immunosuppression (median CD4 count of 25 cells/mm³).[232] Thus, evidence from these trials indicates that ART should be initiated within 2 weeks after the start of tuberculosis treatment for patients with a CD4 count less than 50 cells/mm³ and as early as possible within 8 weeks for the other HIV-positive tuberculosis cases.[209] Caution should be given for early initiation of ART in HIV-positive patients with tuberculous meningitis because of its association with higher rate of adverse events compared with initiation of ART 2 months after start of tuberculosis treatment.[233]

ART should be initiated within 2 weeks after the start of tuberculosis treatment for patients with a CD4 count less than 50 cells/mm³ and as early as possible within 8 weeks for the other HIV-positive tuberculosis cases.

There are some important issues associated with concomitant therapy for tuberculosis and HIV infection that should be considered. These include overlapping toxicity profiles for the drugs used, drug-drug interactions (especially with rifampicin and protease inhibitors), potential problems with adherence to multiple medications, and immune reconstitution inflammatory reactions.[122,214] There are few drug interactions with tuberculosis drugs and the nucleoside reverse transcriptase inhibitors (NRTIs) and no specific changes are recommended. However, rifampicin reduces drug levels of both non-nucleoside reverse transcriptase inhibitors (NNRTI) and protease inhibitors through induction of the cytochrome P450 liver enzyme system. Therefore, efavirenz should be used as the preferred NNRTI since its interactions with antituberculosis drugs are minimal. In several studies, ART with standard-dose efavirenz and two nucleosides was well tolerated and highly efficacious in achieving viral load suppression.[14] In HIV-positive tuberculosis patients who need an ART regimen containing a boosted protease inhibitor (PI), it is recommended to use a rifabutin-based regimen.[14] Patients should also be closely monitored to identify adverse drug reactions and to observe for immune reconstitution inflammatory syndrome (IRIS). Although some studies reported increased risk of IRIS when ART is started earlier, the mortality benefit of earlier ART initiation outweighs the IRIS risk, which usually is self-limited.[234]

Patients with tuberculosis and HIV infection should also receive cotrimoxazole (trimetho-prim-sulfamethoxazole) as prophylaxis for other infections. Several studies have demonstrated the benefits of cotrimoxazole prophylaxis, and this intervention is currently recommended by the WHO as part of the TB/HIV management package.[209,214,235-239]

STANDARD 16. **Persons with HIV infection who, after careful evaluation, do not have active tuberculosis should be treated for presumed latent tuberculosis infection with isoniazid for at least 6 months.**

Rationale and Evidence Summary

Early identification of symptoms consistent with tuberculosis followed by prompt diagnostic evaluation and appropriate treatment of the disease among people living with HIV increases survival and improves quality of life. Thus, screening for symptoms among persons with HIV infection is crucial for identifying both tuberculosis cases and persons who should receive isoniazid preventive therapy.[46,47,240,241] A comprehensive systematic review and meta-analysis found that the absence of four symptoms: current cough, night sweats, fever, or weight loss identified a large subset of PLHIV who are very unlikely to have active tuberculosis.[47] All persons with HIV infection should be regularly screened for tuberculosis using the clinical algorithm with the four symptoms: current cough, night sweats, fever or weight loss, at every visit to a health facility or contact with a health care worker.[47,209,216,241] PLHIV who report any one of the symptoms should be evaluated for tuberculosis and other diseases. Similarly, children living with HIV who have one of the following symptoms—poor weight gain, fever, current cough, or a history of contact with a person who has infectious tuberculosis should be evaluated for tuberculosis and other conditions.[209,241] The diagnostic evaluation for tuberculosis should be done in accordance with national and international guidelines. In HIV-prevalent settings, Xpert MTB/RIF should be used as the initial test.[59,85] PLHIV who do not have any one of the four screening symptoms cited above or a history of contact with a person who has infectious tuberculosis are unlikely to have active tuberculosis (negative predictive value 97.7%, 95% CI 97.4–98.0) and, therefore, are candidates for IPT.[47,241]

Isoniazid, given to PLHIV in whom tuberculosis has been excluded reduces the risk of tuberculosis by approximately 33% compared with placebo.[242] The protective effect decreases with time after treatment but may persist for 2–3 years. The benefit is most pronounced in persons with a positive tuberculin skin test (~64% reduction) and is substantially less (14%) in persons with negative or unknown tuberculin skin test results. After excluding active tuberculosis, isoniazid (approximately 5 mg/kg/day, 300 mg/day maximum for adults and 10 mg/kg/day up to 300 mg/day for children) should be given to persons with HIV infection who are known to have latent tuberculosis infection or who have been in contact with an infectious tuberculosis case. If performing a tuberculin skin test is not possible, isoniazid is recommended for all PLHIV.[209,241] There is a trend to lower tuberculosis incidence with a longer preventive therapy particularly in settings with high tuberculosis prevalence and transmission and among tuberculin skin test-positive PLHIV.[243,244]

In spite of there having been strong evidence-based recommendations for the use of IPT in PLHIV since 1998, implementation for these recommendations has been very limited.

Screening for symptoms among persons with HIV infection is crucial for identifying both tuberculosis cases and persons who should receive isoniazid preventive therapy.

The reluctance to use IPT is based, particularly, on concerns with creating drug resistance if active tuberculosis is not excluded. In a study conducted in Rio de Janeiro, Brazil, operational training of physicians to screen for tuberculosis in public HIV clinics combined with the use of tuberculin skin testing led to improved implementation of IPT.[245] There was a modest population level reduction in the incidence of tuberculosis (13% reduction) and death (24% reduction). After adjustment for important covariates (age, CD4 count, antiretroviral treatment), there was a 27% reduction in incidence and a 31% reduction in deaths. Adverse effects were minimal.

Treatment of latent tuberculosis infection with a regimen of once weekly rifapentine and isoniazid given for 3 months (12 doses) under direct observation has been shown in low tuberculosis incidence settings to be as effective as a 9-month isoniazid regimen in preventing tuberculosis.[246] Moreover, the treatment completion rate was significantly higher. The weekly rifapentine/isoniazid regimen also showed less toxicity than other drug combination or continuous isoniazid regimens.[244,247] However, this regimen has not been evaluated in high-prevalence settings and thus cannot be recommended at this time in those settings.

The combined use of IPT and antiretroviral therapy (ART) among PLHIV significantly reduces the incidence of tuberculosis. The combined use of ART and IPT can reduce tuberculosis incidence among PLHIV by up to 97% particularly among persons with positive tuberculin skin tests.[248,249] Earlier initiation of ART at a CD4 cell count of more than 350/µl can reduce tuberculosis incidence by 60% and the reduction is 84% if ART is started when the CD4 cell count is less than 200/µl.[250] A recent clinical trial among PLHIV who received ART showed that at 12 months isoniazid resulted in a 40% reduction of tuberculosis incidence regardless of the tuberculin skin test result.[251]

STANDARD 17. All providers should conduct a thorough assessment for co-morbid conditions and other factors that could affect tuberculosis treatment response or outcome and identify additional services that would support an optimal outcome for each patient. These services should be incorporated into an individualized plan of care that includes assessment of and referrals for treatment of other illnesses. Particular attention should be paid to diseases or conditions known to affect treatment outcome, for example, diabetes mellitus, drug and alcohol abuse, undernutrition, and tobacco smoking. Referrals to other psychosocial support services, or to such services as antenatal or well-baby care should also be provided.

Rationale and Evidence Summary

In addition to the location, severity, and extent of tuberculosis, a number of other factors can affect the response to and outcome of treatment. These factors include concomitant illnesses (such as diabetes mellitus), psychosocial issues, and socioeconomic barriers to treatment completion. In working with a patient to treat tuberculosis, the provider must assess and address other contributing factors to ensure that there is the greatest chance of cure. Addressing co-morbid conditions commonly associated with tuberculosis can decrease treatment default, prevent drug resistance, and decrease treatment failures and deaths.

There are a number of conditions that are either risk factors for tuberculosis or are common in patients with the disease. Many of these can adversely affect treatment outcome. These include HIV (discussed previously), other immunosuppressive disorders, diabetes mellitus, malnutrition, alcoholism, other substance abuse, and tobacco use.[252-256]

Clinicians should take individual risk factors into account and carry out the necessary tests to evaluate co-morbid conditions relevant to tuberculosis treatment response and outcome. These should be provided free of charge to the patient.

Because of its increasing prevalence, diabetes mellitus is a particular concern.[257] Diabetes triples the risk of developing tuberculosis and can increase the severity of tuberculosis.[258] Conversely, tuberculosis can worsen blood glucose control in persons with diabetes. Tuberculosis must be considered in people with diabetes, and diabetes must be considered in people with tuberculosis. Individuals with both conditions require careful clinical management to ensure that optimal care is provided for both diseases.[259]

The same tuberculosis treatment regimen should be prescribed for patients with diabetes as for those without diabetes. However, because of the potential for reduced concentrations of rifampicin, careful observation of clinical response is necessary.[260] Where possible, patients with tuberculosis should be screened for diabetes at the start of their treatment. Management of diabetes in patients with tuberculosis should be provided in line with existing management guidelines.[261]

Coexisting non-infectious lung diseases, such as chronic obstructive pulmonary disease (COPD), may increase the risk for tuberculosis and complicate management. Both clinical and radiographic assessment of response may be confounded by coexisting lung disease. Tuberculosis is also a risk for the development of COPD and may be a major contributor to this emerging problem in low–resource settings.[262]

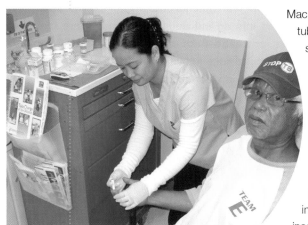

Having a diagnosis of tuberculosis may serve as an entry point to health care and psychosocial services that can enhance treatment completion.

Macro- and micronutritional deficiencies are both causes and consequences of tuberculosis and therefore very common at the time of tuberculosis diagnosis. All tuberculosis patients should have a nutritional assessment including weight and height in order to determine body mass index. Nutritional care should be provided according to the nutritional status of the patient in line with guidelines on nutritional care for people with tuberculosis. Nutritional support, for example a food package, should be considered for patients who do not have the financial means to meet their nutritional needs during tuberculosis treatment.[263]

Social factors[13,142] may also be important in influencing treatment response and outcome, and interventions should be considered to mitigate their impact. Homelessness, social isolation, migration for work, a history of incarceration, and unemployment have all been cited as barriers to treatment adherence and risk factors for poor treatment outcome.[13,142] Having a diagnosis of tuberculosis may serve as an entry point to health care and psychosocial services that can enhance treatment completion. Treatment support including psychosocial support is a cornerstone of the best practices for tuberculosis treatment described in detail in *Best Practice for the Care of Patients with Tuberculosis: a Guide for Low-income Countries*.[16] By providing patients with referrals to accessible services for co-morbid conditions of any kind, the provider enhances their chances for cure in the shortest possible time and contributes to increasing the overall health of the community.

It is recognized that not all necessary services are currently available in the areas most in need of this support. To the extent these services are available, they should be fully utilized to support tuberculosis patient treatment. Where they are not available, plans to enhance relevant capacities should be incorporated into local, regional, and national tuberculosis control strategies.

Other diseases and treatments, especially immunosuppressive treatments such as corticosteroids and tumor necrosis factor (TNF) alpha inhibitors, increase the risk of tuberculosis and may alter the clinical features of the disease.[264,265] Clinicians caring for patients with diseases or taking drugs that alter immune responsiveness must be aware of the increased risk of tuberculosis and be alert for symptoms that may indicate the presence of tuberculosis. Isoniazid preventive treatment may be considered for such patients if active tuberculosis is excluded.

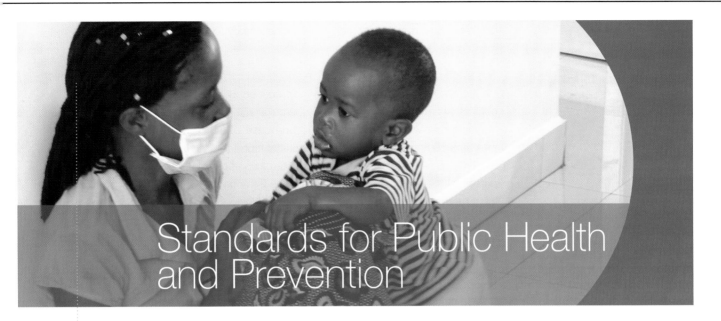

Standards for Public Health and Prevention

STANDARD 18. All providers should ensure that persons in close contact with patients who have infectious tuberculosis are evaluated and managed in line with international recommendations. The highest priority contacts for evaluation are:

- Persons with symptoms suggestive of tuberculosis
- Children aged <5 years
- Contacts with known or suspected immunocompromised states, particularly HIV infection
- Contacts of patients with MDR/XDR tuberculosis

This inability to conduct targeted contact investigations results in missed opportunities to prevent additional cases of tuberculosis, especially among children.

Rationale and Evidence Summary

The determination of priorities for contact investigation is based on the likelihood that a contact: 1) has undiagnosed tuberculosis; 2) is at high risk of developing tuberculosis if infected; 3) is at risk of having severe tuberculosis if the disease develops; and 4) is at high risk of having been infected by the index case. The risk of acquiring infection with *M. tuberculosis* is correlated with intensity and duration of exposure to a person with infectious tuberculosis, generally called an index case. A contact is any person who has been exposed to an index case. Commonly contacts are divided into two groups, household and non-household. A person who shared the same enclosed living space for one or more nights, or for frequent or extended periods during the day with the index case during the 3 months before commencement of the current treatment episode, is defined as a household contact. Non-household contacts may also share an enclosed space, such as a social gathering place, workplace, or facility, for extended periods during the day with the index case during the 3 months before commencement of the current treatment episode and thus also be at risk of having acquired infection with *M. tuberculosis*. Contact investigation is considered an important activity, both to find persons with previously undetected tuberculosis and persons who are candidates for treatment of latent tuberculosis infection.[266-268]

Unfortunately, lack of adequate staff and resources in many areas makes contact investigation a challenging task. This inability to conduct targeted contact investigations results in missed opportunities to prevent additional cases of tuberculosis, especially among children. Thus, more energetic efforts are necessary to overcome these barriers to optimum tuberculosis control practices.

Two systematic reviews of studies on household contact investigations in low- and middle-income settings showed that, on average, about 4.5% and 3.1% respectively of the contacts were found to have active tuberculosis.[269,270] The median number of household contacts that were evaluated to find one case of active tuberculosis was 19 (range 14–300). The median proportion of contacts found to have latent infection was just over 50% in both studies. The median number of contacts that were evaluated to find one person with latent tuberculosis infection was 2 (range 1–14). In the review by Fox et al,[270] longer term follow up demonstrated that the incidence of tuberculosis remained above the background rate for at least 5 years. Evidence from these reviews suggests that contact investigation in high-incidence settings is a high-yield strategy for case finding. Based on the evidence from the reviews, WHO developed recommendations for contact investigation in low resource settings.[8]

A systematic review and meta-analysis of the yield of investigation of contacts of persons with MDR/XDR tuberculosis found a pooled yield of 6.5% of contacts also had active tuberculosis.[271] Latent tuberculosis infection was found in 50.7%.

The main benefit of contact investigation for contacts of MDR/XDR index cases is early detection of active tuberculosis that should result in decreasing transmission of MDR/XDR organisms. In the systematic review, just over 50% of contacts with active tuberculosis had drug susceptibility profiles that were concordant with the index case. Unfortunately, there are no current recommendations for treatment of latent infection that is presumed to be with MDR/XDR organisms.

STANDARD 19. **Children <5 years of age and persons of any age with HIV infection who are close contacts of a person with infectious tuberculosis, and who, after careful evaluation, do not have active tuberculosis, should be treated for presumed latent tuberculosis infection with isoniazid for at least six months.**

Rationale and Evidence Summary

Children (particularly those under the age of five years) are a vulnerable group because of the high likelihood of progressing from latent infection to active tuberculosis. Children, especially if very young, are also more likely to develop disseminated and serious forms of tuberculosis such as meningitis. For these reasons it is recommended that, after active tuberculosis is excluded, children under the age of five years living in the same household as a sputum smear-positive tuberculosis patient should be treated with isoniazid, 10 mg/kg/day (up to a maximum of 300 mg), for 6 months on the presumption that they have been infected by the index case. The screening of children for active tuberculosis can be accomplished by a careful medical history and physical examination, as illustrated in Figure 1.[114]

Likewise, PLHIV are highly vulnerable to developing tuberculosis if infected and, thus, should be carefully evaluated for the presence of active tuberculosis. Persons with HIV infection should be evaluated and treated as described in Standard 16.[241] Monitoring and evaluation of IPT as a programmatic intervention should be undertaken as described in *Recommendations for Investigating Contacts of Persons with Infectious Tuberculosis in Low- and Middle-income Countries.*[8]

In persons other than children <5 years of age and PLHIV, the tuberculin skin test and interferon-gamma release assays may be used to identify those at increased risk for developing active tuberculosis and who are therefore candidates for treatment of latent infection once active tuberculosis is excluded.[8] Because the public health benefit of treatment for latent tuberculosis infection, other than for children and PLHIV, in low- and middle-income countries is not proven, it is not recommended as a programmatic approach. However, as a part of care for individuals with risk factors for tuberculosis who are exposed to a person with infectious tuberculosis, clinicians may choose to test for latent infection with a tuberculin skin test or interferon-gamma release assay and, if the test is positive and active tuberculosis is excluded, give treatment for latent tuberculosis infection as a preventive intervention.[8]

FIGURE 1.

Approach to evaluation and management of children in contact with an infectious case of tuberculosis when a tuberculin skin test and chest radiograph are not available

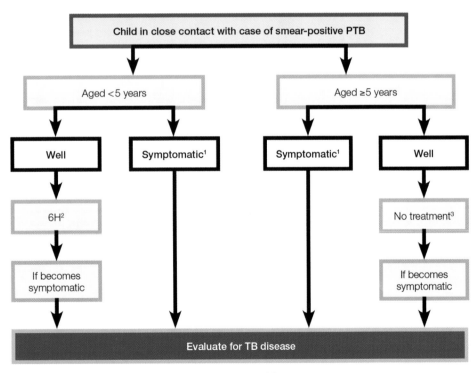

1. If tuberculosis is suspected evaluate as described in Standard 6
2. Treat with isoniazid 10 mg/kg/day for six months
3. No treatment should be given unless the child is HIV-infected in which case give isoniazid 10 mg/kg/day

STANDARD 20. Each health care facility caring for patients who have, or are suspected of having, infectious tuberculosis should develop and implement an appropriate tuberculosis infection control plan to minimize possible transmission of *M. tuberculosis* to patients and health care workers.

Rationale and Evidence Summary

M. tuberculosis is spread nearly exclusively via the air, thus, the simple act of sharing air with a person who has infectious tuberculosis may result in transmission of the infection. There have been a number of well-documented outbreaks of tuberculosis including MDR and XDR tuberculosis that have occurred in health care facilities. Because of the concern with transmission of both drug-resistant and drug susceptible *M. tuberculosis* to patients and health care workers in facilities providing care for patients with tuberculosis, infection control is now recognized to be of considerable importance.[17-19,272-274]

Infection control for tuberculosis consists of managerial activities at the facility level and a hierarchy of three categories of control measures including administrative controls (most important), environmental controls, and the use of respirators (special masks designed to protect the wearer).

Managerial Controls: Facility-level managerial activities constitute the framework for setting up and implementing the other two categories of controls and should include the following: identification and strengthening of local coordinating bodies; development of a facility plan (including human resources) for implementation of infection control measures; and policies and procedures to ensure proper implementation of the control measures. In addition, policies that minimize the use of health care facilities, both for inpatients and outpatients, should be developed and implemented. Community approaches to providing care for persons with, or suspected of having, tuberculosis should be emphasized as a means of reducing visits to health care facilities.

Implementation of the control measures as a group reduces transmission of *M. tuberculosis* in health care facilities.[275] However, in health care facilities, administrative controls should be implemented as the first priority because they have been shown to be the most important measures in reducing transmission of tuberculosis. Consequently, all facilities, public and private, caring for patients with, or suspected of having, infectious tuberculosis should implement the set of measures in a manner that is best suited to the conditions that prevail in the facility, particularly local programmatic, climatic, and socioeconomic conditions. For example, infection control requirements will be less in programs that manage most patients with tuberculosis in the community compared with programs that routinely utilize hospitalization. The interventions should be consistent with and complement overall general infection control efforts and, particularly, those efforts targeting other airborne infections.

Administrative Controls: There are several administrative controls that are feasible in all settings that, taken together, could be predicted to minimize the likelihood of transmission occurring in the facility.[275-278] Administrative measures include careful screening and early identification of patients with, or suspected of having, tuberculosis and separating them from other patients, especially from patients who are highly susceptible to tuberculosis. Organizing patient flow through sections of facilities, for example, rapid identification of coughing patients, systematic use of surgical masks for coughing patients, and directing these patients away from crowded waiting areas (fast-tracking) can minimize the potential for exposure and transmission. Separation of patients who are suspected of having tuberculosis will decrease risks to other patients and will enable health workers to take appropriate precautions. Patients with HIV infection and other forms of immunosuppression, in particular, should be physically separated from patients with suspected or confirmed infectious tuberculosis. Patients who have or are at risk of having MDR tuberculosis should be separated from other patients, including other patients with tuberculosis. Having a universally applied program in which patients taught proper cough etiquette will serve to reduce dissemination of infectious aerosols.

Prompt collection of sputum specimens for microscopy or other microbiological evaluations is an important step in infection control. Early identification of tuberculosis leads to early initiation of treatment and a consequent prompt major reduction in infectiousness, if the organisms causing the disease are not resistant to the drugs being used. In areas in which there is a high prevalence of drug resistance, rapid drug susceptibility/resistance testing would enable identification and appropriate treatment.[276] Diagnostic delays can be further minimized by using rapid molecular tests (including rapid drug susceptibility tests), by reducing the laboratory turnaround time for sputum examination, and by carrying out diagnostic investigations in parallel rather than in sequence.

All health workers should be given appropriate information and encouraged to undergo regular screening for tuberculosis and HIV testing and counseling. Those who are HIV-infected should be offered appropriate prevention and care services. Health workers with HIV infection should not work in areas where exposure to untreated tuberculosis is likely and especially should not be caring for patients with known MDR and XDR tuberculosis, or in settings where drug resistance is likely. Such workers should be provided with jobs in a lower risk area.

Environmental Controls: The choice of environmental controls is largely determined by building design and intended use, construction details, local climatic and socioeconomic conditions, and available resources. Effective ventilation should be given a high priority. Ventilation effectively reduces the number of infectious particles in the air and may be achieved by natural ventilation in some settings, by mixed natural and mechanical ventilation, and by mechanical ventilation systems. The obvious benefit of natural ventilation as an approach to infection control is that can be applied to all areas that have windows and doors that open to the outside.[277] However, around the clock natural ventilation cannot be applied other than in tropical climates, and even in these areas, windows may be closed during the night for security or comfort negating the effect of natural ventilation, thus, it is of limited utility. In settings where optimal natural ventilation cannot be achieved, properly placed and shielded upper room ultraviolet germicidal irradiation fixtures should be considered as a complementary control. This may be especially useful in cold climates where outdoor ventilation is limited.

Disposable Particulate Respirators (masks): Particulate respirators protect the person wearing the device by filtering particles out of the inspired air.[278] Respirators that meet or exceed Centers for Disease Control and Prevention/National Institute for Occupational Services and Health (CDC/NIOSH)-certified N95 or CE-certified FFP2 standards (filter at least 95% of airborne particles $\geq$ 0.3 μm in diameter) should be worn by health care providers in areas where the risk of transmission is high after appropriate training.[17,19]

Indications for using a respirator should be defined by the facility, but commonly include procedures in which aerosols are generated, such as bronchoscopy, or exposure to persons with untreated or ineffectively treated tuberculosis. In areas where drug resistance is common, however, every patient with tuberculosis should be considered potentially to have drug-resistant disease for purposes of infection control.

STANDARD 21. All providers must report both new and re-treatment tuberculosis cases and their treatment outcomes to local public health authorities, in conformance with applicable legal requirements, regulations, and policies.

Rationale and Evidence Summary

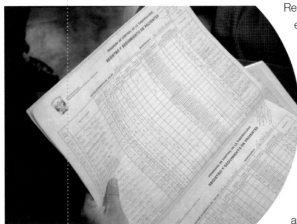

Reporting tuberculosis cases to the local tuberculosis control program is an essential public health function and in many countries is legally mandated. Ideally, the reporting system design, supported by a legal framework, should be capable of receiving and integrating data from several sources including laboratories and health care institutions, as well as from individual practitioners.

An effective reporting system that includes all providers enables a determination of the overall effectiveness of tuberculosis control programs, of resource needs, and of the true distribution and dynamics of the disease within the population as a whole, not just the population served by the government tuberculosis control program. In most countries tuberculosis is a notifiable disease. Such a system is useful not only to monitor progress and treatment outcomes of individual patients, but also to evaluate the overall performance of the tuberculosis control programs at the local, national, and global levels, and to indicate programmatic weaknesses.

A regularly updated recording and reporting system allows for targeted, individualized follow-up to help patients who are not making adequate progress (i.e., failing therapy).[279] The system also allows for evaluation of the performance of the practitioner, the hospital or institution, local health system, and the country as a whole. Finally, a system of recording and reporting ensures accountability.

An additional important function of a recording and reporting system is to identify serious adverse events resulting from antituberculosis drugs.[280] This surveillance is especially important as new drugs and regimens are introduced. In both the WHO and CDC recommendations regarding the use of bedaquiline, it is strongly recommended that there be ongoing surveillance and reporting of adverse events.[200,281] Clinical experience with the drug is limited, but because of the pressing need for new drugs to treat MDR TB,

An effective reporting system that includes all providers enables a determination of the overall effectiveness of tuberculosis control programs, of resource needs, and of the true distribution and dynamics of the disease.

bedaquiline was released for use under specific conditions. There are many instances of serious adverse effects of drugs being identified by post-marketing surveillance (phase IV studies). Similarly there is little systematic information on the adverse effects of many of the drugs and regimens used in treating MDR TB, thus pharmacovigilance is important in this group as well.

Although, on the one hand reporting to public health authorities is essential, on the other hand it is also essential that patient confidentiality be maintained. Thus, reporting must follow predefined channels using standard procedures that guarantee that only authorized persons see the information. Such safeguards must be developed by local and national tuberculosis control programs to ensure the confidentiality of patient information.

References

1. World Health Organization. Systematic screening for active tuberculosis: Principles and recommendations. Geneva: World Health Organization, 2013. WHO/HTM/TB/2013.04.

2. World Health Organization. Global strategy and targets for tuberculosis prevention, care and control after 2015. Geneva: World Health Organization 2014.

3. Hopewell PC, Pai M. Tuberculosis, vulnerability, and access to quality care. *JAMA.* 2005; **293**(22): 2790-3.

4. Hopewell PC, Pai M, Maher D, et al. International standards for tuberculosis care. *Lancet Infect Dis.* 2006; **6**(11): 710-25.

5. World Health Organization. Handbook for guideline development. Geneva: World Health Organization, 2012.

6. World Health Organization. Public-private mix for TB care and control: A toolkit. Geneva: World Health Organization, 2010. WHO/HTM/TB/2010.12.

7. Chakaya J, Uplekar M, Mansoer J, et al. Public-private mix for control of tuberculosis and TB-HIV in Nairobi, Kenya: outcomes, opportunities and obstacles. *Int J Tuberc Lung Dis.* 2008; **12**(11): 1274-8.

8. World Health Organization. Recommendations for investigating contacts of persons with infectious tuberculosis in low- and middle-income countries. Geneva: World Health Organization, 2012. WHO/HTM/TB/2012.9.

9. World Health Organization. Integrating community-based tuberculosis activities into the work of nongovernmental and other civil society organizations. Geneva: World Health Organization, 2012. WHO/HTM/TB/2012/8.

10. World Health Organization. Definitions and reporting framework for tuberculosis. Geneva: World Health Organization, 2013. WHO/HTM/TB/2013.2.

11. Migliori GB, Zellweger JP, Abubakar I, et al. European Union standards for tuberculosis care. *Eur Resp J.* 2012; **39**(4): 807-19.

12. Pai M, Das J. Management of Tuberculosis in India: Time for a deeper dive into quality. *Nat Med J India.* 2013; **26**(2): 65-8.

13. World Health Organization. Adherence to long-term therapies: Evidence for action. Geneva: World Health Organization, 2003. WHO/MNC/03.01.

14. World Health Organization. Treatment of uberculosis guidelines (Fourth edition). Geneva: World Health Organization, 2009. WHO/HTM/TB/2009.420.

15. American Thoracic Society, Centers for Disease Control and Prevention, Infectious Diseases Society of America. Controlling Tuberculosis in the United States. *MMWR* 2005; **54**(RR12): 1-81.

16. Ait-Khaled N, Alarcon E, Armengol R, et al. Management of tuberculosis: A guide to the essentials of good practice. Paris: International Union Against Tuberculosis and Lung Disease; 2010.

17. Centers for Disease Control and Prevention. Guidelines for preventing the transmission of Mycobacterium tuberculosis in health care settings, 2005. MMWR 2005; **54**(RR17):1-141.

18. World Health Organization. WHO policy on TB infection control in health-care facilities, congregate settings and households. Geneva: World Health Organization, 2009. WHO/HTM/TB/2009.419.

19. Sotgiu G, D'Ambrosio L, Centis R, et al. TB and M/XDR TB infection control in European TB reference centres: the Achilles' heel? *Eur Respir J.* 2011; **38**(5): 1221-3.

20. Lönnroth K, Raviglione M. Global epidemiology of tuberculosis: prospects for control. *Semin Respir Crit Care Med.* 2008; **29**(5): 481-91.

21. World Health Organization. Global Tuberculosis Report, 2013. Geneva: World Health Organization; 2013.

22. World Health Organization. Multidrug and extensively drug-resistant TB (M/XDR TB): 2010 global report on surveillance and response. Geneva: World Health Organization, 2010. WHO/HTM/TB/2010.3.

23. Malmborg R, Mann G, Squire SB. A systematic assessment of the concept and practice of public-private mix for tuberculosis care and control. *Int J Equity Health.* 2011; **10**(1): 49.

24. Dewan PK, Lal SS, Lönnroth K, et al. Improving tuberculosis control through public-private collaboration in India: literature review. *BMJ.* 2006; **332**(7541): 574-8.

25. van der Werf MJ, Langendam MW, Huitric E, Manissero D. Multidrug resistance after inappropriate tuberculosis treatment: a meta-analysis. *Eur Respir J.* 2012; **39**(6): 1511-9.

26. World Health Organization. Involving private practitioners in tuberculosis control: issues, interventions, and emerging policy framework. Geneva: World Health Organization, 2001. WHO/CDS/TB/2001.285.

27. Storla DG, Yimer S, Bjune GA. A systematic review of delay in the diagnosis and treatment of tuberculosis. *BMC Public Health.* 2008; **8**: 15.

28. Sreeramareddy CT, Panduru KV, Menten J, Van den Ende J. Time delays in diagnosis of pulmonary tuberculosis: a systematic review of literature. *BMC Infect Dis.* 2009; **9**: 91.

29. Davis J, Katamba A, Vasquez J, et al. Evaluating tuberculosis case detection via real-time monitoring of tuberculosis diagnostic services. *Am J Respir Crit Care Med*. 2011; **184**(3): 362-7.

30. Uplekar M, Pathania V, Raviglione M. Private practitioners and public health: weak links in tuberculosis control. *Lancet.* 2001; **358**(9285): 912-6.

31. Olle-Goig JE, Cullity JE, Vargas R. A survey of prescribing patterns for tuberculosis treatment amongst doctors in a Bolivian city. *Int J Tuberc Lung Dis.* 1999; **3**(1): 74-8.

32. Shah SK, Sadiq H, Khalil M, et al. Do private doctors follow national guidelines for managing pulmonary tuberculosis in Pakistan? *East Mediterr Health J.* 2003; **9**(4): 776-88.

33. Prasad R, Nautiyal RG, Mukherji PK, et al. Diagnostic evaluation of pulmonary tuberculosis: what do doctors of modern medicine do in India? *Int J Tuberc Lung Dis.* 2003; **7**(1): 52-7.

34. Lönnroth K, Thuong LM, Linh PD, Diwan VK. Delay and discontinuity--a survey of TB patients' search of a diagnosis in a diversified health care system. *Int J Tuberc Lung Dis.* 1999; **3**(11): 992-1000.

35. Cheng G, Tolhurst R, Li RZ, Meng QY, Tang S. Factors affecting delays in tuberculosis diagnosis in rural China: a case study in four counties in Shandong Province. *Trans R Soc Trop Med Hyg.* 2005; **99**(5): 355-62.

36. Uplekar M. Involving private health care providers in delivery of TB care: global strategy. *Tuberculosis.* 2003; **83**(1): 156-64.

37. Grenier J, Pinto L, Nair D, et al. Widespread use of serological tests for tuberculosis: data from 22 high-burden countries. *Eur Resp J.* 2012; **39**(2): 502-5.

38. World Health Organization. Commercial serodiagnostic tests for diagnosis of tuberculosis: Policy statement. Geneva, World Health Organization, 2011. WHO/HTM/TB/2011.5.

39. World Health Organization. Guidance on ethics of tuberculosis prevention, care, and control. Geneva: World Health Organization, 2010. WHO/HTM/TB/2010.16.

40. Ukwaja KN, Alobu I, Abimbola S, Hopewell PC. Household catastrophic payments for tuberculosis care in Nigeria: incidence, determinants, and policy implications for universal health coverage. *Infect Dis Poverty.* 2013; **2**: 21.

41. Ukwaja KN, Alobu I, Lgwenyi C, Hopewell PC. The high cost of free tuberculosis services: patient and household costs associated with tuberculosis care in ebonyi state, Nigeria. *PLoS One.* 2013; **8**: e73134.

42. World Health Organization. Early detection of tuberculosis: An overview of approaches, guidelines, and tools. Geneva, World health Organization, 2011. WHO/HTM/STB/PSI/2011.21.

43. Miller CR, Davis JL, Katamba A, et al. Sex disparities in tuberculosis suspect evaluation: a cross-sectional analysis in rural Uganda. *Int J Tuberc Lung Dis.* 2013; **17**(4): 480-5.

44. Ministry of Health, Cambodia. National tuberculosis prevalence survey, 2002. Phnom Penh: Royal Government of Cambodia, 2005.

45. Hoa NB, Sy DN, Nhung NV, Tiemersma EW, Borgdorff MW, Cobelens FG. National survey of tuberculosis prevalence in Viet Nam. *Bull World Health Organ.* 2010; **88**(4): 273-80.

46. Ayles H, Schaap A, Nota A, et al. Prevalence of tuberculosis, HIV and respiratory symptoms in two Zambian communities: implications for tuberculosis control in the era of HIV. *PLoS One.* 2009; **4**(5): e5602.

47. Getahun H, Kittikraisak W, Heilig CM, et al. Development of a standardized screening rule for tuberculosis in people living with HIV in resource-constrained settings: individual participant data meta-analysis of observational studies. *PLoS Med.* 2011; **8**(1): e1000391.

48. World Health Organization. Practical approach to lung health: Manual on initiating PAL implementation. Geneva, World Health Organization, 2008. WHO/HTM/TB/2008.410.

49. World Health Organization. Implementing the Stop TB strategy: A handbook for national tuberculosis control programmes. Geneva: World Health Organization, 2008. WHO/HTM/TB/2008.401.

50. World Health Organization. Toman's tuberculosis: Case detection, treatment, and monitoring. Geneva: World Health Organization, 2004. WHO/HTM/TB/2004.334.

51. World Health Organization. Respiratory care in primary care services: A survey in 9 countries. Geneva, World health Organization, 2004. WHO/HTM/TB/2004.333.

52. Santha T, Garg R, Subramani R, et al. Comparison of cough of 2 and 3 weeks to improve detection of smear-positive tuberculosis cases among out-patients in India. *Int J Tuberc Lung Dis.* 2005; **9**(1): 61-8.

53. Nyamande K, Laloo UG, John M. TB presenting as community-acquired pneumonia in a setting of high TB incidence and high HIV prevalence. *Int J Tuberc Lung Dis.* 2007; **11**(12): 308-13.

54. Cavallazzi R, Wiemken T, Christensen D, et al. Predicting Mycobacterium tuberculosis in patients with community-acquired pneumonia. *Eur Respir J. 2014;* **43**(1):178-84.

55. Lienhardt C, Rowley J, Manneh K, et al. Factors affecting time delay to treatment in a tuberculosis control programme in a sub-Saharan African country: the experience of The Gambia. *Int J Tuberc Lung Di*s. 2001, **5**(3):233-239.

56. Khan J, Malik A, Hussain H, et al. Tuberculosis diagnosis and treatment practices of private physicians in Karachi, Pakistan. *East Mediterr Health J.* 2003; **9**(4): 769-75.

57. Singla N, Sharma PP, Singla R, Jain RC. Survey of knowledge, attitudes and practices for tuberculosis among general practitioners in Delhi, India. *Int J Tuberc Lung Dis.* 1998; **2**(5): 384-9.

58. Suleiman BA, Houssein AI, Mehta F, Hinderaker SG. Do doctors in north-western Somalia follow the national guidelines for tuberculosis management? *East Mediterr Health J.* 2003; **9**(4): 789-95.

59. World Health Organization. Policy statement: Automated real-time nucleic acid amplification technology for rapid and simultaneous detection of tuberculosis and rifampicin resistance: Xpert MTB/RIF system. Geneva: World Health Organization, 2011. WHO/HTM/TB/2011.4.

60. Centers for Disease Control and Prevention. Updated Guidelines for the Use of Nucleic Acid Amplification Tests in the Diagnosis of Tuberculosis. *MMWR.* 2009; **58**: 7-10.

61. Pinto L, Pai M, Dheda K, et al Scoring systems using chest radiographic features for the diagnosis of pulmonary tuberculosis in adults: A systematic review *Eur Respir J. 2013;* **42**(2):480-94.

62. Steingart KR, Henry M, Ng V, et al. Fluorescence versus conventional sputum smear microscopy for tuberculosis: a systematic review. *Lancet Infect Dis.* 2006; **6**(9): 570-81.

63. Steingart KR, Ng V, Henry M, et al. Sputum processing methods to improve the sensitivity of smear microscopy for tuberculosis: a systematic review. *Lancet Infect Dis.* 2006; **6**(10): 664-74.

64. Mase SR, Ramsay A, Ng V, et al. Yield of serial sputum specimen examinations in the diagnosis of pulmonary tuberculosis: a systematic review. *Int J Tuberc Lung Dis.* 2007; **11**(5): 485-95.

65. Davis JL, Cattamanchi A, Cuevas LE, et al. Diagnostic accuracy of same-day microscopy versus standard microscopy for pulmonary tuberculosis: a systematic review and meta-analysis. *Lancet Infect Dis.* 2013; **13**(2): 147-54.

66. Ling DI, Flores LL, Riley LW, Pai M. Commercial nucleic-acid amplification tests for diagnosis of pulmonary tuberculosis in respiratory specimens: Meta-analysis and meta-regression. *PLoS One.* 2008; **3**(2): e1536.

67. Greco S, Girardi E, Navarra S, Saltini C. The current evidence on diagnostic accuracy of commercial based nucleic acid amplification tests for the diagnosis of pulmonary tuberculosis. *Thorax.* 2006; **61**(9): 783-90.

68. Pai M, Flores LL, Hubbard A, et al. Nucleic acid amplification tests in the diagnosis of tuberculous pleuritis: a systematic review and meta-analysis. *BMC Infect Dis.* 2004; **4**(1): 6.

69. Pai M, Flores LL, Pai N, et al. Diagnostic accuracy of nucleic acid amplification tests for tuberculous meningitis: a systematic review and meta-analysis. *Lancet Infect Dis.* 2003; **3**(10): 633-43.

70. Daley P, Thomas S, Pai M. Nucleic acid amplification tests for the diagnosis of tuberculous lymphadenitis: a systematic review. *Int J Tuberc Lung Dis.* 2007; **11**(11): 1166-76.

71. Sarmiento OL, Weigle KA, Alexander J, et al. Assessment by meta-analysis of PCR for diagnosis of smear-negative pulmonary tuberculosis. *J Clin Microbiol.* 2003; **41**(7): 3233-40.

72. Dinnes J, Deeks J, Kunst H, et al. A systematic review of rapid diagnostic tests for the detection of tuberculosis infection. *Health technology assessment (Winchester, England)* 2007; **11**(3): 1-196.

73. Steingart KR, Schiller I, Horne DJ, et al. Xpert® MTB/RIF assay for pulmonary tuberculosis and rifampicin resistance in adults (Review). *Cochrane Database Syst Rev.* 2014; Issue 1. Art. No.: CD009593.

74. Cruciani M, Scarparo C, Malena M, et al. Meta-analysis of BACTEC MGIT 960 and BACTEC 460 TB, with or without solid media, for detection of mycobacteria. *J Clin Microbiol.* 2004; **42**(5): 2321-5.

75. Brent AJ, Mugo D, Musyimi R, et al. Performance of the MGIT TBc identification test and meta-analysis of MPT64 assays for identification of the Mycobacterium tuberculosis complex in liquid culture. *J Clin Microbiol.* 2011; **49**(12): 4343-6.

76. Parsons LM, Somoskövi A, Gutierrez C, et al. Laboratory diagnosis of tuberculosis in resource-poor countries: challenges and opportunities. *Clin. Microbiol. Rev.* 2011; **24**(2): 314-50.

77. World Health Organization. The use of the Xpert MTB/RIF® assay for the detection of pulmonary, extrapulmonary tuberculosis and rifampicin resistance in adults and children. Geneva; World health Organization, 2013, WHO/HTM/TB/2013.14.

78. Harries AD, Hargreaves NJ, Kemp J, et al. Deaths from tuberculosis in sub-Saharan African countries with a high prevalence of HIV-1. *Lancet.* 2001; **357**(9267): 519-23.

79. Maher D, Harries A, Getahun H. Tuberculosis and HIV interaction in sub-Saharan Africa: impact on patients and programmes; implications for policies. *Trop Med Int Health.* 2005; **10**(8): 734-42.

80. Rieder HL, Chiang CY, Rusen ID. A method to determine the utility of the third diagnostic and the second follow-up sputum smear examinations to diagnose tuberculosis cases and failures. *Int J Tuberc Lung Dis.* 2005; **9**(4): 384-91.

81. Steingart KR, Ramsay A, Pai M. Optimizing sputum smear microscopy for the diagnosis of pulmonary tuberculosis. *Expert Rev Anti Infect Ther.* 2007; **5**(3): 327-31.

82. World Health Organization. Fluorescent light-emitting diode (LED) microscopy for diagnosis of tuberculosis: Policy statement. Geneva, World health Organization, 2011. WHO/HTM/TB/2011.8.

83. World Health Organization. Automated real-time nucleic acid amplification technology for rapid and simultaneous detection of tuberculosis and rifampicin resistance: Xpert MTB/RIF system: Policy statement. Geneva: World Health Organization, 2011. WHO/HTM/TB/2011.4.

84. Weyer K, Mirzayev F, Migliori G, et al. Rapid molecular TB diagnosis: evidence, policy-making and global implementation of Xpert(R)MTB/RIF. *Eur Respir J.* 2012; **42**(1): 252-71.

85. World Health Organization. Rapid implementation of the Xpert MTB/RIF diagnostic test: Technical and operational 'how-to' practical considerations. Geneva: World Health Organization, 2011. WHO/HTM/TB/2011.2.

86. World Health Organization. Molecular line probe assays for rapid screening of patients at risk of multidrug-resistant tuberculosis (MDR TB): Policy statement. Geneva: World Health Organization, 2008.

87. Metcalfe JZ, Everett CK, Steingart KR, et al. Interferon-gamma release assays for active pulmonary tuberculosis diagnosis in adults in low- and middle-income countries: systematic review and meta-analysis. *J Infect Dis.* 2011; **204 Suppl 4**: S1120-9.

88. Steingart KR, Flores LL, Dendukuri N, et al. Commercial serological tests for the diagnosis of active pulmonary and extrapulmonary tuberculosis: an updated systematic review and meta-analysis. *PLoS Med.* 2011; **8**(8): e1001062.

89. Sandgren A, Hollo V, van der Werf MJ. Extrapulmonary tuberculosis in the European Union and European Economic Area, 2002 to 2011. *Euro Surveill.* 2013 Mar 21;**18**(12). pii: 20431.

90. Udwadia ZF, Sen T. Pleural tuberculosis: an update. *Curr Opin Pulm Med.* 2010; **16**(4): 399-406.

91. Thwaites GE, Caws M, Chau TT, et al. Comparison of conventional bacteriology with nucleic acid amplification (amplified mycobacterium direct test) for diagnosis of tuberculous meningitis before and after inception of antituberculosis chemotherapy. *J Clin Microbiol.* 2004; **42**(3): 996-1002.

92. Mtei L, Matee M, Herfort O, et al. High rates of clinical and subclinical tuberculosis among HIV-infected ambulatory subjects in Tanzania. *Clin Infect Dis.* 2005; **40**(10): 1500-7.

93. Corbett EL, Bandason T, Duong T, et al. Comparison of two active case-finding strategies for community-based diagnosis of symptomatic smear-positive tuberculosis and control of infectious tuberculosis in Harare, Zimbabwe (DETECTB):a cluster-randomised trial. *Lancet.* 2010; **376**(9748): 1244-52.

94. World Health Organization. Improving the diagnosis and treatment of smear-negative pulmonary and extrapulmonary tuberculosis among adults and adolescents: Recommendations for HIV-prevalent and resource-constrained settings. Geneva, World Health Organization, 2007. WHO/HTM/TB/2007.379 & WHO/HIV/2007.1.

95. Wilson D, Mbhele L, Badri M, et al. Evaluation of the World Health Organization algorithm for the diagnosis of HIV-associated sputum smear-negative tuberculosis. *Int J Tuberc Lung Dis.* 2011; **15** (7): 819-24.

96. Alamo ST Kunutsor S, Walley J et al. Performance of the new WHO diagnostic algorithm for smear-negative pulmonary tuberculosis in HIV prevalent settings: a multisite study in Uganda. *Trop Med Int Health.* 2012; **17**: 884-95.

97. Huerga H Varaine F, Okwaro E. Performance of the 2007 WHO algorithm to diagnose smear-negative pulmonary tuberculosis in a HIV prevalent setting. *PLoS One.* 2012; **7**: e51336.

98. Bah B, Massari V, Sow O, et al. Useful clues to the presence of smear-negative pulmonary tuberculosis in a West African city. *Int J Tuberc Lung Dis.* 2002; **6**(7): 592-8.

99. Wilkinson D, De Cock KM, Sturm AW. Diagnosing tuberculosis in a resource-poor setting: the value of a trial of antibiotics. *Trans R Soc Trop Med Hyg.* 1997; **91**(4): 422-4.

100. Sterling TR. The WHO/IUATLD diagnostic algorithm for tuberculosis and empiric fluoroquinolone use: potential pitfalls. *Int J Tuberc Lung Dis.* 2004; **8**(12): 1396-400.

101. Migliori GB, Langendam MW, D'Ambrosio L, et al. Protecting the tuberculosis drug pipeline: stating the case for the rational use of fluoroquinolones. *Eur Resp J.* 2012; **40**(4): 814-22.

102. Chen TC, Lu PL, Lin CY, et al. Fluoroquinolones are associated with delayed treatment and resistance in tuberculosis: a systematic review and meta-analysis. *Int J Infect Dis.* 2011; **15**(3): 211-16.

103. Dowdy DW, Chaisson RE, Maartens G, et al. Impact of enhanced tuberculosis diagnosis in South Africa: a mathematical model of expanded culture and drug susceptibility testing. *Proc Natl Acad Sci U S A.* 2008; **105**(32):11293-8.

104. van Deun A. What is the role of mycobacterial culture in diagnosis and case finding? In: Frieden TR, ed. Toman's tuberculosis: Case detection, treatment and monitoring, 2nd Edition. Geneva: World Health Organization; 2004: 35-43.

105. Toman K. How many bacilli are present in a sputum specimen found positive by smear microscopy? In: Frieden TR, ed. Toman's tuberculosis: Case detection, treatment and monitoring, 2nd Edition. Geneva: World Health Organization; 2004: 11-3.

106. Toman K. How reliable is smear microscopy? In: Frieden TR, ed. Toman's tuberculosis: Case detection, treatment and monitoring, 2nd Edition. Geneva: World Health Organization; 2004: 14-22.

107. Pai M, Ramsay A, O'Brien R. Evidence-based tuberculosis diagnosis. *PLoS Med.* 2008; **5**(7): e156.

108. World Health Organization. Use of liquid TB culture and drug susceptibility testing (DST) in low and medium income settings. Geneva: World Health Organization, 2007.

109. Daley CL, Gotway MB, Jasmer RM. Radiographic Manifestations of Tuberculosis: A Primer for Clinicians. Second Edition. San Francisco: Curry International Tuberculosis Center, 2011. http://www.currytbcenter.ucsf.edu/radiographic/.

110. Ellis S M, Flower C, Ostensen H, Pettersson H. The WHO manual of diagnostic imaging: Radiographic anatomy and interpretation of the chest and the pulmonary system. Geneva: World health Organization, 2006. http://www.who.int/iris/handle/10665/43293.

111. Tuberculosis Coalition for Technical Assistance/Japan Antituberculosis Association. Handbook for District Hospitals in Resource Constrained Settings on Quality Assurance of Chest Radiography. http://pdf.usaid.gov/pdf_docs/Pnadp465.pdf.

112. Hesseling AC, Schaaf HS, Gie RP, et al. A critical review of diagnostic approaches used in the diagnosis of childhood tuberculosis. *Int J Tuberc Lung Dis.* 2002; **6**(12): 1038-45.

113. Gie RP, Beyers N, Schaaf HS, Goussard P. The challenge of diagnosing tuberculosis in children: a perspective from a high incidence area. *Paediatr Respir Rev.* 2004; **5 Suppl A**: S147-9.

114. World Health Organization. Guidance for national tuberculosis programmes on the management of tuberculosis in children. Geneva: World Health Organization, 2006. WHO/HTM/TB/2006.371.

115. Shingadia D, Novelli V. Diagnosis and treatment of tuberculosis in children. *Lancet Infect Dis.* 2003; **3**(10): 624-32.

116. Nicol MP Zar HJ. New specimens and laboratory diagnostics for childhood pulmonary TB: progress and prospects. *Paediatr Respir Rev.* 2011; **12**(1): 16-21.

117. Nelson LJ, Wells CD. Tuberculosis in children: considerations for children from developing countries. *Semin Pediatr Infect Dis.* 2004; **15**(3): 150-4.

118. Marais BJ, Gie RP, Hesseling AC, et al. A refined symptom-based approach to diagnose pulmonary tuberculosis in children. *Pediatrics.* 2006; **118**(5): e1350-9.

119. Graham SM. The use of diagnostic systems for tuberculosis in children. *Indian J Pediatr.* 2011; **78**(3): 334-9.

120. Pearce EC, Woodward JF, Nyandiko WM, Vreeman RC, Ayaya SO. A systematic review of clinical diagnostic systems used in the diagnosis of tuberculosis in children. *AIDS Res Treat.* 2012; **2012**: 401896.

121. World Health Organization. Management of the child with a serious infection or severe malnutrition: Guidelines for care at the first-referral level in developing countries. Geneva: World Health Organization, 2000. WHO/FCH/CAH/00.1.

122. American Thoracic Society/Centers for Disease Control and Prevention/Infectious Diseases Society of America. Treatment of tuberculosis. *Am J Respir Crit Care Med.* 2003; **167**(4): 603-62.

123. Gelband H. Regimens of less than six months for treating tuberculosis. *Cochrane Database Syst Rev.* 2000; (2): CD001362.

124. Lew W, Pai M, Oxlade O, et al. Initial drug resistance and tuberculosis treatment outcomes: systematic review and meta-analysis. *Ann Intern Med.* 2008; **149**(2): 123-34.

125. Korenromp EL, Scano F, Williams BG, et al. Effects of human immunodeficiency virus infection on recurrence of tuberculosis after rifampin-based treatment: an analytical review. *Clin Infect Dis.* 2003; **37**(1): 101-12.

126. Ahmad Khan F, Minion J, Al-Motairi A, et al. An updated systematic review and meta-analysis on the treatment of active tuberculosis in patients with HIV infection. *Clin Infect Dis.* 2012; **55**(8): 1154-63.

127. Menzies D, Benedetti A, Paydar A, et al. . Effect of duration and intermittency of rifampin on tuberculosis treatment outcomes: a systematic review and meta-analysis. *PLoS Med.* 2009; **6**(9): e1000146.

128. Mitchison DA. Antimicrobial therapy for tuberculosis: justification for currently recommended treatment regimens. *Semin Respir Crit Care Med.* 2004; **25**(3): 307-15.

129. Mwandumba H, Squire S. Fully intermittent dosing with drugs for treating tuberculosis in adults. *Cochrane Database Syst Rev.* 2001; (4).

130. British Medical Research Council. Controlled trial of 4 three-times-weekly regimens and a daily regimen all given for 6 months for pulmonary tuberculosis. Second report: the results up to 24 months. Hong Kong Chest Service/British Medical Research Council. *Tubercle.* 1982; **63**(2): 89-98.

131. British Medical Research Council. Controlled trial of 2, 4, and 6 months of pyrazinamide in 6-month, three-times-weekly regimens for smear-positive pulmonary tuberculosis, including an assessment of a combined preparation of isoniazid, rifampin, and pyrazinamide. Results at 30 months. Hong Kong Chest Service/British Medical Research Council. *Am Rev Respir Dis.* 1991; **143**(4 Pt 1): 700-6.

132. Cao JP, Zhang LY, Zhu JQ, Chin DP. Two-year follow-up of directly-observed intermittent regimens for smear-positive pulmonary tuberculosis in China. *Int J Tuberc Lung Dis.* 1998; **2**(5): 360-4.

133. Caminero JA, Pavon JM, Rodriguez de Castro F, et al. Evaluation of a directly observed six months fully intermittent treatment regimen for tuberculosis in patients suspected of poor compliance. *Thorax.* 1996; **51**(11): 1130-3.

134. Bechan S, Connolly C, Short GM, et al. Directly observed therapy for tuberculosis given twice weekly in the workplace in urban South Africa. *Trans R Soc Trop Med Hyg.* 1997; **91**(6): 704-7.

135. Benator D, Bhattacharya M, Bozeman L, et al. Rifapentine and isoniazid once a week versus rifampicin and isoniazid twice a week for treatment of drug-susceptible pulmonary tuberculosis in HIV-negative patients: a randomised clinical trial. *Lancet.* 2002; **360**(9332): 528-34.

136. Vernon A, Burman W, Benator D, et al. Acquired rifamycin monoresistance in patients with HIV-related tuberculosis treated with once-weekly rifapentine and isoniazid. Tuberculosis Trials Consortium. *Lancet.* 1999; **353**(9167): 1843-7.

137. Lienhardt C, Cook SV, Burgos M, et al. Efficacy and safety of a 4-drug fixed-dose combination regimen compared with separate drugs for treatment of pulmonary tuberculosis: the Study C randomized controlled trial. *JAMA.* 2011; **305**(14): 1415-23.

138. Albanna AS, Smith BM, Cowan D, Menzies D. Fixed Dose Combination Anti-tuberculosis Therapy: A Systematic Review and Meta-Analysis. *ERJ Express.* 2013.

139. Blomberg B, Spinaci S, Fourie B, Laing R. The rationale for recommending fixed-dose combination tablets for treatment of tuberculosis. *Bull World Health Organ.* 2001; **79**(1): 61-8.

140. Panchagnula R, Agrawal S, Ashokraj Y, et al. Fixed dose combinations for tuberculosis: Lessons learned from clinical, formulation and regulatory perspective. *Methods Find Exp Clin Pharmacol.* 2004; **26**(9): 703-21.

141. Monedero I, Caminero JA. Evidence for promoting fixed-dose combination drugs in tuberculosis treatment and control: a review. *Int J Tuberc Lung Dis.* 2011; **15**(4): 433-9.

142. Munro SA, Lewin SA, Smith HJ, et al. Patient adherence to tuberculosis treatment: a systematic review of qualitative research. *PLoS Med.* 2007; **4**(7): e238.

143. Volmink J, Matchaba P, Garner P. Directly observed therapy and treatment adherence. *Lancet.* 2000; **355**(9212): 1345-50.

144. Volmink J, Garner P. Directly observed therapy for treating tuberculosis. *Cochrane Database Syst Rev.* 2003; (1): CD003343.

145. Pope DS, Chaisson RE. TB treatment: as simple as DOT? *Int J Tuberc Lung Dis.* 2003; **7**(7): 611-5.

146. Pasipanodya JG Gumbo T. A meta-analysis of self-administered vs directly observed therapy effect on microbiologic failure, relapse, and acquired drug resistance in tuberculosis patients. *Clin Infect Dis.* 2013; **57**(1): 21-31.

147. Chaulk CP, Kazandjian VA. Directly observed therapy for treatment completion of pulmonary tuberculosis: Consensus Statement of the Public Health Tuberculosis Guidelines Panel. *JAMA.* 1998; **279**(12): 943-8.

148. Frieden TR. Can tuberculosis be controlled? *Int J Epidemiol.* 2002; **31**(5): 894-9.

149. Suarez PG, Watt CJ, Alarcon E, et al. The dynamics of tuberculosis in response to 10 years of intensive control effort in Peru. *J Infect Dis.* 2001; **184**(4): 473-8.

150. Tang S, Squire SB. What lessons can be drawn from tuberculosis (TB) control in China in the 1990s? An analysis from a health system perspective. *Health Policy.* 2005; **72**(1): 93-104.

151. World Health Organization. Integrated Management of Adolescent and Adult Illness (IMAI): General principles of good chronic care. Geneva: World Health Organization, 2004. WHO/CDS/IMAI/2004.3.

152. World Health Organization. Integrated Management of Adolescent and Adult Illness (IMAI): Chronic HIV care with ARV therapy and prevention. Geneva: World Health Organization, 2007. WHO/HTM/2007.02.

153. Hadley M, Maher D. Community involvement in tuberculosis control: lessons from other health care programmes. *Int J Tuberc Lung Dis.* 2000; **4**(5): 401-8.

154. Friedrich SO, Rachow A, Saathoff E. Evaluation of the Xpert® MTB/RIF assay as a rapid sputum biomarker of response to tuberculosis treatment: a prospective cohort study. *Lancet Respir Med.* 2013; **1**(6)462-70.

155. World Health Organization. Guidelines for the programmatic management of drug-resistant tuberculosis. Geneva: World Health Organization, 2008. WHO/HTM/TB/2008.402.

156. World Health Organization. Guidelines for the programmatic management of drug-resistant tuberculosis: A 2011 update. Geneva: World Health Organization, 2011. WHO/HTM/TB/2011.6.

157. Hirpa S, Medhin G, Girma B, et al. Determinants of multidrug-resistant tuberculosis in patients who underwent first-line treatment in Addis Ababa: a case control study. *BMC Public Health.* 2013; **13**: 782.

158. Coninx R, Mathieu C, Debacker M, et al. First-line tuberculosis therapy and drug-resistant Mycobacterium tuberculosis in prisons. *Lancet.* 1999; **353**(9157): 969-73.

159. Edlin BR, Tokars JI, Grieco MH, et al. An outbreak of multidrug-resistant tuberculosis among hospitalized patients with the acquired immunodeficiency syndrome. *N Engl J Med.* 1992; **326**(23): 1514-21.

160. Fischl MA, Uttamchandani RB, Daikos GL, et al. An outbreak of tuberculosis caused by multiple-drug-resistant tubercle bacilli among patients with HIV infection. *Ann Intern Med.* 1992; **117**(3): 177-83.

161. Schaaf HS, Van Rie A, Gie RP, et al. Transmission of multidrug-resistant tuberculosis. *Pediatr Infect Dis J.* 2000; **19**(8): 695-9.

162. Small PM, Shafer RW, Hopewell PC, et al. Exogenous reinfection with multidrug- resistant *Mycobacterium tuberculosis* in patients with advanced HIV infection. *N Engl J Med.* 1993; **328**(16): 1137-44.

163. Zhao Y, Xu S, Wang L, et al. National survey of drug-resistant tuberculosis in China. *N Engl J Med.* 2012; **366**(23): 2161-70.

164. Royce S, Falzon D, van Weezenbeek C, et al. Multidrug resistance in new tuberculosis patients: burden and implications. *Int J Tuberc Lung Dis.* 2013; **17**(4): 511-3.

165. Skrahina A HH, Zalutskaya A, et al. Alarming levels of drug-resistant tuberculosis in Belarus: results of a survey in Minsk. *Eur Respir J.* 2012; **39**(6): 1425-35.

166. World Health Organization. Anti-tuberculosis drug resistance in the world. Fourth global report. Geneva: World Health Organization, 2008. WHO/HTM/TB/2008.394.

167. Caminero JA. Likelihood of generating MDR TB and XDR TB under adequate National Tuberculosis Control Programme implementation. *Int J Tuberc Lung Dis.* 2008; **12**(8): 869-77.

168. Gandhi NR, Moll A, Sturm AW, et al. Extensively drug-resistant tuberculosis as a cause of death in patients co-infected with tuberculosis and HIV in a rural area of South Africa. *Lancet.* 2006; **368**(9547): 1575-80.

169. Kim HR, Hwang SS, Kim HJ, et al. Impact of extensive drug resistance on treatment outcomes in non-HIV-infected patients with multidrug-resistant tuberculosis. *Clin Infect Dis.* 2007; **45**(10): 1290-5.

170. Migliori GB, Ortmann J, Girardi E, et al. Extensively drug-resistant tuberculosis, Italy and Germany. *Emerg Infect Dis.* 2007; **13**(5): 780-2.

171. Shah NS, Wright A, Bai GH, et al. Worldwide emergence of extensively drug-resistant tuberculosis. *Emerg Infect Dis.* 2007; **13**(3): 380-7.

172. Migliori GB, Sotgiu G, Gandhi NR, et al. Drug resistance beyond extensively drug-resistant tuberculosis: individual patient data meta-analysis. *Eur Respir J.* 2013; **42**(1): 169-79.

173. World Health Organization. "Totally drug-resistant" tuberculosis: A WHO consultation on the diagnostic definition and treatment options (21-22 March 2012). Geneva, 2012. http://www.who.int/tb/challenges/xdr/xdrconsultation/en/.

174. Falzon D, Gandhi N, Migliori GB, et al. Resistance to fluoroquinolones and second-line injectable drugs: impact on multidrug-resistant TB outcomes. *Eur Respir J.* 2013; **42**(1): 156-68.

175. Williamson DA, Basu I, Bower J,. An evaluation of the Xpert MTB/RIF assay and detection of false-positive rifampicin resistance in Mycobacterium tuberculosis. *Diagn Microbiol Infect Dis.* 2012; **74**: 207-09.

176. van Deun A, Barrera L, Bastian I, et al. Mycobacterium tuberculosis strains with highly discordant rifampin susceptibility test results. *J Clin Microbiol.* 2009; **47**: 3501-6.

177. Ling DI, Zwerling A, Pai M. GenoType MTBDR assays for the diagnosis of multidrug-resistant tuberculosis: a meta-analysis. *Eur Respir J.* 2008; **32**: 1165-74.

178. Martin A, Portaels F, Palomino JC. Colorimetric redox-indicator methods for the rapid detection of multidrug resistance in Mycobacterium tuberculosis: a systematic review and meta-analysis. *J Antimicrob Chemother.* 2007; **59**(2): 175-83.

179. Martin A, Panaiotov S, Portaels F, et al. The nitrate reductase assay for the rapid detection of isoniazid and rifampicin resistance in Mycobacterium tuberculosis: a systematic review and meta-analysis. *J Antimicrob Chemother.* 2008; **62**(1): 56-64.

180. Minion J, Leung E, Menzies D, Pai M. Microscopic-observation drug susceptibility and thin layer agar assays for the detection of drug resistant tuberculosis: a systematic review and meta-analysis. *Lancet Infect Dis.* 2010; **10**(10): 688-98.

181. Horne DJ, Pinto LM, Arentz M, et al. Diagnostic accuracy and reproducibility of WHO-endorsed phenotypic drug susceptibility testing methods for first-line and second-line anti-tuberculosis drugs: a systematic review and meta-analysis. *J Clin Microbiol.* 2013; **51**(2): 393-401.

182. Feng Y, Liu S, Wang Q, et al. Rapid diagnosis of drug resistance to fluoroquinolones, amikacin, capreomycin, kanamycin and ethambutol using genotype MTBDRsl assay: a meta-analysis. *PLoS One.* 2013; **8**(2): e55292.

183. Guo Q, Zheng RJ, Zhu CT, et al. Pyrosequencing for the rapid detection of rifampicin resistance in Mycobacterium tuberculosis: a meta-analysis [Review article]. *Int J Tuberc Lung Dis.* 2013; **17**(8): 1008-13.

184. Mitnick CD, Castro KG, Harrington M, et al. Randomized trials to optimize treatment of multidrug-resistant tuberculosis. *PLoS Med.* 2007; **4**(11): e292.

185. Caminero JA. Management of multidrug-resistant tuberculosis and patients in retreatment. *Eur Respir J.* 2005; **25**(5): 928-36.

186. Caminero JA. Treatment of multidrug-resistant tuberculosis: evidence and controversies. *Int J Tuberc Lung Dis.* 2006; **10**(8): 829-37.

187. Francis J. Curry National Tuberculosis Center and California Department of Public Health. Drug-Resistant Tuberculosis: A Survival Guide for Clinicians, 2008. www.currytbcenter.ucsf.edu/drtb.

188. Keshavjee S, Gelmanova IY, Pasechnikov AD, et al. Treating multidrug-resistant tuberculosis in Tomsk, Russia: developing programs that address the linkage between poverty and disease. *Ann N Y Acad Sci.* 2008; **1136**: 1-11.

189. Kim DH, Kim HJ, Park SK, et al. Treatment outcomes and long-term survival in patients with extensively drug-resistant tuberculosis. *Am J Respir Crit Care Med.* 2008; **178**(10): 1075-82.

190. Mitnick CD, Shin SS, Seung KJ, et al. Comprehensive treatment of extensively drug-resistant tuberculosis. *N Engl J Med.* 2008; **359**(6): 563-74.

191. Mukherjee JS, Rich ML, Socci AR, et al. Programmes and principles in treatment of multidrug-resistant tuberculosis. *Lancet.* 2004; **363**(9407): 474-81.

192. Johnston JC, Shahidi NC, Sadatsafavi M, Fitzgerald JM (2009) Treatment Outcomes of Multidrug-Resistant Tuberculosis: A Systematic Review and Meta-Analysis. *PLoS One.* 2009; (9): e6914.

193. Caminero JA. Guidelines for Clinical and Operational Management of Drug-Resistant Tuberculosis. Paris: International Union Against Tuberculosis and Lung Disease; 2013.

194. Ahuja SD, Ashkin D, Avendano M, et al. Multidrug resistant pulmonary tuberculosis treatment regimens and patient outcomes: an individual patient data meta-analysis of 9,153 patients. *PLoS Med.* 2012; **9**(8): e1001300.

195. Kim SJ. Drug-susceptibility testing in tuberculosis: methods and reliability of results. *Eur Respir J.* 2005; **25**(3): 564-9.

196. van Deun A, Maug AK, Salim MA, et al. Short, highly effective, and inexpensive standardized treatment of multidrug-resistant tuberculosis. *Am J Respir Crit Care Med.* 2010; **182**(5): 684-92.

197. World Health Organization. The use of short regimens for treatment of multidrug-resistant tuberculosis. Geneva: World Health Organization, 2012.

198. Toczek A, Cox H, du Cros P, et al. Strategies for reducing treatment default in drug-resistant tuberculosis: systematic review and meta-analysis. *Int J Tuberc Lung Dis.* 2013; **17**(3): 299-307.

199. Skripconoka V Danilovits M, Pehme L, et al. Delamanid improves outcomes and reduces mortality in multidrug-resistant tuberculosis. *Eur Respir J.* 2013; **41**(6): 1393-400.

200. World Health Organization. The use of bedaquiline to treat MDR TB: Interim policy guidance. Geneva, World Health Organization, 2013. WHO/HTM/TB/2013.6.

201. Diacon AH, Dawson R, von Groote-Bidlingmaier F, et al. 14-day bactericidal activity of PA-824, bedaquiline, pyrazinamide, and moxifloxacin combinations: a randomised trial. *Lancet.* 2012; **380**(9846): 986-93.

202. Udwadia ZF, Amale RA, Ajbani KK, Rodrigues C. Totally drug resistant tuberculosis in India. *Clin Infect Dis.* 2012; **54**: 579-81.

203. World Health Organization. "Totally drug-resistant" tuberculosis: a WHO consultation on the diagnostic definition and treatment options. (meeting report, 21-22 March 2012) http://www.who.int/tb/challenges/xdr/xdrconsultation/en/.

204. World Health Organization. Electronic recording and reporting for tuberculosis care and control. Geneva: World Health Organization, 2012. WHO/HTM/TB/2011.22.

205. Munsiff S, Ahuja SD, King L, et al. Ensuring accountability: the contribution of the cohort review method to tuberculosis control in New York City. *Int J Tuberc Lung Dis.* 2006; **10**: 1133-39.

206. Getahun H, Gunneberg C, Granich R, Nunn P. HIV infection-associated tuberculosis: the epidemiology and the response. *Clin Infect Dis.* 2010; **50 Suppl 3**: S201-7.

207. Martinson N, Omar T, Lebina L, et al. Post mortem pulmonary pathology in adults dying at home: South Africa Conference on retroviruses and opportunistic infections. Atlanta, GA; 2013.

208. Some F, Mwangi A. Burden of tuberculosis among persons dying with HIV/AIDS while on antiretroviral ltherapy in Western Kenya. Conference on retroviruses and opportunistic infections. Atlanta, GA; 2013.

209. World Health Organization. WHO policy on collaborative TB/HIV activities: Guidelines for national programmes and other stakeholders. Geneva: World Health Organization, 2012. WHO/HTM/TB/2012.1.

210. Odhiambo J, Kizito W, Njoroge A, et al. Provider-initiated HIV testing and counselling for TB patients and suspects in Nairobi, Kenya. *Int J Tuberc Lung Dis.* 2008; **12**(3 Suppl 1): 63-8.

211. Srikantiah P, Lin R, Walusimbi M, et al. Elevated HIV seroprevalence and risk behavior among Ugandan TB suspects: implications for HIV testing and prevention. *Int J Tuberc Lung Dis.* 2007; **11**(2): 168-74.

212. Shapiro AE, Variava E, Rakgokong MH, et al. Community-based targeted case finding for tuberculosis and HIV in household contacts of patients with tuberculosis in South Africa. *Am J Respir Crit Care Med.* 2012; **185**: 1110-16.

213. Suggaravetsiri P, Yanai H, Chongsuvivatwong V, et al. Integrated counseling and screening for tuberculosis and HIV among household contacts of tuberculosis patients in an endemic area of HIV infection: Chiang Rai, Thailand. *Int J Tuberc Lung Dis.* 2003; **7**(12 Suppl 3): S424-31.

214. Harries AD, Zachariah R, Lawn SD. Providing HIV care for co-infected tuberculosis patients: a perspective from sub-Saharan Africa. *Int J Tuberc Lung Dis.* 2009; **13**(1): 6-16.

215. Maher D, Harries A, Getahun H. Tuberculosis and HIV interaction in sub-Saharan Africa: impact on patients and programmes; implications for policies. *Trop Med Int Health.* 2005; **10**(8): 734-42.

216. Getahun H, Harrington M, O'Brien R, Nunn P. Diagnosis of smear-negative pulmonary tuberculosis in people with HIV infection or AIDS in resource-constrained settings: informing urgent policy changes. *Lancet.* 2007; **369**(9578): 2042-9.

217. UNAIDS/WHO. Guidance on provider-initiated HIV testing and counseling in health facilities. Geneva: World Health Organization; 2007.

218. World Health Organization. WHO case definitions of HIV for surveillance and revised clinical staging and immunological classification of HIV-related disease in adults and children. Geneva: World Health Organization, 2007.

219. Lawn SD, Campbell L, Kaplan R, et al. Delays in starting antiretroviral therapy in patients with HIV-associated tuberculosis accessing non-integrated clinical services in a South African township. *BMC Infect Dis.* 2011; **11**: 258.

220. Pevzner ES, Vandebriel G, Lowrance DW, et al. Evaluation of the rapid scale-up of collaborative TB/HIV activities in TB facilities in Rwanda, 2005-2009. *BMC Public Health.* 2011; **11**: 550.

221. Phiri S, Khan PY, Grant AD, et al. Integrated tuberculosis and HIV care in a resource-limited setting: experience from the Martin Preuss centre, Malawi. *Trop Med Int Health.* 2011; **16**(11): 1397-403.

222. Louwagie G, Girdler-Brown B, Odendaal R, et al. Missed opportunities for accessing HIV care among Tshwane tuberculosis patients under different models of care. *Int J Tuberc Lung Dis.* 2012; **16**(8): 1052-8.

223. Legido-Quigley H, Montgomery CM, Khan P, et al. Integrating tuberculosis and HIV services in low- and middle-income countries: a systematic review. *Trop Med Int Health.* 2013; **18**(2):199-211.

224. Dlodlo RA, Fujiwara PI, Enarson DA. Should tuberculosis treatment and control be addressed differently in HIV-infected and -uninfected individuals? *Eur Respir J.* 2005; **25**(4): 751-7.

225. El-Sadr WM, Perlman DC, Denning E, et al. A review of efficacy studies of 6-month short-course therapy for tuberculosis among patients infected with human immunodeficiency virus: differences in study outcomes. *Clin Infect Dis.* 2001; **32**(4): 623-32.

226. Harries A. How does treatment of tuberculosis differ in persons infected with HIV? In: Frieden TR, ed. Toman's tuberculosis: Case detection, treatment and monitoring, 2nd Edition. Geneva: World Health Organization; 2004: 169-72.

227. Page K, Godfrey Faussett P, Chaisson R. Tuberculosis-HIV coinfection: Epidemiology, Clinical Aspects, and Interventions. In: Raviglione M, ed. Tuberculosis: A Comprehensive International Approach. 3rd ed. New York: Informa Healthcare; 2006.

228. World Health Organization. The use of antiretroviral drugs for treating and preventing HIV infection. Geneva, World Health Organization, 2013.

229. Lawn SD, Kranzer K, Wood R. Antiretroviral therapy for control of the HIV-associated tuberculosis epidemic in resource-limited settings. *Clin Chest Med.* 2009; **30**(4):685-99.

230. Havlir DV, Kendall MA, Ive P, et al. Timing of antiretroviral therapy for HIV-1 infection and tuberculosis. *N Engl J Med.* 2011; **365**(16): 1482-91.

231. Abdool Karim SS, Naidoo K, Grobler A, et al. Integration of antiretroviral therapy with tuberculosis treatment. *N Engl J Med.* 2011; **365**(16): 1492-501.

232. Blanc FX, Sok T, Laureillard D, et al. Earlier versus later start of antiretroviral therapy in HIV-infected adults with tuberculosis. *N Engl J Med.* 2011; **365**(16): 1471-81.

233. Torok ME, Yen NT, Chau TT, et al. Timing of initiation of antiretroviral therapy in human immunodeficiency virus (HIV)-associated tuberculous meningitis. *Clin Infect Dis.* 2011; **52**(11):1374-83.

234. Laureillard D, Marcy O, Madec Y, et al. Paradoxical tuberculosis-associated immune reconstitution inflammatory syndrome after early initiation of antiretroviral therapy in the camelia randomized trial. *AIDS.* 2013; **27**(16):2577-86.

235. Chimzizi R, Gausi F, Bwanali A, et al. Voluntary counselling, HIV testing and adjunctive cotrimoxazole are associated with improved TB treatment outcomes under routine conditions in Thyolo District, Malawi. *Int J Tuberc Lung Dis.* 2004; **8**(5): 579-85.

236. Chimzizi RB, Harries AD, Manda E, et al. Counselling, HIV testing and adjunctive cotrimoxazole for TB patients in Malawi: from research to routine implementation. *Int J Tuberc Lung Dis.* 2004; **8**(8): 938-44.

237. Grimwade K, Sturm AW, Nunn AJ, et al. Effectiveness of cotrimoxazole prophylaxis on mortality in adults with tuberculosis in rural South Africa. *AIDS.* 2005; **19**(2): 163-8.

238. Nunn P, Williams B, Floyd K, et al. Tuberculosis control in the era of HIV. *Nat Rev Immunol.* 2005; **5**(10): 819-26.

239. World Health Organization. TB/HIV: A clinical manual. Geneva: World Health Organization, 2004. WHO/HTM/T/2004.329.

240. Wood R, Middelkoop K, Myer L, et al. Undiagnosed tuberculosis in a community with high HIV prevalence: implications for tuberculosis control. *Am J Respir Crit Care Med.* 2007; **175**(1):87-93.

241. World Health Organization. Guidelines for intensified tuberculosis case-finding and isoniazid preventive therapy for people living with HIV in resource-constrained settings. Geneva: World Health Organization, 2011. WHO/HTM/TB/2011.11.

242. Woldebanna S, Volmink J. Treatment of Latent tuberculosis infection in HIV infected persons. *Cochrane Database Syst Rev.* 2010 Jan 20;(1):CD000171.

243. Samandari T, Agizew TB, Nyirenda S, et al. 6-month versus 36-month isoniazid preventive treatment for tuberculosis in adults with HIV infection in Botswana: a randomised, double-blind, placebo-controlled trial. *Lancet.* 2011; **377**(9777):1588-98.

244. Martinson NA, Barnes GL, Moulton LH, et al. New regimens to prevent tuberculosis in adults with HIV infection. *N Engl J Med.* 2011; **365**(1): 11-20.

245. Durovni B, Saraceni V, Moulton LH, et al. Effect of improved tuberculosis screening and isoniazid preventive therapy on incidence of tuberculosis and death in patients with HIV in clinics in Rio de Janeiro, Brazil: a stepped wedge, cluster-randomised trial. *Lancet Infect Dis.* 2013; **13**(10): 852-8.

246. Sterling TR, Villarino ME, Borisov AS, et al. Three months of rifapentine and isoniazid for latent tuberculosis infection. *N Engl J Med.* 2011; **365**(23): 2155-66.

247. Schechter M, Zajdenverg R, Falco G, et al. Weekly rifapentine/isoniazid or daily rifampin/pyrazinamide for latent tuberculosis in household contacts. *Am J Respir Crit Care Med.* 2006; **173**(8):922-6.

248. Golub JE, Saraceni V, Cavalcante SC, et al. The impact of antiretroviral therapy and isoniazid preventive therapy on tuberculosis incidence in HIV-infected patients in Rio de Janeiro, Brazil. *AIDS.* 2007; **21**(11): 1441-8.

249. Golub JE, Pronyk P, Mohapi L, et al. Isoniazid preventive therapy, HAART and tuberculosis risk in HIV-infected adults in South Africa: a prospective cohort. *AIDS.* 2009; **23**(5): 631-6.

250. Suthar AB, Lawn SD, del Amo J, et al. Antiretroviral therapy for prevention of tuberculosis in adults with HIV: a systematic review and meta-analysis. *PLoS Med.* 2012; **9**(7): e1001270.

251. Rangaka MX, Wilkinson RJ. **Isoniazid prevention of HIV-associated tuberculosis.** *Lancet Infect Dis.* 2013; **13**(10):825-7.

252. Lönnroth K, Jaramillo EE, Williams BG, et al. Drivers of tuberculosis epidemics: role of risk factors and social determinants. *Soc Sci Med.* 2009; **68**(12): 2240-6.

253. Jeon CY, Murray MB. Diabetes mellitus increases the risk of active tuberculosis: a systematic review of 13 observational studies. *PLoS Med.* 2008; **5**(7): e152.

254. World Health Organization/The International Union Against Tuberculosis and Lung Disease. Monograph on TB and tobacco control: Joining efforts to control two related global epidemics. Geneva: World Health Organization, 2007. WHO/HTM/TB/2007.390.

255. Wang CS, Yang CJ, Chen HC, et al. Impact of type 2 diabetes on manifestations and treatment outcome of pulmonary tuberculosis. *Epidemiol Infect.* 2009; **137**(2): 203-10.

256. Creswell J, Raviglione M, Ottmani S, et al. Tuberculosis and noncommunicable diseases: neglected links and missed opportunities. *Eur Respir J.* 2011; **37**(5): 1269-82.

257. Shaw JE, Sicree RA, Zimmet PZ. Global estimates of the prevalence of diabetes for 2010 and 2030. *Diabetes Res Clin Pract.* 2010; **87**(1): 4-14.

258. Baker MA, Harries AD, Jeon CY, et al. The impact of diabetes on tuberculosis treatment outcomes: a systematic review. *BMC Med.* 2011; **9**: 81.

259. World Health Organization. Collaborative framework for care and control of tuberculosis and diabetes. Geneva: World Health Organization, 2011. WHO/HTM/TB/2011.15.

260. Nijland HM, Ruslami R, Stalenhoef JE, et al. Exposure to rifampicin is strongly reduced in patients with tuberculosis and type 2 diabetes. *Clin Infect Dis.* 2006; **43**(7): 848-54.

261. American Diabetes Association. Standards of medical care in diabetes-2013. *Diabetes Care.* 2013; **36**(suppl): S 11-66.

262. Allwood BW Meyer L, Bateman ED. A systematic review of the association between pulmonary tuberculosis and the development of chronic airflow obstruction in adults. *Respiration.* 2013; **86**(1): 76-85.

263. World Health Organization. Nutritional care and support for people with tuberculosis. Geneva: World Health Organization, 2013.

264. Winthrop KL. Infections and biologic therapy in rheumatoid arthritis: our changing understanding of risk and prevention. *Rheumatic Dis Clin North Am.* 2012; **38**(4): 727-45.

265. Solovic I, Sester M, Gomez-Reino JJ, et al. The risk of tuberculosis related to tumour necrosis factor antagonist therapies: a TBNET consensus statement. *Eur Respir J.* 2010; **36**(5): 1185-206.

266. Etkind SC, Veen J. Contact follow-up in high and low-prevalence countries. In: Raviglione M, ed. Tuberculosis: a comprehensive international approach, 3rd Edition. New York: Informa Healthcare; 2006: 555-82.

267. Rieder HL. Contacts of tuberculosis patients in high-incidence countries. *Int J Tuberc Lung Dis.* 2003; **7**(12 Suppl 3): S333-6.

268. Erkens CG, Kamphorst M, Abubakar I, et al. Tuberculosis contact investigation in low prevalence countries: a European consensus. *Eur Respir J.* 2010; **36**(4): 925-49.

269. Morrison JL, Pai M, Hopewell P. Tuberculosis and latent tuberculosis infection in close contacts of people with pulmonary tuberculosis in low-income and middle-income countries: a systematic review and meta-analysis. *Lancet Infect Dis.* 2008; **8**(6):359-68.

270. Fox GJ, Barry SE, Britton WJ, Marks GB. Contact investigation for tuberculosis: a systematic review and meta-analysis. *Eur Respir J.* 2013; **41**(1): 140-56.

271. Shah NS Yuen C, Heo M, et al. Yield of Contact Investigations in Households of Drug-Resistant Tuberculosis Patients: Systematic Review and Meta-Analysis. *Clin Infect Dis. 2013.* Epub 2013 24 Sep.

272. Basu S, Andrews JR, Poolman EM, et al. Prevention of nosocomial transmission of extensively drug-resistant tuberculosis in rural South African district hospitals: an epidemiological modelling study. *Lancet.* 2007; **370**(9597): 1500-7.

273. Nardell E, Dharmadhikari A. Turning off the spigot: reducing drug-resistant tuberculosis transmission in resource-limited settings. *Int J Tuberc Lung Dis.* 2010; **14**(10): 1233-43.

274. Ling D, Menzies D. Occupation-related respiratory infections revisited. *Infect Dis Clin North Am.* 2010; **24**(3): 655-80.

275. Blumberg HM, Watkins DL, Berschling JD, et al. Preventing the nosocomial transmission of tuberculosis. *Ann Intern Med.* 1995; **122**(9): 658-63.

276. Escombe AR, Moore DA, Gilman RH, et al. The Infectiousness of tuberculosis patients coinfected with HIV. *PLoS Med.* 2008; **5**(9): e188.

277. Escombe AR, Oeser CC, Gilman RH, et al. Natural ventilation for the prevention of airborne contagion. *PLoS Med.* 2007; **4**(2): e68.

278. Dharmadhikari AS, Mphahlele M, Stoltz A, et al. Surgical face masks worn by patients with multi-drug-resistant tuberculosis: impact on infectivity of air on a hospital ward. *Am J Respir Crit Care Med.* 2012; **185**(10): 1104-9.

279. Maher D, Raviglione MC. Why is a recording and reporting system needed, and what system is recommended? In: Frieden TR, ed. Toman's tuberculosis: Case detection, treatment and monitoring, 2nd Edition. Geneva: World Health Organization; 2004: 270-3.

280. World Health Organization. A Practical Handbook on the Pharmacovigilance of Medicines Used in the treatment of Tuberculosis. Geneva; World Health Organization 2013.

281. Centers for Disease Control and Prevention. Provisional CDC Guidelines for the Use and Safety Monitoring of Bedaquiline Fumarate (Sirturo TM) for the Treatment of Multidrug-Resistant Tuberculosis. *MMWR Recomm Rep.* 2013 Oct 25; **62**(RR-09):1-12.

Annex 1

The steering committees responsible for editions 1 and 2 of the *ISTC* are listed below.

Edition 1

- **Edith Alarcón** (nurse, international technical agency, NGO)
- **R. V. Asokan** (professional society)
- **Jaap Broekmans** (international technical agency, NGO)
- **Jose Caminero** (academic institution, care provider)
- **Kenneth Castro** (national tuberculosis program director)
- **Lakbir Singh Chauhan** (national tuberculosis program director)
- **David Coetzee** (TB/HIV care provider)
- **Sandra Dudereva** (medical student)
- **Saidi Egwaga** (national tuberculosis program director)
- **Paula Fujiwara** (international technical agency, NGO)
- **Robert Gie** (pediatrics, care provider)
- **Case Gordon** (patient advocate)
- **Philip Hopewell, Co-Chair** (professional society, academic institution, care provider)
- **Umesh Lalloo** (academic institution, care provider)
- **Dermot Maher** (global tuberculosis control)
- **G. B. Migliori** (professional society)
- **Richard O'Brien** (new tools development, private foundation)
- **Mario Raviglione, Co-Chair** (global tuberculosis control)
- **D'Arcy Richardson** (nurse, funding agency)
- **Papa Salif Sow** (HIV care provider)
- **Thelma Tupasi** (multiple drug-resistant tuberculosis, private sector, care provider)
- **Mukund Uplekar** (global tuberculosis control)
- **Diana Weil** (global tuberculosis control)
- **Charles Wells** (technical agency, national tuberculosis program)
- **Karin Weyer** (laboratory)
- **Wang Xie Xiu** (national public health agency)

Edition 2

- **Edith Alarcón** (nurse, international technical agency, NGO)
- **R. V. Asokan** (professional society)
- **Carmelia Basri** (national tuberculosis program)
- **Henry Blumberg** (infection control, academic institution)
- **Martien Borgdorff** (international technical agency)
- **Jose Caminero** (training, academic institution, care provider)
- **Martin Castellanos** (national tuberculosis program director)
- **Kenneth Castro** (national tuberculosis program director)
- **Richard Chaisson** (prevention, academic institution)
- **Jeremiah Chakaya** (professional society)
- **Lakbir Singh Chauhan** (national tuberculosis program director)
- **Lucy Chesire** (patient advocate)
- **Daniel Chin** (donor agency)
- **David Cohn** (prevention, academic institution)
- **Charles Daley** (role of radiographic evaluation, academic institution)

- **Saidi Egwaga** (national tuberculosis program director)
- **Elizabeth Fair** (case finding and contact investigation, academic institution)
- **Paula Fujiwara** (international technical agency, NGO)
- **Haileyesus Getahun** (TB/HIV, global tuberculosis control)
- **Robert Gie** (pediatrics, care provider)
- **Case Gordon** (patient advocate)
- **Ruben Granich** (TB/HIV, global tuberculosis control)
- **Malgosia Grzemska** (policy and liaison with WHO, global tuberculosis control)
- **Mark Herrington** (TB/HIV, NGO)
- **Philip Hopewell, Co-Chair** (professional society, academic institution, care provider)
- **Ernesto Jaramillo** (drug resistance, global tuberculosis control)
- **Anwar Jusuf** (professional society)
- **Salmaan Keshavjee** (drug resistance)
- **Umesh Lalloo** (drug resistance, professional society)
- **Kitty Lambregts** (drug resistance, international technical agency)
- **Hadiarto Mangunnegoro** (professional society)
- **Divide Manissero** (pediatric tuberculosis, regional tuberculosis control)
- **Eugene McCray (**TB/HIV, national tuberculosis control program)
- **G. B. Migliori** (professional society)
- **Ed Nardell** (infection control)
- **Paul Nunn** (drug resistance, global tuberculosis control)
- **Rick O'Brien** (diagnosis of smear-negative TB/role of new diagnostics, private foundation)
- **Madhukar Pai** (diagnosis of smear-negative TB/role of new diagnostics, academic institution)
- **Mario Raviglione, Co-Chair** (global tuberculosis control)
- **D'Arcy Richardson** (nursing, funding agency)
- **KJ Seung** (infection control)
- **Joseph Sitienei** (national tuberculosis program director)
- **Pedro Suarez** (role of radiographic evaluation)
- **Thelma Tupasi** (drug resistance, private sector, care provider)
- **Mukund Uplekar** (public private mix, global tuberculosis control)
- **Maarten Van Cleef** (international technical agency)
- **Cheri Vincent** (donor agency)
- **Diana Weil** (policy, global tuberculosis control)
- **Karin Weyer** (laboratory)
- **Wang Xie Xiu** (national public health agency)

Annex 2

Utilization of the ISTC

The *ISTC* is potentially a very powerful tool to improve the quality of tuberculosis care globally. Because of the way in which the *ISTC* was developed and the international endorsements it has received through the two previous editions, the document is broadly credible across categories of practitioners and, thus, carries substantial authority. This credibility and authority are major strengths of the *ISTC* and should be capitalized upon in its utilization.

Based on experience with the first (2006) and second (2009) editions of the ISTC, there are multiple uses for the document by both the public and private sectors. Many of these are described in the *Handbook for Utilizing the International Standards for Tuberculosis Care* which described utilization of the first edition of the ISTC (available at http://www. istcweb.org). Some of the more frequent uses are summarized below:

Unifying Approaches to Tuberculosis Care Between the Public and Private Sectors

One of the intended uses of the *ISTC* is as a tool to unify approaches to diagnosis and treatment between the public and private sectors, especially in countries in which there is a strong private sector. The *ISTC*, by articulating widely accepted, authoritative approaches to tuberculosis care, can serve as a vehicle for bringing the two sectors together. As a product of the collaboration fostered by the *ISTC*, several countries and regions have utilized the ISTC as the framework for developing more local adaptations of the document.

Activities aimed at fostering public-private collaborations may be initiated by organizations representing either sector. Prior to developing activities based on the *ISTC*, the initiating organization must have a sound understanding of the individual standards and assess their ability to be in compliance with the standards. This likely will require internal assessment of capacity, planning, and development of specific strategies to address the standards. For example, if the goal is to involve the private sector more effectively, the NTP must be willing to adjust and accommodate, where necessary, to the needs of private providers. Planned *ISTC* activities should be clearly linked with the identified gaps to be filled. Overall objectives should also be formulated in relation to national tuberculosis control objectives and targets.

Obtaining endorsements by influential local organizations, including governments and professional societies, serves as a way of obtaining buy-in and commitment to the principles in the *ISTC*. Moreover, the influence of the *ISTC* is amplified with each endorsement received, and local endorsement paves the way for further *ISTC*-related activities, as described subsequently.

Mobilizing Professional Societies

Professional societies and their leaders are often influential members of the private medical community, have direct access to a large number of practicing clinicians, and have influence that extends beyond their membership. The societies often include academic physicians who are influential in their own right. Professional societies can provide a convenient means, sometimes the only means, to access the private sector systematically by utilizing society journals, newsletters, and other communications. Strategic thinking needs to be applied in determining the reasons for seeking professional society support, but the *ISTC* can serve as a means to identify and focus on common goals and objectives and can provide a framework for addressing and improving the quality of care delivered by private providers.

Providing the Framework for Conducting a Feasibility Analysis

Because each of the major components of tuberculosis care is included in the *ISTC*, the standards provide a broad framework for a systematic "feasibility analysis" of local capabilities, and can serve as a vehicle for addressing any shortcomings. Conceptually, the *ISTC* feasibility analysis is a way for programs and providers to take stock of the standards that are or are not being met in their country. The feasibility analysis can be applied at any level in the health system national, state/provincial, district, or individual institutional level. The level at which the analysis is performed depends in part on the organization and funding of tuberculosis services. Conducting the analysis at a national level can provide an overall mapping and assessment of tuberculosis services across the country; this can be useful for general NTP planning purposes, for informing policy makers, and for advocacy efforts. Conducting the analysis at a district or local level may enable those participating to discuss more specific problems and to devise more specific solutions. For example, if the problem is limited access to laboratories, specific sharing of resources can be suggested. Within an individual institution, the *ISTC* may be used to assess the availability and quality of essential tuberculosis services provided by the institution and by the clinicians practicing within the institution.

Quality and Performance Assessment

Similar to the feasibility analysis, the *ISTC* can serve as a means for assessing the quality of care. The individual standards within the *ISTC* can be utilized to measure the quality of tuberculosis services delivered by any provider, program, or sector. A major purpose of the *ISTC* is to improve the quality of tuberculosis care. Any or all of the standards may be used as tools for monitoring and evaluation of quality. Such assessments, just as with the feasibility analysis, can identify weaknesses in programs, institutions, or individual providers. Tailored interventions can then be employed to correct the weaknesses and improve quality.

ISTC as an Advocacy Tool

Political commitment is a critical component of tuberculosis control, and its absence limits implementation of control measures. There has been considerable success in bringing high-level government attention and commitment to tuberculosis control. However, in most countries, at all levels of government, there has been a failure to translate this high-level political commitment into effective, country-level public policies that provide a framework for sustained tuberculosis control programs and activities. The *ISTC* provides a set of internationally recognized standards any government should seek to meet. In using the *ISTC* feasibility analysis tools, NTPs can identify gaps in meeting the standards, providing a powerful advocacy tool to seek improved tuberculosis care and control.

Engaging Patients and Communities

The *ISTC* relates to this component in two ways: First, because the *ISTC* is backed by an international consensus and describes agreed upon elements of tuberculosis care that should be available everywhere, patients worldwide should expect that their care is in compliance with the *ISTC*. The *ISTC*, thus, provides patients with the backing they need to insist that they receive high quality care. Similarly, communities should expect that the care provided within their boundaries meets the standards, and thus is of high quality.

Second, the *Patients' Charter for Tuberculosis Care* was developed in tandem with the *ISTC* with the intent that they would be complimentary documents. The *PCTC* relies on the *ISTC* as its technical support. The *PCTC* describes both patients' rights and responsibilities. Implicit in both the statements of patients' rights and their responsibilities is that they will receive care that is in conformance with the *ISTC*. Patients' awareness of and support for the *ISTC* and the *PCTC* can be used to provide leverage in dealings with policy makers and funding agencies, empowering them to be effective advocates for high quality tuberculosis care.

Annex 3

ISTC Tuberculosis Training Modules

The *ISTC Tuberculosis Training Modules* are educational resource tools developed to assist in the incorporation of the *ISTC* into training courses and curricula on tuberculosis. The modules currently available are based on edition 2 of the *ISTC*. Updates modules based on edition 3 will be available in September, 2014. However, the descriptions based on the 2009 update will be equally applicable to the modules based on edition 3. All training material can be downloaded at www.istcweb.org.

The modules are comprehensive in their coverage of core topics in the clinical evaluation and management of tuberculosis and the material is presented in a format that is flexible and adaptable to various training needs. While the modules may be used as core presentations for courses on tuberculosis, the *ISTC Tuberculosis Training Modules* material should also be viewed as a tuberculosis "training resource library" offering easy access to specific *ISTC* material, individual slides, images, or graphics as needed to update or augment existing tuberculosis training materials.

The planning and development of the *ISTC Tuberculosis Training Modules* was guided by members of the original *ISTC* steering committee and through significant input from *ISTC* implementation pilot countries. Through an informal assessment of needs from country-level input and steering committee members, a didactic PowerPoint slide format was chosen as most useful for easy adaptation for general training needs across a spectrum of capacity-building activities. The target audience is practicing physicians, both public and private. The modules may be adapted for pre-service trainees, nursing, and other health care providers.

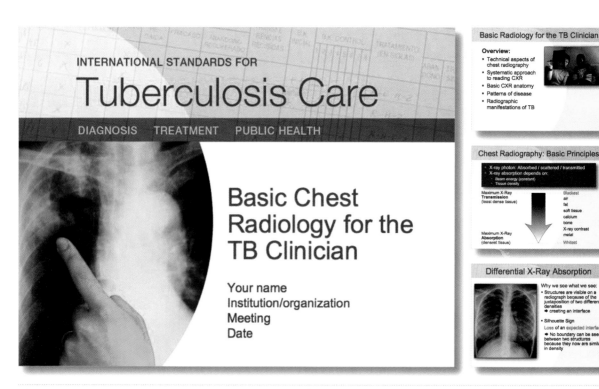

Organization of Modules

Core topics in tuberculosis diagnosis, treatment, and public health responsibilities are covered in the modules, highlighting the relevant *ISTC* standards as they address the basic principles of care for persons with, or suspected of having, tuberculosis.

ISTC Tuberculosis Training Modules cover the following content areas:

Training Module Slide Sets 2009	
Standards for Diagnosis	
Clinical Presentation and Diagnosis of Tuberculosis	Standards 1, 2, 3, 4, 5, 6
Microbiological Evaluation of Tuberculosis	Standards 2, 3, 4, 5, 6, 10, 11
Pediatric Tuberculosis	Standards 2, 3, 4, 6
Standards for Treatment	
Initial Treatment of Tuberculosis	Standards 7, 8, 9, 10, 12,13
Fostering and Assessing Adherence to Treatment	Standard 9,17
Drug-resistant Tuberculosis	Standard 11, 12
Standards for Addressing HIV Infection and other Co-morbid Conditions	
TB and HIV infection: Introduction and Diagnosis	Standards 2, 3, 14
TB and HIV infection: Treatment	Standards 8, 15,16
Standards for Public Health	
Contact Evaluation	Standards 18
Isoniazid Preventive Therapy	Standards 16, 19
Tuberculosis Infection Control	Standards 20
Additional Training Modules/Slides	
Basic Chest Radiology for the TB Clinician	
Introduction to the ISTC Standards	

Additional Training and Evaluation Tools

Additional materials provided with the slidesets include instructor Teaching Notes, a Facilitator's Guide (includes sample *ISTC* course agendas), instructions for producing Participant Manuals, and Evaluation and Training Tools (includes Training Module Test Questions).

Teaching Notes: Each *ISTC Tuberculosis Training Module* contains Teaching Notes to assist instructors by offering speaking points, background material, and interactive tips. The Teaching Note Summary serves as a quick reference document containing a complete set of Teaching Notes with "thumbnail" slide images for all modules.

Facilitator's Guide: The *Facilitator's Guide* explains the organization of the *ISTC Tuberculosis Training Modules* and includes suggestions for effective course development and facilitation, including:

- Sample course agendas
- Participant manual instructions

Test Questions: Questions based on module objectives are included which may be used as Pre- and Post- test evaluation or alternately as interactive discussion tools for module presentations.

Other Evaluation and Training Tools: Template forms for course evaluations and training course administrative tools for registration and certification are also available.

Pilot Testing of the Training Modules

Draft versions of the *ISTC Tuberculosis Training Modules* have been pilot-tested in a variety of settings. The successful adaptation and incorporation of the ISTC material by these pilot groups offers examples of how the *ISTC* Training Modules may be used.

Training curriculum for practicing physicians (private and public): Materials from the *ISTC Tuberculosis Training Modules* were adapted for use in a comprehensive set of training material developed to teach providers about new national tuberculosis guidelines (which incorporated the *ISTC*) in the Caribbean. In-country educators piloted the material in three separate trainings sessions.

Specialty workforce training: Select materials from the *ISTC Tuberculosis Training Modules* were used by outside experts as part of a training course for physicians, nurses, and clinical staff at a new national MDR-referral hospital in Tanzania.

Pre-service training: Collaboration between the National Tuberculosis and Leprosy Program (NTLP) and six medical schools and Allied Health Sciences in Tanzania resulted in a unified curriculum on tuberculosis integrating the *ISTC*. Materials from the *ISTC Tuberculosis Training Modules* were used in the development of the final curriculum.

Professional Societies: *ISTC Tuberculosis Training Modules* were adapted for use as core material for an extensive country-wide training plan developed by a collaborative effort of professional society members and the NTP as part of the *ISTC* task force mission in Indonesia.

2009 Revisions and Online Access

The first version of the training material was released in 2008. The current 2009 version has been updated to reflect the revisions within this document. New modules (radiology, pediatrics, isoniazid preventive therapy, and infection control) have been added as well. All training material can be downloaded at www.istcweb.org.

Index-TB Guidelines
[Guidelines on Extra-pulmonary
Tuberculosis for India]

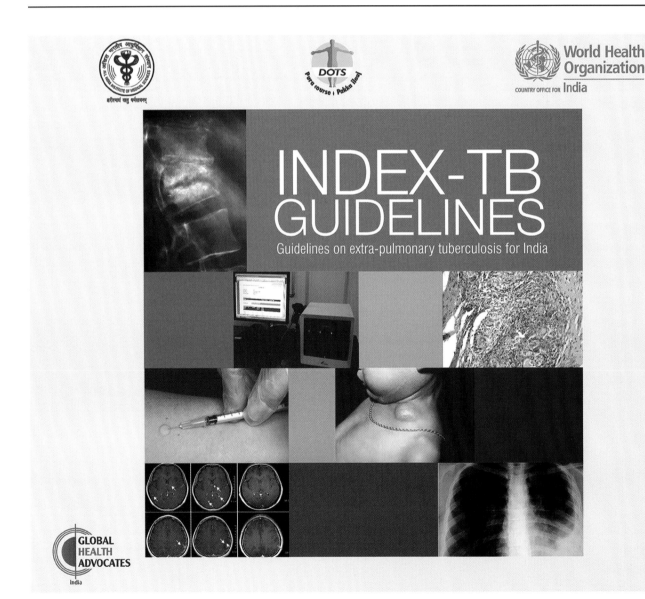

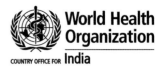

COUNTRY OFFICE FOR India

INDEX-TB
GUIDELINES

Guidelines on extra-pulmonary tuberculosis for India

Initiative of
Central TB Division
Ministry of Health and Family Welfare, Government of India

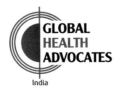

GLOBAL
HEALTH
ADVOCATES

India

Convenors

Department of Medicine, All India Institute of Medical Sciences, New Delhi
WHO Collaborating Centre (WHO-CC) for Training and Research in Tuberculosis
Centre of Excellence for Extra-Pulmonary Tuberculosis, Ministry of Health and Family Welfare, Government of India

Partners

Global Health Advocates, India
Cochrane Infectious Diseases Group
Cochrane South Asia
World Health Organization Country Office for India

Abbreviations

ADA	adenosine deaminase, or adenosine aminohydrolase
AFB	acid-fast bacilli
AIIMS	All India Institute of Medical Sciences
ART	antiretroviral therapy
ATT	anti-tuberculosis therapy
CNS	central nervous system
CoE	Centre of Excellence
CSF	cerebrospinal fluid
CT	computed tomography
CXR	chest X-ray
DGHS	Directorate General of Health Services
ECG	electrocardiogram
ENT	ear, nose and throat
EPTB	extra-pulmonary tuberculosis
ESR	erythrocyte sedimentation rate
FGTB	female genital TB
FNAC	fine-needle aspiration cytology
GHA	Global Health Advocates
GI	gastrointestinal
GRADE	Grading of Recommendations Assessment, Development and Evaluation
HIV	human immunodeficiency virus
ICP	intra cranial pressure
IGRA	interferon-gamma release assay
INDEX-TB	Indian extra-pulmonary tuberculosis
IRIS	immune reconstitution inflammatory syndrome
LDH	lactate dehydrogenase
LNTB	lymph node tuberculosis
MRI	magnetic resonance imaging
Mtb	Mycobacterium tuberculosis (referring to the organism causing tuberculosis disease)
PCR	polymerase chain reaction
PET-CT	positron emission tomography–computed tomography
PGIMER	Post Graduate Institute of Medical Education and Research
RNTCP	Revised National Tuberculosis Control Programme
TAC	Technical Advisory Committee
TB	tuberculosis (referring to the disease caused by Mycobacterium tuberculosis)
TBM	tuberculous meningitis
TST	tuberculin skin testing (also referred to as Mantoux test)
VCT	voluntary counselling and testing
WHO	World Health Organization
WHO-CC	World Health Organization Collaborating Centre

Treatment nomenclature

The first-line anti-tuberculosis drugs are referred to by single-letter abbreviations, as follows:

R – rifampicin
H – isoniazid
Z – pyrazinamide
E – ethambutol
S – streptomycin

Regimens are described using shorthand, with numbers to denote the number of months the treatment should be given for. So, 2RHZE/4RHE refers to 2 months' treatment with rifampicin, isoniazid, pyrazinamide and ethambutol, followed by 4 months' treatment with rifampicin, isoniazid and ethambutol.

Clinicians should refer to the current RNTCP guidelines for dosing of ATT drugs in adults and children. At the time of publication, daily dosing regimens are being introduced in five states with a view to all TB patients nationwide receiving daily ATT.

Executive summary

The main objective of these guidelines is to provide guidance on up-to-date, uniform, evidence-informed practices for suspecting, diagnosing and managing various forms of extra-pulmonary tuberculosis (EPTB) at all levels of healthcare delivery. They can then contribute to the National Programme to improve detection, care and outcomes in EPTB; to help the programme with initiation of treatment, adherence and completion whilst minimizing drug toxicity and overtreatment; and contribute to practices that minimize the development of drug resistance.

The Core Committee, commissioned by the Central TB Division (CTD) and Directorate of Health Services of the Ministry of Health and Family Welfare, Government of India, with the assistance of 10 Technical Advisory Subcommittees representing the different organ systems affected by EPTB, in partnership with the Methodology Support Team, initiated a process of evidence-informed guidelines development in December 2014 drawing on best international practices. This group produced three outputs:

a. Agreed principles relevant to EPTB care, and complementary to the existing 2014 country standards;
b. Agreed recommendations developed using current international evidenceinformed methods on priority areas for EPTB, in Xpert MTB/RIF, use of steroids and length of treatment; and
c. Clinical practice points for each organ system, based on accumulated knowledge in the country and in the working groups.

Principles

In line with the International Standards of TB Care (TB CARE I, 2014), the Guidelines Group as a whole agreed on a set of principles about what every EPTB patient in India needs as a basic standard of care. These principles are a complementary set to the Standards for TB Care in India 2014 (Sreenivas, 2014).

Principle 1	Patients first
	The provider should adopt a patient-centred approach to managing EPTB, to promote well-being and adherence to treatment and to relieve suffering. Patients have the right to be fully informed about their care at every stage, to be able to make decisions about their treatment and to be treated with dignity and respect.
Principle 2	Promoting early diagnosis
	Providers should be informed of the clinical features and risk factors for various forms of EPTB and carry out prompt clinical evaluation and appropriate early diagnostic investigation.
Principle 3	Access to a tissue-based diagnosis
	Where facilities exist, all patients suspected of having EPTB should have appropriate samples taken for microbiological and histological testing, unless diagnostic sampling is deemed to risk undue harm.

Principle 4	Addressing drug resistance
	All patients with a diagnosis of EPTB should be risk-assessed for drug resistance prior to starting treatment, and drug susceptibility testing should be available for all patients at risk of drug-resistant tuberculosis.
Principle 5	Avoiding unnecessary invasive and costly tests
	Providers should consider the impact of diagnostic tests on patient management before referring patients for costly or invasive tests, or repeating these tests.
Principle 6	Access to HIV testing
	As EPTB is particularly associated with HIV, integrated counselling and testing should be made available to all patients suspected of having EPTB.
Principle 7	Identifying patients with concurrent active pulmonary TB
	All patients suspected of having EPTB should have clinical assessment for pulmonary TB in line with RNTCP guidance for investigating suspected pulmonary TB.
Principle 8	Ensuring effective treatment
	All patients should receive an appropriate treatment regimen.
Principle 9	Promoting adherence
	Providers should monitor adherence to treatment and address factors leading to interruption or discontinuation of treatment. Services should promote retention of patients in care.
Principle 10	Record keeping and public health promotion
	A reliable, well-maintained record of all diagnostic tests, treatments given, treatment monitoring, outcomes and adverse events should be kept for each patient, and data should be collected at the national programme level for the purposes of health-care system planning and development.

Recommendations

The Core Committee and Technical Advisory Subcommittees initially considered the first draft of the clinical guides prepared by each of the organ system subcommittees. This raised many potential points of equipoise that could be subject to formal evidence-informed guideline development using the Grading of Recommendations Assessment Development and Evaluation (GRADE) process. From this process, the Core Committee and Methodology Support Team identified priority topics cutting across several organ systems in EPTB for development of guidelines. These were areas where systematic review of the evidence was feasible given the available study data and time and resource constraints, where there were current important dilemmas in what to recommend and where decisions could improve patient care, patient outcomes, or had important resource implications. For example, agreeing on length of treatment has substantive effects on drugs cost and resource use. The committee viewed this guideline process as an essential step in embedding evidence-based processes in the guidelines development and part of a long-term vision for the country. While the topics appeared clinical, all the decisions had potentially profound public health expenditure and management implications. In addition, the guidelines could have an impact towards improving public health outcomes.

The questions addressed were:
1. Should Xpert MTB/RIF be recommended for use in the diagnosis of: a) lymph node TB; b) TB meningitis; c) pleural TB?
2. Should corticosteroids be recommended for use in the treatment of: a) TB pericarditis; b) TB meningitis; c) pleural TB?
3. How long should ATT be given in the treatment of: a) lymph node TB; b) abdominal TB; c) TB meningitis?

Evidence summaries were then produced by members of the Technical Advisory Subcommittees and the Methodology Support Team, and presented to the Guidelines Panel. The Guidelines Panel considered the evidence in accordance with GRADE criteria and decided on recommendations by consensus.

The guidelines process has adhered to the GRADE criteria (GRADE Working Group, 2008) to produce a set of recommendations that are explicitly linked to the evidence they are based on, with consideration given to the various healthcare settings across India. The use of GRADE is in line with the WHO Handbook for Guideline Development (WHO, 2014).

The GRADE criteria require that:
- quality of evidence, as well as the effect estimate, is clearly defined;
- risk of bias of the relevant studies, directness of evidence, consistency of results, precision and other sources of bias in the available evidence are considered and reported for each important outcome;
- evidence summaries are used as the basis for judgements about the quality of the evidence and the strength of recommendations;
- the balance of desirable and undesirable consequences, quality of evidence, values and preferences should be considered and reported when deciding on the strength of a recommendation;
- the strength of recommendations is clearly reported and defined.

Recommendations: Diagnosis of EPTB using the Xpert MTB/RIF test
Lymph node TB
Xpert MTB/RIF should be used as an additional test to conventional smear microscopy, culture and cytology in fine-needle aspiration cytology (FNAC) specimens.
Strong recommendation, low quality evidence for sensitivity estimate, high quality evidence for specificity estimate.
TB meningitis
Xpert MTB/RIF may be used as an adjunctive test for tuberculous meningitis (TBM). A negative Xpert MTB/RIF result on a cerebrospinal fluid (CSF) specimen does not rule out TBM. The decision to give anti-tuberculosis treatment (ATT) should be based on clinical features and CSF profile.
Conditional recommendation, low quality evidence for sensitivity estimate, high quality evidence for specificity estimate.
Pleural TB
Xpert MTB/RIF should not be routinely used to diagnose pleural TB.
Strong recommendation, low quality evidence for sensitivity estimate, high quality evidence for specificity estimate.
Recommendations: Adjunctive steroids in the treatment of EPTB
TB meningitis
Steroids are recommended for TB meningitis in HIV-negative people. Duration of steroid treatment should be for at least 4 weeks with tapering as appropriate.
Strong recommendation, high quality evidence.
Steroids may be used for TB meningitis in HIV-positive people, where other life-threatening opportunistic infections are absent.
Conditional recommendation, very low quality evidence.
TB pericarditis
Steroids are recommended for HIV-negative patients with TB pericarditis with pericardial effusion.
Conditional, low quality evidence.
Steroids are recommended for HIV-positive patients with TB pericarditis with pericardial effusion.
Conditional, low quality evidence.
Pleural TB
Steroids are not routinely recommended in pleural TB.
Conditional, low quality evidence.

Recommendations: length of treatment for EPTB
Lymph node TB
Six months ATT standard first-line regimen is recommended for peripheral lymph node TB.
Strong recommendation, low quality evidence.
Abdominal TB
Six months ATT standard first-line regimen is recommended for abdominal TB.
Strong recommendation, very low quality evidence.
TB meningitis
TB meningitis should be treated with standard first-line ATT for at least 9 months.
Conditional recommendation, very low quality evidence.

Clinical practice points

EPTB takes many forms, and evidence regarding best practice for many aspects of case finding, diagnosis and treatment is lacking. In order to reflect the needs of health-care providers and develop a platform for future guidelines and research, the Technical Advisory Subcommittees produced clinical practice points on each aspect of EPTB care. These are summarized in Part 2. These are based on the expert opinion of senior clinicians in medicine and surgery from across India, and provide a basis for further refinement in evidence-informed guideline development in future. This section of the guidelines seeks to address all aspects of diagnosis and treatment of EPTB, and should be used as a reference.

Part 1
Guidelines

1 Introduction

1.1 EPTB and Revised National Tuberculosis Control Programme

The Revised National Tuberculosis Control Programme (RNTCP) has developed comprehensive guidelines for diagnosis and treatment of pulmonary TB. However, management of extra-pulmonary TB (EPTB) under the programme continues to be a challenge.

The burden of EPTB is high, ranging from 15–20% of all TB cases in HIV-negative patients, while in HIV-positive people it accounts for 40–50% of new TB cases (Sharma S.K., 2004).

The programme has identified the need to expand support for diagnosis and treatment of EPTB and has outlined the following issues:
- lack of evidence-based guidelines on diagnosis and treatment of various types of EPTB;
- absence of adequate infrastructure and resources up to the peripheral level of health facilities to identify, diagnose and treat EPTB;
- lack of skilled and trained staff for appropriate sample collection, transportation and diagnosis;
- uncertainty among clinicians about the optimum duration of treatment and treatment end-points;
- lack of data on EPTB, as most of the cases are being treated outside the public sector.

In response, the Department of Medicine at the All India Institute of Medical Sciences (AIIMS), New Delhi, which is the WHO Collaborating Centre (WHO-CC) for Training and Research in Tuberculosis and also the Centre of Excellence (CoE) for Extra-Pulmonary Tuberculosis in collaboration with Central TB Division and Directorate General of Health Services (DGHS) of the Ministry of Health and Family Welfare (MoHFW), Government of India (GoI), with support from Global Health Advocates India (GHA India) has taken an initiative to develop Indian extra-pulmonary TB (INDEX-TB) guidelines.

1.2 National planning for universal access in EPTB

The public health emphasis on infectious pulmonary TB is central to the health of the Indian people. Nevertheless, EPTB remains extremely common and is probably underrecognized and treated. These guidelines aim to help improve awareness, diagnosis and proper treatment of EPTB, thus promoting universal access to appropriate, effective care.

1.3 Objectives

The main objective of these guidelines is to provide guidance on up-to-date, uniform, evidence-based practices for suspecting, diagnosing and managing various forms of EPTB at all levels of delivery.

A subsidiary objective is to help direct further research by identifying knowledge gaps.

These guidelines will contribute to the programme to improve detection, care and outcomes in EBTP; to provide guidance on initiation of treatment, adherence and completion whilst minimizing drug toxicity and overtreatment; and contribute to practices that minimize the development of drug resistance.

1.4 Scope

The main purpose of the guidelines is to inform national treatment protocols. The major part of the document is concerned with primary and secondary level health care, i.e. at district hospitals and places that have sufficient expertise, clinical capacity and resources to care for EPTB patients. The aim is to standardize practice across the country. The guidelines address diagnosis and treatment in all forms of EPTB, providing recommendations based on systematic reviews of the evidence where possible. The guidelines are intended to be synergistic with existing RNTCP policy.

The guidelines focus on important current areas of debate in EPTB policy and practice. This helps identify priorities and guide resource use and helps policy makers, clinical managers and clinicians implement best practice in these critical areas in the first instance as part of continuous quality improvement in the detection and treatment of EPTB.

1.5 Target audience

The main document is for public and private sector clinicians in primary, secondary and tertiary care, and associated field-level health workers. Suggested points of referral are included to guide general practitioners and field health workers. The guidelines are also intended to inform health-care providers, TB programme managers and policy makers about best practice based on a review of the current evidence.

1.6 Updating the guidelines

The Core Committee and GoI recognized that this guideline represented the start of a process of developing evidence-informed EPTB guidelines in India that would be further developed over time. There was a commitment to updating aspects of these guidelines in the next 3 to 6 years, at which time these topics would be revisited and additional priority topics considered.

2 Methods used to reach recommendations

Representatives from the RNTCP and the Central TB Division of the Ministry of Health and Family Welfare, GoI, worked with representatives from the Department of Medicine at AIIMS New Delhi and other technical advisors to establish a Core Committee for the development of the guidelines (see Annex 1) and a Technical Advisory Committee (TAC), with subcommittees of specialists in each of the organ systems. The Core Committee recruited a Methodology Support Team to provide guidance in the development of the guidelines.

The Core Committee prepared a document that outlined the methods, teams, management of the process and how conflicts of interest would be handled. This was termed the Scoping Document and was approved by representatives from the Central TB Division. The Scoping Document set out the purpose and objectives of the guidelines. This was circulated to members of the TAC along with a suggested framework for identifying key questions for each form of EPTB around diagnosis, treatment and follow-up. During February and March 2015, each TAC subcommittee performed a scoping exercise to identify key questions, and began literature reviews. Each subcommittee carried out a consultation across institutions with experts in every relevant medical specialty to identify topics of interest and key questions relating to the diagnosis and management of all forms of EPTB. Each TAC then prepared a comprehensive state-of-the-art summary of knowledge and opinion about each organ system. This was done using traditional narrative approaches to reviewing. The Methodology Support Team provided advice on taking a systematic approach wherever possible, with training courses organised by Cochrane South Asia.

During the meeting of the guidelines group in March 2015, TAC subcommittees presented their findings for discussion with the Core Committee and Methodology Support Team. This meeting concluded with plans to refine the questions addressed by each subcommittee and outline cross-cutting themes requiring more detailed evidence review. These questions were identified as key policy and clinical questions facing the providers at this point in time.

These questions were around:
- use of tuberculin skin testing
- the role of the Xpert MTB/RIF test in diagnosing EPTB
- the role of other polymerase chain reaction (PCR)-based tests in diagnosing EPTB
- empirical treatment of EPTB in the absence of a laboratory diagnosis, including therapeutic trials and the use of corticosteroids in EPTB
- the duration of anti-tuberculosis treatment (ATT) in EPTB
- the definition of treatment failure in terms of clinical parameters prompting extended treatment, revised diagnosis, or consideration of drug resistance.

The Core Committee and Methodology Support Team selected themes to take forward to systematic evidence review. These were selected on the basis of: a) clinical importance as expressed by the TAC subcommittees; b) current availability of evidence; and c) feasibility of assembling up-to-date evidence within the time frame required.

2.1 Evidence review

The Methodology Support Team, along with members from TAC subcommittees, prepared the evidence summaries for review by the guidelines panel between March and July 2015. As part of this process, existing systematic reviews were updated; and where no review was available, new systematic reviews were developed and carried out. Given the time, three topic areas were prioritised:

1. The use of Xpert MTB/RIF in diagnosing EPTB
2. The use of corticosteroids in EPTB
3. The duration of treatment in EPTB

We intended to summarize the available evidence for all forms of EPTB within each of these topic areas, but due to time and resource constraints, we limited our systematic reviews to areas where there is substantive evidence available or there is urgent priority for evidence-based clinical policy. Hence, the questions covered in the evidence review were as follows:

1. Should Xpert MTB/RIF be recommended for use in the diagnosis of:
   - lymph node TB
   - TB meningitis
   - pleural TB?

2. Should corticosteroids be recommended for use in the treatment of:
   - TB pericarditis;
   - TB meningitis;
   - pleural TB?

3. How long should ATT be given in the treatment of:
   - lymph node TB;
   - abdominal TB;
   - TB meningitis?

The Core Committee recognised the need to revisit many of the topic areas identified in the scoping process for systematic evidence review to inform the next iteration of these guidelines.

Details of the methods used in the preparation of each review are summarised in Annex 2, which will be made available in the supplementary materials on-line on CTD website as well as ICMR website. The general principles of systematic review followed those set out in the Cochrane Handbook (Higgins, 2011) (Panel 1).

Panel 1. Steps in synthesising the evidence used for the main guidelines
1. Identify the question (or objective) of the review
2. Identify the outcomes that are most important – to patients, to clinicians, to policy makers
3. Write a protocol setting out the inclusion criteria for the review – what studies will help to answer the question?
4. Two researchers then carry out steps 5 and 6 independently, to limit bias in the review process.
5. Perform a structured search of the literature and screen the results using the inclusion criteria set out in the protocol. Only include studies that can address the review question.
6. Perform data extraction from each study using a pre-defined tool – find the data in the included studies that answers the question and describe each of the studies and their populations.
7. Perform a risk of bias assessment of each study using a pre-defined tool – how reliable are the data from each study?
8. Resolve any discrepancies between the two researchers' data collection by discussion.
9. Perform data synthesis that is appropriate – this could include performing a meta-analysis across studies, or simply describing the findings, depending on the level of heterogeneity between the studies and the types of studies included in the review.
10. Summarize the findings in a table, and apply the GRADE criteria to assess the level of certainty and the applicability of the effects estimates.

2.2 Making recommendations

The recommendations were made during a meeting of the INDEX-TB guidelines group in July 2015 at AIIMS, New Delhi. The Methodology Support Team apprised the guidelines panel of the methods used in conducting the systematic reviews, and advised on the interpretation of the evidence in the summaries. Each evidence summary was presented by the author, and the guidelines group had time to consider the methods and results of the review before considering the GRADE assessment of the main effects estimates, guided by the Methodology Support Team.

2.3 Quality of the evidence

GRADE assessments were appraised in detail, and revised where appropriate to reflect applicability to the Indian context.

The quality of the evidence from systematic reviews was assessed for each outcome and rated on a four-point scale, after consideration of the risk for bias (including publication bias) and the consistency, directness and precision of the effect estimates. The terms used in the quality assessments refer to the confidence that the guideline development group had in the estimate and not solely to the scientific quality of the investigations reviewed, as follows:

Quality of evidence	Interpretation
High	The group is very confident in the estimates of effect and considers that further research is very unlikely to change this confidence.
Moderate	The group has moderate confidence in the estimate of effect but considers that further research is likely to have an important impact on their confidence and may change the estimate.
Low	The group has low confidence in the estimate of effect and considers that further research is very likely to have an important impact on their confidence and is likely to change the estimate.
Very low	The group is very uncertain about the estimate of effect.

2.4 Strength of the recommendation

The group considered the trade-offs between benefits and harms, the implications for primary, secondary and tertiary health-care contexts and values and preferences relevant to the question. A recommendation was then formulated by the group based on consensus decision-making. Each recommendation was qualified as either "strong" or "conditional" based on the level of certainty in the effects and the degree of concordance among the group.

Recommendations were formulated after considering the quality of the evidence, the balance of benefits and harms and the feasibility of the intervention. Although cost is a critical factor in setting national treatment policies, cost was not formally considered. Areas of disagreement were extensively discussed and consensus reached. Voting was not required.

Factor considered	Rationale
Balance of benefits and harm	The more the expected benefits outweigh the expected risks, the more likely it is that a strong recommendation will be made. When the balance of benefits and harm is likely to vary by setting or is a fine balance, a conditional recommendation is more likely.
Values and preferences	If the recommendation is likely to be widely accepted or highly valued, a strong recommendation is more likely.
Feasibility	If an intervention is achievable in the settings in which the greatest impact is expected, a strong recommendation is more likely.

2.5 Strong and conditional recommendations

There was careful discussion about whether recommendations were strong, where very few people would argue against the recommendation; or conditional, where most people would recommend, but it would not be everyone, or that the intervention may be used in some circumstances and not others, or where some may choose a different management option.

	For patients	For clinicians	For programme managers and policy makers
Strong	Most people would want the recommended test or treatment and only a small proportion would not.	Most patients should receive the recommended test or treatment.	The recommendation can be adopted as standard policy and practice in most situations.
Conditional	Most people would want the recommended test or treatment, but many would not.	Clinicians need to be prepared to help patients make a decision that is consistent with their own values, as this test or treatment might not be right for everybody.	There is need for substantial debate and involvement of stakeholders when considering adopting this policy and practice.

2.6 Drafting the guidelines

Following the meeting of the guidelines group in July 2015, the guidelines were drafted under the supervision of the Core Committee and Methodology Support Team.

The recommendations as drafted and agreed by the Guideline Panel are outlined with accompanying summaries of the evidence and decision-making process.

Each TAC subcommittee drafted a report on current best practice in their specialist field, supported by review of the literature. The Methodology Support Team extracted the Clinical Practice Points from the submitted TAC reports, in dialogue with the TAC leads.

The guidelines, supporting evidence summaries and Clinical Practice Points were submitted for peer review by national and international experts. The Core Committee appraised the results of the peer review process, made necessary changes, if any, and submitted the completed document to the CTD for consideration.

The recommendations laid out in this guidelines document are the result of the process of systematic review and critical appraisal described above, and were agreed upon by the entire guidelines panel. The Clinical Practice Points include these recommendations, but also include other information relevant to clinicians and policy makers on each form of EPTB. The Clinical Practice Points were formulated by the expert clinicians who formed each TAC subcommittee, and reflect the consensus opinions of these experts, rather than the guidelines group as a whole.

In future iterations of these guidelines, it is hoped that time and resources will again be committed to producing transparent, evidence-based recommendations to address more of the many questions that remain in tackling EPTB.

2.7 Panel members and organization

The INDEX-TB Guidelines Core Committee comprises major stakeholders from scientific bodies pertaining to EPTB, and was responsible for recruiting the members of the other committees. The Core Committee prepared the Scoping Document for the guidelines and oversaw the guidelines development process from start to finish.

The Technical Advisory Committee (TAC) is comprised of expert clinicians, public health officials, GoI officials and WHO Regional Office for South-East Asia representatives. Members of the TAC were selected in order to maximize diversity, relevant expertise and representation of both stakeholders and patient groups. TAC subcommittees of expert clinicians generated the key questions to be addressed in the guidelines for each form of EPTB, prepared literature reviews and participated in the appraisal of the evidence summaries and formulation of the main recommendations.

The Methodology Support Team is comprised of staff from the Cochrane South Asia centre at the Christian Medical College in Vellore and from the Cochrane Infectious Diseases Group at the Liverpool School of Tropical Medicine, United Kingdom. The Methodology Support Team was recruited to advise the Core Committee and TAC subcommittees on best practice in terms of the selection of priority questions, production of evidence summaries and systematic reviews, use of evidence summaries to generate recommendations and the drafting of the guidelines document.

The Coordinating Committee organised logistics and periodic meetings as deemed essential by the Central TB Division.

The Peer Review Committee is comprised of national and international experts chosen by the Core Committee and the TACs to appraise the final guidelines document and supply corrections.

2.8 Declaration of interests

Declarations of interest were required from every member of the guidelines group. These were submitted to the CTD. At the commencement of the final guidelines meeting in July 2015, all members of the guideline panel verbally stated any financial or intellectual interests to the rest of the group. The participants and their declarations of interests are published in Annex 1.

2.9 Funding

The preparation of the guidelines was funded exclusively by the National TB Programme through a grant from Global Health Advocates. The WHO Country Office, India, funded the printing of the guidelines. A grant to the Liverpool School of Tropical Medicine from the UK Government Department for International Development for evidenceinformed policy development helped support the Methodology Support Team. No external source of funding from industry was solicited or used.

3 Principles

In line with the International Standards of TB Care (TB CARE I, 2014), the guidelines group as a whole agreed on a set of principles about what every EPTB patient in India needs as a basic standard of care. These principles relate to a basic standard of care that all providers should seek to achieve, a complementary set to the Standards for TB Care in India (Central TB Division and WHO Country Office for India, 2014).

Principle 1	Patients first
	The provider should adopt a patient-centred approach to managing EPTB, to promote well-being and adherence to treatment and to relieve suffering. Patients have the right to be fully informed about their care at every stage, to be able to make decisions about their treatment and to be treated with dignity and respect.
Principle 2	Promoting early diagnosis
	Providers should be informed of the clinical features and risk factors for various forms of EPTB and carry out prompt clinical evaluation and appropriate early diagnostic investigation.
Principle 3	Access to a tissue-based diagnosis
	Where facilities exist, all patients suspected of having EPTB should have appropriate samples taken for microbiological and histological testing, unless diagnostic sampling is deemed to risk undue harm.
Principle 4	Addressing drug resistance
	All patients with a diagnosis of EPTB should be risk-assessed for drug resistance prior to starting treatment, and drug susceptibility testing should be available for all patients at risk of drug-resistant tuberculosis.
Principle 5	Avoiding unnecessary invasive and costly tests
	Providers should consider the impact of diagnostic tests on patient management before referring patients for costly or invasive tests, or repeating these tests.
Principle 6	Access to HIV testing
	As EPTB is particularly associated with HIV, integrated counselling and testing should be made available to all patients suspected of having EPTB.
Principle 7	Identifying patients with concurrent active pulmonary TB
	All patients suspected of having EPTB should have clinical assessment for pulmonary TB in line with RNTCP guidance for investigating suspected pulmonary TB.
Principle 8	Ensuring effective treatment
	All patients should receive an appropriate treatment regimen.
Principle 9	Promoting adherence
	Providers should monitor adherence to treatment and address factors leading to interruption or discontinuation of treatment. Services should promote retention of patients in care.
Principle 10	Record keeping and public health promotion
	A reliable, well-maintained record of all diagnostic tests, treatments given, treatment monitoring, outcomes and adverse events should be kept for each patient, and data should be collected at the national programme level for the purposes of health-care system planning and development.

4 Working definitions of cases and outcomes

4.1 Purpose of defining a TB case

The RNTCP has developed clear definitions for pulmonary TB cases that allow clinicians to categorize patients in terms of their diagnostic status and outcomes of treatment. This provides common terminology that practitioners treating TB patients and policy makers can understand.

Many TB patients never have their diagnosis confirmed by a positive microbiological test due to the limitations of the diagnostic tests currently available, or lack of access to a microbiological test. These patients are often treated based on the clinician's suspicion alone (empirical treatment). Defining EPTB cases by diagnostic status enables clinicians to be clear about treatment decisions, and is essential to facilitate accurate national reporting within the RNTCP.

During the guidelines development process, it became clear that the panels were all using the terms used in pulmonary TB for EPTB. However, because the disease is different for each organ system, individuals were using the terms loosely, and the lack of clarity around treatment end-points and when to classify an EPTB patient as successfully treated or requiring further treatment sometimes caused confusion during discussions.

Creating outcome definitions to guide treatment decisions in EPTB and aid reporting is challenging due to the uncertainty around diagnostic test accuracy, the fact that diagnostic sampling often requires an invasive procedure and the lack of surrogate markers for microbiological cure. However, the Core Committee appreciated that there was a need to agree on a provisional set of definitions for outcomes to assist the panel with decisionmaking.

A comprehensive classification of EPTB case definitions and outcome definitions has not previously been attempted, and the Core Committee was aware that given the nature of EPTB, these outcomes will not directly map on to pulmonary TB outcomes. Nevertheless, these definitions are required for transparent and clear decision-making. Each TAC subcommittee worked with the Methodology Support Team to formulate these definitions with reference to the RNTCP's definitions for pulmonary TB cases. The committee appreciated that this was a pragmatic approach to help decision-making and used these outcomes in the development of guidelines.

The Core Committee proposed these working definitions be used to help transparent guidance in the clinical guides. The Core Committee discussed that there needed to be refinements in national reporting for EPTB to capture more detailed information about the epidemiology of the disease and patient outcomes. It is proposed to examine the approach and utility of these working definitions with user guidelines users in 2017, and continue dialogue with the RNTCP in relation to improved reporting for EPTB.

Standardized outcome definitions specific to each form of EPTB have not been established internationally. The guidelines group recognized that this creates problems in the treatment of EPTB patients, particularly when a patient still has on-going symptoms after several months of treatment. Recognizing when first-line treatment is failing is not always straightforward, and uncertainty around what clinical, radiological, biochemical/haematological markers suggest successful treatment probably leads to some patients receiving excessively long or repeated treatment courses, or being switched to second-line drugs unnecessarily. Conversely, other patients who are likely to have drugresistant EPTB may not be recognized as early as they could be, and may not receive the optimum treatment. The TAC subcommittees have attempted to produce outcome definitions that they felt were appropriate through consensus in their expert groups, and some of these are included in the Clinical Practice Points. The setting of standardized outcome definitions for each form of EPTB requires an extensive evidence review and consultation process, and is beyond the scope of this guidelines project. However, the guidelines group recognizes the importance of this task, and supports efforts to achieve this internationally.

Working case definitions[1]

Presumptive case: A patient with symptoms and signs of EPTB who needs to be investigated.

Bacteriologically confirmed case: A patient who has a microbiological diagnosis of EPTB, based on positive microscopy, culture or a validated PCR-based test.

Clinically diagnosed case: A patient with negative microbiological tests for TB (microscopy, culture and validated PCR-based tests), but with strong clinical suspicion and other evidence of EPTB, such as compatible imaging findings, histological findings, ancillary diagnostic tests or response to anti-TB treatment.*

A presumptive case started on ATT empirically, without microbiological testing, should also be considered a clinically diagnosed case (empirically treated). A clinically diagnosed case subsequently found to be bacteriologically positive (before or after starting treatment) should be reclassified as bacteriologically confirmed.

Non-EPTB case: A patient who has been investigated for EPTB and has been diagnosed with a different condition, with no microbiological evidence of EPTB found.

Presumptive relapse: A patient who was declared successfully treated at the end of ATT and now presents again with symptoms and signs of any form of TB.

Bacteriologically confirmed relapse: A patient with presumptive relapse who has microbiological evidence of persisting *Mycobacterium tuberculosis (Mtb)* infection on subsequent diagnostic sampling.

Clinically diagnosed relapse: A patient with presumptive relapse who does not have microbiological evidence of persisting *Mtb* infection on repeat diagnostic sampling, and has no evidence of another disease process.

A patient with presumptive relapse who is started on ATT empirically without repeat microbiological tests should also be considered a clinically diagnosed relapse (empirically treated). A clinically diagnosed relapse subsequently found to be bacteriologically positive (before or after starting treatment) should be reclassified as bacteriologically confirmed relapse.

"Ancillary diagnostic tests" refer to organ system-specific tests such as pleural fluid adenosine deaminase activity (ADA) in pleural TB, or CSF biochemistry and differential cell count in TB meningitis.

Working outcome definitions[1]

Successfully treated: A TB patient who has clinical and radiological evidence of resolution of active TB at the end of ATT.

It is recognized that some people have residual tissue damage that causes on-going symptoms or radiological change (sequelae) despite resolution of TB infection.

Completed treatment: A TB patient who completed treatment without clinical evidence of failure but with no record to show complete resolution by radiological or bacteriological evidence of persisting infection by the last month of treatment, either because tests were not done or because results are unavailable.

Presumptive treatment failure: A patient who has no satisfactory clinical or imaging response to treatment after completing 3–6 months ATT.

At what point in the course of treatment clinicians should consider a patient to have presumptive treatment failure is uncertain, and is likely to vary between forms of EPTB. For example, in TB meningitis it may not be acceptable to wait longer than 3 months before taking action for presumptive treatment failure, whereas persisting with first-line treatment for up to 6 months may be more acceptable in lymph node TB. Further research is necessary to help inform clinical judgement on treatment endpoints.

Bacteriologically confirmed treatment failure: A patient with presumptive treatment failure who has microbiological evidence of persisting *Mtb* infection on repeat diagnostic sampling.

Clinically diagnosed treatment failure: A presumptive treatment failure case who does not have microbiological evidence of persisting *Mtb* infection on repeat diagnostic sampling and has no evidence of another disease process, but has strong clinical suspicion of treatment failure and other evidence of active TB, such as imaging findings.

---

[1] These definitions from the Core Committee are provisional, working definitions to help people use these guidelines. Appraisal of their usefulness is anticipated in 2017.

* Compatible histological findings include AFB-negative granuloma. If histological examination reveals AFB-positive histological changes, this is consistent with bacteriological confirmation, and the case should be classified as bacteriologically confirmed.

Sequelae of EPTB

Part of the difficulty in defining treatment end-points in EPTB relates to the development of sequelae as a result of the inflammation and subsequent fibrosis produced in different tissues by *Mtb* infection. Patients with sequelae may have complete microbiological cure following ATT, but continue to have symptoms. In many forms of EPTB, sequelae can mimic the signs and symptoms of active TB infection, making the decision to stop treatment and declare the patient successfully treated difficult. Examples of sequelae include:

- small volume fibrotic lymph nodes following lymph node TB
- neurological deficits following TB meningitis
- intestinal strictures leading to abdominal pain and vomiting following gastrointestinal (GI) TB
- deformity and back pain following spinal TB.

The clinician must balance the risks of possibly terminating treatment prematurely with the risks of continuing treatment with drugs that have well characterised adverse effects. The INDEX-TB Guideline Group acknowledge that this is an area where further research is needed to provide clinicians with better information and tools to guide their decision-making. New diagnostic technologies may be helpful in future, but at present involvement of experienced specialists is suggested in cases where uncertainty exists.

4.2 Paradoxical reactions and IRIS in EPTB

The phenomenon of paradoxical reaction in TB infection has long been observed in both HIV-positive and HIV-negative TB patients. Multiple definitions of paradoxical reaction exist in the literature, but essentially this term refers to the phenomenon of clinical (or radiological) deterioration of TB lesions, or the development of new lesions in a patient with TB who has initially improved on ATT occurring in the early phase of treatment (during the first 3 months). Paradoxical reactions manifest in a wide variety of ways, and can sometimes be life-threatening or lead to increased disability in EPTB survivors. A review of case reports detailing paradoxical reactions in HIV-negative patients found 122 episodes with 17 different clinical and radiological presentations (Cheng, 2002). In this review, the paradoxical reaction occurred in a different organ system to the initial TB lesion in 25.4% of cases. Pathogenesis of paradoxical reaction is not yet fully understood, and may occur due to a variety of mechanisms. The predominant theory is that it occurs as a result of an excessive immune response to *Mtb* antigens in patients on effective ATT, involving dysregulation in innate and acquired immune pathways (Garg, 2014).

Immune reconstitution inflammatory syndrome (IRIS) refers to a clinical syndrome observed in HIV-positive people after starting antiretroviral therapy (ART) caused by an inflammatory response to an antigen, thought to be due to the reconstitution of the immune response to that antigen. While extensive research has been done and is ongoing, pathogenetic mechanisms and the best strategies to prevent and treat IRIS are not fully understood. IRIS involving TB infection is common, and can manifest in two principal ways: paradoxical TBIRIS, where an inflammatory exacerbation of TB symptoms occurs after commencing ATT in patients being treated for TB; and unmasking TB-IRIS, where active TB presents in a patient who has commenced ART (Bell, 2015).

Both paradoxical reaction and IRIS pose significant challenges to physicians treating TB patients in India. Worsening of clinical and radiological features of EPTB in both HIV-positive and HIV-negative patients raises several questions:

- Does the patient have treatment failure due to drug-resistant TB?
- Does the patient have drug-sensitive TB that is not responding to ATT for some reason, such as malabsorption or inadequate adherence to treatment?
- Does the patient have another ongoing disease process?
- Does the patient have a drug fever?
- Should the regimen be changed?
- Should the patient be admitted for inpatient care?
- Are adjunctive treatments required to manage the inflammation?

The INDEX-TB guidelines group acknowledge that these are important questions in EPTB, and that detailed evidence review and further research is needed to support recommendations around these issues. Guidance on the initiation of ART in HIV–TB co-infected patients exists elsewhere (see Section 19 Special groups).

5

Recommendations for the use of Xpert MTB/RIF in EPTB diagnosis

What is Xpert MTB/RIF?

Xpert MTB/RIF is a commercially available diagnostic test for Mycobacterium tuberculosis complex, which uses polymerase chain reaction (PCR) to test specimens for genetic material specific to Mtb, and simultaneously detects a gene which confers resistance to rifampicin, rpoB (Blakemore, 2010). It is manufactured by Cepheid, Sunnyvale, California, USA. Unlike other commercial PCR based tests, it is a fully automated test using the GeneXpert® platform. The specimen is loaded into a cartridge and all the steps in the assay are then fully automated and contained within the unit. One of the reagents is powerfully tuberculocidal, making the used test cartridges safe to handle outside of a specialist laboratory environment. This allows the test to be brought closer to the clinical setting.

Xpert MTB/RIF was originally designed to test sputum samples from patients with active pulmonary TB, and has been shown to have high accuracy for diagnosing TB in these patients (Steingart, 2014).

What makes the use of Xpert MTB/RIF in EPTB different?

Since its introduction to research settings in 2010, several investigators have tested the accuracy of this test in non-respiratory samples for the diagnosis of various forms of EPTB. There are several a priori reasons why the Xpert MTB/RIF may perform differently with non-sputum samples: Xpert MTB/RIF has a specimen treatment step which is designed to liquefy sputum but this may not be an optimum pre-test processing for nonsputum samples; although the test has a limit of detection of 131 colony forming units per mL, it has been shown to perform less well in paucibacillary disease; as many forms of EPTB require invasive sampling methods, the size and quality of the specimens may affect the sensitivity of the test. In 2016, a new version of Xpert MTB/RIF, Xpert MTB/RIF Ultra, will be introduced with a lower limit of detection. We anticipate that roll-out and accumulation of efficacy data will take time, and so we have summarized the available evidence for the current version of the test.

Why is this a priority question for these guidelines?

MoHFW has engaged with international partners to roll out Xpert MTB/RIF for the diagnosis of pulmonary TB as part of the RNTCP. Members of the INDEX-TB TAC subcommittees recognized the need for evidence-informed guidance on the use of Xpert MTB/RIF for the diagnosis of EPTB in India, because as this test becomes more widely available, clinicians will need to know when to use and how to interpret this test in different forms of EPTB. The advantages of having a rapid test for EPTB must be weighed against the accuracy of the test and the possible harms from misdiagnosis when considering the use of this test.

The evidence considered by the guideline group in making these recommendations was based on a systematic review carried out by Denkinger et al. In this review, diagnostic test accuracy studies using Xpert MTB/RIF and culture for the diagnosis of M. tuberculosis infection in three forms of EPTB were summarized, with pooled estimates of sensitivity and specificity (Denkinger, 2014). As there was little data on sensitivity and specificity of Xpert MTB/RIF for the diagnosis of rifampicin resistance, this was not addressed in this review, and hence has not been addressed within these recommendations. To ensure the guideline group was able to make recommendations based on the most up-to-date information, a summary of studies published since this review was undertaken in 2013 was also presented to the guidelines group (See Annex 2, online supplementary materials).

WHO has endorsed standard operating procedures for the use of Xpert MTB/RIF for non-respiratory specimens (https://www. ghdonline.org/uploads/GeneXpert_SOP_Xpert_processing_EPTB_specimens_DRAFT. pdf).

5.1 Lymph node TB

Recommendation	Xpert MTB/RIF should be used as an additional test to conventional smear microscopy, culture and cytology in FNAC specimens.
Strength of recommendation	Strong
Evidence	Pooled sensitivity against culture 83.1% (95% CI 71.4–90.7%) (13 studies, 955 specimens with 362 culture positive, low quality evidence)
	Pooled specificity against culture 93.6% (05% CI 87.9–96.8%) (13 studies, 955 specimens with 362 culture positive, high quality evidence)
	In a population of 1000 patients with presumptive lymph node tuberculosis (LNTB) where 200 truly have the disease, if treatment was determined only by Xpert MTB/RIF: • 166 (142 to 182) would be correctly treated for TB (low quality evidence) • 34 (58 to 18) with TB would be missed (low quality evidence) • 48 (96 to 24) without TB would be treated (high quality evidence)
Panel's view on advantages of using the test	Quicker diagnosis
	May lead to fewer patients being treated with ATT when they do not have LNTB (no direct evidence available)
	Reduced stigma from reduction in overtreatment
	May identify rifampicin resistance (evidence not formally reviewed)
Panel's view on disadvantages of using the test	Patients with false negative Xpert results may have ATT withheld or stopped inappropriately
	False negatives may go on to develop disseminated disease
	False positives exposed to ATT unnecessarily
	May falsely diagnose rifampicin resistance – harm to patient from side effects of second line drugs, and high cost
	Cost implications of managing missed cases (repeat diagnostic sampling, repeat hospital/clinic visits)
	Stigma for patients given a false positive diagnosis
	Litigation for misdiagnosis

Explanatory notes

The guidelines group considered the evidence for the diagnostic accuracy of Xpert MTB/RIF in lymph node specimens obtained by fine needle aspiration and biopsy. In making the recommendation, the group considered the context of a district level health-care centre, acknowledging that the current basis for diagnosis of lymph node TB under the RNTCP is cytological examination and smear microscopy for acid-fast bacilli of fine needle aspirate from an affected lymph node (FNAC). The group considered whether there was sufficient evidence to recommend that Xpert MTB/RIF replace FNAC as the principal diagnostic test, and concluded that this would be inappropriate given the fact that one in five patients are missed by Xpert MTB/RIF. The group agreed that Xpert MTB/RIF can be useful in confirming a diagnosis in patients suspected of LNTB when considered alongside the results of FNAC, noting that a negative Xpert MTB/RIF test does not rule out LNTB.

Diagnostic investigations should be carried out in the context of quality of care that can assure patient safety, in line with the Guideline's Principles 3 and 4. Xpert MTB/RIF is of use where clinicians have appropriate expertise in carrying out diagnostic sampling from lymph nodes safely and accurately, and where there is access to Xpert MTB/RIF testing in a laboratory with adequate quality assurance.

5.2 TB meningitis

Recommendation	Xpert may be used as an adjunctive test for tuberculous meningitis (TBM). A negative Xpert result does not rule out TBM. Decision to give ATT should be based on clinical features and CSF profile.
Strength of recommendation	Conditional

Evidence	Pooled sensitivity against culture 80.5% (95% CI 59.0–92.2%) (13 studies, 839 specimens with 159 culture positive, low quality evidence)
	Pooled specificity against culture 97.8% (05% CI 95.2–99.0%) (13 studies, 839 specimens with 159 culture positive, high quality evidence)
	In a population of 1000 patients with presumptive TB meningitis where 100 truly have the disease, if treatment was determined only by Xpert MTB/RIF result: • 81 (59 to 92) would be correctly treated for TB (low quality evidence) • 19 (41 to 8) with TB would be missed (low quality evidence) • 18 (45 to 9) without TB would be treated (high quality evidence)
Panel's view on advantages of using the test	If Xpert MTB/RIF is positive it is highly likely to be TBM – this could increase access to a reliable diagnosis
	Quick result
	Already widely available
Panel's view on disadvantages of using the test	High number of false negatives – significant concern that this could lead to missed or delayed diagnosis, although direct evidence of the impact of Xpert MTB/RIF test results on patient outcomes in TBM is lacking
	Delayed diagnosis leads to worse outcomes (death)
	Additional costs

Explanatory notes

The group noted that the stakes are high in the diagnosis of TBM due to the high mortality associated with this disease, particularly when the diagnosis is delayed. Although the sensitivity of smear microscopy of CSF specimens is extremely low and Xpert MTB/RIF has a higher sensitivity than this test, the fact that one in five patients with TBM are missed by Xpert MTB/RIF raised concerns that patients could be harmed by delayed treatment if clinicians relied on a negative result. The guidelines panel concluded that as Xpert MTB/RIF is not sufficiently sensitive for TB meningitis, the decision to give or withhold ATT should not be based on a negative Xpert result alone. A positive Xpert MTB/RIF result may be reassuring due to the high specificity of the test, but it should only be used as an adjunct to other diagnostic methods.

A concentration step in the processing of CSF before using Xpert MTB/RIF appears to increase the sensitivity of the test. In a subgroup analysis, a concentration step involving centrifugation and resuspension of the sample appeared to enhance the sensitivity of Xpert (84.2% (95% CI 78.3–90.1%) versus 51.3% (95% CI 35.5–67.1%) for unconcentrated samples; specificity 98.0% (95% CI 96.7–99.2%) versus 94.6% (95% CI 90.9–98.2%) for unconcentrated samples (Denkinger, 2014).

5.3 Pleural TB

Recommendation	Xpert MTB/RIF should not be used to diagnose pleural TB
Strength of recommendation	Strong
Evidence	Pooled sensitivity against culture 46.4% (95% CI 26.3–67.8%) (14 studies, 841 specimens with 92 culture positive, low quality evidence)
	Pooled specificity against culture 99.1% (95% CI 95.2–99.8%) (14 studies, 841 specimens with 92 culture positive, high quality evidence)
	In a population of 1000 patients with presumptive pleural TB where 200 truly have the disease, if treatment was determined only by Xpert MTB/RIF results: • 92 (52 to 136) would be correctly treated for TB (low quality evidence) • 108 (148 to 64) with TB would be missed (low quality evidence) • 8 (40 to 0) without TB would be treated (high quality evidence)

Panel's view on advantages of using the test	• If Xpert is positive it is highly likely to be pleural TB – this could increase access to a reliable diagnosis, although direct evidence of the impact of Xpert MTB/RIF test results on patient outcomes in pleural TB is lacking • May help in avoiding invasive procedures like pleural biopsy (closed and thoracoscopic) • Quick result • Already widely available
Panel's view on disadvantages of using the test	• High number of false negatives – significant concern that this could lead to missed or delayed diagnosis, although direct evidence of the impact of Xpert MTB/RIF test results on patient outcomes in pleural TB is lacking • Delayed diagnosis leads to worse outcomes (pleural thickening, impaired lung function, active pulmonary TB) • Additional costs

Explanatory notes

Although the pooled estimate of specificity was high, the sensitivity of Xpert MTB/RIF in pleural fluid specimens was very low, with more than half of all pleural TB patients being missed by this test. The guidelines panel felt that although a positive Xpert result might help if the diagnosis was unclear, there were concerns regarding possible harm to patients associated with reliance on this test, whether the result is positive or negative. Anecdotally, some group members described patients they had treated who had positive Xpert results and were started on ATT, but also had malignancy, diagnosis of which was delayed as the positive Xpert test had led to a diagnosis of pleural TB

6 Recommendations for use of corticosteroids in EPTB

6.1 In treating tuberculous meningitis in HIV-negative people

Tuberculous meningitis (TBM) is a lifethreatening condition affecting adults and children, which can leave survivors with a range of neurological disabilities. The causes of death and disability in TBM are multifactorial. The main pathological mechanisms are persistent or progressive raised intracranial pressure with or without hydrocephalus, arachnoiditis and involvement of optic nerves or optic chiasma leading to visual deficit, cranial neuropathies and vasculitis of the cerebral blood vessels, leading to stroke.

Steroids are thought to reduce inflammation, improve blood flow and reduce cerebral oedema and intracranial pressure. However, the risks associated with steroids include immunosuppression, which is a major concern in the context of an infectious disease, GI bleeding, hyperglycaemia and hypertension, among others. Several randomized controlled trials have been conducted on the effect of corticosteroids in managing TBM. The conclusions from these trials, seen individually, appear inconsistent. One trial (Thwaites G.E., 2004) showed that dexamethasone increases survival rate, but it also raised two questions; do patients who survive because of dexamethasone therapy tend to be left with severe disability, and are there differential effects among subgroups of patients with different degrees of disease severity?

The guideline group reviewed evidence from the updated Cochrane review "Corticosteroids for managing tuberculous meningitis" (Prasad, 2016).

Recommendation	Steroids are recommended for TBM in HIV-negative people. Duration of steroid treatment should be for at least 4 weeks, with tapering as appropriate.
Strength of recommendation	Strong
Evidence	Corticosteroids reduce death from TBM from 41 per 100 people to 31 (27 to 36) per 100 people (nine studies, 1318 participants, high quality evidence). These studies were conducted in a variety of settings, and only one included HIV-positive people (n = 98).
	Disabling neurological deficit is not common in survivors, and steroids may have little or no effect on this outcome (RR 0.92, 95% CI 0.71 to 1.20; eight trials, 1295 participants, low quality evidence).
Panel's view on advantages of using steroids	Reduced mortality from TBM
Panel's view on disadvantages of using steroids	Adverse effects of steroids such as GI bleeding, bacterial infection, high blood pressure, high blood sugar
	Increased numbers of survivors with severe disability, although the evidence from the review does not support this

> **Explanatory notes**
>
> The panel considered the evidence in the systematic review relevant and applicable to the Indian context, noting that three of the eight studies included were carried out in India, while three others were carried out in South-East Asia.
>
> The group noted that the effects may be greater for patients with British Medical Research Council (MRC) Stage I and II, which indicate mild and moderate severity in TBM, but the recommendation should stand for all TBM patients (MRC, 1948). MRC staging is explained in the Clinical Practice Points, Section 2 - CNS TB.
>
> Duration of corticosteroids was discussed. The group agreed that there is no clear evidence for any one regimen of steroids and debated what the best option would be. The expert group agreed that steroids should be given for at least 4 weeks and then tapered. Some patients may need longer treatment with steroids, of up to 6–8 weeks, and decision to extend the course of steroids should be made based on disease severity and complications of TBM.

6.2 In treating tuberculous meningitis in HIV-positive people

The guideline group considered the evidence separately for HIV-negative and HIV-positive people because HIV co-infection is associated with particular complications of TBM disease, and particular adverse events associated with steroid use.

Recommendation	Steroids may be used for TB meningitis in HIV-positive people, where other life-threatening opportunistic infections are absent.
Strength of recommendation	Conditional
Evidence	Corticosteroids reduce death from TB meningitis from 41 per 100 people to 31 (27 to 36) per 100 people (nine studies, 1318 participants, high quality evidence). Eight out of the nine studies either excluded HIV-positive people or did not report HIV status. One study included 98 HIV-positive people out of 545 participants (Thwaites G.E., 2004). A subgroup analysis showed that corticosteroids had no effect on mortality in this group (RR 0.90, 95% CI 0.67 to 1.20), although this result should be interpreted with caution as the authors did not stratify the randomization by HIV status, and the number of HIV-positive participants was small. The very small numbers of events reported in this single study for the outcome disabling neurological deficit mean that we do not know what the effect of corticosteroids is in HIV-positive people for this outcome.
Panel's view on advantages of using steroids	Reduced mortality from TBM
Panel's view on disadvantages of using steroids	• Adverse effects of steroids such as GI bleeding, bacterial infection, high blood pressure, high blood sugar • Increased numbers of survivors with severe disability • Increased morbidity and mortality from opportunistic infections and HIV-associated cancers • Increased adverse drug reactions and interactions with ARVs
Explanatory notes	The group was concerned about the lack of evidence for the use of steroids in people with HIV and TBM. The group noted that there are circumstances where steroids are clearly indicated, for example in cases of raised intracranial pressure/mass effect from a tuberculoma. Steroids are associated with increased risk of serious, lifethreatening opportunistic infections in patients with advanced HIV disease. The criteria to be taken into account are stage of TBM disease, evidence of raised intracranial pressure or mass effect, CD4 cell count and presence or absence of other opportunistic infections. Giving long courses of steroids in patients with HIV may be undesirable, especially in patients with advanced HIV disease. Specialist advice in managing such cases is warranted. Important opportunistic infections to rule out include cryptococcal meningitis and cerebral toxoplasmosis. There is evidence that steroids are associated with increased adverse events and disability in patients with HIV-associated cryptococcal meningitis (Beardsley J, 2016).

6.3 In treating TB pericarditis in HIV-negative people

TB pericarditis is a potentially life-threatening form of EPTB, which can also lead to disability in survivors. TB pericarditis is generally characterized by pericardial effusion, which can be immediately life-threatening. Some patients go on to develop constrictive pericardial disease which causes cardiac disability and may be life-threatening, despite the resolution of TB infection. Corticosteroids have long been used to relieve the inflammation that causes the pericardial effusion, although their effect on reducing mortality and rates of long-term constrictive pericardial disease have been controversial. Corticosteroids are associated with certain risks, including immunosuppression, which is a major concern in the context of an infectious disease like TB and in HIV coinfection, as well as gastrointestinal bleeding, hyperglycaemia and hypertension, among others.

The guideline group reviewed evidence summarised from the draft updated Cochrane review "Corticosteroids and other interventions for treating tuberculous pericarditis" (Wiysonge, 2016).

Recommendation	Steroids are recommended for HIV-negative patients with TB pericarditis with pericardial effusion.
Strength of recommendation	Conditional
Evidence	The review included six studies, all from sub-Saharan Africa.
	The majority of the participants in these trials were HIV-positive; these estimates are based on disaggregated data for HIV-negative participants where possible.
	Corticosteroids may have no effect on all-cause mortality (RR 0.85, 95% CI 0.64 to 1.11, 810 participants, three studies, low quality evidence), but probably reduce death from pericarditis (RR 0.55, 95% CI 0.31 to 0.98, 810 participants, three studies, moderate quality evidence).
	Corticosteroids may have no effect on progression to constrictive pericarditis (RR 0.62, 95% CI 0.35 to 1.1, 431 participants, 1 study, low quality evidence).
	The guideline group further downgraded the quality of the evidence by 1 for indirectness as all the studies took place in sub-Saharan Africa, and because the HIV status of some participants was uncertain.
	Most of the data comes from one large trial in mainly HIV-positive patients. Steroids were associated with more people developing cancer, mainly HIV-related cancers. The authors note this some of these patients also received immunotherapy with M. indicus pranii. The review team is currently clarifying whether there is an interaction between M. indicus pranii and corticosteroids in relation to cancer with the trial authors.
Panel's view on advantages of using steroids	• Increased survival, although the results of the systematic review do not support this • Reduced incidence of constrictive pericarditis • Reduced need for pericardectomy, although the review did not find clear evidence of this • Reduction of ATT-associated adverse effects, although the results of the systematic review do not support this
Panel's view on disadvantages of using steroids	• Adverse effects of steroids such as GI bleeding, bacterial infection, high blood pressure, high blood sugar • Increased numbers of survivors with severe disability due to constrictive pericarditis

Explanatory notes

The group noted that the effects estimates in the review suggest that steroids have little or no effect on all-cause mortality, but probably do reduce mortality from TB pericarditis. The largest study (which had one-third HIV-negative participants) showed a reduction in the number of participants with constrictive pericarditis at the end of treatment in the analysis of all patients. The GRADE tables are based on data disaggregated into people that are HIV-positive and HIV-negative. Both these analyses give point estimates that show reduced risk of constrictive pericarditis with corticosteroids, although disaggregation means that in the smaller group of participants who were HIV-negative the result is not statistically significant. The group felt that it was likely that the result for HIV-negative participants did not reach statistical significance due to the meta-analysis being underpowered, rather than because corticosteroids had no effect on progression to constrictive pericarditis. The group felt that risk of constrictive pericarditis and associated morbidity was the most important outcome for consideration in making this recommendation. The recommendation therefore only relates to steroid use in patients who present with pericardial effusion caused by TB pericarditis; the group did not recommend steroids for patients presenting with constrictive TB pericarditis.

6.4 In treating TB pericarditis in HIV-positive people

The group considered the evidence for HIV-positive people with TB pericarditis separately, principally because there is a concern about corticosteroids leading to increased risk of HIV associated adverse events.

Recommendation	Steroids are recommended for HIV-positive patients with TB pericarditis with pericardial effusion.
Strength of recommendation	Conditional
Evidence	The review included four studies, all from sub-Saharan Africa.
	The majority of the participants in these trials were HIV-positive; these estimates are based on disaggregated data for HIV-positive participants where possible.
	Corticosteroids may have no effect on all-cause mortality (RR 1.14, 95% CI 0.88 to 1.49, 997 participants, two studies, low quality evidence), or on death from pericarditis (RR 1.33, 95% CI 0.68 to 2.62, 939 participants, 1 study, low quality evidence).
	Corticosteroids probably reduce progression to constrictive pericarditis (RR 0.51, 95% CI 0.28 to 0.94, 997 participants, two studies, moderate quality evidence).
	Corticosteroids may have no effect on HIV-associated opportunistic infections over 2 years' follow-up (RR 1.12, 95% CI 0.82 to 1.53, 939 participants, 1 study, low quality evidence). There may increase the risk of HIV-associated cancer over two years follow-up, but this was from one trial and participants also received M. indicus pranii which may have confounded the result.
Panel's view on advantages of using steroids	• Increased survival, although the results of the systematic review do not support this • Reduced incidence of constrictive pericarditis • Reduced need for pericardectomy, although the review did not find clear evidence of this • Reduction of ATT-associated adverse effects, although the review did not find clear evidence of this
Panel's view on disadvantages of using steroids	• Adverse effects of steroids such as GI bleeding, bacterial infection, high blood pressure, high blood sugar • Increased adverse events associated with HIV such as opportunistic infections and cancer • Increased numbers of survivors with severe disability

Explanatory notes

As for HIV-negative people, the group considered the outcome of greatest clinical significance to be the risk of constrictive pericardial disease following TB pericarditis. Again, the group recognized that there was a lack of evidence of effect on mortality. The evidence for steroids increasing the risk of HIV-associated cancers was also considered. The group felt that this may be of less concern in India as the epidemiology of HIV-associated diseases is different compared with Africa, notably, the prevalence of Kaposi's sarcoma is low. The group concluded that the priority was to reduce rates of constrictive pericardial disease, as this is associated with long-term morbidity and the need for invasive surgery (pericardectomy) for patients, and high cost and resource use for the health-care system. Therefore they made a conditional recommendation to use steroids in HIV-positive people with TB pericarditis with pericardial effusion. Steroids may be even more risky in patients with advanced HIV disease with low CD4 cell counts, and may increase the risk of opportunistic infections and HIV associated cancers. This risk needs to be balanced with the risk of constrictive pericarditis in HIV-positive people with TB pericarditis.

6.5 In treating pleural TB (irrespective of HIV status)

Pleural TB is one of the most common forms of EPTB. Characterized by pleural effusion, it usually resolves without treatment of any kind, but untreated patients may experience longer duration of the acute symptoms and risk recurrence of active TB at a later point in time (Light, 2010). Pleural TB can be complicated by massive effusion leading to respiratory compromise in the short term; pleural thickening, fibrosis and pleural adhesions causing impaired respiratory function in the medium to long term.

It is though that pleural TB is caused by a delayed-type (type IV) hypersensitivity reaction following mycobacterial infection of the pleura (Rossi, 1987). This explains the tendency towards resolution of the effusion and associated symptoms with or without treatment of the TB infection. There appears to be a spectrum of disease in pleural TB in terms of the extent of the underlying lung infection, which could be important in terms of patient outcomes and the potential for corticosteroids to be effective. The extent of underlying lung infection seems to be an important determinant of outcome (Shu, 2011).

The guideline panel considered evidence based on a rapid update of an existing Cochrane review "Corticosteroids for tuberculous pleurisy" (Engel, 2007). This review was conducted because there was uncertainty about the efficacy of corticosteroids in reducing the short-term and long-term effects on the acute symptoms of pleural TB and the long-term sequelae. Steroids are associated with several adverse effects, especially in people with HIV, and administering them in the absence of evidence of efficacy may be exposing patients to unnecessary risk.

Recommendation	Steroids are not routinely recommended in pleural TB.
Strength of recommendation	Conditional
Evidence	The review included four studies, all from sub-Saharan Africa.
	The majority of the participants in these trials were HIV-positive.
	Corticosteroids may reduce pleural effusions at 4 weeks (RR 0.76, 95% CI 0.62 to 0.94, 394 participants, three studies, low quality evidence), but we don't know whether corticosteroids have an effect on resolution of pleural effusion at 8 weeks (RR 0.72, 95% CI 0.46 to 1.12, 399 participants, four studies, very low quality evidence).
Evidence	Corticosteroids may reduce pleural thickening at the end of follow up (RR 0.69, 95% CI 0.51 to 0.94, 309 participants, four studies, low quality evidence).
	Corticosteroids may increase the risk of adverse events (RR 2.80, 95% CI 1.12 to 6.98, 586 participants, six studies, low quality evidence).
	This review found insufficient data to estimate the effect of corticosteroids on respiratory function.
	The reviewers deemed it inappropriate in this case to attempt to generate separate estimates for HIV-positive and HIV-negative people due to a lack of disaggregated data.
Panel's view on advantages of using steroids	• Faster recovery • Reduced chest X-ray changes at the end of treatment • Return to baseline lung function • Reduced long-term pulmonary disability
Panel's view on disadvantages of using steroids	• Adverse effects of steroids such as GI bleeding, bacterial infection, high blood pressure, high blood sugar • Risk of adverse events, such as HIV-related cancer due to further immunosuppression in HIV-positive people

Explanatory notes

Pleural TB is not associated with high mortality; therefore the group felt that the most important outcome to consider was respiratory function. The review found insufficient data addressing this outcome, and the panel felt that the outcomes reported in the review were not appropriate proxy measures for this outcome. The panel noted that chest X-ray appearance at the end of treatment may be important to some patients for social or financial reasons, but otherwise pleural thickening causing chest X-ray changes was not a clinically relevant outcome. Given the lack of evidence of effect on respiratory function, and the risks associated with steroid use, the group made a conditional recommendation against the use of steroids for pleural TB.

7 Recommendations for duration of treatment in EPTB

There are variations in existing guidelines and in clinical practice around the world about the optimum duration of ATT in the various forms of EPTB. While the 6-month regimen using the first-line drugs rifampicin, isoniazid, pyrazinamide and ethambutol has long been in use for pulmonary TB, there has been considerable uncertainty about duration of treatment for some forms of EPTB. The guidelines group considered the evidence for the optimum length of treatment for three forms of EPTB – lymph node TB, abdominal TB and TB meningitis.

7.1 In peripheral lymph node TB

Lymph node tuberculosis (LNTB) can present with involvement of peripheral, mediastinal and/or abdominal lymph nodes. As well as enlarged lymph nodes perceivable clinically or visualized on chest X-ray, abdominal ultrasound scan or computed tomography (CT) scan, clinical features sometimes include weight loss, fever and night sweats. The problem of persistently enlarged lymph nodes at the end of treatment has vexed clinicians and some practitioners extend treatment duration in such patients, fearing relapse of active TB disease in this group.

Recommendation	Six months ATT standard first-line regimen (2RHZE/4RHE) is recommended for peripheral lymph node TB.
Strength of recommendation	Strong
Evidence	The review included two randomised controlled trials, one from multiple secondary care hospitals in the United Kingdom and another from a single tertiary care hospital in Hong Kong, China. Participants were adults and adolescents with newly diagnosed peripheral and mediastinal LNTB, and HIV status was not reported in either study.
Evidence	There may be no difference between 6-month and 9-month ATT regimens in terms of relapse rates (RR 0.89, 95% CI 0.37 to 2.16, 253 participants, two studies, low quality evidence). There is probably no difference between 6-month and 9-month ATT regimens in terms of successful treatment at the end of follow up (21–55 months) (RR 1.11, 95% CI 0.97 to 1.26, 312 participants, two studies, moderate quality evidence). A review of five prospective cohort studies (706 participants) where patients with residual lymphadenopathy at the end of ATT were followed up demonstrated that relapse in this subgroup of patients was uncommon – 6 cases of relapse were reported across all studies.
Committee's view on advantages of 6-month treatment	• Cure rates and relapse rates are similar in the data collected for 6 months and 9 months (low quality evidence) • Patients more likely to complete shorter regimens • Less exposure to adverse effects of ATT
Committee's view on disadvantages of 6-month treatment	Theoretically, risk of relapse is higher with shorter regimens, but existing evidence is unclear

Explanatory notes

The guidelines group considered evidence from randomized controlled trials comparing 6 months' with 9 months' ATT in terms of outcomes such as relapse after completion of ATT, treatment completion and default. The group noted that the rates of relapse in the 6-month and 9-month groups were similarly very low, although there were concerns that the pooled data was still not sufficiently powered to detect a difference in this uncommon event.

The group noted that all the evidence pertained to peripheral LNTB, and that other factors needed to be taken into consideration for patients with mediastinal or abdominal LNTB, or disseminated TB. No recommendation was made regarding treatment duration in these patients.

A subgroup of patients, dubbed partial responders, have persisting small volume lymphadenopathy (<1 cm) at the end of treatment. The group agreed that the available evidence suggests that few partial responders appear to relapse, and that these patients generally do not require extension of ATT and can be managed by observation only. Further evidence is required to make firm recommendations for this particular group.

While this recommendation applied to adults and children with LNTB, the group noted that the evidence only relates to adults and adolescents, and so providers treating children should bear in mind that this recommendation is based on indirect evidence for children.

7.2 In abdominal TB

Abdominal TB can present with isolated involvement of any of the following sites: peritoneal, intestinal, upper GI (oesophageal, gastroduodenal), hepatobiliary, pancreatic and perianal. The clinical features as well as diagnostic modalities depend on the site of involvement. Internationally, most guidelines recommend treating all types of abdominal TB with the same regimen as for pulmonary TB – a 2-month intensive phase with four drugs (isoniazid, rifampicin, pyrazinamide and ethambutol) followed by a 4-month continuation phase with isoniazid and rifampicin. However, the evidence base for this practice is extrapolated from studies of pulmonary TB cases, and direct evidence for the optimum duration of treatment in abdominal TB has been lacking.

Shorter duration of treatment may increase compliance, leading to reduced numbers of relapses as well as the emergence of drug-resistance strains. Furthermore, shorter regimens decrease the risk of anti-TB drug toxicity. Whether a 6-month regimen achieves successful treatment rates as good as with a 9-month regimen without significantly increasing the number of relapses is the key concern for accepting a shorter ATT regimen. The present review aims to evaluate the effects of treatment with the 6-month regimen compared to the 9-month regimen for abdominal TB.

Recommendation	Six months ATT standard first-line regimen is recommended for abdominal TB.
Strength of recommendation	Strong
Evidence	The review included three randomised controlled trials, two from India and one from South Korea, with 328 participants. One trial included both GI TB and peritoneal TB patients, and the other two included GI TB patients only. None of the studies included children, or HIV-positive people.
	We do not know whether there is a difference in relapse rates in patients treated for 6 months and those treated for 9 months (RD 0.01, 95% CI -0.01 to 0.04, 328 participants, three studies, very low quality evidence).
Committee's view on advantages of 6-month treatment	• Patients more likely to complete shorter regimens • Less exposure to adverse effects of ATT
Committee's view on disadvantages of 6-month treatment	• Theoretically, risk of relapse is higher with shorter regimens, but existing evidence does not support this

Explanatory notes

The guidelines group reviewed the evidence and felt that for new patients with abdominal TB and with low risk of drug resistance, 6 months ATT followed by a period of observation was appropriate. The group recognized the paucity of data to answer this question, but noted particularly that there were very few relapses in both arms across all studies. The group noted that the available evidence came from patients with GI and peritoneal TB, and were concerned that other forms of abdominal TB, while comparatively rare, may require different management. The group agreed that some patients may require extension of ATT and the need for this should be assessed by the treating clinician, with particular regard to the patient's total ATT dosing.

The gastroenterologists in the group pointed out that some patients have lasting sequelae which may cause symptoms mimicking relapse of abdominal TB or failed treatment. It is important to differentiate these patients, who have peritoneal adhesions or luminal strictures from patients with active TB disease. Giving continued ATT in these patients is not required and could be harmful.

7.3 Duration of treatment in TB meningitis

Tuberculous meningitis (TBM) constitutes a medical emergency, and it is essential to start ATT as soon as it is suspected, in order to reduce rapidly progressing, life-threatening outcomes. In contrast to pulmonary TB, there is a lack of standardized international recommendations for treating TBM. This is partly due to the limited existing evidence regarding the optimal choice and dose of anti-TB drugs, as well as the most appropriate duration of treatment for this form of extrapulmonary TB.

Two main arguments have led to the perception that longer treatment (than for pulmonary TB) is needed for TBM to bring about microbiological cure and prevent relapse. The first one is that the blood-brain barrier hinders the penetration of anti-TB drugs to reach adequate drug concentration in the infected site. The second one concerns relapse rates. When assessing pulmonary TB regimens, relapse rates of 5% are generally considered acceptable (Donald, 2010). However, relapse of TBM is fearsome as it is a life-threatening condition and can lead to severe neurodisability. Thus, whether any risk of relapse is tolerable for TBM is to be considered when establishing TBM regimens. However, longer anti-TB treatments reduce compliance and increase drug toxicity and costs (Van Loenhout-Rooyackers, 2001).

The standard first-line regimen for drug sensitive TBM, according to WHO guidelines, is a 2-month intensive phase with isoniazid, rifampicin, pyrazinamide and ethambutol or streptomycin followed by a 10-month continuation phase with isoniazid and rifampicin – 2 HRZE or S/10 HR (WHO, 2014). Several different regimens are used in current practice, with variations regarding doses, selection of the fourth drug and duration of treatment from 6 to more than 24 months. There are variations in practice regarding the number of drugs used in both the intensive and continuation phases. As an example, the South African regimen consists of a 6-month intensive course with four drugs (isoniazid, rifampicin, pyrazinamide and ethambutol) with no continuation phase. A study reviewing the duration of treatment for TBM by comparing case series of both adults and children showed similar completion and relapse rates for 6-month treatment regimens including at least isoniazid, rifampicin and pyrazinamide and longer treatment (van Loenhout-Rooyackers et al., 2001).

Given the potentially devastating outcomes of relapse on the one hand, and the disadvantages of long therapy on the other hand, we performed a systematic review of the literature in an attempt to establish the most appropriate duration of treatment for TBM.

Recommendation	TB meningitis should be treated with standard first-line ATT for at least 9 months.
Strength of recommendation	Conditional
Evidence	The review included six observational (cohort) studies, with two reporting a comparison between short (6 to 9 month regimens) and long (12 months or more) regimens. The studies were from a variety of settings: Turkey, Ecuador, Papua New Guinea, South Africa and two from Thailand. None reported the HIV status of the participants, who were a mix of adults and children.
	As the data were from a highly heterogeneous set of observational studies, a meta-analysis was not performed. The data were presented to the group in a table demonstrating the absolute numbers of relapsed cases, defaulters, all-cause deaths and deaths after 6 months' treatment across all studies. The evidence was graded as very low quality.

Committee's view on advantages of shorter treatment	• Patients are more likely to complete shorter regimens • Less exposure to adverse effects of ATT • Low numbers of relapses • Good cure rates
Committee's view on disadvantages of shorter treatment	• Longer ATT regimens are associated with poor compliance • Longer regimens expose patients to increased risk of adverse effects of ATT • Concern that shorter regimens may increase the risk of relapse, leading to death or disability
Explanatory notes	The group recognized that there is very low quality evidence for the use of 6 to 9 months versus 12 months or longer ATT in TB meningitis. There is considerable variation in existing guidelines, with the WHO currently recommending 12 months and the RNTCP recommending 9 months for adults and 12 months for children. There is also considerable variation in current clinical practice, with some clinicians present reporting that they are happy to treat for 9 months while others are treating for 12 or 18 months as a minimum. The neurologists in the group were particularly concerned about this question, highlighting that this is an area of clinical equipoise. The paediatricians present were also concerned, as TBM disproportionately affects children and is an important cause of childhood mortality and disability.
	The key factors dictating mortality in TB meningitis may be early treatment and the use of corticosteroids, and the role of treatment duration remains unclear. Extension of ATT may sometimes be indicated, and this should be assessed by the treating clinician on a case-by-case basis. There was disagreement about the optimum duration of treatment, with some group members arguing that 12 months should be the minimum duration recommended; however, the final recommendation was the consensus view of the group. All group members recognized that there is a need for high-quality, large scale randomized trials to answer this question.

8 Research priorities

Relative to pulmonary TB, there is much less research into EPTB. There are several reasons for this, most notably that PTB is transmissible and accounts for four-fifths of all TB disease. However, EPTB remains an important public health problem in India and around the world, and is likely to remain so in the future, especially given the association with HIV co-infection and other forms of immunosuppression.

Several research gaps have been identified during the INDEX-TB guidelines process. Here, we summarize:

a. Some aspects of research priorities related to the specific areas of EBTP addressed by formal GRADE assessment and recommendations in these guidelines;

b. Topics raised during the scoping stage that have not been subject to formal evidence review in this iteration of the guidelines, but may be a priority in subsequent editions.

We also reflect on the type of evidence that would help to answer these questions.

8.1 Key questions from Index-TB 2015 recommendations

The duration of ATT in EPTB

Research into the optimum duration of treatment for all forms of EPTB is lacking. Randomized trials comparing 6-month and 9-month regimens have been carried out for lymph node TB and abdominal TB, but no randomized comparative studies have been conducted directly comparing regimens of different durations containing rifampicin, isoniazid and pyrazinamide (RHZ) for most forms of EPTB. In settings such as India where there are variations in practice, it might be possible to answer these questions using well-conducted prospective cohort studies rather than randomized controlled trials. Lifethreatening forms of EPTB, particularly TB meningitis, require particular attention. As the most important concern when determining the length of ATT is the risk of relapse of TB infection, future cohort studies need to recruit large numbers and have follow-up periods lasting several years to determine relapse rates.

Treatment end-points

A crucial area for further research, closely related to duration of treatment, is establishing clear treatment end-points in EPTB. Each TAC subcommittee identified a group of patients in every form of EPTB who have an equivocal response to treatment, and the clinicians in each group described the uncertainty on how to proceed with these patients—whether to continue ATT for longer or to observe. Newer diagnostic modalities such as PCR-based tests and positron emission tomography–computed tomography (PET-CT) are potentially useful in such cases, but further research is needed to establish their role.

Again, long-term follow-up data from cohort studies would help to address some of these questions. With the widespread use of mobile phones and increasing numbers of Indians having access to the Internet, new ways of keeping track of participants in large cohort studies need to be investigated.

The role of the Xpert MTB/RIF test in diagnosing EPTB

As Xpert MTB/RIF is rolled out across high TB burden countries, further diagnostic test accuracy studies in EPTB are required to better inform the use of this test. The data used to inform the recommendations made in this guideline are based on diagnostic test accuracy studies from a variety of settings using a variety of diagnostic samples and sample processing techniques.

Changes to the test, and the introduction of diagnostic sample processing standard operating procedures endorsed by WHO (WHO, 2014), mean that the accuracy of Xpert MTB/RIF is likely to improve. However, this may not be true for all specimen types and all settings. Future studies are needed to:

- provide estimates of sensitivity and specificity in moderate and high TB burden settings for the latest version of Xpert MTB/RIF;
- provide estimates of sensitivity and specificity in HIV-positive and HIV-negative people with EPTB;
- provide estimates of sensitivity and specificity in forms of EPTB where study data are currently lacking—bone and joint TB, TB pericarditis, urogenital TB, abdominal TB, ENT TB and ocular TB.

There is also an emerging research agenda on how use of Xpert MTB/RIF may improve patient outcomes. Operational and evaluation studies related to its deployment and use in general health services are needed.

The use of corticosteroids in EPTB

In people with TB pericarditis

The updated Cochrane review which informed the recommendation for steroids in TB pericarditis attempted to disaggregate all data by HIV status, because HIV-positive people may be more at risk of adverse events due to pre-existing immunosuppression. The guideline group agreed that rather than reduced mortality during the acute illness with pericardial effusion, the principal goal of giving steroids was to reduce progression to constrictive pericardial disease. Further studies powered to detect an effect of steroids on risk of developing constrictive pericardial disease due to TB pericarditis, with HIV-positive and negative participants, would be useful to inform future recommendations. The largest trial in the systematic review supporting the recommendations included another intervention. M. indicus pranii, an immunotherapy used in the treatment of leprosy, was tested alongside prednisolone in a 2x2 factorial design. In this trial, the number of people developing cancer was higher in the group receiving both prednisolone and M. indicus pranii. These findings are still being discussed with the authors of the review and the investigator of the trial as it seems uncertain whether this effect is attributable to prednisolone, M. indicus pranii, or a synergy between the two.

In people with pleural TB

The studies included in the Cochrane review informing the recommendation against the routine use of steroids in people with pleural TB looked at a variety of short-term outcomes (such as resolution of pleural effusion) as well as some proxy outcomes for lasting lung damage (pleural thickening, pleural adhesions). Future studies investigating the effects of steroids on long-term lung function and disability, as well as adverse events related to steroids and to HIV, are needed to inform future recommendations.

In people with TB meningitis

The Cochrane review update that informed the recommendation in this guideline concluded that there was high quality evidence of reduced mortality in HIV-negative TBM patients who received corticosteroids, and that there was low quality evidence of no effect on disability among survivors. Given this clear benefit in terms of reduced mortality, further placebo-controlled studies of corticosteroid use in TBM would not be ethical. However, further research would be beneficial to address the following:

- Effects of corticosteroids in HIV-positive people with TBM, with long-term follow up of survivors to identify HIV-related adverse events;
- Optimum choice of corticosteroid and dosing regimen. As some corticosteroid related adverse effects are dose-dependent, it would be helpful to know the optimum regimen for effectiveness and reduced adverse events.

8.2 Key questions identified during INDEX-TB scoping

Several topics were identified during the scoping phase for this guideline that we did not have the time to address with formal evidence review. These include the following:

- Empirical treatment of EPTB
- Tuberculin skin testing in EPTB
- PCR-based diagnostics for EPTB
- Radiological imaging for diagnosis in EPTB (including USS, CT, MR and PET)
- Interventions to improve diagnosis in children with suspected EPTB

- Duration of treatment in EPTB (TBM, abdominal TB and LNTB in progress)
- Diagnostic algorithms in EPTB – impact on patient-important outcomes
- Diagnosis of EPTB in people living with HIV, including EPTB immune reconstitution
- Diagnosis and management of drugresistant EPTB
- Interventions to improve adherence to treatment in EPTB
- Diagnosis and management of paradoxical reactions in EPTB
- Treatment end-points in EPTB
- Radiological imaging for assessing treatment success in EPTB
- Markers of treatment failure in EPTB
- Surgical management in EPBT (particularly in bone and joint, pericardial and urogenital TB)
- Treatment of EBPT in people with chronic kidney and liver disease
- Operational interventions to improve pharmacovigilance and promote safe prescribing in EPTB.

The TAC subcommittees also identified research topics that were specific to particular forms of EPTB.

Several of these topics could be addressed through collaborative efforts between the RNTCP, the medical colleges and specialist centres and international partners such as the Union and the WHO. The RNTCP is well placed to initiate collaborative projects across India to further this research agenda in a coordinated fashion. The guideline group recognized that enhanced operational data collection through the RNTCP could provide evidence to assist with some of these questions, and establishing large-scale cohort studies in collaboration with providers across India could prove fruitful, but would require significant systems strengthening and planning to be successful. One important factor in addressing the burden of EPTB in India is establishing reliable baseline data collection for all forms of EPTB, so that priorities can be set in accordance with accurate prevalence data.

Working case and outcome definitions in EPTB

Throughout the guidelines process, all members of the guidelines group noted the difficulties arising from a lack of standardized case definitions and outcome definitions in EPTB (see Section 4). This is a challenging task, given the difficulties with diagnosis and determining treatment end-points in each form of EPTB; however, inconsistencies in definitions compound the problems in carrying out research and interpreting research findings, reporting cases to the national programme and treating patients. In Section 4 of this document, generic case and outcome definitions for EPTB were laid out in order to standardize the language in the guidelines.

Further evidence review and consultation work is required internationally to establish definitions that clinicians, researchers, policy makers and patients can recognize and use.

An evaluation of the experiences of the working definitions with clinicians is anticipated in 2017.

Beardsley J, Wolbers M, Kibengo FM, Ggayi AM, Kamali A, Cuc NTK, et al. for the CryptoDex Investigators (2016). Adjunctive Dexamethasone in HIV-Associated Cryptococcal Meningitis. N Engl J Med. 374:542–54.

Bell LCK, Breen R, Miller RF, Noursadeghi M, Lipman M (2015). Paradoxical reactions and immune reconstitution inflammatory syndrome in tuberculosis. Intl J Infect Dis. 32:39 –45.

Blakemore R, Story E, Helb D, Kop J, Banada P, Owens MR, et al.(2010). Evaluation of the analytical performance of the Xpert MTB/RIF assay. J Clin Microbiol. 48(7):2495–501.

Cheng VC (2002). Clinical spectrum of paradoxical deterioration during antituberculosis therapy in non-HIV-infected patients. Eur J Clin Microbiol Infect Dis. 21(11):803–9.

Denkinger CM, Schumacher SG, Boehme CC, Dendukuri N, Pai M, Steingart KR, et al. (2014). Xpert MTB/RIF assay for the diagnosis of extrapulmonary tuberculosis: a systematic review and meta-analysis. Eur Respir J. 44(2):435–46.

Donald P (2010). The chemotherapy of tuberculous meningitis in children and adults. Tuberculosis (Edinburgh), 90(6):375–92.

Garg RK, Malhotra HS, Kumar N (2014). Paradoxical reaction in HIV-negative tuberculous meningitis. J Neurol Sci. 340 (1–2):26–36.

Guyatt Gordon H, O. A.-Y. (2008). Going from evidence to recommendations. British Medical Journal, 336, 1049. http://www.gradeworkinggroup.org/publications/. Retrieved July 2015

Higgins JPT, Altman DG, Sternen JAC (2011). Chapter 8: Assessing risk of bias in included studies. In: Higgins JPT, Green S, editors. Cochrane Handbook for Systematic Reviews of Interventions Version 5.1.0. The Cochrane Collaboration.

Light R (2010). Update on tuberculous pleural effusion. Respirology. 15(3):451–8.

MRC. (1948). Medical Research Council Report. Streptomycin treatment of tuberculous meningitis. Lancet. 1:582–96.

Prasad K, Singh MB, Ryan H. (2016). Corticosteroids for managing tuberculous meningitis. Cochrane Database of Systematic Reviews 2016, Issue 4. Art. No.: CD002244. DOI: 10.1002/14651858.CD002244.pub4.

Rossi GA, Balbi B, Manca F (1987). Tuberculous pleural effusions. Evidence for selective presence of PPD-specific T-lymphocytes at site of inflammation in the early phase of the infection. American Review of Respiratory Disease. 136(3):575–9.

Sharma SK, Mohan A (2004). Extrapulmonary tuberculosis. Ind J Med Res. 120(4):316–53.

Shu CC, Wang JT, Wang JY, Lee L, Yu C (2011). In-hospital outcome of patients with cultureconfirmed tuberculous pleurisy: clinical impact of pulmonary involvement . BMC Infectious Diseases. 11:46.

Sreenivas A, Rade K, Sachdeva KS, Ghedia M, Parmar M, Ramachandran R, et al. (2014). Standards for TB Care in India. New Delhi: World Health Organization Country Office for India.

Steingart KR, Schiller I, Horne DJ, Pai M, Boehme CC, Dendukuri N (2014). Xpert® MTB/RIF assay for pulmonary tuberculosis and rifampicin resistance in adults. Cochrane Database Systematic Rev. (1):CD009593. doi: 10.1002/14651858.CD009593.pub3.

TB CARE I (2014). International Standards for Tuberculosis Care, third edition. The Hague: TB CARE I.

The Task Force for the Diagnosis and Management of Pericardial Diseases of the European Society of Cardiology (ESC) (2015). 2015 ESC Guidelines for the diagnosis and management of pericardial diseases. European Heart Journal. 36:2921–64.

Thwaites GE, Nguyen Duc Bang ND, Nguyen Huy Dung NH, Hoang Thi Quy HT, Do Thi Tuong Oanh DTT, Nguyen Thi Cam Thoa NTC, et al. (2004). Dexamethasone for the treatment of tuberculous meningitis in adolescents and adults. N Engl J Med. 351(17):1741–51.

Van Loenhout-Rooyackers JH, Keyser A, Laheij RJ, Verbeek AL, van der Meer JW (2001). Tuberculous meningitis: is a 6-month treatment regimen sufficient? Int J Tuberc Lung Dis. 5(11):1028–35.

WHO (2010). Treatment of Tuberculosis: Guidelines, fourth edition. Geneva: World Health Organization.

WHO (2014). Guidance for national tuberculosis programmes on the management of tuberculosis in children, second edition. Geneva: World Health Organization.

WHO (2014). WHO Handbook for Guideline Development, second edition. Geneva: World Health Organization.

Wiysonge, C. N. (2016). Corticosteroids and other interventions for treating tuberculous pericarditis. Cochrane Database of Systematic Reviews , publication pending

Part 2
Clinical practice points

9 Ocular TB

Ocular infection with M. tuberculosis is uncommon, but the difficulty of diagnosing it means that prevalence estimates may not be reliable. Incidence of TB as a cause among patients presenting with uveitis has been reported at 10.1% in north India (Singh, 2004), but much lower in south India at 0.6% (Biswas, 1996-1997). This discrepancy may be due to several factors, including access to ophthalmology services, evolution of diagnostic criteria, description of new diagnostic entities and improvement in diagnostic tools.

Ocular TB can cause moderate to severe visual impairment in up to 40% of affected eyes (Basu, 2014). Delay in diagnosis and treatment can result in chronic inflammation and loss of vision. Improving access to a diagnosis is therefore a high priority.

9.1 Patients who should be referred for assessment by an ophthalmologist

Patients with symptoms consistent with anterior, intermediate, posterior or pan-uveitis, including the following:
- Red eye
- Blurred vision
- Photophobia
- Irregular pupil
- Eye pain
- Floaters
- Flashing lights (photopsia).

9.2 Patients who should be investigated for ocular TB

Presumptive ocular TB	A patient with one of the following clinical presentations: • Granulomatous anterior uveitis • Non-granulomatous anterior uveitis, not associated with any other known clinical entity, e.g. HLA-B27 • Intermediate uveitis, with/without healed/active focal lesions • Posterior uveitis, including subretinal abscess, choroidal/disc granuloma, multifocal choroiditis, retinal periphlebitis and multifocal serpiginous choroiditis • Panuveitis • Rarely, scleritis (anterior and posterior), interstitial and disciform keratitis *Note:* Extraocular TB disease is often absent in ocular TB patients, and patients do not usually have systemic symptoms of fever and weight loss.

9.3 Diagnosis

Test	Patients	Comments
X-ray of chest	All	All patients presenting with symptoms consistent with TB should have a chest X-ray. CT of the chest may also be useful as this test is more sensitive for evidence of current or previous pulmonary TB infection. Evaluation by a TB specialist or general physician as well as the ophthalmology team is advised.

Test	Patients	Comments
HIV test	All	EPTB is associated with HIV infection. All patients should be offered integrated counselling and testing.
Ocular imaging	All	Depending on the presentation, imaging is required to assess extent or complications of disease, and to monitor response to treatment. Fundus photography, fluorescein angiography, optical coherence tomography, or multimodal imaging may be required.
Tuberculin skin testing (Mantoux test)	All	Although usually not recommended in active TB disease, tuberculin skin testing (TST) may be useful in establishing supporting evidence of TB infection. While a positive result may support the diagnosis of TB, a negative test cannot rule out TB. Clinical evaluation by a TB specialist or general physician as well as the ophthalmology team is advised.
PCR testing of vitreous or aqueous specimens	Selected	Various PCR-based tests exist for TB, but evidence of diagnostic test accuracy for the diagnosis of ocular TB is highly variable. Whilst the accuracy of these tests seems to vary significantly, they are often the only specific test that may identify ocular TB. Further evidence is needed to determine which tests are the most accurate, and when they are best used. Vitreous/aqueous humour sampling must only be carried out by a trained practitioner.
Biopsy	Highly selected	Biopsy of the structures of the eye is highly invasive and carries the risk of exacerbating visual loss. However, in rare cases such as scleral or iris granuloma, it may be the only way to make a diagnosis and ensure effective treatment. Specimens should be sent for histopathology with staining for acid-fast bacilli (AFB) and culture.

9.4 Diagnostic categories

Possible ocular TB: Patients with the following (1, 2 and 3 together or 1 and 4) are diagnosed as having possible ocular TB:

1. At least one clinical sign suggestive of ocular TB (see Presumptive ocular TB), and other aetiology excluded
2. X-ray/CT chest not consistent with TB infection and no clinical evidence of extraocular TB
3. At least one of the following:
   - Documented exposure to TB
   - Immunological evidence of TB infection
4. Molecular evidence of Mtb infection.

Clinically diagnosed ocular TB: Patients with all the following (1, 2 and 3 together) are diagnosed as having probable ocular TB:

1. At least one clinical sign suggestive of ocular TB (see presumptive ocular TB), and other aetiologies excluded
2. Evidence of chest X-ray consistent with TB infection or clinical evidence of extraocular TB or microbiological confirmation from sputum or extraocular sites
3. Documented exposure to TB and/or immunological evidence of TB infection.

Bacteriologically confirmed ocular TB: A patient with at least one clinical sign of ocular TB, along with microbiological (smear/culture) or histopathological confirmation of Mtb from ocular fluids/tissues.

9.5 Treatment

Treatment of ocular TB

All patients with possible ocular TB, clinically diagnosed ocular TB or bacteriologically confirmed ocular TB need treatment with ATT with or without other adjuvant therapy.

Aims

1. Protect visual function
2. Control ocular inflammation
3. Prevent recurrence of inflammation.

First line treatment for adults and children with ocular TB	**Drugs**	RHZE/4RHE Corticosteroids (local or systemic) and other immunosuppressants are often used as adjunctive treatments. There is insufficient evidence currently to make specific recommendations regarding their use.
	Duration	Total treatment duration: 6 to 9 months
	Referral	All patients with presumptive ocular TB must be referred to an ophthalmologist for assessment and treatment.
	Follow up	Regular review during and after treatment. Suggested methods for monitoring treatment: • Clinical evaluation (slit-lamp biomicroscopy and indirect ophthalmoscopy) • Fundus photography • Fundus autofluorescence • Optical coherence tomography
	Response to treatment	Treatment outcomes in ocular TB need to be defined differently, as microbiological confirmation of TB is rarely possible in ocular tissues. Thus, treatment success or failure is primarily guided by the level of inflammation seen inside the eye. • *Remission*: Inactive disease for at least 3 months after discontinuing all therapy based on the Standardization of Uveitis Nomenclature recommendations (Jabs, 2005). • *Treatment failure*: No decrease in inflammation, or less than a two-step decrease in level of inflammation after 3 months of ATT (inflammatory scores of fundus lesions such as retinal perivasculitis or multifocal serpiginous choroiditis are not yet defined and are left to the judgment of treating physicians). • *Relapse*: An increase in the level of inflammation after complete remission (at least two-step increase).
	Approach to treatment failure	1. Rule out non-TB aetiology: detailed ocular and systemic evaluation, ancillary tests 2. Rule out paradoxical reaction: usually occurs within 2 months of starting ATT; responds to continuation or escalation of corticosteroid therapy 3. Rule out drug resistance: once previous two points have been ruled out, check contact with MDR TB patient; if facilities exist, consider ocular fluid sampling for molecular diagnosis of drug resistance
	Surgery	The main indications for surgery in ocular TB are as follows: • Complications of retinal vasculitis—retinal neovascularization, vitreous haemorrhage, tractional or combined retinal detachment, epiretinal membrane • Diagnostic vitrectomy when conventional methods fail to establish diagnosis • Non-resolving vitreous inflammation • Visually significant vitreous floaters after completion of medical therapy • Management of complications of uveitis such as cataract and glaucoma

10 Central nervous system TB

10.1 Background

TB can cause meningitis (TBM), cerebral and spinal tuberculoma, myelitis and arachnoiditis. These are all severe forms of TB associated with high incidence of death or disability.

Exact prevalence of CNS TB in India is not known, but it accounts for an estimated 1% of all cases of TB, which equates to around 17 000 cases in India in 2014 (WHO, 2015). Case fatality rates for the most common form of CNS TB, i.e. TB meningitis, are high. All forms of CNS TB can leave survivors with long-term disabilities.

10.2 Patients who should be investigated for TBM

TBM is a medical emergency. Early diagnosis and prompt treatment with ATT saves lives.

TBM classically presents as subacute or chronic meningitis with symptoms developing over days or weeks. Evidence suggests that patients presenting with less than 5 days of symptoms are more likely to have bacterial or viral meningitis than TBM (Thwaites, 2009). However, it should be noted that TBM can present acutely with a short duration of illness, and this acute presentation is not uncommon.

Presumptive TBM	Any patient with clinical features of meningitis in the form of fever, headache, neck rigidity and vomiting, with or without altered sensorium and associated focal neurological deficits for a period of 5 days or more

Common symptoms	Less frequent symptoms	Uncommon symptoms
Headache	Confusion	Photophobia
Fever	Cranial nerve palsy	Paraparesis
Vomiting	Hemiparesis	Seizures
Neck stiffness	Coma	
Weight loss		

10.3 Diagnosis

The most important aspect of TBM diagnosis is to suspect TBM and act quickly to refer the patient to a centre where they will receive:
- rapid access to CSF examination
- rapid access to neuroimaging
- prompt treatment with ATT and supportive care.

Diagnostic workup

Test	Patients	Comments
Lumbar puncture for CSF	All (unless absolutely contraindicated)	CSF findings typical of TBM: lymphocytic (more rarely neutrophilic) pleocytosis with low serum:CSF glucose ratio and high protein. Additional tests on CSF are summarized in the table below.
HIV testing	All	HIV infection predisposes people to CNS infections, including TBM. All patients should be offered integrated counselling and testing.
Chest X-ray	All	Chest X-ray may assist the diagnosis with evidence of current or previous pulmonary TB infection.
CT brain with contrast	All	High priority for comatose or deteriorating patients helps to diagnose hydrocephalus, which may require neurosurgical intervention.
MRI brain with contrast	Selected	Magnetic resonance imaging (MRI) provides more detailed information than CT. May be of assistance where diagnosis is uncertain, in complex cases, and in HIV-positive patients.

CSF sampling and testing

Lumbar puncture should be performed in every patient (unless there are contraindications to the procedure) and CSF should be analysed with the following tests given in the table below. Other tests may also be indicated in some circumstances.

At least 6 mL of CSF should be collected for adults, 2–3 mL for children.

Results available	Tests
Hours to days	• Cell count and differentiation • Protein • CSF:serum glucose ratio (serum samples need to be taken alongside the CSF) • Gram stain for bacterial meningitis (e.g. N. meningitidis, S. pneumonia) • AFB stain for TB • India ink and cryptococcal antigen testing for cryptococcal meningitis • Xpert MTB/RIF can be used as an adjunctive test in the diagnosis of TBM, but a negative test does not rule out a diagnosis of TBM. If it is safe to obtain, 1 mL of CSF is optimal for this test (Nhu, 2014). • Other PCR-based tests for Mtb are available, but diagnostic accuracy is highly variable. • PCR-based tests for viral pathogens, as appropriate
Days	• Bacterial culture, speciation and drug susceptibility testing • Cytological examination for malignant cells
Days to weeks	• Fungal culture, speciation and drug susceptibility testing • Mycobacterial culture, speciation and drug susceptibility testing

Recommendation
Xpert may be used as an adjunctive test for TBM. A negative Xpert result does not rule out TBM. The decision to give ATT should be based on clinical features and CSF profile.
(Conditional recommendation, high quality evidence for specificity estimate, low quality evidence for sensitivity estimate).

Other tests

Interferon-gamma release assays such as ELISPOT and Quantiferon Gold are designed for the diagnosis of latent TB, and are not indicated in the diagnosis of TBM. Currently, the use of these tests is restricted in India.

Adenosine deaminase (ADA) is not useful in the diagnosis of TBM.

MRC staging

The British Medical Research Council (MRC) staging is a widely recognized system for classifying disease severity in TBM (MRC, 1948).

Stage I   Mild cases, for those without altered consciousness or focal neurological signs

Stage II   Moderate cases, for those with altered consciousness who are not comatose and those with moderate neurological signs, e.g. single cranial nerve palsies, paraparesis, and hemiparesis

Stage III   Severe cases, for comatose patients and those with multiple cranial nerve palsies, hemiplegia or paraplegia, or both.

10.4 Treatment

Aims

- Microbiological cure
- Prevention of complications, morbidity and mortality
- Management of treatment complications

First line treatment for adults and children with TB meningitis	Drugs	Intensive phase: 2 months RHZE
		The was the recommendation made by the INDEX-TB Guidelines Panel at the INDEX-TB meeting in 2015, based on the evidence summarized in Annex 2 in the online supplementary materials, as follows:
		Continuation phase: at least 7 months RHE
		The Technical Advisory Sub-committee for CNS TB, who drafted these clinical practice points, expressed a preference for an alternative approach to the continuation phase that differs from the INDEX TB recommendation in two ways: a) recommend the use of pyrazinamide instead of ethambutol; and b) treatment to be continued in all patients for a total of at least 12 months.
		The current RNTCP guidance is to use ethambutol in the continuation phase because of the risk of isoniazid mono-resistance. The variations in expert opinion reflect the uncertainty regarding the optimum choice of regimen, and further research is required.
		If vision is impaired or cannot be assessed, use streptomycin instead of ethambutol in the intensive phase. Use of streptomycin in pregnant women, and patients with kidney impairment or hearing loss should be avoided.
	Duration	Recommendation:
		TB meningitis should be treated with standard first-line ATT for at least 9 months (conditional recommendation, very low quality evidence)
		Note: see Drugs section above.
	Referral	ATT should be started as early as possible in all cases of TBM.
		Presumptive TBM patients should be referred to a secondary/tertiary care centre immediately.
		If referral and transfer is likely to take more than 24 h, or if the patient is critically ill, treatment with ATT may be started prior to transfer. Where possible, CSF sampling prior to initiation of treatment is preferred, as ATT reduces the accuracy of the diagnostic tests for TB, but this should not unduly delay initiation of ATT.
	Follow up	Patients should be assessed for clinical response at the end of the treatment period and at intervals for 2 years. Sustained resolution of clinical features including headache and fever should guide stopping of ATT. Residual neurological deficits may be permanent and should not be used to assess for active TB infection.

Drug-resistant cases		Drug-resistant TBM should be suspected in patients with poor response to standard ATT and history of exposure to MDR-TB.
Steroids	HIV-negative patients	Recommendation: Steroids are recommended for TB meningitis in HIV-negative people. Duration of steroid treatment should be for at least 4 weeks, with tapering as appropriate (strong recommendation, high quality evidence)
	HIV-positive patients	Recommendation: Steroids may be used for TB meningitis in HIV-positive people, where other life-threatening opportunistic infections are absent (conditional recommendation, low quality evidence) Important opportunistic infections to consider include cryptococcal meningitis and cerebral toxoplasmosis. There is evidence that steroids are associated with increased adverse events and disability in patients with HIV-associated cryptococcal meningitis (Beardsley J, 2016).
	Suggested regimen	In hospital: intravenous dexamethasone 0.4 mg/kg/24 h in 3–4 divided doses may be preferred with a slow switch to oral therapy and taper. Currently, there is insufficient evidence to recommend one formulation/regimen of steroids over any other.
Surgery		Patients who develop hydrocephalus with raised intracranial pressure may require CSF diversion by ventriculo-peritoneal shunt insertion. Such patients should be managed in settings with neurosurgical services.

10.5 Complications

Complication	Clinical features	Management
Hydrocephalus	Symptoms and signs of raised intracranial pressure (ICP) such as worsening headache, vomiting, ocular palsies, decreasing conscious level, papilloedema Urgent neuroimaging is needed to assess cause of raised ICP if patient is deteriorating	Ventriculo-peritoneal shunt insertion is indicated for patients at all stages of severity with hydrocephalus or raised ICP not responding to ATT and steroids. Early shunt insertion may be beneficial. Treatment with diuretics such as mannitol should be limited to emergency management, aimed at decreasing ICP until shunt insertion can be performed. External ventricular drainage is not usually recommended, unless surgery is contraindicated or urgent CSF diversion is indicated to buy time before a shunt can be inserted.
Stroke	Focal neurological deficit consistent with a stroke syndrome. Stroke in TBM may not be clinically apparent and may be diagnosed on neuroimaging. Stroke is a significant contributor to disability following TBM.	Most effective treatment strategy is uncertain and evidence is lacking. Acute stroke or evidence of on-going vasculopathy may warrant continuation of steroids, usually intravenously. There is some evidence that aspirin may prevent stroke in TBM in adults. Further trials in adults and children are on-going.
Optico-chiasmatic arachnoiditis	Visual loss, which may arise during treatment with ATT, or on the withdrawal of corticosteroids Characteristic CT and MRI findings	Most effective treatment strategy uncertain Steroid therapy is the first-line treatment, using intravenous dexamethasone. Pulsed methylprednisolone or oral thalidomide has been used in some case series for patients not responding to steroids. Microsurgical intervention and intrathecal hyaluronidase are controversial and not currently recommended.

Complication	Clinical features	Management
Seizures	Generalized seizures secondary to encephalopathy Tuberculoma or infarction may cause secondary generalized seizure	Acute management with anti-epileptic drugs as per local protocol for seizure The use of anti-epileptic drugs alongside ATT must be carefully managed due to the potential for drug interactions and increased risk of liver dysfunction with multiple hepatotoxic agents. Prophylactic anti-epileptic drugs are not required in TBM patients who have not had seizures during their clinical course. Continued treatment with anti-epileptic drugs may be necessary in patients with recurrent seizure and decisions about duration and withdrawal should be individualized to the patient by the treating specialist.

10.6 CNS tuberculoma

Tuberculoma of the central nervous system (CNS) is less common than TBM and has lower morbidity and mortality, but remains an important cause of intracranial space-occupying lesions. Tuberculoma can arise anywhere in the brain or spinal cord, and may present as a mass lesion causing focal neurological deficits depending on anatomical location and/or seizure, or may be found in concurrence with TBM.

Presumptive CNS tuberculoma	Any patient presenting with seizures, headache, fever or focal neurological deficits with neuroimaging features consistent with a mass lesion of inflammatory nature.

Patients with presumptive CNS tuberculoma should be referred for investigation and treatment by a specialist. Neuroimaging, particularly multimodal MRI, with interpretation by a specialist is indicated to characterize the lesion(s).

Diagnosis

Diagnosis is based on the following:
- Patient history – previous TB disease and contact with a pulmonary TB patient make tuberculoma more likely.
- Clinical findings – active TB elsewhere in the body makes tuberculoma more likely. Chest X-ray should be performed. Other imaging such as CT chest should be considered to look for TB, identify other lesions amenable to biopsy, and look for features suggestive of other pathology such as malignancy.
- HIV status – HIV testing is important as HIV-positive people are at increased risk, not only of tuberculoma, but also other diagnoses such as coccidiomycosis and toxoplasmosis. Other causes of immunosuppression are also important.
- MRI/CT scan findings consistent with tuberculoma
- CSF findings – CSF can be normal, or show features similar to TBM. The sensitivity of culture for Mtb is low, and PCR-based tests require further investigation in tuberculoma.

Stereotactic or open biopsy is rarely performed as this is a highly invasive procedure, but it may be indicated in patients where the diagnosis remains very uncertain after non-invasive tests, or there is no response to ATT.

The differential diagnosis for tuberculoma includes, but is not limited to:
- neurocysticercosis
- pyogenic abscess
- metastatic lesions from a primary malignancy elsewhere in the body, e.g. lung cancer
- glioma
- demyelinating lesion.

Treatment

The aims of treatment are:
- Resolution of neurological and constitutional symptoms
- Resolution of the lesion on neuroimaging.

There is a lack of evidence as to the optimum duration of treatment in CNS tuberculoma. The expert group suggested that ATT should be given for 9 to 12 months initially, with repeat neuroimaging at 3 months and 9–12 months to monitor response to treatment. Treatment should then be tailored to the clinical and radiological response of the patient.

Paradoxical reaction with increase in the size and number of lesions can occur, usually in the first 3 months of treatment, and requires treatment with steroids as well as continued ATT.

Treatment failure should be suspected when lesions either increase in size or fail to reduce in size after 3 to 6 months ATT despite appropriate dosing and good adherence. The treating clinician needs to weigh the benefits and risks of biopsy against those of commencing second-line treatment empirically for suspected MDR-TB, or persisting with first-line treatment for suspected paradoxical reaction. If a biopsy is performed due to strong consideration of an alternative diagnosis, the specimens should be sent for: a) histopathology with staining for AFB; b) Mtb culture and drug susceptibility testing; c) other microbiological tests as indicated by the case history.

Ear, nose and throat TB

Head and neck TB constitutes 10–15% of all EPTB cases, with the majority of these cases being cervical lymph node TB, and <1% extra-nodal head and neck TB cases. Malignancy is the most important differential diagnosis in ear, nose and throat (ENT) TB and diagnostic approaches must take this into account.

11.1 Presentation

Laryngeal TB

Presents with hoarse voice and pain on swallowing, mimicking non-specific laryngitis or laryngeal carcinoma. Can be infectious, unlike other forms of EPTB.

Ear TB

Usually presents with chronic suppurative otitis media – painless discharging ear not responding to antibiotics, with hearing loss disproportionate to the clinical appearance. Can be complicated by facial paralysis, promontorial fistulae and inner ear involvement, which may also occur in TB meningitis.

Oral TB

Multiple presentations as TB can affect any part of the mouth. Lesions are usually ulcerative and painless, sometimes with a necrotic base and discharge.

Oropharyngeal TB

TB of the tonsils presents with asymmetrical enlargement with ulceration, mimicking carcinoma. TB of the cervical spine can extend to cause retropharyngeal abscess presenting with pain on swallowing, and complicated by airway compromise which requires emergency intervention.

Sinonasal TB

Very rare, usually presents with nasal obstruction, bleeding and runny nose and lymphadenopathy

Salivary gland TB

Very rare; usually associated with immunosuppression. Presents with swelling

Thyroid gland TB

Very rare; multiple presentations from isolated nodules to thyrotoxicosis.

11.2 Diagnosis

Test	Patients	Comments
X-ray of chest	All	All patients presenting with symptoms consistent with TB should have a chest X-ray.
HIV test	All	EPTB is associated with HIV infection. All patients should be offered integrated counselling and testing.

Test	Patients	Comments
Incisional or punch biopsy from the affected site	All	Incisional or punch biopsy from the affected site, carried out by a trained specialist practitioner is the preferred method of diagnostic sampling for ENT lesions, and should be sent for: • histopathology • staining for acid-fast bacilli (fluorochrome or ZN staining) • culture for *Mtb*
Fine needle aspiration cytology (FNAC)	Selected	FNAC may also be used, particularly where there is lymph node involvement or an abscess, with aspirate sent for: • microscopy for AFB • Xpert MTB/RIF • cytology • culture for *Mtb*
CT or MR imaging of the head and neck	Selected	May be required to further characterize the disease, look for involvement of bone/deep structures, and aid in diagnosis. This should be requested and interpreted by a specialist.

11.3 Treatment

First line treatment for adults and children with ENT TB	Drugs	2RHZE/4–7RHE Steroids have no role in the treatment of ENT TB, and should be avoided as they may do harm.
	Duration	Total treatment duration: 6 to 9 months All cases involving bone, including all TB otitis media cases, should receive 9 months treatment.
	Referral	All patients with ENT TB, except those who have accessible cervical lymph nodes which are amenable to FNAC, will need referral to ENT specialists for diagnosis.
	Follow up	Monthly follow-up for patients with sinonasal and ear/temporal bone TB is suggested during treatment to assess response and monitor adherence, and after treatment to assess resolution and detect recurrence.
	Surgery	May be indicated in some circumstances to treat complications or for reconstruction of the ear or nose. Where facial nerve palsy complicates tuberculous otitis media, surgical decompression should be considered if there is no improvement after 3 to 4 weeks of ATT (good practice statement). Surgical drainage of retropharyngeal abscess complicating TB of the cervical spine may be considered, but requires specialist judgement. Surgery should be avoided in TB of the salivary glands or thyroid; medical treatment is usually sufficient.

There is little evidence to guide recommendations about the duration of treatment in ENT TB, and so this outline is based on the consensus of the ENT expert group.

11.4 Sequelae

Sequelae are related to tissue destruction. Serious complications result from resorption of facial bone. Airway compromise resulting from ankylosis is a lifethreatening complication, which requires emergency surgical treatment.

TB of the ear can lead to permanent hearing loss, facial nerve palsy and balance problems (vestibulopathy). It can be complicated by infection of the underlying bone and meningitis from spread into the central nervous system.

Sinonasal TB can lead to deformity of the nose, and can be complicated by involvement of the eye socket.

12 Lymph node TB

Lymph node TB (LNTB, also called TB lymphadenitis) refers to Mtb infection of the lymph nodes, and may occur as the sole manifestation of TB infection, or alongside pulmonary or miliary TB. LNTB is the most common form of EPTB in India, accounting for around 35% of EPTB cases (Sharma S.K., 2004). Total estimated incidence of LNTB was 30.8 per 100 000 population in India in 2013 (RNTCP, 2014).

Care should be taken to identify patients who need to be investigated for LNTB, as there are multiple differential diagnoses for chronic lymphadenopathy.

TB of the deep lymph nodes in the chest (mediastinal TB) may present with cough or shortness of breath. Abdominal LNTB patients may have abdominal pain or distension.

12.1 Patients who should be investigated for LNTB

Presumptive peripheral LNTB	Patients with enlarged lymph nodes (over 1 cm across) in the neck, armpit or groin. Patients may also present with symptoms of fever, weight loss, night sweats and cough
Presumptive mediastinal LNTB	Patients with cough, fever, shortness of breath, weight loss or night sweats who have hilar widening on chest X-ray and/or mediastinal lymphadenopathy on chest CT in the absence of evidence of active pulmonary TB
Presumptive abdominal LNTB	Patients with dull or colicky abdominal pain, abdominal distension, weight loss, night sweats or fever, and evidence of abdominal lymphadenopathy on abdominal ultrasound scan, CT or MR

12.2 Diagnosis

Test	Patients	Comments
X-ray of chest	All	All patients presenting with symptoms consistent with LNTB, to seek for active or previous pulmonary TB
HIV test	All	EPTB is associated with HIV infection. All patients should be offered integrated counselling and testing.
Ultrasound or CT scans of chest and abdomen	Selected	Indicated when diagnosis is not clear, and in HIV-positive people Finding abdominal lymphadenopathy should prompt biopsy to rule out lymphoma as a differential diagnosis.
Fine needle aspiration cytology (FNAC)	All	Send specimen for: a) Xpert MTB/RIF test; b) microscopy and culture for Mtb with drug susceptibility testing; c) Cytology
Excision biopsy	Selected	IF FNAC has been inconclusive, or where malignancy is suspected. Send specimen for: a) Xpert MTB/RIF test; b) microscopy and culture for Mtb with drug susceptibility testing; c) histopathology
Specimens should be taken from the affected lymph nodes prior to commencing ATT.		
A non-dependent aspiration with Z-technique for manipulating overlying skin by an appropriately trained operator is suggested for superficial lymph nodes. Deep lymph nodes require radiologically-guided sampling. In abdominal LNTB, ultrasound/CT-guided percutaneous FNAC or biopsy is required. In mediastinal LNTB, endobronchial ultrasoundguided FNAC is preferred where facilities exist.		

Recommendation:

Xpert MTB/RIF may be used as additional test to cytology for LNTB (strong recommendation, high quality evidence for specificity, low quality evidence for sensitivity).

Diagnostic definitions

Bacteriologically Confirmed LNTB case	A patient with symptoms and signs of LNTB and has at least one of the following: • positive microscopy for AFB on examination of lymph node fluid or tissue • positive culture of Mtb from lymph node fluid or tissue • positive validated PCR-based test (such as Xpert MTB/RIF)
Clinically diagnosed LNTB case	A presumptive LNTB patient who undergoes diagnostic testing and has all of: • negative microscopy, negative culture and negative PCR-based tests • no other diagnosis made to explain signs and symptoms • strongly suggestive evidence on other tests, such as radiological findings, histopathological findings, clinical course

12.3 Treatment

First line treatment for adults and children with LNTB	Drugs	2RHZE/4RHE
	Duration	Recommendation Six months ATT standard first-line regimen is recommended for peripheral lymph node TB (strong recommendation, low quality evidence).
	Referral	Generally, LNTB patients can be managed at primary care level. Referral to secondary care for specialist diagnostic sampling may be required.
	Follow up	Assess response to treatment at 4 months. Consider possible treatment failure in patients who have worsened or deteriorated after initial improvement – this requires diagnostic investigation and possibly a change of treatment. Deterioration in the first 3 months may be due to paradoxical reaction – this does not require repeat diagnostic tests or change of treatment. Some patients with LNTB have residual lymphadenopathy at the end of treatment. This is not usually due to continued active TB infection where the largest node is less than 1 cm in size. Some patients have residual nodes more than 1 cm in size, and these patients are classified as partial responders. There is uncertainty about whether continued ATT in these patients is beneficial. The expert group suggested these patients should receive an additional 3 months of RHE, followed by a biopsy sent for histology and TB culture in patients who fail to respond to that. While some evidence suggests that these patients may not require further ATT, the data is insufficient at this stage. For mediastinal TB, progress on ATT can be monitored with chest X-ray, but CT scan may be indicated if lymph nodes do not reduce in size after 4 months. In patients who fail to improve on ATT, the alternative diagnoses of lung cancer, lymphoma, sarcoidosis and fungal infection should be considered. Current expert opinion on when to stop ATT in patients with persistently enlarged mediastinal lymph nodes is to stop when there is documentation of absence of interval change in CT/MRI of mediastinal lymph nodes for more than 4 months, with resolution of all other signs and symptoms.

13 Pleural TB

The second most common form of EPTB, pleural TB is a common cause of pleural effusion in India. Pleural TB usually presents with pleural effusion caused by the immune system's response to the presence of mycobacterial antigens in the pleural space, generating inflammation and causing fluid to accumulate. The effusion will usually resolve spontaneously even without ATT, but patients who are not treated are at risk of recurrent active TB infection.

13.1 Patients who should be investigated for Pleural TB

Presumptive pleural TB	A patient with cough, chest pain or shortness of breath, with or without fever and weight loss, with evidence of a pleural effusion on examination or CXR

13.2 Diagnosis

Test	Patients	Comments
X-ray of chest	All	To confirm presence of a pleural effusion and look for underlying pulmonary disease. Progress may be monitored using CXR.
HIV test	All	EPTB is associated with HIV infection. All patients should be offered integrated counselling and testing.
CT scans of chest and abdomen	Selected	Useful when diagnosis is not clear, particularly if malignancy is suspected; or in in HIV-positive patients who are at higher risk of disseminated TB More sensitive than CXR for identifying underlying pulmonary disease
Ultrasound of chest	Selected	Alternative to CXR to identify pleural effusion, and is more sensitive in picking up pleural effusion than CXR
Pleural aspiration/ thoracocentesis	All	Most patients do not require complete therapeutic drainage of their pleural effusion, unless it is causing respiratory compromise; in which case, specialist monitoring is required during and following drainage. All patients should have a diagnostic sample of pleural fluid taken.
Pleural aspiration/ thoracocentesis	All	Send specimen for: a) glucose, protein, ADA and lactate dehydrogenase (LDH) levels (send concurrent blood sample for serum protein and LDH); b) differential cell count; c) microscopy and culture for Mtb; and d) cytology Pleural TB usually causes an exudative effusion, defined on the basis of Light's criteria (pleural fluid/serum protein >0.5; pleural fluid/serum LDH >0.6; pleural fluid LDH > two-thirds the upper limit of serum LDH) (Light R.W., 1972) Test for adenosine deaminase activity (ADA) level performed on pleural fluid can help support a diagnosis of pleural TB (Greco, 2003) (Liang, 2008). It should be noted that other causes of pleural effusion such as empyema, rheumatoid serositis and lymphoma can occasionally also lead to elevated ADA (Porcel, 2010). > 70 U/L – highly likely to be pleural TB 40–70 U/L – indeterminate level, other risk factors need to be considered <40 U/L – low likelihood of pleural TB, investigate for other causes

Test	Patients	Comments
		Because the most common differential diagnosis in children is partially treated parapneumonic effusion, ADA may yield a higher proportion of false positives in this group. Further investigation is required as to the utility of ADA in the diagnosis of pleural TB in children.
Sputum samples	Selected	Send sputum for Xpert MTB/RIF, microscopy and culture as per pulmonary TB guidelines whenever concurrent pulmonary and pleural TB is suspected.
Pleural biopsy (closed or thorascopic)	Selected	Much higher yield than pleural fluid when subjected to microscopy and culture for Mtb; also, histopathological examination can be performed
		Thoracoscopically-obtained specimens have a higher diagnostic yield than closed pleural biopsy.
		Indicated where diagnosis is uncertain despite other tests, or where pleural malignancy is a significant differential diagnosis.

Recommendation:

Xpert MTB/RIF should not be used to diagnose pleural TB (strong recommendation, high quality evidence for specificity, low quality evidence for sensitivity).

13.3 Treatment

First line treatment for adults and children with pleural TB	Drugs	2RHZE/4RHE
		Recommendation: Corticosteroids are not routinely recommended in pleural TB (conditional recommendation, low quality evidence).
	Duration	Total duration of treatment: 6 months
	Referral	Uncomplicated cases do not require referral to specialist centres.
	Follow up	Most patients who respond to treatment will have improvement in their general condition by 2 weeks, and significant improvement in pleural effusion by 6–8 weeks. A follow up CXR at 8 weeks after starting ATT is useful to assess progress. Increasing size of effusion despite treatment may be due to paradoxical reaction, or an alternative diagnosis requiring further investigation.

14 TB of the heart

TB infection of the heart most commonly manifests as TB pericarditis. TB myocarditis is a recognized form of EPTB, but is very rare. In this summary, the main practice points for the diagnosis and management of TB pericarditis are covered.

While it has a low prevalence overall, TB pericarditis accounts for 60–80% of cases of acute pericarditis in high TB burden countries, and 75% of cases of constrictive pericarditis (Fowler, 1991). TB pericarditis has a high mortality if untreated in the acute phase of illness, and survivors can develop constrictive pericardial disease as the acute inflammation resolves, which can cause disability and death later on. ATT greatly reduces both death in the acute phase of illness and the development of constrictive pericardial disease.

14.1 Patients who should be investigated for TB pericarditis

Presumptive TB pericarditis	A patient with chest pain, shortness of breath, with or without fever and weight loss or haemodynamic abnormalities, who has evidence of pericardial effusion or constriction on chest X-ray (CXR) electrocardiogram (ECG) or echocardiogram

14.2 Diagnosis

Test	Patients	Comments
X-ray of chest	All	All patients presenting with symptoms consistent with TB should have a chest X-ray. Features suggestive of pericardial disease include hilar widening, and a globular or "water bottle" heart shadow, although the cardiac shadow may appear normal. Evidence of pulmonary TB or pleural effusions may be noted.
HIV test	All	EPTB is associated with HIV infection. All patients should be offered integrated counselling and testing.
ECG	All	May reveal evidence of pericardial effusion (low voltage trace, T wave flattering or inversion). Patients are at risk of atrial arrhythmia.
Echocardiogram (transthoracic)	All	Reveals or confirms pericardial effusion and/or constriction, and can detect signs of impending tamponade which requires urgent intervention.
CT of the chest	Selected	Useful for demonstrating pericardial thickening or calcification, or associated lung/mediastinal abnormalities. Not routinely required.
Cardiac MRI	Highly selected	Only required in patients where a diagnosis of restrictive cardiomyopathy is being considered as a significant differential diagnosis.

Cardiac tamponade

Cardiac tamponade occurs when fluid accumulating in the pericardial sac impedes ventricular filling, causing cardio-vascular compromise, which can progress to cardiac arrest. Pericardiocentesis is urgently required to relieve the pressure in the pericardial sac and allow normal ventricular filling.

Pericardiocentesis

The European Society of Cardiology guidelines give recommendations about pericardiocentesis (The Task Force for the Diagnosis and Management of Pericardial Diseases of the European Society of Cardiology (ESC), 2015). If the patient does not have signs of cardiac tamponade, pericardiocentesis can be considered for diagnostic purposes, but should only be carried out by trained personnel using ultrasound guidance.

Microbiological tests

Microscopy and culture of pericardial fluid for Mtb have very low sensitivity, meaning that few cases have a microbiologically confirmed diagnosis. In patients with concurrent pulmonary disease, smear and culture of serial sputum samples may yield a diagnosis.

Very few studies have assessed the diagnostic accuracy of Xpert MTB/RIF in pericardial fluid, and so the INDEX-TB guidelines panel did not make a recommendation regarding the use of Xpert MTB/RIF on pericardial specimens.

If pericardial fluid is obtained, it should be sent for culture for Mtb, despite low sensitivity of this test. A differential cell count and raised ADA level may support the diagnosis.

14.3 Treatment

First line treatment for adults and children with TB pericarditis	Drugs	2RHZE/4RHE Recommendation: Corticosteroids are recommended for all patients with TB pericarditis who have pericardial effusion (conditional recommendation, low quality evidence for HIV-positive people, very low quality evidence for HIV-negative people).
	Duration	Total treatment duration: 6 months
	Referral	Patients who develop cardiovascular compromise require urgent management in a specialist setting. Patients who develop constrictive pericardial disease as a late complication may benefit from assessment by a cardiologist.
	Follow up	Assess response to treatment at 4 months. Consider possible treatment failure in patients who have worsened or deteriorated after initial improvement – this requires diagnostic investigation and possibly a change of treatment. Deterioration in the first 3 months may be due to paradoxical reaction; this does not require repeat diagnostic tests or change of treatment.
	Surgery	Pericardiocentesis is indicated as an urgent intervention in cardiac tamponade resulting from pericardial effusion. Pericardectomy is sometimes indicated in patients who develop constrictive pericardial disease as a late complication. Some of these patients will improve without surgery, but others may require pericardectomy too for progressive cardiac failure.

15 Abdominal TB

Abdominal TB refers to TB infection of any organ in the abdominal cavity, including the gut and peritoneum. Abdominal TB cases make up about 3% of all EPTB cases in India (Sharma S.K., 2004).

Abdominal TB causes a variety of presentations relating to the site of disease within the abdomen, stage of disease and complications. When treated with appropriate ATT, mortality is low, but some patients experience ongoing complications which can affect their long-term health, such as strictures in the bowel and adhesions. The most commonly affected sites in the abdomen are the GI tract distal to the duodenum (the ileum, jejunum and colon) and the peritoneum. The other organs are more rarely affected.

15.1 Patients who should be investigated for abdominal TB

Site	Typical presentation
Peritoneal	Abdominal distension, abdominal pain, fever
Intestinal	Recurrent intestinal colic, partial or complete intestinal obstruction, chronic diarrhoea, unexplained weight loss, palpable mass in lower abdomen, lower GI bleeding
Oesophageal*	Dysphagia, odynophagia, hematemesis, constitutional symptoms
Gastroduodenal*	Gastric outlet obstruction, upper GI bleeding
Hepatobiliary*	Fever of unknown origin, hepatomegaly with or without space occupying lesions, abnormal LFTs (especially elevated alkaline phosphatase), abnormal imaging (abscess, space occupying lesions), jaundice
Pancreatic*	Abdominal pain, and/or obstructive jaundice, and/or dilated pancreatic and/or bile ducts with evidence of (peri)-pancreatic mass or cyst with or without constitutional symptoms
Perianal	Complex perianal fistulae, persistent discharge from the fistula, fistulae which recur after multiple surgical excisions

* Sites where other differential diagnoses like malignancy are more common than TB infection

Presumptive abdominal TB	A patient with abdominal pain, distension, fever, unexplained weight loss, chronic diarrhoea or an abdominal mass.

15.2 Diagnosis

All patients with presumptive abdominal TB

Test	Patients	Comments
X-ray of chest	All	All patients presenting with symptoms consistent with TB should have a chest X-ray.
HIV test	All	EPTB is associated with HIV infection. All patients should be offered integrated counselling and testing.

Patients with presumptive peritoneal TB

Ascitic fluid sampling	All	Simple percutaneous sampling of ascitic fluid can aid in the diagnosis of peritoneal TB. Specimens should be sent for: a) cytology; b) albumin and protein; c) adenosine deaminase (ADA); d) microscopy for AFB; e) culture for Mtb and other organisms
		A serum albumin:ascitic fluid albumin ratio (SAAG) of <1.1 with a high protein (>2.5 g/mL) is suggestive of an exudative process, in keeping with abdominal TB (although several other conditions also cause this).
		ADA >39 IU/mL in ascitic fluid is suggestive of abdominal TB (Riquelme A, 2006).
		Sensitivity of smear microscopy and culture for Mtb on ascitic fluid samples is low; however, culture is required to confirm the diagnosis and test for drug susceptibility.
		PCR-based methods for identifying Mtb in ascitic fluid samples are highly variable in terms of diagnostic accuracy, and so no recommendation on the use of these tests has been made.
Ultrasound of abdomen	All	Many abnormal features may be noted, including intra-abdominal fluid (free or loculated), inter-loop ascites, mesenteric lymphadenopathy, bowel wall thickening, enlarged lymph nodes with central necrosis and peripheral enhancement and peritoneal and omental thickening.
US-guided FNAC or core biopsy of mesenteric or retro-peritoneal lymph nodes, omentum or peritoneum	Selected	Microscopy and culture of FNAC/biopsy specimens of affected structures is more sensitive than ascitic fluid testing alone.
		Requires a trained practitioner. Specimens should be sent for: a) histology; b) microscopy for AFB; c) culture for Mtb and other organisms.
CT or MR scan of abdomen	Selected	Many abnormal features may be noted, but as with ultrasound, none are diagnostic for peritoneal TB. These tests may be useful when other differential diagnoses are being considered. Not routinely suggested. Radiation exposure should be considered when deciding to perform a CT.
Laparoscopy	Selected	Visual appearance on laparoscopy can be highly suggestive of peritoneal TB. Typical appearances include: • Thickened peritoneum with tubercles: multiple, yellowish white, uniform sized (about 4–5 mm) tubercles diffusely distributed on the parietal peritoneum. The peritoneum is thickened, hyperaemic and lacks its usual shiny lustre. The omentum, liver and spleen can also be studded with tubercles. • Thickened peritoneum without tubercles. • Fibro-adhesive peritonitis with markedly thickened peritoneum and multiple thick adhesions fixing the viscera. Targeted diagnostic sampling at laparoscopy may improve the yield from biopsy specimens sent for microscopy and culture for Mtb and histopathology. Laparoscopy is not routinely recommended due to the high cost and invasive nature of the procedure, and is usually reserved for cases where the diagnosis remains unclear after other tests.

Patients with presumptive peritoneal TB

Ileocolonoscopy	All	Unless contraindicated, all patients suspected of TB affecting the lower GI tract should be offered endoscopic examination with appropriate biopsy sampling.
		Examination of the ileum by retrograde ileoscopy is important, as this is the commonest site of involvement in GI TB.
		Appearances vary considerably, and differentiating GI TB from other bowel diseases such as Crohn's disease is often challenging.
		Biopsy specimens should be sent for: a) histology and staining for AFBs; b) culture for Mtb PCR-based methods for identifying Mtb in biopsy specimens from the GI tract are highly variable in terms of diagnostic accuracy, and so no recommendation on the use of these tests has been made.
CT/MR enterography/ enteroclysis	Selected	Assessment of the small intestine may require specialist imaging to identify and characterise lesions. Selecting the appropriate test depends on what pathology is suspected, and should be at the discretion of a specialist clinician and/or radiologist.
		Common findings include short segment strictures and ileocecal wall thickening with enlarged necrotic lymph nodes.
Upper GI endoscopy	Selected	If symptoms suggest involvement of the upper GI tract, endoscopy with biopsy is indicated.
Barium studies	Selected	Barium studies of the upper GI tract and small bowel may be indicated where endoscopy is not available or not possible, or where small bowel stricture is suspected.

Diagnosis of other forms of abdominal TB

The principal differential diagnosis in biliary and pancreatic TB patients is usually malignancy, and some patients are diagnosed post-operatively after surgery to resect a suspected tumour. Specialist imaging and image-guided diagnostic sampling techniques are required in cases of suspected biliary and pancreatic TB, and patients should be referred to centres providing these services.

Perianal TB is relatively uncommon, and the differential diagnosis includes a variety of conditions such as Crohn's disease, foreign body reactions, malignancy and sexually transmitted diseases. Careful assessment by specialists is advised.

15.3 Treatment

First line treatment for adults and children with abdominal TB	Drugs	2RHZE/4RHE
		Recommendation: 6 months ATT standard first-line regimen is recommended for abdominal TB.
		Strong recommendation, very low quality evidence
	Duration	Total treatment duration: 6 months, extended at the discretion of the treating clinician
	Referral	Patients with presumptive GI, hepatobiliary, pancreatic or perianal TB will require referral to a gastroenterologist for clinical assessment and diagnosis.
		Patients with presumptive peritoneal TB where the diagnosis is uncertain also require referral.
	Follow up	Assess response to treatment at 3 months and 6 months. Consider possible treatment failure in patients who have worsened or deteriorated after initial improvement – this requires diagnostic investigation and possibly a change of treatment. Deterioration in the first 3 months may be due to paradoxical reaction – this does not require repeat diagnostic tests or change of treatment.
	Surgery	Complications of GI TB include strictures that can cause acute and recurrent partial obstruction, and perforation in some cases.
		Strictures can be managed with endoscopic dilatation, but some cases require resection of the stricture or hemicolectomy.
		Oesophageal and gastroduodenal TB patients rarely require surgery; ATT alone is usually adequate. Duodenal strictures may be treated with balloon dilatation. Bypass surgery may be required if this is not successful.
		Hepatobiliary or pancreatic TB patients who develop biliary obstruction may require endoscopic or percutaneous biliary stenting. Liver abscess which fails to respond to treatment, or ruptured abscesses may require surgical intervention.
		Perianal TB cases with complex fistula may require surgical intervention.

16 Urogenital TB

Urogenital TB refers to TB of the female and male genital tract and the urinary tract. It is usually an insidious disease, and can lead to a variety of presentations depending on the affected site and stage of disease. Serious adverse outcomes include infertility in both women and men, chronic pelvic pain, dysmenorrhoea, bladder dysfunction, renal failure and death. Some (particularly female) patients may experience no symptoms at all other than infertility, meaning that a high index of suspicion and careful clinical evaluation are needed to make the diagnosis.

Urogenital TB makes up approximately 4% of all EPTB cases annually in India. This may be an underestimate of the true number of cases, as the difficulty of diagnosing the condition and lack of clear case definitions may be hampering reporting of cases.

In this summary of the key practice points, forms of urogenital TB are divided into three broad categories:
- Urinary TB – referring to TB of the kidney, ureters and/or bladder
- Female genital TB – referring to TB of the uterus, fallopian tubes and/or ovaries
- Male genital TB – referring to TB of the epididymis and/or testes

16.1 Urinary TB

Patients who should be investigated for urinary TB

Presumptive urinary TB	A patient with lower urinary tract symptoms (frequency, urgency and nocturia) associated with dysuria and/or haematuria for at least 2 weeks, which has not responded to a 3–7 day course of antibiotics. Some patients have systemic symptoms of fever, weight loss and night sweats.
	Note: The use of fluoroquinolones in the treatment of UTI can reduce the sensitivity of subsequent tests for Mtb in the urinary tract, and should therefore be avoided, unless an organism is identified in urine cultures and antibiotic susceptibility test results support fluoroquinolone use.

Diagnosis

Test	Patients	Comments
X-ray of chest	All	All patients presenting with symptoms consistent with TB should have a chest X-ray to look for evidence of previous or active pulmonary TB.
HIV test	All	EPTB is associated with HIV infection. All patients should be offered integrated counselling and testing.
Renal function tests	All	An important complication of urinary TB is renal impairment. All patients should have blood tests and calculation of estimated glomerular filtration rate (eGFR) to detect this.
		Renal impairment should prompt rapid assessment of the urinary tract using ultrasound to look for outflow tract obstruction as a cause. This requires urgent intervention with urinary catheterisation; or in the instance of hydronephrosis, percutaneous nephrostomy or double J stent insertion to decompress the affected kidney.

Test	Patients	Comments
Urine microscopy and culture for non-mycobacterial organisms	All	To identify sterile pyuria, which may suggest urinary TB
		To diagnose active infection with other bacteria. The patient should be reassessed after appropriate antibiotic treatment for symptom resolution. Superadded bacterial infection can occur with urinary TB.
Early morning urine sampling	All	Three to five early morning urine samples collected for staining and microscopy for AFBs and culture for Mtb. While the sensitivity of these tests is low, culture remains the most reliable way to confirm a diagnosis of urinary TB and allows drug susceptibility testing to be carried out.
Ultrasound of the kidneys, ureters and bladder (US KUB)	All	This scan may be normal in early disease. It can help identify structural abnormalities such as hydronephrosis which can either suggest a diagnosis or guide further tests. It is non-invasive and well-tolerated.
Intravenous urography (using plain X-ray)	Selected	This test also helps identify lesions in the urinary tract and has the advantage of being widely available and cheap; however, it has low sensitivity for early lesions.
		Risks include contrast nephropathy (patients with renal impairment are at particular risk), and contrast reaction (asthmatic patients and patients with cardiac failure may be at higher risk).
Contrast-enhanced CT urography	Selected	This test is more sensitive than IV urography using plain X-rays for identifying and characterising TB lesions in the urinary tract.
		Risks include contrast nephropathy and contrast reaction. The relatively high dose of ionizing radiation involved must be taken into account when considering this test, particularly for children and women of childbearing age. It is contraindicated in pregnant women.
MR urography without contrast	Selected	This test is also gives structural information about the urinary tract, and is sensitive for identifying and characterising TB lesions.
		It is more expensive and less accessible than plain X-ray and CT urography, but has the advantage of not requiring intravenous contrast and not necessitating a dose of radiation.
		Pregnant women, children and patients with preexisting renal function may benefit from this test.
FNAC	Selected	Where accessible mass lesions or fluid collections are identified on imaging, radiologically guided aspiration with specimens subjected to staining and microscopy for AFBs, culture and cytology may confirm the diagnosis of TB.
Urethrocystoscopy with/without bladder biopsy	Selected	Indicated when • other less invasive tests are inconclusive • bladder malignancy is also suspected
		Although this is an invasive test, risk to the patient is low when carried out by an experienced practitioner. Has the advantage of allowing visualisation of lesions and targeted biopsy
Biopsy	Most	Biopsy of lesions in the urinary tract is required when • other less invasive tests are inconclusive • malignancy is also suspected
		Specimens should be subject to: a) staining and microscopy for AFBs; b) culture and drug susceptibility testing; c) histopathology

Treatment

Aims of treatment are:
- to achieve TB cure
- to prevent the long term sequelae
- to restore normal anatomy if it has been distorted.

First line treatment for adults and children with urinary TB	Drugs	2RHZE/4RHE
	Duration	Six months
	Referral	Requires assessment by a urology team to perform specialist diagnostic tests and treat structural urinary tract complications.
		Urgent referral is required for patients presenting with renal failure secondary to bilateral hydronephrosis.
	Follow up	Assess response to treatment at 8 weeks – resolution of systemic symptoms, improvement in urinary symptoms, check renal function.
		Repeat imaging may be indicated, especially if partial or impending ureteric stricture was identified at diagnosis. Obstruction can occur as a late complication as the healing of the lesion results in fibrotic stricture.
		If early morning urine culture is positive at diagnosis, this may be repeated at 8 weeks, and at the end of ATT.
	Surgery	Urgent surgical intervention is required when ureteric obstruction prevents drainage of urine from the kidney, to prevent renal damage.
		Reconstructive procedures are required when there are ureteric strictures or small capacity bladder complicates urinary TB. Nephrectomy is rarely indicated, except where chronic pain, hypertension, nephrocutaneous fistula or stone formation complicates a poorly- or non-functioning kidney.

16.2 Female genital TB

Presentation is varied and a high index of clinical suspicion is required to make the diagnosis. Most cases of female genital TB (FGTB) are found in premenopausal women, theoretically because an atrophic endometrium provides a poor milieu for mycobacterial growth. Around 11% of patients present with no symptoms other than infertility, and these patients require a diagnostic workup to look for all common causes of infertility. In patients with pelvic symptoms or vaginal bleeding post menopause, malignancy is an important differential diagnosis to consider.

Patients who should be investigated for female genital TB

Presumptive FGTB	A premenopausal woman presenting with infertility, menstrual problems, unexplained abdominal pain or pelvic mass. Rarely, patients have systemic symptoms of fever, weight loss and night sweats. Ectopic pregnancy and cervical/vulval lesions are rare presenting features.
	A postmenopausal woman presenting with vaginal bleeding

Diagnosis

Test	Patients	Comments
X-ray of chest	All	All patients presenting with symptoms consistent with TB should have a chest X-ray to look for evidence of previous or active pulmonary TB.
HIV test	All	EPTB is associated with HIV infection. All patients should be offered integrated counseling and testing.
Pregnancy test	All of childbearing age	To rule out pregnancy as possible cause of symptoms, and to ensure further testing is safe and appropriate
Pelvic ultrasound	All	Part of the initial assessment of most patients presenting with gynaecological symptoms
Hysterosalpingogram	Selected	May be done as part of the investigation of infertility, but many women with FGTB will have a normal HSG
CT pelvis or MRI pelvis	Selected	To further characterize lesions and plan surgical intervention in selected patients. Disadvantage of CT is exposure to ionising radiation, which is particularly a concern in women of childbearing age

Test	Patients	Comments
FDG-PET CT	Selected	Although not widely available, PET scans may give more information about the presence and activity of tubercular tubo-ovarian mass lesions. Further evidence about the diagnostic accuracy of PET CT for detecting and monitoring the progression of FGTB is needed.
Endometrial aspirate	Selected	Where facilities exist, endometrial aspirate can be obtained and sent for: a) staining and microscopy for AFB; b) culture and drug susceptibility testing. Sensitivity is low, and negative results cannot rule out FGTB.
Laparoscopy	Selected	Laparoscopy with biopsy of lesions is required when • other less invasive tests are inconclusive • malignancy is also suspected • as part of infertility investigations when less invasive tests are inconclusive Laparoscopy offers the dual advantage of pelvic organ visualization and specimen collection from otherwise inaccessible sites. Specimens should be subject to: a) staining and microscopy for AFBs; b) culture and drug susceptibility testing; and c) histopathology.

Making a diagnosis

The group concluded that the diagnosis of FGTB should be made based on any one of:
• laparoscopic appearance typical for FGTB
• any gynaecological specimen positive for AFBs on microscopy or positive for Mtb on culture
• any gynaecological specimen with findings consistent with FGTB on histopathological examination.

Treatment

Aims of treatment:
• To achieve TB cure
• To prevent the long term sequelae
• To restore normal anatomy if has been distorted

First-line treatment for adults and children with urinary TB	Drugs	2RHZE/4RHE
	Duration	Six months
	Referral	Requires assessment by a gynaecologist to make the diagnosis and treat complications. Empirical ATT in women presenting with infertility alone should only be started following assessment by a specialist.
	Follow up	Assess response to treatment at completion of 6 months' ATT
	Surgery	Surgery is not part of primary treatment in FGTB; however, it is sometimes needed for large, residual tubo-ovarian abscesses. Surgery in FGTB is associated with higher complication rates as there are a lot of adhesions as well as the possibility of infection recurrence. Tubal anatomy can sometimes be restored surgically in infertile women following a course of ATT. However, infertility may be an irreversible long-term consequence of FGTB. Giving repeated courses of ATT to women who remain infertile following completed ATT for FGTB is not necessary.

16.3 Male genital TB

Patients who should be investigated for male genital TB (MGTB)

Presumptive MGTB	A patient with scrotal pain or swelling for 2 weeks or more not responding to a 7–14 day course of antibiotics, or with discharging sinuses in the scrotum. Rarely, patients have systemic symptoms of fever, weight loss and night sweats.

Diagnosis

Test	Patients	Comments
X-ray of chest	All	All patients presenting with symptoms consistent with TB should have a chest X-ray to look for evidence of previous or active pulmonary TB.
HIV test	All	EPTB is associated with HIV infection. All patients should be offered integrated counselling and testing.
Renal function tests Urine microscopy and culture for nonmycobacterial organisms Early morning urine sampling Ultrasound of the kidneys, ureters and bladder (US KUB)	All	All patients with suspected MGTB must be evaluated for co-existent urinary TB (see above).
Ultrasound scan of the scrotum	All	To evaluate swelling/mass lesions and guide FNAC
FNAC epididymal mass	All	Specimens should be subject to: a. staining and microscopy for AFB; b. culture and drug susceptibility testing; and c. cytology There is a risk of damaging the epididymis and causing infertility.
Biopsy	Selected	If FNAC does not confirm the diagnosis or malignancy is suspected, biopsy of the lesion is indicated. Specimens should be subject to: a. staining and microscopy for AFBs; b. culture and drug susceptibility testing; c. histopathology

Treatment

First-line treatment for adults and children with MGTB	Drugs	2RHZE/4RHE
	Duration	Six months
	Referral	All cases need evaluation by an urologist to make the diagnosis.
	Follow up	Assess at 8 weeks to assess for response to treatment. Repeat FNAC/biopsy may be required for mass lesions which continue to grow despite treatment (specialist assessment required).
	Surgery	Surgery is not usually required, and is not a routine part of treatment. Epididymectomy may be required if there is a caseating abscess which persists despite completing a course of ATT.
	Sequelae	Infertility is a possible long-term complication of MGTB. Infertility following completed treatment for MGTB should not be interpreted as indicative of treatment failure or recurrence of infection.

PCR-based tests in urogenital TB

Confirming the diagnosis in urogenital TB is very difficult. Often, invasive procedures must be done to obtain specimens. Conventional diagnostic methods (microscopy and culture) have low sensitivity.

PCR-based tests (either commercially available or in-house assays) are increasingly used to diagnose FGTB. A literature review prepared for this guideline found that estimates of sensitivity and specificity varied widely across reports in the literature, and the Technical Advisory Subcommittee for FGTB raised concerns about their experience of high rates of false positives when these tests are applied to peritoneal/gynaecological specimens. There were no data at the time of publication looking at the use of Xpert MTB/RIF for the diagnosis of FGTB. The guideline group decided that a recommendation was not possible at this time regarding the use of PCR-based tests in FGTB, and noted that high quality diagnostic test accuracy studies are needed to address this question.

Similarly, further evidence is needed on the diagnostic test accuracy of Xpert MTB/RIF and other PCR-based tests on urine, FNA aspirates and biopsy specimens for the diagnosis of urinary TB or MGTB. Again, the expert group acknowledged that while these tests are in current use, the guideline group could not make a recommendation about their use at the present time.

17 Spinal TB and other forms of bone and joint TB

TB infection of the bones and joints causes chronic pain, deformity and disability, and TB of the cervical spine can be life threatening. Bone and joint TB makes up around 10% of all EPTB cases, with spinal TB being the most common form (Sharma S.K., 2004). Around 1–2% of all TB cases worldwide are spinal TB cases (Watts, 1996). Both adults and children can be affected.

Since it is the most common and most disabling form, spinal TB is covered in detail here, with key practice points at the end about TB affecting other parts of the skeletal system.

17.1 TB of the spine

Presumptive spinal TB	A patient with localized back pain for more than 6 weeks with tenderness on examination of the spinous processes, fever and weight loss, with or without signs of spinal cord compression. Patients with advanced disease may have severe pain, spinal deformity, paraspinal muscle wasting and neurological deficit.
	In addition in children, failure to thrive, night cries, inability to walk/cautious gait, and use of hands to support the head or trunk are important signs.

Diagnosis

Test	Patients	Comments
X-ray of chest	All	All patients presenting with symptoms consistent with TB should have a chest X-ray.
HIV test	All	EPTB is associated with HIV infection. All patients should be offered VCT.
X-ray of spine	Limited use	Spinal lesions take 3 to 6 months to appear on plain X-ray, so this test is of limited use in the early stages of the disease. However, X-rays are useful to evaluate treatment response on follow up.
MRI spine	All	All patients with suspected TB spine require an MRI to assess the extent of disease and the degree of bony destruction, and confirm spinal cord involvement in patients with neurological signs. MRI is useful in making a diagnosis in the early stages of disease while some MRI appearances are highly suggestive of a diagnosis of spinal TB (Jain, 2012).
CT spine	Selected	Some patients may require CT of the spine in addition to MRI, although CT cannot be used to detect early spinal cord involvement.
Biopsy of the lesion	All	The INDEX-TB guidelines TAC subcommittee for bone and joint TB assert that in TB endemic areas, it is reasonable to start ATT in patients with strong clinical and radiological/MRI evidence of TB of the spine and monitor their progress. Where possible, all patients should have a biopsy of the lesion to provide a specimen for culture to confirm the diagnosis and perform drug susceptibility testing, and to rule out other diagnoses. Percutaneous CT-guided biopsy is preferred, but some patients may require open biopsy. The risks and benefits of obtaining a biopsy must be considered.
		Specimens should be sent for: a) Microscopy and culture for pyogenic bacteria; b) Microscopy and culture for Mtb; and c) histopathology/cytology.
		There is currently insufficient evidence surrounding the use of PCR-based tests such as Xpert MTB/RIF in the diagnosis of TB of the bones and joints.

Treatment

There is uncertainty surrounding the optimum duration of treatment for TB of the bones and joints. Some older trials suggested that 6 months treatment may be sufficient, but more advanced diagnostic imaging has led to uncertainty whether these patients are cured for spinal TB at the end of that time. The TAC subcommittee performed a brief review of the literature to inform their decision regarding duration of treatment in bone and joint TB; a systematic review was not performed. The group found that there is a lack of consensus about what constitutes healed status in the literature.

The expert group agreed that all cases of bone and joint TB should be treated with extended courses of ATT with a 2-month intensive phase consisting of four drugs (isoniazid, rifampicin, pyrazinamide and ethambutol), followed by a continuation phase lasting 10–16 months, depending on the site of disease and the patient's clinical course.

Drugs	2RHZE/10RHE
	All patients require close monitoring for development or progression of neurological deficit in the first 4 weeks of treatment.
	Some patients require surgical intervention.
Duration	Total treatment duration: 12 months (extendable to 18 months on a case-bycase basis)
Referral	Optimum management of spinal TB requires the involvement of multiple specialists including a spinal orthopaedic surgeon, microbiologist/infectious diseases specialist and spinal radiologist, as well as physiotherapists and orthotists. All presumptive spinal TB cases should be referred and managed in specialist centres.
Follow up	Patients without neurological deficit should be advised to return to the clinic immediately if new symptoms develop, and all ambulant patients should be assessed weekly for neurological signs.
	Patients with neurological deficit require staging and grading of their deficit. These patients should be assessed weekly with neural charting to detect neural recovery or deterioration.
	Repeat X-rays of the spine are suggested every 3 months following initiation of treatment to assess for radiological healing.
	Repeat MRI scans are suggested at 6, 9, 12 and 18 months following initiation of treatment to assess healing.
	At the end of treatment, all patients require follow up every 6 months for at least 2 years, and should be told to return to the clinic promptly if they develop new symptoms in the interim.
Surgery	While some require early surgical intervention, most patients can be managed with ATT alone in the initial phase of treatment.
	Surgery may be required for two principal purposes in spinal TB-to establish diagnosis, or to treat spinal deformity, instability and neurological deficit.
	Where available, percutaneous biopsy under CT guidance reduces the need for open biopsy, but this may still be required in some cases, particularly where imaging results are atypical for spinal TB and the diagnosis is uncertain.
	Patients with large, fluctuant cold abscesses may require therapeutic aspiration to relieve symptoms and promote healing.
	Indications for surgery in TB spine with neurological deficit: • Neural complications developing or getting worse or remaining stationary during the course of non-operative treatment (3–4 weeks) • Paraplegia of rapid onset • Spinal tumour syndrome • Neural arch disease • Severe paraplegia – flaccid paraplegia, paraplegia in flexion, complete sensory loss and complete loss of motor power for more than 6 months • Painful paraplegia in elderly patients.

	Indications for surgery in spinal TB without neurological deficit: • When diagnosis is uncertain and open biopsy is indicated • Mechanical instability – panvertebral disease, where bony involvement of both the vertebral body and posterior complex is seen on imaging, or disease affects facet joints bilaterally • Suspected drug resistance – where patients show inadequate clinical improvement or deterioration on ATT • Spinal deformity – severe kyphotic deformity at presentation, or in children at high risk of progression of kyphosis with growth after healing of disease.
Surgery	• Indications for instrumented stabilization: • Panvertebral disease • Long segment disease where a > 4–5 cm long graft is required to bridge the gap after surgical decompression in dorsal spine • In lumbar and cervical spine • When kyphosis correction surgery is contemplated • Lesion in a junctional area.
Sequelae	Early onset paraplegia: Some patients have paraplegia secondary to acute inflammation in and around the cord in early disease. This generally carries a good prognosis with prompt treatment with ATT. MRI and intraoperative findings suggestive of extradural fluid compressing the cord, cord oedema or myelitis generally correlate with neural recovery. Late onset paraplegia: This is defined as the reappearance of neural deficit after a disease-free period of at least 2 years in patients who completed ATT and achieved healed status with a residual kyphotic deformity. This can occur as a result of progression of deformity in healed patients, or as a result of relapse of active TB infection. These two scenarios necessitate different treatment and carry different prognoses. Expert management is required. Deformity: Bony destruction and subsequent healing leads to deformity, which will depend on the site and extent of infection. Some deformity requires surgical correction to prevent further progression or restore function. There is debate over the optimum timing of surgery to correct deformity, but the group agreed that surgery should preferably take place during treatment with ATT for active TB infection.

17.2 TB of the appendicular skeleton

TB of the bones and joints can affect people of any age, but some forms are seen more frequently in children.

Risk factors include previous TB infection, immunosuppression caused by conditions such as HIV, diabetes mellitus and chronic liver or kidney failure, among others; or by immunosuppressive drugs such as long-term corticosteroids.

Key principles of diagnosing TB of the bones and joints are:
• Suspect TB as a possible cause in people with signs of joint infection with an insidious onset
• Refer to an orthopaedic team who can assess the joint and perform a biopsy for culture (for M. tuberculosis as well as other organisms) and histopathology
• All patients should have specimens taken for microscopy and culture where possible

Invasive diagnostic procedures are not always practicable, and in such circumstances the treating clinician must use his judgement as to whether treatment with ATT should be started without a microbiological/histopathological diagnosis, or whether a period of observation is appropriate. The INDEX-TB guidelines TAC subcommittee for bone and joint TB assert that in TB-endemic areas, it is reasonable to start ATT in patients with strong clinical and radiological evidence of TB of the bones and joints and monitor their progress. Where the diagnosis is uncertain, tissue specimens are required before giving ATT.

Where possible and safe for the patient, getting specimens for microscopy, culture and histopathology prior to starting ATT is beneficial because:

- positive culture confirms the diagnosis
- drug susceptibility testing can be carried out to guide ATT
- false negative culture results are more likely if specimens are taken after ATT has been started
- alternative diagnoses can be picked up.

When taking specimens for microbiological testing and histopathology, the following principles are important:

- Early in the course of TB joint infection, aspiration of fluid from the joint will not usually yield a diagnosis, and so tissue biopsy of the affected structures is preferred. This may be done under radiological guidance, using arthroscopy, or via open surgical biopsy. Arthroscopy with biopsy offers the advantage of visualization of the lesion with excision of affected tissue for diagnostic testing, and simultaneous therapeutic intervention if required.
- Fluid or pus from joint aspirates, and pus from collections/cold abscesses should also be sent for microscopy and culture.
- Enlarged lymph nodes regional to the infected site may also be considered for biopsy/FNAC.
- Sinus tract curettage/edge biopsy may also be sent for culture and histopathology, but microbiological results should be interpreted with caution as contamination/colonization/secondary infection with skin commensals or coliforms is common.
- As a general principle, specimens for culture should be collected whenever a therapeutic invasive procedure is carried out, e.g. when a joint is debrided following unsuccessful non-operative management.
- Specimens should be sent for
  - microscopy and culture for non-mycobacterial pathogens (pyogenic bacteria, *Brucella*, fungal species)
  - microscopy and culture for TB
  - histopathology.

This table lists the presenting features of TB of the joints, with basic information about diagnosis and treatment. This section is based on the expert opinion of the INDEX-TB TAC subcommittee for bone and joint TB.

Hand and wrist Hand and wrist	*Identify:* More common in children under 5 years, but can affect any age group Patients present with a variety of features depending on the site of infection. The hand or wrist gradually becomes painful and/or swollen with joint effusions and synovial thickening, causing boggy swelling with restricted range of motion. Systemic symptoms such as fever, weight loss, anorexia and regional lymphadenopathy may be present. In advanced disease, wasting of the muscles of the hand and forearm, deformity, enlargement of digits/metacarpals (sausage finger/spina ventosa), discharging sinuses, cold abscess and compound palmar ganglia may be present. Rarely, patients have carpal tunnel syndrome, or nail involvement. *Diagnose:* Early X-ray changes are subtle and easily missed, but later in the disease sequential X-ray changes are seen which can be used to classify the disease (Martini M, 1986). USS, CT and MRI features are non-specific but these modalities may be used to assess extent of disease or identify biopsy sites or drainable collections. *Treat:* 2RHZE/10–16RHE with rest to the joint provided by immobilisation in plaster/brace for 4 to 6 weeks followed by gradual mobilisation as tolerated (specialist management by upper limb orthopaedic surgeon required). Surgery is rarely needed, but may be indicated for nerve compression, impending bone collapse, joint debridement, drainage of large abscesses and correction of deformity in healed disease.

Elbow	**Identify:** Can affect any age group Patients present with a variety of features depending on the site of infection. The elbow gradually becomes painful and/or swollen with joint effusions and synovial thickening, causing boggy swelling with restricted range of motion. Systemic symptoms such as fever, weight loss, anorexia and regional lymphadenopathy may be present. Rarely, ulnar nerve or posterior interosseous nerve palsies may be the presenting feature. In advanced disease, wasting of the arm and forearm muscles, deformity on flexion/extension, pathological dislocation, discharging sinuses and cold abscesses may develop. **Diagnose:** See Hand and wrist TB **Treat:** See Hand and wrist TB
Shoulder	**Identify:** Can affect all ages, but is more common in adults than children. Relatively rare, it usually presents in the advanced stage with disabling symptoms that may mimic more common pathologies such as neuropathic shoulder, rheumatoid arthritis, and adhesive capsulitis. A high index of suspicion and careful clinical evaluation are required to make the diagnosis. Patients present with pain in the shoulder and restricted range of motion (particularly limited external rotation and abduction), with muscle wasting (particularly deltoid and supraspinatus). Systemic symptoms such as fever, weight loss, anorexia and lymphadenopathy are uncommon, as is swelling of the joint. In advanced disease, there may be marked destruction of the humeral head and glenoid with muscle atrophy, or deformity (particularly, fibrous ankylosis with humeral head pulled up against the glenoid and the arm fixed in adduction and internal rotation). Discharging sinuses around shoulder, arm and scapula and cold abscess are uncommon. "Caries sicca" is the most common form – which is a dry arthropathy (rather than exudative). **Diagnose:** See Hand and wrist TB. In early disease, arthroscopic biopsy offers the advantage of direct visualization of joint, allowing excision of tubercular synovium, granulation tissue, rice bodies and pannus over cartilage. However, in advanced disease where arthroscopy is not feasible, an open debridement and biopsy is indicated. **Treat:** 2RHZE/10-16RHE with rest in sling or brace and gentle mobilization as tolerated. Prolonged immobilisation with spica is no longer widely advocated. Surgery is rarely needed, but may be indicated for drainage of large abscess, excision of persistent sinuses, joint debridement to remove loose bodies and pannus, arthrodesis to relieve a painful fibrous ankylosis, or joint replacement in healed disease with severe joint destruction. Resection arthroplasty has not been shown to improve outcomes, and should be avoided in favour of nonoperative treatment even in cases with severe bony destruction at diagnosis.
Hip	**Identify:** Can affect any age, but most common in children and young adults There are three stages in the course of the disease: 1. **Synovitis.** Characterized by gradual onset of hip pain and limping (antalgic gait) with fullness around the hip caused by joint effusion, restricted range of movement and deformity (the affected limb is flexed, abducted and externally rotated with apparent lengthening of the extremity).

	2. **Early arthritis.** Characterized by progression of bony destruction leading to deformity with the limb flexed, adducted and internally rotated with apparent limb shortening. There is pain with every hip movement, with muscle spasm and atrophy.
	3. **Advanced arthritis.** Characterized by very painful joint movements and grossly restricted range of movement with shortening of the limb. Pathological dislocation or subluxation may occur due to bony destruction at the acetabulum/femoral head. The attitude of the limb and deformity does not always correlate with the stage of arthritis.
Hip	*Diagnose:* 1. **Synovitis stage.** X-ray changes and US appearance, with aspiration of the joint effusion for microscopy, AFB smear and culture may provide sufficient information in high TB burden areas to start treatment. MRI scan can give more information about the extent of the disease. Biopsy should be carried out if there is uncertainty about diagnosis. 2. **Early arthritis.** Radiographic changes with biopsy 3. **Advanced arthritis.** Radiographic changes with biopsy *Treat:* 1. **Synovitis.** 2RHZE/10–16RHE with appropriate analgesia and rest to the joint in above-knee skin traction or skeletal traction for around 4 weeks. Active assisted exercises to mobilize thereafter. Surgery is rarely required. 2. **Early arthritis.** 2RHZE/10–16RHE with appropriate analgesia and rest to the joint in above-knee skin traction or skeletal traction until spasm is relieved, and non-weight bearing exercises as tolerated. Synovectomy and joint debridement are sometimes indicated if the response to nonoperative treatment is inadequate at 6 to 8 weeks. Drainage of large joint effusions or abscesses may be required. Send specimens for culture. 3. **Advanced arthritis.** 2RHZE/10-16RHE with appropriate analgesia and rest to the joint in traction. Arthrolysis with joint debridement is usually indicated, followed by a period of skeletal traction, with early supervised mobilization of the hip as tolerated. 4. **Advanced arthritis with subluxation/dislocation.** 2RHZE/10–16RHE with appropriate analgesia and rest to the joint in traction. Gross bony destruction at this stage requires surgical management with excision arthroplasty, arthrodesis or total hip replacement.
Knee	*Identify:* Can affect any age group Patients present with a painful, swollen, tender knee which may be warm to touch, with limping and reduced range of motion. Systemic symptoms of fever, weight loss and anorexia may be present, with regional lymphadenopathy on examination. In advanced disease, the joint may feel boggy due to synovial thickening, with joint effusion and wasting of the thigh muscles. Discharging sinuses or cold abscess may be seen. Deformity ranging from a mild flexion deformity to severe triple deformity consisting of flexion, posterior subluxation, external rotation and valgus may be present. *Diagnose:* X-ray changes are non-specific in early disease, with progressive changes in late disease, which can be used to classify the stage of disease. MRI changes can be highly suggestive of TB of the knee. Diagnosis is confirmed with microscopy, culture and histopathological examination of US-guided/arthroscopic/open surgical biopsy of the synovium. *Treat:* 1. **Synovitis stage.** 2RHZE/10–16RHE with rest to the joint in traction to prevent flexion deformity with gentle mobilization for 6 weeks, and then reassess. Arthroscopic or open joint debridement may be necessary in some cases if there is little improvement with nonoperative treatment.

	2. **Early arthritis stage.** 2RHZE/10–16RHE with rest to the joint in double traction to prevent triple deformity. Joint debridement is usually necessary, with corrective plaster/bracing following surgery if joint is unstable.
	3. **Advanced arthritis stage.** In children, 2RHZE/10– 16RHE with rest to the joint in double traction, followed by corrective plaster, with arthrodesis deferred until growth is complete. In adults, with painful arthritic knee or fibrous ankylosis, arthrodesis by compression is often necessary.
	4. **Healed tubercular knee with deformity.** Corrective osteotomy or total knee replacement may be necessary to restore normal alignment and improve function.
Ankle	*Identify:* More common in children and young adults, but can affect any age group Patients present with a slow-onset painful, swollen ankle with pain on weight bearing causing a limp, and a history of weight loss, anorexia and fever. On examination, the joint may be warm, red and tender, boggy to palpate due to synovial thickening, with regional lymphadenopathy and restricted range of motion. In advanced disease, calf muscle wasting, effusion, deformity and discharging sinuses may be seen. Differential diagnoses: non-mycobacterial septic joint, neoplastic lesion, e.g. chondroblastoma in children. *Diagnose:* X-ray features are non-specific, and are subtle in early disease. MRI and CT scan may demonstrate changes, but these are not specific to TB. *Treat:* 2RHZE/10–16RHE with rest to the joint in a functional position (in plaster/ankle-foot orthoses) for 4–6 weeks followed by gentle non weight-bearing mobilization as tolerated. Surgery is rarely required, but is indicated for impending bone collapse, large abscess, or correction of deformity in healed patients.
Foot	*Identify:* More common in children and young adults, but can affect any age group Patients present with slow-onset pain, swelling of the foot and a limp. Specific features depend on which bones are involved, e.g. TB of the calcaneus causing heel-up limp and tenderness over heel. Systemic features such as fever, weight loss and lymphadenopathy are uncommon. In advanced disease, there may be effusion, synovial thickening, deformity (caused by collapse of tarsal bone), discharging sinuses or a cold abscess. **Diagnose:** As for Ankle TB **Treat:** As for Ankle TB

Outcomes

Healed status

For patients with a diagnosis of confirmed/probable bone TB, healed status is determined by:
- completion of ATT and no relapse of disease at 2 years' follow up
- resolution of fever, night sweats, weight loss (if initially present)
- resolution of sinuses/ulcers (if initially present)
- radiological signs of bone healing, including remineralisation of affected bone, sharpening of joint/vertebral margins. On MRI, resolution of marrow oedema, fatty replacement in marrow and no contrast enhancement

Presumptive treatment failure

For patients with a diagnosis of bacteriologically confirmed or clinically diagnosed bone TB, treatment failure should be suspected when they have any of the following after completing at least 5 months' ATT:
- Persisting or worsening local and systemic symptoms and signs
- No improvement, or deterioration of the lesion on repeat imaging
- Appearance of new lesion(s)
- Non-healing ulcer/sinus
- New abscesses/lymphadenopathy
- Wound dehiscence post-operatively.

Possible causes of deterioration on treatment or failure to improve on treatment:
- Poor adherence to ATT – inadequately treated skeletal TB
- Drug resistance
- Paradoxical reaction
- Immune reconstitution syndrome associated with HIV
- Alternative diagnosis – patient does not have TB or has two diagnoses.

Suggested investigations in patients with presumptive treatment failure:
- Complete blood count and inflammatory markers such as ESR, liver enzymes, urea and electrolytes, fasting blood glucose/HbA1c and HIV test
- Repeat imaging and repeat diagnostic sampling, for example CT-guided biopsy of the lesion
- Send tissue for: a) staining for AFB and culture for Mtb with drug susceptibility testing; b) Gram's stain and bacterial and fungal culture; c) histopathology. PCR-based diagnostic tests are of variable sensitivity in bone TB, and there is uncertainty about specificity in previously treated TB patients.

The expert group suggests that patients with bacteriologically confirmed or clinically diagnosed treatment failure be treated with second-line drugs. For patients with bacteriologically confirmed treatment failure, treatment should be guided by drug susceptibility testing. For clinically diagnosed treatment failure, the specialist team should carefully monitor empirical treatment with second-line drugs.

Paradoxical reaction

A patient with confirmed or probable skeletal TB on ATT who initially improves and then subsequently has worsening constitutional symptoms or signs of TB in the absence of another diagnosis or drug resistance. Features include increased size of lesion, appearance of new lesions, recurrent fever and night sweats, or development of another form of TB.

In drug-resistant cases, the patient will usually fail to improve from the start of ATT, or deteriorate from the start of ATT. There will be no improvement until an effective second-line ATT regimen is started.

In paradoxical reaction, there is usually an initial improvement, followed by deterioration. The patient will usually begin to improve again without changes to the ATT regimen; ATT should not be stopped or altered. NSAIDs and other supportive treatment are usually sufficient.

18 Cutaneous TB

Cutaneous TB is caused by M. tuberculosis, M. bovis, and, rarely, Bacille Calmette-Guerin (BCG). TB of the skin is uncommon, accounting for around 1.5% of EPTB cases. Cutaneous TB often coexists with other forms of TB, especially pulmonary TB and lymph node TB.

Scrofuloderma and lupus vulgaris are the most common manifestations of cutaneous TB, and are particularly prevalent in children. The manifestations of cutaneous TB are summarized in the table below (Tappeiner, 2008).

Although it is not life threatening, cutaneous TB can cause profound distress to the patient due discomfort and disfigurement if not adequately treated. As some manifestations mimic other skin diseases, it can be difficult to diagnose, and patients may have received unnecessary or inappropriate treatment from several practitioners before the correct diagnosis is made. Evaluation by an experienced dermatologist is crucial if the diagnosis is not clear.

Clinical disease	Aetiology	Host immune status
Lupus vulgaris Scrofuloderma	Haematogenous spread	Can affect immunocompetent or immunocompromised people
Acute miliary TB Orificial TB Metastatic tuberculous abscess (tuberculous gumma)	Haematogenous spread	Usually seen in immunocompromised people
Primary Inoculation TB	Inoculation of the skin with Mtb, e.g. by needle stick injury, or at site of trauma	No previous TB infection, immunocompetent
Tuberculosis verrucosa cutis	Inoculation of the skin with Mtb, e.g. by needle stick injury, or at site of trauma	Previous TB infection, immunocompetent
Normal primary complex-like reaction Post-vaccination lupus vulgaris Perforating regional adenitis	BCG innoculation	No previous TB infection
Lichen scrofulosorum Papulonecrotic tuberculid	True tuberculids – thought to represent hypersensitivity reactions, rather than local TB infection of the skin	Not clear; likely some immunity due to previous exposure
Nodular vasculitis (erythema induratum of Bazin) Erythema nodosum	Facultative tuberculids – Mtb may be one of several aetiological agents causing this pathology	Not clear; likely some immunity due to previous exposure

18.1 Patients who should be investigated for cutaneous TB

Presumptive cutaneous TB	Patients with the following clinical presentations: • Ulcers or discharging sinuses over the sites of lymph nodes, bones and joints • Persistent, asymptomatic raised reddish/reddish brown skin lesion of more than 6 months' duration, which may show scarring at one end • Persistent warty skin lesion of more than 6 months' duration

18.2 Diagnosis

Test	Patients	Comments
X-ray of chest	All	All patients presenting with symptoms consistent with TB should have a chest X-ray to look for previous or active pulmonary TB.
HIV test	All	EPTB is associated with HIV infection. All patients should be offered integrated counselling and testing.
Further radiological tests	Selected	All patients require clinical assessment for TB affecting other organ systems such as the chest, abdomen, lymph nodes, bones and joints and CNS. Radiological evaluation should be focused according to the history and examination findings.
Skin biopsy	All	Skin biopsy is required to determine the aetiology of the lesion. Histopathological examination by an experienced specialist remains the most reliable way of making the diagnosis. Staining and microscopy for AFB has very low sensitivity. Culture has low sensitivity; but if positive, confirms the diagnosis of cutaneous TB and facilitates drug susceptibility testing PCR-based tests are in use with variable diagnostic accuracy, but a lack of evidence from high quality studies means they cannot be recommended for routine use currently.
Mantoux test (tuberculin skin testing)	Selected	The Mantoux test is not usually part of the diagnosis of active TB infection. However, the Cutaneous TB Group agreed that in selected cases where diagnosis was equivocal, it might be used as an ancillary test. However, only a strongly positive result (with a diameter of 22 mm or more at reading) supports a diagnosis of cutaneous TB (Ramam, 2011). A negative or weakly positive result does not rule out TB. Sensitivity and specificity estimates for this test vary widely across case series, and the result must be interpreted in the context of the other clinical findings.

18.3 Treatment

All patients with the following results should be treated for cutaneous TB:
- Patients with histology diagnostic of cutaneous TB
- Patients with positive culture of Mtb or microscopy for AFBs from skin biopsy
- Patients with equivocal histology findings and negative microscopy and culture, but strongly positive Mantoux test

First line treatment for adults and children with TB pericarditis	Drugs	2RHZE/4RHE
	Duration	6 months
	Referral	Referral to a dermatologist for diagnosis and management is encouraged. Physicians in primary or secondary care can used teledermatology services to guide referral decisions. Complex cases where the diagnosis is uncertain or the response to ATT is inadequate may require referral to a specialist centre.
	Follow up	Assess response to treatment at 4–6 weeks. Most patients will show significant improvement by this time. Failure to improve or deterioration may be due to misdiagnosis or drug resistance. Specialist referral is advised for such patients. Subsequent follow up of patients responding to treatment can continue at 8 weekly intervals until treatment is completed.
	Sequelae	Scarring caused by the initial infection and then healing of the skin can cause disfigurement. There is an increased risk of squamous cell carcinoma in patients with long-standing untreated disease.

19 Special groups

Pregnant and breast-feeding women may be treated with RHZE with pyridoxine 10 mg daily, as for other patients. There is no need to cease breast feeding. Some drugs used in secondary regimens such as streptomycin, prothionamide, ethionamide and the quinolones are contraindicated due to teratogenicity.

Women who need contraception should be counselled on the use of oral contraceptives while receiving rifampicin. Women should be offered an oral contraceptive pill containing a higher dose of oestrogen (50 μg) after consultation with a clinician, or a non-hormonal method of contraception while taking rifampicin and for 1 month after the end of treatment.

Patients with kidney impairment may need dose titration of some ATT drugs, and may not tolerate certain drugs at all. Specialist guidance is recommended. There are specialist guidelines for patients with chronic kidney disease elsewhere, such as the British Thoracic Society Guidelines for the Prevention and Management of TB infection in Adult Patients with Chronic Kidney Disease (British Thoracic Society Standards of Care Committee and Joint TB Committee, 2010).

Patients with previous liver disease such as history of acute hepatitis or current alcoholic or non-alcoholic fatty liver disease do not require changes to standard first-line treatment. Patients with acute hepatitis and a non-life-threatening form of EPTB should have treatment with ATT deferred until liver function tests normalize. If EPTB is life threatening, e.g. TB meningitis, specialist advice to select an ATT regimen, which contains the least hepatotoxic drugs, is required.

There is uncertainty around the safety of the standard first-line regimen in patients with liver cirrhosis. People with more advanced liver cirrhosis (Child's B and C liver disease) may be at increased risk of drug-induced hepatoxicity (Sharma, 2015).

The WHO guidelines recommend that the number of hepatotoxic drugs used in this setting should depend on the severity of liver disease (WHO, 2010). The following possible regimens are suggested, after consultation with expert clinicians. The choice of regimen depends on the balance of risks and harms relating to effective treatment of TB and prevention of liver injury.

Regimens containing two hepatotoxic drugs (rather than the three in the standard regimen):
* Nine months of isoniazid and rifampicin, plus ethambutol (until or unless isoniazid susceptibility is documented)
* Two months of isoniazid, rifampicin, streptomycin and ethambutol, followed by 6 months of isoniazid and rifampicin
* Six to nine months of rifampicin, pyrazinamide and ethambutol

Regimens containing one hepatotoxic drug:
* Two months of isoniazid, ethambutol and streptomycin, followed by 10 months of isoniazid and ethambutol.

Regimens containing no hepatotoxic drugs:
* Eighteen to twenty-four months of streptomycin, ethambutol and a fluoroquinolone

People with HIV

TB and HIV disease are linked, and identifying people who have both conditions is important to improve outcomes. All EPTB patients should be offered an HIV test as part of their diagnostic process. People with HIV require specialist advice and support pertaining to their diagnosis and treatment options.

HIV-positive people are more likely to have disseminated TB infection at presentation. More detailed diagnostic tests to look for other opportunistic infections and to assess the extent of disease may be useful.

There is increasing evidence that newer diagnostic tests for TB, including Xpert MTB/RIF, have different diagnostic test accuracy in people with advanced HIV and low CD4 counts. These guidelines have not addressed this issue in detail, but information about this can be found elsewhere in the literature.

HIV-positive people are at higher risk of paradoxical reactions, or immune reconstitution inflammatory syndrome (IRIS), and these reactions may be lifethreatening. The decision to commence ART must also be considered in patients who are not already receiving it. Guidance on initiation of ART can be found elsewhere at: BHIVA guidelines 2011 (Pozniak, 2011); Rapid Advice on ART for HIV infection in adolescents and adults (WHO, 2009); Guideline on when to start ART and on pre-exposure prophylaxis for HIV (WHO, 2015).

Part 2 References

Basu, S. M. (2014). Degree, duration and causes of visual impairment in eyes affected with ocular tuberculosis. *J Ophthalmic Inflamm Infect.* , 4 (1), 10.

Beardsley J, W. M. (2016). Adjunctive Dexamethasone in HIV-Associated Cryptococcal Meningitis. *New England Journal of Medicine* , 374 (6), 542-54.

Bell, L. B. (2015). Paradoxical reactions and immune reconstitution inflammatory syndrome in tuberculosis. *International Journal of Infectious Diseases* , 32, 39-45.

Biswas, J. N. (1996-1997). Pattern of uveitis in a referral uveitis clinic in India. *International Ophthalmology* , 20 (4), 223-8.

Blakemore, R. S. (2010). Evaluation of the analytical performance of the Xpert MTB/RIF assay. *Journal of Clinical Microbiology* , 48 (7), 2495-2501.

British Thoracic Society Standards of Care Committee and Joint TB Committee. (2010). Guidelines for the prevention and management of Mycobacterium tuberculosis infection and disease in adult patients with chronic kidney disease. *Thorax* , 65, 559-570.

Cheng, V. H. (2002). Clinical spectrum of paradoxical deterioration during antituberculosis therapy in non-HIV-infected patients. *European Journal of Clinical Microbiology and Infectious Diseases* , 21 (11), 803-9.

Denkinger, C. S. (2014). Xpert MTB/RIF assay for the diagnosis of extrapulmonary tuberculosis: a systematic review and meta-analysis. *European Respiratory Journal* , 44 (2), 435-46.

Donald, P. (2010). The chemotherapy of tuberculous meningitis in children and adults. *Tuberculosis (Edinburgh)* , 90 (6), 375-392.

Fowler, N. (1991). Tuberculous pericarditis. *Journal of the American Medical Association* , 266, 99-103.

Garg, R. M. (2014). Paradoxical reaction in HIV negative tuberculous meningitis. *Journal of the Neurological Sciences* , 340 (1-2), 26-36.

GRADE Working Group. (2008). *http://www.gradeworkinggroup.org/publications/* . Retrieved July 2015

Greco, S. G. (2003). Adenosine deaminase and interferon gamma measurements for the diagnosis of tuberculous pleurisy: a meta-analysis. Int. J. *Tuberc. Lung Dis.* , 7 (8), 777-786.

Guyatt Gordon H, O. A.-Y. (2008). Going from evidence to recommendations. *British Medical Journal* , 336, 1049.

Higgins, J. A. (2011). Chapter 8: Assessing risk of bias in included studies. In G. S. Higgins JPT, *Cochrane Handbook for Systematic Reviews of Interventions Version 5.1.0.* The Cochrane Collaboration.

Jabs, D. N. (2005). Standardization of uveitis nomenclature for reporting clinical data. Results of the First International Workshop. *American Journal of Ophthalmology* , 140, 509-161.

Jain, A. S. (2012). Magnetic resonance evaluation of tubercular lesion in spine. *International Orthopaedics* , 36 (2), 261-9.

Liang, Q. S. (2008). Diagnostic accuracy of adenosine deaminase in tuberculous pleurisy: a metaanalysis. *Respiratory Medicine* , 102 (5), 744-754.

Light R.W., M. M. (1972). Pleural effusions: the diagnostic separation of transudates and exudates. *Annals of Internal Medicine* , 77 (4), 507-513.

Light, R. (2010). Update on tuberculous pleural effusion. *Respirology* , 15 (3), 451-458.

MRC. (1948). Medical Research Council Report. Streptomycin treatment of tuberculous meningitis. *Lancet* , 1, 582-96.

Nhu, N. H. (2014). Evaluation of GeneXpert MTB/RIF for diagnosis of tuberculous meningitis. *Journal of Clinical Microbiology* , 52 (1), 226-33.

Porcel, J. E. (2010). Diagnostic performance of adenosine deaminase activity in pleural fluid: a singlecenter experience with over 2100 consecutive patients. *European Journal of Internal Medicine* , 21 (5), 419-423.

Pozniak, A. C. (2011). British HIV Association guidelines for the treatment of TB/HIV coninfection. *HIV Medicine* , 12, 517-524.

Prasad, K. S. (2016). Corticosteroids for managing tuberculous meningitis. *The Cochrane Library* (4), 1-64.

Ramam, M. M. (2011). How useful is the Mantoux test in the diagnosis of doubtful cases of cutaneous tuberculosis? *International Journal of Dermatology* , 50 (11), 1379-82.

RNTCP. (2014). *TB India 2014 Revised National TB Control Programme Annual Status Report*. Ministry of Health and Family Welfare, Central TB Division, Directorate General of Health Services. New Delhi: Central TB Division.

Rossi, G. B. (1987). Tuberculous pleural effusions. Evidence for selective presence of PPD-specific T-lymphocytes at site of inflammation in the early phase of the infection. *American Review of Respiratory Disease* , 136 (3), 575-579.

Sharma S.K., M. A. (2004). Extrapulmonary tuberculosis. *Indian Journal of Medical Research* , 120 (4), 316-353.

Sharma, P. T. (2015). Clinical and biochemical profile of tuberculosis in patients with liver cirrhosis. *Journal of Clinical and Experimental Hepatology* , 5, 8-13.

Shu, C. W.-T.-Y.-N.-J. (2011). In-hospital outcome of patients with culture-confirmed tuberculous pleurisy: clinical impact of pulmonary involvement. *BMC Infectious Diseases* , 11, 46.

Singh, R. G. (2004). Pattern of uveitis in a referral eye clinic in north India. *Indian Journal of Ophthalmology* , 52, 121-5.

Sreenivas, A. R. (2014). *Standards for TB Care in India*. New Delhi: World Health Organisation Country Office for India.

Steingart K.R., H. M. (2006). Fluorescence versus conventional sputum smear microscopy for tuberculosis: a systematic review. *Lancet Infectious Diseases* , 6 (9), 570-81.

Steingart, K. S. (2014). Xpert® MTB/RIF assay for pulmonary tuberculosis and rifampicin resistance in adults. *The Cochrane Database of Systematic Reviews* , 1, 1-66.

Tappeiner. (2008). Tuberculosis and Infections with atypical mycobacteria. In G. L. Wolff K, *Fitzpatrick's Dermatology in General Medicine*, 7th ed. (p. 1768). New York: McGraw Hill Medical.

TB CARE I. (2014). *International Standards for Tuberculosis Care* (3rd ed.). The Hague: TB CARE I.

The Task Force for the Diagnosis and Management of Pericardial Diseases of the European Society of Cardiology (ESC). (2015). 2015 ESC Guidelines for the diagnosis and management of pericardial diseases. *European Heart Journal* , 36, 2921–2964.

Thwaites G.E., N. D. (2004). Dexamethasone for the treatment of tuberculous meningitis in adolescents and adults. *New England Journal of Medicine* , 351 (17), 1741-1751.

Thwaites, G. F. (2009). British Infection Society guidelines for the diagnosis and treatment of tuberculosis of the central nervous system in adults and children. *Journal of Infection* , 59, 167-187.

Van Loenhout-Rooyackers, J. K. (2001). Tuberculous meningitis: is a 6-month treatment regimen sufficient? *International Journal of Tuberculosis and Lung Disease* , 5 (11), 1028–35.

Watts, H. L. (1996). Current concepts review: tuberculosis of bone and joints. *The Journal of Bone and Joint Surgery [Am]* , 78 (A), 288-98.

WHO. (2015). *Global Tuberculosis Report* (20th ed.). Geneva: World Health Organisation.

WHO. (2014). *Guidance for national tuberculosis programmes on the management of tuberculosis in children* (2nd ed.). Geneva: World Health Organisation.

WHO. (2015). *Guideline on when to start antiretroviral therapy and on pre-exposure prophylaxis for HIV*. Geneva: World Health Organisation.

WHO. (2009). *Rapid Advice: Antiretroviral therapy for HIV infection in adults and adolescents*. Geneva: WHO.

WHO. (2010). *Treatment of tuberculosis: Guidelines Fourth Edition*. Geneva: WHO.

WHO. (2014). *WHO Handbook for Guideline Development*. Geneva: World Health Organisation.

Wiysonge, C. N. (2016). Corticosteroids and other interventions for treating tuberculous pericarditis. *Cochrane Database of Systematic Reviews*, publication pending.

Index

Page numbers followed by *f* refer to figure and *t* refer to table.